Drug Information Handbook for Dentistry

4th Edition | 1998-99

lexi-comp

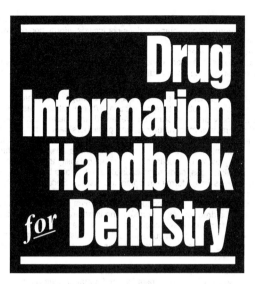

Drug Information Handbook *for* Dentistry

4th Edition | **1998-99**

Richard L. Wynn, BSPharm, PhD
Professor of Pharmacology
Baltimore College of Dental Surgery
Dental School
University of Maryland at Baltimore
Baltimore, Maryland

Timothy F. Meiller, DDS, PhD
Professor
Oral Medicine and Diagnostic Sciences
Baltimore College of Dental Surgery
Professor of Oncology
Greenebaum Cancer Center
University of Maryland at Baltimore
Baltimore, Maryland

Harold L. Crossley, DDS, PhD
Associate Professor of Pharmacology
Dental School
University of Maryland at Baltimore
Baltimore, Maryland

LEXI-COMP INC
Hudson (Cleveland)

NOTICE

This handbook is intended to serve the user as a handy reference and not as a complete drug information resource. It does not include information on every therapeutic agent available. The publication covers a combination of commonly used drugs in dentistry and medicine and is specifically designed to present important aspects of drug data in a more concise format than is typically found in medical literature, exhaustive drug compendia, or product material supplied by manufacturers.

Drug information is constantly evolving because of ongoing research and clinical experience and is often subject to interpretation. While great care has been taken to ensure the accuracy of the information presented, the reader is advised that the authors, editors, reviewers, contributors, and publishers cannot be responsible for the continued currency of the information or for any errors, omissions, or the application of this information, or for any consequences arising therefrom. Therefore, the author(s) and/or the publisher shall have no liability to any person or entity with regard to claims, loss, or damage caused, or alleged to be caused, directly or indirectly, by the use of information contained herein. Because of the dynamic nature of drug information, readers are advised that decisions regarding drug therapy must be based on the independent judgment of the clinician, changing information about a drug (eg, as reflected in the literature and manufacturer's most current product information), and changing medical practices. The editors are not responsible for any inaccuracy of quotation or for any false or misleading implication that may arise due to the text or formulas as used or due to the quotation of revisions no longer official.

The editors, authors, and contributors have written this book in their private capacities. No official support or endorsement by any federal or state agency or pharmaceutical company is intended or inferred.

The publishers have made every effort to trace the copyright holders for borrowed material. If they have inadvertently overlooked any, they will be pleased to make the necessary arrangements at the first opportunity.

If you have any suggestions or questions regarding any information presented in this handbook, please contact our drug information pharmacist at

1-800-837-LEXI (5394)

This manual was produced using the FormuLex™ Program —
A complete publishing service of Lexi-Comp Inc.

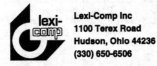

Lexi-Comp Inc
1100 Terex Road
Hudson, Ohio 44236
(330) 650-6506

TABLE OF CONTENTS

ABOUT THE AUTHORS

Richard L. Wynn, BSPharm, PhD

Richard L. Wynn, PhD, is Professor of Pharmacology at the Baltimore College of Dental Surgery, Dental School, University of Maryland at Baltimore. Dr Wynn has served as a dental educator, researcher, and teacher of dental pharmacology and dental hygiene pharmacology for his entire professional career. He holds a BS (pharmacy; registered pharmacist, Maryland), an MS (physiology) and a PhD (pharmacology) from the University of Maryland. Dr Wynn chaired the Department of Pharmacology at the University of Maryland Dental School from 1980 to 1995. Previously, he chaired the Department of Oral Biology at the University of Kentucky College of Dentistry. He has to his credit over 160 publications including original research articles, textbooks, textbook chapters, monographs, and articles in continuing education journals. He has given over 300 continuing education seminars to dental professionals in the U.S., Canada, and Europe. Dr Wynn has been a consultant to drug industry for 16 years. His research laboratories have contributed to the development of new analgesics and anesthetics. He is a consultant to the U.S. Pharmacopeia, Dental Drugs and Products section, a consultant to the Academy of General Dentistry, and a former consultant to the Council on Dental Education, Commission on Accreditation. He is a featured columnist and his drug review articles, entitled *Pharmacology Today*, appear in each issue of General Dentistry, a journal published by the Academy. He is currently funded by drug industry and government agencies for research on the emetogenic nature of pain, mechanisms of postoperative nausea, and animal models of acupuncture. One of his primary interests continues to be keeping dental professionals informed on all aspects of drug use in dental practice.

Timothy F. Meiller, DDS, PhD

Dr Meiller is Professor of Oral Medicine and Diagnostic Sciences at the Baltimore College of Dental Surgery and Professor of Oncology in the Program of Oncology at the Greenebaum Cancer Center, University of Maryland at Baltimore.

Dr Meiller teaches Oral Medicine at the Dental School and serves as an attending faculty at the Greenebaum Cancer Center. He is a Diplomate of the American Board of Oral Medicine. He is a graduate of Johns Hopkins University and the University of Maryland Dental and Graduate Schools, holding a DDS and a PhD in Immunology/Virology. He maintains an active general dental practice and is a consultant to the National Institutes of Health. He is currently engaged in ongoing investigations into cellular immune dysfunction in oral diseases associated with AIDS and in other medically compromised patients.

Harold L. Crossley, DDS, PhD

Dr Crossley is Associate Professor of Pharmacology at the Baltimore College of Dental Surgery, Dental School, University of Maryland at Baltimore. A native of Rhode Island, Hal received a Bachelor of Science degree in Pharmacy from the University of Rhode Island in 1964. He later was awarded the Master of Science (1970) and Doctorate degrees (1972) in the area of Pharmacology. The University of Maryland Dental School in Baltimore awarded Dr Crossley the DDS degree in 1980. He is the Director of Conjoint Sciences and Preclinical Studies at the School of Dentistry and maintains an intramural part-time private dental practice. Dr Crossley has co-authored a number of articles dealing with law enforcement on both a local and federal level. This liaison with law enforcement agencies keeps him well-acquainted with the "drug culture". He has been appointed to the Governor's Commission on Prescription Drug Abuse and the Maryland State Dental Association's Well-Being Committee.

Drawing on this unique background, Dr Crossley has become nationally and internationally recognized as an expert on street drugs and chemical dependency as well as the clinical pharmacology of dental drugs.

EDITORIAL ADVISORY PANEL

Carlos M. Isada, MD
Department of Infectious Disease
Cleveland Clinic Foundation
Cleveland, Ohio

David S. Jacobs, MD
President, Pathologists Chartered
Overland Park, Kansas

John E. Janosik, PharmD
Clinical Pharmacist
Lexi-Comp Inc.
Hudson, Ohio

Bernard L. Kasten, Jr, MD, FCAP
Vice President - Medical Director
Corning Clinical Laboratories
Teterboro, New Jersey

Donna M. Kraus, PharmD
Associate Professor of Pharmacy Practice
Departments of Pharmacy Practice and Pediatrics
Clinical Pharmacist
Pediatric Intensive Care Unit
University of Illinois at Chicago
Chicago, Illinois

Charles Lacy, RPh, PharmD
Drug Information Pharmacist
Cedars-Sinai Medical Center
Los Angeles, California

Leonard L. Lance, RPh, BSPharm
Pharmacist
Lexi-Comp Inc.
Hudson, Ohio

Jerrold B. Leikin, MD
Associate Director
Emergency Services
Medical Director
Rush Poison Control Center
Rush Presbyterian-St. Luke's Medical Center
Chicago, Illinois

Eugene S. Olsowka, MD, PhD
Pathologist
Institute of Pathology
Saginaw, Michigan

Frank P. Paloucek, PharmD
Clinical Associate Professor
University of Illinois
Chicago, Illinois

Christopher J. Papasian, PhD
Director of Diagnostic Microbiology and Immunology Laboratories
Truman Medical Center
Kansas City, Missouri

Todd P. Semla, PharmD
Clinical Pharmacist
St Francis Hospital of Evanston
Evanston, Illinois

Carol K. Taketomo, PharmD
Pharmacy Manager
Children's Hospital of Los Angeles
Los Angeles, California

Lowell L. Tilzer MD
Associate Medical Director
Community Blood Center of Greater Kansas City
Kansas City, Missouri

PREFACE TO THE FOURTH EDITION

The authors of the *Drug Information Handbook for Dentistry* are gratified that the text has received many indicators of success over these last several years. We wish to congratulate and thank the practitioners and students that have made each of the previous editions a success. Each of us have endeavored to respond to all of the comments and creative suggestions from our readership and as a result have incorporated many of these ideas into this new 4th edition.

The goals and the philosophy of the handbook remain the same as in all previous editions. Complete cross-referencing of generic, brand names, medical and oral conditions along with the therapeutic indication and example prescribing guidelines have been the basis of the text. We know the practitioners and staff members can easily access needed information.

The drug monographs now number well over 1400 and the complete alphabetical index exceeds 3600 drug names. This indexing system has been the key to much of the success of this book. Clinicians can cross-reference between an oral medicine problem, a suggested drug regimen, and the important pharmacologic information necessary to move ahead with a treatment selection.

This 4th edition includes easy-to-use algorithms to help the clinician make treatment decisions in evolving areas of patient care including preprocedural antibiotics related to endocarditis and joint prostheses. New drugs have been added to further explain the available combinations for pain control and treatment of common conditions such as temporomandibular dysfunction. Other topics in the text have been edited as appropriate. One very key area has been an entire chapter now dedicated to management of the human immunodeficiency virus infected (AIDS) patient. Also, the chapter on chemical dependency has been updated to include new information. Many chapters now have a section called "Frequently Asked Questions" to help us focus on real-life scenarios. The chapter on herbals and natural products has been expanded to present information on many of the most popular dietary supplements. A new chapter on drug interactions and metabolism along with sections on effects of smoking and smoking cessation products has been added.

We know that our text remains an excellent companion to complete oral medicine and medical reference libraries that each clinician should have available. We hope that it compliments the sound foundation that each dental clinician has received during their education and by building on their knowledge of oral and systemic disease we have helped them with this text to focus on therapeutic considerations. Dental office management protocols, along with prescribing guidelines, should aid the busy practitioner. The active general practitioner, the specialist, the dental hygienist, and the advanced student of dentistry or dental hygiene will be better prepared for patient care with this new 4th edition.

Timothy F. Meiller

Richard L. Wynn

Harold L. Crossley

ACKNOWLEDGMENTS

This handbook exists in its present form as a result of the concerted efforts of many individuals, including Jack D. Bolinski, DDS, and Brad F. Bolinski who recognized the need for a comprehensive dental and medical drug compendium; the publisher and president of Lexi-Comp Inc, Robert D. Kerscher; Lynn D. Coppinger, managing editor; John E. Janosik, PharmD; and Leonard L. Lance, RPh.

Other members of the Lexi-Comp staff include Diane Harbart, MT (ASCP), medical editor; Barbara F. Kerscher, production manager; Jeanne Wilson, Jennifer Rocky, Leslie Ruggles, and Julie Katzen, project managers; Alexandra Hart, composition specialist; Jacqueline L. Mizer, production assistant; Tracey J. Reinecke, graphics; Brian B. Vossler, Jerry M. Reeves, and Marc L. Long, sales managers; Jay L. Katzen, product manager; Kenneth J. Hughes, manager, authoring systems; Kristin M. Thompson, Matthew C. Kerscher, Tina L. Collins, and Mary M. Murphy, sales and marketing representatives; Edmund A. Harbart, vice-president, custom publishing division; Jack L. Stones, vice-president, reference publishing division; David C. Marcus, Dennis P. Smithers and Sean Conrad, system analysts; and Thury L. O'Connor, vice-president of technology.

In addition, the authors wish to thank their families, friends, and colleagues who supported them in their efforts to complete this handbook.

USE OF THE DRUG INFORMATION HANDBOOK FOR DENTISTRY

The *Drug Information Handbook for Dentistry, 4th Edition* is organized into six sections: Introductory text, drug monographs, oral medicine topics, appendix, therapeutic category index, and alphabetical index

INTRODUCTORY TEXT

The first section is a compilation of information pertinent to the use of this handbook.

ALPHABETICAL LISTING OF DRUG MONOGRAPHS

The drug information section of the handbook, in which over 1300 drugs are listed alphabetically, incorporates drugs commonly prescribed in dentistry as well as medications that dental patients may currently be taking. Extensive cross-referencing is provided by brand names and synonyms.

Each monograph is consistent in its format and may include all or some of the following fields:

Generic Name	U.S. Adopted Name
Pronunciation Guide	Phonetic listing of generic name
Related Information	Cross-reference to other pertinent drug information found elsewhere in the book
Brand Names	Common trade names
Canadian/Mexican Brand Names	Trade names found in Canada and Mexico if different from the U.S.; complete listing is located in the Alphabetical Index
Therapeutic Category	Unique systematic classification of medications
Synonyms	Other names or accepted abbreviations of the drug in the U.S., Canada, and Mexico
Use	Information pertaining to appropriate dental and medical indications of the drug
Restrictions	DEA classification for federally scheduled controlled substances and their associated prescribing limits
Usual Dosage	The amount of the drug to be typically given or taken during therapy
Mechanism of Action	How the drug works in the body to elicit a response
Local Anesthetic/Vasoconstrictor Precautions	Specific information to prevent potential drug interactions related to anesthesia
Effects on Dental Treatment	How drug therapy affects the dental treatment/diagnosis with suggested management approaches
Other Adverse Effects	Side effects grouped by percentage of incidence
Contraindications	Information pertaining to inappropriate use of the drug
Warnings/Precautions	Cautions and hazardous conditions related to use of the drug
Drug Interactions	A list of agents that when combined may affect the therapy
Drug Uptake	Information includes onset and duration of effect, absorption, time to peak serum concentration, and serum half-life
Pregnancy Risk Factor	Five categories established by the FDA to indicate the potential of a systemically absorbed drug for causing birth defects
Breast-feeding Considerations	Information pertaining to drug administration while breast-feeding
Dosage Forms	Information with regard to form, strength, and availability of the drug
Dietary Considerations	Information regarding effect of food with drug
Generic Available	Indicated by a "yes" or "no"
Comments	Additional pertinent information

Selected Readings   Sources and literature where the user may find additional information

ORAL MEDICINE TOPICS

The third section contains text on Oral Medicine topics and is divided into two major parts.

In each of the two major parts, the systemic condition or the oral disease state is described briefly, followed by the pharmacologic considerations, with which the dentist must be familiar. Selected readings have been listed for further inquiry.

Part I: **Dental Management and Therapeutic Considerations in Medically Compromised Patients** focuses on common medical conditions and their associated drug therapies with which the dentist must be familiar. Patient profiles with commonly associated drug regimens are described.

Part II: **Dental Management and Therapeutic Considerations in Patients With Specific Oral Conditions and Other Oral Medicine Topics** focus on therapies the dentist may choose to prescribe for patients suffering from oral disease or are in need of special care. Some overlap between these sections has resulted from systemic conditions that have oral manifestations and vice-versa. Cross-references to the descriptions and the monographs for individual drugs described elsewhere in this handbook allow for easy retrieval of information. Example prescriptions of selected drug therapies for each condition are presented so that the clinician can evaluate alternate approaches to treatment. Seldom is there a single drug of choice.

Those drug prescriptions listed represent prototype drugs and popular prescriptions and are examples only. The therapeutic index is available for cross-referencing if alternatives or additional drugs are sought.

APPENDIX

The Appendix section offers a compilation of tables, guidelines, and conversion information which can often be helpful when considering patient care. This section is broken down into various sections for ease of use. The Appendix also includes descriptions of most over-the-counter drugs and oral care products. There are also presentations of drug interactions and drugs under development.

THERAPEUTIC CATEGORY INDEX

The Therapeutic Category Index provides a useful listing by an easy-to-use therapeutic classification system.

ALPHABETICAL INDEX

The Alphabetical Index provides a quick reference for generic, American/Canadian/Mexican brand names, and major headings from the chapters. From this index, the reader can cross-reference to the drug monographs and to Oral Medicine topics.

FDA PREGNANCY CATEGORIES

Throughout this book there is a field labeled Pregnancy Risk Factor (PRF) and the letter A, B, C, D, or X immediately following which signifies a category. The FDA has established these five categories to indicate the potential of a systemically absorbed drug for causing birth defects. The key differentiation among the categories rests upon the reliability of documentation and the risk:benefit ratio. Pregnancy Category X is particularly notable in that if any data exists that may implicate a drug as a teratogen and the risk:benefit ratio is clearly negative, the drug is contraindicated during pregnancy.

These categories are summarized as follows:

A   Controlled studies in pregnant women fail to demonstrate a risk to the fetus in the first trimester with no evidence of risk in later trimesters. The possibility of fetal harm appears remote.

B   Either animal-reproduction studies have not demonstrated a fetal risk but there are no controlled studies in pregnant women, or animal-reproduction studies have shown an adverse effect (other than a decrease in fertility) that was not confirmed in controlled studies in women in the first trimester and there is no evidence of a risk in later trimesters.

C   Either studies in animals have revealed adverse effects on the fetus (teratogenic or embryocidal effects or other) and there are no controlled studies in women, or studies in women and animals are not available. Drugs should be given only if the potential benefits justify the potential risk to the fetus.

D   There is positive evidence of human fetal risk, but the benefits from use in pregnant women may be acceptable despite the risk (eg, if the drug is needed in a life-threatening situation or for a serious disease for which safer drugs cannot be used or are ineffective).

X   Studies in animals or human beings have demonstrated fetal abnormalities or there is evidence of fetal risk based on human experience, or both, and the risk of the use of the drug in pregnant women clearly outweighs any possible benefit. The drug is contraindicated in women who are or may become pregnant.

PHARMACOLOGY OF DRUG METABOLISM AND INTERACTIONS

Most drugs undergo metabolic transformation in the body prior to excretion. Drug metabolism is an enzyme-dependent process that developed as an adaptation to life on earth. Unlike fish, terrestrial vertebrates are unable to excrete lipid soluble compounds because kidney tubular reabsorption favors their retention. Excretion of these substances is accomplished in fish into the surrounding water. Although drug metabolism in humans results in the formation of compounds that are more polar in nature, it does not always result in the initial production of biologically inactive compounds. This means that a drug may stay active for some time during this metabolic process. Enzymatic modification of a parent drug can be distinguished by three basic patterns. First, an inactive parent drug may be transformed to an active compound. Second, an active parent drug may be converted to a second active compound which is subsequently converted to an inactive metabolite or by-product. Third, an inactive compound may be formed directly from an active parent drug.

The most common reaction in drug metabolism is an oxidation reaction in which oxygen in the form of a hydroxyl group is attached to the drug molecule. With oxidation, the original drug molecule is changed just enough so that the drug metabolite won't attach to the receptor that is specific for the original molecule. This chemical change may render the drug inactive and is one mechanism of terminating drug activity. The overall process is called hydroxylation and is the direct incorporation of oxygen into the substrate drug molecule. Although the liver is the primary site for these hydroxylation enzyme reactions, these systems are also present in the kidney and gastrointestinal epithelium. This process is also called oxidative drug metabolism by an oxidative enzyme system.

This oxidative enzyme system relies on a particular cytochrome and numerous isoforms known as the cytochrome P-450 system with designations CYP. Cytochrome P-450 is a complex of protein and heme that contains an iron atom in its oxidized state. Through an energy transfer cascade, cytochrome P-450 is reduced utilizing energy and reducing the iron to a ferrous form. This then binds with molecular oxygen and the cytochrome P-450 eventually reverts to its oxidized form. The oxidized drug bound through this process to the cytochrome P-450 is then released and the cytochrome is regenerated. The rate of drug biotransformation or metabolism appears to be directly related to the amounts of cytochrome P-450 in the microsomal and enzyme cascade. In fact, there is a direct correlation between these systems.

Many drugs that are currently on the market now have associated with them their relationship to the cytochrome P-450 system and a system of analyses has been developed to identify drugs that tend to interfere with the availability of cytochrome P-450 more readily than others. Also, there are numerous isoforms of these enzymes that have been identified within the system. The specific interaction of one drug with another drug's metabolism has now been elucidated through analyses of reactions. Many of the drugs that our patients may be taking may slow the metabolism of another drug. It is important to be aware that our knowledge regarding these systems is increasing on a daily basis. An example of several isoform interactions of this system is found in Tables 2-4. Drugs of common importance in dentistry are in bold. Many of the drugs used as antivirals, for instance, interfere with specific isoforms of the cytochrome P-450 system and may, therefore, interact adversely with the metabolism of other drugs which the patient may be taking.

Another area of intense interest involves smoking effects on drug's metabolism as well as the effects of smoking cessation drugs (Table 5). A review of the literature suggests that at least a dozen drugs interact with cigarette smoke in a clinically significant manner. Polycyclic aromatic hydrocarbons (PAHs) are largely responsible for enhancing drug metabolism. Cigarette smoke induces increased concentrations of the isoenzyme CYP1A2, which is responsible for the metabolism of theophylline. Theophylline is, therefore, eliminated more quickly in smokers than in nonsmokers. Cigarette smoke induces an increase in the concentration of CYP1A2, the isoenzyme responsible for the metabolism of theophylline. As a result of hepatic induction of CYP1A2, serum concentrations of theophylline have been shown to be reduced in smokers. Cigarette smoking may reduce substantially the plasma concentrations of tacrine. The manufacturer states that mean plasma tacrine concentrations in smokers are about one-third of the concentration in nonsmokers (presumably after multiple doses of tacrine).

Patients with insulin-dependent diabetes who smoke heavily may require a higher dosage of insulin than nonsmokers. Cigarette smoking may also reduce serum concentrations of flecainide. Although the mechanism of this interaction is unknown, enhanced hepatic metabolism is a possibility. Propoxyphene, a pain reliever, has

PHARMACOLOGY OF DRUG METABOLISM AND INTERACTIONS *(Continued)*

been found to be less effective in heavy smokers than in nonsmokers. The mechanism for the inefficacy of propoxyphene in smokers compared with nonsmokers may be enhanced biotransformation.

Frankl and Soloff reported in a study of five young, health chronic smokers that propranolol followed by smoking significantly decreased cardiac output and significantly increased blood pressure and peripheral resistance compared with smoking alone. Steady-state concentrations of propranolol were found to be lower in smokers than in nonsmokers. Lastly, the incidence of drowsiness associated with the use of diazepam and chloridazepoxide showed that drowsiness was less likely to occur in smokers than in nonsmokers. Smoking probably acts by producing arousal of the central nervous system rather than be accelerating metabolism and reducing the concentrations of these drugs in the brain. Finally, the interaction between smoking and oral contraceptives is complex and may be deadly. Women older than 35 years of age who smoke more than 15 cigarettes daily may be at increased risk of myocardial infarction.

The norepinephrine and serotonin reuptake inhibitors as a new class of smoking cessation drugs have also received attention relative to metabolic interactions. *In vitro* studies indicate that bupropion is primarily metabolized to hydroxybupropion by the CYP2B6 isoenzyme. Therefore, the potential exists for a drug interaction between Zyban® and drugs that affect the CYP2B6 isoenzyme metabolism (eg, orphenadrine and cyclophosphamide). The threohydrobupropion metabolite of bupropion does not appear to be metabolized by the cytochrome P-450 isoenzymes. No systemic data have been collected on the metabolism of Zyban® following concomitant administration with other drugs, or alternatively, the effect of concomitant administration of Zyban® on the metabolism of other drugs.

Animal data, however, indicated that bupropion may be an inducer of drug metabolizing enzymes in humans. However, following chronic administration of bupropion, 100 3 times daily to 8 healthy male volunteers for 14 days, there was no evidence of induction of its own metabolism. Because bupropion is extensively metabolized, the coadministration of other drugs may affects its clinical activity. In particular, certain drugs may induce the metabolism of bupropion (eg, carbamazepine, phenobarbital, phenytoin), while other drugs may inhibit the metabolism of bupropion (eg, cimetidine). Studies in animals demonstrate that the acute toxicity of bupropion is enhanced by the MAO inhibitor phenelzine.

Limited clinical data suggest a higher incidence of adverse experiences in patients receiving concurrent administration of bupropion and levodopa. Administration of Zyban® to patients receiving levodopa concurrently should be undertaken with caution, using small initial doses and gradual dose increases. Concurrent administration of Zyban® and agents (eg, abrupt discontinuation of benzodiazepines) that lower seizure threshold, should be undertaken only with extreme caution. Physiological changes resulting from smoking cessation itself, with or without treatment with Zyban®, may alter the pharmacokinetics of some concomitant medications, which may require dosage adjustment.

Once a drug has been metabolized in the liver, it is eliminated through several different mechanisms. One is directly through the bile and into the intestine and eventually excreted in feces. More commonly, however, the metabolites and the original drug themselves pass back into the liver from the general circulation and are carried to other organs and tissues. Eventually, these metabolites are excreted through the kidney. In the kidney, the drug and its metabolites may be filtered by the glomerulus or secreted by the renal tubules into the urine. From the kidney, some of the drug may be reabsorbed and pass back into the blood. Another organ to which the drug may be carried is the lung. If the drug or its metabolite is volatile, it can pass from the blood into the alveolar air and be eliminated in the breath. To a minor extent, drugs and metabolites can also be excreted by sweat and by the saliva. In nursing mothers, drugs are also excreted into the mother's milk.

The clinical considerations of drug metabolism may affect which other drugs can and should be administered. Drug tolerance may be a consideration in that larger doses of a drug may be necessary to obtain effect in patients in which the metabolism is extremely rapid. These interactions via cytochrome P-450 or its isoforms can be occasionally used beneficially to increase/maintain blood levels of one drug by administering a second drug. Dental clinicians should attempt to stay current on this topic of drug interactions as our knowledge evolves.

Table 1.
DRUG METABOLIZING CYTOCHROME P-450 ISOZYMES

Isoform	Substrates	Inhibitors
CYP1A2	Caffeine Clozapine Tacrine Theophylline R-Warfarin	Cimetidine **Ciprofloxacin** Diltiazem Enoxacin **Erythromycin** Fluvoxamine Mexiletine Norfloxacin Tacrine
CYP2C9	**Amitriptyline** (demethylation) Diclofenac **Ibuprofen** Imipramine Phenytoin Tolbutamide S-Warfarin	Amiodarone Cimetidine **Co-trimoxazole** Disulfiram **Fluconazole** Fluvastatin **Metronidazole** Phenylbutazone Sulfaphenazole
CYP2C19	**Diazepam** Mephenytoin Omeprazole Phenytoin (minor pathway)	Felbamate Fluoxetine Fluvoxamine Omeprazole
CYP2E1	**Acetaminophen** Alcohol Isoniazid	Disulfiram
CYP2D6	Clomipramine **Codeine -> morphine** Desipramine Dextromethorphan Flecainide Haloperidol Imipramine (OH) Metoprolol Nortriptyline (OH) Paroxetine Perhexiline Propafenone Propranolol (4-OH) Risperidone Thioridazine Venlafaxine	Amiodarone Fluoxetine Haloperidol Paroxetine Propafenone **Quinidine** Thioridazine
CYP3A4	Alprazolam Astemizole **Carbamazepine** Cisapride **Corticosteroids** Cyclosporine **Diazepam** Diltiazem **Erythromycin** Felodipine **Lidocaine** Lovastatin Midazolam Nifedipine Quinidine Simvastatin **Triazolam** Verapamil	Cimetidine **Clarithromycin** Danazol Diltiazem **Erythromycin** **Fluconazole** (large doses) Fluoxetine (norfluoxetine) Grapefruit juice **Itraconazole** **Ketoconazole** **Miconazole** Nefazodone Omeprazole Propoxyphene? **Quinidine** Troleandomycin

PHARMACOLOGY OF DRUG METABOLISM AND INTERACTIONS *(Continued)*

Table 2.
CONTRAINDICATED MEDICATIONS AND POTENTIAL ALTERNATIVES*
WHEN A PATIENT IS TAKING RITONAVIR (Norvir®)

Contraindicated Medications[a]			Potential Alternatives[b] (these alternatives may not be therapeutically equivalent)		
Drug Class	Generic Name	Brand Name	Generic Name	Brand Name	Exposed Patients
Analgesic	Meperidine	Demerol®	Acetaminophen	Tylenol®	N=135
	Piroxicam	Feldene®	Aspirin		N=43
Cardiovascular (antiarrhythmic)	Amiodarone	Cordarone®	Very limited clinical experience		
	Encainide	Enkaid®			
	Flecainide	Tambocor®			
	Propafenone	Rythmol®			
Antimycobacterial	Rifabutin	Mycobutin®	Clarithromycin	Biaxin®	N=156[c]
			Ethambutol	Myambutol®	N=66
Cardiovascular (calcium channel blocker)	Bepridil	Vascor®	Very limited clinical experience		
Cold and allergy (antihistamine)	Astemizole	Hismanal®	Loratadine	Claritin®	N=36
Ergot alkaloid (vasoconstrictor)	Dihydroergotamine	D.H.E. 45®	Very limited clinical experience		
	Ergotamine	Various			
Gastrointestinal	Cisapride	Propulsid®	Very limited clinical experience		
Psychotropic (antidepressant)	Bupropion	Wellbutrin®	Desipramine	Norpramin®[d]	
Psychotropic (neuroleptic)	Clozapine	Clozaril®	Very limited clinical experience		
	Pimozide	Orap®			
Psychotropic (sedative/ hypnotic)	Alprazolam	Xanax®	Temazepam	Restoril®	N=40
	Clorazepate	Tranxene®	Lorazepam	Ativan®	N=33
	Diazepam	Valium®			
	Estazolam	ProSom™			
	Flurazepam	Dalmane®			
	Midazolam	Versed®			
	Triazolam	Halcion®			
	Zolpidem	Ambien™			

[a] See the CONTRAINDICATIONS section of the Norvir® package insert.

[b] See the PRECAUTIONS-DRUG INTERACTIONS section of the Norvir® package insert for more information.

*During clinical trials, Norvir® was given to patients concomitantly taking a variety of medications. These medications were not evaluated in drug interaction studies. The number of Norvir®-treated patients exposed to each drug is provided in the last column.

[c] Also evaluated in drug interaction study (N=22). See "Results of Drug Interaction Studies."

[d] No clinical experience with combination. Only evaluated in drug interaction study (N=14). See "Results of Drug Interaction Studies."

Norvir® has high affinity for several cytochrome P-450 (CYP) isoenzymes including CYP3A, CYP2D6, and CYP2C9. Large dose reductions (>50%) and increased therapeutic drug concentration monitoring of therapeutic and adverse effects is recommended when drugs extensively metabolized are used concomitantly with Norvir®.

Table 3.
DRUG INTERACTIONS WITH HIV ANTIVIRAL DRUGS

Indinavir	Nelfinavir	Ritonavir	Saquinavir
•Inhibits cytochrome P-450 (less than ritonavir)	•Inhibits cytochrome P-450 (less than ritonavir)	•Inhibits cytochrome P-450 (potent inhibitor)	•Inhibits cytochrome P-450
•Not recommended for concurrent use: rifampin, terfenadine, astemizole, cisapride, triazolam, midazolam, ergot alkaloids	•Nelfinavir levels reduced by rifampin, rifabutin	•Ritonavir increases levels of multiple drugs that are not recommended for current use	•Saquinavir levels increased by: ritonavir, ketoconazole, grapefruit juice, nelfinavir, delavirdine
•Indinavir levels increased by: ketoconazole, delavirdine	•Not recommended for concurrent use: rifampin, triazolam, midazolam, ergot alkaloids, terfenadine, astemizole, cisapride	•Didanosine: reduced absorption of both drugs; take >2 hours apart	•Saquinavir levels reduced by: rifampin, rifabutin, phenobarbital, phenytoin, dexamethasone, carbamazepine, and nevirapine
•Indinavir levels reduced by rifampin, rifabutin, nevirapine, grapefruit juice	•Nelfinavir decreases levels of ethinyl estradiol and norethindrone	•Ritonavir decreases levels of ethinyl estradiol, theophylline, sulfamethoxazole, and zidovudine	•Not recommended for concurrent use: terfenadine, astemizole, cisapride, ergot alkaloids
•Didanosine: reduces indinavir absorption unless taken >2 hours apart	•Nelfinavir increases levels of rifabutin, saquinavir, and indinavir	•Ritonavir increases levels of clarithromycin and desipramine	

Table 4.
INTERACTIONS BETWEEN CIGARETTE SMOKE AND DRUGS

Drug	Mechanism	Effect on Cigarette Smokers
Theophylline	Induction of the CYP1A2 isozyme	Smoking may lead to reduced theophylline serum concentrations and decreased clinical effect; the elimination of theophylline is considerably more rapid in smokers
Tacrine	Induction of the CYP1A2 isozyme	Effectiveness of tacrine in smokers may be decreased
Insulin	Decreased insulin absorption, which may be related to peripheral vasoconstriction	Insulin-dependent diabetics who smoke heavily may require a 15% to 30% higher dose of insulin than nonsmokers
Flecainide	Unknown	Smoking may reduce flecainide serum concentrations
Propoxyphene	Unknown	Smokers may require a higher dosage of propoxyphene to achieve analgesic effects
Propranolol	Increased release of catecholamines (eg, epinephrine) in smokers	Smokers taking propranolol may have increased blood pressure and heart rate relative to nonsmokers. Effects on prevention of angina pectoris and stroke should be considered
Diazepam; Chlordiazepoxide	Unknown; whether pharmacokinetics is altered or end-organ responsiveness is decreased is unclear	Smokers may require larger doses of diazepam and chlordiazepoxide to achieve sedative effects

Adapted from Schein, JR, "Cigarette Smoking and Clinically Significant Drug Interactions," *Ann Pharmacother*, 1995, 29(11):1139-47.

ALPHABETICAL LISTING OF DRUGS

A-200™ Shampoo [OTC] *see* Pyrethrins *on page 824*
A and D™ Ointment [OTC] *see* Vitamin A and Vitamin D *on page 993*
Abbokinase® *see* Urokinase *on page 979*

Abciximab (ab SIK si mab)
Brand Names ReoPro™
Therapeutic Category Platelet Aggregation Inhibitor
Synonyms C7E3; 7E3
Use Adjunct to percutaneous transluminal coronary angioplasty or atherectomy (PTCA) for the prevention of acute cardiac ischemic complications in patients at high risk for abrupt closure of the treated coronary vessel
Usual Dosage I.V.: 0.25 mg/kg bolus followed by an infusion of 10 mcg/minute for 12 hours
Mechanism of Action Abciximab binds to the glycoprotein GPIIb/IIIa receptor, a major receptor involved in the common pathway for platelet aggregation. Platelet aggregation is, therefore, inhibited.
Local Anesthetic/Vasoconstrictor Precautions No information available to require special precautions
Effects on Dental Treatment No effects or complications reported
Other Adverse Effects
>10%:
Cardiovascular: Hypotension
Central nervous system: Pain
Gastrointestinal: Nausea
Hematologic: Major bleeding episodes
1% to 10%:
Cardiovascular: Bradycardia, peripheral edema
Hematologic: Minor bleeding episodes, thrombocytopenia, anemia
Respiratory: Pleural effusion
Drug Interactions
Increased toxicity:
Bleeding: Heparin, other anticoagulants, thrombolytics, and antiplatelet drugs
Allergic reactions: Diagnostic or therapeutic monoclonal antibodies
Pregnancy Risk Factor C
Dosage Forms Injection: 2 mg/mL (5 mL)
Generic Available No

Abelcet™ Injection *see* Amphotericin B Lipid Complex *on page 73*
ABLC *see* Amphotericin B Lipid Complex *on page 73*
Absorbine® Antifungal [OTC] *see* Tolnaftate *on page 943*
Absorbine® Antifungal Foot Powder [OTC] *see* Miconazole *on page 635*
Absorbine® Jock Itch [OTC] *see* Tolnaftate *on page 943*
Absorbine Jr.® Antifungal [OTC] *see* Tolnaftate *on page 943*

Acarbose (AY car bose)
Related Information
Endocrine Disorders & Pregnancy *on page 1021*
Brand Names Precose®
Therapeutic Category Alpha-Glucosidase Inhibitor; Hypoglycemic Agent, Oral
Use Treatment of noninsulin-dependent diabetes mellitus (NIDDM); as monotherapy or in combination with a sulfonylurea when diet plus acarbose or a sulfonylurea does not result in adequate glycemic control
Usual Dosage Oral:
Adults: Dosage must be individualized on the basis of effectiveness and tolerance while not exceeding the maximum recommended dose of 100 mg 3 times/day
Initial dose: 25 mg 3 times/day with the first bite of each main meal
Maintenance dose: Should be adjusted at 4- to 8-week intervals based on 1-hour postprandial glucose levels and tolerance. Dosage may be increased from 25 mg 3 times/day to 50 mg 3 times/day. Some patients may benefit from increasing the dose to 100 mg 3 times/day. Maintenance dose ranges: 50-100 mg 3 times/day.
Maximum dose:
≤60 kg: 50 mg 3 times/day
>60 kg: 100 mg 3 times/day
Patients receiving sulfonylureas: Acarbose given in combination with a sulfonylurea will cause a further lowering of blood glucose and may increase the hypoglycemic potential of the sulfonylurea. If hypoglycemia occurs, appropriate adjustments in the dosage of these agents should be made.

Elderly: Mean steady-state AUC and maximum concentrations of acarbose were 1.5 times higher in elderly compared to young volunteers; however, these differences were not statistically significant

Dosing adjustment in renal impairment: Cl_{cr} <25 mL/minute: Peak plasma concentrations were 5 times higher and AUCs were 6 times larger than in volunteers with normal renal function; however, long term clinical trials in diabetic patients with significant renal dysfunction have not been conducted and treatment of these patients with acarbose is not recommended

Mechanism of Action Competitive, reversible inhibition of pancreatic alpha-amylase and membrane-bound intestinal alpha-glucoside hydrolase enzymes to result in delayed glucose absorption and a lowering of postprandial hyperglycemia

Local Anesthetic/Vasoconstrictor Precautions No information available to require special precautions

Effects on Dental Treatment No effects or complications reported

Drug Interactions Decreased effect: Thiazides and other diuretics, corticosteroids, phenothiazines, thyroid products, estrogens, oral contraceptives, phenytoin, nicotinic acid, sympathomimetics, calcium channel-blocking drugs, isoniazid, intestinal adsorbents (eg, charcoal), digestive enzyme preparations (eg, amylase, pancreatin)

Drug Uptake

Absorption: <2% absorbed as active drug

Pregnancy Risk Factor B

Dosage Forms Tablet: 50 mg, 100 mg

Generic Available No

Accolate® see Zafirlukast on page 1000

Accupril® see Quinapril on page 827

Accutane® see Isotretinoin on page 526

Acebutolol (a se BYOO toe lole)

Brand Names Sectral®

Canadian/Mexican Brand Names Monitan® (Canada); Rhotral® (Canada)

Therapeutic Category Antiarrhythmic Agent, Class II; Antiarrhythmic Agent (Supraventricular & Ventricular); Beta-adrenergic Blocker, Cardioselective

Use Treatment of hypertension, ventricular arrhythmias, angina

Usual Dosage Oral:

Adults: 400-800 mg/day in 2 divided doses; maximum: 1200 mg/day

Elderly: Initial: 200-400 mg/day; dose reduction due to age related decrease in Cl_{cr} will be necessary; do not exceed 800 mg/day

Mechanism of Action Competitively blocks beta$_1$-adrenergic receptors with little or no effect on beta$_2$-receptors except at high doses; exhibits membrane stabilizing and intrinsic sympathomimetic activity

Local Anesthetic/Vasoconstrictor Precautions No information available to require special precautions

Effects on Dental Treatment Noncardioselective beta-blockers (ie, propranolol, nadolol) enhance the pressor response to epinephrine, resulting in hypertension and bradycardia. This has not been reported for acebutolol, a cardioselective beta-blocker. Therefore, local anesthetic with vasoconstrictor can be safely used in patients medicated with acebutolol. Many nonsteroidal anti-inflammatory drugs such as ibuprofen and indomethacin can reduce the hypotensive effect of beta-blockers after 3 or more weeks of therapy with the NSAID. Short-term NSAID use (ie, 3 days) requires no special precautions in patients taking beta-blockers.

Other Adverse Effects

>10%: Central nervous system: Fatigue

1% to 10%:

Cardiovascular: Chest pain, edema, bradycardia, hypotension

Central nervous system: Headache, dizziness, insomnia, depression, abnormal dreams

Dermatologic: Rash

Gastrointestinal: Constipation, diarrhea, dyspepsia, nausea, flatulence

Genitourinary: Micturition (frequency)

Neuromuscular & skeletal: Arthralgia, myalgia

Ocular: Abnormal vision

Respiratory: Dyspnea, rhinitis, cough

<1%:

Cardiovascular: Ventricular arrhythmias, heart block, heart failure, facial swelling

Gastrointestinal: Dry mouth, anorexia

Genitourinary: Impotence, urinary retention

Miscellaneous: Cold extremities

(Continued)

Acebutolol *(Continued)*

Drug Interactions
Decreased effect of beta-blockers:
  Barbiturates (increased liver metabolism of beta-blockers to result in lower serum levels)
  NSAIDs (attenuate the hypotensive therapeutic effects of beta-blockers)
  Rifampin (increased liver metabolism of beta-blockers to result in lower serum levels)
Increased effects of beta-blockers:
  Calcium channel blockers (increase serum levels of beta-blockers by unknown mechanism to enhance hypotension)
Beta-blockers increase the effects of:
  Epinephrine (vasoconstrictor; initial hypertensive episode followed by bradycardia) only from noncardioselective type beta-blockers
  Phenylephrine (Neosynephrine®; enhanced pressor response)
  Theophylline (inhibit theophylline metabolism causing increase in serum concentrations)

Drug Uptake
Absorption: Oral: Well absorbed (40%)
Serum half-life: 6-7 hours average
Time to peak: 2-4 hours

Pregnancy Risk Factor B
Generic Available Yes
Selected Readings
Foster CA and Aston SJ, "Propranolol-Epinephrine Interaction: A Potential Disaster," *Plast Reconstr Surg*, 1983, 72(1):74-8.
Wong DG, Spence JD, Lamki L, et al, "Effect of Nonsteroidal Anti-inflammatory Drugs on Control of Hypertension of Beta-Blockers and Diuretics," *Lancet*, 1986, 1(8488):997-1001.
Wynn RL, "Dental Nonsteroidal Anti-inflammatory Drugs and Prostaglandin-Based Drug Interactions, Part Two," *Gen Dent*, 1992, 40(2):104, 106, 108.
Wynn RL, "Epinephrine Interactions With Beta-Blockers," *Gen Dent*, 1994, 42(1):16, 18.

Aceon® *see* Perindopril Erbumine *on page 742*
Acephen® [OTC] *see* Acetaminophen *on this page*
Aceta® [OTC] *see* Acetaminophen *on this page*
Acetaminofen (Mexico) *see* Acetaminophen *on this page*

Acetaminophen (a seet a MIN oh fen)

Related Information
Acetaminophen and Pseudoephedrine *on page 24*
Acetaminophen, Dextromethorphan, and Pseudoephedrine *on page 25*
Butalbital Compound and Acetaminophen *on page 155*
Oral Pain *on page 1053*

Brand Names Acephen® [OTC]; Aceta® [OTC]; Apacet® [OTC]; Arthritis Foundation® Pain Reliever, Aspirin Free [OTC]; Aspirin Free Anacin® Maximum Strength [OTC]; Children's Silapap® [OTC]; Feverall™ [OTC]; Feverall™ Sprinkle Caps [OTC]; Genapap® [OTC]; Halenol® Childrens [OTC]; Infants Feverall™ [OTC]; Infants' Silapap® [OTC]; Junior Strength Panadol® [OTC]; Liquiprin® [OTC]; Mapap® [OTC]; Maranox® [OTC]; Neopap® [OTC]; Panadol® [OTC]; Redutemp® [OTC]; Ridenol® [OTC]; Tempra® [OTC]; Tylenol® [OTC]; Tylenol® Extended Relief [OTC]; Uni-Ace® [OTC]

Canadian/Mexican Brand Names 222 AF® (Canada); Algitrin® (Mexico); Analphen® (Mexico); Atasol® (Canada); Cilag® (Mexico); Febrin® (Mexico); Minofen® (Mexico); Neodol® (Mexico); Pediatrix® (Canada); Sinedol®. 500 (Mexico); Sinedol® (Mexico); Tantaphen® (Canada); Temperal® (Mexico); Tylex® 750 (Mexico); Winasorb® (Mexico)

Therapeutic Category Analgesic, Non-narcotic; Antipyretic
Synonyms Acetaminofen (Mexico); Paracetamol (Mexico)
Use
Dental: Treatment of postoperative pain
Medical: Treatment of pain and fever; does not have anti-inflammatory effects
Usual Dosage Oral:
Children <12 years: 10-15 mg/kg/dose every 4-6 hours as needed; do not exceed 5 doses (2.6 g) in 24 hours
Adults: 325-650 mg (1-2 tablets) every 4-6 hours or 1000 mg 3-4 times/day; do not exceed 4 g/day (4000 mg)
Mechanism of Action Inhibits the synthesis of prostaglandins in the CNS and peripherally blocks pain impulse generation; produces antipyresis by inhibition of hypothalamic heat-regulating center
Local Anesthetic/Vasoconstrictor Precautions No information available to require special precautions
Effects on Dental Treatment No effects or complications reported
Other Adverse Effects No data reported

Contraindications Patients with known Glucose-6-phosphate dehydrogenase (G-6-PD) deficiency; hypersensitivity to acetaminophen

Warnings/Precautions May cause severe hepatic toxicity on overdose; use with caution in patients with alcoholic liver disease; chronic daily dosing in adults of 5-8 g of acetaminophen over several weeks or 3-4 g/day of acetaminophen for 1 year have resulted in liver damage

Drug Interactions

Alcohol: Chronic excessive alcohol ingestion increases the liver toxicity of high doses of acetaminophen

Cholestyramine: Cholestyramine reduces the plasma acetaminophen concentrations and probably reduces acetaminophen response

Isoniazid (INH): Acetaminophen blood levels are increased by INH; hepatotoxicity has been reported with combination of acetaminophen and INH

Phenobarbital: Barbiturates such as phenobarbital may enhance the hepatotoxic effect of large doses of acetaminophen

Phenytoin: Phenytoin may enhance the hepatotoxic potential of large doses of acetaminophen

Drug Uptake

Onset: 1-3 hours

Duration: 3-4 hours

Serum half-life: 1-4 hours

Time to peak serum concentration: 0.5-2 hours

Pregnancy Risk Factor B

Breast-feeding Considerations May be taken while breast-feeding

Dosage Forms

Caplet: 160 mg, 325 mg, 500 mg

Caplet, extended: 650 mg

Capsule: 80 mg

Drops: 48 mg/mL (15 mL); 60 mg/0.6 mL (15 mL); 80 mg/0.8 mL (15 mL); 100 mg/mL (15 mL, 30 mL)

Elixir: 80 mg/5 mL, 120 mg/5 mL, 160 mg/5 mL, 167 mg/5 mL, 325 mg/5 mL

Liquid, oral: 160 mg/5 mL, 500 mg/15 mL

Solution: 100 mg/mL (15 mL); 120 mg/2.5 mL

Suppository, rectal: 80 mg, 120 mg, 125 mg, 300 mg, 325 mg, 650 mg

Suspension, oral: 160 mg/5 mL

Suspension, oral drops: 80 mg/0.8 mL

Tablet: 325 mg, 500 mg, 650 mg

Tablet, chewable: 80 mg, 160 mg

Dietary Considerations May be taken with food

Generic Available Yes

Comments Doses of acetaminophen >5 g/day for several weeks can produce severe, often fatal liver damage. Hepatotoxicity caused by acetaminophen is potentiated by chronic alcohol consumption. It has been reported that a combination of two quarts of whiskey a day with 8-10 acetaminophen tablets daily resulted in severe liver toxicity. People who consume alcohol at the same time that they use acetaminophen, even in therapeutic doses, are at risk of developing hepatotoxicity.

Selected Readings

Barker JD Jr, de Carle DJ, and Anuras S, "Chronic Excessive Acetaminophen Use in Liver Damage," *Ann Intern Med*, 1977, 87(3):299-301.

Dionne RA, Campbell RA, Cooper SA, et al, "Suppression of Postoperative Pain by Preoperative Administration of Ibuprofen in Comparison to Placebo, Acetaminophen, and Acetaminophen Plus Codeine," *J Clin Pharmacol*, 1983, 23(1):37-43.

Lee WM, "Drug-Induced Hepatotoxicity," *N Engl J Med*, 1995, 333(17):1118-27.

Licht H, Seeff LB, and Zimmerman HJ, "Apparent Potentiation of Acetaminophen Hepatotoxicity by Alcohol," *Ann Intern Med*, 1980, 92(4):511.

McClain CJ, et al, "Potentiation of Acetaminophen Hepatotoxicity by Alcohol," *JAMA*, 1980, 244:251.

Murphy R, Swartz R, and Watkins PB, "Severe Acetaminophen Toxicity in a Patient Receiving Isoniazid," *Ann Intern Med*, 1990, 113(110):799-800.

Acetaminophen and Butalbital Compound see Butalbital Compound and Acetaminophen *on page 155*

Acetaminophen and Codeine (a seet a MIN oh fen & KOE deen)

Brand Names Capital® and Codeine; Phenaphen® With Codeine; Tylenol® With Codeine

Canadian/Mexican Brand Names Lenoltec® With Codeine (Canada); Novo-Gesic-C8® (Canada); Novo-Gesic-C15® (Canada); Novo-Gesic-C30® (Canada); Tylex® CD (Mexico)

Therapeutic Category Analgesic, Narcotic

Use

Dental: Treatment of postoperative pain

Medical: Relief of pain

Restrictions C-III; C-V; Refillable up to 5 times in 6 months

(Continued)

Acetaminophen and Codeine *(Continued)*

Usual Dosage
   Children: Not recommended in pediatric dental patients
   Adults: Based on codeine (30-60 mg/dose) every 4-6 hours; 1-2 tablets every 4
      hours to a maximum of 12 tablets/24 hours

Mechanism of Action
   Acetaminophen: Inhibits the synthesis of prostaglandins in the CNS and periph-
      erally blocks pain impulse generation; produces antipyresis by inhibition of
      hypothalamic heat-regulating center
   Codeine: Binds to opiate receptors (mu and kappa subtypes) in the CNS causing
      inhibition of ascending pain pathways, altering the perception of and response
      to pain

Local Anesthetic/Vasoconstrictor Precautions No information available to
   require special precautions

Effects on Dental Treatment <1% of patients may experience dry mouth

Other Adverse Effects
   >10%:
      Central nervous system: Lightheadedness, dizziness, sedation
      Gastrointestinal: Nausea, vomiting
   1% to 10%: Gastrointestinal: Constipation

Contraindications Patients with known G-6-PD deficiency; hypersensitivity to
   acetaminophen; hypersensitivity to codeine

Warnings/Precautions Use with caution in patients with hypersensitivity reactions to other phenanthrene derivative opioid agonists (morphine, hydrocodone,
   hydromorphone, levorphanol, oxycodone, oxymorphone); respiratory diseases
   including asthma, emphysema, COPD, or severe liver or renal insufficiency;
   some preparations contain sulfites which may cause allergic reactions; may be
   habit-forming

   Enhanced analgesia has been seen in elderly patients on therapeutic doses of
   narcotics; duration of action may be increased in the elderly; the elderly may be
   particularly susceptible to the CNS depressant and constipating effects of
   narcotics

Drug Interactions
   With codeine component: Increased toxicity of CNS depressants, phenothi-
      azines, tricyclic antidepressants, guanabenz, MAO inhibitors (may also lead to
      a decrease in blood pressure)
   With acetaminophen component: Refer to Acetaminophen monograph

Drug Uptake
   Acetaminophen:
      Onset: 1-3 hours
      Duration: 3-4 hours
      Serum half-life: 1-4 hours
      Time to peak serum concentration: 0.5-2 hours
   Codeine:
      Onset (analgesia): Oral: 30-45 minutes
      Duration: 4-6 hours
      Serum half-life: 2.5-3.5 hours
      Time to peak serum concentration: 1-2 hours

Pregnancy Risk Factor C

Breast-feeding Considerations Both acetaminophen and codeine may be
   taken while breast-feeding

Dosage Forms
   Capsule:
      #2: Acetaminophen 325 mg and codeine phosphate 15 mg (C-III)
      #3: Acetaminophen 325 mg and codeine phosphate 30 mg (C-III)
      #4: Acetaminophen 325 mg and codeine phosphate 60 mg (C-III)
   Elixir: Acetaminophen 120 mg and codeine phosphate 12 mg per 5 mL with
      alcohol 7% (C-V)
   Suspension, oral, alcohol free: Acetaminophen 120 mg and codeine phosphate
      12 mg per 5 mL (C-V)
   Tablet: Acetaminophen 500 mg and codeine phosphate 30 mg (C-III); acetamin-
      ophen 650 mg and codeine phosphate 30 mg (C-III)
   Tablet:
      #1: Acetaminophen 300 mg and codeine phosphate 7.5 mg (C-III)
      #2: Acetaminophen 300 mg and codeine phosphate 15 mg (C-III)
      #3: Acetaminophen 300 mg and codeine phosphate 30 mg (C-III)
      #4: Acetaminophen 300 mg and codeine phosphate 60 mg (C-III)

Dietary Considerations May be taken with food

Generic Available Yes

Comments Codeine products, as with other narcotic analgesics, are recommended only for acute dosing (ie, 3 days or less). The most common adverse

effect you will see in your dental patients from codeine is nausea, followed by sedation and constipation. Codeine has narcotic addiction liability, especially when given long term. Because of the acetaminophen component, this product should be used with caution in patients with alcoholic liver disease.

Selected Readings

Dionne RA, "New Approaches to Preventing and Treating Postoperative Pain," *J Am Dent Assoc*, 1992, 123(6):26-34.

Dionne RA, Campbell RA, Cooper SA, et al, "Suppression of Postoperative Pain by Preoperative Administration of Ibuprofen in Comparison to Placebo, Acetaminophen, and Acetaminophen Plus Codeine," *J Clin Pharmacol*, 1983, 23(1):37-43.

Forbes JA, Butterworth GA, Burchfield WH, et al, "Evaluation of Ketorolac, Aspirin, and an Acetamino-phen-Codeine Combination in Postoperative Oral Surgery Pain," *Pharmacotherapy*, 1990, 10(6 Pt 2):77S-93S.

Gobetti JP, "Controlling Dental Pain," *J Am Dent Assoc*, 1992, 123(6):47-52.

Acetaminophen and Dextromethorphan

(a seet a MIN oh fen & dex troe meth OR fan)

Brand Names Bayer® Select® Chest Cold Caplets [OTC]; Drixoral® Cough & Sore Throat Liquid Caps [OTC]

Therapeutic Category Analgesic, Non-narcotic; Antipyretic; Antitussive

Use Treatment of mild to moderate pain and fever; symptomatic relief of coughs caused by minor viral upper respiratory tract infections or inhaled irritants; most effective for a chronic nonproductive cough

Local Anesthetic/Vasoconstrictor Precautions No information available to require special precautions

Effects on Dental Treatment No effects or complications reported

Warnings/Precautions Research on chicken embryos exposed to concentrations of dextromethorphan relative to those typically taken by humans has shown to cause birth defects and fetal death; more study is needed, but it is suggested that pregnant women should be advised not to use dextromethorphan-containing medications

Generic Available Yes

Selected Readings

Barker JD Jr, de Carle DJ, and Anuras S, "Chronic Excessive Acetaminophen Use in Liver Damage," *Ann Intern Med*, 1977, 87(3):299-301.

Dionne RA, Campbell RA, Cooper SA, et al, "Suppression of Postoperative Pain by Preoperative Administration of Ibuprofen in Comparison to Placebo, Acetaminophen, and Acetaminophen Plus Codeine," *J Clin Pharmacol*, 1983, 23(1):37-43.

Licht H, Seeff LB, and Zimmerman HJ, "Apparent Potentiation of Acetaminophen Hepatotoxicity by Alcohol," *Ann Intern Med*, 1980, 92(4):511.

Acetaminophen and Diphenhydramine

(a seet a MIN oh fen & dye fen HYE dra meen)

Brand Names Arthritis Foundation® Nighttime [OTC]; Excedrin® P.M. [OTC]; Midol® PM [OTC]

Therapeutic Category Analgesic, Non-narcotic

Use Relief of mild to moderate pain; sinus headache

Local Anesthetic/Vasoconstrictor Precautions No information available to require special precautions

Effects on Dental Treatment 1% to 10%: Dry mouth

Generic Available Yes

Selected Readings

Barker JD Jr, de Carle DJ, and Anuras S, "Chronic Excessive Acetaminophen Use in Liver Damage," *Ann Intern Med*, 1977, 87(3):299-301.

Dionne RA, Campbell RA, Cooper SA, et al, "Suppression of Postoperative Pain by Preoperative Administration of Ibuprofen in Comparison to Placebo, Acetaminophen, and Acetaminophen Plus Codeine," *J Clin Pharmacol*, 1983, 23(1):37-43.

Licht H, Seeff LB, and Zimmerman HJ, "Apparent Potentiation of Acetaminophen Hepatotoxicity by Alcohol," *Ann Intern Med*, 1980, 92(4):511.

Acetaminophen and Phenyltoloxamine

(a seet a MIN oh fen & fen il to LOKS a meen)

Brand Names Percogesic® [OTC]

Therapeutic Category Analgesic, Non-narcotic

Use Relief of mild to moderate pain

Local Anesthetic/Vasoconstrictor Precautions No information available to require special precautions

Effects on Dental Treatment No effects or complications reported

Pregnancy Risk Factor B

Generic Available Yes

Selected Readings

Barker JD Jr, de Carle DJ, and Anuras S, "Chronic Excessive Acetaminophen Use in Liver Damage," *Ann Intern Med*, 1977, 87(3):299-301.

Dionne RA, Campbell RA, Cooper SA, et al, "Suppression of Postoperative Pain by Preoperative Administration of Ibuprofen in Comparison to Placebo, Acetaminophen, and Acetaminophen Plus Codeine," *J Clin Pharmacol*, 1983, 23(1):37-43.

(Continued)

Acetaminophen and Phenyltoloxamine *(Continued)*

Licht H, Seeff LB, and Zimmerman HJ, "Apparent Potentiation of Acetaminophen Hepatotoxicity by Alcohol," *Ann Intern Med*, 1980, 92(4):511.

Acetaminophen and Pseudoephedrine

(a seet a MIN oh fen & soo doe e FED rin)

Brand Names Allerest® No Drowsiness [OTC]; Bayer® Select Head Cold Caplets [OTC]; Coldrine® [OTC]; Dristan® Cold Caplets [OTC]; Dynafed®, Maximum Strength *New Brand* [OTC]; Ornex® No Drowsiness [OTC]; Sinarest®, No Drowsiness [OTC]; Sine-Aid®, Maximum Strength [OTC]; Sine-Off® Maximum Strength No Drowsiness Formula [OTC]; Sinus Excedrin® Extra Strength [OTC]; Sinus-Relief® [OTC]; Sinutab® Without Drowsiness [OTC]; Tylenol® Sinus, Maximum Strength [OTC]

Therapeutic Category Decongestant/Analgesic

Synonyms Pseudoephedrine and Acetaminophen

Use Relief of mild to moderate pain; relief of congestion

Usual Dosage Adults: Oral: 2 tablets every 4-6 hours

Local Anesthetic/Vasoconstrictor Precautions No information available to require special precautions

Effects on Dental Treatment No effects or complications reported

Other Adverse Effects See individual agents

Dosage Forms Tablet:

Allerest® No Drowsiness; Coldrine®, Tylenol® Sinus, Maximum Strength; Ornex® No Drowsiness, Sinus-Relief®: Acetaminophen 325 mg and pseudoephedrine hydrochloride 30 mg

Bayer® Select Head Cold; Dristan® Cold; Dynafed®, Maximum Strength; Sinarest®, No Drowsiness; Sine-Aid®, Maximum Strength; Sine-Off® Maximum Strength No Drowsiness Formula; Sinus Excedrin® Extra Strength; Sinutab® Without Drowsiness; Tylenol® Sinus, Maximum Strength: Acetaminophen 500 mg and pseudoephedrine hydrochloride 30 mg

Generic Available Yes

Acetaminophen, Aspirin, and Caffeine

(a seet a MIN oh fen, AS pir in, & KAF een)

Brand Names Excedrin®, Extra Strength [OTC]; Excedrin® Migraine [OTC]; Gelpirin® [OTC]; Goody's® Headache Powders

Therapeutic Category Analgesic, Non-narcotic

Use Relief of mild to moderate pain

Local Anesthetic/Vasoconstrictor Precautions No information available to require special precautions

Effects on Dental Treatment No effects or complications reported

Other Adverse Effects See individual agents

Pregnancy Risk Factor D

Generic Available Yes

Selected Readings

Barker JD Jr, de Carle DJ, and Anuras S, "Chronic Excessive Acetaminophen Use in Liver Damage," *Ann Intern Med*, 1977, 87(3):299-301.

Desjardins PJ, Cooper SA, Gallegos TL, et al, "The Relative Analgesic Efficacy of Propiram Fumarate, Codeine Aspirin, and Placebo in Post-Impaction Dental Pain," *J Clin Pharmacol*, 1984, 24(1):35-42.

Dionne RA, Campbell RA, Cooper SA, et al, "Suppression of Postoperative Pain by Preoperative Administration of Ibuprofen in Comparison to Placebo, Acetaminophen, and Acetaminophen Plus Codeine," *J Clin Pharmacol*, 1983, 23(1):37-43.

Forbes JA, Butterworth GA, Burchfield WH, et al, "Evaluation of Ketorolac, Aspirin, and an Acetaminophen-Codeine Combination in Postoperative Oral Surgery Pain," *Pharmacotherapy*, 1990, 10(6 Pt 2):77S-93S.

Forbes JA, Keller CK, Smith JW, et al, "Analgesic Effect of Naproxen Sodium, Codeine, a Naproxen-Codeine Combination and Aspirin on the Postoperative Pain of Oral Surgery," *Pharmacotherapy*, 1986, 6(5):211-8.

Licht H, Seeff LB, and Zimmerman HJ, "Apparent Potentiation of Acetaminophen Hepatotoxicity by Alcohol," *Ann Intern Med*, 1980, 92(4):511.

Acetaminophen, Chlorpheniramine, and Pseudoephedrine

(a seet a MIN oh fen, klor fen IR a meen, & soo doe e FED rin)

Brand Names Alka-Seltzer® Plus Cold Liqui-Gels Capsules [OTC]; Aspirin-Free Bayer® Select® Allergy Sinus Caplets [OTC]; Co-Hist® [OTC]; Sinutab® Tablets [OTC]

Therapeutic Category Analgesic, Non-narcotic; Antihistamine/Decongestant Combination

Use Temporary relief of sinus symptoms

Local Anesthetic/Vasoconstrictor Precautions Use with caution since pseudoephedrine is a sympathomimetic amine which could interact with epinephrine to cause a pressor response

Effects on Dental Treatment
Chlorpheniramine: Prolonged use will cause significant xerostomia
Pseudoephedrine: Up to 10% of patients could experience tachycardia, palpitations, and dry mouth; use vasoconstrictor with caution
Other Adverse Effects See individual agents
Pregnancy Risk Factor B
Generic Available Yes
Selected Readings
Barker JD Jr, de Carle DJ, and Anuras S, "Chronic Excessive Acetaminophen Use in Liver Damage," *Ann Intern Med*, 1977, 87(3):299-301.
Dionne RA, Campbell RA, Cooper SA, et al, "Suppression of Postoperative Pain by Preoperative Administration of Ibuprofen in Comparison to Placebo, Acetaminophen, and Acetaminophen Plus Codeine," *J Clin Pharmacol*, 1983, 23(1):37-43.
Licht H, Seeff LB, and Zimmerman HJ, "Apparent Potentiation of Acetaminophen Hepatotoxicity by Alcohol," *Ann Intern Med*, 1980, 92(4):511.

Acetaminophen, Dextromethorphan, and Pseudoephedrine
(a seet a MIN oh fen, deks troe meth OR fan, & soo doe e FED rin)
Brand Names Alka-Seltzer® Plus Flu & Body Aches Non-Drowsy Liqui-Gels [OTC]; Comtrex® Maximum Strength Non-Drowsy [OTC]; Sudafed® Severe Cold [OTC]; Theraflu® Non-Drowsy Formula Maximum Strength [OTC]; Tylenol® Cold No Drowsiness [OTC]; Tylenol® Flu Maximum Strength [OTC]
Therapeutic Category Cold Preparation
Synonyms Dextromethorphan, Acetaminophen, and Pseudoephedrine; Pseudoephedrine, Acetaminophen, and Dextromethorphan; Pseudoephedrine, Dextromethorphan, and Acetaminophen
Use Treatment of mild to moderate pain and fever; symptomatic relief of cough and congestion
Usual Dosage Oral: Adults: Two every 6 hours
Local Anesthetic/Vasoconstrictor Precautions No information available to require special precautions
Effects on Dental Treatment No effects or complications reported
Other Adverse Effects See individual agents
Warnings/Precautions Research on chicken embryos exposed to concentrations of dextromethorphan relative to those typically taken by humans has shown to cause birth defects and fetal death; more study is needed, but it is suggested that pregnant women should be advised not to use dextromethorphan-containing medications
Dosage Forms Tablet:
Alka-Seltzer® Plus Flu & Body Aches Non-Drowsy: Acetaminophen 500 mg, dextromethorphan hydrobromide 10 mg, and pseudoephedrine hydrochloride 30 mg
Tylenol® Cold No Drowsiness: Acetaminophen 325 mg, dextromethorphan hydrobromide 15 mg, and pseudoephedrine hydrochloride 30 mg
Comtrex® Maximum Strength Non-Drowsy; Sudafed® Severe Cold; Theraflu® Non-Drowsy Formula Maximum Strength; Tylenol® Flu Maximum Strength: Acetaminophen 500 mg, dextromethorphan hydrobromide 15 mg, and pseudoephedrine hydrochloride 30 mg
Generic Available Yes

Acetaminophen, Isometheptene, and Dichloralphenazone
(a seet a MIN oh fen, eye soe me THEP teen, & dye KLOR al FEN a zone)
Brand Names Isocom®; Isopap®; Midchlor®; Midrin®; Migratine®
Therapeutic Category Analgesic, Non-narcotic; Antimigraine Agent
Use Relief of migraine and tension headache
Local Anesthetic/Vasoconstrictor Precautions No information available to require special precautions
Effects on Dental Treatment No effects or complications reported
Pregnancy Risk Factor B
Generic Available Yes
Comments Should not exceed 5 g in 12 hours; may cause drowsiness; avoid alcohol and other CNS depressants
Selected Readings
Barker JD Jr, de Carle DJ, and Anuras S, "Chronic Excessive Acetaminophen Use in Liver Damage," *Ann Intern Med*, 1977, 87(3):299-301.
Dionne RA, Campbell RA, Cooper SA, et al, "Suppression of Postoperative Pain by Preoperative Administration of Ibuprofen in Comparison to Placebo, Acetaminophen, and Acetaminophen Plus Codeine," *J Clin Pharmacol*, 1983, 23(1):37-43.
Licht H, Seeff LB, and Zimmerman HJ, "Apparent Potentiation of Acetaminophen Hepatotoxicity by Alcohol," *Ann Intern Med*, 1980, 92(4):511.

Acetasol® HC Otic *see* Acetic Acid, Propylene Glycol Diacetate, and Hydrocortisone *on next page*

Acetazolamide (a set a ZOLE a mide)

Brand Names Diamox®; Diamox Sequels®

Canadian/Mexican Brand Names Acetazolam® (Canada); Apo®-Acetazolamide (Canada); Novo-Zolamide® (Canada)

Therapeutic Category Anticonvulsant, Miscellaneous; Antiglaucoma Agent; Carbonic Anhydrase Inhibitor; Diuretic, Carbonic Anhydrase Inhibitor

Use Lowers intraocular pressure to treat glaucoma, also as a diuretic, adjunct treatment of refractory seizures and acute altitude sickness; centrencephalic epilepsies (sustained release not recommended for anticonvulsant)

Usual Dosage Note: I.M. administration is not recommended because of pain secondary to the alkaline pH

Children:

Glaucoma:

Oral: 8-30 mg/kg/day or 300-900 mg/m²/day divided every 8 hours

I.M., I.V.: 20-40 mg/kg/24 hours divided every 6 hours, not to exceed 1 g/day

Edema: Oral, I.M., I.V.: 5 mg/kg or 150 mg/m² once every day

Epilepsy: Oral: 8-30 mg/kg/day in 1-4 divided doses, not to exceed 1 g/day; sustained release capsule is not recommended for treatment of epilepsy

Adults:

Glaucoma:

Chronic simple (open-angle): Oral: 250 mg 1-4 times/day or 500 mg sustained release capsule twice daily

Secondary, acute (closed-angle): I.M., I.V.: 250-500 mg, may repeat in 2-4 hours to a maximum of 1 g/day

Edema: Oral, I.M., I.V.: 250-375 mg once daily

Epilepsy: Oral: 8-30 mg/kg/day in 1-4 divided doses, not to exceed 1 g/day; **sustained release capsule is not recommended for treatment of epilepsy**

Altitude sickness: Oral: 250 mg every 8-12 hours (or 500 mg extended release capsules every 12-24 hours). Therapy should begin 24-48 hours before and continue during ascent and for at least 48 hours after arrival at the high altitude.

Urine alkalinization: Oral: 5 mg/kg/dose repeated 2-3 times over 24 hours

Elderly: Oral: Initial: 250 mg twice daily; use lowest effective dose

Mechanism of Action Reversible inhibition of the enzyme carbonic anhydrase resulting in reduction of hydrogen ion secretion at renal tubule and an increased renal excretion of sodium, potassium, bicarbonate, and water to decrease production of aqueous humor; also inhibits carbonic anhydrase in central nervous system to retard abnormal and excessive discharge from CNS neurons

Local Anesthetic/Vasoconstrictor Precautions No information available to require special precautions

Effects on Dental Treatment Metallic taste in >10% of patients; disappears upon drug withdrawal

Other Adverse Effects

>10%:

Central nervous system: Malaise

Gastrointestinal: Anorexia, diarrhea, metallic taste

Renal: Polyuria

<1%:

Central nervous system: Fever, fatigue, mental depression, drowsiness

Dermatologic: Rash

Endocrine & metabolic: Hyperchloremic metabolic acidosis, hypokalemia, hyperglycemia

Gastrointestinal: GI irritation, dryness of mouth, black stools

Genitourinary: Dysuria

Hematologic: Bone marrow suppression, blood dyscrasias

Neuromuscular & skeletal: Paresthesia, weakness

Ocular: Myopia

Renal: Renal calculi

Drug Interactions Acetazolamide increases lithium excretion and alters excretion of other drugs by alkalinization of urine (such as amphetamines, quinidine, procainamide, methenamine, phenobarbital, salicylates)

Drug Uptake

Onset of action:

Extended release capsule: 2 hours

I.V.: 2 minutes

Peak effect:

Extended release capsule: 3-6 hours

Tablet: 1-4 hours
I.V.: 15 minutes
Duration:
Extended release capsule: 18-24 hours
Tablet: 8-12 hours
I.V.: 4-5 hours
Serum half-life: 2.4-5.8 hours
Pregnancy Risk Factor C
Generic Available Yes

Acetic Acid and Aluminum Acetate Otic *see* Aluminum Acetate and Acetic Acid *on page 47*

Acetic Acid, Propylene Glycol Diacetate, and Hydrocortisone
(a SEE tik AS id, PRO pa leen GLY kole dye AS e tate, & hye droe KOR ti sone)
Brand Names Acetasol® HC Otic; VōSol® HC Otic
Therapeutic Category Otic Agent, Anti-infective
Use Treatment of superficial infections of the external auditory canal caused by organisms susceptible to the action of the antimicrobial, complicated by swelling
Local Anesthetic/Vasoconstrictor Precautions No information available to require special precautions
Effects on Dental Treatment No effects or complications reported
Other Adverse Effects Transient burning or stinging may be noticed occasionally when the solution is first instilled into the acutely inflamed ear
Generic Available Yes

Acetohexamide (a set oh HEKS a mide)
Related Information
Endocrine Disorders & Pregnancy *on page 1021*
Brand Names Dymelor®
Therapeutic Category Antidiabetic Agent; Hypoglycemic Agent, Oral; Sulfonylurea Agent
Use Adjunct to diet for the management of mild to moderately severe, stable, noninsulin-dependent (type II) diabetes mellitus
Usual Dosage Adults: Oral (elderly patients may be more sensitive and should be started at a lower dosage initially): 250 mg to 1.5 g/day in 1-2 divided doses; doses >1.5 g/day are not recommended; if dose is ≤1 g, administer as a single daily dose
Mechanism of Action Believed to cause hypoglycemia by stimulating insulin release from the pancreatic beta cells; reduces glucose output from the liver (decreases gluconeogenesis); insulin sensitivity is increased at peripheral target sites (alters receptor sensitivity/receptor density); potentiates effects of ADH; may produce mild diuresis and significant uricosuric activity
Local Anesthetic/Vasoconstrictor Precautions No information available to require special precautions
Effects on Dental Treatment Use salicylates with caution in patients taking acetohexamide because of potential increased hypoglycemia. NSAIDs such as ibuprofen, naproxen and others may be safely used. Acetohexamide-dependent diabetics (noninsulin-dependent, type II) should be appointed for dental treatment in mornings to minimize chance of stress-induced hypoglycemia.
Other Adverse Effects
>10%:
Central nervous system: Headache, dizziness
Gastrointestinal: Constipation, diarrhea, heartburn, anorexia, epigastric fullness
1% to 10%: Dermatologic: Rash, urticaria, photosensitivity
<1%:
Endocrine & metabolic: Hypoglycemia
Hematologic: Aplastic anemia, hemolytic anemia, bone marrow suppression, thrombocytopenia, agranulocytosis
Drug Interactions
Monitor patient closely; large number of drugs interact with sulfonylureas
Decreased effect: Decreased hypoglycemic effect when acetohexamide is coadministered with cholestyramine, diazoxide, hydantoins, rifampin, thiazides, loop or thiazide diuretics
Increased effect: Increased hypoglycemia when acetohexamide is coadministered with salicylates or beta-adrenergic blockers; MAO inhibitors; oral anticoagulants, NSAIDs, sulfonamides, insulin, clofibrate, fenfluramine, fluconazole, gemfibrozil, H_2 antagonists, methyldopa, tricyclic antidepressants
(Continued)

Acetohexamide *(Continued)*

Drug Uptake
Onset of effect: 1 hour
Peak hypoglycemic effects: 8-10 hours
Duration: 12-24 hours, prolonged with renal impairment
Serum half-life:
    Parent compound: 0.8-2.4 hours
    Metabolite: 5-6 hours
Pregnancy Risk Factor D
Generic Available Yes

Acetohydroxamic Acid *(a SEE toe hye droks am ik AS id)*
Brand Names Lithostat®
Therapeutic Category Urinary Tract Product
Synonyms AHA
Use Adjunctive therapy in chronic urea-splitting urinary infection
Local Anesthetic/Vasoconstrictor Precautions No information available to require special precautions
Effects on Dental Treatment No effects or complications reported
Pregnancy Risk Factor X
Generic Available No

Acetophenazine *(a set oh FEN a zeen)*
Brand Names Tindal®
Therapeutic Category Antipsychotic Agent
Use Management of manifestations of psychotic disorders
Usual Dosage Adults: Oral: 20 mg 3 times/day up to 60-120 mg/day
Hospitalized schizophrenic patients may require doses as high as 400-600 mg/day

Not dialyzable (0% to 5%)
Mechanism of Action Antagonizes the effects of dopamine in the basal ganglia and limbic areas of the forebrain; this activity appears responsible for the antipsychotic efficacy, as well as the production of extrapyramidal symptoms; increases the secretion of prolactin and has a marked suppressive effect on the chemoreceptor trigger zone; also produces peripheral blockade of cholinergic neurons
Local Anesthetic/Vasoconstrictor Precautions No information available to require special precautions
Effects on Dental Treatment Orthostatic hypotension and nasal congestion possible in dental patients. Since the drug is a dopamine antagonist, extrapyramidal symptoms of the TMJ is a possibility; increased motor activity of head, face, and neck may occur. This drug is also an anticholinergic causing xerostomia.
Other Adverse Effects
>10%:
    Cardiovascular: Hypotension, orthostatic hypotension
    Central nervous system: Pseudoparkinsonism, akathisia, dystonias, tardive dyskinesia (persistent), dizziness
    Gastrointestinal: Constipation
    Ocular: Pigmentary retinopathy
    Respiratory: Nasal congestion
    Miscellaneous: Decreased sweating
1% to 10%:
    Dermatologic: Photosensitivity, skin rash
    Endocrine & metabolic: Changes in menstrual cycle, changes in libido, pain in breasts
    Gastrointestinal: Weight gain, nausea, vomiting, stomach pain
    Genitourinary: Dysuria, ejaculatory disturbances
    Neuromuscular & skeletal: Trembling of fingers
<1%:
    Central nervous system: Neuroleptic malignant syndrome (NMS), impairment of temperature regulation, lowering of seizures threshold
    Dermatologic: Discoloration of skin (blue-gray)
    Endocrine & metabolic: Galactorrhea
    Genitourinary: Priapism
    Hematologic: Agranulocytosis, leukopenia
    Hepatic: Cholestatic jaundice, hepatotoxicity
    Ocular: Cornea and lens changes
Drug Interactions No data reported
Drug Uptake
Duration: ~24 hours, permitting daily dosing

Absorption: Tissue saturation, particularly in high lipid tissues such as the central nervous system

Serum half-life: Range: 20-40 hours

Pregnancy Risk Factor C

Generic Available No

Acetylcholine (a se teel KOE leen)

Brand Names Miochol-E®

Therapeutic Category Cholinergic Agent, Ophthalmic; Ophthalmic Agent, Miotic

Use Produces complete miosis in cataract surgery, keratoplasty, iridectomy and other anterior segment surgery where rapid miosis is required

Usual Dosage Adults: Intraocular: 0.5-2 mL of 1% injection (5-20 mg) instilled into anterior chamber before or after securing one or more sutures

Mechanism of Action Causes contraction of the sphincter muscles of the iris, resulting in miosis and contraction of the ciliary muscle, leading to accommodation spasm

Local Anesthetic/Vasoconstrictor Precautions None

Effects on Dental Treatment Ophthalmic use of acetylcholine has no effect on dental treatment

Other Adverse Effects <1%:

Cardiovascular: Bradycardia, hypotension, flushing

Central nervous system: Headache

Ocular: Altered distance vision, decreased night vision, transient lenticular opacities

Respiratory: Dyspnea

Miscellaneous: Sweating

Drug Interactions No data reported

Drug Uptake

Onset of miosis: Occurs promptly

Duration: ~10 minutes

Pregnancy Risk Factor C

Generic Available No

Acetylcysteine (a se teel SIS teen)

Brand Names Mucomyst®; Mucosil™

Therapeutic Category Antidote, Acetaminophen; Mucolytic Agent

Use Adjunctive mucolytic therapy in patients with abnormal or viscid mucous secretions in acute and chronic bronchopulmonary diseases; pulmonary complications of surgery and cystic fibrosis; diagnostic bronchial studies; antidote for acute acetaminophen toxicity

Usual Dosage

Acetaminophen poisoning: Children and Adults: Oral: 140 mg/kg; followed by 17 doses of 70 mg/kg every 4 hours; repeat dose if emesis occurs within 1 hour of administration; therapy should continue until all doses are administered even though the acetaminophen plasma level has dropped below the toxic range

Inhalation: Acetylcysteine 10% and 20% solution (Mucomyst®) (dilute 20% solution with sodium chloride or sterile water for inhalation); 10% solution may be used undiluted

Children: 3-5 mL of 20% solution or 6-10 mL of 10% solution until nebulized given 3-4 times/day

Adolescents: 5-10 mL of 10% to 20% solution until nebulized given 3-4 times/day

Note: Patients should receive an aerosolized bronchodilator 10-15 minutes prior to acetylcysteine

Meconium ileus equivalent: Children and Adults: 100-300 mL of 4% to 10% solution by irrigation or orally

Mechanism of Action Exerts mucolytic action through its free sulfhydryl group which opens up the disulfide bonds in the mucoproteins thus lowering mucous viscosity. The exact mechanism of action in acetaminophen toxicity is unknown; thought to act by providing substrate for conjugation with the toxic metabolite.

Local Anesthetic/Vasoconstrictor Precautions No information available to require special precautions

Effects on Dental Treatment Stomatitis has been reported in 1% to 10% of patients

Other Adverse Effects

>10%:

Gastrointestinal: Vomiting

Miscellaneous: Unpleasant odor during administration

1% to 10%:

Central nervous system: Drowsiness, chills, clamminess

(Continued)

Acetylcysteine *(Continued)*

    Gastrointestinal: Stomatitis, nausea
    Local: Irritation
    Respiratory: Bronchospasm, rhinorrhea, hemoptysis
    <1%: Dermatologic: Skin rash
Drug Interactions No data reported
Drug Uptake
    Oral:
    Peak plasma levels: 1-2 hours
    Onset of action: Inhalation: Mucus liquefaction occurs maximally within 5-10 minutes
    Duration: Can persist for >1 hour
    Serum half-life:
      Reduced acetylcysteine: 2 hours
      Total acetylcysteine: 5.5 hours
Pregnancy Risk Factor B
Generic Available Yes

Achromycin® *see* Tetracycline *on page 914*

Achromycin® V *see* Tetracycline *on page 914*

Aciclovir (Mexico) *see* Acyclovir *on next page*

Acidulated Phosphate Fluoride *see* Fluoride *on page 415*

Aclovate® *see* Alclometasone *on page 36*

Acrivastine and Pseudoephedrine

    (AK ri vas teen & soo doe e FED rin)
Brand Names Semprex-D®
Therapeutic Category Antihistamine/Decongestant Combination
Use Temporary relief of nasal congestion, decongest sinus openings, running nose, itching of nose or throat, and itchy, watery eyes due to hay fever or other upper respiratory allergies
Usual Dosage Adults: 1 capsule 3-4 times/day
    Dosing comments in renal impairment: Do not use
Mechanism of Action Acrivastine is an analogue of triprolidine and it is considered to be relatively less sedating than traditional antihistamines; believed to involve competitive blockade of H_1-receptor sites resulting in the inability of histamine to combine with its receptor sites and exert its usual effects on target cells

    Pseudoephedrine: Directly stimulates alpha-adrenergic receptors of respiratory mucosa causing vasoconstriction; directly stimulates beta-adrenergic receptors causing bronchial relaxation, increased heart rate and contractility
Local Anesthetic/Vasoconstrictor Precautions Use with caution since pseudoephedrine is a sympathomimetic amine which could interact with epinephrine to cause a pressor response
Effects on Dental Treatment Up to 10% of patients could experience tachycardia, palpitations, and dry mouth; use vasoconstrictor with caution
Other Adverse Effects
    >10%: Central nervous system: Drowsiness, headache
    1% to 10%:
      Cardiovascular: Tachycardia, palpitations
      Central nervous system: Nervousness, dizziness, insomnia, vertigo, lightheadedness, fatigue
      Gastrointestinal: Nausea, vomiting, dry mouth, diarrhea
      Genitourinary: Dysuria
      Neuromuscular & skeletal: Weakness
      Respiratory: Pharyngitis, cough increase
      Miscellaneous: Sweating
    <1%:
      Endocrine & metabolic: Dysmenorrhea
      Gastrointestinal: Dyspepsia
Drug Interactions Increased toxicity with MAO inhibitors (hypertensive crisis) sympathomimetics, CNS depressants, alcohol (sedation)
Pregnancy Risk Factor B
Generic Available No

ACT *see* Dactinomycin *on page 277*

ACT® [OTC] *see* Fluoride *on page 415*

Actagen-C® *see* Triprolidine, Pseudoephedrine, and Codeine *on page 970*

Actagen® Syrup [OTC] *see* Triprolidine and Pseudoephedrine *on page 969*

Actagen® Tablet [OTC] *see* Triprolidine and Pseudoephedrine *on page 969*

Acthar® *see* Corticotropin *on page 262*

Actidose-Aqua® [OTC] *see* Charcoal *on page 206*

Actidose® With Sorbitol [OTC] *see* Charcoal *on page 206*

Actifed® Allergy Tablet (Day) [OTC] *see* Pseudoephedrine *on page 820*

Actifed® Allergy Tablet (Night) [OTC] *see* Diphenhydramine and Pseudoephedrine *on page 324*

Actifed® With Codeine *see* Triprolidine, Pseudoephedrine, and Codeine *on page 970*

Actigall™ *see* Ursodiol *on page 980*

Actimmune® *see* Interferon Gamma-1b *on page 515*

Actinex® *see* Masoprocol *on page 580*

Actinomycin D *see* Dactinomycin *on page 277*

Actisite® *see* Tetracycline Periodontal Fibers *on page 915*

Activase® *see* Alteplase *on page 45*

Actron® [OTC] *see* Ketoprofen *on page 534*

Acular® Ophthalmic *see* Ketorolac Tromethamine *on page 535*

Acutrim® 16 Hours [OTC] *see* Phenylpropanolamine *on page 754*

Acutrim® II, Maximum Strength [OTC] *see* Phenylpropanolamine *on page 754*

Acutrim® Late Day [OTC] *see* Phenylpropanolamine *on page 754*

Acyclovir (ay SYE kloe veer)

Related Information
Oral Viral Infections *on page 1066*
Systemic Viral Diseases *on page 1047*

Brand Names Zovirax®

Canadian/Mexican Brand Names Acifur® (Mexico); Avirax® (Canada)

Therapeutic Category Antiviral Agent, Oral; Antiviral Agent, Parenteral; Antiviral Agent, Topical

Synonyms Aciclovir (Mexico)

Use
Dental: Treatment of initial and prophylaxis of recurrent mucosal and cutaneous herpes simplex (HSV-1 and HSV-2) infections

Medical: In medicine, herpes simplex encephalitis, herpes zoster, genital herpes infection, varicella-zoster infections in healthy, nonpregnant persons >13 years of age, children <12 months of age who have a chronic skin or lung disorder or are receiving long-term aspirin therapy, and immunocompromised patients; for herpes zoster, acyclovir should be started within 72 hours of the appearance of the rash to be effective; acyclovir will not prevent postherpetic neuralgias

Usual Dosage
Dosing weight should be based on the smaller of lean body weight or total body weight

Adult determination of lean body weight (LBW) in kg:
LBW males: 50 kg + (2.3 kg x inches >5 feet)
LBW females: 45 kg + (2.3 kg x inches >5 feet)

Treatment of herpes simplex virus infections: I.V.
Children and Adults:
Mucocutaneous HSV infection 750 mg/m^2/day divided every 8 hours or 5 mg/kg/dose every 8 hours for 5-10 days
HSV encephalitis: 1500 mg/m^2/day divided every 8 hours for 5-10 days
I.V.: 5 mg/kg/dose every 8 hours for 5-10 days

Treatment of herpes simplex virus infections: Adults:
Oral: Treatment: 200 mg every 4 hours while awake (5 times/day)
Topical: ½" ribbon of ointment for a 4" square surface area every 3 hours (6 times/day)

Treatment of varicella-zoster virus (chickenpox) infections:
Oral:
Adults: 600-800 mg/dose every 4 hours while awake (5 times/day) for 7-10 days or 1000 mg every 6 hours for 5 days
Children: 10-20 mg/kg/dose (up to 800 mg) 4 times/day for 5 days; begin treatment within the first 24 hours of rash onset
I.V.: Children and Adults: 1500 mg/m^2/day divided every 8 hours or 10 mg/kg/dose every 8 hours for 7 days

Treatment of herpes zoster infections:
Oral:
Adults (immunocompromised): 800 mg every 4 hours (5 times/day) for 7-10 days
Children (immunocompromised): 250-600 mg/m^2/dose 4-5 times/day for 7-10 days
I.V.: Children and Adults (immunocompromised): 7.5 mg/kg/dose every 8 hours
(Continued)

Acyclovir *(Continued)*

Prophylaxis in immunocompromised patients:
Varicella zoster or herpes zoster in HIV-positive patients: Adults: Oral: 400 mg every 4 hours (5 times/day) for 7-10 days
Bone marrow transplant recipients: Children and Adults: I.V.:
Autologous patients who are HSV seropositive: 150 mg/m^2/dose (5 mg/kg) every 12 hours; with clinical symptoms of herpes simplex: 150 mg/m^2/dose every 8 hours
Autologous patients who are CMV seropositive: 500 mg/m^2/dose (10 mg/kg) every 8 hours; for clinically symptomatic CMV infection, consider replacing acyclovir with ganciclovir

Prophylaxis of herpes simplex virus infections: Adults: 200 mg 3-4 times/day or 400 mg twice daily

Mechanism of Action Inhibits DNA synthesis and viral replication by competing with deoxyguanosine triphosphate for viral DNA polymerase and incorporation into viral DNA

Local Anesthetic/Vasoconstrictor Precautions No information available to require special precautions

Effects on Dental Treatment No effects or complications reported

Other Adverse Effects 1% to 10%:
Central nervous system: Lethargy, dizziness, seizures, confusion, agitation, coma, headache
Dermatologic: Rash
Gastrointestinal: Nausea, vomiting
Neuromuscular & skeletal: Tremor
Renal: Elevated creatinine

Contraindications Hypersensitivity to acyclovir

Warnings/Precautions
Systemic: Use with caution in patients with pre-existing renal disease or in those receiving other nephrotoxic drugs concurrently; use with caution in patients with underlying neurologic abnormalities, serious hepatic or electrolyte abnormalities, or substantial hypoxia
Topical: No data reported

Drug Interactions Systemic: Increased CNS side effects with zidovudine and probenecid

Drug Uptake
Absorption: Oral: 15% to 30%
Time to peak serum concentration:
Oral: 1.5-2 hours
I.V.: Within 1 hour
Serum half-life:
Adults: 3.3 hours
Children 1-12 years: 2-3 hours

Pregnancy Risk Factor C

Breast-feeding Considerations May be taken while breast-feeding

Dosage Forms
Capsule: 200 mg
Powder for Injection: 500 mg (10 mL); 1000 mg (20 mL)
Ointment, topical: 5% [50 mg/g] (3 g, 15 g)
Suspension, oral (banana flavor): 200 mg/5 mL
Tablet: 400 mg, 800 mg

Dietary Considerations May be taken with food; food does not appear to affect absorption

Generic Available Yes

Adagen™ *see* Pegademase Bovine *on page 727*

Adalat® *see* Nifedipine *on page 680*

Adalat® **CC** *see* Nifedipine *on page 680*

Adapalene *(a DAP a leen)*

Brand Names Differin®

Therapeutic Category Acne Products

Use Topical treatment of acne vulgaris

Usual Dosage Children >12 years and Adults: Topical: Apply once daily before retiring; therapeutic results should be noticed after 8-12 weeks of treatment

Mechanism of Action Retinoid-like compound which is a modulator of cellular differentiation, keratinization and inflammatory processes, all of which represent important features in the pathology of acne vulgaris

Local Anesthetic/Vasoconstrictor Precautions No information available to require special precautions

Effects on Dental Treatment No effects or complications reported

Other Adverse Effects
>10%: Dermatologic: Erythema, scaling, dryness, pruritus, burning, pruritus or burning immediately after application
≤1% Dermatologic: Skin irritation, stinging sunburn, acne flares
Drug Uptake
Absorption: Topical: Minimum absorption occurs
Pregnancy Risk Factor C
Dosage Forms Gel, topical (alcohol free): 0.1% (15 g, 45 g)
Generic Available No

Adapin® *see* Doxepin *on page 335*

Adderall® *see* Dextroamphetamine and Amphetamine *on page 297*

Adeflor® *see* Vitamins, Multiple *on page 995*

Adenocard® *see* Adenosine *on this page*

Adenosine (a DEN oh seen)

Brand Names Adenocard®
Therapeutic Category Antiarrhythmic Agent (Supraventricular); Antiarrhythmic Agent, Miscellaneous
Synonyms 9-Beta-D-ribofuranosyladenine
Use Treatment of paroxysmal supraventricular tachycardia (PSVT)
Usual Dosage Rapid I.V. push (over 1-2 seconds) via peripheral line:
Children: Pediatric advanced life support (PALS): Treatment of SVT: 0.1 mg/kg; if not effective, give 0.2 mg/kg
Alternatively: Initial dose: 0.05 mg/kg; if not effective within 2 minutes, increase dose by 0.05 mg/kg increments every 2 minutes to a maximum dose of 0.25 mg/kg or until termination of PSVT; medium dose required: 0.15 mg/kg
Maximum single dose: 12 mg

Adults: 6 mg; if not effective within 1-2 minutes, 12 mg may be given; may repeat 12 mg bolus if needed
Maximum single dose: 12 mg

Note: Patients who are receiving concomitant theophylline therapy may be less likely to respond to adenosine therapy
Note: Higher doses may be needed for administration via peripheral versus central vein
Mechanism of Action Slows conduction time through the A-V node, interrupting the re-entry pathways through the A-V node, restoring normal sinus rhythm
Local Anesthetic/Vasoconstrictor Precautions No information available to require special precautions
Effects on Dental Treatment No effects or complications reported
Other Adverse Effects
>10%:
Cardiovascular: Flushing of face, arrhythmias, palpitations
Respiratory: Dyspnea
1% to 10%:
Cardiovascular: Chest pain
Central nervous system: Dizziness
Gastrointestinal: Nausea
Neuromuscular & skeletal: Numbness
Respiratory: Cough
<1%:
Cardiovascular: Hypotension, tightness of chest
Central nervous system: Lightheadedness, headache, apprehension, pressure in head
Dermatologic: Burning sensation
Gastrointestinal: Metallic taste, pressure in groin
Neuromuscular & skeletal: Heaviness in arms, neck and back pain
Ocular: Blurred vision
Respiratory: Hypoventilation
Miscellaneous: Sweating, tightness in throat
Drug Uptake
Duration: Very brief
Serum half-life: <10 seconds, thus adverse effects are usually rapidly self-limiting
Pregnancy Risk Factor C
Generic Available No
Comments Short action an advantage; not effective in atrial flutter, atrial fibrillation, or ventricular tachycardia

Adipex-P® *see* Phentermine *on page 750*

Adlone® *see* Methylprednisolone *on page 624*

ADR *see* Doxorubicin *on page 336*

Adrenalin® *see* Epinephrine (Dental) *on page 353*
Adriamycin® PFS *see* Doxorubicin *on page 336*
Adriamycin® RDF *see* Doxorubicin *on page 336*
Adrucil® Injection *see* Fluorouracil *on page 417*
Adsorbocarpine® *see* Pilocarpine *on page 759*
Adsorbonac® Ophthalmic [OTC] *see* Sodium Chloride *on page 870*
Adsorbotear® Ophthalmic Solution [OTC] *see* Artificial Tears *on page 87*
Advanced Formula Oxy® Sensitive Gel [OTC] *see* Benzoyl Peroxide *on page 120*
Advil® [OTC] *see* Ibuprofen *on page 495*
Advil® Cold & Sinus Caplets [OTC] *see* Pseudoephedrine and Ibuprofen *on page 821*
Aeroaid® [OTC] *see* Thimerosal *on page 925*
AeroBid®-M Oral Aerosol Inhaler *see* Flunisolide *on page 413*
AeroBid® Oral Aerosol Inhaler *see* Flunisolide *on page 413*
Aerolate III® *see* Theophylline *on page 917*
Aerolate JR® *see* Theophylline *on page 917*
Aerolate SR® S *see* Theophylline *on page 917*
Aerosporin® *see* Polymyxin B *on page 772*
AeroZoin® [OTC] *see* Benzoin *on page 120*
Afrin® Children's Nose Drops [OTC] *see* Oxymetazoline *on page 714*
Afrin® Saline Mist [OTC] *see* Sodium Chloride *on page 870*
Afrin® Sinus [OTC] *see* Oxymetazoline *on page 714*
Afrin® Tablet [OTC] *see* Pseudoephedrine *on page 820*
Aftate® for Athlete's Foot [OTC] *see* Tolnaftate *on page 943*
Aftate® for Jock Itch [OTC] *see* Tolnaftate *on page 943*
AgNO₃ *see* Silver Nitrate *on page 864*
Agrylin® *see* Anagrelide *on page 77*
AHA *see* Acetohydroxamic Acid *on page 28*
AHF *see* Antihemophilic Factor (Human) *on page 80*
Airet® *see* Albuterol *on next page*
Akarpine® *see* Pilocarpine *on page 759*
AKBeta® *see* Levobunolol *on page 546*
AK-Chlor® *see* Chloramphenicol *on page 209*
AK-Cide® Ophthalmic *see* Sulfacetamide Sodium and Prednisolone *on page 891*
AK-Con® Ophthalmic *see* Naphazoline *on page 664*
AK-Dilate® Ophthalmic Solution *see* Phenylephrine *on page 752*
AK-Homatropine® Ophthalmic *see* Homatropine *on page 472*
Akineton® *see* Biperiden *on page 130*
AK-NaCl® [OTC] *see* Sodium Chloride *on page 870*
AK-Nefrin® Ophthalmic Solution *see* Phenylephrine *on page 752*
Akne-Mycin® Topical *see* Erythromycin, Topical *on page 364*
AK-Neo-Dex® Ophthalmic *see* Neomycin and Dexamethasone *on page 671*
AK-Pentolate® *see* Cyclopentolate *on page 269*
AK-Poly-Bac® Ophthalmic *see* Bacitracin and Polymyxin B *on page 108*
AK-Pred® *see* Prednisolone *on page 788*
AKPro® Ophthalmic *see* Dipivefrin *on page 325*
AK-Spore H.C.® Ophthalmic Ointment *see* Bacitracin, Neomycin, Polymyxin B, and Hydrocortisone *on page 108*
AK-Spore H.C.® Ophthalmic Suspension *see* Neomycin, Polymyxin B, and Hydrocortisone *on page 672*
AK-Spore H.C.® Otic *see* Neomycin, Polymyxin B, and Hydrocortisone *on page 672*
AK-Spore® Ophthalmic Ointment *see* Bacitracin, Neomycin, and Polymyxin B *on page 108*
AK-Spore® Ophthalmic Solution *see* Neomycin, Polymyxin B, and Gramicidin *on page 672*
AK-Sulf® Ophthalmic *see* Sulfacetamide Sodium *on page 890*
AK-Taine® *see* Proparacaine *on page 808*
AKTob® Ophthalmic *see* Tobramycin *on page 937*
AK-Tracin® *see* Bacitracin *on page 107*
AK-Trol® *see* Neomycin, Polymyxin B, and Dexamethasone *on page 672*
Akwa Tears® Solution [OTC] *see* Artificial Tears *on page 87*
Alazide® *see* Hydrochlorothiazide and Spironolactone *on page 477*
Albalon-A® Ophthalmic *see* Naphazoline and Antazoline *on page 665*
Albalon® Liquifilm® Ophthalmic *see* Naphazoline *on page 664*

Albendazole (al BEN da zole)

Brand Names Albenza®

Therapeutic Category Anthelmintic

Use Treatment of parenchymal neurocysticerosis and cystic hydatid disease of the liver, lung, and peritoneum; albendazole may also be useful in the treatment of ascariasis, trichuriasis, enterobiasis, hookworm, strongyloidiasis, giardiasis, and microsporidiosis in AIDS

Usual Dosage Oral:

Children ≤2 years:

Neurocysticerosis: 15 mg/kg for 8 days; repeat as necessary

Hookworm, pinworm, roundworm: 200 mg as a single dose; treatment may be repeated in 3 weeks

Strongyloidiasis and tapeworm: 200 mg/day for 3 days; treatment may be repeated in 3 weeks

Children >2 years and Adults:

Hydatid disease: 800-1200 mg/day in divided doses for 28 days followed by a 2-week drug-free period, then repeated for a duration of therapy ranging from 1-12 months determined by the size, number, and location of cysts

Neurocysticerosis: 15 mg/kg for 8-30 days; repeat as necessary

Roundworm, pinworm, hookworm: 400 mg as a single dose; treatment may be repeated in 3 weeks

Giardiasis: Strongyloidiasis and tapeworm: 400 mg/day for 3 days; treatment may be repeated in 3 weeks (giardiasis is a single course)

Mechanism of Action Albendazole appears to cause selective degeneration of cytoplasmic microtubules in intestinal and tegmental cells of intestinal helminths, and larvae; glycogen is depleted, glucose uptake and cholinesterase secretion are impaired, and desecratory substances accumulate intracellularly. ATP production decreases causing energy depletion, immobilization, and worm death.

Local Anesthetic/Vasoconstrictor Precautions No information available to require special precautions

Effects on Dental Treatment No effects or complications reported

Other Adverse Effects (Percentages of occurrence were not available for all adverse effects at the time of this writing)

Central nervous system: Dizziness, headache, fever

Dermatologic: Alopecia, rash, pruritus

Gastrointestinal: Abdominal pain, anorexia, constipation, diarrhea, dry mouth, epigastric pain, nausea, vomiting

Hematologic: Eosinophilia, neutropenia

Hepatic: Elevated LFTs, jaundice

Drug Interactions Carbamazepine may accelerate albendazole metabolism; dexamethasone increases plasma levels of albendazole metabolites

Drug Uptake

Absorption: Oral absorption is poor (<5%); may increase up to 4.5 times when administered with a fatty meal; albendazole itself is essentially undetectable in plasma; albendazole sulfoxide is probably the active agent

Serum half-life: ~8.5 hours

Pregnancy Risk Factor X

Generic Available No

Albenza® see Albendazole on this page

Albuterol (al BYOO ter ole)

Related Information

Ipratropium and Albuterol on page 518

Respiratory Diseases on page 1018

Brand Names Airet®; Proventil®; Proventil® HFA; Ventolin®; Ventolin® Rotocaps®; Volmax®

Canadian/Mexican Brand Names Apo®-Salvent (Canada); Novo-Salmol® (Canada); Sabulin® (Canada); Salbulin® (Mexico); Salbutalan® (Mexico); Volmax® (Canada)

Therapeutic Category Adrenergic Agonist Agent; Antiasthmatic; Beta$_2$-Adrenergic Agonist Agent; Bronchodilator

Synonyms Salbutamol (Mexico)

Use Bronchodilator in reversible airway obstruction due to asthma or COPD

Usual Dosage

Oral:

Children:

2-6 years: 0.1-0.2 mg/kg/dose 3 times/day; maximum dose not to exceed 12 mg/day (divided doses)

6-12 years: 2 mg/dose 3-4 times/day; maximum dose not to exceed 24 mg/day (divided doses)

(Continued)

Albuterol *(Continued)*

Children >12 years and Adults: 2-4 mg/dose 3-4 times/day; maximum dose not to exceed 32 mg/day (divided doses)
Elderly: 2 mg 3-4 times/day; maximum: 8 mg 4 times/day

Inhalation MDI: 90 mcg/spray:
Children <12 years: 1-2 inhalations 4 times/day using a tube spacer
Children ≥12 years and Adults: 1-2 inhalations every 4-6 hours; maximum: 12 inhalations/day
Exercise-induced bronchospasm: 2 inhalations 15 minutes before exercising

Inhalation: Nebulization: 2.5 mg = 0.5 mL of the 0.5% inhalation solution to be diluted in 1-2.5 mL of NS **or** 0.01-0.05 mL/kg of 0.5% solution every 4-6 hours; intensive care patients may require more frequent administration; minimum dose: 0.1 mL; maximum dose: 1 mL diluted in 1-2 mL normal saline
<5 years: 1.25-2.5 mg every 4-6 hours as needed
>5 years: 2.5-5 mg every 4-6 hours as needed

Hemodialysis effects: Not removed by hemodialysis

Mechanism of Action Relaxes bronchial smooth muscle by action on beta$_2$-adrenergic receptors with little effect on heart rate

Local Anesthetic/Vasoconstrictor Precautions No information available to require special precautions

Effects on Dental Treatment No effects or complications reported

Other Adverse Effects
>10%:
Cardiovascular: Tachycardia, palpitations, pounding heartbeat
Gastrointestinal: GI upset, nausea
1% to 10%:
Cardiovascular: Flushing of face, hypertension or hypotension
Central nervous system: Nervousness, CNS stimulation, hyperactivity, insomnia, dizziness, lightheadedness, drowsiness, headache
Gastrointestinal: Dry mouth, heartburn, vomiting, unusual taste
Genitourinary: Dysuria
Neuromuscular & skeletal: Muscle cramping, tremor, weakness
Respiratory: Coughing
Miscellaneous: Increased sweating
<1%:
Cardiovascular: Chest pain, unusual pallor
Gastrointestinal: Loss of appetite
Respiratory: Paradoxical bronchospasm

Drug Interactions Increased toxicity: Cardiovascular effects are potentiated in patients also receiving MAO inhibitors, tricyclic antidepressants, sympathomimetic agents (eg, amphetamine, dopamine, dobutamine), inhaled anesthetics (eg, enflurane)

Drug Uptake
Time to peak: 2-3 hours
Duration of action: 4-6 hours
Serum half-life: 2.7-5 hours

Pregnancy Risk Factor C
Generic Available Yes

Alcaine® *see* Proparacaine *on page 808*
Alclometasona (Mexico) *see* Alclometasone *on this page*

Alclometasone (al kloe MET a sone)

Brand Names Aclovate®
Canadian/Mexican Brand Names Logoderm® (Mexico)
Therapeutic Category Corticosteroid, Topical (Low Potency)
Synonyms Alclometasona (Mexico)
Use Treats inflammation of corticosteroid-responsive dermatosis (low potency topical corticosteroid)
Usual Dosage Topical: Apply a thin film to the affected area 2-3 times/day
Mechanism of Action Stimulates the synthesis of enzymes needed to decrease inflammation, suppress mitotic activity, and cause vasoconstriction
Local Anesthetic/Vasoconstrictor Precautions No information available to require special precautions
Effects on Dental Treatment No effects or complications reported
Other Adverse Effects
1% to 10%:
Dermatologic: Itching, erythema, dryness papular rashes
Local: Burning, irritation

<1%: Dermatologic: Hypertrichosis, acneiform eruptions, hypopigmentation, perioral dermatitis, maceration of skin, skin atrophy, striae, miliaria

Drug Interactions No data reported

Pregnancy Risk Factor C

Dosage Forms

Cream, as dipropionate: 0.05% (15 g, 45 g, 60 g)

Ointment, topical, as dipropionate: 0.05% (15 g, 45 g, 60 g)

Generic Available No

Alconefrin® Nasal Solution [OTC] see Phenylephrine on page 752

Aldactazide® see Hydrochlorothiazide and Spironolactone on page 477

Aldactone® see Spironolactone on page 881

Aldara® see Imiquimod on page 502

Aldesleukin (al des LOO kin)

Brand Names Proleukin®

Therapeutic Category Antineoplastic Agent, Miscellaneous; Biological Response Modulator

Synonyms IL-2; Interleukin-2

Use Primarily investigated in tumors known to have a response to immunotherapy, such as melanoma and renal cell carcinoma; has been used in conjunction with LAK cells, TIL cells, IL-1, and interferon

Usual Dosage All orders should be written in million International units (million IU) (refer to individual protocols)

Adults: Metastatic renal cell carcinoma:

Treatment consists of two 5-day treatment cycles separated by a rest period. 600,000 units/kg (0.037 mg/kg)/dose administered every 8 hours by a 15-minute I.V. infusion for a total of 14 doses; following 9 days of rest, the schedule is repeated for another 14 doses, for a maximum of 28 doses per course.

Investigational regimen: I.V. continuous infusion: 4.5 million units/m^2/day in 250-1000 mL of D$_5$W for 5 days

Dose modification: Hold or interrupt a dose rather than reducing dose; refer to protocol

Retreatment: Patients should be evaluated for response ~4 weeks after completion of a course of therapy and again immediately prior to the scheduled start of the next treatment course. Additional courses of treatment may be given to patients only if there is some tumor shrinkage following the last course and retreatment is not contraindicated. Each treatment course should be separated by a rest period of at least 7 weeks from the date of hospital discharge. Tumors have continued to regress up to 12 months following the initiation of therapy.

Mechanism of Action IL-2 promotes proliferation, differentiation, and recruitment of T and B cells, natural killer (NK) cells, and thymocytes; IL-2 also causes cytolytic activity in a subset of lymphocytes and subsequent interactions between the immune system and malignant cells; IL-2 can stimulate lymphokine-activated killer (LAK) cells and tumor-infiltrating lymphocytes (TIL) cells. LAK cells (which are derived from lymphocytes from a patient and incubated in IL-2) have the ability to lyse cells which are resistant to NK cells; TIL cells (which are derived from cancerous tissue from a patient and incubated in IL-2) have been shown to be 50% more effective than LAK cells.

Local Anesthetic/Vasoconstrictor Precautions No information available to require special precautions

Effects on Dental Treatment Stomatitis in >10% of patients

Other Adverse Effects

>10%:

Cardiovascular: Hypotension, sensory dysfunction, sinus tachycardia, arrhythmias, edema

Central nervous system: Dizziness, fever, mental status changes, fatigue, malaise, pain, chills

Dermatological: Pruritus, erythema, rash, dry skin, exfoliative dermatitis

Endocrine & metabolic: Acidosis, hypocalcemia, hypophosphatemia, hypomagnesemia

Gastrointestinal: Nausea, vomiting, weight gain, diarrhea, stomatitis, anorexia, GI bleeding

Hematological: Anemia, thrombocytopenia, leukopenia, coagulation disorders, elevated transaminases

Hepatic: Jaundice, elevated bilirubin, alkaline phosphatase, transaminases

Neuromuscular & skeletal: Weakness

Renal: Oliguria, anuria, proteinuria, elevated BUN, serum creatinine

Respiratory: Pulmonary congestion, dyspnea, pulmonary edema

(Continued)

Aldesleukin *(Continued)*

1% to 10%:
Cardiovascular: Bradycardia, premature ventricular contractions (PVCs), myocardial ischemia, myocardial infarction, cardiac arrest, syncope
Central nervous system: Sensory disorders
Dermatologic: Purpura
Endocrine & metabolic: Hypokalemia, hypoproteinemia, hyponatremia, alkalosis, hypocholesterolemia
Gastrointestinal: Dyspepsia, constipation, weight loss
Hepatic: Ascites
Hematologic: Leukocytosis, eosinophilia
Local: Injection site reactions
Neuromuscular & skeletal: Arthralgia, myalgia
Renal: Hematuria, renal impairment
Respiratory: Respiratory failure, tachypnea, wheezing

<1%:
Cardiovascular: Congestive heart failure
Central nervous system: Coma, seizures
Dermatologic: Alopecia
Endocrine & metabolic: Hypothyroidism, hypercalcemia
Gastrointestinal: Pancreatitis
Neuromuscular & skeletal: Arthritis, muscle spasm
Renal: Polyuria
Miscellaneous: Allergic reactions

Drug Uptake
Absorption: Oral: Not absorbed
Serum half-life:
Initial: 6-13 minutes
Terminal: 20-120 minutes

Pregnancy Risk Factor C

Generic Available No

Comments 22 million units = 1.3 mg
1 Cetus Unit = 6 International Units
1.1 mg = 18 x 10^6 International Units (or 3 x 10^6 Cetus Units)
1 Roche Unit (Teceleukin) = 3 International Units

Aldoclor® *see* Chlorothiazide and Methyldopa *on page 216*

Aldomet® *see* Methyldopa *on page 621*

Aldoril® *see* Methyldopa and Hydrochlorothiazide *on page 622*

Alendronate *(a LEN droe nate)*

Brand Names Fosamax®

Therapeutic Category Bisphosphonate Derivative

Use FDA-approved: Osteoporosis in postmenopausal women; Paget's disease of the bone

Usual Dosage Oral:
Adults: Patients with osteoporosis or Paget's disease should receive supplemental calcium and vitamin D if dietary intake is inadequate
Osteoporosis in postmenopausal women: 10 mg once daily. Safety of treatment for >4 years has not been studied (extension studies are ongoing).
Paget's disease of bone: 40 mg once daily for 6 months
Retreatment: Relapses during the 12 months following therapy occurred in 9% of patients who responded to treatment. Specific retreatment data are not available. Retreatment with alendronate may be considered, following a 6-month post-treatment evaluation period, in patients who have relapsed based on increases in serum alkaline phosphatase, which should be measured periodically. Retreatment may also be considered in those who failed to normalize their serum alkaline phosphatase.
Elderly: No dosage adjustment is necessary

Mechanism of Action A bisphosphonate which inhibits bone resorption via actions on osteoclasts or on osteoclast precursors; decreases the rate of bone resorption direction, leading to an indirect decrease in bone formation

Local Anesthetic/Vasoconstrictor Precautions No information available to require special precautions

Effects on Dental Treatment No effects or complications reported

Other Adverse Effects Note: Incidence of adverse effects increases significantly in patients treated for Paget's disease at 40 mg/day, mostly GI adverse effects
1% to 10%:
Central nervous system: Headache (2.6%); pain (4.1%)
Gastrointestinal: Flatulence (2.6%); acid regurgitation (2%); esophagitis ulcer (1.5%); dysphagia, abdominal distention (1%)

<1%:
  Dermatologic: Rash, erythema (rare)
  Gastrointestinal: Gastritis (0.5%)
Drug Uptake
  Absorption: Oral:
    Male: 0.6% given in a fasting state
    Female: 0.7%
  Bioavailability: Reduced up to 60% with food or drink
  Half-life: Terminal: Exceeds 10 years; serum concentrations cleared >95% in 6 hours
Pregnancy Risk Factor C
Dosage Forms Tablet, as sodium: 10 mg, 40 mg
Generic Available No

Alersule Forte® *see* Chlorpheniramine, Phenylephrine, and Methscopolamine *on page 220*
Alesse® *see* Ethinyl Estradiol and Levonorgestrel *on page 377*
Aleve® (Naproxen Sodium) (OTC) *see* Naproxen *on page 665*
Alfenta® *see* Alfentanil *on this page*

Alfentanil (al FEN ta nil)
Related Information
  Narcotic Agonists *on page 1141*
Brand Names Alfenta®
Canadian/Mexican Brand Names Alfenta® (Canada); Rapifen® (Mexico)
Therapeutic Category Analgesic, Narcotic; General Anesthetic, Intravenous
Use Analgesic adjunct given by continuous infusion or in incremental doses in maintenance of anesthesia with barbiturate or nitrous oxide (NO₂) or a primary anesthetic agent for the induction of anesthesia in patients undergoing general surgery in which endotracheal intubation and mechanical ventilation are required
Usual Dosage Doses should be titrated to appropriate effects; wide range of doses is dependent upon desired degree of analgesia/anesthesia

Children <12 years: Dose not established
Adults: Dose should be based on ideal body weight; see table.

Alfentanil

Indication	Approximate Duration of Anesthesia (min)	Induction Period (Initial Dose) (mcg/kg)	Maintenance Period (Increments/ Infusion)	Total Dose (mcg/kg)	Effects
Incremental injection	≤30	8-20	3-5 mcg/kg or 0.5-1 mcg/kg/ min	8-40	Spontaneously breathing or assisted ventilation when required.
	30-60	20-50	5-15 mcg/kg	Up to 75	Assisted or controlled ventilation required. Attenuation of response to laryngoscopy and intubation.
Continuous infusion	>45	50-75	0.5-3.0 mcg/ min average infusion rate 1-1.5 mcg/kg/min	Dependent on duration of procedure	Assisted or controlled ventilation required. Some attenuation of response to intubation and incision, with intraoperative stability.
Anesthetic induction	>45	130-245	0.5-1.5 mcg/kg/ min or general anesthetic	Dependent on duration of procedure	Assisted or controlled ventilation required. Administer slowly (over three minutes). Concentration of inhalation agents reduced by 30%-50% for initial hour.

Mechanism of Action Binds to opiate receptors (mu and kappa subtypes) in the CNS causing inhibition of ascending pain pathways, altering the perception of and response to pain; produces generalized CNS depression
Local Anesthetic/Vasoconstrictor Precautions No information available to require special precautions
Effects on Dental Treatment Erythromycin inhibits the liver metabolism of alfentanil resulting in increased sedation and prolonged respiratory depression
Other Adverse Effects
  Endocrine & metabolic: Antidiuretic hormone release
  Ocular: Miosis
  (Continued)

Alfentanil *(Continued)*

>10%:
Cardiovascular: Bradycardia, peripheral vasodilation
Central nervous system: Drowsiness, sedation, increased intracranial pressure
Gastrointestinal: Nausea, vomiting, constipation
1% to 10%:
Cardiovascular: Cardiac arrhythmias, orthostatic hypotension
Central nervous system: Confusion, CNS depression
Ocular: Blurred vision
<1%:
Central nervous system: Convulsions, mental depression, paradoxical CNS
excitation or delirium, dizziness, dysesthesia
Dermatologic: Skin rash, urticaria, itching
Gastrointestinal: Biliary tract spasm
Genitourinary: Urinary tract spasm
Respiratory: Respiratory depression, bronchospasm, laryngospasm
Miscellaneous: Physical and psychological dependence with prolonged use,
cold, clammy skin
Drug Interactions Increased toxicity: CNS depressants (eg, benzodiazepines,
barbiturates, phenothiazines, tricyclic antidepressants), erythromycin, reserpine,
beta-blockers
Drug Uptake
Serum half-life: Adults: 83-97 minutes
Pregnancy Risk Factor C
Generic Available No
Selected Readings
Bartkowski RR, Goldberg ME, Larijani GE, et al, "Inhibition of Alfentanil Metabolism by Erythromycin,"
Clin Pharmacol Ther, 1989, 46(1):99-102.
Bartkowski RR and McDonnell TE, "Prolonged Alfentanil Effect Following Erythromycin Administra-
tion," *Anesthesiology*, 1990, 73(3):566-8.

Alferon® N *see* Interferon Alfa-n3 *on page 513*

Alglucerase *(al GLOO ser ase)*
Brand Names Ceredase® Injection
Therapeutic Category Enzyme, Glucocerebrosidase
Synonyms Glucocerebrosidase
Use Orphan drug for treatment of Gaucher's disease
Usual Dosage Usually administered as a 20-60 units/kg I.V. infusion given with a
frequency ranging from 3 times/week to once every 2 weeks
Mechanism of Action Glucocerebrosidase is an enzyme prepared from human
placental tissue. Gaucher's disease is an inherited metabolic disorder caused by
the defective activity of beta-glucosidase and the resultant accumulation of
glucosyl ceramide laden macrophages in the liver, bone, and spleen; acts by
replacing the missing enzyme associated with Gaucher's disease.
Local Anesthetic/Vasoconstrictor Precautions No information available to
require special precautions
Effects on Dental Treatment No effects or complications reported
Other Adverse Effects
>10%: Local: Discomfort, burning, and edema at the site of injection
<1%:
Central nervous system: Fever, chills
Gastrointestinal: Abdominal discomfort, nausea, vomiting
Pregnancy Risk Factor C
Generic Available No

Alkaban-AQ® *see* Vinblastine *on page 989*

Alka-Mints® [OTC] *see* Calcium Carbonate *on page 162*

Alka-Seltzer® Plus Cold Liqui-Gels Capsules [OTC] *see* Acetaminophen, Chlorpheniramine, and Pseudoephedrine *on page 24*

Alka-Seltzer® Plus Flu & Body Aches Non-Drowsy Liqui-Gels [OTC] *see* Acetaminophen, Dextromethorphan, and Pseudoephedrine *on page 25*

Alkeran® *see* Melphalan *on page 590*

Allbee® With C [OTC] *see* Vitamin B Complex With Vitamin C *on page 994*

Allbee® With C *see* Vitamins, Multiple *on page 995*

Allegra® *see* Fexofenadine *on page 403*

Aller-Chlor® [OTC] *see* Chlorpheniramine *on page 217*

Allercon® Tablet [OTC] *see* Triprolidine and Pseudoephedrine *on page 969*

Allerest® 12 Hour Capsule [OTC] *see* Chlorpheniramine and Phenylpropanolamine
on page 219

Allerest® 12 Hour Nasal Solution [OTC] *see* Oxymetazoline *on page 714*

Allerest® Eye Drops [OTC] *see* Naphazoline *on page 664*

Allerest® Maximum Strength [OTC] *see* Chlorpheniramine and Pseudoephedrine *on page 219*

Allerest® No Drowsiness [OTC] *see* Acetaminophen and Pseudoephedrine *on page 24*

Allerfrin® Syrup [OTC] *see* Triprolidine and Pseudoephedrine *on page 969*

Allerfrin® Tablet [OTC] *see* Triprolidine and Pseudoephedrine *on page 969*

Allerfrin® w/Codeine *see* Triprolidine, Pseudoephedrine, and Codeine *on page 970*

Allergan® Ear Drops *see* Antipyrine and Benzocaine *on page 82*

Allergic Skin Reactions to Drugs *see page 1196*

AllerMax® Oral [OTC] *see* Diphenhydramine *on page 323*

Allerphed Syrup [OTC] *see* Triprolidine and Pseudoephedrine *on page 969*

Allopurinol (al oh PURE i nole)

Brand Names Zyloprim®

Canadian/Mexican Brand Names Apo®-Allopurinol (Canada); Atisuril® (Mexico); Novo-purol® (Canada); Purinol® (Canada); Unizuric® 300 (Mexico)

Therapeutic Category Uric Acid Lowering Agent; Uricosuric Agent

Synonyms Alopurinol (Mexico)

Use Prevention of attacks of gouty arthritis and nephropathy; also used to treat secondary hyperuricemia which may occur during treatment of tumors or leukemia; prevent recurrent calcium oxalate calculi

Usual Dosage Oral:

Children ≤10 years: 10 mg/kg/day in 2-3 divided doses **or** 200-300 mg/m^2/day in 2-4 divided doses, maximum: 800 mg/24 hours

Alternative:

<6 years: 150 mg/day in 3 divided doses

6-10 years: 300 mg/day in 2-3 divided doses

Children >10 years and Adults: Daily doses >300 mg should be administered in divided doses

Myeloproliferative neoplastic disorders: 600-800 mg/day in 2-3 divided doses for prevention of acute uric acid nephropathy for 2-3 days starting 1-2 days before chemotherapy

Gout:

Mild: 200-300 mg/day

Severe: 400-600 mg/day

Dosing adjustment in renal impairment: Must be adjusted due to accumulation of allopurinol and metabolites; removed by hemodialysis. See table.

Adult Maintenance Doses of Allopurinol*

Creatinine Clearance (mL/min)	Maintenance Dose of Allopurinol (mg)
140	400 qd
120	350 qd
100	300 qd
80	250 qd
60	200 qd
40	150 qd
20	100 qd
10	100 q2d
0	100 q3d

*This table is based on a standard maintenance dose of 300 mg of allopurinol per day for a patient with a creatinine clearance of 100 mL/min.

Hemodialysis: Administer dose posthemodialysis or administer 50% supplemental dose

Mechanism of Action Allopurinol inhibits xanthine oxidase, the enzyme responsible for the conversion of hypoxanthine to xanthine to uric acid. Allopurinol is metabolized to oxypurinol which is also an inhibitor of xanthine oxidase; allopurinol acts on purine catabolism, reducing the production of uric acid without disrupting the biosynthesis of vital purines.

Local Anesthetic/Vasoconstrictor Precautions No information available to require special precautions

Effects on Dental Treatment No effects or complications reported

Other Adverse Effects

>10%: Dermatologic: Skin rash (usually maculopapular), exfoliative, urticarial or purpuric lesions

(Continued)

41

Allopurinol *(Continued)*

1% to 10%:

Central nervous system: Drowsiness, chills, fever

Dermatologic: Alopecia

Gastrointestinal: Nausea, vomiting, diarrhea, abdominal pain, abdominal pain, dyspepsia

Hepatic: Elevated alkaline phosphatase, AST, and ALT, hepatomegaly, hyperbilirubinemia, and jaundice; hepatic necrosis has been reported

<1%:

Cardiovascular: Vasculitis

Central nervous system: Headache, neuritis

Dermatologic: Toxic epidermal necrolysis and Stevens-Johnson syndrome have been reported

Hematologic: Bone marrow suppression has been reported in patients receiving allopurinol with other myelosuppressive agents

Idiosyncratic: Reaction characterized by fever, chills, eosinophilia, arthralgia, nausea, and vomiting, leukopenia, leukocytosis

Local: Thrombophlebitis

Neuromuscular & skeletal: Peripheral neuropathy, paresthesia

Ocular: Cataracts

Renal: Renal impairment

Respiratory: Epistaxis

Drug Interactions

Decreased effect with alcohol

Increased toxicity:

Allopurinol prolongs half-life of oral anticoagulants

Allopurinol increases serum half-life of theophylline

Allopurinol may compete for excretion in renal tubule with chlorpropamide and increase chlorpropamide's serum half-life

Allopurinol inhibits metabolism of azathioprine and mercaptopurine

Thiazide diuretics enhance toxicity of allopurinol

Use with ampicillin may increase the incidence of skin rash

Urinary acidification with large amounts of vitamin C may increase kidney stone formation

Drug Uptake

Decreases in serum uric acid occur in 1-2 days with nadir achieved in 1-2 weeks

Absorption:

Oral: ~80% of dose absorbed from GI tract; peak plasma concentrations are seen 30-120 minutes after administration

Rectal: Poor and erratic

Serum half-life:

Normal renal function:

Parent drug: 1-3 hours

Oxypurinol: 18-30 hours

Pregnancy Risk Factor C

Generic Available Yes

All-*trans*-Retinoic Acid *see* Tretinoin, Oral *on page 952*

Alomide® *see* Lodoxamide Tromethamine *on page 563*

Alopurinol (Mexico) *see* Allopurinol *on previous page*

Alor® 5/500 *see* Hydrocodone and Aspirin *on page 480*

Alora® Transdermal *see* Estradiol *on page 365*

Alpha₁-PI *see* Alpha₁-Proteinase Inhibitor *on this page*

Alpha₁-Proteinase Inhibitor (al fa won PRO tee in ase in HI bi tor)

Brand Names Prolastin® Injection

Therapeutic Category Antitrypsin Deficiency Agent

Synonyms Alpha₁-PI; Alpha₁-Proteinase Inhibitor, Human

Use Congenital alpha₁-antitrypsin deficiency

Usual Dosage Adults: I.V.: 60 mg/kg once weekly (at a rate ≥0.08 mL/kg/minute)

Mechanism of Action Human alpha₁-proteinase inhibitor is prepared from the pooled human plasma of normal donors and is intended for use in the therapy of congenital alpha₁-antitrypsin deficiency. Alpha₁-antitrypsin (AAT) is the principal protease inhibitor in the serum and exists as a single polypeptide glycoprotein. Production of AAT occurs in the liver hepatocyte and secretion occurs at a rate to maintain serum concentrations of 150-200 mg/dL. The major physiologic role of the antiprotease is that of combining with proteolytic enzymes to render them inactive. Several proteases can be inactivated by AAT including trypsin, chymotrypsin, coagulation factor XI, plasmin, thrombin, and neutrophil elastase.

Local Anesthetic/Vasoconstrictor Precautions No information available to require special precautions

Effects on Dental Treatment No effects or complications reported
Other Adverse Effects <1%:
> Central nervous system: Dizziness, lightheadedness, fever <102°F (delayed up to 12 hours after treatment)
> Hematologic: Leukocytosis

Drug Uptake Serum half-life, elimination (parent compound): 4.5-5.2 days
Pregnancy Risk Factor C
Generic Available No
Comments Sodium content of 1 L after reconstitution: 100-210 mEq

Alpha₁-Proteinase Inhibitor, Human *see* Alpha₁-Proteinase Inhibitor *on previous page*

Alphagan® *see* Brimonidine *on page 139*

Alphamul® [OTC] *see* Castor Oil *on page 184*

AlphaNine® SD *see* Factor IX Complex (Human) *on page 391*

Alphatrex® *see* Betamethasone *on page 126*

Alprazolam (al PRAY zoe lam)

Related Information
> Patients Requiring Sedation *on page 1081*
> Temporomandibular Dysfunction (TMD) *on page 1078*

Brand Names Xanax®
Canadian/Mexican Brand Names Apo®-Alpraz (Canada); Novo-Aloprazol® (Canada); Nu-Alprax® (Canada); Tafil® (Mexico)
Therapeutic Category Antianxiety Agent; Benzodiazepine; Tranquilizer, Minor
Use Treatment of anxiety; adjunct in the treatment of depression; management of panic attacks
Usual Dosage Oral:
> Children <18 years: Safety and dose have not been established
> Adults: 0.25-0.5 mg 2-3 times/day, titrate dose upward; maximum: 4 mg/day

Mechanism of Action Binds at stereospecific receptors at several sites within the central nervous system, including the limbic system, reticular formation; effects may be mediated through GABA
Local Anesthetic/Vasoconstrictor Precautions No information available to require special precautions
Effects on Dental Treatment Significant dry mouth will occur in over 10% of patients; normal salivary flow occurs with cessation of drug therapy
Other Adverse Effects
Treatment of anxiety:
> >10%:
>> Central nervous system: Drowsiness, lightheadedness, depression, headache
>> Gastrointestinal: Xerostomia, constipation, diarrhea
>
> 1& to 10%:
>> Cardiovascular: Hypotension, tachycardia/palpitations
>> Central nervous system: Confusion, nervousness, dizziness, akathisia, insomnia, memory impairment
>> Gastrointestinal: Nausea, vomiting, weight gain/loss, increased salivation
>> Neuromuscular & skeletal: Rigidity, tremor
>> Ocular: Blurred vision
>> Respiratory: Nasal congestion

Treatment of panic disorder:
> >10%:
>> Cardiovascular: Tachycardia, chest pain
>> Central nervous system: Insomnia, lightheadedness, headache, anxiety, fatigue, irritability, cognitive disorder, dizziness, impaired coordination
>> Dermatologic: Rash
>> Endocrine & metabolic: Decreased libido
>> Gastrointestinal: Nausea, vomiting, diarrhea, decreased salivation, weight loss, decreased appetite, constipation
>> Neuromuscular & skeletal: Dysarthria, abnormal involuntary movement
>> Ocular: Blurred vision
>> Respiratory: Nasal congestion
>
> Miscellaneous: Diaphoresis
> 1% to 10%:
>> Cardiovascular: Syncope
>> Central nervous system: Confusion, memory impairment, depression
>> Endocrine & metabolic: Increased libido, sexual dysfunction
>> Gastrointestinal: Increased salivation
>> Neuromuscular & skeletal: Muscle stiffness, cramps, muscular twitching, weakness, muscle tone disorders
>> Otic: Tinnitus

(Continued)

lprazolam *(Continued)*

Respiratory: Hyperventilation

<1%:

Central nervous system: Seizures, hallucinations, depersonalization

Gastrointestinal: Taste alteration

Hepatic: Elevated bilirubin, elevated hepatic enzymes, jaundice

Ocular: Diplopia

Drug Interactions Alprazolam will produce an additive CNS depressant effect when co-administered with other psychotropic medications, anticonvulsants and antihistamines; the blood level of alprazolam can be increased by cimetidine (Tagamet®) and by oral contraceptives; the clinical significance of this effect is unclear; fluvoxamine (Luvox®) can increase alprazolam plasma concentrations resulting in increased psychomotor impairment

Drug Uptake

Serum half-life: 12-15 hours

Time to peak serum concentration: Within 1-2 hours

Pregnancy Risk Factor D

Dosage Forms Tablet: 0.25 mg, 0.5 mg, 1 mg, 2 mg

Dietary Considerations May be taken with food or water to avoid gastrointestinal upset

Generic Available Yes

Alprostadil *(al PROS ta dill)*

Brand Names Caverject® Injection; Edex® Injection; Muse® Pellet; Prostin VR Pediatric® Injection

Therapeutic Category Prostaglandin

Synonyms PGE_1; Prostaglandin E_1

Use Temporary maintenance of patency of ductus arteriosus in neonates with ductal-dependent congenital heart disease until surgery can be performed. These defects include cyanotic (eg, pulmonary atresia, pulmonary stenosis, tricuspid atresia, Fallot's tetralogy, transposition of the great vessels) and acyanotic (eg, interruption of aortic arch, coarctation of aorta, hypoplastic left ventricle) heart disease; diagnosis and treatment of erectile dysfunction of vasculogenic, psychogenic, or neurogenic etiology; adjunct in the diagnosis of erectile dysfunction

Investigational: Treatment of pulmonary hypertension in infants and children with congenital heart defects with left-to-right shunts

Usual Dosage

Patent ductus arteriosus (Prostin VR Pediatric®):

I.V. continuous infusion into a large vein, or alternatively through an umbilical artery catheter placed at the ductal opening: 0.05-0.1 mcg/kg/minute with therapeutic response, rate is reduced to lowest effective dosage; with unsatisfactory response, rate is increased gradually; maintenance: 0.01-0.4 mcg/kg/minute

PGE_1 is usually given at an infusion rate of 0.1 mcg/kg/minute, but it is often possible to reduce the dosage to $1/2$ or even $1/10$ without losing the therapeutic effect. The mixing schedule is shown in the table.

Add 1 Ampul (500 mcg) to:	Concentration (mcg/mL)	Infusion Rate	
		mL/min/kg Needed to Infuse 0.1 mcg/kg/min	mL/kg/24 h
250 mL	2	0.05	72
100 mL	5	0.02	28.8
50 mL	10	0.01	14.4
25 mL	20	0.005	7.2

Therapeutic response is indicated by increased pH in those with acidosis or by an increase in oxygenation (pO_2) usually evident within 30 minutes

Erectile dysfunction (Caverject®):

Vasculogenic, psychogenic, or mixed etiology: Individualize dose by careful titration; usual dose: 2.5-60 mcg (doses >60 mcg are not recommended); initiate dosage titration at 2.5 mcg, increasing by 2.5 mcg to a dose of 5 mcg and then in increments of 5-10 mcg depending on the erectile response until the dose produces an erection suitable for intercourse, not lasting >1 hour; if there is absolutely no response to initial 2.5 mcg dose, the second dose may increased to 7.5 mcg, followed by increments of 5-10 mcg

Neurogenic etiology (eg, spinal cord injury): Initiate dosage titration at 1.25 mcg, increasing to a doses of 2.5 mcg and then 5 mcg; increase further in increments 5 mcg until the dose is reached that produces an erection suitable for intercourse, not lasting >1 hour

Note: Patient must stay in the physician's office until complete detumescence occurs; if there is no response, then the next higher dose may be given within 1 hour; if there is still no response, a 1-day interval before giving the next dose is recommended; increasing the dose or concentration in the treatment of impotence results in increasing pain and discomfort

Mechanism of Action Causes vasodilation by means of direct effect on vascular and ductus arteriosus smooth muscle

Local Anesthetic/Vasoconstrictor Precautions No information available to require special precautions

Effects on Dental Treatment No effects or complications reported

Other Adverse Effects

>10%:
  Cardiovascular: Flushing
  Central nervous system: Fever
  Genitourinary: Penile pain
  Respiratory: Apnea

1% to 10%:
  Cardiovascular: Bradycardia, hypotension, hypertension, tachycardia, cardiac arrest, edema
  Central nervous system: Seizures, headache, dizziness
  Endocrine & metabolic: Hypokalemia
  Gastrointestinal: Diarrhea
  Genitourinary: Prolonged erection, penile fibrosis, penis disorder, penile rash, penile edema
  Hematologic: Disseminated intravascular coagulation
  Local: Injection site hematoma, injection site bruising
  Neuromuscular & skeletal: Back pain
  Respiratory: Upper respiratory infection, sinusitis, nasal congestion, cough
  Miscellaneous: Sepsis, localized pain in structures other than the injection site, flu syndrome

Drug Uptake
  Serum half-life: 5-10 minutes

Pregnancy Risk Factor X

Generic Available No

AL-R® [OTC] *see* Chlorpheniramine *on page 217*

Altace™ *see* Ramipril *on page 834*

Alteplase (AL te plase)

Brand Names Activase®

Canadian/Mexican Brand Names Lysatec-rt-PA® (Canada)

Therapeutic Category Thrombolytic Agent

Use Management of acute myocardial infarction for the lysis of thrombi in coronary arteries; management of acute massive pulmonary embolism (PE) in adults; to improve neurologic recovery and decrease disability in adults following acute ischemic stroke, and most common type of stroke, caused by blood clots that block blood flow, treatment must start within 3 hours of the start of the stroke and only after bleeding in the brain has been ruled out by a cranial computerized tomography (CT) scan

Usual Dosage

Coronary artery thrombi: I.V.: Front loading dose: Total dose is 100 mg over 1.5 hours (for patients who weigh <65 kg, use 1.25 mg/kg/total dose). Add this dose to a 100 mL bag of 0.9% sodium chloride for a total volume of 200 mL. Infuse 15 mg (30 mL) over 1-2 minutes; infuse 50 mg (100 mL) over 30 minutes. Begin heparin 5000-10,000 unit bolus followed by continuous infusion of 1000 units/hour. Infuse 35 mg/hour (70 mL) for next 2 hours.

Acute pulmonary embolism: 100 mg over 2 hours

Mechanism of Action Initiates local fibrinolysis by binding to fibrin in a thrombus (clot) and converts entrapped plasminogen to plasmin

Local Anesthetic/Vasoconstrictor Precautions No information available to require special precautions

Effects on Dental Treatment No effects or complications reported

Other Adverse Effects

1% to 10%:
  Cardiovascular: Hypotension
  Central nervous system: Fever
  Dermatologic: Bruising
  Gastrointestinal: GI hemorrhage, nausea, vomiting
  Genitourinary: GU hemorrhage

(Continued)

Alteplase *(Continued)*

<1%:
Central nervous system: Intracranial hemorrhage
Gastrointestinal: Gingival hemorrhage
Hematologic: Retroperitoneal hemorrhage, rapid lysis of coronary artery thrombi by thrombolytic agents may be associated with reperfusion-related atrial and/or ventricular arrhythmias
Respiratory: Epistaxis

Drug Interactions Increased effect: Anticoagulants, aspirin, ticlopidine, dipyridamole, and heparin are at least additive

Pregnancy Risk Factor C

Generic Available No

ALternaGEL® [OTC] *see* Aluminum Hydroxide *on next page*

Altretamine (al TRET a meen)

Brand Names Hexalen®

Therapeutic Category Antineoplastic Agent, Alkylating Agent

Use Palliative treatment of persistent or recurrent ovarian cancer following first-line therapy with a cisplatin- or alkylating agent-based combination

Usual Dosage Oral (refer to protocol):
Adults: 4-12 mg/kg/day in 3-4 divided doses for 21-90 days
Alternatively: 240-320 mg/m²/day in 3-4 divided doses for 21 days, repeated every 6 weeks
Alternatively: 260 mg/m²/day for 14-21 days of a 28-day cycle in 4 divided doses

Temporarily discontinue (for ≥14 days) & subsequently restart at 200 mg/m²/day if any of the following occurs:
if GI intolerance unresponsive to symptom measures
WBC <2000/mm³
granulocyte count <1000/mm³
platelet count <75,000/mm³
progressive neurotoxicity

Mechanism of Action Although altretamine clinical antitumor spectrum resembles that of alkylating agents, the drug has demonstrated activity in alkylator-resistant patients; probably requires hepatic microsomal mixed-function oxidase enzyme activation to become cytotoxic. The drug selectively inhibits the incorporation of radioactive thymidine and uridine into DNA and RNA, inhibiting DNA and RNA synthesis; metabolized to reactive intermediates which covalently bind to microsomal proteins and DNA. These reactive intermediates can spontaneously degrade to demethylated melamines and formaldehyde which are also cytotoxic.

Local Anesthetic/Vasoconstrictor Precautions No information available to require special precautions

Effects on Dental Treatment No effects or complications reported

Other Adverse Effects
>10%:
Central nervous system: Neurotoxicity
Gastrointestinal: Nausea, vomiting
Hematologic: Anemia, thrombocytopenia, leukopenia
Neuromuscular & skeletal: Peripheral sensory neuropathy
1% to 10%:
Central nervous system: Seizures
Gastrointestinal: Anorexia, diarrhea, stomach cramps
Hepatic: Elevated alkaline phosphatase
<1%:
Central nervous system: Dizziness, depression
Dermatologic: Rash, alopecia
Hematologic: Myelosuppression
Hepatic: Hepatotoxicity
Neuromuscular & skeletal: Tremor

Drug Interactions
Decreased effect: Phenobarbital may increase metabolism of altretamine
Increased toxicity: May cause severe orthostatic hypotension when administered with MAO inhibitors; cimetidine may decrease metabolism of altretamine

Drug Uptake
Absorption: Oral: Well absorbed (75% to 89%)
Serum half-life: 13 hours
Peak plasma levels: 0.5-3 hours after dose

Pregnancy Risk Factor D

Generic Available No

Alu-Cap® [OTC] *see* Aluminum Hydroxide *on next page*

Aludrox® [OTC] *see* Aluminum Hydroxide and Magnesium Hydroxide *on next page*

Aluminio, Hidroxido De (Mexico) *see* Aluminum Hydroxide *on this page*

Aluminum Acetate and Acetic Acid
(a LOO mi num AS e tate & a SEE tik AS id)

Brand Names Otic Domeboro®

Therapeutic Category Otic Agent, Anti-infective

Synonyms Acetic Acid and Aluminum Acetate Otic; Burow's Otic

Use Treatment of superficial infections of the external auditory canal

Local Anesthetic/Vasoconstrictor Precautions No information available to require special precautions

Effects on Dental Treatment No effects or complications reported

Other Adverse Effects 1% to 10%: Irritation

Generic Available Yes

Aluminum Carbonate (a LOO mi num KAR bun ate)

Brand Names Basaljel® [OTC]

Therapeutic Category Antacid

Use Hyperacidity; hyperphosphatemia

Local Anesthetic/Vasoconstrictor Precautions No information available to require special precautions

Effects on Dental Treatment Aluminum carbonate prevents gastrointestinal absorption of tetracycline by forming a large ionized chelated molecule with the aluminum ion and tetracyclines in the stomach. Aluminum carbonate prevents GI absorption of ketoconazole and itraconazole by increasing the pH in the GI tract. Any of these drugs should be administered at least 1 hour before aluminum carbonate.

Other Adverse Effects

>10%: Gastrointestinal: Constipation, chalky taste, stomach cramps, fecal impaction

1% to 10%: Gastrointestinal: Nausea, vomiting, discoloration of feces (white speckles)

<1%: Endocrine & metabolic: Hypophosphatemia, hypomagnesemia

Pregnancy Risk Factor C

Generic Available Yes

Aluminum Chloride (a LOO mi num KLOR ide)

Brand Names Gingi-Aid® Gingival Retraction Cord; Gingi-Aid® Solution; Hemodent® Gingival Retraction Cord

Therapeutic Category Astringent

Use

Dental: Hemostatic; gingival retraction

Medical: Hemostatic

Mechanism of Action Precipitates tissue and blood proteins causing a mechanical obstruction to hemorrhage from injured blood vessels

Local Anesthetic/Vasoconstrictor Precautions No information available to require special precautions

Effects on Dental Treatment No effects or complications reported

Other Adverse Effects No data reported

Contraindications No data reported

Warnings/Precautions Since large amounts of astringents may cause tissue irritation and possible damage, only small amounts should be applied

Drug Interactions No data reported

Breast-feeding Considerations May be taken while breast-feeding

Dosage Forms

Retraction cord impregnated with aqueous solution of aluminum chloride containing 1.0 mg or 2.0 mg/inch in lengths of 72 inches

Retraction cord impregnated with an aqueous 10% solution of aluminum chloride and dried, containing 0.9 mg/inch or 1.8 mg/inch in lengths of 84 inches

Aqueous solution, 10 g aluminum chloride/100 mL water packaged in 15 and 30 mL bottles

Dietary Considerations No data reported

Generic Available Yes

Aluminum Hydroxide (a LOO mi num hye DROKS ide)

Brand Names ALternaGEL® [OTC]; Alu-Cap® [OTC]; Alu-Tab® [OTC]; Amphojel® [OTC]; Dialume® [OTC]; Nephrox Suspension [OTC]

Therapeutic Category Antacid; Antidote, Hyperphosphatemia

Synonyms Aluminio, Hidroxido De (Mexico)

Use Treatment of hyperacidity; hyperphosphatemia

(Continued)

Aluminum Hydroxide *(Continued)*

Usual Dosage Oral:

Peptic ulcer disease:

Children: 5-15 mL/dose every 3-6 hours or 1 and 3 hours after meals and at bedtime

Adults: 15-45 mL every 3-6 hours or 1 and 3 hours after meals and at bedtime

Prophylaxis against gastrointestinal bleeding:

Children: 5-15 mL/dose every 1-2 hours

Adults: 30-60 mL/dose every hour

Titrate to maintain the gastric pH >5

Hyperphosphatemia:

Children: 50-150 mg/kg/24 hours in divided doses every 4-6 hours, titrate dosage to maintain serum phosphorus within normal range

Adults: 500-1800 mg, 3-6 times/day, between meals and at bedtime

Antacid: Adults: 30 mL 1 and 3 hours postprandial and at bedtime

Mechanism of Action Neutralizes hydrochloride in stomach to form Al (Cl)$_3$ salt + H$_2$O

Local Anesthetic/Vasoconstrictor Precautions No information available to require special precautions

Effects on Dental Treatment Aluminum OH prevents gastrointestinal absorption of tetracycline by forming a large ionized chelated molecule with the aluminum ion and tetracyclines in the stomach. Aluminum OH prevents GI absorption of ketoconazole and itraconazole by increasing the pH in the GI tract. Any of these drugs should be administered at least 1 hour before Al(OH)$_3$.

Other Adverse Effects:

>10%: Gastrointestinal: Constipation, chalky taste, stomach cramps, fecal impaction

1% to 10%: Gastrointestinal: Nausea, vomiting, discoloration of feces (white speckles)

<1%: Endocrine & metabolic: Hypophosphatemia, hypomagnesemia

Drug Interactions Decreased effect: Tetracyclines, digoxin, indomethacin, or iron salts, isoniazid, allopurinol, benzodiazepines, corticosteroids, penicillamine, phenothiazines, ranitidine, ketoconazole, itraconazole

Pregnancy Risk Factor C

Generic Available Yes

Aluminum Hydroxide and Magnesium Carbonate

(a LOO mi num hye DROKS ide & mag NEE zhum KAR bun nate)

Brand Names Gaviscon® Liquid [OTC]

Therapeutic Category Antacid

Use Temporary relief of symptoms associated with gastric acidity

Local Anesthetic/Vasoconstrictor Precautions No information available to require special precautions

Effects on Dental Treatment Aluminum and magnesium ions prevent gastrointestinal absorption of tetracycline by forming a large ionized chelated molecule with the tetracyclines in the stomach. Aluminum hydroxide prevents GI absorption of ketoconazole and itraconazole by increasing the pH in the GI tract. Any of these drugs should be administered at least 1 hour before aluminum hydroxide.

Other Adverse Effects 1% to 10%:

Endocrine & metabolic: Hypermagnesemia, aluminum intoxication (prolonged use and concomitant renal failure), hypophosphatemia

Gastrointestinal: Constipation, diarrhea

Neuromuscular & skeletal: Osteomalacia

Generic Available Yes

Comments Sodium content per 5 mL Gaviscon® liquid: 0.6 mEq

Aluminum Hydroxide and Magnesium Hydroxide

(a LOO mi num hye DROKS ide & mag NEE zhum hye DROK side)

Brand Names Aludrox® [OTC]; Maalox® [OTC]; Maalox® Therapeutic Concentrate [OTC]

Therapeutic Category Antacid

Synonyms Magnesium Hydroxide and Aluminum Hydroxide

Use Antacid, hyperphosphatemia in renal failure

Local Anesthetic/Vasoconstrictor Precautions No information available to require special precautions

Effects on Dental Treatment Aluminum and magnesium ions prevent gastrointestinal absorption of tetracycline by forming a large ionized chelated molecule with the tetracyclines in the stomach. Aluminum hydroxide prevents GI absorption of ketoconazole and itraconazole by increasing the pH in the GI tract. Any of these drugs should be administered at least 1 hour before aluminum hydroxide.

Other Adverse Effects
>10%: Gastrointestinal: Constipation, chalky taste, stomach cramps, fecal impaction
1% to 10%: Gastrointestinal: Nausea, vomiting, discoloration of feces (white speckles)
<1%: Endocrine & metabolic: Hypophosphatemia, hypomagnesemia
Pregnancy Risk Factor C
Generic Available Yes
Comments Sodium content of 5 mL (Maalox®): 1.3 mg (0.06 mEq)

Aluminum Hydroxide and Magnesium Trisilicate
(a LOO mi num hye DROKS ide & mag NEE zhum trye SIL i kate)
Brand Names Gaviscon®-2 Tablet [OTC]; Gaviscon® Tablet [OTC]
Therapeutic Category Antacid
Use Temporary relief of hyperacidity
Local Anesthetic/Vasoconstrictor Precautions No information available to require special precautions
Effects on Dental Treatment Aluminum and magnesium ions prevent gastrointestinal absorption of tetracycline by forming a large ionized chelated molecule with the tetracyclines in the stomach. Aluminum hydroxide prevents GI absorption of ketoconazole and itraconazole by increasing the pH in the GI tract. Any of these drugs should be administered at least 1 hour before aluminum hydroxide.
Pregnancy Risk Factor C
Generic Available Yes
Comments Sodium content per tablet:
Gaviscon®: 0.8 mEq
Gaviscon®-2: 1.6 mEq

Aluminum Hydroxide, Magnesium Hydroxide, and Simethicone
(a LOO mi num hye DROKS ide, mag NEE zhum hye DROKS ide, & sye METH i kone)
Brand Names Di-Gel® [OTC]; Gas-Ban DS® [OTC]; Gelusil® [OTC]; Maalox® Plus [OTC]; Magalox Plus® [OTC]; Mylanta® [OTC]; Mylanta®-II [OTC]
Therapeutic Category Antacid; Antiflatulent
Use Temporary relief of hyperacidity associated with gas; may also be used for indications associated with other antacids
Local Anesthetic/Vasoconstrictor Precautions No information available to require special precautions
Effects on Dental Treatment Aluminum and magnesium ions prevent gastrointestinal absorption of tetracycline by forming a large ionized chelated molecule with the tetracyclines in the stomach. Aluminum hydroxide prevents GI absorption of ketoconazole and itraconazole by increasing the pH in the GI tract. Any of these drugs should be administered at least 1 hour before aluminum hydroxide.
Other Adverse Effects
>10%: Gastrointestinal: Chalky taste, stomach cramps, constipation, decreased bowel motility, fecal impaction, hemorrhoids
1% to 10%: Gastrointestinal: Nausea, vomiting, discoloration of feces (white speckles)
<1%: Endocrine & metabolic: Hypophosphatemia, hypomagnesemia, dehydration or fluid restriction
Pregnancy Risk Factor C
Generic Available Yes
Comments Sodium content of 5 mL:
Maalox® Plus: 1.3 mg (0.06 mEq)
Mylanta®: 0.7 mg (0.03 mEq)
Mylanta®-II: 1.14 mg (0.05 mEq)

Aluminum Sulfate and Calcium Acetate
(a LOO mi num SUL fate & KAL see um AS e tate)
Brand Names Bluboro® [OTC]; Boropak® [OTC]; Domeboro® Topical [OTC]; Pedi-Boro® [OTC]
Therapeutic Category Topical Skin Product
Use Astringent wet dressing for relief of inflammatory conditions of the skin and to reduce weeping that may occur in dermatitis
Local Anesthetic/Vasoconstrictor Precautions No information available to require special precautions
Effects on Dental Treatment No effects or complications reported
Generic Available Yes

Alupent® see Metaproterenol on page 605

Alu-Tab® [OTC] *see* Aluminum Hydroxide *on page 47*
Amantadina, Clorhidrato De (Mexico) *see* Amantadine *on this page*

Amantadine (a MAN ta deen)
Related Information
Respiratory Diseases *on page 1018*
Systemic Viral Diseases *on page 1047*
Brand Names Symmetrel®
Canadian/Mexican Brand Names Endantadine® (Canada); PMS-Amantadine® (Canada)
Therapeutic Category Anti-Parkinson's Agent; Antiviral Agent, Oral
Synonyms Amantadina, Clorhidrato De (Mexico)
Use Symptomatic and adjunct treatment of parkinsonism; prophylaxis and treatment of influenza A viral infection; treatment of drug-induced extrapyramidal symptoms
Usual Dosage
Children:
> 1-9 years: (<45 kg): 5-9 mg/kg/day in 1-2 divided doses to a maximum of 150 mg/day
> 10-12 years: 100-200 mg/day in 1-2 divided doses
> Prophylaxis: Administer for 10-21 days following exposure if the vaccine is concurrently given or for 90 days following exposure if the vaccine is unavailable or contraindicated and re-exposure is possible

Adults:
> Parkinson's disease: 100 mg twice daily
> Influenza A viral infection: 200 mg/day in 1-2 divided doses
> Prophylaxis: Minimum 10-day course of therapy following exposure if the vaccine is concurrently give or for 90 following exposure if the vaccine is unavailable or contraindicated and re-exposure is possible

Elderly patients should take the drug in 2 daily doses rather than a single dose to avoid adverse neurologic reactions
Mechanism of Action As an antiviral, blocks the uncoating of influenza A virus preventing penetration of virus into host; antiparkinsonian activity may be due to its blocking the reuptake of dopamine into presynaptic neurons and causing direct stimulation of postsynaptic receptors
Local Anesthetic/Vasoconstrictor Precautions No information available to require special precautions
Effects on Dental Treatment >10% of patient experience dry mouth; prolonged use of amantadine may cause significant xerostomia
Other Adverse Effects
1% to 10%:
> Cardiovascular: Orthostatic hypotension, peripheral edema
> Central nervous system: Insomnia, depression, anxiety, irritability, dizziness, hallucinations, ataxia, headache, somnolence, nervousness, dream abnormality, agitation, fatigue
> Dermatologic: Livedo reticularis
> Gastrointestinal: Nausea, anorexia, constipation, diarrhea
> Respiratory: Dry nose

<1%:
> Cardiovascular: Congestive heart failure, hypertension
> Central nervous system: Psychosis, slurred speech, euphoria, confusion, amnesia, instances of convulsions
> Dermatologic: Skin rash, eczematoid dermatitis
> Endocrine & metabolic: Decreased libido
> Gastrointestinal: Vomiting
> Genitourinary: Urinary retention
> Hematologic: Leukopenia, neutropenia
> Neuromuscular & skeletal: Hyperkinesis, weakness
> Ocular: Visual disturbances, oculogyric episodes
> Respiratory: Dyspnea
Drug Interactions Anticholinergic drugs may potentiate CNS side effects of amantadine; these include trihexyphenidyl (Artane®) and benztropine (Cogentin®)
Drug Uptake
Onset of antidyskinetic action: Within 48 hours
Absorption: Well absorbed from GI tract
Serum half-life:
> Normal renal function: 2-7 hours
> End stage renal disease: 7-10 days
Time to peak: 1-4 hours
Pregnancy Risk Factor C

Generic Available Yes

Amaphen® *see* Butalbital Compound *on page 154*

Amaphen® *see* Butalbital Compound and Acetaminophen *on page 155*

Amaryl® *see* Glimepiride *on page 442*

Ambenonium (am be NOE nee um)

Brand Names Mytelase® Caplets®

Therapeutic Category Cholinergic Agent

Use Treatment of myasthenia gravis

Local Anesthetic/Vasoconstrictor Precautions No information available to require special precautions

Effects on Dental Treatment Increased salivation

Other Adverse Effects
>10%:
  Gastrointestinal: Diarrhea, nausea, stomach cramps, increased mouth watering
  Miscellaneous: Increased sweating
1% to 10%:
  Genitourinary: Urge to urinate
  Ocular: Small pupils, lacrimation
  Respiratory: Increased bronchial secretions
<1%:
  Cardiovascular: Bradycardia, A-V block
  Central nervous system: Seizures, headache, dysphoria, somnolence
  Local: Thrombophlebitis
  Neuromuscular & skeletal: Muscle spasms, weakness
  Ocular: Miosis, diplopia
  Respiratory: Laryngospasm, respiratory paralysis
  Miscellaneous: Hypersensitivity, hyper-reactive cholinergic responses

Pregnancy Risk Factor C

Generic Available No

Ambenyl® Cough Syrup *see* Bromodiphenhydramine and Codeine *on page 141*

Ambi 10® [OTC] *see* Benzoyl Peroxide *on page 120*

Ambien™ *see* Zolpidem *on page 1006*

Ambi® Skin Tone [OTC] *see* Hydroquinone *on page 487*

AmBisome® *see* Amphotericin B Lipid Complex *on page 73*

Amcill® *see* Ampicillin *on page 73*

Amcinonida (Mexico) *see* Amcinonide *on this page*

Amcinonide (am SIN oh nide)

Related Information
  Corticosteroids, Topical Comparison *on page 1140*

Brand Names Cyclocort®

Canadian/Mexican Brand Names Visderm® (Mexico)

Therapeutic Category Corticosteroid, Topical (Medium/High Potency)

Synonyms Amcinonida (Mexico)

Use Relief of the inflammatory and pruritic manifestations of corticosteroid-responsive dermatoses (high potency corticosteroid)

Usual Dosage Adults: Topical: Apply in a thin film 2-3 times/day

Mechanism of Action Stimulates the synthesis of enzymes needed to decrease inflammation, suppress mitotic activity, and cause vasoconstriction

Local Anesthetic/Vasoconstrictor Precautions No information available to require special precautions

Effects on Dental Treatment No effects or complications reported

Other Adverse Effects
1% to 10%: Topical: Itching, maceration of skin, skin atrophy, burning, erythema, dryness, irritation, papular rashes
<1%: Topical: Hypertrichosis, acneiform eruptions, hypopigmentation, perioral dermatitis, striae, miliaria

Drug Interactions No data reported

Drug Uptake
  Absorption: Adequate through intact skin; increases with skin inflammation or occlusion

Pregnancy Risk Factor C

Generic Available No

Amcort® *see* Triamcinolone *on page 954*

Amen® *see* Medroxyprogesterone Acetate *on page 587*

Amerge® *see* Naratriptan *on page 667*

Americaine [OTC] *see* Benzocaine *on page 118*

Amesec® [OTC] see Aminophylline, Amobarbital, and Ephedrine on page 57

A-Methapred® see Methylprednisolone on page 624

Amfepramone (Canada) see Diethylpropion on page 309

Amgenal® Cough Syrup see Bromodiphenhydramine and Codeine on page 141

Amicar® see Aminocaproic Acid on page 54

Amidate® Injection see Etomidate on page 388

Amifostine (am i FOS teen)
Brand Names Ethyol®

Therapeutic Category Antidote

Synonyms Ethiofos; Gammaphos; WR2721

Use Protection against cisplatin-induced nephrotoxicity in advanced ovarian cancer patients; it may also provide protection from cisplatin-induced peripheral neuropathy

Usual Dosage Adults: I.V. (refer to individual protocols): 910 mg/m^2 administered once daily as a 15-minute I.V. infusion, starting 30 minutes prior to chemotherapy

Mechanism of Action Prodrug that is dephosphorylated by alkaline phosphatase in tissues to a pharmacologically active free thiol metabolite that can reduce the toxic effects of cisplatin. The free thiol is available to bind to, and detoxify, reactive metabolites of cisplatin; and can also act as a scavenger of free radicals that may be generated in tissues exposed to cisplatin.

Local Anesthetic/Vasoconstrictor Precautions No information available to require special precautions

Effects on Dental Treatment Nausea/vomiting (may be severe)

Other Adverse Effects

>10%:
Cardiovascular: Flushing; hypotension (62%)
Central nervous system: Chills, dizziness, somnolence
Gastrointestinal: Nausea/vomiting (may be severe)
Respiratory: Sneezing
Miscellaneous: Feeling of warmth/coldness, hiccups

<1%:
Dermatologic: Mild rashes
Endocrine & metabolic: Hypocalcemia
Neuromuscular & skeletal: Rigors

Drug Interactions Increased toxicity: Special consideration should be given to patients receiving antihypertensive medications or other drugs that could potentiate hypotension

Drug Uptake
Absorption: Oral: Poor
Serum half-life: 9 minutes

Pregnancy Risk Factor C; amifostine at doses of 50 mg/kg has been shown to be embryotoxic in rabbits

Generic Available No

Amikacin (am i KAY sin)
Brand Names Amikin®

Canadian/Mexican Brand Names Amikafur® (Mexico); Amikayect® (Mexico); Amikin® (Canada); Amikin® (Mexico); Biclin® (Mexico); Gamikal® (Mexico); Yectamid® (Mexico)

Therapeutic Category Antibiotic, Aminoglycoside

Synonyms Amikacina, Sulfato De (Mexico)

Use Treatment of documented gram-negative enteric infection resistant to gentamicin and tobramycin (bone infections, respiratory tract infections, endocarditis, and septicemia); documented infection of mycobacterial organisms susceptible to amikacin including Pseudomonas, Proteus, Serratia, and gram-positive Staphylococcus

Usual Dosage Individualization is critical because of the low therapeutic index

Use of ideal body weight (IBW) for determining the mg/kg/dose appears to be more accurate than dosing on the basis of total body weight (TBW)

In morbid obesity, dosage requirement may best be estimated using a dosing weight of IBW + 0.4 (TBW - IBW)

Initial and periodic peak and trough plasma drug levels should be determined, particularly in critically ill patients with serious infections or in disease states known to significantly alter aminoglycoside pharmacokinetics (eg, cystic fibrosis, burns, or major surgery)

Once daily dosing: Higher peak serum drug concentration to MIC ratios, demonstrated aminoglycoside postantibiotic effect, decreased renal cortex drug uptake, and improved cost-time efficiency are supportive reasons for the use of once daily dosing regimens for aminoglycosides. Current research indicates these regimens to be as effective for nonlife-threatening infections, with no higher incidence of nephrotoxicity, than those requiring multiple daily doses. Doses are determined by calculating the entire day's dose via usual multiple dose calculation techniques and administering this quantity as a single dose. Doses are then adjusted to maintain mean serum concentrations above the MIC(s) of the causative organism(s). (Example: 14-35 mg/kg as a single dose/ 24 hours; peak (maximum) serum concentration may approximate 40-55 mcg/ mL and trough (minimum) serum concentration <3 mcg/L). Further research is needed for universal recommendation in all patient populations and gram-negative disease; exceptions may include those with known high clearance (eg, children, patients with cystic fibrosis or burns who may require shorter dosage intervals) and patients with renal function impairment for whom longer than conventional dosage intervals are usually required.

Children and Adults: I.M., I.V.: 5-7.5 mg/kg/dose every 8 hours

Mechanism of Action Inhibits protein synthesis in susceptible bacteria by binding to ribosomal subunits

Local Anesthetic/Vasoconstrictor Precautions No information available to require special precautions

Effects on Dental Treatment No effects or complications reported

Other Adverse Effects
1% to 10%:
Central nervous system: Neurotoxicity
Otic: Ototoxicity (auditory), ototoxicity (vestibular)
Renal: Nephrotoxicity
<1%:
Cardiovascular: Hypotension
Central nervous system: Headache, drowsiness, drug fever
Dermatologic: Rash
Gastrointestinal: Nausea, vomiting
Hematologic: Eosinophilia
Neuromuscular & skeletal: Paresthesia, tremor, arthralgia, weakness
Respiratory: Dyspnea

Drug Interactions
Increased toxicity of aminoglycoside: Indomethacin I.V., amphotericin, loop diuretics, vancomycin, enflurane, methoxyflurane, cephalosporins
Increased toxicity of depolarizing and nondepolarizing neuromuscular blocking agents and polypeptide antibiotics with administration of aminoglycosides

Drug Uptake
Absorption: I.M.: May be delayed in the bedridden patient
Serum half-life (dependent on renal function):
Adults:
Normal renal function: 1.4-2.3 hours
Anuria: End stage renal disease: 28-86 hours
Time to peak serum concentration:
I.M.: Within 45-120 minutes
I.V.: Within 30 minutes following 30-minute infusion

Pregnancy Risk Factor C
Generic Available Yes

Amikacina, Sulfato De (Mexico) *see* Amikacin *on previous page*
Amikin® *see* Amikacin *on previous page*
Amilorida Clorhidrato De (Mexico) *see* Amiloride *on this page*

Amiloride (a MIL oh ride)

Brand Names Midamor®
Therapeutic Category Diuretic, Potassium Sparing
Synonyms Amilorida Clorhidrato De (Mexico)
Use Counteracts potassium loss induced by other diuretics in the treatment of hypertension or edematous conditions including CHF, hepatic cirrhosis, and hypoaldosteronism; usually used in conjunction with more potent diuretics such as thiazides or loop diuretics; investigational solution for cystic fibrosis

Usual Dosage Oral:
Children: Although safety and efficacy have not been established by the FDA in children, a dosage of 0.625 mg/kg/day has been used in children weighing 6-20 kg
Adults: 5-10 mg/day (up to 20 mg)
Elderly: Initial: 5 mg once daily or every other day

Mechanism of Action Interferes with potassium/sodium exchange (active transport) in the distal tubule, cortical collecting tubule and collecting duct by inhibiting sodium, potassium-ATPase; decreases calcium excretion; increases magnesium loss

(Continued)

Amiloride (Continued)

Local Anesthetic/Vasoconstrictor Precautions No information available to require special precautions

Effects on Dental Treatment No effects or complications reported

Other Adverse Effects

1% to 10%:

Central nervous system: Headache, fatigue, dizziness

Endocrine & metabolic: Hyperkalemia, hyperchloremic metabolic acidosis, dehydration, hyponatremia, gynecomastia

Gastrointestinal: Nausea, diarrhea, vomiting, abdominal pain, gas pain, appetite changes, constipation

Genitourinary: Impotence

Neuromuscular & skeletal: Muscle cramps, weakness

Respiratory: Cough, dyspnea

<1%:

Cardiovascular: Angina pectoris, orthostatic hypotension, arrhythmias, palpitations, chest pain

Central nervous system: Vertigo, nervousness, insomnia, depression

Dermatologic: Skin rash or dryness, pruritus, alopecia

Endocrine & metabolic: Decreased libido

Gastrointestinal: GI bleeding, thirst, heartburn, flatulence, dyspepsia

Genitourinary: Bladder spasms, dysuria

Hepatic: Jaundice

Neuromuscular & skeletal: Arthralgia, tremor, neck/shoulder pain, back pain

Ocular: Increased intraocular pressure

Renal: Polyuria

Drug Interactions Increased risk of amiloride-associated hyperkalemia: Triamterene, spironolactone, angiotensin-converting enzyme (ACE) inhibitors, potassium preparations, indomethacin

Drug Uptake

Absorption: Oral: ~15% to 25%

Onset: 2 hours

Duration: 24 hours

Serum half-life:

Normal renal function: 6-9 hours

End stage renal disease: 8-144 hours

Peak serum concentration: 6-10 hours

Pregnancy Risk Factor B

Generic Available Yes

Amiloride and Hydrochlorothiazide

(a MIL oh ride & hye droe klor oh THYE a zide)

Brand Names Moduretic®

Therapeutic Category Diuretic, Combination

Synonyms Hydrochlorothiazide and Amiloride

Use Antikaliuretic diuretic, antihypertensive

Local Anesthetic/Vasoconstrictor Precautions No information available to require special precautions

Effects on Dental Treatment No effects or complications reported

Other Adverse Effects See individual agents

Pregnancy Risk Factor B

Generic Available Yes

Amin-Aid® [OTC] *see* Enteral Nutritional Products *on page 350*

2-Amino-6-Mercaptopurine *see* Thioguanine *on page 925*

Aminocaproic Acid (a mee noe ka PROE ik AS id)

Brand Names Amicar®

Therapeutic Category Hemostatic Agent

Synonyms Aminocaproico, Acido (Mexico)

Use Treatment of excessive bleeding from fibrinolysis

Usual Dosage In the management of acute bleeding syndromes, oral dosage regimens are the same as the I.V. dosage regimens in adults and children

Chronic bleeding: Oral, I.V.: 5-30 g/day in divided doses at 3- to 6-hour intervals

Acute bleeding syndrome:

Children: Oral, I.V.: 100 mg/kg or 3 g/m² during the first hour, followed by continuous infusion at the rate of 33.3 mg/kg/hour or 1 g/m²/hour; total dosage should not exceed 18 g/m²/24 hours

Traumatic hyphema: Oral: 100 mg/kg/dose every 6-8 hours

Adults:
  Oral: For elevated fibrinolytic activity, give 5 g during first hour, followed by 1-1.25 g/hour for approximately 8 hours or until bleeding stops
  I.V.: Give 4-5 g in 250 mL of diluent during first hour followed by continuous infusion at the rate of 1-1.25 g/hour in 50 mL of diluent, continue for 8 hours or until bleeding stops
  Maximum daily dose: Oral, I.V.: 30 g
Mechanism of Action Competitively inhibits activation of plasminogen to plasmin, also, a lesser antiplasmin effect
Local Anesthetic/Vasoconstrictor Precautions No information available to require special precautions
Effects on Dental Treatment No effects or complications reported
Other Adverse Effects
1% to 10%:
  Cardiovascular: Hypotension, bradycardia, arrhythmia
  Central nervous system: Dizziness, headache, malaise, fatigue
  Dermatologic: Rash
  Gastrointestinal: GI irritation, nausea, cramps, diarrhea
  Hematologic: Decreased platelet function, elevated serum enzymes
  Neuromuscular & skeletal: Myopathy, weakness
  Otic: Tinnitus
  Respiratory: Nasal congestion
<1%:
  Central nervous system: Convulsions
  Genitourinary: Ejaculation problems
  Neuromuscular & skeletal: Rhabdomyolysis
  Renal: Renal failure
Drug Interactions No data reported
Drug Uptake Serum half-life: 1-2 hours
Pregnancy Risk Factor C
Generic Available Yes: Injection

Aminocaproico, Acido (Mexico) *see Aminocaproic Acid on previous page*
Amino-Cerv™ Vaginal Cream *see Urea on page 977*

Aminoglutethimide (a mee noe gloo TETH i mide)
Brand Names Cytadren®
Therapeutic Category Antiadrenal Agent; Antineoplastic Agent, Adjuvant
Use Suppression of adrenal function in selected patients with Cushing's syndrome; also used successfully in postmenopausal patients with advanced breast carcinoma and in patients with metastatic prostate carcinoma as salvage (third-line hormonal agent)
Usual Dosage Adults: Oral: 250 mg every 6 hours may be increased at 1- to 2-week intervals to a total of 2 g/day; give in divided doses, 2-3 times/day to reduce incidence of nausea and vomiting
Mechanism of Action Blocks the enzymatic conversion of cholesterol to delta-5-pregnenolone, thereby reducing the synthesis of adrenal glucocorticoids, mineralocorticoids, estrogens, aldosterone, and androgens
Local Anesthetic/Vasoconstrictor Precautions No information available to require special precautions
Effects on Dental Treatment Over 10% of patients likely to experience nausea; approximately 10% may experience orthostatic hypotension
Other Adverse Effects Most adverse effects will diminish in incidence and severity after the first 2-6 weeks

>10%:
  Central nervous system: Headache, dizziness, drowsiness, and lethargy are frequent at the start of therapy, clumsiness
  Dermatologic: Systemic lupus erythematosus, skin rash
  Gastrointestinal: Nausea, vomiting, anorexia
  Hepatic: Cholestatic jaundice
  Neuromuscular & skeletal: Myalgia
  Renal: Nephrotoxicity
  Respiratory: Pulmonary alveolar damage
1% to 10%:
  Cardiovascular: Hypotension and tachycardia, orthostatic hypotension
  Dermatologic: Hirsutism in females
  Endocrine & metabolic: Adrenocortical insufficiency
  Hematologic: Rare cases of neutropenia, leukopenia, thrombocytopenia, pancytopenia, and agranulocytosis have been reported
<1%: Endocrine & metabolic: Adrenal suppression, lipid abnormalities (hypercholesterolemia), hyperkalemia, hypothyroidism, goiter
(Continued)

Aminoglutethimide *(Continued)*

Drug Interactions Aminoglutethimide enhances elimination of dexamethasone resulting in reduction of steroid response; increased clearance of digitoxin after 3-8 weeks of aminoglutethimide therapy resulting in decreased effect of digitoxin; aminoglutethimide increases the metabolism of theophylline; decrease in anticoagulant response to warfarin

Drug Uptake

Onset of action (adrenal suppression): 3-5 days

Serum half-life: 7-15 hours; shorter following multiple administrations than following single doses (induces hepatic enzymes increasing its own metabolism)

Pregnancy Risk Factor D

Generic Available No

Amino-Opti-E® [OTC] *see* Vitamin E *on page 994*

Aminophylline *(am in OFF i lin)*

Related Information

Dental Drug Interactions: Update on Drug Combinations Requiring Special Considerations *on page 1144*

Respiratory Diseases *on page 1018*

Theophylline *on page 917*

Brand Names Phyllocontin®; Truphylline®

Therapeutic Category Theophylline Derivative

Synonyms Theophylline Ethylenediamine

Use Bronchodilator in reversible airway obstruction due to asthma or COPD; increase diaphragmatic contractility; neonatal idiopathic apnea of prematurity

Usual Dosage

Neonates: Apnea of prematurity:

Loading dose: 5 mg/kg for one dose

Maintenance: I.V.:

0-24 days: Begin at 2 mg/kg/day divided every 12 hours and titrate to desired levels and effects

>24 days: 3 mg/kg/day divided every 12 hours; increased dosages may be indicated as liver metabolism matures (usually >30 days of life); monitor serum levels to determine appropriate dosages

Theophylline levels should be initially drawn after 3 days of therapy; repeat levels are indicated 3 days after each increase in dosage or weekly if on a stabilized dosage

Treatment of acute bronchospasm:

Loading dose (in patients not currently receiving aminophylline or theophylline): 6 mg/kg (based on aminophylline) administered I.V. over 20-30 minutes; administration rate should not exceed 25 mg/minute (aminophylline)

Approximate I.V. maintenance dosages are based upon **continuous infusions**; bolus dosing (often used in children <6 months of age) may be determined by multiplying the hourly infusion rate by 24 hours and dividing by the desired number of doses/day

6 weeks to 6 months: 0.5 mg/kg/hour

6 months to 1 year: 0.6-0.7 mg/kg/hour

1-9 years: 1-1.2 mg/kg/hour

9-12 years and young adult smokers: 0.9 mg/kg/hour

12-16 years: 0.7 mg/kg/hour

Adults (healthy, nonsmoking): 0.7 mg/kg/hour

Older patients and patients with cor pulmonale, patients with congestive heart failure or liver failure: 0.25 mg/kg/hour

Dosage should be adjusted according to serum level measurements during the first 12- to 24-hour period; avoid using suppositories due to erratic, unreliable absorption

Rectal: Adults: 500 mg 3 times/day

Mechanism of Action Causes bronchodilatation, diuresis, CNS and cardiac stimulation, and gastric acid secretion by blocking phosphodiesterase which increases tissue concentrations of cyclic adenine monophosphate (cAMP) which in turn promotes catecholamine stimulation of lipolysis, glycogenolysis, and gluconeogenesis and induces release of epinephrine from adrenal medulla cells

Local Anesthetic/Vasoconstrictor Precautions No information available to require special precautions

Effects on Dental Treatment Prescribe erythromycin with caution to patients taking theophylline products. Erythromycin will delay the normal metabolic inactivation of theophyllines leading to increased blood levels; this has resulted in nausea, vomiting and CNS restlessness

Other Adverse Effects

Uncommon at serum theophylline concentrations ≤20 mcg/mL

1% to 10%:

Cardiovascular: Tachycardia

Central nervous system: Nervousness, restlessness

Gastrointestinal: Nausea, vomiting

<1%:

Central nervous system: Insomnia, irritability, seizures

Dermatologic: Skin rash

Gastrointestinal: Gastric irritation

Neuromuscular & skeletal: Tremor

Miscellaneous: Allergic reactions

Drug Interactions Decreased effect/increased toxicity: Changes in diet may affect the elimination of theophylline; charcoal-broiled foods may increase elimination, reducing half-life by 50%; see table for factors affecting serum levels.

Factors Reported to Affect Theophylline Serum Levels

Decreased Theophylline Level	Increased Theophylline Level
Smoking (cigarettes, marijuana)	Hepatic cirrhosis
High protein/low carbohydrate diet	Cor pulmonale
Charcoal	CHF
Phenytoin	Fever/viral illness
Phenobarbital	Propranolol
Carbamazepine	Allopurinol (>600 mg/d)
Rifampin	Erythromycin
I.V. isoproterenol	Cimetidine
Aminoglutethimide	Troleandomycin
Barbiturates	Ciprofloxacin
Hydantoins	Oral contraceptives
Ketoconazole	Beta blockers
Sulfinpyrazone	Calcium channel blockers
Isoniazid	Corticosteroids
Loop diuretics	Disulfiram
Sympathomimetics	Ephedrine
	Influenza virus vaccine
	Interferon
	Macrolides
	Mexiletine
	Quinolones
	Thiabendazole
	Thyroid hormones
	Carbamazepine
	Isoniazid
	Loop diuretics

Pregnancy Risk Factor C

Dietary Considerations Food does not appreciably affect absorption; avoid extremes of dietary protein and carbohydrate intake; limit charcoal-broiled foods

Generic Available Yes

Selected Readings

Cummins LH, et al, "Erythromycin's Effect on Theophylline Blood Levels. Correspondence," *Pediatrics*, 1977, 59:144-5.

Delaforge M and Sartori E, "In Vivo Effects of Erythromycin, Oleandomycin, and Erythralosamine Derivatives on Hepatic Cytochrome P-450," *Biochem Pharmacol*, 1990, 40(2):223-8.

Ludden TM, "Pharmacokinetic Interactions of the Macrolide Antibiotics," *Clin Pharmacokinet*, 1985, 10(1):63-79.

Aminophylline, Amobarbital, and Ephedrine

(am in OFF i lin, am oh BAR bi tal, & e FED rin)

Brand Names Amesec® [OTC]

Therapeutic Category Antiasthmatic; Bronchodilator

Use Symptomatic relief of asthma

Local Anesthetic/Vasoconstrictor Precautions Use vasoconstrictors with caution since ephedrine may enhance cardiostimulation and vasopressor effects of sympathomimetics

(Continued)

Aminophylline, Amobarbital, and Ephedrine *(Continued)*

Effects on Dental Treatment Prescribe erythromycin with caution to patients taking theophylline products. Erythromycin will delay the normal metabolic inactivation of theophyllines leading to increased blood levels; this has resulted in nausea, vomiting and CNS restlessness

Other Adverse Effects See individual agents

Pregnancy Risk Factor C

Generic Available No

Aminosalicilico, Acido *see* Aminosalicylate Sodium *on this page*

Aminosalicylate Sodium (a MEE noe sa LIS i late SOW dee um)

Brand Names Sodium P.A.S.

Canadian/Mexican Brand Names Salofalk® (Mexico); Tubasal® (Canada)

Therapeutic Category Antitubercular Agent; Nonsteroidal Anti-inflammatory Agent (NSAID), Oral

Synonyms Aminosalicilico, Acido

Use Treatment of tuberculosis with combination drugs

Usual Dosage Oral:

    Children: 150-300 mg/kg/day in 3-4 equally divided doses

    Adults: 150 mg/kg/day in 2-3 equally divided doses (usually 12-14 g/day)

Mechanism of Action Aminosalicylic acid (PAS) is a highly specific bacteriostatic agent active against *M. tuberculosis*. Most strains of *M. tuberculosis* are sensitive to a concentration of 1 µg/mL; structurally related to para-aminobenzoic acid (PABA) and its mechanism of action is thought to be similar to the sulfonamides, a competitive antagonism with PABA; disrupts plate biosynthesis in sensitive organisms

Local Anesthetic/Vasoconstrictor Precautions No information available to require special precautions

Effects on Dental Treatment No effects or complications reported

Other Adverse Effects

    1% to 10%: Gastrointestinal: Nausea, vomiting, diarrhea, abdominal pain

    <1%:

        Cardiovascular: Vasculitis

        Central nervous system: Fever

        Dermatologic: Skin eruptions

        Endocrine & metabolic: Goiter with or without myxedema

        Hematologic: Leukopenia, agranulocytosis, thrombocytopenia, hemolytic anemia

        Hepatic: Jaundice, hepatitis

Drug Interactions A small reduction in digoxin (Lanoxin®) plasma levels may result from coadministration with aminosalicylate sodium; probenecid increases the serum concentration of aminosalicylate sodium

Drug Uptake

    Absorption: Readily absorbed >90%

Pregnancy Risk Factor C

Generic Available Yes

Aminosalicylate Sodium *see* Para-Aminosalicylate Sodium *on page 723*

Amiodarona, Clorhidrato De (Mexico) *see* Amiodarone *on this page*

Amiodarone (a MEE oh da rone)

Related Information

    Cardiovascular Diseases *on page 1010*

Brand Names Cordarone®

Canadian/Mexican Brand Names Braxan® (Mexico); Cardiorona® (Mexico)

Therapeutic Category Antiarrhythmic Agent, Class III; Antiarrhythmic Agent (Supraventricular & Ventricular)

Synonyms Amiodarona, Clorhidrato De (Mexico)

Use Management of resistant, life-threatening ventricular arrhythmias or supraventricular arrhythmias unresponsive to conventional therapy with less toxic agents

Usual Dosage Oral:

    Children (calculate doses for children <1 year on body surface area):

        Loading dose: 10-15 mg/kg/day or 600-800 mg/1.73 m²/day for 4-14 days or until adequate control of arrhythmia or prominent adverse effects occur (this loading dose may be given in 1-2 divided doses/day); dosage should then be reduced to 5 mg/kg/day or 200-400 mg/1.73 m²/day given once daily for several weeks; if arrhythmia does not recur, reduce to lowest effective dosage possible; usual daily minimal dose: 2.5 mg/kg/day; maintenance doses may be given for 5 of 7 days/week

Adults: Ventricular arrhythmias: 800-1600 mg/day in 1-2 doses for 1-3 weeks, then 600-800 mg/day in 1-2 doses for 1 month; maintenance: 400 mg/day; lower doses are recommended for supraventricular arrhythmias

Mechanism of Action Class III antiarrhythmic agent which inhibits adrenergic stimulation, prolongs the action potential and refractory period in myocardial tissue; decreases A-V conduction and sinus node function

Local Anesthetic/Vasoconstrictor Precautions No information available to require special precautions

Effects on Dental Treatment This drug is indicated only for life-threatening arrhythmias; dental treatment would not be a consideration during these emergencies

Other Adverse Effects With large dosages (≥400 mg/day), adverse reactions occur in ~75% patients and require discontinuance in 5% to 20%

>10%:
Central nervous system: Ataxia, fatigue, malaise, dizziness, headache, insomnia, nightmares
Dermatologic: Photosensitivity
Gastrointestinal: Nausea, vomiting
Neuromuscular & skeletal: Tremor, paresthesia, weakness
Respiratory: Pulmonary fibrosis (cough, fever, dyspnea, malaise), interstitial pneumonitis
Miscellaneous: Alveolitis

1% to 10%:
Cardiovascular: Congestive heart failure, cardiac arrhythmias (atropine-resistant bradycardia, heart block, sinus arrest, paroxysmal ventricular tachycardia), myocardial depression, flushing, edema
Endocrine & metabolic: Hypothyroidism or hyperthyroidism (less common), decreased libido
Gastrointestinal: Constipation, anorexia, abdominal pain, abnormal salivation, dysgeusia
Hematologic: Coagulation abnormalities
Hepatic: Abnormal liver function tests
Ocular: Visual disturbances
Miscellaneous: Abnormal smell

<1%:
Cardiovascular: Hypotension, vasculitis
Central nervous system: Pseudotumor cerebri
Dermatologic: Skin rash, alopecia, slate blue discoloration of skin
Endocrine & metabolic: Hyperglycemia, hypertriglyceridemia
Genitourinary: Epididymitis
Hematologic: Thrombocytopenia
Hepatic: Cirrhosis, severe hepatic toxicity (potentially fatal hepatitis)
Ocular: Optic neuritis, corneal microdeposits, photophobia

Amiodarone Common Drug Interactions

Drug	Interaction
Anticoagulants, oral	The effects of the anticoagulant is increased due to inhibition of its metabolism
β-adrenergic receptor antagonists	β-blocker effects are enhanced by amiodarone's inhibition of the β-blocker's hepatic metabolism
Calcium channel antagonists	Additive effects of both drugs resulting in a reduction in cardiac sinus conduction, atrioventricular nodal conduction and myocardial contractility
Digoxin	Digoxin concentrations may be increased with resultant increases in activity and potential for toxicity
Flecainide	Flecainide plasma concentrations are increased
Phenytoin	Phenytoin serum concentrations are increased due to reduction in phenytoin metabolism, with possible symptoms of phenytoin toxicity
Procainamide	Procainamide serum concentrations may be increased
Quinidine	Quinidine serum concentrations may be increased and can potentially cause fatal cardiac dysrhythmias

(Continued)

Amiodarone *(Continued)*

Drug Interactions Cytochrome P-450 3A enzyme inhibitor

Amiodarone appears to interfere with the hepatic metabolism of several drugs resulting in significantly increased plasma concentrations; see table.

Drug Uptake

Onset of effect: 3 days to 3 weeks after starting therapy

Peak effect: 1 week to 5 months

Duration of effect after discontinuation of therapy: 7-50 days

Note: Mean onset of effect and duration after discontinuation may be shorter in children versus adults

Serum half-life: Oral chronic therapy: 40-55 days (range: 26-107 days); shortened in children versus adults

Pregnancy Risk Factor C

Generic Available No

Ami-Tex LA® *see* Guaifenesin and Phenylpropanolamine *on page 454*

Amitone® [OTC] *see* Calcium Carbonate *on page 162*

Amitriptilina Clorhidrato De (Mexico) *see* Amitriptyline *on this page*

Amitriptyline *(a mee TRIP ti leen)*

Brand Names Elavil®

Canadian/Mexican Brand Names Anapsique® (Mexico); Apo®-Amitriptyline (Canada); Levate® (Canada); Novo-Tryptin® (Canada); Tryptanol® (Mexico)

Therapeutic Category Antidepressant, Tricyclic

Synonyms Amitriptilina Clorhidrato De (Mexico)

Use Treatment of various forms of depression, often in conjunction with psychotherapy; analgesic for certain chronic and neuropathic pain, prophylaxis against migraine headaches

Usual Dosage

Children: Pain management: Oral: Initial: 0.1 mg/kg at bedtime, may advance as tolerated over 2-3 weeks to 0.5-2 mg/day at bedtime

Adolescents: Oral: Initial: 25-50 mg/day; may give in divided doses; increase gradually to 100 mg/day in divided doses

Adults:

Oral: 30-100 mg/day single dose at bedtime or in divided doses; dose may be gradually increased up to 300 mg/day; once symptoms are controlled, decrease gradually to lowest effective dose

I.M.: 20-30 mg 4 times/day

Mechanism of Action Increases the synaptic concentration of serotonin and/or norepinephrine in the central nervous system by inhibition of their reuptake at the presynaptic neuronal membrane

Local Anesthetic/Vasoconstrictor Precautions Use with caution; epinephrine, norepinephrine and levonordefrin have been shown to have an increased pressor response in combination with TCAs

Effects on Dental Treatment >10% of patients experience dry mouth; amitriptyline is the most anticholinergic and sedating of the antidepressants; pronounced effects on the cardiovascular system; long-term treatment with TCAs such as amitriptyline increases the risk of caries by reducing salivation and salivary buffer capacity. In a study by Rundergren, et al, pathological alterations were observed in the oral mucosa of 72% of 58 patients; 55% had new carious lesions after taking TCAs for a median of 5½ years. Current research is investigating the use of the salivary stimulant pilocarpine (Salagen®) to overcome the xerostomia from amitriptyline.

Other Adverse Effects Anticholinergic effects may be pronounced; moderate to marked sedation can occur (tolerance to these effects usually occurs)

>10%:

Central nervous system: Dizziness, drowsiness, headache

Gastrointestinal: Constipation, increased appetite, nausea, unpleasant taste, weight gain

Neuromuscular & skeletal: Weakness

1% to 10%:

Cardiovascular: Hypotension, postural hypotension, arrhythmias, tachycardia, sudden death

Central nervous system: Nervousness, restlessness, parkinsonian syndrome, insomnia, sedation, fatigue, anxiety, impaired cognitive function, seizures have occurred occasionally, extrapyramidal symptoms are possible

Gastrointestinal: Diarrhea, heartburn

Genitourinary: Sexual dysfunction, urinary retention

Neuromuscular & skeletal: Tremor

Ocular: Eye pain, blurred vision

Miscellaneous: Excessive sweating
<1%:
Central nervous system: Anxiety, seizures
Dermatologic: Alopecia, photosensitivity
Endocrine & metabolic: Breast enlargement, galactorrhea, rarely SIADH
Genitourinary: Testicular swelling
Hematologic: Leukopenia, eosinophilia, rarely agranulocytosis
Hepatic: Cholestatic jaundice, elevated liver enzymes
Ocular: Increased intraocular pressure
Otic: Tinnitus
Miscellaneous: Trouble with gums, decreased lower esophageal sphincter tone may cause GE reflux; allergic reactions

Drug Interactions

Decreased effect: Phenobarbital may increase the metabolism of amitriptyline; amitriptyline blocks the uptake of guanethidine and thus prevents the hypotensive effect of guanethidine

Increased toxicity: Clonidine has caused hypertensive crisis; amitriptyline may be additive with or may potentiate the action of other CNS depressants such as sedatives or hypnotics; with MAO inhibitors, hyperpyrexia, hypertension, tachycardia, confusion, seizures, and **deaths have been reported**; amitriptyline may increase the prothrombin time in patients stabilized on warfarin; amitriptyline potentiates the pressor and cardiac effects of sympathomimetic agents such as isoproterenol, epinephrine, etc; cimetidine and methylphenidate may decrease the metabolism of amitriptyline

Additive anticholinergic effects seen with other anticholinergic agents

Drug Uptake

Onset of action: 7-21 days
Serum half-life: Adults: 9-25 hours (15-hour average)
Time to peak serum concentration: Within 4 hours

Pregnancy Risk Factor D

Generic Available Yes

Selected Readings

Boakes AJ, Laurence DR, Teoh PC, et al, "Interactions Between Sympathomimetic Amines and Antidepressant Agents in Man," Br Med J, 1973, 1(849):311-5.

Jastak JT and Yagiela JA, "Vasoconstrictors and Local Anesthesia: A Review and Rationale for Use," J Am Dent Assoc, 1983, 107(4):623-30.

Larochelle P, Hamet P, and Enjalbert M, "Responses to Tyramine and Norepinephrine After Imipramine and Trazodone," Clin Pharmacol Ther, 1979, 26(1):24-30.

Mitchell JR, "Guanethidine and Related Agents. III Antagonism by Drugs Which Inhibit the Norepinephrine Pump in Man," J Clin Invest, 1970, 49(8):1596-604.

Rundegren J, van Dijken J, Mörnstad H, et al, "Oral Conditions in Patients Receiving Long-Term Treatment With Cyclic Antidepressant Drugs," Swed Dent J, 1985, 9(2):55-64.

Svedmyr N, "The Influence of a Tricyclic Antidepressive Agent (Protriptyline) on Some of the Circulatory Effects of Noradrenaline and Adrenalin® in Man," Life Sci, 1968, 7(1):77-84.

Amitriptyline and Chlordiazepoxide

(a mee TRIP ti leen & klor dye az e POKS ide)

Brand Names Limbitrol® DS 10-25

Therapeutic Category Antidepressant, Tricyclic; Antipsychotic Agent

Synonyms Chlordiazepoxide and Amitriptyline

Use Treatment of moderate to severe anxiety and/or agitation and depression

Local Anesthetic/Vasoconstrictor Precautions Use with caution; epinephrine, norepinephrine and levonordefrin have been shown to have an increased pressor response in combination with TCAs

Effects on Dental Treatment

Amitriptyline: The most anticholinergic and sedating of the antidepressants; pronounced effects on the cardiovascular system; long-term treatment with TCAs such as amitriptyline increases the risk of caries by reducing salivation and salivary buffer capacity. In a study by Rundergren, et al, pathological alterations were observed in the oral mucosa of 72% of 58 patients; 55% had new carious lesions after taking TCAs for a median of 5½ years. Current research is investigating the use of the salivary stimulant pilocarpine (Salagen®) to overcome the xerostomia from amitriptyline.

Chlordiazepoxide: Over 10% of patients will experience dry mouth which disappears with cessation of drug therapy

Other Adverse Effects See individual agents

Pregnancy Risk Factor D

Generic Available Yes

Selected Readings

Boakes AJ, Laurence DR, Teoh PC, et al, "Interactions Between Sympathomimetic Amines and Antidepressant Agents in Man," Br Med J, 1973, 1(849):311-5.

Jastak JT and Yagiela JA, "Vasoconstrictors and Local Anesthesia: A Review and Rationale for Use," J Am Dent Assoc, 1983, 107(4):623-30.

Larochelle P, Hamet P, and Enjalbert M, "Responses to Tyramine and Norepinephrine After Imipramine and Trazodone," Clin Pharmacol Ther, 1979, 26(1):24-30.

(Continued)

Amitriptyline and Chlordiazepoxide *(Continued)*

Mitchell JR, "Guanethidine and Related Agents. III Antagonism by Drugs Which Inhibit the Norepinephrine Pump in Man," *J Clin Invest*, 1970, 49(8):1596-604.

Rundegren J, van Dijken J, Mörnstad H, et al, "Oral Conditions in Patients Receiving Long-Term Treatment With Cyclic Antidepressant Drugs," *Swed Dent J*, 1985, 9(2):55-64.

Svedmyr N, "The Influence of a Tricyclic Antidepressive Agent (Protriptyline) on Some of the Circulatory Effects of Noradrenaline and Adrenaline in Man," *Life Sci*, 1968, 7(1):77-84.

Amitriptyline and Perphenazine

(a mee TRIP ti leen & per FEN a zeen)

Brand Names Etrafon®; Triavil®

Therapeutic Category Antidepressant, Tricyclic; Phenothiazine Derivative

Synonyms Perphenazine and Amitriptyline

Use Treatment of patients with moderate to severe anxiety and depression

Local Anesthetic/Vasoconstrictor Precautions

Amitriptyline: Use with caution; epinephrine, norepinephrine and levonordefrin have been shown to have an increased pressor response in combination with TCAs

Perphenazine: No information available to require special precautions

Effects on Dental Treatment >10% of patients experience dry mouth

Amitriptyline: The most anticholinergic and sedating of the antidepressants; pronounced effects on the cardiovascular system; long-term treatment with TCAs such as amitriptyline increases the risk of caries by reducing salivation and salivary buffer capacity. In a study by Rundergren, et al, pathological alterations were observed in the oral mucosa of 72% of 58 patients; 55% had new carious lesions after taking TCAs for a median of $5^{1}/_{2}$ years. Current research is investigating the use of the salivary stimulant pilocarpine (Salagen®) to overcome the xerostomia from amitriptyline.

Perphenazine: Significant hypotension may occur, especially when the drug is administered parenterally; orthostatic hypotension is due to alpha-receptor blockade, the elderly are at greater risk for orthostatic hypotension

Tardive dyskinesia: Prevalence rate may be 40% in elderly; development of the syndrome and the irreversible nature are proportional to duration and total cumulative dose over time

Extrapyramidal reactions are more common in elderly with up to 50% developing these reactions after 60 years of age; drug-induced **Parkinson's syndrome** occurs often; **Akathisia** is the most common extrapyramidal reaction in elderly

Increased confusion, memory loss, psychotic behavior, and agitation frequently occur as a consequence of anticholinergic effects

Antipsychotic associated sedation in nonpsychotic patients is extremely unpleasant due to feelings of depersonalization, derealization, and dysphoria

Other Adverse Effects

>10%:

Central nervous system: Dizziness, drowsiness, headache

Gastrointestinal: Constipation, increased appetite, nausea, unpleasant taste, weight gain

Neuromuscular & skeletal: Weakness

1% to 10%:

Cardiovascular: Arrhythmias, hypotension

Central nervous system: Confusion, delirium, hallucinations, nervousness, restlessness, Parkinsonian syndrome, insomnia

Endocrine & metabolic: Sexual dysfunction

Gastrointestinal: Diarrhea, heartburn

Genitourinary: Dysuria

Neuromuscular & skeletal: Fine muscle tremors

Ocular: Blurred vision, eye pain

Miscellaneous: Excessive sweating

<1%:

Central nervous system: Anxiety, seizures

Dermatologic: Alopecia, photosensitivity

Endocrine & metabolic: Breast enlargement, galactorrhea, SIADH

Gastrointestinal: Trouble with gums, decreased lower esophageal sphincter tone may cause GE reflux

Genitourinary: Testicular swelling

Hematologic: Agranulocytosis, leukopenia, eosinophilia

Hepatic: Cholestatic jaundice, elevated liver enzymes

Ocular: Increased intraocular pressure

Otic: Tinnitus

Miscellaneous: Allergic reactions

Pregnancy Risk Factor D

Generic Available Yes

Selected Readings

Boakes AJ, Laurence DR, Teoh PC, et al, "Interactions Between Sympathomimetic Amines and Antidepressant Agents in Man," *Br Med J*, 1973, 1(849):311-5.

Jastak JT and Yagiela JA, "Vasoconstrictors and Local Anesthesia: A Review and Rationale for Use," *J Am Dent Assoc*, 1983, 107(4):623-30.

Larochelle P, Hamet P, and Enjalbert M, "Responses to Tyramine and Norepinephrine After Imipramine and Trazodone," *Clin Pharmacol Ther*, 1979, 26(1):24-30.

Mitchell JR, "Guanethidine and Related Agents. III Antagonism by Drugs Which Inhibit the Norepinephrine Pump in Man," *J Clin Invest*, 1970, 49(8):1596-604.

Rundegren J, van Dijken J, Mörnstad H, et al, "Oral Conditions in Patients Receiving Long-Term Treatment With Cyclic Antidepressant Drugs," *Swed Dent J*, 1985, 9(2):55-64.

Svedmyr N, "The Influence of a Tricyclic Antidepressive Agent (Protriptyline) on Some of the Circulatory Effects of Noradrenaline and Adrenalin in Man," *Life Sci*, 1968, 7(1):77-84.

Amlexanox (am LEKS an oks)

Related Information

Oral Nonvital Soft Tissue Ulcerations or Erosions *on page 1070*

Brand Names Aphthasol®

Therapeutic Category Anti-inflammatory, Locally Applied

Use Treatment of aphthous ulcers (ie, canker sores); has been investigated in many allergic disorders

Usual Dosage Administer (0.5 cm - ¼") directly on ulcers 4 times/day following oral hygiene, after meals, and at bedtime

Mechanism of Action As a benzopyrano-bipyridine carboxylic acid derivative, amlexanox has anti-inflammatory and antiallergic properties; it inhibits chemical mediatory release of the slow-reacting substance of anaphylaxis (SRS-A) and may have antagonistic effect son interleukin-3

Local Anesthetic/Vasoconstrictor Precautions Discontinue therapy if rash or contact mucositis develops

Effects on Dental Treatment No effects or complications reported

Other Adverse Effects

>1%:

Dermatologic: Allergic contact dermatitis

Gastrointestinal: Oral irritation

<1%: Gastrointestinal: Contact mucositis

Contraindications Hypersensitivity to amlexanox or components

Drug Uptake

Absorption: Systemic absorption with swallowing of topical application of oral paste

Serum half-life: 3.5 hours

Time to peak serum concentration: 2 hours

Pregnancy Risk Factor B

Dosage Forms Paste: 5% (5 g)

Generic Available No

Comments Treatment of canker sores with amlexanox showed a 76% median reduction in ulcer size compared to a 40% reduction with placebo. Greer, et al, reported an overall mean reduction in ulcer size of 1.82 mm² for patients treated with 5% amlexanox versus an average reduction of 0.52 mm² for the control group.

Selected Readings

Greer RO Jr, Lindenmuth JE, Juarez T, et al, "A Double-Blind Study of Topically Applied 5% Amlexanox in the Treatment of Aphthous Ulcers," *J Oral Maxillofac Surg*, 1993, 51(3):243-8.

Amlodipina, Besilato De (Mexico) *see* Amlodipine *on this page*

Amlodipine (am LOE di peen)

Related Information

Calcium Channel Blockers & Gingival Hyperplasia *on page 1132*

Cardiovascular Diseases *on page 1010*

Brand Names Norvasc®

Canadian/Mexican Brand Names Norvas® (Mexico)

Therapeutic Category Antianginal Agent; Calcium Channel Blocker

Synonyms Amlodipina, Besilato De (Mexico)

Use Treatment of hypertension and angina

Usual Dosage Adults: Oral: Initial dose: 2.5-5 mg once daily; usual dose: 5-10 mg once daily; maximum dose: 10 mg once daily

Hemodialysis effects: Hemodialysis and peritoneal dialysis does not enhance elimination; supplemental dose is not necessary

Dosage adjustment in hepatic impairment: 2.5 mg once daily

Mechanism of Action Inhibits calcium ion from entering the "slow channels" or select voltage-sensitive areas of vascular smooth muscle and myocardium during depolarization, producing a relaxation of coronary vascular smooth muscle and coronary vasodilation; increases myocardial oxygen delivery in patients with vasospastic angina

(Continued)

Amlodipine *(Continued)*

Local Anesthetic/Vasoconstrictor Precautions No information available to require special precautions

Effects on Dental Treatment Other drugs of this class can cause gingival hyperplasia (ie, nifedipine) but there have been no reports for amlodipine

Other Adverse Effects

>10%: Cardiovascular: Peripheral edema

1% to 10%:

Cardiovascular: Edema, flushing, palpitations

Central nervous system: Headache, fatigue, dizziness, somnolence

Dermatologic: Dermatitis, rash

Endocrine & metabolic: Sexual dysfunction

Gastrointestinal: Nausea, abdominal pain

Neuromuscular & skeletal: Muscle cramps

Respiratory: Dyspnea

<1%:

Cardiovascular: Hypotension, bradycardia, arrhythmias, abnormal EKG, ventricular extrasystoles

Dermatologic: Alopecia, petechiae

Gastrointestinal: Weight gain, anorexia

Neuromuscular & skeletal: Joint stiffness

Respiratory: Nasal congestion, cough, epistaxis

Miscellaneous: Sweating

Drug Interactions Hepatic enzyme inhibitor

Increased effect:

Amlodipine and benazepril may increase hypotensive effect

Amlodipine and cyclosporine may increase cyclosporine levels

Drug Uptake

Onset of action: 30-50 minutes

Peak effect: 6-12 hours

Duration: 24 hours

Absorption: Oral: Well absorbed

Serum half-life: 30-50 hours

Pregnancy Risk Factor C

Generic Available No

Selected Readings

Jorgensen MG, "Prevalence of Amlodipine-Related Gingival Hyperplasia," *J Periodontol*, 1997, 68(7):676-8.

Wynn RL, "An Update on Calcium Channel Blocker-Induced Gingival Hyperplasia," *Gen Dent*, 1995, 43(3):218-22.

Wynn RL, "Calcium Channel Blockers and Gingival Hyperplasia," *Gen Dent*, 1991, 39(4):240-3.

Amlodipine and Benazepril *(am LOE di peen & ben AY ze pril)*

Brand Names Lotrel™

Therapeutic Category Angiotensin-Converting Enzyme (ACE) Inhibitors; Calcium Channel Blocker

Use Treatment of hypertension

Local Anesthetic/Vasoconstrictor Precautions No information available to require special precautions

Effects on Dental Treatment Other drugs of this class can cause gingival hyperplasia (ie, nifedipine) but there have been no reports for amlodipine

Pregnancy Risk Factor C (first trimester); D (second and third trimesters)

Generic Available No

Selected Readings

Wynn RL, "An Update on Calcium Channel Blocker-Induced Gingival Hyperplasia," *Gen Dent*, 1995, 43(3):218-22.

Wynn RL, "Calcium Channel Blockers and Gingival Hyperplasia," *Gen Dent*, 1991, 39(4):240-3.

Ammonapse *see* Sodium Phenylbutyrate *on page 873*

Ammonia Spirit, Aromatic *(a MOE nee ah SPEAR it, air oh MAT ik)*

Brand Names Aromatic Ammonia Aspirols®

Therapeutic Category Respiratory Stimulant

Use Respiratory and circulatory stimulant, treatment of fainting

Usual Dosage Used as "smelling salts" to treat or prevent fainting

Local Anesthetic/Vasoconstrictor Precautions No information available to require special precautions

Effects on Dental Treatment No effects or complications reported

Other Adverse Effects 1% to 10%:

Gastrointestinal: Nausea, vomiting

Respiratory: Irritation to nasal mucosa, coughing

Contraindications Hypersensitivity to ammonia or any component

Drug Interactions No data reported

Pregnancy Risk Factor C
Breast-feeding Considerations No data reported
Dosage Forms
    Inhalant, crushable glass perles: 0.33 mL, 0.4 mL
    Solution: 30 mL, 60 mL, 120 mL
Dietary Considerations No data reported
Generic Available Yes

Ammonium Chloride (a MOE nee um KLOR ide)

Therapeutic Category Metabolic Alkalosis Agent; Urinary Acidifying Agent
Use Diuretic or systemic and urinary acidifying agent; treatment of hypochloremic states
Mechanism of Action Increases acidity by increasing free hydrogen ion concentration
Local Anesthetic/Vasoconstrictor Precautions No information available to require special precautions
Effects on Dental Treatment No effects or complications reported
Other Adverse Effects 1% to 10%:
    Cardiovascular: Bradycardia
    Central nervous system: Mental confusion, coma, headache
    Dermatologic: Rash
    Endocrine & metabolic: Metabolic acidosis secondary to hyperchloremia
    Gastrointestinal: Gastric irritation, nausea, vomiting
    Local: Pain at site of injection
    Respiratory: Hyperventilation
Drug Uptake Absorption: Rapid from GI tract, complete within 3-6 hours
Pregnancy Risk Factor C
Dosage Forms
    Injection: 26.75% [5 mEq/mL] (20 mL)
    Tablet: 500 mg
    Tablet, enteric coated: 500 mg
Generic Available Yes

Ammonium Lactate *see* Lactic Acid With Ammonium Hydroxide *on page 539*

Amobarbital (am oh BAR bi tal)

Brand Names Amytal®
Canadian/Mexican Brand Names Amobarbital® (Canada)
Therapeutic Category Barbiturate; Hypnotic; Sedative
Use
    Oral: Hypnotic in short-term treatment of insomnia, to reduce anxiety and provide sedation preoperatively
    I.M., I.V.: Control status epilepticus or acute seizure episodes. Also used in catatonic, negativistic, or manic reactions and in "Amytal® Interviewing" for narcoanalysis
Usual Dosage
    Children: Oral:
        Sedation: 6 mg/kg/day divided every 6-8 hours
        Insomnia: 2 mg/kg or 70 mg/m^2/day in 4 equally divided doses
        Hypnotic: 2-3 mg/kg

    Adults:
        Insomnia: Oral: 65-200 mg at bedtime
        Sedation: Oral: 30-50 mg 2-3 times/day
        Preanesthetic: Oral: 200 mg 1-2 hours before surgery
        Hypnotic:
            Oral: 65-200 mg at bedtime
            I.M., I.V.: 65-500 mg, should not exceed 500 mg I.M. or 1000 mg I.V.
Mechanism of Action Interferes with transmission of impulses from the thalamus to the cortex of the brain resulting in an imbalance in central inhibitory and facilitatory mechanisms
Local Anesthetic/Vasoconstrictor Precautions No information available to require special precautions
Effects on Dental Treatment No effects or complications reported
Other Adverse Effects
    >10%:
        Central nervous system: Dizziness, lightheadedness, "hangover" effect, drowsiness, CNS depression, fever
        Local: Pain at injection site
    1% to 10%:
        Central nervous system: Confusion, mental depression, unusual excitement, nervousness, faint feeling, headache, insomnia, nightmares
        Gastrointestinal: Nausea, vomiting, constipation
(Continued)

Amobarbital *(Continued)*

<1%:
Cardiovascular: Hypotension
Central nervous system: Hallucinations
Dermatologic: Skin rash, exfoliative dermatitis urticaria, Stevens-Johnson syndrome
Hematologic: Agranulocytosis, megaloblastic anemia, thrombocytopenia
Local: Thrombophlebitis
Respiratory: Respiratory depression, apnea, laryngospasm

Drug Interactions
Barbiturates can induce hepatic microsomal enzymes resulting in increased metabolism and, therefore, decreased effects of anticoagulants, corticosteroids, doxycycline
Increased toxicity when combined with other CNS depressants or antidepressants, respiratory and CNS depression may be additive

Drug Uptake
Onset of action:
I.V.: Within 5 minutes
Oral: Within 1 hour
Serum half-life, biphasic:
Initial: 40 minutes
Terminal: 20 hours

Pregnancy Risk Factor D
Generic Available Yes: Capsule

Amobarbital and Secobarbital
(am oh BAR bi tal & see koe BAR bi tal)

Brand Names Tuinal®
Therapeutic Category Barbiturate; Hypnotic
Synonyms Secobarbital and Amobarbital
Use Short-term treatment of insomnia
Local Anesthetic/Vasoconstrictor Precautions No information available to require special precautions
Effects on Dental Treatment No effects or complications reported
Other Adverse Effects
>10%:
Central nervous system: Dizziness, lightheadedness, drowsiness, "hangover" effect
Local: Pain at injection site
1% to 10%:
Central nervous system: Confusion, mental depression, unusual excitement, nervousness, faint feeling, headache, insomnia, nightmares
Gastrointestinal: Constipation, nausea, vomiting
<1%:
Central nervous system: Hallucinations
Cardiovascular: Hypotension
Dermatologic: Skin rash, exfoliative dermatitis, Stevens-Johnson syndrome
Hematologic: Agranulocytosis, megaloblastic anemia, thrombocytopenia
Local: Thrombophlebitis
Respiratory: Respiratory depression

Pregnancy Risk Factor D
Generic Available No

AMO Vitrax® *see* Sodium Hyaluronate *on page 873*
Amoxapina (Mexico) *see* Amoxapine *on this page*

Amoxapine (a MOKS a peen)

Brand Names Asendin®
Canadian/Mexican Brand Names Demolox® (Mexico)
Therapeutic Category Antidepressant, Tricyclic
Synonyms Amoxapina (Mexico)
Use Treatment of neurotic and endogenous depression and mixed symptoms of anxiety and depression
Usual Dosage Once symptoms are controlled, decrease gradually to lowest effective dose. Maintenance dose is usually given at bedtime to reduce daytime sedation. Oral:

Children: Not established in children <16 years of age
Adolescents: Initial: 25-50 mg/day; increase gradually to 100 mg/day; may give as divided doses or as a single dose at bedtime

Adults: Initial: 25 mg 2-3 times/day, if tolerated, dosage may be increased to 100 mg 2-3 times/day; may be given in a single bedtime dose when dosage <300 mg/day

Elderly: Initial: 25 mg at bedtime increased by 25 mg weekly for outpatients and every 3 days for inpatients if tolerated; usual dose: 50-150 mg/day, but doses up to 300 mg may be necessary

Maximum daily dose:
Inpatient: 600 mg
Outpatient: 400 mg

Mechanism of Action Reduces the reuptake of serotonin and norepinephrine and blocks the response of dopamine receptors to dopamine

Local Anesthetic/Vasoconstrictor Precautions Use with caution; epinephrine, norepinephrine and levonordefrin have been shown to have an increased pressor response in combination with TCAs

Effects on Dental Treatment >10% of patients experience dry mouth; long-term treatment with TCAs such as amoxapine increases the risk of caries by reducing salivation and salivary buffer capacity

Other Adverse Effects

>10%:
Central nervous system: Dizziness, drowsiness, headache
Gastrointestinal: Constipation, increased appetite, nausea, unpleasant taste, weight gain
Neuromuscular & skeletal: Weakness

1% to 10%:
Cardiovascular: Arrhythmias, hypotension
Central nervous system: Confusion, delirium, hallucinations, nervousness, restlessness, parkinsonian syndrome, insomnia, tardive dyskinesia
Endocrine & metabolic: Sexual dysfunction
Gastrointestinal: Diarrhea, heartburn
Genitourinary: Dysuria
Neuromuscular & skeletal: Fine muscle tremors
Ocular: Blurred vision, eye pain
Miscellaneous: Excessive sweating

<1%:
Central nervous system: Anxiety, seizures, neuroleptic malignant syndrome
Dermatologic: Photosensitivity, alopecia
Endocrine & metabolic: Breast enlargement, galactorrhea, SIADH
Gastrointestinal: Trouble with gums, decreased lower esophageal sphincter tone may cause GE reflex
Genitourinary: Testicular swelling
Hematologic: Agranulocytosis, leukopenia, eosinophilia
Hepatic: Cholestatic jaundice, elevated liver enzymes
Ocular: Increased intraocular pressure
Otic: Tinnitus
Miscellaneous: Allergic reactions

Drug Interactions
Decreased effect of clonidine, guanethidine
Increased effect of CNS depressants, sympathomimetics, anticholinergic agents
Increased toxicity of MAO inhibitors (hyperpyrexia, tachycardia, hypertension, seizures and death may occur); similar interactions as with other tricyclics may occur

Drug Uptake
Onset of antidepressant effect: Usually occurs after 1-2 weeks
Absorption: Oral: Rapidly and well absorbed
Serum half-life:
Parent drug: 11-16 hours
Active metabolite (8-hydroxy): Adults: 30 hours
Time to peak serum concentration: Within 1-2 hours

Pregnancy Risk Factor C

Generic Available Yes

Selected Readings
Boakes AJ, Laurence DR, Teoh PC, et al, "Interactions Between Sympathomimetic Amines and Antidepressant Agents in Man," Br Med J, 1973, 1(849):311-5.

Jastak JT and Yagiela JA, "Vasoconstrictors and Local Anesthesia: A Review and Rationale for Use," J Am Dent Assoc, 1983, 107:623-30.

Larochelle P, Hamet P, and Enjalbert M, "Responses to Tyramine and Norepinephrine After Imipramine and Trazodone," Clin Pharmacol Ther, 1979, 26(1):24-30.

Mitchell JR, "Guanethidine and Related Agents. III Antagonism by Drugs Which Inhibit the Norepinephrine Pump in Man," J Clin Invest, 1970, 49(8):1596-604.

Rundegren J, van Dijken J, Mörnstad H, et al, "Oral Conditions in Patients Receiving Long-Term Treatment With Cyclic Antidepressant Drugs," Swed Dent J, 1985, 9(2):55-64.

Svedmyr N, "The Influence of a Tricyclic Antidepressive Agent (Protriptyline) on Some of the Circulatory Effects of Noradrenaline and Adrenalin* in Man," Life Sci, 1968, 7(1):77-84.

Amoxicillin (a moks i SIL in)

Related Information
Animal and Human Bites Guidelines *on page 1093*
Antibiotic Prophylaxis, Preprocedural Guidelines for Dental Patients *on page 1034*
Cardiovascular Diseases *on page 1010*
Dentin Hypersensitivity; High Caries Index; Xerostomia *on page 1074*
Oral Bacterial Infections *on page 1059*

Brand Names Amoxil®; Biomox®; Larotid®; Polymox®; Trimox®; Utimox®; Wymox®

Canadian/Mexican Brand Names Acimox® (Mexico); Amoxifur® (Mexico); Amoxisol® (Mexico); Amoxivet® (Mexico); Apo®-Amoxi (Canada); Gimalxina® (Mexico); Grunicina® (Mexico); Hidramox® (Mexico); Novamoxin® (Canada); Nu-Amoxi (Canada); Pro-Amox® (Canada)

Therapeutic Category Antibiotic, Penicillin

Use
Dental: Antibiotic for standard prophylactic regimen for dental patients who are at risk

Medical: Treatment of sinusitis, otitis media, and infections caused by susceptible organisms involving the respiratory tract, skin, and urinary tract

Usual Dosage Subacute bacterial endocarditis prophylaxis (standard regimen):
Children: 50 mg/kg 1 hour before dental procedure; total children's dose should not exceed adult dose
Adults: 2 g 1 hour before dental procedure

Mechanism of Action Interferes with bacterial cell wall synthesis during active multiplication, causing cell wall death and resultant bactericidal activity against susceptible bacteria

Local Anesthetic/Vasoconstrictor Precautions No information available to require special precautions

Effects on Dental Treatment Prolonged use of penicillins may lead to development of oral candidiasis

Other Adverse Effects 1% to 10%:
Central nervous system: Seizures, fever
Dermatologic: Rash (especially patients with mononucleosis)
Gastrointestinal: Diarrhea
Miscellaneous: Superinfection

Contraindications Hypersensitivity to amoxicillin, penicillin, or any component

Warnings/Precautions In patients with renal impairment, doses and/or frequency of administration should be modified in response to the degree of renal impairment; a high percentage of patients with infectious mononucleosis have developed rash during therapy with amoxicillin; a low incidence of cross-allergy with other beta-lactams and cephalosporins exists

Drug Interactions Efficacy of oral contraceptives may be reduced with amoxicillin; disulfiram, probenecid may cause increased amoxicillin levels; allopurinol may increase the potential for amoxicillin rash

Drug Uptake
Onset: Oral: Rapid and nearly complete
Time to peak serum concentration: 2 hours (capsule) and 1 hour (suspension)
Serum half-life:
Adults with normal renal function: 0.7-1.4 hours
Children: 1-2 hours

Pregnancy Risk Factor B

Breast-feeding Considerations May be taken while breast-feeding

Dosage Forms
Capsule, as trihydrate: 250 mg, 500 mg
Powder for oral suspension, as trihydrate: 125 mg/5 mL (5 mL, 80 mL, 100 mL, 150 mL, 200 mL); 250 mg/5 mL (5 mL, 80 mL, 100 mL, 150 mL, 200 mL)
Powder for oral suspension, drops, as trihydrate: 50 mg/mL (15 mL, 30 mL)
Tablet, chewable, as trihydrate: 125 mg, 250 mg

Dietary Considerations Peak concentrations may be delayed with food; may be taken with food; may be mixed with formula, milk, or juice

Generic Available Yes

Selected Readings
Dajani AS, Taubert KA, Wilson W, et al, "Prevention of Bacterial Endocarditis Recommendations by the American Heart Association," *JAMA* 1997, 277(22):1794-801.
Dajani AS, Taubert KA, Wilson W, et al, "Prevention of Bacterial Endocarditis: Recommendations by the American Heart Association," *J Am Dent Assoc* 1997, 128(8):1142-51.
Wynn RL, "Amoxicillin Update," *Gen Dent*, 1991, 39(5):322,4,6.

Amoxicillin and Clavulanate Potassium
(a moks i SIL in & klav yoo LAN ate poe TASS ee um)

Related Information
Animal and Human Bites Guidelines *on page 1093*
Dentin Hypersensitivity; High Caries Index; Xerostomia *on page 1074*
Oral Bacterial Infections *on page 1059*

Brand Names Augmentin®

Canadian/Mexican Brand Names Clavulan® (Canada); Clavulin® (Mexico)

Therapeutic Category Antibiotic, Penicillin

Use
Dental: Treatment of orofacial infections when beta-lactamase-producing staphylococci and beta-lactamase-producing *Bacteroides* are present
Medical: Treatment of otitis media, sinusitis, and infections caused by susceptible organisms involving the lower respiratory tract, skin and skin structure, and urinary tract; spectrum same as amoxicillin with additional coverage of beta-lactamase producing *B. catarrhalis, H. influenzae, N. gonorrhoeae,* and *S. aureus* (not MRSA). The expanded coverage of this combination makes it a useful alternative when penicillinase-producing bacteria are present and patients cannot tolerate alternative treatments.

Usual Dosage Oral:
Children <40 kg: 20-40 mg (amoxicillin)/kg/day in divided doses every 8 hours
Children >40 kg and Adults: 250-500 mg every 8 hours or 875 mg every 12 hours for at least 7 days; maximum dose: 2 g/day

Mechanism of Action Interferes with bacterial cell wall synthesis during active multiplication, causing cell wall death and resultant bactericidal activity against susceptible bacteria. Clavulanic acid binds and inhibits beta-lactamases that inactivate amoxicillin resulting in an antibiotic combination having an expanded spectrum of activity.

Local Anesthetic/Vasoconstrictor Precautions No information available to require special precautions

Effects on Dental Treatment Prolonged use of penicillins may lead to development of oral candidiasis

Other Adverse Effects <1%:
Dermatologic: Rash, urticaria
Gastrointestinal: Nausea, vomiting, diarrhea
Genitourinary: Vaginitis

Contraindications Known hypersensitivity to amoxicillin, clavulanic acid, or penicillin

Warnings/Precautions In patients with renal impairment, doses and/or frequency of administration should be modified in response to the degree of renal impairment; high percentage of patients with infectious mononucleosis have developed rash during therapy; a low incidence of cross-allergy with cephalosporins exists; incidence of diarrhea is higher than with amoxicillin alone

Drug Interactions Efficacy of oral contraceptives may be reduced; probenecid may cause increased amoxicillin levels; amoxicillin may increase the effect of anticoagulants

Drug Uptake Amoxicillin pharmacokinetics are not affected by clavulanic acid
Onset: Rapid and nearly complete
Time to peak serum concentration:
Capsule: 2 hours
Suspension: 1 hour
Serum half-life:
Adults with normal renal function: ~1 hour for both agents
Children: 1-2 hours

Pregnancy Risk Factor B

Breast-feeding Considerations
Amoxicillin: May be taken while breast-feeding
Clavulanic acid: No data reported

Dosage Forms
Suspension, oral:
125 (banana flavor): Amoxicillin trihydrate 125 mg and clavulanate potassium 31.25 mg per 5 mL (75 mL, 150 mL)
200: Amoxicillin 200 mg and clavulanate potassium 28.5 mg per 5 mL (50 mL, 75 mL, 100 mL)
250 (orange flavor): Amoxicillin trihydrate 250 mg and clavulanate potassium 62.5 mg per 5 mL (75 mL, 150 mL)
400: Amoxicillin 400 mg and clavulanate potassium 57 mg per 5 mL (50 mL, 75 mL, 100 mL)
Tablet:
250: Amoxicillin trihydrate 250 mg and clavulanate potassium 125 mg
500: Amoxicillin trihydrate 500 mg and clavulanate potassium 125 mg
(Continued)

Amoxicillin and Clavulanate Potassium *(Continued)*

875: Amoxicillin trihydrate 875 mg and clavulanate potassium 125 mg
Tablet, chewable:
125: Amoxicillin trihydrate 125 mg and clavulanate potassium 31.25 mg
250: Amoxicillin trihydrate 250 mg and clavulanate potassium 62.5 mg

Dietary Considerations May be taken with meals or on an empty stomach; may mix with milk, formula, or juice

Generic Available No

Comments In maxillary sinus, anterior nasal cavity, and deep neck infections, beta-lactamase-producing staphylococci and beta-lactamase-producing *Bacteroides* usually are present. In these situations, antibiotics that resist the beta-lactamase enzyme are indicated. Amoxicillin and clavulanic acid is administered orally for moderate infections. Ampicillin sodium and sulbactam sodium (Unasyn®) is administered parenterally for more severe infections.

Selected Readings
Wynn RL and Bergman SA, "Antibiotics and Their Use in the Treatment of Orofacial Infections, Part I and Part II," *Gen Dent*, 1994, 42(5):398-402, 498-502.

Amoxil® *see* Amoxicillin *on page 68*

Amphetamine *(am FET a meen)*

Related Information
Dextroamphetamine and Amphetamine *on page 297*

Therapeutic Category Amphetamine; Central Nervous System Stimulant, Amphetamine

Use Treatment of narcolepsy; exogenous obesity; abnormal behavioral syndrome in children (minimal brain dysfunction); attention deficit hyperactive disorder (ADHD)

Usual Dosage Oral:
Narcolepsy:
Children:
6-12 years: 5 mg/day, increase by 5 mg at weekly intervals
>12 years: 10 mg/day, increase by 10 mg at weekly intervals
Adults: 5-60 mg/day in 2-3 divided doses

Attention deficit disorder: Children:
3-5 years: 2.5 mg/day, increase by 2.5 mg at weekly intervals
>6 years: 5 mg/day, increase by 5 mg at weekly intervals not to exceed 40 mg/day

Short-term adjunct to exogenous obesity: Children >12 years and Adults: 10 mg or 15 mg long-acting capsule daily, up to 30 mg/day; or 5-30 mg/day in divided doses (immediate release tablets only)

Mechanism of Action The amphetamines are noncatechol sympathomimetic amines with pharmacologic actions similar to ephedrine. They require breakdown by monoamine oxidase for inactivation; produce central nervous system and respiratory stimulation, a pressor response, mydriasis, bronchodilation, and contraction of the urinary sphincter; thought to have a direct effect on both alpha- and beta-receptor sites in the peripheral system, as well as release stores of norepinephrine in adrenergic nerve terminals. The central nervous system action is thought to occur in the cerebral cortex and reticular-activating system. The anorexigenic effect is probably secondary to the CNS-stimulating effect; the site of action is probably the hypothalamic feeding center

Local Anesthetic/Vasoconstrictor Precautions Use vasoconstriction with caution in patients taking amphetamine sulfate. Amphetamines enhance the sympathomimetic response of epinephrine and norepinephrine leading to potential hypertension and cardiotoxicity.

Effects on Dental Treatment No effects or complications reported

Other Adverse Effects
>10%:
Cardiovascular: Arrhythmia
Central nervous system: False feeling of well being, nervousness, restlessness, insomnia
1% to 10%:
Cardiovascular: Hypertension
Central nervous system: Mood or mental changes, dizziness, lightheadedness, headache
Endocrine & metabolic: Changes in libido
Gastrointestinal: Diarrhea, nausea, vomiting, stomach cramps, constipation, anorexia, weight loss, dry mouth
Ocular: Blurred vision
Miscellaneous: Increased sweating

<1%:
  Cardiovascular: Chest pain
  Central nervous system: CNS stimulation (severe), Tourette's syndrome, hyperthermia, seizures, paranoia
  Dermatologic: Skin rash, urticaria
  Miscellaneous: Tolerance and withdrawal with prolonged use
Drug Interactions Increased toxicity of MAO inhibitors (hyperpyrexia, hypertension, arrhythmias, seizures, cerebral hemorrhage, and death has occurred)
Pregnancy Risk Factor C
Generic Available Yes

Amphojel® [OTC] *see* Aluminum Hydroxide *on page 47*

Amphotec® *see* Amphotericin B Colloidal Dispersion *on next page*

Amphotericin B (am foe TER i sin bee)
Related Information
  Oral Fungal Infections *on page 1063*
Brand Names Fungizone®
Therapeutic Category Antifungal Agent, Oral Nonabsorbed; Antifungal Agent, Systemic; Antifungal Agent, Topical
Use Treatment of severe systemic infections and meningitis caused by susceptible fungi such as *Candida* species, *Histoplasma capsulatum*, *Cryptococcus neoformans*, *Aspergillus* species, *Blastomyces dermatitidis*, *Torulopsis glabrata*, and *Coccidioides immitis*; fungal peritonitis; irrigant for bladder fungal infections; topically for cutaneous and mucocutaneous candidal infections; orally for the treatment of oral candidiasis caused by susceptible strains of *Candida albicans*
Usual Dosage
  I.V.:
    Children:
      Test dose (not required): I.V.: 0.1 mg/kg/dose to a maximum of 1 mg; infuse over 30-60 minutes
      Initial therapeutic dose: 0.25 mg/kg gradually increased, usually in 0.25 mg/kg increments on each subsequent day, until the desired daily dose is reached
      Maintenance dose: 0.25-1 mg/kg/day given once daily; infuse over 2-6 hours. Once therapy has been established, amphotericin B can be administered on an every other day basis at 1-1.5 mg/kg/dose; cumulative dose: 1.5-2 g over 6-10 weeks
    Adults:
      Test dose (not required).: 1 mg infused over 20-30 minutes
      Initial dose: 0.25 mg/kg administered over 2-6 hours, gradually increased on subsequent days to the desired level by 0.25 mg/kg increments per day; in critically ill patients, may initiate with 1-1.5 mg/kg/day with close observation
      Maintenance dose: 0.25-1 mg/kg/day or 1.5 mg/kg over 4-6 hours every other day; do not exceed 1.5 mg/kg/day; cumulative dose: 1-4 g over 4-10 weeks
      Duration of therapy varies with nature of infection: Histoplasmosis, *Cryptococcus*, or blastomycosis may be treated with total dose of 2-4 g
  I.T.:
    Children.: 25-100 mcg every 48-72 hours; increase to 500 mcg as tolerated
    Adults: 25-300 mcg every 48-72 hours; increase to 500 mcg to 1 mg as tolerated
  Oral: 1 mL (100 mg) 4 times/day
  Topical: Apply to affected areas 2-4 times/day for 1-4 weeks of therapy depending on nature and severity of infection
Mechanism of Action Binds to ergosterol altering cell membrane permeability in susceptible fungi and causing leakage of cell components with subsequent cell death
Local Anesthetic/Vasoconstrictor Precautions No information available to require special precautions
Effects on Dental Treatment No effects or complications reported
Other Adverse Effects
  >10%:
    Central nervous system: Fever, chills, headache, malaise, generalized pain
    Endocrine & metabolic: Hypokalemia, hypomagnesemia
    Gastrointestinal: Anorexia
    Hematologic: Anemia
    Renal: Nephrotoxicity
  1% to 10%:
    Cardiovascular: Hypotension, hypertension, flushing
    Central nervous system: Delirium, arachnoiditis, pain along lumbar nerves
(Continued)

Amphotericin B *(Continued)*

    Gastrointestinal: Nausea, vomiting
    Genitourinary: Urinary retention
    Hematologic: Leukocytosis, bone marrow suppression
    Local: Thrombophlebitis
    Neuromuscular & skeletal: Paresthesia (especially with I.T. therapy)
    Renal: Renal tubular acidosis, renal failure
<1%:
    Cardiovascular: Cardiac arrest
    Central nervous system: Convulsions
    Dermatologic: Maculopapular rash
    Hematologic: Coagulation defects, thrombocytopenia, agranulocytosis, leuko-
      penia
    Hepatic: Acute liver failure
    Ocular: Vision changes
    Otic: Hearing loss
    Renal: Anuria
    Respiratory: Dyspnea
Drug Interactions Increased toxicity: Cyclosporine and aminoglycosides (neph-
rotoxicity), corticosteroids (hypokalemia)
Drug Uptake
Serum half-life, biphasic:
    Initial: 15-48 hours
    Terminal: 15 days
Time to peak: Within 1 hour following a 4- to 6-hour dose
Pregnancy Risk Factor B
Dosage Forms
    Cream: 3% (20 g)
    Lotion: 3% (30 mL)
    Ointment, topical: 3% (20 g)
    Powder for injection, lyophilized: 50 mg
    Suspension, oral: 100 mg/mL (24 mL with dropper)
Generic Available Yes

Amphotericin B Colloidal Dispersion

(am foe TER i sin bee koe LOY dal dis PER shun)
Brand Names Amphotec®
Therapeutic Category Antifungal Agent
Use Effective in the treatment of invasive mycoses in patient refractory to or
intolerant of conventional amphotericin B
Usual Dosage Children and Adults: 3-4 mg/kg/day I.V. (infusion of 1 mg/kg/hour);
maximum: 7.5 mg/kg/day; duration of therapy is often <6 weeks
Mechanism of Action Binds to ergosterol altering cll membrane permeability in
susceptible fungi and causing leakage of cell components with subsequent cell
death
Local Anesthetic/Vasoconstrictor Precautions No information available to
require special precautions
Effects on Dental Treatment No effects or complications reported
Other Adverse Effects
1% to 10%:
    Cardiovascular: Hypotension, tachycardia
    Central nervous system: Headache, chills, fever
    Dermatologic: Rash
    Endocrine & metabolic: Hypokalemia, hypomagnesemia
    Gastrointestinal: Nausea, diarrhea, abdominal pain
    Hematologic: Thrombocytopenia
    Hepatic: LFT change
    Neuromuscular & skeletal: Rigors
    Respiratory: Dyspnea

Note: Amphotericin B colloidal dispersion has an improved therapeutic index
compared to conventional amphotericin B, and has been used safely in patients
with amphotericin B-related nephrotoxicity; however, continued decline of renal
function has occurred in some patients
Warnings/Precautions Anaphylaxis has been reported; facilities for cardiopulmonary resuscitation should be available; infusion reactions, sometimes, severe,
usually subside with continued therapy
Drug Interactions Increased toxicity: Cyclosporine and aminoglycosides (nephrotoxicity), corticosteroids (hypokalemia)
Drug Uptake Serum half-life: 28-29 hours
Pregnancy Risk Factor B

Amphotericin B Lipid Complex
(am foe TER i sin bee LIP id KOM pleks)

Brand Names Abelcet™ Injection; AmBisome®

Therapeutic Category Antifungal Agent, Systemic

Synonyms ABLC

Use Treatment of aspergillosis in patients who are refractory to or intolerant of conventional amphotericin B therapy. This indication is based on results obtained primarily from emergency use studies for the treatment of aspergillosis; orphan drug status for cryptococcal meningitis

Usual Dosage

Children and Adults: I.V.: 2.5-5 mg/kg/day as a single infusion **Note:** Significantly higher dose of ABLC are tolerated; it appears that attaining higher doses with ABLC produce more rapid fungicidal activity *in vivo* than standard amphotericin B preparations

Dosing adjustment in renal impairment: None necessary; effects of renal impairment are not currently known

Hemodialysis: No supplemental dosage necessary

Peritoneal dialysis effects: No supplemental dosage necessary

Continuous arterio-venous or veno-venous hemofiltration (CAVH/CAVHD): No supplemental dosage necessary

Local Anesthetic/Vasoconstrictor Precautions No information available to require special precautions

Effects on Dental Treatment No effects or complications reported

Other Adverse Effects

>10%:

Central nervous system: Chills, fever

Renal: Elevated serum creatinine

Miscellaneous: Multiple organ failure

1% to 10%:

Cardiovascular: Hypotension, cardiac arrest

Central nervous system: Headache, pain

Dermatologic: Rash

Endocrine & metabolic: Hypokalemia, acidosis

Gastrointestinal: Nausea, vomiting, diarrhea, gastrointestinal hemorrhage, abdominal pain

Hepatic: Bilirubinemia

Renal: Renal failure

Respiratory: Respiratory failure, dyspnea, pneumonia

Warnings/Precautions Anaphylaxis has been reported with amphotericin B desoxycholate and other amphotericin B-containing drugs. Facilities for cardio-pulmonary resuscitation should be available during administration due to the possibility of anaphylactic reaction. If severe respiratory distress occurs, the infusion should be immediately discontinued and the patient should not receive further infusions. During the initial dosing, the drug should be administered intravenously and under close clinical observation by medically trained personnel. Acute reactions (including fever and chills) may occur 1-2 hours after starting an intravenous infusion. These reactions are usually more common with the first few doses and generally diminish with subsequent doses.

Pregnancy Risk Factor B

Dosage Forms Injection: 50 mg; 5 mg/mL (20 mL)

Generic Available No

Ampicillin (am pi SIL in)

Related Information

Antibiotic Prophylaxis, Preprocedural Guidelines for Dental Patients *on page 1034*

Cardiovascular Diseases *on page 1010*

Dental Drug Interactions: Update on Drug Combinations Requiring Special Considerations *on page 1144*

Brand Names Amcill®; Marcillin®; Omnipen®; Omnipen®-N; Polycillin®; Polycillin-N®; Principen®; Totacillin®; Totacillin-N

Canadian/Mexican Brand Names Ampicin® [Sodium] (Canada); Anglopen® (Mexico); Apo®-Ampi [Trihydrate] (Canada); Binotal® (Mexico); Dibacilina® (Mexico); Flamicina® (Mexico); Jaa Amp® [Trihydrate] (Canada); Lampicin® (Mexico); Marovilina® (Mexico); Nu-Ampi [Trihydrate] (Canada); Pentrexyl® (Mexico); Pro-Ampi® [Trihydrate] (Canada); Sinaplin® (Mexico); Taro-Ampicillin® [Trihydrate] (Canada)

Therapeutic Category Antibiotic, Penicillin

(Continued)

Ampicillin *(Continued)*

Use

Dental: Alternate antibiotic for the prevention of bacterial endocarditis in patients undergoing dental procedures. It is used in those patients unable to take oral medications

Medical: Treatment of susceptible bacterial infections (nonbeta-lactamase-producing organisms); susceptible bacterial infections caused by streptococci, pneumococci, nonpenicillinase-producing staphylococci, *Listeria*, meningococci; some strains of *H. influenzae*, *Salmonella*, *Shigella*, *E. coli*, *Enterobacter*, and *Klebsiella*

Usual Dosage Prevention of bacterial endocarditis in patients unable to take oral medications:

Children: 50 mg/kg I.M. or I.V. within 30 minutes before procedure; total children's dose should not exceed adult dose

Adults: I.M., I.V.: 2 g 30 minutes before procedure

Mechanism of Action Interferes with bacterial cell wall synthesis during active multiplication, causing cell wall death and resultant bactericidal activity against susceptible bacteria

Local Anesthetic/Vasoconstrictor Precautions No information available to require special precautions

Effects on Dental Treatment Prolonged use of penicillins may lead to development of oral candidiasis

Other Adverse Effects

>10%:

Dermatologic: Rash (appearance of a rash should be carefully evaluated to differentiate a nonallergic ampicillin rash from a hypersensitivity reaction; incidence is higher in patients with viral infections, *Salmonella* infections, lymphocytic leukemia, or patients that have hyperuricemia)

Gastrointestinal: Diarrhea, vomiting

1% to 10%: Gastrointestinal: Severe abdominal cramps and/or pain

Contraindications Known hypersensitivity to ampicillin or other penicillins

Warnings/Precautions Dosage adjustment may be necessary in patients with renal impairment; a low incidence of cross-allergy with other beta-lactams exists; high percentage of patients with infectious mononucleosis have developed rash during therapy with ampicillin. Appearance of a rash should be carefully evaluated to differentiate a nonallergic ampicillin rash from a hypersensitivity reaction. Ampicillin rash occurs in 5% to 10% of children receiving ampicillin and is a generalized dull red, maculopapular rash, generally appearing 3-14 days after the start of therapy. It normally begins on the trunk and spreads over most of the body. It may be most intense at pressure areas, elbows, and knees.

Drug Interactions Efficacy of oral contraceptives may be reduced with ampicillin; probenecid may cause increased penicillin levels; ampicillin may increase the effect of anticoagulants; allopurinol may increase the potential for amoxicillin (ampicillin) rash

Drug Uptake

Absorption: Oral: 50%

Serum half-life: Adults and Children: 1-1.8 hours

Time to peak serum concentration: Oral: Within 1-2 hours

Pregnancy Risk Factor B

Breast-feeding Considerations Excreted into breast milk in small amounts like amoxicillin which is compatible with breast-feeding

Dosage Forms

Capsule, as anhydrous: 250 mg, 500 mg

Capsule, as trihydrate: 250 mg, 500 mg

Powder for injection, as sodium: 125 mg, 250 mg, 500 mg, 1 g, 2 g, 10 g

Powder for oral suspension, as trihydrate: 125 mg/5 mL (5 mL unit dose, 80 mL, 100 mL, 150 mL, 200 mL); 250 mg/5 mL (5 mL unit dose, 80 mL, 100 mL, 150 mL, 200 mL); 500 mg/5 mL (5 mL unit dose, 100 mL)

Powder for oral suspension, drops, as trihydrate: 100 mg/mL (20 mL)

Dietary Considerations Should be taken on an empty stomach; food decreases rate and extent of absorption

Generic Available Yes

Selected Readings

Dajani AS, Taubert KA, Wilson W, et al, "Prevention of Bacterial Endocarditis Recommendations by the American Heart Association," *JAMA* 1997, 277(22):1794-801.

Dajani AS, Taubert KA, Wilson W, et al, "Prevention of Bacterial Endocarditis: Recommendations by the American Heart Association," *J Am Dent Assoc* 1997, 128(8):1142-51.

Ampicillin and Probenecid *(am pi SIL in & proe BEN e sid)*

Brand Names Polycillin-PRB®; Probampacin®

Therapeutic Category Antibiotic, Penicillin

Use Uncomplicated infections caused by susceptible strains of *Neisseria gonor-rhoeae* in adults

Local Anesthetic/Vasoconstrictor Precautions No information available to require special precautions

Effects on Dental Treatment >10% oral candidiasis after chronic dosing

Other Adverse Effects

>10%:
  Central nervous system: Headache
  Dermatologic: Rash
  Gastrointestinal: Anorexia, nausea, vomiting, diarrhea, oral candidiasis
  Neuromuscular & skeletal: Gouty arthritis (acute)

1% to 10%:
  Cardiovascular: Flushing of face
  Central nervous system: Dizziness
  Dermatologic: Skin rash, itching
  Gastrointestinal: Sore gums, severe abdominal or stomach cramps and pain
  Genitourinary: Dysuria
  Renal: Renal calculi

<1%:
  Central nervous system: Seizures
  Hematologic: Leukopenia, hemolytic anemia, aplastic anemia
  Hepatic: Hepatic necrosis
  Renal: Urate nephropathy, nephrotic syndrome
  Miscellaneous: Anaphylaxis, penicillin encephalopathy, lymphocytic leukemia

Drug Interactions Avoid concomitant use with ketorolac since its half-life is increased two-fold and levels and toxicity are significantly increased by proben-ecid; allopurinol theoretically has an additional potential for ampicillin rash

Pregnancy Risk Factor B

Generic Available Yes

Ampicillin and Sulbactam (am pi SIL in & SUL bak tam)

Related Information

Dental Drug Interactions: Update on Drug Combinations Requiring Special Considerations *on page 1144*

Brand Names Unasyn®

Canadian/Mexican Brand Names Unasyna® (Mexico); Unasyna® Oral (Mexico)

Therapeutic Category Antibiotic, Penicillin

Use

Dental: Parenteral beta-lactamase-resistant antibiotic combination to treat more severe orofacial infections where beta-lactamase-producing staphylococci and beta-lactamase-producing *Bacteroides* are present

Medical: Treatment of susceptible bacterial infections involved with skin and skin structure, intra-abdominal infections, gynecological infections; spectrum is that of ampicillin plus organisms producing beta-lactamases such as *S. aureus*, *H. influenzae*, *E. coli*, *Klebsiella*, *Acinetobacter*, *Enterobacter*, and anaerobes

Usual Dosage Unasyn® (ampicillin/sulbactam) is a combination product. Each 3 g vial contains 2 g of ampicillin and 1 g of sulbactam. Sulbactam has very little antibacterial activity by itself, but effectively extends the spectrum of ampicillin to include beta-lactamase producing strains that are resistant to ampicillin alone. Therefore, dosage recommendations for Unasyn® are based on the ampicillin component.

I.M., I.V.:
  Children: 100-200 mg ampicillin/kg/day divided every 6 hours; maximum dose: 8 g ampicillin/day
  Adults: 1-2 g ampicillin every 6-8 hours; maximum dose: 8 g ampicillin/day

Mechanism of Action Interferes with bacterial cell wall synthesis during active multiplication, causing cell wall death and resultant bactericidal activity against susceptible bacteria; addition of sulbactam, a beta-lactamase inhibitor, to ampi-cillin extends the spectrum of ampicillin to include beta-lactamase producing organisms

Local Anesthetic/Vasoconstrictor Precautions No information available to require special precautions

Effects on Dental Treatment Prolonged use of penicillins may lead to develop-ment of oral candidiasis, some patients may experience hairy tongue

Other Adverse Effects

>10%: Local: Pain at injection site (I.M.)

1% to 10%:
  Dermatologic: Rash
  Gastrointestinal: Diarrhea
  Local: Pain at injection site (I.V.)

(Continued)

Ampicillin and Sulbactam *(Continued)*

Contraindications Hypersensitivity to ampicillin, sulbactam or any component, or penicillins

Warnings/Precautions Dosage adjustment may be necessary in patients with renal impairment; a low incidence of cross-allergy with other beta-lactams exists; high percentage of patients with infectious mononucleosis have developed rash during therapy with ampicillin. Appearance of a rash should be carefully evaluated to differentiate a nonallergic ampicillin rash from a hypersensitivity reaction. Ampicillin rash occurs in 5% to 10% of children receiving ampicillin and is a generalized dull red, maculopapular rash, generally appearing 3-14 days after the start of therapy. It normally begins on the trunk and spreads over most of the body. It may be most intense at pressure areas, elbows, and knees.

Drug Interactions Efficacy of oral contraceptives may be reduced with ampicillin and sulbactam; probenecid results in increased amoxicillin levels; allopurinol may increase the potential for amoxicillin/ampicillin rash

Drug Uptake
Absorption: Oral: 50%
Duration: Ampicillin: 6 hours
Serum half-life:
 Ampicillin: 1-1.8 hours
 Sulbactam: 1-1.3 hours
Time to peak serum concentration: Ampicillin: 1-2 hours

Pregnancy Risk Factor B

Breast-feeding Considerations
Ampicillin: Excreted into breast milk in small amounts like amoxicillin which is compatible with breast-feeding
Sulbactam sodium: No data reported

Dosage Forms Powder for injection: 1.5 g [ampicillin sodium 1 g and sulbactam sodium 0.5 g]; 3 g [ampicillin sodium 2 g and sulbactam sodium 1 g]

Dietary Considerations No data reported

Generic Available No

Comments In maxillary sinus, anterior nasal cavity, and deep neck infections, beta-lactamase-producing staphylococci and beta-lactamase-producing *Bacteroides* usually are present. In these situations, antibiotics that resist the beta-lactamase enzyme should be administered. Amoxicillin and clavulanic acid is administered orally for moderate infections. Ampicillin sodium and sulbactam sodium (Unasyn®) is administered parenterally for more severe infections.

Selected Readings
Wynn RL and Bergman SA, "Antibiotics and Their Use in the Treatment of Orofacial Infections, Part I and Part II," *Gen Dent*, 1994, 42(5):398-402, 498-502.

AMPT *see* Metyrosine *on page 632*

Amrinona, Lactato De (Mexico) *see* Amrinone *on this page*

Amrinone *(AM ri none)*

Brand Names Inocor®

Therapeutic Category Adrenergic Agonist Agent

Synonyms Amrinona, Lactato De (Mexico)

Use Treatment of low cardiac output states (sepsis, congestive heart failure); adjunctive therapy of pulmonary hypertension; normally prescribed for patients who have not responded well to therapy with digitalis, diuretics, and vasodilators

Usual Dosage Dosage is based on clinical response
Note: Dose should not exceed 10 mg/kg/24 hours

Children and Adults: 0.75 mg/kg I.V. bolus over 2-3 minutes followed by maintenance infusion of 5-10 mcg/kg/minute; I.V. bolus may need to be repeated in 30 minutes

Mechanism of Action Inhibits myocardial cyclic adenosine monophosphate (cAMP) phosphodiesterase activity and increases cellular levels of cAMP resulting in a positive inotropic effect and increased cardiac output; also possesses systemic and pulmonary vasodilator effects resulting in pre- and afterload reduction; slightly increases atrioventricular conduction

Local Anesthetic/Vasoconstrictor Precautions No information available to require special precautions

Effects on Dental Treatment No effects or complications reported

Other Adverse Effects
1% to 10%:
Cardiovascular: Arrhythmias, hypotension (may be infusion rate-related), ventricular and supraventricular arrhythmias
Gastrointestinal: Nausea
Hematologic: Thrombocytopenia (may be dose-related)

<1%:
   Cardiovascular: Chest pain
   Central nervous system: Fever
   Gastrointestinal: Vomiting, abdominal pain, anorexia
   Hepatic: Hepatotoxicity
   Local: Pain or burning at injection site
Drug Interactions No data reported
Drug Uptake
   Onset of action: I.V.: Within 2-5 minutes
   Peak effect: Within 10 minutes
   Duration: Dose dependent (~30 minutes low dose, ~2 hours higher doses)
   Serum half-life:
      Adults, normal volunteers: 3.6 hours
      Adults with CHF: 5.8 hours
Pregnancy Risk Factor C
Generic Available No

Amvisc® *see* Sodium Hyaluronate *on page 873*
Amvisc® Plus *see* Sodium Hyaluronate *on page 873*
Amytal® *see* Amobarbital *on page 65*
Anabolin® Injection *see* Nandrolone *on page 663*
Anacin® [OTC] *see* Aspirin *on page 90*
Anadrol® *see* Oxymetholone *on page 715*
Anafranil® *see* Clomipramine *on page 248*

Anagrelide (an AG gre lide)
Brand Names Agrylin®
Therapeutic Category Platelet Aggregation Inhibitor
Synonyms Anagrelide Hydrochloride
Use Agent for essential thrombocythemia (ET)
Usual Dosage Adults: Oral: 0.5 mg 4 times/day or 1 mg twice daily, maintain for ≥1 week, then adjust to the lowest effective dose to reduce and maintain platelet count <600,000 µL ideally to the normal range
Local Anesthetic/Vasoconstrictor Precautions No information available to require special precautions
Effects on Dental Treatment No effects or complications reported
Dosage Forms Capsule: 0.5 mg, 1 mg

Anagrelide Hydrochloride *see* Anagrelide *on this page*
Ana-Kit® *see* Insect Sting Kit *on page 508*
Anamine® Syrup [OTC] *see* Chlorpheniramine and Pseudoephedrine *on page 219*
Anaplex® Liquid [OTC] *see* Chlorpheniramine and Pseudoephedrine *on page 219*
Anaprox® (Naproxen Sodium) *see* Naproxen *on page 665*
Anaspaz® *see* Hyoscyamine *on page 492*

Anastrozole (an AS troe zole)
Brand Names Arimidex®
Therapeutic Category Antineoplastic Agent, Miscellaneous
Use Treatment of advanced breast cancer in postmenopausal women with disease progression following tamoxifen therapy. Patients with ER-negative disease and patients who did not respond to tamoxifen therapy rarely responded to anastrozole.
Usual Dosage Breast cancer: Adults: Oral (refer to individual protocols): 1 mg once daily
Mechanism of Action Potent and selective nonsteroidal aromatase inhibitor. It significantly lowers serum estradiol concentrations and has not detectable effect on formation of adrenal corticosteroids or aldosterone. In postmenopausal women, the principal source of circulating estrogen is conversion of adrenally generated androstenedione to estrone by aromatase in peripheral tissues.
Local Anesthetic/Vasoconstrictor Precautions No information available to require special precautions
Effects on Dental Treatment No effects or complications reported
Other Adverse Effects
   >5%:
      Cardiovascular: Flushing
      Gastrointestinal: Little to mild nausea (10%), vomiting
      Neuromuscular & skeletal: Increased bone and tumor pain
   2% to 5%:
      Cardiovascular: Hypertension
(Continued)

Anastrozole *(Continued)*

Central nervous system: Somnolence, confusion, insomnia, anxiety, nervousness, fever, malaise, accidental injury

Dermatologic: Hair thinning, pruritus

Endocrine & metabolic: Breast pain

Gastrointestinal: Weight loss

Genitourinary: Urinary tract infection

Local: Thrombophlebitis

Neuromuscular & skeletal: Myalgia, arthralgia, pathological fracture, neck pain

Respiratory: Sinusitis, bronchitis, rhinitis

Miscellaneous: Flu-like syndrome, infection

Drug Interactions Anastrozole inhibited *in vitro* metabolic reactions catalyzed by cytochromes P-450 1A2, 2C8/9, and 3A4, but only at relatively high concentrations. It is unlikely that coadministration of anastrozole with other drugs will result in clinically significant inhibition of cytochrome P-450-mediated metabolism of other drugs.

Drug Uptake

Absorption: Well absorbed from GI tract; food does not affect absorption

Serum half-life: 50 hours

Pregnancy Risk Factor C

Generic Available No

Anatuss® [OTC] *see* Guaifenesin, Phenylpropanolamine, and Dextromethorphan *on page 455*

Anatuss® DM [OTC] *see* Guaifenesin, Pseudoephedrine, and Dextromethorphan *on page 456*

Anbesol® [OTC] *see* Benzocaine *on page 118*

Anbesol® Maximum Strength [OTC] *see* Benzocaine *on page 118*

Ancef® *see* Cefazolin *on page 188*

Ancobon® *see* Flucytosine *on page 409*

Androderm® Transdermal System *see* Testosterone *on page 910*

Andro/Fem® Injection *see* Estradiol and Testosterone *on page 366*

Android-25® *see* Methyltestosterone *on page 626*

Andro-L.A.® Injection *see* Testosterone *on page 910*

Androlone®-D Injection *see* Nandrolone *on page 663*

Androlone® Injection *see* Nandrolone *on page 663*

Andropository® Injection *see* Testosterone *on page 910*

Anergan® *see* Promethazine *on page 804*

Anexsia® 5/500 *see* Hydrocodone and Acetaminophen *on page 478*

Anexsia® 7.5/650 *see* Hydrocodone and Acetaminophen *on page 478*

Anexsia® 10/660 *see* Hydrocodone and Acetaminophen *on page 478*

Animal and Human Bites Guidelines *see page 1093*

Anisotropine *(an iss oh TROE peen)*

Brand Names Valpin® 50

Canadian/Mexican Brand Names Miradon® (Canada)

Therapeutic Category Anticholinergic Agent; Antispasmodic Agent, Gastrointestinal

Use Adjunctive treatment of peptic ulcer

Usual Dosage Adults: Oral: 50 mg 3 times/day

Mechanism of Action Blocks the action of acetylcholine at parasympathetic sites in smooth muscle, secretory glands, and the CNS; increases cardiac output, dries secretions, antagonizes histamine and serotonin

Local Anesthetic/Vasoconstrictor Precautions No information available to require special precautions

Effects on Dental Treatment >10% of patients experience dry mouth; orthostatic hypotension possible

Other Adverse Effects

>10%:

Cardiovascular: Palpitations

Dermatologic: Dry skin

Gastrointestinal: Constipation

Respiratory: Dry nose/throat

Miscellaneous: Decreased sweating

1% to 10%:

Endocrine & metabolic: Decreased flow of breast milk

Gastrointestinal: Decreased salivary secretion

<1%:

Cardiovascular: Orthostatic hypotension

Central nervous system: Confusion, drowsiness, headache, loss of memory, fatigue

Dermatologic: Skin rash, photosensitivity

Gastrointestinal: Bloated feeling, nausea, vomiting

Genitourinary: Decreased urination

Neuromuscular & skeletal: Weakness

Ocular: Increased intraocular pain, blurred vision

Drug Interactions No data reported

Drug Uptake

Absorption: Poor (~10%) from GI tract

Pregnancy Risk Factor C

Generic Available Yes

Anistreplase (a NISS tre plase)

Related Information

Cardiovascular Diseases *on page 1010*

Brand Names Eminase®

Therapeutic Category Thrombolytic Agent

Use Management of acute myocardial infarction (AMI) in adults; lysis of thrombi obstructing coronary arteries, reduction of infarct size; and reduction of mortality associated with AMI

Usual Dosage Adults: I.V.: 30 units injected over 2-5 minutes as soon as possible after onset of symptoms

Mechanism of Action Activates the conversion of plasminogen to plasmin by forming a complex exposing plasminogen-activating site and cleavage of a peptide bond that converts plasminogen to plasmin; plasmin being capable of thrombolysis, by degrading fibrin, fibrinogen and other procoagulant proteins into soluble fragments, effective both outside and within the formed thrombus/ embolus

Local Anesthetic/Vasoconstrictor Precautions No information available to require special precautions

Effects on Dental Treatment No effects or complications reported

Other Adverse Effects

>10%:

Cardiovascular: Arrhythmias, hypotension, perfusion arrhythmias

Hematologic: Bleeding or oozing from cuts

1% to 10%: Anaphylactic reaction

<1%:

Central nervous system: Headache, chills

Dermatologic: Rash

Gastrointestinal: Nausea, vomiting

Hematologic: Anemia

Ocular: Eye hemorrhage

Respiratory: Bronchospasm, epistaxis

Miscellaneous: Sweating

Drug Interactions Increased efficacy and bleeding potential: Anticoagulants (heparin, warfarin), antiplatelet agents (aspirin)

Drug Uptake

Duration: Fibrinolytic effect persists for 4-6 hours following administration

Serum half-life: 70-120 minutes

Pregnancy Risk Factor C

Generic Available No

Anodynos-DHC® [5/500] *see* Hydrocodone and Acetaminophen *on page 478*

Anoquan® *see* Butalbital Compound *on page 154*

Anoquan® *see* Butalbital Compound and Acetaminophen *on page 155*

Ansaid® *see* Flurbiprofen *on page 423*

Antabuse® *see* Disulfiram *on page 328*

Antazoline-V® Ophthalmic *see* Naphazoline and Antazoline *on page 665*

Anthra-Derm® *see* Anthralin *on this page*

Anthralin (AN thra lin)

Brand Names Anthra-Derm®; Drithocreme®; Drithocreme® HP 1%; Dritho-Scalp®; Micanol® Cream

Canadian/Mexican Brand Names Anthraforte® (Canada); Anthranol® (Canada); Anthranol® (Mexico); Anthrascalp® (Canada)

Therapeutic Category Antipsoriatic Agent, Topical; Keratolytic Agent

Synonyms Antralina (Mexico)

Use Treatment of psoriasis (quiescent or chronic psoriasis)

Usual Dosage Adults: Topical: Generally, apply once a day or as directed. The irritant potential of anthralin is directly related to the strength being used and (Continued)

Anthralin *(Continued)*

each patient's individual tolerance. Always commence treatment for at least one week using the lowest strength possible.

Skin application: Apply sparingly only to psoriatic lesions and rub gently and carefully into the skin until absorbed. Avoid applying an excessive quantity which may cause unnecessary soiling and staining of the clothing or bed linen.

Scalp application: Comb hair to remove scalar debris and, after suitably parting, rub cream well into the lesions, taking care to prevent the cream from spreading onto the forehead

Remove by washing or showering; optimal period of contact will vary according to the strength used and the patient's response to treatment. Continue treatment until the skin is entirely clear (ie, when there is nothing to feel with the fingers and the texture is normal)

Mechanism of Action Reduction of the mitotic rate and proliferation of epidermal cells in psoriasis by inhibiting synthesis of nucleic protein from inhibition of DNA synthesis to affected areas

Local Anesthetic/Vasoconstrictor Precautions No information available to require special precautions

Effects on Dental Treatment No effects or complications reported

Other Adverse Effects

1% to 10%: Topical: Transient primary irritation of uninvolved skin; temporary discoloration of hair and fingernails, may stain skin, hair, or fabrics

<1%: Topical: Skin rash, excessive irritation

Drug Interactions Increased toxicity: Long-term use of topical corticosteroids may destabilize psoriasis, and withdrawal may also give rise to a "rebound" phenomenon, allow an interval of at least 1 week between the discontinuation of topical corticosteroids and the commencement of therapy

Pregnancy Risk Factor C

Generic Available Yes

AntibiOtic® Otic *see* Neomycin, Polymyxin B, and Hydrocortisone *on page 672*

Antibiotic Prophylaxis, Preprocedural Guidelines for Dental Patients *see page 1034*

Antidigoxin Fab Fragments *see* Digoxin Immune Fab *on page 315*

Antihemophilic Factor (Human)

(an tee hee moe FIL ik FAK tor HYU man)

Brand Names Hemofil® M; Humate-P®; Koāte®-HP; Koāte®-HS; Monoclate-P®; Profilate® OSD; Profilate® SD

Therapeutic Category Antihemophilic Agent; Blood Product Derivative

Synonyms AHF; Factor VIII

Use Management of hemophilia A in patients whom a deficiency in factor VIII has been demonstrated

Usual Dosage I.V.: Individualize dosage based on coagulation studies performed prior to and during treatment at regular intervals. One AHF unit is the activity present in 1 mL of normal pooled human plasma; dosage should be adjusted to actual vial size currently stocked in the pharmacy.

Hospitalized patients: 20-50 units/kg/dose; may be higher for special circumstances. Dose can be given every 12-24 hours and more frequently in special circumstances.

Formula to approximate percentage increase in plasma antihemophilic factor:

Units required = desired level increase (desired level - actual level) x plasma volume (mL)

Total blood volume (mL blood/kg) = 70 mL/kg (adults); 80 mL/kg (children)

Plasma volume = total blood volume (mL) x [1 - Hct (in decimals)]

Example: For a 70 kg adult with a Hct = 40% : plasma volume = [70 kg x 70 mL/kg] x [1 - 0.4] = 2940 mL

To calculate number of units of factor VIII needed to increase level to desired range (highly individualized and dependent on patient's condition):

Number of units = desired level increase [desired level - actual level] x plasma volume (in mL)

Example: For a 100% level in the above patient who has an actual level of 20% the number of units needed = [1 (for a 100% level) - 0.2] x 2940 mL = 2352 units

Mechanism of Action Protein (factor VIII) in normal plasma which is necessary for clot formation and maintenance of hemostasis; activates factor X in conjunction with activated factor IX; activated factor X converts prothrombin to thrombin, which converts fibrinogen to fibrin and with factor XIII forms a stable clot

Local Anesthetic/Vasoconstrictor Precautions No information available to require special precautions

Effects on Dental Treatment No effects or complications reported

Other Adverse Effects <1%:
Cardiovascular: Flushing, tachycardia
Central nervous system: Headache
Gastrointestinal: Nausea, vomiting
Neuromuscular & skeletal: Paresthesia
Miscellaneous: Allergic vasomotor reactions, tightness in neck or chest

Drug Uptake
Serum half-life, biphasic: 4-24 hours with a mean of 12 hours (biphasic: 12 hours is usually used for dosing interval estimates)

Pregnancy Risk Factor C

Generic Available Yes

Antihemophilic Factor (Porcine)
(an tee hee moe FIL ik FAK ter POR seen)

Brand Names Hyate®:C

Therapeutic Category Antihemophilic Agent

Use Treatment of congenital hemophiliacs with antibodies to human factor VIII:C and also for previously nonhemophiliac patients with spontaneously acquired inhibitors to human factor VIII:C; patients with inhibitors who are bleeding or who are to undergo surgery

Usual Dosage Clinical response should be used to assess efficacy rather than relying upon a particular laboratory value for recovery of factor VIII:C.

Initial dose:
Antibody level to human factor VIII:C <50 Bethesda units/mL: 100-150 porcine units/kg (body weight) is recommended

Antibody level to human factor VIII:C >50 Bethesda units/mL: Activity of the antibody to porcine factor VIII:C should be determined; **an antiporcine antibody level** >20 Bethesda units/mL indicates that the patient is unlikely to benefit from treatment; for lower titers, a dose of 100-150 porcine units/kg is recommended

If a patient has previously been treated with Hyate®:C, this may provide a guide to his likely response and, therefore, assist in estimation of the preliminary dose

Subsequent doses: Following administration of the initial dose, if the recovery of factor VIII:C in the patient's plasma is not sufficient, a further higher dose should be administered; if recovery after the second dose is still insufficient, a third and higher dose may prove effective

Mechanism of Action Factor VIII:C is the coagulation portion of the factor VIII complex in plasma. Factor VIII:C acts as a cofactor for factor IX to activate factor X in the intrinsic pathway of blood coagulation.

Local Anesthetic/Vasoconstrictor Precautions No information available to require special precautions

Effects on Dental Treatment No effects or complications reported

Other Adverse Effects 1% to 10%:
Central nervous system: Fever, headache, chills
Dermatologic: Skin rashes
Gastrointestinal: Nausea, vomiting

Pregnancy Risk Factor C

Generic Available No

Comments Sodium ion concentration is not more than 200 mmol/L; the assayed amount of activity is stated on the label, but may vary depending on the type of assay and hemophilic substrate plasma used

Antihemophilic Factor (Recombinant)
(an tee hee moe FIL ik FAK tor ree KOM be nant)

Brand Names Bioclate®; Helixate®; Kogenate®; Recombinate®

Therapeutic Category Antihemophilic Agent

Synonyms Factor VIII Recombinant

Use Management of hemophilia A in patients whom a deficiency in factor VIII has been demonstrated

Local Anesthetic/Vasoconstrictor Precautions No information available to require special precautions

Effects on Dental Treatment No effects or complications reported

Other Adverse Effects <1%:
Cardiovascular: Flushing, tachycardia
Central nervous system: Headache
Gastrointestinal: Nausea, vomiting
Neuromuscular & skeletal: Paresthesia, tightness in neck or chest

(Continued)

Antihemophilic Factor (Recombinant) *(Continued)*

Miscellaneous: Allergic vasomotor reactions
Pregnancy Risk Factor C
Generic Available No

Antihist-1® [OTC] *see Clemastine on page 242*

Anti-inhibitor Coagulant Complex

(an tee-in HI bi tor coe AG yoo lant KOM pleks)
Brand Names Autoplex® T; Feiba VH Immuno®
Therapeutic Category Hemophilic Agent
Use Patients with factor VIII inhibitors who are to undergo surgery or those who are bleeding
Usual Dosage Dosage range: 25-100 factor VIII correctional units per kg depending on the severity of hemorrhage
Local Anesthetic/Vasoconstrictor Precautions No information available to require special precautions
Effects on Dental Treatment No effects or complications reported
Other Adverse Effects <1%:
Cardiovascular: Hypotension, flushing
Central nervous system: Fever, headache, chills
Dermatologic: Rash, urticaria
Hematologic: Disseminated intravascular coagulation
Miscellaneous: Anaphylaxis, indications of protein sensitivity
Pregnancy Risk Factor C
Generic Available No

Antilirium® *see Physostigmine on page 758*
Antimicrobial Prophylaxis in Surgical Patients *see page 1163*
Antiminth® [OTC] *see Pyrantel Pamoate on page 822*

Antipyrine and Benzocaine (an tee PYE reen & BEN zoe kane)

Brand Names Allergan® Ear Drops; Auralgan®; Auroto®; Otocalm® Ear
Therapeutic Category Otic Agent, Analgesic; Otic Agent, Cerumenolytic
Synonyms Benzocaine and Antipyrine
Use Temporary relief of pain and reduction of swelling associated with acute congestive and serous otitis media, swimmer's ear, otitis externa; facilitates ear wax removal
Local Anesthetic/Vasoconstrictor Precautions Information available to require special precautions
Effects on Dental Treatment No effects or complications reported
Other Adverse Effects <1%:
Cardiovascular: Local edema
Local: Burning, stinging, tenderness
Miscellaneous: Hypersensitivity reactions
Pregnancy Risk Factor C
Generic Available Yes

Antirabies Serum (Equine) (an tee RAY beez SEER um EE kwine)

Therapeutic Category Serum
Synonyms ARS
Use Rabies prophylaxis
Local Anesthetic/Vasoconstrictor Precautions No information available to require special precautions
Effects on Dental Treatment No effects or complications reported
Other Adverse Effects 1% to 10%:
Dermatologic: Urticaria
Local: Pain at injection site
Miscellaneous: Serum sickness
Pregnancy Risk Factor C
Generic Available No
Comments Because of a significantly lower incidence of adverse reactions, Rabies Immune Globulin, Human is preferred over Antirabies Serum Equine

Antispas® Injection *see Dicyclomine on page 307*

Antithrombin III (an tee THROM bin three)

Brand Names ATnativ®; Thrombate III™
Therapeutic Category Blood Product Derivative
Synonyms ATIII; Heparin Cofactor I
Use Agent for hereditary antithrombin III deficiency

Usual Dosage After first dose of antithrombin III, level should increase to 120% of normal; thereafter maintain at levels >80%. Generally, achieved by administration of maintenance doses once every 24 hours; initially and until patient is stabilized, measure antithrombin III level at least twice daily, thereafter once daily and always immediately before next infusion. 1 unit = quantity of antithrombin III in 1 mL of normal pooled human plasma; administration of 1 unit/1 kg raises AT-III level by 1% to 2%; assume plasma volume of 40 mL/kg

Initial dosage (units) = [desired AT-III level % - baseline AT-III level %] x body weight (kg) divided by 1%/units/kg, eg, if a 70 kg adult patient had a baseline AT-III level of 57%, the initial dose would be (120% - 57%) x 70/1%/units/kg = 4,410 units

Measure antithrombin III preceding and 30 minutes after dose to calculate *in vivo* recovery rate; maintain level within normal range for 2-8 days depending on type of surgery or procedure

Mechanism of Action Antithrombin III is the primary physiologic inhibitor of *in vivo* coagulation. It is an alpha$_2$-globulin. Its principal actions are the inactivation of thrombin, plasmin, and other active serine proteases of coagulation, including factors IXa, Xa, XIa, XIIa, and VIIa. The inactivation of proteases is a major step in the normal clotting process. The strong activation of clotting enzymes at the site of every bleeding injury facilitates fibrin formation and maintains normal hemostasis. Thrombosis in the circulation would be caused by active serine proteases if they were not inhibited by antithrombin III after the localized clotting process. Patients with congenital deficiency are in a prethrombotic state, even if asymptomatic, as evidenced by elevated plasma levels of prothrombin activation fragment, which are normalized following infusions of antithrombin III concentrate.

Local Anesthetic/Vasoconstrictor Precautions No information available to require special precautions

Effects on Dental Treatment No effects or complications reported

Other Adverse Effects <1%:
Central nervous system: Dizziness, lightheadedness, fever
Cardiovascular: Chest tightness, chest pain, vasodilatory effects, edema
Dermatologic: Urticaria
Endocrine & metabolic: Fluid overload
Gastrointestinal: Nausea, foul taste in mouth, cramps, bowel fullness
Hematologic: Hematoma formation
Ocular: Film over eye
Renal: Diuretic effects
Respiratory: Dyspnea

Pregnancy Risk Factor C

Generic Available No

Antithymocyte Globulin (Equine) see Lymphocyte Immune Globulin *on page 572*

Antithymocyte Immunoglobulin see Lymphocyte Immune Globulin *on page 572*

Anti-Tuss® Expectorant [OTC] see Guaifenesin *on page 452*

Antivert® see Meclizine *on page 584*

Antizol® see Fomepizole *on page 428*

Antralina (Mexico) see Anthralin *on page 79*

Antrizine® see Meclizine *on page 584*

Anturane® see Sulfinpyrazone *on page 896*

Anusol® Ointment [OTC] see Pramoxine *on page 784*

Anxanil® see Hydroxyzine *on page 491*

Anzemet® see Dolasetron *on page 331*

Apacet® [OTC] see Acetaminophen *on page 20*

Apatate® [OTC] see Vitamin B Complex *on page 993*

Aphrodyne™ see Yohimbine *on page 999*

Aphthasol® see Amlexanox *on page 63*

A.P.L.® see Chorionic Gonadotropin *on page 231*

Aplisol® see Tuberculin Purified Protein Derivative *on page 975*

Aplitest® see Tuberculin Purified Protein Derivative *on page 975*

Aplonidine see Apraclonidine *on this page*

Apraclonidine (a pra KLOE ni deen)
Brand Names Iopidine®
Therapeutic Category Alpha$_2$-Adrenergic Agonist Agent, Ophthalmic
Synonyms Aplonidine; Apraclonidine Hydrochloride; p-Aminoclonidine
Use Prevention and treatment of postsurgical intraocular pressure elevation
(Continued)

Apraclonidine *(Continued)*

Usual Dosage Adults: Ophthalmic: Instill 1 drop in operative eye 1 hour prior to laser surgery, second drop in eye upon completion of procedure

Mechanism of Action Apraclonidine is a potent alpha-adrenergic agent similar to clonidine; relatively selective for alpha$_2$-receptors but does retain some binding to alpha$_1$-receptors; appears to result in reduction of aqueous humor formation; its penetration through the blood-brain barrier is more polar than clonidine which reduces its penetration through the blood-brain barrier and suggests that its pharmacological profile is characterized by peripheral rather than central effects.

Local Anesthetic/Vasoconstrictor Precautions No information available to require special precautions

Effects on Dental Treatment No effects or complications reported

Other Adverse Effects
1% to 10%:
Central nervous system: Lethargy
Gastrointestinal: Dry mouth
Ocular: Upper lid elevation, conjunctival blanching, mydriasis, burning and itching eyes, discomfort, conjunctival microhemorrhage, blurred vision
Respiratory: Dry nose
<1%: Miscellaneous: Allergic response; some systemic effects have also been reported including GI, CNS, and cardiovascular symptoms (arrhythmias)

Drug Uptake
Onset of action: 1 hour
Maximum IOP: 3-5 hours

Pregnancy Risk Factor C

Generic Available Yes

Apraclonidine Hydrochloride *see* Apraclonidine *on previous page*

Apresazide® *see* Hydralazine and Hydrochlorothiazide *on page 476*

Apresoline® *see* Hydralazine *on page 475*

Aprodine® Syrup [OTC] *see* Triprolidine and Pseudoephedrine *on page 969*

Aprodine® Tablet [OTC] *see* Triprolidine and Pseudoephedrine *on page 969*

Aprodine® w/C *see* Triprolidine, Pseudoephedrine, and Codeine *on page 970*

Aprotinin *(a proe TYE nin)*

Brand Names Trasylol®

Therapeutic Category Hemostatic Agent

Use Reduction or prevention of blood loss in patients undergoing coronary artery bypass surgery when a high index of suspicion of excessive bleeding potential exists; this includes open heart reoperation, pre-existing coagulopathy, operations on the great vessels, and patients whose religious beliefs prohibit blood transfusions

Usual Dosage
Test dose: **All** patients should receive a 1 mL I.V. test dose at least 10 minutes prior to the loading dose to assess the potential for allergic reactions

Regimen A (standard dose):
2 million units (280 mg) loading dose I.V. over 20-30 minutes
2 million units (280 mg) into pump prime volume
500,000 units/hour (70 mg/hour) I.V. during operation

Regimen B (low dose):
1 million units (140 mg) loading dose I.V. over 20-30 minutes
1 million units (140 mg) into pump prime volume
250,000 units/hour (35 mg/hour) I.V. during operation

Mechanism of Action Serine protease inhibitor; inhibits plasmin, kallikrein, and platelet activation producing antifibrinolytic effects; a weak inhibitor of plasma pseudocholinesterase. It also inhibits the contact phase activation of coagulation and preserves adhesive platelet glycoproteins making them resistant to damage from increased circulating plasmin or mechanical injury occurring during bypass

Local Anesthetic/Vasoconstrictor Precautions No information available to require special precautions

Effects on Dental Treatment No effects or complications reported

Other Adverse Effects Increase in postoperative renal dysfunction compared to placebo; anaphylactic reactions have been reported in <0.5% of cases; such reactions are more likely to occur with repeated administration

Drug Uptake
Serum half-life: 150 minutes

Pregnancy Risk Factor C

Generic Available No

Aquacare® [OTC] *see* Urea *on page 977*

Aquachloral® Supprettes® *see* Chloral Hydrate *on page 207*

AquaMEPHYTON® *see* Phytonadione *on page 758*

Aquaphyllin® *see* Theophylline *on page 917*

AquaSite® Ophthalmic Solution [OTC] *see* Artificial Tears *on page 87*

Aquasol A® [OTC] *see* Vitamin A *on page 992*

Aquasol E® [OTC] *see* Vitamin E *on page 994*

AquaTar® [OTC] *see* Coal Tar *on page 254*

Aquatensen® *see* Methyclothiazide *on page 620*

Aquest® *see* Estrone *on page 369*

Aralen® Phosphate *see* Chloroquine Phosphate *on page 214*

Aralen® Phosphate With Primaquine Phosphate *see* Chloroquine and Primaquine *on page 213*

Ardeparin (ar dee PA rin)

Brand Names Normiflo®

Therapeutic Category Anticoagulant

Synonyms Ardeparin Sodium

Use Prevention of deep vein thrombosis (DVT) which may lead to pulmonary embolism following knee replacement surgery

Usual Dosage Adults: S.C.: 50 anti-Xa units every 12 hours

Local Anesthetic/Vasoconstrictor Precautions No information available to require special precautions

Effects on Dental Treatment No effects or complications reported

Dosage Forms Injection, as sodium: Anti-Xa units 5000 (0.5 mL); Anti-Xa units 10,000 (0.5 mL)

Ardeparin Sodium *see* Ardeparin *on this page*

Aredia™ *see* Pamidronate *on page 720*

Arfonad® *see* Trimethaphan Camsylate (Discontinued 4/96) *on page 963*

Argesic®-SA *see* Salsalate *on page 855*

Arginine (AR ji neen)

Brand Names R-Gene®

Therapeutic Category Metabolic Alkalosis Agent

Use Pituitary function test (growth hormone); management of severe, uncompensated, metabolic alkalosis (pH ≥7.55) **after** optimizing therapy with sodium, potassium, or ammonium chloride supplements

Usual Dosage I.V.:

Growth hormone (pituitary function) reserve test:

Children: 500 mg (5 mL) kg/dose administered over 30 minutes

Adults: 30 g (300 mL) administered over 30 minutes

Metabolic alkalosis: Children and Adults: Usual dose: 10 g/hour

Acid required (mEq) =

[1] 0.2 (L/kg) x wt (kg) x [103 - serum chloride] (mEq/L) **or**

[2] 0.3 (L/kg) x wt (kg) x base excess (mEq/L) **or**

[3] 0.5 (L/kg) x wt (kg) x [serum HCO_3 - 24] (mEq/L)

Give $^1/_2$ to $^2/_3$ of calculated dose and re-evaluate

Note: Arginine hydrochloride should never be used as an alternative to chloride supplementation but used in the patient who is unresponsive to sodium chloride or potassium chloride supplementation

Mechanism of Action

Stimulates pituitary release of growth hormone and prolactin through origins in the hypothalamus; patients with impaired pituitary function have lower or no increase in plasma concentrations of growth hormone after administration of arginine. Arginine hydrochloride has been used for severe metabolic alkalosis due to its high chloride content.

Arginine hydrochloride has been used investigationally to treat metabolic alkalosis. Arginine contains 475 mEq of hydrogen ions and 475 mEq of chloride ions/L. Arginine is metabolized by the liver to produce hydrogen ions. It may be used in patients with relative hepatic insufficiency because arginine combines with ammonia in the body to produce urea.

Local Anesthetic/Vasoconstrictor Precautions No information available to require special precautions

Effects on Dental Treatment No effects or complications reported

Other Adverse Effects

1% to 10%: Rapid I.V. infusion may produce flushing, local irritation, nausea & vomiting

Central nervous system: Headache

Neuromuscular & skeletal: Numbness

<1%:

Endocrine & metabolic: Hyperglycemia, hyperkalemia, elevated serum gastrin concentration, hyperchloremia

(Continued)

85

Arginine *(Continued)*

Gastrointestinal: Abdominal pain, bloating

Drug Uptake

Absorption: Oral: Well absorbed

Time to peak serum concentration: Within 2 hours

Pregnancy Risk Factor C

Generic Available Yes

Argyrol® S.S. 20% *see* Silver Protein, Mild *on page 865*

Aricept® *see* Donepezil *on page 332*

Arimidex® *see* Anastrozole *on page 77*

Aristocort® *see* Triamcinolone *on page 954*

Aristocort® A *see* Triamcinolone *on page 954*

Aristocort® Forte *see* Triamcinolone *on page 954*

Aristocort® Intralesional *see* Triamcinolone *on page 954*

Aristospan® Intra-Articular *see* Triamcinolone *on page 954*

Aristospan® Intralesional *see* Triamcinolone *on page 954*

Arlidin® *see* Nylidrin *on page 694*

Arm-a-Med® Isoetharine *see* Isoetharine *on page 521*

Arm-a-Med® Isoproterenol *see* Isoproterenol *on page 523*

Arm-a-Med® Metaproterenol *see* Metaproterenol *on page 605*

A.R.M.® Caplet [OTC] *see* Chlorpheniramine and Phenylpropanolamine *on page 219*

Armour® Thyroid *see* Thyroid *on page 930*

Aromatic Ammonia Aspirols® *see* Ammonia Spirit, Aromatic *on page 64*

Arrestin® *see* Trimethobenzamide *on page 964*

ARS *see* Antirabies Serum (Equine) *on page 82*

Artane® *see* Trihexyphenidyl *on page 962*

Artha-G® *see* Salsalate *on page 855*

Arthritis Foundation® Nighttime [OTC] *see* Acetaminophen and Diphenhydramine *on page 23*

Arthritis Foundation® Pain Reliever [OTC] *see* Aspirin *on page 90*

Arthritis Foundation® Pain Reliever, Aspirin Free [OTC] *see* Acetaminophen *on page 20*

Arthropan® [OTC] *see* Choline Salicylate *on page 230*

Arthrotec® *see* Diclofenac and Misoprostol *on page 305*

Articaine Hydrochloride and Epinephrine

Canadian/Mexican Brand Names Ultracaine DS® (Canada); Ultracaine DS Forte® (Canada)

Therapeutic Category Local Anesthetic, Injectable

Use Anesthesia for infiltration and nerve block anesthesia in clinical dentistry

Usual Dosage Adults:

Ultracaine DS® Forte:

Infiltration:

Volume: 0.5-2.5 mL

Total dose: 20-100 mg

Nerve block:

Volume: 0.5-3.4 mL

Total dose: 20-136 mg

Oral surgery:

Volume: 1-5.1 mL

Total dose: 40-204 mg

Ultracaine DS®:

Infiltration:

Volume: 0.5-2.5 mL

Total dose: 20-100 mg

Nerve block:

Volume: 0.5-3.4 mL

Total dose: 20-136 mg

Oral surgery:

Volume: 1-5.1 mL

Total dose: 40-204 mg

Maximum dose: 7 mg/kg

To date, Ultracaine® has not been administered to children <4 years of age, nor in doses >5 mg/kg in children between the ages of 4 and 12

Mechanism of Action Blocks nerve conduction by interfering with the permeability of the nerve axonal membrane to sodium ions; this results in the loss of the generation of the nerve axon potential

Local Anesthetic/Vasoconstrictor Precautions No information available to require special precautions

Effects on Dental Treatment No effects or complications reported

Other Adverse Effects

Cardiovascular: Myocardial depression, arrhythmias, tachycardia, bradycardia, blood pressure changes, edema

Central nervous system: Excitation, depression, nervousness, dizziness, headache, somnolence, unconsciousness, convulsions, chills

Dermal: Allergic reactions include cutaneous lesions, urticaria, itching, reddening of skin

Gastrointestinal: Vomiting, allergic reactions include nausea and diarrhea

Local: Reactions at the site of injection, swelling, burning, ischemia, tissue necrosis

Neuromuscular & skeletal: Tremors

Ocular: Visual disturbances, blurred vision, blindness, diplopia, pupillary constriction

Otic: Tinnitus

Respiratory: Allergic reactions include wheezing, acute asthmatic attacks

Contraindications Known hypersensitivity to any of its components and/or local anesthetics of the amide group; in the presence of inflammation and/or sepsis near the injection site; in patients with severe shock, any degree of heart block, paroxysmal tachycardia, known arrhythmia with rapid heart rate, narrow-angle glaucoma, cholinesterase deficiency, existing neurologic disease, severe hypertension; when articaine with epinephrine is used, the caution required of any vasopressor drug should be followed

Warnings/Precautions Articaine should be used cautiously in persons with known drug allergies or sensitivities, or suspected sensitivity to the amide-type local anesthetics. Avoid excessive premedications with sedatives, tranquilizers, and antiemetic agents. Inject slowly with frequent aspirations and if blood is aspirated, relocate needle. Articaine should be used with extreme caution in patients having a history of thyrotoxicosis or diabetes. Due to the sulfite component of the articaine preparation, hypersensitivity reactions may occur occasionally in patients with bronchial asthma.

Drug Interactions Solutions containing epinephrine should be used with caution, if at all, in patients taking MAO inhibitors or tricyclic antidepressants because severe prolonged hypertension may result

Breast-feeding Considerations Articaine is unlikely to be transferred to mother's milk since it is rapidly metabolized and eliminated

Dosage Forms Injection:

Ultracaine DS®: Articaine hydrochloride with epinephrine [1:200,000] and sodium metabisulfite [0.5 mg/mL] and an antioxidant and water for injection (1.7 mL [50s])

Ultracaine DS Forte®: Articaine hydrochloride 4% with epinephrine [1:100,000] and sodium metabisulfite [0.5 mg/mL] and an antioxidant and water for injection (1.7 mL) [50s]

Articulose-50® see Prednisolone on page 788

Artificial Saliva Products see page 1171

Artificial Tears (ar ti FISH il tears)

Brand Names Adsorbotear® Ophthalmic Solution [OTC]; Akwa Tears® Solution [OTC]; AquaSite® Ophthalmic Solution [OTC]; Bion® Tears Solution [OTC]; Comfort® Tears Solution [OTC]; Dakrina® Ophthalmic Solution [OTC]; Dry Eyes® Solution [OTC]; Dry Eye® Therapy Solution [OTC]; Dwelle® Ophthalmic Solution [OTC]; Eye-Lube-A® Solution [OTC]; HypoTears PF Solution [OTC]; HypoTears Solution [OTC]; Isopto® Plain Solution [OTC]; Isopto® Tears Solution [OTC]; Just Tears® Solution [OTC]; Lacril® Ophthalmic Solution [OTC]; Liquifilm® Forte Solution [OTC]; Liquifilm® Tears Solution [OTC]; LubriTears® Solution [OTC]; Moisture® Ophthalmic Drops [OTC]; Murine® Solution [OTC]; Murocel® Ophthalmic Solution [OTC]; Nature's Tears® Solution [OTC]; Nu-Tears® II Solution [OTC]; Nu-Tears® Solution [OTC]; OcuCoat® Ophthalmic Solution [OTC]; OcuCoat® PF Ophthalmic Solution [OTC]; Puralube® Tears Solution [OTC]; Refresh® Ophthalmic Solution [OTC]; Refresh® Plus Ophthalmic Solution [OTC]; Tear Drop® Solution [OTC]; TearGard® Ophthalmic Solution [OTC]; Teargen® Ophthalmic Solution [OTC]; Tearisol® Solution [OTC]; Tears Naturale® Free Solution [OTC]; Tears Naturale® II Solution [OTC]; Tears Naturale® Solution [OTC]; Tears Plus® Solution [OTC]; Tears Renewed® Solution [OTC]; Ultra Tears® Solution [OTC]; Viva-Drops® Solution [OTC]

Therapeutic Category Ophthalmic Agent, Miscellaneous

Synonyms Hydroxyethylcellulose; Polyvinyl Alcohol

Use Ophthalmic lubricant; for relief of dry eyes and eye irritation

(Continued)

Artificial Tears *(Continued)*

Local Anesthetic/Vasoconstrictor Precautions No information available to require special precautions

Effects on Dental Treatment No effects or complications reported

Other Adverse Effects 1% to 10%: Ocular: May cause mild stinging or temporary blurred vision

Pregnancy Risk Factor C

Generic Available Yes

A.S.A. [OTC] *see* Aspirin *on page 90*

Asacol® *see* Mesalamine *on page 602*

Ascorbic Acid *(a SKOR bik AS id)*

Brand Names Ascorbicap® [OTC]; C-Crystals® [OTC]; Cebid® Timecelles® [OTC]; Cecon® [OTC]; Cevalin® [OTC]; Cevi-Bid® [OTC]; Ce-Vi-Sol® [OTC]; Dull-C® [OTC]; Flavorcee® [OTC]; N'ice® Vitamin C Drops [OTC]; Vita-C® [OTC]

Canadian/Mexican Brand Names Apo®-C (Canada); Ascorbic® 500 (Canada); Ce-Vi-Sol® (Mexico); Redoxon® (Canada); Redoxon® Forte (Mexico); Revitalose® C-1000® (Canada)

Therapeutic Category Urinary Acidifying Agent; Vitamin, Water Soluble

Synonyms Ascorbico, Acido (Mexico); Cevitamic Acid (Canada)

Use Prevention and treatment of scurvy and to acidify the urine

Investigational use: In large doses to decrease the severity of "colds"; dietary supplementation

Usual Dosage Oral, I.M., I.V., S.C.:

Recommended daily allowance (RDA):
<6 months: 30 mg
6 months to 1 year: 35 mg
1-3 years: 40 mg
4-10 years: 45 mg
11-14 years: 50 mg
>14 years and Adults: 60 mg

Children:
Scurvy: 100-300 mg/day in divided doses for at least 2 weeks
Urinary acidification: 500 mg every 6-8 hours
Dietary supplement: 35-100 mg/day

Adults:
Scurvy: 100-250 mg 1-2 times/day for at least 2 weeks
Urinary acidification: 4-12 g/day in 3-4 divided doses
Prevention and treatment of colds: 1-3 g/day
Dietary supplement: 50-200 mg/day

Mechanism of Action Not fully understood; necessary for collagen formation and tissue repair; involved in some oxidation-reduction reactions as well as other metabolic pathways, such as synthesis of carnitine, steroids, and catecholamines and conversion of folic acid to folinic acid

Local Anesthetic/Vasoconstrictor Precautions No information available to require special precautions

Effects on Dental Treatment No effects or complications reported

Other Adverse Effects
1% to 10%: Renal: Hyperoxaluria
<1%:
Cardiovascular: Flushing, faintness
Central nervous system: Dizziness, headache, fatigue, flank pain
Gastrointestinal: Nausea, vomiting, heartburn, diarrhea

Contraindications Large doses during pregnancy

Warnings/Precautions Diabetics and patients prone to recurrent renal calculi (eg, dialysis patients) should not take excessive doses for extended periods of time

Drug Interactions
Decreased effect:
Aspirin decreases ascorbate levels, increases aspirin
Fluphenazine decreases fluphenazine levels
Warfarin decreases effect
Increased effect: Iron enhances absorption; oral contraceptives increase contraceptive effect

Drug Uptake
Absorption: Oral: Readily absorbed; an active process and is thought to be dose-dependent

Pregnancy Risk Factor A (C if used in doses above RDA recommendation)

Breast-feeding Considerations Compatible

Dosage Forms
  Capsule, timed release: 500 mg
  Crystals: 4 g/teaspoonful (100 g, 500 g); 5 g/teaspoonful (180 g)
  Injection: 250 mg/mL (2 mL, 30 mL); 500 mg/mL (2 mL, 50 mL)
  Liquid, oral: 35 mg/0.6 mL (50 mL)
  Lozenges: 60 mg
  Powder: 4 g/teaspoonful (100 g, 500 g)
  Solution, oral: 100 mg/mL (50 mL)
  Syrup: 500 mg/5 mL (5 mL, 10 mL, 120 mL, 480 mL)
  Tablet: 25 mg, 50 mg, 100 mg, 250 mg, 500 mg, 1000 mg
  Tablet:
    Chewable: 100 mg, 250 mg, 500 mg
    Timed release: 500 mg, 1000 mg, 1500 mg
Generic Available Yes

Ascorbic Acid and Ferrous Sulfate *see* Ferrous Sulfate and Ascorbic Acid *on page 402*

Ascorbicap® [OTC] *see* Ascorbic Acid *on previous page*

Ascorbico, Acido (Mexico) *see* Ascorbic Acid *on previous page*

Ascriptin® [OTC] *see* Aspirin *on next page*

Asendin® *see* Amoxapine *on page 66*

Asmalix® *see* Theophylline *on page 917*

Asparaginase (a SPIR a ji nase)
Brand Names Elspar®; Erwiniar®
Canadian/Mexican Brand Names Leunase® (Mexico)
Therapeutic Category Antineoplastic Agent, Miscellaneous
Synonyms L-asparaginase
Use Treatment of acute lymphocytic leukemia, lymphoma; used for induction therapy
Usual Dosage Refer to individual protocols; dose must be individualized based upon clinical response and tolerance of the patient

  I.M. administration is **preferred** over I.V. administration; I.M. administration may decrease the risk of anaphylaxis

  Asparaginase is available from two different microbiological sources: One is from *Escherichia coli* and the other is from *Erwinia carotovora*. The *Erwinia* is restricted to patients who have sustained anaphylaxis to the *E. coli* preparation.

  I.M., I.V.: 6000 units/m² every other day for 3-4 weeks or daily doses of 1000-20,000 units/m² for 10-20 days; other induction regimens have been utilized

  Desensitization should be performed before administering the first dose of asparaginase to patients who developed a positive reaction to the intradermal skin test or who are being retreated. One schedule begins with a total of 1 unit given i.V. and doubles the dose every 10 minutes until the total amount given in the planned dose for that day.

Asparaginase Desensitization

Injection No.	Elspar Dose (IU)	Accumulated Total Dose
1	1	1
2	2	3
3	4	7
4	8	15
5	16	31
6	32	63
7	64	127
8	128	255
9	256	511
10	512	1,023
11	1,024	2,047
12	2,048	4,095
13	4,096	8,191
14	8,192	16,383
15	16,384	32,767
16	32,768	65,535
17	65,536	131,071
18	131,072	262,143

(Continued)

Asparaginase (Continued)

For example, if a patient was to receive a total dose of 4000 units, he/she would receive injections 1 through 12 during the desensitization

Mechanism of Action Some malignant cells (ie, lymphoblastic leukemia cells and those of lymphocyte derivation) must acquire the amino acid asparagine from surrounding fluid such as blood, whereas normal cells can synthesize their own asparagine. asparaginase is an enzyme that deaminates asparagine to aspartic acid and ammonia in the plasma and extracellular fluid and therefore deprives tumor cells of the amino acid for protein synthesis.

There are two purified preparations of the enzyme, one from *Escherichia coli* and one from *Erwinia carotovora*. These two preparations vary slightly in the gene sequencing and have slight differences in enzyme characteristics. Both are highly specific for asparagine and have less than 10% activity for the D-isomer. The preparation from *E. coli* has had the most use in clinical and research practice.

Local Anesthetic/Vasoconstrictor Precautions No information available to require special precautions

Effects on Dental Treatment No effects or complications reported

Other Adverse Effects

>10%:
   Gastrointestinal: Pancreatitis occurs in <15% of patients but may progress to severe hemorrhagic pancreatitis
   Miscellaneous: Hypersensitivity and anaphylactic reactions occur in ~10% to 40% of patients and can be fatal. This reaction is more common in patients receiving asparaginase alone or by I.V. administration. Hypersensitivity appears rarely with the first dose and more commonly after the second or third treatment. Hypersensitivity may be treated with antihistamines and/or steroids. If an anaphylactic reaction occurs, a change in treatment to the *Erwinia* preparation may be made, since this preparation does not share antigenic cross-reactivity with the *E. coli* preparation. Note that allergic reactions to the *Erwinia* preparation may also occur and ultimately develop in 5% to 20% of patients.

1% to 10%:
   Endocrine & metabolic: Hyperuricemia
   Gastrointestinal: Mouth sores

<1%:
   Cardiovascular: Hypotension
   Central nervous system: Disorientation, drowsiness, seizures, and coma which may be due to elevated NH_4 levels, hyperthermia, fever, malaise, chills
   Dermatologic: Urticaria, rash, pruritus
   Endocrine & metabolic: Transient diabetes mellitus
   Gastrointestinal: Weight loss
   Hematologic: Inhibition of protein synthesis will cause a decrease in production of albumin, insulin (resulting in hyperglycemia), serum lipoprotein, antithrombin III, and clotting factors II, V, VII, VIII, IX, and X. Leg vein thrombosis. The loss of the later two proteins may result in either thrombotic or hemorrhagic events; these protein losses occur in 100% of patients.
   Hepatic: Elevated serum bilirubin, ST, alkaline phosphatase, and possible decrease in mobilization of lipids
   Renal: Azotemia
   Respiratory: Coughing, laryngeal spasm

Drug Uptake
   Absorption: Not absorbed from GI tract, therefore, requires parenteral administration; I.M. administration produces peak blood levels 50% lower than those from I.V. administration (I.M. may be less immunogenic)
   Serum half-life: 8-30 hours

Pregnancy Risk Factor C

Generic Available No

Comments Myelosuppressive effects:
   WBC: Mild
   Platelets: Mild
   Onset (days): 7
   Nadir (days): 14
   Recovery (days): 21

A-Spas® S/L see Hyoscyamine on page 492

Aspergum® [OTC] see Aspirin on this page

Aspirin (AS pir in)

Related Information

Butalbital Compound and Aspirin on page 156
Cardiovascular Diseases on page 1010

Carisoprodol and Aspirin *on page 180*
Dental Drug Interactions: Update on Drug Combinations Requiring Special Considerations *on page 1144*
Oral Pain *on page 1053*
Rheumatoid Arthritis and Osteoarthritis *on page 1030*

Brand Names Anacin® [OTC]; Arthritis Foundation® Pain Reliever [OTC]; A.S.A. [OTC]; Ascriptin® [OTC]; Aspergum® [OTC]; Asprimox® [OTC]; Bayer® Aspirin [OTC]; Bayer® Buffered Aspirin [OTC]; Bayer® Low Adult Strength [OTC]; Bufferin® [OTC]; Buffex® [OTC]; Cama® Arthritis Pain Reliever [OTC]; Easprin®; Ecotrin® [OTC]; Ecotrin® Low Adult Strength [OTC]; Empirin® [OTC]; Extra Strength Adprin-B® [OTC]; Extra Strength Bayer® Enteric 500 Aspirin [OTC]; Extra Strength Bayer® Plus [OTC]; Halfprin® 81® [OTC]; Regular Strength Bayer® Enteric 500 Aspirin [OTC]; St Joseph® Adult Chewable Aspirin [OTC]; ZORprin®

Canadian/Mexican Brand Names Apo®-ASA (Canada); ASA® (Canada); Asaphen® (Canada); Entrophen® (Canada); Novasen® (Canada)

Therapeutic Category Analgesic, Non-narcotic; Anti-inflammatory Agent; Anti-platelet Agent; Antipyretic

Use

Dental: Treatment of postoperative pain

Medical: Treatment of pain and fever; may be used as prophylaxis of myocardial infarction and transient ischemic episodes; management of rheumatoid arthritis, rheumatic fever, osteoarthritis, and gout (high dose)

Usual Dosage Analgesic: Oral:

Children: 10-15 mg/kg/dose every 4-6 hours, up to a total of 60-80 mg/kg/24 hours

Adults: 325-650 mg (1-2 tablets) every 4-6 hours, up to 4 g/day

Mechanism of Action Inhibits prostaglandin synthesis by decreasing the activity of the enzyme, cyclo-oxygenase, which results in decreased formation of prosta-glandin precursors, acts on the hypothalamic heat-regulating center to reduce fever, blocks thromboxane synthetase action which prevents formation of the platelet-aggregating substance thromboxane A_2

Local Anesthetic/Vasoconstrictor Precautions No information available to require special precautions

Effects on Dental Treatment Avoid aspirin if possible, for 1 week prior to surgery because of the possibility of postoperative bleeding

Other Adverse Effects

>10%: Gastrointestinal: Nausea, vomiting, dyspepsia, epigastric discomfort, heartburn, stomach pains

1% to 10%: Gastrointestinal: Ulceration

Aspirin allergy (incidence is 0.2%): Asthmatic syndrome, wheezing, bronchiolar constriction

Contraindications Bleeding disorders (factor VII or IX deficiencies), hypersensi-tivity to salicylates or other NSAIDs, tartrazine dye and asthma

Warnings/Precautions Use with caution in patients with platelet and bleeding disorders, renal dysfunction, erosive gastritis, or peptic ulcer disease, previous nonreaction does not guarantee future safe taking of medication; do not use aspirin in children <16 years of age for chickenpox or flu symptoms due to the association with Reye's syndrome

Avoid aspirin if possible, for 1 week prior to surgery because of the possibility of postoperative bleeding; use with caution in impaired hepatic function

Elderly are a high-risk population for adverse effects from nonsteroidal anti-inflammatory agents. As much as 60% of elderly with GI complications to NSAIDs can develop peptic ulceration and/or hemorrhage asymptomatically. Also, concomitant disease and drug use contribute to the risk for GI adverse effects. Use lowest effective dose for shortest period possible. Consider renal function decline with age. Use with caution in patients with history of asthma

Drug Interactions

Aspirin:

Warfarin (Coumadin®): Aspirin in normal doses increases the risk of bleeding in anticoagulate patients by inhibition of platelet function; larger doses of aspirin enhance the hypoprothrombinemic response to warfarin

Acetazolamide (Diamox®): Aspirin increases the plasma concentration of acet-azolamide by displacement from plasma protein binding sites. These have resulted in central nervous system toxicity due to higher levels of acetazola-mide

Methotrexate: Salicylates block the renal tubular secretion of methotrexate to result in methotrexate toxicity (hepatotoxicity)

NSAIDs: Aspirin may cause a reduction in serum levels of NSAIDs

Drug Uptake

Absorption: Rapid

(Continued)

Aspirin *(Continued)*

Serum half-life:
Parent drug: 15-20 minutes
Salicylates (dose-dependent): From 3 hours at lower doses (300-600 mg), to 5-6 hours (after 1 g) to 10 hours with higher doses
Time to peak serum concentration: ~1-2 hours

Pregnancy Risk Factor C (D if full-dose aspirin in 3rd trimester)

Breast-feeding Considerations Use cautiously due to potential adverse effects in nursing infants

Dosage Forms

Capsule: 356.4 mg and caffeine 30 mg
Suppository, rectal: 60 mg, 120 mg, 125 mg, 130 mg, 195 mg, 200 mg, 300 mg, 325 mg, 600 mg, 650 mg, 1.2 g
Tablet: 65 mg, 75 mg, 81 mg, 325 mg, 500 mg
Tablet: 400 mg and caffeine 32 mg
Tablet:
Buffered: 325 mg and magnesium-aluminum hydroxide 150 mg; 325 mg, magnesium hydroxide 75 mg, aluminum hydroxide 75 mg, buffered with calcium carbonate; 325 mg and magnesium-aluminum hydroxide 75 mg
Chewable: 81 mg
Controlled release: 800 mg
Delayed release: 81 mg
Enteric coated: 81 mg, 325 mg, 500 mg, 650 mg, 975 mg
Gum: 227.5 mg
Timed release: 650 mg

Dietary Considerations Should be taken with water, food, or milk to decrease GI effects; food decreases rate but not extent of absorption (oral)

Generic Available Yes

Comments Anti-inflammatory actions of aspirin are not seen clinically at doses <3500 mg/day. Patients taking one aspirin tablet daily as an antithrombotic and who require dental surgery should be given special consideration in consultation with the physician before removal of the aspirin relative to prevention of postoperative bleeding.

Selected Readings

Desjardins PJ, Cooper SA, Gallegos TL, et al, "The Relative Analgesic Efficacy of Propiram Fumarate, Codeine Aspirin, and Placebo in Post-Impaction Dental Pain," *J Clin Pharmacol*, 1984, 24(1):35-42.
Forbes JA, Butterworth GA, Burchfield WH, et al, "Evaluation of Ketorolac, Aspirin, and an Acetaminophen-Codeine Combination in Postoperative Oral Surgery Pain," *Pharmacotherapy*, 1990, 10(6 Pt 2):77S-93S.
Forbes JA, Keller CK, Smith JW, et al, "Analgesic Effect of Naproxen Sodium, Codeine, a Naproxen-Codeine Combination and Aspirin on the Postoperative Pain of Oral Surgery," *Pharmacotherapy*, 1986, 6(5):211-8.
Hurlen M, Erikssen J, Smith P, et al, "Comparison of Bleeding Complications of Warfarin and Warfarin Plus Acetylsalicylic Acid: A Study in 3166 Outpatients," *J Intern Med*, 1994, 236(3):299-304.

Aspirin and Codeine *(AS pir in & KOE deen)*

Related Information

Dental Drug Interactions: Update on Drug Combinations Requiring Special Considerations *on page 1144*
Oral Pain *on page 1053*

Brand Names Empirin® With Codeine

Canadian/Mexican Brand Names Coryphen® Codeine (Canada)

Therapeutic Category Analgesic, Narcotic

Use

Dental: Treatment of postoperative pain
Medical: Relief of pain

Restrictions C-III; Refillable up to 5 times in 6 months

Usual Dosage Oral:

Children: Not recommended in pediatric dental patients
Adults: 1-2 tablets every 4-6 hours as needed for pain; maximum: 12 tablets over 24 hours

Mechanism of Action Aspirin inhibits prostaglandin synthesis, acts on the hypothalamus heat-regulating center to reduce fever, blocks prostaglandin synthetase action which prevents formation of the platelet-aggregating substance thromboxane A_2; codeine binds to opiate receptors (mu and kappa subtypes) in the CNS causing inhibition of ascending pain pathways, altering the perception of and response to pain

Local Anesthetic/Vasoconstrictor Precautions No information available to require special precautions

Effects on Dental Treatment <1% of patients may experience dry mouth; avoid aspirin, if possible, for 1 week prior to surgery because of the possibility of postoperative bleeding

Use with caution in impaired hepatic function; use with caution in patients with platelet and bleeding disorders, renal dysfunction, erosive gastritis, or peptic ulcer disease, previous nonreaction does not guarantee future safe taking of medication; do not use aspirin in children <16 years of age for chickenpox or flu symptoms due to the association with Reye's syndrome

Avoid aspirin if possible, for 1 week prior to surgery because of the possibility of postoperative bleeding; use with caution in impaired hepatic function

Elderly are a high-risk population for adverse effects from nonsteroidal anti-inflammatory agents. As much as 60% of elderly with GI complications to NSAIDs can develop peptic ulceration and/or hemorrhage asymptomatically. Also, concomitant disease and drug use contribute to the risk for GI adverse effects. Use lowest effective dose for shortest period possible. Consider renal function decline with age. Use with caution in patients with history of asthma.

Other Adverse Effects

>10%:
    Central nervous system: Lightheadedness, dizziness, sedation, depression
    Gastrointestinal: Nausea, heartburn, stomach pains, dyspepsia, epigastric discomfort, vomiting
1% to 10%: Gastrointestinal: Ulceration, constipation
Aspirin allergy (incidence is 0.2%): Asthmatic syndrome, wheezing, bronchiolar constriction

Contraindications Hypersensitivity to aspirin or codeine

Warnings/Precautions Use with caution in patients with impaired renal function, erosive gastritis, or peptic ulcer disease

Enhanced analgesia has been seen in elderly patients on therapeutic doses of narcotics; duration of action may be increased in the elderly; the elderly may be particularly susceptible to the CNS depressant and constipating effects of narcotics

Drug Interactions

Aspirin:
    Warfarin (Coumadin®): Aspirin in normal doses increases the risk of bleeding in anticoagulate patients by inhibition of platelet function; larger doses of aspirin enhance the hypoprothrombinemic response to warfarin
    Acetazolamide (Diamox®): Aspirin increases the plasma concentration of acetazolamide by displacement from plasma protein binding sites. These have resulted in central nervous system toxicity due to higher levels of acetazolamide
    Methotrexate: Salicylates block the renal tubular secretion of methotrexate to result in methotrexate toxicity (hepatotoxicity)
    NSAIDs: Aspirin may cause a reduction in serum levels of NSAIDs
Codeine: Increased toxicity when given with CNS depressants, phenothiazines, tricyclic antidepressants (TCAs), other narcotic analgesics, MAO inhibitors

Drug Uptake

Aspirin:
    Absorption: Rapid
    Serum half-life:
    Parent drug: 15-20 minutes
    Salicylates (dose-dependent): From 3 hours at lower doses (300-600 mg), to 5-6 hours (after 1 g) to 10 hours with higher doses
    Time to peak serum concentration: ~1-2 hours
Codeine:
    Onset of effect: 0.5-1 hour
    Duration of effect: 4-6 hours
    Serum half-life: 2.5-3.5 hours
    Time to peak serum concentration: 1-1.5 hours

Pregnancy Risk Factor D

Breast-feeding Considerations

Aspirin: Cautious use due to potential adverse effects in nursing infants
Codeine: Codeine not contraindicated with breast-feeding

Dosage Forms Tablet:
#2: Aspirin 325 mg and codeine phosphate 15 mg
#3: Aspirin 325 mg and codeine phosphate 30 mg
#4: Aspirin 325 mg and codeine phosphate 60 mg

Dietary Considerations May be taken with food or milk to minimize GI distress; food decreases rate but not extent of absorption (oral)

Generic Available Yes

Comments Codeine products, as with other narcotic analgesics, are recommended only for limited acute dosing (ie, 3 days or less). The most common adverse effect you will see in your dental patients from codeine is nausea, followed by sedation and constipation. Codeine has narcotic addiction liability, (Continued)

Aspirin and Codeine *(Continued)*

especially when given long term. The aspirin component has anticoagulant effects and can affect bleeding times.

Selected Readings

Dionne RA, "New Approaches to Preventing and Treating Postoperative Pain," *J Am Dent Assoc*, 1992, 123(6):26-34.

Gobetti JP, "Controlling Dental Pain," *J Am Dent Assoc*, 1992, 123(6):47-52.

Aspirin and Meprobamate *(AS pir in & me proe BA mate)*

Brand Names Equagesic®

Therapeutic Category Skeletal Muscle Relaxant

Synonyms Meprobamate and Aspirin

Use Adjunct to treatment of skeletal muscular disease in patients exhibiting tension and/or anxiety

Local Anesthetic/Vasoconstrictor Precautions No information available to require special precautions

Effects on Dental Treatment Avoid aspirin if possible, for 1 week prior to surgery because of the possibility of postoperative bleeding

Use with caution in impaired hepatic function; use with caution in patients with platelet and bleeding disorders, renal dysfunction, erosive gastritis, or peptic ulcer disease, previous nonreaction does not guarantee future safe taking of medication; do not use aspirin in children <16 years of age for chickenpox or flu symptoms due to the association with Reye's syndrome

Elderly are a high-risk population for adverse effects from nonsteroidal anti-inflammatory agents. As much as 60% of elderly with GI complications to NSAIDs can develop peptic ulceration and/or hemorrhage asymptomatically. Also, concomitant disease and drug use contribute to the risk for GI adverse effects. Use lowest effective dose for shortest period possible. Consider renal function decline with age. Use with caution in patients with history of asthma

Other Adverse Effects See individual agents

Pregnancy Risk Factor D

Generic Available Yes

Comments Abrupt discontinuation after sustained use (generally >10 days) may cause withdrawal symptoms

Selected Readings

Desjardins PJ, Cooper SA, Gallegos TL, et al, "The Relative Analgesic Efficacy of Propiram Fumarate, Codeine Aspirin, and Placebo in Post-Impaction Dental Pain," *J Clin Pharmacol*, 1984, 24(1):35-42.

Forbes JA, Butterworth GA, Burchfield WH, et al, "Evaluation of Ketorolac, Aspirin, and an Acetaminophen-Codeine Combination in Postoperative Oral Surgery Pain," *Pharmacotherapy*, 1990, 10(6 Pt 2):77S-93S.

Forbes JA, Keller CK, Smith JW, et al, "Analgesic Effect of Naproxen Sodium, Codeine, a Naproxen-Codeine Combination and Aspirin on the Postoperative Pain of Oral Surgery," *Pharmacotherapy*, 1986, 6(5):211-8.

Aspirin Free Anacin® Maximum Strength [OTC] *see* Acetaminophen *on page 20*

Aspirin-Free Bayer® Select® Allergy Sinus Caplets [OTC] *see* Acetaminophen, Chlorpheniramine, and Pseudoephedrine *on page 24*

Asprimox® [OTC] *see* Aspirin *on page 90*

Astelin® *see* Azelastine *on page 104*

Astemizole *(a STEM mi zole)*

Brand Names Hismanal®

Canadian/Mexican Brand Names Adistan® (Mexico); Antagon-1® (Mexico); Astemina® (Mexico)

Therapeutic Category Antihistamine

Use Perennial and seasonal allergic rhinitis and other allergic symptoms including urticaria

Usual Dosage Oral:

Children:

<6 years: 0.2 mg/kg/day

6-12 years: 5 mg/day

Children >12 years and Adults: 10-30 mg/day; give 30 mg on first day, 20 mg on second day, then 10 mg/day in a single dose

Mechanism of Action Competes with histamine for H_1-receptor sites on effector cells in the gastrointestinal tract, blood vessels, and respiratory tract; binds to lung receptors significantly greater than it binds to cerebellar receptors, resulting in a reduced sedative potential

Local Anesthetic/Vasoconstrictor Precautions No information available to require special precautions

Effects on Dental Treatment Up to 10% of patients taking astemizole may have significant dry mouth which will disappear with cessation of drug therapy;

no erythromycin products or antifungals (ketoconazole, itraconazole) should be given since cardiotoxicities could occur (See respective monographs in Dental Drug Monographs section)

Other Adverse Effects

1% to 10%:

Central nervous system: Drowsiness, headache, fatigue, nervousness, dizziness

Gastrointestinal: Appetite increase, weight increase, nausea, diarrhea, abdominal pain, dry mouth

Neuromuscular & skeletal: Arthralgia

Respiratory: Pharyngitis

<1%:

Cardiovascular: Palpitations, edema

Central nervous system: Depression

Dermatologic: Angioedema, photosensitivity, rash

Hepatic: Hepatitis

Neuromuscular & skeletal: Myalgia, paresthesia

Respiratory: Bronchospasm, epistaxis, thickening of mucous

Contraindications Patients with severe hepatic impairment; contraindicated with coadministration of clarithromycin, troleandomycin, mibefradil, serotonin reuptake inhibitors, protease inhibitors, zileuton, and grapefruit juice

Drug Interactions Increased toxicity: CNS depressants (sedation), triazole antifungals (torsade de pointes and other cardiotoxicities have been reported), macrolide antibiotics (cardiotoxicity)

Drug Uptake Long-acting, with steady-state plasma levels seen within 4-8 weeks following initiation of chronic therapy

Serum half-life: 20 hours

Time to peak serum concentration: Oral: Long-acting, with steady-state plasma levels of parent compound and metabolites seen within 4-8 weeks following initiation of chronic therapy; peak plasma levels appear in 1-4 hours following administration

Pregnancy Risk Factor C

Dosage Forms Tablet: 10 mg

Dietary Considerations Should be taken on an empty stomach; do not take with grapefruit juice

Generic Available No

AsthmaNefrin® *see* Epinephrine, Racemic *on page 354*

Astramorph™ PF Injection *see* Morphine Sulfate *on page 648*

Atarax® *see* Hydroxyzine *on page 491*

Atenolol (a TEN oh lole)

Related Information

Cardiovascular Diseases *on page 1010*

Brand Names Tenormin®

Canadian/Mexican Brand Names Apo®-Atenol (Canada); Novo-Atenol® (Canada); Nu-Atenol® (Canada); Taro-Atenol® (Canada)

Therapeutic Category Antianginal Agent; Beta-adrenergic Blocker, Cardioselective

Use Treatment of hypertension, alone or in combination with other agents; management of angina pectoris, postmyocardial infarction patients

Unlabeled use: Acute alcohol withdrawal, supraventricular and ventricular arrhythmias, and migraine headache prophylaxis

Usual Dosage

Oral:

Children: 1-2 mg/kg/dose given daily

Adults:

Hypertension: 50 mg once daily, may increase to 100 mg/day; doses >100 mg are unlikely to produce any further benefit

Angina pectoris: 50 mg once daily, may increase to 100 mg/day; some patients may require 200 mg/day

Postmyocardial infarction: Follow I.V. dose with 100 mg/day or 50 mg twice daily for 6-9 days postmyocardial infarction

I.V.: Postmyocardial infarction: Early treatment: 5 mg slow I.V. over 5 minutes; may repeat in 10 minutes; if both doses are tolerated, may start oral atenolol 50 mg every 12 hours or 100 mg/day for 6-9 days postmyocardial infarction

Mechanism of Action Competitively blocks response to beta-adrenergic stimulation, selectively blocks beta$_1$-receptors with little or no effect on beta$_2$-receptors except at high doses

Local Anesthetic/Vasoconstrictor Precautions No information available to require special precautions

(Continued)

Atenolol *(Continued)*

Effects on Dental Treatment Noncardioselective beta-blockers (ie, propranolol, nadolol) enhance the pressor response to epinephrine, resulting in hypertension and bradycardia. This has not been reported for atenolol, a cardioselective beta-blocker. Therefore local anesthetic with vasoconstrictor can be safely used in patients medicated with atenolol. Many nonsteroidal anti-inflammatory drugs such as ibuprofen and indometacin can reduce the hypotensive effect of beta-blockers after 3 or more weeks of therapy with the NSAID. Short-term NSAID use (ie, 3 days) requires no special precautions in patients taking beta-blockers.

Other Adverse Effects

1% to 10%:

Cardiovascular: Persistent bradycardia, hypotension, chest pain, edema, heart failure, second or third degree A-V block, Raynaud's phenomenon

Central nervous system: Dizziness, fatigue, insomnia, lethargy, confusion, mental impairment, depression, headache, nightmares

Gastrointestinal: Constipation, diarrhea, nausea

Genitourinary: Impotence

<1%:

Respiratory: Dyspnea (especially with large doses), wheezing

Miscellaneous: Cold extremities

Drug Interactions

Decreased effect of beta-blockers:

Barbiturates (increased liver metabolism of beta-blockers to result in lower serum levels)

NSAIDs (attenuate the hypotensive therapeutic effects of beta-blockers)

Rifampin (increased liver metabolism of beta-blockers to result in lower serum levels)

Increased effects of beta-blockers:

Calcium channel blockers (increase serum levels by unknown mechanism to enhance hypotension)

Beta-blockers increase the effects of:

Epinephrine (vasoconstrictor; initial hypotensive episode followed by brady-cardia) only from noncardioselective type beta-blockers

Phenylephrine (Neosynephrine®; enhanced pressor response)

Theophylline (inhibit theophylline metabolism causing increase in serum concentrations)

Drug Uptake

Absorption: Incomplete from GI tract

Serum half-life, beta:

Adults:

Normal renal function: 6-9 hours, longer in those with renal impairment

End stage renal disease: 15-35 hours

Time to peak: Oral: Within 2-4 hours

Pregnancy Risk Factor C

Generic Available Yes

Selected Readings

Foster CA and Aston SJ, "Propranolol-Epinephrine Interaction: A Potential Disaster," *Plast Reconstr Surg*, 1983, 72(1):74-8.

Wong DG, Spence JD, Lamki L, et al, "Effect of Nonsteroidal Anti-inflammatory Drugs on Control of Hypertension of Beta-Blockers and Diuretics," *Lancet*, 1986, 1(8488):997-1001.

Wynn RL, "Dental Nonsteroidal Anti-inflammatory Drugs and Prostaglandin-Based Drug Interactions-Part Two," *Gen Dent*, 1992, 40(2):104, 106, 108.

Wynn RL, "Epinephrine Interactions With Beta-Blockers," *Gen Dent*, 1994, 42(1):16, 18.

Atenolol and Chlorthalidone *(a TEN oh lole & klor THAL i done)*

Brand Names Tenoretic®

Therapeutic Category Antihypertensive Agent, Combination

Use Treatment of hypertension with a cardioselective beta-blocker and a diuretic

Local Anesthetic/Vasoconstrictor Precautions No information available to require special precautions

Effects on Dental Treatment Noncardioselective beta-blockers (ie, propranolol, nadolol) enhance the pressor response to epinephrine, resulting in hypertension and bradycardia. This has not been reported for atenolol, a cardioselective beta-blocker. Therefore local anesthetic with vasoconstrictor can be safely used in patients medicated with atenolol. Many nonsteroidal anti-inflammatory drugs such as ibuprofen and indometacin can reduce the hypotensive effect of beta-blockers after 3 or more weeks of therapy with the NSAID. Short-term NSAID use (ie, 3 days) requires no special precautions in patients taking beta-blockers.

Other Adverse Effects See individual agents

Pregnancy Risk Factor D

Generic Available Yes

Comments May contain povidone as inactive ingredient

Selected Readings
Foster CA and Aston SJ, "Propranolol-Epinephrine Interaction: A Potential Disaster," *Plast Reconstr Surg*, 1983, 72(1):74-8.
Wong DG, Spence JD, Lamki L, et al, "Effect of Nonsteroidal Anti-inflammatory Drugs on Control of Hypertension of Beta-Blockers and Diuretics," *Lancet*, 1986, 1(8488):997-1001.
Wynn RL, "Dental Nonsteroidal Anti-inflammatory Drugs and Prostaglandin-Based Drug Interactions-Part Two," *Gen Dent*, 1992, 40(2):104, 106, 108.
Wynn RL, "Epinephrine Interactions With Beta-Blockers," *Gen Dent*, 1994, 42(1):16, 18.

ATG *see* Lymphocyte Immune Globulin *on page 572*

Atgam® *see* Lymphocyte Immune Globulin *on page 572*

ATIII *see* Antithrombin III *on page 82*

Ativan® *see* Lorazepam *on page 567*

ATnativ® *see* Antithrombin III *on page 82*

Atolone® *see* Triamcinolone *on page 954*

Atorvastatin (a TORE va sta tin)
Brand Names Lipitor®
Therapeutic Category HMG-CoA Reductase Inhibitor
Use Adjunct to diet for the reduction of elevated total and LDL-cholesterol levels in patients with hypercholesterolemia (Type IIa, IIb, and IIc); used in hypercholesterolemic patients without clinically evident heart disease to reduce the risk of myocardial infarction, to reduce the risk for revascularization, and reduce the risk of death due to cardiovascular causes with no increase in death from noncardiovascular diseases
Usual Dosage Adults: Oral: Initial: 10 mg once daily, titrate up to 80 mg/day if needed
Mechanism of Action Inhibitor of 3-hydroxy-3-methylglutaryl coenzyme A (HMG-CoA) reductase, the rate limiting enzyme in cholesterol synthesis (reduces the production of mevalonic acid from HMG-CoA); this then results in a compensatory increase in the expression of LDL receptors on hepatocyte membranes and a stimulation of LDL catabolism
Local Anesthetic/Vasoconstrictor Precautions No information available to require special precautions
Effects on Dental Treatment No effects or complications reported
Other Adverse Effects
>1%:
Central nervous system: Headache
Gastrointestinal: Diarrhea, flatulence, abdominal pain (2% to 3%)
Neuromuscular & skeletal: Myalgia (1% to 5%)
<1%:
Central nervous system: Giddiness, euphoria, mild confusion, impaired short-term memory
Hepatic: Mild LFT increases
Respiratory: Pharyngitis, rhinitis
Drug Interactions
Increased toxicity: Gemfibrozil (musculoskeletal effects such as myopathy, myalgia and/or muscle weakness accompanied by markedly elevated CK concentrations, rash and/or pruritus); clofibrate, niacin (myopathy), erythromycin, cyclosporine, oral anticoagulants (elevated PT)
Increased effect/toxicity of levothyroxine
Concurrent use of erythromycin and atorvastatin may result in rhabdomyolysis
According to manufacturer's information, there is an increased risk of muscle weakness and breakdown when using erythromycin and azole antifungals with atorvastatin
Drug Uptake
Serum half-life: 14 hours (parent)
Time to peak serum concentration: 1-2 hours (maximal reduction in plasma cholesterol and triglycerides in 2 weeks)
Pregnancy Risk Factor X
Generic Available No

Atovaquone (a TOE va kwone)
Related Information
Systemic Viral Diseases *on page 1047*
Brand Names Mepron™
Therapeutic Category Antiprotozoal
Use Acute oral treatment of mild to moderate *Pneumocystis carinii* pneumonia (PCP) in patients who are intolerant to co-trimoxazole
Usual Dosage Adults: Oral: 750 mg 2 times/day with food for 21 days
Mechanism of Action Mechanism has not been fully elucidated; may inhibit electron transport in mitochondria inhibiting metabolic enzymes
(Continued)

Atovaquone *(Continued)*

Local Anesthetic/Vasoconstrictor Precautions No information available to require special precautions

Effects on Dental Treatment No effects or complications reported

Other Adverse Effects

>10%:
 Central nervous system: Headache, fever, insomnia, anxiety
 Dermatologic: Rash
 Gastrointestinal: Nausea, diarrhea, vomiting
 Respiratory: Cough

1% to 10%:
 Central nervous system: Dizziness
 Dermatologic: Pruritus
 Endocrine & metabolic: Hypoglycemia, hyponatremia
 Gastrointestinal: Abdominal pain, constipation, anorexia, dyspepsia
 Hematologic: Anemia, neutropenia, leukopenia
 Hepatic: Elevated amylase and liver enzymes
 Neuromuscular & skeletal: Weakness
 Renal: Elevated creatinine and BUN
 Miscellaneous: Oral *Monilia*

Drug Interactions No data reported

Drug Uptake
 Absorption: Decreased significantly in single doses >750 mg; increased threefold when administered with a high-fat meal
 Serum half-life: 2.9 days

Pregnancy Risk Factor C

Generic Available No

Atrohist® Plus *see* Chlorpheniramine, Phenylephrine, Phenylpropanolamine, and Belladonna Alkaloids *on page 221*

Atromid-S® *see* Clofibrate *on page 246*

Atropair® *see* Atropine *on this page*

Atropine (A troe peen)

Related Information
 Cardiovascular Diseases *on page 1010*

Brand Names Atropair®; Atropine-Care®; Atropisol®; Isopto® Atropine; I-Tropine®

Canadian/Mexican Brand Names Tropyn® Z (Mexico)

Therapeutic Category Anticholinergic Agent; Anticholinergic Agent, Ophthalmic; Antidote, Organophosphate Poisoning; Antispasmodic Agent, Gastrointestinal; Bronchodilator; Ophthalmic Agent, Mydriatic

Use Medical: Treatment of sinus bradycardia; management of peptic ulcer; treat exercise-induced bronchospasm; antidote for organophosphate pesticide poisoning; produce mydriasis and cycloplegia for examination of the retina and optic disc and accurate measurement of refractive errors; uveitis

Usual Dosage

Children:
 Preanesthetic: I.M., I.V., S.C.:
  <5 kg: 0.02 mg/kg/dose 30-60 minutes preop then every 4-6 hours as needed
  >5 kg: 0.01-0.02 mg/kg/dose to a maximum 0.4 mg 30-60 minutes preop; minimum dose: 0.1 mg

Adults:
 Preanesthetic: I.M., I.V., S.C.: 0.4-0.6 mg 30-60 minutes preop and repeat every 4-6 hours as needed

Mechanism of Action Blocks the action of acetylcholine at parasympathetic sites in smooth muscle, secretory glands, and the CNS; increases cardiac output, dries secretions, antagonizes histamine and serotonin

Local Anesthetic/Vasoconstrictor Precautions No information available to require special precautions

Effects on Dental Treatment >10% of patients experience dry mouth

Other Adverse Effects

>10%:
 Dermatologic: Dry skin
 Gastrointestinal: Constipation, dry throat
 Local: Irritation at injection site
 Respiratory: Dry nose
 Miscellaneous: Decreased sweating

1% to 10%:
 Endocrine & metabolic: Decreased flow of breast milk
 Gastrointestinal: Dysphagia

Ocular: Photosensitivity

Contraindications Hypersensitivity to atropine sulfate or any component; angle-closure glaucoma; tachycardia; thyrotoxicosis; obstructive disease of the GI tract; obstructive uropathy

Warnings/Precautions Use with caution in children with spastic paralysis; use with caution in elderly patients. Low doses cause a paradoxical decrease in heart rates. Some commercial products contain sodium metabisulfite, which can cause allergic-type reactions. May accumulate with multiple inhalational administration, particularly in the elderly. Heat prostration may occur in hot weather. Use with caution in patients with autonomic neuropathy, prostatic hypertrophy, hyperthyroidism, congestive heart failure, cardiac arrhythmias, chronic lung disease, biliary tract disease.

Drug Interactions Decreased effect of phenothiazines, levodopa, cisapride, methacholine, haloperidol; increased anticholinergic effects of amantadine, phenothiazines, TCAs, meperidine, antihistamines, quinidine, MAO inhibitors

Drug Uptake
Absorption: Well absorbed from all dosage forms
Serum half-life: 2-3 hours

Pregnancy Risk Factor C

Breast-feeding Considerations May be taken while breast-feeding

Dosage Forms Injection: 0.05 mg/mL (5 mL); 0.1 mg/mL (5 mL, 10 mL); 0.3 mg/mL (1 mL, 30 mL); 0.4 mg/mL (1 mL, 20 mL, 30 mL); 0.5 mg/mL (1 mL, 5 mL, 30 mL); 0.8 mg/mL (0.5 mL, 1 mL); 1 mg/mL (1 mL, 10 mL)

Dietary Considerations No data reported

Generic Available Yes

Atropine-Care® see Atropine on previous page

Atropisol® see Atropine on previous page

Atrovent® see Ipratropium on page 517

A/T/S® Topical see Erythromycin, Topical on page 364

Attapulgite (at a PULL gite)

Related Information
Oral Nonviral Soft Tissue Ulcerations or Erosions on page 1070

Brand Names Children's Kaopectate® [OTC]; Diasorb® [OTC]; Kaopectate® Advanced Formula [OTC]; Kaopectate® Maximum Strength Caplets; Rheaban® [OTC]

Therapeutic Category Antidiarrheal

Use Symptomatic treatment of diarrhea

Usual Dosage Oral:
Children:
<3 years: Not recommended
3-6 years: 750 mg/dose up to 2250 mg/24 hours
6-12 years: 1200-1500 mg/dose up to 4500 mg/24 hours

Adults: 1200-1500 mg after each loose bowel movement or every 2 hours; 15-30 mL up to 8 times/day, up to 9000 mg/24 hours

Mechanism of Action Controls diarrhea because of its absorbent action

Local Anesthetic/Vasoconstrictor Precautions No information available to require special precautions

Effects on Dental Treatment Do not give oral drugs concomitantly with Kaopectate® due to decreased GI absorption

Other Adverse Effects The powder, if chronically inhaled, can cause pneumoconiosis, since it contains large amounts of silica
1% to 10%: Constipation (dose related)
<1%: Fecal impaction

Drug Interactions Decreased GI absorption of orally administered clindamycin, tetracyclines, penicillamine, digoxin

Drug Uptake Absorption: Not absorbed from GI tract

Pregnancy Risk Factor B

Generic Available Yes

Attenuvax® see Measles Virus Vaccine, Live on page 583

Augmentin® see Amoxicillin and Clavulanate Potassium on page 69

Auralgan® see Antipyrine and Benzocaine on page 82

Auranofin (au RANE oh fin)

Related Information
Rheumatoid Arthritis and Osteoarthritis on page 1030

Brand Names Ridaura®

Therapeutic Category Gold Compound
(Continued)

Auranofin (Continued)

Use Management of active stage of classic or definite rheumatoid arthritis in patients that do not respond to or tolerate other agents; psoriatic arthritis; adjunctive or alternative therapy for pemphigus

Usual Dosage Oral:

Children: Initial: 0.1 mg/kg/day divided daily; usual maintenance: 0.15 mg/kg/day in 1-2 divided doses; maximum: 0.2 mg/kg/day in 1-2 divided doses

Adults: 6 mg/day in 1-2 divided doses; after 3 months may be increased to 9 mg/day in 3 divided doses; if still no response after 3 months at 9 mg/day, discontinue drug

Mechanism of Action The exact mechanism of action of gold is unknown; gold is taken up by macrophages which results in inhibition of phagocytosis and lysosomal membrane stabilization; other actions observed are decreased serum rheumatoid factor and alterations in immunoglobulins. Additionally, complement activation is decreased, prostaglandin synthesis is inhibited, and lysosomal enzyme activity is decreased.

Local Anesthetic/Vasoconstrictor Precautions No information available to require special precautions

Effects on Dental Treatment No effects or complications reported

Other Adverse Effects

>10%:
Dermatologic: Itching, skin rash
Gastrointestinal: Stomatitis
Ocular: Conjunctivitis
Renal: Proteinuria

1% to 10%:
Dermatologic: Urticaria, alopecia
Gastrointestinal: Glossitis
Hematologic: Eosinophilia, leukopenia, thrombocytopenia
Renal: Hematuria

<1%:
Dermatologic: Angioedema
Gastrointestinal: Ulcerative enterocolitis, GI hemorrhage, gingivitis, metallic taste, dysphagia
Hematologic: Agranulocytosis, anemia, aplastic anemia
Hepatic: Hepatotoxicity
Neuromuscular & skeletal: Peripheral neuropathy
Respiratory: Interstitial pneumonitis

Drug Interactions Increased toxicity: Penicillamine, antimalarials, hydroxychloroquine, cytotoxic agents, immunosuppressants

Pregnancy Risk Factor C

Generic Available No

Aureomycin® see Chlortetracycline on page 226
Auro® Ear Drops [OTC] see Carbamide Peroxide on page 175
Aurolate® see Gold Sodium Thiomalate on page 448

Aurothioglucose (aur oh thye oh GLOO kose)

Related Information
Rheumatoid Arthritis and Osteoarthritis on page 1030

Brand Names Solganal®

Therapeutic Category Gold Compound

Use Adjunctive treatment in adult and juvenile active rheumatoid arthritis; alternative or adjunct in treatment of pemphigus; psoriatic patients who do not respond to NSAIDs

Usual Dosage I.M.: Doses should initially be given at weekly intervals

Children 6-12 years: Initial: 0.25 mg/kg/dose first week; increment at 0.25 mg/kg/dose increasing with each weekly dose; maintenance: 0.75-1 mg/kg/dose weekly not to exceed 25 mg/dose to a total of 20 doses, then every 2-4 weeks

Adults: 10 mg first week; 25 mg second and third week; then 50 mg/week until 800 mg to 1 g cumulative dose has been given; if improvement occurs without adverse reactions, give 25-50 mg every 2-3 weeks, then every 3-4 weeks

Mechanism of Action Unknown, may decrease prostaglandin synthesis or may alter cellular mechanisms by inhibiting sulfhydryl systems

Local Anesthetic/Vasoconstrictor Precautions No information available to require special precautions

Effects on Dental Treatment No effects or complications reported

Other Adverse Effects

>10%:
Dermatologic: Itching, skin rash, exfoliative dermatitis, reddened skin
Gastrointestinal: Gingivitis, glossitis, metallic taste, stomatitis

1% to 10%: Renal: Proteinuria
<1%:
    Cardiovascular: EKG abnormalities
    Central nervous system: Encephalitis, fever
    Dermatologic: Alopecia
    Gastrointestinal: Ulcerative enterocolitis
    Genitourinary: Vaginitis
    Hematologic: Agranulocytosis, aplastic anemia, eosinophilia, leukopenia, thrombocytopenia
    Hepatic: Hepatotoxicity
    Neuromuscular & skeletal: Peripheral neuropathy
    Ocular: Conjunctivitis, corneal ulcers, iritis
    Renal: Glomerulitis, hematuria, nephrotic syndrome
    Respiratory: Pharyngitis, bronchitis, pulmonary fibrosis, interstitial pneumonitis
    Miscellaneous: Anaphylactic shock, allergic reaction (severe)
Drug Interactions Increased toxicity: Penicillamine, antimalarials, hydroxychloroquine, cytotoxic agents, immunosuppressants
Drug Uptake
  Absorption: I.M.: Erratic and slow
  Serum half-life: 3-27 days (half-life dependent upon single or multiple dosing)
  Time to peak serum concentration: Within 4-6 hours
Pregnancy Risk Factor C
Generic Available No

Auroto® *see* Antipyrine and Benzocaine *on page 82*
Autoplex® **T** *see* Anti-inhibitor Coagulant Complex *on page 82*
Avapro® *see* Irbesartan *on page 518*
AVC™ **Cream** *see* Sulfanilamide *on page 895*
AVC™ **Suppository** *see* Sulfanilamide *on page 895*
Aveeno® **Cleansing Bar [OTC]** *see* Sulfur and Salicylic Acid *on page 898*
Aventyl® **Hydrochloride** *see* Nortriptyline *on page 692*
Avita® **Topical** *see* Tretinoin, Topical *on page 953*
Avitene® *see* Microfibrillar Collagen Hemostat *on page 636*
Avlosulfon® *see* Dapsone *on page 281*
Avonex® *see* Interferon Beta-1a *on page 514*
Axid® *see* Nizatidine *on page 688*
Axid® **AR [OTC]** *see* Nizatidine *on page 688*
Axotal® *see* Butalbital Compound *on page 154*
Aygestin® *see* Norethindrone *on page 690*
Ayr® **Saline [OTC]** *see* Sodium Chloride *on page 870*

Azacitidine (ay za SYE ti deen)
Brand Names Mylosar®
Therapeutic Category Antineoplastic Agent, Miscellaneous
Synonyms AZA-CR; 5-Azacytidine; 5-AZC; Ladakamycin; NSC-102816
Use Refractory acute lymphocytic and myelogenous leukemia
Local Anesthetic/Vasoconstrictor Precautions No information available to require special precautions
Effects on Dental Treatment No effects or complications reported
Other Adverse Effects 1% to 10%:
  Cardiovascular: Hypotension with rapid infusion
  Central nervous system: Fever
  Dermatologic: Rash
  Gastrointestinal: Nausea, vomiting, diarrhea
  Hematologic: Myelosuppression (granulocyte nadir: 14-17 days)
  Hepatic: Hepatotoxicity
  Neuromuscular & skeletal: Neuropathies (dose dependent) and neurologic toxicity
Pregnancy Risk Factor C
Generic Available No

AZA-CR *see* Azacitidine *on this page*
Azactam® *see* Aztreonam *on page 106*
5-Azacytidine *see* Azacitidine *on this page*
Azatadina, Maleato De (Mexico) *see* Azatadine *on this page*

Azatadine (a ZA ta deen)
Brand Names Optimine®
Canadian/Mexican Brand Names Idulamine® (Mexico)
Therapeutic Category Antihistamine
Synonyms Azatadina, Maleato De (Mexico)
(Continued)

Azatadine *(Continued)*

Use Treatment of perennial and seasonal allergic rhinitis and chronic urticaria

Usual Dosage Children >12 years and Adults: Oral: 1-2 mg twice daily

Mechanism of Action Azatadine is a piperidine-derivative antihistamine; has both anticholinergic and antiserotonin activity; has been demonstrated to inhibit mediator release from human mast cells *in vitro*; mechanism of this action is suggested to prevent calcium entry into the mast cell through voltage-dependent calcium channels

Local Anesthetic/Vasoconstrictor Precautions No information available to require special precautions

Effects on Dental Treatment This drug has atropine-like effects and the patient may experience drowsiness, dry mouth, nose and throat

Other Adverse Effects

>10%:
  Central nervous system: Slight to moderate drowsiness
  Respiratory: Thickening of bronchial secretions

1% to 10%:
  Central nervous system: Headache, fatigue, nervousness, dizziness
  Gastrointestinal: Appetite increase, weight increase, nausea, diarrhea, abdominal pain, dry mouth
  Neuromuscular & skeletal: Arthralgia
  Respiratory: Pharyngitis

<1%:
  Cardiovascular: Palpitations, edema
  Central nervous system: Depression
  Dermatologic: Angioedema, photosensitivity, rash
  Hepatic: Hepatitis
  Neuromuscular & skeletal: Myalgia, paresthesia
  Respiratory: Bronchospasm, epistaxis

Drug Interactions Increased effect/toxicity: Procarbazine, CNS depressants, tricyclic antidepressants, alcohol

Drug Uptake
  Absorption: Oral: Rapid and extensive
  Serum half-life: ~8.7 hours

Pregnancy Risk Factor B

Generic Available No

Azatadine and Pseudoephedrine

(a ZA ta deen & soo doe e FED rin)

Brand Names Trinalin®

Therapeutic Category Antihistamine/Decongestant Combination

Synonyms Pseudoephedrine and Azatadine

Use Perennial and seasonal allergic rhinitis and other allergic symptoms including urticaria

Local Anesthetic/Vasoconstrictor Precautions
  Azatadine: No information available to require special precautions
  Pseudoephedrine: Use with caution since pseudoephedrine is a sympathomimetic amine which could interact with epinephrine to cause a pressor response

Effects on Dental Treatment
  Azatadine: This drug has atropine-like effects and the patient may experience drowsiness, dry mouth, nose and throat
  Pseudoephedrine: Up to 10% of patients could experience tachycardia, palpitations, and dry mouth; use vasoconstrictor with caution

Other Adverse Effects See individual agents

Pregnancy Risk Factor C

Generic Available No

Azathioprine (ay za THYE oh preen)

Brand Names Imuran®

Canadian/Mexican Brand Names Azatrilem® (Mexico)

Therapeutic Category Immunosuppressant Agent

Synonyms Azatioprina (Mexico)

Use Adjunct with other agents in prevention of rejection of solid organ transplants; also used in severe active rheumatoid arthritis unresponsive to other agents; **azathioprine is an imidazolyl derivative of 6-mercaptopurine**

Usual Dosage I.V. dose is equivalent to oral dose
  Children and Adults: Renal transplantation: Oral, I.V.: 2-5 mg/kg/day to start, then 1-3 mg/kg/day maintenance
  Adults: Rheumatoid arthritis: Oral: 1 mg/kg/day for 6-8 weeks; increase by 0.5 mg/kg every 4 weeks until response or up to 2.5 mg/kg/day

Mechanism of Action Antagonizes purine metabolism and may inhibit synthesis of DNA, RNA, and proteins; may also interfere with cellular metabolism and inhibit mitosis

Local Anesthetic/Vasoconstrictor Precautions No information available to require special precautions

Effects on Dental Treatment No effects or complications reported

Other Adverse Effects Dose reduction or temporary withdrawal allows reversal

>10%:
  Central nervous system: Fever, chills
  Gastrointestinal: Nausea, vomiting, anorexia, diarrhea
  Hematologic: Thrombocytopenia, leukopenia, anemia
  Miscellaneous: Secondary infection

1% to 10%:
  Dermatologic: Skin rash
  Hematologic: Pancytopenia
  Hepatic: Hepatotoxicity

<1%:
  Cardiovascular: Hypotension
  Dermatologic: Alopecia, rash, maculopapular rash, aphthous stomatitis
  Neuromuscular & skeletal: Arthralgias, which include myalgias, rigors
  Ocular: Retinopathy
  Respiratory: Dyspnea
  Miscellaneous: Rare hypersensitivity reactions

Drug Interactions Increased toxicity: Allopurinol (reduce azathioprine dose to $\frac{1}{3}$ to $\frac{1}{4}$ of normal dose). The use of angiotensin-converting enzyme inhibitors to control hypertension in patients on azathioprine has been reported to induce severe leukopenia.

Drug Uptake
Serum half-life:
  Parent drug: 12 minutes
  6-mercaptopurine: 0.7-3 hours
  End stage renal disease: Slightly prolonged

Pregnancy Risk Factor D

Generic Available No

Azatioprina (Mexico) *see* Azathioprine *on previous page*

5-AZC *see* Azacitidine *on page 101*

Azdone® *see* Hydrocodone and Aspirin *on page 480*

Azelaic Acid (a zeh LAY ik AS id)

Brand Names Azelex®

Therapeutic Category Topical Skin Product, Acne

Use *Acne vulgaris*: Topical treatment of mild to moderate inflammatory acne vulgaris

Usual Dosage Adults: Topical: After skin is thoroughly washed and patted dry, gently but thoroughly massage a thin film of azelaic acid cream into the affected areas twice daily, in the morning and evening. The duration of use can vary and depends on the severity of the acne. In the majority of patients with inflammatory lesions, improvement of the condition occurs within 4 weeks.

Mechanism of Action Exact mechanism is not known; *in vitro*, azelaic acid possesses antimicrobial activity against *Propionibacteriaceae acnes* and *Staphylococcus epidermis*; may decrease micromedo formation

Local Anesthetic/Vasoconstrictor Precautions No information available to require special precautions

Effects on Dental Treatment No effects or complications reported

Other Adverse Effects
1% to 10%:
  Dermatologic: Pruritus, stinging
  Local: Burning
  Neuromuscular & skeletal: Paresthesia

<1%:
  Dermatologic: Erythema, dryness, rash, peeling, dermatitis, contact dermatitis
  Local: Irritation

Drug Uptake
Absorption: ~3% to 5% penetrates the stratum corneum; up to 10% is found in the epidermis and dermis; 4% is systemically absorbed
Serum half-life: Healthy subjects: 12 hours after topical dosing

Pregnancy Risk Factor B

Generic Available No

Azelastine (a ZEL as teen)

Brand Names Astelin®

Therapeutic Category Antihistamine

Synonyms Azelastine Hydrochloride

Use Treatment of symptoms of seasonal allergic rhinitis (ie, rhinorrhea, sneezing, nasal pruritus) in adults and children >12 years of age

Usual Dosage Two sprays (137 mcg/spray) per nostril twice daily. Before initial use, the delivery system should be primed with 4 sprays or until a fine mist appears. If three or more days have elapsed since last use, the delivery system should be reprimed.

Mechanism of Action Azelastine competes with histamine for histamine$_1$-receptor sites on effector cells in the GI tract, blood vessels, and respiratory tract. This action inhibits the symptoms associated with seasonal allergic rhinitis (ie, sneezing, pruritus, increased mucus production).

Local Anesthetic/Vasoconstrictor Precautions No information available to require special precautions

Effects on Dental Treatment 2% to 10% of patients experience dry mouth; chronic use of antihistamines will inhibit salivary flows particularly in elderly patients; this may contribute to periodontal disease and oral discomfort

Other Adverse Effects

>10%:

Central nervous system: Headache (14.8%), somnolence (11.5%)

Gastrointestinal: Bitter taste (19.7%)

2% to 10%:

Central nervous system: Fatigue (2.3%), dizziness (2.0%)

Gastrointestinal: Dry mouth (2.8%), nausea (2.8%), weight increase (2.0%)

Respiratory: Nasal burning (4.1%), pharyngitis (3.8%), paroxysmal sneezing (3.1%), rhinitis (2.3%), epistaxis (2.0%)

<2%:

Cardiovascular: Flushing, hypertension, tachycardia

Central nervous system: Malaise, vertigo, hypoesthesia, anxiety, depersonalization, depression, nervousness, sleep disorder, abnormal thinking

Dermatological: Contact dermatitis, eczema, hair and follicle infection, furunculosis

Endocrine & metabolic: Amenorrhea, breast pain

Gastrointestinal: Constipation, gastroenteritis, glossitis, increased appetite, ulcerative stomatitis, vomiting, increased ALT, aphthous stomatitis, loss of taste perception, abdominal pain

Genitourinary: Albuminuria, polyuria

Neuromuscular & skeletal: Myalgia, temporomandibular dislocation, hyperkinesis, pain in extremities, back pain

Ocular: Conjunctivitis, eye abnormality, eye pain, water eyes

Renal: Hematuria

Respiratory: Bronchospasm, coughing, throat burning, laryngitis

Miscellaneous: Allergic reaction, herpes simplex, viral infection

Contraindications Patients with a known hypersensitivity to any of the components of Astelin®

Warnings/Precautions Azelastine causes somnolence. Caution should be exercised when performing activities that require mental alertness. Concurrent use of alcohol or other CNS depressants with azelastine should be avoided. Avoid use of azelastine with other antihistamines unless advised by a physician.

Drug Interactions Increased effect: Alcohol and CNS depressants cause additive somnolence and CNS impairment

Drug Uptake

Serum half-life: Azelastine 22 hours, desmethylazelastine 54 hours

Time to peak: 2 to 3 hours

Pregnancy Risk Factor C

Dosage Forms Spray, nasal: 137 mcg/actuation [100 actuations/bottle]

Comments Azelastine is absorbed systemically will cause sedation in some patients. Although this agent is clinically effective, the side effects of sedation, bitter taste, and high cost will limits its use in many patients.

Azelastine Hydrochloride *see Azelastine on this page*

Azelex® *see Azelaic Acid on previous page*

Azithromycin (az ith roe MYE sin)

Related Information

Antibiotic Prophylaxis, Preprocedural Guidelines for Dental Patients *on page 1034*

Brand Names Zithromax™

Therapeutic Category Antibiotic, Macrolide

Synonyms Z-PAKS™

Use

Dental: Alternate antibiotic in the treatment of common orofacial infections caused by aerobic gram-positive cocci and susceptible anaerobes; alternate antibiotic for the prevention of bacterial endocarditis in patients undergoing dental procedures

Medical: Treatment against most respiratory pathogens (eg, *S. pyogenes*, *S. pneumoniae*, *S. agalactiae*, viridans *Streptococcus*, *M. catarrhalis*, *C. trachomatis*, *Legionella* sp, *Mycoplasma pneumoniae*, *S. aureus*)

Usual Dosage Oral:

Children: Prevention of bacterial endocarditis: 15 mg/kg 1 hour before procedure; total children's dose should not exceed adult dose

Adults: 250 mg twice daily first day then 250 mg/day for 4 days; prevention of bacterial endocarditis: 500 mg 1 hour before procedure

Mechanism of Action Inhibits RNA-dependent protein synthesis at the chain elongation step; binds to the 50S ribosomal subunit resulting in blockage of transpeptidation

Local Anesthetic/Vasoconstrictor Precautions No information available to require special precautions

Effects on Dental Treatment No effects or complications reported

Other Adverse Effects 1% to 10%: Gastrointestinal: Diarrhea, nausea, abdominal pain, cramping, vomiting

Contraindications Hepatic impairment, known hypersensitivity to azithromycin, other macrolide antibiotics, or any Zithromax™ components; use with pimozide

Warnings/Precautions Use with caution in patients with hepatic dysfunction; hepatic impairment with or without jaundice has occurred chiefly in older children and adults; it may be accompanied by malaise, nausea, vomiting, abdominal colic, and fever; discontinue use if these occur; may mask or delay symptoms of incubating gonorrhea or syphilis, so appropriate culture and susceptibility tests should be performed prior to initiating azithromycin; pseudomembranous colitis has been reported with use of macrolide antibiotics

Drug Interactions Aluminum- and magnesium-containing antacids decrease serum levels of azithromycin by 24% but not total absorption; manufacturer recommends that when antacids are used, azithromycin should be taken 1-2 hours later

Drug Uptake

Absorption: Rapid from the GI tract

Serum half-life, terminal: 68 hours

Time to peak serum concentration: 2.3-4 hours

Pregnancy Risk Factor B

Breast-feeding Considerations No data reported

Dosage Forms

Capsule, as dihydrate: 250 mg

Capsule (Z-PAKS™): 6 capsules/box

Suspension, oral (single-dose packets): 1 g

Dietary Considerations Should be taken at least 1 hour prior to or 2 hours after a meal; should not be taken with food; food decreases rate and extent of absorption

Generic Available No

Comments Although the erythromycins inhibit the hepatic metabolism of theophylline and carbamazepine to enhance their effects, azithromycin has not been shown to inhibit the hepatic metabolism of these drugs. Clauzel, et al, reported that erythromycin did not inhibit the metabolism of theophylline after a standard 5-day regimen (500 mg on day one followed by 250 mg daily). Rapeport, et al, reported that azithromycin did not affect the blood levels of carbamazepine.

Selected Readings

Clauzel AM, Visier S, and Michel FB, "Efficacy and Safety of Azithromycin in Lower Respiratory Tract Infections," *Eur Respir J*, 1990, 3(suppl 10):89S.

Dajani AS, Taubert KA, Wilson W, et al, "Prevention of Bacterial Endocarditis Recommendations by the American Heart Association," *JAMA*, 1997, 277(22):1794-801.

Dajani AS, Taubert KA, Wilson W, et al, "Prevention of Bacterial Endocarditis: Recommendations by the American Heart Association," *J Am Dent Assoc*, 1997, 128(8):1142-51.

Rapeport WG, Dewland PM, Muirhead DC, et al, "Lack of Interaction Between Azithromycin and Carbamazepine," *Br J Clin Pharmacol*, 1992, 30:551P.

Wynn RL, "New Erythromycins," *Gen Dent*, 1996, 44(4):304-7.

Azmacort™ *see* Triamcinolone *on page 954*

Azo Gantanol® *see* Sulfamethoxazole and Phenazopyridine *on page 894*

Azo Gantrisin® *see* Sulfisoxazole and Phenazopyridine *on page 897*

Azo-Standard® [OTC] *see* Phenazopyridine *on page 746*

AZT + 3TC *see* Zidovudine and Lamivudine *on page 1003*

Aztreonam (AZ tree oh nam)

Brand Names Azactam®

Therapeutic Category Antibiotic, Miscellaneous

Use Treatment of patients with documented aerobic gram-negative bacillary infection in which beta-lactam therapy is contraindicated (eg, penicillin or cephalosporin allergy); used for urinary tract infections, lower respiratory tract infections, septicemia, skin/skin structure infections, intra-abdominal infections, and gynecological infections; as part of a multiple-drug regimen for the empirical treatment of neutropenic fever in persons with a history of beta-lactam allergy or with known multidrug-resistant organisms

Usual Dosage

Children >1 month: I.M., I.V.: 90-120 mg/kg/day divided every 6-8 hours

Cystic fibrosis: 50 mg/kg/dose every 6-8 hours (ie, up to 200 mg/kg/day); maximum: 6-8 g/day

Adults:

Urinary tract infection: I.M., I.V.: 500 mg to 1 g every 8-12 hours

Moderately severe systemic infections: 1 g I.V. or I.M. or 2 g I.V. every 8-12 hours

Severe systemic or life-threatening infections (especially caused by *Pseudomonas aeruginosa*): I.V.: 2 g every 6-8 hours; maximum: 8 g/day

Mechanism of Action Monobactam which is active only against gram-negative bacilli (unlikely cross-allergenicity with other beta-lactams); inhibits bacterial cell wall synthesis during active multiplication, causing cell wall destruction

Local Anesthetic/Vasoconstrictor Precautions No information available to require special precautions

Effects on Dental Treatment No effects or complications reported

Other Adverse Effects

1% to 10%:

Dermatologic: Rash

Gastrointestinal: Diarrhea, nausea, vomiting

Local: Thrombophlebitis, pain at injection site

<1%:

Cardiovascular: Hypotension

Central nervous system: Seizures, confusion, headache, vertigo, insomnia, dizziness, fever

Endocrine & metabolic: Breast tenderness

Gastrointestinal: Pseudomembranous colitis, aphthous ulcer, dysgeusia, halitosis, numb tongue

Genitourinary: Vaginitis

Hepatic: Hepatitis, jaundice, elevation of liver enzymes

Hematologic: Thrombocytopenia, eosinophilia, leukopenia, neutropenia

Neuromuscular & skeletal: Myalgia, weakness

Ocular: Diplopia

Otic: Tinnitus

Respiratory: Sneezing

Miscellaneous: Anaphylaxis

Drug Interactions No data reported

Drug Uptake

Absorption: I.M.: Well absorbed; I.M. and I.V. doses produce comparable serum concentrations

Serum half-life:

Normal renal function: 1.7-2.9 hours

End stage renal disease: 6-8 hours

Time to peak: Within 60 minutes (I.M., I.V. push) and 90 minutes (I.V. infusion)

Pregnancy Risk Factor B

Generic Available No

Bacampicillin (ba kam pi SIL in)

Brand Names Spectrobid®

Canadian/Mexican Brand Names Penglobe®

Therapeutic Category Antibiotic, Penicillin

Synonyms Bacampicillin Hydrochloride; Carampicillin Hydrochloride

Use Treatment of susceptible bacterial infections involving the urinary tract, skin structure, upper and lower respiratory tract; activity is identical to that of ampicillin

Mechanism of Action Interferes with bacterial cell wall synthesis during active multiplication causing cell wall death and resultant bactericidal activity against susceptible bacteria

Local Anesthetic/Vasoconstrictor Precautions No information available to require special precautions

Effects on Dental Treatment No effects or complications reported

Other Adverse Effects

1% to 10%: Gastrointestinal: Gastric upset, diarrhea, nausea

<1%:

Dermatologic: Rash

Gastrointestinal: Pseudomembranous colitis

Hematologic: Agranulocytosis

Hepatic: Mild elevation in AST

Miscellaneous: Hypersensitivity reactions

Drug Interactions

Decreased effect of oral contraceptives

Increased levels with probenecid; allopurinol theoretically has has an additive potential for amoxicillin/ampicillin rash

Drug Uptake

Serum half-life: 65 minutes, prolonged in patients with impaired renal function

Time to peak serum concentration: Area under the serum concentration time curve is 40% higher for bacampicillin than after equivalent ampicillin doses

Pregnancy Risk Factor B

Generic Available No

Comments Each mg of bacampicillin is equivalent to ampicillin 700 mcg

Bacampicillin Hydrochloride see Bacampicillin on previous page

Bacid® [OTC] see Lactobacillus acidophilus and Lactobacillus bulgaricus on page 539

Baciguent® [OTC] see Bacitracin on this page

Baci-IM® see Bacitracin on this page

Bacillus Calmette-Guérin (BCG) Live see BCG Vaccine on page 111

Bacitracin (bas i TRAY sin)

Brand Names AK-Tracin®; Baciguent® [OTC]; Baci-IM®

Canadian/Mexican Brand Names Bacitin® (Canada)

Therapeutic Category Antibiotic, Ophthalmic; Antibiotic, Topical; Antibiotic, Miscellaneous

Use Treatment of susceptible bacterial infections (staphylococcal pneumonia and empyema); due to toxicity risks, systemic and irrigant uses of bacitracin should be limited to situations where less toxic alternatives would not be effective; oral administration has been successful in antibiotic-associated colitis

Usual Dosage Do not administer I.V.:

Children: I.M.: 800-1200 units/kg/day divided every 8 hours

Adults: Antibiotic-associated colitis: Oral: 25,000 units 4 times/day for 7-10 days

Topical: Apply 1-5 times/day

Ophthalmic, ointment: Instill 1/4" to 1/2" ribbon every 3-4 hours into conjunctival sac for acute infections, or 2-3 times/day for mild to moderate infections for 7-10 days

Irrigation, solution: 50-100 units/mL in normal saline, lactated Ringer's, or sterile water for irrigation; soak sponges in solution for topical compresses 1-5 times/ day or as needed during surgical procedures

Mechanism of Action Inhibits bacterial cell wall synthesis by preventing transfer of mucopeptides into the growing cell wall

Local Anesthetic/Vasoconstrictor Precautions No information available to require special precautions

Effects on Dental Treatment No effects or complications reported

Other Adverse Effects 1% to 10%:

Cardiovascular: Hypotension, tightness of chest, swelling of lips and face

Central nervous system: Pain

Dermatologic: Rash, itching

Gastrointestinal: Anorexia, nausea, vomiting, diarrhea, rectal itching and burning

Hematologic: Blood dyscrasias

Miscellaneous: Sweating

Drug Interactions Increased toxicity: Nephrotoxic drugs, neuromuscular blocking agents, and anesthetics (increased neuromuscular blockade)

Drug Uptake

Duration of action: 6-8 hours

(Continued)

Bacitracin *(Continued)*

Absorption: Poor from mucous membranes and intact or denuded skin; rapidly absorbed following I.M. administration; not absorbed by bladder irrigation, but absorption can occur from peritoneal or mediastinal lavage

Time to peak serum concentration: I.M.: Within 1-2 hours

Pregnancy Risk Factor C

Generic Available Yes

Bacitracin and Polymyxin B (bas i TRAY sin & pol i MIKS in bee)

Brand Names AK-Poly-Bac® Ophthalmic; Betadine® First Aid Antibiotics + Moisturizer [OTC]; Polysporin® Ophthalmic; Polysporin® Topical

Canadian/Mexican Brand Names Bioderm® (Canada); Polytopic® (Canada)

Therapeutic Category Antibiotic, Ophthalmic; Antibiotic, Topical

Use Treatment of superficial infections caused by susceptible organisms

Usual Dosage Children and Adults:

Ophthalmic ointment: Instill ½" ribbon in the affected eye(s) every 3-4 hours for acute infections or 2-3 times/day for mild to moderate infections for 7-10 days

Topical ointment/powder: Apply to affected area 1-4 times/day; may cover with sterile bandage if needed

Mechanism of Action Refer to individual monographs for Bacitracin and Polymyxin B

Local Anesthetic/Vasoconstrictor Precautions No information available to require special precautions

Effects on Dental Treatment No effects or complications reported

Other Adverse Effects 1% to 10%: Local: Rash, itching, burning, anaphylactoid reactions, swelling and conjunctival erythema

Drug Interactions No data reported

Pregnancy Risk Factor C

Generic Available Yes

Bacitracin, Neomycin, and Polymyxin B

(bas i TRAY sin, nee oh MYE sin & pol i MIKS in bee)

Brand Names AK-Spore® Ophthalmic Ointment; Medi-Quick® Topical Ointment [OTC]; Mycitracin® Topical [OTC]; Neomixin® Topical [OTC]; Neosporin® Ophthalmic Ointment; Neosporin® Topical Ointment [OTC]; Ocutricin® Topical Ointment; Septa® Topical Ointment [OTC]; Triple Antibiotic® Topical

Canadian/Mexican Brand Names Neotopic® (Canada)

Therapeutic Category Antibiotic, Ophthalmic; Antibiotic, Topical

Use Helps prevent infection in minor cuts, scrapes and burns; short-term treatment of superficial external ocular infections caused by susceptible organisms

Usual Dosage Children and Adults:

Ophthalmic ointment: Instill ½" ribbon into the conjunctival sac every 3-4 hours for acute infections or 2-3 times/day for mild to moderate infections for 7-10 days

Topical: Apply 1-4 times/day to affected areas and cover with sterile bandage if necessary

Mechanism of Action Refer to individual monographs for Bacitracin; Neomycin Sulfate; and Polymyxin B Sulfate

Local Anesthetic/Vasoconstrictor Precautions No information available to require special precautions

Effects on Dental Treatment No effects or complications reported

Other Adverse Effects 1% to 10%:

Dermatologic: Allergic contact dermatitis

Local: Itching, reddening, failure to heal

Drug Interactions No data reported

Pregnancy Risk Factor C

Generic Available Yes

Bacitracin, Neomycin, Polymyxin B, and Hydrocortisone

(bas i TRAY sin, nee oh MYE sin, pol i MIKS in bee & hye droe KOR ti sone)

Brand Names AK-Spore H.C.® Ophthalmic Ointment; Cortisporin® Ophthalmic Ointment; Cortisporin® Topical Ointment; Neotricin HC® Ophthalmic Ointment

Therapeutic Category Antibiotic, Ophthalmic; Antibiotic, Otic; Antibiotic, Topical; Corticosteroid, Ophthalmic; Corticosteroid, Otic; Corticosteroid, Topical (Low Potency)

Use Prevention and treatment of susceptible superficial topical infections

Usual Dosage Children and Adults:
Ophthalmic:
Ointment: Instill ½" ribbon to inside of lower lid every 3-4 hours until improvement occurs
Topical: Apply sparingly 2-4 times/day
Mechanism of Action Refer to individual monographs for Bacitracin, Neomycin, Polymyxin B, and Hydrocortisone
Local Anesthetic/Vasoconstrictor Precautions No information available to require special precautions
Effects on Dental Treatment No effects or complications reported
Other Adverse Effects 1% to 10%:
Dermatologic: Rash, generalized itching
Respiratory: Apnea
Drug Interactions No data reported
Pregnancy Risk Factor C
Generic Available Yes

Bacitracin, Neomycin, Polymyxin B, and Lidocaine
(bas i TRAY sin, nee oh MYE sin, pol i MIKS in bee & LYE doe kane)
Brand Names Clomycin® [OTC]
Therapeutic Category Antibiotic, Topical
Use Prevention and treatment of susceptible superficial topical infections
Local Anesthetic/Vasoconstrictor Precautions No information available to require special precautions
Effects on Dental Treatment No effects or complications reported
Generic Available No

Baclofen (BAK loe fen)
Brand Names Lioresal®
Canadian/Mexican Brand Names Alpha-Baclofen® (Canada); PMS-Baclofen® (Canada)
Therapeutic Category Muscle Relaxant; Skeletal Muscle Relaxant
Use Treatment of reversible spasticity associated with multiple sclerosis or spinal cord lesions; intrathecal baclofen for the treatment of cerebral spasticity

There are a number of unlabeled uses for baclofen including, intractable hiccups, intractable pain relief, and bladder spasticity
Usual Dosage
Oral:
Children:
2-7 years: Initial: 10-15 mg/24 hours divided every 8 hours; titrate dose every 3 days in increments of 5-15 mg/day to a maximum of 40 mg/day
≥8 years: Maximum: 60 mg/day in 3 divided doses
Adults: 5 mg 3 times/day, may increase 5 mg/dose every 3 days to a maximum of 80 mg/day
Intrathecal:
Test dose: 50-100 mcg, doses >50 mcg should be given in 25 mcg increments, separated by 24 hours
Maintenance: After positive response to test dose, a maintenance intrathecal infusion can be administered via an implanted intrathecal pump. Initial dose via pump: Infusion at a 24-hourly rate dosed at twice the test dose.
Mechanism of Action Inhibits the transmission of both monosynaptic and polysynaptic reflexes at the spinal cord level, possibly by hyperpolarization of primary afferent fiber terminals, with resultant relief of muscle spasticity
Local Anesthetic/Vasoconstrictor Precautions No information available to require special precautions
Effects on Dental Treatment No effects or complications reported
Other Adverse Effects
>10%:
Central nervous system: Drowsiness, vertigo, dizziness, psychiatric disturbances, insomnia, slurred speech, ataxia, hypotonia
Neuromuscular & skeletal: Weakness
1% to 10%:
Cardiovascular: Hypotension
Central nervous system: Fatigue, confusion, headache, insomnia
Dermatologic: Rash
Gastrointestinal: Nausea, constipation
Renal: Polyuria
<1%:
Cardiovascular: Palpitations, chest pain, syncope
Central nervous system: Euphoria, excitement, depression, hallucinations
(Continued)

Baclofen (Continued)

Gastrointestinal: Dry mouth, anorexia, taste disorder, abdominal pain, vomiting, diarrhea

Genitourinary: Enuresis, urinary retention, dysuria, impotence, inability to ejaculate, nocturia

Neuromuscular & skeletal: Paresthesia

Renal: Hematuria

Respiratory: Dyspnea

Drug Interactions

Increased effect of baclofen has been caused by opiate analgesics, benzodiazepines, hypertensive agents

Increased toxicity: CNS depressants and alcohol (sedation), tricyclic antidepressants (short-term memory loss), guanabenz (sedation), MAO inhibitors (decreased blood pressure, CNS, and respiratory effects)

Drug Uptake

Onset of action: Muscle relaxation effect requires 3-4 days

Absorption: Oral: Rapid; absorption from GI tract is thought to be dose dependent

Serum half-life: 3.5 hours

Time to peak serum concentration: Oral: Within 2-3 hours

Pregnancy Risk Factor C

Dosage Forms

Injection, intrathecal: 0.5 mg/mL, 2 mg/mL

Tablet: 10 mg, 20 mg

Generic Available Yes: Tablets only

Bactocill® see Oxacillin on page 705

BactoShield® Topical [OTC] see Chlorhexidine Gluconate on page 211

Bactrim™ see Trimethoprim and Sulfamethoxazole on page 965

Bactrim™ DS see Trimethoprim and Sulfamethoxazole on page 965

Bactroban® see Mupirocin on page 652

Bactroban® Nasal see Mupirocin on page 652

Baker's P&S Topical [OTC] see Phenol on page 749

Baking Soda see Sodium Bicarbonate on page 869

Balanced Salt Solution (BAL anced salt soe LOO shun)

Brand Names BSS® Ophthalmic

Therapeutic Category Ophthalmic Agent, Miscellaneous

Use Intraocular irrigating solution; also used to soothe and cleanse the eye in conjunction with hard contact lenses

Local Anesthetic/Vasoconstrictor Precautions No information available to require special precautions

Effects on Dental Treatment No effects or complications reported

Generic Available Yes

BAL in Oil® see Dimercaprol on page 321

Balnetar® [OTC] see Coal Tar, Lanolin, and Mineral Oil on page 255

Bancap® see Butalbital Compound on page 154

Bancap® see Butalbital Compound and Acetaminophen on page 155

Bancap HC® [5/500] see Hydrocodone and Acetaminophen on page 478

Banophen® Decongestant Capsule [OTC] see Diphenhydramine and Pseudoephedrine on page 324

Banophen® Oral [OTC] see Diphenhydramine on page 323

Banthine® see Methantheline on page 609

Barbidonna® see Hyoscyamine, Atropine, Scopolamine, and Phenobarbital on page 493

Barbita® see Phenobarbital on page 747

Barc® Liquid [OTC] see Pyrethrins on page 824

Baridium® [OTC] see Phenazopyridine on page 746

Basaljel® [OTC] see Aluminum Carbonate on page 47

Base Ointment see Zinc Oxide on page 1004

Baycol® see Cerivastatin on page 204

Bayer® Aspirin [OTC] see Aspirin on page 90

Bayer® Buffered Aspirin [OTC] see Aspirin on page 90

Bayer® Low Adult Strength [OTC] see Aspirin on page 90

Bayer® Select® Chest Cold Caplets [OTC] see Acetaminophen and Dextromethorphan on page 23

Bayer® Select Head Cold Caplets [OTC] see Acetaminophen and Pseudoephedrine on page 24

Bayer® Select® Pain Relief Formula [OTC] *see Ibuprofen on page 495*

BCG Vaccine (bee see jee vak SEEN)
Brand Names TheraCys™; TICE® BCG
Therapeutic Category Biological Response Modulator; Vaccine, Live Bacteria
Synonyms Bacillus Calmette-Guérin (BCG) Live
Use BCG vaccine is no longer recommended for adults at high risk for tuberculosis in the United States. BCG vaccination may be considered for infants and children who are skin test-negative to 5 tuberculin units of tuberculin and who cannot be given isoniazid preventive therapy but have close contact with untreated or ineffectively treated active tuberculosis patients or who belong to groups which other control measures have not been successful.

In the United States, tuberculosis control efforts are directed toward early identification, treatment of cases, and preventive therapy with isoniazid.
Usual Dosage Children >1 month and Adults:
Immunization against tuberculosis: 0.2-0.3 mL percutaneous; initial lesion usually appears after 10-14 days consisting of small red papule at injection site and reaches maximum diameter of 3 mm in 4-6 weeks; conduct postvaccinal tuberculin test in 2-3 months; if test is negative, repeat vaccination
Immunotherapy for bladder cancer: TICE® BCG vaccine 6×10^8 viable organisms in 50 mL NS (preservative free) instilled into bladder and retained for 2 hours weekly for 6 weeks
Mechanism of Action BCG live is an attenuated strain of Bacillus Calmette-Guérin used as a biological response modifier; BCG live, when used intravesicular for treatment of bladder carcinoma *in situ*, is thought to cause a local, chronic inflammatory response involving macrophage and leukocyte infiltration of the bladder. By a mechanism not fully understood, this local inflammatory response leads to destruction of superficial tumor cells of the urothelium. Evidence of systemic immune response is also commonly seen, manifested by a positive PPD tuberculin skin test reaction, however, its relationship to clinical efficacy is not well-established. BCG is active immunotherapy which stimulates the host's immune mechanism to reject the tumor.
Local Anesthetic/Vasoconstrictor Precautions No information available to require special precautions
Effects on Dental Treatment No effects or complications reported
Other Adverse Effects
1% to 10%:
Genitourinary: Bladder infection, dysuria, prostatitis
Renal: Polyuria
Miscellaneous: Flu-like syndrome
<1%:
Dermatologic: Skin ulceration, abscesses
Renal: Hematuria
Miscellaneous: Rarely anaphylactic shock in infants, lymphadenitis, tuberculosis in immunosuppressed patients
Pregnancy Risk Factor C
Generic Available No
Comments
Live, attenuated vaccine
Live culture preparation of bacillus Calmette-Guérin (BCG) strain of *Mycobacterium bovis* and is a substrain of Pasteur Institute strain designed for use as active immunizing agent against tuberculosis

BCNU *see Carmustine on page 181*
B Complex *see Vitamins, Multiple on page 995*
B Complex With C *see Vitamins, Multiple on page 995*
B-D Glucose® [OTC] *see Glucose on page 444*

Becaplermin (be KAP ler min)
Brand Names Regranex®
Therapeutic Category Topical Skin Product
Use Treatment of diabetic ulcers that occur on the lower limbs and feet
Usual Dosage Adults: Topical: Apply once daily; applied with a cotton swab or similar tool, as a coating over the ulcer
Mechanism of Action A genetically engineered form of platelet-derived growth factor, a naturally occurring protein in the body that stimulates wound healing.
Local Anesthetic/Vasoconstrictor Precautions No information available to require special precautions
Effects on Dental Treatment No effects or complications reported
Dosage Forms Gel, topical: 0.01%

Because® [OTC] *see Nonoxynol 9 on page 689*

Beclometasona (Mexico) *see* Beclomethasone *on this page*

Beclomethasone (be kloe METH a sone)

Related Information
Respiratory Diseases *on page 1018*

Brand Names Beclovent®; Beconase®; Beconase AQ®; Vancenase®; Vancenase® AQ; Vanceril®

Canadian/Mexican Brand Names Aerobec® (Mexico); Beclodisk® (Canada); Becloforte® (Canada); Beconase® Aqua (Mexico); Becotide® 100 (Mexico); Becotide® 250 (Mexico); Becotide® Aerosol (Mexico); Propaderm® (Canada)

Therapeutic Category Anti-inflammatory Agent; Corticosteroid, Inhalant

Synonyms Beclometasona (Mexico)

Use
Oral inhalation: Treatment of bronchial asthma in patients who require chronic administration of corticosteroids

Nasal aerosol: Symptomatic treatment of seasonal or perennial rhinitis and nasal polyposis

Usual Dosage Nasal inhalation and oral inhalation dosage forms are not to be used interchangeably

Nasal:
Children 6-12 years: 1 spray in each nostril 3 times/day
Adults: 1 spray in each nostril 2-4 times/day

Oral inhalation:
Children 6-12 years: 1-2 inhalations 3-4 times/day; alternatively 2-4 inhalations twice daily; do not exceed 10 inhalations/day
Adults: 2 inhalations 3-4 times/day; alternatively 2-4 inhalations twice daily; do not exceed 20 inhalations/day; patients with severe asthma should be started on 12-16 inhalations/day (divided 3-4 times/day) and dose should be adjusted downward according to the patient's response

Mechanism of Action Controls the rate of protein synthesis, depresses the migration of polymorphonuclear leukocytes, fibroblasts, reverses capillary permeability, and lysosomal stabilization at the cellular level to prevent or control inflammation

Local Anesthetic/Vasoconstrictor Precautions No information available to require special precautions

Effects on Dental Treatment Localized infections with *Candida albicans* or *Aspergillus niger* have occurred frequently in the mouth and pharynx with repetitive use of oral inhaler of beclomethasone. Positive cultures for oral *Candida* may be present in up to 75% of patients. These infections may require treatment with appropriate antifungal therapy or discontinuance of treatment with beclomethasone inhaler.

Other Adverse Effects
>10%:
Local: Growth of *Candida* in the mouth, irritation and burning of the nasal mucosa
Respiratory: Cough, hoarseness
1% to 10%:
Gastrointestinal: Dry mouth
Respiratory: Epistaxis, nasal ulceration
<1%:
Central nervous system: Headache
Dermatologic: Skin rash
Gastrointestinal: Dysphagia
Respiratory: Bronchospasm, rhinorrhea, nasal congestion, sneezing, nasal septal perforations

Drug Interactions No data reported

Drug Uptake
Therapeutic effect: Within 1-4 weeks of use
Inhalation:
Absorption: Readily absorbed; quickly hydrolyzed by pulmonary esterases prior to absorption
Absorption: 90%
Serum half-life:
Initial: 3 hours
Terminal: 15 hours

Pregnancy Risk Factor C

Generic Available No

Beclovent® *see* Beclomethasone *on this page*
Beconase® *see* Beclomethasone *on this page*
Beconase AQ® *see* Beclomethasone *on this page*

Becotin® Pulvules® *see* Vitamins, Multiple *on page 995*

Beepen-VK® *see* Penicillin V Potassium *on page 734*

Belix® Oral [OTC] *see* Diphenhydramine *on page 323*

Belladonna (bel a DON a)

Therapeutic Category Anticholinergic Agent; Antispasmodic Agent, Gastrointestinal

Use Decrease gastrointestinal activity in functional bowel disorders and to delay gastric emptying as well as decrease gastric secretion

Mechanism of Action Belladonna is a mixture of the anticholinergic alkaloids atropine, hyoscyamine, and scopolamine (hyoscine). The belladonna alkaloids act primarily by competitive inhibition of the muscarinic actions of acetylcholine on structures innervated by postganglionic cholinergic neurons and on smooth muscle. The resulting effects include antisecretory activity on exocrine glands and intestinal mucosa and smooth muscle relaxation. The anticholinergic properties of scopolamine and atropine differ in that scopolamine has a more potent activity on the iris, ciliary body, and certain secretory glands; has more potent activity on the heart, intestine, and bronchial muscle, and a more prolonged duration of action; in contrast, hyoscyamine has actions similar to those of atropine, but is more potent in both its central and peripheral effects

Local Anesthetic/Vasoconstrictor Precautions No information available to require special precautions

Effects on Dental Treatment >10% of patients experience dry mouth

Other Adverse Effects

>10%:

Dermatologic: Dry skin

Gastrointestinal: Constipation

Respiratory: Dry nose, throat

Miscellaneous: Decreased sweating

1% to 10%:

Dermatologic: Increased photosensitivity

Endocrine & metabolic: Decreased flow of breast milk

Gastrointestinal: Dysphagia

<1%:

Cardiovascular: Ventricular fibrillation, tachycardia, palpitations, orthostatic hypotension

Central nervous system: Confusion, drowsiness, headache, loss of memory, fatigue, ataxia

Dermatologic: Skin rash

Gastrointestinal: Bloated feeling, nausea, vomiting

Genitourinary: Dysuria

Neuromuscular & skeletal: Weakness

Ocular: Increased intraocular pain, blurred vision

Pregnancy Risk Factor C

Generic Available Yes

Belladonna and Opium (bel a DON a & OH pee um)

Brand Names B&O Supprettes®

Canadian/Mexican Brand Names PMS-Opium & Beladonna (Canada)

Therapeutic Category Analgesic, Narcotic

Use Relief of moderate to severe pain associated with rectal or bladder tenesmus that may occur in postoperative states and neoplastic situations; pain associated with ureteral spasms not responsive to non-narcotic analgesics and to space intervals between injections of opiates

Usual Dosage Adults: Rectal: 1 suppository 1-2 times/day, up to 4 doses/day

Mechanism of Action Anticholinergic alkaloids act primarily by competitive inhibition of the muscarinic actions of acetylcholine on structures innervated by postganglionic cholinergic neurons and on smooth muscle; resulting effects include antisecretory activity on exocrine glands and intestinal mucosa and smooth muscle relaxation. The opium component contains many narcotic alkaloids including morphine; its mechanism for gastric motility inhibition is primarily due to this morphine content; it results in a decrease in digestive secretions, an increase in GI muscle tone, and therefore a reduction in GI propulsion.

Local Anesthetic/Vasoconstrictor Precautions No information available to require special precautions

Effects on Dental Treatment This drug has atropine-like effects and the patient may experience drowsiness, dry mouth, nose and throat

Other Adverse Effects

>10%:

Dermatologic: Dry skin

Gastrointestinal: Constipation, dry mouth

(Continued)

Belladonna and Opium *(Continued)*

   Respiratory: Dry nose, throat
   Miscellaneous: Decreased sweating
  1% to 10%:
   Dermatologic: Photosensitivity
   Endocrine & metabolic: Decreased flow of breast milk
   Gastrointestinal: Dysphagia
  <1%:
   Cardiovascular: Orthostatic hypotension, ventricular fibrillation, tachycardia, palpitations
   Central nervous system: Confusion, drowsiness, headache, loss of memory, fatigue, ataxia, CNS depression
   Dermatologic: Skin rash
   Endocrine & metabolic: Antidiuretic hormone release
   Gastrointestinal: Bloated feeling, nausea, vomiting, constipation, biliary tract spasm
   Genitourinary: Dysuria, urinary retention, urinary tract spasm
   Neuromuscular & skeletal: Weakness
   Ocular: Increased intraocular pain, blurred vision
   Respiratory: Respiratory depression
   Miscellaneous: Histamine release, physical and psychological dependence, sweating
Drug Interactions Increased effect/toxicity: CNS depressants, tricyclic antidepressants
Drug Uptake
  Onset of action:
   Belladonna: 1-2 hours
   Opium: Within 30 minutes
Pregnancy Risk Factor C
Dosage Forms Suppository:
  #15 A: Belladonna extract 15 mg and opium 30 mg
  #16 A: Belladonna extract 15 mg and opium 60 mg
Generic Available Yes

Belladonna, Phenobarbital, and Ergotamine Tartrate

  (bel a DON a, fee noe BAR bi tal, & er GOT a meen TAR trate)
Brand Names Bellergal-S®; Bel-Phen-Ergot S®; Phenerbel-S®
Therapeutic Category Ergot Alkaloid
Use Management and treatment of menopausal disorders, gastrointestinal disorders and recurrent throbbing headache
Local Anesthetic/Vasoconstrictor Precautions No information available to require special precautions
Effects on Dental Treatment >10% of patients experience dry mouth
Other Adverse Effects
  >10%:
   Cardiovascular: Peripheral vascular effects, local edema
   Central nervous system: Drowsiness, dizziness
   Dermatologic: Dry skin
   Gastrointestinal: Constipation, diarrhea, nausea, vomiting
   Local: Irritation at injection site
   Neuromuscular & skeletal: Paresthesia
   Respiratory: Dry nose, throat
   Miscellaneous: Decreased sweating
  1% to 10%:
   Cardiovascular: Precordial distress and pain, transient tachycardia or bradycardia
   Dermatologic: Photosensitivity
   Endocrine & metabolic: Decreased flow of breast milk
   Gastrointestinal: Dysphagia
   Neuromuscular & skeletal: Myalgia, weakness in the legs
  <1%:
   Cardiovascular: Orthostatic hypotension, ventricular fibrillation, tachycardia, palpitations
   Central nervous system: Confusion, headache, loss of memory, fatigue, ataxia
   Dermatologic: Skin rash
   Gastrointestinal: Bloated feeling, nausea, vomiting
   Genitourinary: Dysuria
   Neuromuscular & skeletal: Weakness
   Ocular: Increased intraocular pain, blurred vision
Drug Interactions CNS depressants
Pregnancy Risk Factor X

Generic Available Yes

Bellergal-S® *see* Belladonna, Phenobarbital, and Ergotamine Tartrate *on previous page*

Bel-Phen-Ergot S® *see* Belladonna, Phenobarbital, and Ergotamine Tartrate *on previous page*

Benadryl® Decongestant Allergy Tablet [OTC] *see* Diphenhydramine and Pseudo-ephedrine *on page 324*

Benadryl® Injection *see* Diphenhydramine *on page 323*

Benadryl® Oral [OTC] *see* Diphenhydramine *on page 323*

Benadryl® Topical *see* Diphenhydramine *on page 323*

Ben-Allergin-50® Injection *see* Diphenhydramine *on page 323*

Ben-Aqua® [OTC] *see* Benzoyl Peroxide *on page 120*

Benazepril (ben AY ze pril)
Related Information
Cardiovascular Diseases *on page 1010*
Brand Names Lotensin®
Therapeutic Category Angiotensin-Converting Enzyme (ACE) Inhibitors
Synonyms Benazepril Clorhidrato De (Mexico)
Use Treatment of hypertension, either alone or in combination with other antihypertensive agents
Usual Dosage Adults: Oral: 20-40 mg/day as a single dose or 2 divided doses; maximum daily dose: 80 mg
Mechanism of Action Competitive inhibition of angiotensin I being converted to angiotensin II, a potent vasoconstrictor, through the angiotensin I-converting enzyme (ACE) activity, with resultant lower levels of angiotensin II which causes an increase in plasma renin activity and a reduction in aldosterone secretion
Local Anesthetic/Vasoconstrictor Precautions No information available to require special precautions
Effects on Dental Treatment No effects or complications reported
Other Adverse Effects
1% to 10%:
Central nervous system: Headache, dizziness, fatigue, somnolence, postural dizziness
Gastrointestinal: Nausea
Respiratory: Transient cough
<1%:
Cardiovascular: Hypotension, tachycardia
Central nervous system: Anxiety, insomnia, nervousness
Dermatologic: Rash, photosensitivity, angioedema
Endocrine & metabolic: Hyperkalemia
Gastrointestinal: Constipation, gastritis, vomiting, melena
Genitourinary: Impotence, urinary tract infection
Neuromuscular & skeletal: Hypertonia, paresthesia, arthralgia, arthritis, myalgia, weakness
Respiratory: Asthma, bronchitis, dyspnea, sinusitis
Miscellaneous: Sweating

Drug-Drug Interactions With ACEIs

Precipitant Drug	Drug (Category) and Effect	Description
Antacids	ACE Inhibitors: decreased	Decreased bioavailability of ACEIs. May be more likely with captopril. Separate administration times by 1-2 hours.
NSAIDs (indomethacin)	ACEIs: decreased	Reduced hypotensive effects of ACEIs. More prominent in low renin or volume dependent hypertensive patients.
Phenothiazines	ACEIs: increased	Pharmacologic effects of ACEIs may be increased.
ACEIs	Allopurinol: increased	Higher risk of hypersensitivity reaction possible when given concurrently. Three case reports of Stevens-Johnson syndrome with captopril.
ACEIs	Digoxin: increased	Increased plasma digoxin levels.
ACEIs	Lithium: increased	Increased serum lithium levels and symptoms of toxicity may occur.
ACEIs	Potassium preps/ potassium sparing diuretics increased	Coadministration may result in elevated potassium levels.

(Continued)

Benazepril *(Continued)*

Drug Interactions See table.

Drug Uptake

Reduction in plasma angiotensin-converting enzyme activity: Oral:

Peak effect: 1-2 hours after administration of 2-20 mg dose

Duration of action: >90% inhibition for 24 hours has been observed after 5-20 mg dose

Reduction in blood pressure:

Peak effect after single oral dose: 2-6 hours

Maximum response With continuous therapy: 2 weeks

Absorption: Rapid (37% of each oral dose); food does not alter significantly; metabolite (benazeprilat) itself unsuitable for oral administration due to poor absorption

Serum half-life:

Parent drug: 0.6 hour

Metabolite elimination: 22 hours (from 24 hours after dosing onward)

Metabolite: 1.5-2 hours after fasting or 2-4 hours after a meal

Time to peak: 1-1.5 hours (unchanged parent drug)

Pregnancy Risk Factor C (first trimester); D (second and third trimesters)

Generic Available No

Benazepril and Hydrochlorothiazide

(ben AY ze pril & hye droe klor oh THYE a zide)

Brand Names Lotensin HCT®

Therapeutic Category Antihypertensive Agent, Combination

Use Treatment of hypertension

Usual Dosage Dose is individualized

Local Anesthetic/Vasoconstrictor Precautions No information available to require special precautions

Effects on Dental Treatment No effects or complications reported

Generic Available No

Benazepril Clorhidrato De (Mexico) *see Benazepril on previous page*

Bendroflumethiazide (ben droe floo meth EYE a zide)

Related Information

Cardiovascular Diseases *on page 1010*

Brand Names Naturetin®

Therapeutic Category Diuretic, Thiazide

Synonyms Bendroflumetiacida (Mexico)

Use Management of mild to moderate hypertension; treatment of edema associated with congestive heart failure, pregnancy, or nephrotic syndrome

Mechanism of Action Like other thiazide diuretics, it inhibits sodium, chloride, and water reabsorption in the renal distal tubules, thereby producing diuresis with a resultant reduction in plasma volume; hypothetically may reduce peripheral resistance through increased prostacyclin synthesis

Local Anesthetic/Vasoconstrictor Precautions No information available to require special precautions

Effects on Dental Treatment No effects or complications reported

Other Adverse Effects

1% to 10%:

Cardiovascular: Orthostatic hypotension

Endocrine & metabolic: Hyponatremia, hypokalemia

Gastrointestinal: Anorexia, gastritis, diarrhea

<1%:

Central nervous system: Somnolence

Endocrine & metabolic: Hyperuricemia

Gastrointestinal: Nausea, vomiting

Hematologic: Aplastic anemia, hemolytic anemia, leukopenia, agranulocytosis, thrombocytopenia

Hepatic: Hepatitis, hepatic function impairment

Neuromuscular & skeletal: Paresthesia

Renal: Polyuria, uremia

Miscellaneous: Allergic reactions

Drug Interactions

Thiazides tend to elevate blood glucose in diabetics and thus may antagonize the hypoglycemic effect of antidiabetic drugs.

GI tract absorption of thiazides are impaired by cholestyramine (Questran®) and colestipol (Colestid®).

Thiazides increase plasma lithium concentrations; lithium toxicity may occur

Pregnancy Risk Factor D

Generic Available Yes

Bendroflumetiacida (Mexico) *see* Bendroflumethiazide *on previous page*

Benemid® *see* Probenecid *on page 795*

Benoquin® *see* Monobenzone *on page 647*

Benoxyl® *see* Benzoyl Peroxide *on page 120*

Bentiromide (ben TEER oh mide)

Brand Names Chymex®

Therapeutic Category Diagnostic Agent, Pancreatic Exocrine Insufficiency

Synonyms BTPABA

Use Screening test for pancreatic exocrine insufficiency

Usual Dosage Oral:

Children 6-12 years: 14 mg/kg (maximum dose: 500 mg) followed with 8 oz of water immediately and 2 hours postdosing and an additional 16 oz of water during hours 2-6 postdosing

Children >12 years and Adults: Administer following an overnight fast and morning void, single 500 mg dose and follow with 8 oz of water immediately and 2 hours postdosing and an additional 16 oz of water during hours 2-6 postdosing

Mechanism of Action Cleaved by the pancreatic enzyme chymotrypsin causing a release of para-aminobenzoic acid (PABA), percentage of PABA metabolites recovered in urine reflects enzymatic activity of chymotrypsin providing a way of determining pancreatic function

Local Anesthetic/Vasoconstrictor Precautions No information available to require special precautions

Effects on Dental Treatment No effects or complications reported

Other Adverse Effects

1% to 10%:

Central nervous system: Headache

Gastrointestinal: Diarrhea

<1%:

Central nervous system: Drowsiness

Gastrointestinal: Flatulence, nausea, vomiting, heartburn

Hepatic: Elevations in liver function tests

Neuromuscular & skeletal: Weakness

Drug Uptake

Time to peak serum concentration: Oral: Within 2-3 hours

Pregnancy Risk Factor B

Generic Available No

Bentoquatam (ben to KWA tam)

Brand Names IvyBlock®

Therapeutic Category Protectant, Topical

Use To protect the skin from rash due to exposure to poison sumac, poison ivy or poison oak

Usual Dosage Topical: Apply to exposed skin at least 15 minutes before potential contact and reapply every 4 hours

Local Anesthetic/Vasoconstrictor Precautions No information available to require special precautions

Effects on Dental Treatment No effects or complications reported

Dosage Forms Lotion: 5% (120 mL)

Generic Available No

Bentyl® Hydrochloride Injection *see* Dicyclomine *on page 307*

Bentyl® Hydrochloride Oral *see* Dicyclomine *on page 307*

Benylin® Cough Syrup [OTC] *see* Diphenhydramine *on page 323*

Benylin DM® [OTC] *see* Dextromethorphan *on page 298*

Benylin® Expectorant [OTC] *see* Guaifenesin and Dextromethorphan *on page 453*

Benylin® Pediatric [OTC] *see* Dextromethorphan *on page 298*

Benza® [OTC] *see* Benzalkonium Chloride *on next page*

Benzac AC® Gel *see* Benzoyl Peroxide *on page 120*

Benzac AC® Wash *see* Benzoyl Peroxide *on page 120*

Benzac W® Gel *see* Benzoyl Peroxide *on page 120*

Benzac W® Wash *see* Benzoyl Peroxide *on page 120*

5-Benzagel® *see* Benzoyl Peroxide *on page 120*

10-Benzagel® *see* Benzoyl Peroxide *on page 120*

Benzalkonium Chloride (benz al KOE nee um KLOR ide)
Brand Names Benza® [OTC]; Zephiran® [OTC]
Therapeutic Category Antibacterial, Topical
Synonyms BAC
Use Surface antiseptic and germicidal preservative
Local Anesthetic/Vasoconstrictor Precautions No information available to require special precautions
Effects on Dental Treatment No effects or complications reported
Other Adverse Effects 1% to 10%: Hypersensitivity
Pregnancy Risk Factor C
Generic Available Yes

Benzamycin® *see* Erythromycin and Benzoyl Peroxide *on page 363*
Benzashave® Cream *see* Benzoyl Peroxide *on page 120*
Benzedrex® [OTC] *see* Propylhexedrine *on page 816*
Benzmethyzin *see* Procarbazine *on page 798*

Benzocaine (BEN zoe kane)
Related Information
  Mouth Pain, Cold Sore, Canker Sore Products *on page 1183*
Brand Names Americaine [OTC]; Anbesol® [OTC]; Anbesol® Maximum Strength [OTC]; Babee Teething® [OTC]; Benzocol® [OTC]; Benzodent® [OTC]; Chiggertox® [OTC]; Cylex® [OTC]; Dermoplast® [OTC]; Foille® [OTC]; Foille® Medicated First Aid [OTC]; Hurricaine®; Lanacane® [OTC]; Maximum Strength Anbesol® [OTC]; Maximum Strength Orajel® [OTC]; Mycinettes® [OTC]; Numzitdent® [OTC]; Numzit Teething® [OTC]; Orabase®-B [OTC]; Orabase®-O [OTC]; Orajel® Brace-Aid Oral Anesthetic [OTC]; Orajel® Maximum Strength [OTC]; Orajel® Mouth-Aid [OTC]; Orasept® [OTC]; Orasol® [OTC]; Rhulicaine® [OTC]; Rid-A-Pain® [OTC]; Slim-Mint® [OTC]; Solarcaine® [OTC]; Spec-T® [OTC]; Tanac® [OTC]; Trocaine® [OTC]; Unguentine® [OTC]; Vicks Children's Chloraseptic® [OTC]; Vicks Chloraseptic® Sore Throat [OTC]; Zilactin-B® Medicated [OTC]; ZilaDent® [OTC]
Canadian/Mexican Brand Names Graneodin-B® (Mexico)
Therapeutic Category Local Anesthetic, Topical
Use
  Dental: Ester-type local anesthetic for temporary relief of pain associated with toothache, minor sore throat pain and canker sore
  Medical: Local anesthetic (ester derivative); temporary relief of pain associated with pruritic dermatosis, pruritus, minor burns, acute congestive and serious otitis media, swimmer's ear, otitis externa, hemorrhoids, rectal fissures, anesthetic lubricant for passage of catheters and endoscopic tubes
Usual Dosage Children and Adults:
  Mucous membranes: Dosage varies depending on area to be anesthetized and vascularity of tissues
  Oral mouth/throat preparations: Do not administer for >2 days or in children <2 years of age, unless directed by a physician; refer to specific package labeling
Mechanism of Action Local anesthetics bind selectively to the intracellular surface of sodium channels to block influx of sodium into the axon. As a result, depolarization necessary for action potential propagation and subsequent nerve function is prevented. The block at the sodium channel is reversible. When drug diffuses away from the axon, sodium channel function is restored and nerve propagation returns.
Local Anesthetic/Vasoconstrictor Precautions No information available to require special precautions
Effects on Dental Treatment No effects or complications reported
Other Adverse Effects 1% to 10%:
  Dermatologic: Angioedema, contact dermatitis
  Local: Burning, stinging
Contraindications Known hypersensitivity to benzocaine, other ester-type local anesthetics, or other components in the formulation; ophthalmic use
Warnings/Precautions Not intended for use when infections are present
Drug Interactions May antagonize actions of sulfonamides
Drug Uptake
  Onset: ~1 minute
  Duration: 15-20 minutes
  Absorption: Topical: Poorly absorbed after administration to intact skin, but well absorbed from mucous membranes and traumatized skin
Pregnancy Risk Factor C
Breast-feeding Considerations No data reported

Dosage Forms
Mouth/throat preparations:
Cream: 5% (10 g)
Gel: 6.3% (7.5 g); 7.5% (7.2 g, 9.45 g, 14.1 g); 10% (6 g, 9.45 g, 10 g, 15 g); 15% (10.5 g); 20% (9.45 g, 14.1 g)
Liquid: (3.7 mL); 5% (8.8 mL); 6.3% (9 mL, 22 mL, 14.79 mL); 10% (13 mL); 20% (13.3 mL)
Lotion: 0.2% (15 mL); 2.5% (15 mL)
Lozenges: 5 mg, 6 mg, 10 mg, 15 mg
Ointment: 20% (5 g, 15 g)
Topical for mucous membranes:
Gel: 6% (7.5 g); 20% (2.5 g, 3.75 g, 7.5 g, 30 g)
Liquid: 20% (3.75 mL, 9 mL, 13.3 mL, 30 mL)
Generic Available Yes

Benzocaine and Antipyrine *see* Antipyrine and Benzocaine *on page 82*

Benzocaine and Cetylpyridinium Chloride *see* Cetylpyridinium and Benzocaine *on page 206*

Benzocaine, Butyl Aminobenzoate, Tetracaine, and Benzalkonium Chloride

(BEN zoe kane, BYOO til a meen oh BENZ oh ate, TET ra kane, & benz al KOE nee um KLOR ide)
Brand Names Cetacaine®
Therapeutic Category Local Anesthetic, Topical
Synonyms Tetracaine Hydrochloride, Benzocaine Butyl Aminobenzoate and Benzalkonium Chloride
Use Topical anesthetic to control pain or gagging
Usual Dosage Apply to affected area for approximately 1 second or less
Local Anesthetic/Vasoconstrictor Precautions No information available to require special precautions
Effects on Dental Treatment No effects or complications reported
Other Adverse Effects Dose related and may result from high plasma levels
1% to 10%:
Dermatologic: Contact dermatitis, angioedema
Local: Burning, stinging
<1%:
Cardiovascular: Edema
Dermatologic: Urticaria
Genitourinary: Urethritis
Hematologic: Methemoglobinemia in infants
Local: Tenderness
Pregnancy Risk Factor C
Generic Available No

Benzocaine, Gelatin, Pectin, and Sodium Carboxymethylcellulose

(BEN zoe kane, JEL a tin, PEK tin, & SOW dee um kar box ee meth il SEL yoo lose)
Brand Names Orabase® With Benzocaine [OTC]
Therapeutic Category Local Anesthetic, Topical
Use Topical anesthetic and emollient for oral lesions
Local Anesthetic/Vasoconstrictor Precautions No information available to require special precautions
Effects on Dental Treatment No effects or complications reported
Other Adverse Effects Dose related and may result from high plasma levels
1% to 10%:
Dermatologic: Contact dermatitis, angioedema
Local: Burning, stinging
<1%:
Cardiovascular: Edema
Dermatologic: Urticaria
Gastrointestinal: Urethritis
Hematologic: Methemoglobinemia in infants
Local: Tenderness
Pregnancy Risk Factor C
Generic Available No

Benzocol® [OTC] *see* Benzocaine *on previous page*
Benzodent® [OTC] *see* Benzocaine *on previous page*

Benzoic Acid and Salicylic Acid
(ben ZOE ik AS id & sal i SIL ik AS id)
Brand Names Whitfield's Ointment [OTC]
Therapeutic Category Antifungal Agent, Topical
Synonyms Salicylic Acid and Benzoic Acid
Use Treatment of athlete's foot and ringworm of the scalp
Local Anesthetic/Vasoconstrictor Precautions No information available to require special precautions
Effects on Dental Treatment No effects or complications reported
Generic Available Yes

Benzoin (BEN zoyn)
Brand Names AeroZoin® [OTC]; TinBen® [OTC]; TinCoBen® [OTC]
Therapeutic Category Pharmaceutical Aid; Protectant, Topical
Synonyms Gum Benjamin
Use Protective application for irritations of the skin; sometimes used in boiling water as steam inhalants for their expectorant and soothing action
Local Anesthetic/Vasoconstrictor Precautions No information available to require special precautions
Effects on Dental Treatment No effects or complications reported
Generic Available Yes

Benzonatate (ben ZOE na tate)
Related Information
Patients Undergoing Cancer Therapy *on page 1083*
Brand Names Tessalon® Perles
Canadian/Mexican Brand Names Beknol® (Mexico); Pebegal® (Mexico); Tesalon® (Mexico)
Therapeutic Category Antitussive; Local Anesthetic, Oral
Synonyms Benzonatato (Mexico)
Use Symptomatic relief of nonproductive cough
Usual Dosage Children >10 years and Adults: Oral: 100 mg 3 times/day or every 4 hours up to 600 mg/day
Mechanism of Action Tetracaine congener with antitussive properties; suppresses cough by topical anesthetic action on the respiratory stretch receptors
Local Anesthetic/Vasoconstrictor Precautions No information available to require special precautions
Effects on Dental Treatment No effects or complications reported
Other Adverse Effects 1% to 10%:
Central nervous system: Sedation, headache, dizziness
Dermatologic: Skin rash
Gastrointestinal: GI upset
Neuromuscular & skeletal: Numbness in chest
Ocular: Burning sensation in eyes
Respiratory: Nasal congestion
Drug Interactions No data reported
Drug Uptake
Onset of action: Therapeutic: Within 15-20 minutes
Duration: 3-8 hours
Pregnancy Risk Factor C
Generic Available Yes

Benzonatato (Mexico) *see* Benzonatate *on this page*

Benzoyl Peroxide (BEN zoe il peer OKS ide)
Brand Names Advanced Formula Oxy® Sensitive Gel [OTC]; Ambi 10® [OTC]; Ben-Aqua® [OTC]; Benoxyl®; Benzac AC® Gel; Benzac AC® Wash; Benzac W® Gel; Benzac W® Wash; 5-Benzagel®; 10-Benzagel®; Benzashave® Cream; BlemErase® Lotion [OTC]; Brevoxyl® Gel; Clear By Design® Gel [OTC]; Clearsil® Maximum Strength [OTC]; Del Aqua-5® Gel; Del Aqua-10® Gel; Desquam-E® Gel; Desquam-X® Gel; Desquam-X® Wash; Dryox® Gel [OTC]; Dryox® Wash [OTC]; Exact® Cream [OTC]; Fostex® 10% BPO Gel [OTC]; Fostex® 10% Wash [OTC]; Fostex® Bar [OTC]; Loroxide® [OTC]; Neutrogena® Acne Mask [OTC]; Oxy-5® Advanced Formula for Sensitive Skin [OTC]; Oxy-5® Tinted [OTC]; Oxy-10® Advanced Formula for Sensitive Skin [OTC]; Oxy 10® Wash [OTC]; PanOxyl®-AQ; PanOxyl® Bar [OTC]; Perfectoderm® Gel [OTC]; Peroxin A5®; Peroxin A10®; Persa-Gel®; Theroxide® Wash [OTC]; Vanoxide® [OTC]
Canadian/Mexican Brand Names Acetoxyl® (Canada); Acnomel® B.P.5 (Canada); H₂Oxyl® (Canada); Oxyderm® (Canada); Solugel® (Canada)
Therapeutic Category Acne Products; Topical Skin Product

Use Adjunctive treatment of mild to moderate acne vulgaris and acne rosacea

Usual Dosage Children and Adults:

Cleansers: Wash once or twice daily; control amount of drying or peeling by modifying dose frequency or concentration

Topical: Apply sparingly once daily; gradually increase to 2-3 times/day if needed. If excessive dryness or peeling occurs, reduce dose frequency or concentration; if excessive stinging or burning occurs, remove with mild soap and water; resume use the next day.

Mechanism of Action Releases free-radical oxygen which oxidizes bacterial proteins in the sebaceous follicles decreasing the number of anaerobic bacteria and decreasing irritating-type free fatty acids

Local Anesthetic/Vasoconstrictor Precautions No information available to require special precautions

Effects on Dental Treatment No effects or complications reported

Other Adverse Effects 1% to 10%: Dermatologic: Irritation, contact dermatitis, dryness, erythema, peeling, stinging

Drug Interactions Increased toxicity: Benzoyl peroxide potentiates adverse reactions seen with tretinoin

Drug Uptake

Absorption: ~5% through the skin; gels are more penetrating than creams

Pregnancy Risk Factor C

Generic Available Yes

Benzoyl Peroxide and Hydrocortisone

(BEN zoe il peer OKS ide & hye droe KOR ti sone)

Brand Names Vanoxide-HC®

Therapeutic Category Acne Products; Corticosteroid, Topical (Low Potency); Topical Skin Product

Use Treatment of acne vulgaris and oily skin

Usual Dosage Shake well; apply thin film 1-3 times/day, gently massage into skin

Local Anesthetic/Vasoconstrictor Precautions No information available to require special precautions

Effects on Dental Treatment No effects or complications reported

Other Adverse Effects See individual agents

Pregnancy Risk Factor C

Generic Available No

Benzphetamine (benz FET a meen)

Brand Names Didrex®

Therapeutic Category Anorexiant

Use Short-term adjunct in exogenous obesity

Usual Dosage Adults: Oral: 25-50 mg 2-3 times/day, preferably twice daily, midmorning and midafternoon; maximum dose: 50 mg 3 times/day

Mechanism of Action Noncatechol sympathomimetic amines with pharmacologic actions similar to ephedrine; require breakdown by monoamine oxidase for inactivation; produce central nervous system and respiratory stimulation, a pressor response, mydriasis, bronchodilation, and contraction of the urinary sphincter; thought to have a direct effect on both alpha- and beta-receptor sites in the peripheral system, as well as release stores of norepinephrine in adrenergic nerve terminals; central nervous system action is thought to occur in the cerebral cortex and reticular-activating system; anorexigenic effect is probably secondary to the CNS-stimulating effect; the site of action is probably the hypothalamic feeding center

Local Anesthetic/Vasoconstrictor Precautions Use with caution since amphetamines have actions similar to epinephrine and norepinephrine

Effects on Dental Treatment No effects or complications reported

Other Adverse Effects

>10%:

Cardiovascular: Arrhythmia

Central nervous system: False feeling of well being, nervousness, restlessness, insomnia

1% to 10%:

Cardiovascular: Hypertension

Central nervous system: Mood or mental changes, dizziness, lightheadedness, headache

Endocrine & metabolic: Changes in libido

Gastrointestinal: Diarrhea, nausea, vomiting, stomach cramps, constipation, anorexia, weight loss, dry mouth

Ocular: Blurred vision

Miscellaneous: Increased sweating

(Continued)

Benzphetamine *(Continued)*

<1%:
Cardiovascular: Chest pain
Central nervous system: CNS stimulation (severe), Tourette's syndrome, hyperthermia, seizures, paranoia, tolerance and withdrawal with prolonged use
Dermatologic: Skin rash, urticaria

Pregnancy Risk Factor X
Generic Available No

Benzthiazide (benz THYE a zide)

Related Information
Cardiovascular Diseases *on page 1010*
Brand Names Exna®
Therapeutic Category Diuretic, Thiazide
Use Management of mild to moderate hypertension; treatment of edema in congestive heart failure and nephrotic syndrome
Usual Dosage Oral:
Children: 1-4 mg/kg/day in 3 divided doses
Adults: 50-200 mg/day
Mechanism of Action Like other thiazide diuretics, it inhibits sodium, chloride, and water reabsorption in the renal distal tubules, thereby producing diuresis with a resultant reduction in plasma volume; hypothetically may reduce peripheral resistance through increased prostacyclin synthesis
Local Anesthetic/Vasoconstrictor Precautions No information available to require special precautions
Effects on Dental Treatment No effects or complications reported
Other Adverse Effects
1% to 10%:
Cardiovascular: Orthostatic hypotension
Endocrine & metabolic: Hyponatremia, hypokalemia
Gastrointestinal: Anorexia, upset stomach, diarrhea
<1%:
Central nervous system: Drowsiness
Endocrine & metabolic: Hyperuricemia
Gastrointestinal: Nausea, vomiting
Hematologic: Aplastic anemia, hemolytic anemia, leukopenia, agranulocytosis, thrombocytopenia
Hepatic: Hepatitis, hepatic function impairment
Neuromuscular & skeletal: Paresthesia
Renal: Polyuria, uremia
Miscellaneous: Allergic reactions
Drug Interactions
Thiazides tend to elevate blood glucose in diabetics and thus may antagonize the hypoglycemic effect of antidiabetic drugs.
GI tract absorption of thiazides are impaired by cholestyramine (Questran®) and colestipol (Colestid®).
Thiazides increase plasma lithium concentrations; lithium toxicity may occur.
Drug Uptake
Onset of action: Within 2 hours
Duration: 12 hours
Pregnancy Risk Factor D
Generic Available Yes

Benztropine (BENZ troe peen)

Brand Names Cogentin®
Canadian/Mexican Brand Names PMS-Benztropine® (Canada)
Therapeutic Category Anticholinergic Agent; Anti-Parkinson's Agent
Use Adjunctive treatment of Parkinson's disease; also used in treatment of drug-induced extrapyramidal effects (except tardive dyskinesia) and acute dystonic reactions
Usual Dosage Use in children <3 years of age should be reserved for life-threatening emergencies
Drug-induced extrapyramidal reaction: Oral, I.M., I.V.:
Children >3 years: 0.02-0.05 mg/kg/dose 1-2 times/day
Adults: 1-4 mg/dose 1-2 times/day

Acute dystonia: Adults: I.M., I.V.: 1-2 mg
Parkinsonism: Oral:
Adults: 0.5-6 mg/day in 1-2 divided doses; if one dose is greater, give at bedtime; titrate dose in 0.5 mg increments at 5- to 6-day intervals

Elderly: Initial: 0.5 mg once or twice daily; increase by 0.5 mg as needed at 5-6 days; maximum: 6 mg/day

Mechanism of Action Thought to partially block striatal cholinergic receptors to help balance cholinergic and dopaminergic activity

Local Anesthetic/Vasoconstrictor Precautions No information available to require special precautions

Effects on Dental Treatment Dry mouth, nose and throat very prevalent in patients taking this drug

Other Adverse Effects
>10%:
Dermatologic: Dry skin
Gastrointestinal: Constipation
Respiratory: Dry nose, throat
Miscellaneous: Decreased sweating
1% to 10%:
Dermatologic: Photosensitivity
Endocrine & metabolic: Decreased flow of breast milk
Gastrointestinal: Dysphagia
<1%:
Cardiovascular: Coma, tachycardia, orthostatic hypotension, ventricular fibrillation, palpitations
Central nervous system: Drowsiness, nervousness, hallucinations; the elderly may be at increased risk for confusion and hallucinations, headache, loss of memory, fatigue, ataxia
Dermatologic: Skin rash
Gastrointestinal: Nausea, vomiting, bloated feeling
Genitourinary: Dysuria
Neuromuscular & skeletal: Weakness
Ocular: Blurred vision, mydriasis, increased intraocular pain

Drug Interactions
Decreased effect: May increase gastric degradation of levodopa and decrease the amount of levodopa absorbed by delaying gastric emptying - the opposite may be true for digoxin
Increased toxicity: Central anticholinergic syndrome can occur when administered with narcotic analgesics, phenothiazines and other antipsychotics, tricyclic antidepressants, quinidine and some other antiarrhythmics, and antihistamines

Drug Uptake
Onset of action:
Oral: Within 1 hour
Parenteral: Within 15 minutes
Duration of action: 6-48 hours (wide range)

Pregnancy Risk Factor C

Generic Available Yes: Tablet

Benzylpenicilloyl-polylysine (BEN zil pen i SIL oyl pol i LIE seen)

Brand Names Pre-Pen®

Therapeutic Category Diagnostic Agent, Penicillin Allergy Skin Test

Use Adjunct in assessing the risk of administering penicillin (penicillin or benzylpenicillin) in adults with a history of clinical penicillin hypersensitivity

Usual Dosage PPL is administered by a scratch technique or by intradermal injection. For initial testing, PPL should always be applied via the scratch technique. **Do not give intradermally to patients who have positive reactions to a scratch test.** PPL test alone does not identify those patients who react to a minor antigenic determinant and does not appear to predict reliably the occurrence of late reactions.

Scratch test: Use scratch technique with a 20-gauge needle to make 3-5 mm nonbleeding scratch on epidermis, apply a small drop of solution to scratch, rub in gently with applicator or toothpick. A positive reaction consists of a pale wheal surrounding the scratch site which develops within 10 minutes and ranges from 5-15 mm or more in diameter.

Intradermal test: Use intradermal test with a tuberculin syringe with a 26- to 30-gauge short bevel needle; a dose of 0.01-0.02 mL is injected intradermally. A control of 0.9% sodium chloride should be injected at least 1.5" from the PPL test site. Most skin responses to the intradermal test will develop within 5-15 minutes.

Interpretation:
(-) Negative: No reaction
(±) Ambiguous: Wheal only slightly larger than original bleb with or without erythematous flare and larger than control site
(+) Positive: Itching and marked increase in size of original bleb
Control site should be reactionless

(Continued)

Benzylpenicilloyl-polylysine *(Continued)*

Mechanism of Action Elicits IgE antibodies which produce type I accelerate urticarial reactions to penicillins

Local Anesthetic/Vasoconstrictor Precautions No information available to require special precautions

Effects on Dental Treatment No effects or complications reported

Other Adverse Effects
1% to 10%: Local: Intense local inflammatory response at skin test site
<1%:
Cardiovascular: Local edema
Local: Pruritus, erythema, wheal, urticaria
Miscellaneous: Systemic allergic reactions occur rarely

Drug Interactions Decreased effect: Corticosteroids and other immunosuppressive agents may inhibit the immune response to the skin test

Pregnancy Risk Factor C

Generic Available No

Bepridil *(BE pri dil)*

Related Information
Calcium Channel Blockers & Gingival Hyperplasia *on page 1132*
Cardiovascular Diseases *on page 1010*

Brand Names Vascor®

Canadian/Mexican Brand Names Bapadin® (Canada)

Therapeutic Category Antianginal Agent; Calcium Channel Blocker

Use Treatment of chronic stable angina; due to side effect profile, reserve for patients who have been intolerant of other antianginal therapy; bepridil may be used alone or in combination with nitrates or beta-blockers

Usual Dosage Adults: Oral: Initial: 200 mg/day, then adjust dose at 10-day intervals until optimal response is achieved; maximum daily dose: 400 mg

Mechanism of Action Bepridil, a type 4 calcium antagonist, possesses characteristics of the traditional calcium antagonist, inhibiting calcium ion from entering the "slow channels" or select voltage-sensitive areas of vascular smooth muscle and myocardium during depolarization and producing a relaxation of coronary vascular smooth muscle and coronary vasodilation. However, bepridil may also inhibit fast sodium channels (inward) which may account for some of its side effects (eg, arrhythmias); a direct bradycardia effect of bepridil has been postulated via direct action on the S-A node.

Local Anesthetic/Vasoconstrictor Precautions No information available to require special precautions

Effects on Dental Treatment Other drugs of this class can cause gingival hyperplasia (ie, nifedipine) but there have been no reports for bepridil

Other Adverse Effects
>10%:
Central nervous system: Dizziness, headache
Gastrointestinal: Nausea, dyspepsia, abdominal pain, GI distress
Neuromuscular & skeletal: Weakness
1% to 10%:
Cardiovascular: Bradycardia, palpitations
Central nervous system: Nervousness
Gastrointestinal: Diarrhea, anorexia, dry mouth
Miscellaneous: Flu syndrome
<1%:
Cardiovascular: Ventricular premature contractions, hypertension, torsade de pointes, edema, syncope, prolonged Q-T intervals
Central nervous system: Fever, psychotic behavior, akathisia
Dermatologic: Rash
Endocrine & metabolic: Sexual dysfunction
Gastrointestinal: Taste change
Hematologic: Agranulocytosis
Neuromuscular & skeletal: Tremor, myalgia, arthritis
Ocular: Blurred vision
Respiratory: Nasal congestion, cough, pharyngitis
Miscellaneous: Sweating

Drug Interactions Bepridil increases digoxin serum concentrations by over 30% and enhances the cardiac effects of digoxin

Drug Uptake
Onset of action: 1 hour
Absorption: Oral: 100%
Serum half-life: 24 hours
Time to peak: 2-3 hours

Pregnancy Risk Factor C

Generic Available No

Beractant (ber AKT ant)

Brand Names Survanta®

Therapeutic Category Lung Surfactant

Use Prevention and treatment of respiratory distress syndrome (RDS) in premature infants

Prophylactic therapy: Body weight <1250 g in infants at risk for developing or with evidence of surfactant deficiency

Rescue therapy: Treatment of infants with RDS confirmed by x-ray and requiring mechanical ventilation (administer as soon as possible - within 8 hours of age)

Usual Dosage

Prophylactic treatment: Give 100 mg phospholipids (4 mL/kg) intratracheally as soon as possible; as many as 4 doses may be administered during the first 48 hours of life, no more frequently than 6 hours apart. The need for additional doses is determined by evidence of continuing respiratory distress; if the infant is still intubated and requiring at least 30% inspired oxygen to maintain a PAO_2 ≤80 torr.

Rescue treatment: Administer 100 mg phospholipids (4 mL/kg) as soon as the diagnosis of RDS is made

Mechanism of Action Replaces deficient or ineffective endogenous lung surfactant in neonates with respiratory distress syndrome (RDS) or in neonates at risk of developing RDS. Surfactant prevents the alveoli from collapsing during expiration by lowering surface tension between air and alveolar surfaces.

Local Anesthetic/Vasoconstrictor Precautions No information available to require special precautions

Effects on Dental Treatment No effects or complications reported

Other Adverse Effects During the dosing procedure:

Cardiovascular: Transient bradycardia, vasoconstriction, hypotension, hypertension, pallor

Respiratory: Oxygen desaturation, endotracheal tube blockage, hypocarbia, hypercarbia, apnea, pulmonary air leaks, pulmonary interstitial emphysema

Miscellaneous: Increased probability of post-treatment nosocomial sepsis

Drug Interactions No data reported

Generic Available No

Berocca® see Vitamin B Complex With Vitamin C and Folic Acid *on page 994*

Beta-2® see Isoetharine *on page 521*

Beta-Carotene (BAY tah KARE oh teen)

Brand Names Max-Caro® [OTC]; Provatene® [OTC]; Solatene®

Therapeutic Category Vitamin, Fat Soluble

Use Reduces severity of photosensitivity reactions in patients with erythropoietic protoporphyria (EPP)

Usual Dosage Oral:

Children <14 years: 30-150 mg/day

Adults: 30-300 mg/day

Mechanism of Action The exact mechanism of action in erythropoietic protoporphyria has not as yet been elucidated; although patient must become carotenemic before effects are observed, there appears to be more than a simple internal light screen responsible for the drug's action. A protective effect was achieved when beta-carotene was added to blood samples. The concentrations of solutions used were similar to those achieved in treated patients. Topically applied beta-carotene is considerably less effective than systemic therapy.

Local Anesthetic/Vasoconstrictor Precautions No information available to require special precautions

Effects on Dental Treatment No effects or complications reported

Other Adverse Effects

>10%: Dermatologic: Carotenodermia (yellowing of palms, hands, or soles of feet, and to a lesser extent the face)

<1%:

Central nervous system: Dizziness

Dermatologic: Ecchymoses

Gastrointestinal: Diarrhea

Neuromuscular & skeletal: Arthralgia

Drug Interactions Fulfills vitamin A requirements, do not prescribe additional vitamin A

Pregnancy Risk Factor C

Dosage Forms Capsule: 15 mg, 30 mg

Generic Available Yes

Betachron E-R® Capsule see Propranolol *on page 814*

Betadine® [OTC] *see* Povidone-Iodine *on page 783*

Betadine® First Aid Antibiotics + Moisturizer [OTC] *see* Bacitracin and Polymyxin B *on page 108*

9-Beta-D-ribofuranosyladenine *see* Adenosine *on page 33*

Betagan® *see* Levobunolol *on page 546*

Betaine Anhydrous (BAY tayne an HY drus)
Brand Names Cystadane®
Therapeutic Category Urinary Tract Product
Use Treatment of homocystinuria
Usual Dosage Oral: 6 g/day, usually give in two 3 g doses
Local Anesthetic/Vasoconstrictor Precautions No information available to require special precautions
Effects on Dental Treatment No effects or complications reported
Pregnancy Risk Factor C
Generic Available No

Betalin®S *see* Thiamine *on page 924*

Betamethasone (bay ta METH a sone)
Related Information
Corticosteroid Equivalencies Comparison *on page 1139*
Corticosteroids, Topical Comparison *on page 1140*
Respiratory Diseases *on page 1018*
Brand Names Alphatrex®; Betatrex®; Beta-Val®; Celestone®; Celestone® Soluspan®; Cel-U-Jec®; Diprolene®; Diprolene® AF; Diprosone®; Maxivate®; Teladar®; Valisone®
Canadian/Mexican Brand Names Betnesol® [Disodium Phosphate] (Canada); Diprolene™ Glycol [Dipropionate] (Canada); Occlucort® (Canada); Rhoprolene® (Canada); Rhoprosone® (Canada); Selestoject® [Sodium Phosphate] (Canada); Taro-Sone (Canada); Topilene (Canada); Topisone (Canada)
Therapeutic Category Anti-inflammatory Agent; Corticosteroid, Systemic; Corticosteroid, Topical (Medium/High Potency)
Use
Dental: Treatment of a variety of oral diseases of allergic, inflammatory or auto-immune origin
Medical: Inflammatory dermatoses such as seborrheic or atopic dermatitis, neurodermatitis, anogenital pruritus, psoriasis, inflammatory phase of xerosis
Usual Dosage
Children:
Oral: 0.0175-0.25 mg/kg/day divided every 6-8 hours **or** 0.5-7.5 mg/m^2/day divided every 6-8 hours
I.M.: 0.0175-0.125 mg base/kg/day divided every 6-12 hours **or** 0.5-7.5 mg base/m^2/day divided every 6-12 hours
Adults:
Oral: 0.6-7.2 mg/day in 2-4 doses
I.M., I.V.: Betamethasone sodium phosphate: 0.6-9 mg/day divided every 12-24 hours
Mechanism of Action Controls the rate of protein synthesis, depresses the migration of polymorphonuclear leukocytes, fibroblasts, reverses capillary permeability, and lysosomal stabilization at the cellular level to prevent or control inflammation
Local Anesthetic/Vasoconstrictor Precautions No information available to require special precautions
Effects on Dental Treatment No effects or complications reported
Other Adverse Effects >10%:
Central nervous system: Insomnia
Gastrointestinal: Increased appetite, indigestion
Contraindications Systemic fungal infections; hypersensitivity to betamethasone or any component
Warnings/Precautions Use with caution in patients with hypothyroidism, cirrhosis, ulcerative colitis; do not use occlusive dressings on weeping or exudative lesions and general caution with occlusive dressings should be observed; discontinue if skin irritation or contact dermatitis should occur; do not use in patients with decreased skin circulation.
Drug Interactions Decreased effect of any systemic corticosteroid by barbiturates, phenytoin, rifampin
Drug Uptake
Absorption: Oral: Rapid
Serum half-life: Oral: 6.5 hours
Time to peak serum concentration: I.V.: Within 10-36 minutes
Pregnancy Risk Factor C

Breast-feeding Considerations No data reported

Dosage Forms

Base (Celestone®), Oral:
　Syrup: 0.6 mg/5 mL (118 mL)
　Tablet: 0.6 mg
Dipropionate (Diprosone®)
　Aerosol: 0.1% (85 g)
　Cream: 0.05% (15 g, 45 g)
　Lotion: 0.05% (20 mL, 30 mL, 60 mL)
　Ointment: 0.05% (15 g, 45 g)
Dipropionate augmented (Diprolene®)
　Cream: 0.05% (15 g, 45 g)
　Gel: 0.05% (15 g, 45 g)
　Lotion: 0.05% (30 mL, 60 mL)
　Ointment, topical: 0.05% (15 g, 45 g)
Valerate (Betatrex®, Valisone®)
　Cream: 0.01% (15 g, 60 g); 0.1% (15 g, 45 g, 110 g, 430 g)
　Lotion: 0.1% (20 mL, 60 mL)
　Ointment: 0.1% (15 g, 45 g)
Valerate (Beta-Val®)
　Cream: 0.01% (15 g, 60 g); 0.1% (15 g, 45 g, 110 g, 430 g)
　Lotion: 0.1% (20 mL, 60 mL)
Injection: Sodium phosphate (Celestone® Phosphate, Cel-U-Jec®): 4 mg beta-methasone phosphate/mL (equivalent to 3 mg betamethasone/mL) (5 mL)
Injection, suspension: Sodium phosphate and acetate (Celestone® Soluspan®): 6 mg/mL (3 mg of betamethasone sodium phosphate and 3 mg of betamethasone acetate per mL) (5 mL)

Dietary Considerations May be taken with food to decrease GI distress

Generic Available Yes

Betamethasone and Clotrimazole

(bay ta METH a sone & kloe TRIM a zole)

Brand Names Lotrisone®

Canadian/Mexican Brand Names Lotriderm®

Therapeutic Category Antifungal Agent, Topical; Corticosteroid, Topical (Medium/High Potency)

Use Topical treatment of various dermal fungal infections

Local Anesthetic/Vasoconstrictor Precautions No information available to require special precautions

Effects on Dental Treatment No effects or complications reported

Other Adverse Effects See individual agents

Pregnancy Risk Factor C

Generic Available No

Betapace® *see* Sotalol *on page 878*

Betapen®-VK *see* Penicillin V Potassium *on page 734*

Betasept® [OTC] *see* Chlorhexidine Gluconate *on page 211*

Betaseron® *see* Interferon Beta-1b *on page 514*

Betatrex® *see* Betamethasone *on previous page*

Beta-Val® *see* Betamethasone *on previous page*

Betaxolol (be TAKS oh lol)

Related Information
Cardiovascular Diseases *on page 1010*

Brand Names Betoptic®; Betoptic® S; Kerlone®

Therapeutic Category Antiglaucoma Agent; Beta-adrenergic Blocker, Cardioselective; Beta-Adrenergic Blocker, Ophthalmic

Use Treatment of chronic open-angle glaucoma and ocular hypertension; management of hypertension

Usual Dosage Adults:
Ophthalmic: Instill 1 drop twice daily
Oral: 10 mg/day; may increase dose to 20 mg/day after 7-14 days if desired response is not achieved; initial dose in elderly patients: 5 mg/day

Mechanism of Action Competitively blocks beta$_1$-receptors, with little or no effect on beta$_2$-receptors; ophthalmic reduces intraocular pressure by reducing the production of aqueous humor

Local Anesthetic/Vasoconstrictor Precautions No information available to require special precautions

Effects on Dental Treatment Noncardioselective beta-blockers (ie, propranolol, nadolol) enhance the pressor response to epinephrine, resulting in hypertension and bradycardia. This has not been reported for betaxolol, a cardioselective beta-
(Continued)

Betaxolol *(Continued)*

blocker. Therefore local anesthetic with vasoconstrictor can be safely used in patients medicated with betaxolol. Many nonsteroidal anti-inflammatory drugs such as ibuprofen and indomethacin can reduce the hypotensive effect of beta-blockers after 3 or more weeks of therapy with the NSAID. Short-term NSAID use (ie, 3 days) requires no special precautions in patients taking beta-blockers.

Other Adverse Effects
1% to 10%:
Cardiovascular: Bradycardia, palpitations, edema, congestive heart failure
Central nervous system: Dizziness, fatigue, lethargy, headache
Dermatologic: Erythema, itching
Ocular: Mild ocular stinging and discomfort, tearing, photophobia, decreased corneal sensitivity, keratitis
Miscellaneous: Cold extremities
<1%:
Cardiovascular: Chest pain
Central nervous system: Nervousness, depression, hallucinations
Hematologic: Thrombocytopenia

Drug Interactions
Decreased effects of beta-blockers:
Barbiturates (increased liver metabolism of beta-blockers to result in lower serum levels)
NSAIDs (attenuate the hypotensive therapeutic effects of beta-blockers)
Rifampin (increased liver metabolism of beta-blockers to result in lower serum levels)
Increased effects of beta-blockers:
Calcium channel blockers (increase serum levels by unknown mechanism to enhance hypotension)
Beta-blockers increase the effects of:
Epinephrine (vasoconstrictor; initial hypertensive episode followed by brady-cardia)
Phenylephrine (Neosynephrine®; enhanced pressor response)
Theophylline (inhibit theophylline metabolism causing increase in serum concentrations)

Drug Uptake
Onset of action: 1-1.5 hours
Duration: ≥12 hours
Absorption: Systemically absorbed
Serum half-life: 12-22 hours
Time to peak: Within 2 hours

Pregnancy Risk Factor C

Generic Available No

Selected Readings
Foster CA and Aston SJ, "Propranolol-Epinephrine Interaction: A Potential Disaster," *Plast Reconstr Surg*, 1983, 72(1):74-8.
Wong DG, Spence JD, Lamki L, et al, "Effect of Nonsteroidal Anti-inflammatory Drugs on Control of Hypertension of Beta-Blockers and Diuretics," *Lancet*, 1986, 1(8488):997-1001.
Wynn RL, "Dental Nonsteroidal Anti-inflammatory Drugs and Prostaglandin-Based Drug Interactions, Part Two," *Gen Dent*, 1992, 40(2):104, 106, 108.
Wynn RL, "Epinephrine Interactions With Beta-Blockers," *Gen Dent*, 1994, 42(1):16, 18.

Bethanechol *(be THAN e kole)*

Brand Names Duvoid®; Myotonachol™; Urecholine®

Canadian/Mexican Brand Names PMS-Bethanechol® Chloride (Canada)

Therapeutic Category Cholinergic Agent

Use Nonobstructive urinary retention and retention due to neurogenic bladder; treatment and prevention of bladder dysfunction caused by phenothiazines; diagnosis of flaccid or atonic neurogenic bladder; gastroesophageal reflux

Usual Dosage
Children:
Oral:
Abdominal distention or urinary retention: 0.6 mg/kg/day divided 3-4 times/day
Gastroesophageal reflux: 0.1-0.2 mg/kg/dose given 30 minutes to 1 hour before each meal to a maximum of 4 times/day
S.C.: 0.15-0.2 mg/kg/day divided 3-4 times/day

Adults:
Oral: 10-50 mg 2-4 times/day
S.C.: 2.5-5 mg 3-4 times/day, up to 7.5-10 mg every 4 hours for neurogenic bladder

Mechanism of Action Stimulates cholinergic receptors in the smooth muscle of the urinary bladder and gastrointestinal tract resulting in increased peristalsis, increased GI and pancreatic secretions, bladder muscle contraction, and increased ureteral peristaltic waves

Local Anesthetic/Vasoconstrictor Precautions No information available to require special precautions

Effects on Dental Treatment This is a cholinergic agent similar to pilocarpine and expect to see salivation and sweating in patients

Other Adverse Effects
Oral: <1%:
  Cardiovascular: Hypotension, cardiac arrest, flushed skin
  Gastrointestinal: Abdominal cramps, diarrhea, nausea, vomiting, salivation
  Neuromuscular & skeletal: Vasomotor response
  Respiratory: Bronchial constriction
  Miscellaneous: Sweating
Subcutaneous: 1% to 10%:
  Cardiovascular: Hypotension, cardiac arrest, flushed skin
  Gastrointestinal: Abdominal cramps, diarrhea, nausea, vomiting, salivation
  Neuromuscular & skeletal: Vasomotor response
  Respiratory: Bronchial constriction
  Miscellaneous: Sweating

Drug Interactions
Decreased effect: Procainamide, quinidine
Increased toxicity: Bethanechol and ganglionic blockers cause critical fall in blood pressure; cholinergic drugs or anticholinesterase agents

Drug Uptake
Onset of action:
  Oral: 30-90 minutes
  S.C.: 5-15 minutes
Duration of action:
  Oral: Up to 6 hours
  S.C.: 2 hours
Absorption: Oral: Variable

Pregnancy Risk Factor C

Generic Available Yes: Tablet

Betimol® Ophthalmic *see* Timolol *on page 935*

Betoptic® *see* Betaxolol *on page 127*

Betoptic® S *see* Betaxolol *on page 127*

Bexophene® *see* Propoxyphene and Aspirin *on page 813*

Biamine® *see* Thiamine *on page 924*

Biavax® II *see* Rubella and Mumps Vaccines, Combined *on page 851*

Biaxin™ *see* Clarithromycin *on page 241*

Bicalutamide (bye ka LOO ta mide)

Brand Names Casodex®

Therapeutic Category Androgen; Antineoplastic Agent, Hormone

Use Combination therapy with a luteinizing hormone-releasing hormone (LHRH) analog for the treatment of advanced prostate cancer

Usual Dosage Adults: Oral: 1 tablet once daily (morning or evening), with or without food. It is recommended that bicalutamide be taken at the same time each day; start treatment with bicalutamide at the same time as treatment with an LHRH analog.

Mechanism of Action Pure nonsteroidal antiandrogen that binds to androgen receptors; specifically a competitive inhibitor for the binding of dihydrotestosterone and testosterone; prevents testosterone stimulation of cell growth in prostate cancer

Local Anesthetic/Vasoconstrictor Precautions No information available to require special precautions

Effects on Dental Treatment No effects or complications reported

Other Adverse Effects
>10%: Endocrine & metabolic: Hot flashes (49%)

≥2% to <5%:
  Cardiovascular: Angina pectoris, congestive heart failure, edema
  Central nervous system: Anxiety, depression, confusion, somnolence, nervousness, fever, chills
  Dermatologic: Dry skin, pruritus, alopecia
  Endocrine & metabolic: Breast pain, diabetes mellitus, decreased libido, dehydration, gout
  Gastrointestinal: Anorexia, dyspepsia, rectal hemorrhage, xerostomia, melena, weight gain
  Genitourinary: Polyuria, urinary impairment, dysuria, urinary retention, urinary urgency
(Continued)

Bicalutamide *(Continued)*

Hepatic: Alkaline phosphatase increased
Neuromuscular & skeletal: Myasthenia, arthritis, myalgia, leg cramps, pathological fracture, neck pain, hypertonia, neuropathy
Renal: Creatinine increased
Respiratory: Cough increased, pharyngitis, bronchitis, pneumonia, rhinitis, lung disorder
Miscellaneous: Sepsis, neoplasma

Drug Uptake
Absorption: Rapid and complete
Serum half-life: Active enantiomer is 5.8 days

Pregnancy Risk Factor X

Dosage Forms Tablet: 50 mg

Generic Available No

Bicillin® C-R 900/300 Injection *see* Penicillin G Benzathine and Procaine Combined *on page 732*

Bicillin® C-R Injection *see* Penicillin G Benzathine and Procaine Combined *on page 732*

Bicillin® L-A *see* Penicillin G Benzathine *on page 731*

Bicitra® *see* Sodium Citrate and Citric Acid *on page 872*

BiCNU® *see* Carmustine *on page 181*

Biltricide® *see* Praziquantel *on page 786*

Biocef® *see* Cephalexin *on page 201*

Bioclate® *see* Antihemophilic Factor (Recombinant) *on page 81*

Biohist®-LA *see* Carbinoxamine and Pseudoephedrine *on page 177*

Biomox® *see* Amoxicillin *on page 68*

Bion® Tears Solution [OTC] *see* Artificial Tears *on page 87*

Biozyme-C® *see* Collagenase *on page 260*

Biperiden *(bye PER i den)*

Brand Names Akineton®

Therapeutic Category Anti-Parkinson's Agent

Use Treatment of all forms of Parkinsonism including drug induced type (extrapyramidal symptoms)

Usual Dosage Adults:
Parkinsonism: Oral: 2 mg 3-4 times/day

Extrapyramidal:
Oral: 2 mg 1-3 times/day
I.M., I.V.: 2 mg every 30 minutes up to 4 doses or 8 mg/day

Mechanism of Action Biperiden is a weak anticholinergic agent. The beneficial effects in Parkinson's disease and neuroleptic-induced extrapyramidal reactions are believed to be due to the inhibition of striatal cholinergic receptors.

Local Anesthetic/Vasoconstrictor Precautions No information available to require special precautions

Effects on Dental Treatment Dry mouth, nose and throat very prevalent in patients taking this drug

Other Adverse Effects
>10%:
Dermatologic: Dry skin
Gastrointestinal: Constipation, dry mouth
Respiratory: Dry nose, throat
Miscellaneous: Decreased sweating
1% to 10%:
Dermatologic: Photosensitivity
Endocrine & metabolic: Decreased flow of breast milk
Gastrointestinal: Dysphagia
<1%:
Cardiovascular: Orthostatic hypotension, ventricular fibrillation, tachycardia, palpitations
Central nervous system: Confusion, drowsiness, headache, loss of memory, fatigue, ataxia
Dermatologic: Skin rash
Gastrointestinal: Bloated feeling, nausea, vomiting
Genitourinary: Dysuria
Neuromuscular & skeletal: Weakness
Ocular: Increased intraocular pain, blurred vision

Drug Interactions
Decreased effect of levodopa (↓ absorption)

Increased toxicity (central anticholinergic syndrome): Narcotic analgesics, phenothiazines, and other antipsychotics, tricyclic antidepressants, some antihistamines, quinidine, disopyramide

Drug Uptake
Serum half-life: 18.4-24.3 hours
Time to peak serum concentration: 1-1.5 hours

Pregnancy Risk Factor C

Generic Available No

Bisac-Evac® [OTC] see Bisacodyl on this page

Bisacodilo (Mexico) see Bisacodyl on this page

Bisacodyl (bis a KOE dil)

Brand Names Bisac-Evac® [OTC]; Bisacodyl Uniserts®; Bisco-Lax® [OTC]; Carter's Little Pills® [OTC]; Clysodrast®; Dacodyl® [OTC]; Deficol® [OTC]; Dulcolax® [OTC]; Fleet® Laxative [OTC]

Canadian/Mexican Brand Names Apo®-Bisacodyl (Canada); Dulcolan® (Mexico); PMS-Bisacodyl® (Canada)

Therapeutic Category Laxative, Stimulant

Synonyms Bisacodilo (Mexico)

Use Treatment of constipation; colonic evacuation prior to procedures or examination

Usual Dosage
Children:
Oral: >6 years: 5-10 mg (0.3 mg/kg) at bedtime or before breakfast
Rectal suppository:
<2 years: 5 mg as a single dose
>2 years: 10 mg
Adults:
Oral: 5-15 mg as single dose (up to 30 mg when complete evacuation of bowel is required)
Rectal suppository: 10 mg as single dose
Tannex:
Enema: 2.5 g in 1000 mL warm water
Barium enema: 2.5-5 g in 1000 mL barium suspension
Do not give >10 g within 72-hour period

Mechanism of Action Stimulates peristalsis by directly irritating the smooth muscle of the intestine, possibly the colonic intramural plexus; alters water and electrolyte secretion producing net intestinal fluid accumulation and laxation

Local Anesthetic/Vasoconstrictor Precautions No information available to require special precautions

Effects on Dental Treatment No effects or complications reported

Other Adverse Effects <1%:
Central nervous system: Vertigo
Endocrine & metabolic: Electrolyte and fluid imbalance (metabolic acidosis or alkalosis, hypocalcemia)
Gastrointestinal: Mild abdominal cramps, nausea, vomiting, rectal burning

Drug Interactions Decreased effect: Milk, antacids; decreased effect of warfarin

Drug Uptake
Onset of action:
Oral: 6-10 hours
Rectal: 0.25-1 hour
Absorption: Oral, rectal: <5% absorbed systemically

Pregnancy Risk Factor C

Generic Available Yes

Bisacodyl Uniserts® see Bisacodyl on this page

Bisco-Lax® [OTC] see Bisacodyl on this page

Bishydroxycoumarin see Dicumarol on page 306

Bismatrol® (subsalicylate) [OTC] see Bismuth on this page

Bismuth (BIZ muth)

Related Information
Ranitidine Bismuth Citrate on page 835

Brand Names Bismatrol® (subsalicylate) [OTC]; Devrom® (subgallate) [OTC]; Pepto-Bismol® (subsalicylate) [OTC]; Pink Bismuth® (subsalicylate) [OTC]

Therapeutic Category Antidiarrheal

Synonyms Bismuth Subgallate; Bismuth Subsalicylate

Use Symptomatic treatment of mild, nonspecific diarrhea; indigestion, nausea, control of traveler's diarrhea (enterotoxigenic *Escherichia coli*); as an adjunct in the treatment of *Helicobacter pylori*-associated peptic ulcer disease
(Continued)

Bismuth *(Continued)*

Usual Dosage Oral:

Nonspecific diarrhea: Subsalicylate:

Children: Up to 8 doses/24 hours:

3-6 years: $1/3$ tablet or 5 mL every 30 minutes to 1 hour as needed

6-9 years: $2/3$ tablet or 10 mL every 30 minutes to 1 hour as needed

9-12 years: 1 tablet or 15 mL every 30 minutes to 1 hour as needed

Adults: 2 tablets or 30 mL every 30 minutes to 1 hour as needed up to 8 doses/24 hours

Prevention of traveler's diarrhea: 2.1 g/day or 2 tablets 4 times/day before meals and at bedtime

Subgallate: 1-2 tablets 3 times/day with meals

Mechanism of Action Bismuth subsalicylate exhibits both antisecretory and antimicrobial action. This agent may provide some anti-inflammatory action as well. The salicylate moiety provides antisecretory effect and the bismuth exhibits antimicrobial directly against bacterial and viral gastrointestinal pathogens. Bismuth has some antacid properties.

Local Anesthetic/Vasoconstrictor Precautions No information available to require special precautions

Effects on Dental Treatment No effects or complications reported

Other Adverse Effects

>10%: Discoloration of the tongue (darkening), grayish black stools

<1%:

Central nervous system: Anxiety, confusion, slurred speech, headache, mental depression

Gastrointestinal: Impaction may occur in infants and debilitated patients

Neuromuscular & skeletal: Muscle spasms, weakness

Otic: Loss of hearing, tinnitus

Drug Interactions

Decreased effect: Tetracyclines and uricosurics

Increased toxicity: Aspirin, warfarin, hypoglycemics

Drug Uptake

Absorption: Minimally absorbed across the GI tract while the salt (eg, salicylate) may be readily absorbed

Pregnancy Risk Factor C (D in 3rd trimester)

Generic Available Yes

Bismuth Subgallate *see* Bismuth *on previous page*

Bismuth Subsalicylate *see* Bismuth *on previous page*

Bismuth Subsalicylate, Metronidazole, and Tetracycline

(BIZ muth sub sa LIS i late, me troe NI da zole, & tet ra SYE kleen)

Brand Names Helidac®

Therapeutic Category Antidiarrheal

Use In combination with an H_2-antagonist, used to treat and decrease rate of recurrence of active duodenal ulcer associated with *H. pylori* infection

Usual Dosage Adults: Chew 2 bismuth subsalicylate 262.4 mg tablets, swallow 1 metronidazole 250 mg tablet, and swallow 1 tetracycline 500 mg capsule plus an H_2-antagonist 4 times/day at meals and bedtime for 14 days; follow with 8 oz of water

Mechanism of Action Bismuth subsalicylate, metronidazole, and tetracycline individually have demonstrated *in vitro* activity against most susceptible strains of *H. pylori* isolated from patients with duodenal ulcers. Resistance to metronidazole is increasing in the U.S.; an alternative regimen, not containing metronidazole, if *H. pylori* is not eradicated follow therapy.

Local Anesthetic/Vasoconstrictor Precautions No information available to require special precautions

Effects on Dental Treatment Tetracyclines are not recommended for use during pregnancy since they can cause enamel hypoplasia and permanent teeth discoloration; long-term use associated with oral candidiasis

Other Adverse Effects See individual monographs

>1%:

Central nervous system: Dizziness

Gastrointestinal: Nausea, diarrhea, abdominal pain, vomiting, anal discomfort, anorexia

Neuromuscular & skeletal: Paresthesia

<1%:

Central nervous system: Insomnia

Gastrointestinal: Constipation

Neuromuscular & skeletal: Weakness, pain
Respiratory: Upper respiratory infection

Contraindications Pregnancy or lactation; children; significant renal/hepatic impairment; hypersensitivity to salicylates, bismuth, metronidazole, tetracycline, or any component

Warnings/Precautions See individual monographs

Drug Interactions See individual monographs

Decreased effect: A theoretical reduction in tetracycline systemic absorption due to an interaction with bismuth or calcium carbonate, an excipient of bismuth subsalicylate has, as yet, been unproven to occur or to have any clinical bearing

Drug Uptake No data on combination; see individual monographs

Pregnancy Risk Factor D (tetracycline); B (metronidazole)

Dosage Forms
Tablet:
Bismuth subsalicylate: Chewable: 262.4 mg
Metronidazole: 250 mg
Capsule: Tetracycline: 500 mg

Bisoprolol (bis OH proe lol)

Related Information
Cardiovascular Diseases *on page 1010*

Brand Names Zebeta®

Therapeutic Category Antianginal Agent; Beta-adrenergic Blocker, Cardioselective

Use Treatment of hypertension, alone or in combination with other agents
Unlabeled use: Angina pectoris, supraventricular arrhythmias, PVCs

Usual Dosage Oral:
Adults: 5 mg once daily, may be increased to 10 mg, and then up to 20 mg once daily, if necessary
Elderly: Initial dose: 2.5 mg/day; may be increased by 2.5-5 mg/day; maximum recommended dose: 20 mg/day

Mechanism of Action Selective inhibitor of beta$_1$-adrenergic receptors; competitively blocks beta$_1$-receptors, with little or no effect on beta$_2$-receptors at doses <10 mg

Local Anesthetic/Vasoconstrictor Precautions No information available to require special precautions

Effects on Dental Treatment Noncardioselective beta-blockers (ie, propranolol, nadolol) enhance the pressor response to epinephrine, resulting in hypertension and bradycardia. This has not been reported for bisoprolol, a cardioselective beta-blocker. Therefore local anesthetic with vasoconstrictor can be safely used in patients medicated with bisoprolol. Many nonsteroidal anti-inflammatory drugs such as ibuprofen and indomethacin can reduce the hypotensive effect of beta-blockers after 3 or more weeks of therapy with the NSAID. Short-term NSAID use (ie, 3 days) requires no special precautions in patients taking beta-blockers.

Other Adverse Effects
>10%: Central nervous system: Fatigue, lethargy
1% to 10%:
Cardiovascular: Hypotension, chest pain, heart failure, Raynaud's phenomenon, heart block, edema, bradycardia
Central nervous system: Headache, dizziness, insomnia, confusion, depression, abnormal dreams
Dermatologic: Rash
Gastrointestinal: Constipation, diarrhea, dyspepsia, nausea, flatulence, anorexia
Genitourinary: Micturition (frequency), impotence, urinary retention
Neuromuscular & skeletal: Arthralgia, myalgia
Ocular: Abnormal vision
Respiratory: Dyspnea, rhinitis, cough

Drug Interactions
Decreased effects of beta-blockers:
Barbiturates (increased liver metabolism of beta-blockers to result in lower serum levels)
NSAIDs (attenuate the hypotensive therapeutic effects of beta-blockers)
Rifampin (increased liver metabolism of beta-blockers to result in lower serum levels)
Increased effects of beta-blockers:
Calcium channel blockers (increase serum levels by unknown mechanism to enhance hypotension)
Beta-blockers increase the effects of:
Epinephrine (vasoconstrictor; initial hypertensive episode followed by bradycardia)
(Continued)

Bisoprolol *(Continued)*

Phenylephrine (Neosynephrine®; enhanced pressor response)
Theophylline (inhibit theophylline metabolism causing increase in serum concentrations)

Drug Uptake
Absorption: Rapid and almost complete from GI tract
Serum half-life: 9-12 hours
Time to peak: 1.7-3 hours

Pregnancy Risk Factor C

Generic Available No

Selected Readings
Foster CA and Aston SJ, "Propranolol-Epinephrine Interaction: A Potential Disaster," *Plast Reconstr Surg*, 1983, 72(1):74-8.
Wong DG, Spence JD, Lamki L, et al, "Effect of Nonsteroidal Anti-inflammatory Drugs on Control of Hypertension of Beta-Blockers and Diuretics," *Lancet*, 1986, 1(8488):997-1001.
Wynn RL, "Dental Nonsteroidal Anti-inflammatory Drugs and Prostaglandin-Based Drug Interactions, Part Two," *Gen Dent*, 1992, 40(2):104, 106, 108.
Wynn RL, "Epinephrine Interactions With Beta-Blockers," *Gen Dent*, 1994, 42(1):16, 18.

Bisoprolol and Hydrochlorothiazide

(bis OH proe lol & hye droe klor oh THYE a zide)

Brand Names Ziac™

Therapeutic Category Antihypertensive Agent, Combination; Diuretic, Thiazide

Use Treatment of hypertension

Usual Dosage Adults: Oral: Dose is individualized, given once daily

Local Anesthetic/Vasoconstrictor Precautions No information available to require special precautions

Effects on Dental Treatment Noncardioselective beta-blockers (ie, propranolol, nadolol) enhance the pressor response to epinephrine, resulting in hypertension and bradycardia. This has not been reported for bisoprolol, a cardioselective beta-blocker. Therefore local anesthetic with vasoconstrictor can be safely used in patients medicated with bisoprolol. Many nonsteroidal anti-inflammatory drugs such as ibuprofen and indomethacin can reduce the hypotensive effect of beta-blockers after 3 or more weeks of therapy with the NSAID. Short-term NSAID use (ie, 3 days) requires no special precautions in patients taking beta-blockers.

Other Adverse Effects
>10%: Central nervous system: Fatigue
1% to 10%:
Cardiovascular: Chest pain, edema, bradycardia, hypotension
Central nervous system: Headache, dizziness, depression, abnormal dreams
Dermatologic: Rash, photosensitivity
Endocrine & metabolic: Hypokalemia, fluid and electrolyte imbalances (hypocalcemia, hypomagnesemia, hyponatremia), hyperglycemia
Gastrointestinal: Constipation, diarrhea, dyspepsia, nausea, insomnia, flatulence
Genitourinary: Micturition (frequency)
Hematologic: Rarely blood dyscrasias
Neuromuscular & skeletal: Arthralgia, myalgia
Ocular: Abnormal vision
Renal: Prerenal azotemia
Respiratory: Rhinitis, cough, dyspnea

Drug Interactions
Decreased effect/levels with barbiturates, rifampin, sulfinpyrazone
Decreased effect of oral hypoglycemics; decreased absorption with cholestyramine and colestipol
Increased effect with furosemide and other loop diuretics
Increased toxicity/levels of lithium
Increased effect/toxicity/levels of and with flecainide
Increased levels/toxicity of lidocaine

Pregnancy Risk Factor C

Generic Available No

Bistropamide *see* Tropicamide *on page 973*

Bitolterol *(bye TOLE ter ole)*

Related Information
Respiratory Diseases *on page 1018*

Brand Names Tornalate®

Therapeutic Category Antiasthmatic; Beta$_2$-Adrenergic Agonist Agent; Bronchodilator

Use Prevention and treatment of bronchial asthma and bronchospasm

Usual Dosage Children >12 years and Adults:

Bronchospasm: 2 inhalations at an interval of at least 1-3 minutes, followed by a third inhalation if needed

Prevention of bronchospasm: 2 inhalations every 8 hours; do not exceed 3 inhalations every 6 hours or 2 inhalations every 4 hours

Mechanism of Action Selectively stimulates beta$_2$-adrenergic receptors in the lungs producing bronchial smooth muscle relaxation; minor beta$_1$ activity

Local Anesthetic/Vasoconstrictor Precautions No information available to require special precautions

Effects on Dental Treatment No effects or complications reported

Other Adverse Effects

>10%: Neuromuscular & skeletal: Trembling

1% to 10%:

Cardiovascular: Flushing of face, hypertension, pounding heartbeat

Central nervous system: Dizziness, lightheadedness, nervousness

Gastrointestinal: Dry mouth, nausea, unpleasant taste

Respiratory: Bronchial irritation, coughing

<1%:

Cardiovascular: Chest pain, arrhythmias, tachycardia

Central nervous system: Insomnia

Respiratory: Paradoxical bronchospasm

Drug Interactions Increased toxicity: Cardiovascular effects are potentiated in patients also receiving MAO inhibitors, tricyclic antidepressants, sympathomimetic agents (eg, amphetamine, dopamine, dobutamine), inhaled anesthetics (eg, enflurane)

Drug Uptake

Duration: 4-8 hours

Serum half-life: 3 hours

Time to peak serum concentration (colterol): Inhalation: Within 1 hour

Pregnancy Risk Factor C

Generic Available No

Black Draught® [OTC] *see Senna on page 862*

BlemErase® Lotion [OTC] *see Benzoyl Peroxide on page 120*

Blenoxane® *see Bleomycin on this page*

Bleomycin (blee oh MYE sin)

Brand Names Blenoxane®

Canadian/Mexican Brand Names Bleolem (Mexico)

Therapeutic Category Antineoplastic Agent, Antibiotic

Synonyms BLM; NIM

Use Palliative treatment of squamous cell carcinoma, testicular carcinoma, germ cell tumors, and the following lymphomas: Hodgkin's, lymphosarcoma and reticulum cell sarcoma; sclerosing agent to control malignant effusions

Usual Dosage Refer to individual protocols; 1 unit = 1 mg

May be administered I.M., I.V., S.C., or intracavitary

Children and Adults:

Test dose for lymphoma patients: I.M., I.V., S.C.: 1-5 units of bleomycin before the first dose; monitor vital signs every 15 minutes; wait a minimum of 1 hour before administering remainder of dose

Single agent therapy:

I.M./I.V./S.C.: Squamous cell carcinoma, lymphosarcoma, reticulum cell sarcoma, testicular carcinoma: 0.25-0.5 units/kg (10-20 units/m^2) 1-2 times/week

Continuous intravenous infusion: 15 units/m^2 over 24 hours daily for 4 days

Combination agent therapy:

I.M./I.V.: 3-4 units/m^2

I.V.: ABVD: 10 units/m^2 on days 1 and 15

Maximum cumulative lifetime dose: 400 units

Mechanism of Action Inhibits synthesis of DNA; binds to DNA leading to single- and double-strand breaks; isolated from *Streptomyces verticillus*

Local Anesthetic/Vasoconstrictor Precautions No information available to require special precautions

Effects on Dental Treatment No effects or complications reported

Other Adverse Effects

>10%:

Cardiovascular: Raynaud's phenomenon

Central nervous system: Fever, chills

Dermatologic: Pruritic erythema

Gastrointestinal: Stomatitis, nausea, vomiting, anorexia, weight loss

Emetic potential: Moderately low (10% to 30%)

(Continued)

135

Bleomycin *(Continued)*

Integument: Approximately 50% of patients will develop erythema, induration, hyperkeratosis, and peeling of the skin. Hyperpigmentation, alopecia, nailbed changes may occur; this appears to be dose-related and is reversible after cessation of therapy.

Local: Pain at tumor site, phlebitis

Miscellaneous: Mild febrile reaction, mucocutaneous toxicity, patients may become febrile after intracavitary administration

1% to 10%:

Idiosyncratic: Similar to anaphylaxis and occurs in 1% of lymphoma patients; may include hypotension, confusion, fever, chills, and wheezing. May be immediate or delayed for several hours; symptomatic treatment includes volume expansion, pressor agents, antihistamines, and steroids.

<1%:

Cardiovascular: Myocardial infarction, cerebrovascular accident

Dermatologic: Skin thickening

Hepatic: Hepatotoxicity

Renal: Renal toxicity

Respiratory: Tachypnea, rales; dose-related when total dose is >400 units or with single doses >30 units. Pathogenesis is poorly understood, but may be related to damage of pulmonary, vascular, or connective tissue. Manifested as an acute or chronic interstitial pneumonitis with interstitial fibrosis, hypoxia, and death. Symptoms include cough, dyspnea, and bilateral pulmonary infiltrates noted on CXR. It is controversial whether steroids improve symptoms of bleomycin pulmonary toxicity.

Drug Interactions

Decreased effect:

Digitalis glycosides: May decrease plasma levels and renal excretion of digoxin

Phenytoin: Results in decreased phenytoin levels, possibly due to decreased oral absorption

Increased toxicity:

CCNU: Increased severity of leukopenia

Cisplatin: Results in delayed bleomycin elimination due to decrease in creatinine clearance secondary to cisplatin

Drug Uptake

Absorption: I.M. and intrapleural administration produces serum concentrations of 30% of I.V. administration; intraperitoneal and S.C. routes produce serum concentrations equal to those of I.V.

Serum half-life (biphasic): Dependent upon renal function:

Normal renal function:

Initial: 1.3 hours

Terminal: 9 hours

End stage renal disease:

Initial: 2 hours

Terminal: 30 hours

Time to peak serum concentration: I.M.: Within 30 minutes

Pregnancy Risk Factor D

Generic Available Yes

Bleph®-10 Ophthalmic *see* Sulfacetamide Sodium *on page 890*

Blephamide® Ophthalmic *see* Sulfacetamide Sodium and Prednisolone *on page 891*

Blis-To-Sol® [OTC] *see* Tolnaftate *on page 943*

BLM *see* Bleomycin *on previous page*

Blocadren® Oral *see* Timolol *on page 935*

Bluboro® [OTC] *see* Aluminum Sulfate and Calcium Acetate *on page 49*

Bonine® [OTC] *see* Meclizine *on page 584*

Boric Acid *(BOR ik AS id)*

Brand Names Borofax® Topical [OTC]; Dri-Ear® Otic [OTC]; Swim-Ear® Otic [OTC]

Therapeutic Category Pharmaceutical Aid

Use

Ophthalmic: Mild antiseptic used for inflamed eyelids

Otic: Prophylaxis of swimmer's ear

Topical ointment: Temporary relief of chapped, chafed, or dry skin, diaper rash, abrasions, minor burns, sunburn, insect bites, and other skin irritations

Local Anesthetic/Vasoconstrictor Precautions No information available to require special precautions

Effects on Dental Treatment No effects or complications reported

Generic Available Yes

Comments Not a corrosive substance

Borofax® Topical [OTC] *see* Boric Acid *on previous page*

Boropak® [OTC] *see* Aluminum Sulfate and Calcium Acetate *on page 49*

B&O Supprettes® *see* Belladonna and Opium *on page 113*

Botox® *see* Botulinum Toxin Type A *on this page*

Botulinum Toxin Type A (BOT yoo lin num TOKS in type aye)

Brand Names Botox®

Therapeutic Category Ophthalmic Agent, Toxin

Use

Treatment of strabismus and blepharospasm associated with dystonia (including benign essential blepharospasm or VII nerve disorders in patients ≥12 years of age)

Unlabeled uses: Treatment of hemifacial spasms, spasmodic torticollis (ie, cervical dystonia, clonic twisting of the head), oromandibular dystonia, spasmodic dysphonia (laryngeal dystonia) and other dystonias (ie, writer's cramp, focal task-specific dystonias)

Orphan drug: Treatment of dynamic muscle contracture in pediatric cerebral palsy patients

Usual Dosage

Strabismus: 1.25-5 units (0.05-0.15 mL) injected into any one muscle

Subsequent doses for residual/recurrent strabismus: Re-examine patients 7-14 days after each injection to assess the effect of that dose. Subsequent doses for patients experiencing incomplete paralysis of the target may be increased up to two fold the previously administered dose. Maximum recommended dose as a single injection for any one muscle is 25 units.

Blepharospasm: 1.25-2.5 units (0.05-0.10 mL) injected into the orbicularis oculi muscle

Subsequent doses: Each treatment lasts approximately 3 months. At repeat treatment sessions, the dose may be increased up to twofold if the response from the initial treatment is considered insufficient (usually defined as an effect that does not last >2 months). There appears to be little benefit obtainable from injecting >5 units per site. Some tolerance may be found if treatments are given any more frequently than every 3 months.

The cumulative dose should not exceed 200 units in a 30-day period

Mechanism of Action Botulinum A toxin is a neurotoxin produced by *Clostridium botulinum*, spore-forming anaerobic bacillus, which appears to affect only the presynaptic membrane of the neuromuscular junction in humans, where it prevents calcium-dependent release of acetylcholine and produces a state of denervation. Muscle inactivation persists until new fibrils grow from the nerve and form junction plates on new areas of the muscle-cell walls. The antagonist muscle shortens simultaneously ("contracture"), taking up the slack created by agonist paralysis; following several weeks of paralysis, alignment of the eye is measurably changed, despite return of innervation to the injected muscle.

Local Anesthetic/Vasoconstrictor Precautions No information available to require special precautions

Effects on Dental Treatment No effects or complications reported

Other Adverse Effects

>10%: Ocular: Dry eyes, lagophthalmos, ptosis, photophobia, vertical deviation

1% to 10%:

Dermatologic: Diffuse skin rash

Ocular: Swelling of eyelid, blepharospasm

<1%: Ocular: Ectropion, keratitis, diplopia, entropion

Drug Interactions Increased effect: Botulinum toxin may be potentiated by aminoglycosides

Drug Uptake

Strabismus:

Onset of action: 1-2 days after injection

Duration of paralysis: 2-6 weeks

Blepharospasm:

Onset: 3 days after injection

Peak: 1-2 weeks

Duration of paralysis: 3 months

Pregnancy Risk Factor C

Generic Available No

BQ® Tablet [OTC] *see* Chlorpheniramine, Phenylpropanolamine, and Acetaminophen *on page 222*

Breathe Free® [OTC] *see* Sodium Chloride *on page 870*

Breezee® Mist Antifungal [OTC] *see* Miconazole *on page 635*

Breezee® Mist Antifungal [OTC] *see* Tolnaftate *on page 943*

Breonesin® [OTC] *see Guaifenesin on page 452*
Brethaire® *see Terbutaline on page 908*
Brethine® *see Terbutaline on page 908*

Bretylium (bre TIL ee um)

Related Information
Cardiovascular Diseases *on page 1010*
Brand Names Bretylol®
Canadian/Mexican Brand Names Bretylate® (Canada)
Therapeutic Category Antiarrhythmic Agent, Class III; Antiarrhythmic Agent (Supraventricular & Ventricular)
Use Treatment of ventricular tachycardia and fibrillation; used in the treatment of other serious ventricular arrhythmias resistant to lidocaine
Usual Dosage (**Note:** Patients should undergo defibrillation/cardioversion before and after bretylium doses as necessary)

Children:
I.M.: 2-5 mg/kg as a single dose
I.V.: Initial: 5 mg/kg, then attempt electrical defibrillation; repeat with 10 mg/kg if ventricular fibrillation persists at 15-minute intervals to maximum total of 30 mg/kg
Maintenance dose: I.M., I.V.: 5 mg/kg every 6-8 hours

Adults:
Immediate life-threatening ventricular arrhythmias, ventricular fibrillation, unstable ventricular tachycardia: Initial dose: I.V.: 5 mg/kg (undiluted) over 1 minute; if arrhythmia persists, give 10 mg/kg (undiluted) over 1 minute and repeat as necessary (usually at 15- to 30-minute intervals) up to a total dose of 30-35 mg/kg
Other life-threatening ventricular arrhythmias:
Initial dose: I.M., I.V.: 5-10 mg/kg, may repeat every 1-2 hours if arrhythmia persist; give I.V. dose (diluted) over 8-10 minutes
Maintenance dose: I.M.: 5-10 mg/kg every 6-8 hours; I.V. (diluted): 5-10 mg/kg every 6 hours; I.V. infusion (diluted): 1-2 mg/minute (little experience with doses >40 mg/kg/day)
2 g/250 mL D$_5$W (infusion pump should be used for I.V. infusion administration)
Rate of I.V. infusion: 1-4 mg/minute
1 mg/minute = 7 mL/hour
2 mg/minute = 15 mL/hour
3 mg/minute = 22 mL/hour
4 mg/minute = 30 mL/hour
Mechanism of Action Class II antiarrhythmic; after an initial release of norepinephrine at the peripheral adrenergic nerve terminals, inhibits further release by postganglionic nerve endings in response to sympathetic nerve stimulation
Local Anesthetic/Vasoconstrictor Precautions No information available to require special precautions
Effects on Dental Treatment No effects or complications reported
Other Adverse Effects
>10%: Cardiovascular: Hypotension (both postural and supine)
1% to 10%: Gastrointestinal: Nausea, vomiting
<1%:
Cardiovascular: Transient initial hypertension, increase in PVCs, bradycardia, angina, flushing, syncope
Central nervous system: Vertigo, confusion, hyperthermia
Dermatologic: Rash
Gastrointestinal: Diarrhea, abdominal pain
Neuromuscular & skeletal: Muscle atrophy and necrosis with repeated I.M. injections at same site
Ocular: Conjunctivitis
Renal: Renal impairment
Respiratory: Respiratory depression, nasal congestion
Miscellaneous: Hiccups
Drug Interactions
Increased toxicity: Other antiarrhythmic agents
Additive toxicity or effect by bretylium, pressor catecholamines, digitalis
Drug Uptake
Onset of antiarrhythmic effect:
I.M.: May require 2 hours
I.V.: Within 6-20 minutes
Peak effect: 6-9 hours
Duration: 6-24 hours
Serum half-life: 7-11 hours; average: 4-17 hours

Pregnancy Risk Factor C
Generic Available Yes

Bretylol® see Bretylium on previous page
Brevicon® see Ethinyl Estradiol and Norethindrone on page 379
Brevital® Sodium see Methohexital on page 614
Brevoxyl® Gel see Benzoyl Peroxide on page 120
Bricanyl® see Terbutaline on page 908

Brimonidine (bri MOE ni deen)

Brand Names Alphagan®
Therapeutic Category Alpha$_2$-Adrenergic Agonist Agent, Ophthalmic
Use Lowering of intraocular pressure in patients with open-angle glaucoma or ocular hypertension
Usual Dosage Adults: Ophthalmic: Instill 1 drop in affected eye(s) 3 times/day (approximately every 8 hours)
Mechanism of Action Selective for alpha$_2$-receptors; appears to result in reduction of aqueous humor formation and increase uveoscleral outflow
Local Anesthetic/Vasoconstrictor Precautions No information available to require special precautions
Effects on Dental Treatment No effects or complications reported
Other Adverse Effects
>10%:
Central nervous system: Headache, fatigue/drowsiness
Gastrointestinal: Xerostomia
Ocular: Ocular hyperemia, burning and stinging, blurring, foreign body sensation, conjunctival follicles, ocular allergic reactions and ocular pruritus
1% to 10%:
Central nervous system: Dizziness
Ocular: Corneal staining/erosion, photophobia, eyelid erythema, ocular ache/pain, ocular dryness, tearing, eyelid edema, conjunctival edema, blepharitis, ocular irritation, conjunctival blanching, abnormal vision, lid crusting, conjunctival hemorrhage, abnormal taste, conjunctival discharge
Respiratory: Upper respiratory symptoms
Drug Interactions

Increased effect:
CNS depressants (eg, alcohol, barbiturates, opiates, sedatives, anesthetics): Additive or potentiating effect
Topical beta-blockers, pilocarpine → additive decreased intraocular pressure, antihypertensives, cardiac glycosides

Decreased effect: Tricyclic antidepressants can affect the metabolism and uptake of circulating amines
Drug Uptake
Onset of action: 1-4 hours
Duration: 12 hours
Pregnancy Risk Factor B
Dosage Forms Solution, ophthalmic, as tartrate: 0.2% (5 mL, 10 mL)

Brofed® Elixir [OTC] see Brompheniramine and Pseudoephedrine on page 144
Bromaline® Elixir [OTC] see Brompheniramine and Phenylpropanolamine on page 143
Bromanate® DC see Brompheniramine, Phenylpropanolamine, and Codeine on page 145
Bromanate® Elixir [OTC] see Brompheniramine and Phenylpropanolamine on page 143
Bromanyl® Cough Syrup see Bromodiphenhydramine and Codeine on page 141
Bromarest® [OTC] see Brompheniramine on page 142
Bromatapp® [OTC] see Brompheniramine and Phenylpropanolamine on page 143
Brombay® [OTC] see Brompheniramine on page 142
Bromfed® Syrup [OTC] see Brompheniramine and Pseudoephedrine on page 144
Bromfed® Tablet [OTC] see Brompheniramine and Pseudoephedrine on page 144

Bromfenac (BROME fen ak)

Brand Names Duract™
Therapeutic Category Analgesic, Non-narcotic; Nonsteroidal Anti-inflammatory Agent (NSAID), Oral
Synonyms Bromfenac Sodium
(Continued)

Bromfenac *(Continued)*

Use Short-term (generally less than 10 days) management of pain; not indicated for such conditions as osteoarthritis or rheumatoid arthritis

Usual Dosage Short-term management of pain (generally <10 days): Adults: Oral: 25 mg every 6-8 hours as necessary, except when taken with high fat food, when a total of 50 mg dose may be needed; total daily dose should not exceed 150 mg

Mechanism of Action Inhibits prostaglandin synthesis by decreasing the activity of the enzyme, cyclo-oxygenase, which results in decreased formation of prostaglandin precursors

Local Anesthetic/Vasoconstrictor Precautions No information available to require special precautions

Effects on Dental Treatment No effects or complications reported

Other Adverse Effects The most frequent complaints with bromfenac use relate to minor gastrointestinal problems. In some patients treated with bromfenac therapy, serious gastrointestinal toxicity such as perforation, ulceration, and bleeding can occur. In addition, elevations of liver enzymes have been reported. Therefore, while bromfenac is indicated for the short-term management of pain, generally less than 10 days duration, if a physician chooses to administer bromfenac for a longer duration, it is recommended that liver enzymes should be monitored in patients treated for more than four weeks.

Contraindications Hypersensitivity to bromfenac; patients in whom aspirin or other NSAIDs induce asthma, urticaria, or other allergic-type reactions; severe anaphylactic-like reactions have been reported in patients receiving NSAIDs

Warnings/Precautions Avoid giving bromfenac in patients with chronic hepatitis; elevations of one or more liver tests may occur during therapy; they may progress, remain unchanged, or may be transient despite continued therapy

Hepatic effects severe hepatic reactions, including jaundice, potentially fatal fulminant hepatitis and liver failure (some requiring transplantation), have occurred in patients taking bromfenac for longer than the recommended duration. Bromfenac is a nonsteroidal anti-inflammatory drug (NSAID) indicated only for the short-term (10-days or less) management of acute pain and is not indicated for long-term use. While not recommended, if a practitioner determines that the risk of longer use is justified by the potential benefit, the patient's transaminases (particularly ALT), and bilirubin, must be closely monitored for signs of hepatotoxicity. Patients should be advised to take this medication as directed.

Drug Interactions

Warfarin - (according to the manufacturer) bromfenac has no effect on warfarin anticoagulation; nevertheless, caution is advised when adding any drug that affects platelet function, such as bromfenac, to patients receiving oral anticoagulants

Lithium - other than NSAIDs are known to cause increases in lithium serum levels; there may be an increased possibility of adverse effects from lithium if bromfenac is administered to patients taking lithium

Phenytoin reduced the mean peak plasma levels of bromfenac by 40%; bromfenac had a small effect (11% increase) on the peak serum levels of phenytoin

Cimetidine - concomitant administration of cimetidine with bromfenac caused a moderate increase in bromfenac blood levels; bromfenac has no effect on the pharmacokinetics of cimetidine

Drug Uptake

Serum half-life: 30-54 minutes

Time to peak serum concentration: Within 1 hour

Pregnancy Risk Factor C

Dosage Forms Capsule, as sodium: 25 mg

Generic Available No

Comments In a study using 241 subjects, it has been reported that 25 mg of bromfenac is at least as effective as 400 mg ibuprofen in relieving postoperative pain after the surgical removal of impacted third molars. Also, the same study reported that 5 mg bromfenac was equivalent to 650 mg aspirin in relieving oral surgery pain.

Selected Readings

Forbes JA, Beaver WT, Jones KF, et al, "Analgesic Efficacy of Bromfenac, Ibuprofen, and Aspirin in Postoperative Oral Surgery Pain," *Clin Pharmacol Ther*, 1992, 51(3):343-52.

Forbes JA, Edquist IA, Smith FG, et al, "Evaluation of Bromfenac, Aspirin, and Ibuprofen in Postoperative Oral Surgery Pain," *Pharmacotherapy*, 1991, 11(1):64-70.

Gumbhir-Shah K, Cevallos WH, De Cleene SA, et al, "Evaluation of Pharmacokinetic Interaction Between Bromfenac and Phenytoin in Healthy Males," *J Clin Pharmacol*, 1997, 37(2):160-8.

Bromfenac Sodium *see* Bromfenac *on previous page*

Bromfenex® *see* Brompheniramine and Pseudoephedrine *on page 144*

Bromfenex® PD *see* Brompheniramine and Pseudoephedrine *on page 144*
Bromocriptina (Mexico) *see* Bromocriptine *on this page*

Bromocriptine (broe moe KRIP teen)
Brand Names Parlodel®
Canadian/Mexican Brand Names Apo®-Bromocriptine (Canada); Cryocriptina® (Mexico); Serocryptin® (Mexico)
Therapeutic Category Anti-Parkinson's Agent; Ergot Alkaloid
Synonyms Bromocriptina (Mexico)
Use Usually used with levodopa or levodopa/carbidopa to treat Parkinson's disease - treatment of parkinsonism in patients unresponsive or allergic to levodopa

Prolactin-secreting pituitary adenomas, acromegaly, amenorrhea/galactorrhea secondary to hyperprolactinemia in the absence of primary tumor

The indication for prevention of postpartum lactation has been withdrawn voluntarily by Sandoz Pharmaceuticals Corporation
Usual Dosage Adults: Oral:
Parkinsonism: 1.25 mg 2 times/day, increased by 2.5 mg/day in 2- to 4-week intervals (usual dose range is 30-90 mg/day in 3 divided doses), though elderly patients can usually be managed on lower doses
Hyperprolactinemia: 2.5 mg 2-3 times/day
Acromegaly: Initial: 1.25-2.5 mg increasing as necessary every 3-7 days; usual dose: 20-30 mg/day
Mechanism of Action Semisynthetic ergot alkaloid derivative with dopaminergic properties; inhibits prolactin secretion and can improve symptoms of Parkinson's disease by directly stimulating dopamine receptors in the corpus stratum
Local Anesthetic/Vasoconstrictor Precautions No information available to require special precautions
Effects on Dental Treatment No effects or complications reported
Other Adverse Effects Incidence of adverse effects is high, especially at beginning of treatment and with dosages >20 mg/day

1% to 10%:
Cardiovascular: Hypotension, Raynaud's phenomenon
Central nervous system: Mental depression, confusion, hallucinations
Gastrointestinal: Nausea, constipation, anorexia
Neuromuscular & skeletal: Leg cramps
Respiratory: Nasal congestion
<1%:
Cardiovascular: Hypertension, myocardial infarction, syncope
Central nervous system: Dizziness, drowsiness, fatigue, insomnia, headache, seizures
Gastrointestinal: Vomiting, abdominal cramps
Drug Interactions
Decreased effect: Amitriptyline, butyrophenones, imipramine, methyldopa, phenothiazines, reserpine, may decrease bromocriptine's efficacy at reducing prolactin
Increased toxicity: Ergot alkaloids (increased cardiovascular toxicity)
Drug Uptake
Serum half-life (biphasic):
Initial: 6-8 hours
Terminal: 50 hours
Time to peak serum concentration: Oral: Within 1-2 hours
Pregnancy Risk Factor C (See Contraindications)
Generic Available No

Bromodiphenhydramine and Codeine
(brome oh dye fen HYE dra meen & KOE deen)
Brand Names Ambenyl® Cough Syrup; Amgenal® Cough Syrup; Bromanyl® Cough Syrup; Bromotuss® w/Codeine Cough Syrup
Therapeutic Category Antihistamine; Cough Preparation
Synonyms Codeine and Bromodiphenhydramine
Use Relief of upper respiratory symptoms and cough associated with allergies or common cold
Usual Dosage Adults: Oral: 5-10 mL every 4-6 hours
Local Anesthetic/Vasoconstrictor Precautions No information available to require special precautions
Effects on Dental Treatment
Bromodiphenhydramine: 1% to 10%: Dry mouth
Codeine: <1%: Dry mouth
Pregnancy Risk Factor C
(Continued)

Bromodiphenhydramine and Codeine *(Continued)*

Dosage Forms Liquid: Bromodiphenhydramine hydrochloride 12.5 mg and codeine phosphate 10 mg per 5 mL

Generic Available Yes

Bromofeniramina Maleato De (Mexico) *see* Brompheniramine *on this page*

Bromotuss® w/Codeine Cough Syrup *see* Bromodiphenhydramine and Codeine *on previous page*

Bromphen® [OTC] *see* Brompheniramine *on this page*

Bromphen® DC w/Codeine *see* Brompheniramine, Phenylpropanolamine, and Codeine *on page 145*

Brompheniramine *(brome fen IR a meen)*

Brand Names Bromarest® [OTC]; Brombay® [OTC]; Bromphen® [OTC]; Brotane® [OTC]; Chlorphed® [OTC]; Cophene-B®; Diamine T.D.® [OTC]; Dimetane® Extentabs® [OTC]; Nasahist B®; ND-Stat®

Therapeutic Category Antihistamine

Synonyms Bromofeniramina Maleato De (Mexico)

Use Perennial and seasonal allergic rhinitis and other allergic symptoms including urticaria

Usual Dosage

Oral:

Children:

≤6 years: 0.125 mg/kg/dose given every 6 hours; maximum: 6-8 mg/day

6-12 years: 2-4 mg every 6-8 hours; maximum: 12-16 mg/day

Adults: 4 mg every 4-6 hours or 8 mg of sustained release form every 8-12 hours or 12 mg of sustained release every 12 hours; maximum: 24 mg/day

Elderly: Initial: 4 mg once or twice daily. **Note:** Duration of action may be 36 hours or more, even when serum concentrations are low.

I.M., I.V., S.C.:

Children ≤12 years: 0.5 mg/kg/24 hours divided every 6-8 hours

Adults: 10 mg every 6-12 hours, maximum: 40 mg/24 hours

Mechanism of Action Competes with histamine for H_1-receptor sites on effector cells in the gastrointestinal tract, blood vessels, and respiratory tract

Local Anesthetic/Vasoconstrictor Precautions No information available to require special precautions

Effects on Dental Treatment Chronic use of antihistamines will inhibit salivary flow, particularly in elderly patients; this may contribute to periodontal disease and oral discomfort

Other Adverse Effects

>10%:

Central nervous system: Slight to moderate drowsiness (compared with other first generation antihistamines, brompheniramine is relatively nonsedating)

Respiratory: Thickening of bronchial secretions

1% to 10%:

Central nervous system: Headache, fatigue, nervousness, dizziness

Gastrointestinal: Appetite increase, weight increase, nausea, diarrhea, abdominal pain, dry mouth

Neuromuscular & skeletal: Arthralgia

Respiratory: Pharyngitis

<1%:

Cardiovascular: Palpitations

Central nervous system: Depression

Dermatologic: Photosensitivity, rash, angioedema

Hepatic: Hepatitis

Neuromuscular & skeletal: Myalgia, paresthesia

Respiratory: Bronchospasm, epistaxis

Drug Interactions Increased toxicity: CNS depressants, MAO inhibitors, alcohol, tricyclic antidepressants

Drug Uptake

Duration: Varies with formulation

Serum half-life: 12-34 hours

Time to peak serum concentration: Oral: Within 2-5 hours

Pregnancy Risk Factor C

Dosage Forms

Elixir, as maleate: 2 mg/5 mL with 3% alcohol (120 mL, 480 mL, 4000 mL)

Injection, as maleate: 10 mg/mL (10 mL)

Tablet, as maleate: 4 mg, 8 mg, 12 mg

Tablet, sustained release, as maleate: 8 mg, 12 mg

Generic Available Yes

Brompheniramine and Phenylephrine

(brome fen IR a meen & fen il EF rin)

Brand Names Dimetane® Decongestant Elixir [OTC]

Therapeutic Category Antihistamine/Decongestant Combination

Use Temporary relief of symptoms of seasonal and perennial allergic rhinitis, and vasomotor rhinitis, including nasal obstruction

Usual Dosage Oral: Children >12 years and Adults: 10 mL every 4 hours

Local Anesthetic/Vasoconstrictor Precautions

Brompheniramine: No information available to require special precautions

Phenylephrine: Use with caution since phenylephrine is a sympathomimetic amine which could interact with epinephrine to cause a pressor response

Effects on Dental Treatment

Brompheniramine: Prolonged use may decrease salivary flow

Phenylephrine: Up to 10% of patients could experience tachycardia, palpitations, and dry mouth; use vasoconstrictor with caution

Other Adverse Effects

>10%:

Cardiovascular: Tachycardia

Central nervous system: Slight to moderate drowsiness, nervousness, transient stimulation, insomnia

Respiratory: Thickening of bronchial secretions

1% to 10%:

Central nervous system: Headache, fatigue, nervousness, dizziness

Gastrointestinal: Appetite increase, weight increase, nausea, diarrhea, abdominal pain, dry mouth

Genitourinary: Dysuria

Neuromuscular & skeletal: Arthralgia, weakness

Respiratory: Pharyngitis

Miscellaneous: Sweating

<1%:

Cardiovascular: Edema, palpitations, hypotension

Central nervous system: Depression, sedation, paradoxical excitement, convulsions, hallucinations

Dermatologic: Angioedema, rash, photosensitivity

Genitourinary: Urinary retention

Hepatic: Hepatitis

Neuromuscular & skeletal: Myalgia, paresthesia, tremor

Ocular: Blurred vision

Respiratory: Bronchospasm, epistaxis, dyspnea

Drug Interactions CNS depressants, MAO inhibitors, sympathomimetics, Rauwolfia alkaloids, tricyclic antidepressants, ganglionic blocking agents, propranolol

Pregnancy Risk Factor C

Dosage Forms Elixir: Brompheniramine maleate 4 mg and phenylephrine hydrochloride 5 mg per 5 mL

Generic Available Yes

Brompheniramine and Phenylpropanolamine

(brome fen IR a meen & fen il proe pa NOLE a meen)

Brand Names Bromaline® Elixir [OTC]; Bromanate® Elixir [OTC]; Bromatapp® [OTC]; Bromphen® Tablet [OTC]; Cold & Allergy® Elixir [OTC]; Dimaphen® Elixir [OTC]; Dimaphen® Tablets [OTC]; Dimetapp® 4-Hour Liqui-Gel Capsule [OTC]; Dimetapp® Elixir [OTC]; Dimetapp® Extentabs® [OTC]; Dimetapp® Tablet [OTC]; Genatap® Elixir [OTC]; Tamine® [OTC]; Vicks® DayQuil® Allergy Relief 4 Hour Tablet [OTC]

Therapeutic Category Antihistamine/Decongestant Combination

Synonyms Phenylpropanolamine and Brompheniramine

Use Temporary relief of nasal congestion, running nose, sneezing, and itchy, watery eyes

Usual Dosage Oral:

Children:

1-6 months: 1.25 mL 3-4 times/day

7-24 months: 2.5 mL 3-4 times/day

2-4 years: 3.75 mL 3-4 times/day

4-12 years: 5 mL 3-4 times/day

Adults: 5-10 mL 3-4 times/day or 1 regular tablet every 4 hours; sustained release: 1 tablet every 12 hours

Local Anesthetic/Vasoconstrictor Precautions

Brompheniramine: No information available to require special precautions

(Continued)

Brompheniramine and Phenylpropanolamine
(Continued)

Phenylpropanolamine: Use with caution since phenylpropanolamine is a sympathomimetic amine which could interact with epinephrine to cause a pressor response

Effects on Dental Treatment
Brompheniramine: Prolonged use may decrease salivary flow
Phenylpropanolamine: Up to 10% of patients could experience tachycardia, palpitations, and dry mouth; use vasoconstrictor with caution

Other Adverse Effects
>10%:
Cardiovascular: Tachycardia
Central nervous system: Slight to moderate drowsiness, nervousness, transient stimulation, insomnia
Respiratory: Thickening of bronchial secretions
1% to 10%:
Central nervous system: Headache, fatigue, dizziness
Gastrointestinal: Appetite increase, weight increase, nausea, diarrhea, abdominal pain, dry mouth
Genitourinary: Dysuria
Neuromuscular & skeletal: Arthralgia, weakness
Respiratory: Pharyngitis
Miscellaneous: Sweating
<1%:
Central nervous system: Depression, sedation, paradoxical excitement, convulsions, hallucinations
Cardiovascular: Edema, palpitations, hypotension
Dermatologic: Angioedema, rash, photosensitivity
Genitourinary: Urinary retention
Hepatic: Hepatitis
Neuromuscular & skeletal: Myalgia, paresthesia, tremor
Ocular: Blurred vision
Respiratory: Bronchospasm, epistaxis, dyspnea

Drug Interactions
Increased risk of hypertension: MAO inhibitors (hypertensive crisis, severe headache, hyperpyrexia possible), guanethidine, methyldopa
Increased toxicity with CNS depressants, sympathomimetics, TCAs, anticholinergics
Decreased decongestant activity with phenothiazines, rauwolfia alkaloids

Pregnancy Risk Factor B

Dosage Forms
Capsule (Dimetapp® 4-Hour Liqui-Gel): Brompheniramine maleate 4 mg and phenylpropanolamine hydrochloride 25 mg
Liquid (Bromaline®, Bromanate®, Cold & Allergy®, Dimaphen®, Dimetapp®, Genatap®): Brompheniramine maleate 2 mg and phenylpropanolamine hydrochloride 12.5 mg per 5 mL
Tablet (Dimaphen®, Dimetapp®, Vicks® DayQuil® Allergy Relief 4 Hour): Brompheniramine maleate 4 mg and phenylpropanolamine hydrochloride 25 mg
Tablet, sustained release: Brompheniramine maleate 12 mg and phenylpropanolamine hydrochloride 75 mg

Generic Available Yes

Brompheniramine and Pseudoephedrine
(brome fen IR a meen & soo doe e FED rin)

Brand Names Brofed® Elixir [OTC]; Bromfed® Syrup [OTC]; Bromfed® Tablet [OTC]; Bromfenex®; Bromfenex® PD; Drixoral® Syrup [OTC]; Iofed®; Iofed® PD

Therapeutic Category Antihistamine/Decongestant Combination

Use Temporary relief of symptoms of seasonal and perennial allergic rhinitis, and vasomotor rhinitis, including nasal obstruction

Usual Dosage Oral: Children >12 years and Adults: 10 mL every 4-6 hours, up to 40 mL/day

Local Anesthetic/Vasoconstrictor Precautions Use with caution since pseudoephedrine is a sympathomimetic amine which could interact with epinephrine to cause a pressor response

Effects on Dental Treatment
Brompheniramine: Prolonged use may decrease salivary flow
Pseudoephedrine: Up to 10% of patients could experience tachycardia, palpitations, and dry mouth; use vasoconstrictor with caution

Other Adverse Effects
>10%:
Cardiovascular: Tachycardia

Central nervous system: Slight to moderate drowsiness, nervousness, transient stimulation, insomnia

Respiratory: Thickening of bronchial secretions

1% to 10%:

Central nervous system: Headache, fatigue, dizziness

Gastrointestinal: Appetite increase, weight increase, nausea, diarrhea, abdominal pain, dry mouth

Genitourinary: Dysuria

Neuromuscular & skeletal: Arthralgia, weakness

Respiratory: Pharyngitis

Miscellaneous: Sweating

<1%:

Cardiovascular: Edema, palpitations, hypotension

Central nervous system: Depression, sedation, paradoxical excitement, convulsions, hallucinations

Dermatologic: Angioedema, rash, photosensitivity

Genitourinary: Urinary retention

Hepatic: Hepatitis

Neuromuscular & skeletal: Myalgia, paresthesia, tremor

Ocular: Blurred vision

Respiratory: Bronchospasm, epistaxis, dyspnea

Drug Interactions CNS depressants, MAO inhibitors, sympathomimetics, Rauwolfia alkaloids, tricyclic antidepressants, ganglionic blocking agents, propranolol

Pregnancy Risk Factor C

Dosage Forms

Capsule, extended release:

Bromfenex® PD, Iofed® PD: Brompheniramine maleate 6 mg and pseudoephedrine hydrochloride 60 mg

Bromfenex®, Iofed®: Brompheniramine maleate 12 mg and pseudoephedrine hydrochloride 120 mg

Elixir:

Brofed®: Brompheniramine maleate 4 mg and pseudoephedrine hydrochloride 30 mg per 5 mL

Bromfed®: Brompheniramine maleate 2 mg and pseudoephedrine hydrochloride 30 mg per 5 mL

Drixoral®: Brompheniramine maleate 2 mg and pseudoephedrine sulfate 30 mg per 5 mL

Tablet (Bromfed®): Brompheniramine maleate 4 mg and pseudoephedrine hydrochloride 60 mg

Generic Available Yes

Brompheniramine, Phenylpropanolamine, and Codeine
(brome fen IR a meen, fen il proe pa NOLE a meen, & KOE deen)

Brand Names Bromanate® DC; Bromphen® DC w/Codeine; Dimetane®-DC; Myphetane DC®; Poly-Histine CS®

Therapeutic Category Antihistamine/Decongestant Combination; Cough Preparation

Use Relief of coughs and upper respiratory symptoms, including nasal congestion, associated with allergy or the common cold

Usual Dosage Oral:

Children:

2-6 years: 2.5 mL every 4 hours

6-12 years: 5 mL every 4 hours

Children >12 years and Adults: 10 mL every 4 hours

Local Anesthetic/Vasoconstrictor Precautions

Brompheniramine: No information available to require special precautions

Phenylpropanolamine: Use with caution since phenylpropanolamine is a sympathomimetic amine which could interact with epinephrine to cause a pressor response

Effects on Dental Treatment

Brompheniramine: Prolonged use may decrease salivary flow

Codeine: <1%: Dry mouth

Phenylpropanolamine: Up to 10% of patients could experience tachycardia, palpitations, and dry mouth; use vasoconstrictor with caution

Drug Interactions CNS depressants, MAO inhibitors, sympathomimetics, Rauwolfia alkaloids, tricyclic antidepressants, ganglionic blocking agents, propranolol

Pregnancy Risk Factor C

(Continued)

Brompheniramine, Phenylpropanolamine, and Codeine
(Continued)

Dosage Forms Liquid: Brompheniramine maleate 2 mg, phenylpropanolamine hydrochloride 12.5 mg, and codeine phosphate 10 mg per 5 mL with alcohol 0.95% (480 mL)

Generic Available Yes

Bromphen® Tablet [OTC] see Brompheniramine and Phenylpropanolamine on page 143

Bronchial® see Theophylline and Guaifenesin on page 922

Bronkephrine® Injection see Ethylnorepinephrine on page 384

Bronkodyl® see Theophylline on page 917

Bronkometer® see Isoetharine on page 521

Bronkosol® see Isoetharine on page 521

Brontex® Liquid see Guaifenesin and Codeine on page 452

Brontex® Tablet see Guaifenesin and Codeine on page 452

Brotane® [OTC] see Brompheniramine on page 142

BSS® Ophthalmic see Balanced Salt Solution on page 110

BTPABA see Bentiromide on page 117

Bucladin®-S Softab® see Buclizine on this page

Buclizine (BYOO kli zeen)
Brand Names Bucladin®-S Softab®

Therapeutic Category Antiemetic; Antihistamine

Use Prevention and treatment of motion sickness; symptomatic treatment of vertigo

Usual Dosage Adults: Oral:

Motion sickness (prophylaxis): 50 mg 30 minutes prior to traveling; may repeat 50 mg after 4-6 hours

Vertigo: 50 mg twice daily, up to 150 mg/day

Mechanism of Action Buclizine acts centrally to suppress nausea and vomiting. It is a piperazine antihistamine closely related to cyclizine and meclizine. It also has CNS depressant, anticholinergic, antispasmodic, and local anesthetic effects, and suppresses labyrinthine activity and conduction in vestibular-cerebellar nerve pathways.

Local Anesthetic/Vasoconstrictor Precautions No information available to require special precautions

Effects on Dental Treatment No effects or complications reported

Other Adverse Effects

>10%: Central nervous system: Drowsiness

<1%:

Cardiovascular: Hypotension, palpitations

Central nervous system: Sedation, dizziness, paradoxical excitement, fatigue, insomnia

Gastrointestinal: Nausea, vomiting

Genitourinary: Urinary retention

Neuromuscular & skeletal: Tremor

Ocular: Blurred vision

Drug Interactions Increased toxicity: CNS depressants, MAO inhibitors, tricyclic antidepressants

Pregnancy Risk Factor C

Generic Available Yes

Budesonide (byoo DES oh nide)
Brand Names Rhinocort™

Canadian/Mexican Brand Names Entocort® (Canada); Pulmicort® (Canada)

Therapeutic Category Anti-inflammatory Agent; Corticosteroid, Inhalant; Glucocorticoid

Use Management of symptoms of seasonal or perennial rhinitis in adults and nonallergic perennial rhinitis in adults

Usual Dosage

Children <6 years: Not recommended

Children ≥6 years and Adults: 256 mcg/day, given as either 2 sprays in each nostril in the morning and evening or as 4 sprays in each nostril in the morning

Local Anesthetic/Vasoconstrictor Precautions No information available to require special precautions

Effects on Dental Treatment Localized infections with *Candida albicans* or *Aspergillus niger* have occurred frequently in the mouth and pharynx with repetitive use of oral inhaler of beclomethasone. Positive cultures for oral *Candida* may be present in up to 75% of patients. These infections may require treatment with appropriate antifungal therapy or discontinuance of treatment with beclomethasone inhaler.

Other Adverse Effects
>10%:
    Cardiovascular: Pounding heartbeat
    Central nervous system: Nervousness, headache, dizziness
    Dermatologic: Itching, skin rash
    Gastrointestinal: GI irritation, bitter taste
    Respiratory: Coughing, upper respiratory tract infection, bronchitis, hoarseness
    Miscellaneous: Oral candidiasis, increased susceptibility to infections, sweating
1% to 10%:
    Central nervous system: Insomnia, psychic changes
    Dermatologic: Acne, urticaria
    Endocrine & metabolic: Menstrual problems
    Gastrointestinal: Anorexia, dry mouth/throat, increase in appetite
    Ocular: Cataracts
    Respiratory: Epistaxis
    Miscellaneous: Loss of smell/taste
<1%:
    Gastrointestinal: Abdominal fullness
    Respiratory: Bronchospasm, dyspnea

Drug Interactions No data reported

Drug Uptake
    Absorption: Nasal: 20% of dose delivered reaches systemic circulation

Pregnancy Risk Factor C

Generic Available No

Bufferin® [OTC] *see* Aspirin *on page 90*
Buffex® [OTC] *see* Aspirin *on page 90*
Bumetanida (Mexico) *see* Bumetanide *on this page*

Bumetanide (byoo MET a nide)
Related Information
    Cardiovascular Diseases *on page 1010*
Brand Names Bumex®
Canadian/Mexican Brand Names Bumedyl® (Mexico); Burinex® (Canada)
Therapeutic Category Diuretic, Loop
Synonyms Bumetanida (Mexico)
Use Management of edema secondary to congestive heart failure or hepatic or renal disease including nephrotic syndrome; may be used alone or in combination with antihypertensives in the treatment of hypertension; can be used in furosemide-allergic patients; (1 mg = 40 mg furosemide)
Usual Dosage
Children:
    <6 months: Dose not established
    >6 months:
        Oral: Initial: 0.015 mg/kg/dose once daily or every other day; maximum dose: 0.1 mg/kg/day
        I.M., I.V.: Dose not established
Adults:
    Oral: 0.5-2 mg/dose 1-2 times/day; maximum: 10 mg/day
    I.M., I.V.: 0.5-1 mg/dose; maximum: 10 mg/day
    Continuous I.V. infusions of 0.9-1 mg/hour may be more effective than bolus dosing
Mechanism of Action Inhibits reabsorption of sodium and chloride in the ascending loop of Henle and proximal renal tubule, interfering with the chloride-binding cotransport system, thus causing increased excretion of water, sodium, chloride, magnesium, phosphate and calcium; it does not appear to act on the distal tubule
Local Anesthetic/Vasoconstrictor Precautions No information available to require special precautions
Effects on Dental Treatment No effects or complications reported
Other Adverse Effects
>10%:
    Endocrine & metabolic: Hyperuricemia, hypochloremia, hypokalemia
    Renal: Azotemia
1% to 10%:
    Central nervous system: Dizziness, encephalopathy, headache
    Endocrine & metabolic: Hyponatremia
    Neuromuscular & skeletal: Muscle cramps, weakness
<1%:
    Cardiovascular: Hypotension
(Continued)

Bumetanide *(Continued)*

    Dermatologic: Rash, pruritus
    Endocrine & metabolic: Hyperglycemia
    Gastrointestinal: Cramps, nausea, vomiting
    Hepatic: Alteration of liver function test results
    Otic: Hearing loss
    Renal: Elevated serum creatinine

Drug Interactions
Additive effect: Other antihypertensive agents
Decreased effect: Indomethacin and other NSAIDs, probenecid
Increased effect: Lithium excretion may be decreased

Drug Uptake
Onset of effect:
    Oral, I.M.: 0.5-1 hour
    I.V.: 2-3 minutes
Duration of action: 6 hours
Serum half-life:
    Infants <6 months: Possibly 2.5 hours
    Children and Adults: 1-1.5 hours

Pregnancy Risk Factor D
Generic Available Yes

Bumex® see Bumetanide *on previous page*
Bupap® New Brand see Butalbital Compound and Acetaminophen *on page 155*
Buphenyl® see Sodium Phenylbutyrate *on page 873*

Bupivacaine (byoo PIV a kane)

Related Information
Oral Pain *on page 1053*

Brand Names Marcaine®; Sensorcaine®; Sensorcaine®-MPF
Canadian/Mexican Brand Names Buvacaína® (Mexico)
Therapeutic Category Dental/Local Anesthetics; Local Anesthetic, Injectable
Use Local anesthetic (injectable) for peripheral nerve block, infiltration, sympathetic block, caudal or epidural block, retrobulbar block
Usual Dosage Dose varies with procedure, depth of anesthesia, vascularity of tissues, duration of anesthesia and condition of patient. Metabisulfites (in epinephrine-containing injection); do not use solutions containing preservatives for caudal or epidural block.

Caudal block (with or without epinephrine):
    Children: 1-3.7 mg/kg
    Adults: 15-30 mL of 0.25% or 0.5%

Epidural block (other than caudal block):
    Children: 1.25 mg/kg/dose
    Adults: 10-20 mL of 0.25% or 0.5%

Peripheral nerve block: 5 mL dose of 0.25% or 0.5% (12.5-25 mg); maximum: 2.5 mg/kg (plain); 3 mg/kg (with epinephrine); up to a maximum of 400 mg/day

Sympathetic nerve block: 20-50 mL of 0.25% (no epinephrine) solution

Mechanism of Action Blocks both the initiation and conduction of nerve impulses by decreasing the neuronal membrane's permeability to sodium ions, which results in inhibition of depolarization with resultant blockade of conduction
Local Anesthetic/Vasoconstrictor Precautions No information available to require special precautions
Effects on Dental Treatment No effects or complications reported
Other Adverse Effects 1% to 10% (dose related):
Cardiovascular: Cardiac arrest, hypotension, bradycardia, palpitations
Central nervous system: Seizures, restlessness, anxiety, dizziness
Gastrointestinal: Nausea, vomiting
    Neuromuscular & skeletal: Weakness
Ocular: Blurred vision
Otic: Tinnitus
Respiratory: Apnea
Contraindications Hypersensitivity to bupivacaine hydrochloride or any component, para-aminobenzoic acid or parabens
Warnings/Precautions Use with caution in patients with liver disease. Some commercially available formulations contain sodium metabisulfite, which may cause allergic-type reactions. Pending further data, should not be used in children <12 years of age and the solution for spinal anesthesia should not be used in children <18 years of age. **Do not use solutions containing preservatives for caudal or epidural block**; convulsions due to systemic toxicity leading to

cardiac arrest have been reported, presumably following unintentional intravascular injection. 0.75% is **not** recommended for obstetrical anesthesia.

Drug Interactions

Increased effect: Hyaluronidase

Increased toxicity: Beta-blockers, ergot-type oxytocics, MAO inhibitors, TCAs, phenothiazines, vasopressors

Drug Uptake

Onset of anesthesia (dependent on route administered): Within 4-10 minutes generally

Duration of action: 1.5-8.5 hours

Serum half-life (age dependent): Adults: 1.5-5.5 hours

Pregnancy Risk Factor C

Dosage Forms

Injection: 0.25% (10 mL, 20 mL, 30 mL, 50 mL); 0.5% (10 mL, 20 mL, 30 mL, 50 mL); 0.75% (2 mL, 10 mL, 20 mL, 30 mL)

Injection, with epinephrine (1:200,000): 0.25% (10 mL, 30 mL, 50 mL); 0.5% (1.8 mL, 3 mL, 5 mL, 10 mL, 30 mL, 50 mL); 0.75% (30 mL)

Generic Available Yes

Bupivacaine and Epinephrine (byoo PIV a kane & ep i NEF rin)

Related Information

Oral Pain on page 1053

Brand Names Marcaine® With Epinephrine; Sensorcaine MPF

Canadian/Mexican Brand Names Buvacaina® (Mexico); Sensorcaine® With Epinephrine (Canada)

Therapeutic Category Dental/Local Anesthetics; Local Anesthetic, Injectable

Use Dental and Medical: Local anesthesia

Usual Dosage

Children <10 years: Dosage has not been established

Children >10 years and Adults: Infiltration and nerve block in maxillary and mandibular area: 9 mg (1.8 mL) of bupivacaine as a 0.5% solution with epinephrine 1:200,000 per injection site. A second dose may be administered if necessary to produce adequate anesthesia after allowing up to 10 minutes for onset. Up to a maximum of 90 mg of bupivacaine hydrochloride per dental appointment. The effective anesthetic dose varies with procedure, intensity of anesthesia needed, duration of anesthesia required, and physical condition of the patient; always use the lowest effective dose along with careful aspiration. The following numbers of dental carpules (1.8 mL) provide the indicated amounts of bupivacaine hydrochloride 0.5% and epinephrine 1:200,000.

# of Cartridges	Mg Bupivacaine (0.5%)	Mg Vasoconstrictor (Epinephrine 1:200,000)
1	9	0.009
2	18	0.018
3	27	0.027
4	36	0.036
5	45	0.045
6	54	0.054
7	63	0.063
8	72	0.072
9	81	0.081
10	90	0.090

Note: Adult and children doses of bupivacaine hydrochloride with epinephrine cited from USP Dispensing Information (USP DI), 17th ed, The United States Pharmacopeial Convention, Inc, Rockville, MD, 1997, 134.

Mechanism of Action Local anesthetics bind selectively to the intracellular surface of sodium channels to block influx of sodium into the axon. As a result, depolarization necessary for action potential propagation and subsequent nerve function is prevented. The block at the sodium channel is reversible. When drug diffuses away from the axon, sodium channel function is restored and nerve propagation returns.

Epinephrine prolongs the duration of the anesthetic actions of bupivacaine by causing vasoconstriction (alpha adrenergic receptor agonist) of the vasculature surrounding the nerve axons. This prevents the diffusion of bupivacaine away from the nerves resulting in a longer retention in the axon

Local Anesthetic/Vasoconstrictor Precautions No information available to require special precautions

Effects on Dental Treatment No effects or complications reported

(Continued)

Bupivacaine and Epinephrine *(Continued)*

Other Adverse Effects Degree of adverse effects in the central nervous system and cardiovascular system are directly related to the blood levels of bupivacaine

Cardiovascular: Myocardial effects include a decrease in contraction force as well as a decrease in electrical excitability and myocardial conduction rate resulting in bradycardia and reduction in cardiac output.

Central nervous system: High blood levels result in anxiety, restlessness, disorientation, confusion, dizziness, tremors and seizures. This is followed by depression of CNS resulting in somnolence, unconsciousness and possible respiratory arrest. Nausea and vomiting may also occur. In some cases, symptoms of CNS stimulation may be absent and the primary CNS effects are somnolence and unconsciousness.

Hypersensitivity reactions: Extremely rare, but may be manifest as dermatologic reactions and edema at injection site. Asthmatic syndromes have occurred. Patients may exhibit hypersensitivity to bisulfites contained in local anesthetic solution to prevent oxidation of epinephrine. In general, patients reacting to bisulfites have a history of asthma and their airways are hyper-reactive to asthmatic syndrome.

Psychogenic reactions: It is common to misinterpret psychogenic responses to local anesthetic injection as an allergic reaction. Intraoral injections are perceived by many patients as a stressful procedure in dentistry. Common symptoms to this stress are sweating, palpitations, hyperventilation, generalized pallor and a fainting feeling.

Contraindications Hypersensitivity to bupivacaine

Warnings/Precautions Should be avoided in patients with uncontrolled hyperthyroidism

Drug Interactions Due to epinephrine component: With tricyclic antidepressants or MAO inhibitors could result in increased pressor response; with nonselective beta-blockers (ie, propranolol) could result in serious hypertension and reflex bradycardia

Drug Uptake

Onset of action: Infiltration and nerve block: 2-20 minutes

Duration:

Infiltration: 60 minutes

Nerve block: 5-7 hours

Serum half-life: 1.5-5.5 hours/adult

Pregnancy Risk Factor C

Breast-feeding Considerations Usual infiltration doses of bupivacaine with epinephrine given to nursing mothers has not been shown to affect the health of the nursing infant

Dosage Forms Injection: Bupivacaine hydrochloride 0.5% with epinephrine 1:200,000 (1.8 mL cartridges in boxes of 50)

Dietary Considerations No data reported

Generic Available Yes

Selected Readings

Jastak JT and Yagiela JA, "Vasoconstrictors and Local Anesthesia: A Review and Rationale for Use," *J Am Dent Assoc,* 1983, 107(4):623-30.

MacKenzie TA and Young ER, "Local Anesthetic Update," *Anesth Prog,* 1993, 40(2):29-34.

Wynn RL, "Epinephrine Interactions With Beta-Blockers," *Gen Dent,* 1994, 42(1):16, 18.

Yagiela JA, "Local Anesthetics," *Anesth Prog,* 1991, 38(4-5):128-41.

Buprenex® *see* Buprenorphine *on this page*

Buprenorfina (Mexico) *see* Buprenorphine *on this page*

Buprenorphine *(byoo pre NOR feen)*

Related Information

Narcotic Agonists *on page 1141*

Brand Names Buprenex®

Canadian/Mexican Brand Names Temgesic® (Mexico)

Therapeutic Category Analgesic, Narcotic

Synonyms Buprenorfina (Mexico)

Use Management of moderate to severe pain

Usual Dosage I.M., slow I.V.:

Children ≥13 years and Adults: 0.3-0.6 mg every 6 hours as needed

Elderly: 0.15 mg every 6 hours; elderly patients are more likely to suffer from confusion and drowsiness compared to younger patients

Long-term use is not recommended

Mechanism of Action Opiate agonist/antagonist that produces analgesia by binding to kappa and mu opiate receptors in the CNS

Local Anesthetic/Vasoconstrictor Precautions No information available to require special precautions

Effects on Dental Treatment No effects or complications reported

Other Adverse Effects
>10%: Central nervous system: Drowsiness
1% to 10%:
  Cardiovascular: Hypotension
  Central nervous system: Dizziness, headache
  Gastrointestinal: Vomiting, nausea
  Respiratory: Respiratory depression
<1%:
  Central nervous system: Euphoria, slurred speech, malaise
  Dermatologic: Allergic dermatitis
  Genitourinary: Urinary retention
  Neuromuscular & skeletal: Paresthesia
  Ocular: Blurred vision
Drug Interactions Increased toxicity: Barbiturates, benzodiazepines (increase CNS and respiratory depression)
Drug Uptake
Onset of analgesia: Within 10-30 minutes
Absorption: I.M., S.C.: 30% to 40%
Serum half-life: 2.2-3 hours
Pregnancy Risk Factor C
Generic Available Yes

Bupropion (byoo PROE pee on)
Related Information
Vasoconstrictor Interactions With Antidepressants *on page 1226*
Brand Names Wellbutrin®; Wellbutrin® SR; Zyban®
Therapeutic Category Antidepressant, Miscellaneous
Use Treatment of depression; as an aid to smoking cessation treatment in smokers ≥18 years of age
Usual Dosage Adults: Oral: Begin at 150 mg/day for first 3 days, increase dosage to maximum 300 mg/day (150 mg twice daily) for 7-12 weeks; allow at least 8 hours between successive doses
Mechanism of Action Antidepressant structurally different from all other previously marketed antidepressants; like other antidepressants the mechanism of bupropion's activity is not fully understood; weak blocker of serotonin and norepinephrine re-uptake, inhibits neuronal dopamine re-uptake and is **not** a monoamine oxidase A or B inhibitor
Local Anesthetic/Vasoconstrictor Precautions None; this is not a tricyclic type antidepressant and will not enhance pressor response of epinephrine
Effects on Dental Treatment A common adverse effect is significant dry mouth (>10%); normal salivary flow will occur with cessation of drug therapy
Other Adverse Effects
>10%:
  Central nervous system: Agitation, insomnia, fever, headache, psychosis, confusion, anxiety, restlessness, dizziness, seizures, chills, akathisia
  Gastrointestinal: Nausea, vomiting, constipation, weight loss
  Genitourinary: Impotence
  Neuromuscular & skeletal: Tremor
1% to 10%:
  Central nervous system: Hallucinations, fatigue
  Dermatologic: Skin rash
  Ocular: Blurred vision
<1%:
  Cardiovascular: Syncope
  Central nervous system: Drowsiness
Contraindications In patients with a seizure disorder or with a current profile of bulimia or anorexia nervosa; contraindicated with concurrent administration of an MAO inhibitor
Warnings/Precautions Use of bupropion is associated with dose-dependent risk of seizures; therefore, doses of >300 mg/day should not be prescribed
Drug Interactions
Decreased effects: Increased clearance: Carbamazepine, phenytoin, cimetidine, phenobarbital
Increased effects: Levodopa, MAO inhibitors
Drug Uptake
Absorption: Rapidly absorbed from GI tract
Serum half-life: 14 hours
Time to peak serum concentration: Oral: Within 3 hours
Pregnancy Risk Factor B
Dosage Forms
Tablet (Wellbutrin®): 75 mg, 100 mg
(Continued)

Bupropion *(Continued)*

Tablet, sustained release (Wellbutrin® SR, Zyban®): 100 mg, 150 mg
Generic Available No

Burow's Otic *see* Aluminum Acetate and Acetic Acid *on page 47*
BuSpar® *see* Buspirone *on this page*
Buspirona, Clorhidrato De (Mexico) *see* Buspirone *on this page*

Buspirone (byoo SPYE rone)

Related Information
Patients Requiring Sedation *on page 1081*
Brand Names BuSpar®
Canadian/Mexican Brand Names Neurosine® (Mexico)
Therapeutic Category Antianxiety Agent; Tranquilizer, Minor
Synonyms Buspirona, Clorhidrato De (Mexico)
Use Management of anxiety; has shown little potential for abuse
Unlabeled use: Panic attacks
Usual Dosage Adults: Oral: 15 mg/day (5 mg 3 times/day); may increase in increments of 5 mg/day every 2-4 days to a maximum of 60 mg/day
Mechanism of Action Selectively antagonizes CNS serotonin $5-HT_1A$ receptors without affecting benzodiazepine-GABA receptors; may down-regulate postsynaptic $5-HT_2$ receptors as do antidepressants
Local Anesthetic/Vasoconstrictor Precautions No information available to require special precautions
Effects on Dental Treatment No effects or complications reported
Other Adverse Effects
>10%:
Central nervous system: Dizziness, lightheadedness, headache, restlessness
Gastrointestinal: Nausea
1% to 10%: Central nervous system: Drowsiness
<1%:
Cardiovascular: Chest pain, tachycardia
Central nervous system: Confusion, insomnia, nightmares, sedation, disorientation, excitement, fever, ataxia
Dermatologic: Rash, urticaria
Gastrointestinal: Dry mouth, vomiting, diarrhea, flatulence
Hematologic: Leukopenia, eosinophilia
Neuromuscular & skeletal: Weakness
Ocular: Blurred vision
Otic: Tinnitus
Drug Interactions
Increased effects: Cimetidine, food
Increased toxicity: MAO inhibitors, phenothiazines, CNS depressants; increased toxicity of digoxin and haloperidol
Drug Uptake
Serum half-life: 2-3 hours
Time to peak serum concentration: Oral: Within 40-60 minutes
Pregnancy Risk Factor B
Dosage Forms Tablet, as hydrochloride: 5 mg, 10 mg
Dietary Considerations Food may decrease the absorption of buspirone, but it may also decrease the first-pass metabolism, thereby increasing the bioavailability of buspirone
Generic Available No

Busulfan (byoo SUL fan)

Brand Names Myleran®
Therapeutic Category Antineoplastic Agent, Alkylating Agent
Synonyms Busulfano (Mexico)
Use Chronic myelogenous leukemia and bone marrow disorders, such as polycythemia vera and myeloid metaplasia, conditioning regimens for bone marrow transplantation
Usual Dosage Oral (**refer to individual protocols**):
Children:
For remission induction of CML: 0.06-0.12 mg/kg/day **or** 1.8-4.6 mg/m²/day; titrate dosage to maintain leukocyte count above 40,000/mm³; reduce dosage by 50% if the leukocyte count reaches 30,000-40,000/mm³; discontinue drug if counts fall to ≤20,000/mm³
BMT marrow-ablative conditioning regimen: 1 mg/kg/dose (ideal body weight) every 6 hours for 16 doses

Adults:

BMT marrow-ablative conditioning regimen: 1 mg/kg/dose (ideal body weight) every 6 hours for 16 doses

Remission:

Induction of CML: 4-8 mg/day (may be as high as 12 mg/day)

Maintenance doses: Controversial, range from 1-4 mg/day to 2 mg/week; treatment is continued until WBC reaches 10,000-20,000 cells/mm^3 at which time drug is discontinued; when WBC reaches 50,000/mm^3, maintenance dose is resumed

Unapproved uses:

Polycythemia vera: 2-6 mg/day

Thrombocytosis: 4-6 mg/day

Mechanism of Action Reacts with N-7 position of guanosine and interferes with DNA replication and transcription of RNA. Busulfan has a more marked effect on myeloid cells (and is, therefore, useful in the treatment of CML) than on lymphoid cells. The drug is also very toxic to hematopoietic stem cells (thus its usefulness in high doses in BMT preparative regimens). Busulfan exhibits little immunosuppressive activity. Interferes with the normal function of DNA by alkylation and cross-linking the strands of DNA.

Local Anesthetic/Vasoconstrictor Precautions No information available to require special precautions

Effects on Dental Treatment No effects or complications reported

Other Adverse Effects Fertility/carcinogenesis: Sterility, ovarian suppression, amenorrhea, azoospermia, and testicular atrophy; malignant tumors have been reported in patients on busulfan therapy

>10%:

Hematologic: Severe pancytopenia, leukopenia, thrombocytopenia, anemia, and bone marrow suppression are common and patients should be monitored closely while on therapy. Since this is a delayed effect (busulfan affects the stem cells), the drug should be discontinued temporarily at the first sign of a large or rapid fall in any blood element. Some patients may develop bone marrow fibrosis or chronic aplasia which is probably due to the busulfan toxicity. In large doses, busulfan is myeloablative and is used for this reason in BMT.

Myelosuppressive: WBC: Moderate; Platelets: Moderate; Onset (days): 7-10; Nadir (days): 14-21; Recovery (days): 28

1% to 10%:

Cardiovascular: Endocardial fibrosis

Dermatologic: Hyperpigmentation skin (busulfan tan), urticaria, erythema, alopecia

Endocrine & metabolic: Amenorrhea

Gastrointestinal: Nausea, vomiting, diarrhea; drug has little effect on the GI mucosal lining

Emetic potential: Low (<10%)

Neuromuscular & skeletal: Weakness

<1%:

Central nervous system: Generalized or myoclonic seizures and loss of consciousness have been associated with high-dose busulfan (4 mg/kg/day), blurred vision

Endocrine & metabolic: Adrenal suppression, gynecomastia, hyperuricemia

Genitourinary: Isolated cases of hemorrhagic cystitis have been reported

Hepatic: Hepatic dysfunction

Ocular: Cataracts

Respiratory: After long-term or high-dose therapy, a syndrome known as busulfan lung may occur. This syndrome is manifested by a diffuse interstitial pulmonary fibrosis and persistent cough, fever, rales, and dyspnea. May be relieved by corticosteroids.

Drug Interactions No data reported

Drug Uptake

Absorption: Rapidly and completely from the GI tract

Serum half-life:

After first dose: 3.4 hours

After last dose: 2.3 hours

Time to peak serum concentration:

Oral: Within 4 hours

I.V.: Within 5 minutes

Pregnancy Risk Factor D

Generic Available No

Busulfano (Mexico) *see* Busulfan *on previous page*

Butabarbital Sodium (byoo ta BAR bi tal SOW dee um)
Brand Names Butalan®; Buticaps®; Butisol Sodium®
Therapeutic Category Barbiturate; Hypnotic; Sedative
Use Sedative, hypnotic
Usual Dosage Oral:
  Children: Preop: 2-6 mg/kg/dose; maximum: 100 mg

  Adults:
    Sedative: 15-30 mg 3-4 times/day
    Hypnotic: 50-100 mg
    Preop: 50-100 mg 1-1½ hours before surgery
Mechanism of Action Interferes with transmission of impulses from the thalamus to the cortex of the brain resulting in an imbalance in central inhibitory and facilitatory mechanisms
Local Anesthetic/Vasoconstrictor Precautions No information available to require special precautions
Effects on Dental Treatment No effects or complications reported
Other Adverse Effects
  >10%: Central nervous system: Dizziness, lightheadedness, drowsiness, "hangover" effect
  1% to 10%:
    Central nervous system: Confusion, mental depression, unusual excitement, nervousness, faint feeling, headache, insomnia, nightmares
    Gastrointestinal: Constipation, nausea, vomiting
  <1%:
    Cardiovascular: Hypotension
    Central nervous system: Hallucinations
    Dermatologic: Skin rash, exfoliative dermatitis, Stevens-Johnson syndrome, angioedema
    Hematologic: Agranulocytosis, megaloblastic anemia, thrombocytopenia
    Local: Thrombophlebitis
    Respiratory: Respiratory depression
    Miscellaneous: Dependence
Drug Interactions
  Barbiturates can induce hepatic microsomal enzymes resulting in increased metabolism and therefore decreased effects of anticoagulants, corticosteroids, doxycycline
  Increased toxicity when combined with other CNS depressants or antidepressants, respiratory and CNS depression may be additive
Drug Uptake
  Serum half-life: 40-140 hours
  Time to peak serum concentration: Oral: Within 40-60 minutes
Pregnancy Risk Factor D
Generic Available Yes

Butace® *see* Butalbital Compound *on this page*
Butalan® *see* Butabarbital Sodium *on this page*

Butalbital Compound (byoo TAL bi tal KOM pound)
Related Information
  Butalbital Compound and Acetaminophen *on next page*
  Butalbital Compound and Aspirin *on page 156*
Brand Names Amaphen®; Anoquan®; Axotal®; B-A-C®; Bancap®; Butace®; Endolor®; Esgic®; Femcet®; Fiorgen PF®; Fioricet®; Fiorinal®; G-1®; Isollyl Improved®; Lanorinal®; Marnal®; Medigesic®; Phrenilin®; Phrenilin® Forte®; Repan®; Sedapap-10®; Triapin®; Two-Dyne®
Canadian/Mexican Brand Names Tecnal® (Canada)
Therapeutic Category Analgesic, Non-narcotic; Barbiturate
Use Relief of symptomatic complex of tension or muscle contraction headache
Usual Dosage Adults: Oral: 1-2 tablets or capsules every 4 hours; not to exceed 6/day
Mechanism of Action Butalbital, like other barbiturates, has a generalized depressant effect on the central nervous system (CNS). Barbiturates have little effect on peripheral nerves or muscle at usual therapeutic doses. However, at toxic doses serious effects on the cardiovascular system and other peripheral systems may be observed. These effects may result in hypotension or skeletal muscle weakness. While all areas of the central nervous system are acted on by barbiturates, the mesencephalic reticular activating system is extremely sensitive to their effects. Barbiturates act at synapses where gamma-aminobenzoic acid is a neurotransmitter, but they may act in other areas as well.
Local Anesthetic/Vasoconstrictor Precautions No information available to require special precautions

Effects on Dental Treatment No effects or complications reported

Other Adverse Effects

>10%:

Central nervous system: Dizziness, lightheadedness, drowsiness, "hangover" effect

Gastrointestinal: Nausea, heartburn, stomach pains, dyspepsia, epigastric discomfort

1% to 10%:

Central nervous system: Confusion, mental depression, unusual excitement, nervousness, faint feeling, headache, insomnia, nightmares, fatigue

Dermatologic: Skin rash

Gastrointestinal: Constipation, vomiting, gastrointestinal ulceration

Hematologic: Hemolytic anemia

Neuromuscular & skeletal: Weakness

Respiratory: Dyspnea

Miscellaneous: Anaphylactic shock

<1%:

Cardiovascular: Hypotension

Central nervous system: Hallucinations, jitters

Dermatologic: Exfoliative dermatitis, Stevens-Johnson syndrome

Hematologic: Agranulocytosis, megaloblastic anemia, occult bleeding, prolongation of bleeding time, leukopenia, thrombocytopenia, iron deficiency anemia

Hepatic: Hepatotoxicity

Local: Thrombophlebitis

Renal: Impaired renal function

Respiratory: Respiratory depression, bronchospasm

Drug Interactions

Decreased effect: Phenothiazines, haloperidol, quinidine, cyclosporine, tricyclic antidepressants, corticosteroids, theophylline, ethosuximide, warfarin, oral contraceptives, chloramphenicol, griseofulvin, doxycycline, beta-blockers

Increased effect/toxicity: Propoxyphene, benzodiazepines, CNS depressants, valproic acid, methylphenidate, chloramphenicol

Drug Uptake Serum half-life: 61 hours in healthy volunteers

Pregnancy Risk Factor D

Dosage Forms

Capsule, with acetaminophen:

Amaphen®, Anoquan®, Butace®, Endolor®, Esgic®, Femcet®, G-1®, Medigesic®, Repan®, Two-Dyne®: Butalbital 50 mg, caffeine 40 mg, and acetaminophen 325 mg

Bancap®, Triapin®: Butalbital 50 mg and acetaminophen 325 mg

Phrenilin Forte®: Butalbital 50 mg and acetaminophen 650 mg

Capsule, with aspirin: (Fiorgen PF®, Fiorinal®, Isollyl Improved®, Lanorinal®, Marnal®): Butalbital 50 mg, caffeine 40 mg, and aspirin 325 mg

Tablet, with acetaminophen:

Esgic®, Fioricet®, Repan®: Butalbital 50 mg, caffeine 40 mg, and acetaminophen 325 mg

Phrenilin®: Butalbital 50 mg and acetaminophen 325 mg

Sedapap-10®: Butalbital 50 mg and acetaminophen 650 mg

Tablet, with aspirin:

Axotal®: Butalbital 50 mg and aspirin 650 mg

B-A-C®: Butalbital 50 mg, caffeine 40 mg, and aspirin 650 mg

Fiorinal®, Isollyl Improved®, Lanorinal®, Marnal®: Butalbital 50 mg, caffeine 40 mg, and aspirin 325 mg

Generic Available Yes

Butalbital Compound and Acetaminophen

(byoo TAL bi tal KOM pound & a seet a MIN oh fen)

Brand Names Amaphen®; Anoquan®; Bancap®; Bupap® *New Brand*; Endolor®; Esgic®; Esgic-Plus®; Femcet®; Fioricet®; G-1®; Medigesic®; Phrenilin®; Phrenilin Forte®; Repan®; Sedapap-10®; Triapin®; Two-Dyne®

Therapeutic Category Barbiturate/Analgesic

Synonyms Acetaminophen and Butalbital Compound

Use Relief of the symptomatic complex of tension or muscle contraction headache

Restrictions C-III

Usual Dosage Adults: Oral: 1-2 tablets or capsules every 4 hours; not to exceed 6/day

Local Anesthetic/Vasoconstrictor Precautions No information available to require special precautions

Effects on Dental Treatment No effects or complications reported

Drug Interactions See individual agents

Pregnancy Risk Factor D

(Continued)

Butalbital Compound and Acetaminophen *(Continued)*

Dosage Forms
Capsule:
 Amaphen®, Anoquan®, Butace®, Endolor®, Esgic®, Femcet®, G-1®, Medigesic®, Repan®, Two-Dyne®: Butalbital 50 mg, caffeine 40 mg, and acetaminophen 325 mg

Bancap®, Triapin®: Butalbital 50 mg and acetaminophen 325 mg

Phrenilin Forte®: Butalbital 50 mg and acetaminophen 650 mg

Tablet:
 Esgic®, Fioricet®, Repan®: Butalbital 50 mg, caffeine 40 mg, and acetaminophen 325 mg

Phrenilin®: Butalbital 50 mg and acetaminophen 325 mg

Sedapap-10®: Butalbital 50 mg and acetaminophen 650 mg

Generic Available Yes

Butalbital Compound and Aspirin
(byoo TAL bi tal KOM pound & AS pir in)

Brand Names Fiorgen PF®; Fiorinal®; Isollyl® Improved; Lanorinal®

Therapeutic Category Barbiturate/Analgesic

Use Relief of the symptomatic complex of tension or muscle contraction headache

Restrictions C-III (Fiorinal®)

Usual Dosage Adults: Oral: 1-2 tablets or capsules every 4 hours; not to exceed 6/day

Local Anesthetic/Vasoconstrictor Precautions No information available to require special precautions

Effects on Dental Treatment No effects or complications reported

Drug Interactions See individual agents

Pregnancy Risk Factor D

Dosage Forms
Capsule: (Fiorgen PF®, Fiorinal®, Isollyl Improved®, Lanorinal®, Marnal®): Butalbital 50 mg, caffeine 40 mg, and aspirin 325 mg

Tablet:
 B-A-C®: Butalbital 50 mg, caffeine 40 mg, and aspirin 650 mg

Fiorinal®, Isollyl Improved®, Lanorinal®, Marnal®: Butalbital 50 mg, caffeine 40 mg, and aspirin 325 mg

Generic Available Yes

Butalbital Compound and Codeine
(byoo TAL bi tal KOM pound & KOE deen)

Brand Names Fiorinal® With Codeine

Therapeutic Category Analgesic, Narcotic; Barbiturate

Synonyms Codeine and Butalbital Compound

Use Mild to moderate pain when sedation is needed

Usual Dosage Adults: Oral: 1-2 capsules every 4 hours as needed for pain; up to 6/day

Local Anesthetic/Vasoconstrictor Precautions No information available to require special precautions

Effects on Dental Treatment <1%: Dry mouth

Other Adverse Effects
>10%:
 Central nervous system: Dizziness, lightheadedness, drowsiness, "hangover" effect
 Gastrointestinal: Nausea, heartburn, stomach pains, dyspepsia, epigastric discomfort

1% to 10%:
 Central nervous system: Confusion, mental depression, unusual excitement, nervousness, faint feeling, headache, insomnia, nightmares, fatigue
 Dermatologic: Skin rash
 Gastrointestinal: Constipation, vomiting, gastrointestinal ulceration
 Hematologic: Hemolytic anemia
 Neuromuscular & skeletal: Weakness
 Respiratory: Dyspnea
 Miscellaneous: Anaphylactic shock

<1%:
 Cardiovascular: Hypotension
 Central nervous system: Hallucinations, jitters
 Dermatologic: Skin rash, exfoliative dermatitis, Stevens-Johnson syndrome
 Hematologic: Agranulocytosis, megaloblastic anemia, thrombocytopenia, occult bleeding, prolongation of bleeding time, leukopenia, iron deficiency anemia
 Hepatic: Hepatotoxicity

Local: Thrombophlebitis

Renal: Impaired renal function

Respiratory: Respiratory depression, bronchospasm

Warnings/Precautions Children and teenagers should not use for chickenpox or flu symptoms before a physician is consulted about Reye's syndrome

Pregnancy Risk Factor C (D if used for prolonged periods or in high doses at term)

Dosage Forms Capsule: Butalbital 50 mg, caffeine 40 mg, aspirin 325 mg and codeine phosphate 30 mg

Generic Available Yes

Comments Abrupt discontinuation after sustained use (generally >10 days) may cause withdrawal symptoms

Butenafine (byoo TEN a fine)

Brand Names Mentax®

Therapeutic Category Antifungal Agent, Topical

Use Topical treatment of tinea pedis (athlete's foot)

Usual Dosage Adults: Topical: Apply once daily for 4 weeks

Mechanism of Action Butenafine exerts antifungal activity by blocking squalene epoxidation, resulting in inhibition of ergosterol synthesis (antidermatophyte and *Sporothrix schenckii* activity). In higher concentrations, the drug disrupts fungal cell membranes (anticandidal activity).

Local Anesthetic/Vasoconstrictor Precautions No information available to require special precautions

Effects on Dental Treatment No effects or complications reported

Other Adverse Effects

>1%: Dermatologic: Burning, stinging, irritation, erythema, pruritus (2%)

<1%: Dermatologic: Contact dermatitis

Drug Uptake

Absorption: Minimal systemic absorption when topically applied

Serum half-life: 35 hours

Time to peak serum concentration: 6 hours (10 ng/mL)

Pregnancy Risk Factor B

Dosage Forms Cream, as hydrochloride: 1% (2 g, 15 g, 30 g)

Buticaps® *see* Butabarbital Sodium *on page 154*

Butisol Sodium® *see* Butabarbital Sodium *on page 154*

Butoconazole (byoo toe KOE na zole)

Brand Names Femstat®

Canadian/Mexican Brand Names Femstal® (Mexico)

Therapeutic Category Antifungal Agent, Vaginal

Synonyms Butoconazol (Mexico)

Use Local treatment of vulvovaginal candidiasis

Usual Dosage Adults:

Nonpregnant: Insert 1 applicatorful (~5 g) intravaginally at bedtime for 3 days, may extend for up to 6 days if necessary

Pregnant: **Use only during second or third trimesters**

Mechanism of Action Increases cell membrane permeability in susceptible fungi (*Candida*)

Local Anesthetic/Vasoconstrictor Precautions No information available to require special precautions

Effects on Dental Treatment No effects or complications reported

Other Adverse Effects

1% to 10%: Genitourinary: Vulvar/vaginal burning

<1%:

Genitourinary: Vulvar itching, soreness, swelling, or discharge

Renal: Polyuria

Drug Interactions No data reported

Drug Uptake

Absorption: Following intravaginal application small amounts of drug are absorbed systemically (25%) within 2-8 hours

Serum half-life: 21-24 hours

Pregnancy Risk Factor C (For use only in 2nd or 3rd trimester)

Dosage Forms Cream, vaginal, as nitrate: 2% with applicator (28 g)

Generic Available No

Butoconazol (Mexico) *see* Butoconazole *on this page*

Butorfanol (Mexico) *see* Butorphanol *on next page*

Butorphanol (byoo TOR fa nole)

Related Information
Narcotic Agonists *on page 1141*

Brand Names Stadol®; Stadol® NS

Therapeutic Category Analgesic, Narcotic

Synonyms Butorfanol (Mexico)

Use Management of moderate to severe pain

Restrictions C-IV

Usual Dosage Adults:
I.M.: 1-4 mg every 3-4 hours as needed
I.V.: 0.5-2 mg every 3-4 hours as needed
Nasal spray: Headache: 1 spray in 1 nostril; if adequate pain relief is not achieved within 60-90 minutes, an additional 1 spray in 1 nostril may be given (each spray gives ~1 mg of butorphanol)

Mechanism of Action Mixed narcotic agonist-antagonist with central analgesic actions; binds to opiate receptors in the CNS, causing inhibition of ascending pain pathways, altering the perception of and response to pain; produces generalized CNS depression

Local Anesthetic/Vasoconstrictor Precautions No information available to require special precautions

Effects on Dental Treatment No effects or complications reported

Other Adverse Effects
>10%: Central nervous system: Drowsiness
1% to 10%:
Cardiovascular: Flushing of the face, hypotension
Central nervous system: Dizziness, lightheadedness, headache
Gastrointestinal: Anorexia, nausea, vomiting
Genitourinary: Decreased urination
Miscellaneous: Increased sweating
<1%:
Cardiovascular: Bradycardia or tachycardia, hypertension
Central nervous system: Paradoxical CNS stimulation, confusion, hallucinations, mental depression, false sense of well being, malaise, restlessness, nightmares, CNS depression
Dermatologic: Skin rash
Gastrointestinal: Stomach cramps, constipation, dry mouth
Genitourinary: Painful urination
Neuromuscular & skeletal: Weakness
Ocular: Blurred vision
Otic: Tinnitus
Respiratory: Dyspnea, respiratory depression
Miscellaneous: Dependence with prolonged use

Drug Interactions Increased toxicity: CNS depressants, phenothiazines, barbiturates, skeletal muscle relaxants, alfentanil, guanabenz, MAO inhibitors

Drug Uptake
Absorption: Rapidly and well absorbed
Serum half-life: 2.5-4 hours

Pregnancy Risk Factor B (D if used for prolonged periods or in high doses at term)

Generic Available No

Byclomine® Injection *see* Dicyclomine *on page 307*

Bydramine® Cough Syrup [OTC] *see* Diphenhydramine *on page 323*

C2B8 *see* Rituximab *on page 848*

C7E3 *see* Abciximab *on page 18*

C8-CCK *see* Sincalide *on page 866*

311C90 *see* Zolmitriptan *on page 1006*

Cabergoline (ca BER go leen)

Brand Names Dostinex®

Therapeutic Category Ergot-like Derivative

Use Treatment of hyperprolactinemia

Usual Dosage Oral: Adults: 0.25 mg twice a week; dosage may be increased by 0.25 mg twice weekly to a dose of up to 1 mg twice a week (according to the patient's prolactin level)

Local Anesthetic/Vasoconstrictor Precautions No information available to require special precautions

Effects on Dental Treatment No effects or complications reported

Pregnancy Risk Factor B

Cafatine® *see* Ergotamine *on page 360*

Cafergot® *see* Ergotamine *on page 360*
Cafetrate® *see* Ergotamine *on page 360*

Caffeine and Sodium Benzoate
(KAF een & SOW dee um BEN zoe ate)
Therapeutic Category Diuretic, Miscellaneous
Synonyms Sodium Benzoate and Caffeine
Use Emergency stimulant in acute circulatory failure; as a diuretic; and to relieve spinal puncture headache
Local Anesthetic/Vasoconstrictor Precautions No information available to require special precautions
Effects on Dental Treatment No effects or complications reported
Other Adverse Effects 1% to 10%:
　Cardiovascular: Tachycardia, extrasystoles, palpitations
　Central nervous system: Insomnia, restlessness, nervousness, mild delirium, headache, anxiety
　Gastrointestinal: Nausea, vomiting, gastric irritation
　Neuromuscular & skeletal: Muscle tension following abrupt cessation of drug after regular consumption of 500-600 mg/day
　Renal: Diuresis
Pregnancy Risk Factor C
Generic Available Yes

Caffeine, Citrated (KAF een, SIT rated)
Therapeutic Category Central Nervous System Stimulant, Nonamphetamine; Respiratory Stimulant
Use Central nervous system stimulant; used in the treatment of idiopathic apnea of prematurity
Local Anesthetic/Vasoconstrictor Precautions No information available to require special precautions
Effects on Dental Treatment No effects or complications reported
Pregnancy Risk Factor B
Generic Available Yes
Comments Has several advantages over theophylline in the treatment of neonatal apnea, its half-life is about 3 times as long, allowing once daily dosing, drug levels do not need to be drawn at peak and trough; has a wider therapeutic window, allowing more room between an effective concentration and toxicity; 2 mg caffeine citrate = 1 mg caffeine base

Calan® *see* Verapamil *on page 987*
Calan® SR *see* Verapamil *on page 987*
Cal Carb-HD® [OTC] *see* Calcium Carbonate *on page 162*
Calcibind® *see* Cellulose Sodium Phosphate *on page 201*
Calci-Chew™ [OTC] *see* Calcium Carbonate *on page 162*
Calciday-667® [OTC] *see* Calcium Carbonate *on page 162*

Calcifediol (kal si fe DYE ole)
Brand Names Calderol®
Therapeutic Category Vitamin D Analog
Use Treatment and management of metabolic bone disease associated with chronic renal failure
Usual Dosage Children and Adults: Hepatic osteodystrophy: Oral: 20-100 mcg/day or every other day; titrate to obtain normal serum calcium/phosphate levels; increase dose at 4-week intervals
Mechanism of Action Vitamin D analog that (along with calcitonin and parathyroid hormone) regulates serum calcium homeostasis by promoting absorption of calcium and phosphorus in the small intestine; promotes renal tubule resorption of phosphate; increases rate of accretion and resorption in bone minerals
Local Anesthetic/Vasoconstrictor Precautions No information available to require special precautions
Effects on Dental Treatment No effects or complications reported
Other Adverse Effects
　1% to 10%:
　　Cardiovascular: Hypotension, cardiac arrhythmias, hypertension
　　Central nervous system: Irritability, headache
　　Dermatologic: Pruritus
　　Endocrine & metabolic: Polydipsia, hypermagnesemia
　　Gastrointestinal: Nausea, vomiting, constipation, anorexia, pancreatitis, metallic taste
　　Neuromuscular & skeletal: Muscle/bone pain
　　Ocular: Conjunctivitis, photophobia
(Continued)

159

Calcifediol *(Continued)*

Renal: Polyuria

<1%:

Central nervous system: Overt psychosis, seizures

Endocrine & metabolic: Calcification

Gastrointestinal: Weight loss

Hepatic: Elevated AST/ALT

Drug Interactions

Cholestyramine reduces intestinal absorption of fat-soluble vitamins; may impair intestinal absorption of calcifediol

Magnesium-containing antacids and calcifediol should not be used concomitantly in patients on chronic renal dialysis due to potential for hypermagnesemia

Drug Uptake

Absorption: Rapid from the small intestines

Serum half-life: 12-22 days

Time to peak: Within 4 hours (oral)

Pregnancy Risk Factor A (D if used in doses above the recommended daily allowance)

Generic Available No

Calciferol™ *see Ergocalciferol on page 358*

Calcijex™ *see Calcitriol on next page*

Calcimar® Injection *see Calcitonin on this page*

Calci-Mix™ [OTC] *see Calcium Carbonate on page 162*

Calcipotriene *(kal si POE try een)*

Brand Names Dovonex®

Therapeutic Category Antipsoriatic Agent, Topical

Use Treatment of moderate plaque psoriasis

Usual Dosage Adults: Topical: Apply in a thin film to the affected skin twice daily and rub in gently and completely

Mechanism of Action Synthetic vitamin D_3 analog which regulates skin cell production and proliferation

Local Anesthetic/Vasoconstrictor Precautions No information available to require special precautions

Effects on Dental Treatment No effects or complications reported

Other Adverse Effects

>10%: Dermatologic: Burning, itching, skin irritation, erythema, dry skin, peeling, rash, worsening of psoriasis

1% to 10%: Dermatologic: Dermatitis

<1%:

Dermatologic: Skin atrophy, hyperpigmentation, folliculitis

Endocrine & metabolic: Hypercalcemia

Drug Interactions No data reported

Pregnancy Risk Factor C

Dosage Forms

Cream: 0.005% (30 g, 60 g, 100 g)

Ointment, topical: 0.005% (30 g, 60 g, 100 g)

Solution, topical: 0.005%

Generic Available No

Calcitonin *(kal si TOE nin)*

Brand Names Calcimar® Injection; Cibacalcin® Injection; Miacalcin® Injection; Miacalcin® Nasal Spray; Osteocalcin® Injection; Salmonine® Injection

Canadian/Mexican Brand Names Caltine® (Canada)

Therapeutic Category Antidote, Hypercalcemia

Use

Calcitonin (salmon): Treatment of Paget's disease of bone and as adjunctive therapy for hypercalcemia; also used in postmenopausal osteoporosis

Calcitonin (human): Treatment of Paget's disease of bone

Usual Dosage

Children: Dosage not established

Adults:

Paget's disease:

Salmon calcitonin: I.M., S.C.: 100 units/day to start, 50 units/day or 50-100 units every 1-3 days maintenance dose; Intranasal: 200-400 units (1-2 sprays)/day

Human calcitonin: S.C.: Initial: 0.5 mg/day (maximum: 0.5 mg twice daily); maintenance: 0.5 mg 2-3 times/week or 0.25 mg/day

Hypercalcemia: Initial: Salmon calcitonin: I.M., S.C.: 4 units/kg every 12 hours; may increase up to 8 units/kg every 12 hours to a maximum of every 6 hours

Osteogenesis imperfecta: Salmon calcitonin: I.M., S.C.: 2 units/kg 3 times/week

Postmenopausal osteoporosis: Salmon calcitonin:
I.M., S.C.: 100 units/day
Intranasal: 200 units (1 spray)/day

Mechanism of Action Structurally similar to human calcitonin; it directly inhibits osteoclastic bone resorption; promotes the renal excretion of calcium, phosphate, sodium, magnesium and potassium by decreasing tubular reabsorption; increases the jejunal secretion of water, sodium, potassium, and chloride

Local Anesthetic/Vasoconstrictor Precautions No information available to require special precautions

Effects on Dental Treatment No effects or complications reported

Other Adverse Effects
>10%:
Cardiovascular: Facial flushing
Gastrointestinal: Nausea, diarrhea, anorexia
Local: Swelling at injection site
1% to 10%: Genitourinary: Frequency of urination
<1%:
Cardiovascular: Edema
Central nervous system: Chills, headache, dizziness
Dermatologic: Skin rash, urticaria
Neuromuscular & skeletal: Paresthesia, weakness
Respiratory: Dyspnea, nasal congestion, nasal congestion

Drug Interactions No data reported

Drug Uptake
Hypercalcemia:
Onset of reduction in calcium: 2 hours
Duration of effect: 6-8 hours
Serum half-life: S.C.: 1.2 hours

Pregnancy Risk Factor C

Generic Available No

Calcitriol (kal si TRYE ole)

Brand Names Calcijex™; Rocaltrol®

Therapeutic Category Vitamin D Analog

Use Management of hypocalcemia in patients on chronic renal dialysis; reduce elevated parathyroid hormone levels; decrease severity of psoriatic lesions in psoriatic vulgaris

Usual Dosage Individualize dosage to maintain calcium levels of 9-10 mg/dL
Renal failure:
Oral:
Children: Initial: 15 ng/kg/day; maintenance: 5-40 ng/kg/day
Adults: 0.25 mcg/day or every other day (may require 0.5-1 mcg/day)
I.V.: Adults: 0.5 mcg (0.01 mcg/kg) 3 times/week; most doses in the range of 0.5-3 mcg (0.01-0.05 mcg/kg) 3 times/week

Hypoparathyroidism/pseudohypoparathyroidism: Oral:
Children:
<1 year: 0.04-0.08 mcg/kg/day
1-6 years: Initial: 0.25 mcg/day, increase at 2- to 4-week intervals
Children >6 years and Adults: 0.5-2 mcg/day

Vitamin D-resistant rickets (familial hypophosphatemia): Oral: 2 mcg/day; initial: 15-20 ng/kg/day; maintenance: 30-60 ng/kg/day

Mechanism of Action Promotes absorption of calcium in the intestines and retention at the kidneys thereby increasing calcium levels in the serum; decreases excessive serum phosphatase levels, parathyroid hormone levels, and decreases bone resorption; increases renal tubule phosphate resorption

Local Anesthetic/Vasoconstrictor Precautions No information available to require special precautions

Effects on Dental Treatment No effects or complications reported

Other Adverse Effects
1% to 10%:
Cardiovascular: Hypotension, cardiac arrhythmias, hypertension
Central nervous system: Irritability, headache
Dermatologic: Pruritus
Endocrine & metabolic: Polydipsia
Gastrointestinal: Nausea, vomiting, constipation, anorexia, pancreatitis, metallic taste
Neuromuscular & skeletal: Muscle/bone pain
Ocular: Conjunctivitis, photophobia
Renal: Polyuria
(Continued)

Calcitriol *(Continued)*

<1%:
Central nervous system: Overt psychosis, hyperthermia
Endocrine & metabolic: Hypercalcemia, hypercholesterolemia
Gastrointestinal: Weight loss
Hepatic: Elevated LFTs
Respiratory: Rhinorrhea

Drug Interactions
Cholestyramine reduces intestinal absorption of fat-soluble vitamins; may impair intestinal absorption of calcitriol
Magnesium-containing antacids and calcitriol should not be used concomitantly in patients on chronic renal dialysis due to potential for hypermagnesemia

Drug Uptake
Onset of action: ~2-6 hours
Duration: 3-5 days
Absorption: Oral: Rapid
Serum half-life: 3-8 hours

Pregnancy Risk Factor A (D if used in doses above the recommended daily allowance)

Generic Available No

Calcium Acetate (KAL see um AS e tate)

Brand Names Calphron®; PhosLo®

Therapeutic Category Calcium Salt

Use Control of hyperphosphatemia in end stage renal failure; calcium acetate binds phosphorus in the GI tract better than other calcium salts due to its lower solubility and subsequent reduced absorption and increased formation of calcium phosphate; calcium acetate does not promote aluminum absorption

Usual Dosage Adults: Oral: 2 tablets with each meal; dosage may be increased to bring serum phosphate value to <6 mg/dL; most patients require 3-4 tablets with each meal

Mechanism of Action Moderates nerve and muscle performance via action potential excitation threshold regulation; combines with dietary phosphate to form insoluble calcium phosphate which is excreted in feces

Local Anesthetic/Vasoconstrictor Precautions No information available to require special precautions

Effects on Dental Treatment No effects or complications reported

Other Adverse Effects
Mild hypercalcemia (calcium: >10.5 mg/dL) may be asymptomatic or manifest itself as constipation, anorexia, nausea, and vomiting
More severe hypercalcemia (calcium: >12 mg/dL) is associated with confusion, delirium, stupor, and coma

<1%:
Central nervous system: Headache
Endocrine & metabolic: Hypophosphatemia
Gastrointestinal: Nausea, anorexia, vomiting, abdominal pain, constipation, thirst

Drug Interactions
Decreased effect:
Calcium may antagonize the effects of calcium channel blockers
May decrease the bioavailability of tetracyclines
Renders tetracycline antibiotics inactive
Increased toxicity: Administer cautiously to a digitalized patient, may precipitate arrhythmias

Drug Uptake
Absorption: From the GI tract requires vitamin D

Pregnancy Risk Factor C

Generic Available No

Calcium Carbonate (KAL see um KAR bun ate)

Related Information
Calcium Carbonate and Magnesium Carbonate *on next page*

Brand Names Alka-Mints® [OTC]; Amitone® [OTC]; Cal Carb-HD® [OTC]; Calci-Chew™ [OTC]; Calciday-667® [OTC]; Calci-Mix™ [OTC]; Cal-Plus® [OTC]; Caltrate® 600 [OTC]; Caltrate, Jr.® [OTC]; Chooz® [OTC]; Dicarbosil® [OTC]; Equilet® [OTC]; Florical® [OTC]; Gencalc® 600 [OTC]; Mallamint® [OTC]; Nephro-Calci® [OTC]; Os-Cal® 500 [OTC]; Oyst-Cal 500 [OTC]; Oystercal® 500; Rolaids® Calcium Rich [OTC]; Tums® [OTC]; Tums® E-X Extra Strength Tablet [OTC]; Tums® Extra Strength Liquid [OTC]

Canadian/Mexican Brand Names Apo®-Cal (Canada); Calcite-500® (Canada); Calsan® (Canada); Pharmacal® (Canada)

Therapeutic Category Antacid; Antidote, Hyperphosphatemia; Calcium Salt

Use Adjunct in prevention of postmenopausal osteoporosis, antacid, treatment and prevention of calcium depletion (osteoporosis, osteomalacia, etc); control of hyperphosphatemia in end stage renal disease

Usual Dosage Oral (dosage is in terms of elemental calcium):

Recommended daily allowance (RDA):
<6 months: 360 mg/day
6-12 months: 540 mg/day
1-10 years: 800 mg/day
10-18 years: 1200 mg/day
Adults: 800 mg/day

Hypocalcemia (dose depends on clinical condition and serum calcium level):
Children: 45-65 mg/kg/day in 4 divided doses
Adults: 1-2 g or more/day

Adults:
Dietary supplementation: 500 mg to 2 g divided 2-4 times/day
To reduce bone loss with aging/osteoporosis: 1000-1500 mg/day
Antacid: 2 tablets or 10 mL every 2 hours, up to 12 times/day

Mechanism of Action Moderates nerve and muscle performance via action potential excitation threshold regulation; combines with dietary phosphate to form insoluble calcium phosphate which is excreted in feces; may prevent negative calcium balance when used as a dietary supplement, or for calcium balance when used as a dietary supplement, or as treatment for osteoporosis

Local Anesthetic/Vasoconstrictor Precautions No information available to require special precautions

Effects on Dental Treatment No effects or complications reported

Other Adverse Effects
1% to 10%: Gastrointestinal: Constipation, flatulence
<1%:
Cardiovascular: Hypotension, bradycardia, cardiac arrhythmias
Central nervous system: Mood and mental changes, lethargy
Dermatologic: Erythema
Endocrine & metabolic: Hypercalcemia (with prolonged use), metastatic calcinosis, hypomagnesemia, hypophosphatemia, milk-alkali syndrome
Gastrointestinal: Laxative effect, acid rebound, nausea, vomiting, GI hemorrhage, fecal impaction, elevated serum amylase
Neuromuscular & skeletal: Myalgia
Renal: Polyuria, renal calculi, renal dysfunction, hypercalciuria

Drug Interactions
Decreased effect:
Calcium may antagonize the effects of calcium channel blockers
May decrease the bioavailability of tetracyclines
Renders tetracycline antibiotics inactive
Increased toxicity: Administer cautiously to a digitalized patient, may precipitate arrhythmias

Drug Uptake
Absorption: From the GI tract requires vitamin D; calcium is absorbed in soluble, ionized form; solubility of calcium is increased in an acid environment

Pregnancy Risk Factor C

Generic Available Yes

Calcium Carbonate and Magnesium Carbonate

(KAL see um KAR bun ate & mag NEE zhum KAR bun ate)

Brand Names Mylanta® Gelcaps®

Therapeutic Category Antacid

Use Hyperacidity

Local Anesthetic/Vasoconstrictor Precautions No information available to require special precautions

Effects on Dental Treatment Do not give tetracyclines concomitantly

Drug Interactions See individual agents

Dosage Forms Capsule: Calcium carbonate 311 mg and magnesium carbonate 232 mg

Generic Available No

Calcium Carbonate and Simethicone

(KAL see um KAR bun ate & sye METH i kone)

Brand Names Titralac® Plus Liquid [OTC]

Therapeutic Category Antacid

Synonyms Simethicone and Calcium Carbonate

Use Relief of acid indigestion, heartburn, peptic esophagitis, hiatal hernia, and gas

(Continued)

Calcium Carbonate and Simethicone *(Continued)*

Local Anesthetic/Vasoconstrictor Precautions No information available to require special precautions

Effects on Dental Treatment Do not give tetracycline concomitantly

Pregnancy Risk Factor C

Generic Available Yes

Calcium Channel Blockers & Gingival Hyperplasia *see page 1132*

Calcium Chloride (KAL see um KLOR ide)

Brand Names Cal Plus®

Therapeutic Category Calcium Salt; Electrolyte Supplement, Parenteral

Use Cardiac resuscitation when epinephrine fails to improve myocardial contractions, cardiac disturbances of hyperkalemia, hypocalcemia, or calcium channel blocking agent toxicity; emergent treatment of hypocalcemic tetany, treatment of hypermagnesemia

Usual Dosage Note: Calcium chloride is 3 times as potent as calcium gluconate

Cardiac arrest in the presence of hyperkalemia or hypocalcemia, magnesium toxicity, or calcium antagonist toxicity: I.V.:

Children: 20 mg/kg; may repeat in 10 minutes if necessary

Adults: 2-4 mg/kg (10% solution), repeated every 10 minutes

Hypocalcemia: I.V.:

Children: 10-20 mg/kg/dose (children: 1-7 mEq), repeat every 4-6 hours if needed; doses may be repeated every 1-3 days if needed

Adults: 500 mg to 1 g (7-14 mEq), repeated at 1- to 3-day intervals if necessary

Hypocalcemic tetany: I.V.:

Children: 10 mg/kg (0.5-0.7 mEq/kg) over 5-10 minutes; may repeat after 6-8 hours or follow with an infusion with a maximum dose of 200 mg/kg/day

Adults: 4.5-16 mEq may be administered until response occurs

Hypocalcemia secondary to citrated blood transfusion give 0.45 mEq **elemental** calcium for each 100 mL citrated blood infused

Mechanism of Action Moderates nerve and muscle performance via action potential excitation threshold regulation

Local Anesthetic/Vasoconstrictor Precautions No information available to require special precautions

Effects on Dental Treatment No effects or complications reported

Other Adverse Effects <1%:

Cardiovascular: Vasodilation, hypotension, bradycardia, cardiac arrhythmias, ventricular fibrillation, syncope

Central nervous system: Lethargy, coma, mania

Dermatologic: Erythema

Endocrine & metabolic: Decreased serum magnesium, hypercalcemia

Gastrointestinal: Elevated serum amylase

Local: Tissue necrosis

Neuromuscular & skeletal: Weakness

Renal: Hypercalciuria

Drug Interactions

Decreased effect:

Calcium may antagonize the effects of calcium channel blockers

May decrease the bioavailability of tetracyclines

Renders tetracycline antibiotics inactive

Increased toxicity: Administer cautiously to a digitalized patient, may precipitate arrhythmias

Drug Uptake

Absorption: I.V. calcium salts are absorbed directly into the bloodstream

Pregnancy Risk Factor C

Generic Available Yes

Calcium Citrate (KAL see um SIT rate)

Brand Names Citracal® [OTC]

Therapeutic Category Calcium Salt

Use Adjunct in prevention of postmenopausal osteoporosis; treatment and prevention of calcium depletion

Usual Dosage Dosage is in terms of elemental calcium

Recommended daily allowance (RDA):

<6 months: 360 mg/day

6-12 months: 540 mg/day

1-10 years: 800 mg/day

10-18 years: 1200 mg/day

Adults: 800 mg/day

Adults: Oral: 1-2 g/day

Mechanism of Action Moderates nerve and muscle performance via action potential excitation threshold regulation

Local Anesthetic/Vasoconstrictor Precautions No information available to require special precautions

Effects on Dental Treatment No effects or complications reported

Other Adverse Effects <1%:

Central nervous system: Mental confusion, headache

Endocrine & metabolic: Hypercalcemia, milk-alkali syndrome, hypophosphatemia

Gastrointestinal: Constipation, vomiting, nausea

Drug Interactions

Decreased effect:

Calcium may antagonize the effects of calcium channel blockers

May decrease the bioavailability of tetracyclines

Renders tetracycline antibiotics inactive

Increased toxicity: Administer cautiously to a digitalized patient, may precipitate arrhythmias

Drug Uptake

Absorption: From the GI tract requires vitamin D

Pregnancy Risk Factor C

Generic Available No

Calcium Disodium Edetate *see* Edetate Calcium Disodium *on page 344*

Calcium Disodium Versenate® *see* Edetate Calcium Disodium *on page 344*

Calcium EDTA *see* Edetate Calcium Disodium *on page 344*

Calcium Glubionate (KAL see um gloo BYE oh nate)

Brand Names Neo-Calglucon® [OTC]

Therapeutic Category Calcium Salt

Use Adjunct in prevention of postmenopausal osteoporosis; treatment and prevention of calcium depletion

Usual Dosage Oral:

Recommended daily allowance (RDA) (in terms of elemental calcium):

<6 months: 360 mg/day

6-12 months: 540 mg/day

1-10 years: 800 mg/day

10-18 years: 1200 mg/day

Adults: 800 mg/day

Syrup is a hyperosmolar solution; dosage is in terms of calcium glubionate

Neonatal hypocalcemia: 1200 mg/kg/day in 4-6 divided doses

Maintenance: Children: 600-2000 mg/kg/day in 4 divided doses up to a maximum of 9 g/day

Adults: 6-18 g/day in divided doses

Mechanism of Action Moderates nerve and muscle performance via action potential excitation threshold regulation

Local Anesthetic/Vasoconstrictor Precautions No information available to require special precautions

Effects on Dental Treatment No effects or complications reported

Other Adverse Effects <1%:

Central nervous system: Dizziness, headache, mental confusion

Endocrine & metabolic: Hypercalcemia, hypomagnesemia, hypophosphatemia, milk-alkali syndrome

Gastrointestinal: GI irritation, diarrhea, constipation, dry mouth

Renal: Hypercalciuria

Drug Interactions

Decreased effect:

Calcium may antagonize the effects of calcium channel blockers

May decrease the bioavailability of tetracyclines

Renders tetracycline antibiotics inactive

Increased toxicity: Administer cautiously to a digitalized patient, may precipitate arrhythmias

Drug Uptake

Absorption: From the GI tract requires vitamin D

Pregnancy Risk Factor C

Generic Available No

Calcium Gluceptate (KAL see um gloo SEP tate)

Therapeutic Category Calcium Salt

Use Treatment of cardiac disturbances of hyperkalemia, hypocalcemia, or calcium channel blocker toxicity; cardiac resuscitation when epinephrine fails to improve myocardial contractions; treatment of hypermagnesemia and hypocalcemia

(Continued)

Calcium Gluceptate *(Continued)*

Usual Dosage I.V. (dose expressed in mg of calcium gluceptate):

Cardiac resuscitation in the presence of hypocalcemia, hyperkalemia, magnesium toxicity, or calcium channel blocker toxicity:

Children: 110 mg/kg/dose

Adults: 1.1-1.5 g (5-7 mL)

Hypocalcemia:

Children: 200-500 mg/kg/day divided every 6 hours

Adults: 500 mg to 1.1 g/dose as needed

After citrated blood administration: Children and Adults: 0.4 mEq/100 mL blood infused

Mechanism of Action Moderates nerve and muscle performance via action potential excitation threshold regulation

Local Anesthetic/Vasoconstrictor Precautions No information available to require special precautions

Effects on Dental Treatment No effects or complications reported

Other Adverse Effects <1%:

Cardiovascular: Vasodilation, hypotension, bradycardia, cardiac arrhythmias, ventricular fibrillation, syncope

Central nervous system: Lethargy, mania, coma

Dermatologic: Erythema

Endocrine & metabolic: Hypomagnesemia, hypercalcemia

Gastrointestinal: Elevated serum amylase

Local: Tissue necrosis

Neuromuscular & skeletal: Weakness

Renal: Hypercalciuria

Drug Interactions

Decreased effect:

Calcium may antagonize the effects of calcium channel blockers

May decrease the bioavailability of tetracyclines

Renders tetracycline antibiotics inactive

Increased toxicity: Administer cautiously to digitalized patients, may precipitate arrhythmias

Drug Uptake

Absorption: I.M. and I.V. calcium salts are absorbed directly into the bloodstream

Pregnancy Risk Factor C

Generic Available Yes

Calcium Gluconate (KAL see um GLOO koe nate)

Brand Names Kalcinate®

Therapeutic Category Calcium Salt

Use Treatment and prevention of hypocalcemia; treatment of tetany, cardiac disturbances of hyperkalemia, cardiac resuscitation when epinephrine fails to improve myocardial contractions, hypocalcemia, or calcium channel blocker toxicity; calcium supplementation

Usual Dosage Dosage is in terms of **elemental** calcium

Recommended daily allowance (RDA):

<6 months: 400 mg/day

6-12 months: 600 mg/day

1-10 years: 800 mg/day

10-18 years: 1200 mg/day

Adults: 800 mg/day

Calcium gluconate electrolyte requirement in newborn period:

Premature: 200-1000 mg/kg/24 hours

Term:

0-24 hours: 0-500 mg/kg/24 hours

24-48 hours: 200-500 mg/kg/24 hours

48-72 hours: 200-600 mg/kg/24 hours

>3 days: 200-800 mg/kg/24 hours

Hypocalcemia:

Oral:

Children: 200-500 mg/kg/day divided every 6 hours

Adults: 500 mg to 2 g 2-4 times/day

I.V.:

Children: 200-500 mg/kg/day (children 1-7 mEq/day) as a continuous infusion or in 4 divided doses; doses may be repeated every 1-3 days if necessary

Adults: 2-15 g/24 hours as a continuous infusion or in divided doses, which may be repeated every 1-3 days if necessary

Hypocalcemic tetany: I.V.:
Children: 100-200 mg/kg/dose (0.5-0.7 mEq/kg/dose) over 5-10 minutes; may repeat every 6-8 hours **or** follow with an infusion of 500 mg/kg/day
Adults: 1-3 g (4.5-16 mEq) may be administered until therapeutic response occurs

Osteoporosis/bone loss: Oral: 1000-1500 mg in divided doses/day

Calcium antagonist toxicity, magnesium intoxication, or cardiac arrest in the presence of hyperkalemia or hypocalcemia: I.V.:
Children: Calcium chloride is recommended calcium salt; refer to calcium chloride monograph
Adults: 5-8 mL/dose and repeated as necessary at 10-minute intervals, however, calcium chloride is recommended calcium salt; refer to Calcium Chloride monograph

Hypocalcemia secondary to citrated blood infusion: I.V.: Give 0.45 mEq **elemental** calcium for each 100 mL citrated blood infused

Exchange transfusion:
Adults: 300 mg/100 mL of citrated blood exchanged

Maintenance electrolyte requirements for total parenteral nutrition: I.V.: Daily requirements: Adults: 8-16 mEq/1000 kcals/24 hours

Mechanism of Action Moderates nerve and muscle performance via action potential excitation threshold regulation

Local Anesthetic/Vasoconstrictor Precautions No information available to require special precautions

Effects on Dental Treatment No effects or complications reported

Other Adverse Effects <1%:
Cardiovascular: Vasodilation, hypotension, bradycardia, cardiac arrhythmias, ventricular fibrillation, syncope
Central nervous system: Lethargy, mania, coma
Dermatologic: Erythema
Endocrine & metabolic: Decrease serum magnesium, hypercalcemia
Gastrointestinal: Elevated serum amylase
Local: Tissue necrosis
Neuromuscular & skeletal: Weakness
Renal: Hypercalciuria

Drug Interactions
Decreased effect:
Calcium may antagonize the effects of calcium channel blockers
May decrease the bioavailability of tetracyclines
Renders tetracycline antibiotics inactive
Increased toxicity: Administer cautiously to a digitalized patient, may precipitate arrhythmias

Drug Uptake
Absorption: I.M. and I.V. calcium salts are absorbed directly into the bloodstream; absorption from the GI tract requires vitamin D; calcium is absorbed in soluble, ionized form; solubility of calcium is increased in an acid environment (except calcium lactate)

Pregnancy Risk Factor C
Generic Available Yes

Calcium Lactate (KAL see um LAK tate)

Therapeutic Category Calcium Salt

Use Adjunct in prevention of postmenopausal osteoporosis; treatment and prevention of calcium depletion

Usual Dosage Oral (in terms of calcium lactate)
Recommended daily allowance (RDA) (in terms of elemental calcium):
<6 months: 360 mg/day
6-12 months: 540 mg/day
1-10 years: 800 mg/day
10-18 years: 1200 mg/day
Adults: 800 mg/day
Children: 500 mg/kg/day divided every 6-8 hours
Maximum daily dose: 9 g
Adults: 1.5-3 g divided every 8 hours

Mechanism of Action Moderates nerve and muscle performance via action potential excitation threshold regulation

Local Anesthetic/Vasoconstrictor Precautions No information available to require special precautions

Effects on Dental Treatment No effects or complications reported

Other Adverse Effects <1%:
Central nervous system: Headache, mental confusion, dizziness
Endocrine & metabolic: Hypercalcemia, hypophosphatemia, hypomagnesemia, milk-alkali syndrome

(Continued)

167

Calcium Lactate *(Continued)*

Gastrointestinal: Constipation, nausea, dry mouth, vomiting
Renal: Hypercalciuria

Drug Interactions
Decreased effect:
Calcium may antagonize the effects of calcium channel blockers
May decrease the bioavailability of tetracyclines
Renders tetracycline antibiotics inactive
Increased toxicity: Administer cautiously to a digitalized patient, may precipitate arrhythmias

Drug Uptake
Absorption: From the GI tract requires vitamin D

Pregnancy Risk Factor C

Generic Available Yes

Calcium Leucovorin *see Leucovorin on page 544*

Calcium Pantothenate *see Pantothenic Acid on page 722*

Calcium Phosphate, Tribasic (KAL see um FOS fate tri BAY sik)

Brand Names Posture® [OTC]

Therapeutic Category Calcium Salt

Use Adjunct in prevention of postmenopausal osteoporosis; treatment and prevention of calcium depletion

Usual Dosage Oral (all doses in terms of elemental calcium):
Recommended daily allowance (RDA) (elemental calcium):
<6 months: 360 mg/day
6-12 months: 540 mg/day
1-10 years: 800 mg/day
10-18 years: 1200 mg/day
Adults: 800 mg/day

Children: 45-65 mg/kg/day
Adults: 1-2 g/day

Mechanism of Action Moderates nerve and muscle performance via action potential excitation threshold regulation

Local Anesthetic/Vasoconstrictor Precautions No information available to require special precautions

Effects on Dental Treatment No effects or complications reported

Other Adverse Effects <1%:
Endocrine & metabolic: Hypercalcemia, milk-alkali syndrome, hypophosphatemia
Gastrointestinal: Constipation, nausea, dry mouth

Drug Interactions
Decreased effect:
Calcium may antagonize the effects of calcium channel blockers
May decrease the bioavailability of tetracyclines
Renders tetracycline antibiotics inactive
Increased toxicity: Administer cautiously to a digitalized patient, may precipitate arrhythmias

Pregnancy Risk Factor C

Generic Available Yes

Calcium Polycarbophil (KAL see um pol i KAR boe fil)

Brand Names Equalactin® Chewable Tablet [OTC]; Fiberall® Chewable Tablet [OTC]; FiberCon® Tablet [OTC]; Fiber-Lax® Tablet [OTC]; Mitrolan® Chewable Tablet [OTC]

Therapeutic Category Antidiarrheal; Laxative, Bulk-Producing

Use Treatment of constipation or diarrhea; calcium polycarbophil is supplied as the approved substitute whenever a bulk-forming laxative is ordered in a tablet, capsule, wafer, or other oral solid dosage form

Usual Dosage Oral:
Children:
2-6 years: 500 mg (1 tablet) 1-2 times/day, up to 1.5 g/day
6-12 years: 500 mg (1 tablet) 1-3 times/day, up to 3 g/day
Adults: 1 g 4 times/day, up to 6 g/day

Mechanism of Action Restoring a more normal moisture level and providing bulk in the patient's intestinal tract

Local Anesthetic/Vasoconstrictor Precautions No information available to require special precautions

Effects on Dental Treatment Oral medication should be given at least 1 hour prior to taking the bulk-producing laxative in order to prevent decreased absorption of medication

Other Adverse Effects 1% to 10%: Gastrointestinal: Abdominal fullness

Drug Interactions Decreased absorption of oral anticoagulants, digoxin, potassium-sparing diuretics, salicylates, tetracyclines

Pregnancy Risk Factor C

Generic Available Yes

Calderol® *see* Calcifediol *on page 159*

Caldesene® **Topical [OTC]** *see* Undecylenic Acid and Derivatives *on page 977*

Calm-X® **Oral [OTC]** *see* Dimenhydrinate *on page 320*

Calphron® *see* Calcium Acetate *on page 162*

Cal-Plus® **[OTC]** *see* Calcium Carbonate *on page 162*

Cal Plus® *see* Calcium Chloride *on page 164*

Caltrate® **600 [OTC]** *see* Calcium Carbonate *on page 162*

Caltrate, Jr.® **[OTC]** *see* Calcium Carbonate *on page 162*

Cama® **Arthritis Pain Reliever [OTC]** *see* Aspirin *on page 90*

Campho-Phenique® **[OTC]** *see* Camphor and Phenol *on this page*

Camphor and Phenol (KAM for & FEE nole)

Brand Names Campho-Phenique® [OTC]

Therapeutic Category Topical Skin Product

Use Relief of pain and for minor infections

Local Anesthetic/Vasoconstrictor Precautions No information available to require special precautions

Effects on Dental Treatment No effects or complications reported

Pregnancy Risk Factor C

Generic Available Yes

Camphor, Menthol, and Phenol (KAM for, MEN thol, & FEE nole)

Brand Names Sarna [OTC]

Therapeutic Category Topical Skin Product

Use Relief of dry, itching skin

Local Anesthetic/Vasoconstrictor Precautions No information available to require special precautions

Effects on Dental Treatment No effects or complications reported

Other Adverse Effects 1% to 10%: Dermatologic: Burning sensation, especially on broken skin

Pregnancy Risk Factor C

Generic Available Yes

Camptosar® *see* Irinotecan *on page 518*

Cancer Chemotherapy Regimens *see page 1133*

Cantharidin (kan THAR e din)

Brand Names Verr-Canth™

Therapeutic Category Keratolytic Agent

Use Removal of ordinary and periungual warts

Local Anesthetic/Vasoconstrictor Precautions No information available to require special precautions

Effects on Dental Treatment No effects or complications reported

Pregnancy Risk Factor C

Generic Available No

Cantil® *see* Mepenzolate Bromide *on page 592*

Capastat® **Sulfate** *see* Capreomycin *on this page*

Capital® **and Codeine** *see* Acetaminophen and Codeine *on page 21*

Capitrol® *see* Chloroxine *on page 217*

Capoten® *see* Captopril *on next page*

Capozide® *see* Captopril and Hydrochlorothiazide *on page 172*

Capreomycin (kap ree oh MYE sin)

Related Information

Nonviral Infectious Diseases *on page 1032*

Brand Names Capastat® Sulfate

Therapeutic Category Antibiotic, Miscellaneous; Antitubercular Agent

Use Treatment of tuberculosis in conjunction with at least one other antituberculosis agent

Usual Dosage I.M.:

Children: 15-20 mg/kg/day, up to 1 g/day maximum

Adults: 15-30 mg/kg/day up to 1 g/day for 60-120 days, followed by 1 g 2-3 times/week

(Continued)

Capreomycin *(Continued)*

Mechanism of Action Capreomycin is a cyclic polypeptide antimicrobial. It is administered as a mixture of capreomycin IA and capreomycin IB. The mechanism of action of capreomycin is not well understood. Mycobacterial species that have become resistant to other agents are usually still sensitive to the action of capreomycin. However, significant cross-resistance with viomycin, kanamycin, and neomycin occurs.

Local Anesthetic/Vasoconstrictor Precautions No information available to require special precautions

Effects on Dental Treatment No effects or complications reported

Other Adverse Effects

>10%:
Otic: Ototoxicity
Renal: Nephrotoxicity

1% to 10%: Hematologic: Eosinophilia

<1%:
Central nervous system: Vertigo, fever
Dermatologic: Rash
Hematologic: Leukocytosis, thrombocytopenia
Local: Pain, induration, bleeding at injection site
Otic: Tinnitus

Drug Interactions Additive nephrotoxicity and ototoxicity with other aminoglycosides such as streptomycin

Drug Uptake

Absorption: Oral: Poor absorption necessitates parenteral administration
Serum half-life: Dependent upon renal function and varies with creatinine clearance; 4-6 hours
Time to peak serum concentration: I.M.: Within 1 hour

Pregnancy Risk Factor C

Generic Available No

Capsaicin *(kap SAY sin)*

Brand Names Capsin® [OTC]; Capzasin-P® [OTC]; Dolorac® [OTC]; No Pain-HP® [OTC]; R-Gel® [OTC]; Zostrix® [OTC]; Zostrix-® HP [OTC]

Therapeutic Category Analgesic, Topical; Topical Skin Product

Use FDA approved for the topical treatment of pain associated with postherpetic neuralgia, rheumatoid arthritis, osteoarthritis, diabetic neuropathy, and post-surgical pain.

Unlabeled uses: Treatment of pain associated with psoriasis, chronic neuralgias unresponsive to other forms of therapy, and intractable pruritus

Usual Dosage Children ≥2 years and Adults: Topical: Apply to affected area at least 3-4 times/day; application frequency less than 3-4 times/day prevents the total depletion, inhibition of synthesis, and transport of substance P resulting in decreased clinical efficacy and increased local discomfort

Mechanism of Action Induces release of substance P, the principal chemomediator of pain impulses from the periphery to the CNS, from peripheral sensory neurons; after repeated application, capsaicin depletes the neuron of substance P and prevents reaccumulation

Local Anesthetic/Vasoconstrictor Precautions No information available to require special precautions

Effects on Dental Treatment No effects or complications reported

Other Adverse Effects

>10%: Local: ≥30%: Transient burning on application which usually diminishes with repeated use

1% to 10%:
Local: Itching, stinging sensation, erythema
Respiratory: Cough

Drug Interactions No data reported

Drug Uptake Data following the use of topical capsaicin in humans are lacking
Onset of action: Pain relief is usually seen within 14-28 days of regular topical application; maximal response may require 4-6 weeks of continuous therapy
Duration: Several hours

Pregnancy Risk Factor C

Generic Available No

Capsin® [OTC] *see Capsaicin on this page*

Captopril *(KAP toe pril)*

Related Information

Cardiovascular Diseases *on page 1010*

Brand Names Capoten®

Canadian/Mexican Brand Names Apo®-Capto (Canada); Capitral® (Mexico); Capotena® (Mexico); Cardipril® (Mexico); Cryopril® (Mexico); Ecapresan® (Mexico); Ecaten® (Mexico); Kenolan® (Mexico); Lenpryl® (Mexico); Novo-Captopril® (Canada); Nu-Capto® (Canada); Precaptil® (Mexico); Syn-Captopril® (Canada)

Therapeutic Category Angiotensin-Converting Enzyme (ACE) Inhibitors

Use Management of hypertension and treatment of congestive heart failure

Unlabeled use: Hypertensive crisis, diabetic nephropathy, rheumatoid arthritis, diagnosis of anatomic renal artery stenosis, hypertension secondary to scleroderma renal crisis, diagnosis of aldosteronism, idiopathic edema, Bartter's syndrome, postmyocardial infarction for prevention of ventricular failure; increase circulation in Raynaud's phenomenon

Usual Dosage Note: Dosage must be titrated according to patient's response; use lowest effective dose. Oral:

Children: Initial: 0.5 mg/kg/dose; titrate upward to maximum of 6 mg/kg/day in 2-4 divided doses

Older Children: Initial: 6.25-12.5 mg/dose every 12-24 hours; titrate upward to maximum of 6 mg/kg/day

Adolescents: Initial: 12.5-25 mg/dose given every 8-12 hours; increase by 25 mg/dose to maximum of 450 mg/day

Adults:

Hypertension:

Initial dose: 12.5-25 mg 2-3 times/day; may increase by 12.5-25 mg/dose at 1- to 2-week intervals up to 50 mg 3 times/day; add diuretic before further dosage increases

Maximum dose: 150 mg 3 times/day

Congestive heart failure:

Initial dose: 6.25-12.5 mg 3 times/day in conjunction with cardiac glycoside and diuretic therapy; initial dose depends upon patient's fluid/electrolyte status

Target dose: 50 mg 3 times/day

Maximum dose: 100 mg 3 times/day

Mechanism of Action Competitive inhibitor of angiotensin-converting enzyme (ACE); prevents conversion of angiotensin I to angiotensin II, a potent vasoconstrictor; results in lower levels of angiotensin II which causes an increase in plasma renin activity and a reduction in aldosterone secretion

Local Anesthetic/Vasoconstrictor Precautions No information available to require special precautions

Effects on Dental Treatment No effects or complications reported

Drug-Drug Interactions With ACEIs

Precipitant Drug	Drug (Category) and Effect	Description
Antacids	ACE Inhibitors: decreased	Decreased bioavailability of ACEIs. May be more likely with captopril. Separate administration times by 1-2 hours.
NSAIDs (indomethacin)	ACEIs: decreased	Reduced hypotensive effects of ACEIs. More prominent in low renin or volume dependent hypertensive patients.
Phenothiazines	ACEIs: increased	Pharmacologic effects of ACEIs may be increased.
ACEIs	Allopurinol: increased	Higher risk of hypersensitivity reaction possible when given concurrently. Three case reports of Stevens-Johnson syndrome with captopril.
ACEIs	Digoxin: increased	Increased plasma digoxin levels.
ACEIs	Lithium: increased	Increased serum lithium levels and symptoms of toxicity may occur.
ACEIs	Potassium preps/ potassium sparing diuretics increased	Coadministration may result in elevated potassium levels.

Other Adverse Effects

1% to 10%:

Cardiovascular: Tachycardia, chest pain, palpitations

Central nervous system: Insomnia, headache, dizziness, fatigue, malaise

Dermatologic: Rash, pruritus, alopecia

Gastrointestinal: Abdominal pain, vomiting, nausea, diarrhea, anorexia, constipation, dysgeusia

Neuromuscular & skeletal: Paresthesias

Renal: Oliguria

(Continued)

Captopril *(Continued)*

   Respiratory: Transient cough
   <1%:
   Cardiovascular: Hypotension
   Dermatologic: Angioedema
   Endocrine & metabolic: Hyperkalemia
   Gastrointestinal: Dysgeusia
   Hematologic: Neutropenia, agranulocytosis
   Renal: Proteinuria, elevated BUN, serum creatinine

Drug Interactions
   Increased toxicity:
   Probenecid increases blood levels of captopril
   Captopril and diuretics have additive hypotensive effects; see table.
   Increased serum lithium levels and symptoms of lithium toxicity have been reported in patients receiving concomitant lithium and ACE inhibitor therapy. These drugs should be coadministered with caution.

Drug Uptake
   Onset of effect: Maximal decrease in blood pressure 1-1.5 hours after dose
   Duration: Dose related, may require several weeks of therapy before full hypotensive effect is seen
   Absorption: Oral: 60% to 75%
   Serum half-life (dependent upon renal and cardiac function):
   Adults, normal: 1.9 hours
   Congestive heart failure: 2.06 hours
   Anuria: 20-40 hours
   Time to peak: Within 1-2 hours

Pregnancy Risk Factor C (first trimester); D (second and third trimesters)
Dosage Forms Tablet: 12.5 mg, 25 mg, 50 mg, 100 mg
Generic Available Yes

Captopril and Hydrochlorothiazide
   (KAP toe pril & hye droe klor oh THYE a zide)

Related Information
   Cardiovascular Diseases *on page 1010*
Brand Names Capozide®
Therapeutic Category Antihypertensive Agent, Combination
Use Management of hypertension and treatment of congestive heart failure
Usual Dosage Adults: Oral:
   Hypertension: Initial: 25 mg 2-3 times/day; may increase at 1- to 2-week intervals up to 150 mg 3 times/day (captopril dosages)

   Congestive heart failure: 6.25-25 mg 3 times/day (maximum: 450 mg/day) (captopril dosages)

Mechanism of Action Captopril is a competitive inhibitor of angiotensin-converting enzyme (ACE); prevents conversion of angiotensin I to angiotensin II, a potent vasoconstrictor. This results in lower levels of angiotensin II which causes an increase in plasma renin activity and a reduction in aldosterone secretion. Hydrochlorothiazide inhibits sodium reabsorption in the distal tubules causing increased excretion of sodium and water as well as potassium and hydrogen ions.

Local Anesthetic/Vasoconstrictor Precautions No information available to require special precautions
Effects on Dental Treatment No effects or complications reported
Other Adverse Effects
   Captopril:
   1% to 10%:
   Cardiovascular: Tachycardia, chest pain, palpitations
   Central nervous system: Insomnia, headache, dizziness, fatigue, malaise
   Dermatologic: Rash, pruritus, alopecia
   Gastrointestinal: Abdominal pain, vomiting, nausea, diarrhea, anorexia, constipation, dysgeusia
   Neuromuscular & skeletal: Paresthesias
   Renal: Oliguria
   Respiratory: Transient cough
   <1%:
   Cardiovascular: Hypotension
   Dermatologic: Angioedema
   Endocrine & metabolic: Hyperkalemia
   Gastrointestinal: Dysgeusia
   Hematologic: Neutropenia, agranulocytosis
   Renal: Proteinuria, elevated BUN, serum creatinine

Hydrochlorothiazide:
1% to 10%: Endocrine & metabolic: Hypokalemia
<1%:
Cardiovascular: Hypotension
Dermatologic: Photosensitivity
Endocrine & metabolic: Fluid and electrolyte imbalances (hypocalcemia, hypomagnesemia, hyponatremia), hyperglycemia
Hematologic: Rarely blood dyscrasias
Renal: Prerenal azotemia

Contraindications Hypersensitivity to captopril, hydrochlorothiazide or any component

Drug Interactions Probenecid increases blood levels of captopril. Increased serum lithium levels and symptoms of lithium toxicity have been reported in patients receiving concomitant lithium and ACE inhibitor therapy. Hydrochlorothiazide decreases antidiabetic drug efficacy. Hydrochlorothiazide has been reported to increase digoxin-related cardiac arrhythmias

Pregnancy Risk Factor C

Dosage Forms Tablet:
25/15: Captopril 25 mg and hydrochlorothiazide 15 mg
25/25: Captopril 25 mg and hydrochlorothiazide 25 mg
50/15: Captopril 50 mg and hydrochlorothiazide 15 mg
50/25: Captopril 50 mg and hydrochlorothiazide 25 mg

Generic Available Yes

Capzasin-P® [OTC] *see* Capsaicin *on page 170*

Carafate® *see* Sucralfate *on page 887*

Caramiphen and Phenylpropanolamine
(kar AM i fen & fen il proe pa NOLE a meen)

Brand Names Ordrine AT® Extended Release Capsule; Rescaps-D® S.R. Capsule; Tuss-Allergine® Modified T.D. Capsule; Tussogest® Extended Release Capsule

Therapeutic Category Antihistamine/Decongestant Combination

Synonyms Phenylpropanolamine and Caramiphen

Use Symptomatic relief of cough and nasal congestion associated with the common cold

Local Anesthetic/Vasoconstrictor Precautions Use with caution since phenylpropanolamine is a sympathomimetic amine which could interact with epinephrine to cause a pressor response

Effects on Dental Treatment Up to 10% of patients could experience tachycardia, palpitations, and dry mouth; use vasoconstrictor with caution

Pregnancy Risk Factor C

Generic Available Yes

Carampicillin Hydrochloride *see* Bacampicillin *on page 106*

Carbachol (KAR ba kole)

Brand Names Carbastat® Ophthalmic; Carboptic® Ophthalmic; Isopto® Carbachol Ophthalmic; Miostat® Intraocular

Therapeutic Category Antiglaucoma Agent; Cholinergic Agent, Ophthalmic; Ophthalmic Agent, Miotic

Use Lowers intraocular pressure in the treatment of glaucoma; cause miosis during surgery

Usual Dosage Adults:
Ophthalmic: Instill 1-2 drops up to 3 times/day
Intraocular: 0.5 mL instilled into anterior chamber before or after securing sutures

Mechanism of Action Synthetic direct-acting cholinergic agent that causes miosis by stimulating muscarinic receptors in the eye

Local Anesthetic/Vasoconstrictor Precautions No information available to require special precautions

Effects on Dental Treatment Ophthalmic use of carbachol has no effect on dental treatment

Other Adverse Effects
1% to 10%: Ocular: Blurred vision, eye pain
<1%:
Cardiovascular: Hypotension
Central nervous system: Headache
Gastrointestinal: Stomach cramps, diarrhea, increased peristalsis
Local: Ciliary spasm with temporary decrease of visual acuity
Ocular: Corneal clouding, persistent bullous keratopathy, postoperative keratitis, retinal detachment, transient ciliary and conjunctival injection
Respiratory: Asthma

(Continued)

Carbachol *(Continued)*

Drug Interactions No data reported

Drug Uptake
Ophthalmic instillation:
Onset of miosis: 10-20 minutes
Duration of reduction in intraocular pressure: 4-8 hours
Intraocular administration:
Onset of miosis: Within 2-5 minutes
Duration: 24 hours

Pregnancy Risk Factor C

Generic Available No

Carbamazepine *(kar ba MAZ e peen)*

Related Information
Dental Drug Interactions: Update on Drug Combinations Requiring Special
Considerations *on page 1144*

Brand Names Epitol®; Tegretol®; Tegretol-XR®

Canadian/Mexican Brand Names Apo®-Carbamazepine (Canada); Carbazep®
(Mexico); Carbazina® (Mexico); Mazepine® (Canada); Neugeron® (Mexico);
Novo-Carbamaz® (Canada); Nu-Carbamazepine (Canada); PMS-Carbamaze-
pine® (Canada)

Therapeutic Category Anticonvulsant, Miscellaneous

Use
Dental: Used to relieve pain in trigeminal neuralgia
Medical: Prophylaxis of generalized tonic-clonic, partial (especially complex
partial), and mixed partial or generalized seizure disorder

Unlabeled use: Treat bipolar disorders and other affective disorders; resistant
schizophrenia, alcohol withdrawal, restless leg syndrome, and psychotic
behavior associated with dementia; may be used to relieve pain in trigeminal
neuralgia or diabetic neuropathy

Usual Dosage Oral (dosage must be adjusted according to patient's response
and serum concentrations):
Children >12 years and Adults: 200 mg twice daily to start, increase by 200 mg/
day at weekly intervals until therapeutic levels achieved; usual dose: 800-1200
mg/day in 3-4 divided doses; some patients have required up to 1.6-2.4 g/day;
extended release tablet: 200 mg twice daily for epilepsy, initial dose: 100 mg
for trigeminal neuralgia
Children <12 years: Not used in children for trigeminal neuralgia

Mechanism of Action In addition to anticonvulsant effects, carbamazepine has
anticholinergic, antineuralgic, antidiuretic, muscle relaxant and antiarrhythmic
properties; may depress activity in the nucleus ventralis of the thalamus or
decrease synaptic transmission or decrease summation of temporal stimulation
leading to neural discharge by limiting influx of sodium ions across cell
membrane or other unknown mechanisms; stimulates the release of ADH and
potentiates its action in promoting reabsorption of water; chemically related to
tricyclic antidepressants

Local Anesthetic/Vasoconstrictor Precautions No information available to
require special precautions

Effects on Dental Treatment Some patients may experience sore throat or
mouth ulcers

Other Adverse Effects
Dermatologic: Rash; but does not necessarily mean the drug should be stopped
>10%:
Central nervous system: Sedation, dizziness, fatigue, slurred speech, clumsi-
ness, confusion
Gastrointestinal: Nausea, vomiting
Ocular: Blurred vision, nystagmus

Contraindications Hypersensitivity to carbamazepine or any component; may
have cross-sensitivity with tricyclic antidepressants; should not be used in any
patient with bone marrow depression, or taking MAO inhibitors

Warnings/Precautions MAO inhibitors should be discontinued for a minimum of
14 days before carbamazepine is begun; administer with caution to patients with
history of cardiac damage or hepatic disease; potentially fatal blood cell abnormalities have been reported following treatment; early detection of hematologic
change is important; advise patients of early signs and symptoms including fever,
sore throat, mouth ulcers, infections, easy bruising, petechial or purpuric hemorrhage; carbamazepine is not effective in absence, myoclonic or akinetic seizures;
exacerbation of certain seizure types have been seen after initiation of carbamazepine therapy in children with mixed seizure disorders. Elderly may have
increased risk of SIADH-like syndrome.

Drug Interactions Carbamazepine may induce the metabolism of warfarin, cyclosporine, doxycycline, oral contraceptives, phenytoin, theophylline, benzodiazepines, ethosuximide, valproic acid, corticosteroids, and thyroid hormones; erythromycin, isoniazid, propoxyphene, verapamil, danazol, isoniazid, diltiazem, and cimetidine may inhibit hepatic metabolism of carbamazepine with resultant increase of carbamazepine serum concentrations and toxicity

Drug Uptake
Absorption: Slowly absorbed from GI tract
Serum half-life:
Initial: 18-55 hours
Multiple dosing:
Adults: 12-17 hours
Children: 8-14 hours
Time to peak serum concentration: Unpredictable, within 4-8 hours

Pregnancy Risk Factor C

Breast-feeding Considerations May be taken while breast-feeding

Dosage Forms
Suspension, oral (citrus-vanilla flavor): 100 mg/5 mL (450 mL)
Tablet: 200 mg
Tablet, chewable: 100 mg
Tablet, extended release: 100 mg, 200 mg, 400 mg

Dietary Considerations Food increases absorption

Generic Available Yes: Tablet

Carbamide Peroxide (KAR ba mide per OKS ide)

Related Information
Oral Rinse Products on page 1187

Brand Names Auro® Ear Drops [OTC]; Debrox® Otic [OTC]; E•R•O Ear [OTC]; Gly-Oxide® Oral [OTC]; Mollifene® Ear Wax Removing Formula [OTC]; Murine® Ear Drops [OTC]; Orajel® Perioseptic [OTC]; Proxigel® Oral [OTC]

Canadian/Mexican Brand Names Clamurid® (Canada)

Therapeutic Category Anti-infective Agent, Oral; Otic Agent, Cerumenolytic

Use Relief of minor swelling of gums, oral mucosal surfaces, and lips including canker sores and dental irritation; emulsify and disperse ear wax

Usual Dosage Children and Adults:
Gel: Gently massage on affected area 4 times/day; do not drink or rinse mouth for 5 minutes after use
Oral solution (should not be used for >7 days): Oral preparation should not be used in children <3 years of age; apply several drops undiluted on affected area 4 times/day after meals and at bedtime; expectorate after 2-3 minutes **or** place 10 drops onto tongue, mix with saliva, swish for several minutes, expectorate
Otic solution (should not be used for >4 days): Tilt head sideways and instill 5-10 drops twice daily up to 4 days, tip of applicator should not enter ear canal; keep drops in ear for several minutes by keeping head tilted and placing cotton in ear

Mechanism of Action Carbamide peroxide releases hydrogen peroxide which serves as a source of nascent oxygen upon contact with catalase; deodorant action is probably due to inhibition of odor-causing bacteria; softens impacted cerumen due to its foaming action

Local Anesthetic/Vasoconstrictor Precautions No information available to require special precautions

Effects on Dental Treatment No effects or complications reported

Other Adverse Effects 1% to 10%: Local: Rash, irritation, superinfections, redness

Drug Interactions No data reported

Pregnancy Risk Factor C

Generic Available Yes

Carbastat® Ophthalmic see Carbachol on page 173

Carbenicilina, Disodica (Mexico) see Carbenicillin on this page

Carbenicillin (kar ben i SIL in)

Brand Names Geocillin®

Canadian/Mexican Brand Names Carbecin® Inyectable (Mexico); Geopen® (Canada)

Therapeutic Category Antibiotic, Penicillin

Synonyms Carbenicilina, Disodica (Mexico)

Use Treatment of serious urinary tract infections and prostatitis caused by susceptible gram-negative aerobic bacilli or mixed aerobic-anaerobic bacterial infections excluding those secondary to Klebsiella sp and Serratia marcescens
(Continued)

Carbenicillin *(Continued)*

Usual Dosage Oral:

Children: 30-50 mg/kg/day divided every 6 hours; maximum dose: 2-3 g/day

Adults: 1-2 tablets every 6 hours for urinary tract infections or 2 tablets every 6 hours for prostatitis

Mechanism of Action Interferes with bacterial cell wall synthesis during active multiplication

Local Anesthetic/Vasoconstrictor Precautions No information available to require special precautions

Effects on Dental Treatment Prolonged use of penicillins may lead to development of oral candidiasis

Other Adverse Effects

>10%: Gastrointestinal: Diarrhea

1% to 10%: Gastrointestinal: Nausea, bad taste, vomiting, flatulence, glossitis

<1%:

Central nervous system: Headache, hyperthermia

Dermatologic: Skin rash, urticaria

Endocrine & metabolic: Hypokalemia

Genitourinary: Vaginitis

Hematologic: Anemia, thrombocytopenia, leukopenia, neutropenia, eosinophilia

Hepatic: Elevated LFTs

Local: Thrombophlebitis

Ocular: Itchy eyes

Renal: Hematuria

Miscellaneous: Furry tongue

Drug Interactions

Decreased effect with administration of aminoglycosides within 1 hour; may inactivate both drugs

Increased duration of half-life with probenecid

Drug Uptake

Absorption: Oral: 30% to 40%

Serum half-life:

Children: 0.8-1.8 hours

Adults: 1-1.5 hours, prolonged to 10-20 hours with renal insufficiency

Time to peak serum concentration: Within 0.5-2 hours in patients with normal renal function; serum concentrations following oral absorption are inadequate for treatment of systemic infections

Pregnancy Risk Factor B

Generic Available No

Carbidopa *(kar bi DOE pa)*

Brand Names Lodosyn®

Therapeutic Category Anti-Parkinson's Agent

Use Given with levodopa in the treatment of parkinsonism to enable a lower dosage of levodopa to be used and a more rapid response to be obtained and to decrease side-effects; for details of administration and dosage, see Levodopa; has no effect without levodopa

Usual Dosage Adults: Oral: 70-100 mg/day; maximum daily dose: 200 mg

Mechanism of Action Carbidopa is a peripheral decarboxylase inhibitor with little or no pharmacological activity when given alone in usual doses. It inhibits the peripheral decarboxylation of levodopa to dopamine; and as it does not cross the blood-brain barrier, unlike levodopa, effective brain concentrations of dopamine are produced with lower doses of levodopa. At the same time reduced peripheral formation of dopamine reduces peripheral side-effects, notably nausea and vomiting, and cardiac arrhythmias, although the dyskinesias and adverse mental effects associated with levodopa therapy tend to develop earlier.

Local Anesthetic/Vasoconstrictor Precautions No information available to require special precautions

Effects on Dental Treatment No effects or complications reported

Other Adverse Effects Adverse reactions are associated with concomitant administration with levodopa

>10%: Central nervous system: Anxiety, confusion, nervousness, mental depression

1% to 10%:

Cardiovascular: Orthostatic hypotension, palpitations, cardiac arrhythmias

Central nervous system: Memory loss, insomnia, fatigue, hallucinations, ataxia, dystonic movements

Gastrointestinal: Nausea, vomiting, GI bleeding

Ocular: Blurred vision

<1%:
    Cardiovascular: Hypertension
    Gastrointestinal: Duodenal ulcer
    Hematologic: Hemolytic anemia
Drug Interactions Reports of interaction with tricyclic antidepressants resulting in hypertension and dyskinesias
Drug Uptake
    Absorption: Rapid but incomplete from GI tract
Pregnancy Risk Factor C
Generic Available No

Carbinoxamine and Pseudoephedrine
(kar bi NOKS a meen & soo doe e FED rin)
Brand Names Biohist®-LA; Carbiset® Tablet; Carbiset-TR® Tablet; Carbodec® Syrup; Carbodec® Tablet; Carbodec TR® Tablet; Cardec-S® Syrup; Rondec® Drops; Rondec® Filmtab®; Rondec® Syrup; Rondec-TR®
Therapeutic Category Antihistamine/Decongestant Combination
Use Temporary relief of nasal congestion, running nose, sneezing, itching of nose or throat, and itchy, watery eyes due to the common cold, hay fever, or other respiratory allergies
Usual Dosage Oral:
    Children:
        Drops: 1-18 months: 0.25-1 mL 4 times/day
        Syrup:
            18 months to 6 years: 2.5 mL 3-4 times/day
            >6 years: 5 mL 2-4 times/day
    Adults:
        Liquid: 5 mL 4 times/day
        Tablets: 1 tablet 4 times/day
Mechanism of Action Carbinoxamine competes with histamine for H_1-receptor sites on effector cells in the gastrointestinal tract, blood vessels, and respiratory tract
Local Anesthetic/Vasoconstrictor Precautions Pseudoephedrine is a sympathomimetic which has potential to enhance vasoconstrictor effects of epinephrine; use local anesthetic with vasoconstrictor with caution
Effects on Dental Treatment 1% to 10% of patients will experience dry mouth which disappears with cessation of drug therapy
Other Adverse Effects
>10%:
    Central nervous system: Slight to moderate drowsiness
    Respiratory: Thickening of bronchial secretions
1% to 10%:
    Central nervous system: Headache, fatigue, nervousness, dizziness
    Gastrointestinal: Appetite increase, weight gain, nausea, diarrhea, abdominal pain, dry mouth
    Neuromuscular & skeletal: Arthralgia
    Respiratory: Pharyngitis
<1%:
    Cardiovascular: Edema, palpitations
    Central nervous system: Depression
    Dermatologic: Angioedema, photosensitivity, rash
    Hepatic: Hepatitis
    Neuromuscular & skeletal: Myalgia, paresthesia
    Respiratory: Bronchospasm, epistaxis
Drug Interactions May enhance the effects of barbiturates, TCAs, MAO inhibitors, ethanolamine antihistamines
Pregnancy Risk Factor C
Generic Available Yes

Carbinoxamine, Pseudoephedrine, and Dextromethorphan
(kar bi NOKS a meen, soo doe e FED rin, & deks troe meth OR fan)
Brand Names Carbodec® DM; Cardec® DM; Pseudo-Car® DM; Rondamine®-DM Drops; Rondec®-DM; Tussafed® Drops
Therapeutic Category Antihistamine/Decongestant Combination; Cough Preparation
Use Relief of coughs and upper respiratory symptoms, including nasal congestion, associated with allergy or the common cold
Local Anesthetic/Vasoconstrictor Precautions Use with caution since pseudoephedrine is a sympathomimetic amine which could interact with epinephrine to cause a pressor response
(Continued)

Carbinoxamine, Pseudoephedrine, and Dextromethorphan (Continued)

Effects on Dental Treatment Up to 10% of patients could experience tachycardia, palpitations, and dry mouth; use vasoconstrictor with caution

Warnings/Precautions Research on chicken embryos exposed to concentrations of dextromethorphan relative to those typically taken by humans has shown to cause birth defects and fetal death; more study is needed, but it is suggested that pregnant women should be advised not to use dextromethorphan-containing medications

Pregnancy Risk Factor C (see Warnings)

Generic Available Yes

Carbiset® Tablet *see* Carbinoxamine and Pseudoephedrine *on previous page*

Carbiset-TR® Tablet *see* Carbinoxamine and Pseudoephedrine *on previous page*

Carbocaine® *see* Mepivacaine *on page 595*

Carbocaine® 2% With Neo-Cobefrin® *see* Mepivacaine and Levonordefrin *on page 596*

Carbocaine® 3% *see* Mepivacaine Dental Anesthetic *on page 597*

Carbodec® DM *see* Carbinoxamine, Pseudoephedrine, and Dextromethorphan *on previous page*

Carbodec® Syrup *see* Carbinoxamine and Pseudoephedrine *on previous page*

Carbodec® Tablet *see* Carbinoxamine and Pseudoephedrine *on previous page*

Carbodec TR® Tablet *see* Carbinoxamine and Pseudoephedrine *on previous page*

Carbol-Fuchsin Solution (kar bol-FOOK sin soe LOO shun)

Therapeutic Category Antifungal Agent, Topical

Synonyms Castellani Paint

Use Treatment of superficial mycotic infections

Local Anesthetic/Vasoconstrictor Precautions No information available to require special precautions

Effects on Dental Treatment No effects or complications reported

Generic Available Yes

Carbolic Acid *see* Phenol *on page 749*

Carboplatin (KAR boe pla tin)

Brand Names Paraplatin®

Canadian/Mexican Brand Names Blastocarb (Mexico); Carboplat (Mexico)

Therapeutic Category Antineoplastic Agent, Alkylating Agent

Synonyms CBDCA

Use Palliative treatment of ovarian carcinoma; also used in the treatment of small cell lung cancer, squamous cell carcinoma of the esophagus; solid tumors of the bladder, cervix and testes; pediatric brain tumor, neuroblastoma

Usual Dosage IVPB, I.V. infusion, Intraperitoneal (**refer to individual protocols**):

Children:

Solid tumor: 560 mg/m^2 once every 4 weeks

Brain tumor: 175 mg/m^2 once weekly for 4 weeks with a 2-week recovery period between courses; dose is then adjusted on platelet count and neutrophil count values

Adults:

Ovarian cancer: Usual doses range from 360 mg/m^2 I.V. every 3 weeks single agent therapy to 300 mg/m^2 every 4 weeks as combination therapy

In general, however, single intermittent courses of carboplatin should not be repeated until the neutrophil count is at least 2000/mm^3 and the platelet count is at least 100,000/mm^3

Mechanism of Action Analogue of cisplatin which covalently binds to DNA; possible cross-linking and interference with the function of DNA

Local Anesthetic/Vasoconstrictor Precautions No information available to require special precautions

Effects on Dental Treatment No effects or complications reported

Other Adverse Effects

>10%:

Endocrine & metabolic: Electrolyte abnormalities such as hypocalcemia, hypomagnesemia, hyponatremia, and hypokalemia

Hepatic: Abnormal liver function tests

Hematologic: Neutropenia, leukopenia, thrombocytopenia (platelet count reaches a nadir between 14-21 days), anemia

Myelosuppressive: Dose-limiting toxicity; WBC: Severe (dose-dependent); Platelets: Severe; Nadir: 21-24 days; Recovery: 5-6 weeks

Local: Pain at injection site

Neuromuscular & skeletal: Weakness
1% to 10%:
Central nervous system: Pain
Dermatologic: Urticaria, rash, alopecia
Gastrointestinal: Emetogenic potential low (<10%), stomatitis, diarrhea, anorexia
Hematologic: Hemorrhagic complications
Neuromuscular & skeletal: Peripheral neuropathy
Otic: Ototoxicity in 1% of patients
<1%:
Central nervous system: Neurotoxicity has only been noted in patients previously treated with cisplatin
Ocular: Blurred vision
Renal: Nephrotoxicity (uncommon)

Drug Uptake
Serum half-life, terminal: 22-40 hours

Pregnancy Risk Factor D

Generic Available No

Carboprost Tromethamine (KAR boe prost tro METH a meen)

Brand Names Hemabate™

Therapeutic Category Abortifacient; Prostaglandin

Use Termination of pregnancy

Usual Dosage Adults: I.M.:
Abortion: 250 mcg to start, 250 mcg at 1½-hour to 3½-hour intervals depending on uterine response; a 500 mcg dose may be given if uterine response is not adequate after several 250 mcg doses; do not exceed 12 mg total dose
Refractory postpartum uterine bleeding: Initial: 250 mcg; may repeat at 15- to 90-minute intervals to a total dose of 2 mg
Bladder irrigation for hemorrhagic cystitis (refer to individual protocols): [0.4-1.0 mg/dL as solution] 50 mL instilled into bladder 4 times/day for 1 hour

Mechanism of Action Carboprost tromethamine is a prostaglandin similar to prostaglandin F_2 alpha (dinoprost) except for the addition of a methyl group at the C-15 position. This substitution produces longer duration of activity than dinoprost; carboprost stimulates uterine contractility which usually results in expulsion of the products of conception and is used to induce abortion between 13-20 weeks of pregnancy. Hemostasis at the placentation site is achieved through the myometrial contractions produced by carboprost.

Local Anesthetic/Vasoconstrictor Precautions No information available to require special precautions

Effects on Dental Treatment No effects or complications reported

Other Adverse Effects
>10%: Gastrointestinal: Nausea
1% to 10%: Cardiovascular: Flushing
<1%:
Cardiovascular: Hypertension, hypotension
Central nervous system: Drowsiness, vertigo, nervousness, fever, headache, dystonia, vasovagal syndrome
Endocrine & metabolic: Breast tenderness
Gastrointestinal: Dry mouth, vomiting, diarrhea, hematemesis, taste alterations
Genitourinary: Bladder spasms
Neuromuscular & skeletal: Myalgia
Ocular: Blurred vision
Respiratory: Coughing, asthma, respiratory distress
Miscellaneous: Septic shock, hiccups

Pregnancy Risk Factor X

Generic Available No

Carboptic® Ophthalmic see Carbachol on page 173

Carbose D see Carboxymethylcellulose on this page

Carboxymethylcellulose (kar boks ee meth il SEL yoo lose)

Brand Names Cellufresh® [OTC]; Celluvisc® [OTC]

Therapeutic Category Ophthalmic Agent, Miscellaneous

Synonyms Carbose D

Use Preservative-free artificial tear substitute

Local Anesthetic/Vasoconstrictor Precautions No information available to require special precautions

Effects on Dental Treatment No effects or complications reported

Generic Available Yes

Cardec® DM see Carbinoxamine, Pseudoephedrine, and Dextromethorphan on page 177

Cardec-S® Syrup *see* Carbinoxamine and Pseudoephedrine *on page 177*

Cardene® *see* Nicardipine *on page 677*

Cardene® SR *see* Nicardipine *on page 677*

Cardilate® *see* Erythrityl Tetranitrate *on page 361*

Cardio-Green® *see* Indocyanine Green *on page 506*

Cardioquin® *see* Quinidine *on page 830*

Cardiovascular Diseases *see page 1010*

Cardizem® CD *see* Diltiazem *on page 318*

Cardizem® Injectable *see* Diltiazem *on page 318*

Cardizem® SR *see* Diltiazem *on page 318*

Cardizem® Tablet *see* Diltiazem *on page 318*

Cardura® *see* Doxazosin *on page 334*

Carisoprodate *see* Carisoprodol, Aspirin, and Codeine *on next page*

Carisoprodol (kar i soe PROE dole)

Related Information
Carisoprodol and Aspirin *on this page*

Brand Names Soma®; Soma® Compound

Canadian/Mexican Brand Names Dolaren® (Carisoprodol with Diclofenac) (Mexico); Naxodol® (Carisoprodol with Naproxen) (Mexico)

Therapeutic Category Muscle Relaxant; Skeletal Muscle Relaxant

Synonyms Isomeprobamate (Canada)

Use
Dental: Treatment of muscle spasm associated with acute temporomandibular joint pain
Medical: Skeletal muscle relaxant

Usual Dosage Adults: Oral: 350 mg 3-4 times/day; take last dose at bedtime; compound: 1-2 tablets 4 times/day

Mechanism of Action Precise mechanism is not yet clear, but many effects have been ascribed to its central depressant actions

Local Anesthetic/Vasoconstrictor Precautions No information available to require special precautions

Effects on Dental Treatment No effects or complications reported

Other Adverse Effects
>10%: Central nervous system: Drowsiness
1% to 10%: Central nervous system: Dizziness, lightheadedness

Contraindications Acute intermittent porphyria, hypersensitivity to carisoprodol, meprobamate or any component

Warnings/Precautions Use with caution in renal and hepatic dysfunction

Drug Interactions Alcohol, CNS depressants, phenothiazines, clindamycin, MAO inhibitors

Drug Uptake
Onset of action: Within 30 minutes
Duration: 4-6 hours
Serum half-life: 8 hours
Time to peak serum concentration: 4 hours

Pregnancy Risk Factor C

Breast-feeding Considerations No data reported

Dosage Forms Tablet:
Soma®: 350 mg
Soma® Compound: Carisoprodol 200 mg and aspirin 325 mg

Dietary Considerations No data reported

Generic Available Yes

Carisoprodol and Aspirin (kar i soe PROE dole & AS pir in)

Brand Names Soma® Compound

Therapeutic Category Skeletal Muscle Relaxant

Use Skeletal muscle relaxant

Usual Dosage Adults: Oral: 1-2 tablets 4 times/day

Local Anesthetic/Vasoconstrictor Precautions No information available to require special precautions

Effects on Dental Treatment Avoid aspirin if possible, for 1 week prior to surgery because of the possibility of postoperative bleeding

Use with caution in impaired hepatic function; use with caution in patients with platelet and bleeding disorders, renal dysfunction, erosive gastritis, or peptic ulcer disease, previous nonreaction does not guarantee future safe taking of medication; do not use aspirin in children <16 years of age for chickenpox or flu symptoms due to the association with Reye's syndrome

Elderly are a high-risk population for adverse effects from nonsteroidal anti-inflammatory agents. As much as 60% of elderly with GI complications to NSAIDs can develop peptic ulceration and/or hemorrhage asymptomatically. Also, concomitant disease and drug use contribute to the risk for GI adverse effects. Use lowest effective dose for shortest period possible. Consider renal function decline with age. Use with caution in patients with history of asthma

Drug Interactions See individual agents

Pregnancy Risk Factor C

Dosage Forms Tablet: Carisoprodol 200 mg and aspirin 325 mg

Generic Available Yes

Carisoprodol, Aspirin, and Codeine
(kar i soe PROE dole, AS pir in, and KOE deen)

Brand Names Soma® Compound w/Codeine

Therapeutic Category Skeletal Muscle Relaxant

Synonyms Carisoprodate; Isobamate

Use Skeletal muscle relaxant

Restrictions C-III

Usual Dosage Adults: Oral: 1 or 2 tablets 4 times/day

Local Anesthetic/Vasoconstrictor Precautions No information available to require special precautions

Effects on Dental Treatment Avoid aspirin, if possible, for 1 week prior to surgery because of the possibility of postoperative bleeding

Pregnancy Risk Factor C

Dosage Forms Tablet: Carisoprodol 200 mg, aspirin 325 mg, and codeine phosphate 16 mg

Generic Available No

Carmol® [OTC] see Urea on page 977

Carmol-HC® Topical see Urea and Hydrocortisone on page 978

Carmustine (kar MUS teen)

Brand Names BiCNU®

Therapeutic Category Antineoplastic Agent, Alkylating Agent (Nitrosourea)

Synonyms BCNU

Use Brain tumors, multiple myeloma, Hodgkin's disease, and non-Hodgkin's lymphomas; some activity in malignant melanoma

Usual Dosage I.V. **(refer to individual protocols):**

Children: 200-250 mg/m^2 every 4-6 weeks as a single dose

Adults: 150-200 mg/m^2 every 6 weeks as a single dose or divided into daily injections on 2 successive days; next dose is to be determined based on hematologic response to the previous dose. See table.

Suggested Carmustine Dose Following Initial Dose

Nadir After Prior Dose		% of Prior Dose to Be Given
Leukocytes/mm^3	Platelets/mm^3	
>4000	>100,000	100
3000-3999	75,000-99,999	100
2000-2999	25,000-74,999	70
<2000	<25,000	50

Primary brain cancer: 150-200 mg/m^2 every 6-8 weeks

Autologous BMT: All of the following doses are fatal without BMT

Combination therapy: Up to 300-900 mg/m^2

Single agent therapy: Up to 1200 mg/m^2 (fatal necrosis is associated with doses >2 g/m^2)

Mechanism of Action Interferes with the normal function of DNA by alkylation and cross-linking the strands of DNA, and by possible protein modification

Local Anesthetic/Vasoconstrictor Precautions No information available to require special precautions

Effects on Dental Treatment No effects or complications reported

Other Adverse Effects

>10%:

Gastrointestinal: Nausea and vomiting occur within 2-4 hours after drug injection; dose-related

Emetic potential: <200 mg: Moderately high (60% to 90%); ≥200 mg: High (>90%)

Local: Pain at injection site

(Continued)

181

Carmustine *(Continued)*

1% to 10%:
Cardiovascular: Facial flushing
Dermatologic: Alopecia
Gastrointestinal: Stomatitis, diarrhea, anorexia
Hematologic: Anemia

<1%:
Central nervous system: Ataxia, dizziness
Dermatologic: Hyperpigmentation, dermatitis, facial flushing is probably due to the ethanol used in reconstitution
Hematologic: Myelosuppressive: Delayed, occurs 4-6 weeks after administration and is dose-related; usually persists for 1-2 weeks; thrombocytopenia is usually more severe than leukopenia. Myelofibrosis and preleukemic syndromes are being reported. WBC: Moderate; Platelets: Severe; Onset (days): 14; Nadir (days): 21-35; Recovery (days): 42-50.
Hepatic: Reversible toxicity, elevated LFTs in 20%
Local: Burning at injection site
Ocular: Retinal hemorrhages, ocular toxicity
Pulmonary: Fibrosis occurs mostly in patients treated with prolonged total doses >1400 mg/m² or with bone marrow transplantation doses. Risk factors include a history of lung disease, concomitant bleomycin, or radiation therapy. PFTs should be conducted prior to therapy and monitored. Patients with predicted FVC or DL_{co} <70% are at a higher risk.
Renal: Azotemia, decrease in kidney size, renal failure

Drug Uptake
Absorption: Highly lipid soluble
Serum half-life (biphasic):
Initial: 1.4 minutes
Secondary: 20 minutes (active metabolites may persist for days and have a plasma half-life of 67 hours)

Pregnancy Risk Factor D
Generic Available No

Carnation Instant Breakfast® [OTC] *see* Enteral Nutritional Products *on page 350*

Carnitor® Injection *see* Levocarnitine *on page 547*

Carnitor® Oral *see* Levocarnitine *on page 547*

Carteolol *(KAR tee oh lole)*

Related Information
Cardiovascular Diseases *on page 1010*

Brand Names Cartrol®; Ocupress®

Therapeutic Category Antianginal Agent; Antiglaucoma Agent; Beta-adrenergic Blocker, Noncardioselective; Beta-Adrenergic Blocker, Ophthalmic

Use Management of hypertension; treatment of chronic open-angle glaucoma and intraocular hypertension

Usual Dosage Adults:
Oral: 2.5 mg as a single daily dose, with a maintenance dose normally 2.5-5 mg once daily; maximum daily dose: 10 mg; doses >10 mg do not increase response and may in fact decrease effect
Ophthalmic: Instill 1 drop in affected eye(s) twice daily; see Additional Information

Mechanism of Action Competitively blocks beta₁-adrenergic receptors with little or no effect on beta₂-receptors except at high doses; exhibits membrane stabilizing and intrinsic sympathomimetic activity

Local Anesthetic/Vasoconstrictor Precautions No information available to require special precautions

Effects on Dental Treatment Noncardioselective beta-blockers (ie, propranolol, nadolol) enhance the pressor response to epinephrine, resulting in hypertension and bradycardia. This has not been reported for carteolol, a cardioselective beta-blocker. Therefore, local anesthetic with vasoconstrictor can be safely used in patients medicated with carteolol. Many nonsteroidal anti-inflammatory drugs such as ibuprofen and indomethacin can reduce the hypotensive effect of beta-blockers after 3 or more weeks of therapy with the NSAID. Short-term NSAID use (ie, 3 days) requires no special precautions in patients taking beta-blockers

Other Adverse Effects
1% to 10%:
Cardiovascular: Congestive heart failure, arrhythmia
Central nervous system: Mental depression, headache, dizziness
Neuromuscular & skeletal: Back pain, arthralgia

<1%:
Cardiovascular: Bradycardia, chest pain, mesenteric arterial thrombosis, A-V block, persistent bradycardia, hypotension, edema, Raynaud's phenomenon

Central nervous system: Fatigue, insomnia, lethargy, nightmares, confusion
Dermatologic: Purpura
Endocrine & metabolic: Hyperglycemia
Gastrointestinal: Ischemic colitis, constipation, nausea, diarrhea
Genitourinary: Impotence
Hematologic: Thrombocytopenia
Respiratory: Bronchospasm
Miscellaneous: Cold extremities

Drug Interactions
Decreased effect of beta-blockers:
Barbiturates (increased liver metabolism of beta-blockers to result in lower serum levels)
NSAIDs (attenuate the hypotensive therapeutic effects of beta-blockers)
Rifampin (increased liver metabolism of beta-blockers to result in lower serum levels)
Increased effects of beta-blockers:
Calcium channel blockers (increased serum levels of beta-blockers by unknown mechanism to enhance hypotension)
Beta-blockers increase the effects of:
Epinephrine (vasoconstrictor; initial hypertensive episode followed by bradycardia) only from noncardioselective type beta-blockers
Phenylephrine (Neosynephrine®; enhanced pressor response)
Theophylline (inhibit theophylline metabolism causing increase in serum concentrations)

Drug Uptake
Onset of effect: Oral: 1-1.5 hours
Peak effect: 2 hours
Duration: 12 hours
Absorption: Oral: 80%
Serum half-life: 6 hours

Pregnancy Risk Factor C
Generic Available No
Selected Readings
Foster CA and Aston SJ, "Propranolol-Epinephrine Interaction: A Potential Disaster," *Plast Reconstr Surg*, 1983, 72(1):74-8.
Wong DG, Spence JD, Lamki L, et al, "Effect of Nonsteroidal Anti-inflammatory Drugs on Control of Hypertension of Beta-Blockers and Diuretics," *Lancet*, 1986, 1(8488):997-1001.
Wynn RL, "Dental Nonsteroidal Anti-inflammatory Drugs and Prostaglandin-Based Drug Interactions, Part Two," *Gen Dent*, 1992, 40(2):104, 106, 108.
Wynn RL, "Epinephrine Interactions With Beta-Blockers," *Gen Dent*, 1994, 42(1):16, 18.

Carter's Little Pills® [OTC] *see* Bisacodyl *on page 131*

Cartrol® *see* Carteolol *on previous page*

Carvedilol (KAR ve dil ole)
Related Information
Cardiovascular Diseases *on page 1010*
Brand Names Coreg®
Therapeutic Category Beta-adrenergic Blocker, Noncardioselective
Use Management of hypertension; can be used alone or in combination with other agents, especially thiazide-type diuretics
Usual Dosage Adults: Oral:
Hypertension: 6.25 mg twice daily; if tolerated, dose should be maintained for 1-2 weeks, then increased to 12.5 mg twice daily; dosage may be increased to a maximum of 25 mg twice daily after 1-2 weeks; reduce dosage if heart rate drops <55 beats/minute
Congestive heart failure: 12.5-50 mg twice daily
Angina pectoris: 25-50 mg twice daily
Idiopathic cardiomyopathy: 6.25-25 mg twice daily
Mechanism of Action As a racemic mixture, carvedilol has nonselective beta-adrenoreceptor and alpha-adrenergic blocking activity at equal potency. No intrinsic sympathomimetic activity has been documented. Associated effects include reduction of cardiac output, exercise- or beta agonist-induced tachycardia, reduction of reflex orthostatic tachycardia, vasodilation, decreased peripheral vascular resistance (especially in standing position), decreased renal vascular resistance, reduced plasma renin activity, and increased levels of atrial natriuretic peptide.
Local Anesthetic/Vasoconstrictor Precautions No information available to require special precautions
Effects on Dental Treatment No effects or complications reported
Other Adverse Effects
1% to 10%:
Cardiovascular: Bradycardia, postural hypotension, edema
Central nervous system: Dizziness, somnolence, insomnia, fatigue
(Continued)

Carvedilol *(Continued)*

    Gastrointestinal: Diarrhea, abdominal pain
    Neuromuscular & skeletal: Back pain
    Respiratory: Rhinitis, pharyngitis, dyspnea
  <1%:
    Cardiovascular: A-V block, extrasystoles, hypertension, hypotension, palpitations, peripheral ischemia, syncope
    Central nervous system: Ataxia, vertigo, depression, nervousness, malaise
    Dermatologic: Pruritus, rash
    Endocrine & metabolic: Decreased male libido, hypercholesterolemia, hyperglycemia, hyperuricemia
    Gastrointestinal: Constipation, flatulence, dry mouth
    Genitourinary: Impotence
    Hematologic: Anemia, leukopenia
    Hepatic: Hyperbilirubinemia, elevated LFTs
    Neuromuscular & skeletal: Paresthesia, myalgia, weakness
    Ocular: Abnormal vision
    Otic: Tinnitus
    Respiratory: Asthma, cough
    Miscellaneous: Increased sweating

Drug Uptake
  Absorption: Rapid; food decreases the rate but not the extent of absorption; administration with food minimizes risks of orthostatic hypotension
  Serum half-life: 7-10 hours

Pregnancy Risk Factor C

Generic Available No

Casanthranol and Docusate *see* Docusate and Casanthranol *on page 331*

Cascara Sagrada (kas KAR a sah GRAH dah)

Therapeutic Category Laxative, Stimulant

Use Temporary relief of constipation; sometimes used with milk of magnesia ("black and white" mixture)

Usual Dosage Note: Cascara sagrada fluid extract is 5 times more potent than cascara sagrada aromatic fluid extract.

  Oral (aromatic fluid extract):
    Children 2-11 years: 2.5 mL/day (range: 1-3 mL) as needed
    Children ≥12 years and Adults: 5 mL/day (range: 2-6 mL) as needed at bedtime (1 tablet as needed at bedtime)

Mechanism of Action Direct chemical irritation of the intestinal mucosa resulting in an increased rate of colonic motility and change in fluid and electrolyte secretion

Local Anesthetic/Vasoconstrictor Precautions No information available to require special precautions

Effects on Dental Treatment No effects or complications reported

Other Adverse Effects 1% to 10%:
  Cardiovascular: Faintness
  Endocrine & metabolic: Electrolyte and fluid imbalance
  Gastrointestinal: Abdominal cramps, nausea, diarrhea
  Genitourinary: Discolors urine reddish pink or brown

Drug Interactions Decreased effect of oral anticoagulants

Drug Uptake
  Onset of action: 6-10 hours

Pregnancy Risk Factor C

Generic Available Yes

Casodex® *see* Bicalutamide *on page 129*

Castellani Paint *see* Carbol-Fuchsin Solution *on page 178*

Castor Oil (KAS tor oyl)

Brand Names Alphamul® [OTC]; Emulsoil® [OTC]; Fleet® Flavored Castor Oil [OTC]; Neoloid® [OTC]; Purge® [OTC]

Therapeutic Category Laxative, Stimulant

Use Preparation for rectal or bowel examination or surgery; rarely used to relieve constipation; also applied to skin as emollient and protectant

Usual Dosage Oral:
  Liquid:
    Children 2-11 years: 5-15 mL as a single dose
    Children ≥12 years and Adults: 15-60 mL as a single dose

Emulsified:
36.4%:
Children <2 years: 5-15 mL/dose
Children 2-11 years: 7.5-30 mL/dose
Children ≥12 years and Adults: 30-60 mL/dose
60% to 67%:
Children <2 years: 1.25-5 mL
Children 2-12 years: 5-15 mL
Adults: 15-45 mL
95%, mix with ½ to 1 full glass liquid:
Children: 5-10 mL
Adults: 15-60 mL

Mechanism of Action Acts primarily in the small intestine; hydrolyzed to ricinoleic acid which reduces net absorption of fluid and electrolytes and stimulates peristalsis

Local Anesthetic/Vasoconstrictor Precautions No information available to require special precautions

Effects on Dental Treatment No effects or complications reported

Other Adverse Effects
1% to 10%:
Central nervous system: Dizziness
Endocrine & metabolic: Electrolyte disturbance
Gastrointestinal: Abdominal cramps, nausea, diarrhea
<1%: Pelvic congestion

Drug Interactions No data reported

Drug Uptake Onset of action: Oral: 2-6 hours

Pregnancy Risk Factor X

Generic Available Yes

Cataflam® Oral see Diclofenac on page 304

Catapres® Oral see Clonidine on page 250

Catapres-TTS® Transdermal see Clonidine on page 250

Caverject® Injection see Alprostadil on page 44

CBDCA see Carboplatin on page 178

CCNU see Lomustine on page 564

C-Crystals® [OTC] see Ascorbic Acid on page 88

2-CdA see Cladribine on page 239

CDDP see Cisplatin on page 237

Cebid® Timecelles® [OTC] see Ascorbic Acid on page 88

Ceclor® see Cefaclor on this page

Ceclor® CD see Cefaclor on this page

Cecon® [OTC] see Ascorbic Acid on page 88

Cedax® see Ceftibuten on page 196

CeeNU® Oral see Lomustine on page 564

Ceepryn® [OTC] see Cetylpyridinium on page 205

Cefaclor (SEF a klor)

Brand Names Ceclor®; Ceclor® CD

Therapeutic Category Antibiotic, Cephalosporin (Second Generation)

Use
Dental: An alternate antibiotic to treat orofacial infections in patients allergic to penicillins; susceptible bacteria including aerobic gram-positive bacteria and anaerobes
Medical: Infections in the medical patient caused by susceptible organisms including *Staphylococcus aureus* and *H. influenzae*; treatment of otitis media, sinusitis, and infections involving the respiratory tract, skin and skin structure, bone and joint, and urinary tract

Usual Dosage Oral:
Children >1 month: 20-40 mg/kg/day divided every 8-12 hours; maximum dose: 2 g/day (twice daily option is for treatment of otitis media or pharyngitis)
Adults: 250-500 mg every 8 hours (or daily dose can be given in 2 divided doses) for at least 7 days

Mechanism of Action Inhibits bacterial cell wall synthesis by binding to one or more of the penicillin-binding proteins (PBPs) which in turn inhibits the final transpeptidation step of peptidoglycan synthesis in bacterial cell walls, thus inhibiting cell wall biosynthesis. Bacteria eventually lyse due to ongoing activity of cell wall autolytic enzymes (autolysins and murein hydrolases) while cell wall assembly is arrested.

Local Anesthetic/Vasoconstrictor Precautions No information available to require special precautions
(Continued)

185

Cefaclor *(Continued)*

Effects on Dental Treatment No effects or complications reported

Other Adverse Effects 1% to 10%: Gastrointestinal: Pseudomembranous colitis, diarrhea

Contraindications Hypersensitivity to cefaclor, any component, or cephalosporins

Warnings/Precautions Modify dosage in patients with severe renal impairment; prolonged use may result in superinfection; a low incidence in cross-hypersensitivity to penicillins exists

Drug Interactions Probenecid may decrease cephalosporin elimination; furosemide, aminoglycosides may be a possible additive to nephrotoxicity

Drug Uptake
Absorption: Oral: Well absorbed, acid stable
Serum half-life: 0.5-1 hour
Time to peak serum concentration:
Capsule: 60 minutes
Suspension: 45 minutes

Pregnancy Risk Factor B

Breast-feeding Considerations Excreted into breast milk in small amounts like other cephalosporins

Dosage Forms
Capsule: 250 mg, 500 mg
Powder for oral suspension (strawberry flavor): 125 mg/5 mL (75 mL, 150 mL); 187 mg/5 mL (50 mL, 100 mL); 250 mg/5 mL (75 mL, 150 mL); 375 mg/5 mL (50 mL, 100 mL)
Tablet, extended release: 375 mg, 500 mg

Dietary Considerations May be taken with food, however, there is delayed absorption

Generic Available Yes

Comments Patients allergic to penicillins can use a cephalosporin; the incidence of cross-reactivity between penicillins and cephalosporins is 1% when the allergic reaction to penicillin is delayed. Cefaclor is effective against anaerobic bacteria, but the sensitivity of alpha-hemolytic *Streptococcus* vary; approximately 10% of strains are resistant. Nearly 70% are intermediately sensitive. If the patient has a history of immediate reaction to penicillin, the incidence of cross-reactivity is 20%; cephalosporins are contraindicated in these patients.

Selected Readings
Saxon A, Beall GN, Rohr AS, et al, "Immediate Hypersensitivity Reactions to Beta-Lactam Antibiotics," *Ann Intern Med*, 1987, 107(2):204-15.

Cefadroxil *(sef a DROKS il)*

Related Information
Antibiotic Prophylaxis, Preprocedural Guidelines for Dental Patients *on page 1034*

Brand Names Duricef®

Canadian/Mexican Brand Names Cefamox® (Mexico); Duracef® (Mexico)

Therapeutic Category Antibiotic, Cephalosporin (First Generation)

Use
Dental: Alternative antibiotic for prevention of bacterial endocarditis. Individuals allergic to amoxicillin (penicillins) may receive cefadroxil provided they have not had an immediate, local, or systemic IgE-mediated anaphylactic allergic reaction to penicillin.
Medical: Treatment of susceptible bacterial infections, including those caused by group A beta-hemolytic *Streptococcus*

Usual Dosage Oral:
Children: 30 mg/kg/day divided twice daily up to a maximum of 2 g/day
Prophylaxis: 50 mg/kg orally 1 hour before procedure
Adults: 1-2 g/day in 2 divided doses
Prophylaxis: 2 g 1 hour before procedure

Mechanism of Action Inhibits bacterial cell wall synthesis by binding to one or more of the penicillin-binding proteins (PBPs) which in turn inhibits the final transpeptidation step of peptidoglycan synthesis in bacterial cell walls, thus inhibiting cell wall biosynthesis. Bacteria eventually lyse due to ongoing activity of cell wall autolytic enzymes (autolysins and murein hydrolases) while cell wall assembly is arrested.

Local Anesthetic/Vasoconstrictor Precautions No information available to require special precautions

Effects on Dental Treatment No effects or complications reported

Other Adverse Effects
1% to 10%: Gastrointestinal: Diarrhea

<1%:
- Central nervous system: Fatigue, chills
- Dermatologic: Maculopapular and erythematous rash
- Gastrointestinal: Dyspepsia, pseudomembranous colitis, nausea, vomiting, heartburn, gastritis, bloating
- Hematologic: Neutropenia
- Miscellaneous: Superinfections

Drug Interactions
Increased effect: High-dose probenecid decreases renal clearance of cephalosporins

Drug Uptake
Absorption: Oral: Rapid and well absorbed from GI tract
Serum half-life: 1-2 hours; 20-24 hours in renal failure
Time to peak serum concentration: Within 70-90 minutes

Pregnancy Risk Factor B

Breast-feeding Considerations Excreted into breast milk in small amounts like other cephalosporins

Dosage Forms
Capsule, as monohydrate: 500 mg
Suspension, oral, as monohydrate: 125 mg/5 mL, 250 mg/5 mL, 500 mg/5 mL (50 mL, 100 mL)
Tablet, as monohydrate: 1 g

Generic Available Yes

Selected Readings
"Advisory Statement. Antibiotic Prophylaxis for Dental Patients With Total Joint Replacements. American Dental Association; American Academy of Orthopedic Surgeons," *J Am Dent Assoc*, 1997, 128(7):1004-8.

Dajani AS, Taubert KA, Wilson W, et al, "Prevention of Bacterial Endocarditis Recommendations by the American Heart Association," *JAMA*, 1997, 277(22):1794-801.

Dajani AS, Taubert KA, Wilson W, et al, "Prevention of Bacterial Endocarditis: Recommendations by the American Heart Association," *J Am Dent Assoc*, 1997, 128(8):1142-51.

Donowitz GR and Mandell GL, "Beta-Lactam Antibiotics," *N Engl J Med*, 1988, 318(7):419-26 and 318(8):490-500.

Gustaferro CA and Steckelberg JM, "Cephalosporin Antimicrobial Agents and Related Compounds," *Mayo Clin Proc*, 1991, 66(10):1064-73.

Cefadyl® *see* Cephapirin *on page 203*

Cefalotina Sal Sodica De (Mexico) *see* Cephalothin *on page 202*

Cefamandole (sef a MAN dole)

Brand Names Mandol®

Therapeutic Category Antibiotic, Cephalosporin (Second Generation)

Use Treatment of susceptible bacterial infection; mainly respiratory tract, skin and skin structure, bone and joint, urinary tract and gynecologic, as well as, septicemia

Usual Dosage I.M., I.V.:
Children: 100-150 mg/kg/day in divided doses every 4-6 hours

Adults: 4-12 g/24 hours divided doses every 4-6 hours or 500-1000 mg every 4-8 hours; maximum: 2 g/dose

Mechanism of Action Inhibits bacterial cell wall synthesis by binding to one or more of the penicillin-binding proteins (PBPs) which in turn inhibits the final transpeptidation step of peptidoglycan synthesis in bacterial cell walls, thus inhibiting cell wall biosynthesis. Bacteria eventually lyse due to ongoing activity of cell wall autolytic enzymes (autolysins and murein hydrolases) while cell wall assembly is arrested.

Local Anesthetic/Vasoconstrictor Precautions No information available to require special precautions

Effects on Dental Treatment No effects or complications reported

Other Adverse Effects
1% to 10%: Gastrointestinal: Diarrhea
<1%:
- Central nervous system: CNS irritation, seizures, fever
- Dermatologic: Rash, urticaria
- Gastrointestinal: Abdominal cramps, pseudomembraneous colitis
- Hematologic: Eosinophilia, hypoprothrombinemia, leukopenia, thrombocytopenia
- Hepatic: Transient elevation of liver enzymes, cholestatic jaundice
- Local: Pain at injection site
- Miscellaneous: Superinfections

Drug Interactions
Disulfiram-like reaction has been reported when taken within 72 hours of alcohol consumption
Increased effect: High-dose probenecid decreases renal clearance of cephalosporins
(Continued)

Cefamandole *(Continued)*

Drug Uptake
Serum half-life: 30-60 minutes
Time to peak serum concentration:
I.M.: Within 1-2 hours
I.V.: Within 10 minutes
Pregnancy Risk Factor B
Generic Available No

Cefanex® *see* Cephalexin *on page 201*

Cefazolin (sef A zoe lin)

Related Information
Animal and Human Bites Guidelines *on page 1093*
Antimicrobial Prophylaxis in Surgical Patients *on page 1163*
Brand Names Ancef®; Kefzol®; Zolicef®
Canadian/Mexican Brand Names Cefamezin® (Mexico)
Therapeutic Category Antibiotic, Cephalosporin (First Generation)
Synonyms Cefazolina (Mexico)
Use
Dental: Alternative antibiotic for prevention of bacterial endocarditis when parenteral administration is needed. Individuals allergic to amoxicillin (penicillins)
may receive cefazolin provided they have not had an immediate, local, or
systemic IgE-mediated anaphylactic allergic reaction to penicillin. Alternate
antibiotic for premedication in patients not allergic to penicillin who may be at
potential increased risk of hematogenous total joint infection when parenteral
administration is needed.

Medical: Treatment of gram-positive bacilli and cocci (except enterococcus);
some gram-negative bacilli including *E. coli*, *Proteus*, and *Klebsiella* may be
susceptible

Usual Dosage I.M., I.V.:
Children >1 month: 50-100 mg/kg/day divided every 8 hours; maximum: 6 g/day
SBE prophylaxis: 25 mg/kg I.M. or I.V. within 30 minutes before procedure
Adults: 1-2 g every 8 hours, depending on severity of infection; maximum dose:
12 g/day
SBE prophylaxis: 1 g I.M. or I.V. within 30 minutes before procedure
Joint replacement prophylaxis: I.M., I.V.: 1 g one hour before procedure

Mechanism of Action
Inhibits bacterial cell wall synthesis by binding to one or
more of the penicillin-binding proteins (PBPs) which in turn inhibits the final
transpeptidation step of peptidoglycan synthesis in bacterial cell walls, thus inhibiting cell wall biosynthesis. Bacteria eventually lyse due to ongoing activity of cell
wall autolytic enzymes (autolysins and murein hydrolases) while cell wall
assembly is arrested.

Local Anesthetic/Vasoconstrictor Precautions
No information available to
require special precautions

Effects on Dental Treatment
No effects or complications reported

Other Adverse Effects
1% to 10%: Gastrointestinal: Diarrhea
<1%:
Central nervous system: CNS irritation, seizures, confusion, fever
Dermatologic: Rash, urticaria
Hematologic: Leukopenia, thrombocytopenia, neutropenia
Hepatic: Transient elevation of liver enzymes, cholestatic jaundice
Miscellaneous: Superinfections

Drug Interactions
Increased effect: High-dose probenecid decreases renal clearance of
cephalosporins

Drug Uptake
Serum half-life: 90-150 minutes (prolonged with renal impairment)
Time to peak serum concentration:
I.M.: Within 0.5-2 hours
I.V.: Within 5 minutes

Pregnancy Risk Factor B

Dosage Forms
Infusion, premixed, as sodium, in D_5W (frozen) (Ancef®): 500 mg (50 mL); 1 g (50
mL)
Injection, as sodium (Kefzol®): 500 mg, 1 g
Powder for injection, as sodium (Ancef®, Zolicef®): 250 mg, 500 mg, 1 g, 5 g, 10
g, 20 g

Generic Available Yes

Selected Readings

"Advisory Statement. Antibiotic Prophylaxis for Dental Patients With Total Joint Replacements. American Dental Association; American Academy of Orthopedic Surgeons," *J Am Dent Assoc*, 1997, 128(7):1004-8.

Dajani AS, Taubert KA, Wilson W, et al, "Prevention of Bacterial Endocarditis Recommendations by the American Heart Association," *JAMA*, 1997, 277(22):1794-801.

Dajani AS, Taubert KA, Wilson W, et al, "Prevention of Bacterial Endocarditis: Recommendations by the American Heart Association," *J Am Dent Assoc*, 1997, 128(8):1142-51.

Donowitz GR and Mandell GL, "Beta-Lactam Antibiotics," *N Engl J Med*, 1988, 318(7):419-26 and 318(8):490-500.

Gustaferro CA and Steckelberg JM, "Cephalosporin Antimicrobial Agents and Related Compounds," *Mayo Clin Proc*, 1991, 66(10):1064-73.

Cefazolina (Mexico) *see* Cefazolin *on previous page*

Cefepime (SEF e pim)

Brand Names Maxipime®

Therapeutic Category Antibiotic, Cephalosporin (Fourth Generation)

Use Treatment of respiratory tract infections (including bronchitis and pneumonia), cellulitis and other skin and soft tissue infections, and urinary tract infections; considered a fourth generation cephalosporin because it has good gram-negative coverage similar to third generation cephalosporins, but better gram-positive coverage

Usual Dosage I.V.:

Children: Unlabeled: 50 mg/kg every 8 hours; maximum dose: 2 g

Adults:

Most infections: 1-2 g every 12 hours for 5-10 days; higher doses or more frequent administration may be required in pseudomonal infections

Urinary tract infections, uncomplicated: 500 mg every 12 hours

Dosing adjustment in renal impairment:

Cl_{cr} 10-30 mL/minute: Administer 500 mg every 24 hours

Cl_{cr} <10 mL/minute: Administer 250 mg every 24 hours

Hemodialysis: Removed by dialysis; administer supplemental dose of 250 mg after each dialysis session

Peritoneal dialysis: Removed to a lesser extent than hemodialysis; administer 250 mg every 48 hours

Mechanism of Action Inhibits bacterial cell wall synthesis by binding to one or more of the penicillin-binding proteins (PBPs) which in turn inhibits the final transpeptidation step of peptidoglycan synthesis in bacterial cell walls, thus inhibiting cell wall biosynthesis. Bacterial eventually lyse due to ongoing activity of cell wall autolytic enzymes (autolysis and murein hydrolases) while cell wall assembly is arrested.

Local Anesthetic/Vasoconstrictor Precautions No information available to require special precautions

Effects on Dental Treatment No effects or complications reported

Warnings/Precautions Modify dosage in patients with severe renal impairment; prolonged use may result in superinfection; a low incidence of cross-hypersensitivity to penicillins exists

Drug Interactions

Increased effect: High-dose probenecid decreases clearance

Increased toxicity: Aminoglycosides increase nephrotoxic potential

Drug Uptake

Absorption: I.M.: Rapid and complete; T_{max}: 0.5-1.5 hours

Serum half-life: 2 hours

Pregnancy Risk Factor C

Generic Available No

Cefixima (Mexico) *see* Cefixime *on this page*

Cefixime (sef IKS eem)

Related Information

Nonviral Infectious Diseases *on page 1032*

Brand Names Suprax®

Canadian/Mexican Brand Names Denvar® (Mexico); Novacef® (Mexico)

Therapeutic Category Antibiotic, Cephalosporin (Third Generation)

Synonyms Cefixima (Mexico)

Use Treatment of urinary tract infections, otitis media, respiratory infections due to susceptible organisms including *S. pneumoniae* and *Pyogenes*, *H. influenzae* and many *Enterobacteriaceae*; documented poor compliance with other oral antimicrobials; outpatient therapy of serious soft tissue or skeletal infections due to susceptible organisms; single-dose oral treatment of uncomplicated cervical/urethral gonorrhea due to *N. gonorrhoeae*

Usual Dosage Oral:

Children: 8 mg/kg/day in 1-2 divided doses; maximum dose: 400 mg/day

(Continued)

Cefixime *(Continued)*

Children >50 kg or >12 years and Adults: 400 mg/day in 1-2 divided doses
Uncomplicated cervical/urethral gonorrhea due to *N. gonorrhoeae*: 400 mg as a single dose

Dosing adjustment in renal impairment:
Cl_{cr} 21-60 mL/minute: Administer 75% of the standard dose
Cl_{cr} ≤20 mL/minute: Administer 50% of the standard dose
Moderately dialyzable (10%)

Mechanism of Action Inhibits bacterial cell wall synthesis by binding to one or more of the penicillin-binding proteins (PBPs) which in turn inhibits the final transpeptidation step of peptidoglycan synthesis in bacterial cell walls, thus inhibiting cell wall biosynthesis. Bacteria eventually lyse due to ongoing activity of cell wall autolytic enzymes (autolysins and murein hydrolases) while cell wall assembly is arrested.

Local Anesthetic/Vasoconstrictor Precautions No information available to require special precautions

Effects on Dental Treatment No effects or complications reported

Other Adverse Effects

1% to 10%: Gastrointestinal: Diarrhea (up to 15% of children), abdominal pain, nausea, dyspepsia, flatulence, pseudomembranous colitis

<1%:
Central nervous system: Headache, dizziness, fever
Dermatologic: Rash, urticaria, pruritus
Genitourinary: Vaginitis
Hematologic: Thrombocytopenia, leukopenia, eosinophilia
Hepatic: Transient elevation of LFTs
Renal: Transient elevation of BUN or creatinine

Drug Interactions
Increased effect: High-dose probenecid decreases renal clearance of cephalosporins

Pregnancy Risk Factor B

Generic Available No

Cefizox® *see* Ceftizoxime *on page 197*

Cefmetazole *(sef MET a zole)*

Brand Names Zefazone®

Therapeutic Category Antibiotic, Cephalosporin (Second Generation)

Use Second generation cephalosporin with an antibacterial spectrum similar to cefoxitin, useful on many aerobic and anaerobic gram-positive and gram-negative bacteria

Usual Dosage Adults: I.V.:
Infections: 2 g every 6-12 hours for 5-14 days

Prophylaxis: 2 g 30-90 minutes before surgery **or** 1 g 30-90 minutes before surgery; repeat 8 and 16 hours later

Mechanism of Action Inhibits bacterial cell wall synthesis by binding to one or more of the penicillin-binding proteins (PBPs) which in turn inhibits the final transpeptidation step of peptidoglycan synthesis in bacterial cell walls, thus inhibiting cell wall biosynthesis. Bacteria eventually lyse due to ongoing activity of cell wall autolytic enzymes (autolysins and murein hydrolases) while cell wall assembly is arrested.

Local Anesthetic/Vasoconstrictor Precautions No information available to require special precautions

Effects on Dental Treatment No effects or complications reported

Other Adverse Effects
1% to 10%:
Dermatologic: Rash
Gastrointestinal: Diarrhea, nausea
<1%:
Cardiovascular: Shock, hypotension
Central nervous system: Headache, fever
Endocrine & metabolic: Hot flashes
Gastrointestinal: Epigastric pain, pseudomembraneous colitis
Genitourinary: Vaginitis
Hematologic: Bleeding
Local: Pain at injection site, phlebitis
Respiratory: Respiratory distress, dyspnea, epistaxis
Miscellaneous: Alteration of color, candidiasis

Drug Interactions
Increased effect: High-dose probenecid decreases renal clearance of cephalosporins

Drug Uptake
Serum half-life: 72 minutes
Pregnancy Risk Factor B
Generic Available No

Cefobid® *see* Cefoperazone *on this page*

Cefol® Filmtab® *see* Vitamins, Multiple *on page 995*

Cefonicid (se FON i sid)
Brand Names Monocid®
Canadian/Mexican Brand Names Monocidur® (Mexico)
Therapeutic Category Antibiotic, Cephalosporin (Second Generation)
Synonyms Cefonicidid (Mexico)
Use Treatment of susceptible bacterial infection; mainly respiratory tract, skin and skin structure, bone and joint, urinary tract and gynecologic, as well as, septicemia; second generation cephalosporin
Usual Dosage Adults: I.M., I.V.: 0.5-2 g every 24 hours
Prophylaxis: Preop: 1 g/hour
Mechanism of Action Inhibits bacterial cell wall synthesis by binding to one or more of the penicillin-binding proteins (PBPs) which in turn inhibits the final transpeptidation step of peptidoglycan synthesis in bacterial cell walls, thus inhibiting cell wall biosynthesis. Bacteria eventually lyse due to ongoing activity of cell wall autolytic enzymes (autolysins and murein hydrolases) while cell wall assembly is arrested.
Local Anesthetic/Vasoconstrictor Precautions No information available to require special precautions
Effects on Dental Treatment No effects or complications reported
Other Adverse Effects
1% to 10%:
Hematologic: Elevated platelets and eosinophils
Hepatic: Liver function alterations
Local: Pain at injection site
<1%:
Central nervous system: Fever, headache
Dermatologic: Skin rash
Gastrointestinal: Nausea, diarrhea, abdominal pain, pseudomembranous colitis
Hepatic: Transient elevations in liver enzymes
Renal: Transient elevations in BUN or creatinine
Drug Interactions
Increased effect: High-dose probenecid decreases renal clearance of cephalosporins
Drug Uptake
Serum half-life: 6-7 hours
Pregnancy Risk Factor B
Generic Available No

Cefonicidid (Mexico) *see* Cefonicid *on this page*

Cefoperazona (Mexico) *see* Cefoperazone *on this page*

Cefoperazone (sef oh PER a zone)
Brand Names Cefobid®
Therapeutic Category Antibiotic, Cephalosporin (Third Generation)
Synonyms Cefoperazona (Mexico)
Use Treatment of susceptible bacterial infection; mainly respiratory tract, skin and skin structure, bone and joint, urinary tract and gynecologic, as well as, septicemia
Usual Dosage I.M., I.V.:
Children: 100-150 mg/kg/day divided every 8-12 hours; up to 12 g/day
Adults: 2-4 g/day in divided doses every 12 hours; up to 12 g/day
Mechanism of Action Inhibits bacterial cell wall synthesis by binding to one or more of the penicillin-binding proteins (PBPs) which in turn inhibits the final transpeptidation step of peptidoglycan synthesis in bacterial cell walls, thus inhibiting cell wall biosynthesis. Bacteria eventually lyse due to ongoing activity of cell wall autolytic enzymes (autolysins and murein hydrolases) while cell wall assembly is arrested.
Local Anesthetic/Vasoconstrictor Precautions No information available to require special precautions
Effects on Dental Treatment No effects or complications reported
Other Adverse Effects
1% to 10%: Gastrointestinal: Diarrhea
(Continued)

Cefoperazone *(Continued)*

<1%:
Dermatologic: Maculopapular and erythematous rash
Gastrointestinal: Dyspepsia, pseudomembranous colitis, nausea, vomiting
Hematologic: Bleeding
Local: Pain and induration at injection site

Drug Interactions
Increased effect: High-dose probenecid decreases renal clearance of cephalosporins

Drug Uptake
Serum half-life: 2 hours, higher with hepatic disease or biliary obstruction
Time to peak serum concentration:
I.M.: Within 1-2 hours
I.V.: Within 15-20 minutes (serum levels 2-3 times the serum levels following I.M. administration)

Pregnancy Risk Factor B
Generic Available No

Cefotan® *see Cefotetan on next page*
Cefotaxima (Mexico) *see Cefotaxime on this page*

Cefotaxime *(sef oh TAKS eem)*

Brand Names Claforan®
Canadian/Mexican Brand Names Alfotax® (Mexico); Benaxima® (Mexico); Biosint® (Mexico); Cefaxim® (Mexico); Cefoclin® (Mexico); Fotexina® (Mexico); Taporin® (Mexico); Viken® (Mexico)
Therapeutic Category Antibiotic, Cephalosporin (Third Generation)
Synonyms Cefotaxima (Mexico)
Use Treatment of susceptible infection in respiratory tract, skin and skin structure, bone and joint, urinary tract, gynecologic as well as septicemia, and documented or suspected meningitis
Usual Dosage I.M., I.V.:
Children 1 month to 12 years:
<50 kg: 100-150 mg/kg/day in divided doses every 6-8 hours
Meningitis: 200 mg/kg/day in divided doses every 6 hours
>50 kg: Moderate to severe infection: 1-2 g every 6-8 hours; life-threatening infection: 2 g/dose every 4 hours; maximum dose: 12 g/day

Children >12 years and Adults: 1-2 g every 6-8 hours (up to 12 g/day)

Mechanism of Action Inhibits bacterial cell wall synthesis by binding to one or more of the penicillin-binding proteins (PBPs) which in turn inhibits the final transpeptidation step of peptidoglycan synthesis in bacterial cell walls, thus inhibiting cell wall biosynthesis. Bacteria eventually lyse due to ongoing activity of cell wall autolytic enzymes (autolysins and murein hydrolases) while cell wall assembly is arrested.

Local Anesthetic/Vasoconstrictor Precautions No information available to require special precautions
Effects on Dental Treatment No effects or complications reported
Other Adverse Effects
1% to 10%:
Central nervous system: Fever
Dermatologic: Rash, pruritus
Gastrointestinal: Colitis, diarrhea, nausea, vomiting
Hematologic: Eosinophilia
Local: Pain at injection site
<1%:
Central nervous system: Headache
Gastrointestinal: Pseudomembranous colitis
Hematologic: Transient neutropenia, thrombocytopenia
Hepatic: Transient elevation of liver enzymes
Local: Phlebitis
Renal: Transient elevation of BUN and creatinine

Drug Interactions
Increased effect: High-dose probenecid decreases renal clearance of cephalosporins

Drug Uptake
Serum half-life:
Cefotaxime:
Adults: 1-1.5 hours (prolonged with renal and/or hepatic impairment)
Desacetylcefotaxime: 1.5-1.9 hours (prolonged with renal impairment)
Time to peak serum concentration: I.M.: Within 30 minutes

Pregnancy Risk Factor B

Generic Available No

Cefotetan (SEF oh tee tan)
Related Information
Animal and Human Bites Guidelines *on page 1093*
Antimicrobial Prophylaxis in Surgical Patients *on page 1163*
Brand Names Cefotan®
Therapeutic Category Antibiotic, Cephalosporin (Second Generation)
Use Treatment of susceptible bacterial infection; mainly respiratory tract, skin and skin structure, bone and joint, urinary tract and gynecologic, as well as, septicemia, similar spectrum to cefoxitin
Usual Dosage I.M., I.V.:
Children: 20-40 mg/kg/dose every 12 hours

Adults: 1-6 g/day in divided doses every 12 hours, 1-2 g may be given every 24 hours for urinary tract infection
Mechanism of Action Inhibits bacterial cell wall synthesis by binding to one or more of the penicillin-binding proteins (PBPs) which in turn inhibits the final transpeptidation step of peptidoglycan synthesis in bacterial cell walls, thus inhibiting cell wall biosynthesis. Bacteria eventually lyse due to ongoing activity of cell wall autolytic enzymes (autolysins and murein hydrolases) while cell wall assembly is arrested.
Local Anesthetic/Vasoconstrictor Precautions No information available to require special precautions
Effects on Dental Treatment No effects or complications reported
Other Adverse Effects
1% to 10%:
Gastrointestinal: Diarrhea
Hepatic: Hepatic enzyme elevation
Miscellaneous: Hypersensitivity reactions
<1%:
Central nervous system: Fever
Dermatologic: Rash, pruritus
Gastrointestinal: Nausea, vomiting, antibiotic-associated colitis
Hematologic: Prolongation of bleeding time or prothrombin time, neutropenia, thrombocytopenia
Local: Phlebitis
Drug Interactions
Increased effect: High-dose probenecid decreases renal clearance of cephalosporins
Drug Uptake
Serum half-life: 1.5-3 hours
Time to peak serum concentration: I.M.: Within 1.5-3 hours
Pregnancy Risk Factor B
Generic Available No

Cefoxitin (se FOKS i tin)
Related Information
Antimicrobial Prophylaxis in Surgical Patients *on page 1163*
Brand Names Mefoxin®
Therapeutic Category Antibiotic, Cephalosporin (Second Generation)
Use Less active against staphylococci and streptococci than first generation cephalosporins, but active against anaerobes including *Bacteroides fragilis*; active against gram-negative enteric bacilli including *E. coli*, *Klebsiella*, and *Proteus*; used predominantly for respiratory tract, skin and skin structure, bone and joint, urinary tract and gynecologic as well as septicemia; surgical prophylaxis; intra-abdominal infections and other mixed infections
Usual Dosage I.M., I.V.:
Children >3 months:
Mild-moderate infection: 80-100 mg/kg/day in divided doses every 4-6 hours
Severe infection: 100-160 mg/kg/day in divided doses every 4-6 hours
Maximum dose: 12 g/day

Adults: 1-2 g every 6-8 hours (I.M. injection is painful); up to 12 g/day
Mechanism of Action Inhibits bacterial cell wall synthesis by binding to one or more of the penicillin-binding proteins (PBPs) which in turn inhibits the final transpeptidation step of peptidoglycan synthesis in bacterial cell walls, thus inhibiting cell wall biosynthesis. Bacteria eventually lyse due to ongoing activity of cell wall autolytic enzymes (autolysins and murein hydrolases) while cell wall assembly is arrested.
Local Anesthetic/Vasoconstrictor Precautions No information available to require special precautions
Effects on Dental Treatment No effects or complications reported
(Continued)

Cefoxitin *(Continued)*

Other Adverse Effects
1% to 10%: Gastrointestinal: Diarrhea

<1%:
Cardiovascular: Hypotension
Central nervous system: Fever
Dermatologic: Rash, exfoliative dermatitis
Gastrointestinal: Nausea, vomiting, pseudomembranous colitis
Hematologic: Transient leukopenia, thrombocytopenia, anemia, eosinophilia
Hepatic: Elevation in serum AST concentration
Local: Thrombophlebitis
Renal: Elevations in serum creatinine and/or BUN
Respiratory: Dyspnea

Drug Interactions
Increased effect: High-dose probenecid decreases renal clearance of cephalosporins

Drug Uptake
Serum half-life: 45-60 minutes, increases significantly with renal insufficiency
Time to peak serum concentration:
I.M.: Within 20-30 minutes
I.V.: Within 5 minutes

Pregnancy Risk Factor B
Generic Available No

Cefpodoxime (sef pode OKS eem)

Brand Names Vantin®
Therapeutic Category Antibiotic, Cephalosporin (Second Generation)
Use Treatment of susceptible acute, community-acquired pneumonia caused by *S. pneumoniae* or nonbeta-lactamase producing *H. influenzae*; acute uncomplicated gonorrhea caused by *N. gonorrhoeae*; uncomplicated skin and skin structure infections caused by *S. aureus* or *S. pyogenes*; acute otitis media caused by *S. pneumoniae*, *H. influenzae*, or *M. catarrhalis*; pharyngitis or tonsillitis; and uncomplicated urinary tract infections caused by *E. coli*, *Klebsiella*, and *Proteus*

Usual Dosage Oral:
Children >5 months to 12 years:
Acute otitis media: 10 mg/kg/day as a single dose or divided every 12 hours (400 mg/day)
Pharyngitis/tonsillitis: 10 mg/kg/day in 2 divided doses (maximum: 200 mg/day)
Children ≥13 years and Adults:
Acute community-acquired pneumonia and bacterial exacerbations of chronic bronchitis: 200 mg every 12 hours for 14 days and 10 days, respectively
Skin and skin structure: 400 mg every 12 hours for 7-14 days
Uncomplicated gonorrhea (male and female) and rectal gonococcal infections (female): 200 mg as a single dose
Pharyngitis/tonsillitis: 100 mg every 12 hours for 10 days
Uncomplicated urinary tract infection: 100 mg every 12 hours for 7 days

Mechanism of Action Inhibits bacterial cell wall synthesis by binding to one or more of the penicillin-binding proteins (PBPs) which in turn inhibits the final transpeptidation step of peptidoglycan synthesis in bacterial cell walls, thus inhibiting cell wall biosynthesis. Bacteria eventually lyse due to ongoing activity of cell wall autolytic enzymes (autolysins and murein hydrolases) while cell wall assembly is arrested.

Local Anesthetic/Vasoconstrictor Precautions No information available to require special precautions
Effects on Dental Treatment No effects or complications reported
Other Adverse Effects
1% to 10%: Gastrointestinal: Diarrhea

<1%:
Central nervous system: Headache
Dermatologic: Diaper rash
Gastrointestinal: Nausea, vomiting, abdominal pain, pseudomembranous colitis
Genitourinary: Vaginal fungal infections

Drug Interactions
Decreased effect: Antacids and H₂-receptor antagonists (reduce absorption and serum concentration of cefpodoxime)
Increased effect: Probenecid may decrease cephalosporin elimination

Drug Uptake
Absorption: Oral: Rapidly and well absorbed (50%), acid stable; enhanced in the presence of food or low gastric pH
Serum half-life: 2.2 hours (prolonged with renal impairment)

Pregnancy Risk Factor B

Dosage Forms

Granules for oral suspension, as proxetil (lemon creme flavor): 50 mg/5 mL (100 mL); 100 mg/5 mL (100 mL)

Tablet, film coated, as proxetil: 100 mg, 200 mg

Dietary Considerations May be taken with food, however, there is delayed absorption

Generic Available No

Cefprozil (sef PROE zil)

Brand Names Cefzil®

Therapeutic Category Antibiotic, Cephalosporin (Second Generation)

Use Infections causes by susceptible organisms including *S. pneumoniae, S. aureus, S. pyogenes*; treatment of otitis media and infections involving the respiratory tract and skin and skin structure

Usual Dosage Oral:

Children >6 months to 12 years: 7.5-15 mg/kg every 12 hours for 10 days

Pharyngitis/tonsillitis:

Children 2-12 years: 15 mg/kg/day divided every 12 hours; maximum: 1 g/day

Children >13 years and Adults: 250-500 mg every 12-24 hours for 10-14 days

Mechanism of Action Inhibits bacterial cell wall synthesis by binding to one or more of the penicillin-binding proteins (PBPs) which in turn inhibits the final transpeptidation step of peptidoglycan synthesis in bacterial cell walls, thus inhibiting cell wall biosynthesis. Bacteria eventually lyse due to ongoing activity of cell wall autolytic enzymes (autolysins and murein hydrolases) while cell wall assembly is arrested.

Local Anesthetic/Vasoconstrictor Precautions No information available to require special precautions

Effects on Dental Treatment No effects or complications reported

Other Adverse Effects

1% to 10%:

Central nervous system: Dizziness

Dermatologic: Diaper rash, genital pruritus

Gastrointestinal: Diarrhea, nausea, vomiting, abdominal pain

Genitourinary: Vaginitis

Hematologic: Eosinophilia

Hepatic: Elevation of AST and ALT, elevation of alkaline phosphatase

Miscellaneous: Superinfection

<1%:

Central nervous system: Headache, insomnia, confusion

Dermatologic: Rash, urticaria

Hematologic: Prolonged PT

Hepatic: Cholestatic jaundice

Neuromuscular & skeletal: Arthralgia

Renal: Elevated BUN and serum creatinine

Drug Interactions

Increased effect: Probenecid may decrease cephalosporin elimination

Drug Uptake

Absorption: Oral: Well absorbed (94%)

Serum half-life, elimination: 1.3 hours (normal renal function)

Peak serum levels: 1.5 hours (fasting state)

Pregnancy Risk Factor B

Dosage Forms

Powder for oral suspension, as anhydrous: 125 mg/5 mL (50 mL, 75 mL, 100 mL); 250 mg/5 mL (50 mL, 75 mL, 100 mL)

Tablet, as anhydrous: 250 mg, 500 mg

Dietary Considerations May be taken with food, however, there is delayed absorption

Generic Available No

Cefradina (Mexico) *see* Cephradine *on page 203*

Ceftazidima (Mexico) *see* Ceftazidime *on this page*

Ceftazidime (SEF tay zi deem)

Brand Names Ceptaz™; Fortaz®; Tazicef®; Tazidime®

Canadian/Mexican Brand Names Ceftazim® (Mexico); Ceptaz™ (Canada); Fortum® (Mexico); Tagal® (Mexico); Taloken® (Mexico); Waytrax® (Mexico)

Therapeutic Category Antibiotic, Cephalosporin (Third Generation)

Synonyms Ceftazidima (Mexico)

Use Treatment of documented susceptible *Pseudomonas aeruginosa* infection; *Pseudomonas* infection in patients at risk of developing aminoglycoside-induced

(Continued)

Ceftazidime *(Continued)*

nephrotoxicity and/or ototoxicity; empiric therapy of febrile, granulocytopenic patients

Usual Dosage I.M., I.V.:

Children 1 month to 12 years: 30-50 mg/kg/dose every 8 hours; maximum dose: 6 g/day

Adults: 1-2 g every 8-12 hours

Urinary tract infections: 250-500 mg every 12 hours

Mechanism of Action Inhibits bacterial cell wall synthesis by binding to one or more of the penicillin-binding proteins (PBPs) which in turn inhibits the final transpeptidation step of peptidoglycan synthesis in bacterial cell walls, thus inhibiting cell wall biosynthesis. Bacteria eventually lyse due to ongoing activity of cell wall autolytic enzymes (autolysins and murein hydrolases) while cell wall assembly is arrested.

Local Anesthetic/Vasoconstrictor Precautions No information available to require special precautions

Effects on Dental Treatment No effects or complications reported

Other Adverse Effects

1% to 10%:

Gastrointestinal: Diarrhea

Local: Pain at injection site

<1%:

Central nervous system: Fever, headache, dizziness

Dermatologic: Rash, angioedema

Gastrointestinal: Nausea, vomiting, pseudomembranous colitis

Hematologic: Eosinophilia, thrombocytosis, transient leukopenia, hemolytic anemia

Hepatic: Transient elevation in liver enzymes

Local: Phlebitis

Neuromuscular & skeletal: Paresthesia

Renal: Transient elevation in BUN and creatinine

Miscellaneous: Candidiasis

Drug Interactions

Increased effect: High-dose probenecid decreases renal clearance of cephalosporins

Drug Uptake

Serum half-life: 1-2 hours (prolonged with renal impairment)

Time to peak serum concentration: I.M.: Within 1 hour

Pregnancy Risk Factor B

Generic Available No

Ceftibuten *(sef TYE byoo ten)*

Brand Names Cedax®

Therapeutic Category Antibiotic, Cephalosporin (Third Generation)

Use Oral cephalosporin for bronchitis, otitis media, and strep throat

Usual Dosage Oral:

Children <12 years: 9 mg/kg/day for 10 days; maximum daily dose: 400 mg

Children ≥12 years and Adults: 400 mg once daily for 10 days; maximum: 400 mg

Mechanism of Action Inhibits bacterial cell wall synthesis by binding to one or more of the penicillin-binding proteins (PBPs) which in turn inhibits the final transpeptidation step of peptidoglycan synthesis in bacterial cell walls, thus inhibiting cell wall biosynthesis. Bacteria eventually lyse due to ongoing activity of cell wall autolytic enzymes (autolysins and murein hydrolases) while cell wall assembly is arrested.

Local Anesthetic/Vasoconstrictor Precautions No information available to require special precautions

Effects on Dental Treatment No effects or complications reported

Other Adverse Effects

1% to 10%: Gastrointestinal: Diarrhea

<1%:

Central nervous system: Dizziness, fatigue, headache

Dermatologic: Rash

Gastrointestinal: Nausea, vomiting, pseudomembranous colitis

Hematologic: Transient neutropenia, anemia

Hepatic: Transient elevation in LFTs

Contraindications Hypersensitivity to ceftibuten, any component, or cephalosporins

Warnings/Precautions Modify dosage in patients with severe renal impairment, prolonged use may result in superinfection; a low incidence of cross-hypersensitivity to penicillins exist

Drug Interactions
Increased effect: High-dose probenecid decreases clearance
Increased toxicity: Aminoglycosides increase nephrotoxic potential
Drug Uptake
Absorption: Rapid; food decreases peak concentrations
Serum half-life: 2 hours
Time to peak serum concentration: Within 2-3 hours
Pregnancy Risk Factor B
Dosage Forms
Capsule: 400 mg
Powder for oral suspension (cherry flavor): 90 mg/5 mL (30 mL, 60 mL, 120 mL); 180 mg/5 mL (30 mL, 60 mL, 120 mL)
Dietary Considerations Take without regard to food
Generic Available No
Comments In clinical trials, ceftibuten once or twice daily was at least as effective as cefaclor or ciprofloxacin for treatment of acute bacterial exacerbations of bronchitis, as effective as amoxicillin/clavulanic acid or cefaclor for otitis media, as effective as penicillin for pharyngitis, and as effective as trimethoprim-sulfamethoxazole for urinary tract infections

Ceftin® see Cefuroxime *on page 199*

Ceftizoxima (Mexico) see Ceftizoxime *on this page*

Ceftizoxime (sef ti ZOKS eem)
Brand Names Cefizox®
Canadian/Mexican Brand Names Ultracef® (Mexico)
Therapeutic Category Antibiotic, Cephalosporin (Third Generation)
Synonyms Ceftizoxima (Mexico)
Use Treatment of susceptible nonpseudomonal gram-negative rod infections or mixed gram-negative and anaerobic infections; predominantly respiratory tract, skin and skin structure, bone and joint, urinary tract and gynecologic, as well as septicemia
Usual Dosage I.M., I.V.:
Children ≥6 months: 150-200 mg/kg/day divided every 6-8 hours (maximum of 12 g/24 hours)
Adults: 1-2 g every 8-12 hours, up to 2 g every 4 hours or 4 g every 8 hours for life-threatening infections
Mechanism of Action Inhibits bacterial cell wall synthesis by binding to one or more of the penicillin-binding proteins (PBPs) which in turn inhibits the final transpeptidation step of peptidoglycan synthesis in bacterial cell walls, thus inhibiting cell wall biosynthesis. Bacteria eventually lyse due to ongoing activity of cell wall autolytic enzymes (autolysins and murein hydrolases) while cell wall assembly is arrested.
Local Anesthetic/Vasoconstrictor Precautions No information available to require special precautions
Effects on Dental Treatment No effects or complications reported
Other Adverse Effects
1% to 10%:
Central nervous system: Fever
Dermatologic: Rash, pruritus
Hematologic: Eosinophilia, thrombocytosis
Hepatic: Transient elevation of AST, ALT, and alkaline phosphatase
Local: Pain, burning at injection site
<1%:
Genitourinary: Vaginitis
Hematologic: Anemia, leukopenia, neutropenia, thrombocytopenia
Hepatic: Elevation of bilirubin
Neuromuscular & skeletal: Numbness
Renal: Transient elevations of BUN and creatinine
Drug Interactions
Increased effect: High-dose probenecid decreases renal clearance of cephalosporins
Drug Uptake
Serum half-life: 1.6 hours, increases to 25 hours when Cl$_{cr}$ falls to <10 mL/minute
Time to peak serum concentration: I.M.: Within 0.5-1 hour
Pregnancy Risk Factor B
Generic Available No

Ceftriaxona (Mexico) see Ceftriaxone *on this page*

Ceftriaxone (sef trye AKS one)
Related Information
Animal and Human Bites Guidelines *on page 1093*
(Continued)

Ceftriaxone *(Continued)*

Nonviral Infectious Diseases *on page 1032*

Brand Names Rocephin®

Canadian/Mexican Brand Names Benaxona® (Mexico); Cefaxona® (Mexico); Tacex® (Mexico); Triaken® (Mexico)

Therapeutic Category Antibiotic, Cephalosporin (Third Generation)

Synonyms Ceftriaxona (Mexico)

Use Treatment of lower respiratory tract infections, skin and skin structure infections, bone and joint infections, intra-abdominal and urinary tract infections, sepsis and meningitis due to susceptible organisms; documented or suspected infection due to susceptible organisms in home care patients and patients without I.V. line access; treatment of documented or suspected gonococcal infection or chancroid; emergency room management of patients at high risk for bacteremia, periorbital or buccal cellulitis, salmonellosis or shigellosis, and pneumonia of unestablished etiology (<5 years of age)

Usual Dosage I.M., I.V.:

Children: 50-75 mg/kg/day in 1-2 divided doses every 12-24 hours; maximum: 2 g/24 hours

Meningitis: 100 mg/kg/day divided every 12-24 hours, up to a maximum of 4 g/24 hours; loading dose of 75 mg/kg/dose may be given at start of therapy

Uncomplicated gonococcal infections, sexual assault, and STD prophylaxis: I.M.: 125 mg as a single dose

Complicated gonococcal infections:

<45 kg: 50 mg/kg/day once daily; maximum: 1 g/day; for ophthalmia, peritonitis, arthritis, or bacteremia: 50-100 mg/kg/day divided every 12-24 hours; maximum: 2 g/day for meningitis or endocarditis

>45 kg: 1 g/day once daily for disseminated gonococcal infections; 1-2 g dose every 12 hours for meningitis or endocarditis

Acute epididymitis: I.M.: 250 mg in a single dose

Adults: 1-2 g every 12-24 hours (depending on the type and severity of infection); maximum dose: 2 g every 12 hours for treatment of meningitis

Uncomplicated gonorrhea: I.M.: 250 mg as a single dose

Mechanism of Action Inhibits bacterial cell wall synthesis by binding to one or more of the penicillin-binding proteins (PBPs) which in turn inhibits the final transpeptidation step of peptidoglycan synthesis in bacterial cell walls, thus inhibiting cell wall biosynthesis. Bacteria eventually lyse due to ongoing activity of cell wall autolytic enzymes (autolysins and murein hydrolases) while cell wall assembly is arrested.

Local Anesthetic/Vasoconstrictor Precautions No information available to require special precautions

Effects on Dental Treatment No effects or complications reported

Other Adverse Effects

1% to 10%:
Dermatologic: Rash
Gastrointestinal: Diarrhea
Hematologic: Eosinophilia, thrombocytosis, leukopenia
Hepatic: Elevations of SGOT [AST], SGPT [ALT]
Local: Pain at injection site
Renal: Elevations of BUN

<1%:
Cardiovascular: Flushing
Central nervous system: Fever, chills, headache, dizziness
Dermatologic: Pruritus
Gastrointestinal: Nausea, vomiting, dysgeusia
Genitourinary: Presence of casts in urine, vaginitis
Hematologic: Anemia, hemolytic anemia, neutropenia, lymphopenia, thrombocytopenia
Hepatic: Elevations of alkaline phosphatase and bilirubin
Local: Phlebitis
Renal: Elevation of creatinine
Miscellaneous: Moniliasis, sweating

Drug Interactions

Increased effect: High-dose probenecid decreases renal clearance of cephalosporins

Drug Uptake

Serum half-life: Normal renal and hepatic function: 5-9 hours
Time to peak serum concentration:
I.M.: Within 1-2 hours
I.V.: Within minutes

Pregnancy Risk Factor B

Generic Available No

Cefuroxima (Mexico) *see* Cefuroxime *on this page*

Cefuroxime (se fyoor OKS eem)
Brand Names Ceftin®; Kefurox®; Zinacef®
Canadian/Mexican Brand Names Froxal® (Mexico); Zinnat® (Mexico)
Therapeutic Category Antibiotic, Cephalosporin (Second Generation)
Synonyms Cefuroxima (Mexico)
Use Treatment of infections caused by staphylococci, group B streptococci, *H. influenzae* (type A and B), *E. coli*, *Enterobacter*, *Salmonella*, and *Klebsiella*; treatment of susceptible infections of the lower respiratory tract, otitis media, urinary tract, skin and soft tissue, bone and joint, sepsis and gonorrhea
Usual Dosage
Children:
Pharyngitis, tonsillitis: Oral:
Suspension: 20 mg/kg/day (maximum: 500 mg/day) in 2 divided doses
Tablet: 125 mg every 12 hours
Acute otitis media, impetigo: Oral:
Suspension: 30 mg/kg/day (maximum: 1 g/day) in 2 divided doses
Tablet: 250 mg every 12 hours
I.M., I.V.: 75-150 mg/kg/day divided every 8 hours; maximum dose: 6 g/day
Meningitis: Not recommended (doses of 200-240 mg/kg/day divided every 6-8 hours have been used); maximum dose: 9 g/day
Adults:
Oral: 250-500 mg twice daily; uncomplicated urinary tract infection: 125-250 mg every 12 hours
I.M., I.V.: 750 mg to 1.5 g/dose every 8 hours or 100-150 mg/kg/day in divided doses every 6-8 hours; maximum: 6 g/24 hours
Mechanism of Action Inhibits bacterial cell wall synthesis by binding to one or more of the penicillin-binding proteins (PBPs) which in turn inhibits the final transpeptidation step of peptidoglycan synthesis in bacterial cell walls, thus inhibiting cell wall biosynthesis. Bacteria eventually lyse due to ongoing activity of cell wall autolytic enzymes (autolysins and murein hydrolases) while cell wall assembly is arrested.
Local Anesthetic/Vasoconstrictor Precautions No information available to require special precautions
Effects on Dental Treatment No effects or complications reported
Other Adverse Effects
1% to 10%:
Hematologic: Decreased hemoglobin and hematocrit, eosinophilia
Hepatic: Transient rise in SGOT [AST], SGPT [ALT], and alkaline phosphatase
Local: Thrombophlebitis
<1%:
Central nervous system: Dizziness, fever, headache
Dermatologic: Rash
Gastrointestinal: Nausea, vomiting, diarrhea, stomach cramps, colitis, GI bleeding
Genitourinary: Vaginitis
Hematologic: Transient neutropenia and leukopenia
Hepatic: Transient increase in liver enzymes
Local: Pain at the injection site
Renal: Elevated creatinine and/or BUN
Drug Interactions
Increased effect: High-dose probenecid decreases clearance of cefuroxime
Drug Uptake
Absorption: Increased when given with or shortly after food or infant formula
Serum half-life:
Adults: 1-2 hours (prolonged in renal impairment)
I.M.: Within 15-60 minutes
I.V.: 2-3 minutes
Pregnancy Risk Factor B
Dosage Forms
Infusion, as sodium, premixed (frozen) (Zinacef®): 750 mg (50 mL); 1.5 g (50 mL)
Powder for injection, as sodium: 750 mg, 1.5 g, 7.5 g
Powder for injection, as sodium (Kefurox®, Zinacef®): 750 mg, 1.5 g, 7.5 g
Powder for oral suspension, as axetil (tutti-frutti flavor) (Ceftin®): 125 mg/5 mL (50 mL, 100 mL, 200 mL)
Tablet, as axetil (Ceftin®): 125 mg, 250 mg, 500 mg
Dietary Considerations May be taken with food, however, bioavailability is increased with food
Generic Available Yes

Cefzil® *see* Cefprozil *on page 195*

Celestone® *see* Betamethasone *on page 126*
Celestone® Soluspan® *see* Betamethasone *on page 126*
CellCept® *see* Mycophenolate *on page 653*
Cellufresh® [OTC] *see* Carboxymethylcellulose *on page 179*

Cellulose, Oxidized (SEL yoo lose, OKS i dyzed)

Brand Names Oxycel®; Surgicel®
Therapeutic Category Hemostatic Agent
Use Temporary packing for the control of capillary, venous, or small arterial hemorrhage
Usual Dosage Minimal amounts of an appropriate size are laid on the bleeding site
Local Anesthetic/Vasoconstrictor Precautions No information available to require special precautions
Effects on Dental Treatment No effects or complications reported
Other Adverse Effects
1% to 10%:
Central nervous system: Headache
Respiratory: Nasal burning or stinging, sneezing (rhinological procedures)
Miscellaneous: Encapsulation of fluid, foreign body reactions (with or without) infection
Contraindications Do not apply as packing or wadding as a hemostatic agents; do not use for packing or implantation in fractures or laminectomies; do not use to control hemorrhage from large arteries or on nonhemorrhagic serous oozing surfaces
Warnings/Precautions By swelling, oxidized cellulose may cause nerve damage by pressure in bony confine (ie, optic nerve and chiasm); always remove from these sites of application or do not use at all (see contraindications); do not autoclave, do not moisten with water or saline (lessens hemostatic effect). Avoid wadding or packing tightly; do not use after application of AgNO$_3$ or other escharotic agents.
Drug Interactions No data reported
Pregnancy Risk Factor No data reported
Breast-feeding Considerations No data reported
Dosage Forms
Pad (Oxycel®): 3" x 3", 8 ply
Pledget (Oxycel®): 2" x 1" x 1"
Strip:
Oxycel®:
18" x 2", 4 ply
5" x $\frac{1}{2}$", 4 ply
36" x $\frac{1}{2}$", 4 ply
Surgicel®:
2" x 14"
4" x 8"
2" x 3"
$\frac{1}{2}$" x 2"
Dietary Considerations No data reported
Generic Available No

Cellulose, Oxidized Regenerated

(SEL yoo lose, OKS i dyzed re JEN er ay ted)
Brand Names Surgicel® Absorbable Hemostat
Therapeutic Category Hemostatic Agent
Use
Dental: To control bleeding created during dental surgery
Medical: Hemostatic
Usual Dosage Minimal amounts of the fabric strip are laid on the bleeding site or held firmly against the tissues until hemostasis occurs
Mechanism of Action Cellulose, oxidized regenerated is saturated with blood at the bleeding site and swells into a brownish or black gelatinous mass which aids in the formation of a clot. When used in small amounts, it is absorbed from the sites of implantation with little or no tissue reaction.
Local Anesthetic/Vasoconstrictor Precautions No information available to require special precautions
Effects on Dental Treatment No effects or complications reported
Other Adverse Effects No data reported
Contraindications Not to be used as packing or wadding unless it is removed after hemostasis occurs; not to be used for implantation in bone defects
Warnings/Precautions Autoclaving causes physical breakdown of the product. Closing the material in a contaminated wound without drainage may lead to

complications. The material should not be moistened before insertion since the hemostatic effect is greater when applied dry. The material should not be impregnated with anti-infective agents. Its hemostatic effect is not enhanced by the addition of thrombin. The material may be left in situ when necessary but it is advisable to remove it once hemostasis is achieved.

Drug Interactions No data reported

Breast-feeding Considerations No data reported

Dosage Forms Knitted fabric strips: Envelopes in a size of ½" x 2"

Dietary Considerations No data reported

Generic Available No

Comments Oxidized regenerated cellulose is prepared by the controlled oxidation of regenerated cellulose. The fabric is white with a pale yellow cast and has a faint, caramel-like aroma. A slight discoloration may occur with age but this does not effect its hemostatic actions.

Cellulose Sodium Phosphate (sel yoo lose SOW dee um FOS fate)

Brand Names Calcibind®

Therapeutic Category Urinary Tract Product

Synonyms CSP; Sodium Cellulose Phosphate

Use Adjunct to dietary restriction to reduce renal calculi formation in absorptive hypercalciuria type I

Local Anesthetic/Vasoconstrictor Precautions No information available to require special precautions

Effects on Dental Treatment No effects or complications reported

Pregnancy Risk Factor C

Generic Available No

Celluvisc® [OTC] see Carboxymethylcellulose on page 179

Celontin® see Methsuximide on page 620

Cel-U-Jec® see Betamethasone on page 126

Cenafed® [OTC] see Pseudoephedrine on page 820

Cenafed® Plus Tablet [OTC] see Triprolidine and Pseudoephedrine on page 969

Cena-K® see Potassium Chloride on page 778

Cenolate® see Sodium Ascorbate on page 868

Centrax® see Prazepam on page 785

Cēpacol® Anesthetic Troches [OTC] see Cetylpyridinium and Benzocaine on page 206

Cēpacol® Troches [OTC] see Cetylpyridinium on page 205

Cēpastat® [OTC] see Phenol on page 749

Cephalexin (sef a LEKS in)

Related Information

Antibiotic Prophylaxis, Preprocedural Guidelines for Dental Patients on page 1034

Dental Drug Interactions: Update on Drug Combinations Requiring Special Considerations on page 1144

Oral Bacterial Infections on page 1059

Brand Names Biocef®; Cefanex®; Keflex®; Keftab®

Canadian/Mexican Brand Names Apo®-Cephalex (Canada); Ceporex® (Mexico); Novo-Lexin® (Canada); Nu-Cephalex (Canada)

Therapeutic Category Antibiotic, Cephalosporin (First Generation)

Use

Dental: An alternate antibiotic to treat orofacial infections in patients allergic to penicillins; susceptible bacteria including aerobic gram-positive bacteria and anaerobes. Also, an alternate antibiotic for prevention of bacterial endocarditis; individuals allergic to amoxicillin (penicillins) may receive cephalexin provided they have not had an immediate, local, or systemic IgE-mediated anaphylactic allergic reaction to penicillin. Also, antibiotic for premedication in patients not allergic to penicillin who may be at potential increased risk of hematogenous total joint infection.

Medical: Treatment of susceptible bacterial infections in the medical patient, including those caused by group A beta-hemolytic *Streptococcus*, *Staphylococcus*, *Klebsiella pneumoniae*, *E. coli*, *Proteus mirabilis*, and *Shigella*; predominantly used for lower respiratory tract, urinary tract, skin and soft tissue, and bone and joint

Usual Dosage Oral:

Children: 25-50 mg/kg/day every 6 hours; severe infections: 50-100 mg/kg/day in divided doses every 6 hours; maximum: 3 g/24 hours

SBE prophylaxis: 50 mg/kg orally 1 hour before procedure; total children's dose not to exceed adult dose

(Continued)

Cephalexin *(Continued)*

Adults: 250-1000 mg every 6 hours; maximum: 4 g/day
  SBE prophylaxis: 2 g 1 hour before procedure

Mechanism of Action Inhibits bacterial cell wall synthesis by binding to one or more of the penicillin-binding proteins (PBPs) which in turn inhibits the final transpeptidation step of peptidoglycan synthesis in bacterial cell walls, thus inhibiting cell wall biosynthesis. Bacteria eventually lyse due to ongoing activity of cell wall autolytic enzymes (autolysins and murein hydrolases) while cell wall assembly is arrested.

Local Anesthetic/Vasoconstrictor Precautions No information available to require special precautions

Effects on Dental Treatment No effects or complications reported

Other Adverse Effects 1% to 10%: Gastrointestinal: Diarrhea

Contraindications Hypersensitivity to cephalexin, any component, or cephalosporins

Warnings/Precautions Modify dosage in patients with severe renal impairment; prolonged use may result in superinfection; a low incidence of cross-hypersensitivity to penicillins exists

Drug Interactions
Increased effect: Probenecid may decrease cephalosporin elimination
Increased toxicity: Aminoglycosides may be a possible additive to nephrotoxicity

Drug Uptake
Duration: 6 hours
Absorption:
  Adults: Rapid
  Children: Delayed in young children
Serum half-life: Adults: 0.5-1.2 hours (prolonged with renal impairment)
Time to peak serum concentration: Oral: Within 1 hour

Pregnancy Risk Factor B

Breast-feeding Considerations Excreted into breast milk in small amounts like other cephalosporins

Dosage Forms
Capsule, as monohydrate: 250 mg, 500 mg
Powder for oral suspension, as monohydrate: 125 mg/5 mL (5 mL unit dose, 60 mL, 100 mL, 200 mL); 250 mg/5 mL (5 mL unit dose, 100 mL, 200 mL)
Suspension, oral, as monohydrate, pediatric: 100 mg/mL [5 mg/drop] (10 mL)
Tablet, as monohydrate: 250 mg, 500 mg, 1 g
Tablet, as hydrochloride: 500 mg

Dietary Considerations Should be taken on an empty stomach (ie, 1 hour prior to, or 2 hours after meals) to increase total absorption

Generic Available Yes

Comments Cephalexin is effective against anaerobic bacteria, but the sensitivity of alpha-hemolytic *Streptococcus* vary; approximately 10% of strains are resistant. Nearly 70% are intermediately sensitive. Patients allergic to penicillins can use a cephalosporin; the incidence of cross-reactivity between penicillins and cephalosporins is 1% when the allergic reaction to penicillin is delayed. If the patient has a history of immediate reaction to penicillin, the incidence of cross-reactivity is 20%; cephalosporins are contraindicated in these patients.

Selected Readings
"Advisory Statement. Antibiotic Prophylaxis for Dental Patients With Total Joint Replacements. American Dental Association; American Academy of Orthopedic Surgeons," *J Am Dent Assoc*, 1997, 128(7):1004-8.
Dajani AS, Taubert KA, Wilson W, et al, "Prevention of Bacterial Endocarditis Recommendations by the American Heart Association," *JAMA* 1997, 277(22):1794-801.
Dajani AS, Taubert KA, Wilson W, et al, "Prevention of Bacterial Endocarditis: Recommendations by the American Heart Association," *J Am Dent Assoc* 1997, 128(8):1142-51.
Saxon A, Beall GN, Rohr AS, et al, "Immediate Hypersensitivity Reactions to Beta-Lactam Antibiotics," *Ann Intern Med*, 1987, 107(2):204-15.

Cephalothin *(sef A loe thin)*

Brand Names Keflin®

Canadian/Mexican Brand Names Ceftina® (Mexico); Ceporacin® (Canada)

Therapeutic Category Antibiotic, Cephalosporin (First Generation)

Synonyms Cefalotina Sal Sodica De (Mexico)

Use Treatment of susceptible bacterial infections, including those caused by group A beta-hemolytic *Streptococcus*; respiratory, genitourinary, gastrointestinal, skin and soft tissue, bone and joint infections; septicemia; cephalexin is the oral equivalent

Usual Dosage I.M., I.V.:
Children: 75-125 mg/kg/day divided every 4-6 hours; maximum dose: 10 g in a 24-hour period
Adults: 500 mg to 2 g every 4-6 hours

ALPHABETICAL LISTING OF DRUGS

Mechanism of Action Inhibits bacterial cell wall synthesis by binding to one or more of the penicillin-binding proteins (PBPs) which in turn inhibits the final transpeptidation step of peptidoglycan synthesis in bacterial cell walls, thus inhibiting cell wall biosynthesis. Bacteria eventually lyse due to ongoing activity of cell wall autolytic enzymes (autolysins and murein hydrolases) while cell wall assembly is arrested.

Local Anesthetic/Vasoconstrictor Precautions No information available to require special precautions

Effects on Dental Treatment No effects or complications reported

Other Adverse Effects
1% to 10%: Gastrointestinal: Nausea, vomiting, diarrhea
<1%:
  Dermatologic: Maculopapular and erythematous rash
  Gastrointestinal: Dyspepsia, pseudomembranous colitis
  Hematologic: Bleeding
  Local: Pain and induration at injection site

Drug Interactions
Increased effect: High-dose probenecid decreases renal clearance of cephalothin

Drug Uptake
Serum half-life: 30-60 minutes
Time to peak serum concentration:
  I.M.: Within 30 minutes
  I.V.: Within 15 minutes

Pregnancy Risk Factor B
Generic Available Yes

Cephapirin (sef a PYE rin)
Brand Names Cefadyl®

Therapeutic Category Antibiotic, Cephalosporin (First Generation)

Use Treatment of infections when caused by susceptible strains including group A beta-hemolytic *Streptococcus*; used in serious respiratory, genitourinary, gastrointestinal, skin and soft tissue, bone and joint infections; septicemia; endocarditis; identical to cephalothin

Usual Dosage I.M., I.V.:
Children: 10-20 mg/kg/dose every 6 hours up to 4 g/24 hours
Adults: 500 mg to 1 g every 6 hours up to 12 g/day

Mechanism of Action Inhibits bacterial cell wall synthesis by binding to one or more of the penicillin-binding proteins (PBPs) which in turn inhibits the final transpeptidation step of peptidoglycan synthesis in bacterial cell walls, thus inhibiting cell wall biosynthesis. Bacteria eventually lyse due to ongoing activity of cell wall autolytic enzymes (autolysins and murein hydrolases) while cell wall assembly is arrested.

Local Anesthetic/Vasoconstrictor Precautions No information available to require special precautions

Effects on Dental Treatment No effects or complications reported

Other Adverse Effects
1% to 10%: Gastrointestinal: Diarrhea
<1%:
  Central nervous system: CNS irritation, seizures, fever
  Dermatologic: Rash, urticaria
  Hematologic: Leukopenia, thrombocytopenia
  Hepatic: Transient elevation of liver enzymes

Drug Interactions
Increased effect: High-dose probenecid decreases renal clearance of cephalosporins

Drug Uptake
Serum half-life: 36-60 minutes
Time to peak serum concentration:
  I.M.: Within 30 minutes
  I.V.: Within 5 minutes

Pregnancy Risk Factor B
Generic Available No

Cephradine (SEF ra deen)
Related Information
Antibiotic Prophylaxis, Preprocedural Guidelines for Dental Patients *on page 1034*

Brand Names Velosef®

Canadian/Mexican Brand Names Veracef® (Mexico)

Therapeutic Category Antibiotic, Cephalosporin (First Generation)
(Continued)

Cephradine *(Continued)*

Synonyms Cefradina (Mexico)

Use Treatment of susceptible bacterial infections, including those caused by group A beta-hemolytic *Streptococcus*; used in in respiratory, genitourinary, gastrointestinal, skin and soft tissue, bone and joint infections. Also, antibiotic for premedication in patients not allergic to penicillin who may be at potential increased risk of hematogenous total joint infection.

Usual Dosage Oral:
Children ≥9 months: 25-50 mg/kg/day in divided doses every 6 hours
Adults: 250-500 mg every 6-12 hours

Mechanism of Action Inhibits bacterial cell wall synthesis by binding to one or more of the penicillin-binding proteins (PBPs) which in turn inhibits the final transpeptidation step of peptidoglycan synthesis in bacterial cell walls, thus inhibiting cell wall biosynthesis. Bacteria eventually lyse due to ongoing activity of cell wall autolytic enzymes (autolysins and murein hydrolases) while cell wall assembly is arrested.

Local Anesthetic/Vasoconstrictor Precautions No information available to require special precautions

Effects on Dental Treatment No effects or complications reported

Other Adverse Effects
1% to 10%: Gastrointestinal: Diarrhea
<1%:
Dermatologic: Rash
Gastrointestinal: Nausea, vomiting, pseudomembranous colitis
Renal: Elevated BUN and creatinine

Contraindications Hypersensitivity to cephradine, any component, or cephalosporins

Warnings/Precautions Prolonged use may result in superinfection; use with caution in patients with a history of colitis; reduce dose in patients with renal dysfunction; a low incidence of cross-hypersensitivity with penicillins exists

Drug Interactions No data reported

Drug Uptake
Absorption: Oral is faster than I.M. but well absorbed from all routes
Serum half-life: 1-2 hours
Time to peak serum concentration: Oral, I.M.: Within 1-2 hours

Pregnancy Risk Factor B

Dosage Forms
Capsule: 250 mg, 500 mg
Powder for oral suspension: 125 mg/5 mL (5 mL, 100 mL, 200 mL); 250 mg/5 mL (5 mL, 100 mL, 200 mL)

Generic Available Yes

Selected Readings
"Advisory Statement. Antibiotic Prophylaxis for Dental Patients With Total Joint Replacements. American Dental Association; American Academy of Orthopedic Surgeons," *J Am Dent Assoc*, 1997, 128(7):1004-8.
Donowitz GR and Mandell GL, "Beta-Lactam Antibiotics," *N Engl J Med*, 1988, 318(7):419-26 and 318(8):490-500.
Gustaferro CA and Steckelberg JM, "Cephalosporin Antimicrobial Agents and Related Compounds," *Mayo Clin Proc*, 1991, 66(10):1064-73.

Cephulac® *see* Lactulose *on page 540*

Ceptaz™ *see* Ceftazidime *on page 195*

Cerebyx® *see* Fosphenytoin *on page 432*

Ceredase® Injection *see* Alglucerase *on page 40*

Cerezyme® *see* Imiglucerase *on page 500*

Cerivastatin *(se ree va STAT in)*

Brand Names Baycol®

Therapeutic Category HMG-CoA Reductase Inhibitor

Synonyms Cerivastatin Sodium

Use Adjunct to dietary therapy to for the reduction of elevated total and LDL cholesterol levels in patients with primary hypercholesterolemia and mixed dyslipidemia when the response to dietary restriction of saturated fat and cholesterol and other nonpharmacological measures alone has been inadequate

Usual Dosage Adults: Oral: 0.3 mg once daily in the evening; may be taken with or without food

Local Anesthetic/Vasoconstrictor Precautions No information available to require special precautions

Effects on Dental Treatment No effects or complications reported

Drug Interactions Concurrent use of erythromycin and HMG-CoA reductase inhibitors may result in rhabdomyolysis

Pregnancy Risk Factor X

Dosage Forms Tablet, as sodium: 0.2 mg, 0.3 mg

Cerivastatin Sodium *see* Cerivastatin *on previous page*

Cerose-DM® [OTC] *see* Chlorpheniramine, Phenylephrine, and Dextromethorphan *on page 220*

Cerubidine® *see* Daunorubicin Hydrochloride *on page 283*

Cerumenex® *see* Triethanolamine Polypeptide Oleate-Condensate *on page 959*

Cervidil® Vaginal Insert *see* Dinoprostone *on page 322*

Cesamet® *see* Nabilone *on page 655*

Cetacaine® *see* Benzocaine, Butyl Aminobenzoate, Tetracaine, and Benzalkonium Chloride *on page 119*

Cetamide® Ophthalmic *see* Sulfacetamide Sodium *on page 890*

Cetapred® Ophthalmic *see* Sulfacetamide Sodium and Prednisolone *on page 891*

Cetirizine (se TI ra zeen)

Brand Names Zyrtec™

Therapeutic Category Antihistamine

Synonyms Cetirizine Hydrochloride; P-071; UCB-P071

Use Perennial and seasonal allergic rhinitis and other allergic symptoms including urticaria

Usual Dosage Children ≥12 years and Adults: Oral: 5-10 mg once daily, depending upon symptom severity

Dosing interval in hepatic or renal impairment:
Cl_{cr} ≤31 mL/minute: Administer 5 mg once daily

Mechanism of Action Competes with histamine for H_1-receptor sites on effector cells in the gastrointestinal tract, blood vessels, and respiratory tract

Local Anesthetic/Vasoconstrictor Precautions No information available to require special precautions

Effects on Dental Treatment No effects or complications reported

Other Adverse Effects
>10%: Central nervous system: Headache has been reported to occur in 10% to 12% of patients, drowsiness has been reported in as much as 26% of patients on high doses
1% to 10%:
Central nervous system: Fatigue, dizziness
Gastrointestinal: Dry mouth
<1%: Central nervous system: Depression

Contraindications Hypersensitivity to cetirizine, hydroxyzine, or any component

Warnings/Precautions Cetirizine should be used cautiously in patients with hepatic or renal dysfunction, the elderly and in nursing mothers. Doses >10 mg/day may cause significant drowsiness

Drug Interactions Increased toxicity: CNS depressants, anticholinergics

Drug Uptake
Onset of effect: Within 15-30 minutes
Absorption: Oral: Rapid
Serum half-life: 8-11 hours
Time to peak serum concentration: Within 30-60 minutes

Pregnancy Risk Factor B

Generic Available No

Cetirizine Hydrochloride *see* Cetirizine *on this page*

Cetylpyridinium (SEE til peer i DI nee um)

Brand Names Ceepryn® [OTC]; Cēpacol® Troches [OTC]

Therapeutic Category Local Anesthetic

Synonyms Cetylpyridinium Chloride

Use Temporary relief of sore throat

Usual Dosage Children >6 years and Adults: Oral: Dissolve 1 lozenge in the mouth every 2 hours as needed

Local Anesthetic/Vasoconstrictor Precautions No information available to require special precautions

Effects on Dental Treatment No effects or complications reported

Pregnancy Risk Factor C

Dosage Forms
Troches, as chloride: 1:1500 (24s)
Mouthwash, as chloride: 0.05% and alcohol 14% (180 mL)

Generic Available Yes

Cetylpyridinium and Benzocaine
(SEE til peer i DI nee um & BEN zoe kane)
Brand Names Cēpacol® Anesthetic Troches [OTC]
Therapeutic Category Local Anesthetic, Oral
Synonyms Benzocaine and Cetylpyridinium Chloride
Use Symptomatic relief of sore throat
Local Anesthetic/Vasoconstrictor Precautions No information available to require special precautions
Effects on Dental Treatment No effects or complications reported
Pregnancy Risk Factor C
Generic Available Yes

Cetylpyridinium Chloride see Cetylpyridinium on previous page
Cevalin® [OTC] see Ascorbic Acid on page 88
Cevi-Bid® [OTC] see Ascorbic Acid on page 88
Ce-Vi-Sol® [OTC] see Ascorbic Acid on page 88
Cevitamic Acid (Canada) see Ascorbic Acid on page 88
Charcoaid® [OTC] see Charcoal on this page

Charcoal (CHAR kole)
Brand Names Actidose-Aqua® [OTC]; Actidose® With Sorbitol [OTC]; Charcoaid® [OTC]; Charcocaps® [OTC]; Insta-Char® [OTC]; Liqui-Char® [OTC]; SuperChar® [OTC]
Therapeutic Category Antidiarrheal; Antidote, Adsorbent; Antiflatulent
Use Emergency treatment in poisoning by drugs and chemicals; repetitive doses for gastric dialysis in uremia to adsorb various waste products, and repetitive doses have proven useful to enhance the elimination of certain drugs (eg, theophylline, phenobarbital, and aspirin)
Usual Dosage Oral:
Acute poisoning:
Charcoal with sorbitol: Single-dose:
Children 1-12 years: 1-2 g/kg/dose or 15-30 g or approximately 5-10 times the weight of the ingested poison; 1 g adsorbs 100-1000 mg of poison; the use of repeat oral charcoal with sorbitol doses is not recommended. In young children, sorbitol should be repeated no more than 1-2 times/day.
Adults: 30-100 g
Charcoal in water:
Single-dose:
Children 1-12 years: 15-30 g or 1-2 g/kg
Adults: 30-100 g or 1-2 g/kg
Multiple-dose:
Children 1-12 years: 20-60 g or 0.5-1 g/kg every 2-6 hours until clinical observations, serum drug concentration have returned to a subtherapeutic range, or charcoal stool apparent
Adults: 20-60 g or 0.5-1 g/kg every 2-6 hours

Gastric dialysis: Adults: 20-50 g every 6 hours for 1-2 days

Intestinal gas, diarrhea, GI distress: Adults: 520-975 mg after meals or at first sign of discomfort; repeat as needed to a maximum dose of 4.16 g/day
Mechanism of Action Adsorbs toxic substances or irritants, thus inhibiting GI absorption; adsorbs intestinal gas; the addition of sorbitol results in hyperosmotic laxative action causing catharsis
Local Anesthetic/Vasoconstrictor Precautions No information available to require special precautions
Effects on Dental Treatment No effects or complications reported
Other Adverse Effects
>10%: Gastrointestinal: Vomiting, diarrhea with sorbitol, constipation, stools will turn black
<1%: Gastrointestinal: Swelling of abdomen
Drug Interactions Do not administer concomitantly with syrup of ipecac; do not mix with milk, ice cream, or sherbet
Drug Uptake
Absorption: Not absorbed from GI tract
Pregnancy Risk Factor C
Generic Available Yes

Charcocaps® [OTC] see Charcoal on this page
Chealamide® see Edetate Disodium on page 345
Chemical Dependency and Smoking Cessation see page 1087
Chenix® see Chenodiol on next page
Chenodeoxycholic Acid see Chenodiol on next page

Chenodiol (kee noe DYE ole)

Brand Names Chenix®

Therapeutic Category Bile Acid; Gallstone Dissolution Agent

Synonyms Chenodeoxycholic Acid

Use Oral dissolution of cholesterol gallstones in selected patients

Usual Dosage Adults: Oral: 13-16 mg/kg/day in 2 divided doses, starting with 250 mg twice daily the first 2 weeks and increasing by 250 mg/day each week thereafter until the recommended or maximum tolerated dose is achieved

Dosing comments in hepatic impairment: Contraindicated for use in presence of known hepatocyte dysfunction or bile ductal abnormalities

Mechanism of Action Chenodiol is a primary acid excreted into bile, normally constituting one-third of the total biliary bile acids. Synthesis of chenodiol is regulated by the relative composition and flux of cholesterol and bile acids through the hepatocyte by a negative feedback effect on the rate-limiting enzymes for synthesis of cholesterol (HMGCoA reductase) and bile acids (cholesterol 7 alpha-hydroxyl).

Local Anesthetic/Vasoconstrictor Precautions No information available to require special precautions

Effects on Dental Treatment No effects or complications reported

Other Adverse Effects

>10%:
  Gastrointestinal: Diarrhea (mild), biliary pain
  Miscellaneous: Aminotransferase increases

1% to 10%:
  Endocrine & metabolic: Increases in cholesterol and LDL cholesterol
  Gastrointestinal: Dyspepsia

<1%:
  Gastrointestinal: Diarrhea (severe), cramps, nausea, vomiting, flatulence, constipation
  Hematologic: Leukopenia
  Hepatic: Intrahepatic cholestasis, higher cholecystectomy rates

Contraindications Presence of known hepatocyte dysfunction or bile ductal abnormalities; a gallbladder confirmed as nonvisualizing after two consecutive single doses of dye; radiopaque stones; gallstone complications or compelling reasons for gallbladder surgery; inflammatory bowel disease or active gastric or duodenal ulcer; pregnancy

Warnings/Precautions Chenodiol is hepatotoxic in animal models including subhuman Primates; chenodiol should be discontinued if aminotransferases exceed 3 times the upper normal limit; chenodiol may contribute to colon cancer in otherwise susceptible individuals

Drug Interactions Decreased effect: Antacids, cholestyramine, colestipol, oral contraceptives

Pregnancy Risk Factor X

Dosage Forms Tablet, film coated: 250 mg

Generic Available No

Chloral Hydrate (KLOR al HYE drate)

Brand Names Aquachloral® Supprettes®

Canadian/Mexican Brand Names Novo-Chlorhydrate® (Canada); PMS-Chloral Hydrate (Canada)

Therapeutic Category Hypnotic; Sedative

Use

Dental: Sedative/hypnotic for dental procedures

Medical: Short-term sedative and hypnotic (<2 weeks), sedative/hypnotic for diagnostic procedures; sedative prior to EEG evaluations

(Continued)

Chloral Hydrate *(Continued)*

Restrictions C-IV; Refillable up to 5 times in 6 months

Usual Dosage

Children: Preoperative sedation: Oral: 50-75 mg/kg/dose 30-60 minutes prior to procedure with no follow-up dose; dose should not exceed 1000 mg

Adults: Very rarely used in adults as preoperative sedative in dentistry

Sedation, anxiety: 250 mg 3 times/day

Hypnotic: 500-1000 mg at bedtime or 30 minutes prior to procedure, not to exceed 2 g/24 hours

Mechanism of Action Central nervous system depressant effects are due to its active metabolite trichloroethanol, mechanism unknown

Local Anesthetic/Vasoconstrictor Precautions No information available to require special precautions

Effects on Dental Treatment No effects or complications reported

Other Adverse Effects

>10%: Gastrointestinal: Gastric irritation, nausea, vomiting, diarrhea

1% to 10%:

Central nervous system: Clumsiness, hallucinations, drowsiness, "hangover" effect

Dermatologic: Rash, urticaria

Contraindications Hypersensitivity to chloral hydrate or any component; hepatic or renal impairment; gastritis or ulcers; severe cardiac disease

Warnings/Precautions Use with caution in patients with porphyria; use with caution in neonates, drug may accumulate with repeated use, prolonged use in neonates associated with hyperbilirubinemia; tolerance to hypnotic effect develops, therefore, not recommended for use >2 weeks; taper dosage to avoid withdrawal with prolonged use; trichloroethanol (TCE), a metabolite of chloral hydrate, is a carcinogen in mice; there is no data in humans. Chloral hydrate is considered a second line hypnotic agent in adults and elderly.

Drug Interactions May potentiate effects of warfarin, central nervous system depressants, alcohol; vasodilation reaction (flushing, tachycardia, etc) may occur with concurrent use of alcohol; concomitant use of furosemide (I.V.) may result in flushing, sweating, and blood pressure changes

Drug Uptake

Duration of effect: 4-8 hours

Absorption: Oral: Rapid

Serum half-life: Active metabolite: 8-11 hours

Time to peak serum concentration: Within 0.5-1 hour

Pregnancy Risk Factor C

Breast-feeding Considerations May be taken while breast-feeding

Dosage Forms

Capsule: 250 mg, 500 mg

Suppository, rectal: 324 mg, 500 mg, 648 mg

Syrup: 250 mg/5 mL (10 mL); 500 mg/5 mL (5 mL, 10 mL, 480 mL)

Dietary Considerations May be taken with chilled liquid to mask taste

Generic Available Yes

Chlorambucil *(klor AM byoo sil)*

Brand Names Leukeran®

Therapeutic Category Antineoplastic Agent, Alkylating Agent (Nitrogen Mustard)

Use Management of chronic lymphocytic leukemia (CLL), Hodgkin's and non-Hodgkin's lymphoma; breast and ovarian carcinoma, testicular carcinoma, choriocarcinoma; Waldenström's macroglobulinemia, and nephrotic syndrome unresponsive to conventional therapy

Usual Dosage Oral (refer to individual protocols):

Children:

General short courses: 0.1-0.2 mg/kg/day **or** 4.5 mg/m²/day for 3-6 weeks for remission induction (usual: 4-10 mg/day); maintenance therapy: 0.03-0.1 mg/kg/day (usual: 2-4 mg/day)

Nephrotic syndrome: 0.1-0.2 mg/kg/day every day for 5-15 weeks with low-dose prednisone

Chronic lymphocytic leukemia (CLL):

Biweekly regimen: Initial: 0.4 mg/kg/dose every 2 weeks; increase dose by 0.1 mg/kg every 2 weeks until a response occurs and/or myelosuppression occurs

Monthly regimen: Initial: 0.4 mg/kg, increase dose by 0.2 mg/kg every 4 weeks until a response occurs and/or myelosuppression occurs

Malignant lymphomas:

Non-Hodgkin's lymphoma: 0.1 mg/kg/day

Hodgkin's lymphoma: 0.2 mg/kg/day

Adults: 0.1-0.2 mg/kg/day **or** 3-6 mg/m²/day for 3-6 weeks, then adjust dose on basis of blood counts. Pulse dosing has been used in CLL as intermittent, biweekly, or monthly doses of 0.4 mg/kg and increased by 0.1 mg/kg until the disease is under control or toxicity ensues. An alternate regimen is 14 mg/m²/day for 5 days, repeated every 21-28 days.

Mechanism of Action Interferes with DNA replication and RNA transcription by alkylation and cross-linking the strands of DNA

Local Anesthetic/Vasoconstrictor Precautions No information available to require special precautions

Effects on Dental Treatment No effects or complications reported

Other Adverse Effects

>10%:

Hematologic: Myelosuppressive: Use with caution when receiving radiation; bone marrow suppression frequently occurs and occasionally bone marrow failure has occurred; blood counts should be monitored closely while undergoing treatment; leukopenia, thrombocytopenia, anemia. WBC: Moderate; Platelets: Moderate; Onset (days): 7; Nadir (days): 10-14; Recovery (days): 28.

Secondary malignancies: Increased incidence of AML

1% to 10%:

Dermatologic: Skin rashes

Endocrine & metabolic: Menstrual changes, hyperuricemia

Gastrointestinal: Diarrhea, oral ulceration are infrequent

Emetic potential: Low (<10%)

<1%:

Central nervous system: Confusion, agitation, ataxia, hallucination; rarely generalized or focal seizures, drug fever

Dermatologic: Rash, skin hypersensitivity

Fertility impairment: Has caused chromosomal damage in man, oligospermia, both reversible and permanent sterility have occurred in both sexes; can produce amenorrhea in females, oligospermia

Hematologic: Leukopenia, thrombocytopenia

Hepatic: Hepatic necrosis, hepatotoxicity

Neuromuscular & skeletal: Peripheral neuropathy, tremors, muscular twitching, weakness

Ocular: Keratitis

Respiratory: Pulmonary fibrosis

Drug Uptake

Absorption: 70% to 80%

Serum half-life: 90 minutes to 2 hours

Pregnancy Risk Factor D

Generic Available No

Chloramphenicol (klor am FEN i kole)

Brand Names AK-Chlor®; Chloromycetin®; Chloroptic®; Ophthochlor®

Canadian/Mexican Brand Names Cetina® (Mexico); Clorafen® (Mexico); Diochloram® (Canada); Paraxin® (Mexico); Pentamycetin® (Canada); Quemicetina® (Mexico); Sopamycetin® (Canada)

Therapeutic Category Antibiotic, Ophthalmic; Antibiotic, Otic; Antibiotic, Miscellaneous

Synonyms Cloranfenicol (Mexico)

Use Treatment of serious infections due to organisms resistant to other less toxic antibiotics or when its penetrability into the site of infection is clinically superior to other antibiotics to which the organism is sensitive; useful in infections caused by *Bacteroides*, *H. influenzae*, *Neisseria meningitidis*, *Salmonella*, and *Rickettsia*

Usual Dosage

Meningitis: Oral, I.V.: Children: 75-100 mg/kg/day divided every 6 hours

Other infections: Oral, I.V.:

Children: 50-75 mg/kg/day divided every 6 hours; maximum daily dose: 4 g/day

Adults: 50-100 mg/kg/day in divided doses every 6 hours; maximum daily dose: 4 g/day

Ophthalmic: Children and Adults: Instill 1-2 drops or 1.25 cm (½" of ointment every 3-4 hours); increase interval between applications after 48 hours to 2-3 times/day

Otic solution: Instill 2-3 drops into ear 3 times/day

Topical: Gently rub into the affected area 1-4 times/day

Mechanism of Action Reversibly binds to 50S ribosomal subunits of susceptible organisms preventing amino acids from being transferred to growing peptide chains thus inhibiting protein synthesis

Local Anesthetic/Vasoconstrictor Precautions No information available to require special precautions

Effects on Dental Treatment No effects or complications reported

(Continued)

Chloramphenicol *(Continued)*

Other Adverse Effects

<1%:

Central nervous system: Nightmares, headache

Dermatologic: Rash

Gastrointestinal: Diarrhea, stomatitis, enterocolitis, nausea, vomiting

Hematologic: Bone marrow suppression, aplastic anemia

Neuromuscular & skeletal: Peripheral neuropathy

Ocular: Optic neuritis

Miscellaneous: Gray baby syndrome

Three (3) major toxicities associated with chloramphenicol include:

Aplastic anemia, an idiosyncratic reaction which can occur with any route of administration; usually occurs 3 weeks to 12 months after initial exposure to chloramphenicol

Bone marrow suppression is thought to be dose-related with serum concentrations >25 µg/mL and reversible once chloramphenicol is discontinued; anemia and neutropenia may occur during the first week of therapy

Gray baby syndrome is characterized by circulatory collapse, cyanosis, acidosis, abdominal distention, myocardial depression, coma, and death; reaction appears to be associated with serum levels ≥50 µg/mL; may result from drug accumulation in patients with impaired hepatic or renal function

Drug Interactions

Decreased effect: Phenobarbital and rifampin may decrease concentration of chloramphenicol

Increased toxicity: Chloramphenicol inhibits the metabolism of chlorpropamide, phenytoin, oral anticoagulants

Drug Uptake

Serum half-life: (Prolonged with markedly reduced liver function or combined liver/kidney dysfunction):

Normal renal function: 1.6-3.3 hours

End stage renal disease: 3-7 hours

Cirrhosis: 10-12 hours

Time to peak serum concentration: Oral: Within 0.5-3 hours

Pregnancy Risk Factor C

Generic Available Yes

Chloramphenicol and Prednisolone

(klor am FEN i kole & pred NIS oh lone)

Brand Names Chloroptic-P® Ophthalmic

Therapeutic Category Antibiotic, Ophthalmic; Corticosteroid, Ophthalmic

Use Topical anti-infective and corticosteroid for treatment of ocular infections

Local Anesthetic/Vasoconstrictor Precautions No information available to require special precautions

Effects on Dental Treatment No effects or complications reported

Pregnancy Risk Factor C

Generic Available No

Chloramphenicol, Polymyxin B, and Hydrocortisone

(klor am FEN i kole, pol i MIKS in bee, & hye droe KOR ti sone)

Brand Names Ophthocort® Ophthalmic

Therapeutic Category Antibiotic, Ophthalmic

Use Topical anti-infective and corticosteroid for treatment of ocular infections

Local Anesthetic/Vasoconstrictor Precautions No information available to require special precautions

Effects on Dental Treatment No effects or complications reported

Pregnancy Risk Factor C

Generic Available No

Chloraseptic® Oral [OTC] *see* Phenol *on page 749*

Chlorate® [OTC] *see* Chlorpheniramine *on page 217*

Chlordiazepoxide (klor dye az e POKS ide)

Brand Names Libritabs®; Librium®; Mitran®; Reposans-10®

Canadian/Mexican Brand Names Apo®-Chlordiazepoxide (Canada); Corax® (Canada); Medilium® (Canada); Novo-Poxide® (Canada); Solium® (Canada)

Therapeutic Category Benzodiazepine; Hypnotic; Sedative

Synonyms Clorodiacepoxido (Mexico)

Use Approved for anxiety, may be useful for acute alcohol withdrawal symptoms

Usual Dosage

Children:

<6 years: Not recommended

>6 years: Anxiety: Oral, I.M.: 0.5 mg/kg/24 hours divided every 6-8 hours

Adults:
Anxiety:
Oral: 15-100 mg divided 3-4 times/day
I.M., I.V.: Initial: 50-100 mg followed by 25-50 mg 3-4 times/day as needed
Preoperative anxiety: I.M.: 50-100 mg prior to surgery
Alcohol withdrawal symptoms: Oral, I.V.: 50-100 mg to start, dose may be repeated in 2-4 hours as necessary to a maximum of 300 mg/24 hours

Mechanism of Action Benzodiazepines appear to potentiate the effects of GABA and other inhibitory transmitters by binding to specific benzodiazepine receptor sites; benzodiazepine anxiolytic sedative that produces CNS depression at the subcortical level, except at high doses, whereby it works at the cortical level

Local Anesthetic/Vasoconstrictor Precautions No information available to require special precautions

Effects on Dental Treatment >10% of patients will experience dry mouth which disappears with cessation of drug therapy

Other Adverse Effects
>10%:
Cardiovascular: Chest pain
Central nervous system: Drowsiness, fatigue, lightheadedness, memory impairment, insomnia, anxiety, depression, headache, impaired coordination
Dermatologic: Skin eruptions, rash
Endocrine & metabolic: Decreased libido
Gastrointestinal: Nausea, constipation, vomiting, diarrhea, increased or decreased appetite
Neuromuscular & skeletal: Dysarthria
Ocular: Blurred vision
Miscellaneous: Decreased salivation, sweating
1% to 10%:
Cardiovascular: Hypotension, tachycardia, edema, syncope
Central nervous system: Confusion, mental impairment, nervousness, dizziness, akathisia
Dermatologic: Dermatitis
Gastrointestinal: Weight gain or loss, increased salivation
Neuromuscular & skeletal: Rigidity, tremor, muscle cramps
Otic: Tinnitus
Respiratory: Nasal congestion, hyperventilation
<1%:
Endocrine & metabolic: Menstrual irregularities
Hematologic: Blood dyscrasias
Neuromuscular & skeletal: Depressed reflexes
Miscellaneous: Drug dependence

Drug Interactions Potentiation of chlordiazepoxide-induced sedation may occur with alcohol and sedative-hypnotics

Drug Uptake
Serum half-life: 6.6-25 hours
End stage renal disease: 5-30 hours
Cirrhosis: 30-63 hours
Time to peak serum concentration:
Oral: Within 2 hours
I.M.: Results in lower peak plasma levels than oral

Pregnancy Risk Factor D

Dosage Forms
Capsule, as hydrochloride: 5 mg, 10 mg, 25 mg
Powder for injection, as hydrochloride: 100 mg
Tablet: 5 mg, 10 mg, 25 mg

Generic Available Yes

Chlordiazepoxide and Amitriptyline see Amitriptyline and Chlordiazepoxide on page 61

Chlordiazepoxide and Clidinium see Clidinium and Chlordiazepoxide on page 243

Chloresium® [OTC] see Chlorophyll on next page

Chlorhexidine Gluconate (klor HEKS i deen GLOO koe nate)
Related Information
Dentin Hypersensitivity; High Caries Index; Xerostomia on page 1074
Oral Nonviral Soft Tissue Ulcerations or Erosions on page 1070
Brand Names BactoShield® Topical [OTC]; Betasept® [OTC]; Dyna-Hex® Topical [OTC]; Exidine® Scrub [OTC]; Hibiclens® Topical [OTC]; Hibistat® Topical [OTC]; Peridex® Oral Rinse; PerioGard®
(Continued)

Chlorhexidine Gluconate *(Continued)*

Therapeutic Category Antibacterial, Oral Rinse; Antibiotic, Topical; Antimicrobial Mouth Rinse; Antiplaque Agent

Use

Dental: Antibacterial dental rinse; chlorhexidine is active against gram-positive and gram-negative organisms, facultative anaerobes, aerobes, and yeast

Medical: Skin cleanser for surgical scrub, cleanser for skin wounds, germicidal hand rinse

Mechanism of Action The bactericidal effect of chlorhexidine is a result of the binding of this cationic molecule to negatively charged bacterial cell walls and extramicrobial complexes. At low concentrations, this causes an alteration of bacterial cell osmotic equilibrium and leakage of potassium and phosphorous resulting in a bacteriostatic effect. At high concentrations of chlorhexidine, the cytoplasmic contents of the bacterial cell precipitate and result in cell death.

Local Anesthetic/Vasoconstrictor Precautions No information available to require special precautions

Effects on Dental Treatment Swelling of face has been reported

Other Adverse Effects

>10%: Increase of tartar on teeth, changes in taste. Staining of oral surfaces (mucosa, teeth, dorsum of tongue) may be visible as soon as 1 week after therapy begins and is more pronounced when there is a heavy accumulation of unremoved plaque and when teeth fillings have rough surfaces. Stain does not have a clinically adverse effect but because removal may not be possible, patients with anterior restoration should be advised of the potential permanency of the stain.

1% to 10%: Tongue irritation, oral irritation

<1%: Respiratory: Nasal congestion, dyspnea

Drug Interactions No data reported

Pregnancy Risk Factor B

Breast-feeding Considerations No data reported

Dosage Forms

Foam, topical, with isopropyl alcohol 4% (BactoShield®): 4% (180 mL)

Liquid, topical, with isopropyl alcohol 4%:

Dyna-Hex® Skin Cleanser: 2% (120 mL, 240 mL, 480 mL, 960 mL, 4000 mL); 4% (120 mL, 240 mL, 480 mL, 4000 mL)

BactoShield® 2: 2% (960 mL)

BactoShield®, Betasept®, Exidine® Skin Cleanser, Hibiclens® Skin Cleanser: 4% (15 mL, 120 mL, 240 mL, 480 mL, 960 mL, 4000 mL)

Rinse:

Oral (mint flavor) (Peridex®, PerioGard®): 0.12% with alcohol 11.6% (480 mL)

Topical (Hibistat® Hand Rinse): 0.5% with isopropyl alcohol 70% (120 mL, 240 mL)

Sponge/Brush (Hibiclens®): 4% with isopropyl alcohol 4% (22 mL)

Wipes (Hibistat®): 0.5% (50s)

Generic Available Yes

4-Chloro-1,2-Diphenyl-1(4-[2-(N,N-Dimethylamino)-Ethoxy]-Phenyl)-1-Butene *see* Toremifene *on page 946*

2-Chlorodeoxyadenosine *see* Cladribine *on page 239*

Chloroethane *see* Ethyl Chloride *on page 384*

Chloromycetin® *see* Chloramphenicol *on page 209*

Chlorophyll *(KLOR oh fil)*

Brand Names Chloresium® [OTC]; Derifil® [OTC]; Nullo® [OTC]; PALS® [OTC]

Therapeutic Category Gastrointestinal Agent, Miscellaneous; Topical Skin Product

Synonyms Chlorophyllin

Use Topically promotes normal healing, relieves pain and swelling, and reduces malodors in wounds, burns, surface ulcers, abrasions and skin irritations; used orally to control fecal and urinary odors in colostomy, ileostomy, or incontinence

Local Anesthetic/Vasoconstrictor Precautions No information available to require special precautions

Effects on Dental Treatment No effects or complications reported

Other Adverse Effects 1% to 10%: Gastrointestinal: Mild diarrhea, green stools

Generic Available No

Chlorophyllin *see* Chlorophyll *on this page*

Chloroprocaine *(klor oh PROE kane)*

Related Information

Oral Pain *on page 1053*

Brand Names Nesacaine®; Nesacaine®-MPF

Therapeutic Category Dental/Local Anesthetics; Local Anesthetic, Injectable

Use Infiltration anesthesia and peripheral and epidural anesthesia

Usual Dosage Dosage varies with anesthetic procedure, the area to be anesthetized, the vascularity of the tissues, depth of anesthesia required, degree of muscle relaxation required, and duration of anesthesia; range: 1.5-25 mL of 2% to 3% solution; single adult dose should not exceed 800 mg

Infiltration and peripheral nerve block: 1% to 2%

Infiltration, peripheral and central nerve block, including caudal and epidural block: 2% to 3%, without preservatives

Mechanism of Action Chloroprocaine HCl is benzoic acid, 4-amino-2-chloro-2-(diethylamino) ethyl ester monohydrochloride. Chloroprocaine is an ester-type local anesthetic, which stabilizes the neuronal membranes and prevents initiation and transmission of nerve impulses thereby affecting local anesthetic actions. Local anesthetics including chloroprocaine, reversibly prevent generation and conduction of electrical impulses in neurons by decreasing the transient increase in permeability to sodium. The differential sensitivity generally depends on the size of the fiber; small fibers are more sensitive than larger fibers and require a longer period for recovery. Sensory pain fibers are usually blocked first, followed by fibers that transmit sensations of temperature, touch, and deep pressure. High concentrations block sympathetic somatic sensory and somatic motor fibers. The spread of anesthesia depends upon the distribution of the solution. This is primarily dependent on the volume of drug injected.

Local Anesthetic/Vasoconstrictor Precautions No information available to require special precautions

Effects on Dental Treatment No effects or complications reported

Other Adverse Effects <1%:

Cardiovascular: Myocardial depression, hypotension, bradycardia, cardiovascular collapse, edema

Central nervous system: Anxiety, restlessness, disorientation, confusion, seizures, drowsiness, unconsciousness, chills, shivering

Dermatologic: Urticaria

Gastrointestinal: Nausea, vomiting

Local: Transient stinging or burning at injection site

Neuromuscular & skeletal: Tremor

Ocular: Blurred vision

Otic: Tinnitus

Respiratory: Respiratory arrest

Miscellaneous: Anaphylactoid reactions

Drug Interactions PABA (from ester-type anesthetics) may inhibit sulfonamides

Drug Uptake

Onset of action: 6-12 minutes

Duration: 30-60 minutes

Pregnancy Risk Factor C

Dosage Forms Injection, as hydrochloride:

Preservative free (Nesacaine®-MPF): 2% (30 mL); 3% (30 mL)

With preservative (Nesacaine®): 1% (30 mL); 2% (30 mL)

Generic Available No

Chloroptic® *see* Chloramphenicol *on page 209*

Chloroptic-P® Ophthalmic *see* Chloramphenicol and Prednisolone *on page 210*

Chloroquine and Primaquine (KLOR oh kwin & PRIM a kween)

Brand Names Aralen® Phosphate With Primaquine Phosphate

Therapeutic Category Antimalarial Agent

Use Prophylaxis of malaria, regardless of species, in all areas where the disease is endemic

Weight		Chloroquine Base (mg)	Primaquine Base (mg)	Dose* (mL)
lb	kg			
10-15	4.5-6.8	20	3	2.5
16-25	7.3-11.4	40	6	5
26-35	11.8-15.9	60	9	7.5
36-45	16.4-20.5	80	12	10
46-55	20.9-25	100	15	12.5
56-100	25.4-45.4	150	22.5	½ tablet
100+	>45.4	300	45	1 tablet

*Dose based on liquid containing approximately 40 mg of chloroquine base and 6 mg primaquine base per 5 mL, prepared from chloroquine phosphate with primaquine phosphate tablets.

(Continued)

Chloroquine and Primaquine *(Continued)*

Usual Dosage Oral: Start at least 1 day before entering the endemic area; continue for 8 weeks after leaving the endemic area

Children: For suggested weekly dosage (based on body weight), see table.

Adults: 1 tablet/week on the same day each week

Mechanism of Action Chloroquine concentrates within parasite acid vesicles and raises internal pH resulting in inhibition of parasite growth; may involve aggregates of ferriprotoporphyrin IX acting as chloroquine receptors causing membrane damage; may also interfere with nucleoprotein synthesis. Primaquine eliminates the primary tissue exoerythrocytic forms of *P. falciparum*; disrupts mitochondria and binds to DNA.

Local Anesthetic/Vasoconstrictor Precautions No information available to require special precautions

Effects on Dental Treatment No effects or complications reported

Other Adverse Effects

1% to 10%: Gastrointestinal: Diarrhea, nausea

<1%:

Cardiovascular: Hypotension, EKG changes

Central nervous system: Fatigue, personality changes, headache

Dermatologic: Pruritus, hair bleaching

Gastrointestinal: Anorexia, vomiting, stomatitis

Hematologic: Blood dyscrasias

Ocular: Retinopathy, blurred vision

Drug Interactions

Decreased absorption if administered concomitantly with kaolin and magnesium trisilicate

Increased toxicity/levels with cimetidine

Drug Uptake

Absorption: Oral: Both drugs are readily absorbed

Pregnancy Risk Factor C

Generic Available No

Chloroquine Phosphate (KLOR oh kwin FOS fate)

Brand Names Aralen® Phosphate

Therapeutic Category Amebicide; Antimalarial Agent

Synonyms Cloroquina, Defosfato De (Mexico)

Use Suppression or chemoprophylaxis of malaria; treatment of uncomplicated or mild-moderate malaria; extraintestinal amebiasis; rheumatoid arthritis; discoid lupus erythematosus, scleroderma, pemphigus

Usual Dosage Oral (**dosage expressed in terms of mg of base**):

Suppression or prophylaxis of malaria:

Children: Administer 5 mg base/kg/week on the same day each week (not to exceed 300 mg base/dose); begin 1-2 weeks prior to exposure; continue for 4-6 weeks after leaving endemic area; if suppressive therapy is not begun prior to exposure, double the initial loading dose to 10 mg base/kg and give in 2 divided doses 6 hours apart, followed by the usual dosage regimen

Adults: 300 mg/week (base) on the same day each week; begin 1-2 weeks prior to exposure; continue for 4-6 weeks after leaving endemic area; if suppressive therapy is not begun prior to exposure, double the initial loading dose to 600 mg base and give in 2 divided doses 6 hours apart, followed by the usual dosage regimen

Acute attack:

Children: 10 mg/kg on day 1, followed by 5 mg/kg 6 hours later and 5 mg/kg on days 2 and 3

Adults: 600 mg on day 1, followed by 300 mg 6 hours later, followed by 300 mg on days 2 and 3

Extraintestinal amebiasis:

Children: 10 mg/kg once daily for 2-3 weeks (up to 300 mg base/day)

Adults: 600 mg base/day for 2 days followed by 300 mg base/day for at least 2-3 weeks

Mechanism of Action Binds to and inhibits DNA and RNA polymerase; interferes with metabolism and hemoglobin utilization by parasites; inhibits prostaglandin effects; chloroquine concentrates within parasite acid vesicles and raises internal pH resulting in inhibition of parasite growth; may involve aggregates of ferriprotoporphyrin IX acting as chloroquine receptors causing membrane damage; may also interfere with nucleoprotein synthesis

Local Anesthetic/Vasoconstrictor Precautions No information available to require special precautions

Effects on Dental Treatment No effects or complications reported

Other Adverse Effects
1% to 10%: Gastrointestinal: Nausea, diarrhea
<1%:
Cardiovascular: Hypotension, EKG changes
Central nervous system: Fatigue, personality changes, headache
Dermatologic: Pruritus, hair bleaching
Gastrointestinal: Anorexia, vomiting, stomatitis
Hematologic: Blood dyscrasias
Ocular: Retinopathy, blurred vision

Drug Interactions
Decreased absorption if administered concomitantly with kaolin and magnesium trisilicate
Increased toxicity/levels with cimetidine

Drug Uptake
Absorption: Oral: Rapid (~89%)
Serum half-life: 3-5 days
Time to peak serum concentration: Within 1-2 hours

Pregnancy Risk Factor C
Generic Available Yes

Chlorothiazide (klor oh THYE a zide)
Related Information
Cardiovascular Diseases *on page 1010*
Brand Names Diurigen®; Diuril®
Therapeutic Category Diuretic, Thiazide
Use Management of mild to moderate hypertension, or edema associated with congestive heart failure, pregnancy, or nephrotic syndrome in patients unable to take oral hydrochlorothiazide, when a thiazide is the diuretic of choice
Usual Dosage I.V. form not recommended for children and should only be used in adults if unable to take oral in emergency situations:
Children >6 months:
Oral: 20 mg/kg/day in 2 divided doses
I.V.: 4 mg/kg/day
Adults:
Oral: 500 mg to 2 g/day divided in 1-2 doses
I.V.: 100-500 mg/day
Elderly: Oral: 500 mg once daily **or** 1 g 3 times/week
Mechanism of Action Inhibits sodium reabsorption in the distal tubules causing increased excretion of sodium and water as well as potassium and hydrogen ions, magnesium, phosphate, calcium
Local Anesthetic/Vasoconstrictor Precautions No information available to require special precautions
Effects on Dental Treatment No effects or complications reported
Other Adverse Effects
1% to 10%: Endocrine & metabolic: Hypokalemia, hyponatremia
<1%:
Cardiovascular: Arrhythmia, weak pulse, orthostatic hypotension
Central nervous system: Dizziness, vertigo, headache, fever
Dermatologic: Rash, photosensitivity
Endocrine & metabolic: Hypochloremic alkalosis, hyperglycemia, hyperlipidemia, hyperuricemia
Hematologic: Rarely blood dyscrasias, leukopenia, agranulocytosis, aplastic anemia
Neuromuscular & skeletal: Paresthesias
Renal: Prerenal azotemia

Drug Interactions
Decreased absorption of thiazides with cholestyramine resins; chlorothiazide causes a decreased effect of oral hypoglycemics
Increased toxicity: Digitalis glycosides, lithium (decreased clearance), probenecid

Drug Uptake
Onset of diuresis: Oral: 2 hours
Duration of diuretic action:
Oral: 6-12 hours
I.V.: ~2 hours
Absorption: Oral: Poor
Serum half-life: 1-2 hours

Pregnancy Risk Factor D
Generic Available Yes: Tablet

Chlorothiazide and Methyldopa
(klor oh THYE a zide & meth il DOE pa)
Brand Names Aldoclor®
Therapeutic Category Antihypertensive Agent, Combination
Synonyms Methyldopa and Chlorothiazide
Use Treatment of hypertension
Local Anesthetic/Vasoconstrictor Precautions No information available to require special precautions
Effects on Dental Treatment No effects or complications reported
Pregnancy Risk Factor D
Generic Available No

Chlorothiazide and Reserpine
(klor oh THYE a zide & re SER peen)
Brand Names Diupres-250®; Diupres-500®
Therapeutic Category Antihypertensive Agent, Combination
Synonyms Reserpine and Chlorothiazide
Use Management of hypertension
Local Anesthetic/Vasoconstrictor Precautions No information available to require special precautions
Effects on Dental Treatment No effects or complications reported
Pregnancy Risk Factor D
Generic Available Yes

Chlorotrianisene (klor oh trye AN i seen)
Related Information
Endocrine Disorders & Pregnancy *on page 1021*
Brand Names TACE®
Therapeutic Category Estrogen Derivative
Use Treat inoperable prostatic cancer; management of atrophic vaginitis, female hypogonadism, vasomotor symptoms of menopause
Usual Dosage Adults: Oral:
Atrophic vaginitis: 12-25 mg/day in 28-day cycles (21 days on and 7 days off)
Female hypogonadism: 12-25 mg cyclically for 21 days. May be followed by I.M. progesterone 100 mg or 5 days of oral progestin; next course may begin on day 5 of induced uterine bleeding.
Postpartum breast engorgement: 12 mg 4 times/day for 7 days or 50 mg every 6 hours for 6 doses; give first dose within 8 hours after delivery
Vasomotor symptoms associated with menopause: 12-25 mg cyclically for 30 days; one or more courses may be prescribed
Prostatic cancer (inoperable/progressing): 12-25 mg/day
Mechanism of Action Diethylstilbestrol derivative with similar estrogenic actions
Local Anesthetic/Vasoconstrictor Precautions No information available to require special precautions
Effects on Dental Treatment No effects or complications reported
Other Adverse Effects
>10%:
Cardiovascular: Peripheral edema
Endocrine & metabolic: Enlargement of breasts (female and male), breast tenderness
Gastrointestinal: Nausea, anorexia, bloating
1% to 10%:
Central nervous system: Headache
Endocrine & metabolic: Increased libido (female), decreased libido (male)
Gastrointestinal: Vomiting, diarrhea
<1%:
Cardiovascular: Hypertension, thromboembolism, myocardial infarction, edema
Central nervous system: Depression, dizziness, anxiety, stroke
Dermatologic: Chloasma, melasma, rash
Endocrine & metabolic: Breast tumors, amenorrhea, alterations in frequency and flow of menses, decreased glucose tolerance, hypertriglyceridemia, elevated LDL
Gastrointestinal: GI distress
Hepatic: Cholestatic jaundice
Ocular: Intolerance to contact lenses
Miscellaneous: Increased susceptibility to *Candida* infection
Drug Interactions No data reported
Drug Uptake
Onset of therapeutic effect: Commonly occurs within 14 days of therapy
Pregnancy Risk Factor X

Generic Available No

Chloroxine (klor OKS een)
Brand Names Capitrol®
Therapeutic Category Antiseborrheic Agent, Topical; Shampoos
Use Treatment of dandruff or seborrheic dermatitis of the scalp
Local Anesthetic/Vasoconstrictor Precautions No information available to require special precautions
Effects on Dental Treatment No effects or complications reported
Pregnancy Risk Factor C
Generic Available No

Chlorphed® [OTC] *see* Brompheniramine *on page 142*
Chlorphed®-LA Nasal Solution [OTC] *see* Oxymetazoline *on page 714*

Chlorphenesin (klor FEN e sin)
Brand Names Maolate®
Therapeutic Category Muscle Relaxant; Skeletal Muscle Relaxant
Use Adjunctive treatment of discomfort in short-term, acute, painful musculoskel-etal conditions
Local Anesthetic/Vasoconstrictor Precautions No information available to require special precautions
Effects on Dental Treatment No effects or complications reported
Other Adverse Effects
>10%: Central nervous system: Somnolence
1% to 10%:
Cardiovascular: Tachycardia, flushing of face, tightness in chest, syncope
Central nervous system: Mental depression, dizziness, lightheadedness, head-ache, paradoxical stimulation
Dermatologic: Angioedema
Gastrointestinal: Stomach cramps, nausea, vomiting
Neuromuscular & skeletal: Trembling
Ocular: Burning of eyes
Respiratory: Dyspnea
Miscellaneous: Allergic fever, hiccups
<1%:
Central nervous system: Ataxia
Dermatologic: Skin rash, urticaria, erythema multiforme
Hematologic: Aplastic anemia, leukopenia, eosinophilia
Ocular: Blurred vision
Pregnancy Risk Factor C
Generic Available No

Chlorpheniramine (klor fen IR a meen)
Related Information
Dentin Hypersensitivity; High Caries Index; Xerostomia *on page 1074*
Oral Bacterial Infections *on page 1059*
Brand Names Aller-Chlor® [OTC]; AL-R® [OTC]; Chlo-Amine® [OTC]; Chlorate® [OTC]; Chlor-Pro® [OTC]; Chlor-Trimeton® [OTC]; Phenetron®; Telachlor®; Teldrin® [OTC]
Canadian/Mexican Brand Names Chlor-Tripolon® (Canada)
Therapeutic Category Antihistamine
Synonyms Clorfeniramina, Maleato De (Mexico)
Use Perennial and seasonal allergic rhinitis and other allergic symptoms including urticaria
Usual Dosage
Children: Oral: 0.35 mg/kg/day in divided doses every 4-6 hours
2-6 years: 1 mg every 4-6 hours, not to exceed 6 mg in 24 hours
6-12 years: 2 mg every 4-6 hours, not to exceed 12 mg/day or sustained release 8 mg at bedtime
Children >12 years and Adults: Oral: 4 mg every 4-6 hours, not to exceed 24 mg/day or sustained release 8-12 mg every 8-12 hours, not to exceed 24 mg/day
Adults: Allergic reactions: I.M., I.V., S.C.: 10-20 mg as a single dose; maximum recommended dose: 40 mg/24 hours
Elderly: 4 mg once or twice daily. **Note:** Duration of action may be 36 hours or more when serum concentrations are low.

Hemodialysis effects: Supplemental dose is not necessary
Mechanism of Action Competes with histamine for H_1-receptor sites on effector cells in the gastrointestinal tract, blood vessels, and respiratory tract
Local Anesthetic/Vasoconstrictor Precautions No information available to require special precautions
(Continued)

Chlorpheniramine *(Continued)*

Effects on Dental Treatment Chronic use of antihistamines will inhibit salivary flow, particularly in elderly patients; this may contribute to periodontal disease and oral discomfort

Other Adverse Effects
Genitourinary: Urinary retention
Ocular: Diplopia
Renal: Polyuria

>10%:
Central nervous system: Slight to moderate drowsiness
Respiratory: Thickening of bronchial secretions
1% to 10%:
Central nervous system: Headache, excitability, fatigue, nervousness, dizziness
Gastrointestinal: Nausea, dry mouth, diarrhea, abdominal pain, appetite increase, weight gain
Neuromuscular & skeletal: Arthralgia, weakness
Respiratory: Pharyngitis
<1%:
Cardiovascular: Palpitations
Central nervous system: Depression
Dermatologic: Dermatitis, photosensitivity, angioedema
Hepatic: Hepatitis
Neuromuscular & skeletal: Myalgia, paresthesia
Respiratory: Bronchospasm, epistaxis

Drug Interactions Sedative effects of chlorpheniramine are enhanced by other CNS depressants, MAO inhibitors, alcohol, and tricyclic antidepressants

Drug Uptake
Serum half-life: 20-24 hours

Pregnancy Risk Factor B

Dosage Forms
Capsule, as maleate: 12 mg
Capsule, as maleate, timed release: 8 mg, 12 mg
Injection, as maleate: 10 mg/mL (1 mL, 30 mL); 100 mg/mL (2 mL)
Syrup, as maleate: 2 mg/5 mL (120 mL, 473 mL)
Tablet, as maleate: 4 mg, 8 mg, 12 mg
Tablet, as maleate:
Chewable: 2 mg
Timed release: 8 mg, 12 mg

Dietary Considerations May be taken with food or water

Generic Available Yes

Chlorpheniramine and Acetaminophen
(klor fen IR a meen & a seet a MIN oh fen)

Brand Names Coricidin® [OTC]

Therapeutic Category Analgesic, Non-narcotic; Antihistamine

Use Symptomatic relief of congestion, headache, aches and pains of colds and flu

Local Anesthetic/Vasoconstrictor Precautions No information available to require special precautions

Effects on Dental Treatment Chronic use of antihistamines will inhibit salivary flow, particularly in elderly patients; this may contribute to periodontal disease and oral discomfort

Generic Available Yes

Chlorpheniramine and Phenylephrine
(klor fen IR a meen & fen il EF rin)

Brand Names Dallergy-D® Syrup; Ed A-Hist® Liquid; Histatab® Plus Tablet [OTC]; Histor-D® Syrup; Rolatuss® Plain Liquid; Ru-Tuss® Liquid

Therapeutic Category Antihistamine/Decongestant Combination

Synonyms Phenylephrine and Chlorpheniramine

Use Temporary relief of nasal congestion and eustachian tube congestion as well as runny nose, sneezing, itching of nose or throat, itchy and watery eyes

Local Anesthetic/Vasoconstrictor Precautions Use with caution since phenylephrine is a sympathomimetic amine which could interact with epinephrine to cause a pressor response

Effects on Dental Treatment
Chlorpheniramine: Prolonged use will cause significant xerostomia
Phenylephrine: Up to 10% of patients could experience tachycardia, palpitations, and dry mouth; use vasoconstrictor with caution; prolonged use will cause significant xerostomia

Pregnancy Risk Factor C
Generic Available Yes

Chlorpheniramine and Phenylpropanolamine
(klor fen IR a meen & fen il proe pa NOLE a meen)

Brand Names Allerest® 12 Hour Capsule [OTC]; A.R.M.® Caplet [OTC]; Chlor-Rest® Tablet [OTC]; Demazin® Syrup [OTC]; Genamin® Cold Syrup [OTC]; Ornade® Spansule®; Resaid®; Rescon Liquid [OTC]; Silaminic® Cold Syrup [OTC]; Temazin® Cold Syrup [OTC]; Thera-Hist® Syrup [OTC]; Triaminic® Allergy Tablet [OTC]; Triaminic® Cold Tablet [OTC]; Triaminic® Syrup [OTC]; Tri-Nefrin® Extra Strength Tablet [OTC]; Triphenyl® Syrup [OTC]

Therapeutic Category Antihistamine/Decongestant Combination

Synonyms Phenylpropanolamine and Chlorpheniramine

Use Symptomatic relief of nasal congestion, runny nose, sneezing, itchy nose or throat, and itchy or watery eyes due to the common cold or allergic rhinitis

Local Anesthetic/Vasoconstrictor Precautions Use with caution since phenylpropanolamine is a sympathomimetic amine which could interact with epinephrine to cause a pressor response

Effects on Dental Treatment
Chlorpheniramine: Prolonged use will cause significant xerostomia
Phenylpropanolamine: Up to 10% of patients could experience tachycardia, palpitations, and dry mouth; use vasoconstrictor with caution; prolonged use will cause significant xerostomia

Pregnancy Risk Factor C
Generic Available Yes

Chlorpheniramine and Pseudoephedrine
(klor fen IR a meen & soo doe e FED rin)

Brand Names Allerest® Maximum Strength [OTC]; Anamine® Syrup [OTC]; Anaplex® Liquid [OTC]; Chlorafed® Liquid [OTC]; Chlor-Trimeton® 4 Hour Relief Tablet [OTC]; Co-Pyronil® 2 Pulvules® [OTC]; Deconamine® SR; Deconamine® Syrup [OTC]; Deconamine® Tablet [OTC]; Fedahist® Tablet [OTC]; Hayfebrol® Liquid [OTC]; Histalet® Syrup [OTC]; Klerist-D® Tablet [OTC]; Pseudo-Gest Plus® Tablet [OTC]; Rhinosyn® Liquid [OTC]; Rhinosyn-PD® Liquid [OTC]; Ryna® Liquid [OTC]; Sudafed Plus® Liquid [OTC]; Sudafed Plus® Tablet [OTC]

Therapeutic Category Antihistamine/Decongestant Combination

Synonyms Pseudoephedrine and Chlorpheniramine

Use Relief of nasal congestion associated with the common cold, hay fever, and other allergies, sinusitis, eustachian tube blockage, and vasomotor and allergic rhinitis

Local Anesthetic/Vasoconstrictor Precautions Use with caution since pseudoephedrine is a sympathomimetic amine which could interact with epinephrine to cause a pressor response

Effects on Dental Treatment
Chlorpheniramine: Prolonged use will cause significant xerostomia
Pseudoephedrine: Up to 10% of patients could experience tachycardia, palpitations, and dry mouth; use vasoconstrictor with caution; prolonged use will cause significant xerostomia

Pregnancy Risk Factor C
Generic Available Yes

Chlorpheniramine, Ephedrine, Phenylephrine, and Carbetapentane
(klor fen IR a meen, e FED rin, fen il EF rin, & kar bay ta PEN tane)

Brand Names Rentamine®; Rynatuss® Pediatric Suspension; Tri-Tannate® Plus

Therapeutic Category Antihistamine/Decongestant Combination

Use Symptomatic relief of cough

Local Anesthetic/Vasoconstrictor Precautions
Ephedrine: Use vasoconstrictors with caution since ephedrine may enhance cardiostimulation and vasopressor effects of sympathomimetics
Phenylephrine: Use with caution since phenylephrine is a sympathomimetic amine which could interact with epinephrine to cause a pressor response

Effects on Dental Treatment
Chlorpheniramine: Prolonged use will cause significant xerostomia
Ephedrine: No effects or complications reported
Phenylephrine: Up to 10% of patients could experience tachycardia, palpitations, and dry mouth; use vasoconstrictor with caution

Pregnancy Risk Factor C
Generic Available Yes

Chlorpheniramine, Phenindamine, and Phenylpropanolamine

(klor fen IR a meen, fen IN dah meen, & fen il proe pa NOLE a meen)

Brand Names Nolamine®

Therapeutic Category Antihistamine/Decongestant Combination

Use Upper respiratory and nasal congestion

Local Anesthetic/Vasoconstrictor Precautions Use with caution since phenylpropanolamine is a sympathomimetic amine which could interact with epinephrine to cause a pressor response

Effects on Dental Treatment

Chlorpheniramine: Prolonged use will cause significant xerostomia

Phenylpropanolamine: Up to 10% of patients could experience tachycardia, palpitations, and dry mouth; use vasoconstrictor with caution

Generic Available No

Chlorpheniramine, Phenylephrine, and Codeine

(klor fen IR a meen, fen il EF rin, & KOE deen)

Brand Names Pediacof®; Pedituss®

Therapeutic Category Antihistamine/Decongestant Combination; Cough Preparation

Use Symptomatic relief of rhinitis, nasal congestion and cough due to colds or allergy

Local Anesthetic/Vasoconstrictor Precautions Use with caution since phenylephrine is a sympathomimetic amine which could interact with epinephrine to cause a pressor response

Effects on Dental Treatment

Chlorpheniramine: Prolonged use will cause significant xerostomia

Codeine: <1%: Dry mouth

Phenylephrine: Up to 10% of patients could experience tachycardia, palpitations, and dry mouth; use vasoconstrictor with caution; prolonged use will cause significant xerostomia

Generic Available No

Chlorpheniramine, Phenylephrine, and Dextromethorphan

(klor fen IR a meen, fen il EF rin, & deks troe meth OR fan)

Brand Names Cerose-DM® [OTC]

Therapeutic Category Antihistamine/Decongestant Combination; Cough Preparation

Use Temporary relief of cough due to minor throat and bronchial irritation; relieves nasal congestion, runny nose and sneezing

Local Anesthetic/Vasoconstrictor Precautions

Chlorpheniramine, Dextromethorphan: No information available to require special precautions

Phenylephrine: Use with caution since phenylephrine is a sympathomimetic amine which could interact with epinephrine to cause a pressor response

Effects on Dental Treatment

Chlorpheniramine: Prolonged use will cause significant xerostomia

Dextromethorphan: No effects or complications reported

Phenylephrine: Up to 10% of patients could experience tachycardia, palpitations, and dry mouth; use vasoconstrictor with caution; prolonged use will cause significant xerostomia

Warnings/Precautions Research on chicken embryos exposed to concentrations of dextromethorphan relative to those typically taken by humans has shown to cause birth defects and fetal death; more study is needed, but it is suggested that pregnant women should be advised not to use dextromethorphan-containing medications

Generic Available No

Chlorpheniramine, Phenylephrine, and Methscopolamine

(klor fen IR a meen, fen il EF rin, & meth skoe POL a meen)

Brand Names Alersule Forte®; D.A.II® Tablet; Dallergy®; Dura-Vent/DA®; Extendryl® SR; Histor-D® Timecelles®

Therapeutic Category Antihistamine/Decongestant Combination

Use Relieves nasal congestion, runny nose and sneezing

Local Anesthetic/Vasoconstrictor Precautions Use with caution since phenylephrine is a sympathomimetic amine which could interact with epinephrine to cause a pressor response

Effects on Dental Treatment
   Chlorpheniramine: Prolonged use will cause significant xerostomia
   Methscopolamine: Anticholinergic side effects can cause a reduction of saliva production or secretion contributes to discomfort and dental disease (ie, caries, oral candidiasis and periodontal disease)
   Phenylephrine: Up to 10% of patients could experience tachycardia, palpitations, and dry mouth; use vasoconstrictor with caution
Generic Available Yes

Chlorpheniramine, Phenylephrine, and Phenylpropanolamine
(klor fen IR a meen, fen il EF rin, & fen il proe pa NOLE a meen)
Brand Names Hista-Vadrin® Tablet
Therapeutic Category Antihistamine/Decongestant Combination
Use Symptomatic relief of rhinitis and nasal congestion due to colds or allergy
Local Anesthetic/Vasoconstrictor Precautions Use with caution since phenylephrine and phenylpropanolamine are sympathomimetic amines which could interact with epinephrine to cause a pressor response
Effects on Dental Treatment Up to 10% of patients could experience tachycardia, palpitations, and dry mouth; use vasoconstrictor with caution; prolonged use will cause significant xerostomia
Pregnancy Risk Factor C
Generic Available Yes

Chlorpheniramine, Phenylephrine, and Phenyltoloxamine
(klor fen IR a meen, fen il EF rin, & fen il tole LOKS a meen)
Brand Names Comhist®; Comhist® LA
Therapeutic Category Antihistamine/Decongestant Combination
Use Symptomatic relief of rhinitis and nasal congestion due to colds or allergy
Local Anesthetic/Vasoconstrictor Precautions Use with caution since phenylephrine is a sympathomimetic amine which could interact with epinephrine to cause a pressor response
Effects on Dental Treatment
   Chlorpheniramine: Prolonged use will cause significant xerostomia
   Phenylephrine: Up to 10% of patients could experience tachycardia, palpitations, and dry mouth; use vasoconstrictor with caution
Pregnancy Risk Factor C
Generic Available No

Chlorpheniramine, Phenylephrine, Phenylpropanolamine, and Belladonna Alkaloids
(klor fen IR a meen, fen il EF rin, fen il proe pa NOLE a meen, & bel a DON a AL ka loydz)
Brand Names Atrohist® Plus; Phenahist-TR®; Phenchlor® S.H.A.; Ru-Tuss®; Stahist®
Therapeutic Category Cold Preparation
Synonyms Phenylephrine, Chlorpheniramine, Phenylpropanolamine, and Belladonna Alkaloids; Phenylpropanolamine, Chlorpheniramine, Phenylephrine, and Belladonna Alkaloids
Use Relief of symptoms resulting from irritation of sinus, nasal, and upper respiratory tract tissues, including nasal congestion, watering eyes, and postnasal drip; this product contains anticholinergic agents and should be reserved for patients who do not respond to other antihistamine/decongestants
Usual Dosage Oral: Children ≥12 years and Adults: One tablet morning and evening, swallowed whole
Local Anesthetic/Vasoconstrictor Precautions Use with caution since phenylpropanolamine & phenylephrine are sympathomimetic amines which could interact with epinephrine to cause a pressor response
Effects on Dental Treatment
   Chlorpheniramine: Prolonged use will cause significant xerostomia
   Phenylephrine, Phenylpropanolamine: Up to 10% of patients could experience tachycardia, palpitations, and dry mouth; use vasoconstrictor with caution
Pregnancy Risk Factor C
Dosage Forms Tablet, sustained release: Chlorpheniramine 8 mg, phenylephrine 25 mg, phenylpropanolamine 50 mg, hyoscyamine 0.19 mg, atropine 0.04 mg, and scopolamine 0.01 mg
Generic Available Yes

Chlorpheniramine, Phenylpropanolamine, and Acetaminophen

(klor fen IR a meen, fen il proe pa NOLE a meen, & a seet a MIN oh fen)

Brand Names BQ® Tablet [OTC]; Congestant D® [OTC]; Coricidin ©D'® [OTC]; Dapacin® Cold Capsule [OTC]; Duadacin® Capsule [OTC]; Tylenol® Cold Effervescent Medication Tablet [OTC]

Therapeutic Category Analgesic, Non-narcotic; Antihistamine/Decongestant Combination

Use Symptomatic relief of nasal congestion and headache from colds/sinus congestion

Local Anesthetic/Vasoconstrictor Precautions Use with caution since phenylpropanolamine is a sympathomimetic amine which could interact with epinephrine to cause a pressor response

Effects on Dental Treatment

Acetaminophen: No effects or complications reported

Chlorpheniramine: Prolonged use will cause significant xerostomia

Phenylpropanolamine: Up to 10% of patients could experience tachycardia, palpitations, and dry mouth; use vasoconstrictor with caution

Generic Available Yes

Chlorpheniramine, Phenylpropanolamine, and Dextromethorphan

(klor fen IR a meen, fen il proe pa NOLE a meen, & deks troe meth OR fan)

Brand Names Triaminicol® Multi-Symptom Cold Syrup [OTC]

Therapeutic Category Antihistamine/Decongestant Combination; Cough Preparation

Use Provides relief of runny nose, sneezing, suppresses cough, promotes nasal and sinus drainage

Local Anesthetic/Vasoconstrictor Precautions Use with caution since phenylpropanolamine is a sympathomimetic amine which could interact with epinephrine to cause a pressor response

Effects on Dental Treatment

Chlorpheniramine: Prolonged use will cause significant xerostomia

Dextromethorphan: No effects or complications reported

Phenylpropanolamine: Up to 10% of patients could experience tachycardia, palpitations, and dry mouth; use vasoconstrictor with caution; prolonged use will cause significant xerostomia

Warnings/Precautions Research on chicken embryos exposed to concentrations of dextromethorphan relative to those typically taken by humans has shown to cause birth defects and fetal death; more study is needed, but it is suggested that pregnant women should be advised not to use dextromethorphan-containing medications

Pregnancy Risk Factor C (see Warnings)

Generic Available Yes

Comments Alcohol free

Chlorpheniramine, Phenyltoloxamine, Phenylpropanolamine, and Phenylephrine

(klor fen IR a meen, fen il tole LOKS a meen, fen il proe pa NOLE a meen & fen il EF rin)

Brand Names Naldecon®; Naldelate®; Nalgest®; Nalspan®; New Decongestant®; Par Decon®; Tri-Phen-Chlor®; Uni-Decon®

Therapeutic Category Antihistamine/Decongestant Combination

Use Symptomatic treatment of nasal and eustachian tube congestion associated with sinusitis and acute upper respiratory infection; symptomatic relief of perennial and allergic rhinitis

Local Anesthetic/Vasoconstrictor Precautions Use with caution since phenylpropanolamine & phenylephrine are sympathomimetic amines which could interact with epinephrine to cause a pressor response

Effects on Dental Treatment

Chlorpheniramine: Prolonged use will cause significant xerostomia

Phenylephrine, Phenylpropanolamine: Up to 10% of patients could experience tachycardia, palpitations, and dry mouth; use vasoconstrictor with caution

Pregnancy Risk Factor C

Generic Available Yes

Chlorpheniramine, Pseudoephedrine, and Codeine
(klor fen IR a meen, soo doe e FED rin, & KOE deen)

Brand Names Codehist® DH; Decohistine® DH; Dihistine® DH; Ryna-C® Liquid

Therapeutic Category Antihistamine/Decongestant Combination; Cough Preparation

Use Temporary relief of cough associated with minor throat or bronchial irritation or nasal congestion due to common cold, allergic rhinitis, or sinusitis

Local Anesthetic/Vasoconstrictor Precautions Use with caution since pseudoephedrine is a sympathomimetic amine which could interact with epinephrine to cause a pressor response

Effects on Dental Treatment
Chlorpheniramine: Prolonged use will cause significant xerostomia
Codeine: <1%: Dry mouth
Pseudoephedrine: Up to 10% of patients could experience tachycardia, palpitations, and dry mouth; use vasoconstrictor with caution

Other Adverse Effects 1% to 10%:
Cardiovascular: Hypotension
Central nervous system: Sedation, dizziness, drowsiness, increased intracranial pressure
Gastrointestinal: Constipation, biliary tract spasm
Genitourinary: Urinary tract spasm
Miscellaneous: Physical or psychological dependence with continued use

Pregnancy Risk Factor C

Generic Available Yes

Chlorpheniramine, Pyrilamine, and Phenylephrine
(klor fen IR a meen, pye RIL a meen, & fen il EF rin)

Brand Names Rhinatate® Tablet; R-Tannamine® Tablet; R-Tannate® Tablet; Rynatan® Pediatric Suspension; Rynatan® Tablet; Tanoral® Tablet; Triotann® Tablet; Tri-Tannate® Tablet

Therapeutic Category Antihistamine/Decongestant Combination

Use Symptomatic relief of nasal congestion associated with upper respiratory tract condition

Local Anesthetic/Vasoconstrictor Precautions Use with caution since phenylephrine is a sympathomimetic amine which could interact with epinephrine to cause a pressor response

Effects on Dental Treatment
Chlorpheniramine: Prolonged use will cause significant xerostomia
Phenylephrine: Up to 10% of patients could experience tachycardia, palpitations, and dry mouth; use vasoconstrictor with caution

Pregnancy Risk Factor C

Generic Available Yes

Chlorpheniramine, Pyrilamine, Phenylephrine, and Phenylpropanolamine
(klor fen IR a meen, pye RIL a meen, fen il EF rin, & fen il proe pa NOLE a meen)

Brand Names Histalet Forte® Tablet

Therapeutic Category Antihistamine/Decongestant Combination

Use Symptomatic relief of rhinitis and nasal congestion due to colds or allergy

Local Anesthetic/Vasoconstrictor Precautions Use with caution since phenylephrine & phenylpropanolamine are sympathomimetic amines which could interact with epinephrine to cause a pressor response

Effects on Dental Treatment
Chlorpheniramine: Prolonged use will cause significant xerostomia
Phenylephrine, Phenylpropanolamine: Up to 10% of patients could experience tachycardia, palpitations, and dry mouth; use vasoconstrictor with caution

Pregnancy Risk Factor C

Generic Available Yes

Chlor-Pro® [OTC] *see* Chlorpheniramine *on page 217*

Chlorpromazine (klor PROE ma zeen)

Brand Names Ormazine; Thorazine®

Canadian/Mexican Brand Names Apo®-Chlorpromazine (Canada); Chlorpromanyl® (Canada); Chlorprom® (Canada); Largactil® (Canada); Novo-Chlorpromazine® (Canada)

Therapeutic Category Antiemetic; Antipsychotic Agent; Phenothiazine Derivative

Use Treatment of psychoses, nausea and vomiting; Tourette's syndrome; mania; intractable hiccups (adults); behavioral problems (children)
(Continued)

Chlorpromazine *(Continued)*

Usual Dosage

Children >6 months:

Psychosis:

Oral: 0.5-1 mg/kg/dose every 4-6 hours; older children may require 200 mg/day or higher

I.M., I.V.: 0.5-1 mg/kg/dose every 6-8 hours; maximum dose for <5 years (22.7 kg): 40 mg/day; maximum for 5-12 years (22.7-45.5 kg): 75 mg/day

Nausea and vomiting:

Oral: 0.5-1 mg/kg/dose every 4-6 hours as needed

I.M., I.V.: 0.5-1 mg/kg/dose every 6-8 hours; maximum dose for <5 years (22.7 kg): 40 mg/day; maximum for 5-12 years (22.7-45.5 kg): 75 mg/day

Rectal: 1 mg/kg/dose every 6-8 hours as needed

Adults:

Psychosis:

Oral: Range: 30-800 mg/day in 1-4 divided doses, initiate at lower doses and titrate as needed; usual dose: 200 mg/day; some patients may require 1-2 g/day

I.M., I.V.: Initial: 25 mg, may repeat (25-50 mg) in 1-4 hours, gradually increase to a maximum of 400 mg/dose every 4-6 hours until patient is controlled; usual dose: 300-800 mg/day

Intractable hiccups: Oral, I.M.: 25-50 mg 3-4 times/day

Nausea and vomiting:

Oral: 10-25 mg every 4-6 hours

I.M., I.V.: 25-50 mg every 4-6 hours

Rectal: 50-100 mg every 6-8 hours

Elderly (nonpsychotic patient; dementia behavior): Initial: 10-25 mg 1-2 times/day; increase at 4- to 7-day intervals by 10-25 mg/day. Increase dose intervals (bid, tid, etc) as necessary to control behavior response or side effects; maximum daily dose: 800 mg; gradual increases (titration) may prevent some side effects or decrease their severity.

Not dialyzable (0% to 5%)

Mechanism of Action Blocks postsynaptic mesolimbic dopaminergic receptors in the brain; exhibits a strong alpha-adrenergic blocking effect and depresses the release of hypothalamic and hypophyseal hormones; believed to depress the reticular-activating system, thus affecting basal metabolism, body temperature, wakefulness, vasomotor tone, and emesis

Local Anesthetic/Vasoconstrictor Precautions No information available to require special precautions

Effects on Dental Treatment Significant hypotension may occur, especially when the drug is administered parenterally; orthostatic hypotension is due to alpha-receptor blockade, the elderly are at greater risk for orthostatic hypotension

Tardive dyskinesia: Prevalence rate may be 40% in elderly; development of the syndrome and the irreversible nature are proportional to duration and total cumulative dose over time

Extrapyramidal reactions are more common in elderly with up to 50% developing these reactions after 60 years of age; drug-induced **Parkinson's syndrome** occurs often; **Akathisia** is the most common extrapyramidal reaction in elderly

Increased confusion, memory loss, psychotic behavior, and agitation frequently occur as a consequence of anticholinergic effects

Antipsychotic associated sedation in nonpsychotic patients is extremely unpleasant due to feelings of depersonalization, derealization, and dysphoria

Other Adverse Effects

>10%:

Cardiovascular: Hypotension (especially with I.V. use), tachycardia, arrhythmias, orthostatic hypotension

Central nervous system: Pseudoparkinsonism, akathisia, dystonias, tardive dyskinesia (persistent), dizziness

Gastrointestinal: Constipation

Ocular: Pigmentary retinopathy

Respiratory: Nasal congestion

Miscellaneous: Decreased sweating

1% to 10%:

Dermatologic: Pruritus, rash, photosensitivity

Endocrine & metabolic: Amenorrhea, galactorrhea, gynecomastia, changes in libido, pain in breasts

Gastrointestinal: GI upset, nausea, vomiting, stomach pain, weight gain, dry mouth

Genitourinary: Dysuria, ejaculatory disturbances, urinary retention
Neuromuscular & skeletal: Trembling of fingers
Ocular: Blurred vision
<1%:
Central nervous system: Sedation, drowsiness, restlessness, anxiety, extrapy-ramidal reactions, seizures, altered central temperature regulation, lowering of seizures threshold, neuroleptic malignant syndrome (NMS)
Dermatologic: Discoloration of skin (blue-gray)
Genitourinary: Priapism
Hematologic: Agranulocytosis (more often in women between 4th and 10th weeks of therapy), leukopenia (usually in patients with large doses for prolonged periods)
Hepatic: Cholestatic jaundice, hepatotoxicity
Ocular: Cornea and lens changes
Miscellaneous: Anaphylactoid reactions
Warnings/Precautions Safety in children <6 months of age has not been established; use with caution in patients with seizures, bone marrow depression, or severe liver disease
Drug Interactions Increased toxicity: Additive effects with other CNS-depressants
Drug Uptake
Serum half-life, biphasic:
Initial: 2 hours
Terminal: 30 hours
Pregnancy Risk Factor C
Generic Available Yes

Chlorpropamide (klor PROE pa mide)

Related Information
Endocrine Disorders & Pregnancy *on page 1021*
Brand Names Diabinese®
Canadian/Mexican Brand Names Apo®-Chlorpropamide (Canada); Deavynfar® (Mexico); Insogen® (Mexico); Novo-Propamide® (Canada)
Therapeutic Category Antidiabetic Agent; Hypoglycemic Agent, Oral; Sulfonylurea Agent
Synonyms Clorpropamida (Mexico)
Use Control blood sugar in adult onset, noninsulin-dependent diabetes (type II); **unlabeled use:** Neurogenic diabetes insipidus
Usual Dosage Oral: The dosage of chlorpropamide is variable and should be individualized based upon the patient's response
Initial dose:
Adults: 250 mg/day in mild to moderate diabetes in middle-aged, stable diabetic
Elderly: 100-125 mg/day in older patients
Maintenance dose: 100-250 mg/day; severe diabetics may require 500 mg/day; avoid doses >750 mg/day
Mechanism of Action Stimulates insulin release from the pancreatic beta cells; reduces glucose output from the liver; insulin sensitivity is increased at peripheral target sites
Local Anesthetic/Vasoconstrictor Precautions No information available to require special precautions
Effects on Dental Treatment Chlorpropamide-dependent diabetics (noninsulin dependent, Type II) should be appointed for dental treatment in morning in order to minimize chance of stress-induced hypoglycemia
Other Adverse Effects
>10%:
Central nervous system: Headache, dizziness
Gastrointestinal: Anorexia, constipation, heartburn, epigastric fullness, nausea, vomiting, diarrhea
1% to 10%: Dermatologic: Skin rash, urticaria, photosensitivity
<1%:
Cardiovascular: Edema
Endocrine & metabolic: Hypoglycemia, hyponatremia, SIADH
Hematologic: Blood dyscrasias, aplastic anemia, hemolytic anemia, bone marrow suppression, thrombocytopenia, agranulocytosis
Hepatic: Cholestatic jaundice
Drug Interactions
Excessive ethanol intake may lead to hypoglycemia; "antabuse-like" reaction may occur in patients taking chlorpropamide
Salicylates may enhance the hypoglycemic response to chlorpropamide due to increased plasma levels of chlorpropamide by displacing from plasma proteins
(Continued)

Chlorpropamide *(Continued)*

Thiazide diuretics will increase blood glucose leading to increased requirements of chlorpropamide

Drug Uptake
Peak effect: Oral: Within 6-8 hours
Serum half-life: 30-42 hours; prolonged in the elderly or with renal disease
Time to peak serum concentration: Within 3-4 hours

Pregnancy Risk Factor C
Generic Available Yes

Chlorprothixene *(klor proe THIKS een)*

Brand Names Taractan®
Therapeutic Category Antipsychotic Agent
Use Management of psychotic disorders
Usual Dosage
Children >6 years: Oral: 10-25 mg 3-4 times/day

Adults:
Oral: 25-50 mg 3-4 times/day, to be increased as needed; doses exceeding 600 mg/day are rarely required
I.M.: 25-50 mg up to 3-4 times/day

Not dialyzable (0% to 5%)

Mechanism of Action The mechanism of action for chlorprothixene, like other thioxanthenes and phenothiazines, is not fully understood. The sites of action appear to be the reticular activating system of the midbrain, the limbic system, the hypothalamus, and the globus pallidus and corpus striatum. The mechanism appears to be one or more of a combination of postsynaptic blockade of adrenergic, dopaminergic, or serotonergic receptor sites, metabolic inhibition of oxidative phosphorylation, or decrease in the excitability of neuronal membranes.

Local Anesthetic/Vasoconstrictor Precautions No information available to require special precautions

Effects on Dental Treatment Over 10% of dental patients may experience tardive dyskinesia and Parkinson-like syndromes; orthostatic hypotension is induced by chlorprothixene in over 10% of patients

Other Adverse Effects
>10%:
Cardiovascular: Hypotension, orthostatic hypotension
Central nervous system: Pseudoparkinsonism, akathisia, dystonias, tardive dyskinesia (persistent), dizziness
Gastrointestinal: Constipation
Ocular: Pigmentary retinopathy
Respiratory: Nasal congestion
Miscellaneous: Decreased sweating
1% to 10%:
Dermatologic: Photosensitivity, skin rash
Endocrine & metabolic: Changes in menstrual cycle, changes in libido, pain in breasts
Gastrointestinal: Weight gain, nausea, vomiting, stomach pain
Genitourinary: Dysuria, ejaculatory disturbances
Neuromuscular & skeletal: Trembling of fingers
<1%:
Central nervous system: Neuroleptic malignant syndrome (NMS)
Dermatologic: discoloration of skin (blue-gray)
Endocrine & metabolic: Galactorrhea
Genitourinary: Priapism
Hematologic: Agranulocytosis, leukopenia
Hepatic: Cholestatic jaundice, hepatotoxicity
Ocular: Cornea and lens changes, pigmentary retinopathy
Miscellaneous: Impairment of temperature regulation lowering of seizures threshold

Drug Interactions
Decreased effect of guanethidine
Increased effect/toxicity: Alcohol, CNS depressants

Pregnancy Risk Factor C
Generic Available No

Chlor-Rest® Tablet [OTC] *see* Chlorpheniramine and Phenylpropanolamine *on page 219*

Chlortetracycline *(klor tet ra SYE kleen)*

Brand Names Aureomycin®
Canadian/Mexican Brand Names Aureomicina® (Mexico)

Therapeutic Category Antibiotic, Ophthalmic; Antibiotic, Tetracycline Derivative

Synonyms Clortetraciclina (Mexico)

Use

Ophthalmic: Treatment of superficial ocular infections involving the conjunctiva or cornea due to strains of susceptible microorganisms

Topical: Treatment of superficial infections of the skin due to susceptible organisms, also infection prophylaxis in minor skin abrasions

Usual Dosage

Ophthalmic:

Acute infections: Instill ½" (1.25 cm) every 3-4 hours until improvement

Mild to moderate infections: Instill ½" (1.25 cm) 2-3 times/day

Topical: Apply 1-4 times/day, cover with sterile bandage if needed

Mechanism of Action Inhibits bacterial protein synthesis by binding with the 30S and possibly the 50S ribosomal subunit(s) of susceptible bacteria; may also cause alterations in the cytoplasmic membrane; usually bacteriostatic, may be bactericidal

Local Anesthetic/Vasoconstrictor Precautions No information available to require special precautions

Effects on Dental Treatment No effects or complications reported

Other Adverse Effects

1% to 10%: Dermatologic: Faint yellowing of skin

<1%: Dermatologic: Redness, swelling, irritation, photosensitivity

Drug Interactions No data reported

Pregnancy Risk Factor D

Dosage Forms Ointment:

Ophthalmic: 1% [10 mg/g] (3.5 g)

Topical: 3% (14.2 g, 30 g)

Generic Available Yes

Chlorthalidone (klor THAL i done)

Related Information

Cardiovascular Diseases *on page 1010*

Brand Names Hygroton®; Thalitone®

Canadian/Mexican Brand Names Apo®-Chlorthalidone (Canada); Higroton® 50 (Mexico); Novo-Thalidone® (Canada); Uridon® (Canada)

Therapeutic Category Diuretic, Thiazide

Synonyms Clortalidona (Mexico)

Use Management of mild to moderate hypertension, used alone or in combination with other agents; treatment of edema associated with congestive heart failure, nephrotic syndrome, or pregnancy. Recent studies have found chlorthalidone effective in the treatment of isolated systolic hypertension in the elderly.

Usual Dosage Oral:

Children: 2 mg/kg/dose 3 times/week or 1-2 mg/kg/day

Adults: 25-100 mg/day or 100 mg 3 times/week

Elderly: Initial: 12.5-25 mg/day or every other day; there is little advantage to using doses >25 mg/day

Mechanism of Action Sulfonamide-derived diuretic that inhibits sodium and chloride reabsorption in the cortical-diluting segment of the ascending loop of Henle

Local Anesthetic/Vasoconstrictor Precautions No information available to require special precautions

Effects on Dental Treatment No effects or complications reported

Other Adverse Effects

1% to 10%: Endocrine & metabolic: Hypokalemia

<1%:

Cardiovascular: Hypotension

Dermatologic: Photosensitivity

Endocrine & metabolic: Fluid and electrolyte imbalances (hypocalcemia, hypomagnesemia, hyponatremia), hyperglycemia

Hematologic: Rarely blood dyscrasias

Renal: Prerenal azotemia

Drug Interactions

Decreased absorption of thiazides with cholestyramine resins; chlorthalidone may cause a decreased effect of oral hypoglycemics

Increased toxicity: Digitalis glycosides, lithium (decreased clearance), probenecid

Drug Uptake

Peak effect: 2-6 hours

Absorption: Oral: 65%

(Continued)

Chlorthalidone *(Continued)*

Serum half-life: 35-55 hours; may be prolonged with renal impairment, with anuria: 81 hours

Pregnancy Risk Factor D

Generic Available Yes

Chlor-Trimeton® [OTC] *see* Chlorpheniramine *on page 217*

Chlor-Trimeton® 4 Hour Relief Tablet [OTC] *see* Chlorpheniramine and Pseudoephedrine *on page 219*

Chlorzoxazone *(klor ZOKS a zone)*

Related Information

Temporomandibular Dysfunction (TMD) *on page 1078*

Brand Names Flexaphen®; Paraflex®; Parafon Forte™ DSC

Therapeutic Category Centrally Acting Skeletal Muscle Relaxant; Muscle Relaxant; Skeletal Muscle Relaxant

Use

Dental: Treatment of muscle spasm with acute temporomandibular joint pain

Medical: Treatment of muscle spasm associated with acute painful musculoskeletal conditions

Mechanism of Action Acts on the spinal cord and subcortical levels by depressing polysynaptic reflexes

Local Anesthetic/Vasoconstrictor Precautions No information available to require special precautions

Effects on Dental Treatment No effects or complications reported

Other Adverse Effects

>10%: Central nervous system: Drowsiness

1% to 10%:

Cardiovascular: Tachycardia, tightness in chest, flushing of face, syncope

Central nervous system: Mental depression, dizziness, lightheadedness, headache, paradoxical stimulation

Dermatologic: Angioedema

Gastrointestinal: Nausea, vomiting, stomach cramps

Neuromuscular & skeletal: Trembling

Ocular: Burning of eyes

Respiratory: Dyspnea

Miscellaneous: Hiccups, allergic fever

Drug Interactions Alcohol, CNS depressants

Drug Uptake

Onset of action: Within 1 hour

Pregnancy Risk Factor C

Breast-feeding Considerations No data reported

Dosage Forms

Caplet (Parafon Forte™ DSC): 500 mg

Capsule (Flexaphen®, Mus-Lax®): 250 mg with acetaminophen 300 mg

Tablet: Paraflex®: 250 mg

Dietary Considerations No data reported

Generic Available Yes

Cholac® *see* Lactulose *on page 540*

Cholan-HMB® *see* Dehydrocholic Acid *on page 285*

Cholecalciferol *(kole e kal SI fer ole)*

Brand Names Delta-D®

Therapeutic Category Vitamin D Analog

Synonyms D_3

Use Dietary supplement, treatment of vitamin D deficiency or prophylaxis of deficiency

Local Anesthetic/Vasoconstrictor Precautions No information available to require special precautions

Effects on Dental Treatment No effects or complications reported

Other Adverse Effects

1% to 10%:

Cardiovascular: Hypotension, cardiac arrhythmias, hypertension

Central nervous system: Irritability, headache

Dermatologic: Pruritus

Endocrine & metabolic: Polydypsia

Gastrointestinal: Nausea, vomiting, anorexia, pancreatitis, metallic taste

Neuromuscular & skeletal: Bone pain, myalgia

Ocular: Conjunctivitis, photophobia

Renal: Polyuria

<1%:
  Central nervous system: Overt psychosis
  Gastrointestinal: Weight loss
Pregnancy Risk Factor C
Generic Available No
Comments Cholecalciferol 1 mg = 40,000 units of vitamin D activity

Choledyl® *see* Oxtriphylline *on page 708*

Cholera Vaccine (KOL er a vak SEEN)
Therapeutic Category Vaccine, Inactivated Bacteria
Use Primary immunization for cholera prophylaxis
Usual Dosage
  Children:
    6 months to 4 years: Two 0.2 mL doses I.M./S.C. 1 week to 1 month apart; booster doses (0.2 mL I.M./S.C.) every 6 months
    5-10 years: Two 0.3 mL doses I.M./S.C. or two 0.2 mL intradermal doses 1 week to 1 month apart; booster doses (0.3 mL I.M./S.C. or 0.2 mL I.D.) every 6 months

  Children ≥10 years and Adults: Two 0.5 mL doses given I.M./S.C. or two 0.2 mL doses I.D. 1 week to 1 month apart; booster doses (0.5 mL I.M. or S.C. or 0.2 mL I.D.) every 6 months
Mechanism of Action Inactivated vaccine producing active immunization
Local Anesthetic/Vasoconstrictor Precautions No information available to require special precautions
Effects on Dental Treatment No effects or complications reported
Other Adverse Effects >10%:
  Cardiovascular: Swelling
  Central nervous system: Malaise, fever, headache, pain
  Dermatologic: Tenderness, erythema
  Local: Induration at injection site
Pregnancy Risk Factor C
Generic Available No
Comments Inactivated bacteria vaccine

Cholestyramine Resin (koe LES tir a meen REZ in)
Related Information
  Cardiovascular Diseases *on page 1010*
Brand Names Prevalite®; Questran®; Questran® Light
Canadian/Mexican Brand Names PMS-Cholestyramine® (Canada)
Therapeutic Category Lipid Lowering Drugs
Synonyms Colestiramina (Mexico)
Use Adjunct in the management of primary hypercholesterolemia; pruritus associated with elevated levels of bile acids; diarrhea associated with excess fecal bile acids; binding toxicologic agents; pseudomembraneous colitis
Usual Dosage Oral (dosages are expressed in terms of anhydrous resin):
  Powder:
    Children: 240 mg/kg/day in 3 divided doses; need to titrate dose depending on indication
    Adults: 4 g 1-6 times/day to a maximum of 16-32 g/day
  Tablet: Adults: Initial: 4 g once or twice daily; maintenance: 8-16 g/day in 2 divided doses

  Not removed by hemo- or peritoneal dialysis; supplemental doses not necessary with dialysis or continuous arterio-venous or veno-venous hemofiltration effects
Mechanism of Action Forms a nonabsorbable complex with bile acids in the intestine, releasing chloride ions in the process; inhibits enterohepatic reuptake of intestinal bile salts and thereby increases the fecal loss of bile salt-bound low density lipoprotein cholesterol
Local Anesthetic/Vasoconstrictor Precautions No information available to require special precautions
Effects on Dental Treatment No effects or complications reported
Other Adverse Effects
  1% to 10%: Gastrointestinal: Constipation
  <1%:
    Dermatologic: Rash; irritation of perianal area, skin, or tongue
    Endocrine & metabolic: Hyperchloremic acidosis
    Gastrointestinal: Nausea, vomiting, abdominal distention and pain, malabsorption of fat-soluble vitamins, intestinal obstruction, steatorrhea
    Hematologic: Hypoprothrombinemia (secondary to vitamin K deficiency)
    Renal: Elevated urinary calcium excretion
  (Continued)

Cholestyramine Resin *(Continued)*

Drug Interactions Decreased effect: Decreased absorption (oral) of digitalis glycosides, warfarin, thyroid hormones, thiazide diuretics, propranolol, phenobarbital, amiodarone, methotrexate, NSAIDs, and other drugs by binding to the drug in the intestine

Drug Uptake
Absorption: Not absorbed from the GI tract
Peak effect: 21 days

Pregnancy Risk Factor C

Generic Available Yes

Choline Magnesium Trisalicylate
(KOE leen mag NEE zhum trye sa LIS i late)

Related Information
Rheumatoid Arthritis and Osteoarthritis *on page 1030*

Brand Names Trilisate®

Therapeutic Category Analgesic, Non-narcotic; Anti-inflammatory Agent; Nonsteroidal Anti-inflammatory Agent (NSAID), Oral; Salicylate

Use Management of osteoarthritis, rheumatoid arthritis, and other arthritis; salicylate salts may not inhibit platelet aggregation and, therefore, should not be substituted for aspirin in the prophylaxis of thrombosis

Usual Dosage Oral (based on total salicylate content):
Children <37 kg: 50 mg/kg/day given in 2 divided doses
Adults: 500 mg to 1.5 g 2-3 times/day; usual maintenance dose: 1-4.5 g/day

Mechanism of Action Inhibits prostaglandin synthesis; acts on the hypothalamus heat-regulating center to reduce fever; blocks the generation of pain impulses

Local Anesthetic/Vasoconstrictor Precautions No information available to require special precautions

Effects on Dental Treatment No effects or complications reported

Other Adverse Effects
>10%: Gastrointestinal: Nausea, heartburn, stomach pains, dyspepsia, epigastric discomfort
1% to 10%:
Central nervous system: Fatigue
Dermatologic: Skin rash
Gastrointestinal: Gastrointestinal ulceration
Hematologic: Hemolytic anemia
Neuromuscular & skeletal: Weakness
Respiratory: Dyspnea
Miscellaneous: Anaphylactic shock
<1%:
Central nervous system: Insomnia, nervousness, jitters
Hematologic: Occult bleeding, prolongation of bleeding time, leukopenia, thrombocytopenia, iron deficiency anemia
Hepatic: Hepatotoxicity
Renal: Impaired renal function
Respiratory: Bronchospasm

Drug Interactions
Decreased effect with antacids
Increased effect of warfarin

Drug Uptake
Absorption: Absorbed from the stomach and small intestine
Serum half-life: Dose-dependent ranging from 2-3 hours at low doses to 30 hours at high doses
Time to peak serum concentration: ~2 hours

Pregnancy Risk Factor C

Generic Available Yes

Choline Salicylate (KOE leen sa LIS i late)

Brand Names Arthropan® [OTC]

Canadian/Mexican Brand Names Teejel® (Canada)

Therapeutic Category Analgesic, Non-narcotic; Anti-inflammatory Agent; Nonsteroidal Anti-inflammatory Agent (NSAID), Oral; Salicylate

Use Temporary relief of pain of rheumatoid arthritis, rheumatic fever, osteoarthritis, and other conditions for which oral salicylates are recommended; useful in patients in which there is difficulty in administering doses in a tablet or capsule dosage form, because of the liquid dosage form

Usual Dosage
Children >12 years and Adults: Oral: 5 mL (870 mg) every 3-4 hours, if necessary, but not more than 6 doses in 24 hours

Rheumatoid arthritis: 870-1740 mg (5-10 mL) up to 4 times/day

Mechanism of Action Inhibits prostaglandin synthesis; acts on the hypothalamus heat-regulating center to reduce fever; blocks the generation of pain impulses

Local Anesthetic/Vasoconstrictor Precautions No information available to require special precautions

Effects on Dental Treatment No effects or complications reported

Other Adverse Effects

>10%: Gastrointestinal: Nausea, heartburn, stomach pains, dyspepsia, epigastric discomfort

1% to 10%:
Central nervous system: Fatigue
Dermatologic: Skin rash
Gastrointestinal: Gastrointestinal ulceration
Hematologic: Hemolytic anemia
Neuromuscular & skeletal: Weakness
Respiratory: Dyspnea
Miscellaneous: Anaphylactic shock

<1%:
Central nervous system: Insomnia, nervousness, jitters
Hematologic: Occult bleeding, prolongation of bleeding time, leukopenia, thrombocytopenia, iron deficiency anemia
Hepatic: Hepatotoxicity
Renal: Impaired renal function
Respiratory: Bronchospasm

Drug Interactions
Decreased effect with antacids
Increased effect of warfarin

Drug Uptake
Absorption: From the stomach and small intestine within ~2 hours
Serum half-life: Dose-dependent ranging from 2-3 hours at low doses to 30 hours at high doses
Time to peak serum concentration: 1-2 hours

Pregnancy Risk Factor C

Generic Available No

Choline Theophyllinate *see Oxtriphylline on page 708*

Choloxin® *see Dextrothyroxine on page 299*

Chondroitin Sulfate-Sodium Hyaluronate
(kon DROY tin SUL fate-SOW de um hye a loo ROE nate)

Brand Names Viscoat®

Therapeutic Category Ophthalmic Agent, Viscoelastic

Synonyms Sodium Hyaluronate-Chrondroitin Sulfate

Use Surgical aid in anterior segment procedures, protects corneal endothelium and coats intraocular lens thus protecting it

Usual Dosage Carefully introduce (using a 27-gauge needle or cannula) into anterior chamber after thoroughly cleaning the chamber with a balanced salt solution

Mechanism of Action Functions as a tissue lubricant and is thought to play an important role in modulating the interactions between adjacent tissues

Local Anesthetic/Vasoconstrictor Precautions No information available to require special precautions

Effects on Dental Treatment No effects or complications reported

Other Adverse Effects 1% to 10%: Increased intraocular pressure (transient)

Drug Uptake
Absorption: Following intravitreous injection, diffusion occurs slowly

Pregnancy Risk Factor C

Generic Available No

Chooz® [OTC] *see Calcium Carbonate on page 162*

Chorex® *see Chorionic Gonadotropin on this page*

Chorionic Gonadotropin (kor ee ON ik goe NAD oh troe pin)

Brand Names A.P.L.®; Chorex®; Choron®; Gonic®; Pregnyl®; Profasi® HP

Therapeutic Category Gonadotropin; Ovulation Stimulator

Use Induces ovulation and pregnancy in anovulatory, infertile females; treatment of hypogonadotropic hypogonadism, prepubertal cryptorchidism

Usual Dosage I.M.:
Children:
Prepubertal cryptorchidism (not due to anatomical obstruction): 4000 units 3 times/week for 3 weeks

(Continued)

Chorionic Gonadotropin (Continued)

or

5000 units every other day for 4 injections

or

15 injections of 500-1000 units over a period of 6 weeks

or

500 units 3 times per week for 4-6 weeks. If unsuccessful, start another course 1 month later, giving 1000 units/injection.

Hypogonadotropic hypogonadism in males: 500-1000 units 3 times/week for 3 weeks, followed by the same dose twice weekly for 3 weeks

or

1000-2000 units 3 times/week

or

4000 units 3 times/week for 6-9 months; reduce dose to 2000 units 3 times/week for an additional 3 months

Adults:

Use with menotropins to stimulate spermatogenesis: 5000 units 3 times/week for 4-6 months. With the beginning of menotropins therapy, hCG dose is continued at 2000 2 times/week.

Induction of ovulation and pregnancy: 5000-10,000 units one day following last dose of menotropins

Mechanism of Action Stimulates production of gonadal steroid hormones by causing production of androgen by the testis; as a substitute for luteinizing hormone (LH) to stimulate ovulation

Local Anesthetic/Vasoconstrictor Precautions No information available to require special precautions

Effects on Dental Treatment No effects or complications reported

Other Adverse Effects

1% to 10%:

Central nervous system: Mental depression, fatigue

Endocrine & metabolic: Pelvic pain, ovarian cysts, enlargement of breasts, precocious puberty

Local: Pain at the injection site

Neuromuscular & skeletal: Premature closure of epiphyses

<1%:

Cardiovascular: Peripheral edema

Central nervous system: Irritability, restlessness, headache

Endocrine & metabolic: Ovarian hyperstimulation syndrome, gynecomastia

Drug Interactions No data reported

Drug Uptake

Half-life, biphasic:

Initial: 11 hours

Terminal: 23 hours

Pregnancy Risk Factor C

Generic Available Yes

Choron® see Chorionic Gonadotropin on previous page

Chromagen® OB [OTC] see Vitamins, Multiple on page 995

Chroma-Pak® see Trace Metals on page 948

Chromium see Trace Metals on page 948

Chronulac® see Lactulose on page 540

Chymex® see Bentiromide on page 117

Chymodiactin® see Chymopapain on this page

Chymopapain (KYE moe pa pane)

Brand Names Chymodiactin®

Therapeutic Category Enzyme, Intradiscal; Enzyme, Proteolytic

Use Alternative to surgery in patients with herniated lumbar intervertebral disks

Usual Dosage Adults: 2000-4000 units/disc with a maximum cumulative dose not to exceed 8000 units for patients with multiple disc herniations

Mechanism of Action Chymopapain, when injected into the disc center, causes hydrolysis of the mucal mucopolysaccharide protein complex into acid polysaccharide, polypeptides, and amino acids. Subsequently, the water trapping properties of the nucleus pulposus are destroyed which permanently diminishes the pressure within the disc. The adjacent structures including the annulus fibrosus are not affected by chymopapain.

Local Anesthetic/Vasoconstrictor Precautions No information available to require special precautions

Effects on Dental Treatment No effects or complications reported

Other Adverse Effects
>10%: Neuromuscular & skeletal: Back pain
1% to 10%:
  Central nervous system: Dizziness, headache
  Gastrointestinal: Nausea
  Neuromuscular & skeletal: Weakness in legs
<1%:
  Central nervous system: CNS hemorrhage, seizures
  Dermatologic: Allergic dermatitis
  Gastrointestinal: Paralytic ileus
  Local: Thrombophlebitis
  Ocular: Conjunctivitis
  Respiratory: Rhinorrhea, dyspnea
  Miscellaneous: Anaphylaxis
Pregnancy Risk Factor C
Generic Available No

Cianocobalamina (Mexico) *see* Cyanocobalamin *on page 266*
Cibacalcin® Injection *see* Calcitonin *on page 160*
Ciclofosfamida (Mexico) *see* Cyclophosphamide *on page 269*

Ciclopirox (sye kloe PEER oks)
Brand Names Loprox®
Therapeutic Category Antifungal Agent, Topical
Use Treatment of tinea pedis (athlete's foot), tinea cruris (jock itch), tinea corporis (ringworm), cutaneous candidiasis, and tinea versicolor (pityriasis)
Usual Dosage Children >10 years and Adults: Apply twice daily, gently massage into affected areas; if no improvement after 4 weeks of treatment, re-evaluate the diagnosis
Mechanism of Action Inhibiting transport of essential elements in the fungal cell causing problems in synthesis of DNA, RNA, and protein
Local Anesthetic/Vasoconstrictor Precautions No information available to require special precautions
Effects on Dental Treatment No effects or complications reported
Other Adverse Effects
1% to 10%:
  Central nervous system: Pain
  Local: Irritation, redness, or burning; worsening of clinical condition
Drug Interactions No data reported
Drug Uptake
Absorption: <2% absorbed through intact skin
Serum half-life: 1.7 hours
Pregnancy Risk Factor B
Dosage Forms
Cream, topical, as olamine: 1% (15 g, 30 g, 90 g)
Lotion, as olamine: 1% (30 mL)
Generic Available No

Ciclosporina (Mexico) *see* Cyclosporine *on page 272*

Cidofovir (si DOF o veer)
Brand Names Vistide®
Therapeutic Category Antiviral Agent, Parenteral
Use Treatment of CMV retinitis in patients with acquired immunodeficiency syndrome (AIDS)
Usual Dosage
Induction treatment: 5 mg/kg once weekly for 2 consecutive weeks
Maintenance treatment: 5 mg/kg administered once every 2 weeks
Probenecid must be administered orally with each dose of cidofovir
Probenecid dose: 2 g 3 hours prior to cidofovir dose, 1 g 2 hours and 8 hours after completion of the infusion; patients should also receive 1 L of normal saline intravenously prior to each infusion of cidofovir; saline should be infused over 1-2 hours

Dosing adjustment in renal impairment:
Cl_{cr} 41-55 mL/minute:
  Induction (weekly x 2 doses): 2 mg/kg
  Maintenance (every other week): 2 mg/kg
Cl_{cr} 30-40 mL/minute:
  Induction (weekly x 2 doses): 1.5 mg/kg
  Maintenance (every other week): 1.5 mg/kg
Cl_{cr} 20-29 mL/minute:
  Induction (weekly x 2 doses): 1 mg/kg
(Continued)

Cidofovir *(Continued)*

    Maintenance (every other week): 1 mg/kg
   Cl_{cr} <19 mL/minute:
    Induction (weekly x 2 doses): 0.5 mg/kg
    Maintenance (every other week): 0.5 mg/kg

Patients with clinically significant changes in serum creatinine during therapy: Cidofovir dose should be reduced to 3 mg/kg and discontinued if creatinine rise is >0.5 mg/dL

Data unavailable in patients on dialysis

Mechanism of Action Cidofovir is converted to cidofovir diphosphate which is the active intracellular metabolite; cidofovir diphosphate suppresses CMV replication by selective inhibition of viral DNA synthesis. Incorporation of cidofovir into growing viral DNA chain results in reductions in the rate of viral DNA synthesis.

Local Anesthetic/Vasoconstrictor Precautions No information available to require special precautions

Effects on Dental Treatment No effects or complications reported

Other Adverse Effects

>10%:
  Central nervous system: Fever, headache, chills
  Dermatologic: Rash, alopecia
  Gastrointestinal: Nausea, vomiting, diarrhea, anorexia, abdominal pain
  Hematologic: Neutropenia, anemia
  Neuromuscular & skeletal: Weakness
  Ocular: Ocular hypotony
  Renal: Proteinuria, elevated creatinine
  Respiratory: Dyspnea
  Miscellaneous: Infections

<10%:
  Cardiovascular: Hypotension, tachycardia
  Central nervous system: Anxiety, hallucinations, depression, convulsion, somnolence, malaise
  Dermatologic: Acne, skin discoloration/dryness, pruritus, urticaria
  Endocrine & metabolic: Hyperglycemia, hyperlipidemia, hypocalcemia, hypokalemia, dehydration
  Gastrointestinal: Colitis, GI distress, stomatitis
  Genitourinary: Urinary incontinence, glycosuria
  Hematologic: Thrombocytopenia
  Hepatic: Elevated LFTs
  Neuromuscular & skeletal: Skeletal pain, myalgia, arthralgia, neuropathy
  Ocular: Ocular symptoms
  Renal: Hematuria
  Respiratory: Respiratory symptoms
  Miscellaneous: Allergic reaction, sarcoma, sepsis

Warnings/Precautions Dose-dependent nephrotoxicity is a major dose-limiting toxicity related to cidofovir. Cidofovir is not recommended for use in patients with creatinine >1.5 mg/dL or creatinine clearance <55 mL/minute; in these benefits, consideration should be made of potential benefits vs risks. Dose adjustment or discontinuation may be required for changes in renal function while on therapy; renal function secondary to cidofovir is not always reversible. Neutropenia and metabolic acidosis (Fanconi syndrome) have been reported; administration of cidofovir must be accompanied by oral probenecid and intravenous saline prehydration.

Drug Interactions Probenecid may decrease metabolism or tubular excretion of drugs such as AZT, acyclovir, benzodiazepines, acetaminophen, ACE inhibitors, barbiturates, loop diuretics, famotidine, NSAIDs, and theophylline; avoid concomitant administration with other nephrotoxic agents

Drug Uptake The following pharmacokinetic data is based on a combination of cidofovir administered with probenecid:
Serum half-life: ~2.6 hours (nonintracellular)

Pregnancy Risk Factor C

Generic Available No

Comments Cidofovir preparation should be performed in a class two laminar flow biologic safety cabinet and personnel should be wearing surgical gloves and a closed front surgical gown with knit cuffs; appropriate safety equipment is recommended for preparation, administration, and disposal of cidofovir. If cidofovir contacts skin, wash and flush thoroughly with water.

Selected Readings
Hitchcock MJ, Jaffe HS, Martin JC, et al, "Cidofovir, A New Agent With Potent Anti-Herpes Virus Activity," *Antiviral Chemistry Chemotherapy*, 1996, 7:115-27.

Cimetidina (Mexico) *see* Cimetidine *on next page*

Cimetidine (sye MET i deen)

Related Information

Dental Drug Interactions: Update on Drug Combinations Requiring Special Considerations *on page 1144*

Brand Names Tagamet®; Tagamet® HB [OTC]

Canadian/Mexican Brand Names Apo®-Cimetidine (Canada); Blocan® (Mexico); Cimetase® (Mexico); Cimetigal® (Mexico); Columina® (Mexico); Novo-Cimetidine® (Canada); Nu-Cimet® (Canada); Peptol® (Canada); Ulcedine® (Mexico); Zymerol® (Mexico)

Therapeutic Category Histamine H_2 Antagonist

Synonyms Cimetidina (Mexico)

Use Short-term treatment of active duodenal ulcers and benign gastric ulcers; long-term prophylaxis of duodenal ulcer; gastric hypersecretory states; gastroesophageal reflux; prevention of upper GI bleeding in critically ill patients.

Usual Dosage

Children: Oral, I.M., I.V.: 20-40 mg/kg/day in divided doses every 4 hours

Adults: Short-term treatment of active ulcers:

Oral: 300 mg 4 times/day or 800 mg at bedtime or 400 mg twice daily for up to 8 weeks

I.M., I.V.: 300 mg every 6 hours or 37.5 mg/hour by continuous infusion; I.V. dosage should be adjusted to maintain an intragastric pH ≥5

Patients with an active bleed: Give cimetidine as a continuous infusion (see above)

Duodenal ulcer prophylaxis: Oral: 400-800 mg at bedtime

Gastric hypersecretory conditions: Oral, I.M., I.V.: 300-600 mg every 6 hours; dosage not to exceed 2.4 g/day

Mechanism of Action Competitive inhibition of histamine at H_2-receptors of the gastric parietal cells resulting in reduced gastric acid secretion, gastric volume and hydrogen ion concentration reduced

Local Anesthetic/Vasoconstrictor Precautions No information available to require special precautions

Effects on Dental Treatment No effects or complications reported

Other Adverse Effects

1% to 10%:

Central nervous system: Dizziness, agitation, headache, drowsiness

Gastrointestinal: Diarrhea, nausea, vomiting

<1%:

Cardiovascular: Bradycardia, hypotension, tachycardia

Central nervous system: Confusion, fever

Dermatologic: Rash

Endocrine & metabolic: Gynecomastia, swelling of breasts, decreased sexual ability

Hematologic: Neutropenia, agranulocytosis, thrombocytopenia

Hepatic: Elevated AST and ALT

Neuromuscular & skeletal: Myalgia

Renal: Elevated creatinine

Drug Interactions Inhibits liver metabolism of many drugs resulting in potential for increased toxicity of those drugs; these include warfarin anticoagulants, phenytoin, propranolol, nifedipine, diazepam, tricyclic antidepressants, theophylline, and metronidazole

Drug Uptake

Serum half-life: Adults (with normal renal function): 2 hours

Time to peak serum concentration: Oral: Within 1-2 hours

Pregnancy Risk Factor B

Generic Available Yes

Cinobac® Pulvules® *see* Cinoxacin *on this page*

Cinoxacin (sin OKS a sin)

Brand Names Cinobac® Pulvules®

Canadian/Mexican Brand Names Gugecin® (Mexico)

Therapeutic Category Antibiotic, Quinolone

Synonyms Cinoxacino (Mexico)

Use Treatment of urinary tract infections

Usual Dosage Children >12 years and Adults: 1 g/day in 2-4 doses for 7-14 days

Mechanism of Action Inhibits microbial synthesis of DNA with resultant problems in protein synthesis

Local Anesthetic/Vasoconstrictor Precautions No information available to require special precautions

Effects on Dental Treatment No effects or complications reported

(Continued)

Cinoxacin *(Continued)*

Other Adverse Effects
1% to 10%:
 Central nervous system: Headache, dizziness
 Gastrointestinal: Heartburn, abdominal pain, GI bleeding, belching, flatulence, anorexia, nausea
<1%:
 Central nervous system: Insomnia, confusion
 Gastrointestinal: Diarrhea
 Hematologic: Thrombocytopenia
 Ocular: Photophobia
 Otic: Tinnitus

Drug Interactions
Decreased effect: Decreased urine levels with probenecid; decreased absorption with aluminum-, magnesium-, calcium-containing antacids

Drug Uptake
Absorption: Oral: Rapid and complete; food decreases peak levels by 30% but not total amount absorbed
Serum half-life: 1.5 hours, prolonged in renal impairment
Time to peak serum concentration: Oral: Within 2-3 hours

Pregnancy Risk Factor B
Generic Available Yes

Cinoxacino (Mexico) *see* Cinoxacin *on previous page*

Cipro™ *see* Ciprofloxacin *on this page*

Ciprofloxacin *(sip roe FLOKS a sin)*

Related Information
Nonviral Infectious Diseases *on page 1032*

Brand Names Cipro™

Canadian/Mexican Brand Names Cimogal® (Mexico); Ciproflox® (Mexico); Ciproflur® (Mexico); Ciproxina® (Mexico); Eni® (Mexico); Italnik® (Mexico); Kenzoflex® (Mexico); Microrgan® (Mexico); Mitroken® (Mexico); Nivoflox® (Mexico); Sophixin® Ofteno (Mexico)

Therapeutic Category Antibiotic, Ophthalmic; Antibiotic, Quinolone

Use
Dental: Useful as a single agent or in combination with metronidazole in the treatment of periodontitis associated with the presence of *Actinobacillus actinomycetemcomitans*, (AA) as well as enteric rods/pseudomonads
Medical: Treatment of documented or suspected pseudomonal infection (eg, home care patients); documented multidrug resistant gram-negative organisms; documented infectious diarrhea due to *Campylobacter jejuni*, *Shigella*, or *Salmonella*; osteomyelitis caused by susceptible organisms in which parenteral therapy is not feasible; used ophthalmically for superficial ocular infections (corneal ulcers, conjunctivitis) due to strains of microorganisms susceptible to ciprofloxacin

Usual Dosage Adults: Oral: 250-750 mg every 12 hours, depending on severity of infection and susceptibility; in treatment of periodontitis, ciprofloxacin and metronidazole 500 mg each twice daily for 8 days

Mechanism of Action Inhibits DNA-gyrase in susceptible organisms; inhibits relaxation of supercoiled DNA and promotes breakage of double-stranded DNA

Local Anesthetic/Vasoconstrictor Precautions No information available to require special precautions

Effects on Dental Treatment <1% of patients experience painful oral mucosa, oral candidiasis, oral ulceration, or mouth dryness

Other Adverse Effects 1% to 10%:
Central nervous system: Headache, restlessness
Dermatologic: Rash
Gastrointestinal: Nausea, diarrhea, vomiting, abdominal pain

Contraindications Hypersensitivity to ciprofloxacin, any component or other quinolones

Warnings/Precautions Not recommended in children <18 years of age; has caused transient arthropathy in children; CNS stimulation may occur (tremor, restlessness, confusion, and very rarely hallucinations or seizures). Use with caution in patients with known or suspected CNS disorders.

Drug Interactions Decreased absorption with antacids containing aluminum, magnesium, and/or calcium (by up to 98% if given at the same time); quinolones cause increased levels of caffeine, warfarin, cyclosporine, and theophylline; azlocillin, cimetidine, probenecid increase quinolone levels

Drug Uptake
Absorption: Oral: Rapid

Serum half-life: 3-5 hours in patients with normal renal function
Time to peak serum concentration: Oral: Within 0.5-2 hours
Pregnancy Risk Factor C
Breast-feeding Considerations Not compatible; can resume breast-feeding 48 hours after the last dose
Dosage Forms
Infusion, in D_5W: 400 mg (200 mL)
Infusion, in NS or D_5W: 200 mg (100 mL)
Injection: 200 mg (20 mL); 400 mg (40 mL)
Tablet: 250 mg, 500 mg, 750 mg
Dietary Considerations Dairy foods decrease ciprofloxacin concentration, use caution with xanthine-containing foods and beverages; food delays absorption but total absorption remains unchanged
Generic Available Yes
Selected Readings
Rams TE and Slots J, "Antibiotics in Periodontal Therapy: An Update," *Compendium*, 1992, 13(12):1130, 1132, 1134.

Cisaprida (Mexico) *see* Cisapride on this page

Cisapride (SIS a pride)
Related Information
Endocrine Disorders & Pregnancy *on page 1021*
Brand Names Propulsid®
Canadian/Mexican Brand Names Enteropride® (Mexico); Kinestase® (Mexico); Prepulsid® (Canada); Unamol® (Mexico)
Therapeutic Category Antiemetic; Gastrointestinal Agent, Prokinetic
Synonyms Cisaprida (Mexico)
Use Treatment of nocturnal symptoms of gastroesophageal reflux disease (GERD), also demonstrated effectiveness for gastroparesis, refractory constipation, and nonulcer dyspepsia
Usual Dosage Oral:
Children: 0.15-0.3 mg/kg/dose 3-4 times/day; maximum: 10 mg/dose
Adults: Initial: 10 mg 4 times/day at least 15 minutes before meals and at bedtime; in some patients the dosage will need to be increased to 20 mg to obtain a satisfactory result
Mechanism of Action Enhances the release of acetylcholine at the myenteric plexus. *In vitro* studies have shown cisapride to have serotonin-4 receptor agonistic properties which may increase gastrointestinal motility and cardiac rate; increases lower esophageal sphincter pressure and lower esophageal peristalsis; accelerates gastric emptying of both liquids and solids
Local Anesthetic/Vasoconstrictor Precautions No information available to require special precautions
Effects on Dental Treatment No effects or complications reported
Other Adverse Effects
>5%:
Central nervous system: Headache
Dermatologic: Rash
Gastrointestinal: Diarrhea, GI cramping, dyspepsia, flatulence, nausea, dry mouth
Respiratory: Rhinitis
<5%:
Cardiovascular: Tachycardia
Central nervous system: Extrapyramidal effects, drowsiness, fatigue, seizures, insomnia, anxiety
Hematologic: Thrombocytopenia, pancytopenia, leukopenia, granulocytopenia, aplastic anemia
Hepatic: Elevated LFTs
Respiratory: Sinusitis, coughing, upper respiratory tract infection
Miscellaneous: Increased incidence of viral infection
Drug Interactions Cisapride accelerates gastric emptying; this could affect the absorption of other drugs given simultaneously
Drug Uptake
Onset of action: 0.5-1 hour
Serum half-life: 6-12 hours
Pregnancy Risk Factor C
Generic Available No

Cisplatin (SIS pla tin)
Brand Names Platinol®; Platinol®-AQ
Canadian/Mexican Brand Names Blastolem (Mexico); Medsaplatin (Mexico); Niyaplat (Mexico)
(Continued)

Cisplatin *(Continued)*

Therapeutic Category Antineoplastic Agent, Alkylating Agent

Synonyms CDDP

Use Management of metastatic testicular or ovarian carcinoma, advanced bladder cancer, osteosarcoma, Hodgkin's and non-Hodgkin's lymphoma, head or neck cancer, cervical cancer, lung cancer, brain tumors, neuroblastoma; used alone or in combination with other agents

Usual Dosage I.V. **(refer to individual protocols)**:

An estimated Cl_{cr} should be on all cisplatin chemotherapy orders along with other patient parameters (ie, patient's height, weight, and body surface area). Pharmacy and nursing staff should check the Cl_{cr} on the order and determine the appropriateness of cisplatin dosing.

It is recommended that a 24-hour urine creatinine clearance be checked prior to a patient's first dose of cisplatin and periodically thereafter (ie, after every 2-3 cycles of cisplatin)

Pretreatment hydration with 1-2 L of fluid is recommended prior to cisplatin administration; adequate hydration and urinary output (>100 mL/hour) should be maintained for 24 hours after administration

If the dose prescribed is a reduced dose, then this should be indicated on the chemotherapy order

Children: Various dosage schedules range from 30-100 mg/m^2 once every 2-3 weeks; may also dose similar to adult dosing

Osteogenic sarcoma or neuroblastoma: 90 mg/m^2 once every 3 weeks or 30 mg/m^2 once weekly

Recurrent brain tumors: 60 mg/m^2 once daily for 2 consecutive days every 3-4 weeks

Adults:

Head and neck cancer: 100-150 mg/m^2 every 3-4 weeks

Testicular cancer: 10-20 mg/m^2/day for 5 days repeated every 3-4 weeks

Metastatic ovarian cancer: 50 mg/m^2 every 3 weeks

Intraperitoneal: cisplatin has been administered intraperitoneal with systemic sodium thiosulfate for ovarian cancer; doses up to 90-270 mg/m^2 have been administered and retained for 4 hours before draining

Mechanism of Action Inhibits DNA synthesis by the formation of DNA cross-links; denatures the double helix; covalently binds to DNA bases and disrupts DNA function; may also bind to proteins; the *cis*-isomer is 14 times more cytotoxic than the *trans*-isomer; both forms cross-link DNA but cis-platinum is less easily recognized by cell enzymes and, therefore, not repaired. Cisplatin can also bind two adjacent guanines on the same strand of DNA producing intrastrand cross-linking and breakage

Local Anesthetic/Vasoconstrictor Precautions No information available to require special precautions

Effects on Dental Treatment No effects or complications reported

Other Adverse Effects

>10%:

Endocrine & metabolic: Hyperuricemia

Gastrointestinal: Cisplatin is one of the most emetogenic agents used in cancer chemotherapy; nausea and vomiting occur in 76% to 100% of patients and is dose related. Prophylactic antiemetics should always be prescribed; nausea and vomiting may last up to 1 week after therapy.

Emetic potential: <75 mg: Moderately high (60% to 90%); ≥75 mg: High (>90%)

Hematologic: Myelosuppressive effects: Mild with moderate doses, mild to moderate with high-dose therapy; WBC: Mild; Platelets: Mild; Onset (days): 10; Nadir (days): 14-23; Recovery (days): 21-39

Local: Extravasation: May cause thrombophlebitis and tissue damage if infiltrated; may use sodium thiosulfate as antidote, but consult hospital policy for guidelines

Nephrotoxicity: Related to elimination, protein binding, and uptake of cisplatin. Two types of nephrotoxicity: Acute renal failure and chronic renal insufficiency.

Acute renal failure and azotemia is a dose-dependent process and can be minimized with proper administration and prophylaxis. Damage to the proximal tubules by the aquation products of cisplatin is suspected to cause the toxicity. It is manifested as elevated BUN and creatinine, oliguria, protein wasting, and potassium, calcium, and magnesium wasting.

Chronic renal dysfunction can develop in patients receiving multiple courses of cisplatin. This occurs with slow release of the platinum ion from tissues, which then accumulates in the distal tubules. Manifestations of this toxicity are varied and can include sodium and water wasting, nephropathy, decreased Cl_{cr}, and magnesium wasting.

Recommendations for minimizing nephrotoxicity include:

Prepare cisplatin in saline-containing vehicles

Vigorous hydration (125-150 mL/hour) before, during, and after cisplatin administration

Simultaneous administration of either mannitol or furosemide

Avoid other nephrotoxic agents (aminoglycosides, amphotericin, etc)

Otic: Ototoxicity, manifested as high frequency hearing loss (especially pronounced in children)

Miscellaneous: Anaphylactic reaction occurs within minutes after administration and can be controlled with epinephrine, antihistamines, and steroids

1% to 10%:

Gastrointestinal: Anorexia

Local: Pain at injection site

<1%:

Cardiovascular: Bradycardia, arrhythmias

Dermatologic: Mild alopecia

Endocrine & metabolic: SIADH, hypomagnesemia, hypocalcemia, hypokalemia, hypophosphatemia

Gastrointestinal: Mouth sores

Hepatic: Elevation of liver enzymes

Local: Phlebitis

Neurotoxicity: Peripheral neuropathy is dose- and duration-dependent. The mechanism is through axonal degeneration with subsequent damage to the long sensory nerves. Toxicity can first be noted at doses of 200 mg/m^2, with measurable toxicity at doses >350 mg/m^2. This process is irreversible and progressive with continued therapy. Baseline audiography should be performed.

Ocular: Optic neuritis, blurred vision, papilledema

Drug Uptake

Serum half-life:

Initial: 20-30 minutes

Beta: 1 hour

Terminal: ~24 hours

Secondary half-life: 44-73 hours

Pregnancy Risk Factor D

Generic Available No

Comments Sodium content (10 mg): 35.4 mg (1.54 mEq)

Citanest Forte® With Epinephrine see Prilocaine With Epinephrine on page 792

Citanest Plain 4% Injection see Prilocaine on page 791

Citracal® [OTC] see Calcium Citrate on page 164

Citrate of Magnesia see Magnesium Citrate on page 575

Citric Acid and d-gluconic Acid Irrigant see Citric Acid Bladder Mixture on this page

Citric Acid Bladder Mixture (SI trik AS id BLAD dur MIKS chur)

Brand Names Renacidin®

Therapeutic Category Irrigating Solution

Synonyms Citric Acid and d-gluconic Acid Irrigant; Hemiacidrin

Use Preparing solutions for irrigating indwelling urethral catheters; to dissolve or prevent formation of calcifications

Local Anesthetic/Vasoconstrictor Precautions No information available to require special precautions

Effects on Dental Treatment No effects or complications reported

Pregnancy Risk Factor C

Generic Available Yes

Citrotein® [OTC] see Enteral Nutritional Products on page 350

Citrovorum Factor see Leucovorin on page 544

Citrucel® [OTC] see Methylcellulose on page 621

Cladribine (KLA dri been)

Brand Names Leustatin™

Therapeutic Category Antineoplastic Agent, Antimetabolite

Synonyms 2-CdA; 2-Chlorodeoxyadenosine

Use Hairy cell and chronic lymphocytic leukemias

(Continued)

Cladribine *(Continued)*

Usual Dosage I.V.:

Children:

Acute leukemia:

The safety and effectiveness of cladribine in children have not been established; in a phase I study involving patients 1-21 years of age with relapsed acute leukemia, cladribine was administered by continuous intravenous infusion at doses ranging from 3-10.7 mg/m^2/day for 5 days (0.5-2 times the dose recommended in HCL). Investigators reported beneficial responses in this study; the dose-limiting toxicity was severe myelosuppression with profound neutropenia and thrombocytopenia.

Continuous intravenous infusion: 15-18 mg/m^2/day for 5 days

Adults:

Hairy cell leukemia:

Continuous intravenous infusion: 0.09-0.1 mg/kg/day continuous infusion for 7 consecutive days

Continuous intravenous infusion: 4 mg/m^2/day for 7 days

Non-Hodgkin's lymphoma: Continuous intravenous infusion: 0.1 mg/kg/day for 7 days

Mechanism of Action A purine nucleoside analogue; prodrug which is activated via phosphorylation by deoxycytidine kinase to a 5'-triphosphate derivative. This active form incorporates into susceptible cells and into DNA to result in the breakage of DNA strand and shutdown of DNA synthesis and also results in a depletion of nicotinamide adenine dinucleotide and adenosine triphosphate (ATP). The induction of strand breaks results in a drop in the cofactor nicotinamide adenine dinucleotide and disruption of cell metabolism. ATP is depleted to deprive cells of an important source of energy. Cladribine is able to kill resting as well as dividing cells, unlike most other cytotoxic drugs.

Local Anesthetic/Vasoconstrictor Precautions No information available to require special precautions

Effects on Dental Treatment No effects or complications reported

Other Adverse Effects

>10%:

Bone marrow suppression: Commonly observed in patients treated with cladribine, especially at high doses; at the initiation of treatment, however, most patients in clinical studies had hematologic impairment as a result of HCL. During the first 2 weeks after treatment initiation, mean platelet counts decline and subsequently increased with normalization of mean counts by day 12. Absolute neutrophil counts and hemoglobin declined and subsequently increased with normalization of mean counts by week 5 and week 6.

Central nervous system: Fatigue, headache

Dermatologic: Rash

Fever: Temperature ≥101°F has been associated with the use of cladribine in approximately 66% of patients in the first month of therapy. Although 69% of patients developed fevers, less than 33% of febrile events were associated with documented infection.

Gastrointestinal: Nausea and vomiting are not severe with cladribine at any dose level. Most cases of nausea were mild, not accompanied by vomiting and did not require treatment with antiemetics. In patients requiring antiemetics, nausea was easily controlled most often by chlorpromazine.

Local: Injection site reactions

1% to 10%:

Cardiovascular: Edema, tachycardia

Central nervous system: Dizziness, insomnia, chills, malaise, pain

Dermatologic: Pruritus, erythema

Gastrointestinal: Constipation, abdominal pain

Neuromuscular & skeletal: Arthralgia, myalgia, trunk pain, weakness

Miscellaneous: Sweating

Drug Uptake

Serum half-life: Biphasic:

Alpha: 25 minutes

Beta: 6.7 hours

Terminal, mean (normal renal function): 5.4 hours

Pregnancy Risk Factor D

Generic Available No

Claforan® *see* Cefotaxime *on page 192*

Clarithromycin (kla RITH roe mye sin)

Related Information
Antibiotic Prophylaxis, Preprocedural Guidelines for Dental Patients *on page 1034*
Respiratory Diseases *on page 1018*

Brand Names Biaxin™
Canadian/Mexican Brand Names Klaricid® (Mexico)
Therapeutic Category Antibiotic, Macrolide
Use
Dental: Alternate antibiotic in the treatment of common orofacial infections caused by aerobic gram-positive cocci and susceptible anaerobes; alternate antibiotic for the prevention of bacterial endocarditis in patients undergoing dental procedures

Medical: Treatment against most respiratory pathogens (eg, *S. pyogenes, S. pneumoniae, S. agalactiae*, viridans *Streptococcus, M. catarrhalis, C. trachomatis, Legionella* sp, *Mycoplasma pneumoniae, S. aureus*). Clarithromycin is highly active (MICs ≤0.25 mcg/mL) against *H. influenzae*, the combination of clarithromycin and its metabolite demonstrate an additive effect. Additionally, clarithromycin has shown activity against *C. pneumoniae* (including strain TWAR) and *M. avium* infection.

Usual Dosage Oral:
Children: Prevention of bacterial endocarditis: 15 mg/kg orally 1 hour before procedure; total children's dose should not exceed adult dose
Adults: 250-500 mg every 12 hours for 7 days; prevention of bacterial endocarditis: 500 mg 1 hour before procedure

Mechanism of Action
Exerts its antibacterial action by binding to 50S ribosomal subunit resulting in inhibition of protein synthesis. The 14-OH metabolite of clarithromycin is twice as active as the parent compound.

Local Anesthetic/Vasoconstrictor Precautions
No information available to require special precautions

Effects on Dental Treatment
No effects or complications reported

Other Adverse Effects 1% to 10%:
Central nervous system: Headache
Gastrointestinal: Diarrhea, nausea, dysgeusia, dyspepsia, abdominal pain

Contraindications
Hypersensitivity to clarithromycin, erythromycin, or any macrolide antibiotic; use with pimozide

Warnings/Precautions
In presence of severe renal impairment with or without coexisting hepatic impairment, decreased dosage or prolonged dosing interval may be appropriate; antibiotic associated colitis has been reported with use of clarithromycin; elderly patients have experienced increased incidents of adverse effects due to known age-related decreases in renal function

Drug Interactions
Clarithromycin increases serum theophylline levels by as much as 20% and significantly increases carbamazepine levels

Note: While other drug interactions (digoxin, anticoagulants, ergotamine, triazolam) known to occur with erythromycin have not been reported in clinical trials with clarithromycin, concurrent use of these drugs should be monitored closely

Drug Uptake
Absorption: Rapid; highly stable in the presence of gastric acid (unlike erythromycin)
Serum half-life, elimination: 3-4 hours with a 250 mg dose; 5-7 hours with a 500 mg dose
Time to peak serum concentration: Oral: 2-4 hours

Pregnancy Risk Factor C
Breast-feeding Considerations
No data reported; however, erythromycins may be taken while breast-feeding

Dosage Forms
Granules for oral suspension: 125 mg/5 mL (100 mL, 200 mL); 250 mg/5 mL (100 mL, 200 mL)
Tablet, film coated: 250 mg, 500 mg

Dietary Considerations
May be taken with or without meals; may be taken with milk; food delays absorption; total absorption remains unchanged

Generic Available No
Comments
Helicobacter pylori induced gastric ulcers: Combination regimen with bismuth subsalicylate, tetracycline, clarithromycin, and an H_2 receptor antagonist; or combination of omeprazole and clarithromycin. Adult dosage: Oral: 250 mg twice daily to 500 mg 3 times/day.

Selected Readings
Dajani AS, Taubert KA, Wilson W, et al, "Prevention of Bacterial Endocarditis Recommendations by the American Heart Association," *JAMA* 1997, 277(22):1794-801.
Dajani AS, Taubert KA, Wilson W, et al, "Prevention of Bacterial Endocarditis: Recommendations by the American Heart Association," *J Am Dent Assoc* 1997, 128(8):1142-51.

(Continued)

Clarithromycin *(Continued)*

"Pimozide (Orap) Contraindicated With Clarithromycin (Biaxin) and Other Macrolide Antibiotics," *FDA Medical Bulletin*, October 1996, 3.

Wynn RL, "New Erythromycins," *Gen Dent*, 1996, 44(4):304-7.

Claritin® *see* Loratadine *on page 566*

Claritin-D® *see* Loratadine and Pseudoephedrine *on page 567*

Claritin-D 24-Hour® *see* Loratadine and Pseudoephedrine *on page 567*

Clear Away® Disc [OTC] *see* Salicylic Acid *on page 853*

Clear By Design® Gel [OTC] *see* Benzoyl Peroxide *on page 120*

Clear Eyes® [OTC] *see* Naphazoline *on page 664*

Clearsil® Maximum Strength [OTC] *see* Benzoyl Peroxide *on page 120*

Clear Tussin® 30 *see* Guaifenesin and Dextromethorphan *on page 453*

Clemastina (Mexico) *see* Clemastine *on this page*

Clemastine *(KLEM as teen)*
Brand Names Antihist-1® [OTC]; Tavist®; Tavist®-1 [OTC]
Therapeutic Category Antihistamine
Synonyms Clemastina (Mexico)
Use Perennial and seasonal allergic rhinitis and other allergic symptoms including urticaria
Usual Dosage Oral:

Children: <12 years: 0.4-1 mg twice daily

Children >12 years and Adults: 1.34 mg twice daily to 2.68 mg 3 times/day; do not exceed 8.04 mg/day; lower doses should be considered in patients >60 years

Mechanism of Action Competes with histamine for H_1-receptor sites on effector cells in the gastrointestinal tract, blood vessels, and respiratory tract
Local Anesthetic/Vasoconstrictor Precautions No information available to require special precautions
Effects on Dental Treatment No effects or complications reported
Other Adverse Effects

>10%:
 Central nervous system: Slight to moderate drowsiness
 Respiratory: Thickening of bronchial secretions

1% to 10%:
 Central nervous system: Headache, fatigue, nervousness, increased dizziness
 Gastrointestinal: Appetite increase, nausea, diarrhea, abdominal pain, dry mouth
 Neuromuscular & skeletal: Arthralgia
 Respiratory: Pharyngitis

<1%:
 Cardiovascular: Edema, palpitations
 Central nervous system: Depression
 Dermatologic: Angioedema, photosensitivity, rash
 Hepatic: Hepatitis
 Neuromuscular & skeletal: Myalgia, paresthesia
 Respiratory: Bronchospasm, epistaxis

Drug Interactions May interact with other sedatives to cause drowsiness; these include alcohol and tranquilizers
Drug Uptake Absorption: Almost 100% from GI tract
Pregnancy Risk Factor C
Generic Available Yes

Clemastine and Phenylpropanolamine
(KLEM as teen & fen il proe pa NOLE a meen)
Brand Names Tavist-D®
Therapeutic Category Antihistamine/Decongestant Combination
Use Symptomatic relief of allergic rhinitis; pruritus of the eyes, nose or throat, lacrimation and nasal congestion
Usual Dosage Children >12 years and Adults: Oral: 1 tablet every 12 hours
Local Anesthetic/Vasoconstrictor Precautions Use with caution since phenylpropanolamine is a sympathomimetic amine which could interact with epinephrine to cause a pressor response
Effects on Dental Treatment Up to 10% of patients could experience tachycardia, palpitations, and dry mouth; use vasoconstrictor with caution
Pregnancy Risk Factor B
Dosage Forms Tablet: Clemastine fumarate 1.34 mg and phenylpropanolamine hydrochloride 75 mg
Generic Available No

Cleocin HCl® *see Clindamycin on this page*
Cleocin Pediatric® *see Clindamycin on this page*
Cleocin Phosphate® *see Clindamycin on this page*

Clidinium and Chlordiazepoxide
(kli DI nee um & klor dye a e POKS ide)
Brand Names Clindex®; Librax®
Therapeutic Category Antispasmodic Agent, Gastrointestinal
Synonyms Chlordiazepoxide and Clidinium
Use Adjunct treatment of peptic ulcer, treatment of irritable bowel syndrome
Local Anesthetic/Vasoconstrictor Precautions No information available to require special precautions
Effects on Dental Treatment No effects or complications reported
Pregnancy Risk Factor D
Generic Available Yes
Comments After extended therapy, abrupt discontinuation should be avoided and a gradual dose tapering schedule followed

Climara® Transdermal *see Estradiol on page 365*

Clindamycin (klin da MYE sin)
Related Information
Animal and Human Bites Guidelines *on page 1093*
Antibiotic Prophylaxis, Preprocedural Guidelines for Dental Patients *on page 1034*
Antimicrobial Prophylaxis in Surgical Patients *on page 1163*
Cardiovascular Diseases *on page 1010*
Oral Bacterial Infections *on page 1059*
Brand Names Cleocin HCl®; Cleocin Pediatric®; Cleocin Phosphate®
Canadian/Mexican Brand Names Dalacin® C [Hydrochloride] (Canada); Dalacin® C (Mexico); Galecin® (Mexico); Klyndaken® (Mexico)
Therapeutic Category Acne Products; Antibiotic, Anaerobic; Antibiotic, Miscellaneous
Use
Dental: Alternate antibiotic, when amoxicillin cannot be used, for the standard regimen for prevention of bacterial endocarditis in patients undergoing dental procedures; an alternative to penicillin VK and erythromycin for treating orofacial infections; alternate antibiotic for prophylaxis for dental patients with total joint replacement
Medical: Treatment against aerobic and anaerobic streptococci (except enterococci), most staphylococci, *Bacteroides* sp and *Actinomyces*; used topically in treatment of severe acne, vaginally for *Gardnerella vaginalis*, alternate treatment for toxoplasmosis
Usual Dosage
Children:
Prevention of bacterial endocarditis: 20 mg/kg orally 1 hour before procedure; for patients allergic to penicillin and unable to take oral medications: 20 mg/kg I.V. within 30 minutes before procedure
Orofacial infections: 8-25 mg/kg in 3-4 equally divided doses
Adults:
Prevention of bacterial endocarditis in patients unable to take amoxicillin: Oral: 600 mg 1 hour before procedure; for patients allergic to penicillin and unable to take oral medications: 600 mg I.V. within 30 minutes before procedure
Orofacial infections: 150-450 mg every 6 hours for at least 7 days; maximum dose: 1.8 g/day
Patients with prosthesis allergic to penicillin: Oral: 600 mg 1 hour before procedure
Patients with prosthesis allergic to penicillin and unable to take oral medication: I.V.: 600 mg 1 hour before procedure
Mechanism of Action Reversibly binds to 50S ribosomal subunits preventing peptide bond formation thus inhibiting bacterial protein synthesis; bacteriostatic or bactericidal depending on drug concentration, infection site, and organism
Local Anesthetic/Vasoconstrictor Precautions No information available to require special precautions
Effects on Dental Treatment No effects or complications reported
Other Adverse Effects
>10%: Gastrointestinal: Diarrhea
1% to 10%:
Dermatologic: Rashes
Gastrointestinal: Pseudomembranous colitis, nausea, vomiting
Contraindications Hypersensitivity to clindamycin or any component; previous pseudomembranous colitis, hepatic impairment
(Continued)

Clindamycin *(Continued)*

Warnings/Precautions Dosage adjustment may be necessary in patients with severe hepatic dysfunction; no change necessary with renal insufficiency; can cause severe and possibly fatal colitis; use with caution in patients with a history of pseudomembranous colitis; discontinue drug if significant diarrhea, abdominal cramps, or passage of blood and mucus occurs

Drug Interactions Increased duration of neuromuscular blockade from tubocurarine, pancuronium

Drug Uptake

Absorption: 90% absorbed rapidly from GI tract following oral administration

Serum half-life: Adults: 1.6-5.3 hours, average: 2-3 hours

Time to peak serum concentration: Oral: Within 60 minutes

Pregnancy Risk Factor B

Breast-feeding Considerations May be taken while breast-feeding

Dosage Forms

Capsule, as hydrochloride: 75 mg, 150 mg, 300 mg

Granules for oral solution, as palmitate: 75 mg/5 mL (100 mL)

Infusion, as phosphate, in D_5W: 300 mg (50 mL); 600 mg (50 mL)

Injection, as phosphate: 150 mg/mL (2 mL, 4 mL, 6 mL, 50 mL, 60 mL)

Dietary Considerations Peak concentrations may be delayed with food; may be taken with food

Generic Available Yes

Comments Clindamycin has not been shown to interfere with oral contraceptive activity; however, it reduces GI microflora, thus, oral contraceptive users should be advised to use additional methods of birth control. About 1% of clindamycin users develop pseudomembranous colitis. Symptoms may occur 2-9 days after initiation of therapy; however, it has never occurred with the 1-dose regimen of clindamycin used to prevent bacterial endocarditis.

Selected Readings

"Advisory Statement. Antibiotic Prophylaxis for Dental Patients With Total Joint Replacements. American Dental Association; American Academy of Orthopedic Surgeons," *J Am Dent Assoc*, 1997, 128(7):1004-8.

Dajani AS, Taubert KA, Wilson W, et al, "Prevention of Bacterial Endocarditis Recommendations by the American Heart Association," *JAMA* 1997, 277(22):1794-801.

Dajani AS, Taubert KA, Wilson W, et al, "Prevention of Bacterial Endocarditis: Recommendations by the American Heart Association," *J Am Dent Assoc* 1997, 128(8):1142-51.

Wynn RL and Bergman SA, "Antibiotics and Their Use in the Treatment of Orofacial Infections, Part I and Part II," *Gen Dent*, 1994, 42(5):398-402, 498-502.

Wynn RL, "Clindamycin: An Often Forgotten but Important Antibiotic," *AGD Impact*, 1994, 22:10.

Clindex® *see* Clidinium and Chlordiazepoxide *on previous page*

Clinoril® *see* Sulindac *on page 898*

Clioquinol *(klye oh KWIN ole)*

Brand Names Vioform® [OTC]

Canadian/Mexican Brand Names Clioquinol® (Canada)

Therapeutic Category Antifungal Agent, Topical

Use Used topically in the treatment of tinea pedis, tinea cruris, and skin infections caused by dermatophytic fungi (ring worm)

Usual Dosage Children and Adults: Topical: Apply 2-3 times/day; do not use for longer than 7 days

Mechanism of Action Chelates bacterial surface and trace metals needed for bacterial growth

Local Anesthetic/Vasoconstrictor Precautions No information available to require special precautions

Effects on Dental Treatment No effects or complications reported

Other Adverse Effects 1% to 10%:

Dermatologic: Skin irritation, rash

Neuromuscular & skeletal: Peripheral neuropathy

Ocular: Optic atrophy

Drug Interactions No data reported

Drug Uptake

Absorption: With an occlusive dressing, up to 40% of dose can be absorbed systemically during a 12-hour period; absorption is enhanced when applied under diapers

Serum half-life: 11-14 hours

Pregnancy Risk Factor C

Generic Available Yes: Cream

Clioquinol and Hydrocortisone
(klye oh KWIN ole & hye droe KOR ti sone)

Brand Names Corque® Topical; Pedi-Cort V® Creme

Therapeutic Category Antifungal Agent, Topical; Corticosteroid, Topical (Low Potency)

Synonyms Hydrocortisone and Clioquinol; Iodochlorhydroxyquin and Hydrocortisone

Use Contact or atopic dermatitis; eczema; neurodermatitis; anogenital pruritus; mycotic dermatoses; moniliasis

Local Anesthetic/Vasoconstrictor Precautions No information available to require special precautions

Effects on Dental Treatment No effects or complications reported

Pregnancy Risk Factor C

Generic Available Yes

Clobetasol (kloe BAY ta sol)

Related Information

Corticosteroids, Topical Comparison *on page 1140*
Oral Nonviral Soft Tissue Ulcerations or Erosions *on page 1070*

Brand Names Temovate®

Canadian/Mexican Brand Names Dermasone® (Canada); Dermatovate® (Mexico); Dermovate® (Canada); Gen-Clobetasol® (Canada); Novo-Clobetasol® (Canada)

Therapeutic Category Corticosteroid, Topical (Very High Potency)

Synonyms Clobetasol, Propionato De (Mexico)

Use Short-term relief of inflammation of moderate to severe corticosteroid-responsive dermatosis (very high potency topical corticosteroid)

Usual Dosage Adults: Topical: Apply twice daily for up to 2 weeks with no more than 50 g/week

Mechanism of Action Stimulates the synthesis of enzymes needed to decrease inflammation, suppress mitotic activity, and cause vasoconstriction

Local Anesthetic/Vasoconstrictor Precautions No information available to require special precautions

Effects on Dental Treatment No effects or complications reported

Other Adverse Effects
1% to 10%:
Dermatologic: Erythema, papular rashes
Local: Itching, burning, dryness, irritation
<1%: Dermatologic: Hypertrichosis, acneiform eruptions, hypopigmentation, perioral dermatitis, maceration of skin, skin atrophy, striae, miliaria

Drug Interactions No data reported

Drug Uptake
Absorption: Percutaneous absorption variable and dependent upon many factors including vehicle used, integrity of epidermis, dose, and use of occlusive dressings

Pregnancy Risk Factor C

Generic Available Yes

Clobetasol, Propionato De (Mexico) *see* Clobetasol *on this page*

Clocortolone (kloe KOR toe lone)

Related Information

Corticosteroids, Topical Comparison *on page 1140*

Brand Names Cloderm®

Therapeutic Category Corticosteroid, Topical (Medium Potency)

Use Inflammation of corticosteroid-responsive dermatoses (medium potency topical corticosteroid)

Usual Dosage Adults: Apply sparingly and gently; rub into affected area from 1-4 times/day

Mechanism of Action Stimulates the synthesis of enzymes needed to decrease inflammation, suppress mitotic activity, and cause vasoconstriction

Local Anesthetic/Vasoconstrictor Precautions No information available to require special precautions

Effects on Dental Treatment No effects or complications reported

Other Adverse Effects
1% to 10%:
Dermatologic: Erythema, papular rashes
Local: Itching, burning,
<1%: Dermatologic: Hypertrichosis, acneiform eruptions, hypopigmentation, perioral dermatitis, maceration of skin, skin atrophy, striae, miliaria

Drug Interactions No data reported

(Continued)

Clocortolone *(Continued)*

Drug Uptake
Absorption: Percutaneous absorption is variable and dependent upon many factors including vehicle used, integrity of epidermis, dose, and use of occlusive dressings

Pregnancy Risk Factor C

Generic Available No

Cloderm® *see Clocortolone on previous page*

Clofazimine *(kloe FA zi meen)*

Brand Names Lamprene®

Therapeutic Category Antibiotic, Miscellaneous

Use Treatment of dapsone-resistant leprosy; multibacillary dapsone-sensitive leprosy; erythema nodosum leprosum; *Mycobacterium avium* - intracellular (MAI) infections

Usual Dosage Oral:
Children: Leprosy: 1 mg/kg/day every 24 hours in combination with dapsone and rifampin

Adults:
Dapsone-resistant leprosy: 100 mg/day in combination with one or more antileprosy drugs for 3 years; then alone 100 mg/day
Dapsone-sensitive multibacillary leprosy: 100 mg/day in combination with two or more antileprosy drugs for at least 2 years and continue until negative skin smears are obtained, then institute single drug therapy with appropriate agent
Erythema nodosum leprosum: 100-200 mg/day for up to 3 months or longer then taper dose to 100 mg/day when possible
Pyoderma gangrenosum: 300-400 mg/day for up to 12 months

Mechanism of Action Binds preferentially to mycobacterial DNA to inhibit mycobacterial growth; also has some anti-inflammatory activity through an unknown mechanism

Local Anesthetic/Vasoconstrictor Precautions No information available to require special precautions

Effects on Dental Treatment No effects or complications reported

Other Adverse Effects
>10%:
Dermatologic: Dry skin, pink to brownish-black discoloration of the skin
Gastrointestinal: Abdominal pain, nausea, vomiting, diarrhea
Ocular: Pink to brownish-black discoloration of the conjunctiva
1% to 10%:
Dermatologic: Rash, pruritus
Endocrine & metabolic: Elevated blood sugar
Gastrointestinal: Discoloration of feces/sputum
Genitourinary: Discoloration of urine
Ocular: Irritation of the eyes
Miscellaneous: Discoloration of sweat

Drug Interactions No data reported

Drug Uptake
Absorption: Oral: 45% to 70% absorbed slowly
Serum half-life:
Terminal: 8 days
Tissue: 70 days
Time to peak serum concentration: 1-6 hours with chronic therapy

Pregnancy Risk Factor C

Generic Available No

Clofibrate *(kloe FYE brate)*

Brand Names Atromid-S®

Canadian/Mexican Brand Names Abitrate® (Canada); Claripex® (Canada); Novo-Fibrate® (Canada)

Therapeutic Category Lipid Lowering Drugs

Use Adjunct to dietary therapy in the management of hyperlipidemias associated with high triglyceride levels (types III, IV, V); primarily lowers triglycerides and very low density lipoprotein

Usual Dosage Adults: Oral: 500 mg 4 times/day; some patients may respond to lower doses

Mechanism of Action Mechanism is unclear but thought to reduce cholesterol synthesis and triglyceride hepatic-vascular transference

Local Anesthetic/Vasoconstrictor Precautions No information available to require special precautions

Effects on Dental Treatment No effects or complications reported
Other Adverse Effects
>10%: Gastrointestinal: Nausea
1% to 10%: Gastrointestinal: Diarrhea, vomiting, dyspepsia, flatulence, abdominal distress
<1%:
Cardiovascular: Angina, cardiac arrhythmias
Central nervous system: Headache, dizziness, fatigue
Dermatologic: Skin rash, urticaria, pruritus, alopecia
Gastrointestinal: Gallstones
Genitourinary: Impotence
Hematologic: Leukopenia, anemia, eosinophilia, agranulocytosis
Hepatic: Elevated liver function test
Neuromuscular & skeletal: Muscle cramping, aching, myalgia, weakness
Renal: Renal toxicity, rhabdomyolysis-induced renal failure
Miscellaneous: Dry, brittle hair
Drug Interactions
Increased effect:
Warfarin: Clofibrate increases the hypoprothrombinemic effect of warfarin. The mechanism has not been established, but serious bleeding episodes have occurred in some patients receiving both drugs
Sulfonylureas: Clofibrate may enhance the effects of the sulfonylurea-type oral hypoglycemics by displacement from plasma protein binding sites
Drug Uptake
Absorption: Occurs completely; intestinal transformation is required to activate the drug
Serum half-life: 6-24 hours, increases significantly with reduced renal function; with anuria: 110 hours
Time to peak serum concentration: Within 3-6 hours
Pregnancy Risk Factor C
Generic Available Yes

Clomid® *see* Clomiphene *on this page*

Clomifeno, Citrato De (Mexico) *see* Clomiphene *on this page*

Clomiphene (KLOE mi feen)

Brand Names Clomid®; Milophene®; Serophene®
Canadian/Mexican Brand Names Omifin® (Mexico)
Therapeutic Category Ovulation Stimulator
Synonyms Clomifeno, Citrato De (Mexico)
Use Treatment of ovulatory failure in patients desiring pregnancy

Unlabeled use: Male infertility
Usual Dosage Adults: Oral:
Males (infertility): 25 mg/day for 25 days with 5 days rest, or 100 mg every Monday, Wednesday, Friday
Females (ovulatory failure): Oral: 50 mg/day for 5 days (first course); start the regimen on or about the fifth day of cycle; if ovulation occurs do not increase dosage; if not, increase next course to 100 mg/day for 5 days. Three courses of therapy are an adequate therapeutic trial. Further treatment is not recommended in patients who do not exhibit ovulation.
Mechanism of Action Induces ovulation by stimulating the release of pituitary gonadotropins
Local Anesthetic/Vasoconstrictor Precautions No information available to require special precautions
Effects on Dental Treatment No effects or complications reported
Other Adverse Effects
>10%: Endocrine & metabolic: Hot flashes, ovarian enlargement
1% to 10%:
Cardiovascular: Thromboembolism
Central nervous system: Mental depression, headache
Endocrine & metabolic: Breast enlargement (males), abnormal menstrual flow
Gastrointestinal: Distention, bloating, nausea, vomiting
Hepatic: Hepatotoxicity
Ocular: Blurring of vision, diplopia, floaters, after-images, phosphenes, photophobia
<1%:
Central nervous system: Insomnia, fatigue
Dermatologic: Alopecia (reversible)
Gastrointestinal: Weight gain
Renal: Polyuria
Drug Interactions No data reported
(Continued)

Clomiphene (Continued)

Drug Uptake
Serum half-life: 5-7 days
Pregnancy Risk Factor X
Generic Available No

Clomipramine (kloe MI pra meen)

Brand Names Anafranil®
Canadian/Mexican Brand Names Apo®-Clomipramine (Canada)
Therapeutic Category Antidepressant, Tricyclic
Use Treatment of obsessive-compulsive disorder (OCD); may also relieve depression, panic attacks, and chronic pain
Usual Dosage Oral: Initial:
Children: 25 mg/day and gradually increase, as tolerated, to a maximum of 3 mg/kg/day or 200 mg/day, whichever is smaller
Adults: 25 mg/day and gradually increase, as tolerated, to 100 mg/day the first 2 weeks, may then be increased to a total of 250 mg/day maximum
Mechanism of Action Clomipramine appears to affect serotonin uptake while its active metabolite, desmethylclomipramine, affects norepinephrine uptake
Local Anesthetic/Vasoconstrictor Precautions Use with caution; epinephrine, norepinephrine and levonordefrin have been shown to have an increased pressor response in combination with TCAs
Effects on Dental Treatment >10% of patients experience dry mouth; long-term treatment with TCAs such as clomipramine increases the risk of caries by reducing salivation and salivary buffer capacity
Other Adverse Effects
>10%:
Central nervous system: Dizziness, drowsiness, headache
Gastrointestinal: Constipation, increased appetite, nausea, unpleasant taste, weight gain
Neuromuscular & skeletal: Weakness
1% to 10%:
Cardiovascular: Arrhythmias, hypotension
Central nervous system: Confusion, delirium, hallucinations, nervousness, restlessness, parkinsonian syndrome, insomnia
Endocrine & metabolic: Sexual dysfunction
Gastrointestinal: Diarrhea, heartburn
Genitourinary: Dysuria
Neuromuscular & skeletal: Fine muscle tremors
Ocular: Blurred vision, eye pain
Miscellaneous: Excessive sweating
<1%:
Central nervous system: Anxiety, seizures
Dermatologic: Alopecia, photosensitivity
Endocrine & metabolic: Breast enlargement, galactorrhea, SIADH
Gastrointestinal: Trouble with gums, decreased lower esophageal sphincter tone may cause GE reflux
Genitourinary: Testicular swelling
Hematologic: Agranulocytosis, leukopenia, eosinophilia
Hepatic: Cholestatic jaundice, elevated liver enzymes
Ocular: Increased intraocular pressure
Otic: Tinnitus
Miscellaneous: Allergic reactions
Drug Interactions
Decreased effect: Phenobarbital may increase the metabolism of clomipramine; clomipramine blocks the uptake of guanethidine and thus prevents the hypotensive effect of guanethidine
Increased toxicity: Tricyclic antidepressants, such as clomipramine, can inhibit the antihypertensive to clonidine resulting in hypertension; clomipramine may be additive with or may potentiate the action of other CNS depressants such as sedatives or hypnotics; with MAO inhibitors, hyperpyrexia, hypertension, tachycardia, confusion, and seizures. Clomipramine may increase the prothrombin time in patients stabilized on warfarin; clomipramine may potentiate the pressor and cardiac effects of sympathomimetic agents such as isoproterenol, epinephrine, etc; cimetidine and methylphenidate may decrease the metabolism of clomipramine
Additive anticholinergic effects seen with other anticholinergic agents
Drug Uptake
Absorption: Oral: Rapid
Serum half-life: 20-30 hours
Pregnancy Risk Factor C

Generic Available Yes

Selected Readings

Boakes AJ, Laurence DR, Teoh PC, et al, "Interactions Between Sympathomimetic Amines and Antidepressant Agents in Man," *Br Med J,* 1973, 1(849):311-5.

Jastak JT and Yagiela JA, "Vasoconstrictors and Local Anesthesia: A Review and Rationale for Use," *J Am Dent Assoc,* 1983, 107(4):623-30.

Larochelle P, Hamet P, and Enjalbert M, "Responses to Tyramine and Norepinephrine After Imipramine and Trazodone," *Clin Pharmacol Ther,* 1979, 26(1):24-30.

Mitchell JR, "Guanethidine and Related Agents. III Antagonism by Drugs Which Inhibit the Norepinephrine Pump in Man," *J Clin Invest,* 1970, 49(8):1596-604.

Rundegren J, van Dijken J, Mörnstad H, et al, "Oral Conditions in Patients Receiving Long-Term Treatment With Cyclic Antidepressant Drugs," *Swed Dent J,* 1985, 9(2):55-64.

Svedmyr N, "The Influence of a Tricyclic Antidepressive Agent (Protriptyline) on Some of the Circulatory Effects of Noradrenaline and Adrenalin® in Man," *Life Sci,* 1968, 7(1):77-84.

Clomycin® [OTC] *see* Bacitracin, Neomycin, Polymyxin B, and Lidocaine *on page 109*

Clonacepam (Mexico) *see* Clonazepam *on this page*

Clonazepam (kloe NA ze pam)

Brand Names Klonopin™

Canadian/Mexican Brand Names PMS-Clonazepam® (Canada); Rivotril® (Canada); Rivotril® (Mexico)

Therapeutic Category Anticonvulsant, Benzodiazepine

Synonyms Clonacepam (Mexico)

Use Prophylaxis of petit mal, petit mal variant (Lennox-Gastaut), akinetic, and myoclonic seizures

> **Unlabeled use:** Restless legs syndrome, neuralgia, multifocal tic disorder, parkinsonian dysarthria, acute manic episodes, and adjunct therapy for schizophrenia

Usual Dosage Oral:

Children <10 years or 30 kg:

Initial daily dose: 0.01-0.03 mg/kg/day (maximum: 0.05 mg/kg/day) given in 2-3 divided doses; increase by no more than 0.5 mg every third day until seizures are controlled or adverse effects seen

Usual maintenance dose: 0.1-0.2 mg/kg/day divided 3 times/day; not to exceed 0.2 mg/kg/day

Adults:

Initial daily dose not to exceed 1.5 mg given in 3 divided doses; may increase by 0.5-1 mg every third day until seizures are controlled or adverse effects seen

Usual maintenance dose: 0.05-0.2 mg/kg; do not exceed 20 mg/day

Hemodialysis effects: Supplemental dose is not necessary

Mechanism of Action Suppresses the spike-and-wave discharge in absence seizures by depressing nerve transmission in the motor cortex

Local Anesthetic/Vasoconstrictor Precautions No information available to require special precautions

Effects on Dental Treatment No effects or complications reported

Other Adverse Effects

>10%:

Cardiovascular: Tachycardia

Central nervous system: Somnolence (50%), ataxia (30%), fatigue, depression, amnesia, lightheadedness, insomnia, anxiety, headache

Dermatologic: Rash

Gastrointestinal: Constipation, diarrhea, nausea, vomiting

Neuromuscular & skeletal: Dysarthria

Ocular: Blurred vision

Miscellaneous: Diaphoresis

1% to 10%:

Cardiovascular: Syncope, hypotension

Central nervous system: Confusion

Dermatologic: Dermatitis

Gastrointestinal: Weight gain or loss, increased salivation

Neuromuscular & skeletal: Rigidity, tremor, muscle cramps/weakness

Otic: Tinnitus

Respiratory: Nasal congestion

Drug Interactions No significant interactions have been reported

Drug Uptake

Onset of effect: 20-60 minutes

Duration: Up to 6-8 hours in infants and young children, up to 12 hours in adults

Absorption: Oral: Well absorbed

Serum half-life:

Children: 22-33 hours

(Continued)

Clonazepam *(Continued)*

    Adults: 19-50 hours
    Time to peak serum concentration: Oral: 1-3 hours
        Steady-state: 5-7 days
Pregnancy Risk Factor C
Generic Available Yes

Clonidina (Mexico) *see* Clonidine *on this page*

Clonidine (KLOE ni deen)

Related Information
    Cardiovascular Diseases *on page 1010*
Brand Names Catapres® Oral; Catapres-TTS® Transdermal; Duraclon® Injection
Canadian/Mexican Brand Names Apo®-Clonidine (Canada); Catapresan-100® (Mexico); Dixarit® (Canada); Novo-Clonidine® (Canada); Nu-Clonidine® (Canada)
Therapeutic Category Alpha-Adrenergic Blockers - Peripheral-Acting (Alpha$_1$-Blockers); Antiglaucoma Agent
Synonyms Clonidina (Mexico)
Use Management of mild to moderate hypertension; either used alone or in combination with other antihypertensives; not recommended for first-line therapy for hypertension; also used for heroin withdrawal and in smoking cessation therapy; other uses may include prophylaxis of migraines, glaucoma, paralytic ileus, and diabetes-associated diarrhea
Usual Dosage
    Oral:
        Children: Initial: 5-10 mcg/kg/day in divided doses every 8-12 hours; increase gradually at 5- to 7-day intervals to 25 mcg/kg/day in divided doses every 6 hours; maximum: 0.9 mg/day
            Clonidine tolerance test (test of growth hormone release from pituitary): 0.15 mg/m^2 or 4 mcg/kg as single dose
        Adults: Initial dose: 0.1 mg twice daily, usual maintenance dose: 0.2-1.2 mg/day in 2-4 divided doses; maximum recommended dose: 2.4 mg/day
            Nicotine withdrawal symptoms: 0.1 mg twice daily to maximum of 0.4 mg/day for 3-4 weeks
        Elderly: Initial: 0.1 mg once daily at bedtime, increase gradually as needed
    Transdermal: Apply once every 7 days; for initial therapy start with 0.1 mg and increase by 0.1 mg at 1- to 2-week intervals; dosages >0.6 mg do not improve efficacy
Mechanism of Action Stimulates alpha$_2$-adrenoreceptors in the brain stem, thus activating an inhibitory neuron, resulting in reduced sympathetic outflow, producing a decrease in vasomotor tone and heart rate
Local Anesthetic/Vasoconstrictor Precautions No information available to require special precautions
Effects on Dental Treatment >10% of patients experience significant dry mouth
Other Adverse Effects
  >10%:
    Central nervous system: Drowsiness, dizziness
    Gastrointestinal: Constipation
  1% to 10%:
    Cardiovascular: Orthostatic hypotension
    Central nervous system: Nervousness, agitation, mental depression, headache, fatigue
    Dermatologic: Rash
    Endocrine & metabolic: Decreased sexual activity, loss of libido
    Gastrointestinal: Nausea, vomiting
    Genitourinary: Nocturia, impotence
    Hepatic: Abnormal liver function tests
    Neuromuscular & skeletal: Weakness
  <1%:
    Cardiovascular: Palpitations, tachycardia, bradycardia, Raynaud's phenomenon, congestive heart failure
    Central nervous system: Insomnia, vivid dreams, delirium, fever
    Dermatologic: Pruritus, urticaria, alopecia
    Endocrine & metabolic: Gynecomastia
    Gastrointestinal: Weight gain
    Genitourinary: Difficulty in micturition, urinary retention
    Ocular: Burning of the eyes, blurred vision
Drug Interactions
  Tricyclic antidepressants antagonize hypotensive effects of clonidine; this could result in hypertension

Increased toxicity: Beta-blockers may potentiate bradycardia in patients receiving clonidine and may increase the rebound hypertension of withdrawal; discontinue beta-blocker several days before clonidine is tapered

Drug Uptake
Onset of effect: Oral: 0.5-1 hour; T_{max}: 2-4 hours
Duration: 6-10 hours
Serum half-life: Adults:
Normal renal function: 6-20 hours
Renal impairment: 18-41 hours

Pregnancy Risk Factor C
Generic Available Yes: Tablet

Clonidine and Chlorthalidone (KLOE ni deen & klor THAL i done)
Brand Names Combipres®
Therapeutic Category Antihypertensive Agent, Combination
Use Management of mild to moderate hypertension
Local Anesthetic/Vasoconstrictor Precautions No information available to require special precautions
Effects on Dental Treatment No effects or complications reported
Pregnancy Risk Factor C
Generic Available No

Clopidogrel (kloh PID oh grel)
Brand Names Plavix®
Therapeutic Category Antiplatelet Agent
Synonyms Clopidogrel Bisulfate
Use The reduction of atherosclerotic events (myocardial infarction, stroke, vascular deaths) in patients with atherosclerosis documented by recent myocardial infarctions, recent stroke or established peripheral arterial disease
Mechanism of Action Blocks the ADP receptor and in so doing, prevents the binding of fibrinogen to that site. Clopidrogel, however, does not alter the receptor, which suggests that it prevents the binding of fibrinogen in an indirect manner. This drug reduces the number of functional ADP receptors. The effect of clopidrogel continues for several days after discontinuing the drug and it effects decrease proportionally to platelet renewal.
Local Anesthetic/Vasoconstrictor Precautions No information available to require special precautions
Effects on Dental Treatment No effects or complications reported
Contraindications In patients with active pathologic bleeding or who have shown hypersensitivity to the drug or any component of the drug and should be used with caution in patients with severe liver disease
Dosage Forms Tablet, as bisulfate: 75 mg

Clopidogrel Bisulfate see Clopidogrel *on this page*
Clopra® see Metoclopramide *on page 627*
Cloracepato Dipotasico (Mexico) see Clorazepate *on this page*
Cloranfenicol (Mexico) see Chloramphenicol *on page 209*

Clorazepate (klor AZ e pate)
Brand Names Gen-XENE®; Tranxene®
Canadian/Mexican Brand Names Apo®-Clorazepate (Canada); Novo-Clopate® (Canada)
Therapeutic Category Anticonvulsant, Benzodiazepine; Benzodiazepine; Sedative
Synonyms Cloracepato Dipotasico (Mexico)
Use Treatment of generalized anxiety and panic disorders; management of alcohol withdrawal; adjunct anticonvulsant in management of partial seizures
Usual Dosage Oral:
Children 9-12 years: Anticonvulsant: Initial: 3.75-7.5 mg/dose twice daily; increase dose by 3.75 mg at weekly intervals, not to exceed 60 mg/day in 2-3 divided doses

Children >12 years and Adults: Anticonvulsant: Initial: Up to 7.5 mg/dose 2-3 times/day; increase dose by 7.5 mg at weekly intervals; not to exceed 90 mg/day

Adults:
Anxiety: 7.5-15 mg 2-4 times/day, or given as single dose of 11.25 or 22.5 mg at bedtime
Alcohol withdrawal: Initial: 30 mg, then 15 mg 2-4 times/day on first day; maximum daily dose: 90 mg; gradually decrease dose over subsequent days
(Continued)

Clorazepate *(Continued)*

Mechanism of Action Facilitates gamma aminobutyric acid (GABA)-mediated transmission inhibitory neurotransmitter action, depresses subcortical levels of CNS

Local Anesthetic/Vasoconstrictor Precautions No information available to require special precautions

Effects on Dental Treatment Many patients will experience drowsiness and dry mouth while taking clorazepate which will disappear with cessation of drug therapy; orthostatic hypotension is possible; it is suggested that narcotic analgesics not be given for pain control to patients taking clorazepate because of enhanced sedation

Other Adverse Effects

>10%: Central nervous system: Drowsiness

1% to 10%:

Central nervous system: Confusion, nervousness, dizziness, headache

Gastrointestinal: Xerostomia

Ocular: Blurred vision

<1%:

Cardiovascular: Decreased systolic blood pressure

Hematologic: Decreased hematocrit

Hepatic: Abnormal LFTs

Renal: Abnormal kidney function tests

Drug Interactions Increased effect: Cimetidine, CNS depressants, alcohol

Drug Uptake

Serum half-life: Adults:

Desmethyldiazepam: 48-96 hours

Oxazepam: 6-8 hours

Time to peak serum concentration: Oral: Within 1 hour

Pregnancy Risk Factor D

Generic Available Yes

Clorfeniramina, Maleato De (Mexico) *see* Chlorpheniramine *on page 217*

Clorodiacepoxido (Mexico) *see* Chlordiazepoxide *on page 210*

Cloroquina, Defosfato De (Mexico) *see* Chloroquine Phosphate *on page 214*

Clorpactin® WCS-90 *see* Oxychlorosene *on page 710*

Clorpropamida (Mexico) *see* Chlorpropamide *on page 225*

Clortalidona (Mexico) *see* Chlorthalidone *on page 227*

Clortetraciclina (Mexico) *see* Chlortetracycline *on page 226*

Clotrimazole *(kloe TRIM a zole)*

Related Information

Oral Fungal Infections *on page 1063*

Brand Names Mycelex® Troche

Therapeutic Category Antifungal Agent, Oral Nonabsorbed; Antifungal Agent, Topical; Antifungal Agent, Vaginal

Use

Dental: Treatment of susceptible fungal infections, including oropharyngeal candidiasis; limited data suggests that the use of clotrimazole troches may be effective for prophylaxis against oropharyngeal candidiasis in neutropenic patients

Medical: Treatment of susceptible fungal infections including dermatophytoses, superficial mycoses, and cutaneous candidiasis, as well as vulvovaginal candidiasis

Usual Dosage Children >3 years and Adults: 10 mg troche dissolved slowly 5 times/day for 14 consecutive days

Mechanism of Action Binds to phospholipids in the fungal cell membrane altering cell wall permeability resulting in loss of essential intracellular elements

Local Anesthetic/Vasoconstrictor Precautions No information available to require special precautions

Effects on Dental Treatment No effects or complications reported

Other Adverse Effects

>10%: Hepatic: Abnormal liver function tests

1% to 10%:

Gastrointestinal: Nausea and vomiting may occur in patients on clotrimazole troches

Local: Mild burning, irritation, stinging to skin or vaginal area

Contraindications Hypersensitivity to clotrimazole or any component

Warnings/Precautions Clotrimazole should not be used for treatment of systemic fungal infection; safety and effectiveness of clotrimazole lozenges (troches) in children <3 years of age have not been established

Drug Interactions Increased cyclosporine levels can occur; enhanced hypoglycemic effects with sulfonylureas

Drug Uptake
Duration: Up to 3 hours
Absorption: Oral: Poor
Time to peak serum concentration: Oral topical administration: Salivary levels occur within 3 hours following 30 minutes of dissolution time in the mouth

Pregnancy Risk Factor B; C (oral)

Breast-feeding Considerations No data reported

Dosage Forms Troche, oral (Mycelex®): 10 mg

Dietary Considerations No data reported

Generic Available Yes

Cloxacillin (kloks a SIL in)

Brand Names Cloxapen®; Tegopen®

Canadian/Mexican Brand Names Apo®-Cloxi (Canada); Novo-Cloxin (Canada); Nu-Cloxi (Canada); Orbenin® (Canada); Taro-Cloxacillin® (Canada)

Therapeutic Category Antibiotic, Penicillin

Use
Dental: Treatment of susceptible orofacial infections, notably penicillinase-producing staphylococci
Medical: Treatment of susceptible bacterial infections in the medical patient, notably penicillinase-producing staphylococci causing respiratory tract, skin and skin structure, bone and joint, urinary tract infections, endocarditis, septicemia, and meningitis

Usual Dosage Oral:
Children <20 kg: 50-100 mg/kg/day in divided doses every 6 hours
Children >20 kg and Adults: 250-500 mg every 6 hours for at least 7 days

Mechanism of Action Inhibits bacterial cell wall synthesis by binding to one or more of the penicillin-binding proteins (PBPs) which in turn inhibits the final transpeptidation step of peptidoglycan synthesis in bacterial cell walls, thus inhibiting cell wall biosynthesis. Bacteria eventually lyse due to ongoing activity of cell wall autolytic enzymes (autolysins and murein hydrolases) while cell wall assembly is arrested.

Local Anesthetic/Vasoconstrictor Precautions No information available to require special precautions

Effects on Dental Treatment Prolonged use of penicillins may lead to development of oral candidiasis

Other Adverse Effects 1% to 10%:
Gastrointestinal: Nausea, diarrhea
Hematologic: Agranulocytosis
Hepatic: Elevations of AST and ALT
Renal: Hematuria
Miscellaneous: Serum sickness-like reactions

Contraindications Hypersensitivity to cloxacillin or any component, or penicillins

Warnings/Precautions Monitor PTT if patient concurrently on warfarin, elimination of drug is slow in renally impaired; use with caution in patients allergic to cephalosporins due to a low incidence of cross-hypersensitivity

Drug Interactions Efficacy of oral contraceptives may be reduced; disulfiram, probenecid may increase cloxacillin levels; cloxacillin may increase the effect of anticoagulants

Drug Uptake
Absorption: Oral: ~50%
Serum half-life: 0.5-1.5 hours
Time to peak serum concentration: Oral: Within 0.5-2 hours

Pregnancy Risk Factor B

Breast-feeding Considerations No data reported; however, other penicillins may be taken while breast-feeding

Dosage Forms
Capsule, as sodium: 250 mg, 500 mg
Powder for oral suspension, as sodium: 125 mg/5 mL (100 mL, 200 mL)

Dietary Considerations Should be taken 1 hour before or 2 hours after meals with water

Generic Available Yes

Comments Although cloxacillin is a penicillin antibiotic indicated for infections caused by penicillinase-secreting staph, amoxicillin with clavulanic acid is considered the drug of choice for these types of orofacial infections

Cloxapen® see Cloxacillin on this page

Clozapina (Mexico) see Clozapine on next page

Clozapine (KLOE za peen)
Brand Names Clozaril®
Canadian/Mexican Brand Names Leponex® (Mexico)
Therapeutic Category Antipsychotic Agent
Synonyms Clozapina (Mexico)
Use Management of schizophrenic patients
Usual Dosage Adults: Oral: 25 mg once or twice daily initially and increased, as tolerated to a target dose of 300-450 mg/day after 2 weeks, but may require doses as high as 600-900 mg/day
Mechanism of Action Clozapine is a weak dopamine$_1$ and dopamine$_2$ receptor blocker; in addition, it blocks the serotonin$_2$, alpha-adrenergic, and histamine H$_1$ central nervous system receptors
Local Anesthetic/Vasoconstrictor Precautions No information available to require special precautions
Effects on Dental Treatment Many patients may experience orthostatic hypotension with clozapine; precautions should be taken; do not use atropine-like drugs for xerostomia in patients taking clozapine because of significant potentiation

Other Adverse Effects
>10%:
  Cardiovascular: Tachycardia, hypotension, orthostatic hypotension
  Central nervous system: Fever, headache, drowsiness
  Gastrointestinal: Constipation, nausea, vomiting, unusual weight gain
1% to 10%:
  Cardiovascular: EKG changes, hypertension
  Central nervous system: Agitation, akathisia
  Gastrointestinal: Abdominal discomfort, heartburn, dry mouth
  Ocular: Blurred vision
  Miscellaneous: Increased sweating
<1%:
  Central nervous system: Insomnia, seizures, tardive dyskinesia, neuroleptic malignant syndrome
  Genitourinary: Dysuria, impotence
  Hematologic: Agranulocytosis, eosinophilia, granulocytopenia, leukopenia, thrombocytopenia
  Neuromuscular & skeletal: Rigidity, tremor

Drug Interactions
Decreased effect with phenytoin
Increased effect of CNS depressants, guanabenz, anticholinergics
Increased toxicity with cimetidine, MAO inhibitors, neuroleptics, TCAs

Clozapine may significantly potentiate the hypotensive effects of antihypertensive drugs and the anticholinergic effects of atropine-type drugs. In medical emergencies, the administration of epinephrine should be avoided in the treatment of drug-induced hypotension because of a possible reverse epinephrine effect. There are no data to suggest any interaction between clozapine and the use of vasoconstrictors in local anesthesia.

Pregnancy Risk Factor B
Generic Available No

Clozaril® *see* Clozapine *on this page*

Clysodrast® *see* Bisacodyl *on page 131*

Coal Tar (KOLE tar)
Brand Names AquaTar® [OTC]; Denorex® [OTC]; DHS® Tar [OTC]; Duplex® T [OTC]; Estar® [OTC]; Fototar® [OTC]; Neutrogena® T/Derm; Oxipor® VHC [OTC]; Pentrax® [OTC]; Polytar® [OTC]; psoriGel® [OTC]; T/Gel® [OTC]; Zetar® [OTC]
Therapeutic Category Antipsoriatic Agent, Topical; Antiseborrheic Agent, Topical
Synonyms Crude Coal Tar; LCD; Pix Carbonis
Use Topically for controlling dandruff, seborrheic dermatitis, or psoriasis
Local Anesthetic/Vasoconstrictor Precautions No information available to require special precautions
Effects on Dental Treatment No effects or complications reported
Other Adverse Effects 1% to 10%: Dermatologic: Dermatitis, folliculitis
Pregnancy Risk Factor C
Generic Available Yes
Comments Avoid exposure to sunlight for 24 hours after use; may stain clothing and skin

Coal Tar and Salicylic Acid (KOLE tar & sal i SIL ik AS id)

Brand Names X-seb® T [OTC]

Therapeutic Category Antipsoriatic Agent, Topical; Antiseborrheic Agent, Topical

Use Seborrheal dermatitis; dandruff

Local Anesthetic/Vasoconstrictor Precautions No information available to require special precautions

Effects on Dental Treatment No effects or complications reported

Pregnancy Risk Factor C

Generic Available Yes

Coal Tar, Lanolin, and Mineral Oil

(KOLE tar, LAN oh lin, & MIN er al oyl)

Brand Names Balnetar® [OTC]

Therapeutic Category Antipsoriatic Agent, Topical; Antiseborrheic Agent, Topical

Use Psoriasis; seborrheal dermatitis; atopic dermatitis; eczematoid dermatitis

Local Anesthetic/Vasoconstrictor Precautions No information available to require special precautions

Effects on Dental Treatment No effects or complications reported

Generic Available Yes

Cobalamin (Canada) *see* Cyanocobalamin *on page 266*

Cocaine (koe KANE)

Therapeutic Category Local Anesthetic, Topical

Use Topical anesthesia (ester derivative) for mucous membranes

Usual Dosage Dosage depends on the area to be anesthetized, tissue vascularity, technique of anesthesia, and individual patient tolerance; use the lowest dose necessary to produce adequate anesthesia should be used, not to exceed 1 mg/kg. Use reduced dosages for children, elderly, or debilitated patients.

Topical application (ear, nose, throat, bronchoscopy): Concentrations of 1% to 4% are used; concentrations >4% are not recommended because of potential for increased incidence and severity of systemic toxic reactions

Mechanism of Action Blocks both the initiation and conduction of nerve impulses by decreasing the neuronal membrane's permeability to sodium ions, which results in inhibition of depolarization with resultant blockade of conduction; interferes with the uptake of norepinephrine by adrenergic nerve terminals producing vasoconstriction

Local Anesthetic/Vasoconstrictor Precautions No information available to require special precautions

Effects on Dental Treatment No effects or complications reported

Other Adverse Effects

>10%:
  Central nervous system: CNS stimulation
  Local: Loss of smell/taste, chronic rhinitis, nasal congestion

1% to 10%:
  Cardiovascular: Bradycardia with low doses, tachycardia with moderate doses, hypertension, cardiac arrhythmias
  Central nervous system: Nervousness, restlessness, euphoria, excitement, hallucination, seizures
  Gastrointestinal: Vomiting
  Neuromuscular & skeletal: Tremors and clonic-tonic reactions
  Ocular: Sloughing of the corneal epithelium, ulceration of the cornea
  Respiratory: Tachypnea, respiratory failure

Drug Interactions Increased toxicity: MAO inhibitors

Drug Uptake Following topical administration to mucosa:
  Onset of action: Within 1 minute
  Peak action: Within 5 minutes
  Duration: ≥30 minutes, depending on dosage administered
  Absorption: Well absorbed through mucous membranes; limited by drug-induced vasoconstriction; enhanced by inflammation
  Serum half-life: 75 minutes

Pregnancy Risk Factor C (X if nonmedicinal use)

Dosage Forms
  Powder, as hydrochloride: 5 g, 25 g
  Solution, topical, as hydrochloride: 4% [40 mg/mL] (2 mL, 4 mL, 10 mL); 10% [100 mg/mL] (4 mL, 10 mL)
  Solution, topical, viscous, as hydrochloride: 4% [40 mg/mL] (4 mL, 10 mL); 10% [100 mg/mL] (4 mL, 10 mL)
  Tablet, soluble, for topical solution, as hydrochloride: 135 mg
  (Continued)

Cocaine *(Continued)*

Generic Available Yes

Codafed® Expectorant *see* Guaifenesin, Pseudoephedrine, and Codeine *on page 455*

Codamine® *see* Hydrocodone and Phenylpropanolamine *on page 483*

Codamine® Pediatric *see* Hydrocodone and Phenylpropanolamine *on page 483*

Codehist® DH *see* Chlorpheniramine, Pseudoephedrine, and Codeine *on page 223*

Codeine (KOE deen)

Related Information

Dental Drug Interactions: Update on Drug Combinations Requiring Special Considerations *on page 1144*

Narcotic Agonists *on page 1141*

Canadian/Mexican Brand Names Linctus Codeine Blac (Canada); Linctus With Codeine Phosphate (Canada); Paveral Stanley Syrup With Codeine Phosphate (Canada)

Therapeutic Category Analgesic, Narcotic; Antitussive

Synonyms Methylmorphine (Canada)

Use

Dental: Treatment of postoperative pain

Medical: Relief of pain

Restrictions C-II; Nonrefillable

Usual Dosage Oral:

Children: Not recommended in pediatric dental patients

Adults: 30 mg/dose; range: 15-60 mg every 4-6 hours as needed; maximum: 360 mg/24 hours

Mechanism of Action Binds to opiate receptors (mu and kappa subtypes) in the CNS causing inhibition of ascending pain pathways, altering the perception of and response to pain

Local Anesthetic/Vasoconstrictor Precautions No information available to require special precautions

Effects on Dental Treatment <1% of patients experience dry mouth

Other Adverse Effects

>10%:

Central nervous system: Lightheadedness, dizziness, sedation

Gastrointestinal: Nausea, vomiting

1% to 10%: Gastrointestinal: Constipation

Contraindications Hypersensitivity to codeine

Warnings/Precautions Use with caution in patients with hypersensitivity reactions to other phenanthrene derivative opioid agonists (morphine, hydrocodone, hydromorphone, levorphanol, oxycodone, oxymorphone); respiratory diseases including asthma, emphysema, COPD, or severe liver or renal insufficiency; some preparations contain sulfites which may cause allergic reactions; may be habit-forming

Enhanced analgesia has been seen in elderly patients on therapeutic doses of narcotics; duration of action may be increased in the elderly; the elderly may be particularly susceptible to the CNS depressant and constipating effects of narcotics

Drug Interactions Increased toxicity of CNS depressants, phenothiazines, tricyclic antidepressants, guanabenz, MAO inhibitors (may also lead to a decrease in blood pressure)

Drug Uptake

Onset of effect: Analgesia: 30-45 minutes

Duration of effect: 4-6 hours

Serum half-life: 2.5-3.5 hours

Time to peak serum concentration: 1-2 hours

Pregnancy Risk Factor C (D if used for prolonged periods or in high doses at term)

Breast-feeding Considerations May be taken while breast-feeding

Dosage Forms

Injection, as phosphate: 30 mg (1 mL, 2 mL); 60 mg (1 mL, 2 mL)

Solution, oral: 15 mg/5 mL

Tablet, as sulfate: 15 mg, 30 mg, 60 mg

Tablet, as phosphate, soluble: 30 mg, 60 mg

Tablet, as sulfate, soluble: 15 mg, 30 mg, 60 mg

Dietary Considerations May be taken with food or water to minimize GI distress

Generic Available Yes

Comments It is recommended that codeine not be used as the sole entity for analgesia because of moderate efficacy along with relatively high incidence of nausea, sedation, and constipation. In addition, codeine has some narcotic addiction liability. Codeine in combination with acetaminophen or aspirin is recommended. Maximum effective analgesic dose of codeine is 60 mg (1 grain). Beyond 60 mg increases respiratory depression only.

Selected Readings
Desjardins PJ, Cooper SA, Gallegos TL, et al, "The Relative Analgesic Efficacy of Propiram Fumarate, Codeine, Aspirin, and Placebo in Post-Impaction Dental Pain," *J Clin Pharmacol*, 1984, 24(1):35-42.

Forbes JA, Keller CK, Smith JW, et al, "Analgesic Effect of Naproxen Sodium, Codeine, a Naproxen-Codeine Combination and Aspirin on the Postoperative Pain of Oral Surgery," *Pharmacotherapy*, 1986, 6(5):211-8.

Codeine and Bromodiphenhydramine *see* Bromodiphenhydramine and Codeine *on page 141*

Codeine and Butalbital Compound *see* Butalbital Compound and Codeine *on page 156*

Codiclear® DH *see* Hydrocodone and Guaifenesin *on page 481*

Codoxy® *see* Oxycodone and Aspirin *on page 712*

Cogentin® *see* Benztropine *on page 122*

Co-Gesic® [5/500] *see* Hydrocodone and Acetaminophen *on page 478*

Cognex® *see* Tacrine *on page 901*

Co-Hist® [OTC] *see* Acetaminophen, Chlorpheniramine, and Pseudoephedrine *on page 24*

Colace® [OTC] *see* Docusate *on page 331*

Colchicina (Mexico) *see* Colchicine *on this page*

Colchicine (KOL chi seen)
Canadian/Mexican Brand Names Colchiquim-30® (Mexico); Colchiquim® (Mexico)

Therapeutic Category Anti-inflammatory Agent; Uricosuric Agent

Synonyms Colchicina (Mexico)

Use Treat acute gouty arthritis attacks and to prevent recurrences of such attacks; management of familial Mediterranean fever

Usual Dosage
Prophylaxis of familial Mediterranean fever: Oral:
Children:
≤5 years: 0.5 mg/day
>5 years: 1-1.5 mg/day in 2-3 divided doses
Adults: 1-2 mg/day in 2-3 divided doses

Gouty arthritis, acute attacks: Adults:
Oral: Initial: 0.5-1.2 mg, then 0.5-0.6 mg every 1-2 hours or 1-1.2 mg every 2 hours until relief or GI side effects (nausea, vomiting, or diarrhea) occur to a maximum total dose of 8 mg; wait 3 days before initiating another course of therapy
I.V.: Initial: 1-3 mg, then 0.5 mg every 6 hours until response, not to exceed 4 mg/day; if pain recurs, it may be necessary to administer a daily dose of 1-2 mg for several days, however, do not give more colchicine by any route for at least 7 days after a full course of I.V. therapy (4 mg), transfer to oral colchicine in a dose similar to that being given I.V.

Gouty arthritis, prophylaxis of recurrent attacks: Adults: Oral: 0.5-0.6 mg/day or every other day

Mechanism of Action Decreases leukocyte motility, decreases phagocytosis in joints and lactic acid production, thereby reducing the deposition of urate crystals that perpetuates the inflammatory response

Local Anesthetic/Vasoconstrictor Precautions No information available to require special precautions

Effects on Dental Treatment No effects or complications reported

Other Adverse Effects
>10%: Gastrointestinal: Nausea, vomiting, diarrhea, abdominal pain
1% to 10%:
Dermatologic: Alopecia
Gastrointestinal: Anorexia
<1%:
Dermatologic: Rash
Genitourinary: Azoospermia
Hematologic: Bone marrow suppression, agranulocytosis, aplastic anemia
Hepatic: Hepatotoxicity
Neuromuscular & skeletal: Myopathy, peripheral neuritis

Drug Interactions Decreased effect: Vitamin B_{12} absorption may be reduced

Drug Uptake
Onset of effect:
Oral: Relief of pain and inflammation occurs after 24-48 hours
(Continued)

Colchicine *(Continued)*

I.V.: 6-12 hours

Serum half-life: 12-30 minutes

Time to peak serum concentration: Oral: Within 0.5-2 hours declining for the next 2 hours before increasing again due to enterohepatic recycling

Pregnancy Risk Factor C (oral)/D (parenteral)

Generic Available Yes: Tablet

Colchicine and Probenecid (KOL chi seen & proe BEN e sid)

Therapeutic Category Uricosuric Agent

Synonyms Probenecid and Colchicine

Use Treatment of chronic gouty arthritis when complicated by frequent, recurrent acute attacks of gout

Local Anesthetic/Vasoconstrictor Precautions No information available to require special precautions

Effects on Dental Treatment No effects or complications reported

Other Adverse Effects 1% to 10%:

Cardiovascular: Flushing

Central nervous system: Headache, dizziness

Dermatologic: Rash, alopecia

Gastrointestinal: Anorexia, nausea, vomiting, diarrhea, abdominal pain

Hematologic: Anemia, leukopenia, aplastic anemia, agranulocytosis

Hepatic: Hepatic necrosis, hepatotoxicity

Neuromuscular & skeletal: Peripheral neuritis, myopathy

Renal: Nephrotic syndrome, uric acid stones, polyuria

Miscellaneous: Hypersensitivity reactions

Pregnancy Risk Factor C oral/D parenteral

Generic Available Yes

Comments Do not initiate therapy until an acute gouty attack has subsided

Cold & Allergy® Elixir [OTC] *see* Brompheniramine and Phenylpropanolamine *on page 143*

Coldiac-LA® *see* Guaifenesin and Phenylpropanolamine *on page 454*

Coldloc® *see* Guaifenesin, Phenylpropanolamine, and Phenylephrine *on page 455*

Coldrine® [OTC] *see* Acetaminophen and Pseudoephedrine *on page 24*

Colestid® *see* Colestipol *on this page*

Colestipol (koe LES ti pole)

Related Information

Cardiovascular Diseases *on page 1010*

Brand Names Colestid®

Therapeutic Category Lipid Lowering Drugs

Synonyms Colestipol, Clorhidrato De (Mexico)

Use Adjunct in management of primary hypercholesterolemia; regression of arteri-olosclerosis; relief of pruritus associated with elevated levels of bile acids; possibly used to decrease plasma half-life of digoxin in toxicity

Usual Dosage Adults: Oral: 5-30 g/day in divided doses 2-4 times/day

Mechanism of Action Binds with bile acids to form an insoluble complex that is eliminated in feces; it thereby increases the fecal loss of bile acid-bound low density lipoprotein cholesterol

Local Anesthetic/Vasoconstrictor Precautions No information available to require special precautions

Effects on Dental Treatment No effects or complications reported

Other Adverse Effects

>10%: Gastrointestinal: Constipation

1% to 10%: Gastrointestinal: Abdominal pain and distention, belching, flatulence, nausea, vomiting, diarrhea

<1%:

Central nervous system: Headache, dizziness, anxiety, vertigo, drowsiness, fatigue

Dermatologic: Dermatitis, urticaria

Endocrine & metabolic: Elevated serum phosphorous and chloride with decrease of sodium and potassium

Gastrointestinal: Peptic ulceration, GI irritation and bleeding, anorexia

Hepatic: Cholelithiasis, cholecystitis

Neuromuscular & skeletal: Arthralgia, arthritis, weakness

Respiratory: Dyspnea

Drug Interactions Decreased absorption of tetracycline, vitamins A, D, E and K, digitalis glycosides, warfarin, thyroid hormones, thiazide diuretics, propranolol, phenobarbital, amiodarone, methotrexate, NSAIDs, and other drugs by binding to the drug in the intestine

Drug Uptake Absorption: Oral: Not absorbed
Pregnancy Risk Factor C
Generic Available No

Colestipol, Clorhidrato De (Mexico) *see* Colestipol *on previous page*
Colestiramina (Mexico) *see* Cholestyramine Resin *on page 229*

Colfosceril Palmitate (kole FOS er il PALM i tate)

Brand Names Exosurf® Neonatal™
Therapeutic Category Lung Surfactant
Synonyms Dipalmitoylphosphatidylcholine; DPPC; Synthetic Lung Surfactant
Use Neonatal respiratory distress syndrome (RDS):
  Prophylactic therapy: Infants at risk for developing RDS with body weight <1350 g; infants with evidence of pulmonary immaturity with body weight >1350 g
  Rescue therapy: Treatment of infants with RDS based on respiratory distress not attributable to any other causes and chest radiographic findings consistent with RDS
Usual Dosage For intratracheal use only
  Prophylactic treatment: Give 5 mL/kg (as two 2.5 mL/kg half-doses) as soon as possible; the second and third doses should be administered at 12 and 24 hours later to those infants remaining on ventilators
  Rescue treatment: Give 5 mL/kg (as two 2.5 mL/kg half-doses) as soon as the diagnosis of RDS is made; the second 5 mL/kg (as two 2.5 mL/kg half-doses) dose should be administered 12 hours later
Mechanism of Action Replaces deficient or ineffective endogenous lung surfactant in neonates with respiratory distress syndrome (RDS) or in neonates at risk of developing RDS; reduces surface tension and stabilizes the alveoli from collapsing
Local Anesthetic/Vasoconstrictor Precautions No information available to require special precautions
Effects on Dental Treatment No effects or complications reported
Other Adverse Effects 1% to 10%: Respiratory: Pulmonary hemorrhage, apnea, mucous plugging, decrease in transcutaneous O_2 >20%
Drug Uptake
  Absorption: Intratracheal: Absorbed from the alveolus
Generic Available No

Colistimethate (koe lis ti METH ate)

Brand Names Coly-Mycin® M Parenteral
Therapeutic Category Antibiotic, Miscellaneous
Use Treatment of infections due to sensitive strains of certain gram-negative bacilli
Local Anesthetic/Vasoconstrictor Precautions No information available to require special precautions
Effects on Dental Treatment No effects or complications reported
Other Adverse Effects 1% to 10%:
  Central nervous system: Vertigo, slurring of speech
  Dermatologic: Urticaria
  Gastrointestinal: GI upset
  Renal: Decreased urine output
  Respiratory: Respiratory arrest
Pregnancy Risk Factor B
Generic Available No

Colistin (koe LIS tin)

Brand Names Coly-Mycin® S Oral
Therapeutic Category Antibiotic, Miscellaneous; Antidiarrheal
Synonyms Polymyxin E
Use Treat diarrhea in infants and children caused by susceptible organisms, especially *E. coli* and *Shigella*
Usual Dosage Diarrhea: Children: Oral: 5-15 mg/kg/day in 3 divided doses given every 8 hours
Mechanism of Action A polypeptide antibiotic that binds to and damages the bacterial cell membrane
Local Anesthetic/Vasoconstrictor Precautions No information available to require special precautions
Effects on Dental Treatment No effects or complications reported
Other Adverse Effects <1%:
  Gastrointestinal: Nausea, vomiting
  Neuromuscular & skeletal: Neuromuscular blockade
  Renal: Nephrotoxicity
  Respiratory: Respiratory arrest
  (Continued)

Colistin *(Continued)*

Miscellaneous: Hypersensitivity reactions, superinfections

Drug Uptake

Absorption: Oral: Slightly absorbed from GI tract (adults); unpredictable absorption occurs in infants, can lead to significant serum levels

Serum half-life: 2.8-4.8 hours, prolonged in renal insufficiency; with anuria: 48-72 hours

Pregnancy Risk Factor C

Generic Available No

Colistin, Neomycin, and Hydrocortisone

(koe LIS tin, nee oh MYE sin & hye droe KOR ti sone)

Brand Names Coly-Mycin® S Otic Drops

Therapeutic Category Antibiotic, Miscellaneous; Corticosteroid, Otic; Otic Agent, Anti-infective

Use Treatment of superficial and susceptible bacterial infections of the external auditory canal; for treatment of susceptible bacterial infections of mastoidectomy and fenestration cavities

Local Anesthetic/Vasoconstrictor Precautions No information available to require special precautions

Effects on Dental Treatment No effects or complications reported

Pregnancy Risk Factor C

Generic Available No

CollaCote® *see* Collagen, Absorbable *on this page*

Collagen, Absorbable (KOL la jen, ab SORB able)

Brand Names CollaCote®; CollaPlug®; CollaTape®

Therapeutic Category Hemostatic Agent

Use

Dental: To control bleeding created during dental surgery

Medical: Hemostatic

Usual Dosage Children and Adults: A sufficiently large dressing should be selected so as to completely cover the oral wound

Mechanism of Action The highly porous sponge structure absorbs blood and wound exudate. The collagen component causes aggregation of platelets which bind to collagen fibrils. The aggregated platelets degranulate, releasing coagulation factors that promote the formation of fibrin.

Local Anesthetic/Vasoconstrictor Precautions No information available to require special precautions

Effects on Dental Treatment No effects or complications reported

Other Adverse Effects No data reported

Contraindications No data reported

Warnings/Precautions Should not be used on infected or contaminated wounds

Drug Interactions No data reported

Breast-feeding Considerations May be taken while breast-feeding

Dosage Forms Wound dressings: 1" x 3", 3/4" x 1 1/2", 3/8" x 3/4"

Dietary Considerations No data reported

Generic Available Yes

Comments The dressing should be applied over the wound and held in place with moderate pressure. The period of time necessary to apply pressure will vary with the degree of bleeding. In general, 2-5 minutes should be sufficient to achieve hemostasis. At the end of the procedure, the dressing can be removed, replaced or left in situ, any excess dressing should be removed prior to wound closure.

Collagenase (KOL la je nase)

Brand Names Biozyme-C®; Santyl®

Therapeutic Category Enzyme, Topical Debridement

Use Promotes debridement of necrotic tissue in dermal ulcers and severe burns

Usual Dosage Topical: Apply once daily

Mechanism of Action Collagenase is an enzyme derived from the fermentation of *Clostridium histolyticum* and differs from other proteolytic enzymes in that its enzymatic action has a high specificity for native and denatured collagen. Collagenase will not attack collagen in healthy tissue or newly formed granulation tissue. In addition, it does not act on fat, fibrin, keratin, or muscle.

Local Anesthetic/Vasoconstrictor Precautions No information available to require special precautions

Effects on Dental Treatment No effects or complications reported

Other Adverse Effects

1% to 10%: Local: Irritation

<1%: Local: Pain and burning may occur at site of application

Drug Interactions Decreased effect: Enzymatic activity is inhibited by detergents, benzalkonium chloride, hexachlorophene, nitrofurazone, tincture of iodine, and heavy metal ions (silver and mercury)

Pregnancy Risk Factor C

Generic Available No

CollaPlug® *see Collagen, Absorbable on previous page*

CollaTape® *see Collagen, Absorbable on previous page*

Collyrium Fresh® Ophthalmic [OTC] *see Tetrahydrozoline on page 916*

Colovage® *see Polyethylene Glycol-Electrolyte Solution on page 771*

Coly-Mycin® M Parenteral *see Colistimethate on page 259*

Coly-Mycin® S Oral *see Colistin on page 259*

Coly-Mycin® S Otic Drops *see Colistin, Neomycin, and Hydrocortisone on previous page*

CoLyte® *see Polyethylene Glycol-Electrolyte Solution on page 771*

Combipres® *see Clonidine and Chlorthalidone on page 251*

Combivent® *see Ipratropium and Albuterol on page 518*

Combivir® *see Zidovudine and Lamivudine on page 1003*

Comfort® Ophthalmic [OTC] *see Naphazoline on page 664*

Comfort® Tears Solution [OTC] *see Artificial Tears on page 87*

Comhist® *see Chlorpheniramine, Phenylephrine, and Phenyltoloxamine on page 221*

Comhist® LA *see Chlorpheniramine, Phenylephrine, and Phenyltoloxamine on page 221*

Common Oral-Facial Infections and Antibiotics for Treatment *see page 1197*

Compazine® *see Prochlorperazine on page 799*

Compound W® [OTC] *see Salicylic Acid on page 853*

Compoz® Gel Caps [OTC] *see Diphenhydramine on page 323*

Compoz® Nighttime Sleep Aid [OTC] *see Diphenhydramine on page 323*

Comtrex® Maximum Strength Non-Drowsy [OTC] *see Acetaminophen, Dextromethorphan, and Pseudoephedrine on page 25*

Condylox® *see Podofilox on page 769*

Conex® [OTC] *see Guaifenesin and Phenylpropanolamine on page 454*

Congess® Jr *see Guaifenesin and Pseudoephedrine on page 454*

Congess® Sr *see Guaifenesin and Pseudoephedrine on page 454*

Congestac® *see Guaifenesin and Pseudoephedrine on page 454*

Congestant D® [OTC] *see Chlorpheniramine, Phenylpropanolamine, and Acetaminophen on page 222*

Constilac® *see Lactulose on page 540*

Constulose® *see Lactulose on page 540*

Contac® Cough Formula Liquid [OTC] *see Guaifenesin and Dextromethorphan on page 453*

Control® [OTC] *see Phenylpropanolamine on page 754*

Controlled Substances *see page 1198*

Contuss® *see Guaifenesin, Phenylpropanolamine, and Phenylephrine on page 455*

Contuss® XT *see Guaifenesin and Phenylpropanolamine on page 454*

Cool Mint Listerine® Antiseptic [OTC] *see Mouthwash, Antiseptic on page 650*

Copaxone® *see Glatiramer Acetate on page 442*

Cophene-B® *see Brompheniramine on page 142*

Cophene XP® *see Hydrocodone, Pseudoephedrine, and Guaifenesin on page 484*

Copolymer-1 *see Glatiramer Acetate on page 442*

Copper *see Trace Metals on page 948*

Co-Pyronil® 2 Pulvules® [OTC] *see Chlorpheniramine and Pseudoephedrine on page 219*

Cordarone® *see Amiodarone on page 58*

Cordran® *see Flurandrenolide on page 422*

Cordran® SP *see Flurandrenolide on page 422*

Coreg® *see Carvedilol on page 183*

Corgard® *see Nadolol on page 657*

Coricidin® [OTC] *see Chlorpheniramine and Acetaminophen on page 218*

Coricidin D® [OTC] *see Chlorpheniramine, Phenylpropanolamine, and Acetaminophen on page 222*

Corlopam® *see Fenoldopam on page 397*

Corque® Topical *see Clioquinol and Hydrocortisone on page 245*

Cortatrigen® Otic *see Neomycin, Polymyxin B, and Hydrocortisone on page 672*

Cortef® *see* Hydrocortisone *on page 484*

Corticaine® Topical *see* Dibucaine and Hydrocortisone *on page 303*

Corticosteroid Equivalencies Comparison *see page 1139*

Corticosteroids, Topical Comparison *see page 1140*

Corticotropin (kor ti koe TROE pin)

Brand Names Acthar®; H.P. Acthar® Gel

Therapeutic Category Adrenal Corticosteroid

Use Acute exacerbations of multiple sclerosis; diagnostic aid in adrenocortical insufficiency, severe muscle weakness in myasthenia gravis; cosyntropin is preferred over corticotropin for diagnostic test of adrenocortical insufficiency (cosyntropin is less allergenic and test is shorter in duration)

Mechanism of Action Stimulates the adrenal cortex to secrete adrenal steroids (including hydrocortisone, cortisone), androgenic substances, and a small amount of aldosterone

Local Anesthetic/Vasoconstrictor Precautions No information available to require special precautions

Effects on Dental Treatment No effects or complications reported

Other Adverse Effects

>10%:
  Central nervous system: Insomnia, nervousness
  Gastrointestinal: Increased appetite, indigestion

1% to 10%:
  Endocrine & metabolic: Diabetes mellitus
  Neuromuscular & skeletal: Arthralgia
  Ocular: Cataracts
  Respiratory: Epistaxis

<1%:
  Central nervous system: Seizures, mood swings, headache, delirium, hallucinations, euphoria
  Dermatologic: Skin atrophy, bruising, hyperpigmentation, acne, hirsutism
  Endocrine & metabolic: Amenorrhea, sodium and water retention, Cushing's syndrome, hyperglycemia, bone growth suppression
  Gastrointestinal: Abdominal distention, ulcerative esophagitis, pancreatitis
  Neuromuscular & skeletal: Muscle wasting
  Miscellaneous: Hypersensitivity reactions

Drug Interactions Decreased effect: Spironolactone, hydrocortisone, cortisone; can antagonize the effects of anticholinesterases (eg, neostigmine)

Pregnancy Risk Factor C

Generic Available Yes

Cortisone Acetate (KOR ti sone AS e tate)

Related Information

Corticosteroid Equivalencies Comparison *on page 1139*

Respiratory Diseases *on page 1018*

Brand Names Cortone® Acetate

Therapeutic Category Adrenal Corticosteroid; Anti-inflammatory Agent; Corticosteroid, Systemic

Use Management of adrenocortical insufficiency

Usual Dosage If possible, administer glucocorticoids before 9 AM to minimize adrenocortical suppression; dosing depends upon the condition being treated and the response of the patient; supplemental doses may be warranted during times of stress in the course of withdrawing therapy

Children:
  Anti-inflammatory or immunosuppressive:
    Oral: 2.5-10 mg/kg/day **or** 20-300 mg/m²/day in divided doses every 6-8 hours
    I.M.: 1-5 mg/kg/day **or** 14-375 mg/m²/day in divided doses every 12-24 hours
  Physiologic replacement:
    Oral: 0.5-0.75 mg/kg/day **or** 20-25 mg/m²/day in divided doses every 8 hours
    I.M.: 0.25-0.35 mg/kg/day once daily **or** 12.5 mg/m²/day
  Stress coverage for surgery: I.M.: 1 and 2 days before preanesthesia, and 1-3 days after surgery: 50-62.5 mg/m²/day; 4 days after surgery: 31-50 mg/m²/day; 5 days after surgery, resume presurgical corticosteroid dose.

Adults: Oral, I.M.: 25-300 mg/day in divided doses every 12-24 hours

Hemodialysis effects: Supplemental dose is not necessary

Mechanism of Action Decreases inflammation by suppression of migration of polymorphonuclear leukocytes and reversal of increased capillary permeability

Local Anesthetic/Vasoconstrictor Precautions No information available to require special precautions

Effects on Dental Treatment A compromised immune response may occur if patient has been taking systemic cortisone; the need for corticosteroid coverage in these patients should be considered before any dental treatment; consult with physician

Other Adverse Effects

>10%:

Central nervous system: Insomnia, nervousness

Gastrointestinal: Increased appetite, indigestion

1% to 10%:

Dermatologic: Hirsutism

Endocrine & metabolic: Diabetes mellitus

Gastrointestinal: Peptic ulcer, nausea, vomiting

Neuromuscular & skeletal: Muscle weakness, osteoporosis, fractures, arthralgia

Ocular: Cataracts, glaucoma

Respiratory: Epistaxis

<1%:

Cardiovascular: Edema, hypertension

Central nervous system: Mood swings, vertigo, seizures, headache, psychoses, pseudotumor cerebri, delirium, hallucinations, euphoria

Dermatologic: Acne, skin atrophy, hyperpigmentation, bruising

Endocrine & metabolic: Cushing's syndrome, pituitary-adrenal axis suppression, growth suppression, glucose intolerance, hypokalemia, alkalosis, amenorrhea, sodium and water retention, hyperglycemia

Gastrointestinal: Abdominal distention, ulcerative esophagitis, pancreatitis

Neuromuscular & skeletal: Muscle wasting

Miscellaneous: Hypersensitivity reactions

Drug Interactions

Decreased effect:

Barbiturates, phenytoin, rifampin causes decreased cortisone effects

Cortisone causes decreased warfarin effects

Cortisone causes decreased effects of salicylates

Increased effect: Estrogens (increased cortisone effects)

Increased toxicity:

Cortisone + NSAIDs causes increased ulcerogenic potential

Cortisone causes increased potassium deletion due to diuretics

Drug Uptake

Peak effect:

Oral: Within 2 hours

I.M.: Within 20-48 hours

Duration of action: 30-36 hours

Absorption: Slow rate of absorption

Serum half-life: 30 minutes to 2 hours

End stage renal disease: 3.5 hours

Pregnancy Risk Factor D

Dosage Forms

Injection: 50 mg/mL (10 mL)

Tablet: 5 mg, 10 mg, 25 mg

Dietary Considerations Limit caffeine; may need diet with increased potassium, pyridoxine, vitamin C, vitamin D, folate, calcium, and phosphorus and decreased sodium; may be taken with food to decrease GI distress

Generic Available Yes

Cortisporin® Ophthalmic Ointment *see* Bacitracin, Neomycin, Polymyxin B, and Hydrocortisone *on page 108*

Cortisporin® Ophthalmic Suspension *see* Neomycin, Polymyxin B, and Hydrocortisone *on page 672*

Cortisporin® Otic *see* Neomycin, Polymyxin B, and Hydrocortisone *on page 672*

Cortisporin® Topical Cream *see* Neomycin, Polymyxin B, and Hydrocortisone *on page 672*

Cortisporin® Topical Ointment *see* Bacitracin, Neomycin, Polymyxin B, and Hydrocortisone *on page 108*

Cortone® Acetate *see* Cortisone Acetate *on previous page*

Cortrosyn® *see* Cosyntropin *on this page*

Corvert® *see* Ibutilide *on page 496*

Cosmegen® *see* Dactinomycin *on page 277*

Cosyntropin (koe sin TROE pin)

Brand Names Cortrosyn®

Therapeutic Category Adrenal Corticosteroid

Use Diagnostic test to differentiate primary adrenal from secondary (pituitary) adrenocortical insufficiency

(Continued)

Cosyntropin (Continued)

Usual Dosage

Adrenocortical insufficiency: I.M., I.V. (over 2 minutes): Peak plasma cortisol concentrations usually occur 45-60 minutes after cosyntropin administration

Children <2 years: 0.125 mg

Children >2 years and Adults: 0.25 mg

When greater cortisol stimulation is needed, an I.V. infusion may be used:
Children >2 years and Adults: 0.25 mg administered at 0.04 mg/hour over 6 hours

Congenital adrenal hyperplasia evaluation: 1 mg/m^2/dose up to a maximum of 1 mg

Mechanism of Action Stimulates the adrenal cortex to secrete adrenal steroids (including hydrocortisone, cortisone), androgenic substances, and a small amount of aldosterone

Local Anesthetic/Vasoconstrictor Precautions No information available to require special precautions

Effects on Dental Treatment No effects or complications reported

Other Adverse Effects

1% to 10%:
Cardiovascular: Flushing
Central nervous system: Mild fever
Dermatologic: Pruritus
Gastrointestinal: Chronic pancreatitis

<1%: Hypersensitivity reactions

Drug Interactions No data reported

Drug Uptake

Time to peak serum concentration: Within 1 hour (plasma cortisol levels rise in healthy individuals within 5 minutes of administration I.M. or I.V. push)

Pregnancy Risk Factor C

Generic Available No

Cotazym® *see* Pancrelipase *on page 722*

Cotazym-S® *see* Pancrelipase *on page 722*

Cotrim® *see* Trimethoprim and Sulfamethoxazole *on page 965*

Cotrim® DS *see* Trimethoprim and Sulfamethoxazole *on page 965*

Co-trimoxazole *see* Trimethoprim and Sulfamethoxazole *on page 965*

Coumadin® *see* Warfarin *on page 997*

Covera-HS® *see* Verapamil *on page 987*

Cozaar® *see* Losartan *on page 569*

CP-99,219-27 *see* Trovafloxacin/Alatrofloxacin *on page 974*

Creon® *see* Pancreatin *on page 721*

Creon® 10 *see* Pancrelipase *on page 722*

Creon® 20 *see* Pancrelipase *on page 722*

Creo-Terpin® [OTC] *see* Dextromethorphan *on page 298*

Cresylate® *see* m-Cresyl Acetate *on page 581*

Crinone® Vaginal Gel *see* Progesterone *on page 802*

Criticare HN® [OTC] *see* Enteral Nutritional Products *on page 350*

Crixivan® *see* Indinavir *on page 505*

Cromoglicato Disodico (Mexico) *see* Cromolyn Sodium *on this page*

Cromolyn Sodium (KROE moe lin SOW dee um)

Related Information

Respiratory Diseases *on page 1018*

Brand Names Gastrocrom®; Intal®; Nasalcrom®

Canadian/Mexican Brand Names Novo-Cromolyn® (Canada); Opticrom® (Canada); PMS-Sodium Cromoglycate® (Canada); Rynacrom® (Canada)

Therapeutic Category Inhalation, Miscellaneous

Synonyms Cromoglicato Disodico (Mexico); Sodium Cromoglycate (Canada)

Use Adjunct in the prophylaxis of allergic disorders, including rhinitis, giant papillary conjunctivitis, and asthma; inhalation product may be used for prevention of exercise-induced bronchospasm; systemic mastocytosis, food allergy, and treatment of inflammatory bowel disease; **cromolyn is a prophylactic drug with no benefit for acute situations**

Usual Dosage Not effective for immediate relief of symptoms in acute asthmatic attacks; must be used at regular intervals for 2-4 weeks to be effective

Children:
  Inhalation (taper frequency to the lowest effective dose, ie, 4 times/day → 3 times/day → twice daily):
    Initial dose: Metered spray: >5 years: 2 inhalations 4 times/day by metered spray
    Initial dose: Nebulization solution: >2 years: 20 mg 4 times/day
    Prevention of exercise-induced bronchospasm: Metered spray: >5 years: Single dose of 2 inhalations (aerosol) just prior to (10 minutes to 1 hour) exercise
  Nasal: >6 years: Instill 1 spray in each nostril 3-4 times/day
  Children 2-12 years: Oral: 100 mg 4 times/day 15-20 minutes before meals, not to exceed 40 mg/kg/day
  Children >12 years and Adults: Oral: 200 mg 4 times/day 15-20 minutes before meal, up to 400 mg 4 times/day
Adults:
  Inhalation: Metered spray: 2 inhalations 4 times/day
  Nasal: Instill 1 spray in each nostril 3-4 times/day
  Ophthalmic: Instill 1-2 drops 4-6 times/day into each eye

Mechanism of Action Prevents the mast cell release of histamine, leukotrienes and slow-reacting substance of anaphylaxis by inhibiting degranulation after contact with antigens

Local Anesthetic/Vasoconstrictor Precautions No information available to require special precautions

Effects on Dental Treatment No effects or complications reported

Other Adverse Effects
>10%: Local: Hoarseness, coughing, unpleasant taste (inhalation aerosol)
1% to 10%:
  Dermatologic: Angioedema
  Gastrointestinal: Dry mouth
  Genitourinary: Dysuria
  Respiratory: Sneezing, nasal congestion
<1%:
  Central nervous system: Dizziness, headache
  Dermatologic: Rash, urticaria
  Gastrointestinal: Nausea, vomiting, diarrhea
  Local: Nasal burning
  Neuromuscular & skeletal: Arthralgia
  Ocular: Ocular stinging, lacrimation
  Respiratory: Wheezing, throat irritation, eosinophilic pneumonia, pulmonary infiltrates
  Miscellaneous: Anaphylactic reactions

Drug Interactions No data reported

Drug Uptake
Absorption:
  Inhalation: ~8% of dose reaches the lungs upon inhalation of the powder and is well absorbed
  Oral: Only 0.5% to 2% of dose absorbed
Serum half-life: 80-90 minutes
Time to peak serum concentration: Inhalation: Within 15 minutes

Pregnancy Risk Factor B

Generic Available Yes

Crotamiton (kroe TAM i tonn)

Brand Names Eurax®

Therapeutic Category Antipruritic, Topical; Scabicidal Agent

Synonyms Crotamiton (Mexico)

Use Treatment of scabies and symptomatic treatment of pruritus

Usual Dosage Topical:
  Scabicide: Children and Adults: Wash thoroughly and scrub away loose scales, then towel dry; apply a thin layer and massage drug onto skin of the entire body from the neck to the toes (with special attention to skin folds, creases, and interdigital spaces). Repeat application in 24 hours. Take a cleansing bath 48 hours after the final application. Treatment may be repeated after 7-10 days if live mites are still present.
  Pruritus: Massage into affected areas until medication is completely absorbed; repeat as necessary

Mechanism of Action Crotamiton has scabicidal activity against *Sarcoptes scabiei*; mechanism of action unknown

Local Anesthetic/Vasoconstrictor Precautions No information available to require special precautions

Effects on Dental Treatment No effects or complications reported

(Continued)

Crotamiton *(Continued)*

Other Adverse Effects <1%: Local: Pruritus, irritation, contact dermatitis, warm sensation

Drug Interactions No data reported

Pregnancy Risk Factor C

Generic Available No

Crotamiton (Mexico) *see* Crotamiton *on previous page*

Crude Coal Tar *see* Coal Tar *on page 254*

Crystamine® *see* Cyanocobalamin *on this page*

Crysti 1000® *see* Cyanocobalamin *on this page*

Crysticillin® A.S. *see* Penicillin G Procaine *on page 733*

Crystodigin® *see* Digitoxin *on page 312*

CSP *see* Cellulose Sodium Phosphate *on page 201*

Cuprimine® *see* Penicillamine *on page 730*

Curretab® *see* Medroxyprogesterone Acetate *on page 587*

Cutivate™ *see* Fluticasone *on page 424*

Cyanocobalamin *(sye an oh koe BAL a min)*

Brand Names Crystamine®; Crysti 1000®; Cyanoject®; Cyomin®

Canadian/Mexican Brand Names Rubramin® (Canada)

Therapeutic Category Vitamin, Water Soluble

Synonyms Cianocobalamina (Mexico); Cobalamin (Canada)

Use

Dental: Vitamin B_{12} deficiency

Medical: Treatment of pernicious anemia; increased B_{12} requirements due to pregnancy, thyrotoxicosis, hemorrhage, malignancy, liver or kidney disease

Usual Dosage I.M. or deep S.C. (oral is not generally recommended due to poor absorption and I.V. is not recommended due to more rapid elimination):

Recommended daily allowance (RDA):

Children: 0.3-2 mcg

Adults: 2 mcg

Pernicious anemia, congenital (if evidence of neurologic involvement): 1000 mcg/day for at least 2 weeks; maintenance: 50 mcg/month

Children: 30-50 mcg/day for 2 or more weeks (to a total dose of 1000-5000 mcg), then follow with 100 mcg month as maintenance dosage

Adults: 100 mcg/day for 6-7 days; if improvement, give same dose on alternate days for 7 doses; then every 3-4 days for 2-3 weeks; once hematologic values have returned to normal, maintenance dosage: 100 mcg/month. **Note:** Use only parenteral therapy as oral therapy is not dependable.

Vitamin B_{12} deficiency:

Children: 100 mcg/day for 10-15 days (total dose of 1-1.5 mg), then once or twice weekly for several months; may taper to 60 mcg every month

Adults: Initial: 30 mcg/day for 5-10 days; maintenance: 100-200 mcg/month

Mechanism of Action Coenzyme for various metabolic functions, including fat and carbohydrate metabolism and protein synthesis, used in cell replication and hematopoiesis

Local Anesthetic/Vasoconstrictor Precautions No information available to require special precautions

Effects on Dental Treatment No effects or complications reported

Other Adverse Effects 1% to 10%:

Dermatologic: Itching

Gastrointestinal: Diarrhea

Contraindications Hypersensitivity to cyanocobalamin or any component, cobalt; patients with hereditary optic nerve atrophy

Warnings/Precautions I.M. route used to treat pernicious anemia; vitamin B_{12} deficiency for >3 months results in irreversible degenerative CNS lesions; treatment of vitamin B_{12} megaloblastic anemia may result in severe hypokalemia, sometimes, fatal, when anemia corrects due to cellular potassium requirements. B_{12} deficiency masks signs of polycythemia vera; vegetarian diets may result in B_{12} deficiency; pernicious anemia occurs more often in gastric carcinoma than in general population.

Drug Interactions

Aminosalicylic acid may reduce therapeutic action of vitamin B_{12}

Chloramphenicol may decrease the hematologic effect of vitamin B_{12} in patients with pernicious anemia

Colchicine and prolonged alcohol (>2 weeks) use may decrease absorption of vitamin B_{12}

Drug Uptake

Absorption: Absorbed from the terminal ileum in the presence of calcium; for absorption to occur gastric "intrinsic factor" must be present to transfer the compound across the intestinal mucosa

Pregnancy Risk Factor A (C if dose exceeds RDA recommendation)

Dosage Forms

Gel, nasal (Ener-B®): 400 mcg/0.1 mL

Injection: 30 mcg/mL (30 mL); 100 mcg/mL (1 mL, 10 mL, 30 mL); 1000 mcg/mL (1 mL, 10 mL, 30 mL)

Tablet [OTC]: 25 mcg, 50 mcg, 100 mcg, 250 mcg, 500 mcg, 1000 mcg

Generic Available Yes

Cyanoject® *see* Cyanocobalamin *on previous page*

Cyclan® *see* Cyclandelate *on this page*

Cyclandelate (sye KLAN de late)

Brand Names Cyclan®; Cyclospasmol®

Therapeutic Category Vasodilator, Peripheral

Use Considered as "possibly effective" for adjunctive therapy in peripheral vascular disease and possibly senility due to cerebrovascular disease or multi-infarct dementia; migraine prophylaxis, vertigo, tinnitus, and visual disturbances secondary to cerebrovascular insufficiency and diabetic peripheral polyneuropathy

Usual Dosage Adults: Oral: Initial: 1.2-1.6 g/day in divided doses before meals and at bedtime until response; maintenance therapy: 400-800 mg/day in 2-4 divided doses; start with lowest dose in elderly due to hypotensive potential; decrease dose by 200 mg decrements to achieve minimal maintenance dose; improvement can usually be seen over weeks of therapy and prolonged use; short courses of therapy are usually ineffective and not recommended

Mechanism of Action Cyclandelate, 3,3,5-trimethylcyclohexyl mandelate is a vasodilator that exerts a direct, papaverine-like action on smooth muscles, particularly that found within the blood vessels. Animal data indicate that cyclandelate also has antispasmodic properties; exhibits no adrenergic stimulation or blocking action; action exceeds that of papaverine; mild calcium channel blocking agent, may benefit in mild hypercalcemia; calcium channel blocking activity may explain some of its pharmacologic effects (enhanced blood flow) and inhibition of platelet aggregation.

Local Anesthetic/Vasoconstrictor Precautions No information available to require special precautions

Effects on Dental Treatment No effects or complications reported

Other Adverse Effects <1%:

Cardiovascular: Flushing of face, tachycardia

Central nervous system: Headache, pain, dizziness

Gastrointestinal: Belching, heartburn

Neuromuscular & skeletal: Paresthesia, weakness

Drug Interactions No data reported

Pregnancy Risk Factor C

Generic Available Yes

Cyclizine (SYE kli zeen)

Brand Names Marezine® [OTC]

Therapeutic Category Antiemetic; Antihistamine

Use Prevention and treatment of nausea, vomiting, and vertigo associated with motion sickness; control of postoperative nausea and vomiting

Usual Dosage

Children 6-12 years:

Oral: 25 mg up to 3 times/day

I.M.: Not recommended

Adults:

Oral: 50 mg taken 30 minutes before departure, may repeat in 4-6 hours if needed, up to 200 mg/day

I.M.: 50 mg every 4-6 hours as needed

Mechanism of Action Cyclizine is a piperazine derivative with properties of histamines. The precise mechanism of action in inhibiting the symptoms of motion sickness is not known. It may have effects directly on the labyrinthine apparatus and central actions on the labyrinthine apparatus and on the chemoreceptor trigger zone. Cyclizine exerts a central anticholinergic action.

Local Anesthetic/Vasoconstrictor Precautions No information available to require special precautions

Effects on Dental Treatment >10% of patients will experience dry mouth

(Continued)

Cyclizine *(Continued)*

Other Adverse Effects
>10%: Central nervous system: Drowsiness
1% to 10%:
Central nervous system: Headache
Dermatologic: Dermatitis
Gastrointestinal: Nausea
Ocular: Diplopia
Renal: Polyuria, urinary retention

Drug Interactions Increased effect/toxicity with CNS depressants, alcohol

Pregnancy Risk Factor B

Generic Available No

Cyclobenzaprine (sye kloe BEN za preen)

Related Information
Temporomandibular Dysfunction (TMD) *on page 1078*

Brand Names Flexeril®

Canadian/Mexican Brand Names Novo-Cycloprine (Canada)

Therapeutic Category Muscle Relaxant; Skeletal Muscle Relaxant

Use
Dental: Treatment of muscle spasm associated with acute temporomandibular joint pain
Medical: Treatment of muscle spasm associated with acute painful musculoskeletal conditions; supportive therapy in tetanus

Usual Dosage Oral: **Note:** Do not use longer than 2-3 weeks
Children: Dosage has not been established
Adults: 20-40 mg/day in 2-4 divided doses; maximum dose: 60 mg/day

Mechanism of Action Centrally acting skeletal muscle relaxant pharmacologically related to tricyclic antidepressants; reduces tonic somatic motor activity influencing both alpha and gamma motor neurons

Local Anesthetic/Vasoconstrictor Precautions No information available to require special precautions

Effects on Dental Treatment >10% of patient experience dry mouth

Other Adverse Effects
>10%: Central nervous system: Drowsiness, dizziness, lightheadedness
1% to 10%:
Cardiovascular: Swelling of face, lips, syncope
Gastrointestinal: Bloated feeling
Neuromuscular & skeletal: Problems in speaking, muscle weakness
Ocular: Blurred vision

Contraindications Hypersensitivity to cyclobenzaprine or any component; do not use concomitantly or within 14 days of MAO inhibitors; hyperthyroidism, congestive heart failure, arrhythmias

Warnings/Precautions Cyclobenzaprine shares the toxic potentials of the tricyclic antidepressants and the usual precautions of tricyclic antidepressant therapy should be observed; use with caution in patients with urinary hesitancy or angle-closure glaucoma

Drug Interactions Do not use concomitantly or within 14 days after MAO inhibitors; because of chemical similarities to the tricyclic antidepressants, may have additive toxicities; because of cyclobenzaprine's anticholinergic action, use with caution in patients receiving these agents; alcohol, barbiturates, and other CNS depressants may be enhanced by cyclobenzaprine

Drug Uptake
Absorption: Oral: Completely
Onset of action: Commonly occurs within 1 hour
Duration: 12-24 hours
Serum half-life: 1-3 days
Time to peak serum concentration: Within 3-8 hours

Pregnancy Risk Factor B

Breast-feeding Considerations No data reported

Dosage Forms Tablet, as hydrochloride: 10 mg

Dietary Considerations No data reported

Generic Available Yes

Cyclocort® *see* Amcinonide *on page 51*

Cyclogyl® *see* Cyclopentolate *on next page*

Cyclomydril® Ophthalmic *see* Cyclopentolate and Phenylephrine *on next page*

Cyclopentolate (sye kloe PEN toe late)

Brand Names AK-Pentolate®; Cyclogyl®; I-Pentolate®

Therapeutic Category Anticholinergic Agent, Ophthalmic; Ophthalmic Agent, Mydriatic

Use Diagnostic procedures requiring mydriasis and cycloplegia

Usual Dosage

Children: Instill 1 drop of 0.5%, 1%, or 2% in eye followed by 1 drop of 0.5% or 1% in 5 minutes, if necessary

Adults: Instill 1 drop of 1% followed by another drop in 5 minutes; 2% solution in heavily pigmented iris

Mechanism of Action Prevents the muscle of the ciliary body and the sphincter muscle of the iris from responding to cholinergic stimulation, causing mydriasis and cycloplegia

Local Anesthetic/Vasoconstrictor Precautions No information available to require special precautions

Effects on Dental Treatment No effects or complications reported

Other Adverse Effects 1% to 10%:

Cardiovascular: Tachycardia

Central nervous system: Restlessness, hallucinations, psychosis, hyperactivity, seizures, incoherent speech, ataxia

Dermatologic: Burning sensation

Ocular: Increase in intraocular pressure, loss of visual accommodation

Miscellaneous: Allergic reaction

Drug Uptake

Peak effect:

Cycloplegia: 25-75 minutes

Mydriasis: 30-60 minutes

Duration: Recovery takes up to 24 hours

Pregnancy Risk Factor C

Generic Available Yes

Comments Pilocarpine ophthalmic drops applied after the examination may reduce recovery time to 3-6 hours

Cyclopentolate and Phenylephrine

(sye kloe PEN toe late & fen il EF rin)

Brand Names Cyclomydril® Ophthalmic

Therapeutic Category Anticholinergic/Adrenergic Agonist

Synonyms Phenylephrine and Cyclopentolate

Use Induce mydriasis greater than that produced with cyclopentolate HCl alone

Usual Dosage Ophthalmic: Instill 1 drop every 5-10 minutes, not to exceed 3 instillations

Local Anesthetic/Vasoconstrictor Precautions No information available to require special precautions

Effects on Dental Treatment No effects or complications reported

Pregnancy Risk Factor C

Dosage Forms Solution, ophthalmic: Cyclopentolate hydrochloride 0.2% and phenylephrine hydrochloride 1% (2 mL, 5 mL)

Generic Available No

Cyclophosphamide (sye kloe FOS fa mide)

Brand Names Cytoxan®; Neosar®

Canadian/Mexican Brand Names Genoxal® (Mexico); Ledoxina® (Mexico); Procytox® (Canada)

Therapeutic Category Antineoplastic Agent, Alkylating Agent (Nitrogen Mustard)

Synonyms Ciclofosfamida (Mexico)

Use Treatment of Hodgkin's and non-Hodgkin's lymphoma, Burkitt's lymphoma, chronic lymphocytic leukemia, chronic granulocytic leukemia, AML, ALL, mycosis fungoides, breast cancer, multiple myeloma, neuroblastoma, retinoblastoma, rhabdomyosarcoma, Ewing's sarcoma; testicular, endometrium and ovarian, and lung cancer, and as a conditioning regimen for BMT; prophylaxis of rejection for kidney, heart, liver, and BMT transplants, severe rheumatoid disorders, nephrotic syndrome, Wegener's granulomatosis, idiopathic pulmonary hemosideroses, myasthenia gravis, multiple sclerosis, systemic lupus erythematosus, lupus nephritis, autoimmune hemolytic anemia, idiopathic thrombocytic purpura, macroglobulinemia, and antibody-induced pure red cell aplasia

Usual Dosage Refer to individual protocols

Patients with compromised bone marrow function may require a 33% to 50% reduction in initial loading dose

(Continued)

Cyclophosphamide (Continued)

Children: I.V.:
Neuroblastomas/sarcomas: 3 g/m^2/day for 2 days or 2 g/m^2/day for 3 days
SLE: 500-750 mg/m^2 every month; maximum dose: 1 g/m^2
JRA/vasculitis: 10 mg/kg every 2 weeks

Children and Adults:
Oral: 50-100 mg/m^2/day as continuous therapy or 400-1000 mg/m^2 in divided doses over 4-5 days as intermittent therapy
I.V.:
Single doses: 400-1800 mg/m^2 (30-50 mg/kg) per treatment course (1-5 days) which can be repeated at 2- to 4-week intervals
Maximum single dose without BMT is 7 g/m^2 (190 mg/kg) single agent therapy
Continuous daily doses: 60-120 mg/m^2 (1-2.5 mg/kg) per day
Autologous BMT: IVPB: 50 mg/kg/dose for 4 days or 60 mg/kg/dose for 2 days; total dose is usually divided over 2-4 days

Nephrotic syndrome: Oral: 2-3 mg/kg/day every day for up to 12 weeks when corticosteroids are unsuccessful

Mechanism of Action Interferes with the normal function of DNA by alkylation and cross-linking the strands of DNA, and by possible protein modification; cyclophosphamide also possesses potent immunosuppressive activity; note that cyclophosphamide must be metabolized to its active form in the liver

Local Anesthetic/Vasoconstrictor Precautions No information available to require special precautions

Effects on Dental Treatment No effects or complications reported

Other Adverse Effects

>10%:
Dermatologic: Alopecia is frequent, but hair will regrow although it may be of a different color or texture. Hair loss usually occurs 3 weeks after therapy.
Fertility: May cause sterility; interferes with oogenesis and spermatogenesis; may be irreversible in some patients; gonadal suppression (amenorrhea)
Gastrointestinal: Nausea and vomiting occur more frequently with larger doses, usually beginning 6-10 hours after administration; also seen are anorexia, diarrhea, stomatitis, mucositis
Emetic potential: Oral: Low (<10%); <1 g: Moderate (30% to 60%); ≥1 g: High (>90%)
Hepatic: Jaundice seen occasionally

1% to 10%:
Cardiovascular: Facial flushing
Central nervous system: Headache
Dermatologic: Skin rash
Hematologic: Anemia
Myelosuppressive: Thrombocytopenia occurs less frequently than with mechlorethamine; WBC: Moderate; Platelets: Moderate; Onset (days): 7; Nadir (days): 10-14; Recovery (days): 21

<1%:
Cardiovascular: High-dose therapy may cause cardiac dysfunction manifested as congestive heart failure; cardiac necrosis or hemorrhagic myocarditis has occurred rarely, but is fatal. Cyclophosphamide may also potentiate the cardiac toxicity of anthracyclines.
Central nervous system: Dizziness
Dermatologic: Darkening of skin/fingernails
Endocrine & metabolic: Hyperglycemia, hypokalemia, distortion, hyperuricemia
Genitourinary: Acute hemorrhagic cystitis is believed to be a result of chemical irritation of the bladder by acrolein, a cyclophosphamide metabolite. Acute hemorrhagic cystitis occurs in 7% to 12% of patients, and has been reported in up to 40% of patients. Hemorrhagic cystitis can be severe and even fatal. Patients should be encouraged to drink plenty of fluids (3-4 L/day) during therapy, void frequently, and avoid taking the drug at nighttime. If large I.V. doses are being administered, I.V. hydration should be given during therapy. The administration of mesna or continuous bladder irrigation may also be warranted.
Hepatic: Hepatic toxicity
Renal: SIADH has occurred with I.V. doses >50 mg/kg; renal tubular necrosis has also occurred, but usually resolves after the discontinuation of therapy
Respiratory: Nasal congestion occurs when given in large I.V. doses; patients experience runny eyes, rhinorrhea, sinus congestion, and sneezing during or immediately after the infusion; interstitial pulmonary fibrosis with prolonged high dosage has occurred

Secondary malignancy: Has developed with cyclophosphamide alone or in combination with other antineoplastics; both bladder carcinoma and acute leukemia are well documented

Drug Interactions

Decreased effect: Digoxin: Cyclophosphamide may reduce digoxin serum levels

Increased toxicity:

Allopurinol may cause an increase in bone marrow depression and may result in significant elevations of cyclophosphamide cytotoxic metabolites

Anesthetic agents: Cyclophosphamide reduces serum pseudocholinesterase concentrations and may prolong the neuromuscular blocking activity of succinylcholine; use with caution with halothane, nitrous oxide, and succinylcholine

Chloramphenicol results in prolonged cyclophosphamide half-life to increase toxicity

Cimetidine inhibits hepatic metabolism of drugs and may reduce the activation of cyclophosphamide

Doxorubicin: Cyclophosphamide may enhance cardiac toxicity of anthracyclines

Phenobarbital and phenytoin induce hepatic enzymes and cause a more rapid production of cyclophosphamide metabolites with a concurrent decrease in the serum half-life of the parent compound

Tetrahydrocannabinol results in enhanced immunosuppression in animal studies

Thiazide diuretics: Leukopenia may be prolonged

Pregnancy Risk Factor D

Generic Available No

Cycloserine (sye kloe SER een)

Related Information

Nonviral Infectious Diseases *on page 1032*

Brand Names Seromycin® Pulvules®

Therapeutic Category Antibiotic, Miscellaneous; Antitubercular Agent

Use Adjunctive treatment in pulmonary or extrapulmonary tuberculosis; treatment of acute urinary tract infections caused by *E. coli* or *Enterobacter* sp when less toxic conventional therapy has failed or is contraindicated

Usual Dosage Some of the neurotoxic effects may be relieved or prevented by the concomitant administration of pyridoxine

Tuberculosis: Oral:

Children: 10-20 mg/kg/day in 2 divided doses up to 1000 mg/day for 18-24 months

Adults: Initial: 250 mg every 12 hours for 14 days, then give 500 mg to 1 g/day in 2 divided doses for 18-24 months (maximum daily dose: 1 g)

Mechanism of Action Inhibits bacterial cell wall synthesis by competing with amino acid (D-alanine) for incorporation into the bacterial cell wall; bacteriostatic or bactericidal

Local Anesthetic/Vasoconstrictor Precautions No information available to require special precautions

Effects on Dental Treatment No effects or complications reported

Other Adverse Effects

1% to 10%: Central nervous system: Drowsiness, headache

<1%:

Cardiovascular: Cardiac arrhythmias

Central nervous system: Dizziness, vertigo, seizures, confusion, psychosis, paresis, coma

Dermatologic: Rash

Endocrine & metabolic: Vitamin B_{12} deficiency, folate deficiency

Hepatic: Elevated liver enzymes

Neuromuscular & skeletal: Tremor

Drug Interactions Increased toxicity: Alcohol, isoniazid, ethionamide increase toxicity of cycloserine; cycloserine inhibits the hepatic metabolism of phenytoin

Drug Uptake

Absorption: Oral: ~70% to 90% from the GI tract

Serum half-life: 10 hours in patients with normal renal function

Time to peak serum concentration: Oral: Within 3-4 hours

Pregnancy Risk Factor C

Generic Available No

Cyclospasmol® *see* Cyclandelate *on page 267*

Cyclosporine (SYE kloe spor een)

Brand Names Neoral® Oral; Sandimmune® Injection; Sandimmune® Oral
Canadian/Mexican Brand Names Consupren® (Mexico); Sandimmun® Neoral (Mexico)
Therapeutic Category Immunosuppressant Agent
Synonyms Ciclosporina (Mexico)
Use Immunosuppressant which may be used with azathioprine and/or corticosteroids to prolong organ and patient survival in kidney, liver, heart, and bone marrow transplants
Usual Dosage Children and Adults (oral dosage is ~3 times the I.V. dosage); **dosage should be based on ideal body weight:**

I.V.:
Initial: 5-6 mg/kg/day beginning 4-12 hours prior to organ transplantation; patients should be switched to oral cyclosporine as soon as possible; dose should be infused over 2-24 hours
Maintenance: 2-10 mg/kg/day in divided doses every 8-12 hours; dose should be adjusted to maintain whole blood HPLC trough concentrations in the reference range

Oral: Solution or soft gelatin capsule (Sandimmune®):
Initial: 14-18 mg/kg/day, beginning 4-12 hours prior to organ transplantation
Maintenance: 5-15 mg/kg/day divided every 12-24 hours; maintenance dose is usually tapered to 3-10 mg/kg/day
Focal segmental glomerulosclerosis: Initial: 3 mg/kg/day divided every 12 hours

Dosing considerations of cyclosporine, see table.

Cyclosporine

Condition	Cyclosporine
Switch from I.V. to oral therapy	Threefold increase in dose
T-tube clamping	Decrease dose; increase availability of bile facilitates absorption of CsA
Pediatric patients	About 2-3 times higher dose compared to adults
Liver dysfunction	Decrease I.V. dose; increase oral dose
Renal dysfunction	Decrease dose to decrease levels if renal dysfunction is related to the drug
Dialysis	Not removed
Inhibitors of hepatic metabolism	Decrease dose
Inducers of hepatic metabolism	Monitor drug level; may need to increase dose

Oral: Solution or soft gelatin capsule in a microemulsion (Neoral®): Based on the organ transplant population:
Initial: Same as the initial dose for solution or soft gelatin capsule (listed above)
or
Renal: 9 mg/kg/day (range: 6-12 mg/kg/day)
Liver: 8 mg/kg/day (range: 4-12 mg/kg/day)
Heart: 7 mg/kg/day (range: 4-10 mg/kg/day)

Note: A 1:1 ratio conversion from Sandimmune® to Neoral® has been recommended initially; however, lower doses of Neoral® may be required after conversion to prevent overdose. Total daily doses should be adjusted based on the cyclosporine trough blood concentration and clinical assessment of organ rejection. CsA blood trough levels should be determined prior to conversion. After conversion to Neoral®, CsA trough levels should be monitored every 4-7 days

Hemodialysis effects: Supplemental dose is not necessary
Peritoneal dialysis effects: Supplemental dose is not necessary
Mechanism of Action Inhibition of production and release of interleukin II and inhibits interleukin II-induced activation of resting T-lymphocytes
Local Anesthetic/Vasoconstrictor Precautions No information available to require special precautions
Effects on Dental Treatment Gingival hypertrophy
Other Adverse Effects
>10%:
Cardiovascular: Hypertension
Dermatologic: Hirsutism
Gastrointestinal: Gingival hypertrophy

Neuromuscular & skeletal: Tremor

Renal: Nephrotoxicity

1% to 10%:

Central nervous system: Seizure, headache

Dermatologic: Acne

Gastrointestinal: Abdominal discomfort, nausea, vomiting

Neuromuscular & skeletal: Leg cramps

<1%:

Cardiovascular: Hypotension, tachycardia, flushing

Central nervous system: Sensitivity to temperature extremes

Endocrine & metabolic: Hyperkalemia, hypomagnesemia, hyperuricemia

Gastrointestinal: Pancreatitis

Hepatic: Hepatotoxicity

Neuromuscular & skeletal: Myositis, paresthesias

Respiratory: Respiratory distress, sinusitis

Miscellaneous: Anaphylaxis, warmth, increased susceptibility to infection

Drug Interactions

Decreased effect: Rifampin, phenytoin, phenobarbital decreases plasma concentration of cyclosporine

Increased toxicity: Ketoconazole, fluconazole, and itraconazole increase plasma concentration of cyclosporine

Drug Uptake

Absorption: Oral:

Solution or soft gelatin capsule (Sandimmune®): Erratically and incompletely absorbed; dependent on the presence of food, bile acids, and GI motility; larger oral doses of cyclosporine are needed in pediatric patients versus adults due to a shorter bowel length resulting in limited intestinal absorption

Solution in microemulsion or soft gelatin capsule in a microemulsion are bioequivalent (Neoral®): Erratically and incompletely absorbed; increased absorption, up to 30% when compared to Sandimmune®; absorption is less dependent on food intake, bile, or GI motility when compared to Sandimmune®

Serum half-life:

Solution or soft gelatin capsule (Sandimmune®): Biphasic, alpha phase: 1.4 hours and terminal phase 6-24 hours (prolonged in patients with hepatic dysfunction)

Solution or soft gelatin capsule in a microemulsion (Neoral®): 8.4 hours, lower in pediatric patients versus adults due to the higher metabolism rate

Time to peak serum concentration:

Oral solution or capsule (Sandimmune®): 2-6 hours; some patients have a second peak at 5-6 hours

Oral solution or capsule in a microemulsion (Neoral®): 1.5-2 hours (in renal transplant patients)

Pregnancy Risk Factor C

Generic Available No

Cycofed® Pediatric *see* Guaifenesin, Pseudoephedrine, and Codeine *on page 455*

Cycrin® *see* Medroxyprogesterone Acetate *on page 587*

Cyklokapron® Injection *see* Tranexamic Acid *on page 950*

Cyklokapron® Oral *see* Tranexamic Acid *on page 950*

Cylert® *see* Pemoline *on page 728*

Cylex® [OTC] *see* Benzocaine *on page 118*

Cyomin® *see* Cyanocobalamin *on page 266*

Cyproheptadine (si proe HEP ta deen)

Brand Names Periactin®

Canadian/Mexican Brand Names PMS-Cyproheptadine® (Canada)

Therapeutic Category Antihistamine

Use Perennial and seasonal allergic rhinitis and other allergic symptoms including urticaria; its off-labeled uses have included appetite stimulation, blepharospasm, cluster headaches, migraine headaches, Nelson's syndrome, pruritus, schizophrenia, spinal cord damage associated spasticity, and tardive dyskinesia

Usual Dosage Oral:

Children: 0.25 mg/kg/day in 2-3 divided doses or 8 mg/m²/day in 2-3 divided doses

2-6 years: 2 mg every 8-12 hours (not to exceed 12 mg/day)

7-14 years: 4 mg every 8-12 hours (not to exceed 16 mg/day)

Adults: 4-20 mg/day divided every 8 hours (not to exceed 0.5 mg/kg/day) in patients with significant hepatic dysfunction

(Continued)

Cyproheptadine (Continued)

Mechanism of Action A potent antihistamine and serotonin antagonist, competes with histamine for H_1-receptor sites on effector cells in the gastrointestinal tract, blood vessels, and respiratory tract

Local Anesthetic/Vasoconstrictor Precautions No information available to require special precautions

Effects on Dental Treatment No effects or complications reported

Other Adverse Effects

>10%:

Central nervous system: Slight to moderate drowsiness

Respiratory: Thickening of bronchial secretions

1% to 10%:

Central nervous system: Headache, fatigue, nervousness, dizziness

Gastrointestinal: Appetite stimulation, nausea, diarrhea, abdominal pain, dry mouth

Neuromuscular & skeletal: Arthralgia

Respiratory: Pharyngitis

<1%:

Cardiovascular: Tachycardia, palpitations, edema

Central nervous system: Sedation, CNS stimulation, seizures, depression

Dermatologic: Photosensitivity, rash, angioedema

Hematologic: Hemolytic anemia, leukopenia, thrombocytopenia

Hepatic: Hepatitis

Neuromuscular & skeletal: Myalgia, paresthesia

Respiratory: Bronchospasm, epistaxis

Miscellaneous: Allergic reactions

Drug Interactions Increased toxicity: MAO inhibitors cause hallucinations

Pregnancy Risk Factor B

Generic Available Yes

Cystadane® see Betaine Anhydrous on page 126
Cystagon® see Cysteamine on this page

Cysteamine (sis TEE a meen)

Brand Names Cystagon®

Therapeutic Category Antiurolithic

Use Nephropathic cystinosis in children and adults

Usual Dosage Initiate therapy with $1/4$ to $1/8$ of maintenance dose; titrate slowly upward over 4-6 weeks

Children <12 years: Oral: Maintenance: 1.3 g/m²/day divided into 4 doses

Children >12 years and Adults (>110 lb): 2 g/day in 4 divided doses; dosage may in increased to 1.95 g/m²/day if cystine levels are <1 nmol/$1/2$ cystine/mg protein, although intolerance and incidence of adverse events may be increased

Mechanism of Action Reacts with cystine in the lysosome to convert it to cysteine and to a cysteine-cysteamine mixed disulfide, both of which can then exit the lysosome in patients with cystinosis, an inherited defect of lysosomal transport

Local Anesthetic/Vasoconstrictor Precautions No information available to require special precautions

Effects on Dental Treatment No effects or complications reported

Other Adverse Effects

5% to 10%:

Central nervous system: Fever, lethargy

Dermatologic: Rash

Gastrointestinal: Vomiting, anorexia, diarrhea

<5%:

Cardiovascular: Hypertension

Central nervous system: Somnolence, encephalopathy, headache, seizures, ataxia, confusion, dizziness, jitteriness, nervousness, impaired cognition, emotional changes, hallucinations, nightmares

Dermatologic: Urticaria

Endocrine & metabolic: Dehydration

Gastrointestinal: Bad breath, abdominal pain, dyspepsia, constipation, gastroenteritis, duodenitis, duodenal ulceration

Hematologic: Anemia, leukopenia

Hepatic: Abnormal LFTs

Neuromuscular & skeletal: Tremor, hyperkinesia

Otic: Decreased hearing

Pregnancy Risk Factor C

Generic Available No

Cysteine (SIS teen)

Therapeutic Category Nutritional Supplement

Use Total parenteral nutrition of infants as an additive to meet the I.V. amino acid requirements

Local Anesthetic/Vasoconstrictor Precautions No information available to require special precautions

Effects on Dental Treatment No effects or complications reported

Generic Available Yes

Cystospaz® *see* Hyoscyamine *on page 492*

Cystospaz-M® *see* Hyoscyamine *on page 492*

Cytadren® *see* Aminoglutethimide *on page 55*

Cytarabine (sye TARE a been)

Brand Names Cytosar-U®

Therapeutic Category Antineoplastic Agent, Antimetabolite

Use Ara-C is one of the most active agents in leukemia; also active against lymphoma, meningeal leukemia, and meningeal lymphoma; has little use in the treatment of solid tumors

Usual Dosage I.V. bolus, IVPB, and continuous intravenous infusion doses of cytarabine are very different. Bolus doses are relatively well tolerated since the drug is rapidly metabolized; continuous infusion uniformly results in myelosuppression. Refer to individual protocols.

Children and Adults:

Induction remission:

I.V.: 200 mg/m²/day for 5 days at 2-week intervals

100-200 mg/m²/day for 5- to 10-day therapy course or every day until remission

I.T.: 5-75 mg/m² every 2-7 days until CNS findings normalize

or

<1 year: 20 mg

1-2 years: 30 mg

2-3 years: 50 mg

>3 years: 70 mg

Maintenance remission:

I.V.: 70-200 mg/m²/day for 2-5 days at monthly intervals

I.M., S.C.: 1-1.5 mg/kg single dose for maintenance at 1- to 4-week intervals

High-dose therapies:

Doses as high as 1-3 g/m² have been used for refractory or secondary leukemias or refractory non-Hodgkin's lymphoma

Doses of 3 g/m² every 12 hours for up to 12 doses have been used

Bone marrow transplant: 1.5 g/m² continuous infusion over 48 hours

Mechanism of Action Inhibition of DNA synthesis; cell cycle-specific for the S phase of cell division; cytosine gains entry into cells by a carrier process, and then must be converted to its active compound; cytosine acts as an analog and is incorporated into DNA; however, the primary action is inhibition of DNA polymerase resulting in decreased DNA synthesis and repair; degree of its cytotoxicity correlates linearly with its incorporation into DNA; therefore, incorporation into the DNA is responsible for drug activity and toxicity

Local Anesthetic/Vasoconstrictor Precautions No information available to require special precautions

Effects on Dental Treatment No effects or complications reported

Other Adverse Effects

Central nervous system: Has produced seizures when given I.T.; cerebellar syndrome (or cerebellar toxicity), manifested as ataxia, dysarthria, and dysdiadochokinesia, has been reported to be dose-related. This may or may not be reversible.

High-dose therapy toxicities: Cerebellar toxicity, conjunctivitis (make sure the patient is on steroid eye drops during therapy), corneal keratitis, hyperbilirubinemia, pulmonary edema, pericarditis, and tamponade

>10%:

Central nervous system: Fever, rash

Dermatologic: Oral/anal ulceration

Gastrointestinal: Nausea, vomiting, diarrhea, and mucositis which subside quickly after discontinuing the drug; GI effects may be more pronounced with divided I.V. bolus doses than with continuous infusion

Emetic potential: ≤20 mg: Moderately low (10% to 30%); 250 mg to 1 g: Moderately high (60% to 90%); >1 g: High (>90%)

Hematologic: Bleeding

(Continued)

Cytarabine *(Continued)*

Myelosuppressive: Occurs within the first week of treatment and lasts for 10-14 days; primarily manifested as granulocytopenia, but anemia can also occur. WBC: Severe; Platelets: Severe; Onset (days): 4-7; Nadir (days): 14-18; Recovery (days): 21-28

Hepatic: Hepatic dysfunction, mild jaundice and acute increase in transaminases can be produced

Local: Thrombophlebitis

1% to 10%:

Cardiovascular: Cardiomegaly

Central nervous system: Dizziness, headache, somnolence, confusion, neuritis, malaise

Dermatologic: Skin freckling, itching, alopecia

Genitourinary: Urinary retention

Local: Cellulitis at injection site

Neuromuscular & skeletal: Myalgia, bone pain, peripheral neuropathy

Respiratory: Syndrome of sudden respiratory distress progressing to pulmonary edema, pneumonia

Miscellaneous: Sepsis

Drug Interactions

Decreased effect of gentamicin, flucytosine; decreased digoxin oral tablet absorption

Increased toxicity: Alkylating agents and radiation; purine analogs; methotrexate

Drug Uptake

Absorption: Because high concentrations of cytidine deaminase are in the GI mucosa and liver, three- to tenfold higher doses than I.V. would need to be given orally; therefore, the oral route is not used

Serum half-life:

Initial: 7-20 minutes

Terminal: 0.5-2.6 hours

Pregnancy Risk Factor D

Generic Available Yes

Cytomel® *see Liothyronine on page 558*

Cytosar-U® *see Cytarabine on previous page*

Cytotec® *see Misoprostol on page 641*

Cytovene® *see Ganciclovir on page 436*

Cytoxan® *see Cyclophosphamide on page 269*

D₃ *see Cholecalciferol on page 228*

D-3-Mercaptovaline *see Penicillamine on page 730*

Dacarbazine *(da KAR ba zeen)*

Brand Names DTIC-Dome®

Therapeutic Category Antineoplastic Agent, Miscellaneous

Synonyms DIC; Dimethyl Triazeno Imidazol Carboxamide; DTIC; Imidazole Carboxamide

Use Singly or in various combination therapy to treat malignant melanoma, Hodgkin's disease, soft-tissue sarcomas (fibrosarcomas, rhabdomyosarcoma), islet cell carcinoma, medullary carcinoma of the thyroid, and neuroblastoma

Usual Dosage I.V. (refer to individual protocols):

Children:

Pediatric solid tumors: 200-470 mg/m²/day over 5 days every 21-28 days

Pediatric neuroblastoma: 800-900 mg/m² as a single dose on day 1 of therapy every 3-4 weeks in combination therapy

Hodgkin's disease: 375 mg/m² on days 1 and 15 of treatment course, repeat every 28 days

Adults:

Malignant melanoma: 2-4.5 mg/kg/day for 10 days, repeat in 4 weeks **or** may use 250 mg/m²/day for 5 days, repeat in 3 weeks

Hodgkin's disease: 150 mg/m²/day for 5 days, repeat every 4 weeks **or** 375 mg/m² on day 1, repeat in 15 days of each 28-day cycle in combination with other agents **or** 375 mg/m² repeated in 15 days of each 28-day cycle

Mechanism of Action Alkylating agent which forms methylcarbonium ions that attack nucleophilic groups in DNA; cross-links strands of DNA resulting in the inhibition of DNA, RNA, and protein synthesis, but the exact mechanism of action is still unclear; originally developed as a purine antimetabolite, but it does not interfere with purine synthesis; metabolism by the host is necessary for activation of dacarbazine, then the methylated species acts by alkylation of nucleic acids; dacarbazine is active in all phases of the cell cycle

Local Anesthetic/Vasoconstrictor Precautions No information available to require special precautions

Effects on Dental Treatment No effects or complications reported
Other Adverse Effects
>10%:
Central nervous system: Polyneuropathy, headache, and seizures have been reported
Extravasation: Dacarbazine is a vesicant; may cause tissue necrosis after extravasation; apply ice and consult extravasation policy if this occurs
Gastrointestinal: Moderate to severe nausea and vomiting in 90% of patients and lasting up to 12 hours after administration; nausea and vomiting are dose-related and occur more frequently when given as a one-time dose, as opposed to a less intensive 5-day course; diarrhea may also occur
Emetic potential: <500 mg: Moderately high (60% to 90%); ≥500 mg: High (>90%)
Local: Pain and burning at infusion site
Hematologic: Myelosuppressive effects: Mild to moderate is common and dose-related; leukopenia and thrombocytopenia may be delayed 2-3 weeks and may be the dose-limiting toxicity; WBC: Mild (primarily leukocytes); Platelets: Mild; Onset (days): 7; Nadir (days): 10-14; Recovery (days): 21-28
Neuromuscular & skeletal: Weakness
Ocular: Blurred vision
1% to 10%:
Cardiovascular: Facial flushing
Dermatologic: Alopecia, rash
Gastrointestinal: Anorexia, metallic taste
Hematologic: Myelosuppression
Neuromuscular & skeletal: Paresthesias
Flu-like effects: Fever, malaise, headache, myalgia, and sinus congestion may last up to several days after administration
<1%:
Cardiovascular: Orthostatic hypotension
Dermatologic: Photosensitivity reactions
Gastrointestinal: Stomatitis, diarrhea
Hepatic: Hepatotoxicity, elevated LFTs
Miscellaneous: Mild immunosuppression, anaphylaxis
Drug Uptake
Onset of action: I.V.: 18-24 days
Absorption: Oral administration demonstrates slow and variable absorption; preferable to administer by I.V. route
Serum half-life (biphasic):
Initial: 20-40 minutes
Terminal: 5 hours
Pregnancy Risk Factor C
Generic Available Yes

Dacodyl® [OTC] *see* Bisacodyl *on page 131*

Dactinomycin (dak ti noe MYE sin)
Brand Names Cosmegen®
Therapeutic Category Antineoplastic Agent, Antibiotic
Synonyms ACT; Actinomycin D
Use Management, either alone or in combination with other treatment modalities of Wilms' tumor, rhabdomyosarcoma, neuroblastoma, retinoblastoma, Ewing's sarcoma, trophoblastic neoplasms, testicular carcinoma, and other malignancies
Usual Dosage Refer to individual protocols
Calculation of the dosage for obese or edematous patients should be on the basis of surface area in an effort to relate dosage to lean body mass
Children >6 months and Adults: I.V.:
15 mcg/kg/day **or** 400-600 mcg/m²/day (maximum: 500 mcg) for 5 days, may repeat every 3-6 weeks **or**
2.5 mg/m² given in divided doses over 1-week period and repeated at 2-week intervals **or**
0.75-2 mg/m² as a single dose given at intervals of 1-4 weeks have been used
Mechanism of Action Binds to the guanine portion of DNA intercalating between guanine and cytosine base pairs inhibiting DNA and RNA synthesis and protein synthesis; product of *Streptomyces parvullus* (a yeast species)
Local Anesthetic/Vasoconstrictor Precautions No information available to require special precautions
Effects on Dental Treatment No effects or complications reported
Other Adverse Effects
>10%:
Dermatologic: Alopecia (reversible), hyperpigmentation of skin
Central nervous system: Unusual fatigue
(Continued)

Dactinomycin *(Continued)*

Extravasation: An irritant and should be administered through a rapidly running I.V. line; extravasation can lead to tissue necrosis, pain, and ulceration

Gastrointestinal: Severe nausea and vomiting occur in most patients and persist for up to 24 hours; stomatitis, anorexia, abdominal pain, and diarrhea, esophagitis

Hematologic: Myelosuppressive: Dose-limiting toxicity; anemia, aplastic anemia, agranulocytosis, pancytopenia; WBC: Moderate; Platelets: Moderate; Onset (days): 7; Nadir (days): 14-21; Recovery (days): 21-28

1% to 10%: Gastrointestinal: Mucositis

<1%:

Central nervous system: Fever

Dermatologic: Skin eruptions, acne

Endocrine & metabolic: Hyperuricemia, hypocalcemia

Hepatic: Hepatitis, liver function test abnormalities Anaphylactoid reaction

Drug Uptake

Serum half-life: 36 hours

Time to peak serum concentration: I.V.: Within 2-5 minutes

Pregnancy Risk Factor C

Generic Available No

D.A.II® Tablet *see* Chlorpheniramine, Phenylephrine, and Methscopolamine *on page 220*

Dairy Ease® [OTC] *see* Lactase *on page 539*

Dakin's Solution *see* Sodium Hypochlorite Solution *on page 873*

Dakrina® Ophthalmic Solution [OTC] *see* Artificial Tears *on page 87*

Dalalone L.A.® *see* Dexamethasone *on page 291*

Dalgan® *see* Dezocine *on page 299*

Dallergy® *see* Chlorpheniramine, Phenylephrine, and Methscopolamine *on page 220*

Dallergy-D® Syrup *see* Chlorpheniramine and Phenylephrine *on page 218*

Dalmane® *see* Flurazepam *on page 422*

Dalteparin *(dal TE pa rin)*

Brand Names Fragmin®

Therapeutic Category Anticoagulant

Use Prevention of deep vein thrombosis which may lead to pulmonary embolism, in patients requiring abdominal surgery who are at risk for thromboembolism complications (ie, patients >40 years of age, obese, patients with malignancy, history of deep vein thrombosis or pulmonary embolism, and surgical procedures requiring general anesthesia and lasting longer than 30 minutes)

Usual Dosage Adults: S.C.:

Low-moderate risk patients: 2500 units 1-2 hours prior to surgery, then once daily for 5-10 days postoperatively

High risk patients: 5000 units 1-2 hours prior to surgery and then once daily for 5-10 days postoperatively

Mechanism of Action Low molecular weight heparin analog with a molecular weight of 4000-6000 daltons; the commercial product contains 3% to 15% heparin with a molecular weight <3000 daltons, 65% to 78% with a molecular weight of 3000-8000 daltons and 14% to 26% with a molecular weight >8000 daltons; while dalteparin has been shown to inhibit both factor Xa and factor IIa (thrombin), the antithrombotic effect of dalteparin is characterized by a higher ratio of antifactor Xa to antifactor IIa activity (ratio = 4)

Local Anesthetic/Vasoconstrictor Precautions No information available to require special precautions

Effects on Dental Treatment No effects or complications reported

Other Adverse Effects

1% to 10%:

Central nervous system: Allergic fever

Dermatologic: Pruritus, rash, bullous eruption, skin necrosis

Hematologic: Bleeding, thrombocytopenia, wound hematoma

Local: Pain at injection site, injection site hematoma, injection site reactions

Miscellaneous: Anaphylactoid reactions, allergic reactions

Drug Interactions Increased toxicity: Caution should be used when using aspirin, other platelet inhibitors, and oral anticoagulants in combination with dalteparin due to an increased risk of bleeding

Pregnancy Risk Factor B

Dosage Forms Injection: Prefilled syringe: Anti-Factor Xa 2500 units per 0.2 mL; anti-Factor Xa 5000 units per 0.2 mL

Generic Available No

Damason-P® *see* Hydrocodone and Aspirin *on page 480*

Danaparoid (da NAP a roid)

Brand Names Orgaran®

Therapeutic Category Anticoagulant

Synonyms Danaparoid Sodium

Use Prophylaxis of postoperative deep vein thrombosis (DVT)

Usual Dosage S.C.:

Children: Safety and effectiveness have not been established

Adults: 750 anti-Xa units twice daily; beginning 1-4 hours before surgery and then not sooner than 2 hours after surgery and every 12 hours until the risk of DVT has diminished, the average duration of therapy is 7-10 days

Local Anesthetic/Vasoconstrictor Precautions No information available to require special precautions

Effects on Dental Treatment No effects or complications reported

Other Adverse Effects

1% to 10%:

Cardiovascular: Peripheral edema, generalized edema

Central nervous system: Fever, insomnia, headache, dizziness

Dermatologic: Rash, pruritus

Gastrointestinal: Nausea, constipation, vomiting

Genitourinary: Urinary tract infections, urinary retention

Hematologic: Anemia, hemorrhage, hematoma

Local: Injection site pain

Neuromuscular & skeletal: Joint disorder, weakness

Warnings/Precautions Do not administer intramuscularly; use with extreme caution in patients with a history of bacterial endocarditis, hemorrhagic stroke, recent CNS or ophthalmological surgery, bleeding diathesis, uncontrolled arterial hypertension, or a history of recent gastrointestinal ulceration and hemorrhage. Danaparoid shows a low cross-sensitivity with antiplatelet antibodies in individuals with type II heparin-induced thrombocytopenia. This product contains sodium sulfite which may cause allergic-type reactions, including anaphylactic symptoms and life-threatening asthmatic episodes in susceptible people; this is seen more frequently in asthmatics.

Drug Interactions Increased toxicity with oral anticoagulants, platelet inhibitors

Drug Uptake

Onset of effect: Maximum anti-factor Xa and antithrombin (anti-factor IIa) activities occur 2-5 hours after S.C. administration

Serum half-life, plasma: Mean terminal half-life: ~24 hours

Pregnancy Risk Factor B

Generic Available No

Danaparoid Sodium *see* Danaparoid *on this page*

Danazol (DA na zole)

Brand Names Danocrine®

Canadian/Mexican Brand Names Cyclomen® (Canada); Ladogal® (Mexico); Zoldan-A® (Mexico)

Therapeutic Category Androgen

Use Treatment of endometriosis, fibrocystic breast disease, and hereditary angioedema

Usual Dosage Adults: Oral:

Endometriosis: 100-400 mg twice daily for 3-6 months (may extend to 9 months)

Fibrocystic breast disease: 50-200 mg twice daily for 2-6 months

Hereditary angioedema: 400-600 mg/day in 2-3 divided doses

Mechanism of Action Suppresses pituitary output of follicle-stimulating hormone and luteinizing hormone that causes regression and atrophy of normal and ectopic endometrial tissue; decreases rate of growth of abnormal breast tissue; reduces attacks associated with hereditary angioedema by increasing levels of C4 component of complement

Local Anesthetic/Vasoconstrictor Precautions No information available to require special precautions

Effects on Dental Treatment No effects or complications reported

Other Adverse Effects

>10%:

Cardiovascular: Fluid retention, edema

Dermatologic: Oily skin, acne, hirsutism

Endocrine & metabolic: Irregular menstrual periods, decreased breast size

Gastrointestinal: Weight gain

Hematologic: Breakthrough bleeding

Hepatic: Hepatic impairment

Miscellaneous: Voice deepening

(Continued)

Danazol (Continued)

1% to 10%:
  Endocrine & metabolic: Virilization, androgenic effects, amenorrhea, hypoestrogenism
  Neuromuscular & skeletal: Weakness

<1%:
  Central nervous system: Dizziness, headache
  Dermatologic: Skin rashes, photosensitivity
  Gastrointestinal: Pancreatitis, bleeding gums
  Genitourinary: Monilial vaginitis, testicular atrophy, enlarged clitoris
  Hepatic: Cholestatic jaundice
  Neuromuscular & skeletal: Carpal tunnel syndrome
  Miscellaneous: Benign intracranial hypertension

Drug Interactions Danazol has prolonged the prothrombin times in patients taking warfarin; anticoagulant effects are enhanced; danazol has increased the serum concentrations of carbamazepine (Tegretol®) leading to dizziness, nausea, drowsiness, and ataxia

Drug Uptake
Onset of therapeutic effect: Within 4 weeks following daily doses
Serum half-life: 4.5 hours (variable)
Time to peak serum concentration: Within 2 hours

Pregnancy Risk Factor X
Generic Available Yes

Danocrine® see Danazol on previous page
Dantrium® see Dantrolene on this page

Dantrolene (DAN troe leen)

Brand Names Dantrium®
Therapeutic Category Antidote, Malignant Hyperthermia; Hyperthermia, Treatment; Muscle Relaxant; Skeletal Muscle Relaxant
Use Treatment of spasticity associated with spinal cord injury, stroke, cerebral palsy, or multiple sclerosis; also used as treatment of malignant hyperthermia

Usual Dosage
Spasticity: Oral:
  Children: Initial: 0.5 mg/kg/dose twice daily, increase frequency to 3-4 times/day at 4- to 7-day intervals, then increase dose by 0.5 mg/kg to a maximum of 3 mg/kg/dose 2-4 times/day up to 400 mg/day
  Adults: 25 mg/day to start, increase frequency to 2-4 times/day, then increase dose by 25 mg every 4-7 days to a maximum of 100 mg 2-4 times/day or 400 mg/day

Malignant hyperthermia: Children and Adults:
  Oral: 4-8 mg/kg/day in 4 divided doses
    Preoperative prophylaxis: Begin 1-2 days prior to surgery with last dose 3-4 hours prior to surgery
  I.V.: 1 mg/kg; may repeat dose up to cumulative dose of 10 mg/kg (mean effective dose is 2.5 mg/kg), then switch to oral dosage
    Preoperative: 2.5 mg/kg ~1¼ hours prior to anesthesia and infused over 1 hour with additional doses as needed and individualized

Mechanism of Action Acts directly on skeletal muscle by interfering with release of calcium ion from the sarcoplasmic reticulum; prevents or reduces the increase in myoplasmic calcium ion concentration that activates the acute catabolic processes associated with malignant hyperthermia

Local Anesthetic/Vasoconstrictor Precautions No information available to require special precautions
Effects on Dental Treatment No effects or complications reported
Other Adverse Effects

>10%:
  Central nervous system: Drowsiness, dizziness, lightheadedness, fatigue,
  Dermatologic: Rash
  Gastrointestinal: Diarrhea (mild), nausea, vomiting
  Neuromuscular & skeletal: Weakness

1% to 10%:
  Cardiovascular: Pleural effusion with pericarditis
  Central nervous system: Chills, fever, headache, insomnia, nervousness, mental depression
  Gastrointestinal: Diarrhea (severe), constipation, anorexia, stomach cramps
  Ocular: Blurred vision
  Respiratory: Respiratory depression

<1%:
  Central nervous system: Seizures, confusion

Hepatic: Hepatitis

Drug Interactions When given simultaneously dantrolene has increased the toxicity of the following drugs: Estrogens (hepatotoxicity), CNS depressants (sedation), MAO inhibitors, phenothiazines, clindamycin (increased neuromuscular blockade), verapamil (hyperkalemia and cardiac depression), warfarin, clofibrate and tolbutamide

Drug Uptake
Absorption: Slow and incomplete from GI tract
Serum half-life: 8.7 hours

Pregnancy Risk Factor C

Generic Available No

Dapacin® Cold Capsule [OTC] *see* Chlorpheniramine, Phenylpropanolamine, and Acetaminophen *on page 222*

Dapiprazole (DA pi pray zole)
Brand Names Rēv-Eyes™

Therapeutic Category Alpha-Adrenergic Blocking Agent, Ophthalmic

Use Reverse dilation due to drugs (adrenergic or parasympathomimetic) after eye exams

Usual Dosage Adults: Administer 2 drops followed 5 minutes later by an additional 2 drops applied to the conjunctiva of each eye; should not be used more frequently than once a week in the same patient

Mechanism of Action Dapiprazole is a selective alpha-adrenergic blocking agent, exerting effects primarily on alpha$_1$-adrenoceptors. It induces miosis via relaxation of the smooth dilator (radial) muscle of the iris, which causes pupillary constriction. It is devoid of cholinergic effects. Dapiprazole also partially reverses the cycloplegia induced with parasympatholytic agents such as tropicamide. Although the drug has no significant effect on the ciliary muscle *per se*, it may increase accommodative amplitude, therefore relieving the symptoms of paralysis of accommodation.

Local Anesthetic/Vasoconstrictor Precautions No information available to require special precautions

Effects on Dental Treatment No effects or complications reported

Other Adverse Effects
>10%:
Central nervous system: Headache
Ocular: Conjunctival injection, burning sensation in the eyes, lid edema, ptosis, lid erythema, chemosis, itching, punctate keratitis, corneal edema, photophobia
1% to 10%: Ocular: Dry eyes, blurring of vision, tearing of eye

Drug Interactions No data reported

Pregnancy Risk Factor B

Generic Available No

Dapsone (DAP sone)
Related Information
HIV Infection and AIDS *on page 1024*

Brand Names Avlosulfon®

Therapeutic Category Antibiotic, Sulfone

Use Treatment of leprosy and dermatitis herpetiformis (infections caused by *Mycobacterium leprae*), alternative agent for *Pneumocystis carinii* pneumonia prophylaxis (given alone) and treatment (given with trimethoprim)

Usual Dosage Oral:
Leprosy:
Children: 1-2 mg/kg/24 hours, up to a maximum of 100 mg/day
Adults: 50-100 mg/day for 3-10 years
Dermatitis herpetiformis: Adults: Start at 50 mg/day, increase to 300 mg/day, or higher to achieve full control, reduce dosage to minimum level as soon as possible
Prophylaxis of *Pneumocystis carinii* pneumonia: Children >1 month: 1 mg/kg/day; maximum: 100 mg
Treatment of *Pneumocystis carinii* pneumonia: Adults: 100 mg/day in combination with trimethoprim (20 mg/kg/day) for 21 days

Mechanism of Action Dapsone is a sulfone antimicrobial. The mechanism of action of the sulfones is similar to that of the sulfonamides. Sulfonamides are competitive antagonists of para-aminobenzoic acid (PABA) and prevent normal bacterial utilization of PABA for the synthesis of folic acid.

Local Anesthetic/Vasoconstrictor Precautions No information available to require special precautions

Effects on Dental Treatment No effects or complications reported
(Continued)

281

Dapsone *(Continued)*

Other Adverse Effects

1% to 10%:
    Hematologic: Dose-related hemolysis, methemoglobinemia with cyanosis
    Miscellaneous: Reactional states

<1%:
    Central nervous system: Insomnia, headache
    Dermatologic: Exfoliative dermatitis
    Gastrointestinal: Nausea, vomiting
    Hematologic: Hemolytic anemia, methemoglobinemia, leukopenia, agranulocytosis
    Hepatic: Hepatitis, cholestatic jaundice
    Neuromuscular & skeletal: Peripheral neuropathy
    Ocular: Blurred vision
    Otic: Tinnitus

Drug Interactions

Dapsone has decreased the effects of para-aminobenzoic acid and rifampin
Dapsone has increased the effects of folic acid antagonists

Drug Uptake

Absorption: Oral: Well absorbed
Serum half-life, elimination: 30 hours (range: 10-50 hours)

Pregnancy Risk Factor C

Generic Available Yes

Daranide® *see* Dichlorphenamide *on page 303*

Daraprim® *see* Pyrimethamine *on page 825*

Daricon® *see* Oxyphencyclimine *on page 717*

Darvocet-N® *see* Propoxyphene and Acetaminophen *on page 812*

Darvocet-N® 100 *see* Propoxyphene and Acetaminophen *on page 812*

Darvon® *see* Propoxyphene *on page 811*

Darvon® Compound-65 Pulvules® *see* Propoxyphene and Aspirin *on page 813*

Darvon-N® *see* Propoxyphene *on page 811*

Daunomycin *see* Daunorubicin Hydrochloride *on next page*

Daunorubicin Citrate (Liposomal)

(daw noe ROO bi sin SI trate lip po SOE mal)

Brand Names DaunoXome®

Therapeutic Category Antineoplastic Agent, Anthracycline; Antineoplastic Agent, Antibiotic

Use Advanced HIV-associated Kaposi's sarcoma; first-line cytotoxic therapy for advanced HIV-associated Kaposi's sarcoma

Usual Dosage Adults: I.V.: 40 mg/m^2 over 1 hour; repeat every 2 weeks; continue treatment until there is evidence of progressive disease

Dosing adjustment in renal/hepatic impairment:

Serum Bilirubin	Serum Creatinine	Recommended Dose
1.2-3 mg/dL		¾ normal dose
>3 mg/dL	>3 mg/dL	½ normal dose

Mechanism of Action Liposomal daunorubicin contains an aqueous solution of the citrate salt of daunorubicin encapsulated with lipid vesicles (liposomes) composed of a lipid bilayer of distearoylphosphatidylcholine and cholesterol (2:1 molar ratio). This liposomal daunorubicin is formulated to maximum the selectivity of daunorubicin for solid tumors *in situ*; refer to Daunorubicin monograph.

Local Anesthetic/Vasoconstrictor Precautions No information available to require special precautions

Effects on Dental Treatment No effects or complications reported

Other Adverse Effects

>10%:
    Central nervous system: Fatigue, headache
    Gastrointestinal: Abdominal pain, anorexia, diarrhea, nausea, vomiting
    Hematologic: Neutropenia
    Neuromuscular & skeletal: Neuropathy
    Respiratory: Cough, dyspnea, rhinitis
    Miscellaneous: Infection

5% to 10%:
    Cardiovascular: Hypertension, palpitations, syncope, tachycardia, chest pain, edema
    Central nervous system: Depression, dizziness, insomnia, malaise
    Dermatologic: Alopecia, pruritus

Endocrine & metabolic: Hot flashes
Gastrointestinal: Constipation, stomatitis, tenesmus
Neuromuscular & skeletal: Arthralgia, myalgia
Ocular: Abnormal vision
Respiratory: Sinusitis

Contraindications Hypersensitivity to previous doses or any constituents of the product

Warnings/Precautions

The U.S. Food and Drug Administration (FDA) currently recommends that procedures for proper handling and disposal of antineoplastic agents be considered.

The primary toxicity is myelosuppression, especially off the granulocytic series, which may be severe, with much less marked effects on platelets and erythroid series. Potential cardiac toxicity, particularly in patients who have received prior anthracyclines or who have pre-existing cardiac disease, may occur. Refer to Daunorubicin monograph.

Although grade 3-4 injection site inflammation has been reported in patients treated with the liposomal daunorubicin, no instances of local tissue necrosis were observed with extravasation. However, refer to daunorubicin monograph and avoid extravasation.

Reduce dosage in patients with impaired hepatic function. Hyperuricemia can be induced secondary to rapid lysis of leukemic cells. As a precaution, administer allopurinol prior to initiating antileukemic therapy.

Drug Uptake
Serum half-life: 4.4 hours

Pregnancy Risk Factor D

Dosage Forms Injection: 2 mg/mL (equivalent to 50 mg daunorubicin base) (1 mL, 4 mL, 10 mL unit packs)

Generic Available No

Daunorubicin Hydrochloride

(daw noe ROO bi sin hye droe KLOR ide)

Brand Names Cerubidine®

Canadian/Mexican Brand Names Rubilem (Mexico); Trixilem (Mexico)

Therapeutic Category Antineoplastic Agent, Antibiotic

Synonyms Daunomycin; DNR; Rubidomycin Hydrochloride

Use In combination with other agents in the treatment of leukemias (ALL, AML)

Usual Dosage I.V. (**refer to individual protocols**):

Children:

ALL Combination therapy: Remission induction: 25-45 mg/m^2 on day 1 every week for 4 cycles **or** 30-45 mg/m^2/day for 3 days

In children <2 years or <0.5 m^2, daunorubicin should be based on weight - mg/kg: 1 mg/kg per protocol with frequency dependent on regimen employed

Cumulative dose should not exceed 300 mg/m^2 in children >2 years or 10 mg/kg in children <2 years

Adults: 30-60 mg/m^2/day for 3-5 days, repeat dose in 3-4 weeks

Single agent induction for AML: 60 mg/m^2/day for 3 days; repeat every 3-4 weeks

Combination therapy induction for AML: 45 mg/m^2/day for 3 days of the first course of induction therapy; subsequent courses: Every day for 2 days

ALL combination therapy: 45 mg/m^2/day for 3 days

Cumulative dose should not exceed 400-600 mg/m^2

Mechanism of Action Inhibition of DNA and RNA synthesis, by intercalating between DNA base pairs and by steric obstruction; is not cell cycle-specific for the S phase of cell division; daunomycin is preferred over doxorubicin for the treatment of ANLL because of its dose-limiting toxicity (myelosuppression) is not of concern in the therapy of this disease; has less mucositis associated with its use

Local Anesthetic/Vasoconstrictor Precautions No information available to require special precautions

Effects on Dental Treatment No effects or complications reported

Other Adverse Effects

>10%:

Dermatologic: Alopecia (reversible)

Gastrointestinal: Mild nausea or vomiting occurs in 50% of patients within the first 24 hours; stomatitis may occur 3-7 days after administration, but is not as severe as that caused by doxorubicin

Genitourinary: Discoloration of urine (red)

1% to 10%:

Cardiovascular: Congestive heart failure

Endocrine & metabolic: Hyperuricemia

Gastrointestinal: GI ulceration, diarrhea

(Continued)

Daunorubicin Hydrochloride *(Continued)*

Hematologic: Myelosuppressive: Dose-limiting toxicity, occurs in all patients; leukopenia is more significant than thrombocytopenia; WBC: Severe; Platelets: Severe; Onset (days): 7; Nadir (days): 14; Recovery (days): 21-28

Local: Extravasation: Daunorubicin is a vesicant; infiltration can cause severe inflammation, tissue necrosis, and ulceration; if the drug is infiltrated, consult institutional policy, apply ice to the area, and elevate the limb

<1%:

Cardiovascular: Pericarditis/myocarditis

Central nervous system: Chills

Dermatologic: Skin rash, urticaria

Hepatic: Elevation in serum bilirubin, AST, and alkaline phosphatase

Miscellaneous: Fertility impairment, pigmentation changes in nailbeds

Drug Uptake

Serum half-life: 14-20 hours

Pregnancy Risk Factor D

Generic Available No

DaunoXome® *see Daunorubicin Citrate (Liposomal) on page 282*

Daypro™ *see Oxaprozin on page 706*

Dayto Himbin® *see Yohimbine on page 999*

DC 240® Softgels® [OTC] *see Docusate on page 331*

DCF *see Pentostatin on page 740*

DDAVP® *see Desmopressin Acetate on page 289*

Debrisan® [OTC] *see Dextranomer on page 296*

Debrox® Otic [OTC] *see Carbamide Peroxide on page 175*

Decadron® *see Dexamethasone on page 291*

Decadron®-LA *see Dexamethasone on page 291*

Deca-Durabolin® Injection *see Nandrolone on page 663*

Decaject-L.A.® *see Dexamethasone on page 291*

Decholin® *see Dehydrocholic Acid on next page*

Declomycin® *see Demeclocycline on page 286*

Decofed® Syrup [OTC] *see Pseudoephedrine on page 820*

Decohistine® DH *see Chlorpheniramine, Pseudoephedrine, and Codeine on page 223*

Decohistine® Expectorant *see Guaifenesin, Pseudoephedrine, and Codeine on page 455*

Deconamine® SR *see Chlorpheniramine and Pseudoephedrine on page 219*

Deconamine® Syrup [OTC] *see Chlorpheniramine and Pseudoephedrine on page 219*

Deconamine® Tablet [OTC] *see Chlorpheniramine and Pseudoephedrine on page 219*

Deconsal® II *see Guaifenesin and Pseudoephedrine on page 454*

Deconsal® Sprinkle® *see Guaifenesin and Phenylephrine on page 454*

Defen-LA® *see Guaifenesin and Pseudoephedrine on page 454*

Deferoxamine *(de fer OKS a meen)*

Brand Names Desferal® Mesylate

Therapeutic Category Antidote, Aluminum Toxicity; Antidote, Iron Toxicity

Use Acute iron intoxication; chronic iron overload secondary to multiple transfusions; diagnostic test for iron overload; used investigationally in the treatment of aluminum accumulation in renal failure; iron overload secondary to congenital anemias; hemochromatosis; removal of corneal rust rings following surgical removal of foreign bodies

Usual Dosage

Children:

Acute iron intoxication (I.M. is preferred route for patients not in shock). Treat until urine is no longer pink salmon colored:

I.M.: 50 mg/kg/dose every 6 hours to a maximum of 6 g/day

I.V.: 15 mg/kg/hour; maximum: 6 g/day

Chronic iron overload:

I.M., I.V.: 50 mg/kg/dose to a maximum of 6 g/24 hours or 2 g/dose; do not exceed 15 mg/kg/hour I.V.

S.C.: 20-40 mg/kg/day over 8-12 hours (via a portable, controlled infusion device)

Aluminum-induced bone disease: 20-40 mg/kg every hemodialysis treatment, frequency dependent on clinical status of the patient

Adults:
Acute iron intoxication: (I.M. is preferred route for patients not in shock). Treat until urine is no longer pink salmon colored:
I.M., I.V.: 1 g stat, then 0.5 g every 4 hours for 2 doses, then 0.5 g every 4-12 hours up to 6 g/day; do not exceed 15 mg/kg/hour I.V.
Chronic iron overload:
I.M.: 0.5-1 g every day
I.V.: 2 g after each unit of blood infusion at 15 mg/kg/hour
S.C.: 1-2 g every day over 8-24 hours
Mechanism of Action Complexes with trivalent ions (ferric ions) to form ferrioxamine, which are removed by the kidneys
Local Anesthetic/Vasoconstrictor Precautions No information available to require special precautions
Effects on Dental Treatment No effects or complications reported
Other Adverse Effects
1% to 10%: Local: Pain and induration at injection site
<1%:
Cardiovascular: Flushing, hypotension, tachycardia, shock, swelling
Central nervous system: Fever
Dermatologic: Erythema, urticaria, pruritus, rash, cutaneous wheal formation
Gastrointestinal: Abdominal discomfort, diarrhea
Neuromuscular & skeletal: Leg cramps
Ocular: Blurred vision, cataracts
Otic: Hearing loss
Miscellaneous: Anaphylaxis
Drug Interactions No data reported
Drug Uptake
Absorption: Oral: <15%
Serum half-life:
Parent drug: 6.1 hours
Ferrioxamine: 5.8 hours
Pregnancy Risk Factor C
Generic Available No

Deficol® [OTC] *see* Bisacodyl *on page 131*

Degas® [OTC] *see* Simethicone *on page 865*

Degest® 2 Ophthalmic [OTC] *see* Naphazoline *on page 664*

Dehydrocholic Acid (dee hye droe KOE lik AS id)
Brand Names Cholan-HMB®; Decholin®
Therapeutic Category Bile Acid; Laxative, Hydrocholeretic
Use Relief of constipation; adjunct to various biliary tract conditions
Local Anesthetic/Vasoconstrictor Precautions No information available to require special precautions
Effects on Dental Treatment No effects or complications reported
Other Adverse Effects 1% to 10%: Gastrointestinal: Dehydration, diarrhea, abdominal cramps
Pregnancy Risk Factor C
Generic Available Yes

Dekasol-L.A.® *see* Dexamethasone *on page 291*

Deladumone® Injection *see* Estradiol and Testosterone *on page 366*

Del Aqua-5® Gel *see* Benzoyl Peroxide *on page 120*

Del Aqua-10® Gel *see* Benzoyl Peroxide *on page 120*

Delatest® Injection *see* Testosterone *on page 910*

Delatestryl® Injection *see* Testosterone *on page 910*

Delavirdine (de la VIR deen)
Related Information
HIV Infection and AIDS *on page 1024*
Brand Names Rescriptor™
Therapeutic Category Antiviral Agent, Oral
Synonyms U-90152S
Use Treatment of HIV-1 infection in combination with appropriate antiretrovirals
Usual Dosage Adults: Oral: 400 mg 3 times/day
Local Anesthetic/Vasoconstrictor Precautions No information available to require special precautions
Effects on Dental Treatment No effects or complications reported
Pregnancy Risk Factor C
Dosage Forms Tablet: 100 mg

Delfen® [OTC] *see* Nonoxynol 9 *on page 689*

Del-Mycin® Topical *see* Erythromycin, Topical *on page 364*

Delsym® [OTC] *see* Dextromethorphan *on page 298*

Delta-Cortef® *see* Prednisolone *on page 788*

Delta-D® *see* Cholecalciferol *on page 228*

Deltasone® *see* Prednisone *on page 789*

Delta-Tritex® *see* Triamcinolone *on page 954*

Demadex® *see* Torsemide *on page 946*

Demazin® Syrup [OTC] *see* Chlorpheniramine and Phenylpropanolamine *on page 219*

Demecarium (dem e KARE ee um)
Brand Names Humorsol®

Therapeutic Category Antiglaucoma Agent; Cholinergic Agent, Ophthalmic; Ophthalmic Agent, Miotic

Use Management of chronic simple glaucoma, chronic and acute angle-closure glaucoma; strabismus

Usual Dosage Children and Adults: Ophthalmic:

Glaucoma: Instill 1 drop into eyes twice weekly to a maximum dosage of 1 or 2 drops twice daily for up to 4 months

Strabismus:

Diagnosis: Instill 1 drop daily for 2 weeks, then 1 drop every 2 days for 2-3 weeks. If eyes become straighter, an accommodative factor is demonstrated.

Therapy: Instill not more than 1 drop at a time in both eyes every day for 2-3 weeks. Then reduce dosage to 1 drop every other day for 3-4 weeks and re-evaluate. Continue at 1 drop every 2 days to 1 drop twice a week and evaluate the patient's condition every 4-12 weeks. If improvement continues, reduce dose to 1 drop once a week and eventually off of medication. Discontinue therapy after 4 months if control of the condition still requires 1 drop every 2 days.

Mechanism of Action Cholinesterase inhibitor (anticholinesterase) which causes acetylcholine to accumulate at cholinergic receptor sites and produces effects equivalent to excessive stimulation of cholinergic receptors. Demecarium mainly acts by inhibiting true (erythrocyte) cholinesterase and causes a reduction in intraocular pressure due to facilitation of outflow of aqueous humor; the reduction is likely to be particularly marked in eyes in which the pressure is elevated.

Local Anesthetic/Vasoconstrictor Precautions No information available to require special precautions

Effects on Dental Treatment No effects or complications reported

Other Adverse Effects

1% to 10%: Ocular: Stinging, burning, myopia, visual blurring

<1%:

Cardiovascular: Bradycardia, hypotension, flushing

Gastrointestinal: Nausea, vomiting, diarrhea

Neuromuscular & skeletal: Weakness

Ocular: Retinal detachment, miosis, twitching eyelids, watering eyes

Respiratory: Dyspnea

Miscellaneous: Sweating

Drug Interactions No data reported

Pregnancy Risk Factor C

Generic Available No

Demeclociclina (Mexico) *see* Demeclocycline *on this page*

Demeclocycline (dem e kloe SYE kleen)
Brand Names Declomycin®

Canadian/Mexican Brand Names Ledermicina® (Mexico)

Therapeutic Category Antibiotic, Tetracycline Derivative

Synonyms Demeclociclina (Mexico)

Use Treatment of susceptible bacterial infections (acne, gonorrhea, pertussis and urinary tract infections) caused by both gram-negative and gram-positive organisms; used when penicillin is contraindicated (other agents are preferred); treatment of chronic syndrome of inappropriate secretion of antidiuretic hormone (SIADH)

Usual Dosage Oral:

Children ≥8 years: 8-12 mg/kg/day divided every 6-12 hours

Adults: 150 mg 4 times/day or 300 mg twice daily

Uncomplicated gonorrhea (penicillin sensitive): 600 mg stat, 300 mg every 12 hours for 4 days (3 g total)

SIADH: 900-1200 mg/day or 13-15 mg/kg/day divided every 6-8 hours initially, then decrease to 0.6-0.9 g/day

Mechanism of Action Inhibits protein synthesis by binding with the 30S and possibly the 50S ribosomal subunit(s) of susceptible bacteria; may also cause alterations in the cytoplasmic membrane

Local Anesthetic/Vasoconstrictor Precautions No information available to require special precautions

Effects on Dental Treatment Tetracycline's are not recommended for use during pregnancy or in children ≤8 years of age since they have been reported to cause enamel hypoplasia and permanent teeth discoloration. The use of tetracycline's should only be used in these patients if other agents are contraindicated or alternative antimicrobials will not eradicate the organism. Long-term use associated with oral candidiasis.

Other Adverse Effects
1% to 10%:
Dermatologic: Photosensitivity
Gastrointestinal: Nausea, diarrhea
<1%:
Cardiovascular: Pericarditis
Central nervous system: Increased intracranial pressure, bulging fontanels in infants
Dermatologic: Dermatologic effects, pruritus, exfoliative dermatitis
Endocrine & metabolic: Diabetes insipidus syndrome
Gastrointestinal: Vomiting, esophagitis, anorexia, abdominal cramps
Neuromuscular & skeletal: Paresthesia
Renal: Acute renal failure, azotemia
Miscellaneous: Superinfections, anaphylaxis, pigmentation of nails

Drug Interactions
Decreased effect with antacids (aluminum, calcium, zinc, or magnesium), bismuth salts, sodium bicarbonate, barbiturates, carbamazepine, hydantoins
Decreased effect of oral contraceptives
Increased effect of warfarin

Drug Uptake
Onset of action for diuresis in SIADH: Several days
Absorption: ~50% to 80% from GI tract; food and dairy products reduce absorption
Serum half-life: Reduced renal function: 10-17 hours
Time to peak serum concentration: Oral: Within 3-6 hours

Pregnancy Risk Factor D

Dosage Forms
Capsule, as hydrochloride: 150 mg
Tablet, as hydrochloride: 150 mg, 300 mg

Dietary Considerations Should be taken 1 hour before or 2 hours after food or milk with plenty of fluid

Generic Available No

Demerol® *see* Meperidine *on page 592*

4-demethoxydaunorubicin *see* Idarubicin *on page 497*

Demser® *see* Metyrosine *on page 632*

Demulen® *see* Ethinyl Estradiol and Ethynodiol Diacetate *on page 375*

Denavir® *see* Penciclovir *on page 729*

Denorex® [OTC] *see* Coal Tar *on page 254*

Dental Drug Interactions: Update on Drug Combinations Requiring Special Considerations *see page 1144*

Dental Office Emergencies *see page 1103*

Dentifrice Products *see page 1172*

Dentin Hypersensitivity; High Caries Index; Xerostomia *see page 1074*

Dentipatch® *see* Lidocaine Transoral *on page 556*

Denture Adhesive Products *see page 1180*

Denture Cleanser Products *see page 1182*

Deoxycoformycin *see* Pentostatin *on page 740*

2'-deoxycoformycin *see* Pentostatin *on page 740*

Depacon® *see* Valproic Acid and Derivatives *on page 981*

Depakene® *see* Valproic Acid and Derivatives *on page 981*

Depakote® *see* Valproic Acid and Derivatives *on page 981*

depAndrogyn® Injection *see* Estradiol and Testosterone *on page 366*

depAndro® Injection *see* Testosterone *on page 910*

Depen® *see* Penicillamine *on page 730*

depGynogen® Injection *see* Estradiol *on page 365*

depMedalone® *see* Methylprednisolone *on page 624*

Depo®-Estradiol Injection *see* Estradiol *on page 365*

Depogen® Injection *see* Estradiol *on page 365*

Depoject® see Methylprednisolone on page 624

Depo-Medrol® see Methylprednisolone on page 624

Deponit® see Nitroglycerin on page 685

Depopred® see Methylprednisolone on page 624

Depo-Provera® see Medroxyprogesterone Acetate on page 587

Depo-Testadiol® Injection see Estradiol and Testosterone on page 366

Depotest® Injection see Testosterone on page 910

Depotestogen® Injection see Estradiol and Testosterone on page 366

Depo®-Testosterone Injection see Testosterone on page 910

Deproist® Expectorant with Codeine see Guaifenesin, Pseudoephedrine, and Codeine on page 455

Derifil® [OTC] see Chlorophyll on page 212

Derma-Smoothe/FS® see Fluocinolone on page 414

Dermatop® see Prednicarbate on page 788

Dermoplast® [OTC] see Benzocaine on page 118

Desferal® Mesylate see Deferoxamine on page 284

Desipramina, Clorhidrato De (Mexico) see Desipramine on this page

Desipramine (des IP ra meen)

Brand Names Norpramin®; Pertofrane®

Canadian/Mexican Brand Names PMS-Desipramine® (Canada)

Therapeutic Category Antidepressant, Tricyclic

Synonyms Desipramina, Clorhidrato De (Mexico)

Use Treatment of various forms of depression, often in conjunction with psycho-therapy; analgesic adjunct in chronic pain, peripheral neuropathies

Usual Dosage Oral:

Children 6-12 years: 10-30 mg/day or 1-5 mg/kg/day in divided doses; do not exceed 5 mg/kg/day

Adolescents: Initial: 25-50 mg/day; gradually increase to 100 mg/day in single or divided doses; maximum: 150 mg/day

Adults: Initial: 75 mg/day in divided doses; increase gradually to 150-200 mg/day in divided or single dose; maximum: 300 mg/day

Elderly: Initial dose: 10-25 mg/day; increase by 10-25 mg every 3 days for inpatients and every week for outpatients if tolerated; usual maintenance dose: 75-100 mg/day, but doses up to 300 mg/day may be necessary

Hemodialysis/peritoneal dialysis effects: Supplemental dose is not necessary

Mechanism of Action Traditionally believed to increase the synaptic concentration of norepinephrine in the central nervous system by inhibition of reuptake by the presynaptic neuronal membrane. However, additional receptor effects have been found including desensitization of adenyl cyclase, down regulation of beta-adrenergic receptors, and down regulation of serotonin receptors.

Local Anesthetic/Vasoconstrictor Precautions Use with caution; epinephrine, norepinephrine and levonordefrin have been shown to have an increased pressor response in combination TCAs

Effects on Dental Treatment >10% of patients experience dry mouth; long-term treatment with TCAs increases the risk of caries by reducing salivation and salivary buffer capacity

Other Adverse Effects

>10%:

Central nervous system: Dizziness, drowsiness, headache

Gastrointestinal: Constipation, increased appetite, nausea, unpleasant taste, weight gain

1% to 10%:

Cardiovascular: Arrhythmias, hypotension,

Central nervous system: Confusion, delirium, hallucinations, nervousness, restlessness, parkinsonian syndrome, insomnia

Endocrine & metabolic: Sexual dysfunction

Gastrointestinal: Diarrhea, heartburn

Genitourinary: Dysuria

Neuromuscular & skeletal: Fine muscle tremors, weakness

Ocular: Blurred vision, eye pain

Miscellaneous: Excessive sweating

<1%:

Central nervous system: Anxiety, seizures

Dermatologic: Alopecia, photosensitivity

Endocrine & metabolic: Breast enlargement, galactorrhea, SIADH

Gastrointestinal: Trouble with gums, decreased lower esophageal sphincter tone may cause GE reflux

Genitourinary: Testicular swelling

Hematologic: Agranulocytosis, leukopenia, eosinophilia

Hepatic: Cholestatic jaundice, elevated liver enzymes
Ocular: Increased intraocular pressure
Otic: Tinnitus
Miscellaneous: Allergic reactions

Drug Interactions

Decreased effect: Phenobarbital may increase the metabolism, of desipramine; desipramine blocks the uptake of guanethidine and thus prevents the hypotensive effect of guanethidine

Increased toxicity: Clonidine causes hypertensive crisis; desipramine may be additive with or may potentiate the action of other CNS depressants such as sedatives or hypnotics; with MAO inhibitors, hyperpyrexia, hypertension, tachycardia, confusion, and seizures. Desipramine may increase the prothrombin time in patients stabilized on warfarin; desipramine may potentiate the pressor and cardiac effects of sympathomimetic agents such as isoproterenol, epinephrine, etc; cimetidine and methylphenidate may decrease the metabolism of desipramine

Additive anticholinergic effects seen with other anticholinergic agents

Drug Uptake

Onset of action: 1-3 weeks (maximum antidepressant effects: after >2 weeks)
Absorption: Well absorbed (90%) from GI tract
Serum half-life: Adults: 12-57 hours

Pregnancy Risk Factor C

Generic Available Yes: Tablet

Selected Readings

Boakes AJ, Laurence DR, Teoh PC, et al, "Interactions Between Sympathomimetic Amines and Antidepressant Agents in Man," *Br Med J*, 1973, 1(849):311-5.

Jastak JT and Yagiela JA, "Vasoconstrictors and Local Anesthesia: A Review and Rationale for Use," *J Am Dent Assoc*, 1983, 107(4):623-30.

Larochelle P, Hamet P, and Enjalbert M, "Responses to Tyramine and Norepinephrine After Imipramine and Trazodone," *Clin Pharmacol Ther*, 1979, 26(1):24-30.

Mitchell JR, "Guanethidine and Related Agents. III Antagonism by Drugs Which Inhibit the Norepinephrine Pump in Man," *J Clin Invest*, 1970, 49(8):1596-604.

Rundegren J, van Dijken J, Mörnstad H, et al, "Oral Conditions in Patients Receiving Long-Term Treatment With Cyclic Antidepressant Drugs," *Swed Dent J*, 1985, 9(2):55-64.

Svedmyr N, "The Influence of a Tricyclic Antidepressive Agent (Protriptyline) on Some of the Circulatory Effects of Noradrenaline and Adrenalin® in Man," *Life Sci*, 1968, 7(1):77-84.

Desitin® Topical [OTC] see Zinc Oxide, Cod Liver Oil, and Talc on page 1005

Desmopressin Acetate (des moe PRES in AS e tate)

Brand Names DDAVP®; Stimate™

Canadian/Mexican Brand Names Octostim® (Canada)

Therapeutic Category Antihemophilic Agent; Hemostatic Agent; Vasopressin Analog, Synthetic

Use Treatment of diabetes insipidus and controlling bleeding in mild hemophilia, von Willebrand's disease, and thrombocytopenia (eg, uremia)

Usual Dosage Dilute I.V. dose in 50 mL 0.9% sodium chloride and infuse over 15-30 minutes

Children:
Diabetes insipidus: 3 months to 12 years: Intranasal: Initial: 5 mcg/day divided 1-2 times/day; range: 5-30 mcg/day divided 1-2 times/day
Von Willebrand disease, thrombocytopathies, hemophilia: >3 months:
Intranasal: 2-4 mcg/kg/dose
I.V.: 0.3 mcg/kg by slow infusion over 15-30 minutes; usually tachyphylaxis occurs after 2-3 doses in 24 hours, recovery of response may take 48-72 hours
Nocturnal enuresis: ≥6 years: Intranasal: Initial: 20 mcg at bedtime; range: 10-40 mcg

Adults:
Diabetes insipidus: I.V., S.C.: 2-4 mcg/day in 2 divided doses or $^1/_{10}$ of the maintenance intranasal dose; intranasal: 5-40 mcg/day 1-3 times/day
Von Willebrand disease, thrombocytopathies, hemophilia:
Intranasal: 2-4 mcg/kg/dose
I.V.: 0.3 mcg/kg by slow infusion over 15-30 minutes; usually tachyphylaxis occurs after 2-3 doses in 24 hours; recovery of responsiveness may take 48-72 hours

Oral: Begin therapy 12 hours after the last intranasal dose for patients previously on intranasal therapy
Children: Initial: 0.05 mg; fluid restrictions required in children to prevent hyponatremia and water intoxication
Adults: 0.05 mg twice daily; adjust individually to optimal therapeutic dose. Total daily dose should be increased or decreased (range: 0.1-1.2 mg divided 2-3 times/day) as needed to obtain adequate antidiuresis.

(Continued)

Desmopressin Acetate *(Continued)*

Mechanism of Action Enhances reabsorption of water in the kidneys by increasing cellular permeability of the collecting ducts; possibly causes smooth muscle constriction with resultant vasoconstriction; raises plasma levels of von Willebrand's factor and factor VIII

Local Anesthetic/Vasoconstrictor Precautions No information available to require special precautions

Effects on Dental Treatment No effects or complications reported

Other Adverse Effects

1% to 10%:
Cardiovascular: Facial flushing
Central nervous system: Headache, dizziness
Gastrointestinal: Nausea, abdominal cramps
Genitourinary: Vulval pain
Local: Pain at the injection site
Respiratory: Nasal congestion

<1%:
Cardiovascular: Hypertension
Endocrine & metabolic: Hyponatremia, water intoxication

Drug Interactions No data reported

Drug Uptake

Intranasal administration:
Onset of ADH effects: Within 1 hour
Peak effect: Within 1-5 hours
Duration: 5-21 hours

I.V. infusion:
Onset of increased factor VIII activity: Within 15-30 minutes
Peak effect: 90 minutes to 3 hours

Absorption: Nasal: Slow; 10% to 20%
Serum half-life: Elimination (terminal): 75 minutes

Pregnancy Risk Factor B

Generic Available No

Desogen® *see* Ethinyl Estradiol and Desogestrel *on page 375*

Desogestrel and Ethinyl Estradiol *see* Ethinyl Estradiol and Desogestrel *on page 375*

Desonide *(DES oh nide)*

Brand Names DesOwen®; Tridesilon®

Canadian/Mexican Brand Names Desocort® (Canada)

Therapeutic Category Corticosteroid, Topical (Low Potency)

Use Adjunctive therapy for inflammation in acute and chronic corticosteroid responsive dermatosis (low potency corticosteroid)

Usual Dosage Children and Adults: Topical: Apply 2-4 times/day sparingly

Mechanism of Action Stimulates the synthesis of enzymes needed to decrease inflammation, suppress mitotic activity, and cause vasoconstriction

Local Anesthetic/Vasoconstrictor Precautions No information available to require special precautions

Effects on Dental Treatment No effects or complications reported

Other Adverse Effects

<1%:
Dermatologic: Itching, dry skin, folliculitis, hypertrichosis, acneiform eruptions, hypopigmentation, perioral dermatitis, allergic contact dermatitis, skin maceration, skin atrophy, striae
Local: Burning, irritation, miliaria
Miscellaneous: Secondary infection

Drug Interactions No data reported

Drug Uptake

Onset of effect: Commonly noted within 7 days of continued therapy
Absorption: Topical absorption extensive from the scalp, face, axilla and scrotum; adequate through epidermis on appendages; absorption can be increased with occlusion or the addition of penetrants (eg, urea, DMSO)

Pregnancy Risk Factor C

Dosage Forms

Cream, topical: 0.05% (15 g, 60 g)
Lotion: 0.05% (60 mL, 120 mL)
Ointment, topical: 0.05% (15 g, 60 g)

Generic Available Yes

DesOwen® *see* Desonide *on this page*

Desoximetasone (des oks i MET a sone)
Related Information
Corticosteroids, Topical Comparison *on page 1140*
Brand Names Topicort®; Topicort®-LP
Therapeutic Category Corticosteroid, Topical (High Potency)
Use Relieves inflammation and pruritic symptoms of corticosteroid-responsive dermatosis [medium to high potency topical corticosteroid]
Usual Dosage Topical:
Children: Apply sparingly in a very thin film to affected area 1-2 times/day
Adults: Apply sparingly in a thin film twice daily
Mechanism of Action Stimulates the synthesis of enzymes needed to decrease inflammation, suppress mitotic activity, and cause vasoconstriction
Local Anesthetic/Vasoconstrictor Precautions No information available to require special precautions
Effects on Dental Treatment No effects or complications reported
Other Adverse Effects <1%: Topical: Burning, itching, irritation, dryness, folliculitis, hypertrichosis, acneiform eruptions, hypopigmentation, perioral dermatitis, allergic contact dermatitis, skin maceration, secondary infection, skin atrophy, striae, miliaria
Drug Interactions No data reported
Drug Uptake
Absorption: Topical: Extensive from the scalp, face, axilla, and scrotum and adequate through epidermis on appendages; absorption can be increased with occlusion or the addition of penetrants
Pregnancy Risk Factor C
Generic Available Yes

Desoxyn® *see* Methamphetamine *on page 609*

Desoxyribonuclease and Fibrinolysin *see* Fibrinolysin and Desoxyribonuclease *on page 404*

Desquam-E® Gel *see* Benzoyl Peroxide *on page 120*

Desquam-X® Gel *see* Benzoyl Peroxide *on page 120*

Desquam-X® Wash *see* Benzoyl Peroxide *on page 120*

Desyrel® *see* Trazodone *on page 951*

Detussin® Expectorant *see* Hydrocodone, Pseudoephedrine, and Guaifenesin *on page 484*

Devrom® (subgallate) [OTC] *see* Bismuth *on page 131*

Dexacidin® *see* Neomycin, Polymyxin B, and Dexamethasone *on page 672*

Dexamethasone (deks a METH a sone)
Related Information
Corticosteroid Equivalencies Comparison *on page 1139*
Corticosteroids, Topical Comparison *on page 1140*
Neomycin, Polymyxin B, and Dexamethasone *on page 672*
Oral Nonviral Soft Tissue Ulcerations or Erosions *on page 1070*
Respiratory Diseases *on page 1018*
Brand Names Dalalone L.A.®; Decadron®; Decadron®-LA; Decaject-L.A.®; Dekasol-L.A.®; Dexasone L.A.®; Dexone®; Dexone L.A.®; Hexadrol®; I-Methasone®; Solurex L.A.®
Canadian/Mexican Brand Names Alin® Depot (Mexico); Alin® (Mexico); Decadronal® (Mexico); Decorex® (Mexico); Dibasona® (Mexico)
Therapeutic Category Antiemetic; Anti-inflammatory Agent; Corticosteroid, Inhalant; Corticosteroid, Ophthalmic; Corticosteroid, Systemic; Corticosteroid, Topical (Low Potency)
Use
Dental: Treatment of a variety of oral diseases of allergic, inflammatory or autoimmune origin
Medical: Systemically and locally for chronic swelling, allergic, hematologic, neoplastic, and autoimmune diseases; may be used in management of cerebral edema, septic shock, as a diagnostic agent, antiemetic
Usual Dosage
Children: Anti-inflammatory immunosuppressant: Oral, I.M., I.V. (injections should be given as sodium phosphate): 0.08-0.3 mg/kg/day or 2.5-10 mg/m²/day in divided doses every 6-12 hours
Adults: Anti-inflammatory:
Oral, I.M., I.V. (injections should be given as sodium phosphate): 0.5-9 mg/day in divided doses every 6-12 hours
I.M. (as acetate): 8-16 mg; may repeat in 1-3 weeks
Intralesional (as acetate): 0.8-1.6 mg
(Continued)

Dexamethasone *(Continued)*

Mechanism of Action Decreases inflammation by suppression of migration of polymorphonuclear leukocytes and reversal of increased capillary permeability; suppresses normal immune response

Local Anesthetic/Vasoconstrictor Precautions No information available to require special precautions

Effects on Dental Treatment No effects or complications reported

Other Adverse Effects >10%:
Central nervous system: Insomnia, nervousness
Gastrointestinal: Increased appetite, indigestion

Contraindications Active untreated infections; viral, fungal, or tuberculosis; diseases of the eye

Warnings/Precautions Fatalities have occurred due to adrenal insufficiency in asthmatic patients during and after transfer from systemic corticosteroids to aerosol steroids; aerosol steroids do **not** provide the systemic steroid needed to treat patients having trauma, surgery, or infections; use with caution in patients with hypothyroidism, cirrhosis, hypertension, congestive heart failure, ulcerative colitis, thromboembolic disorders. Because of the risk of adverse effects, systemic corticosteroids should be used cautiously in the elderly in the smallest possible dose and for the shortest possible time.

Drug Interactions Barbiturates, phenytoin, rifampin cause decrease in dexamethasone effects; dexamethasone decreases effect of salicylates, vaccines, toxoids

Drug Uptake
Absorption: Rapid and complete
Duration of metabolic effect: Can last for 72 hours; acetate is a long-acting repository preparation with a prompt onset of action
Serum half-life:
Normal renal function: 1.8-3.5 hours
Biological half-life: 36-54 hours
Time to peak serum concentration:
Oral: Within 1-2 hours
I.M.: Within 8 hours

Pregnancy Risk Factor C

Breast-feeding Considerations No data reported

Dosage Forms
Elixir: 0.5 mg/5 mL (5 mL, 20 mL, 100 mL, 120 mL, 237 mL, 240 mL, 500 mL)
Injection, as acetate suspension: 8 mg/mL (1 mL, 5 mL); 16 mg/mL (1 mL, 5 mL)
Injection, as sodium phosphate: 4 mg/mL (1 mL, 5 mL, 10 mL, 25 mL, 30 mL); 10 mg/mL (1 mL, 10 mL); 20 mg/mL (5 mL); 24 mg/mL (5 mL, 10 mL)
Solution, oral:
Concentrate: 0.5 mg/0.5 mL (30 mL) (30% alcohol)
Oral: 0.5 mg/5 mL (5 mL, 20 mL, 500 mL)
Tablet: 0.25 mg, 0.5 mg, 0.75 mg, 1 mg, 1.5 mg, 2 mg, 4 mg, 6 mg
Tablet, therapeutic pack: 6 x 1.5 mg; 8 x 0.75 mg

Dietary Considerations May be taken with meals to decrease GI upset; limit caffeine; may need diet with increased potassium, pyridoxine, vitamin C, vitamin D, folate, calcium, and phosphorus

Generic Available Yes

Dexamethasone and Neomycin *see* Neomycin and Dexamethasone *on page 671*

Dexasone L.A.® *see* Dexamethasone *on previous page*

Dexasporin® *see* Neomycin, Polymyxin B, and Dexamethasone *on page 672*

Dexatrim® Pre-Meal [OTC] *see* Phenylpropanolamine *on page 754*

Dexbrompheniramine and Pseudoephedrine
(deks brom fen EER a meen & soo doe e FED rin)

Brand Names Disobrom® [OTC]; Disophrol® Chronotabs® [OTC]; Disophrol® Tablet [OTC]; Drixomed®; Drixoral® [OTC]

Therapeutic Category Antihistamine/Decongestant Combination

Synonyms Pseudoephedrine and Dexbrompheniramine

Use Relief of symptoms of upper respiratory mucosal congestion in seasonal and perennial nasal allergies, acute rhinitis, rhinosinusitis and eustachian tube blockage

Local Anesthetic/Vasoconstrictor Precautions Use with caution since pseudoephedrine is a sympathomimetic amine which could interact with epinephrine to cause a pressor response

Effects on Dental Treatment Up to 10% of patients could experience tachycardia, palpitations, and dry mouth; use vasoconstrictor with caution

Pregnancy Risk Factor B

Generic Available Yes

Dexchlor® see Dexchlorpheniramine *on this page*

Dexchlorpheniramine (deks klor fen EER a meen)
Brand Names Dexchlor®; Poladex®; Polaramine®
Therapeutic Category Antihistamine
Synonyms Dextroclorofeniramina (Mexico)
Use Perennial and seasonal allergic rhinitis and other allergic symptoms including urticaria
Usual Dosage Oral:
Children:
2-5 years: 0.5 mg every 4-6 hours (do not use timed release)
6-11 years: 1 mg every 4-6 hours or 4 mg timed release at bedtime
Adults: 2 mg every 4-6 hours or 4-6 mg timed release at bedtime or every 8-10 hours
Mechanism of Action Competes with histamine for H_1-receptor sites on effector cells in the gastrointestinal tract, blood vessels, and respiratory tract
Local Anesthetic/Vasoconstrictor Precautions No information available to require special precautions
Effects on Dental Treatment Up to 10% of patients will complain of significant dry mouth and drowsiness. This will disappear with cessation of drug therapy.
Other Adverse Effects
>10%:
Central nervous system: Slight to moderate drowsiness
Respiratory: Thickening of bronchial secretions
1% to 10%:
Central nervous system: Headache, fatigue, nervousness, dizziness
Gastrointestinal: Appetite increase, weight gain, nausea, diarrhea, abdominal pain, dry mouth
Neuromuscular & skeletal: Arthralgia
Respiratory: Pharyngitis
<1%:
Cardiovascular: Edema, palpitations
Central nervous system: Depression
Dermatologic: Angioedema, photosensitivity, rash
Hepatic: Hepatitis
Neuromuscular & skeletal: Myalgia, paresthesia
Respiratory: Bronchospasm, epistaxis
Drug Interactions Alcohol and other sedative drugs will potentiate the sedative effects of dexchlorpheniramine
Drug Uptake
Duration: 3-6 hours
Absorption: Well absorbed from GI tract
Pregnancy Risk Factor B
Generic Available Yes

Dexedrine® see Dextroamphetamine *on page 296*

Dexfenfluramine Hydrochloride see Dexfenfluramine *Withdrawn from Market 1997 on this page*

Dexfenfluramine *Withdrawn from Market 1997*
(deks fen FLURE a meen)
Brand Names Redux®
Therapeutic Category Anorexiant
Synonyms Dexfenfluramine Hydrochloride; S5614
Use Management of obesity (initial body mass >30 kg/m² or >27 kg/m² with other risk factors such as hypertension, diabetes, or hyperlipidemia); given as an adjunct to dietary restriction
Usual Dosage Oral: Adults: 15 mg 2 times/day with meals
Mechanism of Action Dexfenfluramine is known as a serotonergic appetite suppressant. Increases serotonin levels in the brain are associated with decreased caloric intake. Dexfenfluramine increases serotonin levels by inhibiting the reuptake of serotonin within the nerves that secrete serotonin, and by releasing more serotonin into the synaptic spaces.
Local Anesthetic/Vasoconstrictor Precautions Dexfenfluramine increases serotonin levels and has no effect on norepinephrine and epinephrine levels; therefore, no precautions appear to be necessary to the use of vasoconstrictors in patients taking dexfenfluramine
Effects on Dental Treatment >10% of patients experience dry mouth
Other Adverse Effects
>10%:
Central nervous system: Headache, insomnia
(Continued)

Dexfenfluramine *Withdrawn from Market 1997* (Continued)

Gastrointestinal: Diarrhea, abdominal pain
Neuromuscular & skeletal: Weakness

1% to 10%:
Cardiovascular: Hypertension, angina, palpitations
Central nervous system: Chills, somnolence, dizziness, depression, vertigo, emotional lability, headache, abnormal dreams, abnormal thoughts
Dermatologic: Rash
Endocrine & metabolic: Increased libido, decreased libido
Gastrointestinal: Vomiting, constipation, nausea, dyspepsia, increased appetite, gastritis, flatulence
Neuromuscular & skeletal: Peripheral neuritis, arthralgia, myalgia
Renal: Polyuria
Respiratory: Pharyngitis, rhinitis, cough, bronchitis
Miscellaneous: Thirst

Contraindications Hypersensitivity to dexfenfluramine or fenfluramine or related compounds, glaucoma, pulmonary hypertension or use of monoamine oxidase inhibitors within 2 weeks of dexfenfluramine; children, pregnancy, or nursing women; should not be used with other serotonergic drugs

Warnings/Precautions Use with caution in patients with cardiac disease, renal or hepatic insufficiency, porphyria, drug abuse, psychiatric disorder, or organic causes for obesity

Drug Interactions Not to be used with monoamine oxidase inhibitors or other serotonergic drugs

Drug Uptake
Peak serum levels: 2-4 hours
Serum half-life:
18 hours (dexfenfluramine)
30 hours (d-norfenfluramine)

Pregnancy Risk Factor C
Dosage Forms Capsule, as hydrochloride: 15 mg
Generic Available No

Dexferrum® Injection *see* Iron Dextran Complex *on page 519*
Dexone® *see* Dexamethasone *on page 291*
Dexone L.A.® *see* Dexamethasone *on page 291*

Dexpanthenol (deks PAN the nole)

Brand Names Ilopan®; Ilopan-Choline®; Panthoderm® [OTC]
Therapeutic Category Gastrointestinal Agent, Stimulant
Use Prophylactic use to minimize paralytic ileus, treatment of postoperative distention
Usual Dosage
Children and Adults: Relief of itching and aid in skin healing: Topical: Apply to affected area 1-2 times/day
Adults:
Relief of gas retention: Oral: 2-3 tablets 3 times/day
Prevention of postoperative ileus: I.M.: 250-500 mg stat, repeat in 2 hours, followed by doses every 6 hours until danger passes
Paralyzed ileus: I.M.: 500 mg stat, repeat in 2 hours, followed by doses every 6 hours, if needed
Mechanism of Action A pantothenic acid B vitamin analog that is converted to coenzyme A internally; coenzyme A is essential to normal fatty acid synthesis, amino acid synthesis and acetylation of choline in the production of the neurotransmitter, acetylcholine
Local Anesthetic/Vasoconstrictor Precautions No information available to require special precautions
Effects on Dental Treatment No effects or complications reported
Other Adverse Effects <1%:
Cardiovascular: Slight drop in blood pressure
Dermatologic: Dermatitis, urticaria
Gastrointestinal: Vomiting, diarrhea, hyperperistalsis
Hematologic: Prolonged bleeding time
Local: Irritation
Neuromuscular & skeletal: Paresthesia
Respiratory: Dyspnea
Drug Interactions Increased/prolonged effect of succinylcholine (do not administer within 1 hour)
Drug Uptake
Absorption: Well absorbed

Pregnancy Risk Factor C
Generic Available Yes

Dexrazoxane (deks ray ZOKS ane)

Brand Names Zinecard®

Therapeutic Category Cardioprotectant

Use Reduction of the incidence and severity of cardiomyopathy associated with doxorubicin administration in women with metastatic breast cancer who have received a cumulative doxorubicin dose of 300 mg/m² and who would benefit from continuing therapy with doxorubicin. It is not recommended for use with the initiation of doxorubicin therapy.

Mechanism of Action Derivative of EDTA and potent intracellular chelating agent. The mechanism of cardioprotectant activity is not fully understood. Appears to be converted intracellularly to a ring-opened chelating agent that interferes with iron-mediated free radical generation thought to be responsible, in part, for anthracycline-induced cardiomyopathy.

Local Anesthetic/Vasoconstrictor Precautions No information available to require special precautions

Effects on Dental Treatment No effects or complications reported

Other Adverse Effects The adverse experiences are likely attributable to the FAC regimen, with the exception of pain on injection that was observed mainly with dexrazoxane. Patients receiving FAC with dexrazoxane experienced more severe leukopenia, granulocytopenia, and thrombocytopenia at nadir than patients receiving FAC without dexrazoxane; but recovery counts were similar for the two groups.

1% to 2%: Dermatologic: Urticaria, recall skin reaction, extravasation

Drug Interactions Decreased effect: There is some evidence that the use of dexrazoxane concurrently with the initiation of FAC therapy interferes with the antitumor efficacy of the regimen, and this use is not recommended

Drug Uptake Serum half-life: 2.1-2.5 hours

Pregnancy Risk Factor C

Dosage Forms Powder for injection, lyophilized: 250 mg, 500 mg (10 mg/mL when reconstituted)

Generic Available No

Dextran (DEKS tran)

Brand Names Gentran®; LMD®; Macrodex®; Rheomacrodex®

Canadian/Mexican Brand Names Alpha-Dextrano"40" (Mexico)

Therapeutic Category Plasma Volume Expander

Synonyms Dextran 40; Dextran 70; Dextran, High Molecular Weight; Dextran, Low Molecular Weight

Use Fluid replacement and blood volume expander used in the treatment of hypovolemia, shock, or near shock states

Usual Dosage I.V.: (requires an infusion pump):
Children: Total dose should not be >20 mL/kg during first 24 hours
Adults: 500-1000 mL at rate of 20-40 mL/minute; if therapy continues beyond 24 hours, total daily dosage should not exceed 10 mL/kg and therapy should not continue beyond 5 days

Mechanism of Action Produces plasma volume expansion by virtue of its highly colloidal starch structure, similar to albumin

Local Anesthetic/Vasoconstrictor Precautions No information available to require special precautions

Effects on Dental Treatment No effects or complications reported

Other Adverse Effects <1%:
Cardiovascular: Mild hypotension, tightness of chest
Central nervous system: Fever
Dermatologic: Urticaria
Gastrointestinal: Nausea, vomiting
Neuromuscular & skeletal: Arthralgia
Respiratory: Nasal congestion, wheezing
Miscellaneous: Anaphylaxis

Drug Uptake
Onset of action: I.V.: Within minutes to 1 hour (depending upon the molecular weight polysaccharide administered), infusion volume expansion occurs

Pregnancy Risk Factor C

Generic Available Yes

Comments Dextran 40 is known as low molecular weight dextran (LMD) and has an average molecular weight of 40,000; dextran 75 has an average molecular weight of 75,000

Dextran 1 (DEKS tran won)
Brand Names Promit®
Therapeutic Category Plasma Volume Expander
Use Prophylaxis of serious anaphylactic reactions to I.V. infusion of dextran
Mechanism of Action Binds to dextran-reactive immunoglobulin without bridge formation and no formation of large immune complexes
Local Anesthetic/Vasoconstrictor Precautions No information available to require special precautions
Effects on Dental Treatment No effects or complications reported
Other Adverse Effects <1%:
Cardiovascular: Mild hypotension, tightness of chest
Central nervous system: Fever
Dermatologic: Urticaria
Gastrointestinal: Nausea, vomiting
Local: Cutaneous reactions
Neuromuscular & skeletal: Arthralgia
Respiratory: Nasal congestion, wheezing
Pregnancy Risk Factor C
Dosage Forms Injection: 150 mg/mL (20 mL)
Generic Available No

Dextran 40 see Dextran on previous page
Dextran 70 see Dextran on previous page
Dextran, High Molecular Weight see Dextran on previous page
Dextran, Low Molecular Weight see Dextran on previous page

Dextranomer (deks TRAN oh mer)
Brand Names Debrisan® [OTC]
Therapeutic Category Topical Skin Product
Use Clean exudative ulcers and wounds such as venous stasis ulcers, decubitus ulcers, and infected traumatic and surgical wounds; no controlled studies have found dextranomer to be more effective than conventional therapy
Usual Dosage Debride and clean wound prior to application; apply to affected area once or twice daily in a ¼" layer; apply a dressing and seal on all four sides; removal should be done by irrigation
Mechanism of Action Dextranomer is a network of dextran-sucrose beads possessing a great many exposed hydroxy groups; when this network is applied to an exudative wound surface, the exudate is drawn by capillary forces generated by the swelling of the beads, with vacuum forces producing an upward flow of exudate into the network
Local Anesthetic/Vasoconstrictor Precautions No information available to require special precautions
Effects on Dental Treatment No effects or complications reported
Other Adverse Effects 1% to 10%:
Local: Transitory pain, blistering
Dermatologic: Maceration may occur, erythema
Hematologic: Bleeding
Drug Interactions No data reported
Pregnancy Risk Factor C
Generic Available No

Dextroamphetamine (deks troe am FET a meen)
Related Information
Dextroamphetamine and Amphetamine on next page
Brand Names Dexedrine®
Therapeutic Category Amphetamine; Anorexiant; Central Nervous System Stimulant, Amphetamine
Use Narcolepsy, exogenous obesity, abnormal behavioral syndrome in children (minimal brain dysfunction), attention deficit hyperactive disorder (ADHD)
Usual Dosage Oral:
Children:
Narcolepsy: 6-12 years: Initial: 5 mg/day, may increase at 5 mg increments in weekly intervals until side effects appear; maximum dose: 60 mg/day
Attention deficit disorder:
3-5 years: Initial: 2.5 mg/day given every morning; increase by 2.5 mg/day in weekly intervals until optimal response is obtained, usual range: 0.1-0.5 mg/kg/dose every morning with maximum of 40 mg/day
≥6 years: 5 mg once or twice daily; increase in increments of 5 mg/day at weekly intervals until optimal response is reached, usual range: 0.1-0.5 mg/kg/dose every morning (5-20 mg/day) with maximum of 40 mg/day

Children >12 years and Adults:
  Narcolepsy: Initial: 10 mg/day, may increase at 10 mg increments in weekly
    intervals until side effects appear; maximum: 60 mg/day
  Exogenous obesity: 5-30 mg/day in divided doses of 5-10 mg 30-60 minutes
    before meals
Mechanism of Action Blocks reuptake of dopamine and norepinephrine from
  the synapse, thus increases the amount of circulating dopamine and norepinephrine in cerebral cortex to reticular activating system; inhibits the action of monoamine oxidase and causes catecholamines to be released
Local Anesthetic/Vasoconstrictor Precautions Use vasoconstriction with
  caution in patients taking dextroamphetamine. Amphetamines enhance the
  sympathomimetic response of epinephrine and norepinephrine leading to potential hypertension and cardiotoxicity.
Effects on Dental Treatment Up to 10% of patients taking
  dextroamphetamines may present with hypertension. The use of local anesthetic
  without vasoconstrictor is recommended in these patients.
Other Adverse Effects
  >10%:
    Cardiovascular: Arrhythmia
    Central nervous system: False feeling of well being, nervousness, restless-
      ness, insomnia
  1% to 10%:
    Cardiovascular: Hypertension
    Central nervous system: Mood or mental changes, dizziness, lightheadedness,
      headache
    Endocrine & metabolic: Changes in libido
    Gastrointestinal: Diarrhea, nausea, vomiting, stomach cramps, constipation,
      anorexia, weight loss, dry mouth
    Ocular: Blurred vision
    Miscellaneous: Increased sweating
  <1%:
    Cardiovascular: Chest pain
    Central nervous system: CNS stimulation (severe), Tourette's syndrome,
      hyperthermia, seizures, paranoia
    Dermatologic: Skin rash, urticaria
    Miscellaneous: Tolerance and withdrawal with prolonged use
Drug Interactions
  Adrenergic blockers are inhibited by amphetamines
  Amphetamines enhance the activity of tricyclic or sympathomimetic agents
  MAO Inhibitors slow the metabolism of amphetamines
  Amphetamines will counteract the sedative effects of antihistamines
  Amphetamines potentiate the analgesic effects of meperidine
Drug Uptake
  Onset of action: 1-1.5 hours
  Serum half-life: Adults: 34 hours (pH dependent)
  Time to peak serum concentration: Oral: Within 3 hours
Pregnancy Risk Factor C
Generic Available Yes

Dextroamphetamine and Amphetamine
(deks troe am FET a meen & am FET a meen)
Brand Names Adderall®
Therapeutic Category Amphetamine
Use Treatment of narcolepsy; exogenous obesity; abnormal behavioral syndrome
  in children (minimal brain dysfunction); attention deficit hyperactive disorder
  (ADHD)
Usual Dosage Oral:
  Narcolepsy:
    Children:
      6-12 years: 5 mg/day, increase by 5 mg at weekly intervals
      >12 years: 10 mg/day, increase by 10 mg at weekly intervals
    Adults: 5-60 mg/day in 2-3 divided doses

  Attention deficit disorder: Children:
    3-5 years: 2.5 mg/day, increase by 2.5 mg at weekly intervals
    >6 years: 5 mg/day, increase by 5 mg at weekly intervals not to exceed 40 mg/
      day

  Short-term adjunct to exogenous obesity: Children >12 years and Adults: 5-30
    mg/day in divided doses
Local Anesthetic/Vasoconstrictor Precautions Use vasoconstriction with
  caution in patients taking dextroamphetamine. Amphetamines enhance the
  (Continued)

Dextroamphetamine and Amphetamine *(Continued)*

sympathomimetic response of epinephrine and norepinephrine leading to potential hypertension and cardiotoxicity.

Effects on Dental Treatment Up to 10% of patients taking dextroamphetamines may present with hypertension. The use of local anesthetic without vasoconstrictor is recommended in these patients.

Other Adverse Effects See individual agents

Drug Interactions See individual agents

Dosage Forms Tablet:

10 mg [dextroamphetamine sulfate 2.5 mg, dextroamphetamine saccharate 2.5 mg and amphetamine aspartate 2.5 mg, amphetamine sulfate 2.5 mg]

20 mg [dextroamphetamine sulfate 5 mg, dextroamphetamine saccharate 5 mg and amphetamine aspartate 5 mg, amphetamine sulfate 5 mg]

Generic Available No

Dextroclorofeniramina (Mexico) *see* Dexchlorpheniramine *on page 293*

Dextromethorphan *(deks troe meth OR fan)*

Related Information

Acetaminophen, Dextromethorphan, and Pseudoephedrine *on page 25*
Guaifenesin, Pseudoephedrine, and Dextromethorphan *on page 456*

Brand Names Benylin DM® [OTC]; Benylin® Pediatric [OTC]; Children's Hold® [OTC]; Creo-Terpin® [OTC]; Delsym® [OTC]; Drixoral® Cough Liquid Caps [OTC]; Hold® DM [OTC]; Pertussin® CS [OTC]; Pertussin® ES [OTC]; Robitussin® Cough Calmers [OTC]; Robitussin® Pediatric [OTC]; Scot-Tussin DM® Cough Chasers [OTC]; Silphen DM® [OTC]; St. Joseph® Cough Suppressant [OTC]; Sucrets® Cough Calmers [OTC]; Suppress® [OTC]; Trocal® [OTC]; Vicks Formula 44® [OTC]; Vicks Formula 44® Pediatric Formula [OTC]

Canadian/Mexican Brand Names Balminil-DM® (Canada)

Therapeutic Category Antitussive

Synonyms Dextrometorfano (Mexico)

Use Symptomatic relief of coughs caused by minor viral upper respiratory tract infections or inhaled irritants; most effective for a chronic nonproductive cough

Usual Dosage Oral:

Children:

<2 years: Use only as directed by a physician

2-6 years (syrup): 2.5-7.5 mg every 4-8 hours; extended release is 15 mg twice daily (maximum: 30 mg/24 hours)

6-12 years: 5-10 mg every 4 hours or 15 mg every 6-8 hours; extended release is 30 mg twice daily (maximum: 60 mg/24 hours)

Children >12 years and Adults: 10-30 mg every 4-8 hours or 30 mg every 6-8 hours; extended release is 60 mg twice daily (maximum: 120 mg/24 hours)

Mechanism of Action Chemical relative of morphine lacking narcotic properties except in overdose; controls cough by depressing the medullary cough center

Local Anesthetic/Vasoconstrictor Precautions No information available to require special precautions

Effects on Dental Treatment No effects or complications reported

Other Adverse Effects <1%:

Central nervous system: Drowsiness, dizziness, coma

Gastrointestinal: Nausea, GI upset, constipation

Respiratory: Respiratory depression

Warnings/Precautions Research on chicken embryos exposed to concentrations of dextromethorphan relative to those typically taken by humans has shown to cause birth defects and fetal death; more study is needed, but it is suggested that pregnant women should be advised not to use dextromethorphan-containing medications

Drug Interactions No data reported

Drug Uptake

Onset of antitussive action: Within 15-30 minutes

Duration: Up to 6 hours

Pregnancy Risk Factor C (see Warnings)

Generic Available Yes

Dextromethorphan, Acetaminophen, and Pseudoephedrine *see* Acetaminophen, Dextromethorphan, and Pseudoephedrine *on page 25*

Dextromethorphan, Guaifenesin, and Pseudoephedrine *see* Guaifenesin, Pseudoephedrine, and Dextromethorphan *on page 456*

Dextrometorfano (Mexico) *see* Dextromethorphan *on this page*

Dextrose, Levulose and Phosphoric Acid *see* Phosphorated Carbohydrate Solution *on page 757*

Dextrothyroxine (deks troe thye ROKS een)
Brand Names Choloxin®
Therapeutic Category Lipid Lowering Drugs
Use Reduction of elevated serum cholesterol
Usual Dosage Oral:
Children: 0.05 mg/kg/day, increase at 1-month intervals by 0.05 mg/kg/day to a maximum of 0.4 mg/kg/day or 4 mg/day
Adults: 1-2 mg/day, increase at 1-2 mg at intervals of 4 weeks, up to a maximum of 8 mg/day
Mechanism of Action Unclear mechanism, thought to increase the liver breakdown of cholesterol
Local Anesthetic/Vasoconstrictor Precautions No information available to require special precautions
Effects on Dental Treatment No effects or complications reported
Other Adverse Effects <1%:
Cardiovascular: Myocardial infarction, angina, arrhythmias
Central nervous system: Insomnia, headache
Dermatologic: Alopecia, skin rash
Gastrointestinal: Weight loss
Neuromuscular & skeletal: Tremor, paresthesia
Ocular: Visual disturbances
Otic: Tinnitus
Miscellaneous: Sweating
Drug Interactions
Decreased effect of beta-blockers, digitalis, hypoglycemics; decreased effect with cholestyramine
Increased effect of anticoagulants
Drug Uptake
Absorption: Poorly absorbed from GI tract (25%)
Serum half-life: 18 hours
Pregnancy Risk Factor C
Generic Available No

Dey-Dose® Isoproterenol *see* Isoproterenol *on page 523*

Dey-Dose® Metaproterenol *see* Metaproterenol *on page 605*

Dey-Lute® Isoetharine *see* Isoetharine *on page 521*

Dezocine (DEZ oh seen)
Related Information
Narcotic Agonists *on page 1141*
Brand Names Dalgan®
Therapeutic Category Analgesic, Narcotic
Use Relief of moderate to severe postoperative, acute renal and ureteral colic, and cancer pain
Usual Dosage Adults (not recommended for patients <18 years):
I.M.: Initial: 5-20 mg; may be repeated every 3-6 hours as needed; maximum: 120 mg/day and 20 mg/dose
I.V.: Initial: 2.5-10 mg; may be repeated every 2-4 hours as needed
Mechanism of Action Binds to opiate receptors in the CNS, causing inhibition of ascending pain pathways, altering the perception of and response to pain; produces generalized CNS depression; it is a mixed agonist-antagonist that appears to bind selectively to CNS μ and Δ opiate receptors
Local Anesthetic/Vasoconstrictor Precautions No information available to require special precautions
Effects on Dental Treatment No effects or complications reported
Other Adverse Effects
1% to 10%:
Central nervous system: Sedation, dizziness, vertigo
Gastrointestinal: Nausea, vomiting
Local: Injection site reactions
<1%:
Cardiovascular: Hypotension, palpitations, bradycardia, peripheral vasodilation
Central nervous system: Increased intracranial pressure, CNS depression, drowsiness
Endocrine & metabolic: Antidiuretic hormone release
Gastrointestinal: Constipation, biliary tract spasm
Genitourinary: Urinary tract spasm
Ocular: Miosis
Respiratory: Respiratory depression
Miscellaneous: Histamine release, physical and psychological dependence with prolonged use
(Continued)

Dezocine *(Continued)*

Drug Interactions Increased effect with CNS depressants
Drug Uptake
Onset of analgesia: Within 15-30 minutes
Duration of analgesia: 4-6 hours
Serum half-life: 2.6-2.8 hours
Pregnancy Risk Factor C
Generic Available No

DHAD *see* Mitoxantrone *on page 643*

DHC Plus® *see* Dihydrocodeine Compound *on page 315*

D.H.E. 45® Injection *see* Dihydroergotamine *on page 317*

DHS® Tar [OTC] *see* Coal Tar *on page 254*

DHS Zinc® [OTC] *see* Pyrithione Zinc *on page 826*

DHT™ *see* Dihydrotachysterol *on page 317*

Diaβeta® *see* Glyburide *on page 445*

Diabetic Tussin DM® [OTC] *see* Guaifenesin and Dextromethorphan *on page 453*

Diabetic Tussin® EX [OTC] *see* Guaifenesin *on page 452*

Diabinese® *see* Chlorpropamide *on page 225*

Dialose® [OTC] *see* Docusate *on page 331*

Dialose® Plus Capsule [OTC] *see* Docusate and Casanthranol *on page 331*

Dialume® [OTC] *see* Aluminum Hydroxide *on page 47*

Diamine T.D.® [OTC] *see* Brompheniramine *on page 142*

Diamox® *see* Acetazolamide *on page 26*

Diamox Sequels® *see* Acetazolamide *on page 26*

Diaparene® [OTC] *see* Methylbenzethonium Chloride *on page 621*

Diapid® *see* Lypressin *on page 573*

Diar-aid® [OTC] *see* Loperamide *on page 565*

Diasorb® [OTC] *see* Attapulgite *on page 99*

Diazepam *(dye AZ e pam)*

Related Information
Dental Drug Interactions: Update on Drug Combinations Requiring Special Considerations *on page 1144*
Patients Requiring Sedation *on page 1081*
Temporomandibular Dysfunction (TMD) *on page 1078*
Brand Names Dizac® Injection; Valium®
Canadian/Mexican Brand Names Apo®-Diazepam (Canada); Diazemuls® (Canada); E Pam® (Canada); Meval® (Canada); Novo-Dipam® (Canada); PMS®-Diazepam (Canada); Vivol® (Canada)
Therapeutic Category Antianxiety Agent; Anticonvulsant, Benzodiazepine; Benzodiazepine; Muscle Relaxant; Sedative; Skeletal Muscle Relaxant; Tranquilizer, Minor
Use
Dental: Oral medication for preoperative dental anxiety; sedative component in I.V. conscious sedation in oral surgery patients; skeletal muscle relaxant
Medical: In medicine, management of general anxiety disorders, panic disorders, and provide preoperative sedation, light anesthesia, and amnesia; treatment of status epilepticus, alcohol withdrawal symptoms; used as a skeletal muscle relaxant
Restrictions C-IV; Refillable up to 5 times in 6 months
Usual Dosage
Children: Oral:
Conscious sedation for procedures: 0.2-0.3 mg/kg (maximum: 10 mg) 45-60 minutes prior to procedure
Sedation or muscle relaxation or anxiety: 0.12-0.8 mg/kg/day in divided doses every 6-8 hours the day before the procedure
Adults:
Oral: Preop sedation/antianxiety: 2-10 mg 2 times/day the day before the procedure; 2-10 mg morning of procedure if needed
I.V.: Conscious sedation: 5-15 mg titrated slowly to effect
Mechanism of Action Depresses all levels of the CNS, including the limbic and reticular formation, probably through the increased action of gamma-aminobutyric acid (GABA), which is a major inhibitory neurotransmitter in the brain
Local Anesthetic/Vasoconstrictor Precautions No information available to require special precautions
Effects on Dental Treatment >10% of patients experience dry mouth or changes in salivation

Other Adverse Effects

>10%:

Central nervous system: Drowsiness, ataxia, amnesia, slurred speech, light-headedness

Local: Phlebitis, pain with injection

1% to 10%: Central nervous system: Confusion, dizziness

Contraindications Hypersensitivity to diazepam or any component; there may be a cross-sensitivity with other benzodiazepines; do not use in a comatose patient, in those with pre-existing CNS depression, respiratory depression, narrow-angle glaucoma, or severe uncontrolled pain; do not use in pregnant women

Warnings/Precautions Use with caution in patients receiving other CNS depressants, patients with low albumin, hepatic dysfunction, and in the elderly and young infants. Due to its long-acting metabolite, diazepam is not considered a drug of choice in the elderly; long-acting benzodiazepines have been associated with falls in the elderly.

Drug Interactions Enzyme inducers may increase the metabolism of diazepam; CNS depressants (alcohol, barbiturates, opioids) may enhance sedation and respiratory depression; cimetidine may decrease the metabolism of diazepam; cisapride can significantly increase diazepam levels; valproic acid may displace diazepam from binding sites which may result in an increase in sedative effects; selective serotonin reuptake inhibitors (eg, fluoxetine, sertraline, paroxetine) have greatly increased diazepam levels by altering its clearance

Drug Uptake

Absorption: Oral: 85% to 100%, more reliable than I.M.

Serum half-life:

Parent drug: Adults: 20-50 hours, increased half-life in neonates, elderly, and those with severe hepatic disorders

Active major metabolite (desmethyldiazepam): 50-100 hours, can be prolonged in neonates

Time to peak serum concentration: 0.5-2 hours

Pregnancy Risk Factor D

Breast-feeding Considerations Not compatible

Dosage Forms

Injection: 5 mg/mL (1 mL, 2 mL, 5 mL, 10 mL)

Injection, emulsified (Dizac®): 5 mg/mL (3 mL)

Solution, oral (wintergreen-spice flavor): 5 mg/5 mL (5 mL, 10 mL, 500 mL)

Solution, oral concentrate: 5 mg/mL (30 mL)

Tablet: 2 mg, 5 mg, 10 mg

Dietary Considerations May be taken with food or water

Generic Available Yes

Diazoxide (dye az OKS ide)

Brand Names Hyperstat® I.V.; Proglycem®

Canadian/Mexican Brand Names Sefulken® (Mexico)

Therapeutic Category Antihypertensive; Antihypoglycemic Agent

Synonyms Diazoxido (Mexico)

Use

Oral: Hypoglycemia related to islet cell adenoma, carcinoma, hyperplasia, or adenomatosis, nesidioblastosis, leucine sensitivity, or extrapancreatic malignancy

I.V.: Emergency lowering of blood pressure

Usual Dosage

Hypertension: Children and Adults: I.V.: 1-3 mg/kg up to a maximum of 150 mg in a single injection; repeat dose in 5-15 minutes until blood pressure adequately reduced; repeat administration at intervals of 4-24 hours; monitor the blood pressure closely; do not use longer than 10 days

Hyperinsulinemic hypoglycemia: Oral: **Note:** Use lower dose listed as initial dose

Children and Adults: 3-8 mg/kg/day in divided doses every 8-12 hours

Mechanism of Action Inhibits insulin release from the pancreas; produces direct smooth muscle relaxation of the peripheral arterioles which results in decrease in blood pressure and reflex increase in heart rate and cardiac output

Local Anesthetic/Vasoconstrictor Precautions No information available to require special precautions

Effects on Dental Treatment No effects or complications reported

Other Adverse Effects

1% to 10%:

Cardiovascular: Hypotension

Central nervous system: Dizziness

Gastrointestinal: Nausea, vomiting

Neuromuscular & skeletal: Weakness

(Continued)

Diazoxide (Continued)

<1%:
Cardiovascular: Tachycardia, flushing
Central nervous system: Seizures, headache, extrapyramidal symptoms and development of abnormal facies with chronic oral use
Dermatologic: Rash, hirsutism
Endocrine & metabolic: Hyperglycemia, ketoacidosis, sodium and water retention, hyperuricemia, inhibition of labor
Gastrointestinal: Anorexia, constipation
Hematologic: Leukopenia, thrombocytopenia
Local: Pain, burning, cellulitis/phlebitis upon extravasation

Drug Interactions
Decreased effect: Diazoxide may increase phenytoin metabolism or free fraction
Increased toxicity:
Diuretics and hypotensive agents may potentiate diazoxide adverse effects
Diazoxide may decrease warfarin protein binding

Drug Uptake
Hyperglycemic effect: Oral:
Onset of action: Within 1 hour
Duration (normal renal function): 8 hours
Hypotensive effect: I.V.:
Peak: Within 5 minutes
Duration: Usually 3-12 hours
Serum half-life:
Children: 9-24 hours
Adults: 20-36 hours
End stage renal disease: >30 hours

Pregnancy Risk Factor C
Generic Available Yes: Injection

Diazoxido (Mexico) see Diazoxide on previous page
Dibent® Injection see Dicyclomine on page 307
Dibenzyline® see Phenoxybenzamine on page 749

Dibucaine (DYE byoo kane)

Brand Names Nupercainal® [OTC]
Therapeutic Category Local Anesthetic, Topical
Use
Dental: Amide derivative local anesthetic for minor skin conditions
Medical: Fast, temporary relief of pain and itching due to hemorrhoids, minor burns
Usual Dosage Children and Adults: Topical: Apply gently to the affected areas; no more than 30 g for adults or 7.5 g for children should be used in any 24-hour period
Mechanism of Action Local anesthetics bind selectively to the intracellular surface of sodium channels to block influx of sodium into the axon. As a result, depolarization necessary for action potential propagation and subsequent nerve function is prevented. The block at the sodium channel is reversible. When drug diffuses away from the axon, sodium channel function is restored and nerve propagation returns.
Local Anesthetic/Vasoconstrictor Precautions No information available to require special precautions
Effects on Dental Treatment No effects or complications reported
Other Adverse Effects 1% to 10%:
Local: Burning
Dermatologic: Angioedema, contact dermatitis
Contraindications Known hypersensitivity to amide-type anesthetics, ophthalmic use
Warnings/Precautions Avoid use in sensitive individuals
Drug Interactions No data reported
Drug Uptake
Onset of action: Within 15 minutes
Duration: 2-4 hours
Absorption: Poor through intact skin, but well absorbed through mucous membranes and excoriated skin
Pregnancy Risk Factor C
Breast-feeding Considerations No data reported; however, topical administration is probably compatible
Dosage Forms
Cream, topical: 0.5% (45 g)
Ointment, topical: 1% (30 g, 60 g, 454 g)

Generic Available Yes

Dibucaine and Hydrocortisone
(DYE byoo kane & hye droe KOR ti sone)

Brand Names Corticaine® Topical

Therapeutic Category Corticosteroid, Topical (Low Potency); Local Anesthetic, Topical

Synonyms Hydrocortisone and Dibucaine

Use Relief of the inflammatory and pruritic manifestations of corticosteroid-responsive dermatoses and for external anal itching

Local Anesthetic/Vasoconstrictor Precautions No information available to require special precautions

Effects on Dental Treatment No effects or complications reported

Pregnancy Risk Factor C

Generic Available Yes

DIC see Dacarbazine on page 276

Dicarbosil® [OTC] see Calcium Carbonate on page 162

Dichlorodifluoromethane and Trichloromonofluoromethane
(dye klor oh dye flor oh METH ane & tri klor oh mon oh flor oh METH ane)

Related Information

Temporomandibular Dysfunction (TMD) on page 1078

Brand Names Fluori-Methane®

Therapeutic Category Local Anesthetic, Topical

Use

Dental: Topical application in the management of myofascial pain, restricted motion, and muscle spasm

Medical: For the control of pain associated with injections

Usual Dosage Invert bottle over treatment area approximately 12" away from site of application; open dispenseal spring valve completely, allowing liquid to flow in a stream from the bottle. The rate of spraying is approximately 10 cm/second and should be continued until entire muscle has been covered.

Local Anesthetic/Vasoconstrictor Precautions No information available to require special precautions

Effects on Dental Treatment No effects or complications reported

Other Adverse Effects No data reported

Contraindications In individuals with a history of hypersensitivity to dichlorofluoromethane and/or trichloromonofluoromethane; should not be used on patients having vascular impairment of the extremities

Warnings/Precautions For external use only; care should be taken to minimize inhalation of vapors, especially with application to head and neck; avoid contact with eyes; should not be applied to the point of frost formation

Drug Interactions No data reported

Drug Uptake No data reported

Breast-feeding Considerations No data reported

Dosage Forms Spray: 4 oz amber glass bottles; calibrated fine spray and calibrated medium spray

Generic Available No

Comments Dichlorodifluoromethane and trichloromonofluoromethane are not classified as carcinogens; based on animal studies and human experience, these fluorocarbons pose no hazard to man relative to systemic toxicity, carcinogenicity, mutagenicity, or teratogenicity when occupational exposures are <1000 ppm over an 8-hour time weighted average.

Dichlorotetrafluoroethane and Ethyl Chloride see Ethyl Chloride and Dichlorotetrafluoroethane on page 384

Dichlorphenamide (dye klor FEN a mide)

Brand Names Daranide®

Therapeutic Category Antiglaucoma Agent; Carbonic Anhydrase Inhibitor; Diuretic, Carbonic Anhydrase Inhibitor

Synonyms Diclofenamide

Use Adjunct in treatment of open-angle glaucoma and perioperative treatment for angle-closure glaucoma

Local Anesthetic/Vasoconstrictor Precautions No information available to require special precautions

Effects on Dental Treatment No effects or complications reported

Other Adverse Effects

>10%:

Central nervous system: Fatigue, malaise

(Continued)

Dichlorphenamide *(Continued)*

Gastrointestinal: Diarrhea, anorexia, metallic taste
Renal: Polyuria
1% to 10%:
Central nervous system: Mental depression, somnolence
Renal: Renal calculi
<1%:
Central nervous system: Fever
Dermatologic: Rash
Endocrine & metabolic: Hyperchloremic metabolic acidosis, hypokalemia, hyperglycemia
Gastrointestinal: Black stools, GI irritation, dryness of the mouth
Genitourinary: Dysuria
Hematologic: Blood dyscrasias, bone marrow suppression
Neuromuscular & skeletal: Paresthesias
Ocular: Myopia

Pregnancy Risk Factor C
Generic Available No

Diclofenac *(dye KLOE fen ak)*

Related Information
Nonsteroidal Anti-Inflammatory Agents, Comparative Dosages, and Pharmacokinetics *on page 1143*
Rheumatoid Arthritis and Osteoarthritis *on page 1030*

Brand Names Cataflam® Oral; Voltaren® Ophthalmic; Voltaren® Oral; Voltaren-XR® Oral

Canadian/Mexican Brand Names Apo®-Diclo (Canada); Artrenac® (Mexico); Clonodifen® (Mexico); Dolo Pangavit D® (Mexico); Fustaren® Retard (Mexico); Galedol® (Mexico); Liroken® (Mexico); Novo-Difenac® (Canada); Novo-Difenac-SR® (Canada); Nu-Diclo® (Canada)

Therapeutic Category Analgesic, Non-narcotic; Anti-inflammatory Agent; Nonsteroidal Anti-inflammatory Agent (NSAID), Ophthalmic; Nonsteroidal Anti-inflammatory Agent (NSAID), Oral

Synonyms Diclofenaco (Mexico)

Use Acute treatment of mild to moderate pain; acute and chronic treatment of rheumatoid arthritis, ankylosing spondylitis, and osteoarthritis; used for juvenile rheumatoid arthritis, gout, dysmenorrhea; ophthalmic solution for the treatment of postoperative swelling in patients who have undergone cataract extraction and for the treatment of photophobia in patients undergoing incisional refractive surgery

Usual Dosage Adults:
Oral:
Analgesia (Cataflam®): Starting dose: 50 mg 3 times/day
Rheumatoid arthritis: 150-200 mg/day in 2-4 divided doses (100 mg/day of sustained release product)
Osteoarthritis: 100-150 mg/day in 2-3 divided doses (100-200 mg/day of sustained release product)
Ankylosing spondylitis: 100-125 mg/day in 4-5 divided doses
Ophthalmic: Instill 1 drop into affected eye 4 times/day beginning 24 hours after cataract surgery and continuing for 2 weeks

Mechanism of Action Inhibits prostaglandin synthesis by decreasing the activity of the enzyme, cyclo-oxygenase, which results in decreased formation of prostaglandin precursors

Local Anesthetic/Vasoconstrictor Precautions No information available to require special precautions

Effects on Dental Treatment No effects or complications reported

Other Adverse Effects
>10%:
Dermatologic: Skin rash
Gastrointestinal: Abdominal cramps, heartburn, indigestion, nausea
1% to 10%:
Cardiovascular: Angina pectoris, arrhythmias
Central nervous system: Dizziness, nervousness
Dermatologic: Skin rash, itching
Gastrointestinal: GI ulceration, vomiting
Genitourinary: Vaginal bleeding
Otic: Tinnitus
<1%:
Cardiovascular: Chest pain, congestive heart failure, hypertension, tachycardia
Central nervous system: Convulsions, forgetfulness, mental depression, drowsiness, insomnia

Dermatologic: Urticaria, exfoliative dermatitis, erythema multiforme, Stevens-Johnson syndrome, angioedema
Gastrointestinal: Stomatitis
Genitourinary: Cystitis
Hematologic: Agranulocytosis, anemia, pancytopenia, leukopenia, thrombocytopenia
Hepatic: Hepatitis
Neuromuscular & skeletal: Peripheral neuropathy, trembling, weakness
Ocular: Blurred vision, change in vision
Otic: Decreased hearing
Renal: Interstitial nephritis, nephrotic syndrome, renal impairment
Respiratory: Wheezing, laryngeal edema, dyspnea, epistaxis
Miscellaneous: Anaphylaxis, increased sweating

Drug Interactions
Decreased effect with aspirin; decreased effect of thiazides, furosemide
Increased toxicity of digoxin, methotrexate, cyclosporine, lithium, insulin, sulfonylureas, potassium-sparing diuretics, aspirin

Drug Uptake
Onset of action: Cataflam® has a more rapid onset of action than does the sodium salt (Voltaren®), because it is absorbed in the stomach instead of the duodenum
Serum half-life: 2 hours
Time to peak serum concentration:
Cataflam®: Within 1 hour
Voltaren®: Within 2 hours

Pregnancy Risk Factor B

Dosage Forms
Solution, ophthalmic, as sodium (Voltaren®): 0.1% (2.5 mL, 5 mL)
Tablet, enteric coated, as sodium: 25 mg, 50 mg, 75 mg
Voltaren®: 25 mg, 50 mg, 75 mg
Tablet, extended release, as sodium (Voltaren-XR®): 100 mg
Tablet, as potassium (Cataflam®): 50 mg

Dietary Considerations May be taken with food to decrease GI distress
Generic Available Yes: Tablet

Diclofenac and Misoprostol

Brand Names Arthrotec®
Therapeutic Category Analgesic, Non-narcotic; Prostaglandin
Use The diclofenac component is indicated for the treatment of osteoarthritis and rheumatoid arthritis; the misoprostol component is indicated for the prophylaxis of NSAID-induced gastric and duodenal ulceration
Usual Dosage Adults: Oral: One tablet to be taken with food, two or three times daily; tablets should be swallowed whole, not chewed
Local Anesthetic/Vasoconstrictor Precautions No information available to require special precautions
Effects on Dental Treatment No effects or complications reported
Warnings/Precautions Use in premenopausal women; should not be used in premenopausal women unless they use effective contraception and have been advised of the risks of taking the product if pregnant
Drug Uptake The pharmacokinetic profiles of diclofenac and misoprostol administered as a combination product is similar to the profiles when the two drugs are administered as separate tablets. No pharmacokinetic interaction between the two drugs has been observed following multiple doses.
Pregnancy Risk Factor X
Dosage Forms Tablet: Diclofenac 50 mg and misoprostol 200 mcg; diclofenac 75 mg and misoprostol 200 mcg

Diclofenaco (Mexico) see Diclofenac on previous page
Diclofenamide see Dichlorphenamide on page 303

Dicloxacillin (dye kloks a SIL in)
Related Information
Oral Bacterial Infections on page 1059
Brand Names Dycill®; Dynapen®; Pathocil®
Canadian/Mexican Brand Names Brispen® (Mexico); Posipen® (Mexico)
Therapeutic Category Antibiotic, Penicillin
Use
Dental: Treatment of susceptible orofacial infections, notably penicillinase-producing staph
Medical: Treatment of systemic infections in the medical patient such as pneumonia, skin and soft tissue infections, and osteomyelitis caused by penicillinase-producing staphylococci
(Continued)

Dicloxacillin (Continued)

Usual Dosage Oral:

Children >40 kg and Adults: 250-500 mg every 6 hours for at least 7 days

Children <40 kg: 125-150 mg/kg/day divided every 6 hours

Mechanism of Action Interferes with bacterial cell wall synthesis during active multiplication, causing cell wall death and resultant bactericidal activity against susceptible bacteria

Local Anesthetic/Vasoconstrictor Precautions No information available to require special precautions

Effects on Dental Treatment Prolonged use of penicillins may lead to development of oral candidiasis

Other Adverse Effects 1% to 10%: Gastrointestinal: Diarrhea

Contraindications Known hypersensitivity to dicloxacillin, penicillin, or any components

Warnings/Precautions Monitor PT if patient concurrently on warfarin; elimination of drug is slow in neonates; use with caution in patients allergic to cephalosporins; bad taste of suspension may make compliance difficult

Drug Interactions Efficacy of oral contraceptives may be reduced; disulfiram, probenecid causes increased penicillin levels; increased effect of anticoagulants

Drug Uptake

Absorption: 35% to 76% from GI tract; food decreases rate and extent of absorption

Serum half-life: 0.6-0.8 hours

Time to peak serum concentration: Within 0.5-2 hours

Pregnancy Risk Factor B

Breast-feeding Considerations No data reported; however, other penicillins may be taken while breast-feeding

Dosage Forms

Capsule, as sodium: 125 mg, 250 mg, 500 mg

Powder for oral suspension, as sodium: 62.5 mg/5 mL (80 mL, 100 mL, 200 mL)

Dietary Considerations Should be taken with water 1 hour before or 2 hours after meals on an empty stomach

Generic Available Yes

Comments Although dicloxacillin is a penicillin antibiotic indicated for infections caused by penicillinase secreting staph, amoxicillin with clavulanic acid is considered the drug of choice for these types of orofacial infections

Dicumarol (dye KOO ma role)

Therapeutic Category Anticoagulant

Synonyms Bishydroxycoumarin

Use Prophylaxis and treatment of thromboembolic disorders

Usual Dosage Adults: Oral: 25-200 mg/day based on prothrombin time (PT) determinations

Mechanism of Action Interferes with hepatic synthesis of vitamin K-dependent coagulation factors (II, VII, IX, X)

Local Anesthetic/Vasoconstrictor Precautions No information available to require special precautions

Effects on Dental Treatment Signs of dicumarol overdose may first appear as bleeding from gingival tissue; consultation with prescribing physician is advisable prior to surgery to determine temporary dose reduction or withdrawal of medication

Other Adverse Effects

1% to 10%:

Dermatologic: Skin lesions, alopecia, skin necrosis

Gastrointestinal: Anorexia, nausea, vomiting, stomach cramps, diarrhea

Hematologic: Hemorrhage; leukopenia, unrecognized bleeding sites (eg, colon cancer) may be uncovered by anticoagulation

Respiratory: Hemoptysis

<1%:

Central nervous system: Fever

Dermatologic: Skin rash, discolored toes (blue or purple)

Gastrointestinal: Mouth ulcers

Hematologic: Agranulocytosis

Hepatic: Hepatotoxicity

Renal: Renal damage

Drug Interactions See Warfarin

Pregnancy Risk Factor D

Dosage Forms Tablet: 25 mg, 50 mg, 100 mg

Dietary Considerations Avoid proteolytic enzymes (papain), fried/boiled onions & soybean oil

Generic Available Yes

Dicyclomine (dye SYE kloe meen)
Brand Names Antispas® Injection; Bentyl® Hydrochloride Injection; Bentyl® Hydrochloride Oral; Byclomine® Injection; Dibent® Injection; Di-Spaz® Injection; Di-Spaz® Oral; Or-Tyl® Injection
Canadian/Mexican Brand Names Bentylol® (Canada)
Therapeutic Category Antispasmodic Agent, Gastrointestinal
Synonyms Dicycloverine Hydrochloride
Use Treatment of functional disturbances of GI motility such as irritable bowel syndrome

Unlabeled use: Urinary incontinence
Usual Dosage
Oral:
Children: 10 mg/dose 3-4 times/day
Adults: Begin with 80 mg/day in 4 equally divided doses, then increase up to 160 mg/day
I.M. **(should not be used I.V.):** Adults: 80 mg/day in 4 divided doses (20 mg/dose)
Mechanism of Action Blocks the action of acetylcholine at parasympathetic sites in smooth muscle, secretory glands and the CNS
Local Anesthetic/Vasoconstrictor Precautions No information available to require special precautions
Effects on Dental Treatment >10% of patients experience dry mouth
Other Adverse Effects
>10%:
Dermatologic: Dry skin
Gastrointestinal: Constipation
Local: Injection site reactions
Respiratory: Dry nose, throat
Miscellaneous: Decreased sweating
1% to 10%:
Dermatologic: Photosensitivity
Endocrine & metabolic: Decreased flow of breast milk
Gastrointestinal: Dysphagia
Ocular: Blurred vision
<1%:
Cardiovascular: Orthostatic hypotension, tachycardia, palpitations
Central nervous system: Confusion, drowsiness, headache, lightheadedness, loss of memory, fatigue, seizures, coma, nervousness, excitement, insomnia
Dermatologic: Skin rash
Gastrointestinal: Bloated feeling, nausea, vomiting
Genitourinary: Dysuria, urinary retention
Neuromuscular & skeletal: Muscular hypotonia, weakness
Ocular: Increased intraocular pain
Respiratory: Asphyxia, respiratory distress
Drug Interactions
Decreased effect: Phenothiazines, anti-Parkinson's drugs, haloperidol, sustained release dosage forms; decreased effect with antacids
Increased toxicity: Anticholinergics, amantadine, narcotic analgesics, type I antiarrhythmics, antihistamines, phenothiazines, TCAs
Drug Uptake
Onset of effect: 1-2 hours
Duration: Up to 4 hours
Absorption: Oral: Well absorbed
Serum half-life:
Initial phase: 1.8 hours
Terminal phase: 9-10 hours
Pregnancy Risk Factor B
Generic Available Yes

Dicycloverine Hydrochloride see Dicyclomine on this page
Didanosina (Mexico) see Didanosine on this page

Didanosine (dye DAN oh seen)
Related Information
HIV Infection and AIDS on page 1024
Systemic Viral Diseases on page 1047
Brand Names Videx®
Therapeutic Category Antiviral Agent, Oral
Synonyms Didanosina (Mexico)
(Continued)

Didanosine *(Continued)*

Use Treatment of advanced HIV infection in patients who are intolerant of zidovudine therapy or who have demonstrated significant clinical or immunologic deterioration during zidovudine therapy

Usual Dosage Oral (administer on an empty stomach):

Children: 180 mg/m²/day divided every 12 hours **or** dosing is based on body surface area (m²): See table.

Didanosine — Pediatric Dosing

Body Surface Area (m²)	Dosing (Tablets) (mg bid)
≤0.4	25
0.5-0.7	50
0.8-1	75
1.1-1.4	100

Adults: Dosing is based on patient weight: See table.

Didanosine — Adult Dosing

Patient Weight (kg)	Dosing (Tablets) (mg bid)
35-49	125
50-74	200
≥75	300

Note: Children >1 year and Adults should receive 2 tablets per dose and children <1 year should receive 1 tablet per dose for adequate buffering and absorption; tablets should be chewed

Mechanism of Action Didanosine, a purine nucleoside analogue and the deamination product of dideoxyadenosine (ddA), inhibits HIV replication *in vitro* in both T cells and monocytes. Didanosine is converted within the cell to the mono-, di-, and triphosphates of ddA. These ddA triphosphates act as substrate and inhibitor of HIV reverse transcriptase substrate and inhibitor of HIV reverse transcriptase thereby blocking viral DNA synthesis and suppressing HIV replication.

Local Anesthetic/Vasoconstrictor Precautions No information available to require special precautions

Effects on Dental Treatment No effects or complications reported

Other Adverse Effects

>10%:

Central nervous system: Anxiety, headache, irritability, insomnia, restlessness

Gastrointestinal: Abdominal pain, nausea, diarrhea

Neuromuscular & skeletal: Peripheral neuropathy

1% to 10%:

Central nervous system: Depression

Dermatologic: Rash, pruritus

Gastrointestinal: Pancreatitis

<1%:

Central nervous system: Seizures

Hematologic: Anemia, granulocytopenia, leukopenia, thrombocytopenia

Hepatic: Hepatitis

Ocular: Retinal depigmentation

Renal: Renal impairment

Miscellaneous: Hypersensitivity

Drug Interactions Drugs whose absorption depends on the level of acidity in the stomach such as ketoconazole, itraconazole, and dapsone should be administered at least 2 hours prior to didanosine

Decreased effect: Didanosine may decrease absorption of quinolones or tetracyclines, didanosine should be held during PCP treatment with pentamidine

Increased toxicity: Concomitant administration of other drugs which have the potential to cause peripheral neuropathy or pancreatitis may increase the risk of these toxicities

Drug Uptake

Absorption: Subject to degradation by the acidic pH of the stomach; buffered to resist the acidic pH; as much as 50% reduction in the peak plasma concentration is observed in the presence of food

Serum half-life:

Children and Adolescents: 0.8 hour

Adults:

Normal renal function: 1.5 hours; however, its active metabolite ddATP has an intracellular half-life >12 hours *in vitro*; this permits the drug to be dosed at 12-hour intervals; total body clearance averages 800 mL/minute

Impaired renal function: Half-life is increased, with values ranging from 2.5-5 hours

Pregnancy Risk Factor B

Generic Available No

Didrex® *see* Benzphetamine *on page 121*

Didronel® *see* Etidronate Disodium *on page 386*

Dienestrol (dye en ES trole)

Brand Names DV® Vaginal Cream; Ortho-Dienestrol® Vaginal

Therapeutic Category Estrogen Derivative

Use Symptomatic management of atrophic vaginitis or kraurosis vulvae in post-menopausal women

Usual Dosage Adults: Vaginal: Insert 1 applicatorful once or twice daily for 1-2 weeks and then 1/2 of that dose for 1-2 weeks; maintenance dose: 1 applicatorful 1-3 times/week for 3-6 months

Mechanism of Action Increases the synthesis of DNA, RNA, and various proteins in target tissues; reduces the release of gonadotropin-releasing hormone from the hypothalamus; reduces FSH and LH release from the pituitary

Local Anesthetic/Vasoconstrictor Precautions No information available to require special precautions

Effects on Dental Treatment No effects or complications reported

Other Adverse Effects

1% to 10%:

Cardiovascular: Peripheral edema

Endocrine & metabolic: Breast tenderness, breast enlargement

Gastrointestinal: Anorexia, abdominal cramping

<1%:

Cardiovascular: Hypertension, thromboembolism, myocardial infarction

Central nervous system: Stroke, migraine, dizziness, anxiety, depression, headache

Dermatologic: Chloasma, melasma, rash

Endocrine & metabolic: Decreased glucose tolerance, alterations in frequency and flow of menses, breast tenderness or enlargement, elevated triglycerides and LDL

Gastrointestinal: Nausea, GI distress

Hepatic: Cholestatic jaundice

Miscellaneous: Increased susceptibility to *Candida* infection

Drug Interactions No data reported

Drug Uptake

Time to peak serum concentration: Topical: Within 3-4 hours

Pregnancy Risk Factor X

Generic Available No

Dietary Supplements *see* Enteral Nutritional Products *on page 350*

Diethylpropion (dye eth il PROE pee on)

Brand Names Tenuate®; Tenuate® Dospan®

Canadian/Mexican Brand Names Nobesine® (Canada)

Therapeutic Category Anorexiant

Synonyms Amfepramone (Canada)

Use Short-term adjunct in exogenous obesity

Usual Dosage Adults: Oral:

Tablet: 25 mg 3 times/day before meals or food

Tablet, controlled release: 75 mg at midmorning

Mechanism of Action Diethylpropion is used as an anorexiant agent possessing pharmacological and chemical properties similar to those of amphetamines. The mechanism of action of diethylpropion in reducing appetite appears to be secondary to CNS effects, specifically stimulation of the hypothalamus to release catecholamines into the central nervous system; anorexiant effects are mediated via norepinephrine and dopamine metabolism. An increase in physical activity and metabolic effects (inhibition of lipogenesis and enhancement of lipolysis) may also contribute to weight loss.

Local Anesthetic/Vasoconstrictor Precautions Use vasoconstrictor with caution in patients taking diethylpropion. Amphetamine-like drugs such as diethylpropion enhance the sympathomimetic response of epinephrine and norepinephrine leading to potential hypertension and cardiotoxicity.

(Continued)

Diethylpropion *(Continued)*

Effects on Dental Treatment Up to 10% of patients may present with hypertension. The use of local anesthetic without vasoconstrictor is recommended in these patients.

Other Adverse Effects

>10%:
  Cardiovascular: Hypertension
  Central nervous system: Euphoria, nervousness, insomnia

1% to 10%:
  Central nervous system: Confusion, mental depression
  Endocrine & metabolic: Changes in libido
  Gastrointestinal: Nausea, vomiting, restlessness, constipation
  Hematologic: Blood dyscrasias
  Neuromuscular & skeletal: Tremor
  Ocular: Blurred vision

<1%:
  Cardiovascular: Tachycardia, arrhythmias
  Central nervous system: Depression, headache
  Dermatologic: Alopecia
  Gastrointestinal: Diarrhea, abdominal cramps
  Genitourinary: Dysuria
  Neuromuscular & skeletal: Myalgia
  Renal: Polyuria
  Respiratory: Dyspnea
  Miscellaneous: Increased sweating

Drug Interactions

Decreased effect of guanethidine; decreased effect with phenothiazines
Increased effect/toxicity with MAO inhibitors (hypertensive crisis), CNS depressants, general anesthetics (arrhythmias), sympathomimetics

Pregnancy Risk Factor B

Generic Available Yes

Diethylstilbestrol *(dye eth il stil BES trole)*

Brand Names Stilphostrol®

Canadian/Mexican Brand Names Honvol® (Canada)

Therapeutic Category Estrogen Derivative

Use Palliative treatment of inoperable metastatic prostatic carcinoma and postmenopausal inoperable, progressing breast cancer

Usual Dosage Adults:

Male:
  Prostate carcinoma (inoperable, progressing): Oral: 1-3 mg/day
  Diphosphate: Inoperable progressing prostate cancer:
  Oral: 50 mg 3 times/day; increase up to 200 mg or more 3 times/day; maximum daily dose: 1 g
  I.V.: Give 0.5 g, dissolved in 250 mL of saline or D$_5$W, administer slowly the first 10-15 minutes then adjust rate so that the entire amount is given in 1 hour; repeat for ≥5 days depending on patient response, then repeat 0.25-0.5 g 1-2 times for one week or change to oral therapy
Female: Postmenopausal inoperable, progressing breast carcinoma: Oral: 15 mg/day

Mechanism of Action Competes with estrogenic and androgenic compounds for binding onto tumor cells and thereby inhibits their effects on tumor growth

Local Anesthetic/Vasoconstrictor Precautions No information available to require special precautions

Effects on Dental Treatment No effects or complications reported

Other Adverse Effects

>10%:
  Cardiovascular: Peripheral edema
  Endocrine & metabolic: Enlargement of breasts (female and male), breast tenderness
  Gastrointestinal: Nausea, anorexia, bloating

1% to 10%:
  Central nervous system: Headache
  Endocrine & metabolic: Increased libido (female), decreased libido (male)
  Gastrointestinal: Vomiting, diarrhea

<1%:
  Cardiovascular: Hypertension, thromboembolism, myocardial infarction, edema
  Central nervous system: Stroke, depression, dizziness, anxiety
  Dermatologic: Chloasma, melasma, rash

Endocrine & metabolic: Breast tumors, amenorrhea, alterations in frequency and flow of menses, elevated triglycerides and LDL

Gastrointestinal: GI distress

Hepatic: Cholestatic jaundice

Ocular: Intolerance to contact lenses

Miscellaneous: Decreased glucose tolerance, increased susceptibility to *Candida* infection

Drug Interactions No data reported

Pregnancy Risk Factor X

Generic Available Yes

Difenoxin and Atropine (dye fen OKS in & A troe peen)

Brand Names Motofen®

Therapeutic Category Antidiarrheal

Use Treatment of diarrhea

Local Anesthetic/Vasoconstrictor Precautions No information available to require special precautions

Effects on Dental Treatment No effects or complications reported

Other Adverse Effects

1% to 10%:

Central nervous system: Dizziness, drowsiness, lightheadedness, headache

Gastrointestinal: Nausea, vomiting, dry mouth, epigastric distress

<1%:

Central nervous system: Confusion

Gastrointestinal: Constipation

Ocular: Blurred vision

Pregnancy Risk Factor C

Generic Available No

Differin® *see* Adapalene *on page 32*

Diflorasone (dye FLOR a sone)

Related Information

Corticosteroids, Topical Comparison *on page 1140*

Brand Names Florone®; Florone® E; Maxiflor®; Psorcon™

Therapeutic Category Corticosteroid, Topical (High Potency)

Use Relieves inflammation and pruritic symptoms of corticosteroid-responsive dermatosis (high to very high potency topical corticosteroid)

Maxiflor™: High potency topical corticosteroid

Psorcon™: Very high potency topical corticosteroid

Usual Dosage Topical: Apply ointment sparingly 1-3 times/day; apply cream sparingly 2-4 times/day

Mechanism of Action Decreases inflammation by suppression of migration of polymorphonuclear leukocytes and reversal of increased capillary permeability

Local Anesthetic/Vasoconstrictor Precautions No information available to require special precautions

Effects on Dental Treatment No effects or complications reported

Other Adverse Effects <1%:

Local: Burning, itching, folliculitis, dryness, maceration

Neuromuscular & skeletal: Muscle atrophy, arthralgia

Miscellaneous: Secondary infection

Drug Interactions No data reported

Drug Uptake Absorption: Topical: Negligible, around 1% reaches dermal layers or systemic circulation; occlusive dressings increase absorption percutaneously

Pregnancy Risk Factor C

Dosage Forms

Cream, as diacetate: 0.05% (15 g, 30 g, 60 g)

Ointment, topical, as diacetate: 0.05% (15 g, 30 g, 60 g)

Generic Available No

Diflucan® *see* Fluconazole *on page 408*

Diflunisal (dye FLOO ni sal)

Related Information

Dental Drug Interactions: Update on Drug Combinations Requiring Special Considerations *on page 1144*

Oral Pain *on page 1053*

Rheumatoid Arthritis and Osteoarthritis *on page 1030*

Brand Names Dolobid®

Canadian/Mexican Brand Names Apo®-Diflunisal (Canada); Novo-Diflunisal (Canada); Nu-Diflunisal (Canada)

(Continued)

Diflunisal *(Continued)*

Therapeutic Category Analgesic, Non-narcotic; Nonsteroidal Anti-inflammatory Agent (NSAID), Oral

Use

Dental: Treatment of postoperative pain

Medical: Management of pain and inflammatory disorders usually including rheumatoid arthritis and osteoarthritis

Usual Dosage Adults: Oral: 500-1000 mg followed by 250-500 mg every 8-12 hours; maximum daily dose: 1.5 g

Mechanism of Action Inhibits prostaglandin synthesis by decreasing the activity of the enzyme, cyclo-oxygenase, which results in decreased formation of prostaglandin precursors

Local Anesthetic/Vasoconstrictor Precautions No information available to require special precautions

Effects on Dental Treatment No effects or complications reported

Other Adverse Effects

>10%:

Cardiovascular: Fluid retention

Central nervous system: Headache

1% to 10%: Gastrointestinal: GI ulceration

Contraindications Hypersensitivity to diflunisal or any component, may be a cross-sensitivity with other nonsteroidal anti-inflammatory agents including aspirin; should not be used in patients with active GI bleeding

Warnings/Precautions Peptic ulceration and GI bleeding have been reported; platelet function and bleeding time are inhibited; ophthalmologic effects; impaired renal function, use lower dosage; peripheral edema; possibility of Reye's syndrome; may cause elevated liver function tests

Drug Interactions Decreased effect with antacids; increased effect/toxicity of digoxin, methotrexate, anticoagulants, phenytoin, sulfonylureas, sulfonamides, lithium, indomethacin, hydrochlorothiazide, acetaminophen

Drug Uptake

Absorption: Rapid and complete

Onset of effect: Within 1 hour

Duration of effect: 8-12 hours

Serum half-life: 8-12 hours

Time to peak serum concentration: Within 2-3 hours

Pregnancy Risk Factor C (first and second trimester); D (third trimester)

Breast-feeding Considerations Diflunisal is excreted in breast milk, however, there is no specific data regarding use during lactation

Dosage Forms Tablet: 250 mg, 500 mg

Dietary Considerations Should be taken with food to decrease GI distress

Generic Available Yes

Comments The advantage of diflunisal as a pain reliever is its 12-hour duration of effect. In many cases, this long effect will ensure a full night sleep during the postoperative pain period.

Selected Readings

Brooks PM and Day RO, "Nonsteroidal Anti-inflammatory Drugs-Differences and Similarities," *N Engl J Med*, 1991, 324(24):1716-25.

Dionne RA, "New Approaches to Preventing and Treating Postoperative Pain," *J Am Dent Assoc*, 1992, 123(6):26-34.

Forbes JA, Butterworth GA, Burchfield WH, et al, "A 12-Hour Evaluation of the Analgesic Efficacy of Diflunisal, Zomepirac Sodium, Aspirin, and Placebo in Postoperative Oral Surgery Pain," *Pharmacotherapy*, 1983, 3(2 Pt 2):38S-46S.

Forbes JA, Calderazzo JP, Bowser MW, et al, "A 12-Hour Evaluation of the Analgesic Efficacy of Diflunisal, Aspirin, and Placebo in Postoperative Dental Pain," *J Clin Pharmacol*, 1982, 22(2-3):89-96.

Gobetti JP, "Controlling Dental Pain," *J Am Dent Assoc*, 1992, 123(6):47-52.

Di-Gel® [OTC] *see* Aluminum Hydroxide, Magnesium Hydroxide, and Simethicone *on page 49*

Digepepsin® *see* Pancreatin *on page 721*

Digibind® *see* Digoxin Immune Fab *on page 315*

Digitoxin *(di ji TOKS in)*

Related Information

Cardiovascular Diseases *on page 1010*

Brand Names Crystodigin®

Canadian/Mexican Brand Names Digitaline® (Canada)

Therapeutic Category Antiarrhythmic Agent (Supraventricular); Antiarrhythmic Agent, Miscellaneous; Cardiac Glycoside

Use Treatment of congestive heart failure, atrial fibrillation, atrial flutter, paroxysmal atrial tachycardia, and cardiogenic shock

Usual Dosage Oral:

Children: Doses are very individualized; **when recommended**, digitalizing dose is as follows:

<1 year: 0.045 mg/kg

1-2 years: 0.04 mg/kg

>2 years: 0.03 mg/kg which is equivalent to 0.75 mg/mm^2

Maintenance: Approximately $1/10$ of the digitalizing dose

Adults: Oral:

Rapid loading dose: Initial: 0.6 mg followed by 0.4 mg and then 0.2 mg at intervals of 4-6 hours

Slow loading dose: 0.2 mg twice daily for a period of 4 days followed by a maintenance dose

Maintenance: 0.05-0.3 mg/day

Most common dose: 0.15 mg/day

Mechanism of Action Digitalis binds to and inhibits magnesium and adenosine triphosphate dependent sodium and potassium ATPase thereby increasing the influx of calcium ions, from extracellular to intracellular cytoplasm due to the inhibition of sodium and potassium ion movement across the myocardial membranes; this increase in calcium ions results in a potentiation of the activity of the contractile heart muscle fibers and an increase in the force of myocardial contraction (positive inotropic effect); digitalis may also increase intracellular entry of calcium via slow calcium channel influx; stimulates release and blocks re-uptake of norepinephrine; decreases conduction through the S-A and A-V nodes

Local Anesthetic/Vasoconstrictor Precautions Use vasoconstrictor with caution due to risk of cardiac arrhythmias with digitoxin

Effects on Dental Treatment Sensitive gag reflex may cause difficulty in taking a dental impression

Other Adverse Effects

1% to 10%: Gastrointestinal: Anorexia, nausea, vomiting

<1%:

Cardiovascular: Sinus bradycardia, A-V block, S-A block, atrial or nodal ectopic beats, ventricular arrhythmias, bigeminy, trigeminy, atrial tachycardia with A-V block

Central nervous system: Drowsiness, headache, fatigue, lethargy, vertigo, disorientation

Endocrine & metabolic: Hyperkalemia with acute toxicity

Gastrointestinal: Feeding intolerance, abdominal pain, diarrhea

Neuromuscular & skeletal: Neuralgia

Ocular: Blurred vision, halos, yellow or green vision, diplopia, photophobia, flashing lights

Drug Interactions

Decreased effect/levels of digitoxin/digoxin: Antacids (magnesium, aluminum), cholestyramine, colestipol, kaolin/pectin, aminosalicylic acid, metoclopramide, sulfasalazine

Decreased effect/levels of digitoxin only (eg, increased metabolism): Aminoglutethimide, barbiturates, hydantoins, rifampin, phenylbutazone, thyroid replacement

Increased effect/toxicity/levels of digitoxin/digoxin: Amiodarone, nifedipine, quinidine, quinine, verapamil, nondepolarizing muscle relaxants, succinylcholine, potassium-losing diuretics

Concomitant use of digitoxin and sympathomimetics increases the risk of cardiac arrhythmias

Drug Uptake

Absorption: 90% to 100%

Serum half-life: 7-8 days

Time to peak: 8-12 hours

Pregnancy Risk Factor C

Generic Available Yes

Digoxin (di JOKS in)

Related Information

Cardiovascular Diseases *on page 1010*

Brand Names Lanoxicaps®; Lanoxin®

Canadian/Mexican Brand Names Mapluxin® (Mexico); Novo-Digoxin® (Canada)

Therapeutic Category Antiarrhythmic Agent (Supraventricular); Antiarrhythmic Agent, Miscellaneous; Cardiac Glycoside

Synonyms Digoxina (Mexico)

Use Treatment of congestive heart failure and to slow the ventricular rate in tachyarrhythmias such as atrial fibrillation, atrial flutter, and supraventricular tachycardia (paroxysmal atrial tachycardia); cardiogenic shock

(Continued)

Digoxin (Continued)

Usual Dosage When changing from oral (tablets or liquid) or I.M. to I.V. therapy, dosage should be reduced by 20% to 25%. See table.

Dosage Recommendations for Digoxin

Age	Total Digitalizing Dose† (mcg/kg)*		Daily Maintenance Dose‡ (mcg/kg*)	
	P.O.	I.V. or I.M.	P.O.	I.V. or I.M.
Preterm infant*	20-30	15-25	5-7.5	4-6
Full-term infant*	25-35	20-30	6-10	5-8
1 mo - 2 y*	35-60	30-50	10-15	7.5-12
2-5 y*	30-40	25-35	7.5-10	6-9
5-10 y*	20-35	15-30	5-10	4-8
>10 y*	10-15	8-12	2.5-5	2-3
Adults	0.75-1.5 mg	0.5-1 mg	0.125-0.5 mg	0.1-0.4 mg

†Give one-half of the total digitalizing dose (TDD) in the initial dose, then give one-quarter of the TDD in each of two subsequent doses at 8- to 12-hour intervals. Obtain EKG 6 hours after each dose to assess potential toxicity.

*Based on lean body weight and normal renal function for age. Decrease dose in patients with ↓ renal function; digitalizing dose often not recommended in infants and children.

‡Divided every 12 hours in infants and children <10 years of age. Given once daily to children >10 years of age and adults.

Mechanism of Action

Congestive heart failure: Inhibition of the sodium/potassium ATPase pump which acts to increase the intracellular sodium-calcium exchange to increase intracellular calcium leading to increased contractility

Supraventricular arrhythmias: Direct suppression of the A-V node conduction to increase effective refractory period and decrease conduction velocity - positive inotropic effect, enhanced vagal tone, and decreased ventricular rate to fast atrial arrhythmias. Atrial fibrillation may decrease sensitivity and increase tolerance to higher serum digoxin concentrations.

Local Anesthetic/Vasoconstrictor Precautions Use vasoconstrictor with caution due to risk of cardiac arrhythmias with digoxin

Effects on Dental Treatment Sensitive gag reflex may cause difficulty in taking a dental impression

Other Adverse Effects

1% to 10%: Gastrointestinal: Anorexia, nausea, vomiting

<1%:

Cardiovascular: Sinus bradycardia, A-V block, S-A block, atrial or nodal ectopic beats, ventricular arrhythmias, bigeminy, trigeminy, atrial tachycardia with A-V block

Central nervous system: Drowsiness, headache, fatigue, lethargy, vertigo, disorientation

Endocrine & metabolic: Hyperkalemia with acute toxicity

Gastrointestinal: Feeding intolerance, abdominal pain, diarrhea

Neuromuscular & skeletal: Neuralgia

Ocular: Blurred vision, halos, yellow or green vision, diplopia, photophobia, flashing lights

Drug Interactions

Decreased effect/levels of digitoxin/digoxin: Antacids (magnesium, aluminum), cholestyramine, colestipol, kaolin/pectin, aminosalicylic acid, metoclopramide, sulfasalazine

Decreased effect/levels of digitoxin only (eg, increased metabolism): Aminoglutethimide, barbiturates, hydantoins, rifampin, phenylbutazone, thyroid replacement

Increased effect/toxicity/levels of digitoxin/digoxin: Amiodarone, nifedipine, quinidine, quinine, verapamil, nondepolarizing muscle relaxants, succinylcholine, potassium-losing diuretics

Concomitant use of digitoxin and sympathomimetics increase the risk of cardiac arrhythmias

Drug Uptake

Onset of action:

Oral: 1-2 hours

I.V.: 5-30 minutes

Peak effect:

Oral: 2-8 hours

I.V.: 1-4 hours

Duration: Adults: 3-4 days both forms
Absorption: By passive nonsaturable diffusion in the upper small intestine; food may delay, but does not affect extent of digoxin absorption
Serum half-life: Dependent upon age, renal and cardiac function:
Children: 35 hours
Adults: 38-48 hours
Adults, anephric: 4-6 days
Time to peak serum concentration: Oral: Within 1 hour
Pregnancy Risk Factor C
Generic Available Yes: Tablet

Digoxina (Mexico) *see* Digoxin *on page 313*

Digoxin Immune Fab (di JOKS in i MYUN fab)
Brand Names Digibind®
Therapeutic Category Antidote, Digoxin
Synonyms Antidigoxin Fab Fragments
Use Digoxin immune Fab are specific antibodies for the treatment of digitalis intoxication in carefully selected patients; use in life-threatening ventricular arrhythmias secondary to digoxin, acute digoxin ingestion (ie, >10 mg in adults or >4 mg in children), hyperkalemia (serum potassium >5 mEq/L) in the setting of digoxin toxicity
Usual Dosage Each vial of Digibind® will bind approximately 0.6 mg of digoxin or digitoxin

I.V.: To determine the dose of digoxin immune Fab, first determine the total body load of digoxin (TBL using either an approximation of the amount ingested or a postdistribution serum digoxin concentration). If neither ingestion amount or serum level is known: Adult dosage is 20 vials (800 mg) I.V. infusion.
Mechanism of Action Binds with molecules of digoxin or digitoxin and then is excreted by the kidneys and removed from the body
Local Anesthetic/Vasoconstrictor Precautions No information available to require special precautions
Effects on Dental Treatment No effects or complications reported
Other Adverse Effects
<1%:
Cardiovascular: Worsening of low cardiac output or congestive heart failure, rapid ventricular response in patients with atrial fibrillation as digoxin is withdrawn, facial edema and redness
Endocrine & metabolic: Hypokalemia
Dermatologic: Urticarial rash
Miscellaneous: Allergic reactions
Contraindications Hypersensitivity to sheep products
Drug Uptake
Onset of action: I.V.: Improvement in signs and symptoms occur within 2-30 minutes
Serum half-life: 15-20 hours; prolonged in patients with renal impairment
Pregnancy Risk Factor C
Dosage Forms Powder for injection, lyophilized: 40 mg
Generic Available No

Dihidroergotamina (Mexico) *see* Dihydroergotamine *on page 317*

Dihistine® DH *see* Chlorpheniramine, Pseudoephedrine, and Codeine *on page 223*

Dihistine® Expectorant *see* Guaifenesin, Pseudoephedrine, and Codeine *on page 455*

Dihydrocodeine Compound (dye hye droe KOE deen KOM pound)
Related Information
Oral Pain *on page 1053*
Brand Names DHC Plus®; Synalgos®-DC
Therapeutic Category Analgesic, Narcotic
Use
Dental: Management of postoperative pain
Medical: Management of mild to moderate pain from medical conditions
Restrictions C-III; Refillable up to 5 times in 6 months
Usual Dosage Oral:
Children: Not recommended
Adults: 1-2 capsules every 4-6 hours as needed for pain; maximum dose: 12 capsules/day
Mechanism of Action Dihydrocodeine binds to opiate receptors (mu and kappa subtypes) in the CNS causing inhibition of ascending pain pathways, altering the perception of and response to pain; produces generalized CNS depression; (Continued)

Dihydrocodeine Compound *(Continued)*

causes cough suppression by direct central action in the medulla; produces generalized CNS depression

Acetaminophen inhibits the synthesis of prostaglandins in the CNS and peripherally blocks pain impulse generation; produces antipyresis from inhibition of hypothalamic heat-regulating center

Aspirin inhibits prostaglandin synthesis by decreasing the activity of the enzyme, cyclo-oxygenase, which results in decreased formation of prostaglandin precursors acts on the hypothalamic heat-regulating center to reduce fever, blocks thromboxane synthetase action which prevents formation of the platelet-aggregating substance thromboxane A_2

Local Anesthetic/Vasoconstrictor Precautions No information available to require special precautions

Effects on Dental Treatment Use with caution in patients with platelet and bleeding disorders, renal dysfunction, erosive gastritis, or peptic ulcer disease, previous nonreaction does not guarantee future safe taking of medication; do not use aspirin in children <16 years of age for chickenpox or flu symptoms due to the association with Reye's syndrome

Avoid aspirin if possible, for 1 week prior to surgery because of the possibility of postoperative bleeding; use with caution in impaired hepatic function

Elderly are a high-risk population for adverse effects from nonsteroidal anti-inflammatory agents. As much as 60% of elderly with GI complications to NSAIDs can develop peptic ulceration and/or hemorrhage asymptomatically. Also, concomitant disease and drug use contribute to the risk for GI adverse effects. Use lowest effective dose for shortest period possible. Consider renal function decline with age. Use with caution in patients with history of asthma

Other Adverse Effects
>10%:
Central nervous system: Lightheadedness, dizziness, sedation
Gastrointestinal: Nausea, heartburn, stomach pains, dyspepsia, vomiting
1% to 10%: Gastrointestinal: Ulceration, constipation

Contraindications Hypersensitivity to acetaminophen or aspirin; hypersensitivity to other phenanthrene derivative opioid agonists (morphine, hydrocodone, hydromorphone, levorphanol, oxycodone, oxymorphone)

Warnings/Precautions Respiratory diseases including asthma, emphysema, COPD, or severe liver or renal insufficiency; some preparations contain sulfites which may cause allergic reactions; may be habit-forming; dextromethorphan has equivalent antitussive activity but has much lower toxicity in accidental overdose

Enhanced analgesia has been seen in elderly patients on therapeutic doses of narcotics; duration of action may be increased in the elderly; the elderly may be particularly susceptible to the CNS depressant and constipating effects of narcotics

Drug Interactions
Dihydrocodeine component: MAO inhibitors cause increased adverse symptoms
Acetaminophen component: Refer to Acetaminophen monograph
Aspirin component: Refer to Aspirin monograph

Drug Uptake
Onset of action: 10-30 minutes
Duration: Oral: 4-6 hours
Serum half-life: 3.8 hours
Time to peak serum concentration: 30-60 minutes

Pregnancy Risk Factor B (D if used for prolonged periods or in high doses at term)

Breast-feeding Considerations
Acetaminophen: May be taken while breast-feeding
Aspirin: Use cautiously due to potential adverse effects in nursing infants
Dihydrocodeine: No data reported

Dosage Forms Capsule:
DHC Plus®: Dihydrocodeine bitartrate 16 mg, acetaminophen 356.4 mg, and caffeine 30 mg
Synalgos®-DC: Dihydrocodeine bitartrate 16 mg, aspirin 356.4 mg, and caffeine 30 mg

Dietary Considerations Should be taken with food

Generic Available Yes

Comments Dihydrocodeine products, as with other narcotic analgesics, are recommended only for acute dosing (ie, 3 days or less). The most common adverse effect you will see in your dental patients from dihydrocodeine is nausea, followed by sedation and constipation. Dihydrocodeine has narcotic addiction liability, especially when given long term. Dihydrocodeine with aspirin could have anticoagulant effects and could possibly affect bleeding times. Dihydrocodeine with acetaminophen should be used with caution in patients with alcoholic liver disease.

Dihydroergotamine (dye hye droe er GOT a meen)

Brand Names D.H.E. 45® Injection; Migranal® Nasal Spray

Therapeutic Category Ergot Alkaloid

Synonyms Dihidroergotamina (Mexico)

Use

Injection: Aborts or prevents vascular headaches; also as an adjunct for DVT prophylaxis for hip surgery, for orthostatic hypotension, xerostomia secondary to antidepressant use, and pelvic congestion with pain;

Nasal spray: Acute treatment of migraine headaches with or without aura; is not indicated for prophylactic therapy or for the management of hemiplegic or basilar migraine

Usual Dosage Adults:

I.M.: 1 mg at first sign of headache; repeat hourly to a maximum dose of 3 mg total

I.V.: Up to 2 mg maximum dose for faster effects; maximum dose: 6 mg/week

Mechanism of Action Ergot alkaloid alpha-adrenergic blocker directly stimulates vascular smooth muscle to vasoconstrict peripheral and cerebral vessels; also has effects on serotonin receptors

Local Anesthetic/Vasoconstrictor Precautions No information available to require special precautions

Effects on Dental Treatment >10% of patients experience dry mouth

Other Adverse Effects

>10%:

Cardiovascular: Localized edema, peripheral vascular effects

Central nervous system: Drowsiness, dizziness

Gastrointestinal: Diarrhea, nausea, vomiting

Neuromuscular & skeletal: Paresthesia

1% to 10%:

Cardiovascular: Precordial distress and pain, transient tachycardia or bradycardia

Neuromuscular & skeletal: Myalgia in the extremities, weakness in the legs

Drug Interactions

Increased effect of heparin

Increased toxicity with erythromycin, clarithromycin, nitroglycerin, propranolol, troleandomycin

Drug Uptake

Onset of action: Within 15-30 minutes

Duration: 3-4 hours

Serum half-life: 1.3-3.9 hours

Time to peak serum concentration: I.M.: Within 15-30 minutes

Pregnancy Risk Factor X

Generic Available Yes

Dihydrohydroxycodeinone see Oxycodone on page 710

Dihydrotachysterol (dye hye droe tak IS ter ole)

Brand Names DHT™; Hytakerol®

Therapeutic Category Vitamin D Analog

Use Treatment of hypocalcemia associated with hypoparathyroidism; prophylaxis of hypocalcemic tetany following thyroid surgery

Usual Dosage Oral:

Hypoparathyroidism:

Young Children: Initial: 1-5 mg/day for 4 days, then 0.1-0.5 mg/day

Older Children and Adults: Initial: 0.8-2.4 mg/day for several days followed by maintenance doses of 0.2-1 mg/day

Nutritional rickets: 0.5 mg as a single dose or 13-50 mcg/day until healing occurs

Renal osteodystrophy: Maintenance: 0.25-0.6 mg/24 hours adjusted as necessary to achieve normal serum calcium levels and promote bone healing

Mechanism of Action Synthetic analogue of vitamin D with a faster onset of action; stimulates calcium and phosphate absorption from the small intestine, promotes secretion of calcium from bone to blood; promotes renal tubule resorption of phosphate

Local Anesthetic/Vasoconstrictor Precautions No information available to require special precautions

Effects on Dental Treatment No effects or complications reported

(Continued)

317

Dihydrotachysterol *(Continued)*
Other Adverse Effects
>10%:

Endocrine & metabolic: Hypercalcemia, hypercalciuria

Renal: Elevated serum creatinine

<1%:

Central nervous system: Convulsions

Endocrine & metabolic: Polydipsia

Gastrointestinal: Nausea, vomiting, anorexia, weight loss

Hematologic: Anemia

Neuromuscular & skeletal: Metastatic calcification, weakness

Renal: Renal damage, polyuria

Drug Interactions
Decreased effect/levels of vitamin D: Cholestyramine, colestipol, mineral oil

Increased toxicity: Thiazide diuretics increase calcium

Drug Uptake
Peak hypercalcemic effect: Within 2-4 weeks

Duration: Can be as long as 9 weeks

Absorption: Well absorbed from the GI tract

Pregnancy Risk Factor A (D if used in doses above the recommended daily allowance)

Generic Available Yes

Dihydroxyaluminum Sodium Carbonate
(dye hye DROKS i a LOO mi num SOW dee um KAR bun ate)

Brand Names Rolaids® [OTC]

Therapeutic Category Antacid

Use Symptomatic relief of upset stomach associated with hyperacidity

Usual Dosage Oral: Chew 1-2 tablets as needed

Local Anesthetic/Vasoconstrictor Precautions No information available to require special precautions

Effects on Dental Treatment No effects or complications reported

Dosage Forms Tablet, chewable: 334 mg

Generic Available Yes

Dihydroxypropyl Theophylline *see* Dyphylline *on page 342*

Dilacor™ XR *see* Diltiazem *on this page*

Dilantin® *see* Phenytoin *on page 756*

Dilantin® With Phenobarbital *see* Phenytoin With Phenobarbital *on page 757*

Dilatrate®-SR *see* Isosorbide Dinitrate *on page 525*

Dilaudid® *see* Hydromorphone *on page 486*

Dilaudid-5® *see* Hydromorphone *on page 486*

Dilaudid-HP® *see* Hydromorphone *on page 486*

Dilocaine® *see* Lidocaine *on page 553*

Dilor® *see* Dyphylline *on page 342*

Diltiazem (dil TYE a zem)
Related Information
Calcium Channel Blockers & Gingival Hyperplasia *on page 1132*

Cardiovascular Diseases *on page 1010*

Enalapril and Diltiazem *on page 347*

Brand Names Cardizem® CD; Cardizem® Injectable; Cardizem® SR; Cardizem® Tablet; Dilacor™ XR; Tiamate®; Tiazac®

Canadian/Mexican Brand Names Angiotrofen A.P.® (Mexico); Angiotrofen® (Mexico); Angiotrofen® Retard (Mexico); Apo®-Diltiaz (Canada); Novo-Diltazem® (Canada); Nu-Diltiaz® (Canada); Presoken® (Mexico); Presoquim® (Mexico); Syn-Diltiazem® (Canada); Tilazem® (Mexico)

Therapeutic Category Antianginal Agent; Calcium Channel Blocker

Synonyms Diltiazem, Clorhidrato De (Mexico)

Use
Capsule: Hypertension (alone or in combination); chronic stable angina or angina from coronary artery spasm

Injection: Atrial fibrillation or atrial flutter; paroxysmal supraventricular tachycardias (PSVT)

Usual Dosage Adults:

Oral: 30-120 mg 3-4 times/day; dosage should be increased gradually, at 1- to 2-day intervals until optimum response is obtained; usual maintenance dose: 240-360 mg/day

Sustained-release capsules:

Cardizem SR®: Initial: 60-120 mg twice daily; adjust to maximum antihypertensive effect (usually within 14 days); usual range: 240-360 mg/day

Cardizem® CD, Tiazac®: Hypertension: Total daily dose of short-acting administered once daily or initially 180 or 240 mg once daily; adjust to maximum effect (usually within 14 days); maximum: 360 mg/day; usual range: 240-360 mg/day

Cardizem® CD: Angina: Initial: 120-180 mg once daily; maximum: 480 mg once/day

Dilacor™ XR:

Hypertension: 180-240 mg once daily; maximum: 540 mg/day; usual range: 180-480 mg/day; use lower dose in elderly

Angina: Initial: 120 mg/day; titrate slowly over 7-14 days up to 480 mg/day, as needed

Note: Hypertensive or anginal patients treated with other formulations of diltiazem sustained release can be safely switched to Dilacor™ XR at the nearest equivalent total daily dose; subsequent titration may be needed

I.V. (requires an infusion pump): See table.

Diltiazem — I.V. Dosage and Administration

Initial Bolus Dose	0.25 mg/kg actual body weight over 2 min (average adult dose: 20 mg)
Repeat Bolus Dose may be administered after 15 min if the response is inadequate	0.35 mg/kg actual body weight over 2 min (average adult dose: 25 mg)
Continuous Infusion Infusions >24 h or infusion rates >15 mg/h are not recommended due to potential accumulation of metabolites and increased toxicity	Initial infusion rate of 10 mg/h; rate may be increased in 5 mg/h increments up to 15 mg/h as needed; some patients may respond to an initial rate of 5 mg/h

If Cardizem® injectable is administered by continuous infusion for >24 hours, the possibility of decreased diltiazem clearance, prolonged elimination half-life, and increased diltiazem and/or diltiazem metabolite plasma concentrations should be considered

Conversion from I.V. diltiazem to oral diltiazem: Start oral approximately 3 hours after bolus dose

Oral dose (mg/day) is approximately equal to [rate (mg/hour) x 3 + 3] x 10

3 mg/hour = 120 mg/day

5 mg/hour = 180 mg/day

7 mg/hour = 240 mg/day

11 mg/hour = 360 mg/day (maximum recommended dose)

Mechanism of Action Inhibits calcium ion from entering the "slow channels" or select voltage-sensitive areas of vascular smooth muscle and myocardium during depolarization, producing a relaxation of coronary vascular smooth muscle and coronary vasodilation; increases myocardial oxygen delivery in patients with vasospastic angina

Local Anesthetic/Vasoconstrictor Precautions No information available to require special precautions

Effects on Dental Treatment Calcium channel blockers cause gingival hyperplasia in approximately 1% of patients. There have been fewer reports with diltiazem than with other CCBs. The hyperplasia will disappear with cessation of drug therapy. Consultation with physician is suggested.

Other Adverse Effects

>10%: Central nervous system: Headache

1% to 10%:

Cardiovascular: Bradycardia, A-V block (first degree), edema, EKG abnormality

Central nervous system: Dizziness

Gastrointestinal: Nausea, vomiting

Neuromuscular & skeletal: Weakness

<1%:

Cardiovascular: A-V block (second degree), angina

Central nervous system: Abnormal dreams, amnesia, depression, insomnia, nervousness

Dermatologic: Urticaria, photosensitivity, alopecia, purpura

Gastrointestinal: Anorexia, constipation, diarrhea, dysgeusia, dyspepsia

Hematologic: Hemolytic anemia, leukopenia thrombocytopenia

Neuromuscular & skeletal: Paresthesia, tremor, gait abnormality

Ocular: Amblyopia, retinopathy

Respiratory: Pharyngitis, cough increase

Miscellaneous: Flu syndrome

(Continued)

Diltiazem *(Continued)*

Drug Interactions Increased toxicity/effect/levels:
H_2-blockers cause increased bioavailability of diltiazem
Beta-blockers cause increased cardiac depressant effects on A-V conduction
Diltiazem increases serum levels and effects/toxicity of carbamazepine, cyclosporin, digitalis, quinidine, and theophylline

Drug Uptake
Onset of action: Oral: 30-60 minutes (including sustained release)
Absorption: 80% to 90%
Time to peak serum concentration:
Short-acting tablets: Within 2-3 hours
Sustained release: 6-11 hours

Pregnancy Risk Factor C
Generic Available Yes

Diltiazem, Clorhidrato De (Mexico) *see* Diltiazem *on page 318*

Dimacol® Caplets [OTC] *see* Guaifenesin, Pseudoephedrine, and Dextromethorphan *on page 456*

Dimaphen® Elixir [OTC] *see* Brompheniramine and Phenylpropanolamine *on page 143*

Dimaphen® Tablets [OTC] *see* Brompheniramine and Phenylpropanolamine *on page 143*

Dimenhidrinato (Mexico) *see* Dimenhydrinate *on this page*

Dimenhydrinate *(dye men HYE dri nate)*

Brand Names Calm-X® Oral [OTC]; Dimetabs® Oral; Dinate® Injection; Dramamine® Oral [OTC]; Dymenate® Injection; Hydrate® Injection; TripTone® Caplets® [OTC]

Canadian/Mexican Brand Names Apo®-Dimenhydrinate (Canada); Gravol® (Canada); PMS-Dimenhydrinate® (Canada); Travel Aid® (Canada); Travel Tabs® (Canada); Vomisen® (Mexico)

Therapeutic Category Antiemetic; Antihistamine

Synonyms Dimenhidrinato (Mexico)

Use Treatment and prevention of nausea, vertigo, and vomiting associated with motion sickness

Usual Dosage
Children:
Oral:
2-5 years: 12.5-25 mg every 6-8 hours, maximum: 75 mg/day
6-12 years: 25-50 mg every 6-8 hours, maximum: 150 mg/day
I.M.: 1.25 mg/kg or 37.5 mg/m² 4 times/day, not to exceed 300 mg/day

Adults: Oral, I.M., I.V.: 50-100 mg every 4-6 hours, not to exceed 400 mg/day

Mechanism of Action Competes with histamine for H_1-receptor sites on effector cells in the gastrointestinal tract, blood vessels, and respiratory tract; blocks chemoreceptor trigger zone, diminishes vestibular stimulation, and depresses labyrinthine function through its central anticholinergic activity

Local Anesthetic/Vasoconstrictor Precautions No information available to require special precautions

Effects on Dental Treatment Up to 10% of patients will complain of significant dry mouth and drowsiness. This will disappear with cessation of drug therapy.

Other Adverse Effects
>10%:
Central nervous system: Slight to moderate drowsiness
Respiratory: Thickening of bronchial secretions
1% to 10%:
Central nervous system: Headache, fatigue, nervousness, dizziness
Gastrointestinal: Appetite increase, weight gain, nausea, diarrhea, abdominal pain, dry mouth
Neuromuscular & skeletal: Arthralgia
Respiratory: Pharyngitis
<1%:
Cardiovascular: Edema, palpitations, hypotension
Central nervous system: Depression, paradoxical CNS stimulation
Dermatologic: Angioedema, photosensitivity, rash
Gastrointestinal: Anorexia
Hepatic: Hepatitis,
Local: Pain at the injection site
Neuromuscular & skeletal: Myalgia, paresthesia
Ocular: Blurred vision
Otic: Tinnitus
Renal: Polyuria

Respiratory: Bronchospasm, epistaxis

Drug Interactions
Increased effect/toxicity with CNS depressants, anticholinergics, TCAs, MAO inhibitors
Increased toxicity of antibiotics, especially aminoglycosides (ototoxicity)

Drug Uptake
Onset of action: Oral: Within 15-30 minutes
Absorption: Well absorbed from GI tract

Pregnancy Risk Factor B
Generic Available Yes

Dimercaprol (dye mer KAP role)

Brand Names BAL in Oil®

Therapeutic Category Antidote, Arsenic Toxicity; Antidote, Gold Toxicity; Antidote, Lead Toxicity; Antidote, Mercury Toxicity

Use Antidote to gold, arsenic, and mercury poisoning; adjunct to edetate calcium disodium in lead poisoning

Usual Dosage Children and Adults: Deep I.M.:
Mild arsenic and gold poisoning: 2.5 mg/kg/dose every 6 hours for 2 days, then every 12 hours on the third day, and once daily thereafter for 10 days
Severe arsenic and gold poisoning: 3 mg/kg/dose every 4 hours for 2 days then every 6 hours on the third day, then every 12 hours thereafter for 10 days
Mercury poisoning: Initial: 5 mg/kg followed by 2.5 mg/kg/dose 1-2 times/day for 10 days
Lead poisoning (use with edetate calcium disodium):
Mild: 3 mg/kg/dose every 4 hours for 5-7 days
Severe and acute encephalopathy: 4 mg/kg/dose initially alone then every 4 hours in combination of edetate calcium disodium

Mechanism of Action Sulfhydryl group combines with ions of various heavy metals to form relatively stable, nontoxic, soluble chelates which are excreted in urine

Local Anesthetic/Vasoconstrictor Precautions No information available to require special precautions

Effects on Dental Treatment No effects or complications reported

Other Adverse Effects
>10%:
Cardiovascular: Hypertension, tachycardia
Central nervous system: Convulsions
1% to 10%: Gastrointestinal: Nausea, vomiting
<1%:
Central nervous system: Nervousness, fever, headache
Gastrointestinal: Salivation
Hematologic: Transient neutropenia
Local: Pain at the injection site
Ocular: Blepharospasm
Renal: Nephrotoxicity
Miscellaneous: Burning sensation of the lips, mouth, throat, eyes, and penis

Drug Interactions Toxic complexes with iron, cadmium, selenium, or uranium

Drug Uptake
Time to peak serum concentration: 0.5-1 hour

Pregnancy Risk Factor C
Generic Available No

Dimetabs® Oral see Dimenhydrinate on previous page

Dimetane®-DC see Brompheniramine, Phenylpropanolamine, and Codeine on page 145

Dimetane® Decongestant Elixir [OTC] see Brompheniramine and Phenylephrine on page 143

Dimetane® Extentabs® [OTC] see Brompheniramine on page 142

Dimetapp® 4-Hour Liqui-Gel Capsule [OTC] see Brompheniramine and Phenylpropanolamine on page 143

Dimetapp® Elixir [OTC] see Brompheniramine and Phenylpropanolamine on page 143

Dimetapp® Extentabs® [OTC] see Brompheniramine and Phenylpropanolamine on page 143

Dimetapp® Sinus Caplets [OTC] see Pseudoephedrine and Ibuprofen on page 821

Dimetapp® Tablet [OTC] see Brompheniramine and Phenylpropanolamine on page 143

β,β-Dimethylcysteine see Penicillamine on page 730

Dimethyl Triazeno Imidazol Carboxamide see Dacarbazine on page 276

Dinate® Injection see Dimenhydrinate on previous page

Dinoprostone (dye noe PROST one)

Brand Names Cervidil® Vaginal Insert; Prepidil® Vaginal Gel; Prostin E$_2$® Vaginal Suppository

Therapeutic Category Abortifacient; Prostaglandin

Synonyms PGE$_2$; Prostaglandin E$_2$

Use

Gel: Promote cervical ripening prior to labor induction; usage for gel include any patient undergoing induction of labor with an unripe cervix, most commonly for pre-eclampsia, eclampsia, postdates, diabetes, intrauterine growth retardation, and chronic hypertension

Suppositories: Terminate pregnancy from 12th through 28th week of gestation; evacuate uterus in cases of missed abortion or intrauterine fetal death; manage benign hydatidiform mole

Usual Dosage

Abortifacient: Insert 1 suppository high in vagina, repeat at 3- to 5-hour intervals until abortion occurs up to 240 mg (maximum dose); continued administration for longer than 2 days is not advisable

Cervical ripening:

Gel:

Intracervical: 0.25-1 mg

Intravaginal: 2.5 mg

Suppositories: Intracervical: 2-3 mg

Mechanism of Action A synthetic prostaglandin E$_2$ abortifacient that stimulates uterine contractions similar to those seen during natural labor

Local Anesthetic/Vasoconstrictor Precautions No information available to require special precautions

Effects on Dental Treatment No effects or complications reported

Other Adverse Effects

>10%:

Central nervous system: Headache

Gastrointestinal: Vomiting, diarrhea, nausea

1% to 10%:

Cardiovascular: Bradycardia

Central nervous system: Fever

Neuromuscular & skeletal: Back pain

<1%:

Cardiovascular: Hypotension, cardiac arrhythmias, syncope, flushing, tightness of the chest

Central nervous system: Vasomotor and vasovagal reactions, dizziness, chills, pain

Endocrine & metabolic: Hot flashes

Respiratory: Wheezing, dyspnea, coughing, bronchospasm

Miscellaneous: Shivering

Drug Interactions Increased effect of oxytocics

Drug Uptake

Onset of effect (uterine contractions): Within 10 minutes

Duration: Up to 2-3 hours

Absorption: Vaginal: Slow following administration

Pregnancy Risk Factor X

Dosage Forms

Insert, vaginal (Cervidil®): 10 mg

Gel, endocervical: 0.5 mg in 3 g syringes [each package contains a 10-mm and 20-mm shielded catheter]

Suppository, vaginal: 20 mg

Generic Available No

Dinoprost Tromethamine (DYE noe prost tro METH a meen)

Brand Names Prostin F$_2$ Alpha®

Therapeutic Category Prostaglandin

Synonyms PGF$_{2\alpha}$; Prostaglandin F$_2$ Alpha

Use Abort 2nd trimester pregnancy

Usual Dosage 40 mg (8 mL) via transabdominal tap; if abortion not completed in 24 hours, another 10-40 mg may be administered

Local Anesthetic/Vasoconstrictor Precautions No information available to require special precautions

Effects on Dental Treatment No effects or complications reported

Pregnancy Risk Factor X

Dosage Forms Injection: 5 mg/mL (4 mL, 8 mL)

Generic Available No

Diocto® [OTC] *see* Docusate *on page 331*

Diocto C® [OTC] *see Docusate and Casanthranol on page 331*

Diocto-K® [OTC] *see Docusate on page 331*

Diocto-K Plus® [OTC] *see Docusate and Casanthranol on page 331*

Dioctolose Plus® [OTC] *see Docusate and Casanthranol on page 331*

Dioeze® [OTC] *see Docusate on page 331*

Dioval® Injection *see Estradiol on page 365*

Diovan® *see Valsartan on page 982*

Dipalmitoylphosphatidylcholine *see Colfosceril Palmitate on page 259*

Dipentum® *see Olsalazine on page 699*

Diphen® Cough [OTC] *see Diphenhydramine on this page*

Diphenhist® [OTC] *see Diphenhydramine on this page*

Diphenhydramine (dye fen HYE dra meen)

Related Information

Diphenhydramine and Pseudoephedrine *on next page*
Oral Nonviral Soft Tissue Ulcerations or Erosions *on page 1070*
Oral Viral Infections *on page 1066*
Patients Undergoing Cancer Therapy *on page 1083*

Brand Names AllerMax® Oral [OTC]; Banophen® Oral [OTC]; Belix® Oral [OTC]; Benadryl® Injection; Benadryl® Oral [OTC]; Benadryl® Topical; Ben-Allergin-50® Injection; Benylin® Cough Syrup [OTC]; Bydramine® Cough Syrup [OTC]; Compoz® Gel Caps [OTC]; Compoz® Nighttime Sleep Aid [OTC]; Diphen® Cough [OTC]; Diphenhist® [OTC]; Dormarex® 2 Oral [OTC]; Dormin® Oral [OTC]; Genahist® Oral; Hydramyn® Syrup [OTC]; Hyrexin-50® Injection; Maximum Strength Nytol® [OTC]; Miles Nervine® Caplets [OTC]; Nytol® Oral [OTC]; Phendry® Oral [OTC]; Siladryl® Oral [OTC]; Silphen® Cough [OTC]; Sleep-eze 3® Oral [OTC]; Sleepinal® [OTC]; Sleepwell 2-nite® [OTC]; Sominex® Oral [OTC]; Tusstat® Syrup; Twilite® Oral [OTC]; Uni-Bent® Cough Syrup; 40 Winks® [OTC]

Canadian/Mexican Brand Names Allerdryl (Canada); Allernix (Canada)

Therapeutic Category Antidote, Hypersensitivity Reactions; Antihistamine; Sedative

Use

Dental: Symptomatic relief of allergic symptoms caused by histamine release which include nasal allergies and allergic dermatosis; also to produce local anesthesia through infiltration of mucous membranes

Medical: Can be used for mild nighttime sedation; prevention of motion sickness and as an antitussive; has antinauseant and topical anesthetic properties; treatment of phenothiazine-induced dystonic reactions

Usual Dosage Oral:

Children >10 kg: 12.5-25 mg 3-4 times/day; maximum daily dose: 300 mg
Adults: 25-50 mg every 6-8 hours

Mechanism of Action Competes with histamine for H_1-receptor sites on effector cells in the gastrointestinal tract, blood vessels, and respiratory tract

Local Anesthetic/Vasoconstrictor Precautions No information available to require special precautions

Effects on Dental Treatment Chronic use of antihistamines will inhibit salivary flow, particularly in elderly patients; this may contribute to periodontal disease and oral discomfort

Other Adverse Effects >10%: Central nervous system: Slight to moderate drowsiness

Contraindications Hypersensitivity to diphenhydramine or any component; should not be used in acute attacks of asthma

Warnings/Precautions Use with caution in patients with angle-closure glaucoma, peptic ulcer, urinary tract obstruction, hyperthyroidism; some preparations contain sodium bisulfite; syrup contains alcohol; diphenhydramine has high sedative and anticholinergic properties, so it may not be considered the antihistamine of choice for prolonged use in the elderly

Drug Interactions CNS depressants worsens CNS and respiratory depression, monoamine oxidase inhibitors may cause increased anticholinergic effects; syrup should not be given to patients taking drugs that can cause disulfiram reactions (ie, metronidazole, chlorpropamide) due to high alcohol content

Drug Uptake

Absorption: Oral: 40% to 60% reaches systemic circulation due to first-pass metabolism

Maximum sedative effect: 1-3 hours

Duration of action: 4-7 hours

Serum half-life:
Elderly: 13.5 hours
Adults: 2-8 hours

Time to peak serum concentration: 2-4 hours

(Continued)

323

Diphenhydramine *(Continued)*

Pregnancy Risk Factor C
Breast-feeding Considerations No data reported
Dosage Forms
Capsule, as hydrochloride: 25 mg, 50 mg
Cream, as hydrochloride: 1%, 2%
Elixir, as hydrochloride: 12.5 mg/5 mL (5 mL, 10 mL, 20 mL, 120 mL, 480 mL, 3780 mL)
Injection, as hydrochloride: 10 mg/mL (10 mL, 30 mL); 50 mg/mL (1 mL, 10 mL)
Lotion, as hydrochloride: 1% (75 mL)
Solution, topical spray, as hydrochloride: 1% (60 mL)
Syrup, as hydrochloride: 12.5 mg/5 mL (5 mL, 120 mL, 240 mL, 480 mL, 3780 mL)
Tablet, as hydrochloride: 25 mg, 50 mg
Dietary Considerations May be taken with food or water
Generic Available Yes
Comments 25-50 mg of diphenhydramine orally every 4-6 hours can be used to treat mild dermatologic manifestations of allergic reactions to penicillin and other antibiotics; used as local anesthetic in patients allergic to all other local anesthetics; used for infiltration only; should never be used for block anesthesia because of irritative qualities of vehicle

Diphenhydramine and Pseudoephedrine

(dye fen HYE dra meen & soo doe e FED rin)
Brand Names Actifed® Allergy Tablet (Night) [OTC]; Banophen® Decongestant Capsule [OTC]; Benadryl® Decongestant Allergy Tablet [OTC]
Therapeutic Category Antihistamine/Decongestant Combination
Use Relief of symptoms of upper respiratory mucosal congestion in seasonal and perennial nasal allergies, acute rhinitis, rhinosinusitis, and eustachian tube blockage
Usual Dosage Adults: Oral: 1 capsule or tablet every 4-6 hours, up to 4/day
Local Anesthetic/Vasoconstrictor Precautions Use with caution since pseudoephedrine is a sympathomimetic amine which could interact with epinephrine to cause a pressor response
Effects on Dental Treatment Chronic use of antihistamines will inhibit salivary flow, particularly in elderly patients; this may contribute to periodontal disease and oral discomfort
Other Adverse Effects See individual agents
Drug Interactions See individual agents
Dosage Forms
Capsule: Diphenhydramine hydrochloride 25 mg and pseudoephedrine hydrochloride 60 mg
Tablet:
Actifed® Allergy (Night): Diphenhydramine hydrochloride 25 mg and pseudoephedrine hydrochloride 30 mg
Benadryl® Decongestant Allergy: Diphenhydramine hydrochloride 25 mg and pseudoephedrine hydrochloride 60 mg
Generic Available Yes

Diphenidol *(dye FEN i dole)*

Brand Names Vontrol®
Therapeutic Category Antiemetic
Use Control of nausea and vomiting; peripheral vertigo and associated nausea and vomiting, Ménière's disease, and middle and inner ear surgery
Local Anesthetic/Vasoconstrictor Precautions No information available to require special precautions
Effects on Dental Treatment No effects or complications reported
Other Adverse Effects
>10%: Central nervous system: Drowsiness
1% to 10%:
Central nervous system: Dizziness, headache, nervousness, insomnia
Gastrointestinal: Dry mouth, heartburn
Neuromuscular & skeletal: Weakness
Ocular: Blurred vision
<1%: Central nervous system: Confusion, hallucinations
Pregnancy Risk Factor C
Generic Available No

Diphenoxylate and Atropine *(dye fen OKS i late & A troe peen)*

Brand Names Logen®; Lomanate®; Lomotil®; Lonox®
Therapeutic Category Antidiarrheal

Use Treatment of diarrhea

Usual Dosage Oral:

Children (use with caution in young children due to variable responses): Liquid: 0.3-0.4 mg of diphenoxylate/kg/day in 2-4 divided doses **or**

<2 years: Not recommended

2-5 years: 2 mg of diphenoxylate 3 times/day

5-8 years: 2 mg of diphenoxylate 4 times/day

8-12 years: 2 mg of diphenoxylate 5 times/day

Adults: 15-20 mg/day of diphenoxylate in 3-4 divided doses; maintenance: 5-15 mg/day in 2-3 divided doses

Mechanism of Action Diphenoxylate inhibits excessive GI motility and GI propulsion; commercial preparations contain a subtherapeutic amount of atropine to discourage abuse

Local Anesthetic/Vasoconstrictor Precautions No information available to require special precautions

Effects on Dental Treatment Up to 10% of patients will complain of significant dry mouth and drowsiness. This will disappear with cessation of drug therapy.

Other Adverse Effects

1% to 10%:

Central nervous system: Nervousness, restlessness, dizziness, drowsiness, headache, mental depression

Gastrointestinal: Paralytic ileus, dry mouth

Genitourinary: Urinary retention, dysuria

Ocular: Blurred vision

Respiratory: Respiratory depression

<1%:

Cardiovascular: Tachycardia

Central nervous system: Sedation, euphoria, hyperthermia

Dermatologic: Pruritus, urticaria

Gastrointestinal: Nausea, vomiting, abdominal discomfort, pancreatitis, stomach cramps

Neuromuscular & skeletal: Muscle cramps, weakness

Miscellaneous: Increased sweating

Drug Interactions Increased toxicity: MAO inhibitors (hypertensive crisis), CNS depressants, antimuscarinics (paralytic ileus); may prolong half-life of drugs metabolized in liver

Drug Uptake

Onset of action: Within 45-60 minutes

Duration: 3-4 hours

Absorption: Oral: Well absorbed

Serum half-life: Diphenoxylate: 2.5 hours

Time to peak serum concentration: 2 hours

Pregnancy Risk Factor C

Generic Available Yes

Diphenylan Sodium® see Phenytoin on page 756

Diphtheria CRM₁₉₇ Protein Conjugate see Haemophilus b Conjugate Vaccine on page 460

Diphtheria Toxoid Conjugate see Haemophilus b Conjugate Vaccine on page 460

Dipiridamol (Mexico) see Dipyridamole on next page

Dipivefrin (dye PI ve frin)

Brand Names AKPro® Ophthalmic; Propine® Ophthalmic

Therapeutic Category Adrenergic Agonist Agent, Ophthalmic; Antiglaucoma Agent; Ophthalmic Agent, Vasoconstrictor

Use Reduces elevated intraocular pressure in chronic open-angle glaucoma; also used to treat ocular hypertension, low tension, and secondary glaucomas

Usual Dosage Adults: Ophthalmic: Instill 1 drop every 12 hours into the eyes

Mechanism of Action Dipivefrin is a prodrug of epinephrine which is the active agent that stimulates alpha- and/or beta-adrenergic receptors increasing aqueous humor outflow

Local Anesthetic/Vasoconstrictor Precautions No information available to require special precautions

Effects on Dental Treatment No effects or complications reported

Other Adverse Effects

1% to 10%:

Central nervous system: Headache

Local: Burning, stinging

Ocular: Ocular congestion, photophobia, mydriasis, blurred vision, ocular pain, bulbar conjunctival follicles, blepharoconjunctivitis, cystoid macular edema

<1%: Cardiovascular: Arrhythmias, hypertension

(Continued)

Dipivefrin *(Continued)*

Drug Interactions Increased or synergistic effect when used with other agents to lower intraocular pressure

Drug Uptake

Ocular pressure effect:
Onset of action: Within 30 minutes
Duration: ≥12 hours
Mydriasis:
Onset of action: May occur within 30 minutes
Duration: Several hours
Absorption: Rapid into the aqueous humor

Pregnancy Risk Factor B

Generic Available Yes

Diprivan® Injection *see* Propofol *on page 809*

Diprolene® *see* Betamethasone *on page 126*

Diprolene® AF *see* Betamethasone *on page 126*

Diprosone® *see* Betamethasone *on page 126*

Dipyridamole *(dye peer ID a mole)*

Brand Names Persantine®

Canadian/Mexican Brand Names Apo®-Dipyridamole FC (Canada); Apo®-Dipyridamole SC (Canada); Dirinol® (Mexico); Lodimol® (Mexico); Novo-Dipiradol® (Canada); Trompersantin® (Mexico)

Therapeutic Category Antiplatelet Agent

Synonyms Dipiridamol (Mexico)

Use Maintains patency after surgical grafting procedures including coronary artery bypass; used with warfarin to decrease thrombosis in patients after artificial heart valve replacement; used with aspirin to prevent coronary artery thrombosis; in combination with aspirin or warfarin to prevent other thromboembolic disorders. Dipyridamole may also be given 2 days prior to open heart surgery to prevent platelet activation by extracorporeal bypass pump and as a diagnostic agent in CAD.

Usual Dosage

Oral:
Children: 3-6 mg/kg/day in 3 divided doses
Doses of 4-10 mg/kg/day have been used investigationally to treat proteinuria in pediatric renal disease
Adults: 75-400 mg/day in 3-4 divided doses
I.V.: 0.14 mg/kg/minute for 4 minutes; maximum dose: 60 mg

Mechanism of Action Inhibits the activity of adenosine deaminase and phosphodiesterase, which causes an accumulation of adenosine, adenine nucleotides, and cyclic AMP; these mediators then inhibit platelet aggregation and may cause vasodilation; may also stimulate release of prostacyclin or PGD_2; causes coronary vasodilation

Local Anesthetic/Vasoconstrictor Precautions No information available to require special precautions

Effects on Dental Treatment No effects or complications reported

Other Adverse Effects

>10%:
Cardiovascular: Exacerbation of angina pectoris
Central nervous system: Dizziness
1% to 10%:
Cardiovascular: Hypotension, hypertension, tachycardia
Central nervous system: Headache
Dermatologic: Rash
Gastrointestinal: Abdominal distress
Respiratory: Dyspnea
<1%:
Cardiovascular: Vasodilatation, flushing, syncope, edema
Central nervous system: Migraine
Neuromuscular & skeletal: Hypertonia, weakness
Respiratory: Rhinitis, hyperventilation, pleural pain
Miscellaneous: Allergic reaction

Drug Interactions No data reported

Drug Uptake

Absorption: Readily absorbed from GI tract but variable
Serum half-life, terminal: 10-12 hours
Time to peak serum concentration: 2-2.5 hours

Pregnancy Risk Factor C

Generic Available Yes

Dirithromycin (dye RITH roe mye sin)

Brand Names Dynabac®

Therapeutic Category Antibiotic, Macrolide

Use Treatment of mild to moderate upper and lower respiratory tract infections, infections of the skin and skin structure, and sexually transmitted diseases due to susceptible strains

Usual Dosage Adults: Oral: 500 mg once daily for 7-14 days (14 days required for treatment of community-acquired pneumonia due to *Legionella, Mycoplasma,* or *S. pneumoniae;* 10 days is recommended for treatment of *S. pyogenes* pharyngitis/tonsillitis)

Mechanism of Action After being converted during intestinal absorption to its active form, erthromycylamine, dirithromycin inhibits protein synthesis by binding to the 50S ribosomal subunits of susceptible microorganisms

Local Anesthetic/Vasoconstrictor Precautions No information available to require special precautions

Effects on Dental Treatment No effects or complications reported

Other Adverse Effects

Central nervous system: Headache, dizziness

Dermatologic: Skin rash, urticaria

Gastrointestinal: Abdominal pain, nausea, diarrhea, vomiting, dyspepsia, flatulence

Hepatic: Elevated LFTs, alkaline phosphatase

Neuromuscular & skeletal: Weakness

Renal: Nephrotoxicity

Contraindications Hypersensitivity to any macrolide or component of dirithromycin; the FDA has issued a contraindication with pimozide (Orap®), clarithromycin, and other macrolide antibiotics

Warnings/Precautions Contrary to potential serious consequences with other macrolides (eg, cardiac arrhythmias), the combination of terfenadine and dirithromycin has not shown alteration of terfenadine metabolism; however, caution should be taken during coadministration of dirithromycin and terfenadine

Drug Interactions Increased effect: Absorption of dirithromycin is slightly enhanced with concomitant antacids and H_2 antagonists; dirithromycin may, like erythromycin, increase the effect of alfentanil, anticoagulants, bromocriptine, carbamazepine, cyclosporine, digoxin, disopyramide, ergots, methylprednisolone, and triazolam

Drug Uptake

Absorption: Rapidly absorbed and nonenzymatically hydrolyzed to erythromycylamine; T_{max}: 4 hours

Serum half-life: 8 hours (range: 2-36 hours)

Pregnancy Risk Factor C

Dosage Forms Tablet, enteric coated: 250 mg

Generic Available No

Selected Readings

"Pimozide (Orap) Contraindicated With Clarithromycin (Biaxin) and Other Macrolide Antibiotics," *FDA Medical Bulletin,* October 1996, 3.

Disalcid® *see* Salsalate *on page 855*

Disanthrol® [OTC] *see* Docusate and Casanthranol *on page 331*

Disobrom® [OTC] *see* Dexbrompheniramine and Pseudoephedrine *on page 292*

Disonate® [OTC] *see* Docusate *on page 331*

Disophrol® Chronotabs® [OTC] *see* Dexbrompheniramine and Pseudoephedrine *on page 292*

Disophrol® Tablet [OTC] *see* Dexbrompheniramine and Pseudoephedrine *on page 292*

Disopiramida (Mexico) *see* Disopyramide *on this page*

Disopyramide (dye soe PEER a mide)

Related Information

Cardiovascular Diseases *on page 1010*

Brand Names Norpace®

Canadian/Mexican Brand Names Dimodan® (Mexico)

Therapeutic Category Antiarrhythmic Agent, Class I-A; Antiarrhythmic Agent (Supraventricular & Ventricular)

Synonyms Disopiramida (Mexico)

Use Suppression and prevention of unifocal and multifocal premature, ventricular premature complexes, coupled ventricular tachycardia; effective in the conversion of atrial fibrillation, atrial flutter, and paroxysmal atrial tachycardia to normal sinus rhythm and prevention of the reoccurrence of these arrhythmias after conversion by other methods

(Continued)

Disopyramide *(Continued)*

Usual Dosage Oral:

Children:

<1 year: 10-30 mg/kg/24 hours in 4 divided doses

1-4 years: 10-20 mg/kg/24 hours in 4 divided doses

4-12 years: 10-15 mg/kg/24 hours in 4 divided doses

12-18 years: 6-15 mg/kg/24 hours in 4 divided doses

Adults:

<50 kg: 100 mg every 6 hours or 200 mg every 12 hours (controlled release)

>50 kg: 150 mg every 6 hours or 300 mg every 12 hours (controlled release); if no response, may increase to 200 mg every 6 hours; maximum dose required for patients with severe refractory ventricular tachycardia is 400 mg every 6 hours

Mechanism of Action Class IA antiarrhythmic: Decreases myocardial excitability and conduction velocity; reduces disparity in refractory between normal and infarcted myocardium; possesses anticholinergic, peripheral vasoconstrictive, and negative inotropic effects

Local Anesthetic/Vasoconstrictor Precautions No information available to require special precautions

Effects on Dental Treatment No effects or complications reported

Other Adverse Effects

>10%: Genitourinary: Urinary retention/hesitancy

1% to 10%:

Cardiovascular: Chest pains, congestive heart failure, hypotension

Endocrine & metabolic: Hypokalemia

Gastrointestinal: Stomach pain, bloating, dry mouth

Neuromuscular & skeletal: Muscle weakness

Ocular: Blurred vision

<1%:

Cardiovascular: Syncope and conduction disturbances including A-V block, widening QRS complex and lengthening of Q-T interval

Central nervous system: Fatigue, malaise, nervousness, acute psychosis, depression, dizziness, headache, pain

Dermatologic: Generalized rashes

Endocrine & metabolic: Hypoglycemia, may initiate contractions of pregnant uterus, hyperkalemia may enhance toxicities, elevated cholesterol and triglycerides

Gastrointestinal: Constipation, nausea, vomiting, diarrhea, gas, anorexia, weight gain

Hepatic: Hepatic cholestasis, elevated liver enzymes

Neuromuscular & skeletal: Weakness

Ocular: Dry eyes

Respiratory: Dyspnea, dry nose, throat

Drug Interactions

Decreased effect with hepatic microsomal enzyme-inducing agents (ie, phenytoin, phenobarbital, rifampin)

Increased effect/levels/toxicity with erythromycin; increased levels of digoxin

Drug Uptake

Onset of action: 0.5-3.5 hours

Duration of effect: 1.5-8.5 hours

Absorption: 60% to 83%

Serum half-life: Adults: 4-10 hours, increased half-life with hepatic or renal disease

Pregnancy Risk Factor C

Generic Available Yes

Disotate® *see* Edetate Disodium *on page 345*

Di-Spaz® Injection *see* Dicyclomine *on page 307*

Di-Spaz® Oral *see* Dicyclomine *on page 307*

Disulfiram *(dye SUL fi ram)*

Brand Names Antabuse®

Therapeutic Category Aldehyde Dehydrogenase Inhibitor Agent; Antialcoholic Agent

Use Management of chronic alcoholism

Usual Dosage Adults: Oral: Do not administer until the patient has abstained from alcohol for at least 12 hours

Initial: 500 mg/day as a single dose for 1-2 weeks; maximum daily dose is 500 mg

Average maintenance dose: 250 mg/day; range: 125-500 mg; duration of therapy is to continue until the patient is fully recovered socially and a basis for permanent self control has been established; maintenance therapy may be required for months or even years

Mechanism of Action Disulfiram is a thiuram derivative which interferes with aldehyde dehydrogenase. When taken concomitantly with alcohol, there is an increase in serum acetaldehyde levels. High acetaldehyde causes uncomfortable symptoms including flushing, nausea, thirst, palpitations, chest pain, vertigo, and hypotension. This reaction is the basis for disulfiram use in postwithdrawal long-term care of alcoholism.

Local Anesthetic/Vasoconstrictor Precautions No information available to require special precautions

Effects on Dental Treatment No effects or complications reported

Other Adverse Effects
>10%: Central nervous system: Drowsiness
1% to 10%:
Central nervous system: Headache, fatigue, mood changes, neurotoxicity
Dermatologic: Skin rash
Gastrointestinal: Metallic or garlic-like aftertaste
Genitourinary: Impotence
<1%:
Endocrine & metabolic: Disulfiram reaction with alcohol (flushing, sweating, cardiovascular collapse, myocardial infarction, vertigo, seizures, headache, nausea, vomiting, dyspnea, chest pain, death)
Hepatic: Hepatitis, encephalopathy

Drug Interactions
Increased effect: Diazepam, chlordiazepoxide
Increased toxicity:
Alcohol and disulfiram: Antabuse® reaction
Tricyclic antidepressants, metronidazole, isoniazid: Encephalopathy
Disulfiram has caused increases in serum levels of phenytoin and warfarin leading to phenytoin toxicity and enhanced anticoagulation

Drug Uptake
Full effect: 12 hours
Duration: May persist for 1-2 weeks after last dose
Absorption: Rapid from GI tract

Pregnancy Risk Factor C
Generic Available Yes

Ditropan® see Oxybutynin on page 709

Diucardin® see Hydroflumethiazide on page 485

Diupres-250® see Chlorothiazide and Reserpine on page 216

Diupres-500® see Chlorothiazide and Reserpine on page 216

Diurigen® see Chlorothiazide on page 215

Diuril® see Chlorothiazide on page 215

Dizac® Injection see Diazepam on page 300

Dizmiss® [OTC] see Meclizine on page 584

DNR see Daunorubicin Hydrochloride on page 283

Doan's®, Original [OTC] see Magnesium Salicylate on page 577

Dobutamina, Clorhidrato De (Mexico) see Dobutamine on this page

Dobutamine (doe BYOO ta meen)
Brand Names Dobutrex®
Canadian/Mexican Brand Names Dobuject® (Mexico); Oxiken® (Mexico)
Therapeutic Category Adrenergic Agonist Agent
Synonyms Dobutamina, Clorhidrato De (Mexico)

Infusion Rates of Various Dilutions of Dobutamine

Desired Delivery Rate (mcg/kg/min)	Infusion Rate (mL/kg/min)	
	500 mcg/mL*	1000 mcg/mL†
2.5	0.005	0.0025
5.0	0.01	0.005
7.5	0.015	0.0075
10.0	0.02	0.01
12.5	0.025	0.0125
15.0	0.03	0.015

* 500 mg per liter or 250 mg per 500 mL of diluent.

†1000 mg per liter or 250 mg per 250 mL of diluent.

(Continued)

Dobutamine *(Continued)*

Use Short-term management of patients with cardiac decompensation

Usual Dosage I.V. infusion:

Children: 2.5-15 mcg/kg/minute, titrate to desired response

Adults: 2.5-15 mcg/kg/minute; maximum: 40 mcg/kg/minute, titrate to desired response

Mechanism of Action Stimulates beta$_1$-adrenergic receptors, causing increased contractility and heart rate, with little effect on beta$_2$- or alpha-receptors

Local Anesthetic/Vasoconstrictor Precautions No information available to require special precautions

Effects on Dental Treatment No effects or complications reported

Other Adverse Effects

>10%:

Cardiovascular: Ectopic heartbeats, tachycardia, chest pain, angina, palpitations, hypertension; in higher doses ventricular tachycardia or arrhythmias may be seen; patients with atrial fibrillation or flutter are at risk of developing a rapid ventricular response

1% to 10%:

Cardiovascular: Premature ventricular beats, chest pain, angina, palpitations

Central nervous system: Headache

Gastrointestinal: Nausea, vomiting

Neuromuscular & skeletal: Mild leg cramps, paresthesia

Respiratory: Dyspnea

Drug Interactions

Decreased effect: Beta-adrenergic blockers (increased peripheral resistance)

Increased toxicity: General anesthetics (ie, halothane or cyclopropane) and usual doses of dobutamine have resulted in ventricular arrhythmias in animals

Drug Uptake

Onset of action: I.V.: 1-10 minutes

Serum half-life: 2 minutes

Pregnancy Risk Factor C

Generic Available Yes

Dobutrex® *see Dobutamine on previous page*

Docetaxel *(doe se TAKS el)*

Brand Names Taxotere®

Therapeutic Category Antineoplastic Agent, Miscellaneous

Use FDA-approved: Treatment of patients with locally advanced or metastatic breast cancer who have progressed during anthracycline-based therapy or have relapsed during anthracycline-based adjuvant therapy

Investigational: Treatment of nonsmall cell lung cancer, gastric, pancreatic, head and neck, ovarian, soft tissue sarcoma, and melanoma

Usual Dosage Adults: I.V.: 60-100 mg/m^2 administered over 1 hour every 3 weeks

Local Anesthetic/Vasoconstrictor Precautions No information available to require special precautions

Effects on Dental Treatment No effects or complications reported

Other Adverse Effects

Irritant chemotherapy

>10%:

Central nervous system: Fever

Dermatologic: Alopecia

Gastrointestinal: Nausea, vomiting, diarrhea, stomatitis

Hematologic: Neutropenia, leukopenia, thrombocytopenia, anemia

Neuromuscular & skeletal: Myalgia

1% to 10%: Cardiovascular: Severe fluid retention: poorly tolerated peripheral edema, generalized edema, pleural effusion requiring urgent drainage, dyspnea at rest, cardiac tamponade or pronounced abdominal distention (due to ascites)

>1%: Miscellaneous: Hypersensitivity reactions

Drug Interactions Cytochrome P-450 substrate

Increased toxicity: Possibility of an inhibition of metabolism in patients treated with ketoconazole, erythromycin, and cyclosporine

Drug Uptake Administered by I.V. infusion and exhibits linear pharmacokinetics at the recommended dosage range

Half-lifes: α, β, and γ phases are 4 minutes, 36 minutes, and 11.1 hours, respectively

Pregnancy Risk Factor D

Dosage Forms Injection: 40 mg/mL (0.5 mL, 2 mL)

Generic Available No

Docusate (DOK yoo sate)
Brand Names Colace® [OTC]; DC 240® Softgels® [OTC]; Dialose® [OTC]; Diocto® [OTC]; Diocto-K® [OTC]; Dioeze® [OTC]; Disonate® [OTC]; DOK® [OTC]; DOS® Softgel® [OTC]; D-S-S® [OTC]; Kasof® [OTC]; Modane® Soft [OTC]; Pro-Cal-Sof® [OTC]; Regulax SS® [OTC]; Sulfalax® [OTC]; Surfak® [OTC]

Canadian/Mexican Brand Names Albert Docusate® (Canada); Colax-C® (Canada); PMS-Docusate Calcium® (Canada)

Therapeutic Category Laxative, Surfactant; Stool Softener

Use Stool softener in patients who should avoid straining during defecation and constipation associated with hard, dry stools; prophylaxis for straining (Valsalva) following myocardial infarction. A safe agent to be used in elderly; some evidence that doses <200 mg are ineffective; stool softeners are unnecessary if stool is well hydrated or "mushy" and soft; shown to be ineffective used long-term.

Usual Dosage Docusate salts are interchangeable; the amount of sodium, calcium, or potassium per dosage unit is clinically insignificant

Children <3 years: Oral: 10-40 mg/day in 1-4 divided doses
Children: Oral:
   3-6 years: 20-60 mg/day in 1-4 divided doses
   6-12 years: 40-150 mg/day in 1-4 divided doses
Adolescents and Adults: Oral: 50-500 mg/day in 1-4 divided doses
Older Children and Adults: Rectal: Add 50-100 mg of docusate liquid to enema fluid (saline or water); give as retention or flushing enema

Mechanism of Action Reduces surface tension of the oil-water interface of the stool resulting in enhanced incorporation of water and fat allowing for stool softening

Local Anesthetic/Vasoconstrictor Precautions No information available to require special precautions

Effects on Dental Treatment No effects or complications reported

Other Adverse Effects 1% to 10%: Gastrointestinal: Intestinal obstruction, diarrhea, abdominal cramping, throat irritation

Drug Interactions
   Decreased effect of Coumadin®, aspirin
   Increased toxicity with mineral oil

Drug Uptake Onset of action: 12-72 hours

Pregnancy Risk Factor C

Generic Available Yes

Docusate and Casanthranol (DOK yoo sate & ka SAN thra nole)
Brand Names Dialose® Plus Capsule [OTC]; Diocto C® [OTC]; Diocto-K Plus® [OTC]; Dioctolose Plus® [OTC]; Disanthrol® [OTC]; DSMC Plus® [OTC]; Genasoft® Plus [OTC]; Peri-Colace® [OTC]; Pro-Sof® Plus [OTC]; Regulace® [OTC]; Silace-C® [OTC]

Therapeutic Category Laxative, Surfactant; Stool Softener

Synonyms Casanthranol and Docusate; DSS With Casanthranol

Use Treatment of constipation generally associated with dry, hard stools and decreased intestinal motility

Local Anesthetic/Vasoconstrictor Precautions No information available to require special precautions

Effects on Dental Treatment No effects or complications reported

Other Adverse Effects 1% to 10%:
   Dermatologic: Rash
   Gastrointestinal: Intestinal obstruction, diarrhea, abdominal cramping, throat irritation

Pregnancy Risk Factor C

Generic Available Yes

DOK® [OTC] see Docusate on this page

Dolacet® [5/500] see Hydrocodone and Acetaminophen on page 478

Dolasetron (dol A se tron)
Brand Names Anzemet®
Therapeutic Category Antiemetic
Synonyms Dolasetron Mesylate
Use
   Oral: The prevention of nausea and vomiting associated with moderately-emetogenic cancer chemotherapy, including initial and repeat courses; the prevention of postoperative nausea and vomiting.
   Parenteral: The prevention of nausea and vomiting associated with initial and repeat courses of emetogenic cancer chemotherapy, including high dose cisplatin; the prevention of postoperative nausea and vomiting; as with other
(Continued)

Dolasetron *(Continued)*

antiemetics, routine prophylaxis is not recommended for patients in whom there is little expectation that nausea and/or vomiting will occur postoperatively; in patients where nausea and/or vomiting must be avoided postoperatively; injection is recommended even where the incidence of postoperative nausea and/or vomiting is low; the treatment of postoperative nausea and/or vomiting

Mechanism of Action Dolasetron is a pseudopelletierine derived serotonin antagonist. Serotonin antagonists block the serotonin receptors in the chemoreceptor trigger zone and in the gastrointestinal tract. Once the receptor site is blocked, antagonism of the chemotherapy induced nausea and vomiting that occurs.

Local Anesthetic/Vasoconstrictor Precautions No information available to require special precautions

Effects on Dental Treatment No effects or complications reported

Comments A single I.V. dose of dolasetron mesylate (1.8 or 2.4 mg/kg) has comparable safety and efficacy to a single 32-mg IV dose of ondansetron in patients receiving cisplatin chemotherapy.

Dolasetron Mesylate *see* Dolasetron *on previous page*

Dolene® *see* Propoxyphene *on page 811*

Dolobid® *see* Diflunisal *on page 311*

Dolophine® *see* Methadone *on page 608*

Dolorac® [OTC] *see* Capsaicin *on page 170*

Domeboro® Topical [OTC] *see* Aluminum Sulfate and Calcium Acetate *on page 49*

Dome Paste Bandage *see* Zinc Gelatin *on page 1004*

Donepezil *(don EH pa zil)*

Brand Names Aricept®

Therapeutic Category Acetylcholinesterase Inhibitor

Use Treatment of mild to moderate dementia of the Alzheimer's type

Usual Dosage Adults: Initial: 5 mg/day at bedtime; may increase to 10 mg/day at bedtime after 4-6 weeks

Local Anesthetic/Vasoconstrictor Precautions No information available to require special precautions

Effects on Dental Treatment No effects or complications reported

Other Adverse Effects

>10%:

Central nervous system: Headache

Gastrointestinal: Nausea, diarrhea

1% to 10%:

Cardiovascular: Syncope, chest pain

Central nervous system: Fatigue, insomnia, dizziness, depression, abnormal dreams, somnolence

Dermatologic: Bruising

Gastrointestinal: Anorexia, vomiting, weight loss

Genitourinary: Polyuria

Neuromuscular & skeletal: Muscle cramps, arthritis, body pain

Warnings/Precautions Use with caution in patients with sick sinus syndrome or other supraventricular cardiac conduction abnormalities, in patients with seizures or asthma; avoid use in nursing mothers

Drug Interactions Increased effects of succinylcholine, cholinesterase inhibitors, or cholinergic agonists (bethanechol). Concomitant NSAIDs may increase the risk of gastrointestinal bleeding.

Pregnancy Risk Factor C

Dosage Forms Tablet: 5 mg, 10 mg

Generic Available No

Donnamar® *see* Hyoscyamine *on page 492*

Donnapectolin-PG® *see* Hyoscyamine, Atropine, Scopolamine, Kaolin, Pectin, and Opium *on page 494*

Donnatal® *see* Hyoscyamine, Atropine, Scopolamine, and Phenobarbital *on page 493*

Donnazyme® *see* Pancreatin *on page 721*

Dopar® *see* Levodopa *on page 547*

Dopram® Injection *see* Doxapram *on page 334*

Doral® *see* Quazepam *on page 826*

Dormarex® 2 Oral [OTC] *see* Diphenhydramine *on page 323*

Dormin® Oral [OTC] *see* Diphenhydramine *on page 323*

Dornase Alfa (DOOR nase AL fa)

Brand Names Pulmozyme®

Therapeutic Category Enzyme

Use Management of cystic fibrosis patients to reduce the frequency of respiratory infections that require parenteral antibiotics, and to improve pulmonary function

Usual Dosage Children >5 years and Adults: Inhalation: 2.5 mg once daily through selected nebulizers in conjunction with a Pulmo-Aide® or a Pari-Proneb® compressor

Mechanism of Action The hallmark of cystic fibrosis lung disease is the presence of abundant, purulent airway secretions composed primarily of highly polymerized DNA. The principal source of this DNA is the nuclei of degenerating neutrophils, which is present in large concentrations in infected lung secretions. The presence of this DNA produces a viscous mucous that may contribute to the decreased mucociliary transport and persistent infections that are commonly seen in this population. Dornase alfa is a deoxyribonuclease (DNA) enzyme produced by recombinant gene technology. Dornase selectively cleaves DNA, thus reducing mucous viscosity and as a result, airflow in the lung is improved and the risk of bacterial infection may be decreased.

Local Anesthetic/Vasoconstrictor Precautions No information available to require special precautions

Effects on Dental Treatment No effects or complications reported

Other Adverse Effects

>10%:
  Respiratory: Pharyngitis
  Miscellaneous: Voice alteration
1% to 10%:
  Cardiovascular: Chest pain
  Dermatologic: Rash
  Ocular: Conjunctivitis
  Respiratory: Laryngitis, cough, dyspnea, hemoptysis, rhinitis, hoarse throat, wheezing

Drug Interactions No data reported

Drug Uptake Following nebulization, enzyme levels are measurable in the sputum within 15 minutes and decline rapidly thereafter

Pregnancy Risk Factor B

Generic Available No

Doryx® *see Doxycycline on page 338*

Dorzolamide (dor ZOLE a mide)

Brand Names Trusopt®

Therapeutic Category Antiglaucoma Agent; Carbonic Anhydrase Inhibitor

Use Lower intraocular pressure to treat glaucoma

Usual Dosage Adults: Glaucoma: Instill 1 drop in the affected eye(s) 3 times/day

Local Anesthetic/Vasoconstrictor Precautions No information available to require special precautions

Effects on Dental Treatment No effects or complications reported

Other Adverse Effects

Central nervous system: Headache, fatigue (infrequent)
Dermatologic: Rash
Gastrointestinal: Bitter taste (~25%), nausea
Genitourinary: Urolithiasis
Neuromuscular & skeletal: Weakness (infrequent)
Ocular: Burning, stinging, or discomfort immediately following administration (~33%); iridocyclitis (rare); superficial punctate keratitis (10% to 15%); signs and symptoms of ocular allergic reaction (~10%); blurred vision, tearing, dryness (1% to 5%); photophobia (~1% to 5%)

Drug Uptake

Peak effect: 2 hours
Duration: 8-12 hours
Absorption: Systemically absorbed, however, detailed absorption characteristics and pharmacokinetic data are unavailable
Serum half-life: Terminal RBC half-life of 147 days

Pregnancy Risk Factor C

Generic Available No

DOS® Softgel® [OTC] *see Docusate on page 331*

Dostinex® *see Cabergoline on page 158*

Dovonex® *see Calcipotriene on page 160*

Doxapram (DOKS a pram)

Brand Names Dopram® Injection

Therapeutic Category Central Nervous System Stimulant, Nonamphetamine; Respiratory Stimulant

Use Respiratory and CNS stimulant; idiopathic apnea of prematurity refractory to xanthines

Usual Dosage Not for use in newborns since doxapram contains a significant amount of benzyl alcohol (0.9%)

Neonatal apnea (apnea of prematurity): I.V.:
Initial: 1-1.5 mg/kg/hour
Maintenance: 0.5-2.5 mg/kg/hour, titrated to the lowest rate at which apnea is controlled

Adults: Respiratory depression following anesthesia: I.V.:
Initial: 0.5-1 mg/kg; may repeat at 5-minute intervals; maximum total dose: 2 mg/kg
I.V. infusion: Initial: 5 mg/minute until adequate response or adverse effects seen; decrease to 1-3 mg/minute; usual total dose: 0.5-4 mg/kg; maximum: 300 mg

Not dialyzable

Mechanism of Action Stimulates respiration through action on respiratory center in medulla or indirectly on peripheral carotid chemoreceptors

Local Anesthetic/Vasoconstrictor Precautions No information available to require special precautions

Effects on Dental Treatment No effects or complications reported

Other Adverse Effects

1% to 10%:
Cardiovascular: Ectopic beats, hypotension, vasoconstriction, tachycardia, anginal pain, palpitations
Central nervous system: Headache
Gastrointestinal: Nausea, vomiting
Respiratory: Dyspnea

<1%:
Cardiovascular: Hypertension (dose related), arrhythmias, flushing
Central nervous system: CNS stimulation, restlessness, lightheadedness, jitters, hallucinations, irritability, seizures, extremely high fever
Gastrointestinal: Abdominal distention, retching
Hematologic: Hemolysis
Local: Phlebitis
Neuromuscular & skeletal: Tremor, hyper-reflexia
Ocular: Mydriasis, lacrimation
Respiratory: Coughing, laryngospasm
Miscellaneous: Sweating, feeling of warmth

Drug Uptake
Onset of action (respiratory stimulation): I.V.: Within 20-40 seconds
Peak effect: Within 1-2 minutes
Duration: 5-12 minutes
Serum half-life: Adults: 3.4 hours (mean half-life)

Pregnancy Risk Factor B

Generic Available No

Comments Initial studies suggest a therapeutic range of at least 1.5 mg/L; toxicity becomes frequent at serum levels >5 mg/L

Doxazosin (doks AYE zoe sin)

Related Information
Cardiovascular Diseases *on page 1010*

Brand Names Cardura®

Therapeutic Category Alpha-Adrenergic Blockers - Peripheral-Acting (Alpha$_1$-Blockers)

Use Treatment of hypertension, severe congestive heart failure (in conjunction with diuretics and cardiac glycosides)

Unlabeled use: Symptoms of benign prostatic hypertrophy

Usual Dosage Oral:
Adults: 1 mg once daily in morning or evening; may be increased to 2 mg once daily; thereafter titrate upwards, if needed, over several weeks, balancing therapeutic benefit with doxazosin-induced postural hypotension; maximum dose for hypertension: 16 mg/day, for BPH: 8 mg/day
Elderly: Initial: 0.5 mg once daily

Mechanism of Action Competitively inhibits postsynaptic alpha-adrenergic receptors which results in vasodilation of veins and arterioles and a decrease in total peripheral resistance and blood pressure; approximately 50% as potent on a weight by weight basis as prazosin

Local Anesthetic/Vasoconstrictor Precautions No information available to require special precautions

Effects on Dental Treatment No effects or complications reported

Other Adverse Effects
>10%: Central nervous system: Dizziness
1% to 10%:
Cardiovascular: Palpitations, arrhythmia
Central nervous system: Vertigo, nervousness, somnolence, anxiety
Endocrine & metabolic: Decreased libido
Gastrointestinal: Nausea, vomiting, dry mouth, diarrhea, constipation
Neuromuscular & skeletal: Shoulder, neck, back pain
Ocular: Abnormal vision
Respiratory: Rhinitis
<1%:
Cardiovascular: Hypotension, tachycardia
Central nervous system: Depression
Gastrointestinal: Abdominal discomfort, flatulence
Genitourinary: Incontinence
Ocular: Conjunctivitis
Otic: Tinnitus
Renal: Polyuria
Respiratory: Dyspnea, sinusitis, epistaxis

Drug Interactions Increased effect with diuretics and antihypertensive medications (especially beta-blockers)

Pregnancy Risk Factor B

Generic Available No

Doxepin (DOKS e pin)

Brand Names Adapin®; Sinequan®

Canadian/Mexican Brand Names Apo®-Doxepin (Canada); Novo-Doxepin® (Canada); Triadapin® (Canada)

Therapeutic Category Antianxiety Agent; Antidepressant, Tricyclic; Tranquilizer, Minor

Use Treatment of various forms of depression, usually in conjunction with psychotherapy; treatment of anxiety disorders; analgesic for certain chronic and neuropathic pain

Usual Dosage
Oral (entire daily dose may be given at bedtime):
Adolescents: Initial: 25-50 mg/day in single or divided doses; gradually increase to 100 mg/day

Adults: Initial: 30-150 mg/day at bedtime or in 2-3 divided doses; may gradually increase up to 300 mg/day; single dose should not exceed 150 mg; select patients may respond to 25-50 mg/day

Mechanism of Action Increases the synaptic concentration of serotonin and/or norepinephrine in the central nervous system by inhibition of their reuptake by the presynaptic neuronal membrane

Local Anesthetic/Vasoconstrictor Precautions Use with caution; epinephrine, norepinephrine and levonordefrin have been shown to have an increased pressor response in combination with TCAs

Effects on Dental Treatment >10% of patients experience dry mouth; long-term treatment with TCAs increases the risk of caries by reducing salivation and salivary buffer capacity

Other Adverse Effects
>10%:
Central nervous system: Sedation, drowsiness, dizziness, headache
Gastrointestinal: Constipation, increased appetite, nausea, unpleasant taste, weight gain
1% to 10%:
Cardiovascular: Hypotension, arrhythmias
Central nervous system: Confusion, delirium, hallucinations, nervousness, restlessness, parkinsonian syndrome, insomnia
Endocrine & metabolic: Sexual dysfunction
Gastrointestinal: Diarrhea, heartburn
Genitourinary: Dysuria
Neuromuscular & skeletal: Fine muscle tremors, weakness
Ocular: Blurred vision, eye pain
Miscellaneous: Excessive sweating
<1%:
Central nervous system: Anxiety, seizures
(Continued)

Doxepin *(Continued)*

Dermatologic: Alopecia, dermal photosensitivity

Endocrine & metabolic: Breast enlargement, galactorrhea, SIADH

Gastrointestinal: Trouble with gums, decreased lower esophageal sphincter tone may cause GE reflux

Genitourinary: Urinary retention, testicular swelling

Hematologic: Agranulocytosis, leukopenia, eosinophilia

Hepatic: Hepatitis, cholestatic jaundice and elevated liver enzymes

Ocular: Increased intraocular pressure

Otic: Tinnitus

Miscellaneous: Allergic reactions

Drug Interactions

Decreased effect: Phenobarbital may increase the metabolism of doxepin; doxepin blocks the uptake of guanethidine and thus prevents the hypotensive effect of guanethidine

Increased toxicity: Clonidine causes hypertensive crisis; doxepin may be additive with or may potentiate the action of other CNS depressants such as sedatives or hypnotics; with MAO inhibitors, hyperpyrexia, hypertension, tachycardia, confusion, and seizures. Doxepin may increase the prothrombin time in patients stabilized on warfarin; doxepin may potentiate the pressor and cardiac effects of sympathomimetic agents such as isoproterenol, epinephrine, etc; cimetidine and methylphenidate may decrease the metabolism of doxepin

Additive anticholinergic effects seen with other anticholinergic agents

Drug Uptake

Serum half-life: Adults: 6-8 hours

Pregnancy Risk Factor C (oral); (B topical)

Generic Available Yes

Selected Readings

Boakes AJ, Laurence DR, Teoh PC, et al, "Interactions Between Sympathomimetic Amines and Antidepressant Agents in Man," *Br Med J*, 1973, 1(849):311-5.

Jastak JT and Yagiela JA, "Vasoconstrictors and Local Anesthesia: A Review and Rationale for Use," *J Am Dent Assoc*, 1983, 107(4):623-30.

Larochelle P, Hamet P, and Enjalbert M, "Responses to Tyramine and Norepinephrine After Imipramine and Trazodone," *Clin Pharmacol Ther*, 1979, 26(1):24-30.

Mitchell JR, "Guanethidine and Related Agents. III Antagonism by Drugs Which Inhibit the Norepinephrine Pump in Man," *J Clin Invest*, 1970, 49(8):1596-604.

Rundegren J, van Dijken J, Mörnstad H, et al, "Oral Conditions in Patients Receiving Long-Term Treatment With Cyclic Antidepressant Drugs," *Swed Dent J*, 1985, 9(2):55-64.

Svedmyr N, "The Influence of a Tricyclic Antidepressive Agent (Protriptyline) on Some of the Circulatory Effects of Noradrenaline and Adrenalin® in Man," *Life Sci*, 1968, 7(1):77-84.

Doxil™ *see* Doxorubicin (Liposomal) *on next page*

Doxil® Injection *see* Doxorubicin *on this page*

Doxorubicin *(doks oh ROO bi sin)*

Brand Names Adriamycin® PFS; Adriamycin® RDF; Doxil® Injection; Rubex®

Canadian/Mexican Brand Names Doxolem (Mexico)

Therapeutic Category Antineoplastic Agent, Antibiotic

Synonyms ADR; Hydroxydaunomycin Hydrochloride

Use Treatment of various solid tumors including ovarian, breast, and bladder tumors; various lymphomas and leukemias (ANL, ALL), soft tissue sarcomas, neuroblastoma, osteosarcoma

Usual Dosage Refer to individual protocols

I.V. (patient's ideal weight should be used to calculate body surface area):

Children: 35-75 mg/m^2 as a single dose, repeat every 21 days; **or** 20-30 mg/m^2 once weekly; **or** 60-90 mg/m^2 given as a continuous infusion over 96 hours every 3-4 weeks

Adults: 60-75 mg/m^2 as a single dose, repeat every 21 days **or** other dosage regimens like 20-30 mg/m^2/day for 2-3 days, repeat in 4 weeks **or** 20 mg/m^2 once weekly

The lower dose regimen should be given to patients with decreased bone marrow reserve, prior therapy or marrow infiltration with malignant cells

Currently the maximum cumulative dose is 550 mg/m^2 or 450 mg/m^2 in patients who have received RT to the mediastinal areas; a baseline MUGA should be performed prior to initiating treatment. If the LVEF is <30% to 40%, therapy should not be instituted; LVEF should be monitored during therapy.

Doxorubicin has also been administered intraperitoneal (phase I in refractory ovarian cancer patients) and intra-arterially.

Mechanism of Action Doxorubicin works through inhibition of topoisomerase-II at the point of DNA cleavage. A second mechanism of action is the production of free radicals (the hydroxy radical OH) by doxorubicin, which in turn can destroy DNA and cancerous cells. Doxorubicin is also a very powerful iron chelator, equal to deferoxamine. The iron-doxorubicin complex can bind DNA and cell membranes rapidly and produce free radicals that immediately cleave the DNA and cell membranes. Inhibits DNA and RNA synthesis by intercalating between DNA base pairs and by steric obstruction; active throughout entire cell cycle.

Local Anesthetic/Vasoconstrictor Precautions No information available to require special precautions

Effects on Dental Treatment No effects or complications reported

Other Adverse Effects

>10%:

Dermatologic: Alopecia

Gastrointestinal: Acute nausea and vomiting may be seen in 21% to 55% of patients; mucositis, ulceration, and necrosis of the colon, anorexia, and diarrhea

Emetic potential: ≤20 mg: Moderately low (10% to 30%); >20 mg or <75 mg: Moderate (30% to 60%); ≥75 mg: Moderately high (60% to 90%)

Hematologic: Myelosuppressive: 60% to 80% of patients will have leukopenia; dose-limiting toxicity; WBC: Moderate; Platelets: Moderate; Onset (days): 7; Nadir (days): 10-14; Recovery (days): 21-28

Local: Extravasation: Doxorubicin is one of the most notorious vesicants. Infiltration can cause severe inflammation, tissue necrosis, and ulceration. If the drug is infiltrated, consult institutional policy, apply ice to the area, and elevate the limb. Can have ongoing tissue destruction secondary to propagation of free radicals; may require debridement.

Radiation recall: Noticed in patients who have had prior irradiation; reactions include redness, warmth, erythema, and dermatitis in the radiation port. Can progress to severe desquamation and ulceration. Occurs 5-7 days after doxorubicin administration; local therapy with topical corticosteroids and cooling have given the best relief.

1% to 10%: Erythematous streaking along the vein if administered too rapidly

Cardiac toxicity: Dose-limiting and related to cumulative dose; usually a maximum total lifetime dose of 450-550 mg/m^2 is administered; although, it has been demonstrated that if given by continuous infusion in breast cancer patients, higher doses may be tolerated. Cardiac tissue seems to be very sensitive to damage from free radicals produced by doxorubicin. Patients may present with acute toxicity (arrhythmias, heart block, pericarditis-myocarditis) which may be fatal. More commonly, chronic toxicity is seen, in which patients present with signs of congestive heart failure. Several methods of monitoring cardiac toxicity have been utilized, including myocardial biopsy (expensive and hazardous procedure).

<1%: Allergic reaction, anaphylaxis

Miscellaneous: Fever, chills, urticaria, conjunctivitis

Drug Uptake

Absorption: Oral: Poor, <50%

Serum half-life, triphasic:

Primary: 30 minutes

Secondary: 3-3.5 hours for metabolites

Terminal: 17-30 hours for doxorubicin and its metabolites

Pregnancy Risk Factor D

Generic Available Yes

Doxorubicin Hydrochloride (Liposomal) *see* Doxorubicin (Liposomal) *on this page*

Doxorubicin (Liposomal) (doks oh ROO bi sin lip pah SOW mal)

Brand Names Doxil™

Therapeutic Category Antineoplastic Agent, Anthracycline; Antineoplastic Agent, Antibiotic

Synonyms Doxorubicin Hydrochloride (Liposomal)

Use Treatment of AIDS-related Kaposi's sarcoma in patients with disease that has progressed on prior combination chemotherapy or in patients who are intolerant to such therapy

Off-label use: Breast cancer, ovarian cancer, and solid tumors

Mechanism of Action Doxil® is doxorubicin hydrochloride encapsulated in long-circulating STEALTH® liposomes. Liposomes are microscopic vesicles composed of a phospholipid bilayer that are capable of encapsulating active drugs. Doxorubicin works through inhibition of topoisomerase-II at the point of DNA cleavage. A second mechanism of action is the production of free radicals (the hydroxy radical OH) by doxorubicin, which in turn can destroy DNA and cancerous cells. Doxorubicin is also a very powerful iron chelator, equal to deferoxamine. The iron-doxorubicin complex can bind DNA and cell membranes rapidly and produce free radicals that immediately cleave the DNA and cell membranes. Inhibits DNA and RNA synthesis by intercalating between DNA base pairs and by steric obstruction; active throughout entire cell cycle.

(Continued)

Doxorubicin (Liposomal) *(Continued)*

Local Anesthetic/Vasoconstrictor Precautions No information available to require special precautions

Effects on Dental Treatment No effects or complications reported

Other Adverse Effects Information on adverse events is based on the experience reported in 753 patients with AIDS-related Kaposi's sarcoma enrolled in four studies

>10%:

Extravasation: Doxorubicin is one of the most notorious vesicants. Infiltration can cause severe inflammation, tissue necrosis, and ulceration. If the drug is infiltrated, consult institutional policy, apply ice to the area, and elevate the limb. Can have ongoing tissue destruction secondary to propagation of free radicals; may require debridement.

1% to 10%:

Cardiovascular: Cardiac toxicity (9.7%): Cardiomyopathy, congestive heart failure, arrhythmia, pericardial effusion, tachycardia, facial flushing

Dermatologic: Hyperpigmentation of nail beds, erythematous streaking along the vein if administered too rapidly

Endocrine & metabolic: Hyperuricemia

<1%:

Hypersensitivity: Allergic reaction, anaphylaxis, fever, chills, urticaria

Ocular: Conjunctivitis

Contraindications Hypersensitivity to doxorubicin or the components of Doxil®

Drug Interactions

No formal drug interaction studies have been conducted with doxorubicin hydrochloride liposome injection, however, may interact with drugs known to interact with the conventional formulation of doxorubicin hydrochloride

Decreased effect: Doxorubicin may decrease digoxin plasma levels and renal excretion

Increased effect: Allopurinol may enhance the antitumor activity of doxorubicin (animal data only)

Increased toxicity:

Cyclophosphamide enhances the cardiac toxicity of doxorubicin by producing additional myocardial cell damage

Mercaptopurine enhances toxicities

Streptozocin greatly enhances leukopenia and thrombocytopenia

Verapamil alters the cellular distribution of doxorubicin; may result in increased cell toxicity by inhibition of the P-glycoprotein pump

Pregnancy Risk Factor D

Dosage Forms Injection, as hydrochloride: 2 mg/mL (10 mL)

Generic Available No

Doxy® *see* Doxycycline *on this page*

Doxychel® *see* Doxycycline *on this page*

Doxycycline (doks i SYE kleen)

Related Information

Animal and Human Bites Guidelines *on page 1093*

Antimicrobial Prophylaxis in Surgical Patients *on page 1163*

Nonviral Infectious Diseases *on page 1032*

Brand Names Doryx®; Doxy®; Doxychel®; Vibramycin®; Vibra-Tabs®

Canadian/Mexican Brand Names Apo®-Doxy (Canada); Apo®-Doxy Tabs (Canada); Doxycin (Canada); Doxytec (Canada); Novo-Doxylin (Canada); Nu-Doxycycline (Canada); Vibramicina® (Mexico)

Therapeutic Category Antibiotic, Tetracycline Derivative

Use

Dental: Treatment of periodontitis associated with presence of *Actinobacillus actinomycetemcomitans* (AA)

Medical: In medicine, principally in the treatment of infections caused by susceptible *Rickettsia*, *Chlamydia*, and *Mycoplasma* along with uncommon susceptible gram-negative and gram-positive organisms; alternative to mefloquine for malaria prophylaxis

Unapproved use: Treatment for syphilis in penicillin-allergic patients; sclerosing agent for pleural effusions

Usual Dosage Adults: 100 mg/day for 21 days or until improvement

Mechanism of Action Inhibits protein synthesis by binding with the 30S and possibly the 50S ribosomal subunit(s) of susceptible bacteria; may also cause alterations in the cytoplasmic membrane

Local Anesthetic/Vasoconstrictor Precautions No information available to require special precautions

Effects on Dental Treatment Opportunistic "superinfection" with *Candida albicans*; tetracycline's are not recommended for use during pregnancy or in children ≤8 years of age since they have been reported to cause enamel hypoplasia and permanent teeth discoloration. The use of tetracycline's should only be used in these patients if other agents are contraindicated or alternative antimicrobials will not eradicate the organism. Long-term use associated with oral candidiasis.

Other Adverse Effects
>10%: Discoloration of teeth in children
<1%: Gastrointestinal: Nausea, diarrhea

Contraindications Hypersensitivity to doxycycline, tetracycline or any component; children <8 years of age; severe hepatic dysfunction

Warnings/Precautions Use of tetracyclines during tooth development may cause permanent discoloration of the teeth and enamel hypoplasia; prolonged use may result in superinfection; photosensitivity reaction may occur with this drug; avoid prolonged exposure to sunlight or tanning equipment

Drug Interactions Iron and bismuth subsalicylate may decrease doxycycline bioavailability; barbiturates, phenytoin, and carbamazepine decrease doxycycline's half-life; increased effect of warfarin

Drug Uptake
Absorption: Oral: 90% to 100%
Serum half-life: 12-15 hours (usually increases to 22-24 hours with multiple dosing)
Time to peak serum concentration: Within 1.5-4 hours

Pregnancy Risk Factor D

Breast-feeding Considerations May be taken while breast-feeding

Dosage Forms
Capsule, as hyclate:
Doxychel®, Vibramycin®: 50 mg
Doxy®, Doxychel®, Vibramycin®: 100 mg
Capsule, coated pellets, as hyclate (Doryx®): 100 mg
Powder for injection, as hyclate (Doxy®, Doxychel®, Vibramycin® IV): 100 mg, 200 mg
Powder for oral suspension, as monohydrate (raspberry flavor) (Vibramycin®): 25 mg/5 mL (60 mL)
Syrup, as calcium (raspberry-apple flavor) (Vibramycin®): 50 mg/5 mL (30 mL, 473 mL)
Tablet, as hyclate
Doxychel®: 50 mg
Doxychel®, Vibra-Tabs®: 100 mg

Dietary Considerations May be taken with food, milk, or water

Generic Available Yes

Selected Readings
Rams TE and Slots J, "Antibiotics in Periodontal Therapy: An Update," *Compendium*, 1992, 13(12):1130, 1132, 1134.

Dronabinol (droe NAB i nol)

Related Information
Chemical Dependency and Smoking Cessation *on page 1087*

Brand Names Marinol®

Therapeutic Category Antiemetic

Use When conventional antiemetics fail to relieve the nausea and vomiting associated with cancer chemotherapy, AIDS-related anorexia

Usual Dosage Oral:

Children: NCI protocol recommends 5 mg/m^2 starting 6-8 hours before chemotherapy and every 4-6 hours after to be continued for 12 hours after chemotherapy is discontinued

Adults: 5 mg/m^2 1-3 hours before chemotherapy, then give 5 mg/m^2/dose every 2-4 hours after chemotherapy for a total of 4-6 doses/day; dose may be increased up to a maximum of 15 mg/m^2/dose if needed (dosage may be increased by 2.5 mg/m^2 increments)

Appetite stimulant (AIDS-related): Initial: 2.5 mg twice daily (before lunch and dinner); titrate up to a maximum of 20 mg/day

Mechanism of Action Not well defined, probably inhibits the vomiting center in the medulla oblongata

Local Anesthetic/Vasoconstrictor Precautions No information available to require special precautions

Effects on Dental Treatment No effects or complications reported

Other Adverse Effects

>10%: Central nervous system: Drowsiness, dizziness, detachment, anxiety, difficulty concentrating, mood change

1% to 10%:

Cardiovascular: Orthostatic hypotension, tachycardia

Central nervous system: Depression, headache, vertigo, hallucinations, memory lapse, ataxia

Gastrointestinal: Dry mouth

Neuromuscular & skeletal: Paresthesia, weakness

<1%:

Cardiovascular: Syncope

Central nervous system: Nightmares, speech difficulties

Gastrointestinal: Diarrhea

Neuromuscular & skeletal: Muscular pains

Otic: Tinnitus

Miscellaneous: Sweating

Drug Interactions Increased toxicity (drowsiness) with alcohol, barbiturates, benzodiazepines

Drug Uptake

Absorption: Oral: Erratic

Serum half-life: 19-24 hours

Time to peak serum concentration: Within 2-3 hours

Pregnancy Risk Factor B

Generic Available Yes

Droperidol (droe PER i dole)

Brand Names Inapsine®

Canadian/Mexican Brand Names Dehydrobenzperidol® (Mexico)

Therapeutic Category Antiemetic; Antipsychotic Agent

Use Tranquilizer and antiemetic in surgical and diagnostic procedures; antiemetic for cancer chemotherapy; preoperative medication; has good antiemetic effect as well as sedative and antianxiety effects

Usual Dosage Titrate carefully to desired effect

Children 2-12 years:

Premedication: I.M.: 0.1-0.15 mg/kg; smaller doses may be sufficient for control of nausea or vomiting

Adjunct to general anesthesia: I.V. induction: 0.088-0.165 mg/kg

Nausea and vomiting: I.M., I.V.: 0.05-0.06 mg/kg/dose every 4-6 hours as needed

Adults:

Premedication: I.M.: 2.5-10 mg 30 minutes to 1 hour preoperatively

Adjunct to general anesthesia: I.V. induction: 0.22-0.275 mg/kg; maintenance: 1.25-2.5 mg/dose

Alone in diagnostic procedures: I.M.: Initial: 2.5-10 mg 30 minutes to 1 hour before; then 1.25-2.5 mg if needed

Nausea and vomiting: I.M., I.V.: 2.5-5 mg/dose every 3-4 hours as needed

Mechanism of Action Alters the action of dopamine in the CNS, at subcortical levels, to produce sedation; reduces emesis by blocking dopamine stimulation of the chemotrigger zone

Local Anesthetic/Vasoconstrictor Precautions No information available to require special precautions

Effects on Dental Treatment Significant hypotension may occur, especially when the drug is administered parenterally; orthostatic hypotension is due to alpha-receptor blockade, the elderly are at greater risk for orthostatic hypotension

Tardive dyskinesia: Prevalence rate may be 40% in elderly; development of the syndrome and the irreversible nature are proportional to duration and total cumulative dose over time

Extrapyramidal reactions are more common in elderly with up to 50% developing these reactions after 60 years of age; drug-induced **Parkinson's syndrome** occurs often; **akathisia** is the most common extrapyramidal reaction in elderly

Increased confusion, memory loss, psychotic behavior, and agitation frequently occur as a consequence of anticholinergic effects

Antipsychotic associated sedation in nonpsychotic patients is extremely unpleasant due to feelings of depersonalization, derealization, and dysphoria

Other Adverse Effects
>10%:
   Cardiovascular: Mild to moderate hypotension, tachycardia
   Central nervous system: Postoperative drowsiness
1% to 10%:
   Cardiovascular: Hypertension
   Central nervous system: Extrapyramidal reactions
   Respiratory: Respiratory depression
<1%:
   Central nervous system: Dizziness, chills, shivering, postoperative hallucinations
   Respiratory: Laryngospasm, bronchospasm

Drug Interactions Increased toxicity: CNS depressants, fentanyl and other analgesics increased blood pressure; conduction anesthesia decreased blood pressure; epinephrine decreased blood pressure; atropine, lithium

Drug Uptake Following parenteral administration:
   Duration: 2-4 hours, may extend to 12 hours
   Serum half-life: Adults: 2.3 hours

Pregnancy Risk Factor C
Generic Available Yes

Droxia® *see* Hydroxyurea *on page 490*
Dr Scholl's Athlete's Foot [OTC] *see* Tolnaftate *on page 943*
Dr Scholl's® Disk [OTC] *see* Salicylic Acid *on page 853*
Dr Scholl's Maximum Strength Tritin [OTC] *see* Tolnaftate *on page 943*
Dr Scholl's® Wart Remover [OTC] *see* Salicylic Acid *on page 853*
Drugs Associated With Adverse Hematologic Effects *see page 1199*
Dry Eyes® Solution [OTC] *see* Artificial Tears *on page 87*
Dry Eye® Therapy Solution [OTC] *see* Artificial Tears *on page 87*
Dryox® Gel [OTC] *see* Benzoyl Peroxide *on page 120*
Dryox® Wash [OTC] *see* Benzoyl Peroxide *on page 120*
DSMC Plus® [OTC] *see* Docusate and Casanthranol *on page 331*
D-S-S® [OTC] *see* Docusate *on page 331*
DSS With Casanthranol *see* Docusate and Casanthranol *on page 331*
DTIC *see* Dacarbazine *on page 276*
DTIC-Dome® *see* Dacarbazine *on page 276*
Duadacin® Capsule [OTC] *see* Chlorpheniramine, Phenylpropanolamine, and Acetaminophen *on page 222*
Dulcolax® [OTC] *see* Bisacodyl *on page 131*
Dull-C® [OTC] *see* Ascorbic Acid *on page 88*
DuoCet™ [5/500] *see* Hydrocodone and Acetaminophen *on page 478*
Duo-Cyp® Injection *see* Estradiol and Testosterone *on page 366*
DuoFilm® [OTC] *see* Salicylic Acid *on page 853*
Duofilm® Solution *see* Salicylic Acid and Lactic Acid *on page 853*
Duo-Medihaler® Aerosol *see* Isoproterenol and Phenylephrine *on page 524*
DuoPlant® Gel [OTC] *see* Salicylic Acid *on page 853*
Duo-Trach® *see* Lidocaine *on page 553*
Duotrate® *see* Pentaerythritol Tetranitrate *on page 735*
DuP 753 *see* Losartan *on page 569*
Duphalac® *see* Lactulose *on page 540*
Duplex® T [OTC] *see* Coal Tar *on page 254*
Duraclon® Injection *see* Clonidine *on page 250*

Duract™ see Bromfenac on page 139

Duradyne DHC® [5/500] see Hydrocodone and Acetaminophen on page 478

Duraflor® Cavity Varnish see Fluoride on page 415

Duragesic™ see Fentanyl on page 398

Dura-Gest® see Guaifenesin, Phenylpropanolamine, and Phenylephrine on page 455

Duralone® see Methylprednisolone on page 624

Duramist® Plus [OTC] see Oxymetazoline on page 714

Duramorph® Injection see Morphine Sulfate on page 648

Duranest® With Epinephrine see Etidocaine With Epinephrine on page 385

Duratest® Injection see Testosterone on page 910

Duratestrin® Injection see Estradiol and Testosterone on page 366

Durathate® Injection see Testosterone on page 910

Duration® Nasal Solution [OTC] see Oxymetazoline on page 714

Duratuss-G® see Guaifenesin on page 452

Dura-Vent® see Guaifenesin and Phenylpropanolamine on page 454

Dura-Vent/DA® see Chlorpheniramine, Phenylephrine, and Methscopolamine on page 220

Duricef® see Cefadroxil on page 186

Duvoid® see Bethanechol on page 128

DV® Vaginal Cream see Dienestrol on page 309

Dwelle® Ophthalmic Solution [OTC] see Artificial Tears on page 87

Dyazide® see Hydrochlorothiazide and Triamterene on page 478

Dycill® see Dicloxacillin on page 305

Dyclone® see Dyclonine on this page

Dyclonine (DYE kloe neen)

Related Information
Oral Viral Infections on page 1066

Brand Names Dyclone®

Therapeutic Category Local Anesthetic, Oral

Use
Dental: Use topically for temporary relief of pain associated with oral mucosa
Medical: Local anesthetic prior to laryngoscopy, bronchoscopy, or endotracheal intubation

Mechanism of Action Blocks impulses at peripheral nerve endings in skin and mucous membranes by altering cell membrane permeability to ionic transfer

Local Anesthetic/Vasoconstrictor Precautions No information available to require special precautions

Effects on Dental Treatment No effects or complications reported

Other Adverse Effects <1%:
Cardiovascular: Hypotension, bradycardia, cardiac arrest
Central nervous system: Excitation, drowsiness, nervousness, dizziness, seizures
Local: Slight irritation and stinging may occur when applied
Ocular: Blurred vision
Respiratory: Respiratory arrest
Miscellaneous: Allergic reactions

Drug Interactions No data reported

Pregnancy Risk Factor C

Breast-feeding Considerations No data reported

Generic Available No

Dymelor® see Acetohexamide on page 27

Dymenate® Injection see Dimenhydrinate on page 320

Dynabac® see Dirithromycin on page 327

Dynacin® Oral see Minocycline on page 639

DynaCirc® see Isradipine on page 528

Dynafed®, Maximum Strength New Brand [OTC] see Acetaminophen and Pseudoephedrine on page 24

Dyna-Hex® Topical [OTC] see Chlorhexidine Gluconate on page 211

Dynapen® see Dicloxacillin on page 305

Dyphylline (DYE fi lin)

Brand Names Dilor®; Lufyllin®

Therapeutic Category Bronchodilator; Theophylline Derivative

Synonyms Dihydroxypropyl Theophylline

Use Bronchodilator in reversible airway obstruction due to asthma or COPD

Local Anesthetic/Vasoconstrictor Precautions No information available to require special precautions

Effects on Dental Treatment Do not prescribe any erythromycin product to patients taking theophylline products. Erythromycin will delay the normal metabolic inactivation of theophyllines leading to increased blood levels; this has resulted in nausea, vomiting and CNS restlessness

Other Adverse Effects

Uncommon at serum theophylline concentrations ≤20 mcg/mL

1% to 10%:

    Cardiovascular: Tachycardia

    Central nervous system: Nervousness, restlessness

    Gastrointestinal: Nausea, vomiting

<1%:

    Central nervous system: Insomnia, irritability, seizures

    Dermatologic: Skin rash

    Gastrointestinal: Gastric irritation

    Neuromuscular & skeletal: Tremor

    Miscellaneous: Allergic reactions

Pregnancy Risk Factor C

Generic Available Yes

Comments This drug is rarely used today. Requires a special laboratory measuring procedure rather than the standard theophylline assay. Saliva levels are approximately equal to 60% of plasma levels; charcoal-broiled foods may increase elimination, reducing half-life by 50%; cigarette smoking may require an increase of dosage by 50% to 100%. Because different salts of theophylline have different theophylline content, various salts are not equivalent.

Dyrenium® *see* Triamterene *on page 956*

7E3 *see* Abciximab *on page 18*

Easprin® *see* Aspirin *on page 90*

Echothiophate Iodide (ek oh THYE oh fate EYE oh dide)

Brand Names Phospholine Iodide®

Therapeutic Category Antiglaucoma Agent; Ophthalmic Agent, Miotic

Use Reverses toxic CNS effects caused by anticholinergic drugs; used as miotic in treatment of glaucoma; accommodative esotropia

Usual Dosage Adults:

Ophthalmic: Glaucoma: Instill 1 drop twice daily into eyes with 1 dose just prior to bedtime; some patients have been treated with 1 dose daily or every other day

Accommodative esotropia:

Diagnosis: Instill 1 drop of 0.125% once daily into both eyes at bedtime for 2-3 weeks

Treatment: Use lowest concentration and frequency which gives satisfactory response, with a maximum dose of 0.125% once daily, although more intensive therapy may be used for short periods of time

Mechanism of Action Produces miosis and changes in accommodation by inhibiting cholinesterase, thereby preventing the breakdown of acetylcholine; acetylcholine is, therefore, allowed to continuously stimulate the iris and ciliary muscles of the eye

Local Anesthetic/Vasoconstrictor Precautions No information available to require special precautions

Effects on Dental Treatment No effects or complications reported

Other Adverse Effects

1% to 10%: Ocular: Stinging, burning, myopia, visual blurring

<1%:

    Cardiovascular: Bradycardia, hypotension, flushing

    Gastrointestinal: Nausea, vomiting, diarrhea

    Ocular: Retinal detachment, muscle weakness, browache, miosis, twitching eyelids, watering eyes

    Respiratory: Dyspnea

    Miscellaneous: Sweating

Drug Interactions Increased toxicity: Carbamate or organophosphate insecticides and pesticides; succinylcholine; systemic acetylcholinesterases may increase neuromuscular effects

Drug Uptake

Onset of action:

    Miosis: 10-30 minutes

    Intraocular pressure decrease: 4-8 hours

Peak intraocular pressure decrease: 24 hours

Duration: Up to 1-4 weeks

Pregnancy Risk Factor C

Generic Available No

E-Complex-600® [OTC] *see* Vitamin E *on page 994*

Econazole (e KONE a zole)

Brand Names Spectazole™

Canadian/Mexican Brand Names Ecostatin® (Canada); Micostyl® (Mexico)

Therapeutic Category Antifungal Agent, Topical

Use Topical treatment of tinea pedis (athlete's foot), tinea cruris (jock itch), tinea corporis (ringworm), tinea versicolor, and cutaneous candidiasis

Usual Dosage Children and Adults: Topical:

Tinea pedis, tinea cruris, tinea corporis, tinea versicolor: Apply sufficient amount to cover affected areas once daily

Cutaneous candidiasis: Apply sufficient quantity twice daily (morning and evening)

Duration of treatment: Candidal infections and tinea cruris, versicolor, and corporis should be treated for 2 weeks and tinea pedis for 1 month; occasionally, longer treatment periods may be required

Mechanism of Action Alters fungal cell wall membrane permeability; may interfere with RNA and protein synthesis, and lipid metabolism

Local Anesthetic/Vasoconstrictor Precautions No information available to require special precautions

Effects on Dental Treatment No effects or complications reported

Other Adverse Effects 1% to 10%: Local: Pruritus, erythema, burning, stinging

Drug Interactions No data reported

Drug Uptake

Absorption: Topical: <10%

Pregnancy Risk Factor C

Dosage Forms Cream: 1% in water miscible base (15 g, 30 g, 85 g)

Generic Available No

Econopred® *see* Prednisolone *on page 788*

Econopred® Plus *see* Prednisolone *on page 788*

Ecotrin® [OTC] *see* Aspirin *on page 90*

Ecotrin® Low Adult Strength [OTC] *see* Aspirin *on page 90*

Ed A-Hist® Liquid *see* Chlorpheniramine and Phenylephrine *on page 218*

Edathamil Disodium *see* Edetate Disodium *on next page*

Edecrin® *see* Ethacrynic Acid *on page 371*

Edetate Calcium Disodium

(ED e tate KAL see um dye SOW dee um)

Brand Names Calcium Disodium Versenate®

Therapeutic Category Antidote, Lead Toxicity

Synonyms Calcium Disodium Edetate; Calcium EDTA

Use Treatment of acute and chronic lead poisoning; used as an aid in the diagnosis of lead poisoning

Mechanism of Action Calcium is displaced by divalent and trivalent heavy metals, forming a nonionizing soluble complex that is excreted in urine

Local Anesthetic/Vasoconstrictor Precautions No information available to require special precautions

Effects on Dental Treatment No effects or complications reported

Other Adverse Effects

1% to 10%: Renal: Renal tubular necrosis

<1%:

Cardiovascular: Hypotension, arrhythmias

Central nervous system: Fever, headache, chills

Dermatologic: Skin lesions

Endocrine & metabolic: Hypercalcemia

Gastrointestinal: Nausea, vomiting

Hematologic: Transient marrow suppression

Local: Pain at injection site following I.M. injection, thrombophlebitis following I.V. infusion (when concentration >0.5%)

Neuromuscular & skeletal: Numbness, paresthesia

Ocular: Lacrimation

Renal: Proteinuria, microscopic hematuria

Respiratory: Sneezing, nasal congestion

Contraindications Severe renal disease, anuria

Drug Interactions Decreased effect: Do not use simultaneously with zinc insulin preparations; do not mix in the same syringe with dimercaprol

Drug Uptake

Absorption: I.M., S.C.: Well absorbed

Serum half-life:

I.M.: 1.5 hours

I.V.: 20 minutes
Pregnancy Risk Factor C
Dosage Forms Injection: 200 mg/mL (5 mL)
Generic Available No

Edetate Disodium (ED e tate dye SOW dee um)

Brand Names Chealamide®; Disotate®; Endrate®
Therapeutic Category Antidote, Hypercalcemia; Chelating Agent, Parenteral
Synonyms Edathamil Disodium; EDTA; Sodium Edetate
Use Emergency treatment of hypercalcemia; control digitalis-induced cardiac dysrhythmias (ventricular arrhythmias)
Mechanism of Action Chelates with divalent or trivalent metals to form a soluble complex that is then eliminated in urine
Local Anesthetic/Vasoconstrictor Precautions No information available to require special precautions
Effects on Dental Treatment No effects or complications reported
Other Adverse Effects

Rapid I.V. administration or excessive doses may cause a sudden drop in serum calcium concentration which may lead to hypocalcemic tetany, seizures, arrhythmias, and death from respiratory arrest. Do **not** exceed recommended dosage and rate of administration.

1% to 10%: Gastrointestinal: Nausea, vomiting, abdominal cramps, diarrhea
<1%:
Cardiovascular: Arrhythmias, transient hypotension, acute tubular necrosis
Central nervous system: Seizures, fever, headache, tetany, chills
Dermatologic: Eruptions, dermatologic lesions
Endocrine & metabolic: Hypomagnesemia, hypokalemia
Hematologic: Anemia
Local: Thrombophlebitis, pain at the site of injection
Neuromuscular & skeletal: Paresthesia may occur, back pain, muscle cramps
Renal: Nephrotoxicity
Respiratory: Death from respiratory arrest

Contraindications Severe renal failure or anuria
Drug Interactions Increased effect of insulin (edetate disodium may decrease blood glucose concentrations and reduce insulin requirements in diabetic patients treated with insulin)
Drug Uptake Serum half-life: 20-60 minutes
Pregnancy Risk Factor C
Dosage Forms Injection: 150 mg/mL (20 mL)
Generic Available Yes
Comments Sodium content of 1 g: 5.4 mEq

Elocon® see Mometasone Furoate on page 646

Elspar® see Asparaginase on page 89

Eltroxin™ see Levothyroxine on page 552

Emcyt® see Estramustine on page 366

Emecheck® [OTC] see Phosphorated Carbohydrate Solution on page 757

Emetrol® [OTC] see Phosphorated Carbohydrate Solution on page 757

Emgel™ Topical see Erythromycin, Topical on page 364

Eminase® see Anistreplase on page 79

Emko® [OTC] see Nonoxynol 9 on page 689

EMLA® Cream see Lidocaine and Prilocaine on page 556

EMLA® Disc see Lidocaine and Prilocaine on page 556

Empirin® [OTC] see Aspirin on page 90

Empirin® With Codeine see Aspirin and Codeine on page 92

Emulsoil® [OTC] see Castor Oil on page 184

E-Mycin® Oral see Erythromycin on page 361

Enalapril (e NAL a pril)

Related Information
Cardiovascular Diseases on page 1010
Enalapril and Diltiazem on next page
Enalapril and Felodipine on page 348

Brand Names Vasotec®

Canadian/Mexican Brand Names Apo®-Enalapril (Canada); Enaladil® (Mexico); Glioten® (Mexico); Renitec® (Mexico)

Therapeutic Category Angiotensin-Converting Enzyme (ACE) Inhibitors

Use Management of mild to severe hypertension and congestive heart failure

Unlabeled use: Hypertensive crisis, diabetic nephropathy, rheumatoid arthritis, diagnosis of anatomic renal artery stenosis, hypertension secondary to scleroderma renal crisis, diagnosis of aldosteronism, idiopathic edema, Bartter's syndrome, postmyocardial infarction for prevention of ventricular failure

Usual Dosage Use lower listed initial dose in patients with hyponatremia, hypovolemia, severe congestive heart failure, decreased renal function, or in those receiving diuretics

Children:
Investigational initial oral doses of **enalapril**: 0.1 mg/kg/day increasing as needed over 2 weeks to 0.5 mg/kg/day have been used to treat severe congestive heart failure in infants
Investigational I.V. doses of **enalaprilat**: 5-10 mcg/kg/dose administered every 8-24 hours have been used for the treatment of neonatal hypertension; monitor patients carefully; select patients may require higher doses

Adults:
Oral: **Enalapril**
Hypertension: 2.5-5 mg/day then increase as required, usual therapeutic dose for hypertension: 10-40 mg/day in 1-2 divided doses; usual therapeutic dose for heart failure: 5-20 mg/day
Heart failure: As adjunct with diuretics and digitalis, initiate with 2.5 mg once or twice daily (usual range: 5-20 mg/day in 2 divided doses; maximum: 40 mg)
Asymptomatic left ventricular dysfunction: 2.5 mg twice daily, titrated as tolerated to 20 mg/day

I.V.: **Enalaprilat**
Hypertension: 1.25 mg/dose, given over 5 minutes every 6 hours; doses as high as 5 mg/dose every 6 hours have been tolerated for up to 36 hours. **Note:** If patients are concomitantly receiving diuretic therapy, begin with 0.625 mg I.V. over 5 minutes; if the effect is not adequate after 1 hour, repeat the dose and administer 1.25 mg at 6-hour intervals thereafter; if adequate, administer 0.625 mg I.V. every 6 hours
Conversion from I.V. to oral therapy if not concurrently on diuretics: 5 mg once daily; subsequent titration as needed; if concurrently receiving diuretics and responding to 0.625 mg I.V. every 6 hours, initiate with 2.5 mg/day

Mechanism of Action Competitive inhibitor of angiotensin-converting enzyme (ACE); prevents conversion of angiotensin I to angiotensin II, a potent vasoconstrictor; results in lower levels of angiotensin II which causes an increase in plasma renin activity and a reduction in aldosterone secretion

Local Anesthetic/Vasoconstrictor Precautions No information available to require special precautions

Effects on Dental Treatment No effects or complications reported

Other Adverse Effects

1% to 10%:

Cardiovascular: Chest pain, palpitations, tachycardia, syncope

Central nervous system: Insomnia, headache dizziness, fatigue, malaise

Dermatologic: Rash

Gastrointestinal: Dysgeusia, abdominal pain, vomiting, nausea, diarrhea, anorexia, constipation

Neuromuscular & skeletal: Paresthesia, weakness

Respiratory: Bronchitis, cough, dyspnea

<1%:

Cardiovascular: Angina pectoris, flushing

Dermatologic: Alopecia, erythema multiforme, pruritus, Stevens-Johnson syndrome, urticaria, angioedema

Endocrine & metabolic: Hypoglycemia, hyperkalemia

Genitourinary: Impotence

Hematologic: Agranulocytosis, neutropenia, anemia

Neuromuscular & skeletal: Myalgia

Ocular: Blurred vision

Otic: Tinnitus

Renal: Oliguria

Respiratory: Asthma, bronchospasm

Miscellaneous: Sweating

Drug Interactions See table.

Drug-Drug Interactions With ACEIs

Precipitant Drug	Drug (Category) and Effect	Description
Antacids	ACE Inhibitors: decreased	Decreased bioavailability of ACEIs. May be more likely with captopril. Separate administration times by 1-2 hours.
NSAIDs (indomethacin)	ACEIs: decreased	Reduced hypotensive effects of ACEIs. More prominent in low renin or volume dependent hypertensive patients.
Phenothiazines	ACEIs: increased	Pharmacologic effects of ACEIs may be increased.
ACEIs	Allopurinol: increased	Higher risk of hypersensitivity reaction possible when given concurrently. Three case reports of Stevens-Johnson syndrome with captopril.
ACEIs	Digoxin: increased	Increased plasma digoxin levels.
ACEIs	Lithium: increased	Increased serum lithium levels and symptoms of toxicity may occur.
ACEIs	Potassium preps/ potassium sparing diuretics increased	Coadministration may result in elevated potassium levels.

Drug Uptake

Oral:

Onset of action: ~1 hour

Duration: 12-24 hours

Absorption: Oral: 55% to 75%

Serum half-life:

Enalapril: Adults:

Healthy: 2 hours

With congestive heart failure: 3.4-5.8 hours

Enalaprilat:

Infants 6 weeks to 8 months: 6-10 hours

Adults: 35-38 hours

Time to peak serum concentration: Oral:

Enalapril: Within 0.5-1.5 hours

Enalaprilat (active): Within 3-4.5 hours

Pregnancy Risk Factor C (first trimester); D (second and third trimesters)

Generic Available No

Enalapril and Diltiazem (e NAL a pril & dil TYE a zem)

Brand Names Teczem®

Therapeutic Category Antihypertensive Agent, Combination

Use Combination drug for treatment of hypertension

Local Anesthetic/Vasoconstrictor Precautions No information available to require special precautions

Effects on Dental Treatment No effects or complications reported

(Continued)

Enalapril and Diltiazem *(Continued)*

Dosage Forms Tablet, extended release: Enalapril maleate 5 mg and diltiazem maleate 180 mg

Generic Available No

Enalapril and Felodipine (e NAL a pril & fe LOE di peen)

Brand Names Lexxel®

Therapeutic Category Antihypertensive Agent, Combination

Use Treatment of hypertension

Usual Dosage Adults: Oral: One tablet daily

Mechanism of Action See individual agents

Local Anesthetic/Vasoconstrictor Precautions No information available to require special precautions

Effects on Dental Treatment Calcium channel blockers cause gingival hyperplasia in approximately 1% of patients. There have been fewer reports with felodipine than with other CCBs. The hyperplasia will disappear with cessation of drug therapy. Consultation with physician is suggested.

Other Adverse Effects See individual agents

Drug Interactions See individual agents

Dosage Forms Tablet, extended release: Enalapril maleate 5 mg and felodipine 5 mg

Enalapril and Hydrochlorothiazide

(e NAL a pril & hye droe klor oh THYE a zide)

Related Information

Cardiovascular Diseases *on page 1010*

Brand Names Vaseretic® 5-12.5; Vaseretic® 10-25

Therapeutic Category Antihypertensive Agent, Combination

Use Treatment of hypertension

Usual Dosage Oral: Dose is individualized

Local Anesthetic/Vasoconstrictor Precautions No information available to require special precautions

Effects on Dental Treatment No effects or complications reported

Pregnancy Risk Factor C (first trimester); D (second and third trimesters)

Generic Available No

Encainide (en KAY nide)

Related Information

Cardiovascular Diseases *on page 1010*

Brand Names Enkaid®

Therapeutic Category Antiarrhythmic Agent, Class I-C; Antiarrhythmic Agent (Supraventricular & Ventricular)

Use Ventricular arrhythmias; supraventricular arrhythmias

Local Anesthetic/Vasoconstrictor Precautions No information available to require special precautions

Effects on Dental Treatment No effects or complications reported

Other Adverse Effects

>10%:

Central nervous system: Dizziness

Ocular: Blurred vision

1% to 10%:

Central nervous system: Headache

Cardiovascular: Chest pain congestive heart failure, ventricular tachycardia

Gastrointestinal: Vomiting

Neuromuscular & skeletal: Weakness

Otic: Tinnitus

<1%: Neuromuscular & skeletal: Tremor

Pregnancy Risk Factor B

Generic Available No

Comments Based on adverse outcomes noted with encainide in the CAST trial, the FDA recommends that use of encainide be limited to patients with life-threatening ventricular arrhythmias

Encare® [OTC] *see Nonoxynol 9 on page 689*

Endal® *see Guaifenesin and Phenylephrine on page 454*

End Lice® Liquid [OTC] *see Pyrethrins on page 824*

Endocrine Disorders & Pregnancy *see page 1021*

Endolor® *see Butalbital Compound on page 154*

Endolor® *see Butalbital Compound and Acetaminophen on page 155*

Endrate® *see Edetate Disodium on page 345*

Enduron® *see* Methyclothiazide *on page 620*

Enduronyl® *see* Methyclothiazide and Deserpidine *on page 621*

Enduronyl® Forte *see* Methyclothiazide and Deserpidine *on page 621*

Engerix-B® *see* Hepatitis B Vaccine *on page 468*

Enhanced-potency Inactivated Poliovirus Vaccine *see* Poliovirus Vaccine, Inactivated *on page 770*

Enisyl® [OTC] *see* L-Lysine *on page 562*

Enkaid® *see* Encainide *on previous page*

Enomine® *see* Guaifenesin, Phenylpropanolamine, and Phenylephrine *on page 455*

Enovid® *see* Mestranol and Norethynodrel *on page 604*

Enoxacin (en OKS a sin)
Brand Names Penetrex™
Canadian/Mexican Brand Names Comprecin® (Mexico)
Therapeutic Category Antibiotic, Quinolone
Synonyms Enoxacina (Mexico)
Use Treatment of complicated and uncomplicated urinary tract infections caused by susceptible gram-negative and gram-positive bacteria
Usual Dosage Adults: Oral: 400 mg twice daily
Dosing adjustment in renal impairment:
    Cl$_{cr}$ <50 mL/minute: Administer 50% of dose
Mechanism of Action Exerts a broad spectrum antimicrobial effect. The primary target of the fluoroquinolones is DNA gyrase (topoisomerase II) an essential bacterial enzyme that maintains the superhelical structure of DNA. DNA gyrase is required for DNA replication and transcription, DNA repair, recombination, and transposition.
Local Anesthetic/Vasoconstrictor Precautions No information available to require special precautions
Effects on Dental Treatment No effects or complications reported
Other Adverse Effects
    1% to 10%: Gastrointestinal: Nausea, vomiting
    <1%:
        Central nervous system: Restlessness, dizziness, confusion, seizures, headache
        Dermatologic: Rash
        Gastrointestinal: Diarrhea, GI bleeding
        Hematologic: Anemia
        Hepatic: Elevated liver enzymes
        Neuromuscular & skeletal: Tremor, arthralgia
        Renal: Elevated serum creatinine and BUN, acute renal failure
Drug Interactions
    Decreased effect with antacids (magnesium, aluminum), iron and zinc salts, sucralfate, bismuth salts
    Increased toxicity/levels of warfarin, cyclosporine, digoxin, caffeine; increased levels with cimetidine
Drug Uptake
    Absorption: 98%
    Serum half-life: 3-6 hours (average)
Pregnancy Risk Factor C
Generic Available No

Enoxacina (Mexico) *see* Enoxacin *on this page*

Enoxaparin (e noks ah PAIR in)
Brand Names Lovenox®
Therapeutic Category Anticoagulant
Synonyms Enoxaparin Sodium
Use Prevention of deep vein thrombosis following orthopedic or abdominal surgery; has demonstrated effectiveness in the treatment of existing deep vein thromboses and pulmonary embolus
Usual Dosage S.C.:
    Children: In one dose-finding study, children >2 months of age required 1 mg/kg twice daily for treatment of thrombotic disease
    Adults:
        Prophylaxis: 30 mg twice daily; first dose within 12 hours after orthopedic surgery and every 12 hours for 3 days (including day of surgery); after 3 days, switch to adjusted dose heparin
        A single daily dose of 40 mg has been found to be equally effective in patients undergoing orthopedic or gynecologic surgical procedures
    (Continued)

Enoxaparin *(Continued)*

Abdominal surgery: 40 mg once daily; first dose beginning 2 hours before surgery and continuing for a maximum of 12 days (usual: 10 days)

Treatment of DVT: 1 mg/kg twice daily

Local Anesthetic/Vasoconstrictor Precautions No information available to require special precautions

Effects on Dental Treatment No effects or complications reported

Other Adverse Effects

1% to 10%:

Central nervous system: Fever, confusion, pain

Dermatologic: Erythema, bruising

Gastrointestinal: Nausea

Hematologic: Hemorrhage, thrombocytopenia, hypochromic anemia, hematoma

Local: Irritation

At the recommended doses, single injections of enoxaparin do not significantly influence platelet aggregation or affect global clotting time (ie, prothrombin time or activated partial thromboplastin time)

Warnings/Precautions Do not administer intramuscularly; use with extreme caution in patients with a history of heparin-induced thrombocytopenia; bacterial endocarditis, hemorrhagic stroke, recent CNS or ophthalmological surgery, bleeding diathesis, uncontrolled arterial hypertension, or a history of recent gastrointestinal ulceration and hemorrhage. Elderly and patients with renal insufficiency may show delayed elimination of enoxaparin; avoid use in lactation.

Drug Interactions Increased toxicity with oral anticoagulants, platelet inhibitors

Drug Uptake

Onset of effect: Maximum antifactor Xa and antithrombin (antifactor IIa) activities occur 3-5 hours after S.C. administration

Duration: Following a 40 mg dose, significant antifactor Xa activity persists in plasma for ~12 hours

Half-life, plasma: Low molecular weight heparin is 2-4 times longer than standard heparin independent of the dose

Pregnancy Risk Factor B

Dosage Forms Injection, as sodium, preservative free: 30 mg/0.3 mL; 40 mg/0.4 mL

Generic Available No

Enoxaparin Sodium *see Enoxaparin on previous page*

Ensure® [OTC] *see Enteral Nutritional Products on this page*

Ensure Plus® [OTC] *see Enteral Nutritional Products on this page*

Enteral Nutritional Products

Brand Names Amin-Aid® [OTC]; Carnation Instant Breakfast® [OTC]; Citrotein® [OTC]; Criticare HN® [OTC]; Ensure® [OTC]; Ensure Plus® [OTC]; Isocal® [OTC]; Magnacal® [OTC]; Microlipid™ [OTC]; Osmolite® HN [OTC]; Pedialyte® [OTC]; Polycose® [OTC]; Portagen® [OTC]; Pregestimil® [OTC]; Propac™ [OTC]; Soyalac® [OTC]; Vital HN® [OTC]; Vitaneed™ [OTC]; Vivonex® [OTC]; Vivonex® T.E.N. [OTC]

Canadian/Mexican Brand Names Citrisource® (Canada); Citrotein® (Canada); Glucerna™ (Canada); Isocal® with Fibre (Canada): Isosource® (Canada); Nutrisource™ (Canada); Optifast® 900 (Canada); Palmocare® (Canada); Pediasure™ (Canada); Resource® (Canada); Sandosource® Peptide (Canada), Sustacal® (Canada); Tolerex® (Canada); Travasol® (Canada); Vital® HN (Canada); Vivonex® Plus (Canada)

Therapeutic Category Nutritional Supplement

Synonyms Dietary Supplements

Local Anesthetic/Vasoconstrictor Precautions No information available to require special precautions

Effects on Dental Treatment No effects or complications reported

Dosage Forms

Liquid (Magnacal®): Calcium and sodium caseinate, maltodextrin, sucrose, partially hydrogenated soy oil, soy lecithin

Powder (Vivonex® T.E.N.): Amino acids, predigested carbohydrates, safflower oil

Generic Available Yes

Entertainer's Secret® Spray [OTC] *see Saliva Substitute on page 854*

Entex® *see Guaifenesin, Phenylpropanolamine, and Phenylephrine on page 455*

Entex® LA *see Guaifenesin and Phenylpropanolamine on page 454*

Entex® PSE *see Guaifenesin and Pseudoephedrine on page 454*

Enulose® *see Lactulose on page 540*

Enzone® *see Pramoxine and Hydrocortisone on page 784*

Ephedrine (e FED rin)

Brand Names Kondon's Nasal® [OTC]; Pretz-D® [OTC]

Therapeutic Category Adrenergic Agonist Agent

Synonyms Efedrina (Mexico)

Use Treatment of bronchial asthma, nasal congestion, acute bronchospasm, idiopathic orthostatic hypotension

Usual Dosage

Children:

Oral, S.C.: 3 mg/kg/day or 25-100 mg/m²/day in 4-6 divided doses every 4-6 hours

I.M., slow I.V. push: 0.2-0.3 mg/kg/dose every 4-6 hours

Adults:

Oral: 25-50 mg every 3-4 hours as needed

I.M., S.C.: 25-50 mg, parenteral adult dose should not exceed 150 mg in 24 hours

I.V.: 5-25 mg/dose slow I.V. push repeated after 5-10 minutes as needed, then every 3-4 hours not to exceed 150 mg/24 hours

Mechanism of Action Releases tissue stores of epinephrine and thereby produces an alpha- and beta-adrenergic stimulation; longer acting and less potent than epinephrine

Local Anesthetic/Vasoconstrictor Precautions Use vasoconstrictors with caution since ephedrine may enhance cardiostimulation and vasopressor effects of sympathomimetics such as epinephrine

Effects on Dental Treatment No effects or complications reported

Other Adverse Effects

>10%: Central nervous system: CNS stimulating effects, nervousness, anxiety, apprehension, fear, tension, agitation, excitation, restlessness, irritability, insomnia, hyperactivity

1% to 10%:

Cardiovascular: Hypertension, tachycardia, palpitations, elevation or depression of blood pressure, unusual pallor

Central nervous system: Dizziness, headache

Gastrointestinal: Dry mouth, nausea, anorexia, GI upset, vomiting

Genitourinary: Painful urination

Neuromuscular & skeletal: Trembling, tremor (more common in the elderly), weakness

Miscellaneous: Increased sweating

<1%:

Cardiovascular: Chest pain, arrhythmias

Respiratory: Dyspnea

Drug Interactions

Decreased effect: Alpha- and beta-adrenergic blocking agents decrease ephedrine vasopressor effects

Increased toxicity: Additive cardiostimulation with other sympathomimetic agents; theophylline leads to cardiostimulation; MAO inhibitors or atropine lead to increased blood pressure; cardiac glycosides or general anesthetics lead to increased cardiac stimulation

Drug Uptake Oral:

Duration of action: 3-6 hours

Serum half-life: 2.5-3.6 hours

Pregnancy Risk Factor C

Generic Available Yes

Ephedrine, Theophylline and Phenobarbital see Theophylline, Ephedrine, and Phenobarbital on page 922

E-Pilo-x® Ophthalmic see Pilocarpine and Epinephrine on page 761

Epinal® see Epinephryl Borate on page 355

Epinephrine (ep i NEF rin)

Related Information

Dental Drug Interactions: Update on Drug Combinations Requiring Special Considerations on page 1144

Respiratory Diseases on page 1018

Therapeutic Category Adrenergic Agonist Agent; Antidote, Hypersensitivity Reactions; Antiglaucoma Agent; Bronchodilator

Use Treatment of bronchospasms, anaphylactic reactions, cardiac arrest, management of open-angle (chronic simple) glaucoma

Usual Dosage

Bronchodilator:

Children: S.C.: 10 mcg/kg (0.01 mL/kg of 1:1000) (single doses not to exceed 0.5 mg); injection suspension (1:200): 0.005 mL/kg/dose (0.025 mg/kg/dose) to a maximum of 0.15 mL (0.75 mg for single dose) every 8-12 hours

(Continued)

Epinephrine *(Continued)*

Adults:
I.M., S.C. (1:1000): 0.1-0.5 mg every 10-15 minutes to 4 hours
Suspension (1:200) S.C.: 0.1-0.3 mL (0.5-1.5 mg)
I.V.: 0.1-0.25 mg (single dose maximum: 1 mg)

Cardiac arrest:
Children: Asystole or pulseless arrest:
I.V., intraosseous: First dose: 0.01 mg/kg (0.1 mL/kg of a 1:10,000 solution); subsequent doses: 0.1 mg/kg (0.1 mL/kg of a 1:1000 solution); doses as high as 0.2 mg/kg may be effective; repeat every 3-5 minutes
Intratracheal: 0.1 mg/kg (0.1 mL/kg of a 1:1000 solution); doses as high as 0.2 mg/kg may be effective
Adults: Asystole:
I.V.: 1 mg every 3-5 minutes; if this approach fails, alternative regimens include: Intermediate: 2-5 mg every 3-5 minutes; Escalating: 1 mg, 3 mg, 5 mg at 3-minute intervals; High: 0.1 mg/kg every 3-5 minutes
Intratracheal: Although optimal dose is unknown, doses of 2-2.5 times the I.V. dose may be needed

Bradycardia: Children:
I.V.: 0.01 mg/kg (0.1 mL/kg of 1:10,000 solution) every 3-5 minutes as needed (maximum: 1 mg/10 mL)
Intratracheal: 0.1 mg/kg (0.1 mL/kg of 1:1000 solution every 3-5 minutes); doses as high as 0.2 mg/kg may be effective

Refractory hypotension (refractory to dopamine/dobutamine): I.V. infusion administration requires the use of an infusion pump:
Children: Infusion rate 0.1-4 mcg/kg/minute
Adults: I.V. infusion: 1 mg in 250 mL NS/D_5W at 0.1-1 mcg/kg/minute; titrate to desired effect

Hypersensitivity reaction:
Children: S.C.: 0.01 mg/kg every 15 minutes for 2 doses then every 4 hours as needed (single doses not to exceed 0.5 mg)
Adults: I.M., S.C.: 0.2-0.5 mg every 20 minutes to 4 hours (single dose maximum: 1 mg)

Nebulization:
Children <2 years: 0.25 mL of 1:1000 diluted in 3 mL NS with treatments ordered individually
Children >2 years and Adolescents: 0.5 mL of 1:1000 concentration diluted in 3 mL NS
Children >2 years and Adults (racemic epinephrine):
<10 kg: 2 mL of 1:8 dilution over 15 minutes every 1-4 hours
10-15 kg: 2 mL of 1:6 dilution over 15 minutes every 1-4 hours
15-20 kg: 2 mL of 1:4 dilution over 15 minutes every 1-4 hours
>20 kg: 2 mL of 1:3 dilution over 15 minutes every 1-4 hours
Adults: Instill 8-15 drops into nebulizer reservoirs; administer 1-3 inhalations 4-6 times/day

Ophthalmic: Instill 1-2 drops in eye(s) once or twice daily

Intranasal: Children ≥6 years and Adults: Apply locally as drops or spray or with sterile swab

Mechanism of Action Stimulates alpha-, beta$_1$-, and beta$_2$-adrenergic receptors resulting in relaxation of smooth muscle of the bronchial tree, cardiac stimulation, and dilation of skeletal muscle vasculature; small doses can cause vasodilation via beta$_2$-vascular receptors; large doses may produce constriction of skeletal and vascular smooth muscle; decreases production of aqueous humor and increases aqueous outflow; dilates the pupil by contracting the dilator muscle

Local Anesthetic/Vasoconstrictor Precautions No information available to require special precautions

Effects on Dental Treatment No effects or complications reported

Other Adverse Effects
>10%:
Cardiovascular: Tachycardia (parenteral), pounding heartbeat
Central nervous system: Nervousness, restlessness
1% to 10%:
Cardiovascular: Flushing, hypertension, unusual pallor
Central nervous system: Headache, dizziness, lightheadedness, insomnia
Gastrointestinal: Nausea, vomiting
Neuromuscular & skeletal: Trembling, weakness
Miscellaneous: Increased sweating

Contraindications Hypersensitivity to epinephrine or any component; cardiac arrhythmias, angle-closure glaucoma

Warnings/Precautions Use with caution in elderly patients, patients with diabetes mellitus, cardiovascular diseases (angina, tachycardia, myocardial infarction), thyroid disease, or cerebral arteriosclerosis, Parkinson's; some products contain sulfites as antioxidants. Rapid I.V. infusion may cause death from cerebrovascular hemorrhage or cardiac arrhythmias. Oral inhalation of epinephrine is **not** the preferred route of administration.

Drug Interactions Increased cardiac irritability if administered concurrently with halogenated inhalational anesthetics, beta-blocking agents, alpha-blocking agents

Drug Uptake
Onset of bronchodilation:
Subcutaneous: Within 5-10 minutes
Inhalation: Within 1 minute
Conjunctival instillation:
Onset of effect: Intraocular pressures fall within 1 hour
Peak effect: Within 4-8 hours
Duration of ocular effect: 12-24 hours
Absorption: Orally ingested doses are rapidly metabolized in the GI tract and liver; pharmacologically active concentrations are not achieved

Pregnancy Risk Factor C

Breast-feeding Considerations No data reported

Dosage Forms
Aerosol, oral:
Bitartrate (AsthmaHaler®, Bronitin®, Medihaler-Epi®, Primatene® Suspension): 0.3 mg/spray [epinephrine base 0.16 mg/spray] (10 mL, 15 mL, 22.5 mL)
Bronkaid®: 0.5% (10 mL, 15 mL, 22.5 mL)
Primatene®: 0.2 mg/spray (15 mL, 22.5 mL)
Auto-injector:
EpiPen®: Delivers 0.3 mg I.M. of epinephrine 1:1000 (2 mL)
EpiPen® Jr.: Delivers 0.15 mg I.M. of epinephrine 1:2000 (2 mL)
Injection (Adrenalin®): 0.01 mg/mL [1:100,000] (5 mL); 0.1 mg/mL [1:10,000] (3 mL, 10 mL); 1 mg/mL [1:1000] (1 mL, 2 mL, 30 mL)
Solution:
Inhalation:
Adrenalin®: 1% [10 mg/mL, 1:100] (7.5 mL)
AsthmaNefrin®, microNefrin®, Nephron®: Racepinephrine 2% [epinephrine base 1.125%] (7.5 mL, 15 mL, 30 mL)
Vaponefrin®: Racepinephrine 2% [epinephrine base 1%] (15 mL, 30 mL)
Nasal (Adrenalin®): 0.1% [1 mg/mL, 1:1000] (30 mL)
Ophthalmic, as base (Epifrin®): 0.5% (15 mL); 1% (15 mL); 2% (15 mL)
Ophthalmic, as hydrochloride: 0.1% (1 mL)
Glaucon®: 1% (10 mL); 2% (10 mL)
Topical (Adrenalin®): 0.1% [1 mg/mL, 1:1000] (30 mL, 10 mL)
Suspension for injection (Sus-Phrine®): 5 mg/mL [1:200] (0.3 mL, 5 mL)

Dietary Considerations No data reported

Generic Available Yes

Epinephrine (Dental) (ep i NEF rin DEN tal)
Related Information
Dental Drug Interactions: Update on Drug Combinations Requiring Special Considerations *on page 1144*
Respiratory Diseases *on page 1018*

Brand Names Adrenalin®; Sus-Phrine®

Therapeutic Category Adrenergic Agonist Agent; Antidote, Hypersensitivity Reactions

Use
Dental: Emergency drug for treatment of anaphylactic reactions; used as vasoconstrictor to prolong local anesthesia

Usual Dosage
Hypersensitivity reaction:
Children: S.C.: 0.01 mg/kg every 15 minutes for 2 doses then every 4 hours as needed (single doses not to exceed 0.5 mg)
Adults: I.M., S.C.: 0.2-0.5 mg every 20 minutes to 4 hours (single dose maximum: 1 mg)

Mechanism of Action Stimulates alpha-, beta$_1$-, and beta$_2$-adrenergic receptors resulting in relaxation of smooth muscle of the bronchial tree, cardiac stimulation, and dilation of skeletal muscle vasculature; small doses can cause vasodilation via beta$_2$-vascular receptors; large doses may produce constriction of skeletal and vascular smooth muscle; decreases production of aqueous humor and increases aqueous outflow; dilates the pupil by contracting the dilator muscle

Local Anesthetic/Vasoconstrictor Precautions No information available to require special precautions
(Continued)

Epinephrine (Dental) *(Continued)*

Effects on Dental Treatment No effects or complications reported

Other Adverse Effects No data reported

Contraindications Hypersensitivity to epinephrine or any component; cardiac arrhythmias, angle-closure glaucoma

Warnings/Precautions Use with caution in elderly patients, patients with diabetes mellitus, cardiovascular diseases (angina, tachycardia, myocardial infarction), thyroid disease, or cerebral arteriosclerosis, Parkinson's; some products contain sulfites as antioxidants. Rapid I.V. infusion may cause death from cerebrovascular hemorrhage or cardiac arrhythmias. Oral inhalation of epinephrine is **not** the preferred route of administration.

Drug Interactions Increased cardiac irritability if administered concurrently with halogenated inhalational anesthetics, beta-blocking agents, alpha-blocking agents

Drug Uptake
Absorption: Not absorbed orally

Pregnancy Risk Factor C

Breast-feeding Considerations Usual infiltration doses of epinephrine given to nursing mothers has not been shown to affect the health of the nursing infant

Dosage Forms
Injection:
Adrenalin®: 0.01 mg/mL [1:100,000] (5 mL); 0.1 mg/mL [1:10,000] (3 mL, 10 mL); 1 mg/mL [1:1000] (1 mL, 2 mL, 30 mL)
Suspension (Sus-Phrine®): 5 mg/mL [1:200] (0.3 mL, 5 mL)
Solution, topical (Adrenalin®): 0.1% [1 mg/mL, 1:1000] (30 mL, 10 mL)

Dietary Considerations No data reported

Generic Available Yes

Epinephrine, Racemic *(ep i NEF rin, ra SEE mik)*

Brand Names AsthmaNefrin®; microNefrin®; Nephron®; S-2®; Vaponefrin®

Therapeutic Category Vasoconstrictor

Local Anesthetic/Vasoconstrictor Precautions No information available to require special precautions

Effects on Dental Treatment No effects or complications reported

Other Adverse Effects No data reported

Drug Interactions No data reported

Drug Uptake
Absorption: Not absorbed orally
Onset of bronchodilation:
Subcutaneous: Within 5-10 minutes
Inhalation: Within 1 minute

Breast-feeding Considerations No data reported

Dosage Forms
Solution, inhalation:
AsthmaNefrin®, microNefrin®, Nephron®, S-2®: Racepinephrine 2.25% [epinephrine base 1.125%] (7.5 mL, 15 mL, 30 mL)
Vaponefrin®: Racepinephrine 2% [epinephrine base 1%] (15 mL, 30 mL)

Dietary Considerations No data reported

Generic Available Yes

Epinephrine, Racemic and Aluminum Potassium Sulfate

(ep i NEF rin, ra SEE mik and a LOO mi num poe TASS ee um SUL fate)

Brand Names Van R Gingibraid®

Therapeutic Category Astringent; Vasoconstrictor

Use
Dental: Gingival retraction
Medical: None

Usual Dosage Pass the impregnated yarn around the neck of the tooth and place into gingival sulcus; normal tissue moisture, water, or gingival retraction solutions activate impregnated yarn. Limit use to one quadrant of the mouth at a time; recommended use is for 3-8 minutes in the mouth.

Mechanism of Action Epinephrine stimulates alpha, adrenergic receptors to cause vasoconstriction in blood vessels in gingiva; aluminum potassium sulfate, precipitates tissue and blood proteins

Local Anesthetic/Vasoconstrictor Precautions No information available to require special precautions

Effects on Dental Treatment Tissue retraction around base of the tooth (therapeutic effect)

Other Adverse Effects No data reported

Contraindications Patients with cardiovascular disease, hyperthyroidism, or diabetes; patients sensitive to epinephrine; do not apply to areas of heavy or deep bleeding or over exposed bone

Warnings/Precautions Caution should be exercised whenever using gingival retraction cords with epinephrine since it delivers vasoconstrictor doses of racemic epinephrine to patients; the general medical history should be thoroughly evaluated before using in any patient

Drug Interactions No data reported

Drug Uptake No data reported

Breast-feeding Considerations No data reported

Dosage Forms Yarn, saturated in solution of 8% racemic epinephrine and 7% aluminum potassium sulfate; yarn labeled type "0e" contains 0.20±0.10 mg epinephrine per inch; "1e" contains 0.40±0.20 mg per inch; "2e" contains 0.60±0.20 mg per inch

Dietary Considerations No data reported

Generic Available No

Epinephryl Borate (ep i NEF ril BOR ate)

Brand Names Epinal®

Therapeutic Category Adrenergic Agonist Agent, Ophthalmic; Antiglaucoma Agent; Ophthalmic Agent, Vasoconstrictor

Use Reduces elevated intraocular pressure in chronic open-angle glaucoma

Local Anesthetic/Vasoconstrictor Precautions No information available to require special precautions

Effects on Dental Treatment No effects or complications reported

Generic Available No

Epitol® *see* Carbamazepine *on page 174*

Epivir® *see* Lamivudine *on page 541*

EPO *see* Epoetin Alfa *on this page*

Epoetin Alfa (e POE e tin AL fa)

Brand Names Epogen®; Procrit®

Canadian/Mexican Brand Names Eprex® (Mexico)

Therapeutic Category Recombinant Human Erythropoietin

Synonyms EPO; Erythropoietin; rHuEPO-α

Use Anemia associated with end stage renal disease; anemia related to therapy with AZT-treated HIV-infected patients; anemia in cancer patients receiving chemotherapy; anemia of prematurity

Usual Dosage

Individuals with anemia due to iron deficiency, sickle cell disease, autoimmune hemolytic anemia, and bleeding, generally have appropriate endogenous EPO levels to drive erythropoiesis and would not ordinarily be candidates for EPO therapy.

In patients on dialysis, epoetin alfa usually has been administered as an IVP 3 times/week. While the administration is independent of the dialysis procedure, it may be administered into the venous line at the end of the dialysis procedure to obviate the need for additional venous access; in patients with CRF not on dialysis, epoetin alfa may be given either as an IVP or S.C. injection.

Children and Adults: Dosing recommendations:

Dosing schedules need to be individualized and careful monitoring of patients receiving the drug is mandatory

rHuEPO-α may be ineffective if other factors such as iron or B₁₂/folate deficiency limit marrow response

IVP, S.C.:

Chronic renal failure patients:

Initial dose: 50-100 units/kg 3 times/week

Dose should be reduced when the hematocrit reaches the target range of 30% to 36% or a hematocrit increase >4% points over any 2-week period

Dose should be held if the hematocrit exceeds 36% and until the hematocrit decreases to the target range (30% to 36%).

Dose should be increased not more frequently than once a month, unless clinically indicated. After any dose adjustment, the hematocrit should be determined twice weekly for at least 2-6 weeks. If a hematocrit increase of 5-6 points is not achieved after a 8-week period and iron stores are adequate, the dose may be incrementally increased. Further increases may be made at 4-6 week intervals until the desired response is obtained.

Maintenance dose: Should be individualized to maintain the hematocrit within the 30% to 33% target range. The median maintenance dose in phase III studies in chronic renal failure patients on dialysis was 75 units/kg 3 times/week (range 12.5-525 units/kg 3 times/week).

(Continued)

Epoetin Alfa *(Continued)*

Epoetin doses of 75-150 units/kg/week have been shown to maintain hematocrits of 36% to 38% for up to 6 months in patients with chronic renal failure not requiring dialysis

Zidovudine-treated HIV patients: Prior to beginning epoetin alfa, serum erythropoietin levels should be determined. Available evidence suggest that patients receiving zidovudine with endogenous serum erythropoietin levels >500 mIU/mL are unlikely to respond to therapy with epoetin alfa.

Initial dose: For patients with serum erythropoietin levels <500 mIU/mL who are receiving a dose of zidovudine ≤4,200 mg/week: 100 units/kg 3 times/week for 8 weeks.

Dose should be held if the hematocrit is >40% until the hematocrit drops to 36%. The dose should be reduced by 25% when the treatment is resumed and then titrated to maintain the desired hematocrit.

Dose should be reduced if the initial dose of epoetin alfa includes a rapid rise in hematocrit (>4% points in any 2-week period).

Increase dose by 50-100 units/kg if the response is not satisfactory in terms of reducing transfusion requirements or increasing hematocrit after 8 weeks of therapy. Response should be evaluated every 4-8 weeks thereafter and the dose adjusted and the dose adjusted accordingly by 50-100 units/kg increments 3 times/week. If patients have not responded satisfactorily to a dose of 300 units/kg 3 times/week, it is unlikely that they will respond to higher doses.

Maintenance dose: Dose should be titrated to maintain target hematocrit range: 36% to 40%

Cancer patients on chemotherapy: Although no specific serum erythropoietin level can be stipulated above which patients would be unlikely to respond to epoetin alfa therapy, treatment of patients with grossly elevated serum erythropoietin levels (>200 mIU/mL) is not recommended

Initial dose: 150 units/kg 3 times/week

Increase dose: Response should be evaluated every 8 weeks thereafter and the dose adjusted and the dose adjusted accordingly by 50-100 units/kg increments 3 times/week up to 300 units/kg 3 times/week if the response is not satisfactory. If patients have not responded satisfactorily to a dose of 300 units/kg 3 times/week, it is unlikely that they will respond to higher doses.

Dose should be held if the hematocrit is >40% until the hematocrit drops to 36%. The dose should be reduced by 25% when the treatment is resumed and then titrated to maintain the desired hematocrit.

Dose should be reduced if the initial dose of epoetin alfa includes a rapid rise in hematocrit (>4% points in any 2-week period), the dose should be reduced

Maintenance dose: Dose should be titrated to maintain target hematocrit range: 36% to 40%

Mechanism of Action Induces erythropoiesis by stimulating the division and differentiation of committed erythroid progenitor cells; induces the release of reticulocytes from the bone marrow into the blood stream, where they mature to erythrocytes. There is a dose response relationship with this effect. This results in an increase in reticulocyte counts followed by a rise in hematocrit and hemoglobin levels.

Local Anesthetic/Vasoconstrictor Precautions No information available to require special precautions

Effects on Dental Treatment No effects or complications reported

Other Adverse Effects

1% to 10%:
 Cardiovascular: Hypertension, chest pain, edema
 Central nervous system: Fatigue, headache, dizziness, seizures
 Dermatologic: Rash
 Gastrointestinal: Nausea, vomiting, diarrhea
 Hematologic: Clotted access
 Neuromuscular & skeletal: Arthralgias, weakness

<1%:
 Cardiovascular: Myocardial infarction, CVA/TIA
 Miscellaneous: Hypersensitivity reactions

Drug Uptake

Onset of action: Several days
Peak effect: 2-3 weeks
Serum half-life: Circulating: 4-13 hours in patients with chronic renal failure; 20% shorter in patients with normal renal function
Time to peak serum concentrations: S.C.: 2-8 hours

Pregnancy Risk Factor C

Generic Available No

Comments Epogen® reimbursement hotline number for information regarding coverage of epoetin alfa is 1-800-2-PAY-EPO. ProCrit™ reimbursement hotline is 1-800-441-1366.

Epogen® *see* Epoetin Alfa *on page 355*

Epoprostenol (e poe PROST en ole)
Brand Names Flolan® Injection
Therapeutic Category Platelet Inhibitor
Use Long-term intravenous treatment of primary pulmonary hypertension (PPH)
Usual Dosage I.V.: The drug is administered by continuous intravenous infusion via a central venous catheter using an ambulatory infusion pump; during dose ranging it may be administered peripherally
  Acute dose ranging: The initial infusion rate should be 2 ng/kg/minute by continuous I.V. and increased in increments of 2 ng/kg/minute every 15 minutes or longer until dose-limiting effects are elicited (such as chest pain, anxiety, dizziness, changes in heart rate, dyspnea, nausea, vomiting, headache, hypotension and/or flushing)
  Continuous chronic infusion: Initial: 4 ng/kg/minute **less** than the maximum-tolerated infusion rate determined during acute dose ranging.
  If maximum-tolerated infusion rate is <5 ng/kg/minute the chronic infusion rate should be ½ the maximum-tolerated acute infusion rate
  Dosage adjustments: Dose adjustments in the chronic infusion rate should be based on persistence, recurrence or worsening of patient symptoms of pulmonary hypertension
  If symptoms persist or recur after improving, the infusion rate should be increased by 1-2 ng/kg/minute increments, every 15 minutes or greater; following establishment of a new chronic infusion rate, the patient should be observed and vital signs monitored.

Preparation of Infusion

To make 100 mL of solution with concentration:	Directions:
3000 ng/mL	Dissolve one 0.5 mg vial with 6 mL supplied diluent, withdraw 3 mL and add to sufficient diluent to make a total of 100 mL
5000 ng/mL	Dissolve one 0.5 mg vial with 5 mL supplied diluent, withdraw entire vial contents and add a sufficient volume of diluent to make a total of 100 mL
10,000 ng/mL	Dissolve two 0.5 mg vials each with 5 mL supplied diluent, withdraw entire vial contents and add a sufficient volume of diluent to make a total of 100 mL
15,000 ng/mL	Dissolve one 1.5 mg vial with 5 mL supplied diluent, withdraw entire vial contents and add a sufficient volume of diluent to make a total of 100 mL

Local Anesthetic/Vasoconstrictor Precautions No information available to require special precautions
Effects on Dental Treatment No effects or complications reported
Drug Uptake
  Steady state levels are reached in about 15 minutes with continuous infusions
  Serum half-life: 2.7-6 minutes
Pregnancy Risk Factor X
Generic Available No

Eprosartan (ep roe SAR tan)
Brand Names Teveten®
Therapeutic Category Angiotensin II Antagonists
Use For use in the management of essential hypertension
Local Anesthetic/Vasoconstrictor Precautions No information available to require special precautions
Effects on Dental Treatment No effects or complications reported

Epsom Salts *see* Magnesium Sulfate *on page 577*

EPT *see* Teniposide *on page 906*

Equagesic® *see* Aspirin and Meprobamate *on page 94*

Equalactin® Chewable Tablet [OTC] *see* Calcium Polycarbophil *on page 168*

Equanil® *see* Meprobamate *on page 599*

Equilet® [OTC] *see* Calcium Carbonate *on page 162*

Ercaf® *see* Ergotamine *on page 360*
Ergamisol® *see* Levamisole *on page 546*

Ergocalciferol (er goe kal SIF e role)

Brand Names Calciferol™; Drisdol®
Canadian/Mexican Brand Names Ostoforte®(Canada); Radiostol® (Canada)
Therapeutic Category Vitamin D Analog
Synonyms Ergocalciferol (Mexico)
Use Treatment of refractory rickets, hypophosphatemia, hypoparathyroidism
Usual Dosage Oral dosing is preferred
  Dietary supplementation (each mcg = 40 USP units):
    Healthy Children: 10 mcg/day (400 units)
    Adults: 10 mcg/day (400 units)
  Renal failure:
    Children: 100-1000 mcg/day (4000-40,000 units)
    Adults: 500 mcg/day (20,000 units)
  Hypoparathyroidism:
    Children: 1.25-5 mg/day (50,000-200,000 units) and calcium supplements
    Adults: 625 mcg to 5 mg/day (25,000-200,000 units) and calcium supplements
  Vitamin D-dependent rickets:
    Children: 75-125 mcg/day (3000-5000 units); maximum: 1500 mcg/day
    Adults: 250 mcg to 1.5 mg/day (10,000-60,000 units)
  Nutritional rickets and osteomalacia:
    Children and Adults (with normal absorption): 25-125 mcg/day (1000-5000 units)
    Children with malabsorption: 250-625 mcg/day (10,000-25,000 units)
    Adults with malabsorption: 250-7500 mcg (10,000-300,000 units)
  Vitamin D-resistant rickets:
    Children: Initial: 1000-2000 mcg/day (400,000-800,000 units) with phosphate supplements; daily dosage is increased at 3- to 4-month intervals in 250-500 mcg (10,000-20,000 units) increments
    Adults: 250-1500 mcg/day (10,000-60,000 units) with phosphate supplements
Mechanism of Action Stimulates calcium and phosphate absorption from the small intestine, promotes secretion of calcium from bone to blood; promotes renal tubule phosphate resorption
Local Anesthetic/Vasoconstrictor Precautions No information available to require special precautions
Effects on Dental Treatment No effects or complications reported
Other Adverse Effects
  1% to 10%:
    Cardiovascular: Hypotension, cardiac arrhythmias, hypertension
    Central nervous system: Irritability, headache
    Dermatologic: Pruritus
    Endocrine & metabolic: Polydipsia
    Gastrointestinal: Nausea, vomiting, anorexia, pancreatitis, metallic taste
    Neuromuscular & skeletal: Bone pain, myalgia
    Ocular: Conjunctivitis, photophobia
    Renal: Polyuria
  <1%:
    Central nervous system: Overt psychosis
    Gastrointestinal: Weight loss
Drug Interactions
  Decreased effect: Cholestyramine, colestipol, mineral oil causes decreased oral absorption
  Increased effect: Thiazide diuretics causes increased vitamin D effects
  Increased toxicity: Cardiac glycosides causes increased toxicity
Drug Uptake
  Peak effect: In ~1 month following daily doses
  Absorption: Readily absorbed from GI tract; absorption requires intestinal presence of bile
Pregnancy Risk Factor A (C if dose exceeds RDA recommendation)
Generic Available Yes

Ergocalciferol (Mexico) *see* Ergocalciferol *on this page*

Ergoloid Mesylates (ER goe loid MES i lates)

Brand Names Germinal®; Hydergine®; Hydergine® LC
Therapeutic Category Ergot Alkaloid
Use Treatment of cerebrovascular insufficiency in primary progressive dementia, Alzheimer's dementia, and senile onset
Usual Dosage Adults: Oral: 1 mg 3 times/day up to 4.5-12 mg/day; up to 6 months of therapy may be necessary

Mechanism of Action Ergoloid mesylates do not have the vasoconstrictor effects of the natural ergot alkaloids; exact mechanism in dementia is unknown; originally classed as peripheral and cerebral vasodilator, now considered a "metabolic enhancer"; there is no specific evidence which clearly establishes the mechanism by which ergoloid mesylate preparations produce mental effects, nor is there conclusive evidence that the drug particularly affects cerebral arteriosclerosis or cerebrovascular insufficiency

Local Anesthetic/Vasoconstrictor Precautions No information available to require special precautions

Effects on Dental Treatment No effects or complications reported

Other Adverse Effects
1% to 10%:
Gastrointestinal: Transient nausea
Miscellaneous: Sublingual irritation
<1%:
Cardiovascular: Bradycardia, orthostatic hypotension, flushing, syncope
Central nervous system: Headache
Dermatologic: Skin rash
Gastrointestinal: Anorexia, nausea, vomiting, stomach cramps
Ocular: Blurred vision
Respiratory: Nasal congestion

Drug Interactions Increased toxicity with dopamine

Drug Uptake
Absorption: Rapid yet incomplete
Serum half-life: 3.5 hours
Time to peak serum concentration: Within 1 hour

Pregnancy Risk Factor C

Generic Available Yes

Ergomar® *see* Ergotamine *on next page*

Ergometrine Maleate (Canada) *see* Ergonovine *on this page*

Ergonovina (Mexico) *see* Ergonovine *on this page*

Ergonovine (er goe NOE veen)

Brand Names Ergotrate® Maleate

Therapeutic Category Ergot Alkaloid

Synonyms Ergometrine Maleate (Canada); Ergonovina (Mexico)

Use Prevention and treatment of postpartum and postabortion hemorrhage caused by uterine atony or subinvolution

Usual Dosage Adults:
Oral: 1-2 tablets (0.2-0.4 mg) every 6-12 hours for up to 48 hours
I.M., I.V. (I.V. should be reserved for emergency use only): 0.2 mg, repeat dose in 2-4 hours as needed

Mechanism of Action Ergot alkaloid alpha-adrenergic agonist directly stimulates vascular smooth muscle to vasoconstrict peripheral and cerebral vessels; may also have antagonist effects on serotonin

Local Anesthetic/Vasoconstrictor Precautions No information available to require special precautions

Effects on Dental Treatment No effects or complications reported

Other Adverse Effects
1% to 10%: Gastrointestinal: Nausea, vomiting
<1%:
Cardiovascular: Palpitations, bradycardia, transient chest pain, hypertension, cerebrovascular accidents
Central nervous system: Seizures, dizziness, headache
Local: Thrombophlebitis
Otic: Tinnitus
Respiratory: Dyspnea
Miscellaneous: Sweating

Drug Interactions No data reported

Drug Uptake
Onset of effect:
Oral: Within 5-15 minutes
I.M.: Within 2-5 minutes
Duration: Uterine effects persist for 3 hours, except when given I.V., then effects persist for ~45 minutes

Pregnancy Risk Factor X

Generic Available No

Ergotamina Tartrato De (Mexico) *see* Ergotamine *on next page*

Ergotamine (er GOT a meen)

Brand Names Cafatine®; Cafergot®; Cafetrate®; Ercaf®; Ergomar®; Wigraine®

Canadian/Mexican Brand Names Ergocaf® (Mexico); Ergomar® (Canada); Gynergen® (Canada); Sydolil® (Mexico)

Therapeutic Category Adrenergic Blocking Agent; Ergot Alkaloid

Synonyms Ergotamina Tartrato De (Mexico)

Use Abort or prevent vascular headaches, such as migraine or cluster

Usual Dosage Adults:

Oral:

Cafergot®: 2 tablets at onset of attack; then 1 tablet every 30 minutes as needed; maximum: 6 tablets per attack; do not exceed 10 tablets/week

Ergostat®: 1 tablet under tongue at first sign, then 1 tablet every 30 minutes, 3 tablets/24 hours, 5 tablets/week

Rectal (Cafergot® suppositories, Wigraine® suppositories, Cafatine® suppositories): 1 at first sign of an attack; follow with second dose after 1 hour, if needed; maximum dose: 2 per attack; do not exceed 5/week

Mechanism of Action Has partial agonist and/or antagonist activity against tryptaminergic, dopaminergic and alpha-adrenergic receptors depending upon their site; is a highly active uterine stimulant; it causes constriction of peripheral and cranial blood vessels and produces depression of central vasomotor centers

Local Anesthetic/Vasoconstrictor Precautions No information available to require special precautions

Effects on Dental Treatment >10% of patients experience dry mouth

Other Adverse Effects

>10%:

Cardiovascular: Tachycardia, bradycardia, arterial spasm, claudication and vasoconstriction; rebound headache may occur with sudden withdrawal of the drug in patients on prolonged therapy; localized edema, peripheral vascular effects

Central nervous system: Drowsiness, dizziness

Gastrointestinal: Nausea, vomiting, diarrhea

1% to 10%:

Cardiovascular: Transient tachycardia or bradycardia, precordial distress and pain

Gastrointestinal: Abdominal pain

Neuromuscular & skeletal: Weakness in the legs, myalgia, muscle pains in the extremities, paresthesia

Drug Interactions Increased toxicity:

Propranolol: One case of severe vasoconstriction with pain and cyanosis has been reported

Erythromycin, troleandomycin and other macrolide antibiotics: Monitor for signs of ergot toxicity

Drug Uptake

Absorption: Oral, rectal: Erratic; enhanced by caffeine coadministration

Time to peak serum concentration: Within 0.5-3 hours following co-administration with caffeine

Pregnancy Risk Factor X

Generic Available Yes

Ergotrate® Maleate see Ergonovine on previous page

Eritromicina y Sulfisoxasol (Mexico) see Erythromycin and Sulfisoxazole on page 363

E•R•O Ear [OTC] see Carbamide Peroxide on page 175

Erwinia Asparaginase (ehr WIN ee ah a SPAIR a ji nase)

Therapeutic Category Antineoplastic Agent, Miscellaneous

Synonyms NSC-106977; Porton Asparaginase

Use Acute lymphocytic leukemia (ALL) in patients sensitive to E. coli L-asparaginase

Local Anesthetic/Vasoconstrictor Precautions No information available to require special precautions

Effects on Dental Treatment No effects or complications reported

Dosage Forms Injection: 10,000 units

Generic Available No

Erwiniar® see Asparaginase on page 89

Eryc® Oral see Erythromycin on next page

Eryderm® Topical see Erythromycin, Topical on page 364

Erygel® Topical see Erythromycin, Topical on page 364

Erymax® Topical see Erythromycin, Topical on page 364

EryPed® Oral see Erythromycin on next page

Ery-Tab® Oral *see* Erythromycin *on this page*

Erythrityl Tetranitrate (e RI thri til te tra NYE trate)

Related Information

Cardiovascular Diseases *on page 1010*

Brand Names Cardilate®

Therapeutic Category Antianginal Agent; Nitrate; Vasodilator, Coronary

Use Prophylaxis and long-term treatment of frequent or recurrent anginal pain and reduced exercise tolerance associated with angina pectoris

Usual Dosage Adults: Oral: 5 mg under the tongue or in the buccal pouch 3 times/day or 10 mg before meals or food, chewed 3 times/day, increasing in 2-3 days if needed; dosages of up to 100 mg/day are tolerated; some patients may need bedtime doses if they experience nocturnal symptoms

Mechanism of Action Erythrityl tetranitrate, like other organic nitrates, induces vasodilation by dephosphorylation of the myosin light chain in smooth muscles. This is accomplished by activation of guanylate cyclase, which eventually stimulates a cyclic GMP-dependent protein kinase that alters the phosphorylation of the myosin. Venodilation causes peripheral blood pooling, which decreases venous return to the heart, central venous pressure, and pulmonary capillary wedge pressure. A reduction in pulmonary vascular resistance occurs secondary to pulmonary arteriolar dilation and afterload may be decreased by a lowering of systemic arterial pressure.

Local Anesthetic/Vasoconstrictor Precautions No information available to require special precautions

Effects on Dental Treatment No effects or complications reported

Other Adverse Effects

>10%: Central nervous system: Headache

1% to 10%: Cardiovascular: Tachycardia, hypotension, flushing

<1%:

Central nervous system: Restlessness, dizziness

Gastrointestinal: Nausea, vomiting, diarrhea

Hematologic: Methemoglobinemia

Neuromuscular & skeletal: Weakness

Pregnancy Risk Factor C

Generic Available No

Comments Doses up to 100 mg are generally well tolerated; headache may occur when increasing doses; should headache occur, reduce dose for 2-3 days; may use analgesics to treat headache

Erythrocin® Oral *see* Erythromycin *on this page*

Erythromycin (er ith roe MYE sin)

Related Information

Cardiovascular Diseases *on page 1010*

Dental Drug Interactions: Update on Drug Combinations Requiring Special Considerations *on page 1144*

Oral Bacterial Infections *on page 1059*

Oral Viral Infections *on page 1066*

Respiratory Diseases *on page 1018*

Brand Names E.E.S.® Oral; E-Mycin® Oral; Eryc® Oral; EryPed® Oral; Ery-Tab® Oral; Erythrocin® Oral; Ilosone® Oral; PCE® Oral

Canadian/Mexican Brand Names Apo®-Erythro E-C (Canada); Diomycin (Canada); Eritroquim® (Mexico); Erybid™ (Canada); Erythro-Base® (Canada); Latotryd® (Mexico); Lauricin® (Mexico); Lederpax® (Mexico); Luritran® (Mexico); Novo-Rythro Encap (Canada); Pantomicina® (Mexico); PMS-Erythromycin (Canada); Tromigal® (Mexico)

Therapeutic Category Antibiotic, Macrolide; Antibiotic, Ophthalmic

Use

Dental: An alternative to penicillin VK for treating orofacial infections

Medical: Treatment of susceptible bacterial infections in the medical patient including *M. pneumoniae*, *Legionella pneumophila*, diphtheria, pertussis, chancroid, *Chlamydia*, and *Campylobacter* gastroenteritis; used in conjunction with neomycin for decontaminating the bowel

Unlabeled use: Gastroparesis

Usual Dosage Orofacial infections:

Adults:

Stearate or base: 250-500 mg every 6 hours for at least 7 days

Ethylsuccinate: 400-800 mg every 6 hours for at least 7 days

Children: Base and ethylsuccinate: 30-50 mg/kg/day divided every 6-8 hours; do not exceed 2 g/day

(Continued)

Erythromycin *(Continued)*

Mechanism of Action Inhibits RNA-dependent protein synthesis at the chain elongation step; binds to the 50S ribosomal subunit resulting in blockage of transpeptidation

Local Anesthetic/Vasoconstrictor Precautions No information available to require special precautions

Effects on Dental Treatment 1% to 10% of patients experience oral candidiasis

Other Adverse Effects

>10%: Gastrointestinal: Abdominal pain, cramping, nausea, vomiting

1% to 10%:

Gastrointestinal: Oral candidiasis

Hepatic: Cholestatic jaundice

Local: Phlebitis at the injection site

Miscellaneous: Hypersensitivity reactions

Contraindications Hepatic impairment, known hypersensitivity to erythromycin or its components; use with pimozide

Warnings/Precautions Hepatic impairment with or without jaundice has occurred, it may be accompanied by malaise, nausea, vomiting, abdominal colic, and fever; discontinue use if these occur; avoid using erythromycin lactobionate in neonates since formulations may contain benzyl alcohol which is associated with toxicity in neonates

Drug Interactions Cytochrome P-450 IIIA enzyme inhibitor

Increased toxicity:

Erythromycin decreases clearance of carbamazepine, cyclosporine, and triazolam

Erythromycin may decrease theophylline clearance and increase theophylline's half-life by up to 60% (patients on high-dose theophylline and erythromycin or who have received erythromycin for >5 days may be at higher risk)

Terfenadine increases Q-T interval

May potentiate anticoagulant effect of warfarin

Concurrent use of erythromycin and lovastatin may result in rhabdomyolysis

Drug Uptake

Absorption: Variable but better with salt forms than with base form; 18% to 45% absorbed orally; due to differences in absorption, **200 mg erythromycin ethylsuccinate produces the same serum levels as 125 mg of erythromycin base** hours for the ethylsuccinate

Serum half-life: 1.5-2 hours (peak)

Time to peak serum concentration: 4 hours for the base, 30 minutes to 2.5

Pregnancy Risk Factor B

Breast-feeding Considerations May be taken while breast-feeding

Dosage Forms

Erythromycin base:

Capsule, delayed release: 250 mg

Capsule, delayed release, enteric coated pellets (Eryc®): 250 mg

Tablet, delayed release: 333 mg

Tablet, enteric coated (E-Mycin®, Ery-Tab®, E-Base®): 250 mg, 333 mg, 500 mg

Tablet, film coated: 250 mg, 500 mg

Tablet, polymer coated particles (PCE®): 333 mg, 500 mg

Erythromycin estolate:

Capsule (Ilosone® Pulvules®): 250 mg

Suspension, oral (Ilosone®): 125 mg/5 mL (480 mL); 250 mg/5 mL (480 mL)

Tablet (Ilosone®): 500 mg

Erythromycin ethylsuccinate:

Granules for oral suspension (EryPed®): 400 mg/5 mL (60 mL, 100 mL, 200 mL)

Powder for oral suspension (E.E.S.®): 200 mg/5 mL (100 mL, 200 mL)

Suspension, oral (E.E.S.®, EryPed®): 200 mg/5 mL (5 mL, 100 mL, 200 mL, 480 mL); 400 mg/5 mL (5 mL, 60 mL, 100 mL, 200 mL, 480 mL)

Suspension, oral [drops] (EryPed®): 100 mg/2.5 mL (50 mL)

Tablet (E.E.S.®): 400 mg

Tablet, chewable (EryPed®): 200 mg

Erythromycin gluceptate:

Injection: 1000 mg (30 mL)

Erythromycin lactobionate:

Powder for injection: 500 mg, 1000 mg

Erythromycin stearate:

Tablet, film coated (Eramycin®, Erythrocin®): 250 mg, 500 mg

Dietary Considerations Erythromycin has decreased absorption with food; avoid milk and acidic beverages 1 hour before or after a dose; ethylsuccinate, estolate, and enteric coated products are **not** affected by food; ethylsuccinate may be better absorbed with food

Generic Available Yes

Comments Many patients cannot tolerate erythromycin because of abdominal pain and nausea; the mechanism of this adverse effect appears to be the motilin agonistic properties of erythromycin in the GI tract. For these patients, clindamycin is indicated as the alternative antibiotic for treatment of orofacial infections.

Erythromycin has been used as a prokinetic agent to improve gastric emptying time and intestinal motility. In adults, 200 mg was infused I.V. initially followed by 250 mg orally 3 times/day 30 minutes before meals. In children, erythromycin 3 mg/kg I.V. has been infused over 60 minutes initially followed by 20 mg/kg/day orally in 3-4 divided doses before meals or before meals and at bedtime.

Selected Readings

Council on Dental Therapeutics, American Heart Association, "Preventing Bacterial Endocarditis," *J Am Dent Assoc*, 1991, 122(2):87-92.

Dajani AS, Bisno AL, Chung KJ, et al, "Prevention of Bacterial Endocarditis. Recommendations by the American Heart Association," *JAMA*, 1990, 264(22):2919-22.

"Pimozide (Orap) Contraindicated With Clarithromycin (Biaxin) and Other Macrolide Antibiotics," *FDA Medical Bulletin*, October 1996, 3.

Wynn RL and Bergman SA, "Antibiotics and Their Use in the Treatment of Orofacial Infections, Part I and Part II," *Gen Dent*, 1994, 42(5):398-402, 498-502.

Wynn RL, "Current Concepts of the Erythromycins," *Gen Dent*, 1991, 39(6):408,10-1.

Erythromycin and Benzoyl Peroxide

(er ith roe MYE sin & BEN zoe il per OKS ide)

Brand Names Benzamycin®

Therapeutic Category Acne Products

Use Topical control of acne vulgaris

Local Anesthetic/Vasoconstrictor Precautions No information available to require special precautions

Effects on Dental Treatment No effects or complications reported

Pregnancy Risk Factor C

Generic Available No

Erythromycin and Sulfisoxazole

(er ith roe MYE sin & sul fi SOKS a zole)

Brand Names Eryzole®; Pediazole®

Therapeutic Category Antibiotic, Macrolide; Antibiotic, Sulfonamide Derivative

Synonyms Eritromicina y Sulfisoxasol (Mexico)

Use Treatment of susceptible bacterial infections of the upper and lower respiratory tract, otitis media in children caused by susceptible strains of *Haemophilus influenzae*, and other infections in patients allergic to penicillin

Usual Dosage Oral (dosage recommendation is based on the product's erythromycin content):

Children ≥2 months: 50 mg/kg/day erythromycin and 150 mg/kg/day sulfisoxazole in divided doses every 6 hours; not to exceed 2 g erythromycin/day or 6 g sulfisoxazole/day for 10 days

Adults: 400 mg erythromycin and 1200 mg sulfisoxazole every 6 hours

Mechanism of Action Erythromycin inhibits bacterial protein synthesis; sulfisoxazole competitively inhibits bacterial synthesis of folic acid from para-aminobenzoic acid

Local Anesthetic/Vasoconstrictor Precautions No information available to require special precautions

Effects on Dental Treatment No effects or complications reported

Other Adverse Effects

>10%: Gastrointestinal: Abdominal pain, cramping, nausea, vomiting

1% to 10%:

Gastrointestinal: Oral candidiasis

Hepatic: Cholestatic jaundice

Local: Phlebitis at the injection site

Miscellaneous: Hypersensitivity reactions

<1%:

Cardiovascular: Ventricular arrhythmias

Central nervous system: Fever, headache

Dermatologic: Skin rash, Stevens-Johnson syndrome, toxic epidermal necrolysis

Gastrointestinal: Hypertrophic pyloric stenosis, diarrhea

Hematologic: Eosinophilia, agranulocytosis, aplastic anemia

Hepatic: Hepatic necrosis

Local: Thrombophlebitis

(Continued)

Erythromycin and Sulfisoxazole *(Continued)*
Renal: Toxic nephrosis, crystalluria
Drug Interactions Increased effect/toxicity/levels of alfentanil, anticoagulants, astemizole, terfenadine, loratadine, bromocriptine, carbamazepine, cyclosporine, digoxin, disopyramide, theophylline, triazolam, and warfarin
Drug Uptake
Erythromycin ethylsuccinate:
Absorption: Well absorbed from GI tract
Serum half-life: 1-1.5 hours

Sulfisoxazole acetyl:
Absorption: Readily absorbed
Serum half-life: 6 hours, prolonged in renal impairment
Pregnancy Risk Factor C
Generic Available Yes

Erythromycin, Topical *(er ith roe MYE sin TOP i kal)*
Brand Names Akne-Mycin® Topical; A/T/S® Topical; Del-Mycin® Topical; Emgel™ Topical; Eryderm® Topical; Erygel® Topical; Erymax® Topical; E-Solve-2® Topical; ETS-2%® Topical; Ilotycin® Ophthalmic; Staticin® Topical; T-Stat® Topical
Therapeutic Category Acne Products; Antibiotic, Topical
Use Topical treatment of acne vulgaris
Local Anesthetic/Vasoconstrictor Precautions No information available to require special precautions
Effects on Dental Treatment No effects or complications reported
Other Adverse Effects 1% to 10%: Dermatologic: Erythema, desquamation, dryness, pruritus
Pregnancy Risk Factor B
Generic Available Yes

Estazolam *(es TA zoe lam)*
Brand Names ProSom™
Canadian/Mexican Brand Names Tasedan® (Mexico)
Therapeutic Category Benzodiazepine; Hypnotic; Sedative
Use Short-term management of insomnia; there has been little experience with this drug in the elderly, but because of its lack of active metabolites, it is a reasonable choice when a benzodiazepine hypnotic is indicated
Usual Dosage Adults: Oral: 1 mg at bedtime, some patients may require 2 mg; start at doses of 0.5 mg in debilitated or small elderly patients
Mechanism of Action Benzodiazepines may exert their pharmacologic effect through potentiation of the inhibitory activity of GABA. Benzodiazepines do not alter the synthesis, release, reuptake, or enzymatic degradation of GABA.
Local Anesthetic/Vasoconstrictor Precautions No information available to require special precautions
Effects on Dental Treatment Significant xerostomia occurs in up to 10% of patients. Disappears with cessation of drug therapy.
Other Adverse Effects
>10%:
Central nervous system: Somnolence
Neuromuscular & skeletal: Weakness
1% to 10%:
Central nervous system: "Hangover" feeling, abnormal thinking, anxiety
Gastrointestinal: Dyspepsia
Neuromuscular & skeletal: Hypokinesis
Respiratory: Cold symptoms, pharyngitis, asthma, cough, dyspnea, rhinitis

<1%:
 Cardiovascular: Syncope
 Central nervous system: Agitation, amnesia, apathy, seizure, sleep disorder, stupor, ataxia, neuritis
 Dermatologic: Urticaria, acne, dry skin, photosensitivity
 Endocrine & metabolic: Decreased libido
 Gastrointestinal: Increased/decreased appetite, flatulence, gastritis, enterocolitis, melena, mouth ulceration
 Genitourinary: Nocturia, urinary incontinence
 Hematologic: Agranulocytosis
 Hepatic: Elevated AST
 Neuromuscular & skeletal: Twitching, decreased reflexes
 Renal: Hematuria, oliguria
 Respiratory: Epistaxis, laryngitis

Drug Interactions
 Decreased effect: Enzyme inducers may increase the metabolism of estazolam
 Increased toxicity: CNS depressants may increase CNS adverse effects; cimetidine may decrease metabolism of estazolam

Pregnancy Risk Factor X
Generic Available Yes

Estinyl® *see* Ethinyl Estradiol *on page 374*

Estivin® II Ophthalmic [OTC] *see* Naphazoline *on page 664*

Estrace® Oral *see* Estradiol *on this page*

Estraderm® Transdermal *see* Estradiol *on this page*

Estradiol (es tra DYE ole)
Related Information
 Endocrine Disorders & Pregnancy *on page 1021*
Brand Names Alora® Transdermal; Climara® Transdermal; depGynogen® Injection; Depo®-Estradiol Injection; Depogen® Injection; Dioval® Injection; Estrace® Oral; Estraderm® Transdermal; Estra-L® Injection; Estring®; Estro-Cyp® Injection; Gynogen L.A.® Injection; Valergen® Injection; Vivelle™ Transdermal
Canadian/Mexican Brand Names Ginedisc® (Mexico); Oestrogel® (Mexico); Systen® (Mexico)
Therapeutic Category Estrogen Derivative
Use Treatment of atrophic vaginitis, atrophic dystrophy of vulva, menopausal symptoms, female hypogonadism, ovariectomy, primary ovarian failure, inoperable breast cancer, inoperable prostatic cancer, mild to severe vasomotor symptoms associated with menopause
Usual Dosage Adults (all dosage needs to be adjusted based upon the patient's response):
 Male:
  Prostate cancer: Valerate: I.M.: ≥30 mg or more every 1-2 weeks
  Prostate cancer (androgen-dependent, inoperable, progressing): Oral: 10 mg 3 times/day for at least 3 months
 Female:
  Breast cancer (inoperable, progressing): Oral: 10 mg 3 times/day for at least 3 months
  Osteoporosis prevention: Oral: 0.5 mg/day in a cyclic regimen (3 weeks on and 1 week off of drug)
  Hypogonadism, moderate to severe vasomotor symptoms:
   Oral: 1-2 mg/day in a cyclic regimen for 3 weeks on drug, then 1 week off drug
  Moderate to severe vasomotor symptoms:
   I.M.: Cypionate: 1-5 mg every 3-4 weeks
   I.M.: Valerate: 10-20 mg every 4 weeks
  Postpartum breast engorgement: I.M.: Valerate: 10-25 mg at end of first stage of labor
  Transdermal: Apply 0.05 mg patch initially (titrate dosage to response) applied twice weekly in a cyclic regimen, for 3 weeks on drug and 1 week off drug in patients with an intact uterus and continuously in patients without a uterus
  Atrophic vaginitis, kraurosis vulvae: Vaginal: Insert 2-4 g/day for 2 weeks then gradually reduce to ¹/₂ the initial dose for 2 weeks followed by a maintenance dose of 1 g 1-3 times/week
Mechanism of Action Increases the synthesis of DNA, RNA, and various proteins in target tissues; reduces the release of gonadotropin-releasing hormone from the hypothalamus; reduces FSH and LH release from the pituitary
Local Anesthetic/Vasoconstrictor Precautions No information available to require special precautions
Effects on Dental Treatment No effects or complications reported
(Continued)

Estradiol *(Continued)*

Other Adverse Effects

>10%:
- Cardiovascular: Peripheral edema
- Endocrine & metabolic: Enlargement of breasts (female and male), breast tenderness
- Gastrointestinal: Nausea, anorexia, bloating

1% to 10%:
- Central nervous system: Headache
- Endocrine & metabolic: Increased libido (female), decreased libido (male)
- Gastrointestinal: Vomiting, diarrhea

<1%:
- Cardiovascular: Hypertension, edema, thromboembolic disorders, myocardial infarction
- Central nervous system: Depression, dizziness, anxiety, stroke
- Dermatologic: Chloasma, melasma, rash
- Endocrine & metabolic: Hypercalcemia, folate deficiency, change in menstrual flow, breast tumors, amenorrhea, decreased glucose tolerance, elevated triglycerides and LDL
- Gastrointestinal: GI distress
- Hepatic: Cholestatic jaundice
- Local: Pain at injection site
- Ocular: Intolerance to contact lenses
- Miscellaneous: Increased susceptibility to *Candida* infection

Drug Interactions
Decreased effect: Rifampin decreases estrogen serum concentrations
Increased toxicity: Hydrocortisone increases corticosteroid toxic potential; increases potential for thromboembolic events with anticoagulants

Drug Uptake
Absorption: Readily absorbed through skin and GI tract; reabsorbed from bile in GI tract and enterohepatically recycled
Serum half-life: 50-60 minutes

Pregnancy Risk Factor X
Generic Available Yes

Estradiol and Testosterone *(es tra DYE ole & tes TOS ter one)*

Brand Names Andro/Fem® Injection; Deladumone® Injection; depAndrogyn® Injection; Depo-Testadiol® Injection; Depotestogen® Injection; Duo-Cyp® Injection; Duratestrin® Injection; Valertest No.1® Injection

Therapeutic Category Estrogen and Androgen Combination

Synonyms Testosterone and Estradiol

Use Vasomotor symptoms associated with menopause; postpartum breast engorgement

Local Anesthetic/Vasoconstrictor Precautions No information available to require special precautions

Effects on Dental Treatment No effects or complications reported

Pregnancy Risk Factor X

Generic Available No

Estradurin® *see* Polyestradiol *on page 771*

Estra-L® Injection *see* Estradiol *on previous page*

Estramustine *(es tra MUS teen)*

Brand Names Emcyt®

Therapeutic Category Antineoplastic Agent, Hormone (Estrogen/Nitrogen Mustard)

Use Palliative treatment of prostatic carcinoma (progressive or metastatic)

Usual Dosage Adults: Oral: 14 mg/kg/day (range: 10-16 mg/kg/day) in 3-4 divided doses for 30-90 days; some patients have been maintained for >3 years on therapy

Mechanism of Action Mechanism is not completely clear, thought to act as an alkylating agent and as estrogen

Local Anesthetic/Vasoconstrictor Precautions No information available to require special precautions

Effects on Dental Treatment No effects or complications reported

Other Adverse Effects

>10%:
- Cardiovascular: Edema
- Endocrine & metabolic: Decreased libido, breast tenderness, breast enlargement
- Gastrointestinal: Diarrhea, nausea

    Hepatic: Mild elevations in AST (SGOT) or LDH
    Respiratory: Dyspnea
1% to 10%:
    Cardiovascular: Myocardial infarction
    Central nervous system: Insomnia, lethargy
    Gastrointestinal: Anorexia, flatulence
    Hematologic: Leukopenia
    Local: Thrombophlebitis
    Neuromuscular & skeletal: Leg cramps
    Respiratory: Pulmonary embolism
<1%:
    Cardiovascular: Cardiac arrest
    Central nervous system: Night sweats, depression
    Dermatologic: Pigment changes
    Endocrine & metabolic: Hypercalcemia, hot flashes
    Otic: Tinnitus

Drug Interactions Decreased effect: Milk products and calcium-rich foods/drugs may impair the oral absorption of estramustine phosphate sodium

Drug Uptake
    Absorption: Oral: Well absorbed (75%)
    Serum half-life: 20 hours
    Time to peak serum concentration: Within 2-3 hours

Pregnancy Risk Factor C

Generic Available No

Estratab® see Estrogens, Esterified *on page 369*

Estratest® H.S. Oral see Estrogens and Methyltestosterone *on next page*

Estratest® Oral see Estrogens and Methyltestosterone *on next page*

Estring® see Estradiol *on page 365*

Estro-Cyp® Injection see Estradiol *on page 365*

Estrogenos Conjugados (Mexico) see Estrogens, Conjugated *on next page*

Estrogens and Medroxyprogesterone
(ES troe jenz & me DROKS ee proe JES te rone)

Related Information
    Endocrine Disorders & Pregnancy *on page 1021*

Brand Names Premphase™; Prempro™

Therapeutic Category Estrogen and Progestin Combination

Use Women with an intact uterus for the treatment of moderate to severe vasomotor symptoms associated with the menopause; treatment of atrophic vaginitis; primary ovarian failure; osteoporosis prophylactic

Local Anesthetic/Vasoconstrictor Precautions No information available to require special precautions

Effects on Dental Treatment No effects or complications reported

Other Adverse Effects
>10%:
    Cardiovascular: Peripheral edema
    Endocrine & metabolic: Changes in menstrual flow, amenorrhea, enlargement of breasts, breast tenderness, breakthrough bleeding, spotting
    Gastrointestinal: Anorexia, nausea, bloating
    Local: Pain at injection site
    Neuromuscular & skeletal: Weakness
1% to 10%:
    Cardiovascular: Edema
    Central nervous system: Mental depression, fever, insomnia, headache
    Dermatologic: Melasma or chloasma, allergic rash with or without pruritus
    Endocrine & metabolic: Changes in cervical erosion and secretions, increased libido
    Gastrointestinal: Weight gain or loss, vomiting, diarrhea
    Hepatic: Cholestatic jaundice
    Local: Thrombophlebitis
    Respiratory: Pulmonary thrombosis and embolism
<1%:
    Cardiovascular: Hypertension, thromboembolism, myocardial infarction
    Central nervous system: Dizziness, anxiety, stroke
    Dermatologic: Rash
    Endocrine & metabolic: Breast tumors, amenorrhea, decreased glucose tolerance, elevated triglycerides and LDL
    Gastrointestinal: GI distress
    Ocular: Intolerance to contact lenses
    Miscellaneous: Increased susceptibility to *Candida* infection

Generic Available Yes

Estrogens and Methyltestosterone

(ES troe jenz & meth il tes TOS te rone)

Related Information

Endocrine Disorders & Pregnancy *on page 1021*

Brand Names Estratest® H.S. Oral; Estratest® Oral; Premarin® With Methyltestosterone Oral

Therapeutic Category Estrogen and Androgen Combination

Use Atrophic vaginitis; hypogonadism; primary ovarian failure; vasomotor symptoms of menopause; prostatic carcinoma; osteoporosis prophylactic

Local Anesthetic/Vasoconstrictor Precautions No information available to require special precautions

Effects on Dental Treatment No effects or complications reported

Pregnancy Risk Factor X

Generic Available No

Estrogens, Conjugated (ES troe jenz KON joo gate ed)

Related Information

Dental Drug Interactions: Update on Drug Combinations Requiring Special Considerations *on page 1144*

Endocrine Disorders & Pregnancy *on page 1021*

Brand Names Premarin®

Canadian/Mexican Brand Names C.E.S.® (Canada); Congest® (Canada)

Therapeutic Category Estrogen Derivative

Synonyms Estrogenos Conjugados (Mexico)

Use Atrophic vaginitis; hypogonadism; primary ovarian failure; vasomotor symptoms of menopause; prostatic carcinoma; osteoporosis prophylactic

Usual Dosage Adults:

Male: Prostate cancer: Oral: 1.25-2.5 mg 3 times/day

Female:

Hypogonadism: Oral: 2.5-7.5 mg/day for 20 days, off 10 days and repeat until menses occur

Abnormal uterine bleeding:

Oral: 2.5-5 mg/day for 7-10 days; then decrease to 1.25 mg/day for 2 weeks

I.M., I.V.: 25 mg every 6-12 hours until bleeding stops

Moderate to severe vasomotor symptoms: Oral: 0.625-1.25 mg/day

Postpartum breast engorgement: Oral: 3.75 mg every 4 hours for 5 doses, then 1.25 mg every 4 hours for 5 days

Atrophic vaginitis, kraurosis vulvae: Vaginal: 2-4 g instilled/day 3 weeks on and 1 week off

Osteoporosis: Oral: 0.625 mg/day chronically

Uremic bleeding: I.V.: 0.6 mg/kg/dose daily for 5 days

Mechanism of Action Increases the synthesis of DNA, RNA, and various proteins in target tissues; reduces the release of gonadotropin-releasing hormone from the hypothalamus; reduces FSH and LH release from the pituitary

Local Anesthetic/Vasoconstrictor Precautions No information available to require special precautions

Effects on Dental Treatment No effects or complications reported

Other Adverse Effects

>10%:

Cardiovascular: Peripheral edema

Endocrine & metabolic: Breast tenderness, hypercalcemia, enlargement of breasts

Gastrointestinal: Nausea, anorexia, bloating

1% to 10%:

Central nervous system: Headache

Endocrine & metabolic: Increased libido

Gastrointestinal: Vomiting, diarrhea

Local: Pain at injection site

<1%:

Cardiovascular: Hypertension, edema, thromboembolic disorder, myocardial infarction, hypertension

Central nervous system: Depression, dizziness, anxiety, stroke

Dermatologic: Chloasma, melasma, rash

Endocrine & metabolic: Breast tumors, amenorrhea, alterations in frequency and flow of menses, decreased glucose tolerance, elevated triglycerides and LDL

Gastrointestinal: GI distress

Hepatic: Cholestatic jaundice

Ocular: Intolerance to contact lenses

Miscellaneous: Increased susceptibility to *Candida* infection

Drug Interactions
Decreased effect: Rifampin decreases estrogen serum concentrations
Increased toxicity:
Anticoagulants: Increases potential for thromboembolic events with anticoagulants
Drug Uptake
Absorption: Readily absorbed from GI tract
Pregnancy Risk Factor X
Generic Available No

Estrogens, Esterified (ES troe jenz, es TER i fied)
Related Information
Dental Drug Interactions: Update on Drug Combinations Requiring Special Considerations *on page 1144*
Endocrine Disorders & Pregnancy *on page 1021*
Brand Names Estratab®; Menest®
Canadian/Mexican Brand Names Neo-Estrone® (Canada)
Therapeutic Category Estrogen Derivative
Use Atrophic vaginitis; hypogonadism; primary ovarian failure; vasomotor symptoms of menopause; prostatic carcinoma; osteoporosis prophylactic
Usual Dosage Adults: Oral:
Male: Prostate cancer (inoperable, progressing): 1.25-2.5 mg 3 times/day
Female:
Hypogonadism: 2.5-7.5 mg/day for 20 days, off 10 days and repeat until menses occur
Moderate to severe vasomotor symptoms: 0.3-1.25 mg/day
Breast cancer (inoperable, progressing): 10 mg 3 times/day for at least 3 months
Mechanism of Action Primary effects on the interphase DNA-protein complex (chromatin) by binding to a receptor (usually located in the cytoplasm of a target cell) and initiating translocation of the hormone-receptor complex to the nucleus
Local Anesthetic/Vasoconstrictor Precautions No information available to require special precautions
Effects on Dental Treatment No effects or complications reported
Other Adverse Effects
>10%:
Cardiovascular: Peripheral edema
Endocrine & metabolic: Enlargement of breasts, breast tenderness
Gastrointestinal: Nausea, anorexia, bloating
1% to 10%:
Central nervous system: Headache
Endocrine & metabolic: Increased libido
Gastrointestinal: Vomiting, diarrhea
<1%:
Cardiovascular: Hypertension, thromboembolism, myocardial infarction, edema
Central nervous system: Stroke, depression, dizziness, anxiety
Dermatologic: Chloasma, melasma, rash
Endocrine & metabolic: Breast tumors, amenorrhea, alterations in frequency and flow of menses, decreased glucose tolerance, elevated triglycerides and LDL
Gastrointestinal: GI distress
Hepatic: Cholestatic jaundice
Ocular: Intolerance to contact lenses
Miscellaneous: Increased susceptibility to *Candida* infection
Drug Interactions
Decreased effect: Rifampin decreases estrogen serum concentrations
Increased toxicity:
Anticoagulants: Increases potential for thromboembolic events with anticoagulants
Drug Uptake
Absorption: Readily absorbed from GI tract
Pregnancy Risk Factor X
Generic Available No

Estrone (ES trone)
Related Information
Endocrine Disorders & Pregnancy *on page 1021*
Brand Names Aquest®; Kestrone®
Canadian/Mexican Brand Names Femogen® (Canada); Neo-Estrone® (Canada); Oestrillin® (Canada)
(Continued)

Estrone *(Continued)*

Therapeutic Category Estrogen Derivative

Use Hypogonadism; primary ovarian failure; vasomotor symptoms of menopause; prostatic carcinoma; inoperable breast cancer, kraurosis vulvae, abnormal uterine bleeding due to hormone imbalance

Usual Dosage Adults: I.M.:
Male: Prostatic carcinoma: 2-4 mg 2-3 times/week
Female:
Senile vaginitis and kraurosis vulvae: 0.1-0.5 mg 2-3 times/week
Breast cancer (inoperable, progressing): 5 mg 3 or more times/week
Primary ovarian failure, hypogonadism: 0.1-1 mg/week, up to 2 mg/week in single or divided doses
Abnormal uterine bleeding: 2.5 mg/day for several days

Mechanism of Action Estrone is a natural ovarian estrogenic hormone that is available as an aqueous mixture of water insoluble estrone and water soluble estrone potassium sulfate; all estrogens, including estrone, act in a similar manner; there is no evidence that there are biological differences among various estrogen preparations other than their ability to bind to cellular receptors inside the target cells

Local Anesthetic/Vasoconstrictor Precautions No information available to require special precautions

Effects on Dental Treatment No effects or complications reported

Other Adverse Effects
>10%:
Cardiovascular: Peripheral edema
Endocrine & metabolic: Enlargement of breasts, breast tenderness
Gastrointestinal: Nausea, anorexia, bloating
1% to 10%:
Central nervous system: Headache
Endocrine & metabolic: Increased libido
Gastrointestinal: Vomiting, diarrhea
<1%:
Cardiovascular: Hypertension, thromboembolism, myocardial infarction, edema
Central nervous system: Stroke, depression, dizziness, anxiety
Dermatologic: Chloasma, melasma, rash
Endocrine & metabolic: Breast tumors, amenorrhea, alterations in frequency and flow of menses, decreased glucose tolerance, elevated triglycerides and LDL
Gastrointestinal: GI distress
Hepatic: Cholestatic jaundice
Ocular: Intolerance to contact lenses
Miscellaneous: Increased susceptibility to *Candida* infection

Drug Interactions
Decreased effect: Rifampin decreases estrogen serum concentrations
Increased toxicity:
Anticoagulants: Increases potential for thromboembolic events with anticoagulants

Pregnancy Risk Factor X

Generic Available Yes

Estropipate *(ES troe pih pate)*

Related Information
Endocrine Disorders & Pregnancy *on page 1021*

Brand Names Ogen®; Ortho-Est®

Canadian/Mexican Brand Names Estrouis® (Canada)

Therapeutic Category Estrogen Derivative

Use Atrophic vaginitis; hypogonadism; primary ovarian failure; vasomotor symptoms of menopause; osteoporosis prophylactic

Usual Dosage Adults: Female:
Moderate to severe vasomotor symptoms: Oral: 0.625-5 mg/day
Hypogonadism or primary ovarian failure: Oral: 1.25-7.5 mg/day for 3 weeks followed by an 8- to 10-day rest period
Osteoporosis prevention: Oral: 0.625 mg/day for 25 days of a 31-day cycle
Atrophic vaginitis or kraurosis vulvae: Vaginal: Instill 2-4 g/day 3 weeks on and 1 week off

Mechanism of Action Crystalline estrone that has been solubilized as the sulfate and stabilized with piperazine. Primary effects on the interphase DNA-protein complex (chromatin) by binding to a receptor (usually located in the cytoplasm of a target cell) and initiating translocation of the hormone receptor complex to the nucleus.

Local Anesthetic/Vasoconstrictor Precautions No information available to require special precautions

Effects on Dental Treatment No effects or complications reported

Other Adverse Effects

>10%:
Cardiovascular: Peripheral edema
Endocrine & metabolic: Enlargement of breasts, breast tenderness
Gastrointestinal: Nausea, anorexia, bloating

1% to 10%:
Central nervous system: Headache
Endocrine & metabolic: Increased libido
Gastrointestinal: Vomiting, diarrhea

<1%:
Cardiovascular: Hypertension, thromboembolism, myocardial infarction, edema
Central nervous system: Stroke, depression, dizziness, anxiety
Dermatologic: Chloasma, melasma, rash
Endocrine & metabolic: Breast tumors, amenorrhea, alterations in frequency and flow of menses, decreased glucose tolerance, elevated triglycerides and LDL
Gastrointestinal: GI distress
Hepatic: Cholestatic jaundice
Ocular: Intolerance to contact lenses
Miscellaneous: Increased susceptibility to *Candida* infection

Drug Interactions
Decreased effect: Rifampin decreases estrogen serum concentrations
Increased toxicity:
Anticoagulants: Increases potential for thromboembolic events with anticoagulants

Pregnancy Risk Factor X
Generic Available Yes

Estrostep® 21 *see* Ethinyl Estradiol and Norethindrone *on page 379*
Estrostep® Fe *see* Ethinyl Estradiol and Norethindrone *on page 379*
Estrovis® *see* Quinestrol *on page 829*

Ethacrynic Acid (eth a KRIN ik AS id)

Related Information
Cardiovascular Diseases *on page 1010*

Brand Names Edecrin®

Therapeutic Category Diuretic, Loop

Use Management of edema associated with congestive heart failure; hepatic cirrhosis or renal disease; short-term management of ascites due to malignancy, idiopathic edema, and lymphedema

Usual Dosage I.V. formulation should be diluted in D_5W or NS (1 mg/mL) and infused over several minutes

Children:
Oral: 1 mg/kg/dose once daily; increase at intervals of 2-3 days as needed, to a maximum of 3 mg/kg/day
I.V.: 1 mg/kg/dose, (maximum: 50 mg/dose); repeat doses not routinely recommended; however, if indicated, repeat doses every 8-12 hours

Adults:
Oral: 50-100 mg/day in 1-2 divided doses; may increase in increments of 25-50 mg at intervals of several days to a maximum of 400 mg/24 hours
I.V.: 0.5-1 mg/kg/dose (maximum: 100 mg/dose); repeat doses not routinely recommended; however, if indicated, repeat doses every 8-12 hours

Mechanism of Action Inhibits reabsorption of sodium and chloride in the ascending loop of Henle and distal renal tubule, interfering with the chloride-binding cotransport system, thus causing increased excretion of water, sodium, chloride, magnesium, and calcium

Local Anesthetic/Vasoconstrictor Precautions No information available to require special precautions

Effects on Dental Treatment No effects or complications reported

Other Adverse Effects
>10%: Diarrhea
1% to 10%:
Cardiovascular: Orthostatic hypotension
Central nervous system: Headache
Endocrine & metabolic: Hyponatremia, hypochloremic alkalosis, hypokalemia
Gastrointestinal: Loss of appetite
Ocular: Blurred vision
Otic: Ototoxicity
(Continued)

Ethacrynic Acid *(Continued)*

<1%:
Central nervous system: Nervousness
Dermatologic: Skin rash
Endocrine & metabolic: Hyperuricemia, gout
Gastrointestinal: Gastrointestinal bleeding, pancreatitis, stomach cramps
Hepatic: Hepatic dysfunction, abnormal LFTs
Hematologic: Leukopenia, agranulocytosis, thrombocytopenia
Local: Local irritation
Renal: Renal injury, hematuria

Drug Interactions
Increased effect:
Hypotensive agents causes additive decrease in blood pressure
Drugs affected by or causing potassium depletion cause additive decrease in potassium
Increased nephrotoxic potential with aminoglycosides
Digoxin increases cardiotoxic potential leading to arrhythmias
Increased warfarin anticoagulant effects; increased lithium levels
Decreased effect:
Probenecid decreases diuretic effects
Decreased effectiveness of antidiabetic agents

Drug Uptake
Onset of diuretic effect:
Oral: Within 30 minutes
I.V.: 5 minutes
Peak effect:
Oral: 2 hours
I.V.: 30 minutes
Duration of action:
Oral: 12 hours
I.V.: 2 hours
Absorption: Oral: Rapid
Serum half-life: Normal renal function: 2-4 hours

Pregnancy Risk Factor B
Generic Available No

Ethambutol *(e THAM byoo tole)*

Related Information
Nonviral Infectious Diseases *on page 1032*

Brand Names Myambutol®

Canadian/Mexican Brand Names Etibl® (Canada)

Therapeutic Category Antitubercular Agent

Use Treatment of tuberculosis and other mycobacterial diseases in conjunction with other antituberculosis agents; only indicated when patients are from areas where drug-resistant M. tuberculosis is endemic, in HIV-infected elderly patients, and when drug-resistant M. tuberculosis is suspected

Usual Dosage Oral:

Ethambutol is generally not recommended in children whose visual acuity cannot be monitored (<6 years of age). However, ethambutol should be considered for all children with organisms resistant to other drugs, when susceptibility to ethambutol has been demonstrated, or susceptibility is likely.

Note: A four-drug regimen (isoniazid, rifampin, pyrazinamide, and either streptomycin or ethambutol) is preferred for the initial, empiric treatment of TB. When the drug susceptibility results are available, the regimen should be altered as appropriate.

Patients with tuberculosis and without HIV infection:

OPTION 1: Isoniazid resistance rate <4%: Administer daily isoniazid, rifampin, and pyrazinamide for 8 weeks followed by isoniazid and rifampin daily or directly observed therapy (DOT) 2-3 times/week for 16 weeks. If isoniazid resistance rate is not documented, ethambutol or streptomycin should also be administered until susceptibility to isoniazid or rifampin is demonstrated. Continue treatment for at least 6 months or 3 months beyond culture conversion.

OPTION 2: Administer daily isoniazid, rifampin, pyrazinamide, and either streptomycin or ethambutol for 2 weeks followed by DOT 2 times/week administration of the same drugs for 6 weeks, and subsequently, with isoniazid and rifampin DOT 2 times/week administration for 16 weeks

OPTION 3: Administer isoniazid, rifampin, pyrazinamide, and either ethambutol or streptomycin by DOT 3 times/week for 6 months

Patients with TB and with HIV infection: Administer any of the above OPTIONS 1, 2 or 3; however, treatment should be continued for a total of 9 months and at least 6 months beyond culture conversion

Note: Some experts recommend that the duration of therapy should be extended to 9 months for patients with disseminated disease, miliary disease, disease involving the bones or joints, or tuberculosis lymphadenitis

Children (>6 years) and Adults:
    Daily therapy: 15-25 mg/kg/day (maximum: 2.5 g/day)
    Directly observed therapy (DOT): Twice weekly: 50 mg/kg (maximum: 2.5 g)
    DOT: 3 times/week: 25-30 mg/kg (maximum: 2.5 g)
Mechanism of Action Suppresses mycobacteria multiplication by interfering with RNA synthesis
Local Anesthetic/Vasoconstrictor Precautions No information available to require special precautions
Effects on Dental Treatment No effects or complications reported
Other Adverse Effects
1% to 10%:
    Central nervous system: Headache, confusion, disorientation
    Endocrine & metabolic: Acute gout or hyperuricemia
    Gastrointestinal: Abdominal pain, anorexia, nausea, vomiting
<1%:
    Central nervous system: Malaise, mental confusion, fever
    Dermatologic: Rash, pruritus
    Hepatic: Abnormal liver function tests
    Neuromuscular & skeletal: Peripheral neuritis
    Ocular: Optic neuritis
    Miscellaneous: Anaphylaxis
Drug Interactions Decreased absorption with aluminum salts
Drug Uptake
Absorption: Oral: ~80%
Serum half-life: 2.5-3.6 hours
    End stage renal disease: 7-15 hours
Time to peak serum concentration: 2-4 hours
Pregnancy Risk Factor B
Generic Available No

Ethamolin® see Ethanolamine Oleate *on this page*
ETH and C see Terpin Hydrate and Codeine *on page 909*

Ethanolamine Oleate (ETH a nol a meen OH lee ate)
Brand Names Ethamolin®
Therapeutic Category Sclerosing Agent
Synonyms Monoethanolamine (Canada)
Use Mild sclerosing agent used for bleeding esophageal varices
Usual Dosage Adults: 1.5-5 mL per varix, up to 20 mL total or 0.4 mL/kg; patients with severe hepatic dysfunction should receive less than recommended maximum dose
Mechanism of Action Derived from oleic acid and similar in physical properties to sodium morrhuate; however, the exact mechanism of the hemostatic effect used in endoscopic injection sclerotherapy is not known. Intravenously injected ethanolamine oleate produces a sterile inflammatory response resulting in fibrosis and occlusion of the vein; a dose-related extravascular inflammatory reaction occurs when the drug diffuses through the venous wall. Autopsy results indicate that variceal obliteration occurs secondary to mural necrosis and fibrosis. Thrombosis appears to be a transient reaction.
Local Anesthetic/Vasoconstrictor Precautions No information available to require special precautions
Effects on Dental Treatment No effects or complications reported
Other Adverse Effects
1% to 10%:
    Central nervous system: Fever
    Gastrointestinal: Esophageal ulcer, esophageal stricture
    Neuromuscular & skeletal: Retrosternal pain
    Respiratory: Pleural effusion, pneumonia
<1%:
    Local: Injection necrosis
    Renal: Acute renal failure
    Respiration: Aspiration
    Miscellaneous: Anaphylaxis
Drug Interactions No data reported
Pregnancy Risk Factor C
(Continued)

Ethanolamine Oleate *(Continued)*

Generic Available No

Ethaquin® *see* Ethaverine *on this page*
Ethatab® *see* Ethaverine *on this page*

Ethaverine (eth AV er een)

Brand Names Ethaquin®; Ethatab®; Ethavex-100®; Isovex®
Therapeutic Category Vasodilator
Use Peripheral and cerebral vascular insufficiency associated with arterial spasm
Local Anesthetic/Vasoconstrictor Precautions No information available to require special precautions
Effects on Dental Treatment No effects or complications reported
Other Adverse Effects <1%:
  Cardiovascular: Flushing of the face, tachycardia, hypotension
  Central nervous system: Depression, dizziness, vertigo, drowsiness, sedation, lethargy, headache
  Dermatologic: Pruritus
  Gastrointestinal: Dry mouth, nausea, constipation
  Hepatic: Hepatic hypersensitivity
  Miscellaneous: Sweating
Generic Available Yes

Ethavex-100® *see* Ethaverine *on this page*

Ethchlorvynol (eth klor VI nole)

Brand Names Placidyl®
Therapeutic Category Hypnotic; Sedative
Use Short-term management of insomnia
Usual Dosage Adults: Oral: 500-1000 mg at bedtime
  Dosing adjustment in renal impairment: Cl_{cr} <50 mL/minute: Avoid use
Mechanism of Action Causes nonspecific depression of the reticular activating system
Local Anesthetic/Vasoconstrictor Precautions No information available to require special precautions
Effects on Dental Treatment No effects or complications reported
Other Adverse Effects
  >10%:
    Central nervous system: Dizziness
    Gastrointestinal: Indigestion, nausea, stomach pain, unpleasant aftertaste
    Neuromuscular & skeletal: Weakness
    Ocular: Blurred vision
  1% to 10%:
    Central nervous system: Nervousness, excitement, clumsiness, confusion, drowsiness (daytime)
    Dermatologic: Skin rash
  <1%:
    Cardiovascular: Bradycardia
    Central nervous system: Hyperthermia, slurred speech
    Hepatic: Cholestatic jaundice
    Neuromuscular & skeletal: Trembling, weakness (severe)
    Respiratory: Dyspnea
Drug Interactions
  Decreased effect of oral anticoagulants
  Increased toxicity (CNS depression) with alcohol, CNS depressants, MAO inhibitors, TCAs (delirium)
Drug Uptake
  Onset of action: 15-60 minutes
  Duration: 5 hours
  Absorption: Rapid from GI tract
  Serum half-life: 10-20 hours
  Time to peak serum concentration: 2 hours
Pregnancy Risk Factor C
Generic Available No

Ethinyl Estradiol (ETH in il es tra DYE ole)

Related Information
  Endocrine Disorders & Pregnancy *on page 1021*
Brand Names Estinyl®
Therapeutic Category Estrogen Derivative
Synonyms Etinilestradiol (Mexico)

Use Hypogonadism; primary ovarian failure; vasomotor symptoms of menopause; prostatic carcinoma; breast cancer

Usual Dosage Adults: Oral:

Male: Prostatic cancer (inoperable, progressing): 0.15-2 mg/day for palliation

Female:

Hypogonadism: 0.05 mg 1-3 times/day for 2 weeks of a theoretical menstrual cycle followed by progesterone for 3-6 months

Vasomotor symptoms: 0.02-0.05 mg for 21 days, off 7 days and repeat

Breast cancer (inoperable, progressing): 1 mg 3 times/day for palliation

Mechanism of Action Increases the synthesis of DNA, RNA, and various proteins in target tissues; reduces the release of gonadotropin-releasing hormone from the hypothalamus; reduces FSH and LH release from the pituitary

Local Anesthetic/Vasoconstrictor Precautions No information available to require special precautions

Effects on Dental Treatment No effects or complications reported

Other Adverse Effects

>10%:

Cardiovascular: Peripheral edema

Endocrine & metabolic: Enlargement of breasts, breast tenderness

Gastrointestinal: Nausea, anorexia, bloating

1% to 10%:

Central nervous system: Headache

Endocrine & metabolic: Increased libido

Gastrointestinal: Vomiting, diarrhea

<1%:

Cardiovascular: Hypertension, thromboembolism, myocardial infarction, edema

Central nervous system: Stroke, depression, dizziness, anxiety

Dermatologic: Chloasma, melasma, rash

Endocrine & metabolic: Breast tumors, amenorrhea, alterations in frequency and flow of menses, decreased glucose tolerance, elevated triglycerides and LDL

Gastrointestinal: GI distress

Hepatic: Cholestatic jaundice

Ocular: Intolerance to contact lenses

Miscellaneous: Increased susceptibility to *Candida* infection

Drug Interactions

Decreased effect: Rifampin decreases estrogen serum concentrations

Increased toxicity:

Anticoagulants: Increases potential for thromboembolic events with anticoagulants

Drug Uptake

Absorption: Absorbed well from GI tract

Pregnancy Risk Factor X

Generic Available No

Ethinyl Estradiol and Desogestrel

(ETH in il es tra DYE ole & des oh JES trel)

Brand Names Desogen®; Ortho-Cept®

Therapeutic Category Contraceptive, Oral

Synonyms Desogestrel and Ethinyl Estradiol

Use Prevention of pregnancy

Local Anesthetic/Vasoconstrictor Precautions No information available to require special precautions

Effects on Dental Treatment When prescribing antibiotics, patient must be warned to use supplemental methods of birth control if on oral contraceptives

Pregnancy Risk Factor X

Generic Available No

Ethinyl Estradiol and Ethynodiol Diacetate

(ETH in il es tra DYE ole & e thye noe DYE ole dye AS e tate)

Related Information

Endocrine Disorders & Pregnancy *on page 1021*

Brand Names Demulen®; Zovia®

Therapeutic Category Contraceptive, Oral

Use Prevention of pregnancy; treatment of hypermenorrhea, endometriosis, female hypogonadism

Usual Dosage Adults: Female: Oral:

For 21-tablet cycle packs, with 21 active tablets (28-day packs have 21 active tablets and 7 inert tablets): Take 1 tablet daily starting on the fifth day of menstrual cycle, with day 1 being the first day of menstruation; begin taking a

(Continued)

Ethinyl Estradiol and Ethynodiol Diacetate *(Continued)*

new cycle pack on the eighth day after taking the last tablet from the previous pack

With 28-tablet packages, dosage is 1 tablet daily without interruption; extra tablets are placebos or contain iron. If next menstrual period does not begin on schedule, rule out pregnancy before starting new dosing cycle. If menstrual period begins, start new dosing cycle 7 days after last tablet was taken. If all doses have been taken on schedule and one menstrual period is missed, continue dosing cycle. If two consecutive menstrual periods are missed, pregnancy test is required before new dosing cycle is started.

One dose missed: Take as soon as remembered or take 2 tablets next day

Two doses missed: Take 2 tablets as soon as remembered or 2 tablets next 2 days

Three doses missed: Begin new compact of tablets starting on day 1 of next cycle

Mechanism of Action Combination oral contraceptives inhibit ovulation via a negative feedback mechanism on the hypothalamus, which alters the normal pattern of gonadotropin secretion of a follicle-stimulating hormone (FSH) and luteinizing hormone by the anterior pituitary. The follicular phase FSH and midcycle surge of gonadotropins are inhibited. In addition, oral contraceptives produce alterations in the genital tract, including changes in the cervical mucus, rendering it unfavorable for sperm penetration even if ovulation occurs. Changes in the endometrium may also occur, producing an unfavorable environment for nidation. Oral contraceptive drugs may alter the tubal transport of the ova through the fallopian tubes. Progestational agents may also alter sperm fertility.

Local Anesthetic/Vasoconstrictor Precautions No information available to require special precautions

Effects on Dental Treatment When prescribing antibiotics, patient must be warned to use supplemental methods of birth control if on oral contraceptives

Other Adverse Effects

>10%:

Cardiovascular: Peripheral edema

Endocrine & metabolic: Enlargement of breasts, breast tenderness

Gastrointestinal: Nausea, anorexia, bloating

1% to 10%:

Central nervous system: Headache

Endocrine & metabolic: Increased libido

Gastrointestinal: Vomiting, diarrhea

<1%:

Cardiovascular: Hypertension, thromboembolism, myocardial infarction, edema

Central nervous system: Depression, dizziness, anxiety, stroke

Dermatologic: Chloasma, melasma, rash

Endocrine & metabolic: Decreased glucose tolerance, breast tumors, amenorrhea, alterations in frequency and flow of menses, elevated triglycerides and LDL

Gastrointestinal: GI distress

Hepatic: Cholestatic jaundice

Ocular: Intolerance to contact lenses

Miscellaneous: Increased susceptibility to *Candida* infection

See tables.

Achieving Proper Hormonal Balance in an Oral Contraceptive

Estrogen		Progestin	
Excess	**Deficiency**	**Excess**	**Deficiency**
Nausea, bloating	Early or midcycle breakthrough bleeding	Increased appetite	Late breakthrough bleeding
Cervical mucorrhea, polyposis		Weight gain	
Melasma	Increased spotting	Tiredness, fatigue	Amenorrhea
Migraine headache	Hypomenorrhea	Hypomenorrhea	Hypermenorrhea
		Acne, oily scalp*	
Breast fullness or		Hair loss, hirsutism*	
tenderness		Depression	
Edema		Monilial vaginitis	
Hypertension		Breast regression	

*Result of androgenic activity of progestins.

Pharmacological Effects of Progestins Used in Oral Contraceptives

	Progestin	Estrogen	Antiestrogen	Androgen
Norgestrel/levonorgestrel	+++	0	++	+++
Ethynodiol diacetate	++	+*	+*	+
Norethindrone acetate	+	+	+++	+
Norethindrone	+	+*	+*	+
Norethynodrel	+	+++	0	0

*Has estrogenic effect at low doses; may have antiestrogenic effect at higher doses.

+++ = pronounced effect

++ = moderate effect

+ = slight effect

0 = no effect

Drug Interactions

Decreased effect of oral contraceptives with barbiturates, hydantoins - phenytoin, rifampin, antibiotics - penicillins, tetracyclines, griseofulvin

Increased toxicity of acetaminophen, anticoagulants, benzodiazepines, caffeine, corticosteroids, metoprolol, theophylline, tricyclic antidepressants

Drug Uptake

Ethinyl estradiol:

Absorption: Absorbed well from GI tract

Serum half-life, terminal: 5-14 hours

Pregnancy Risk Factor X

Generic Available Yes

Ethinyl Estradiol and Fluoxymesterone

(eth i nil es tra DYE ole & floo oks i MES te rone)

Therapeutic Category Androgen; Estrogen Derivative

Synonyms Fluoxymesterone and Estradiol

Use Moderate to severe vasomotor symptoms of menopause, postpartum breast engorgement

Local Anesthetic/Vasoconstrictor Precautions No information available to require special precautions

Effects on Dental Treatment When prescribing antibiotics, patient must be warned to use supplemental methods of birth control if on oral contraceptives

Other Adverse Effects 1% to 10%:

Cardiovascular: Hypertension, thromboembolism, myocardial infarction, edema

Central nervous system: Depression, migraine, dizziness, anxiety, headache, stroke

Dermatologic: Chloasma, melasma, rash

Endocrine & metabolic: Decreased glucose tolerance, alterations in frequency and flow of menses, breast tenderness or enlargement, hypertriglyceridemia, elevated LDL

Gastrointestinal: Nausea, GI distress

Hepatic: Cholestatic jaundice

Miscellaneous: Increased susceptibility to *Candida* infection

Pregnancy Risk Factor X

Generic Available No

Ethinyl Estradiol and Levonorgestrel

(ETH in il es tra DYE ole & LEE voe nor jes trel)

Related Information

Endocrine Disorders & Pregnancy *on page 1021*

Brand Names Alesse®; Levlen®; Levora®; Nordette®; Tri-Levlen®; Triphasil®

Canadian/Mexican Brand Names Microgynon® (Mexico); Nordet® (Mexico); Nordiol® (Mexico)

Therapeutic Category Contraceptive, Oral

Use Prevention of pregnancy; treatment of hypermenorrhea, endometriosis, female hypogonadism

Usual Dosage Adults: Female: Oral:

Contraception: 1 tablet daily, beginning on day 5 of menstrual cycle (first day of menstrual flow is day 1). With 20-tablet and 21-tablet packages, new dosing cycle begins 7 days after last tablet taken. With 28-tablet packages, dosage is 1 tablet daily without interruption; extra tablets are placebos or contain iron. If next menstrual period does not begin on schedule, rule out pregnancy before starting new dosing cycle. If menstrual period begins, start new dosing cycle 7 days after last tablet was taken. If all doses have been taken on schedule and one menstrual period is missed, continue dosing cycle. If two consecutive

(Continued)

Ethinyl Estradiol and Levonorgestrel *(Continued)*

menstrual periods are missed, pregnancy test is required before new dosing cycle is started.

One dose missed: Take as soon as remembered or take 2 tablets next day

Two doses missed: Take 2 tablets as soon as remembered or 2 tablets next 2 days

Three doses missed: Begin new compact of tablets starting on day 1 of next cycle

Triphasic oral contraceptive (Tri-Levlen®, Triphasil®): 1 tablet/day in the sequence specified by the manufacturer

Mechanism of Action Combination oral contraceptives inhibit ovulation via a negative feedback mechanism on the hypothalamus, which alters the normal pattern of gonadotropin secretion of a follicle-stimulating hormone (FSH) and luteinizing hormone by the anterior pituitary. The follicular phase FSH and midcycle surge of gonadotropins are inhibited. In addition, oral contraceptives produce alterations in the genital tract, including changes in the cervical mucus, rendering it unfavorable for sperm penetration even if ovulation occurs. Changes in the endometrium may also occur, producing an unfavorable environment for nidation. Oral contraceptive drugs may alter the tubal transport of the ova through the fallopian tubes. Progestational agents may also alter sperm fertility.

Local Anesthetic/Vasoconstrictor Precautions No information available to require special precautions

Effects on Dental Treatment When prescribing antibiotics, patient must be warned to use supplemental methods of birth control if on oral contraceptives

Other Adverse Effects

>10%:
  Cardiovascular: Peripheral edema
  Endocrine & metabolic: Enlargement of breasts, breast tenderness
  Gastrointestinal: Nausea, anorexia, bloating

1% to 10%:
  Central nervous system: Headache
  Endocrine & metabolic: Increased libido
  Gastrointestinal: Vomiting, diarrhea

<1%:
  Cardiovascular: Hypertension, thromboembolism, myocardial infarction, edema
  Central nervous system: Depression, dizziness, anxiety, stroke
  Dermatologic: Chloasma, melasma, rash
  Endocrine & metabolic: Decreased glucose tolerance, breast tumors, amenorrhea, alterations in frequency and flow of menses, hypertriglyceridemia, elevated LDL
  Gastrointestinal: GI distress
  Hepatic: Cholestatic jaundice
  Ocular: Intolerance to contact lenses
  Miscellaneous: Increased susceptibility to *Candida* infection

Drug Interactions

Decreased effect of oral contraceptives with barbiturates, hydantoins - phenytoin, rifampin, antibiotics - penicillins, tetracyclines, griseofulvin

Increased toxicity of acetaminophen, anticoagulants, benzodiazepines, caffeine, corticosteroids, metoprolol, theophylline, tricyclic antidepressants

Drug Uptake

Ethinyl estradiol:
  Absorption: Absorbed well from GI tract

Levonorgestrel:
  Serum half-life, terminal: 11-45 hours
  Time to peak: 0.5-2 hours

Pharmacological Effects of Progestins Used in Oral Contraceptives

	Progestin	Estrogen	Antiestrogen	Androgen
Norgestrel/levonorgestrel	+++	0	++	+++
Ethynodiol diacetate	++	+*	+*	+
Norethindrone acetate	+	+*	+++	+
Norethindrone	+	+*	+*	+
Norethynodrel	+	+++	0	0

*Has estrogenic effect at low doses; may have antiestrogenic effect at higher doses.

+++ = pronounced effect

++ = moderate effect

+ = slight effect

0 = no effect

Achieving Proper Hormonal Balance in an Oral Contraceptive

Estrogen		Progestin	
Excess	**Deficiency**	**Excess**	**Deficiency**
Nausea, bloating	Early or midcycle	Increased appetite	Late breakthrough
Cervical mucorrhea,	breakthrough	Weight gain	bleeding
polyposis	bleeding	Tiredness, fatigue	Amenorrhea
Melasma	Increased spotting	Hypomenorrhea	Hypermenorrhea
Migraine headache	Hypomenorrhea	Acne, oily scalp*	
Breast fullness or		Hair loss,	
		hirsutism*	
tenderness		Depression	
Edema		Monilial vaginitis	
Hypertension		Breast regression	

*Result of androgenic activity of progestins.

Pregnancy Risk Factor X
Generic Available Yes

Ethinyl Estradiol and Norethindrone
(ETH in il es tra DYE ole & nor eth IN drone)
Related Information
   Endocrine Disorders & Pregnancy *on page 1021*
Brand Names Brevicon®; Estrostep® 21; Estrostep® Fe; Genora® 0.5/35; Genora® 1/35; Jenest-28™; Loestrin®; Modicon™; N.E.E.® 1/35; Nelova™ 0.5/35E; Nelova™ 10/11; Norethin™ 1/35E; Norinyl® 1+35; Ortho-Novum® 1/35; Ortho-Novum® 7/7/7; Ortho-Novum® 10/11; Ovcon® 35; Ovcon® 50; Tri-Norinyl®
Canadian/Mexican Brand Names Ortho®0.5/35 (Canada); Synphasic® (Canada); Trinovum® (Mexico)
Therapeutic Category Contraceptive, Oral
Synonyms Etinilestradiol and Noretindrona (Mexico)
Use Prevention of pregnancy; treatment of hypermenorrhea, endometriosis, female hypogonadism
Usual Dosage Adults: Female: Oral:
   For 21-tablet cycle packs, with 21 active tablets (28-day packs have 21 active tablets and 7 inert tablets): Take 1 tablet daily starting on the fifth day of menstrual cycle, with day 1 being the first day of menstruation; begin taking a new cycle pack on the eighth day after taking the last tablet from the previous pack
   With 28-tablet packages, dosage is 1 tablet daily without interruption; extra tablets are placebos or contain iron. If next menstrual period does not begin on schedule, rule out pregnancy before starting new dosing cycle. If menstrual period begins, start new dosing cycle 7 days after last tablet was taken. If all doses have been taken on schedule and one menstrual period is missed, continue dosing cycle. If two consecutive menstrual periods are missed, pregnancy test is required before new dosing cycle is started.
   One dose missed: Take as soon as remembered or take 2 tablets next day
   Two doses missed: Take 2 tablets as soon as remembered or 2 tablets next 2 days
   Three doses missed: Begin new compact of tablets starting on day 1 of next cycle
   Biphasic oral contraceptive (Jenest™-28, Ortho-Novum™ 10/11, Nelova™ 10/11): 1 color tablet/day for 10 days, then next color tablet for 11 days
   Triphasic oral contraceptive (Ortho-Novum™ 7/7/7, Tri-Norinyl®, Triphasil®): 1 tablet/day in the sequence specified by the manufacturer
Mechanism of Action Combination oral contraceptives inhibit ovulation via a negative feedback mechanism on the hypothalamus, which alters the normal pattern of gonadotropin secretion of a follicle-stimulating hormone (FSH) and luteinizing hormone by the anterior pituitary. The follicular phase FSH and midcycle surge of gonadotropins are inhibited. In addition, oral contraceptives produce alterations in the genital tract, including changes in the cervical mucus, rendering it unfavorable for sperm penetration even if ovulation occurs. Changes in the endometrium may also occur, producing an unfavorable environment for nidation. Oral contraceptive drugs may alter the tubal transport of the ova through the fallopian tubes. Progestational agents may also alter sperm fertility.
Local Anesthetic/Vasoconstrictor Precautions No information available to require special precautions
Effects on Dental Treatment When prescribing antibiotics, patient must be warned to use supplemental methods of birth control if on oral contraceptives
(Continued)

Ethinyl Estradiol and Norethindrone *(Continued)*

Other Adverse Effects

>10%:
Cardiovascular: Peripheral edema
Endocrine & metabolic: Enlargement of breasts, breast tenderness
Gastrointestinal: Nausea, anorexia, bloating
1% to 10%:
Central nervous system: Headache
Endocrine & metabolic: Increased libido
Gastrointestinal: Vomiting, diarrhea
<1%:
Cardiovascular: Hypertension, thromboembolism, myocardial infarction, edema
Central nervous system: Depression, dizziness, anxiety, stroke
Dermatologic: Chloasma, melasma, rash
Endocrine & metabolic: Decreased glucose tolerance, breast tumors, amenorrhea, alterations in frequency and flow of menses, elevated triglycerides and LDL
Gastrointestinal: GI distress
Hepatic: Cholestatic jaundice
Ocular: Intolerance to contact lenses
Miscellaneous: Increased susceptibility to *Candida* infection
See tables.

Achieving Proper Hormonal Balance in an Oral Contraceptive

Estrogen		Progestin	
Excess	**Deficiency**	**Excess**	**Deficiency**
Nausea, bloating	Early or midcycle	Increased appetite	Late breakthrough
Cervical mucorrhea,	breakthrough	Weight gain	bleeding
polyposis	bleeding	Tiredness, fatigue	Amenorrhea
Melasma	Increased spotting	Hypomenorrhea	Hypermenorrhea
Migraine headache	Hypomenorrhea	Acne, oily scalp*	
Breast fullness or		Hair loss, hirsutism*	
tenderness		Depression	
Edema		Monilial vaginitis	
Hypertension		Breast regression	

*Result of androgenic activity of progestins.

Pharmacological Effects of Progestins Used in Oral Contraceptives

	Progestin	Estrogen	Antiestrogen	Androgen
Norgestrel/levonorgestrel	+++	0	++	+++
Ethynodiol diacetate	++	+*	+*	+
Norethindrone acetate	+	+	+++	+
Norethindrone	+	+*	+*	+
Norethynodrel	+	+++	0	0

*Has estrogenic effect at low doses; may have antiestrogenic effect at higher doses.

+++ = pronounced effect
++ = moderate effect
+ = slight effect
0 = no effect

Drug Interactions

Decreased effect of oral contraceptives with barbiturates, hydantoins - phenytoin, rifampin, antibiotics - penicillins, tetracyclines, griseofulvin
Increased toxicity of acetaminophen, anticoagulants, benzodiazepines, caffeine, corticosteroids, metoprolol, theophylline, tricyclic antidepressants

Drug Uptake

Ethinyl estradiol:
Absorption: Absorbed well from GI tract
Norethindrone:
Serum half-life, terminal: 5-14 hours
Time to peak: Oral: 0.5-4 hours

Pregnancy Risk Factor X
Generic Available Yes

Ethinyl Estradiol and Norgestimate
(ETH in il es tra DYE ole & nor JES ti mate)

Brand Names Ortho-Cyclen®; Ortho Tri-Cyclen®

Therapeutic Category Contraceptive, Oral

Synonyms Norgestimate and Ethinyl Estradiol

Use Prevention of pregnancy

Local Anesthetic/Vasoconstrictor Precautions No information available to require special precautions

Effects on Dental Treatment When prescribing antibiotics, patient must be warned to use supplemental methods of birth control if on oral contraceptives

Pregnancy Risk Factor X

Generic Available No

Ethinyl Estradiol and Norgestrel
(ETH in il es tra DYE ole & nor JES trel)

Brand Names Lo/Ovral®; Ovral®

Therapeutic Category Contraceptive, Oral

Use Prevention of pregnancy; treatment of hypermenorrhea, endometriosis, female hypogonadism; postcoital contraception

Usual Dosage Adults: Female: Oral: Contraception: 1 tablet daily, beginning on day 5 of menstrual cycle (first day of menstrual flow is day 1). With 20-tablet and 21-tablet packages, new dosing cycle begins 7 days after last tablet taken; with 28-tablet packages, dosage is 1 tablet daily without interruption; extra tablets are placebos or contain iron. If next menstrual period does not begin on schedule, rule out pregnancy before starting new dosing cycle; if menstrual period begins, start new dosing cycle 7 days after last tablet was taken; if all doses have been taken on schedule and one menstrual period is missed, continue dosing cycle; if two consecutive menstrual periods are missed, pregnancy test is required before new dosing cycle is started.

One dose missed: Take as soon as remembered or take 2 tablets next day

Two doses missed: Take 2 tablets as soon as remembered or 2 tablets next 2 days

Three doses missed: Begin new compact of tablets starting on day 1 of next cycle

"Morning After" pill: Postcoital contraception (Ovral®): 2 tablets at initial visit and 2 tablets 12 hours later

Mechanism of Action Combination oral contraceptives inhibit ovulation via a negative feedback mechanism on the hypothalamus, which alters the normal pattern of gonadotropin secretion of a follicle-stimulating hormone (FSH) and luteinizing hormone by the anterior pituitary. The follicular phase FSH and midcycle surge of gonadotropins are inhibited. In addition, oral contraceptives produce alterations in the genital tract, including changes in the cervical mucus, rendering it unfavorable for sperm penetration even if ovulation occurs. Changes in the endometrium may also occur, producing an unfavorable environment for nidation. Oral contraceptive drugs may alter the tubal transport of the ova through the fallopian tubes. Progestational agents may also alter sperm fertility.

Local Anesthetic/Vasoconstrictor Precautions No information available to require special precautions

Effects on Dental Treatment When prescribing antibiotics, patient must be warned to use supplemental methods of birth control if on oral contraceptives

Other Adverse Effects

>10%:
Cardiovascular: Peripheral edema
Endocrine & metabolic: Enlargement of breasts, breast tenderness
Gastrointestinal: Nausea, anorexia, bloating

1% to 10%:
Central nervous system: Headache
Endocrine & metabolic: Increased libido
Gastrointestinal: Vomiting, diarrhea

<1%:
Cardiovascular: Hypertension, thromboembolism, myocardial infarction, edema
Central nervous system: Depression, dizziness, anxiety, stroke
Dermatologic: Chloasma, melasma, rash
Endocrine & metabolic: Decreased glucose tolerance, breast tumors, amenorrhea, alterations in frequency and flow of menses, elevated triglycerides and LDL
Gastrointestinal: GI distress
Hepatic: Cholestatic jaundice
Ocular: Intolerance to contact lenses
Miscellaneous: Increased susceptibility to *Candida* infection

(Continued)

Ethinyl Estradiol and Norgestrel *(Continued)*

See tables.

Achieving Proper Hormonal Balance in an Oral Contraceptive

Estrogen		Progestin	
Excess	**Deficiency**	**Excess**	**Deficiency**
Nausea, bloating	Early or midcycle	Increased appetite	Late breakthrough
Cervical mucorrhea,	breakthrough	Weight gain	bleeding
polyposis	bleeding	Tiredness, fatigue	Amenorrhea
Melasma	Increased spotting	Hypomenorrhea	Hypermenorrhea
Migraine headache	Hypomenorrhea	Acne, oily scalp*	
Breast fullness or		Hair loss,	
tenderness		hirsutism*	
		Depression	
Edema		Monilial vaginitis	
Hypertension		Breast regression	

*Result of androgenic activity of progestins.

Pharmacological Effects of Progestins Used in Oral Contraceptives

	Progestin	Estrogen	Antiestrogen	Androgen
Norgestrel/levonorgestrel	+++	0	++	+++
Ethynodiol diacetate	++	+*	+*	+
Norethindrone acetate	+	+	+++	+
Norethindrone	+	+*	+*	+
Norethynodrel	+	+++	0	0

*Has estrogenic effect at low doses; may have antiestrogenic effect at higher doses.

+++ = pronounced effect

++ = moderate effect

+ = slight effect

0 = no effect

Drug Interactions
Decreased effect of oral contraceptives with barbiturates, hydantoins - phenytoin, rifampin, antibiotics - penicillins, tetracyclines, griseofulvin

Increased toxicity of acetaminophen, anticoagulants, benzodiazepines, caffeine, corticosteroids, metoprolol, theophylline, tricyclic antidepressants

Drug Uptake
Ethinyl estradiol:

Absorption: Absorbed well from GI tract

Norgestrel:

Serum half-life, terminal: 11-45 hours

Time to peak: 0.5-2 hours

Pregnancy Risk Factor X
Generic Available Yes

Ethiofos *see Amifostine on page 52*

Ethionamide (e thye on AM ide)
Related Information
Nonviral Infectious Diseases *on page 1032*
Brand Names Trecator®-SC
Therapeutic Category Antitubercular Agent
Use Treatment of tuberculosis and other mycobacterial diseases, in conjunction with other antituberculosis agents, when first-line agents have failed or resistance has been demonstrated
Usual Dosage Oral:
Children: 15-20 mg/kg/day in 2 divided doses, not to exceed 1 g/day

Adults: 500-1000 mg/day in 1-3 divided doses

Mechanism of Action Inhibits peptide synthesis
Local Anesthetic/Vasoconstrictor Precautions No information available to require special precautions
Effects on Dental Treatment No effects or complications reported
Other Adverse Effects
>10%: Gastrointestinal: Anorexia, nausea, vomiting

1% to 10%:

Cardiovascular: Postural hypotension

Central nervous system: Psychiatric disturbances

Gastrointestinal: Metallic taste
Hepatic: Hepatitis, jaundice
Neuromuscular & skeletal: Peripheral neuritis
<1%:
Central nervous system: Drowsiness, dizziness, seizures, headache
Dermatologic: Rash
Endocrine & metabolic: Hypothyroidism or goiter, hypoglycemia, gynecomastia
Gastrointestinal: Stomatitis, abdominal pain, diarrhea
Hematologic: Thrombocytopenia
Ocular: Optic neuritis
Drug Interactions No data reported
Drug Uptake
Serum half-life: 2-3 hours
Time to peak serum concentration: Oral: Within 3 hours
Pregnancy Risk Factor C
Generic Available No

Ethmozine® *see Moricizine on page 648*

Ethosuximide (eth oh SUKS i mide)

Brand Names Zarontin®
Therapeutic Category Anticonvulsant, Succinimide
Use Management of absence (petit mal) seizures, myoclonic seizures, and akinetic epilepsy; considered to be drug of choice for simple absence seizures
Usual Dosage Oral:
Children 3-6 years: Initial: 250 mg/day (or 15 mg/kg/day) in 2 divided doses; increase every 4-7 days; usual maintenance dose: 15-40 mg/kg/day in 2 divided doses
Children >6 years and Adults: Initial: 250 mg twice daily; increase by 250 mg as needed every 4-7 days up to 1.5 g/day in 2 divided doses; usual maintenance dose: 20-40 mg/kg/day in 2 divided doses
Mechanism of Action Increases the seizure threshold and suppresses paroxysmal spike-and-wave pattern in absence seizures; depresses nerve transmission in the motor cortex
Local Anesthetic/Vasoconstrictor Precautions No information available to require special precautions
Effects on Dental Treatment No effects or complications reported
Other Adverse Effects
>10%:
Central nervous system: Ataxia, drowsiness, sedation, dizziness, lethargy, euphoria, hallucinations, insomnia, agitation, behavioral changes, headache
Dermatologic: Stevens-Johnson syndrome
Gastrointestinal: Weight loss, nausea, vomiting, anorexia, abdominal pain
Miscellaneous: Hiccups, SLE
1% to 10%:
Central nervous system: Aggressiveness, mental depression, nightmares, fatigue
Neuromuscular & skeletal: Weakness
<1%:
Central nervous system: Paranoid psychosis
Dermatologic: Rashes, urticaria, exfoliative dermatitis
Hematologic: Leukopenia, aplastic anemia, thrombocytopenia, agranulocytosis, pancytopenia
Drug Interactions
Decreased effect: Phenytoin, carbamazepine, primidone, phenobarbital may increase the hepatic metabolism of ethosuximide
Increased toxicity: Isoniazid may inhibit hepatic metabolism with a resultant increase in ethosuximide serum concentrations
Drug Uptake
Serum half-life:
Children: 30 hours
Adults: 50-60 hours
Time to peak serum concentration:
Capsule: Within 2-4 hours
Syrup: <2-4 hours
Pregnancy Risk Factor C
Generic Available Yes

Ethotoin (ETH oh toyn)

Brand Names Peganone®
Therapeutic Category Anticonvulsant, Hydantoin
Synonyms Ethylphenylhydantoin
(Continued)

Ethotoin *(Continued)*

Use Generalized tonic-clonic or complex-partial seizures

Local Anesthetic/Vasoconstrictor Precautions No information available to require special precautions

Effects on Dental Treatment No effects or complications reported

Other Adverse Effects

>10%:

Central nervous system: Psychiatric changes, slurred speech, drowsiness, dizziness

Gastrointestinal: Constipation, nausea, vomiting

Neuromuscular & skeletal: Trembling

1% to 10%:

Central nervous system: Headache, insomnia

Dermatologic: Skin rash

Gastrointestinal: Anorexia, weight loss

Hematologic: Leukopenia

Hepatic: Hepatitis

Renal: Elevated serum creatinine

<1%:

Cardiovascular: Hypotension, bradycardia, cardiac arrhythmias, cardiovascular collapse

Central nervous system: Confusion, fever, ataxia

Dermatologic: Stevens-Johnson syndrome

Gastrointestinal: Gingival hyperplasia

Hematologic: Blood dyscrasias

Local: Thrombophlebitis, venous irritation and pain

Neuromuscular & skeletal: Paresthesia, peripheral neuropathy

Ocular: Diplopia, nystagmus, blurred vision

Miscellaneous: Lymphadenopathy, SLE-like syndrome

Pregnancy Risk Factor D

Generic Available No

Ethyl Chloride *(ETH il KLOR ide)*

Therapeutic Category Local Anesthetic, Topical

Synonyms Chloroethane

Use Local anesthetic in minor operative procedures and to relieve pain caused by insect stings and burns, and irritation caused by myofascial and visceral pain syndromes

Local Anesthetic/Vasoconstrictor Precautions No information available to require special precautions

Effects on Dental Treatment No effects or complications reported

Other Adverse Effects 1% to 10%: Mucous membrane irritation, freezing may alter skin pigment

Pregnancy Risk Factor C

Generic Available Yes

Comments Spray for a few seconds to the point of frost formation when the tissue becomes white; avoid prolonged spraying of skin beyond this point

Ethyl Chloride and Dichlorotetrafluoroethane

(ETH il KLOR ide & dye klor oh te tra floo or oh ETH ane)

Brand Names Fluro-Ethyl® Aerosol

Therapeutic Category Local Anesthetic, Topical

Synonyms Dichlorotetrafluoroethane and Ethyl Chloride

Use Topical refrigerant anesthetic to control pain associated with minor surgical procedures, dermabrasion, injections, contusions, and minor strains

Local Anesthetic/Vasoconstrictor Precautions No information available to require special precautions

Effects on Dental Treatment No effects or complications reported

Pregnancy Risk Factor C

Generic Available No

Ethylnorepinephrine *(eth il nor ep i NEF rin)*

Brand Names Bronkephrine® Injection

Therapeutic Category Adrenergic Agonist Agent; Bronchodilator

Use Bronchial asthma and reversible bronchospasm

Local Anesthetic/Vasoconstrictor Precautions No information available to require special precautions

Effects on Dental Treatment No effects or complications reported

Other Adverse Effects

>10%:

Cardiovascular: Tachycardia, pounding heart beat

Central nervous system: Nervousness

Gastrointestinal: Nausea

Neuromuscular & skeletal: Trembling, tremor

1% to 10%:

Cardiovascular: Flushing of face, hypertension or hypotension

Central nervous system: Dizziness, lightheadedness, drowsiness, headache, insomnia

Gastrointestinal: Dry mouth, heartburn, vomiting, unusual taste

Genitourinary: Dysuria

Neuromuscular & skeletal: Muscle cramping, weakness

Respiratory: Coughing

Miscellaneous: Increased sweating

<1%:

Cardiovascular: Chest pain, vasoconstriction, cerebral hemorrhage, cardiac arrhythmias, palpitations, angina, cardiac arrest, sudden death, syncope, unusual pallor

Central nervous system: Fear, anxiety, restlessness, confusion, irritability, psychotic states

Endocrine & metabolic: Altered glucose metabolism

Gastrointestinal: Loss of appetite, hypersalivation

Genitourinary: Urinary retention

Local: Extravasation results in tissue necrosis

Respiratory: Paradoxical bronchospasm, pulmonary edema, dyspnea

Miscellaneous: Sweating

Pregnancy Risk Factor C

Generic Available No

Ethylphenylhydantoin *see* Ethotoin *on page 383*

Ethyol® *see* Amifostine *on page 52*

Etidocaine With Epinephrine (e TI doe kane)

Related Information

Oral Pain *on page 1053*

Brand Names Duranest® With Epinephrine

Therapeutic Category Dental/Local Anesthetics; Local Anesthetic, Injectable

Use Dental: An amide-type local anesthetic for local infiltration anesthesia; injection near nerve trunks to produce nerve block

Usual Dosage

Children <10 years: Dosage has not been established

Children >10 years and Adults: Dental infiltration and nerve block: 15-75 mg (1-5 mL) as a 1.5% solution; up to a maximum of 5.5 mg/kg of body weight but not to exceed 400 mg/injection of etidocaine hydrochloride with epinephrine 1:200,000. The effective anesthetic dose varies with procedure, intensity of anesthesia needed, duration of anesthesia required, and physical condition of the patient. Always use the lowest effective dose along with careful aspiration.

The numbers of dental carpules (1.8 mL) in the table provide the indicated amounts of etidocaine hydrochloride 1.5% and epinephrine 1:200,000.

# of Cartridges	Mg Etidocaine (1.5%)	Mg Vasoconstrictor (Epinephrine 1:200,000)
1	27	0.009
2	54	0.018
3	81	0.027
4	108	0.036
5	135	0.045
6	162	0.054
7	189	0.063
8	216	0.072
9	243	0.081
10	270	0.090

Note: Adult and children doses of etidocaine hydrochloride with epinephrine cited from USP Dispensing Information (USP DI), 17th ed, The United States Pharmacopeial Convention, Inc, Rockville, MD, 1997, 136.

Mechanism of Action Local anesthetics bind selectively to the intracellular surface of sodium channels to block influx of sodium into the axon. As a result, depolarization necessary for action potential propagation and subsequent nerve
(Continued)

385

Etidocaine With Epinephrine *(Continued)*

function is prevented. The block at the sodium channel is reversible. When drug diffuses away from the axon, sodium channel function is restored and nerve propagation is subsequently restored.

Epinephrine prolongs the duration of the anesthetic actions of etidocaine by causing vasoconstriction (alpha adrenergic receptor agonist) of the vasculature surrounding the nerve axons. This prevents the diffusion of lidocaine away from the nerves resulting in a longer retention in the axon.

Local Anesthetic/Vasoconstrictor Precautions No information available to require special precautions

Effects on Dental Treatment No effects or complications reported

Other Adverse Effects Degree of adverse effects in the central nervous system and cardiovascular system are directly related to the blood levels of etidocaine. The effects below are more likely to occur after systemic administration rather than infiltration.

Cardiovascular: Myocardial effects include a decrease in contraction force as well as a decrease in electrical excitability and myocardial conduction rate resulting in bradycardia and reduction in cardiac output.

Central nervous system: High blood levels result in anxiety, restlessness, disorientation, confusion, dizziness, tremors and seizures. This is followed by depression of CNS resulting in somnolence, unconsciousness and possible respiratory arrest. Nausea and vomiting may also occur. In some cases, symptoms of CNS stimulation may be absent and the primary CNS effects are drowsiness and unconsciousness.

Hypersensitivity reactions: Extremely rare, but may be manifest as dermatologic reactions and edema at injection site. Asthmatic syndromes have occurred. Patients may exhibit hypersensitivity to bisulfites contained in local anesthetic solution to prevent oxidation of epinephrine. In general, patients reacting to bisulfites have a history of asthma and their airways are hyper-reactive to asthmatic syndrome

Psychogenic reactions: It is common to misinterpret psychogenic responses to local anesthetic injection as an allergic reaction. Intraoral injections are perceived by many patients as a stressful procedure in dentistry. Common symptoms to this stress are sweating, palpitations, hyperventilation, generalized pallor and a fainting feeling.

Contraindications Hypersensitivity to local anesthetics of the amide-type

Warnings/Precautions Should be avoided in patients with uncontrolled hyperthyroidism. Should be used in minimal amounts in patients with significant cardiovascular problems (because of epinephrine component). Aspirate the syringe after tissue penetration and before injection to minimize chance of direct vascular injection.

Drug Interactions Due to epinephrine component, use with tricyclic antidepressants or MAO inhibitors could result in increased pressor response; use with nonselective beta-blockers (ie, propranolol) could result in serious hypertension and reflex bradycardia

Drug Uptake

Onset of action: Maxillary infiltration and inferior alveolar nerve block: 3-5 minutes

Duration after infiltration or nerve block: 5-10 hours

Serum half-life: 2.7 hours

Pregnancy Risk Factor B

Breast-feeding Considerations Usual infiltration doses of etidocaine hydrochloride with epinephrine given to nursing mothers has not been shown to affect the health of the nursing infant

Dosage Forms Etidocaine Hydrochloride 1.5% with epinephrine 1:200,000 cartridges, 1.8 mL, in 100 cartridge boxes

Dietary Considerations No data reported

Generic Available No

Selected Readings

Jastak JT and Yagiela JA, "Vasoconstrictors and Local Anesthesia: A Review and Rationale for Use," *J Am Dent Assoc*, 1983, 107(4):623-30.

MacKenzie TA and Young ER, "Local Anesthetic Update," *Anesth Prog*, 1993, 40(2):29-34.

Wynn RL, "Epinephrine Interactions With Beta-Blockers," *Gen Dent*, 1994, 42(1):16, 18.

Wynn RL, "Recent Research on Mechanisms of Local Anesthetics," *Gen Dent*, 1995, 43(4):316-8.

Yagiela JA, "Local Anesthetics," *Anesth Prog*, 1991, 38(4-5):128-41.

Etidronate Disodium *(e ti DROE nate dye SOW dee um)*

Brand Names Didronel®

Therapeutic Category Antidote, Hypercalcemia; Bisphosphonate Derivative

Use Symptomatic treatment of Paget's disease and heterotopic ossification due to spinal cord injury or after total hip replacement, hypercalcemia associated with malignancy

Usual Dosage Adults:

Paget's disease: Oral: 5 mg/kg/day given every day for no more than 6 months; may give 10 mg/kg/day for up to 3 months; daily dose may be divided if adverse GI effects occur

Heterotopic ossification with spinal cord injury: 20 mg/kg/day for 2 weeks, then 10 mg/kg/day for 10 weeks (this dosage has been used in children, however, treatment >1 year has been associated with a rachitic syndrome)

Hypercalcemia associated with malignancy:

I.V. (Dilute dose in at least 250 mL NS): 7.5 mg/kg/day for 3 days; there should be at least 7 days between courses of treatment

Oral: Start 20 mg/kg/day on the last day of infusion and continue for 30-90 days

Mechanism of Action Decreases bone resorption by inhibiting osteocystic osteolysis; decreases mineral release and matrix or collagen breakdown in bone

Local Anesthetic/Vasoconstrictor Precautions No information available to require special precautions

Effects on Dental Treatment No effects or complications reported

Other Adverse Effects

1% to 10%:

Central nervous system: Fever, convulsions

Endocrine & metabolic: Hypophosphatemia, hypomagnesemia, fluid overload

Neuromuscular & skeletal: Bone pain

Respiratory: Dyspnea

<1%:

Dermatologic: Angioedema, skin rash

Gastrointestinal: Occult blood in stools, dysgeusia

Neuromuscular & skeletal: Pain, increased risk of fractures

Renal: Nephrotoxicity

Miscellaneous: Hypersensitivity reactions

Drug Interactions No data reported

Drug Uptake

Onset of therapeutic effect: Within 1-3 months of therapy

Duration: Can persist for 12 months without continuous therapy

Absorption: Dependent upon dose administered

Pregnancy Risk Factor B (oral)/C (parenteral)

Generic Available No

Etinilestradiol and Noretindrona (Mexico) see Ethinyl Estradiol and Norethindrone on page 379

Etinilestradiol (Mexico) see Ethinyl Estradiol on page 374

Etodolac (ee toe DOE lak)

Related Information

Nonsteroidal Anti-Inflammatory Agents, Comparative Dosages, and Pharmacokinetics on page 1143

Rheumatoid Arthritis and Osteoarthritis on page 1030

Brand Names Lodine®; Lodine® XL

Canadian/Mexican Brand Names Lodine® Retard (Mexico)

Therapeutic Category Analgesic, Non-narcotic; Nonsteroidal Anti-inflammatory Agent (NSAID), Oral

Use

Dental: Management of postoperative pain

Medical: Acute and long-term use in the management of signs and symptoms of osteoarthritis and management of pain, not approved for use in rheumatoid arthritis

Usual Dosage Adults: Oral: Single dose of 76-100 mg is comparable to the analgesic effect of aspirin 650 mg; in patients ≥65 years, no substantial differences in the pharmacokinetics or side-effects profile were seen compared with the general population

Acute pain: 200-400 mg every 6-8 hours, as needed, not to exceed total daily doses of 1200 mg; for patients weighing <60 kg, total daily dose should not exceed 20 mg/kg/day; extended release dose: one tablet daily

Mechanism of Action Inhibits prostaglandin synthesis by decreasing the activity of the enzyme, cyclo-oxygenase, which results in decreased formation of prostaglandin precursors

Local Anesthetic/Vasoconstrictor Precautions No information available to require special precautions

Effects on Dental Treatment No effects or complications reported

Other Adverse Effects >10%:

Central nervous system: Dizziness

(Continued)

387

Etodolac *(Continued)*

Dermatologic: Rash

Gastrointestinal: Abdominal cramps, heartburn, indigestion, nausea

Contraindications Hypersensitivity to etodolac, aspirin, or other NSAIDs

Warnings/Precautions Use with caution in patients with congestive heart failure, hypertension, decreased renal or hepatic function, history of GI disease, or those receiving anticoagulants

Drug Interactions Decreased effect with aspirin; increased effect/toxicity with aspirin (GI irritation), probenecid; increased effect/toxicity of lithium (nausea), methotrexate, digoxin, cyclosporin (nephrotoxicity), warfarin (bleeding)

Drug Uptake

Onset of effect: 0.5 hours following single dose of 200-400 mg

Duration of effect: 4-6 hours

Serum half-life: 7 hours

Time to peak serum concentration: 1 hour

Pregnancy Risk Factor C

Breast-feeding Considerations No data reported

Dosage Forms

Capsule: 200 mg, 300 mg

Tablet: 400 mg

Tablet, extended release: 400 mg, 600 mg

Dietary Considerations May be taken with food to decrease GI distress

Generic Available Yes

Selected Readings

Brooks PM and Day RO, "Nonsteroidal Anti-inflammatory Drugs-Differences and Similarities," *N Engl J Med*, 1991, 324(24):1716-25.

Tucker PW, Smith JR, and Adams DF, "A Comparison of 2 Analgesic Regimens for the Control of Postoperative Periodontal Discomfort," *J Periodontol*, 1996, 67(2):125-9.

Etomidate (e TOM i date)

Brand Names Amidate® Injection

Canadian/Mexican Brand Names Hypnomidate® (Mex)

Therapeutic Category General Anesthetic, Intravenous

Use Induction of general anesthesia

Usual Dosage Children >10 years and Adults: I.V.: 0.2-0.6 mg/kg over a period of 30-60 seconds for induction of anesthesia

Mechanism of Action Ultrashort-acting nonbarbiturate hypnotic used for the induction of anesthesia; chemically, it is a carboxylated imidazole and has been shown to produce a rapid induction of anesthesia with minimal cardiovascular and respiratory effects

Local Anesthetic/Vasoconstrictor Precautions No information available to require special precautions

Effects on Dental Treatment No effects or complications reported

Other Adverse Effects

>10%:

Gastrointestinal: Nausea, vomiting

Local: Pain at injection site

Neuromuscular & skeletal: Transient skeletal movements

Ocular: Uncontrolled eye movements

1% to 10%: Hiccups

<1%:

Cardiovascular: Hypertension, hypotension, tachycardia, bradycardia, arrhythmias

Respiratory: Hyperventilation, hypoventilation, apnea, laryngospasm

Warnings/Precautions Consider exogenous corticosteroid replacement in patients undergoing severe stress

Pregnancy Risk Factor C

Dosage Forms Injection: 2 mg/mL (10 mL, 20 mL)

Generic Available No

Etopophos® Injection *see* Etoposide *on this page*

Etoposide (e toe POE side)

Brand Names Etopophos® Injection; Toposar® Injection; VePesid® Injection; VePesid® Oral

Canadian/Mexican Brand Names Etopos® (Mexico); Medsaposide® (Mexico); Serozide® (Mexico)

Therapeutic Category Antineoplastic Agent, Mitotic Inhibitor

Use Treatment of lymphomas, ANLL, lung, testicular, bladder, and prostate carcinoma, hepatoma, rhabdomyosarcoma, uterine carcinoma, neuroblastoma, mycosis fungoides, Kaposi's sarcoma, histiocytosis, gestational trophoblastic disease, Ewing's sarcoma, Wilms' tumor, and brain tumors

Usual Dosage Refer to individual protocols

Oral: Twice the I.V. dose rounded to the nearest 50 mg given once daily if total dose ≤400 mg or in divided doses if >400 mg

Children: I.V.: 60-120 mg/m²/day for 3-5 days every 3-6 weeks
AML:
Remission induction: 150 mg/m²/day for 2-3 days for 2-3 cycles
Intensification or consolidation: 250 mg/m²/day for 3 days, courses 2-5
Conditioning regimen for allogeneic BMT: 60 mg/kg/dose as a single dose

Adults:
Small cell lung cancer:
Oral: Twice the I.V. dose rounded to the nearest 50 mg given once daily if
I.V.: 35 mg/m²/day for 4 days or 50 mg/m²/day for 5 days every 3-4 weeks
total dose ≤400 mg/day or in divided doses if >400 mg/day
IVPB: 200-250 mg/m² repeated every 7 weeks
Continuous intravenous infusion: 500 mg/m² over 24 hours every 3 weeks
Testicular cancer:
IVPB: 50-100 mg/m²/day for 5 days repeated every 3-4 weeks
I.V.: 100 mg/m² every other day for 3 doses repeated every 3-4 weeks
BMT/relapsed leukemia: I.V.: 2.4-3.5 g/m² or 25-70 mg/kg administered over 4-36 hours

Mechanism of Action Inhibits mitotic activity; inhibits cells from entering prophase; inhibits DNA synthesis. Initially thought to be mitotic inhibitors similar to podophyllotoxin, but actually have no effect on microtubule assembly. However, later shown to induce DNA strand breakage and inhibition of topoisomerase II (an enzyme which breaks and repairs DNA); etoposide acts in late S or early G2 phases.

Local Anesthetic/Vasoconstrictor Precautions No information available to require special precautions

Effects on Dental Treatment No effects or complications reported

Other Adverse Effects
>10%:
Dermatologic: Alopecia (reversible)
Gastrointestinal: Anorexia; occasional diarrhea and infrequent nausea and vomiting at standard doses; severe mucositis occurs with high (BMT) doses
Emetic potential: Moderately low (10% to 30%)
Hematologic: Myelosuppressive: Principal dose-limiting toxicity of VP-16. White blood cell count nadir is 5-15 days after administration and is more frequent than thrombocytopenia. Recovery is usually within 24-28 days and cumulative toxicity has not been noted with VP-16 as a single agent. No difference in toxicity is seen when VP-16 is administered over a 24-hour period or over 2 hours on 5 consecutive days. WBC: Mild to severe; Platelets: Mild; Onset (days): 10; Nadir (days): 14-16; Recovery (days): 21-28
1% to 10%:
Central nervous system: Unusual fatigue
Gastrointestinal: Stomatitis, diarrhea, abdominal pain, hepatitic dysfunction
Hypotension: Related to drug infusion time; may be related to vehicle used in the I.V. preparation (polysorbate 80 plus polyethylene glycol). Best to administer the drug over 1 hour.
<1%:
Cardiovascular: Tachycardia
Central nervous system: Neurotoxicity, somnolence, fatigue, fever, headache
Irritant chemotherapy; thrombophlebitis has been reported
Hepatic: Toxic hepatitis (with high-dose therapy)
Neuromuscular & skeletal: Peripheral neuropathy
Miscellaneous: Reports of flushing or bronchospasm, which did not reoccur in one report if patients were pretreated with corticosteroids and antihistamines

Drug Interactions Increased toxicity:
Warfarin may cause increases prothrombin time with concurrent use
Methotrexate: Alteration of MTX transport has been found as a slow efflux of MTX and its polyglutamated form out of the cell, leading to intercellular accumulation of MTX
Calcium antagonists: Increases the rate of VP-16-induced DNA damage and cytotoxicity in vitro
Carmustine: Reports of frequent hepatic dysfunction with hyperbilirubinemia, ascites, and thrombocytopenia
Cyclosporine: Additive cytotoxic effects on tumor cells

Drug Uptake
Absorption: Oral: 32% to 57%
Serum half-life: Terminal: 4-15 hours
Children: 6-8 hours with normal renal and hepatic function
Time to peak serum concentration: Oral: 1-1.5 hours
(Continued)

Etoposide *(Continued)*
Pregnancy Risk Factor D
Generic Available Yes

Etrafon® *see Amitriptyline and Perphenazine on page 62*

Etretinate (e TRET i nate)
Brand Names Tegison®
Therapeutic Category Antipsoriatic Agent, Systemic
Use Treatment of severe recalcitrant psoriasis in patients intolerant of or unresponsive to standard therapies
Usual Dosage Adults: Oral: Individualized; Initial: 0.75-1 mg/kg/day in divided doses, increase by 0.25 mg/kg/day at weekly intervals up to 1.5 mg/kg/day; maintenance dose established after 8-10 weeks of therapy 0.5-0.75 mg/kg/day
Mechanism of Action Unknown; related to retinoic acid and retinol (vitamin A)
Local Anesthetic/Vasoconstrictor Precautions No information available to require special precautions
Effects on Dental Treatment >10% of patients experience dry mouth
Other Adverse Effects
>10%:
  Central nervous system: Fatigue, headache, fever
  Dermatologic: Chapped lips, alopecia
  Endocrine & metabolic: Hypercholesterolemia, hypertriglyceridemia
  Gastrointestinal: Nausea, appetite change, sore tongue
  Neuromuscular & skeletal: Hyperostosis, bone pain, arthralgia
  Ocular: Eye irritation
  Respiratory: Epistaxis
1% to 10%:
  Cardiovascular: Edema
  Central nervous system: Dizziness, lethargy
  Hepatic: Hepatitis
  Neuromuscular & skeletal: Myalgia
  Ocular: Blurred vision
  Otic: Otitis externa
  Respiratory: Dyspnea
<1%:
  Cardiovascular: Syncope
  Central nervous system: Amnesia, confusion, pseudotumor cerebri, depression
  Dermatologic: Urticaria
  Gastrointestinal: Mouth ulcers, diarrhea, constipation, flatulence, weight loss, gingival bleeding
  Endocrine & metabolic: Gout
  Genitourinary: Dysuria
  Local: Phlebitis
  Neuromuscular & skeletal: Hyperkinesia, hypertonia
  Ocular: Photophobia
  Otic: Ear infection
  Renal: Polyuria, kidney stones
  Respiratory: Rhinorrhea
Drug Interactions
  Increased effect: Milk increases absorption of etretinate
  Increased toxicity: Additive toxicity with vitamin A
Drug Uptake
  Absorption: Oral: Absorbed from small intestine; absorption enhanced when coadministered with whole milk or a high lipid meal (highly lipophilic)
  Serum half-life: 4-8 days (with multiple doses)
Pregnancy Risk Factor X
Generic Available No

ETS-2%® **Topical** *see Erythromycin, Topical on page 364*
Eudal-SR® *see Guaifenesin and Pseudoephedrine on page 454*
Eulexin® *see Flutamide on page 424*
Eurax® *see Crotamiton on page 265*
Eutron® *see Methyclothiazide and Pargyline on page 621*
Evac-Q-Mag® **[OTC]** *see Magnesium Citrate on page 575*
Evalose® *see Lactulose on page 540*
Everone® **Injection** *see Testosterone on page 910*
E-Vista® *see Hydroxyzine on page 491*
Evista® *see Raloxifene on page 833*
E-Vitamin® **[OTC]** *see Vitamin E on page 994*
Exact® **Cream [OTC]** *see Benzoyl Peroxide on page 120*

Excedrin®, Extra Strength [OTC] see Acetaminophen, Aspirin, and Caffeine on page 24

Excedrin® Migraine [OTC] see Acetaminophen, Aspirin, and Caffeine on page 24

Excedrin® P.M. [OTC] see Acetaminophen and Diphenhydramine on page 23

Exelderm® see Sulconazole on page 889

Exidine® Scrub [OTC] see Chlorhexidine Gluconate on page 211

Exna® see Benzthiazide on page 122

Exosurf® Neonatal™ see Colfosceril Palmitate on page 259

Exsel® see Selenium Sulfide on page 861

Extendryl® SR see Chlorpheniramine, Phenylephrine, and Methscopolamine on page 220

Extra Action Cough Syrup [OTC] see Guaifenesin and Dextromethorphan on page 453

Extra Strength Adprin-B® [OTC] see Aspirin on page 90

Extra Strength Bayer® Enteric 500 Aspirin [OTC] see Aspirin on page 90

Extra Strength Bayer® Plus [OTC] see Aspirin on page 90

Extra Strength Doan's® [OTC] see Magnesium Salicylate on page 577

Eye-Lube-A® Solution [OTC] see Artificial Tears on page 87

Eye-Sed® [OTC] see Zinc Supplements on page 1005

Eye-Sed® Ophthalmic [OTC] see Zinc Sulfate on page 1005

Eyesine® Ophthalmic [OTC] see Tetrahydrozoline on page 916

Ezide® see Hydrochlorothiazide on page 476

Factor IX Complex (Human) (FAK ter nyne KOM pleks HYU man)

Brand Names AlphaNine® SD; Konÿne® 80; Mononine®; Profilnine® Heat-Treated; Proplex® SX-T; Proplex® T

Therapeutic Category Antihemophilic Agent; Blood Product Derivative

Use To control bleeding in patients with Factor IX deficiency (Hemophilia B or Christmas Disease); prevention/control of bleeding in hemophilia A patients with inhibitors to factor VIII; Proplex® T is indicated to prevent or control bleeding due to factor VII deficiency

Usual Dosage Children and Adults: Dosage is expressed in units of factor IX activity and must be individualized. I.V. only:

Factor VII deficiency: Highly individualized
0.5 unit/kg x body weight (kg) x desired increase (%)
For example, for a 70 kg adult to increase level by 25%:
0.5 unit/kg x 70 kg x 25 = 875 units

Factor IX deficiency: Highly individualized
1 unit/kg x body weight (in kg) x desired increase (%)
For example, to increase the level by 25% in a 70 kg adult:
1 unit x 70 kg x 25 = 1,750 units

Formula for units required to raise blood level %:
Total blood volume (mL blood/kg) = 70 mL/kg (adults), 80 mL/kg (children)
Plasma volume = total blood volume (mL) x [1 - Hct (in decimals)]
For example, for a 70 kg adult with a Hct = 40%: Plasma volume = [70 kg x 70 mL/kg] x [1 - 0.4] = 2940 mL
To calculate number of units needed to increase level to desired range (highly individualized and dependent on patient's condition):
Number of units = desired level increase [desired level - actual level] x plasma volume (in mL)
For example, for a 100% level in the above patient who has an actual level of 20%: Number of units needed = [1 (for a 100% level) - 0.2] x 2940 mL = 2,352 units

	Minor Spontaneous Hemorrhage, Prophylaxis	Major Trauma or Surgery
Desired levels of factor IX for hemostasis	15%-25%	25%-50%
Initial loading dose to achieve desired level	<20-30 units/kg	<75 units/kg
Frequency of dosing	Once; repeated in 24 h if necessary	q18-30h, depending on half-life and measured factor IX levels
Duration of treatment	Once; repeated if necessary	Up to 10 days, depending upon nature of insult

(Continued)

Factor IX Complex (Human) *(Continued)*

As a general rule, the level of factor IX required for treatment of different conditions is shown in the table.

Factor VIII inhibitor patients: 75 units/kg/dose; may be given every 6-12 hours

Anticoagulant overdosage: I.V.: 15 units/kg

Mechanism of Action Replaces deficient clotting factor including factor X; hemophilia B, or Christmas disease, is an X-linked recessively inherited disorder of blood coagulation characterized by insufficient or abnormal synthesis of the clotting protein factor IX. Factor IX is a vitamin K-dependent coagulation factor which is synthesized in the liver. Factor IX is activated by factor XIa in the intrinsic coagulation pathway. Activated factor IX (IXa), in combination with factor VII:C activates factor X to Xa, resulting ultimately in the conversion of prothrombin to thrombin and the formation of a fibrin clot. The infusion of exogenous factor IX to replace the deficiency present in hemophilia B temporarily restores hemostasis.

Local Anesthetic/Vasoconstrictor Precautions No information available to require special precautions

Effects on Dental Treatment No effects or complications reported

Other Adverse Effects

1% to 10%: Following rapid administration: Transient fever, chills, headache, flushing, paresthesia

<1%:
Cardiovascular: Thrombosis following high dosages in hemophilia B patients
Central nervous system: Somnolence
Dermatologic: Urticaria
Hematologic: Disseminated intravascular coagulation
Miscellaneous: Tightness in chest and neck

Drug Uptake

Serum half-life:
VII component: Cleared rapidly from the serum in two phases; initial: 4-6 hours; terminal: 22.5 hours
IX component: 24 hours

Pregnancy Risk Factor C

Generic Available No

Comments Factor VII and IX units are listed per vial and per lot to lot variation

Factor VIII *see* Antihemophilic Factor (Human) *on page 80*

Factor VIII Recombinant *see* Antihemophilic Factor (Recombinant) *on page 81*

Famciclovir (fam SYE kloe veer)

Related Information
Systemic Viral Diseases *on page 1047*

Brand Names Famvir™

Therapeutic Category Antiviral Agent, Oral

Use Management of acute herpes zoster (shingles)

Usual Dosage Adults: Oral:
Acute herpes zoster: 500 mg every 8 hours for 7 days
Recurrent herpes simplex in immunocompetent patients: 125 mg twice daily for 5 days

Mechanism of Action After undergoing rapid biotransformation to the active compound, penciclovir, famciclovir is phosphorylated by viral thymidine kinase in HSV-1, HSV-2, and VZV-infected cells to a monophosphate form; this is then converted to penciclovir triphosphate and competes with deoxyguanosine triphosphate to inhibit HSV-2 polymerase (ie, herpes viral DNA synthesis/replication is selectively inhibited)

Local Anesthetic/Vasoconstrictor Precautions No information available to require special precautions

Effects on Dental Treatment No effects or complications reported

Other Adverse Effects

>10%:
Central nervous system: Headache
Gastrointestinal: Nausea

1% to 10%:
Central nervous system: Fatigue, fever, dizziness, somnolence
Gastrointestinal: Diarrhea, vomiting, constipation, anorexia, abdominal pain
Neuromuscular & skeletal: Rigors, paresthesia

Drug Interactions No data reported

Drug Uptake

Absorption: Food decreases the maximum peak concentration and delays the time to peak; AUC remains the same

Serum half-life: Penciclovir: 2-3 hours (10, 20, and 7 hours in HSV-1, HSV-2, and VZV-infected cells); linearly decreased with reductions in renal failure
Pregnancy Risk Factor B
Dosage Forms Tablet: 125 mg, 250 mg, 500 mg
Dietary Considerations May be taken with food or on an empty stomach
Generic Available No

Famotidina (Mexico) *see* Famotidine *on this page*

Famotidine (fa MOE ti deen)
Brand Names Pepcid®; Pepcid® AC Acid Controller [OTC]
Canadian/Mexican Brand Names Apo®-Famotidine (Canada); Durater® (Mexico); Famoxal® (Mexico); Farmotex® (Mexico); Novo-Famotidine® (Canada); Nu-Famotidine® (Canada); Pepcidine® (Mexico); Sigafam® (Mexico)
Therapeutic Category Histamine H$_2$ Antagonist
Synonyms Famotidina (Mexico)
Use Therapy and treatment of duodenal ulcer, gastric ulcer, control gastric pH in critically ill patients, symptomatic relief in gastritis, gastroesophageal reflux, active benign ulcer, and pathological hypersecretory conditions
Usual Dosage
Children: Oral, I.V.: Doses of 1-2 mg/kg/day have been used; maximum dose: 40 mg
Adults:
Oral:
Duodenal ulcer, gastric ulcer: 40 mg/day at bedtime for 4-8 weeks
Hypersecretory conditions: Initial: 20 mg every 6 hours, may increase up to 160 mg every 6 hours
GERD: 20 mg twice daily for 6 weeks
I.V.: 20 mg every 12 hours
Mechanism of Action Competitive inhibition of histamine at H$_2$ receptors of the gastric parietal cells, which inhibits gastric acid secretion
Local Anesthetic/Vasoconstrictor Precautions No information available to require special precautions
Effects on Dental Treatment No effects or complications reported
Other Adverse Effects
1% to 10%:
Central nervous system: Dizziness, headache
Gastrointestinal: Constipation, diarrhea
<1%:
Cardiovascular: Bradycardia, tachycardia, palpitations, hypertension
Central nervous system: Fever, fatigue, seizures, insomnia, drowsiness
Dermatologic: Acne, pruritus, urticaria, dry skin
Gastrointestinal: Abdominal discomfort, flatulence, belching, anorexia
Hematologic: Agranulocytosis, neutropenia, thrombocytopenia
Hepatic: Elevated AST, ALT
Neuromuscular & skeletal: Paresthesia, weakness
Renal: Elevated BUN, creatinine, proteinuria
Respiratory: Bronchospasm
Miscellaneous: Allergic reaction
Drug Interactions Decreased effect of ketoconazole, itraconazole
Drug Uptake
Onset of GI effect: Oral: Within 1 hour
Duration: 10-12 hours
Serum half-life: 2.5-3.5 hours; increases with renal impairment, oliguric patients: 20 hours
Time to peak serum concentration: Oral: Within 1-3 hours
Pregnancy Risk Factor B
Generic Available No

Famvir™ *see* Famciclovir *on previous page*
Fansidar® *see* Sulfadoxine and Pyrimethamine *on page 892*
Fareston® *see* Toremifene *on page 946*
Fastin® *see* Phentermine *on page 750*

Fat Emulsion (fat e MUL shun)
Brand Names Intralipid®; Liposyn®; Nutrilipid®; Soyacal®
Canadian/Mexican Brand Names Emulsan 20% (Mexico); Lipocin (Mexico); Lyposyn (Mexico)
Therapeutic Category Caloric Agent; Intravenous Nutritional Therapy
Synonyms Intravenous Fat Emulsion
Use Source of calories and essential fatty acids for patients requiring parenteral nutrition of extended duration
(Continued)

Fat Emulsion *(Continued)*

Usual Dosage Fat emulsion should not exceed 60% of the total daily calories

Children: Initial dose: 0.5-1 g/kg/day, increase by 0.5 g/kg/day to a maximum of 3-4 g/kg/day; maximum rate of infusion: 0.25 g/kg/hour (1.25 mL/kg/hour of 20% solution)

Adolescents and Adults: Initial dose: 1 g/kg/day, increase by 0.5-1 g/kg/day to a maximum of 2.5 g/kg/day of 10% and 3 g/kg/day of 20%; maximum rate of infusion: 0.25 g/kg/hour (1.25 mL/kg/hour of 20% solution); do not exceed 50 mL/hour (20%) or 100 mL/hour (10%)

Note: At the onset of therapy, the patient should be observed for any immediate allergic reactions such as dyspnea, cyanosis, and fever. Slower initial rates of infusion may be used for the first 10-15 minutes of the infusion (eg, 0.1 mL/minute of 10% or 0.05 mL/minute of 20% solution).

Prevention of fatty acid deficiency (8% to 10% of total caloric intake): 0.5-1 g/kg/24 hours

Children: 5-10 mL/kg/day at 0.1 mL/minute then up to 100 mL/hour

Adults: 500 mL twice weekly at rate of 1 mL/minute for 30 minutes, then increase to 500 mL over 4-6 hours

Can be used in both children and adults on a daily basis as a caloric source in TPN

Mechanism of Action Essential for normal structure and function of cell membranes

Local Anesthetic/Vasoconstrictor Precautions No information available to require special precautions

Effects on Dental Treatment No effects or complications reported

Other Adverse Effects

>10%: Local: Thrombophlebitis

1% to 10%: Endocrine & metabolic: Hyperlipemia

<1%:

Cardiovascular: Cyanosis, flushing, chest pain

Gastrointestinal: Nausea, vomiting, diarrhea

Hepatic: Hepatomegaly

Respiratory: Dyspnea

Miscellaneous: Sepsis

Drug Uptake

Serum half-life: 0.5-1 hour

Pregnancy Risk Factor B/C

Generic Available Yes

FC1157a *see* Toremifene *on page 946*

Fedahist® Expectorant [OTC] *see* Guaifenesin and Pseudoephedrine *on page 454*

Fedahist® Expectorant Pediatric [OTC] *see* Guaifenesin and Pseudoephedrine *on page 454*

Fedahist® Tablet [OTC] *see* Chlorpheniramine and Pseudoephedrine *on page 219*

Feiba VH Immuno® *see* Anti-inhibitor Coagulant Complex *on page 82*

Felbamate *(FEL ba mate)*

Brand Names Felbatol™

Therapeutic Category Anticonvulsant, Miscellaneous

Use Not a first-line agent; reserved for patients who do not adequately respond to alternative agents and whose epilepsy is so severe that benefit outweighs risk of liver failure or aplastic anemia; used as monotherapy and adjunctive therapy in patients ≥14 years of age with partial seizures with and without secondary generalization; adjunctive therapy in children ≥2 years of age who have partial and generalized seizures associated with Lennox-Gastaut syndrome

Local Anesthetic/Vasoconstrictor Precautions No information available to require special precautions

Effects on Dental Treatment No effects or complications reported

Other Adverse Effects

>10%:

Central nervous system: Anxiety, headache, fatigue, dizziness

Gastrointestinal: Nausea, diarrhea, anorexia, vomiting, constipation

Respiratory: Cough

1% to 10%:

Central nervous system: Somnolence, insomnia, ataxia, depression or behavior changes, clouded sensorium, lethargy, slurred speech

Dermatologic: Acne, skin rash

Gastrointestinal: Weight gain

Neuromuscular & skeletal: Muscle twitches

Ocular: Blurred vision, diplopia, uncontrollable eye movements
<1%:
Dermatologic: Alopecia
Gastrointestinal: Gum bleeding or hyperplasia
Pregnancy Risk Factor C
Generic Available No
Comments Monotherapy has not been associated with gingival hyperplasia, impaired concentration, weight gain, or abnormal thinking

Felbatol™ *see Felbamate on previous page*

Feldene® *see Piroxicam on page 767*

Felodipina (Mexico) *see Felodipine on this page*

Felodipine (fe LOE di peen)
Related Information
Calcium Channel Blockers & Gingival Hyperplasia *on page 1132*
Cardiovascular Diseases *on page 1010*
Enalapril and Felodipine *on page 348*
Brand Names Plendil®
Canadian/Mexican Brand Names Munobal® (Mexico); Renedil® (Canada)
Therapeutic Category Calcium Channel Blocker
Synonyms Felodipina (Mexico)
Use Treatment of hypertension, congestive heart failure
Usual Dosage Adults: Oral: 5-10 mg once daily; increase by 5 mg at 2-week intervals, as needed, to a maximum of 20 mg/day (Elderly: Begin with 2.5 mg/day)
Mechanism of Action Inhibits calcium ions from entering the select voltage-sensitive areas or "slow channels" of vascular smooth muscle and myocardium during depolarization, producing a relaxation of coronary vascular smooth muscle and coronary vasodilation; increases myocardial oxygen delivery in patients with vasospastic angina
Local Anesthetic/Vasoconstrictor Precautions No information available to require special precautions
Effects on Dental Treatment Calcium channel blockers cause gingival hyperplasia in approximately 1% of patients. There have been fewer reports with felodipine than with other CCBs. The hyperplasia will disappear with cessation of drug therapy. Consultation with physician is suggested.
Other Adverse Effects
>10%: Cardiovascular: Peripheral edema
1% to 10%:
Cardiovascular: Chest pain, tachycardia
Central nervous system: Dizziness, lightheadedness
Dermatologic: Skin rash
Gastrointestinal: Constipation, diarrhea
<1%:
Cardiovascular: Hypotension, arrhythmia, bradycardia, palpitations
Central nervous system: Mental depression, headache
Gastrointestinal: Gingival hyperplasia, dry mouth, nausea
Hepatic: Marked elevations in liver function tests
Ocular: Blurred vision
Respiratory: Dyspnea
Drug Interactions Increased toxicity/effect/levels:
Calcium channel blockers (CCB) and H₂-blockers such as cimetidine cause increased bioavailability CCB
Beta-blockers cause increased depressant effects on A-V conduction
Drug Uptake
Onset of effect: 2-5 hours
Duration: 16-24 hours
Absorption: 100%; absolute: 20% due to first-pass effect
Serum half-life: 11-16 hours
Pregnancy Risk Factor C
Generic Available No

Femara® *see Letrozole on page 543*

Femcet® *see Butalbital Compound on page 154*

Femcet® *see Butalbital Compound and Acetaminophen on page 155*

Femguard® *see Sulfabenzamide, Sulfacetamide, and Sulfathiazole on page 889*

Femiron® [OTC] *see Ferrous Fumarate on page 400*

Femizol-M® [OTC] *see Miconazole on page 635*

Femstat® *see Butoconazole on page 157*

Fenazopiridina (Mexico) *see Phenazopyridine on page 746*

enesin™ *see* Guaifenesin *on page 452*
Fenesin DM® *see* Guaifenesin and Dextromethorphan *on page 453*

Fenfluramine *Withdrawn from Market 1997*
(fen FLURE a meen)

Brand Names Pondimin®

Canadian/Mexican Brand Names Ponderal® (Canada)

Therapeutic Category Adrenergic Agonist Agent; Anorexiant

Use Short-term adjunct in exogenous obesity

Usual Dosage Adults: Oral: 20 mg 3 times/day before meals or food, up to 40 mg 3 times/day; maximum daily dose: 120 mg

Mechanism of Action Fenfluramine hydrochloride is a phenethylamine structurally related to amphetamine; central nervous system depression is more common than stimulation, which makes fenfluramine pharmacologically different from amphetamine. Fenfluramine's exact mechanism of action is not well understood; the drug's appetite suppressing action may be due to the stimulation of the hypothalamus; the anorectic effect may also be due to delayed gastric emptying.

Local Anesthetic/Vasoconstrictor Precautions Use vasoconstrictor with caution in patients taking fenfluramine; amphetamine like drugs enhance the sympathomimetic response of epinephrine and norepinephrine leading to potential hypertension and cardiotoxicity.

Effects on Dental Treatment Up to 10% of patients may present with hypertension. The use of local anesthetic without vasoconstrictor is recommended in these patients.

Other Adverse Effects
>10%:
  Cardiovascular: Hypertension
  Central nervous system: Euphoria, nervousness, insomnia
1% to 10%:
  Central nervous system: Confusion, mental depression, restlessness
  Endocrine & metabolic: Changes in libido
  Gastrointestinal: Nausea, vomiting, constipation
  Hematologic: Blood dyscrasias
  Neuromuscular & skeletal: Tremor
  Ocular: Blurred vision
<1%:
  Cardiovascular: Tachycardia, arrhythmias
  Central nervous system: Headache
  Dermatologic: Alopecia
  Gastrointestinal: Diarrhea, abdominal cramps
  Genitourinary: Dysuria
  Neuromuscular & skeletal: Myalgia
  Renal: Polyuria
  Respiratory: Dyspnea
  Miscellaneous: Increased sweating

Drug Interactions
  Adrenergic blockers are inhibited by amphetamines
  Amphetamines enhance the activity of tricyclic or sympathomimetic agents
  MAO inhibitors slow the metabolism of amphetamines
  Amphetamines will counteract the sedative effects of antihistamines
  Amphetamines potentiate the analgesic effects of meperidine

Pregnancy Risk Factor C

Generic Available No

Fenilefrina (Mexico) *see* Phenylephrine *on page 752*
Fenilpropanolamina (Mexico) *see* Phenylpropanolamine *on page 754*
Fenobarbital (Mexico) *see* Phenobarbital *on page 747*

Fenofibrate (fen oh FYE brate)

Brand Names Lipidil®; Tricor®

Canadian/Mexican Brand Names Controlip® (Mexico)

Therapeutic Category Lipid Lowering Drugs

Synonyms Fenofibrato (Mexico)

Use Adjunct to dietary therapy for the treatment of adults with very high elevations of serum triglyceride levels (types IV and V hyperlipidemia) who are at risk of pancreatitis and who do not respond adequately to a determined dietary effort; its efficacy can be enhanced by combination with other hypolipidemic agents that have a different mechanism of action; safety and efficacy may be greater than that of clofibrate

Usual Dosage Oral:
Children >10 years: 5 mg/kg/day

Adults: 100 mg 3 times/day with meals or 200 mg in the morning and 100 mg in the evening

Mechanism of Action Fenofibric acid is believed to increase VLDL catabolism by enhancing the synthesis of lipoprotein lipase; as a result of a decrease in VLDL levels, total plasma triglycerides are reduced by 30% to 60% (VLDL contains ~60% triglycerides and 10% to 15% cholesterol); apolipoprotein B, which stabilizes the structure of VLDL and LDL, decreases in a parallel fashion and plasma cholesterol levels decrease by fenofibrate's effect on LDL levels and cholesterol synthesis; modest increase in HDL occurs in some hypertriglyceridemic patients since it is involved in the storage and transport of cholesterol ester and apolipoproteins

Local Anesthetic/Vasoconstrictor Precautions No information available to require special precautions

Effects on Dental Treatment No effects or complications reported

Other Adverse Effects
>10%: Gastrointestinal: Nausea, gastric discomfort
1% to 10%:
    Dermatologic: Skin reactions
    Gastrointestinal: Constipation, diarrhea
<1%:
    Central nervous system: Dizziness, headache, fatigue, insomnia
    Hepatic: Transient elevation in LFTs
    Neuromuscular & skeletal: Arthralgia, myalgia

Drug Interactions
Increased hypolipidemic effect: Cholestyramine, colestipol will add to the hypolipidemic effect of fenofibrate

Drug Uptake
Peak effect: 4-6 hours
Absorption: 60% to 90% when given with meals
Serum half-life: Fenofibrate: 21 hours (30 hours in elderly, 44-54 hours in hepatic impairment)

Pregnancy Risk Factor C
Generic Available No

Fenofibrato (Mexico) *see* Fenofibrate *on previous page*

Fenoldopam (fe NOL doe pam)

Brand Names Corlopam®
Therapeutic Category Antihypertensive
Synonyms Fenoldopam Mesylate
Use Investigational in U.S.: Severe hypertension; congestive heart failure
Usual Dosage
Oral: 100 mg 2-4 times daily
I.V.: Severe hypertension: Initial: 0.1 mcg/kg/minute; may be increased in increments of 0.05-0.2 mcg/kg/minute; maximal infusion rate: 1.6 mcg/kg/minute

Mechanism of Action A selective dopamine agonist (D_1-receptors) with vasodilitary properties; 6 times as potent as dopamine in producing vasodilitation

Local Anesthetic/Vasoconstrictor Precautions No information available to require special precautions

Effects on Dental Treatment No effects or complications reported

Other Adverse Effects
Cardiovascular: Fibrillation (atrial), hypotension, edema, tachycardia, facial flushing, asymptomatic T wave flattening on EKG, flutter (atrial), chest pain, angina
Central nervous system: Headache, dizziness
Gastrointestinal: Nausea, vomiting, diarrhea
Ocular: Intraocular pressure (increased)

Contraindications Previous hypersensitive reaction to fenoldopam

Warnings/Precautions Use with caution in patients with cirrhosis, unstable angina or glaucoma

Drug Uptake
Onset of action: I.V.: 15 minutes
Duration:
    Oral: 2-4 hours
    I.V.: 1 hour
Absorption: Oral: Poor
Distribution: V_d: 0.6 L/kg
Half-life: I.V.: 9.8 minutes
Metabolism: Hepatic to multiple metabolites; the 8-sulfate metabolite may have some activity
Elimination: Renal

Fenoldopam Mesylate *see* Fenoldopam *on this page*

Fenoprofen (fen oh PROE fen)

Related Information

Nonsteroidal Anti-Inflammatory Agents, Comparative Dosages, and Pharmacokinetics *on page 1143*

Rheumatoid Arthritis and Osteoarthritis *on page 1030*

Brand Names Nalfon®

Therapeutic Category Analgesic, Non-narcotic; Anti-inflammatory Agent; Nonsteroidal Anti-inflammatory Agent (NSAID), Oral

Synonyms Fenoprofeno Calcio (Mexico)

Use Symptomatic treatment of acute and chronic rheumatoid arthritis and osteoarthritis; relief of mild to moderate pain

Usual Dosage Adults: Oral:

Rheumatoid arthritis: 300-600 mg 3-4 times/day up to 3.2 g/day

Mild to moderate pain: 200 mg every 4-6 hours as needed

Mechanism of Action Inhibits prostaglandin synthesis by decreasing the activity of the enzyme, cyclo-oxygenase, which results in decreased formation of prostaglandin precursors

Local Anesthetic/Vasoconstrictor Precautions No information available to require special precautions

Effects on Dental Treatment No effects or complications reported

Other Adverse Effects

>10%:

Central nervous system: Dizziness

Dermatologic: Skin rash

Gastrointestinal: Abdominal cramps, heartburn, indigestion, nausea

1% to 10%:

Central nervous system: Headache, nervousness

Dermatologic: Itching

Endocrine & metabolic: Fluid retention

Gastrointestinal: Vomiting

Otic: Tinnitus

<1%:

Cardiovascular: Congestive heart failure, hypertension, arrhythmias, tachycardia

Central nervous system: Confusion, hallucinations, aseptic meningitis, mental depression, drowsiness, insomnia

Dermatologic: Urticaria, erythema multiforme, toxic epidermal necrolysis, Stevens-Johnson syndrome, angioedema

Endocrine & metabolic: Polydipsia, hot flashes

Gastrointestinal: Gastritis, GI ulceration

Genitourinary: Cystitis

Hematologic: Agranulocytosis, anemia, hemolytic anemia, bone marrow suppression, leukopenia, thrombocytopenia

Hepatic: Hepatitis

Neuromuscular & skeletal: Peripheral neuropathy

Ocular: Toxic amblyopia, blurred vision, conjunctivitis, dry eyes

Otic: Decreased hearing

Renal: Polyuria, acute renal failure

Respiratory: Allergic rhinitis, dyspnea, epistaxis

Drug Interactions

Decreased effect with phenobarbital

Increased effect/toxicity of phenytoin, sulfonamides, sulfonylureas

Increased toxicity with salicylates, oral anticoagulants

Drug Uptake

Absorption: Rapid (to 80%) from upper GI tract

Serum half-life: 2.5-3 hours

Time to peak serum concentration: Within 2 hours

Pregnancy Risk Factor B (D if used in the 3rd trimester or near delivery)

Generic Available Yes

Fenoprofeno Calcico (Mexico) *see* Fenoprofen *on this page*

Fentanyl (FEN ta nil)

Related Information

Narcotic Agonists *on page 1141*

Brand Names Duragesic™; Fentanyl Oralet®; Sublimaze®

Canadian/Mexican Brand Names Durogesic® (Mexico); Fentanest® (Mexico)

Therapeutic Category Analgesic, Narcotic; General Anesthetic, Intravenous

Use

Dental: Adjunct in preoperative intravenous conscious sedation in patients undergoing dental surgery

Medical: In medicine, adjunct to general or regional anesthesia; management of chronic pain (transdermal product)

Restrictions C-II; Nonrefillable

Usual Dosage

Children 1-12 years:

Sedation for minor procedures/analgesia:

I.M., I.V.: 1-2 mcg/kg/dose

Transmucosal (lozenge): 5 mcg/kg if child is not fearful; fearful children and some younger children may require doses of 5-15 mcg/kg (which also carries an increased risk of hypoventilation); drug effect begins within 10 minutes, with sedation beginning shortly thereafter

Children >12 years and Adults:

Sedation for minor procedures/analgesia:

I.M., I.V.: 0.5-1 mcg/kg/dose; higher doses are used for major procedures

Transmucosal (lozenge): 5 mcg/kg, suck on lozenge vigorously approximately 20-40 minutes before the start of procedure, drug effect begins within 10 minutes, with sedation beginning shortly thereafter

Preoperative sedation: I.M., I.V.: 50-100 mcg/dose

Pain control: Transdermal fentanyl is not to be used for acute dosing in treatment of dental pain

Mechanism of Action Binds to opiate receptors (mu and kappa subtypes) in the CNS causing inhibition of ascending pain pathways, altering the perception of and response to pain; produces generalized CNS depression

Local Anesthetic/Vasoconstrictor Precautions No information available to require special precautions

Effects on Dental Treatment No effects or complications reported

Other Adverse Effects >10%:

Cardiovascular: Hypotension, bradycardia

Central nervous system: CNS depression, drowsiness, sedation

Gastrointestinal: Nausea, vomiting, constipation

Respiratory: Respiratory depression

1% to 10%:

Cardiovascular: Cardiac arrhythmias, orthostatic hypotension

Central nervous system: Confusion, CNS depression

Gastrointestinal: Biliary tract spasm

Ocular: Miosis

<1%:

Cardiovascular: Circulatory depression

Central nervous system: Convulsions, dysesthesia, paradoxical CNS excitation or delirium, dizziness

Dermatologic: Erythema, pruritus, rash, hives, itching, cold, clammy skin

Endocrine & metabolic: ADH release

Gastrointestinal: Biliary tract spasm

Genitourinary: Urinary tract spasm

Respiratory: Bronchospasm, laryngospasm

Miscellaneous: Physical and psychological dependence with prolonged use

Contraindications Hypersensitivity to fentanyl or any component; increased intracranial pressure; severe respiratory depression; severe liver or renal insufficiency;

Transmucosal is contraindicated in unmonitored settings where a risk of unrecognized hypoventilation exists or in treating acute or chronic pain

Warnings/Precautions Fentanyl shares the toxic potentials of opiate agonists, and precautions of opiate agonist therapy should be observed; use with caution in patients with bradycardia; rapid I.V. infusion may result in skeletal muscle and chest wall rigidity → impaired ventilation → respiratory distress → apnea, bronchoconstriction, laryngospasm; inject slowly over 3-5 minutes; nondepolarizing skeletal muscle relaxant may be required.

Enhanced analgesia has been seen in elderly patients on therapeutic doses of narcotics; duration of action may be increased in the elderly; the elderly may be particularly susceptible to the CNS depressant and constipating effects of narcotics

Drug Interactions Increased toxicity of CNS depressants, phenothiazines, tricyclic antidepressants may potentiate fentanyl's adverse effects

Drug Uptake

Onset of effect (respiratory depressant effect may last longer than analgesic effect):

I.M.: Analgesia: 7-15 minutes

I.V.: Analgesia: Almost immediate

Transmucosal (lozenge): 5-15 minutes with a maximum reduction in activity/apprehension

Duration of effect:

I.M.: 1-2 hours

(Continued)

399

Fentanyl *(Continued)*

    I.V.: 0.5-1 hour
    Transmucosal: Related to blood level of drug
   Serum half-life: 2-4 hours; transmucosal: 5-15 hours

Pregnancy Risk Factor B (D if used for prolonged periods or in high doses at term)

Breast-feeding Considerations Not contraindicated

Dosage Forms
    Injection, as citrate: 0.05 mg/mL (2 mL, 5 mL, 10 mL, 20 mL, 50 mL)
    Lozenge, oral transmucosal (raspberry flavored): 200 mcg, 300 mcg, 400 mcg
    Transdermal system: 25 mcg/hour [10 cm^2]; 50 mcg/hour [20 cm^2]; 75 mcg/hour [30 cm^2]; 100 mcg/hour [40 cm^2] (all available in 5s)

Dietary Considerations No data reported

Generic Available Injection: Yes

Comments Transdermal fentanyl should not be used as a pain reliever in dentistry due to danger of hypoventilation

Fentanyl Oralet® *see* Fentanyl *on page 398*

Fentermina (Mexico) *see* Phentermine *on page 750*

Feosol® [OTC] *see* Ferrous Sulfate *on next page*

Feostat® [OTC] *see* Ferrous Fumarate *on this page*

Ferancee® [OTC] *see* Ferrous Sulfate and Ascorbic Acid *on page 402*

Feratab® [OTC] *see* Ferrous Sulfate *on next page*

Fergon® [OTC] *see* Ferrous Gluconate *on next page*

Fer-In-Sol® [OTC] *see* Ferrous Sulfate *on next page*

Fer-Iron® [OTC] *see* Ferrous Sulfate *on next page*

Fero-Grad 500® [OTC] *see* Ferrous Sulfate and Ascorbic Acid *on page 402*

Fero-Gradumet® [OTC] *see* Ferrous Sulfate *on next page*

Ferospace® [OTC] *see* Ferrous Sulfate *on next page*

Ferralet® [OTC] *see* Ferrous Gluconate *on next page*

Ferralyn® Lanacaps® [OTC] *see* Ferrous Sulfate *on next page*

Ferra-TD® [OTC] *see* Ferrous Sulfate *on next page*

Ferromar® [OTC] *see* Ferrous Sulfate and Ascorbic Acid *on page 402*

Ferro-Sequels® [OTC] *see* Ferrous Fumarate *on this page*

Ferrous Fumarate *(FER us FYOO ma rate)*

Brand Names Femiron® [OTC]; Feostat® [OTC]; Ferro-Sequels® [OTC]; Fuma-sorb® [OTC]; Fumerin® [OTC]; Hemocyte® [OTC]; Ircon® [OTC]; Nephro-Fer™ [OTC]; Span-FF® [OTC]

Canadian/Mexican Brand Names Ferval® Ferroso (Mexico); Palafer® (Canada)

Therapeutic Category Iron Salt

Use Prevention and treatment of iron deficiency anemias

Usual Dosage Oral (dose expressed in terms of elemental iron):
    Children:
        Severe iron deficiency anemia: 4-6 mg Fe/kg/day in 3 divided doses
        Mild to moderate iron deficiency anemia: 3 mg Fe/kg/day in 1-2 divided doses
        Prophylaxis: 1-2 mg Fe/kg/day
    Adults:
        Iron deficiency: 60-100 mg twice daily up to 60 mg 2 times/day
        Prophylaxis: 60-100 mg/day
        To avoid GI upset, start with a single daily dose and increase by 1 tablet/day each week or as tolerated until desired daily dose is achieved
    Elderly: 200 mg 3-4 times/day

Mechanism of Action Replaces iron found in hemoglobin, myoglobin, and enzymes; allows the transportation of oxygen via hemoglobin

Local Anesthetic/Vasoconstrictor Precautions No information available to require special precautions

Effects on Dental Treatment Do not prescribe tetracyclines simultaneously with iron since GI tract absorption of both tetracycline and iron may be inhibited

Other Adverse Effects
    >10%: Gastrointestinal: Stomach cramping, constipation, nausea, vomiting, dark stools
    1% to 10%:
        Gastrointestinal: Heartburn, diarrhea, staining of teeth
        Genitourinary: Discolored urine
    <1%: Ocular: Contact irritation

Drug Interactions

Decreased effect: Absorption of oral preparation of iron and tetracyclines are decreased when both of these drugs are given together; concurrent administration of antacids may decrease iron absorption; iron may decrease absorption of penicillamine when given at the same time; response to iron therapy may be delayed in patients receiving chloramphenicol

Milk may decrease absorption of iron

Increased effect: Current administration of ≥200 mg vitamin C per 30 mg elemental iron increases absorption of oral iron

Drug Uptake

Onset of hematologic response (essentially the same to either oral or parenteral iron salts): Red blood cell form and color changes within 3-10 days

Peak reticulocytosis: Within 5-10 days; hemoglobin values increase within 2-4 weeks

Absorption: Iron is absorbed in the duodenum and upper jejunum; in persons with normal iron stores 10% of an oral dose is absorbed, this is increased to 20% to 30% in persons with inadequate iron stores; food and achlorhydria will decrease absorption

Pregnancy Risk Factor A

Generic Available Yes

Ferrous Gluconate (FER us GLOO koe nate)

Brand Names Fergon® [OTC]; Ferralet® [OTC]; Simron® [OTC]

Canadian/Mexican Brand Names Apo®-Ferrous Gluconate (Canada)

Therapeutic Category Iron Salt

Use Prevention and treatment of iron deficiency anemias

Usual Dosage Oral **(dose expressed in terms of elemental iron):**

Children:

Severe iron deficiency anemia: 4-6 mg Fe/kg/day in 3 divided doses

Mild to moderate iron deficiency anemia: 3 mg Fe/kg/day in 1-2 divided doses

Prophylaxis: 1-2 mg Fe/kg/day

Adults:

Iron deficiency: 60 mg twice daily up to 60 mg 4 times/day

Prophylaxis: 60 mg/day

Mechanism of Action Replaces iron found in hemoglobin, myoglobin, and enzymes; allows the transportation of oxygen via hemoglobin

Local Anesthetic/Vasoconstrictor Precautions No information available to require special precautions

Effects on Dental Treatment Do not prescribe tetracyclines simultaneously with iron since GI tract absorption of both tetracycline and iron may be inhibited

Other Adverse Effects

>10%: Gastrointestinal: Stomach cramping, constipation, nausea, vomiting, dark stools

1% to 10%:

Gastrointestinal: Heartburn, diarrhea, staining of teeth

Genitourinary: Discolored urine

<1%: Ocular: Contact irritation

Drug Interactions Absorption of oral preparation of iron and tetracyclines is decreased when both of these drugs are given together; concurrent administration of antacids may decrease iron absorption; iron may decrease absorption of penicillamine when given at the same time. Response to iron therapy may be delayed in patients receiving chloramphenicol. Concurrent administration of ≥ 200 mg vitamin C/30 mg elemental iron increases absorption of oral iron; milk may decrease absorption of iron.

Drug Uptake Onset of hematologic response (essentially the same to either oral or parenteral iron salts): Red blood cells form and color changes within 3-10 days, peak reticulocytosis occurs in 5-10 days, and hemoglobin values increase within 2-4 weeks

Pregnancy Risk Factor A

Generic Available Yes

Ferrous Sulfate (FER us SUL fate)

Brand Names Feosol® [OTC]; Feratab® [OTC]; Fer-In-Sol® [OTC]; Fer-Iron® [OTC]; Fero-Gradumet® [OTC]; Ferospace® [OTC]; Ferralyn® Lanacaps® [OTC]; Ferra-TD® [OTC]; Mol-Iron® [OTC]; Slow FE® [OTC]

Canadian/Mexican Brand Names Apo®-Ferrous Sulfate (Canada); Hemobion® 200 (Mexico); Hemobion® 400 (Mexico); Orafer® (Mexico); PMS-Ferrous® Sulfate (Canada)

Therapeutic Category Iron Salt

Use Prevention and treatment of iron deficiency anemias

(Continued)

Ferrous Sulfate *(Continued)*

Usual Dosage Oral:

Children **(dose expressed in terms of elemental iron)**:
Severe iron deficiency anemia: 4-6 mg Fe/kg/day in 3 divided doses
Mild to moderate iron deficiency anemia: 3 mg Fe/kg/day in 1-2 divided doses
Prophylaxis: 1-2 mg Fe/kg/day up to a maximum of 15 mg/day

Adults **(dose expressed in terms of ferrous sulfate)**:
Iron deficiency: 300 mg twice daily up to 300 mg 4 times/day or 250 mg (extended release) 1-2 times/day
Prophylaxis: 300 mg/day

Mechanism of Action Replaces iron, found in hemoglobin, myoglobin, and other enzymes; allows the transportation of oxygen via hemoglobin

Local Anesthetic/Vasoconstrictor Precautions No information available to require special precautions

Effects on Dental Treatment Do not prescribe tetracyclines simultaneously with iron since GI tract absorption of both tetracycline and iron may be inhibited

Other Adverse Effects
>10%: Gastrointestinal: GI irritation, epigastric pain, nausea, dark stool, vomiting, stomach cramping, constipation
1% to 10%:
Gastrointestinal: Heartburn, diarrhea, liquid preparations may temporarily stain the teeth
Genitourinary: Discolored urine
<1%: Ocular: Contact irritation

Drug Interactions
Decreased effect: Absorption of oral preparation of iron and tetracyclines are decreased when both of these drugs are given together; concurrent administration of antacids may decrease iron absorption; iron may decrease absorption of penicillamine when given at the same time; response to iron therapy may be delayed in patients receiving chloramphenicol; milk may decrease absorption of iron
Increased effect: Concurrent administration of ≥200 mg vitamin C per 30 mg elemental Fe increases absorption of oral iron

Drug Uptake
Onset of hematologic response (essentially the same to either oral or parenteral iron salts): Red blood cell form and color changes within 3-10 days
Peak reticulocytosis: Occurs in 5-10 days, and hemoglobin values increase within 2-4 weeks
Absorption: Iron is absorbed in the duodenum and upper jejunum; in persons with normal serum iron stores, 10% of an oral dose is absorbed; this is increased to 20% to 30% in persons with inadequate iron stores. Food and achlorhydria will decrease absorption

Pregnancy Risk Factor A

Generic Available Yes

Ferrous Sulfate and Ascorbic Acid

(FER us SUL fate & a SKOR bik AS id)

Brand Names Ferancee® [OTC]; Fero-Grad 500® [OTC]; Ferromar® [OTC]

Therapeutic Category Iron Salt; Vitamin

Synonyms Ascorbic Acid and Ferrous Sulfate

Use Treatment of iron deficiency in nonpregnant adults; treatment and prevention of iron deficiency in pregnant adults

Local Anesthetic/Vasoconstrictor Precautions No information available to require special precautions

Effects on Dental Treatment Do not prescribe tetracyclines simultaneously with iron since GI tract absorption of both tetracycline and iron may be inhibited

Generic Available Yes

Ferrous Sulfate, Ascorbic Acid, and Vitamin B-Complex

(FER us SUL fate, a SKOR bik AS id, & VYE ta min bee KOM pleks)

Brand Names Iberet®-Liquid [OTC]

Therapeutic Category Iron Salt; Vitamin

Use Conditions of iron deficiency with an increased needed for B-complex vitamins and vitamin C

Local Anesthetic/Vasoconstrictor Precautions No information available to require special precautions

Effects on Dental Treatment Do not prescribe tetracyclines simultaneously with iron since GI tract absorption of both tetracycline and iron may be inhibited

Generic Available Yes

Ferrous Sulfate, Ascorbic Acid, Vitamin B-Complex, and Folic Acid

(FER us SUL fate, a SKOR bik AS id, VYE ta min bee KOM pleks, & FOE lik AS id)

Brand Names Iberet-Folic-500®

Therapeutic Category Iron Salt; Vitamin

Use Treatment of iron deficiency and prevention of concomitant folic acid deficiency where there is an associated deficient intake or increased need for B-complex vitamins

Local Anesthetic/Vasoconstrictor Precautions No information available to require special precautions

Effects on Dental Treatment Do not prescribe tetracyclines simultaneously with iron since GI tract absorption of both tetracycline and iron may be inhibited

Pregnancy Risk Factor A

Generic Available Yes

Fertinex® Injection *see* Urofollitropin *on page 978*

Feverall™ [OTC] *see* Acetaminophen *on page 20*

Feverall™ Sprinkle Caps [OTC] *see* Acetaminophen *on page 20*

Fexofenadine (feks oh FEN a deen)

Brand Names Allegra®

Therapeutic Category Antihistamine

Use Nonsedating antihistamine indicated for the relief of seasonal allergic rhinitis

Usual Dosage Children ≥12 years and Adults: Oral: 1 capsule (60 mg) twice daily

Mechanism of Action Fexofenadine is an active metabolite of terfenadine and like terfenadine it competes with histamine for H_1-receptor sites on effector cells in the gastrointestinal tract, blood vessels and respiratory tract; it appears that fexofenadine does not cross the blood brain barrier to any appreciable degree, resulting in a reduced potential for sedation

Local Anesthetic/Vasoconstrictor Precautions No information available to require special precautions

Effects on Dental Treatment No effects or complications reported

Other Adverse Effects

1% to 10%:
Central nervous system: Drowsiness (1.3%), fatigue (1.3%)
Endocrine & metabolic: Dysmenorrhea (1.5%)
Gastrointestinal: Nausea (1.5%), dyspepsia (1.3%)
Miscellaneous: Viral infection (2.5%)

Contraindications Hypersensitivity to fexofenadine or any components of its formulation

Drug Interactions Fexofenadine levels have increased with erythromycin (82% higher) and with ketoconazole (135% higher); this has not been associated with any increased incidence of side effects

In two separate studies, fexofenadine 120 mg twice daily (high doses) was coadministered with standard doses of erythromycin or ketoconazole to healthy volunteers and although fexofenadine peak plasma concentrations increased, no differences in adverse events or QTc intervals were observed. **It remains unknown if a similar interaction occurs with other azole antifungal agents (eg, itraconazole) or other macrolide antibiotics (eg, clarithromycin).**

Drug Uptake

Onset of action: 60 minutes
Duration of antihistaminic effect: At least 12 hours
Half-life: 14.4 hours
Time to peak serum concentration: ~2.6 hours after oral administration

Pregnancy Risk Factor C

Dosage Forms Capsule, as hydrochloride: 60 mg

Generic Available No

Selected Readings

Day JH, et al, "Onset of Action, Efficacy and Safety of a Single Dose of 60 mg and 120 mg Fexofenadine HCl for Ragweed Allergy Using Controlled Antigen Exposure in an Environmental Exposure Unit," *J Allergy Clin Immunol*, 1996, 97(1 Pt 3):1007.

"Fexofenadine," *Med Lett Drugs Ther*, 1996, 38(986):95-6.

Simons FE, Bergman JN, Watson WT, et al, "The Clinical Pharmacology of Fexofenadine in Children," *J Allergy Clin Immunol*, 1996, 98(6 Pt 1):1062-4.

Fiberall® Chewable Tablet [OTC] *see* Calcium Polycarbophil *on page 168*

Fiberall® Powder [OTC] *see* Psyllium *on page 822*

Fiberall® Wafer [OTC] *see* Psyllium *on page 822*

FiberCon® Tablet [OTC] *see* Calcium Polycarbophil *on page 168*

Fiber-Lax® Tablet [OTC] *see* Calcium Polycarbophil *on page 168*

Fibrinolysin and Desoxyribonuclease
(fye brin oh LYE sin & des oks i rye boe NOO klee ase)

Brand Names Elase-Chloromycetin® Topical; Elase® Topical

Therapeutic Category Enzyme, Topical Debridement

Synonyms Desoxyribonuclease and Fibrinolysin

Use Debriding agent; cervicitis; and irrigating agent in infected wounds

Local Anesthetic/Vasoconstrictor Precautions No information available to require special precautions

Effects on Dental Treatment No effects or complications reported

Pregnancy Risk Factor C

Generic Available No

Filgrastim (fil GRA stim)

Brand Names Neupogen® Injection

Therapeutic Category Colony Stimulating Factor

Synonyms G-CSF; Granulocyte Colony Stimulating Factor

Use To reduce the duration of neutropenia and the associated risk of infection in patients with nonmyeloid malignancies receiving myelosuppressive chemotherapeutic regimens associated with a significant incidence of severe neutropenia with fever; it has also been used in AIDS patients on zidovudine and in patients with noncancer chemotherapy-induced neutropenia

Usual Dosage Children and Adults: administered S.C. or I.V. as a single daily infusion over 20-30 minutes

Myelosuppressive chemotherapy 5 mcg/kg/day S.C. or I.V.

Doses may be increased in increments of 5 mcg/kg for each chemotherapy cycle, according to the duration and severity of the absolute neutrophil count (ANC) nadir. In phase III trials, efficacy was observed at doses of 4-6 mcg/kg/day. Discontinue therapy if the ANC count is >10,000/mm^3 after the ANC nadir has occurred following the expected chemotherapy-induced neutrophil nadir. Some cancer centers are stopping therapy at an ANC of 2500. Duration of therapy needed to attenuate chemotherapy-induced neutropenia may be dependent on the myelosuppressive potential of the chemotherapy regimen employed. Duration of therapy in clinical studies has ranged from 2 weeks to 3 years.

Bone marrow transplant patients

Bone marrow transplant patients: 10 mcg/kg/day as an I.V. infusion of 4 or 24 hours or as continuous 24-hour S.C. infusion. Administer first dose at least 24 hours after cytotoxic chemotherapy and at least 24 hours after bone marrow infusion.

Filgrastim Dose Based on Neutrophil Response

Absolute Neutrophil Count	Filgrastim Dose Adjustment
When ANC >1000/mm^3 for 3 consecutive days	Reduce to 5 mcg/kg/day
If ANC remains >1000/mm^3 for 3 more consecutive days	Discontinue filgrastim
If ANC decreases to <1000/mm^3	Resume at 5 mcg/kg/day

Severe chronic neutropenia:

Congenital neutropenia: 6 mcg/kg twice daily S.C.

Idiopathic/cyclic neutropenia: 5 mcg/kg/day S.C.

Chronic daily administration is required to maintain clinical benefit. Adjust dose based on the patients' clinical course as well as ANC. In phase III studies, the target ANC was 1,500-10,000/mm^3. Reduce the dose of the ANC is persistently >10,000/mm^3.

Premature discontinuation of G-CSF therapy prior to the time of recovery from the expected neutrophil is generally not recommended. A transient increase in neutrophil counts is typically seen 1-2 days after initiation of therapy.

Mechanism of Action Stimulates the production, maturation, and activation of neutrophils, G-CSF activates neutrophils to increase both their migration and

Proliferation/Differentiation	G-CSF (Filgrastim)	GM-CSF (Sargramostim)
Neutrophils	Yes	Yes
Eosinophils	No	Yes
Macrophages	No	Yes
Neutrophil migration	Enhanced	Inhibited

cytotoxicity. Natural proteins which stimulate hematopoietic stem cells to proliferate, prolong cell survival, stimulate cell differentiation, and stimulate functional activity of mature cells. CSFs are produced by a wide variety of cell types. Specific mechanisms of action are not yet fully understood, but possibly work by a second-messenger pathway with resultant protein production. See table.

Local Anesthetic/Vasoconstrictor Precautions No information available to require special precautions

Effects on Dental Treatment No effects or complications reported

Other Adverse Effects Effects are generally mild and dose related

>10%:

Central nervous system: Neutropenic fever

Dermatologic: Alopecia

Gastrointestinal: Nausea, vomiting, diarrhea, mucositis

Medullary bone pain (24% incidence): This occurs most commonly in lower back pain, posterior iliac crest, and sternum and is controlled with non-narcotic analgesics

Splenomegaly: This occurs more commonly in patients with cyclic neutropenia/congenital agranulocytosis who received S.C. injections for a prolonged (>14 days) period of time; ~33% of these patients experience subclinical splenomegaly (detected by MRI or CT scan); ~3% of these patients experience clinical splenomegaly

1% to 10%:

Cardiovascular: Chest pain

Central nervous system: Headache

Dermatologic: Rash

Endocrine & metabolic: Fluid retention

Gastrointestinal: Anorexia, stomatitis, constipation, sore throat

Hematologic: Leukocytosis

Local: Pain at injection site

Neuromuscular & skeletal: Weakness

Respiratory: Dyspnea, cough

<1%:

Cardiovascular: Transient supraventricular arrhythmia, pericarditis

Local: Thrombophlebitis

Hypersensitivity: Anaphylactic reaction

Drug Uptake

Onset of action: Rapid elevation in neutrophil counts within the first 24 hours, reaching a plateau in 3-5 days

Duration: ANC decreases by 50% within 2 days after discontinuing G-CSF; white counts return to the normal range in 4-7 days

Absorption: S.C.: 100% absorbed; peak plasma levels can be maintained for up to 12 hours

Serum half-life: 1.8-3.5 hours

Time to peak serum concentration: S.C.: Within 2-6 hours

Pregnancy Risk Factor C

Generic Available No

Comments Reimbursement hotline: 1-800-28-AMGEN

Filibon® [OTC] see Vitamins, Multiple on page 995

Finasteride (fi NAS teer ide)

Brand Names Propecia®; Proscar®

Therapeutic Category Antiandrogen; Urinary Tract Product

Use Early data indicate that finasteride is useful in the treatment of symptomatic benign prostatic hyperplasia (BPH); male pattern baldness or androgenetic alopecia

Unlabeled use: Adjuvant monotherapy after radical prostatectomy in the treatment of prostatic cancer

Usual Dosage Adults: Male:

Benign prostatic hyperplasia: Oral: 5 mg/day as a single dose; clinical responses occur within 12 weeks to 6 months of initiation of therapy; long-term administration is recommended for maximal response

Male pattern baldness: One tablet daily

Mechanism of Action Finasteride is a 4-azo analog of testosterone and is a competitive inhibitor of both tissue and hepatic 5-alpha reductase. This results in inhibition of the conversion of testosterone to dihydrotestosterone and markedly suppresses serum dihydrotestosterone levels; depending on dose and duration, serum testosterone concentrations may or may not increase. Testosterone-dependent processes such as fertility, muscle strength, potency, and libido are not affected by finasteride.

Local Anesthetic/Vasoconstrictor Precautions No information available to require special precautions

(Continued)

Finasteride *(Continued)*

Effects on Dental Treatment No effects or complications reported

Other Adverse Effects 1% to 10%:

Endocrine & metabolic: Decreased libido

Genitourinary: <4% incidence of impotence, decreased volume of ejaculate

Drug Interactions No data reported

Drug Uptake

Onset of clinical effect: Within 12 weeks to 6 months of ongoing therapy

Duration of action:

After a single oral dose as small as 0.5 mg: 65% depression of plasma dihydro-testosterone levels persists 5-7 days

After 6 months of treatment with 5 mg/day: Circulating dihydrotestosterone levels are reduced to castrate levels without significant effects on circulating testosterone; levels return to normal within 14 days of discontinuation of treatment

Absorption: Oral: Extent may be reduced if administered with food

Time to peak serum concentration: Oral: 2-6 hours

Serum half-life, serum: Parent drug: ~5-17 hours (mean: 1.9 fasting, 4.2 with breakfast)

Serum half-life:

Elderly: 8 hours

Adults: 6 hours (3-16)

Pregnancy Risk Factor X

Generic Available No

Fiorgen PF® *see* Butalbital Compound *on page 154*

Fiorgen PF® *see* Butalbital Compound and Aspirin *on page 156*

Fioricet® *see* Butalbital Compound *on page 154*

Fioricet® *see* Butalbital Compound and Acetaminophen *on page 155*

Fiorinal® *see* Butalbital Compound *on page 154*

Fiorinal® *see* Butalbital Compound and Aspirin *on page 156*

Fiorinal® With Codeine *see* Butalbital Compound and Codeine *on page 156*

Flagyl® *see* Metronidazole *on page 631*

Flarex® *see* Fluorometholone *on page 417*

Flatulex® [OTC] *see* Simethicone *on page 865*

Flavorcee® [OTC] *see* Ascorbic Acid *on page 88*

Flavoxate (fla VOKS ate)

Brand Names Urispas®

Therapeutic Category Antispasmodic Agent, Urinary

Use Antispasmodic used to provide symptomatic relief of dysuria, nocturia, supra-pubic pain, urgency, and incontinence

Usual Dosage Children >12 years and Adults: Oral: 100-200 mg 3-4 times/day; reduce the dose when symptoms improve

Mechanism of Action Synthetic antispasmotic with similar actions to that of propantheline; it exerts a direct relaxant effect on smooth muscles via phosphodi-esterase inhibition, providing relief to a variety of smooth muscle spasms; it is especially useful for the treatment of bladder spasticity, whereby it produces an increase in urinary capacity

Local Anesthetic/Vasoconstrictor Precautions No information available to require special precautions

Effects on Dental Treatment >10% of patients experience dry mouth

Other Adverse Effects

>10%:

Central nervous system: Drowsiness

Respiratory: Dry throat

1% to 10%:

Cardiovascular: Tachycardia, palpitations

Central nervous system: Nervousness, fatigue, vertigo, headache, drowsiness, fever

Gastrointestinal: Constipation, nausea, vomiting

<1%:

Central nervous system: Confusion (especially in the elderly)

Dermatologic: Skin rash

Hematologic: Leukopenia

Ocular: Increased intraocular pressure

Drug Interactions No data reported

Drug Uptake

Onset of action: 55-60 minutes

Pregnancy Risk Factor B

Generic Available No

Flecainida, Acetato De (Mexico) *see Flecainide on this page*

Flecainide (fle KAY nide)
Related Information
Cardiovascular Diseases *on page 1010*
Brand Names Tambocor™
Therapeutic Category Antiarrhythmic Agent, Class I-C; Antiarrhythmic Agent (Supraventricular & Ventricular)
Synonyms Flecainida, Acetato De (Mexico)
Use Prevention and suppression of documented life-threatening ventricular arrhythmias (ie, sustained ventricular tachycardia); controlling symptomatic, disabling supraventricular tachycardias in patients without structural heart disease in whom other agents fail
Usual Dosage Oral:
Children:
Initial: 3 mg/kg/day or 50-100 mg/m²/day in 3 divided doses
Usual: 3-6 mg/kg/day or 100-150 mg/m²/day in 3 divided doses; up to 11 mg/kg/day or 200 mg/m²/day for uncontrolled patients with subtherapeutic levels
Adults:
Life-threatening ventricular arrhythmias:
Initial: 100 mg every 12 hours
Increase by 50-100 mg/day (given in 2 doses/day) every 4 days; maximum: 400 mg/day
For patients receiving 400 mg/day who are not controlled and have trough concentrations <0.6 µg/mL, dosage may be increased to 600 mg/day
Prevention of paroxysmal supraventricular arrhythmias in patients with disabling symptoms but no structural heart disease:
Initial: 50 mg every 12 hours
Increase by 50 mg twice daily at 4-day intervals; maximum: 300 mg/day
Mechanism of Action Class IC antiarrhythmic; slows conduction in cardiac tissue by altering transport of ions across cell membranes; causes slight prolongation of refractory periods; decreases the rate of rise of the action potential without affecting its duration; increases electrical stimulation threshold of ventricle, HIS-Purkinje system; possesses local anesthetic and moderate negative inotropic effects
Local Anesthetic/Vasoconstrictor Precautions No information available to require special precautions
Effects on Dental Treatment No effects or complications reported
Other Adverse Effects
>10%:
Central nervous system: Dizziness
Ocular: Visual disturbances
Respiratory: Dyspnea
1% to 10%:
Cardiovascular: Palpitations, chest pain, edema, tachycardia
Central nervous system: Headache, fatigue, fever
Dermatologic: Rash
Gastrointestinal: Nausea, constipation, abdominal pain
Neuromuscular & skeletal: Tremor, weakness
<1%:
Cardiovascular: Bradycardia, heart block, elevated P-R, QRS duration, worsening ventricular arrhythmias, congestive heart failure
Central nervous system: Nervousness, hypoesthesia
Dermatologic: Alopecia
Hematologic: Blood dyscrasias
Hepatic: Possible hepatic dysfunction
Neuromuscular & skeletal: Paresthesia
Drug Interactions
Increased toxicity:
Alkalinizing agents (high dose antacids, cimetidine, carbonic anhydrase inhibitors or sodium bicarbonate) may decrease flecainide clearance
Beta-adrenergic blockers, disopyramide, verapamil (possible additive negative inotropic effects)
Digoxin, amiodarone (increased plasma concentrations)
Decreased toxicity: Smoking and acid urine (increases flecainide clearance)
Drug Uptake
Absorption: Oral: Rapid
Serum half-life:
Children: 8 hours
Adults: 7-22 hours, increased with congestive heart failure or renal dysfunction
End stage renal disease: 19-26 hours
(Continued)

Flecainide *(Continued)*

Time to peak serum concentration: Within 1.5-3 hours
Pregnancy Risk Factor C
Generic Available No

Fleet® Babylax® Rectal [OTC] *see Glycerin on page 446*
Fleet® Enema [OTC] *see Sodium Phosphates on page 874*
Fleet® Flavored Castor Oil [OTC] *see Castor Oil on page 184*
Fleet® Laxative [OTC] *see Bisacodyl on page 131*
Fleet® Pain Relief [OTC] *see Pramoxine on page 784*
Fleet® Phospho®-Soda [OTC] *see Sodium Phosphates on page 874*
Flexaphen® *see Chlorzoxazone on page 228*
Flexeril® *see Cyclobenzaprine on page 268*
Flolan® Injection *see Epoprostenol on page 357*
Flomax™ *see Tamsulosin on page 904*
Flonase® *see Fluticasone on page 424*
Florical® [OTC] *see Calcium Carbonate on page 162*
Florinef® Acetate *see Fludrocortisone Acetate on page 411*
Florone® *see Diflorasone on page 311*
Florone® E *see Diflorasone on page 311*
Floropryl® *see Isoflurophate on page 522*
Florvite® *see Vitamins, Multiple on page 995*
Flovent® *see Fluticasone on page 424*
Floxin® Oral *see Ofloxacin on page 697*
Floxin® Otic *see Ofloxacin on page 697*

Floxuridine *(floks YOOR i deen)*

Brand Names FUDR®
Therapeutic Category Antineoplastic Agent, Antimetabolite
Synonyms Fluorodeoxyuridine
Use Palliative management of carcinomas of head, neck, and brain as well as liver, gallbladder, and bile ducts
Usual Dosage Adults (refer to individual protocols):
Intra-arterial: Primarily by an implantable pump: 0.1-0.6 mg/kg/day continuous intra-arterial administration for 14 days then heparinized saline is given for 14 days; toxicity requires dose reduction
I.V.: 0.5-1 mg/kg/day for 6-15 days
Mechanism of Action Mechanism of action and pharmacokinetics are very similar to 5-FU; FUDR® is the deoxyribonucleotide of 5-FU. Inhibits DNA and RNA synthesis via formation of carbonium ions; cross-links strands of DNA, causing an imbalance of growth and cell death
Local Anesthetic/Vasoconstrictor Precautions No information available to require special
Effects on Dental Treatment No effects or complications reported
Other Adverse Effects
>10%: Gastrointestinal: GI hemorrhage, stomatitis, esophagopharyngitis, diarrhea, gastritis
1% to 10%:
Gastrointestinal: Anorexia, glossitis
Dermatologic: Alopecia, dermatitis, rash
<1%:
Cardiovascular: Myocardial ischemia, angina
Central nervous system: Lethargy, acute cerebellar syndrome, confusion, euphoria, fever
Hematologic: Severe hematologic toxicity, leukopenia, thrombocytopenia, pancytopenia, agranulocytosis
Neuromuscular & skeletal: Weakness
Ocular: Photophobia
Miscellaneous: Anaphylaxis
Pregnancy Risk Factor D
Generic Available No

Fluconazole *(floo KOE na zole)*

Related Information
Oral Fungal Infections *on page 1063*
Brand Names Diflucan®
Canadian/Mexican Brand Names Oxifungol® (Mexico); Zonal® (Mexico)
Therapeutic Category Antifungal Agent, Systemic

Use Oral fluconazole should be used in persons able to tolerate oral medications; parenteral fluconazole should be reserved for patients who are both unable to take oral medications and are unable to tolerate amphotericin B (eg, due to hypersensitivity or renal insufficiency)

Dental: Treatment of susceptible fungal infections in the oral cavity including candidiasis, oral thrush, and chronic mucocutaneous candidiasis; treatment of esophageal and oropharyngeal candidiasis caused by *Candida* species; treatment of severe, chronic mucocutaneous candidiasis caused by *Candida* species

Medical: Vaginal candidiasis unresponsive to nystatin or clotrimazole; treatment of hepatosplenic candidiasis; treatment of other *Candida* infections in persons unable to tolerate amphotericin B; treatment of cryptococcal infections; secondary prophylaxis for cryptococcal meningitis in persons with AIDS; antifungal prophylaxis in allogeneic bone marrow transplant recipients

Usual Dosage The daily dose of fluconazole is the same for oral and I.V. administration

Children: Efficacy of fluconazole has not been established in children; a small number of patients from 3-13 years of age have been treated with fluconazole using doses of 3-6 mg/kg/day once daily. Doses as high as 12 mg/kg/day once daily have been used to treat candidiasis in immunocompromised children; 10-12 mg/kg/day has been used prophylactically against fungal infections in pediatric bone marrow transplant patients.

Adults: Oral, I.V.: See table for once daily dosing.

Indication	Day 1	Daily Therapy	Minimum Duration of Therapy
Oropharyngeal candidiasis	200 mg	100 mg	14 d
Esophageal candidiasis	200 mg	100 mg	21 d
Systemic candidiasis	400 mg	200 mg	28 d
Cryptococcal meningitis			10-12 wk after CSF culture becomes negative
acute	400 mg	200 mg	
relapse	200 mg	200 mg	

Mechanism of Action Interferes with cytochrome P-450 activity, decreasing ergosterol synthesis (principal sterol in fungal cell membrane) and inhibiting cell membrane formation

Local Anesthetic/Vasoconstrictor Precautions No information available to require special precautions

Effects on Dental Treatment No effects or complications reported

Other Adverse Effects 1% to 10%:
Central nervous system: Headache
Dermatologic: Skin rash
Gastrointestinal: Nausea, vomiting, abdominal pain, diarrhea

Contraindications Known hypersensitivity to fluconazole or other azoles

Warnings/Precautions Should be used with caution in patients with renal and hepatic dysfunction or previous hepatotoxicity from other azole derivatives. Patients who develop abnormal liver function tests during fluconazole therapy should be monitored closely and discontinued if symptoms consistent with liver disease develop.

Drug Interactions Cytochrome P-450 IIIA4 enzyme inhibitor and cytochrome P-450 IIC enzyme inhibitor
Rifampin decreases concentrations of fluconazole; fluconazole may increase cyclosporine levels when high doses used; may increase phenytoin serum concentration; fluconazole may also inhibit warfarin metabolism

Drug Uptake
Absorption: >90%
Serum half-life: 25-30 hours with normal renal function
Time to peak serum concentration: Oral: Within 2-4 hours

Pregnancy Risk Factor C

Breast-feeding Considerations Probably safe (not absorbed orally)

Dosage Forms
Injection: 2 mg/mL (100 mL, 200 mL)
Powder for oral suspension: 10 mg/mL (35 mL); 40 mg/mL (35 mL)
Tablet: 50 mg, 100 mg, 150 mg, 200 mg

Dietary Considerations No data reported

Generic Available No

Flucytosine (floo SYE toe seen)
Brand Names Ancobon®
Canadian/Mexican Brand Names Ancotil® (Canada)
(Continued)

Flucytosine (Continued)

Therapeutic Category Antifungal Agent, Systemic

Synonyms 5-Flurocytosine

Use Adjunctive treatment of susceptible fungal infections (usually *Candida* or *Cryptococcus*); in combination with amphotericin B, fluconazole, or itraconazole; synergy with amphotericin B for fungal infections (*Aspergillus*)

Usual Dosage Children and Adults: Oral: 50-150 mg/kg/day in divided doses every 6 hours

Mechanism of Action Penetrates fungal cells and is converted to fluorouracil which competes with uracil interfering with fungal RNA and protein synthesis

Local Anesthetic/Vasoconstrictor Precautions No information available to require special precautions

Effects on Dental Treatment No effects or complications reported

Other Adverse Effects

1% to 10%:
  Dermatologic: Skin rash
  Gastrointestinal: Abdominal pain, diarrhea, loss of appetite, nausea, vomiting
  Hematologic: Anemia, leukopenia, thrombocytopenia
  Hepatic: Hepatitis, jaundice

<1%:
  Cardiovascular: Cardiac arrest
  Central nervous system: Confusion, hallucinations, dizziness, drowsiness, headache, parkinsonism, psychosis, ataxia
  Dermatologic: Photosensitivity
  Endocrine & metabolic: Temporary growth failure, hypoglycemia, hypokalemia
  Hematologic: Bone marrow suppression
  Hepatic: Elevated liver enzymes
  Neuromuscular & skeletal: Paresthesia
  Otic: Hearing loss
  Respiratory: Respiratory arrest

Drug Interactions Increased effect/toxicity (enterocolitis) with concurrent amphotericin administration

Drug Uptake
  Absorption: Oral: 75% to 90%
  Serum half-life: 3-8 hours
    Anuria: May be as long as 200 hours
    End stage renal disease: 75-200 hours
  Time to peak serum concentration: Within 2-6 hours

Pregnancy Risk Factor C

Generic Available No

Fludara® *see* Fludarabine *on this page*

Fludarabine (floo DARE a been)

Brand Names Fludara®

Therapeutic Category Antineoplastic Agent, Antimetabolite

Use Treatment of B-cell chronic lymphocytic leukemia unresponsive to previous therapy with an alkylating agent containing regimen. Fludarabine has been tested in patients with refractory acute lymphocytic leukemia and acute nonlymphocytic leukemia, but required a highly toxic dose to achieve response.

Usual Dosage I.V.:

Children:
  Acute leukemia: 10 mg/m² bolus over 15 minutes followed by continuous infusion of 30.5 mg/m²/day over 5 days **or**
  10.5 mg/m² bolus over 15 minutes followed by 30.5 mg/m²/day over 48 hours followed by cytarabine has been used in clinical trials
  Solid tumors: 9 mg/m² bolus followed by 27 mg/m²/day continuous infusion over 5 days

Adults:
  Chronic lymphocytic leukemia: 20-25 mg/m²/day over a 30-minute period for 5 days; 5-day courses are repeated every 28-35 days days
  Non-Hodgkin's lymphoma: Loading dose: 20 mg/m² followed by 30 mg/m²/day for 48 hours

Mechanism of Action Fludarabine is analogous to that of Ara-C and Ara-A. Following systemic administration, FAMP is rapidly dephosphorylated to 2-fluoro-Ara-A. 2-Fluoro-Ara-A enters the cell by a carrier-mediated transport process, then is phosphorylated intracellularly by deoxycytidine kinase to form the active metabolite 2-fluoro-Ara-ATP. 2-Fluoro-Ara-ATP inhibits DNA synthesis by inhibition of DNA polymerase and ribonucleotide reductase.

Local Anesthetic/Vasoconstrictor Precautions No information available to require special precautions

Effects on Dental Treatment No effects or complications reported
Other Adverse Effects
>10%:
Cardiovascular: Edema
Central nervous system: Fever, chills, fatigue, pain
Dermatologic: Rash
Gastrointestinal: Mild nausea, vomiting, diarrhea, stomatitis, GI bleeding
Genitourinary: Urinary infection
Hematologic: Myelosuppression: Dose-limiting toxicity; myelosuppression may
not be related to cumulative dose; Granulocyte nadir: 13 days (3-25); Platelet
nadir: 16 days (2-32); WBC nadir: 8 days; Recovery: 5-7 weeks
Neuromuscular & skeletal: Paresthesia, myalgia, weakness
Respiratory: Manifested as dyspnea and a nonproductive cough; lung biopsy
has shown pneumonitis in some patients, pneumonia
Miscellaneous: Infection
1% to 10%:
Cardiovascular: Congestive heart failure
Central nervous system: Malaise, headache
Dermatologic: Alopecia
Endocrine & metabolic: Hyperglycemia
Gastrointestinal: Anorexia
Otic: Hearing loss
<1%:
Central nervous system: Reported with higher dose levels; most patients
shown to have CNS demyelination; somnolence also noted; severe neuro-
toxicity
Endocrine & metabolic: Metabolic acidosis
Gastrointestinal: Metallic taste
Hepatic: Reversible hepatotoxicity
Renal: Renal failure, hematuria, elevated serum creatinine
Respiratory: Interstitial pneumonitis
Miscellaneous: Tumor lysis syndrome
Drug Uptake
Absorption: Oral preparation is under study
Serum half-life, elimination: 2-fluoro-vidarabine: 9 hours
Pregnancy Risk Factor D
Generic Available No

Fludrocortisone Acetate (floo droe KOR ti sone AS e tate)
Brand Names Florinef® Acetate
Therapeutic Category Mineralocorticoid
Use Partial replacement therapy for primary and secondary adrenocortical insuffi-
ciency in Addison's disease; treatment of salt-losing adrenogenital syndrome
Usual Dosage Adults: Oral: 0.1-0.2 mg/day with ranges of 0.1 mg 3 times/week
to 0.2 mg/day
Mechanism of Action Promotes increased reabsorption of sodium and loss of
potassium from renal distal tubules
Local Anesthetic/Vasoconstrictor Precautions No information available to
require special precautions
Effects on Dental Treatment No effects or complications reported
Other Adverse Effects 1% to 10%:
Cardiovascular: Hypertension, edema, congestive heart failure
Central nervous system: Convulsions, headache, dizziness
Dermatologic: Acne, rash, bruising
Endocrine & metabolic: Hypokalemic alkalosis, suppression of growth, hypergly-
cemia, HPA suppression
Gastrointestinal: Peptic ulcer
Neuromuscular & skeletal: Muscle weakness
Ocular: Cataracts
Miscellaneous: Sweating
Drug Interactions
Decreased corticosteroid effects by rifampin, barbiturates, and hydantoins
Drug Uptake
Absorption: Rapid and complete from GI tract, partially absorbed through skin
Serum half-life:
Plasma: 30-35 minutes
Biological: 18-36 hours
Time to peak serum concentration: Within 1.7 hours
Pregnancy Risk Factor C
Generic Available No

Flufenacina (Mexico) see Fluphenazine on page 420

Flumadine® *see Rimantadine on page 845*

Flumazenil (FLO may ze nil)
Brand Names Romazicon™
Canadian/Mexican Brand Names Anexate® (Canada); Lanexat® (Mexico)
Therapeutic Category Antidote, Benzodiazepine
Use Benzodiazepine antagonist - reverses sedative effects of benzodiazepines used in general anesthesia; for management of benzodiazepine overdose; flumazenil does **not** antagonize the CNS effects of other GABA agonists (such as ethanol, barbiturates, or general anesthetics), **does not** reverse narcotics
Usual Dosage See table.

Flumazenil

Pediatric Dosage	
Further studies are needed	
Pediatric dosage for **reversal of conscious sedation:** Intravenously through a freely running intravenous infusion into a large vein to minimize pain at the injection site	
Initial dose	0.01 mg/kg over 15 seconds (maximum dose of 0.2 mg)
Repeat doses	0.005-0.01 mg/kg (maximum dose of 0.2 mg) repeated at 1-minute intervals
Maximum total cumulative dose	1 mg
Pediatric dosage for **management of benzodiazepine overdose** Intravenously through a freely running intravenous infusion into a large vein to minimize pain at the injection site	
Initial dose	0.01 mg/kg (maximum dose: 0.2 mg)
Repeat doses	0.01 mg/kg (maximum dose of 0.2 mg) repeated at 1-minute intervals
Maximum total cumulative dose	1 mg
In place of repeat bolus doses, follow-up continuous infusions of 0.005-0.01 mg/kg/hour have been used; further studies are needed	
Adult Dosage	
Adult dosage for **reversal of conscious sedation:** Intravenously through a freely running intravenous infusion into a large vein to minimize pain at the injection site	
Initial dose	0.2 mg intravenously over 15 seconds
Repeat doses	If desired level of consciousness is not obtained, 0.2 mg may be repeated at 1-minute intervals
Maximum total cumulative dose	1 mg (usual dose 0.6-1 mg) **In the event of resedation:** repeat doses may be given at 20-minute intervals with maximum of 1 mg/dose and 3 mg/hour
Adult dosage for **suspected benzodiazepine overdose:** Intravenously through a freely running intravenous infusion into a large vein to minimize pain at the injection site	
Initial dose	0.2 mg intravenously over 30 seconds
Repeat doses	0.5 mg over 30 seconds repeated at 1-minute intervals
Maximum total cumulative dose	3 mg (usual dose 1-3 mg) Patients with a partial response at 3 mg may require additional titration up to a total dose of 5 mg. If a patient has not responded 5 minutes after cumulative dose of 5 mg, the major cause of sedation is not likely due to benzodiazepines. **In the event of resedation:** may repeat doses at 20-minute intervals with maximum of 1 mg/dose and 3 mg/hour

Resedation: Repeated doses may be given at 20-minute intervals as needed; repeat treatment doses of 1 mg (at a rate of 0.5 mg/minute) should be given at any time and no more than 3 mg should be given in any hour. After intoxication with high doses of benzodiazepines, the duration of a single dose of flumazenil is not expected to exceed 1 hour; if desired, the period of wakefulness may be prolonged with repeated low intravenous doses of flumazenil, or by an infusion of 0.1-0.4 mg/hour. Most patients with benzodiazepine overdose will respond to a cumulative dose of 1-3 mg and doses >3 mg do not reliably produce additional effects. Rarely, patients with a partial response at 3 mg may require additional titration up to a total dose of 5 mg. **If a patient has not responded 5 minutes after receiving a cumulative dose of 5 mg, the major cause of sedation is not likely to be due to benzodiazepines.**

Mechanism of Action Antagonizes the effect of benzodiazepines on the GABA/benzodiazepine receptor complex. Flumazenil is benzodiazepine specific and does not antagonize other nonbenzodiazepine GABA agonists (including ethanol, barbiturates, general anesthetics); flumazenil does not reverse the effects of opiates

Local Anesthetic/Vasoconstrictor Precautions No information available to require special precautions

Effects on Dental Treatment No effects or complications reported

Other Adverse Effects
>10%:
Central nervous system: Dizziness
Gastrointestinal: Vomiting, nausea
1% to 10%:
Central nervous system: Headache, malaise, anxiety, nervousness, insomnia, abnormal crying, euphoria, depression
Endocrine & metabolic: Hot flashes
Gastrointestinal: Dry mouth
Local: Pain at injection site
Neuromuscular & skeletal: Tremor, weakness
Respiratory: Dyspnea, hyperventilation
Miscellaneous: Increased sweating disorders
<1%:
Cardiovascular: Bradycardia, tachycardia, chest pain, hypertension, ventricular extrasystoles, altered blood pressure (increases and decreases)
Central nervous system: Anxiety and sensation of coldness, generalized convulsions, withdrawal syndrome, shivering, somnolence
Otic: Abnormal hearing
Miscellaneous: Thick tongue, hiccups

Drug Interactions Increased toxicity:
Use with caution in overdosage involving mixed drug overdose
Toxic effects may emerge (especially with cyclic antidepressants) with the reversal of the benzodiazepine effect by flumazenil

Drug Uptake
Onset of action: 1-3 minutes; 80% response within 3 minutes
Peak effect: 6-10 minutes
Duration: Resedation occurs usually within 1 hour; duration is related to dose given and benzodiazepine plasma concentrations; reversal effects of flumazenil may wear off before effects of benzodiazepine
Serum half-life, adults:
Alpha: 7-15 minutes
Terminal: 41-79 minutes

Pregnancy Risk Factor C
Dosage Forms Injection: 0.1 mg/mL (5 mL, 10 mL)
Generic Available No

Flunisolide (floo NIS oh lide)
Related Information
Respiratory Diseases *on page 1018*
Brand Names AeroBid®-M Oral Aerosol Inhaler; AeroBid® Oral Aerosol Inhaler; Nasalide® Nasal Aerosol; Nasarel® Nasal Spray
Canadian/Mexican Brand Names Bronalide® (Canada); Rhinalar® (Canada); Rhinaris-F® (Canada); Syn-Flunisolide® (Canada)
Therapeutic Category Anti-inflammatory Agent; Corticosteroid, Inhalant
Use Steroid-dependent asthma; nasal solution is used for seasonal or perennial rhinitis
Usual Dosage
Children >6 years:
Oral inhalation: 2 inhalations twice daily (morning and evening) up to 4 inhalations/day
Nasal: 1 spray each nostril twice daily (morning and evening), not to exceed 4 sprays/day each nostril
Adults:
Oral inhalation: 2 inhalations twice daily (morning and evening) up to 8 inhalations/day maximum
Nasal: 2 sprays each nostril twice daily (morning and evening); maximum dose: 8 sprays/day in each nostril
(Continued)

Flunisolide *(Continued)*

Mechanism of Action Decreases inflammation by suppression of migration of polymorphonuclear leukocytes and reversal of increased capillary permeability; does not depress hypothalamus

Local Anesthetic/Vasoconstrictor Precautions No information available to require special precautions

Effects on Dental Treatment No effects or complications reported

Other Adverse Effects
>10%:
  Cardiovascular: Pounding heartbeat
  Central nervous system: Dizziness, headache, nervousness
  Dermatologic: Itching, skin rash
  Endocrine & metabolic: Adrenal suppression, menstrual problems
  Gastrointestinal: GI irritation, anorexia
  Local: Nasal burning, nasal congestion, nasal dryness, sore throat, bitter taste, *Candida* infections of the nose or pharynx, atrophic rhinitis
  Respiratory: Sneezing, coughing, upper respiratory tract infection, bronchitis
  Miscellaneous: Increased susceptibility to infections
1% to 10%:
  Central nervous system: Insomnia, psychic changes
  Dermatologic: Acne, urticaria
  Gastrointestinal: Increase in appetite, dry mouth/throat, ageusia
  Ocular: Cataracts
  Respiratory: Epistaxis,
  Miscellaneous: Sweating, loss of smell
<1%:
  Gastrointestinal: Abdominal fullness
  Respiratory: Bronchospasm, dyspnea

Drug Interactions No data reported

Drug Uptake
  Absorption: Nasal inhalation: ~50%
  Serum half-life: 1.8 hours

Pregnancy Risk Factor C

Generic Available No

Fluocinolona, Acetonido De (Mexico) *see* Fluocinolone *on this page*

Fluocinolone (floo oh SIN oh lone)

Related Information
  Corticosteroids, Topical Comparison *on page 1140*

Brand Names Derma-Smoothe/FS®; Fluonid®; Flurosyn®; FS Shampoo®; Synalar®; Synalar-HP®; Synemol®

Canadian/Mexican Brand Names Cremisona® (Mexico); Lidemol® (Canada); Synalar® Simple (Mexico)

Therapeutic Category Corticosteroid, Topical (Medium Potency)

Synonyms Fluocinolona, Acetonido De (Mexico)

Use Relief of susceptible inflammatory dermatosis [low, medium, high potency topical corticosteroid]

Usual Dosage Children and Adults: Topical: Apply a thin layer to affected area 2-4 times/day

Mechanism of Action A synthetic corticosteroid which differs structurally from triamcinolone acetonide in the presence of an additional fluorine atom in the 6-alpha position on the steroid nucleus. The mechanism of action for all topical corticosteroids is not well defined, however, is believed to be a combination of three important properties: anti-inflammatory activity, immunosuppressive properties, and antiproliferative actions.

Local Anesthetic/Vasoconstrictor Precautions No information available to require special precautions

Effects on Dental Treatment No effects or complications reported

Other Adverse Effects <1%:
  Dermatologic: Acne, hypopigmentation, allergic dermatitis, maceration of the skin, skin atrophy, folliculitis, hypertrichosis
  Endocrine & metabolic: HPA suppression, Cushing's syndrome, growth retardation
  Local: Burning, itching, irritation, dryness
  Miscellaneous: Secondary infection

Drug Interactions No data reported

Drug Uptake
  Absorption: Dependent on strength of preparation, amount applied, and nature of skin at application site; ranges from ~1% in thick stratum corneum areas (palms, soles, elbows, etc) to 36% in areas of thinnest stratum corneum (face,

eyelids, etc); increased absorption in areas of skin damage, inflammation, or occlusion

Pregnancy Risk Factor C
Generic Available Yes

Fluocinonide (floo oh SIN oh nide)

Related Information
Corticosteroids, Topical Comparison *on page 1140*
Oral Nonviral Soft Tissue Ulcerations or Erosions *on page 1070*
Brand Names Lidex®; Lidex-E®
Canadian/Mexican Brand Names Gelisyn® (Mexico); Lyderm® (Canada); Topactin® (Canada); Topsyn® (Canada)
Therapeutic Category Corticosteroid, Topical (High Potency)
Synonyms Fluocinonido (Mexico)
Use Anti-inflammatory, antipruritic, relief of inflammatory and pruritic manifestations [high potency topical corticosteroid]
Usual Dosage Children and Adults: Topical: Apply thin layer to affected area 2-4 times/day depending on the severity of the condition
Mechanism of Action Not well defined for all topical corticosteroids; however, is felt to be a combination of three important properties: anti-inflammatory activity, immunosuppressive properties, and antiproliferative actions
Local Anesthetic/Vasoconstrictor Precautions No information available to require special precautions
Effects on Dental Treatment No effects or complications reported
Other Adverse Effects <1%:
Central nervous system: Intracranial hypertension
Dermatologic: Acne, hypopigmentation, allergic dermatitis, maceration of the skin, skin atrophy
Endocrine & metabolic: HPA suppression, Cushing's syndrome, growth retardation
Local: Burning, itching, irritation, dryness, folliculitis, hypertrichosis
Miscellaneous: Secondary infection
Drug Interactions No data reported
Drug Uptake
Absorption: Dependent on amount applied and nature of skin at application site; ranges from ~1% in areas of thick stratum corneum (palms, soles, elbows, etc) to 36% in areas of thin stratum corneum (face, eyelids, etc); absorption is increased in areas of skin damage, inflammation, or occlusion
Pregnancy Risk Factor C
Dosage Forms
Cream: 0.05% (15 g, 30 g, 60 g, 120 g)
Anhydrous, emollient (Lidex®): 0.05% (15 g, 30 g, 60 g, 120 g)
Aqueous, emollient (Lidex-E®): 0.05% (15 g, 30 g, 60 g, 120 g)
Gel, topical: 0.05% (15 g, 60 g)
Lidex®: 0.05% (15 g, 30 g, 60 g, 120 g)
Ointment, topical: 0.05% (15 g, 30 g, 60 g)
Lidex®: 0.05% (15 g, 30 g, 60 g, 120 g)
Solution, topical: 0.05% (20 mL, 60 mL)
Lidex®: 0.05% (20 mL, 60 mL)
Generic Available Yes

Fluocinonido (Mexico) *see* Fluocinonide *on this page*

Fluogen® *see* Influenza Virus Vaccine *on page 507*

Fluonid® *see* Fluocinolone *on previous page*

Fluoracaine® Ophthalmic *see* Proparacaine and Fluorescein *on page 808*

Fluor-A-Day® *see* Fluoride *on this page*

Fluoride (FLOR ide)

Related Information
Dentin Hypersensitivity; High Caries Index; Xerostomia *on page 1074*
Patients Undergoing Cancer Therapy *on page 1083*
Brand Names ACT® [OTC]; Duraflor® Cavity Varnish; Fluor-A-Day®; Fluorigard® [OTC]; Fluorinse®; Fluoritab®; Flura-Drops®; Flura-Loz®; Gel-Kam®; Gel-Tin® [OTC]; Karidium®; Karigel®; Karigel®-N; Listermint® with Fluoride [OTC]; Luride®; Luride® Lozi-Tab®; Luride®-SF Lozi-Tab®; Minute-Gel®; Pediaflor®; Pharmaflur®; Phos-Flur®; Point-Two®; PreviDent®; Stop® [OTC]; Thera-Flur®; Thera-Flur-N®
Therapeutic Category Fluoride; Mineral, Oral; Mineral, Oral Topical
Synonyms Acidulated Phosphate Fluoride; Sodium Fluoride; Stannous Fluoride
Use
Dental: Prevention of dental caries
(Continued)

Fluoride *(Continued)*

Usual Dosage Oral:
Recommended daily fluoride supplement (2.2 mg of sodium fluoride is equivalent to 1 mg of fluoride ion): See table.

Fluoride Ion

Fluoride Content of Drinking Water	Daily Dose, Oral (mg)
<0.3 ppm	
Birth - 6 mo	None
6 mo - 3 y	0.25
3-6 y	0.5
6 y	1.0
0.3-0.7 ppm	
Birth - 6 mo	0
6 mo - 3 y	0.125
3-6 y	0.25
6 y	0.5

Dental rinse or gel:
Adults: 10 mL rinse or apply to teeth and spit daily after brushing
Children 6-12 years: 5-10 mL rinse or apply to teeth and spit daily after brushing

Mechanism of Action Promotes remineralization of decalcified enamel; inhibits the cariogenic microbial process in dental plaque; increases tooth resistance to acid dissolution

Local Anesthetic/Vasoconstrictor Precautions No information available to require special precautions

Effects on Dental Treatment No effects or complications reported

Other Adverse Effects <1%:
Dermatologic: Rash
Gastrointestinal: Nausea, vomiting, products containing stannous fluoride may stain the teeth

Contraindications Hypersensitivity to fluoride or any component, or when fluoride content of drinking water exceeds 0.7 ppm

Warnings/Precautions Prolonged ingestion with excessive doses may result in dental fluorosis and osseous changes; do **not** exceed recommended dosage; some products contain tartrazine

Drug Interactions Decreased effect/absorption with magnesium-, aluminum-, and calcium-containing products

Drug Uptake
Absorption: Rapid and complete from GI tract; calcium, iron, or magnesium may delay absorption
Time to peak serum concentration: 30-60 minutes

Pregnancy Risk Factor C

Breast-feeding Considerations No data reported

Dosage Forms Fluoride ion content listed in brackets
Drops, oral, as sodium:
Fluoritab®, Flura-Drops®: 0.55 mg/drop [0.25 mg/drop] (22.8 mL, 24 mL)
Karidium®, Luride®: 0.275 mg/drop [0.125 mg/drop] (30 mL, 60 mL)
Pediaflor®: 1.1 mg/mL [0.5 mg/mL] (50 mL)
Gel, topical:
Acidulated phosphate fluoride (Minute-Gel®): 1.23% (480 mL)
Sodium fluoride (Karigel®, Karigel®-N, PreviDent®): 1.1% [0.5%] (24 g, 30 g, 60 g, 120 g, 130 g, 250 g)
Stannous fluoride (Gel-Kam®, Gel-Tin®, Stop®): 0.4% [0.1%] (60 g, 65 g, 105 g, 120 g)
Lozenge, as sodium (Flura-Loz®) (raspberry flavor): 2.2 mg [1 mg]
Rinse, topical, as sodium:
ACT®, Fluorigard®: 0.05% [0.02%] (90 mL, 180 mL, 300 mL, 360 mL, 480 mL)
Fluorinse®, Point-Two®: 0.2% [0.09%] (240 mL, 480 mL, 3780 mL)
Listermint® with Fluoride: 0.02% [0.01%] (180 mL, 300 mL, 360 mL, 480 mL, 540 mL, 720 mL, 960 mL, 1740 mL)
Solution, oral, as sodium (Phos-Flur®): 0.44 mg/mL [0.2 mg/mL] (250 mL, 500 mL, 3780 mL)
Tablet, as sodium:
Chewable:
Fluor-A-Day®: 0.55 mg [0.25 mg]

Fluor-A-Day®, Fluoritab®, Luride Lozi-Tab®, Pharmaflur®: 1.1 mg [0.5 mg]
Fluor-A-Day®, Fluoritab®, Karidium®, Luride® Lozi-Tab®, Luride®-SF Lozi-Tab®, Pharmaflur®: 2.2 mg [1 mg]
Oral: Flura®, Karidium®: 2.2 mg [1 mg]
Varnish (Duraflor®): 5% [50 mg/mL] (10 mL)

Dietary Considerations Do not administer with milk; do **not** allow eating or drinking for 30 minutes after use

Generic Available Yes

Comments Neutral pH fluoride preparations are preferred in patients with oral mucositis to reduce tissue irritation; long-term use of acidulated fluorides has been associated with enamel demineralization and damage to porcelain crowns

Fluorigard® [OTC] see Fluoride on page 415

Fluori-Methane® see Dichlorodifluoromethane and Trichloromonofluoromethane on page 303

Fluorinse® see Fluoride on page 415

Fluoritab® see Fluoride on page 415

Fluorodeoxyuridine see Floxuridine on page 408

Fluorometholone (flure oh METH oh lone)

Related Information
Corticosteroids, Topical Comparison on page 1140

Brand Names Flarex®; Fluor-Op®; FML®; FML® Forte

Therapeutic Category Anti-inflammatory Agent, Ophthalmic; Corticosteroid, Ophthalmic

Use Inflammatory conditions of the eye, including keratitis, iritis, cyclitis, and conjunctivitis

Usual Dosage Children >2 years and Adults: Ophthalmic:
Ointment: May be applied every 4 hours in severe cases; 1-3 times/day in mild to moderate cases
Solution: Instill 1-2 drops into conjunctival sac every hour during day, every 2 hours at night until favorable response is obtained, then use 1 drop every 4 hours; for mild to moderate inflammation, instill 1-2 drops into conjunctival sac 2-4 times/day

Mechanism of Action Decreases inflammation by suppression of migration of polymorphonuclear leukocytes and reversal of increased capillary permeability

Local Anesthetic/Vasoconstrictor Precautions No information available to require special precautions

Effects on Dental Treatment No effects or complications reported

Other Adverse Effects
1% to 10%: Ocular: Blurred vision
<1%: Ocular: Stinging, burning, increased intraocular pressure, open-angle glaucoma, defect in visual acuity and field of vision, cataracts

Drug Interactions No data reported

Drug Uptake Absorption: Into aqueous humor with slight systemic absorption

Pregnancy Risk Factor C

Generic Available No

Fluor-Op® see Fluorometholone on this page

Fluoroplex® Topical see Fluorouracil on this page

Fluorouracil (flure oh YOOR a sil)

Brand Names Adrucil® Injection; Efudex® Topical; Fluoroplex® Topical

Canadian/Mexican Brand Names Efudix® (Mexico); Fluoro-uracil® (Mexico)

Therapeutic Category Antineoplastic Agent, Antimetabolite

Synonyms 5-Fluorouracil; 5-FU

Use Treatment of carcinoma of stomach, colon, rectum, breast, and pancreas; also used topically for management of multiple actinic keratoses and superficial basal cell carcinomas

Usual Dosage Refer to individual protocols

All dosages are based on the patient's actual weight. However, the estimated lean body mass (dry weight) is used if the patient is obese or if there has been a spurious weight gain due to edema, ascites or other forms of abnormal fluid retention.

Children and Adults:
I.V.: Initial: 400-500 mg/m^2/day (12 mg/kg/day; maximum: 800 mg/day) for 4-5 days either as a single daily I.V. push or 4-day continuous intravenous infusion
I.V.: Maintenance dose regimens:
200-250 mg/m^2 (6 mg/kg) every other day for 4 days repeated in 4 weeks
500-600 mg/m^2 (15 mg/kg) weekly as a continuous intravenous infusion or I.V. push

(Continued)

Fluorouracil *(Continued)*

I.V.: Concomitant with leucovorin:

370 mg/m^2/day for 5 days

500-1000 mg/m^2 every 2 weeks

600 mg/m^2/week for 6 weeks

Although the manufacturer recommends no daily dose >800 mg, higher doses of up to 2 g/day are routinely administered by continuous intravenous infusion; by continuous intravenous infusion, higher daily doses have been successfully used

Hemodialysis: Administer dose posthemodialysis

Dosing adjustment/comments in hepatic impairment: Bilirubin >5 mg/dL: Omit use

Topical:

Actinic or solar keratosis: Apply twice daily for 2-6 weeks

Superficial basal cell carcinomas: Apply 5% twice daily for at least 3-6 weeks and up to 10-12 weeks

Mechanism of Action A pyrimidine antimetabolite that interferes with DNA synthesis by blocking the methylation of deoxyuricytic acid; 5-FU rapidly enters the cell and is activated to the nucleotide level; there it inhibits thymidylate synthetase (TS), or is incorporated into RNA (most evident during the GI phase of the cell cycle). The reduced folate cofactor is required for tight binding to occur between the 5-FdUMP and TS.

Local Anesthetic/Vasoconstrictor Precautions No information available to require special precautions

Effects on Dental Treatment No effects or complications reported

Other Adverse Effects Toxicity depends on route and duration of infusion

Irritant chemotherapy

>10%:

Dermatologic: Dermatitis, alopecia

Gastrointestinal (route and schedule dependent): Heartburn, stomatitis, nausea, vomiting, esophagitis, anorexia, and diarrhea; bolus dosing produces milder GI problems, while continuous infusion tends to produce severe mucositis and diarrhea; emesis is moderate, occurring in 30% to 60% of patients, and responds well to phenothiazines and dexamethasone

Emetic potential: <1000 mg: Moderately low (10% to 30%); ≥1000 mg: Moderate (30% to 60%)

1% to 10%:

Dermatologic: Dry skin

Gastrointestinal: GI ulceration

Hematologic: Myelosuppressive: Granulocytopenia occurs around 9-14 days after 5-FU and thrombocytopenia around 7-17 days. The marrow recovers after 22 days. Myelosuppression tends to be more pronounced in patients receiving bolus dosing of 5-FU. WBC: Mild to moderate; Platelets: Mild; Onset (days): 7-10; Nadir (days): 14; Recovery (days): 21

<1%:

Cardiovascular: Chest pain, EKG changes similar to ischemic changes, and possibly cardiac enzyme abnormalities. Usually occurs within the first 2 days of therapy, and may resolve with nitroglycerin and calcium channel blockers. May be due to coronary vessel vasospasm induced by 5-FU.

Central nervous system: Headache, cerebellar ataxia, tingling of hands, somnolence, and ataxia are seen primarily in intracarotid arterial infusions for head and neck tumors; this is believed to be caused by fluorocitrate, a neurotoxic metabolite of the parent compound

Dermatologic: Hyperpigmentation of nailbeds, face, hands, and veins used in infusion; photosensitization with UV light; palmar-plantar syndrome; hand-foot syndrome, pruritic maculopapular rash

Hematologic: Coagulopathy

Hepatic: Hepatotoxicity

Neuromuscular & skeletal: Paresthesia

Ocular: Conjunctivitis, tear duct stenosis, excessive lacrimation, visual disturbances

Respiratory: Dyspnea

Drug Uptake

Absorption: Oral: Erratic and rarely used

Serum half-life (biphasic): Initial: 6-20 minutes; doses of 400-600 mg/m^2 produce drug concentrations above the threshold for cytotoxicity for normal tissue and remain there for 6 hours; 2 metabolites, FdUMP and FUTP, have prolonged half-lives depending on the type of tissue; the clinical effect of these metabolites has not been determined

Pregnancy Risk Factor D (injection); X (topical)

Generic Available Yes: Injection

Comments Myelosuppressive effects:
WBC: Mild
Platelets: Mild
Onset (days): 7-10
Nadir (days): 9-14
Recovery (days): 21

5-Fluorouracil see Fluorouracil on page 417

Fluoxetina Clorhidrato De (Mexico) see Fluoxetine on this page

Fluoxetine (floo OKS e teen)

Related Information
Vasoconstrictor Interactions With Antidepressants on page 1226

Brand Names Prozac®

Canadian/Mexican Brand Names Fluoxac® (Mexico)

Therapeutic Category Antidepressant, Selective Serotonin Reuptake Inhibitor

Synonyms Fluoxetina Clorhidrato De (Mexico)

Use Treatment of major depression

Usual Dosage Oral:
Children <18 years: Dose and safety not established; preliminary experience in children 6-14 years using initial doses of 20 mg/day have been reported
Adults: 20 mg/day in the morning; may increase after several weeks by 20 mg/day increments; maximum: 80 mg/day; doses >20 mg should be divided into morning and noon doses
Usual dosage range:
20-80 mg/day for depression and OCD
20-60 mg/day for obesity
60-80 mg/day for bulimia nervosa
Note: Lower doses of 5 mg/day have been used for initial treatment
Elderly: Some patients may require an initial dose of 10 mg/day with dosage increases of 10 and 20 mg every several weeks as tolerated; should not be taken at night unless patient experiences sedation

Mechanism of Action Inhibits CNS neuron serotonin uptake; minimal or no effect on reuptake of norepinephrine or dopamine; does not significantly bind to alpha-adrenergic, histamine or cholinergic receptors; may therefore be useful in patients at risk from sedation, hypotension, and anticholinergic effects of tricyclic antidepressants

Local Anesthetic/Vasoconstrictor Precautions Although caution should be used in patients taking tricyclic antidepressants, no interactions have been reported with vasoconstrictors and fluoxetine, a nontricyclic antidepressant which acts to increase serotonin

Effects on Dental Treatment >10% of patients experience dry mouth

Other Adverse Effects Predominant adverse effects are CNS and GI
>10%:
Central nervous system: Headache, nervousness, insomnia, drowsiness
Gastrointestinal: Nausea, diarrhea
1% to 10%:
Central nervous system: Anxiety, dizziness, fatigue, sedation
Dermatologic: Rash, pruritus
Endocrine & metabolic: SIADH, hypoglycemia, hyponatremia (elderly or volume-depleted patients)
Gastrointestinal: Anorexia, dyspepsia, constipation
Neuromuscular & skeletal: Tremor
Miscellaneous: Excessive sweating
<1%:
Central nervous system: Extrapyramidal reactions (rare), suicidal ideation
Ocular: Visual disturbances
Miscellaneous: Anaphylactoid reactions, allergies

Drug Interactions
Increased/decreased effect of lithium (both increases and decreases level has been reported)
Increased toxicity of diazepam, trazodone via decreased clearance; increased toxicity with MAO inhibitors (hyperpyrexia, tremors, seizures, delirium, coma)
Displace protein bound drugs

Drug Uptake
Peak antidepressant effect: After >4 weeks
Absorption: Oral: Well absorbed
Serum half-life: Adults: 2-3 days; due to long half-life, resolution of adverse reactions after discontinuation may be slow
Time to peak serum concentration: Within 4-8 hours

Pregnancy Risk Factor B

Generic Available No

(Continued)

Fluoxetine *(Continued)*

Selected Readings
Wynn RL, "New Antidepressant Medications," *Gen Dent*, 1997, 45(1):24-8.

Fluoximesterona (Mexico) *see* Fluoxymesterone *on this page*

Fluoxymesterone (floo oks i MES te rone)

Brand Names Halotestin®

Canadian/Mexican Brand Names Stenox® (Mexico)

Therapeutic Category Androgen

Synonyms Fluoximesterona (Mexico)

Use Replacement of endogenous testicular hormone; in female used as palliative treatment of breast cancer, postpartum breast engorgement

Usual Dosage Adults: Oral:
  Male:
    Hypogonadism: 5-20 mg/day
    Delayed puberty: 2.5-20 mg/day for 4-6 months
  Female:
    Inoperable breast carcinoma: 10-40 mg/day in divided doses for 1-3 months
    Breast engorgement: 2.5 mg after delivery, 5-10 mg/day in divided doses for 4-5 days

Mechanism of Action Synthetic androgenic anabolic hormone responsible for the normal growth and development of male sex organs and maintenance of secondary sex characteristics; stimulates RNA polymerase activity resulting in an increase in protein production; increases bone development

Local Anesthetic/Vasoconstrictor Precautions No information available to require special precautions

Effects on Dental Treatment No effects or complications reported

Other Adverse Effects
  >10%:
    Males: Priapism
    Females: Menstrual problems (amenorrhea), virilism, breast soreness
    Cardiovascular: Edema
    Dermatologic: Acne
  1% to 10%:
    Males: Prostatic carcinoma, hirsutism (increase in pubic hair growth), impotence, testicular atrophy
    Gastrointestinal: GI irritation, nausea, vomiting, prostatic hypertrophy
    Hepatic: Hepatic dysfunction
  <1%:
    Males: Gynecomastia
    Females: Amenorrhea
    Endocrine & metabolic: Hypercalcemia
    Hematologic: Leukopenia, polycythemia
    Hepatic: Hepatic necrosis, cholestatic hepatitis
    Miscellaneous: Hypersensitivity reactions

Drug Interactions
  Decreased blood glucose concentrations and insulin requirements in patients with diabetes
  Increased effect of oral anticoagulants

Drug Uptake
  Absorption: Oral: Rapid
  Serum half-life: 10-100 minutes

Pregnancy Risk Factor X

Generic Available Yes

Fluoxymesterone and Estradiol *see* Ethinyl Estradiol and Fluoxymesterone *on page 377*

Fluphenazine (floo FEN a zeen)

Brand Names Permitil®; Prolixin®; Prolixin Decanoate®; Prolixin Enanthate®

Canadian/Mexican Brand Names Apo®-Fluphenazine [Hydrochloride] (Canada); Modecate® [Fluphenazine Decanoate] (Canada); Modecate® Enanthate [Fluphenazine Enanthate] (Canada); Moditen® Hydrochloride (Canada); PMS-Fluphenazine® [Hydrochloride] (Canada)

Therapeutic Category Antipsychotic Agent; Phenothiazine Derivative

Synonyms Flufenacina (Mexico)

Use Management of manifestations of psychotic disorders

Usual Dosage Adults:
  Oral: 0.5-10 mg/day in divided doses at 6- to 8-hour intervals; some patients may require up to 40 mg/day

I.M.: 2.5-10 mg/day in divided doses at 6- to 8-hour intervals (parenteral dose is ⅓ to ½ the oral dose for the hydrochloride salts)

I.M., S.C. (decanoate): 12.5 mg every 3 weeks

Conversion from hydrochloride to decanoate I.M. 0.5 mL (12.5 mg) decanoate every 3 weeks is approximately equivalent to 10 mg hydrochloride/day

I.M., S.C. (enanthate): 12.5-25 mg every 3 weeks

Not dialyzable (0% to 5%)

Mechanism of Action Blocks postsynaptic mesolimbic dopaminergic D_1 and D_2 receptors in the brain; exhibits a strong alpha-adrenergic blocking and anticholinergic effect, depresses the release of hypothalamic and hypophyseal hormones; believed to depress the reticular activating system thus affecting basal metabolism, body temperature, wakefulness, vasomotor tone, and emesis

Local Anesthetic/Vasoconstrictor Precautions No information available to require special precautions

Effects on Dental Treatment Orthostatic hypotension and nasal congestion possible in dental patients. Since the drug is a dopamine antagonist, extrapyramidal symptoms of the TMJ a possibility.

Other Adverse Effects

>10%:
Cardiovascular: Orthostatic hypotension, hypotension, tachycardia, arrhythmias
Central nervous system: Parkinsonian symptoms, akathisia, dystonias, tardive dyskinesia (persistent), dizziness
Gastrointestinal: Constipation
Ocular: Pigmentary retinopathy
Respiratory: Nasal congestion
Miscellaneous: Decreased sweating

1% to 10%:
Dermatologic: Photosensitivity, skin rash
Endocrine & metabolic: Changes in menstrual cycle pain in breasts, amenorrhea, galactorrhea, gynecomastia, changes in libido
Gastrointestinal: Weight gain, nausea, vomiting, stomach pain
Genitourinary: Dysuria, ejaculatory disturbances
Neuromuscular & skeletal: Trembling of fingers

<1%:
Central nervous system: Sedation, drowsiness, restlessness, anxiety, extrapyramidal reactions, pseudoparkinsonian signs and symptoms, seizures, altered central temperature regulation
Dermatologic: Hyperpigmentation, pruritus, discoloration of skin (blue-gray)
Endocrine & metabolic: Galactorrhea
Gastrointestinal: Dry mouth
Genitourinary: Priapism, urinary retention
Hematologic: Agranulocytosis (more often in women between 4th and 10th weeks of therapy); leukopenia (usually in patients with large doses for prolonged periods)
Hepatic: Cholestatic jaundice, hepatotoxicity
Ocular: Retinal pigmentation, cornea and lens changes, blurred vision

Drug Interactions

Decreased effect: Barbiturate levels and decreased fluphenazine effectiveness when given together
Increased toxicity: With ethanol, effects of both drugs may be increased; EPSEs and other CNS effects may be increased when coadministered with lithium; may potentiate the effects of narcotics including respiratory depression

Drug Uptake

Following I.M. or S.C. administration (derivative dependent):
Decanoate (lasts the longest and requires more time for onset):
Onset of action: 24-72 hours
Hydrochloride salt (acts quickly and persists briefly):
Onset of action: Within 1 hour
Duration: 6-8 hours
Serum half-life: Derivative dependent:
Enanthate: 84-96 hours
Hydrochloride: 33 hours
Decanoate: 163-232 hours

Pregnancy Risk Factor C
Generic Available Yes

Flura-Drops® see Fluoride on page 415
Flura-Loz® see Fluoride on page 415

Flurandrenolide (flure an DREN oh lide)
Related Information
    Corticosteroids, Topical Comparison *on page 1140*
Brand Names Cordran®; Cordran® SP
Canadian/Mexican Brand Names Drenison® (Canada)
Therapeutic Category Corticosteroid, Topical (Medium Potency)
Use Inflammation of corticosteroid-responsive dermatoses [medium potency topical corticosteroid]
Usual Dosage Topical:
    Children:
        Ointment, cream: Apply sparingly 1-2 times/day
        Tape: Apply once daily
    Adults: Cream, lotion, ointment: Apply sparingly 2-3 times/day
Mechanism of Action Decreases inflammation by suppression of migration of polymorphonuclear leukocytes and reversal of increased capillary permeability
Local Anesthetic/Vasoconstrictor Precautions No information available to require special precautions
Effects on Dental Treatment No effects or complications reported
Other Adverse Effects <1%:
    Systemic: HPA suppression, Cushing's syndrome, growth retardation, burning, secondary infection
    Topical: Burning, itching, irritation, dryness, folliculitis, hypertrichosis, acneiform eruptions, hypopigmentation, perioral dermatitis, allergic contact dermatitis, skin atrophy, striae, miliaria, intracranial hypertension, acne, maceration of the skin
Drug Interactions No data reported
Drug Uptake
    Absorption: Adequate with intact skin
Pregnancy Risk Factor C
Generic Available Yes: Lotion

Flurazepam (flure AZ e pam)
Brand Names Dalmane®
Canadian/Mexican Brand Names Apo®-Flurazepam (Canada); Novo-Flupam® (Canada); PMS-Flupam® (Canada); Somnol® (Canada); Som Pam® (Canada)
Therapeutic Category Benzodiazepine; Hypnotic; Sedative
Use Short-term treatment of insomnia
Usual Dosage Oral:
    Children:
        <15 years: Dose not established
        >15 years: 15 mg at bedtime
    Adults: 15-30 mg at bedtime
Mechanism of Action Depresses all levels of the CNS, including the limbic and reticular formation, probably through the increased action of gamma-aminobutyric acid (GABA), which is a major inhibitory neurotransmitter in the brain
Local Anesthetic/Vasoconstrictor Precautions No information available to require special precautions
Effects on Dental Treatment >10% of patients experience dry mouth
Other Adverse Effects
    >10%:
        Cardiovascular: Tachycardia, chest pain
        Central nervous system: Drowsiness, fatigue, lightheadedness, memory impairment, insomnia, anxiety, depression, headache, impaired coordination
        Dermatologic: Rash
        Endocrine & metabolic: Decreased libido
        Gastrointestinal: Constipation, decreased salivation, nausea, vomiting, diarrhea, increased or decreased appetite
        Neuromuscular & skeletal: Dysarthria
        Ocular: Blurred vision
        Miscellaneous: Sweating
    1% to 10%:
        Cardiovascular: Syncope, hypotension
        Central nervous system: Confusion, nervousness, dizziness, akathisia
        Dermatologic: Dermatitis
        Gastrointestinal: Weight gain or loss, increased salivation
        Neuromuscular & skeletal: Rigidity, tremor, muscle cramps
        Otic: Tinnitus
        Respiratory: Hyperventilation, nasal congestion
    <1%:
        Endocrine & metabolic: Menstrual irregularities
        Hematologic: Blood dyscrasias

Neuromuscular & skeletal: Reflex slowing
Miscellaneous: Drug dependence

Drug Interactions
Decreased effect with enzyme inducers
Increased toxicity with other CNS depressants and cimetidine

Drug Uptake
Onset of hypnotic effect: 15-20 minutes
Peak: 3-6 hours
Duration of action: 7-8 hours
Serum half-life: Adults: 40-114 hours

Pregnancy Risk Factor X

Generic Available Yes

Flurbiprofen (flure BI proe fen)

Related Information
Dental Drug Interactions: Update on Drug Combinations Requiring Special Considerations *on page 1144*
Nonsteroidal Anti-Inflammatory Agents, Comparative Dosages, and Pharmacokinetics *on page 1143*
Rheumatoid Arthritis and Osteoarthritis *on page 1030*
Temporomandibular Dysfunction (TMD) *on page 1078*

Brand Names Ansaid®

Canadian/Mexican Brand Names Apo®-Flurbiprofen® (Canada); Froben® (Canada); Froben-SR® (Canada); Novo-Flurprofen (Canada); Nu-Flurbiprofen (Canada)

Therapeutic Category Analgesic, Non-narcotic; Nonsteroidal Anti-inflammatory Agent (NSAID), Oral

Use
Dental: Management of postoperative pain
Medical: Acute or long-term treatment of signs and symptoms of rheumatoid arthritis and osteoarthritis; ophthalmic preparation indicated for inhibition of intraoperative miosis

Usual Dosage Adults: Oral: 200-300 mg/day in 2, 3, or 4 divided doses

Mechanism of Action Inhibits prostaglandin synthesis by decreasing the activity of the enzyme, cyclo-oxygenase, which results in decreased formation of prostaglandin precursors

Local Anesthetic/Vasoconstrictor Precautions No information available to require special precautions

Effects on Dental Treatment <1% of patients experience dry mouth

Other Adverse Effects >10%:
Central nervous system: Dizziness
Dermatologic: Rash
Gastrointestinal: Abdominal cramps, heartburn, indigestion, nausea

Contraindications Hypersensitivity to flurbiprofen or any component

Warnings/Precautions Should be used with caution in patients affected by inhibition of platelet aggregation

Drug Interactions Has caused bleeding in combination with anticoagulants; when given concurrently with aspirin, has resulted in 50% lower serum levels of flurbiprofen

Drug Uptake
Onset of effect: Within 1 hour
Duration of effect: 6-8 hours
Absorption: Rapid and nearly complete
Serum half-life: 6.5 hours
Time to peak serum concentration: 1.5 hours

Pregnancy Risk Factor C

Breast-feeding Considerations No data reported

Dosage Forms Tablet (Ansaid®): 50 mg, 100 mg

Dietary Considerations Can be taken with food, milk, or antacid to decrease GI effects; food alters rate of absorption but not amount

Generic Available Yes

Comments Flurbiprofen is a chiral NSAID with the S-(+) enantiomer possessing most of the beneficial anti-inflammatory activity; both the S-(+) and R-(-) enantiomers possess analgesic activity. All flurbiprofen preparations are marketed as the racemic mixture (equal parts of each enantiomer). Flurbiprofen may be effective in the treatment of periodontal disease. Animal studies have shown flurbiprofen in topical form to be effective in reducing loss of attachment and bone loss. Flurbiprofen as with other NSAIDs can be administered preoperatively in the patient undergoing dental surgery in order to delay the onset and severity of postoperative pain. Doses which have been used are 100 mg twice daily the day before procedure, and 50-100 mg 30 minutes before the procedure.
(Continued)

Flurbiprofen *(Continued)*

Selected Readings

Bragger U, Muhle T, Fourmousis I, et al, "Effect of the NSAID Flurbiprofen on Remodelling After Periodontal Surgery," *J Periodontal Res*, 1997, 32(7):575-82.

Cooper SA and Kupperman A, "The Analgesic Efficacy of Flurbiprofen Compared to Acetaminophen With Codeine," *J Clin Dent*, 1991, 2(3):70-4.

Cooper SA, Mardirossian G, and Miles M, "Analgesic Relative Potency Assay Comparing Flurbiprofen 50, 100, and 150 mg, Aspirin 600 mg, and Placebo in Postsurgical Dental Pain," *Clin J Pain*, 1988, 4:175-81.

Dionne RA, "Suppression of Dental Pain by the Preoperative Administration of Flurbiprofen," *Am J Med*, 1986, 80(3A):41-9.

Dionne RA, Snyder J, and Hargreaves KM, "Analgesic Efficacy of Flurbiprofen in Comparison With Acetaminophen, Acetaminophen Plus Codeine, and Placebo After Impacted Third Molar Removal," *J Oral Maxillofac Surg*, 1994, 52(9):919-24.

Forbes JA, Yorio CC, Selinger LR, et al, "An Evaluation of Flurbiprofen, Aspirin, and Placebo in Postoperative Oral Surgery Pain," *Pharmacotherapy*, 1989, 9(2):66-73.

Gallardo F and Rossi E, "Analgesic Efficacy of Flurbiprofen as Compared to Acetaminophen and Placebo After Periodontal Surgery," *J Periodontol*, 1990, 61(4):224-7.

Jeffcoat MK, Reddy MS, Haigh S, et al, "A Comparison of Topical Ketorolac, Systemic Flurbiprofen, and Placebo for the Inhibition of Bone Loss in Adult Periodontitis," *J Periodontol*, 1995, 66(5):329-38.

Jeffcoat MK, Reddy MS, Wang IC, et al, "The Effect of Systemic Flurbiprofen on Bone Supporting Dental Implants," *J Am Dent Assoc*, 1995, 126(3):305-11.

Malmberg AB and Yaksh TL, "Antinociception Produced by Spinal Delivery of the S and R Enantiomers of Flurbiprofen in the Formalin Test," *Eur J Pharmacol*, 1994, 256(2):205-9.

5-Flurocytosine *see* Flucytosine *on page 409*

Fluro-Ethyl® Aerosol *see* Ethyl Chloride and Dichlorotetrafluoroethane *on page 384*

Flurosyn® *see* Fluocinolone *on page 414*

Flutamide *(FLOO ta mide)*

Brand Names Eulexin®

Canadian/Mexican Brand Names Eulexin® (Mexico); Fluken® (Mexico); Flulem (Mexico)

Therapeutic Category Antiandrogen

Use In combination with LHRH agonistic analogs for the treatment of metastatic prostatic carcinoma

Usual Dosage Adults: Oral: 2 capsules every 8 hours for a total daily dose of 750 mg

Mechanism of Action Nonsteroidal antiandrogen that inhibits androgen uptake or inhibits binding of androgen in target tissues

Local Anesthetic/Vasoconstrictor Precautions No information available to require special precautions

Effects on Dental Treatment No effects or complications reported

Other Adverse Effects

>10%:
Gastrointestinal: Nausea, vomiting, diarrhea
Genitourinary: Impotence
Endocrine & metabolic: Loss of libido, hot flashes

1% to 10%:
Endocrine & metabolic: Gynecomastia
Gastrointestinal: Anorexia
Neuromuscular & skeletal: Numbness in extremities

<1%:
Cardiovascular: Hypertension, edema
Central nervous system: Drowsiness, nervousness, confusion
Hepatic: Hepatitis

Drug Uptake
Absorption: Rapid and complete
Serum half-life: 5-6 hours

Pregnancy Risk Factor D

Generic Available No

Comments To achieve benefit to combination therapy, both drugs need to be started simultaneously

Flutex® *see* Triamcinolone *on page 954*

Fluticasone *(floo TIK a sone)*

Brand Names Cutivate™; Flonase®; Flovent®

Therapeutic Category Corticosteroid, Topical (Medium Potency)

Use

Intranasal: Management of seasonal and perennial allergic rhinitis in patients ≥12 years of age

Topical: Relief of inflammation and pruritus associated with corticosteroid-responsive dermatoses [medium potency topical corticosteroid]

Usual Dosage

Adolescents:

Topical: Apply sparingly in a thin film twice daily

Intranasal: Initially 1 spray (50 mcg/spray) per nostril once daily. Patients not adequately responding or patients with more severe symptoms may use 2 sprays (200 mcg) per nostril. Depending on response, dosage may be reduced to 100 mcg daily. Total daily dosage should not exceed 4 sprays (200 mcg)/day.

Adults:

Topical: Apply sparingly in a thin film twice daily

Intranasal: Initially 2 sprays (50 mcg/spray) per nostril once daily. After the first few days, dosage may be reduced to 1 spray per nostril once daily for maintenance therapy. Maximum total daily dose should not exceed 4 sprays (200 mcg)/day.

Mechanism of Action Fluticasone belongs to a new group of corticosteroids which utilizes a fluorocarbothioate ester linkage at the 17 carbon position; extremely potent vasoconstrictive and anti-inflammatory activity; has a weak hypothalamic -pituitary- adrenocortical axis (HPA) inhibitory potency when applied topically, which gives the drug a high therapeutic index. The mechanism of action for all topical corticosteroids is not well defined, however, is believed to be a combination of three important properties: anti-inflammatory activity, immunosuppressive properties, and antiproliferative actions.

Local Anesthetic/Vasoconstrictor Precautions No information available to require special precautions

Effects on Dental Treatment No effects or complications reported

Other Adverse Effects <1%:

Dermatologic: Acne, hypopigmentation, allergic dermatitis, maceration of the skin, skin atrophy, folliculitis, hypertrichosis

Endocrine & metabolic: HPA suppression, Cushing's syndrome, growth retardation

Local: Burning, itching, irritation, dryness

Miscellaneous: Secondary infection

Drug Interactions No data reported

Pregnancy Risk Factor C

Dosage Forms

Spray, aerosol, oral inhalation (Flovent®): 44 mcg/actuation (7.9 g = 60 actuations or 13 g = 120 actuations), 110 mcg/actuation (13 g = 120 actuations); 220 mcg/actuation (13 g = 120 actuations)

Spray, intranasal (Flonase®): 50 mcg/actuation (9 g = 60 actuations, 16 g = 120 actuations)

Topical (Cutivate™):

Cream: 0.05% (15 g, 30 g, 60 g)

Ointment: 0.005% (15 g, 60 g)

Generic Available No

Fluvastatin (FLOO va sta tin)

Related Information

Cardiovascular Diseases on page 1010

Brand Names Lescol®

Therapeutic Category HMG-CoA Reductase Inhibitor; Lipid Lowering Drugs

Use Adjunct to dietary therapy to decrease elevated serum total and LDL cholesterol concentrations in primary hypercholesterolemia

Usual Dosage Adults: Oral:

Initial dose: 20 mg at bedtime

Usual dose: 20-40 mg at bedtime

Note: Splitting the 40 mg dose into a twice/daily regimen may provide a modest improvement in LDL response; maximum response occurs within 4-6 weeks; decrease dose and monitor effects carefully in patients with hepatic insufficiency

Mechanism of Action Acts by competitively inhibiting 3-hydroxy-3-methylglutaryl-coenzyme A (HMG-CoA) reductase, the enzyme that catalyzes the reduction of HMG-CoA to mevalonate; this is an early rate-limiting step in cholesterol biosynthesis. HDL is increased while total, LDL and VLDL cholesterols, apolipoprotein B, and plasma triglycerides are decreased

Local Anesthetic/Vasoconstrictor Precautions No information available to require special precautions

Effects on Dental Treatment No effects or complications reported

Other Adverse Effects 1% to 1%:

Central nervous system: Headache, dizziness, insomnia

Dermatologic: Rash

Gastrointestinal: Dyspepsia, diarrhea, nausea, vomiting, constipation, flatulence

(Continued)

Fluvastatin *(Continued)*

Neuromuscular & skeletal: Back pain, abdominal pain, myalgia, arthropathy
Miscellaneous: Cold symptoms

Drug Interactions

Anticoagulant effect of warfarin may be increased

Concurrent use of erythromycin and HMG-CoA reductase inhibitors may result in rhabdomyolysis

Drug Uptake

Serum half-life: 1.2 hours

Pregnancy Risk Factor X

Generic Available No

Fluvoxamine *(floo VOKS ah meen)*

Brand Names Luvox®

Therapeutic Category Antidepressant, Selective Serotonin Reuptake Inhibitor

Use Treatment of obsessive-compulsive disorder (OCD); effective in the treatment of major depression; may be useful for the treatment of panic disorder

Usual Dosage

Adults: Initial: 50 mg at bedtime; adjust in 50 mg increments at 4- to 7-day intervals; usual dose range: 100-300 mg/day; divide total daily dose into 2 doses; give larger portion at bedtime

Elderly or hepatic impairment: Reduce dose, titrate slowly

Mechanism of Action Inhibits CNS neuron serotonin uptake; minimal or no effect on reuptake of norepinephrine or dopamine; does not significantly bind to alpha-adrenergic, histamine or cholinergic receptors

Local Anesthetic/Vasoconstrictor Precautions Although caution should be used in patients taking tricyclic antidepressants, no interactions have been reported with vasoconstrictors and fluvoxamine, a nontricyclic antidepressant which acts to increase serotonin

Effects on Dental Treatment No effects or complications reported

Other Adverse Effects

>10%: Gastrointestinal: Nausea

1% to 10%:

Cardiovascular: Palpitations

Central nervous system: Somnolence, headache, insomnia, dizziness, nervousness, mania, hypomania, vertigo, abnormal thinking, agitation, anxiety, malaise, amnesia

Endocrine & metabolic: Decreased libido

Gastrointestinal: Dry mouth, abdominal pain, vomiting, dyspepsia, constipation, diarrhea, dysgeusia, anorexia

Neuromuscular & skeletal: Tremors, weakness

Miscellaneous: Sweating

<1%:

Central nervous system: Seizures, extrapyramidal reactions

Dermatologic: Toxic epidermal necrolysis

Hematologic: Thrombocytopenia

Hepatic: Hepatic dysfunction

Renal: Elevated serum creatinine

Drug Interactions Because fluvoxamine inhibits cytochrome P-450 isozymes IA2, IIC9, IIIA4, and possibly IID6, it is associated with numerous significant drug interactions

Increased toxicity: Terfenadine and astemizole are both metabolized by the cytochrome P-450 IIIA4 isozyme, increased levels of these drugs have been associated with prolongation of the Q-T interval and potentially fatal, torsade de pointes ventricular arrhythmias. Since fluvoxamine inhibits the enzyme responsible for their clearance, the concomitant use of these agents is contraindicated.

Potentiates triazolam and alprazolam (dose should be reduced by at least 50%), hypertensive crisis with MAO inhibitors, theophylline (doses should be reduced by 1/3 and plasma levels monitored), warfarin (reduce its dose and monitor PT/INR), carbamazepine (monitor levels), tricyclic antidepressants (monitor effects and reduce doses accordingly), methadone, beta-blockers (reduce dose of propranolol or metoprolol), diltiazem. Caution with other benzodiazepines, phenytoin, lithium, clozapine, alcohol, other CNS drugs, quinidine, ketoconazole.

Pregnancy Risk Factor C

Generic Available No

Selected Readings

Wynn RL, "New Antidepressant Medications," *Gen Dent*, 1997, 45(1):24-8.

Fluzone® *see* Influenza Virus Vaccine *on page 507*

FML® *see* Fluorometholone *on page 417*

FML® Forte *see* Fluorometholone *on page 417*

FML-S® Ophthalmic Suspension *see* Sulfacetamide Sodium and Fluorometholone *on page 890*

Foille® [OTC] *see* Benzocaine *on page 118*

Foille® Medicated First Aid [OTC] *see* Benzocaine *on page 118*

Folex® PFS *see* Methotrexate *on page 615*

Folic Acid (FOE lik AS id)

Brand Names Folvite®

Canadian/Mexican Brand Names A.F. Valdecasas® (Mexico); Apo®-Folic (Canada); Dalisol® (Mexico); Flodine® (Canada); Folitab® (Mexico); Novo-Folacid® (Canada)

Therapeutic Category Vitamin, Water Soluble

Synonyms Folico Acido (Mexico)

Use

Dental: Treatment of megaloblastic and macrocytic anemias due to folate deficiency

Medical: Dietary supplement to prevent neural tube defects

Usual Dosage Oral, I.M., I.V., S.C.:

Children: Initial: 1 mg/day

Deficiency: 0.5-1 mg/day

Maintenance dose:

<4 years: Up to 0.3 mg/day

>4 years: 0.4 mg/day

Adults: Initial: 1 mg/day

Deficiency: 1-3 mg/day

Maintenance dose: 0.5 mg/day

Women of childbearing age, pregnant, and lactating women: 0.8 mg/day

Mechanism of Action Folic acid is necessary for formation of a number of coenzymes in many metabolic systems, particularly for purine and pyrimidine synthesis; required for nucleoprotein synthesis and maintenance in erythropoiesis; stimulates WBC and platelet production in folate deficiency anemia

Local Anesthetic/Vasoconstrictor Precautions No information available to require special precautions

Effects on Dental Treatment No effects or complications reported

Other Adverse Effects <1%:

Cardiovascular: Slight flushing

Central nervous system: General malaise

Dermatologic: Pruritus, rash

Respiratory: Bronchospasm

Miscellaneous: Allergic reaction

Contraindications Pernicious, aplastic, or normocytic anemias

Warnings/Precautions Doses <0.1 mg/day may obscure pernicious anemia with continuing irreversible nerve damage progression. Resistance to treatment may occur with depressed hematopoiesis, alcoholism, deficiencies of other vitamins. Injection contains benzyl alcohol (1.5%) as preservative (use care in administration to neonates).

Drug Interactions

Decreased effect: In folate-deficient patients, folic acid therapy may increase phenytoin metabolism. Phenytoin, primidone, para-aminosalicylic acid, and sulfasalazine may decrease serum folate concentrations and cause deficiency. Oral contraceptives may also impair folate metabolism producing depletion, but the effect is unlikely to cause anemia or megaloblastic changes. Concurrent administration of chloramphenicol and folic acid may result in antagonism of the hematopoietic response to folic acid.

Drug Uptake

Peak effect: Oral: Within 0.5-1 hour

Absorption: In the proximal part of the small intestine

Pregnancy Risk Factor A (C if dose exceeds RDA recommendation)

Breast-feeding Considerations May be taken while breast-feeding

Dosage Forms

Injection, as sodium folate: 5 mg/mL (10 mL); 10 mg/mL (10 mL)

Folvite®: 5 mg/mL (10 mL)

Tablet: 0.1 mg, 0.4 mg, 0.8 mg, 1 mg

Folvite®: 1 mg

Generic Available Yes

Folico Acido (Mexico) *see* Folic Acid *on this page*

Folinic Acid *see* Leucovorin *on page 544*

Follitropin Alpha (foe li TRO pin AL fa)
Brand Names Gonal-F®
Therapeutic Category Ovulation Stimulator
Use Induction of ovulation in the anovulatory infertile patient in whom the cause of infertility is functional and not caused by primary ovarian failure
Usual Dosage Adults (women): S.C.: Initially 75 units/day for the first cycle; an incremental dose adjustment of up to 37.5 units may be considered after 14 days; treatment duration should not exceed 35 days unless an E2 rise indicates follicular development
Local Anesthetic/Vasoconstrictor Precautions No information available to require special precautions
Effects on Dental Treatment No effects or complications reported
Dosage Forms Injection: 75 FSH units, 150 FSH units

Folvite® see Folic Acid on previous page

Fomepizole (foe ME pi zole)
Brand Names Antizol®
Therapeutic Category Antidote
Synonyms 4-Methylpyrazole; 4-MP
Use Ethylene glycol and methanol toxicity; may be useful in propylene glycol; unclear whether it is useful in disulfiram-ethanol reactions
Usual Dosage Oral: 15 mg/kg followed by 5 mg/kg in 12 hours and then 10 mg/kg every 12 hours until levels of toxin are not present
One other protocol (from France) suggests an infusion of 10-20 mg/kg before dialysis and intravenous infusion of 1-1.5 mg/kg/hour during hemodialysis
META (methylpyrazole for toxic alcohol) study in U.S. (investigational): Loading I.V. dose of 15 mg/kg followed by 10 mg/kg I.V. every 12 hours for 48 hours; continue treatment until methanol or ethylene glycol levels are <20 mg/dL; supplemental doses required during dialysis; contact your local poison center regarding this study
Mechanism of Action Complexes and inactivates alcohol dehydrogenase thus preventing formation of the toxic metabolites of the alcohols
Local Anesthetic/Vasoconstrictor Precautions No information available to require special precautions
Effects on Dental Treatment No effects or complications reported
Drug Interactions Inhibitory effects on alcohol dehydrogenase are increased in presence of ethanol; ethanol also decreases metabolism of 4-MP; 4-MPO induces cytochrome P-450 mixed function oxidases in vitro; 4-MP may worsen the ethanol-chlorohydrate central nervous system interaction
Drug Uptake
Maximum effect: 1.5-2 hours
Absorption: Oral: Readily absorbed
Distribution: V_d: 0.6-0.7 L/kg; unknown distribution, probably very similar to ethanol
Protein binding: Negligible
Elimination: Nonlinear elimination; at suggested therapeutic doses of 10-20 mg/kg the apparent elimination rate is 4-5 μmol/L/hour; 4-MP is dializable
Selected Readings
Borron SW and Baud FJ, "Intravenous 4-Methylpyrazole as an Antidote for Diethylene Glycol and Triethylene Glycol Poisoning: A Case Report," Vet Hum Toxicol, 1997, 37(1): 26-8.
Brent J, McMartin K, Phillips S, et al, "4-Methylpyrazole (Fomepizole) Therapy of Ethylene Glycol Poisoning: Preliminary Results of the Meta Trial," J Toxicol Clin Toxicol, 1997, 35(5):507.
Brent J, McMartin K, Phillips SP, et al, "4-Methylpyrazole (Fomepizole) Therapy of Methanol Poisoning: Preliminary Results of the Meta Trial," J Toxicol Clin Toxicol, 1997, 35(5):507.
Hung O, Kaplan J, Hoffman R, et al, "Improved Understanding of the Ethanol-Chloral Hydrate Interaction Using 4-MP," J Toxicol Clin Toxicol, 1997, 35(5):507-8.
Jacobsen D and McMartin KE, "Antidotes for Methanol and Ethylene Glycol Poisoning," J Toxicol Clin Toxicol, 1997, 35(2):127-43.
Jacobsen D and McMartin K, "4-Methylpyrazole - Present Status," J Toxicol Clin Toxicol, 1996, 34(4):379-81.
Jacobsen D, Ostensen J, Bredesen L, et al, "4-Methylpyrazole (4-MP) Is Effectively Removed by Haemodialysis in the Pig Model," Hum Exp Toxicol, 1996, 15(6):494-6.
Jacobsen D, Sebastian CS, Barron SK, et al, "Effects of 4-Methylpyrazole, Methanol/Ethylene Glycol Antidote in Healthy Humans," J Emerg Med, 1990, 8(4):455-61.
Jobard E, Harry P, Turcant A, et al, "4-Methylpyrazole and Hemodialysis in Ethylene Glycol Poisoning," J Toxicol Clin Toxicol, 1996, 34(4):373-7.
McMartin KE and Heath A, "Treatment of Ethylene Glycol Poisoning With Intravenous 4-Methylpyrazole," N Engl J Med, 1989, 320(2):125.

Formula Q® [OTC] see Quinine on page 831
5-Formyl Tetrahydrofolate see Leucovorin on page 544
Fortaz® see Ceftazidime on page 195
Fosamax® see Alendronate on page 38

Foscarnet (fos KAR net)
Related Information
Systemic Viral Diseases *on page 1047*
Brand Names Foscavir®
Therapeutic Category Antiviral Agent, Parenteral
Use Approved indications in adult patients:
Herpesvirus infections suspected to be caused by acyclovir (HSV, VZV) or ganci-clovir (CMV) resistant strains (this occurs almost exclusively in persons with advanced AIDS who have received prolonged treatment for a herpesvirus infection)
CMV retinitis in persons with AIDS
Other CMV infections in persons unable to tolerate ganciclovir
Usual Dosage
Adolescents and Adults: I.V.:
Induction treatment: 60 mg/kg/dose every 8 hours for 14-21 days
Maintenance therapy: 90-120 mg/kg/day as a single infusion
See table.

Dose Adjustment for Renal Impairment

The induction dose of foscarnet should be adjusted according to creatinine clearance as follows:

Creatinine Clearance (mL/min/kg)	Foscarnet Induction Dose (mg/kg q8h)
1.6	60
1.5	57
1.4	53
1.3	49
1.2	46
1.1	42
1	39
0.9	35
0.8	32
0.7	28
0.6	25
0.5	21
0.4	18

The maintenance dose of foscarnet should be adjusted according to creatinine clearance as follows:

Creatinine Clearance (mL/min/kg)	Foscarnet Maintenance Dose (mg/kg/day)
1.4	90-120
1.2-1.4	78-104
1-1.2	75-100
0.8-1	71-94
0.6-0.8	63-84
0.4-0.6	57-75

Mechanism of Action
Pyrophosphate analogue which acts as a noncompetitive inhibitor of many viral RNA and DNA polymerases as well as HIV reverse transcriptase. Inhibitory effects occur at concentrations which do not affect host cellular DNA polymerases; however, some human cell growth suppression has been observed with high *in vitro* concentrations. Similar to ganciclovir, foscarnet is a virostatic agent. Foscarnet does not require activation by thymidine kinase.
Local Anesthetic/Vasoconstrictor Precautions
No information available to require special precautions
Effects on Dental Treatment
No effects or complications reported
Other Adverse Effects
>10%:
Central nervous system: Fever, headache, seizures
Gastrointestinal: Nausea, diarrhea, vomiting
Hematologic: Anemia
Renal: Abnormal renal function, decreased creatinine clearance
1% to 10%:
Central nervous system: Fatigue, malaise, dizziness, hypoesthesia, depression, confusion, anxiety
Dermatologic: Rash
(Continued)

Foscarnet *(Continued)*

    Endocrine & metabolic: Electrolyte imbalance
    Gastrointestinal: Anorexia
    Hematologic: Granulocytopenia, leukopenia
    Local: Injection site pain
    Neuromuscular & skeletal: Paresthesia, involuntary muscle contractions, rigors, neuropathy, weakness
    Ocular: Vision abnormalities
    Respiratory: Coughing, dyspnea
    Miscellaneous: Sepsis, increased sweating

  <1%:
    Cardiovascular: Cardiac failure, bradycardia, arrhythmias, cerebral edema, leg edema, peripheral edema, syncope, substernal chest pain
    Central nervous system: Hypothermia, abnormal crying, malignant fever, vertigo, coma, speech disorders
    Endocrine & metabolic: Gynecomastia, decreased gonadotropins
    Hepatic: Cholecystitis, cholelithiasis, hepatitis, hepatosplenomegaly, ascites
    Neuromuscular & skeletal: Abnormal gait, dyskinesia, hypertonia
    Ocular: Nystagmus
    Miscellaneous: Vocal cord paralysis

Drug Interactions No data reported

Drug Uptake
  Absorption: Oral: Poorly absorbed; I.V. therapy is needed for the treatment of viral infections in AIDS patients
  Serum half-life: ~3 hours

Pregnancy Risk Factor C

Generic Available No

Foscavir® *see* Foscarnet *on previous page*

Fosfomycin *(fos foe MYE sin)*

Brand Names Monurol™

Therapeutic Category Antibiotic, Miscellaneous

Synonyms Fosfomycin Tromethamine

Use Treatment of uncomplicated urinary tract infections

Usual Dosage Adults: Urinary tract infections: Oral:
  Female: Single dose of 3 g in 4 oz of water
  Male: 3 g once daily for 2-3 days for complicated urinary tract infections

Mechanism of Action As a phosphonic acid derivative, fosfomycin inhibits bacterial wall synthesis (bactericidal) by inactivating the enzyme, pyruvyl transferase, which is critical in the synthesis of cell walls by bacteria; the tromethamine salt is preferable to the calcium salt due to its superior absorption; many gram-positive and gram-negative organisms are inhibited staphylococci, pneumococci, *E. coli, Salmonella, Shigella, H. influenzae, Neisseria* spp, and some strains of *P. aeruginosa*, indole-negative *Proteus*, and *Providencia*; *B. fragilis*, and anaerobic g (-) cocci are resistant; *in vitro* synergism occurs with penicillins, cephalosporins, aminoglycosides, erythromycin, and tetracyclines

Local Anesthetic/Vasoconstrictor Precautions No information available to require special precautions

Effects on Dental Treatment No effects or complications reported

Other Adverse Effects
  >1%:
    Central nervous system: Headache
    Dermatologic: Rash
    Gastrointestinal: Diarrhea (2% to 8%), nausea, vomiting, epigastric discomfort, anorexia
  <1%:
    Central nervous system: Dizziness, drowsiness, fatigue
    Dermatologic: Pruritus

Drug Interactions Decreased effect: Food decreases absorption significantly; antacids or calcium salts may cause precipitate formation and decrease fosfomycin absorption

Drug Uptake
  Absorption: Well absorbed
  Serum half-life: 4-8 hours; prolonged in renal failure (50 hours with Cl_{cr} <10 mL/minute)
  Time to peak serum concentration: 2 hours

Pregnancy Risk Factor B

Fosfomycin Tromethamine *see* Fosfomycin *on this page*

Fosinopril (foe SIN oh pril)

Related Information
Cardiovascular Diseases on page 1010

Brand Names Monopril®

Therapeutic Category Angiotensin-Converting Enzyme (ACE) Inhibitors

Synonyms Fosinopril Sodico (Mexico)

Use Treatment of hypertension, either alone or in combination with other antihypertensive agents; congestive heart failure

Usual Dosage Adults: Oral:

Hypertension: Initial: 10 mg/day; increase to a maximum dose of 80 mg/day; most patients are maintained on 20-40 mg/day; may need to divide the dose into two if trough effect is inadequate; discontinue the diuretic, if possible 2-3 days before initiation of therapy; resume diuretic therapy carefully, if needed.

Heart failure: Initial: 10 mg/day (5 mg if renal dysfunction present) and increase, as needed, to a maximum of 40 mg once daily over several weeks; usual dose: 20-40 mg/day; if hypotension, orthostasis, or azotemia occur during titration, consider decreasing concomitant diuretic dose, if any

Mechanism of Action Competitive inhibitor of angiotensin-converting enzyme (ACE); prevents conversion of angiotensin I to angiotensin II, a potent vasoconstrictor; results in lower levels of angiotensin II which causes an increase in plasma renin activity and a reduction in aldosterone secretion; a CNS mechanism may also be involved in hypotensive effect as angiotensin II increases adrenergic outflow from CNS; vasoactive kallikreins may be decreased in conversion to active hormones by ACE inhibitors, thus reducing blood pressure

Local Anesthetic/Vasoconstrictor Precautions No information available to require special precautions

Effects on Dental Treatment No effects or complications reported

Other Adverse Effects

1% to 10%:

Cardiovascular: Orthostatic hypotension
Central nervous system: Headache, dizziness, fatigue
Endocrine & metabolic: Sexual dysfunction
Gastrointestinal: Diarrhea, nausea, vomiting
Respiratory: Cough

<1%:

Cardiovascular: Syncope
Central nervous system: Vertigo, insomnia
Dermatologic: Angioedema, rash
Endocrine & metabolic: Hypoglycemia, hyperkalemia
Gastrointestinal: Dysgeusia
Genitourinary: Impotence
Hematologic: Neutropenia, agranulocytosis, anemia
Neuromuscular & skeletal: Muscle cramps
Renal: Deterioration in renal function

Drug Interactions

Fosinopril and diuretics have additive hypotensive effects; see table.

Drug-Drug Interactions With ACEIs

Precipitant Drug	Drug (Category) and Effect	Description
Antacids	ACE Inhibitors: decreased	Decreased bioavailability of ACEIs. May be more likely with captopril. Separate administration times by 1-2 hours.
NSAIDs (indomethacin)	ACEIs: decreased	Reduced hypotensive effects of ACEIs. More prominent in low renin or volume dependent hypertensive patients.
Phenothiazines	ACEIs: increased	Pharmacologic effects of ACEIs may be increased.
ACEIs	Allopurinol: increased	Higher risk of hypersensitivity reaction possible when given concurrently. Three case reports of Stevens-Johnson syndrome with captopril.
ACEIs	Digoxin: increased	Increased plasma digoxin levels.
ACEIs	Lithium: increased	Increased serum lithium levels and symptoms of toxicity may occur.
ACEIs	Potassium preps/ potassium sparing diuretics increased	Coadministration may result in elevated potassium levels.

(Continued)

Fosinopril *(Continued)*

Drug Uptake
Absorption: 36%
Serum half-life, serum (fosinoprilat): 12 hours
Time to peak serum concentration: ~3 hours
Pregnancy Risk Factor C (first trimester); D (second and third trimesters)
Generic Available No

Fosinopril Sodico (Mexico) *see Fosinopril on previous page*

Fosphenytoin *(FOS fen i toyn)*

Brand Names Cerebyx®
Therapeutic Category Anticonvulsant, Hydantoin
Use Indicated for short-term parenteral administration when other means of phenytoin administration are unavailable, inappropriate or deemed less advantageous; the safety and effectiveness of fosphenytoin in this use has not been systematically evaluated for more than 5 days; may be used for the control of generalized convulsive status epilepticus and prevention and treatment of seizures occurring during neurosurgery
Usual Dosage The dose, concentration in solutions, and infusion rates for fosphenytoin are expressed as phenytoin sodium equivalents; fosphenytoin should always be prescribed and dispensed in phenytoin sodium equivalents

Status epilepticus: I.V.: Adults: Loading dose: Phenytoin equivalent 15-20 mg/kg I.V. administered at 100-150 mg/minute

Nonemergent loading and maintenance dosing: I.V. or I.M.: Adults:
Loading dose: Phenytoin equivalent 10-20 mg/kg I.V. or I.M. (max I.V. rate 150 mg/minute)
Initial daily maintenance dose: Phenytoin equivalent 4-6 mg/kg/day I.V. or I.M.

I.M. or I.V. substitution for oral phenytoin therapy: May be substituted for oral phenytoin sodium at the same total daily dose, however, Dilantin® capsules are ~90% bioavailable by the oral route; phenytoin, supplied as fosphenytoin, is 100% bioavailable by both the I.M. and I.V. routes; for this reason, plasma phenytoin concentrations may increase when I.M. or I.V. fosphenytoin is substituted for oral phenytoin sodium therapy; in clinical trials I.M. fosphenytoin was administered as a single daily dose utilizing either 1 or 2 injection sites; some patients may require more frequent dosing

Dosing adjustments in renal and hepatic impairment: Phenytoin clearance may be substantially reduced in cirrhosis and plasma level monitoring with dose adjustment advisable; free phenytoin levels should be monitored closely in patients with renal or hepatic disease or in those with hypoalbumineria; furthermore fosphenytoin clearance to phenytoin may be increased without a similar increase in phenytoin in these patients leading to increase frequency and severity of adverse events

Local Anesthetic/Vasoconstrictor Precautions No information available to require special precautions
Effects on Dental Treatment No effects or complications reported
Other Adverse Effects
I.V. administration (maximum dose/rate):
Body as whole: Pelvic pain (4.4%), weakness (2.2%), back pain (2.2%), headache (2.2%)
Cardiovascular: I.V.: Hypotension (7.7%), vasodilation (5.6%), tachycardia (2.2%)
Central nervous system: Dizziness (31%), drowsiness (20%), ataxia (11%), stupor (7.7%), extrapyramidal syndrome (4.4%), agitation (3.3%), hypesthesia (2.2%), vertigo (2.2%), brain edema (2.2%), impaired coordination (4.4%)
Dermatologic: Pruritus (48.9%)
Gastrointestinal: Nausea (8.9%), tongue disorder (4.4%), dry mouth (4.4%), vomiting (2.2%), taste perversion (3.3%)
Neuromuscular & skeletal: Paresthesia (4.4%), dysarthria (2.2%), tremor (3.3%)
Ocular: Diplopia (3.3%), amblyopia (2.2%), nystagmus (44%)
Otic: Tinnitus (8.9%), deafness (2.2%)

I.M. administration (substitute for oral phenytoin):
Body as a whole: Headache (8.9%), weakness (3.9%), accidental injury (3.4%)
Central nervous system: Ataxia (8.4%), drowsiness (6.7%), dizziness (5%)
Dermatologic: Pruritus (2.8%)
Gastrointestinal: Nausea (4.5%), vomiting (2.8%)
Dermatologic: Bruising (7.3%)

Neuromuscular & skeletal: Tremor (9.5%), paresthesia (3.9%), incoordination (7.8%), reflexes decreased (2.8%)

Ocular: Nystagmus (15%)

Other ≤1%:

Cardiovascular: Hypertension, cardiac arrest, syncope, cerebral hemorrhage, palpitations, sinus bradycardia, atrial flutter, bundle branch block, cardiomegaly, cerebral infarct, postural hypotension, pulmonary embolus, QT interval prolongation, thrombophlebitis, ventricular extrasystoles, congestive heart failure

Central nervous system: Migraine

Dermatologic: Rash, maculopapular rash, urticaria, skin discoloration, contact dermatitis, pustular rash, skin nodule, petechia

Endocrine & metabolic: Hypokalemia, hyperglycemia, hypophosphatemia, alkalosis, acidosis, dehydration, hyperkalemia, ketosis

Hematologic/lymphatic: Thrombocytopenia, anemia, leukocytosis, cyanosis, hypochromic anemia, leukopenia, lymphadenopathy

Hepatic: Acute hepatotoxicity, acute hepatic failure

Miscellaneous: Sweating

Warnings/Precautions Doses of fosphenytoin are expressed as their phenytoin sodium equivalent; antiepileptic drugs should not be abruptly discontinued; hypotension may occur, especially after I.V. administration at high doses and high rates of administration, administration of phenytoin has been associated with atrial and ventricular conduction depression and ventricular fibrillation, careful cardiac monitoring is needed when administering I.V. loading doses of fosphenytoin; use with caution in patients with hypotension and severe myocardial insufficiency; discontinue if skin rash or lymphadenopathy occurs; acute hepatotoxicity associated with a hypersensitivity syndrome characterized by fever, skin eruptions and lymphadenopathy has been reported to occur within the first 2 months of treatment

Drug Interactions No drugs are known to interfere with the conversion of fosphenytoin to phenytoin; phenytoin may decrease the serum concentration or effectiveness of valproic acid, ethosuximide, felbamate, benzodiazepines, carbamazepine, lamotrigine, primidone, warfarin, oral contraceptives, corticosteroids, cyclosporine, theophylline, chloramphenicol, rifampin, doxycycline, quinidine, mexiletine, disopyramide, dopamine, or nondepolarizing skeletal muscle relaxants; phenytoin may increase phenobarbital and primidone levels; protein binding of phenytoin can be affected by valproic acid or salicylates; serum phenytoin concentrations may be increased by cimetidine, felbamate, ethosuximide, methsuximide, chloramphenicol, disulfiram, fluconazole, omeprazole, isoniazid, trimethoprim, or sulfonamides and decreased by rifampin, cisplatin, vinblastine, bleomycin, folic acid

Drug Uptake

Fosphenytoin is a prodrug of phenytoin and its anticonvulsant effects are attributable to phenytoin

Conversion to phenytoin: Following I.V. administration conversion half-life is 15 minutes; following I.M. administration peak phenytoin levels are reached in 3 hours

Pregnancy Risk Factor D

Generic Available No

Fostex® [OTC] see Sulfur and Salicylic Acid on page 898

Fostex® 10% BPO Gel [OTC] see Benzoyl Peroxide on page 120

Fostex® 10% Wash [OTC] see Benzoyl Peroxide on page 120

Fostex® Bar [OTC] see Benzoyl Peroxide on page 120

Fototar® [OTC] see Coal Tar on page 254

Fragmin® see Dalteparin on page 278

Freezone® Solution [OTC] see Salicylic Acid on page 853

Fresh Burst Listerine® Antiseptic [OTC] see Mouthwash, Antiseptic on page 650

FS Shampoo® see Fluocinolone on page 414

5-FU see Fluorouracil on page 417

FUDR® see Floxuridine on page 408

Fulvicin® P/G see Griseofulvin on page 451

Fulvicin-U/F® see Griseofulvin on page 451

Fumasorb® [OTC] see Ferrous Fumarate on page 400

Fumerin® [OTC] see Ferrous Fumarate on page 400

Fungizone® see Amphotericin B on page 71

Fungoid® AF Topical Solution [OTC] see Undecylenic Acid and Derivatives on page 977

Fungoid® Creme see Miconazole on page 635

Fungoid® Tincture *see Miconazole on page 635*

Furacin® *see Nitrofurazone on page 685*

Furadantin® *see Nitrofurantoin on page 684*

Furazolidona (Mexico) *see Furazolidone on this page*

Furazolidone (fyoor a ZOE li done)

Brand Names Furoxone®

Canadian/Mexican Brand Names Furoxona® Gotas (Mexico); Furoxona® Tabletas (Mexico); Fuxol® (Mexico)

Therapeutic Category Antibiotic, Miscellaneous; Antidiarrheal; Antiprotozoal

Synonyms Furazolidona (Mexico)

Use Treatment of bacterial or protozoal diarrhea and enteritis caused by susceptible organisms *Giardia lamblia* and *Vibrio cholerae*

Usual Dosage Oral:

Children >1 month: 5-8 mg/kg/day in 4 divided doses for 7 days, not to exceed 400 mg/day or 8.8 mg/kg/day

Adults: 100 mg 4 times/day for 7 days

Mechanism of Action Inhibits several vital enzymatic reactions causing antibacterial and antiprotozoal action

Local Anesthetic/Vasoconstrictor Precautions No information available to require special precautions

Effects on Dental Treatment No effects or complications reported

Other Adverse Effects

>10%: Genitourinary: Dark yellow to brown discoloration of urine

1% to 10%:

Central nervous system: Headache

Gastrointestinal: Abdominal pain, diarrhea, nausea, vomiting

<1%:

Cardiovascular: Orthostatic hypotension

Central nervous system: Fever, dizziness, drowsiness, malaise

Dermatologic: Skin rash

Endocrine & metabolic: Hypoglycemia, disulfiram-like reaction after alcohol ingestion, leukopenia

Hematologic: Agranulocytosis, hemolysis in patients with G-6-PD deficiency

Neuromuscular & skeletal: Arthralgia

Drug Interactions

Increased effect with indirectly acting sympathomimetic amines such as ephedrine and phenylephrine, tricyclic antidepressants, tyramine-containing foods, MAO inhibitors, meperidine, anorexiants, dextromethorphan, fluoxetine, paroxetine, sertraline, trazodone

Increased effect/toxicity of levodopa

Disulfiram-like reaction with alcohol

Drug Uptake

Absorption: Oral: Poor

Pregnancy Risk Factor C

Generic Available No

Furosemida (Mexico) *see Furosemide on this page*

Furosemide (fyoor OH se mide)

Related Information

Cardiovascular Diseases *on page 1010*

Brand Names Lasix®

Canadian/Mexican Brand Names Apo®-Furosemide (Canada); Edenol® (Mexico); Furoside® (Canada); Henexal® (Mexico); Novo-Semide® (Canada); Uritol® (Canada)

Therapeutic Category Diuretic, Loop

Synonyms Furosemida (Mexico); Fursemide (Canada)

Use Management of edema associated with congestive heart failure and hepatic or renal disease; used alone or in combination with antihypertensives in treatment of hypertension

Usual Dosage

Children:

Oral: 1-2 mg/kg/dose increased in increments of 1 mg/kg/dose with each succeeding dose until a satisfactory effect is achieved to a maximum of 6 mg/kg/dose no more frequently than 6 hours

I.M., I.V.: 1 mg/kg/dose, increasing by each succeeding dose at 1 mg/kg/dose at intervals of 6-12 hours until a satisfactory response up to 6 mg/kg/dose

Adults:

Oral: 20-80 mg/dose initially increased in increments of 20-40 mg/dose at intervals of 6-8 hours; usual maintenance dose interval is twice daily or every day

I.M., I.V.: 20-40 mg/dose, may be repeated in 1-2 hours as needed and increased by 20 mg/dose with each succeeding dose up to 1000 mg/day; usual dosing interval: 6-12 hours

Continuous I.V. infusion: Initial I.V. bolus dose of 0.1 mg/kg followed by continuous I.V. infusion doses of 0.1 mg/kg/hour doubled every 2 hours to a maximum of 0.4 mg/kg/hour if urine output is <1 mL/kg/hour have been found to be effective and result in a lower daily requirement of furosemide than with intermittent dosing. Other studies have used 20-160 mg/hour continuous I.V. infusion

Elderly: Oral, I.M., I.V.: Initial: 20 mg/day; increase slowly to desired response

Mechanism of Action Inhibits reabsorption of sodium and chloride in the ascending loop of Henle and distal renal tubule, interfering with the chloride-binding cotransport system, thus causing increased excretion of water, sodium, chloride, magnesium, and calcium

Local Anesthetic/Vasoconstrictor Precautions No information available to require special precautions

Effects on Dental Treatment No effects or complications reported

Other Adverse Effects

>10%:
  Cardiovascular: Orthostatic hypotension
  Central nervous system: Dizziness

1% to 10%:
  Central nervous system: Headache
  Dermatologic: Photosensitivity
  Endocrine & metabolic: Electrolyte imbalance (hypokalemia, hyponatremia, hypochloremia, hypercalciuria, hyperuricemia), alkalosis, dehydration
  Gastrointestinal: Diarrhea, loss of appetite, stomach cramps or pain
  Ocular: Blurred vision

<1%:
  Dermatologic: Skin rash
  Endocrine & metabolic: Gout
  Gastrointestinal: Pancreatitis, nausea
  Genitourinary: Prerenal azotemia
  Hepatic: Hepatic dysfunction
  Hematologic: Agranulocytosis, leukopenia, anemia, thrombocytopenia
  Local: Redness at injection site
  Ocular: Xanthopsia
  Otic: Ototoxicity
  Renal: Nephrocalcinosis, interstitial nephritis

Drug Interactions

Decreased effect:
  Furosemide interferes with hypoglycemic effect of antidiabetic agents
  Indomethacin may reduce natriuretic and hypotensive effects of furosemide

Increased effect: Effects of antihypertensive agents may be enhanced by furosemide

Increased toxicity:
  Furosemide inhibits renal clearance of lithium resulting in risk of lithium toxicity
  Concomitant use of furosemide with aminoglycoside antibiotics or other ototoxic drugs should be avoided

Drug Uptake

Onset of diuresis:
  Oral: Within 30-60 minutes
  I.M.: 30 minutes
  I.V.: Within 5 minutes
Peak effect: Oral: Within 1-2 hours
Duration:
  Oral: 6-8 hours
  I.V.: 2 hours
Absorption: Oral: 60% to 67%
Serum half-life:
  Normal renal function: 0.5-1.1 hours
  End stage renal disease: 9 hours

Pregnancy Risk Factor C

Generic Available Yes

Furoxone® see Furazolidone on previous page

Fursemide (Canada) see Furosemide on previous page

G-1® see Butalbital Compound on page 154

G-1® see Butalbital Compound and Acetaminophen on page 155

Gabapentin (GA ba pen tin)
Brand Names Neurontin®
Therapeutic Category Anticonvulsant, Miscellaneous
Use Adjunct for treatment of drug-refractory partial and secondarily generalized seizures in adults with epilepsy; not effective for absence seizures
Usual Dosage If gabapentin is discontinued or if another anticonvulsant is added to therapy, it should be done slowly over a minimum of 1 week
  Children >12 years and Adults: Oral:
    Initial: 300 mg on day 1 (at bedtime to minimize sedation), then 300 mg twice daily on day 2, and then 300 mg 3 times/day on day 3
    Total daily dosage range: 900-1800 mg/day administered in 3 divided doses at 8-hour intervals
Mechanism of Action Exact mechanism of action is not known, but does have properties in common with other anticonvulsants; although structurally related to GABA, it does not interact with GABA receptors
Local Anesthetic/Vasoconstrictor Precautions No information available to require special precautions
Effects on Dental Treatment No effects or complications reported
Other Adverse Effects
  >10%: Central nervous system: Somnolence, dizziness, abnormal coordination, fatigue
  1% to 10%:
    Cardiovascular: Peripheral edema
    Central nervous system: Nervousness, amnesia, depression, anxiety
    Dermatologic: Pruritus
    Gastrointestinal: Dyspepsia, dry mouth/throat, nausea, constipation, appetite stimulation (weight gain)
    Genitourinary: Impotence
    Hematologic: Leukopenia
    Neuromuscular & skeletal: Back pain, myalgia, dysarthria, tremor, abnormal coordination
    Ocular: Diplopia, blurred vision, nystagmus
    Respiratory: Rhinitis, bronchospasm
    Miscellaneous: Hiccups
Drug Interactions
  Gabapentin does not modify plasma concentrations of standard anticonvulsant medications (ie, valproic acid, carbamazepine, phenytoin, or phenobarbital)
  Decreased effect: Antacids reduce the bioavailability of gabapentin by 20%
  Increased toxicity: Cimetidine may decrease clearance of gabapentin; gabapentin may increase levels of norethindrone by 13%
Drug Uptake
  Absorption: Oral: 50% to 60%
  Serum half-life: 5-6 hours
Pregnancy Risk Factor C
Generic Available No

Ganciclovir (gan SYE kloe veer)
Related Information
  Systemic Viral Diseases on page 1047
Brand Names Cytovene®; Vitrasert®
Canadian/Mexican Brand Names Cymevene® (Mexico)
Therapeutic Category Antiviral Agent, Parenteral
Synonyms Ganciclovir Sodico (Mexico)
Use Treatment of CMV retinitis in immunocompromised individuals, including patients with acquired immunodeficiency syndrome; treatment of CMV pneumonia in marrow transplant recipients AIDS patients and organ transplant recipients with CMV colitis, pneumonitis, and multiorgan involvement; bone marrow transplant patients when given in combination with IVIG or CMV hyperimmune globulin

Oral: Alternative to the I.V. formulation for maintenance treatment of CMV retinitis in immunocompromised patients, including patients with AIDS, in whom retinitis is stable following appropriate induction therapy and for whom the risk of more rapid progression is balanced by the benefit associated with avoiding daily I.V. infusions

Usual Dosage

Slow I.V. infusion (dosing is based on total body weight):

Children >3 months and Adults:

Induction therapy: 5 mg/kg/dose every 12 hours for 14-21 days followed by maintenance therapy

Maintenance therapy: 5 mg/kg/day as a single daily dose for 7 days/week or 6 mg/kg/day for 5 days/week

Oral: 1000 mg 3 times/day with food **or** 500 mg 6 times/day with food

Mechanism of Action Ganciclovir is phosphorylated to a substrate which competitively inhibits the binding of deoxyguanosine triphosphate to DNA polymerase resulting in inhibition of viral DNA synthesis

Local Anesthetic/Vasoconstrictor Precautions No information available to require special precautions

Effects on Dental Treatment No effects or complications reported

Other Adverse Effects

>10%:

Central nervous system: Headache

Hematologic: Granulocytopenia, thrombocytopenia

1% to 10%:

Central nervous system: Confusion, fever

Dermatologic: Rash

Hematologic: Anemia

Hepatic: Abnormal liver function values

Miscellaneous: Sepsis

<1%:

Cardiovascular: Arrhythmia, hypertension, hypotension, edema

Central nervous system: Ataxia, dizziness, nervousness, psychosis, malaise, coma

Dermatologic: Alopecia, pruritus, urticaria

Gastrointestinal: Nausea, vomiting, diarrhea, abdominal pain

Hematologic: Eosinophilia, hemorrhage

Local: Inflammation or pain at injection site

Neuromuscular & skeletal: Paresthesia, tremor

Ocular: Retinal detachment

Respiratory: Dyspnea

Drug Interactions

Increased toxicity:

Zidovudine, immunosuppressive agents leads to increased hematologic toxicity

Imipenem/cilastatin leads to increased seizure potential

Probenecid: The renal clearance of ganciclovir is decreased in the presence of probenecid

Drug Uptake

Absorption: Oral: Absolute bioavailability under fasting conditions: 5% and following food: 6% to 9%; following fatty meal: 28% to 31%

Serum half-life: 1.7-5.8 hours; increases with impaired renal function

End stage renal disease: 3.6 hours

Pregnancy Risk Factor C

Generic Available No

Ganciclovir Sodico (Mexico) *see* Ganciclovir *on previous page*

Gantanol® *see* Sulfamethoxazole *on page 893*

Gantrisin® *see* Sulfisoxazole *on page 896*

Garamycin® *see* Gentamicin *on page 440*

Gas-Ban DS® [OTC] *see* Aluminum Hydroxide, Magnesium Hydroxide, and Simethicone *on page 49*

Gas Relief® *see* Simethicone *on page 865*

Gastrocrom® *see* Cromolyn Sodium *on page 264*

Gastrosed™ *see* Hyoscyamine *on page 492*

Gas-X® [OTC] *see* Simethicone *on page 865*

Gaviscon®-2 Tablet [OTC] *see* Aluminum Hydroxide and Magnesium Trisilicate *on page 49*

Gaviscon® Liquid [OTC] *see* Aluminum Hydroxide and Magnesium Carbonate *on page 48*

Gaviscon® Tablet [OTC] *see* Aluminum Hydroxide and Magnesium Trisilicate *on page 49*

G-CSF *see* Filgrastim *on page 404*

Gee Gee® [OTC] *see* Guaifenesin *on page 452*

Gelatin, Absorbable (JEL a tin, ab SORB a ble)
Brand Names Gelfoam® Topical
Canadian/Mexican Brand Names Gelafundin® (Mexico); Haemaccel® (Mexico)
Therapeutic Category Hemostatic Agent
Synonyms Gelatina Desdoblada Pulimerizado De (Mexico)
Use
Dental: Adjunct to provide hemostasis in oral and dental surgery
Medical: In medicine, adjunct to provide hemostasis in surgery; open prostatic surgery
Usual Dosage Hemostasis: Apply packs or sponges dry or saturated with sodium chloride. When applied dry, hold in place with moderate pressure. When applied wet, squeeze to remove air bubbles. The powder is applied as a paste prepared by adding approximately 4 mL of sterile saline solution to the powder.
Local Anesthetic/Vasoconstrictor Precautions No information available to require special precautions
Effects on Dental Treatment No effects or complications reported
Other Adverse Effects 1% to 10%: Local: Infection and abscess formation
Contraindications Should not be used in closure of skin incisions since they may interfere with the healing of skin edges
Warnings/Precautions Do not sterilize by heat; do not use in the presence of infection
Drug Interactions No data reported
Pregnancy Risk Factor No data reported
Breast-feeding Considerations No data reported
Dosage Forms
Packs:
Size 2 cm (40 cm x 2 cm) (1s)
Size 6 cm (40 cm x 6 cm) (6s)
Packs, dental:
Size 2 (10 mm x 20 mm x 7 mm) (15s)
Size 4 (20 mm x 20 mm x 7 mm) (15s)
Generic Available No

Gelatina Desdoblada Pulimerizado De (Mexico) *see* Gelatin, Absorbable *on this page*

Gelatin, Pectin, and Methylcellulose
(JEL a tin, PEK tin, & meth il SEL yoo lose)
Brand Names Orabase® Plain [OTC]
Therapeutic Category Protectant, Topical
Use Temporary relief from minor oral irritations
Local Anesthetic/Vasoconstrictor Precautions No information available to require special precautions
Effects on Dental Treatment No effects or complications reported
Generic Available No

Gelfoam® Topical *see* Gelatin, Absorbable *on this page*

Gel-Kam® *see* Fluoride *on page 415*

Gelpirin® [OTC] *see* Acetaminophen, Aspirin, and Caffeine *on page 24*

Gel-Tin® [OTC] *see* Fluoride *on page 415*

Gelucast® *see* Zinc Gelatin *on page 1004*

Gelusil® [OTC] *see* Aluminum Hydroxide, Magnesium Hydroxide, and Simethicone *on page 49*

Gemcitabine (jem SIT a been)
Brand Names Gemzar®
Therapeutic Category Antineoplastic Agent, Miscellaneous
Synonyms Gemcitabine Hydrochloride
Use Treatment of patients with inoperable pancreatic cancer
Usual Dosage Adults: I.V.: 1000 mg/m² once weekly for up to 7 weeks (or until toxicity necessitates reducing or holding a dose), followed by a week of rest from treatment. Subsequent cycles should consist of infusions once weekly for 3 consecutive weeks out of every 4 weeks.
Mechanism of Action Nucleoside analogue that primarily kills cells undergoing DNA synthesis (S-phase) and blocks the progression of cells through the G1/S-phase boundary
Local Anesthetic/Vasoconstrictor Precautions No information available to require special precautions
Effects on Dental Treatment No effects or complications reported

Other Adverse Effects

>10%:

Cardiovascular: Peripheral edema

Central nervous system: Fever

Dermatologic: Rash, alopecia

Gastrointestinal: Nausea, vomiting, constipation, diarrhea, stomatitis

Hematologic: Anemia, leukopenia, neutropenia, thrombocytopenia

Hepatic: Elevated liver enzymes (ALT, AST, alkaline phosphatase) and bilirubin

Neuromuscular & skeletal: Pain

Renal: Proteinuria, hematuria, elevated BUN

Respiratory: Dyspnea

Miscellaneous: Infection

Warnings/Precautions The U.S. Food & Drug Administration (FDA) recommends that procedures for proper handling and disposal of antineoplastic agents be considered. Prolongation of the infusion time >60 minutes and more frequent than weekly dosing have been shown to increase toxicity. Gemcitabine can suppress bone marrow function manifested by leukopenia, thrombocytopenia and anemia, and myelosuppression is usually the dose-limiting ototoxicity. The incidence of fever is 41% and gemcitabine may cause fever in the absence of clinical infection. Rash has been reported in 30% of patients - typically a macular or finely granular maculopapular pruritic eruption of mild-moderate severity involving the trunk and extremities. Gemcitabine should be used with caution in patients with pre-existing renal impairment (mild proteinuria and hematuria were commonly reported; hemolytic uremic syndrome has been reported) and hepatic impairment (associated with transient elevations of serum transaminases in $2/3$ of patients - but no evidence of increasing hepatic toxicity).

Drug Uptake Serum half-life: 42-94 minutes

Pregnancy Risk Factor D

Generic Available No

Gemcitabine Hydrochloride *see* Gemcitabine *on previous page*

Gemfibrozil (jem FI broe zil)

Related Information

Cardiovascular Diseases *on page 1010*

Brand Names Lopid®

Canadian/Mexican Brand Names Apo®-Gemfibrozil (Canada); Nu-Gemfibrozil® (Canada)

Therapeutic Category Lipid Lowering Drugs

Use Treatment of hypertriglyceridemia in types IV and V hyperlipidemia for patients who are at greater risk for pancreatitis and who have not responded to dietary intervention; reduction of coronary heart disease in type IIB patients who have low HDL-cholesterol, increased LDL cholesterol, and increased triglycerides

Usual Dosage Adults: Oral: 1200 mg/day in 2 divided doses, 30 minutes before breakfast and dinner

Hemodialysis effects: Not removed by hemodialysis; supplemental dose is not necessary

Mechanism of Action The exact mechanism of action of gemfibrozil is unknown, however, several theories exist regarding the VLDL effect; it can inhibit lipolysis and decrease subsequent hepatic fatty acid uptake as well as inhibit hepatic secretion of VLDL; together these actions decrease serum VLDL levels; increases HDL cholesterol; the mechanism behind HDL elevation is currently unknown

Local Anesthetic/Vasoconstrictor Precautions No information available to require special precautions

Effects on Dental Treatment No effects or complications reported

Other Adverse Effects

>10%:

Gastrointestinal: Dyspepsia, abdominal pain

Hepatic: Cholelithiasis

1% to 10%:

Central nervous system: Fatigue, vertigo, headache

Dermatologic: Eczema, rash

Gastrointestinal: Diarrhea, nausea, vomiting, constipation, acute appendicitis

<1%:

Cardiovascular: Atrial fibrillation

Central nervous system: Hypesthesia, dizziness, drowsiness, mental depression

Gastrointestinal: Flatulence

Neuromuscular & skeletal: Paresthesia

Ocular: Blurred vision

(Continued)

Gemfibrozil *(Continued)*

Drug Interactions
Increased toxicity:
Gemfibrozil may potentiate the effects of warfarin
Manufacturer warns against the use of gemfibrozil with concomitant lovastatin therapy

Drug Uptake
Absorption: Well absorbed
Serum half-life: 1.4 hours
Time to peak serum concentration: Within 1-2 hours

Pregnancy Risk Factor B
Generic Available Yes

Gemzar® *see* Gemcitabine *on page 438*

Genabid® *see* Papaverine *on page 722*

Genac® Tablet [OTC] *see* Triprolidine and Pseudoephedrine *on page 969*

Genagesic® *see* Guaifenesin and Phenylpropanolamine *on page 454*

Genahist® Oral *see* Diphenhydramine *on page 323*

Genamin® Cold Syrup [OTC] *see* Chlorpheniramine and Phenylpropanolamine *on page 219*

Genamin® Expectorant [OTC] *see* Guaifenesin and Phenylpropanolamine *on page 454*

Genapap® [OTC] *see* Acetaminophen *on page 20*

Genasoft® Plus [OTC] *see* Docusate and Casanthranol *on page 331*

Genaspor® [OTC] *see* Tolnaftate *on page 943*

Genatap® Elixir [OTC] *see* Brompheniramine and Phenylpropanolamine *on page 143*

Genatuss® [OTC] *see* Guaifenesin *on page 452*

Genatuss DM® [OTC] *see* Guaifenesin and Dextromethorphan *on page 453*

Gencalc® 600 [OTC] *see* Calcium Carbonate *on page 162*

Geneye® Ophthalmic [OTC] *see* Tetrahydrozoline *on page 916*

Gen-K® *see* Potassium Chloride *on page 778*

Genora® 0.5/35 *see* Ethinyl Estradiol and Norethindrone *on page 379*

Genora® 1/35 *see* Ethinyl Estradiol and Norethindrone *on page 379*

Genora® 1/50 *see* Mestranol and Norethindrone *on page 603*

Genotropin® Injection *see* Human Growth Hormone *on page 473*

Genpril® [OTC] *see* Ibuprofen *on page 495*

Gentamicin *(jen ta MYE sin)*

Related Information
Antimicrobial Prophylaxis in Surgical Patients *on page 1163*
Cardiovascular Diseases *on page 1010*

Brand Names Garamycin®
Canadian/Mexican Brand Names Garalen® (Mexico); Garamicina® (Mexico); Genenicina® (Mexico); Genkova® (Mexico); Genrex® (Mexico); Gentarim® (Mexico); Nozolon® (Mexico); Quilagen® (Mexico); Yectamicina® (Mexico)
Therapeutic Category Antibiotic, Aminoglycoside; Antibiotic, Ophthalmic; Antibiotic, Topical

Use
Dental: An alternate antibiotic for the prevention of bacterial endocarditis in patients undergoing dental procedures; it is to be used in those patients considered high risk and not candidates for the standard regimen of prevention of bacterial endocarditis
Medical: Treatment of susceptible bacterial infections, normally gram-negative organisms including *Pseudomonas, Proteus, Serratia,* and gram-positive *Staphylococcus;* treatment of bone infections, respiratory tract infections, skin and soft tissue infections, as well as abdominal and urinary tract infections, endocarditis, and septicemia; used topically to treat superficial infections of the skin or ophthalmic infections caused by susceptible bacteria

Usual Dosage
Children: 2 mg/kg with total dose not exceeding total adult dose
Adults; I.M., I.V.: 2 g plus gentamicin 1.5 mg/kg (not to exceed 80 mg) 30 minutes before the procedure, followed by amoxicillin 1.5 g orally 6 hours after initial dose; alternatively, the parenteral regimen may be repeated 8 hours after initial dose

Mechanism of Action Interferes with bacterial protein synthesis by binding to 30S and 50S ribosomal subunits resulting in a defective bacterial cell membrane
Local Anesthetic/Vasoconstrictor Precautions No information available to require special precautions
Effects on Dental Treatment Increased salivation has been reported

Other Adverse Effects
>10%:
Central nervous system: Neurotoxicity (vertigo, ataxia, gait instability)
Otic: Ototoxicity (auditory), ototoxicity (vestibular)
Renal: Nephrotoxicity, decreased creatinine clearance
1% to 10%: Dermatologic: Itching, redness, rash, swelling
Contraindications Hypersensitivity to gentamicin or other aminoglycosides
Warnings/Precautions
Not intended for long-term therapy due to toxic hazards associated with extended administration; pre-existing renal insufficiency, vestibular or cochlear impairment, myasthenia gravis, hypocalcemia, conditions which depress neuromuscular transmission
Parenteral aminoglycosides are associated with significant nephrotoxicity or ototoxicity; the ototoxicity may be directly proportional to the amount of drug given and the duration of treatment; tinnitus or vertigo are indications of vestibular injury and impending hearing loss; renal damage is usually reversible
Drug Interactions Penicillins, cephalosporins, amphotericin B, loop diuretics may increase nephrotoxic potential; neuromuscular blocking agents may increase neuromuscular blockade
Drug Uptake
Absorption: Oral: Not absorbed
Serum half-life: Adults: 1.5-3 hours
Time to peak serum concentration:
I.M.: Within 30-90 minutes
I.V.: 30 minutes after a 30-minute infusion
Pregnancy Risk Factor C
Breast-feeding Considerations No data reported; however, gentamicin is not absorbed orally and other aminoglycosides may be taken while breast-feeding
Dosage Forms
Injection: 40 mg/mL (1 mL, 2 mL, 10 mL, 20 mL)
Injection, pediatric: 10 mg/mL (2 mL)
Generic Available Yes
Selected Readings
Council on Dental Therapeutics, American Heart Association, "Preventing Bacterial Endocarditis," *J Am Dent Assoc*, 1991, 122(2):87-92.
Dajani AS, Bisno AL, Chung KJ, et al, "Prevention of Bacterial Endocarditis, Recommendations by the American Heart Association," *JAMA*, 1990, 264(22):2919-22.
Wynn RL, "Gentamicin for Prophylaxis of Bacterial Endocarditis: A Review for the Dentist," *Oral Surg Oral Med Oral Pathol*, 1985, 60(2):159-65.

Gentamicin and Prednisolone *see* Prednisolone and Gentamicin *on page 789*

Gentian Violet (JEN shun VYE oh let)

Therapeutic Category Antibacterial, Topical; Antifungal Agent, Topical
Use Treatment of cutaneous or mucocutaneous infections caused by *Candida albicans* and other superficial skin infections - antibacterial and antifungal dye
Usual Dosage Children and Adults: Topical: Apply 0.5% to 2% locally with cotton to lesion 2-3 times/day for 3 days, do not swallow and avoid contact with eyes
Mechanism of Action Topical antiseptic/germicide effective against some vegetative gram-positive bacteria, particularly *Staphylococcus* sp, and some yeast; it is much less effective against gram-negative bacteria and is ineffective against acid-fast bacteria
Local Anesthetic/Vasoconstrictor Precautions No information available to require special precautions
Effects on Dental Treatment No effects or complications reported
Other Adverse Effects 1% to 10%:
Local: Esophagitis, burning, irritation, vesicle formation, ulceration of mucous membranes
Systemic: Sensitivity reactions, laryngitis, tracheitis, laryngeal obstruction
Drug Interactions No data reported
Pregnancy Risk Factor C
Generic Available Yes

Gentran® *see* Dextran *on page 295*

Gen-XENE® *see* Clorazepate *on page 251*

Geocillin® *see* Carbenicillin *on page 175*

Geref® Injection *see* Sermorelin Acetate *on page 862*

German Measles Vaccine *see* Rubella Virus Vaccine, Live *on page 851*

Germinal® *see* Ergoloid Mesylates *on page 358*

Gevrabon® [OTC] *see* Vitamin B Complex *on page 993*

GG-Cen® [OTC] *see* Guaifenesin *on page 452*

Gingi-Aid® Gingival Retraction Cord *see* Aluminum Chloride *on page 47*

Gingi-Aid® Solution *see* Aluminum Chloride *on page 47*

Glatiramer Acetate (gla TIR a mer AS e tate)

Brand Names Copaxone®

Therapeutic Category Biological, Miscellaneous

Synonyms Copolymer-1

Use Relapsing-remitting type multiple sclerosis; studies indicate that it reduces the frequency of attacks and the severity of disability; appears to be most effective for patients with minimal disability and has not demonstrated benefits in the chronic progressive form of multiple sclerosis

Usual Dosage Adults: S.C.: 20 mg daily

Mechanism of Action Glatiramer is a mixture of random polymers of four amino acids; L-alanine, L-glutamic acid, L-lysine and L-tyrosine, the resulting mixture is antigenically similar to myelin basic protein, which is an important component of the myelin sheath of nerves; glatiramer is thought to suppress T-lymphocytes specific for a myelin antigen, it is also proposed that glatiramer interferes with the antigen-presenting function of certain immune cells opposing pathogenic T-cell function

Local Anesthetic/Vasoconstrictor Precautions No information available to require special precautions

Effects on Dental Treatment No effects or complications reported

Other Adverse Effects

>10%:

Dermatologic: Erythema

Local: Pain

1% to 10%:

Cardiovascular: Chest pain or tightness, flushing

Central nervous system: Anxiety

Hematologic: Transient eosinophilia

Respiratory: Dyspnea

Miscellaneous: Diaphoresis

Contraindications Previous hypersensitivity to any component of the copolymer formulation

Pregnancy Risk Factor B

Dosage Forms

Injection: Single-use vials containing 20 mg of glatiramer and 40 mg mannitol; packaged in 2 mL vials along with 1 mL vial of diluent (sterile water for injection)

GlaucTabs® *see* Methazolamide *on page 610*

Glibenclamida (Mexico) *see* Glyburide *on page 445*

Glimepiride (GLYE me pye ride)

Related Information

Endocrine Disorders & Pregnancy *on page 1021*

Brand Names Amaryl®

Therapeutic Category Antidiabetic Agent; Hypoglycemic Agent, Oral; Sulfonylurea Agent

Use

Management of noninsulin-dependent diabetes mellitus (type II) as an adjunct to diet and exercise to lower blood glucose

Use in combination with insulin to lower blood glucose in patients whose hyperglycemia cannot be controlled by diet and exercise in conjunction with an oral hypoglycemic agent

Usual Dosage Oral (allow several days between dose titrations):

Adults: Initial: 1-2 mg once daily, administered with breakfast or the first main meal; usual maintenance dose: 1-4 mg once daily; after a dose of 2 mg once daily, increase in increments of 2 mg at 1- to 2-week intervals based upon the patient's blood glucose response to a maximum of 8 mg once daily

Elderly: Initial: 1 mg/day

Combination with insulin therapy (fasting glucose level for instituting combination therapy is in the range of >150 mg/dL in plasma or serum depending on the patient): 8 mg once daily with the first main meal

After starting with low-dose insulin, upward adjustments of insulin can be done approximately weekly as guided by frequent measurements of fasting blood glucose. Once stable, combination-therapy patients should monitor their capillary blood glucose on an ongoing basis, preferably daily.

Dosing adjustment/comments in renal impairment: Cl_{cr} <22 mL/minute: Initial starting dose should be 1 mg and dosage increments should be based on fasting blood glucose levels

Dosing adjustment in hepatic impairment: No data available

Mechanism of Action Stimulates insulin release from the pancreatic beta cells; reduces glucose output from the liver; insulin sensitivity is increased at peripheral target sites

Local Anesthetic/Vasoconstrictor Precautions No information available to require special precautions

Effects on Dental Treatment Glipizide-dependent diabetics (noninsulin dependent, Type II) should be appointed for dental treatment in morning in order to minimize chance of stress-induced hypoglycemia

Contraindications Hypersensitivity to glimepiride or any component, other sulfonamides; diabetic ketoacidosis (with or without coma)

Warnings/Precautions

The administration of oral hypoglycemic drugs (ie, tolbutamide) has been reported to be associated with increased cardiovascular mortality as compared to treatment with diet alone or diet plus insulin

All sulfonylurea drugs are capable of producing severe hypoglycemia. Hypoglycemia is more likely to occur when caloric intake is deficient, after severe or prolonged exercise, when alcohol is ingested, or when more than one glucose-lowering drug is used.

Drug Interactions

Decreased effects: Beta-blockers, cholestyramine, hydantoins, rifampin, thiazide diuretics, urinary alkalines, charcoal

Increased effects: H_2 antagonists, anticoagulants, androgens, fluconazole, salicylates, gemfibrozil, sulfonamides, tricyclic antidepressants, probenecid, MAO inhibitors, methyldopa, digitalis glycosides, urinary acidifiers

Increased toxicity: Cimetidine → ↑ hypoglycemic effects

Drug Uptake

Duration of action: 24 hours

Peak blood glucose reductions: Within 2-3 hours

Absorption: 100% absorbed; delayed when given with food

Serum half-life: 5-9 hours

Pregnancy Risk Factor C

Generic Available No

Glipicida (Mexico) *see* Glipizide *on this page*

Glipizida (Mexico) *see* Glipizide *on this page*

Glipizide (GLIP i zide)

Related Information

Endocrine Disorders & Pregnancy *on page 1021*

Brand Names Glucotrol®; Glucotrol® XL

Canadian/Mexican Brand Names Minodiab® (Mexico)

Therapeutic Category Antidiabetic Agent; Hypoglycemic Agent, Oral; Sulfonylurea Agent

Synonyms Glipicida (Mexico); Glipizida (Mexico)

Use Management of noninsulin-dependent diabetes mellitus (type II)

Usual Dosage Oral (allow several days between dose titrations):

Adults: 2.5-40 mg/day; doses >15-20 mg/day should be divided and given twice daily

Elderly: Initial: 2.5-5 mg/day; increase by 2.5-5 mg/day at 1- to 2-week intervals

Mechanism of Action Stimulates insulin release from the pancreatic beta cells; reduces glucose output from the liver; insulin sensitivity is increased at peripheral target sites

Local Anesthetic/Vasoconstrictor Precautions No information available to require special precautions

Effects on Dental Treatment Glipizide-dependent diabetics (noninsulin dependent, Type II) should be appointed for dental treatment in morning in order to minimize chance of stress-induced hypoglycemia

Other Adverse Effects

>10%:

Central nervous system: Headache

Gastrointestinal: Anorexia, nausea, vomiting, diarrhea, epigastric fullness, constipation, heartburn

1% to 10%: Dermatologic: Rash, urticaria, photosensitivity

<1%:

Cardiovascular: Edema

Endocrine & metabolic: Hypoglycemia, hyponatremia

Hematologic: Blood dyscrasias, aplastic anemia, hemolytic anemia, bone marrow suppression, thrombocytopenia, agranulocytosis

Hepatic: Cholestatic jaundice

Renal: Diuretic effect

(Continued)

Glipizide *(Continued)*

Drug Interactions
Salicylates may enhance the hypoglycemic response to glipizide due to increased plasma levels of glipizide by displacing from plasma proteins
Thiazide diuretics will increase blood glucose leading to increased requirements of glipizide

Drug Uptake
Duration of action: 12-24 hours
Peak blood glucose reductions: Within 1.5-2 hours
Absorption: Delayed when given with food
Serum half-life: 2-4 hours

Pregnancy Risk Factor C

Generic Available Yes

Glucagon (GLOO ka gon)

Therapeutic Category Antihypoglycemic Agent

Use
Hypoglycemia; diagnostic aid in the radiologic examination of GI tract when a hypotonic state is needed; used with some success as a cardiac stimulant in management of severe cases of beta-adrenergic blocking agent overdosage

Usual Dosage
Hypoglycemia or insulin shock therapy: I.M., I.V., S.C.:
Children: 0.025-0.1 mg/kg/dose, not to exceed 1 mg/dose, repeated in 20 minutes as needed
Adults: 0.5-1 mg, may repeat in 20 minutes as needed
If patient fails to respond to glucagon, I.V. dextrose must be given
Diagnostic aid: Adults: I.M., I.V.: 0.25-2 mg 10 minutes prior to procedure

Mechanism of Action
Stimulates adenylate cyclase to produce increased cyclic AMP, which promotes hepatic glycogenolysis and gluconeogenesis, causing a raise in blood glucose levels

Local Anesthetic/Vasoconstrictor Precautions
No information available to require special precautions

Effects on Dental Treatment
No effects or complications reported

Other Adverse Effects 1% to 10%:
Cardiovascular: Hypotension
Dermatologic: Urticaria
Gastrointestinal: Nausea, vomiting
Respiratory: Respiratory distress

Drug Uptake
Peak effect on blood glucose levels: Parenteral: Within 5-20 minutes
Duration of action: 60-90 minutes
Serum half-life, plasma: 3-10 minutes

Pregnancy Risk Factor B

Generic Available No

Comments 1 unit = 1 mg

Glucocerebrosidase *see* Alglucerase *on page 40*

Glucophage® *see* Metformin *on page 607*

Glucose (GLOO kose, IN stant)

Brand Names B-D Glucose® [OTC]; Glutose® [OTC]; Insta-Glucose® [OTC]

Therapeutic Category Antihypoglycemic Agent

Use Management of hypoglycemia

Local Anesthetic/Vasoconstrictor Precautions
No information available to require special precautions

Effects on Dental Treatment No effects or complications reported

Other Adverse Effects 1% to 10%:
Cardiovascular: Syncope
Gastrointestinal: Nausea, vomiting, diarrhea

Pregnancy Risk Factor A

Generic Available Yes

Comments 4 calories/g

Glucose Polymers (GLOO kose POL i merz)

Brand Names Moducal® [OTC]; Polycose® [OTC]; Sumacal® [OTC]

Therapeutic Category Nutritional Supplement

Use
Supplies calories for those persons not able to meet the caloric requirement with usual food intake

Local Anesthetic/Vasoconstrictor Precautions
No information available to require special precautions

Effects on Dental Treatment No effects or complications reported

Generic Available Yes

Glucotrol® *see* Glipizide *on page 443*
Glucotrol® XL *see* Glipizide *on page 443*

Glutamic Acid (gloo TAM ik AS id)
Therapeutic Category Gastrointestinal Agent, Miscellaneous
Use Treatment of hypochlorhydria and achlorhydria
Local Anesthetic/Vasoconstrictor Precautions No information available to require special precautions
Effects on Dental Treatment No effects or complications reported
Other Adverse Effects Systemic acidosis may occur with massive overdosage
Pregnancy Risk Factor C
Generic Available Yes

Glutethimide (gloo TETH i mide)
Therapeutic Category Hypnotic; Sedative
Use Short-term treatment of insomnia
Local Anesthetic/Vasoconstrictor Precautions No information available to require special precautions
Effects on Dental Treatment No effects or complications reported
Other Adverse Effects
>10%: Central nervous system: Daytime drowsiness
1% to 10%:
Central nervous system: Confusion, headache
Dermatologic: Skin rash
Gastrointestinal: Nausea, vomiting
Ocular: Blurred vision
<1%:
Hematologic: Blood dyscrasias
Cardiovascular: Bradycardia
Central nervous system: Paradoxical reaction, convulsions, fever
Pregnancy Risk Factor C
Generic Available Yes

Glutose® [OTC] *see* Glucose *on previous page*
Glyate® [OTC] *see* Guaifenesin *on page 452*

Glyburide (GLYE byoor ide)
Related Information
Endocrine Disorders & Pregnancy *on page 1021*
Brand Names DiaβBeta®; Glynase™ PresTab™; Micronase®
Canadian/Mexican Brand Names Albert® Glyburide (Canada); Apo®-Glyburide (Canada); Daonil® (Mexico); Euglucon® (Canada); Euglucon® (Mexico); Gen-Glybe® (Canada); Glibenil® (Mexico); Glucal® (Mexico); Norboral® (Mexico); Novo-Glyburide® (Canada); Nu-Glyburide® (Canada)
Therapeutic Category Antidiabetic Agent; Hypoglycemic Agent, Oral; Sulfonylurea Agent
Synonyms Glibenclamida (Mexico)
Use Management of noninsulin-dependent diabetes mellitus (type II)
Usual Dosage Oral:
Adults: 1.25-5 mg to start then increase at weekly intervals to 1.25-20 mg maintenance dose/day divided in 1-2 doses
Elderly: Initial: 1.25-2.5 mg/day, increase by 1.25-2.5 mg/day every 1-3 weeks
Prestab™: Initial: 0.75-3 mg/day, increase by 1.5 mg/day in weekly intervals, maximum: 12 mg/day
Mechanism of Action Stimulates insulin release from the pancreatic beta cells; reduces glucose output from the liver; insulin sensitivity is increased at peripheral target sites
Local Anesthetic/Vasoconstrictor Precautions No information available to require special precautions
Effects on Dental Treatment Glyburide-dependent diabetics (noninsulin dependent, Type II) should be appointed for dental treatment in morning in order to minimize chance of stress-induced hypoglycemia
Other Adverse Effects
>10%:
Central nervous system: Headache, dizziness
Gastrointestinal: Nausea, epigastric fullness, heartburn, constipation, diarrhea, anorexia
1% to 10%: Dermatologic: Pruritus, rash, urticaria, photosensitivity reaction
<1%:
Endocrine & metabolic: Hypoglycemia
Genitourinary: Nocturia
(Continued)

Glyburide *(Continued)*

Hematologic: Leukopenia, thrombocytopenia, hemolytic anemia, aplastic anemia, bone marrow suppression, agranulocytosis

Hepatic: Cholestatic jaundice

Neuromuscular & skeletal: arthralgia, paresthesia

Renal: Diuretic effect

Drug Interactions

Salicylates may enhance the hypoglycemic response to glyburide due to increased plasma levels of glyburide by displacing from plasma proteins

Thiazide diuretics will increase blood glucose leading to increased requirements of glyburide

Drug Uptake

Onset of action: Oral: Insulin levels in the serum begin to increase within 15-60 minutes after a single dose

Duration: Up to 24 hours

Serum half-life: 5-16 hours; may be prolonged with renal insufficiency or hepatic insufficiency

Time to peak serum concentration: Adults: Within 2-4 hours

Pregnancy Risk Factor C

Generic Available yes

Glycerin (GLIS er in)

Brand Names Fleet® Babylax® Rectal [OTC]; Ophthalgan® Ophthalmic; Osmoglyn® Ophthalmic; Sani-Supp® Suppository [OTC]

Therapeutic Category Laxative, Hyperosmolar

Synonyms Glycerol

Use Constipation; reduction of intraocular pressure; reduction of corneal edema; glycerin has been administered orally to reduce intracranial pressure

Usual Dosage

Constipation: Rectal:

Children <6 years: 1 infant suppository 1-2 times/day as needed or 2-5 mL as an enema

Children >6 years and Adults: 1 adult suppository 1-2 times/day as needed or 5-15 mL as an enema

Children and Adults:

Reduction of intraocular pressure: Oral: 1-1.8 g/kg 1-1½ hours preoperatively; additional doses may be administered at 5-hour intervals

Reduction of intracranial pressure: Oral: 1.5 g/kg/day divided every 4 hours; 1 g/kg/dose every 6 hours has also been used

Reduction of corneal edema: Ophthalmic solution: Instill 1-2 drops in eye(s) prior to examination OR for lubricant effect, instill 1-2 drops in eye(s) every 3-4 hours

Mechanism of Action Osmotic dehydrating agent which increases osmotic pressure; draws fluid into colon and thus stimulates evacuation

Local Anesthetic/Vasoconstrictor Precautions No information available to require special precautions

Effects on Dental Treatment No effects or complications reported

Other Adverse Effects

>10%:

Central nervous system: Headache

Gastrointestinal: Nausea, vomiting

1% to 10%:

Central nervous system: Confusion, dizziness

Endocrine: Polydipsia

Gastrointestinal: Diarrhea, dry mouth

<1%:

Cardiovascular: Arrhythmias

Endocrine & metabolic: Hyperglycemia

Gastrointestinal: Tenesmus, rectal irritation, cramping pain

Drug Uptake

Absorption:

Oral: Well absorbed

Rectal: Poorly absorbed

Decrease in intraocular pressure: Oral:

Onset of action: Within 10-30 minutes

Peak effect: Within 60-90 minutes

Duration: 4-8 hours

Reduction of intracranial pressure: Oral:

Onset of action: Within 10-60 minutes

Peak effect: Within 60-90 minutes

Duration: ~2-3 hours

Constipation: Suppository: Onset of action: 15-30 minutes
Serum half-life: 30-45 minutes
Pregnancy Risk Factor C
Generic Available Yes

Glycerin, Lanolin, and Peanut Oil

(GLIS er in, LAN oh lin, & PEE nut oyl)
Brand Names Massé® Breast Cream [OTC]
Therapeutic Category Topical Skin Product
Use Nipple care of pregnant and nursing women
Local Anesthetic/Vasoconstrictor Precautions No information available to require special precautions
Effects on Dental Treatment No effects or complications reported
Generic Available Yes

Glycerol see Glycerin on previous page

Glycerol-T® see Theophylline and Guaifenesin on page 922

Glycerol Triacetate see Triacetin on page 954

Glycofed® see Guaifenesin and Pseudoephedrine on page 454

Glycopyrrolate (glye koe PYE roe late)

Brand Names Robinul®; Robinul® Forte
Therapeutic Category Anticholinergic Agent; Antispasmodic Agent, Gastrointestinal
Use Adjunct in treatment of peptic ulcer disease; inhibit salivation and excessive secretions of the respiratory tract preoperatively; reversal of neuromuscular blockade; control of upper airway secretions
Usual Dosage
Children:
Control of secretions:
Oral: 40-100 mcg/kg/dose 3-4 times/day
I.M., I.V.: 4-10 mcg/kg/dose every 3-4 hours; maximum: 0.2 mg/dose or 0.8 mg/24 hours
Intraoperative: I.V.: 4 mcg/kg not to exceed 0.1 mg; repeat at 2- to 3-minute intervals as needed
Preoperative: I.M.:
<2 years: 4.4-8.8 mcg/kg 30-60 minutes before procedure
>2 years: 4.4 mcg/kg 30-60 minutes before procedure

Children and Adults: Reverse neuromuscular blockade: I.V.: 0.2 mg for each 1 mg of neostigmine or 5 mg of pyridostigmine administered

Adults:
Intraoperative: I.V.: 0.1 mg repeated as needed at 2- to 3-minute intervals
Preoperative: I.M.: 4.4 mcg/kg 30-60 minutes before procedure
Peptic ulcer:
Oral: 1-2 mg 2-3 times/day
I.M., I.V.: 0.1-0.2 mg 3-4 times/day
Mechanism of Action Blocks the action of acetylcholine at parasympathetic sites in smooth muscle, secretory glands, and the CNS
Local Anesthetic/Vasoconstrictor Precautions No information available to require special precautions
Effects on Dental Treatment >10% of patients will experience significant dry mouth (reversible with cessation of drug therapy)
Other Adverse Effects
>10%:
Dermatologic: Dry skin
Gastrointestinal: Constipation
Local: Irritation at injection site
Respiratory: Dry nose, throat
Miscellaneous: Decreased sweating
1% to 10%:
Dermatologic: Photosensitivity
Endocrine & metabolic: Decreased flow of breast milk
Gastrointestinal: Dysphagia
<1%:
Cardiovascular: Orthostatic hypotension, ventricular fibrillation, tachycardia, palpitations
Central nervous system: Confusion, drowsiness, headache, loss of memory, fatigue, ataxia
Dermatologic: Skin rash
Gastrointestinal: Bloated feeling, nausea, vomiting
Genitourinary: Dysuria
(Continued)

Glycopyrrolate *(Continued)*

Neuromuscular & skeletal: Weakness
Ocular: Increased intraocular pain, blurred vision

Drug Interactions
Decreased effect of levodopa
Increased toxicity with amantadine

Drug Uptake
Oral:
Onset of action: Within 50 minutes
I.M.: Onset of action: 20-40 minutes
I.V.: Onset of action: 10-15 minutes
Absorption: Oral: Poor and erratic

Pregnancy Risk Factor B
Generic Available Yes

Glycotuss® [OTC] *see* Guaifenesin *on page 452*

Glycotuss-dM® [OTC] *see* Guaifenesin and Dextromethorphan *on page 453*

Glynase™ PresTab™ *see* Glyburide *on page 445*

Gly-Oxide® Oral [OTC] *see* Carbamide Peroxide *on page 175*

Glyset® *see* Miglitol *on page 638*

Glytuss® [OTC] *see* Guaifenesin *on page 452*

GM-CSF *see* Sargramostim *on page 857*

Gold Sodium Thiomalate *(gold SOW dee um thye oh MAL ate)*

Brand Names Aurolate®
Therapeutic Category Gold Compound
Use Treatment of progressive rheumatoid arthritis
Usual Dosage I.M.:
Children: Initial: Test dose of 10 mg is recommended, followed by 1 mg/kg/week for 20 weeks; maintenance: 1 mg/kg/dose at 2- to 4-week intervals thereafter for as long as therapy is clinically beneficial and toxicity does not develop. Administration for 2-4 months is usually required before clinical improvement is observed.
Adults: 10 mg first week; 25 mg second week; then 25-50 mg/week until 1 g cumulative dose has been given; if improvement occurs without adverse reactions, give 25-50 mg every 2-3 weeks for 2-20 weeks, then every 3-4 weeks indefinitely

Mechanism of Action Unknown, may decrease prostaglandin synthesis or may alter cellular mechanisms by inhibiting sulfhydryl systems

Local Anesthetic/Vasoconstrictor Precautions No information available to require special precautions

Effects on Dental Treatment No effects or complications reported

Other Adverse Effects
>10%:
Dermatologic: Itching, skin rash
Gastrointestinal: Stomatitis, gingivitis, glossitis
Ocular: Conjunctivitis
1% to 10%:
Dermatologic: Urticaria, alopecia
Hematologic: Eosinophilia, leukopenia, thrombocytopenia
Renal: Hematuria, proteinuria
<1%:
Dermatologic: Angioedema, gray-to-blue pigmentation
Gastrointestinal: Dysphagia, ulcerative enterocolitis, GI hemorrhage, metallic taste
Hematologic: Agranulocytosis, anemia, aplastic anemia
Hepatic: Hepatotoxicity
Neuromuscular & skeletal: Peripheral neuropathy
Respiratory: Interstitial pneumonitis

Drug Uptake
Serum half-life: 5 days; may lengthen with multiple doses
Time to peak serum concentration: Within 4-6 hours

Pregnancy Risk Factor C
Generic Available Yes
Comments Approximately 50% gold

GoLYTELY® *see* Polyethylene Glycol-Electrolyte Solution *on page 771*

Gonak™ [OTC] *see* Hydroxypropyl Methylcellulose *on page 490*

Gonal-F® *see* Follitropin Alpha *on page 428*

Gonic® *see* Chorionic Gonadotropin *on page 231*

Gonioscopic Ophthalmic Solution *see* Hydroxypropyl Methylcellulose *on page 490*

Goniosol® [OTC] *see* Hydroxypropyl Methylcellulose *on page 490*

Goody's® Headache Powders *see* Acetaminophen, Aspirin, and Caffeine *on page 24*

Gordofilm® Liquid *see* Salicylic Acid *on page 853*

Goserelin (GOE se rel in)

Brand Names Zoladex® Implant

Canadian/Mexican Brand Names Prozoladex® (Mexico)

Therapeutic Category Gonadotropin Releasing Hormone Analog

Use Palliative treatment of advanced prostate cancer

Usual Dosage
Adults: S.C.: 3.6 mg injected into upper abdomen every 28 days; do not try to aspirate with the goserelin syringe, if the needle is in a large vessel, blood will immediately appear in syringe chamber

Prostate carcinoma: Intended for long-term administration

Endometriosis: Recommended duration is 6 months; retreatment is not recommended since safety data is not available

Mechanism of Action LHRH synthetic analog of luteinizing hormone-releasing hormone also known as gonadotropin-releasing hormone (GnRH) incorporated into a biodegradable depot material which allows for continuous slow release over 28 days; mechanism of action is similar to leuprolide

Local Anesthetic/Vasoconstrictor Precautions No information available to require special precautions

Effects on Dental Treatment No effects or complications reported

Other Adverse Effects
General: Worsening of signs and symptoms may occur during the first few weeks of therapy and are usually manifested by an increase in bone pain, increased difficulty in urinating, hot flashes, injection site irritation, and weakness; this will subside, but patients should be aware

>10%:
Endocrine & metabolic: Gynecomastia, postmenopausal symptoms, sexual dysfunction, loss of libido, hot flashes
Genitourinary: Impotence, decreased erection

1% to 10%:
Cardiovascular: Edema
Central nervous system: Headache, spinal cord compression (possible result of tumor flare), lethargy, dizziness, insomnia
Dermatologic: Rash
Endocrine & metabolic: Breast tenderness/enlargement, vaginal spotting and breakthrough bleeding
Gastrointestinal: Nausea and vomiting, anorexia, diarrhea, weight gain
Local: Pain on injection
Neuromuscular & skeletal: Bone loss, increased bone pain
Miscellaneous: Sweating

Drug Uptake
Absorption:
Oral: Inactive when administered orally
S.C.: Rapid and can be detected in the serum in 10 minutes
Time to peak serum concentration: S.C.: 12-15 days
Serum half-life: Following a bolus S.C. dose: 5 hours

Pregnancy Risk Factor X

Generic Available No

Granisetron (gra NI se tron)

Brand Names Kytril®

Therapeutic Category Antiemetic

Use Prophylaxis and treatment of chemotherapy-related emesis; may be prescribed for patients who are refractory to or have severe adverse reactions to standard antiemetic therapy. Granisetron may be prescribed for young patients (ie, <45 years of age who are more likely to develop extrapyramidal reactions to high-dose metoclopramide) who are to receive highly emetogenic chemotherapeutic agents as listed:

Agents with high emetogenic potential (>90%) (dose/m^2):
Carmustine ≥200 mg
Cisplatin ≥75 mg
Cyclophosphamide ≥1000 mg
Cytarabine ≥1000 mg
Dacarbazine ≥500 mg
Ifosfamide ≥1000 mg
(Continued)

Granisetron *(Continued)*

    Lomustine ≥60 mg
    Mechlorethamine
    Pentostatin
    Streptozocin

or two agents classified as having high or moderately high emetogenic potential as listed:

Agents with moderately high emetogenic potential (60% to 90%) (dose/m^2):
    Carmustine <200 mg
    Cisplatin <75 mg
    Cyclophosphamide 1000 mg
    Cytarabine 250-1000 mg
    Dacarbazine <500 mg
    Doxorubicin ≥75 mg
    Ifosfamide
    Lomustine <60 mg
    Methotrexate ≥250 mg
    Mitomycin
    Mitoxantrone
    Procarbazine

Granisetron should not be prescribed for chemotherapeutic agents with a low emetogenic potential (eg, bleomycin, busulfan, cyclophosphamide <1000 mg, etoposide, 5-fluorouracil, vinblastine, vincristine)

Usual Dosage
I.V.: Children and Adults: 10 mcg/kg for 1-3 doses. Doses should be administered as a single IVPB over 5 minutes to 1 hour, given just prior to chemotherapy (15-60 minutes before); as intervention therapy for breakthrough nausea and vomiting, during the first 24 hours following chemotherapy, 2 or 3 repeat infusions (same dose) have been administered, separated by at least 10 minutes

Oral: Adults: 1 mg twice daily; the first 1 mg dose should be given up to 1 hour before chemotherapy, and the second tablet, 12 hours after the first

Note: Granisetron should only be given on the day(s) of chemotherapy

Mechanism of Action Selective 5-HT$_3$ receptor antagonist, blocking serotonin, both peripherally on vagal nerve terminals and centrally in the chemoreceptor trigger zone

Local Anesthetic/Vasoconstrictor Precautions No information available to require special precautions

Effects on Dental Treatment No effects or complications reported

Other Adverse Effects
>10%: Central nervous system: Headache
1% to 10%:
    Cardiovascular: Transient blood pressure changes
    Central nervous system: Dizziness, insomnia, anxiety
    Gastrointestinal: Constipation, abdominal pain, diarrhea
    Neuromuscular & skeletal: Weakness
<1%:
    Cardiovascular: Arrhythmias
    Central nervous system: Somnolence, agitation
    Endocrine & metabolic: Hot flashes
    Hepatic: Liver enzyme elevations

Drug Interactions No data reported

Drug Uptake
Onset of action: Commonly controls emesis within 1-3 minutes of administration
Duration: Effects generally last no more than 24 hours maximum
Serum half-life:
    Cancer patients: 10-12 hours
    Healthy volunteers: 3-4 hours

Pregnancy Risk Factor B
Generic Available No

Granulex *see* Trypsin, Balsam Peru, and Castor Oil *on page 974*

Granulocyte Colony Stimulating Factor *see* Filgrastim *on page 404*

Granulocyte-Macrophage Colony Stimulating Factor *see* Sargramostim *on page 857*

Grepafloxacin (grep a FLOX a sin)

Brand Names Raxar®

Therapeutic Category Antibiotic, Quinolone

Use Treatment of acute bacterial exacerbations of chronic bronchitis caused by *Haemophilus influenzae*, *Streptococcus pneumoniae*, or *Moxaxella catarrhalis*;

community-acquired pneumonia caused by *Mycoplasma pneumoniae* or the organisms previously mentioned; uncomplicated gonorrhea caused by *Neisseria gonorrhoeae*, and nongonococcal cervicitis and urethritis caused by *Chlamydia trachomatis*

Local Anesthetic/Vasoconstrictor Precautions No information available to require special precautions

Effects on Dental Treatment No effects or complications reported

Contraindications In patients with hepatic failure; given concomitantly with class I and III antiarrhythmics or bepridil due to the potential risk of cardiac arrhythmias (including *torsade de pointes*)

Grifulvin® V *see* Griseofulvin *on this page*

Grisactin® *see* Griseofulvin *on this page*

Grisactin® Ultra *see* Griseofulvin *on this page*

Griseofulvin (gri see oh FUL vin)

Brand Names Fulvicin® P/G; Fulvicin-U/F®; Grifulvin® V; Grisactin®; Grisactin® Ultra; Gris-PEG®

Canadian/Mexican Brand Names Fulvina® P/G (Mexico); Grisovin-FP® (Canada); Grisovin-FP® (Mexico)

Therapeutic Category Antifungal Agent, Systemic

Synonyms Griseofulvina (Mexico)

Use Treatment of susceptible tinea infections of the skin, hair, and nails

Usual Dosage Oral:

Children:
Microsize: 10-15 mg/kg/day in single or divided doses
Ultramicrosize: >2 months: 5.5-7.3 mg/kg/day in single or divided doses

Adults:
Microsize: 500-1000 mg/day in single or divided doses
Ultramicrosize: 330-375 mg/day in single or divided doses; doses up to 750 mg/day have been used for infections more difficult to eradicate such as tinea unguium and tinea pedis

Duration of therapy depends on the site of infection:
Tinea corporis: 2-4 weeks
Tinea capitis: 4-6 weeks or longer
Tinea pedis: 4-8 weeks
Tinea unguium: 4-6 months

Mechanism of Action Inhibits fungal cell mitosis at metaphase; binds to human keratin making it resistant to fungal invasion

Local Anesthetic/Vasoconstrictor Precautions No information available to require special precautions

Effects on Dental Treatment Griseofulvin may cause soreness or irritation of mouth or tongue

Other Adverse Effects

>10%: Dermatologic: Skin rash, urticaria

1% to 10%:
Central nervous system: Headache, fatigue, dizziness, insomnia, mental confusion
Dermatologic: Photosensitivity
Gastrointestinal: Nausea, vomiting, epigastric distress, diarrhea
Miscellaneous: Oral thrush

<1%:
Dermatologic: Angioneurotic edema
Endocrine & metabolic: Menstrual toxicity
Gastrointestinal: GI bleeding
Hematologic: Leukopenia
Hepatic: Hepatic toxicity
Renal: Proteinuria, nephrosis

Drug Interactions

Decreased effect:
Barbiturates leads to decreased levels of griseofulvin
Decreased warfarin activity
Decreased oral contraceptive effectiveness
Increased toxicity: With alcohol causes tachycardia and flushing

Drug Uptake

Absorption: Ultramicrosize griseofulvin absorption is almost complete; absorption of microsize griseofulvin is variable (25% to 70% of an oral dose); absorption is enhanced by ingestion of a fatty meal
Serum half-life: 9-22 hours

Pregnancy Risk Factor C

Generic Available Yes

Griseofulvina (Mexico) *see Griseofulvin on previous page*
Gris-PEG® *see Griseofulvin on previous page*
Guaifed® [OTC] *see Guaifenesin and Pseudoephedrine on page 454*
Guaifed®-PD *see Guaifenesin and Pseudoephedrine on page 454*

Guaifenesin (gwye FEN e sin)
Related Information
Guaifenesin and Phenylephrine *on page 454*
Guaifenesin, Pseudoephedrine, and Dextromethorphan *on page 456*
Brand Names Anti-Tuss® Expectorant [OTC]; Breonesin® [OTC]; Diabetic Tussin® EX [OTC]; Duratuss-G®; Fenesin™; Gee Gee® [OTC]; Genatuss® [OTC]; GG-Cen® [OTC]; Glyate® [OTC]; Glycotuss® [OTC]; Glytuss® [OTC]; Guaifenex® LA; GuiaCough® Expectorant [OTC]; Guiatuss® [OTC]; Halotussin® [OTC]; Humibid® L.A.; Humibid® Sprinkle; Hytuss® [OTC]; Hytuss-2X® [OTC]; Liquibid®; Medi-Tuss® [OTC]; Monafed®; Muco-Fen-LA®; Mytussin® [OTC]; Naldecon® Senior EX [OTC]; Organidin® NR; Pneumomist®; Respa-GF®; Robitussin® [OTC]; Scot-Tussin® [OTC]; Siltussin® [OTC]; Sinumist®-SR Capsulets®; Touro Ex®; Tusibron® [OTC]; Uni-tussin® [OTC]
Canadian/Mexican Brand Names Balminil® Expectorant (Canada); Calmylin® Expectorant (Canada)
Therapeutic Category Expectorant
Synonyms Guaifenesina (Mexico)
Use Temporary control of cough due to minor throat and bronchial irritation
Usual Dosage Oral:
Children:
<2 years: 12 mg/kg/day in 6 divided doses
2-5 years: 50-100 mg every 4 hours, not to exceed 600 mg/day
6-11 years: 100-200 mg every 4 hours, not to exceed 1.2 g/day
Children >12 years and Adults: 200-400 mg every 4 hours to a maximum of 2.4 g/day
Mechanism of Action Thought to act as an expectorant by irritating the gastric mucosa and stimulating respiratory tract secretions, thereby increasing respiratory fluid volumes and decreasing phlegm viscosity
Local Anesthetic/Vasoconstrictor Precautions No information available to require special precautions
Effects on Dental Treatment No effects or complications reported
Other Adverse Effects 1% to 10%:
Central nervous system: Drowsiness, headache
Dermatologic: Rash
Gastrointestinal: Nausea, vomiting, stomach pain
Drug Interactions No data reported
Drug Uptake
Absorption: Well absorbed from GI tract
Pregnancy Risk Factor C
Generic Available Yes

Guaifenesina Dextrometorfano (Mexico) *see Guaifenesin and Dextromethorphan on next page*
Guaifenesina (Mexico) *see Guaifenesin on this page*

Guaifenesin and Codeine (gwye FEN e sin & KOE deen)
Brand Names Brontex® Liquid; Brontex® Tablet; Cheracol®; Guaituss AC®; Guiatussin® with Codeine; Mytussin® AC; Robafen® AC; Robitussin® A-C; Tussi-Organidin® NR
Therapeutic Category Antitussive; Cough Preparation; Expectorant
Use Temporary control of cough due to minor throat and bronchial irritation
Usual Dosage Oral:
Children:
2-6 years: 1-1.5 mg/kg codeine/day divided into 4 doses administered every 4-6 hours (maximum: 30 mg/24 hours)
6-12 years: 5 mL every 4 hours, not to exceed 30 mL/24 hours
Children >12 years and Adults: 5-10 mL every 4-8 hours not to exceed 60 mL/24 hours
Mechanism of Action
Guaifenesin is thought to act as an expectorant by irritating the gastric mucosa and stimulating respiratory tract secretions, thereby increasing respiratory fluid volumes and decreasing phlegm viscosity
Codeine is an antitussive that controls cough by depressing the medullary cough center
Local Anesthetic/Vasoconstrictor Precautions No information available to require special precautions
Effects on Dental Treatment No effects or complications reported

Other Adverse Effects

Codeine:

>10%:

Central nervous system: Drowsiness

Gastrointestinal: Constipation

1% to 10%:

Cardiovascular: Hypotension, palpitations, tachycardia or bradycardia, peripheral vasodilation

Central nervous system: CNS depression, sedation, confusion, headache, increased intracranial pressure, dizziness, lightheadedness, false feeling of well being, restlessness, paradoxical CNS stimulation, malaise

Dermatologic: Skin rash, urticaria

Endocrine & metabolic: Antidiuretic hormone release

Gastrointestinal: Nausea, vomiting, anorexia, dry mouth, biliary spasm

Genitourinary: Decreased urination, urinary tract spasm

Neuromuscular & skeletal: Weakness

Ocular: Miosis, blurred vision

Respiratory: Respiratory depression, dyspnea

Miscellaneous: Histamine release, physical and psychological dependence with prolonged use

<1%:

Central nervous system: Convulsions, hallucinations, mental depression, nightmares, insomnia

Gastrointestinal: Stomach cramps, paralytic ileus

Neuromuscular & skeletal: Trembling, muscle rigidity

Guaifenesin:

1% to 10%:

Central nervous system: Drowsiness, headache

Dermatologic: Rash

Gastrointestinal: Nausea, vomiting, stomach pain

Drug Interactions Increased toxicity: CNS depressant medications produce additive sedative properties

Pregnancy Risk Factor C

Generic Available Yes

Guaifenesin and Dextromethorphan

(gwye FEN e sin & deks troe meth OR fan)

Brand Names Benylin® Expectorant [OTC]; Cheracol® D [OTC]; Clear Tussin® 30; Contac® Cough Formula Liquid [OTC]; Diabetic Tussin DM® [OTC]; Extra Action Cough Syrup [OTC]; Fenesin DM®; Genatuss DM® [OTC]; Glycotuss-dM® [OTC]; Guaifenex® DM; GuiaCough® [OTC]; Guiatuss-DM® [OTC]; Halotussin® DM [OTC]; Humibid® DM [OTC]; Iobid DM®; Kolephrin® GG/DM [OTC]; Monafed® DM; Muco-Fen-DM®; Mytussin® DM [OTC]; Naldecon® Senior DX [OTC]; Phanatuss® Cough Syrup [OTC]; Phenadex® Senior [OTC]; Respa-DM®; Rhinosyn-DMX® [OTC]; Robafen DM® [OTC]; Robitussin®-DM [OTC]; Safe Tussin® 30 [OTC]; Scot-Tussin® Senior Clear [OTC]; Siltussin DM® [OTC]; Synacol® CF [OTC]; Syracol-CF® [OTC]; Tolu-Sed® DM [OTC]; Tusibron-DM® [OTC]; Tuss-DM® [OTC]; Tussi-Organidin® DM NR; Uni-tussin® DM [OTC]; Vicks® 44E [OTC]; Vicks® Pediatric Formula 44E [OTC]

Therapeutic Category Antitussive; Cough Preparation; Expectorant

Synonyms Guaifenesina Dextrometorfano (Mexico)

Use Temporary control of cough due to minor throat and bronchial irritation

Usual Dosage Oral:

Children: Dextromethorphan: 1-2 mg/kg/24 hours divided 3-4 times/day

Children >12 years and Adults: 5 mL every 4 hours or 10 mL every 6-8 hours not to exceed 40 mL/24 hours

Mechanism of Action

Guaifenesin is thought to act as an expectorant by irritating the gastric mucosa and stimulating respiratory tract secretions, thereby increasing respiratory fluid volumes and decreasing phlegm viscosity

Dextromethorphan is a chemical relative of morphine lacking narcotic properties except in overdose; controls cough by depressing the medullary cough center

Local Anesthetic/Vasoconstrictor Precautions No information available to require special precautions

Effects on Dental Treatment No effects or complications reported

Other Adverse Effects 1% to 10%:

Central nervous system: Drowsiness, headache

Dermatologic: Rash

Gastrointestinal: Nausea, vomiting

Warnings/Precautions Research on chicken embryos exposed to concentrations of dextromethorphan relative to those typically taken by humans has shown to cause birth defects and fetal death; more study is needed, but it is suggested (Continued)

Guaifenesin and Dextromethorphan *(Continued)*

that pregnant women should be advised not to use dextromethorphan-containing medications

Drug Interactions No data reported

Drug Uptake

Onset of action: Exerts its antitussive effect in 15-30 minutes after oral administration

Pregnancy Risk Factor C (see Warnings)

Generic Available Yes

Guaifenesin and Hydrocodone *see* Hydrocodone and Guaifenesin *on page 481*

Guaifenesin and Phenylephrine (gwye FEN e sin & fen il EF rin)

Brand Names Deconsal® Sprinkle®; Endal®; Sinupan®

Therapeutic Category Cold Preparation

Synonyms Phenylephrine and Guaifenesin

Usual Dosage Oral: Adults: 1 or 2 every 12 hours

Mechanism of Action See individual agents

Local Anesthetic/Vasoconstrictor Precautions Use with caution since phenylephrine is a sympathomimetic amine which could interact with epinephrine to cause a pressor response

Effects on Dental Treatment

Guaifenesin: No effects or complications reported

Phenylephrine: Up to 10% of patients could experience tachycardia, palpitations, and dry mouth; use vasoconstrictor with caution

Other Adverse Effects See individual agents

Drug Interactions See individual agents

Dosage Forms

Capsule, sustained release:

Deconsal® Sprinkle®: Guaifenesin 300 mg and phenylephrine hydrochloride 10 mg

Sinupan®: Guaifenesin 200 mg and phenylephrine hydrochloride 40 mg

Tablet, timed release (Endal®): Guaifenesin 300 mg and phenylephrine hydrochloride 20 mg

Generic Available No

Guaifenesin and Phenylpropanolamine

(gwye FEN e sin & fen il proe pa NOLE a meen)

Brand Names Ami-Tex LA®; Coldlac-LA®; Conex® [OTC]; Contuss® XT; Dura-Vent®; Entex® LA; Genagesic®; Genamin® Expectorant [OTC]; Guaifenex® PPA 75; Guaipax®; Myminic® Expectorant [OTC]; Naldecon-EX® Children's Syrup [OTC]; Nolex® LA; Partuss® LA; Phenylfenesin® L.A.; Profen II®; Profen LA®; Rymed-TR®; Silaminic® Expectorant [OTC]; Sildicon-E® [OTC]; Snaplets-EX® [OTC]; Theramin® Expectorant [OTC]; Triaminic® Expectorant [OTC]; Tri-Clear® Expectorant [OTC]; Triphenyl® Expectorant [OTC]; ULR-LA®; Vicks® DayQuil® Sinus Pressure & Congestion Relief [OTC]

Therapeutic Category Decongestant; Expectorant

Synonyms Phenylpropanolamine and Guaifenesin

Use Symptomatic relief of those respiratory conditions where tenacious mucous plugs and congestion complicate the problem such as sinusitis, pharyngitis, bronchitis, asthma, and as an adjunctive therapy in serous otitis media

Local Anesthetic/Vasoconstrictor Precautions Use with caution since phenylpropanolamine is a sympathomimetic amine which could interact with epinephrine to cause a pressor response

Effects on Dental Treatment

Guaifenesin: No effects or complications reported

Phenylpropanolamine: Up to 10% of patients could experience tachycardia, palpitations, and dry mouth; use vasoconstrictor with caution

Pregnancy Risk Factor C

Generic Available Yes

Guaifenesin and Pseudoephedrine

(gwye FEN e sin & soo doe e FED rin)

Brand Names Congess® Jr; Congess® Sr; Congestac®; Deconsal® II; Defen-LA®; Entex® PSE; Eudal-SR®; Fedahist® Expectorant [OTC]; Fedahist® Expectorant Pediatric [OTC]; Glycofed® [OTC]; Guaifed® [OTC]; Guaifed®-PD; Guaifenex® PSE; GuaiMAX-D®; Guaitab®; Guaivent®; Guai-Vent/PSE®; Guiatuss PE® [OTC]; Halotussin® PE [OTC]; Histalet® X; Nasabid™; Respa-1st®; Respaire®-60 SR; Respaire®-120 SR; Robitussin-PE® [OTC]; Robitussin® Severe Congestion Liqui-Gels [OTC]; Ru-Tuss® DE; Rymed®; Sinufed® Timecelles®; Touro LA®; Tuss-LA®; V-Dec-M®; Versacaps®; Zephrex®; Zephrex LA®

Therapeutic Category Decongestant; Expectorant

Synonyms Pseudoephedrine and Guaifenesin

Use Enhance the output of respiratory tract fluid and reduce mucosal congestion and edema in the nasal passage

Local Anesthetic/Vasoconstrictor Precautions Use with caution since pseudoephedrine is a sympathomimetic amine which could interact with epinephrine to cause a pressor response

Effects on Dental Treatment

Guaifenesin: No effects or complications reported

Pseudoephedrine: Up to 10% of patients could experience tachycardia, palpitations, and dry mouth; use vasoconstrictor with caution

Pregnancy Risk Factor C

Generic Available Yes

Guaifenesin, Phenylpropanolamine, and Dextromethorphan

(gwye FEN e sin, fen il proe pa NOLE a meen, & deks troe meth OR fan)

Brand Names Anatuss® [OTC]; Guiatuss CF® [OTC]; Naldecon® DX Adult Liquid [OTC]; Robafen® CF [OTC]; Robitussin-CF® [OTC]; Siltussin-CF® [OTC]

Therapeutic Category Cough Preparation; Decongestant; Expectorant

Use Temporarily relieves nasal congestion and controls cough due to minor throat and bronchial irritation; helps loosen phlegm and thin bronchial secretions to make coughs more productive

Local Anesthetic/Vasoconstrictor Precautions Use with caution since phenylpropanolamine is a sympathomimetic amine which could interact with epinephrine to cause a pressor response

Effects on Dental Treatment

Dextromethorphan, Guaifenesin: No effects or complications reported

Phenylpropanolamine: Up to 10% of patients could experience tachycardia, palpitations, and dry mouth; use vasoconstrictor with caution

Warnings/Precautions Research on chicken embryos exposed to concentrations of dextromethorphan relative to those typically taken by humans has shown to cause birth defects and fetal death; more study is needed, but it is suggested that pregnant women should be advised not to use dextromethorphan-containing medications

Pregnancy Risk Factor C (see Warnings)

Generic Available Yes

Guaifenesin, Phenylpropanolamine, and Phenylephrine

(gwye FEN e sin, fen il proe pa NOLE a meen, & fen il EF rin)

Brand Names Coldloc®; Contuss®; Dura-Gest®; Enomine®; Entex®; Guaifenex®; Guiatex®

Therapeutic Category Decongestant; Expectorant

Use Temporary relief of nasal congestion, running nose, sneezing, itching of nose and throat, and itchy, watery eyes due to common cold, hay fever, or other upper respiratory allergies

Local Anesthetic/Vasoconstrictor Precautions Use with caution since phenylpropanolamine and phenylephrine are sympathomimetic amines which could interact with epinephrine to cause a pressor response

Effects on Dental Treatment

Guaifenesin: No effects or complications reported

Phenylephrine, Phenylpropanolamine: Up to 10% of patients could experience tachycardia, palpitations, and dry mouth; use vasoconstrictor with caution

Pregnancy Risk Factor C

Generic Available Yes

Guaifenesin, Pseudoephedrine, and Codeine

(gwye FEN e sin, soo doe e FED rin, & KOE deen)

Brand Names Codafed® Expectorant; Cycofed® Pediatric; Decohistine® Expectorant; Deproist® Expectorant with Codeine; Dihistine® Expectorant; Guiatuss DAC®; Guiatussin® DAC; Halotussin® DAC; Isoclor® Expectorant; Mytussin® DAC; Nucofed®; Nucofed® Pediatric Expectorant; Nucotuss®; Phenhist® Expectorant; Robitussin®-DAC; Ryna-CX®; Tussar® SF Syrup

Therapeutic Category Cough Preparation; Decongestant; Expectorant

Use Temporarily relieves nasal congestion and controls cough due to minor throat and bronchial irritation; helps loosen phlegm and thin bronchial secretions to make coughs more productive

Local Anesthetic/Vasoconstrictor Precautions Use with caution since pseudoephedrine is a sympathomimetic amine which could interact with epinephrine to cause a pressor response

(Continued)

Guaifenesin, Pseudoephedrine, and Codeine
(Continued)

Effects on Dental Treatment
Codeine: <1%: Dry mouth
Guaifenesin: No effects or complications reported
Pseudoephedrine: Up to 10% of patients could experience tachycardia, palpitations, and dry mouth; use vasoconstrictor with caution
Pregnancy Risk Factor C
Generic Available Yes

Guaifenesin, Pseudoephedrine, and Dextromethorphan
(gwye FEN e sin, soo doe e FED rin, & deks troe meth OR fan)
Brand Names Anatuss® DM [OTC]; Dimacol® Caplets [OTC]; Novahistine® DMX Liquid [OTC]; Rhinosyn-X® Liquid [OTC]; Ru-Tuss® Expectorant [OTC]; Sudafed® Cold & Cough Liquid Caps [OTC]
Therapeutic Category Cold Preparation
Synonyms Dextromethorphan, Guaifenesin, and Pseudoephedrine; Pseudoephedrine, Dextromethorphan, and Guaifenesin
Use Temporarily relieves nasal congestion and controls cough due to minor throat and bronchial irritation; helps loosen phlegm and thin bronchial secretions to make coughs more productive
Usual Dosage Oral: Adults: 2 capsules (caplets) or 10 mL every 4 hours
Mechanism of Action See individual agents
Local Anesthetic/Vasoconstrictor Precautions Use with caution since pseudoephedrine is a sympathomimetic amine which could interact with epinephrine to cause a pressor response
Effects on Dental Treatment
Guaifenesin: No effects or complications reported
Pseudoephedrine: Up to 10% of patients could experience tachycardia, palpitations, and dry mouth; use vasoconstrictor with caution
Dextromethorphan: No effects or complications reported
Other Adverse Effects See individual agents
Warnings/Precautions Research on chicken embryos exposed to concentrations of dextromethorphan relative to those typically taken by humans has shown to cause birth defects and fetal death; more study is needed, but it is suggested that pregnant women should be advised not to use dextromethorphan-containing medications
Drug Interactions See individual agents
Dosage Forms
Caplets (Dimacol®): Guaifenesin 100 mg, pseudoephedrine hydrochloride 30 mg, and dextromethorphan hydrobromide 10 mg
Capsule (Sudafed® Cold & Cough Liquid Caps): Guaifenesin 100 mg, pseudoephedrine hydrochloride 30 mg, and dextromethorphan hydrobromide 10 mg
Liquid (Anatuss® DM, Novahistine® DMX Liquid, Rhinosyn-X® Liquid, Ru-Tuss® Expectorant): Guaifenesin 100 mg, pseudoephedrine hydrochloride 30 mg, and dextromethorphan hydrobromide 10 mg per 5 mL
Generic Available Yes

Guaifenex® *see* Guaifenesin, Phenylpropanolamine, and Phenylephrine *on previous page*
Guaifenex® DM *see* Guaifenesin and Dextromethorphan *on page 453*
Guaifenex® LA *see* Guaifenesin *on page 452*
Guaifenex® PPA 75 *see* Guaifenesin and Phenylpropanolamine *on page 454*
Guaifenex® PSE *see* Guaifenesin and Pseudoephedrine *on page 454*
GuaiMAX-D® *see* Guaifenesin and Pseudoephedrine *on page 454*
Guaipax® *see* Guaifenesin and Phenylpropanolamine *on page 454*
Guaitab® *see* Guaifenesin and Pseudoephedrine *on page 454*
Guaituss AC® *see* Guaifenesin and Codeine *on page 452*
Guaivent® *see* Guaifenesin and Pseudoephedrine *on page 454*
Guai-Vent/PSE® *see* Guaifenesin and Pseudoephedrine *on page 454*

Guanabenz (GWAHN a benz)
Related Information
Cardiovascular Diseases *on page 1010*
Brand Names Wytensin®
Therapeutic Category Alpha-Adrenergic Blockers - Peripheral-Acting (Alpha$_1$-Blockers)
Use Management of hypertension
Usual Dosage Adults: Oral: Initial: 4 mg twice daily, increase in increments of 4-8 mg/day every 1-2 weeks to a maximum of 32 mg twice daily

Mechanism of Action Stimulates alpha$_2$-adrenoreceptors in the brain stem, thus activating an inhibitory neuron, resulting in reduced sympathetic outflow, producing a decrease in vasomotor tone and heart rate

Local Anesthetic/Vasoconstrictor Precautions No information available to require special precautions

Effects on Dental Treatment >10% of patients will experience significant dry mouth; normal salivation occurs with cessation of drug therapy

Other Adverse Effects
>10%:
Central nervous system: Drowsiness, sedation, dizziness
Neuromuscular & skeletal: Weakness
1% to 10%:
Cardiovascular: Chest pain, edema
Central nervous system: Headache
Endocrine & metabolic: Decreased sexual ability
Gastrointestinal: Nausea
<1%:
Cardiovascular: Arrhythmias, palpitations
Central nervous system: Anxiety, ataxia, depression, sleep disturbances
Dermatologic: Rash, pruritus
Endocrine & metabolic: Sexual dysfunction, gynecomastia
Gastrointestinal: Diarrhea, vomiting, constipation, taste disorders
Neuromuscular & skeletal: Myalgia
Ocular: Blurring of vision
Renal: Polyuria
Respiratory: Nasal congestion, dyspnea

Drug Interactions
Decreased hypotensive effect of guanabenz with tricyclic antidepressants
Increased effect: Other hypotensive agents

Drug Uptake
Onset of antihypertensive effect: Within 1 hour
Absorption: ~75%
Serum half-life: 7-10 hours

Pregnancy Risk Factor C

Generic Available Yes

Guanadrel (GWAHN a drel)

Related Information
Cardiovascular Diseases *on page 1010*

Brand Names Hylorel®

Therapeutic Category Alpha-Adrenergic Blockers - Peripheral-Acting (Alpha$_1$-Blockers)

Use Considered a second line agent in the treatment of hypertension, usually with a diuretic

Usual Dosage
Adults: Oral: Initial: 10 mg/day (5 mg twice daily); adjust dosage until blood pressure is controlled, usual dosage: 20-75 mg/day, given twice daily
Elderly: Initial: 5 mg once daily

Mechanism of Action Acts as a false neurotransmitter that blocks the adrenergic actions of norepinephrine; it displaces norepinephrine from its presynaptic storage granules and thus exposes it to degradation; it thereby produces a reduction in total peripheral resistance and, therefore, blood pressure

Local Anesthetic/Vasoconstrictor Precautions No information available to require special precautions

Effects on Dental Treatment No effects or complications reported

Other Adverse Effects
>10%:
Cardiovascular: Palpitations, chest pain, peripheral edema, faintness
Central nervous system: Fatigue, headache, drowsiness, confusion
Gastrointestinal: Increased bowel movements, gas pain, constipation, anorexia, weight gain/loss
Genitourinary: Nocturia, ejaculation disturbances
Neuromuscular & skeletal: Paresthesia, aching limbs, leg cramps, backache, arthralgia
Ocular: Visual disturbances
Renal: Polyuria
Respiratory: Dyspnea, coughing
1% to 10%:
Cardiovascular: Orthostatic hypotension
Central nervous system: Psychological problems, depression, sleep disorders
Gastrointestinal: Glossitis, nausea, vomiting, dry mouth
Genitourinary: Impotence

(Continued)

Guanadrel *(Continued)*

Renal: Hematuria
<1%: Cardiovascular: Angina
Drug Interactions
Decreased effect with tricyclic antidepressants, indirect-acting amines (ephedrine, phenylpropanolamine), phenothiazines
Increased toxicity of direct-acting amines (epinephrine, norepinephrine)
Increased effect of beta-blockers, vasodilators
Drug Uptake
Peak effect: Within 4-6 hours
Duration: 4-14 hours
Absorption: Oral: Rapid
Serum half-life, biphasic:
Initial: 1-4 hours
Terminal: 5-45 hours
Time to peak serum concentration: Within 1.5-2 hour
Pregnancy Risk Factor B
Generic Available No

Guanethidine (gwahn ETH i deen)

Related Information
Cardiovascular Diseases *on page 1010*
Brand Names Ismelin®
Canadian/Mexican Brand Names Apo®-Guanethidine (Canada)
Therapeutic Category Alpha-Adrenergic Blockers - Peripheral-Acting (Alpha$_1$-Blockers)
Use Treatment of moderate to severe hypertension
Usual Dosage Oral:
Children: Initial: 0.2 mg/kg/day, increase by 0.2 mg/kg/day at 7- to 10-day intervals to a maximum of 3 mg/kg/day
Adults:
Ambulatory patients: Initial: 10 mg/day, increase at 5- to 7-day intervals to a maximum of 25-50 mg/day
Hospitalized patients: Initial: 25-50 mg/day, increase by 25-50 mg/day or every other day to desired therapeutic response
Elderly: Initial: 5 mg once daily
Mechanism of Action Acts as a false neurotransmitter that blocks the adrenergic actions of norepinephrine; it displaces norepinephrine from its presynaptic storage granules and thus exposes it to degradation; it thereby produces a reduction in total peripheral resistance and, therefore, blood pressure
Local Anesthetic/Vasoconstrictor Precautions No information available to require special precautions
Effects on Dental Treatment No effects or complications reported
Other Adverse Effects
>10%:
Cardiovascular: Palpitations, chest pain, peripheral edema, faintness
Central nervous system: Fatigue, headache, drowsiness, confusion
Gastrointestinal: Increased bowel movements, gas pain, constipation, anorexia, weight gain/loss
Genitourinary: Nocturia, impotence, ejaculation disturbances
Neuromuscular & skeletal: Paresthesia, aching limbs, leg cramps, backache, arthralgia
Ocular: Visual disturbances
Renal: Polyuria
Respiratory: Dyspnea, coughing
1% to 10%:
Cardiovascular: Orthostatic hypotension
Central nervous system: Psychological problems, depression, sleep disorders
Gastrointestinal: Glossitis, nausea, vomiting, dry mouth
Renal: Hematuria
<1%: Cardiovascular: Angina
Drug Interactions
Decreased effect with tricyclic antidepressants, indirect-acting amines (ephedrine, phenylpropanolamine)
Increased toxicity of direct-acting amines (epinephrine, norepinephrine)
Drug Uptake
Onset of effect: Within 0.5-2 hours
Peak antihypertensive effect: Within 6-8 hours
Duration: 24-48 hours
Absorption: Irregular (3% to 55%)
Serum half-life: 5-10 days

Pregnancy Risk Factor C
Generic Available Yes

Guanfacine (GWAHN fa seen)

Related Information
Cardiovascular Diseases *on page 1010*

Brand Names Tenex®

Therapeutic Category Alpha-Adrenergic Blockers - Peripheral-Acting (Alpha$_1$-Blockers)

Use Management of hypertension

Usual Dosage Adults: Oral: 1 mg usually at bedtime, may increase if needed at 3- to 4-week intervals to a maximum of 3 mg/day; 1 mg/day is most common dose

Mechanism of Action Stimulates alpha$_2$-adrenoreceptors in the brain stem, thus activating an inhibitory neuron, resulting in reduced sympathetic outflow, producing a decrease in vasomotor tone and heart rate

Local Anesthetic/Vasoconstrictor Precautions No information available to require special precautions

Effects on Dental Treatment >10% of patients experience dry mouth

Other Adverse Effects
>10%:
Central nervous system: Somnolence, dizziness
Gastrointestinal: Constipation
1% to 10%:
Central nervous system: Fatigue, headache, insomnia
Endocrine & metabolic: Decreased sexual ability
Gastrointestinal: Nausea, vomiting
Ocular: Conjunctivitis
<1%:
Cardiovascular: Bradycardia, palpitations, substernal pain
Central nervous system: Amnesia, confusion, depression, malaise
Dermatologic: Dermatitis, pruritus, purpura
Gastrointestinal: Abdominal pain, diarrhea, dyspepsia, dysphagia, taste perversion
Genitourinary: Testicular disorder, urinary incontinence
Neuromuscular & skeletal: Leg cramps, hypokinesia, paresthesia
Otic: Tinnitus
Respiratory: Rhinitis, dyspnea
Miscellaneous: Sweating

Drug Interactions
Decreased hypotensive effect of guanfacine with tricyclic antidepressants
Increased effect: Other hypotensive agents

Drug Uptake
Peak effect: Within 8-11 hours
Duration: 24 hours following a single dose
Serum half-life: 17 hours
Time to peak serum concentration: Within 1-4 hours

Pregnancy Risk Factor B
Generic Available No

GuiaCough® [OTC] *see* Guaifenesin and Dextromethorphan *on page 453*

GuiaCough® Expectorant [OTC] *see* Guaifenesin *on page 452*

Guiatex® *see* Guaifenesin, Phenylpropanolamine, and Phenylephrine *on page 455*

Guiatuss® [OTC] *see* Guaifenesin *on page 452*

Guiatuss CF® [OTC] *see* Guaifenesin, Phenylpropanolamine, and Dextromethorphan *on page 455*

Guiatuss DAC® *see* Guaifenesin, Pseudoephedrine, and Codeine *on page 455*

Guiatuss-DM® [OTC] *see* Guaifenesin and Dextromethorphan *on page 453*

Guiatussin® DAC *see* Guaifenesin, Pseudoephedrine, and Codeine *on page 455*

Guiatussin® with Codeine *see* Guaifenesin and Codeine *on page 452*

Guiatuss PE® [OTC] *see* Guaifenesin and Pseudoephedrine *on page 454*

Gum Benjamin *see* Benzoin *on page 120*

G-well® *see* Lindane *on page 558*

Gyne-Sulf® *see* Sulfabenzamide, Sulfacetamide, and Sulfathiazole *on page 889*

Gynogen L.A.® Injection *see* Estradiol *on page 365*

Gynol II® [OTC] *see* Nonoxynol 9 *on page 689*

Habitrol™ *see* Nicotine *on page 678*

Haemophilus b Conjugate Vaccine
(hem OF fi lus bee KON joo gate vak SEEN)

Brand Names HibTITER®; OmniHIB®; PedvaxHIB™; ProHIBiT®

Therapeutic Category Vaccine, Inactivated Bacteria

Synonyms Diphtheria CRM$_{197}$ Protein Conjugate; Diphtheria Toxoid Conjugate; *Haemophilus* b Oligosaccharide Conjugate Vaccine; *Haemophilus* b Polysaccharide Vaccine; HbCV; Hib Polysaccharide Conjugate; PRP-D

Use Immunization of children 24 months to 6 years of age against diseases caused by *H. influenzae* type b

Usual Dosage Children: I.M.: 0.5 mL as a single dose should be administered according to one of the following "brand-specific" schedules; do not inject I.V.

Vaccination Schedule for Haemophilus b Conjugate Vaccines

Age at 1st Dose (mo)	HibTITER®		PedvaxHIB®		ProHIBiT®	
	Primary Series	Booster	Primary Series	Booster	Primary Series	Booster
2-6*	3 doses, 2 months apart	15 mo†	2 doses, 2 months apart	12 mo†		
7-11	2 doses, 2 months apart	15 mo†	2 doses, 2 months apart	15 mo†		
12-14	1 dose	15 mo†	1 dose	15 mo†		
15-60	1 dose	—	1 dose	—	1 dose	—

*It is not currently recommended that the various Haemophilus b conjugate vaccines be interchanged (ie, the same brand should be used throughout the entire vaccination series). If the health care provider does not know which vaccine was previously used, it is prudent that an infant, 2-6 months of age, be given a primary series of three doses.

†At least 2 months after previous dose.

Mechanism of Action Stimulates production of anticapsular antibodies and provides active immunity to *Haemophilus influenzae*; Hib conjugate vaccines use covalent binding of capsular polysaccharide of *Haemophilus influenzae* type b to diphtheria CRM 197 (HibTITER®) to produce an antigen which is postulated to convert a T-independent antigen into a T-dependent antigen to result in enhanced antibody response and on immunologic memory

Local Anesthetic/Vasoconstrictor Precautions No information available to require special precautions

Effects on Dental Treatment No effects or complications reported

Other Adverse Effects When administered during the same visit that DTP vaccine is given, the rates of systemic reactions do not differ from those observed only when DTP vaccine is administered

25%:
  Cardiovascular: Swelling
  Dermatologic: Local erythema
  Local: Increased risk of *Haemophilus* b infections in the week after vaccination
  Miscellaneous: Warmth
>10%: Acute febrile reactions
1% to 10%:
  Central nervous system: Fever (up to 102.2°F), irritability, lethargy
  Gastrointestinal: Anorexia, diarrhea
  Local: Irritation at injection site
<1%:
  Cardiovascular: Edema of face, eyes
  Central nervous system: Convulsions, fever >102.2°F, unusual fatigue
  Dermatologic: Urticaria, itching
  Gastrointestinal: Vomiting
  Neuromuscular & skeletal: Weakness
  Respiratory: Dyspnea
  Miscellaneous: Allergic or anaphylactic reactions

Drug Uptake
The seroconversion following one dose of Hib vaccine for children 18 months or 24 months of age or older is 75% to 90% respectively
Onset of serum antibody responses: 1-2 weeks after vaccination
Duration: Immunity appears to last 1.5 years

Pregnancy Risk Factor C

Generic Available No

Comments Federal law requires that the date of administration, the vaccine manufacturer, lot number of vaccine, and the administering person's name, title and address be entered into the patient's permanent medical record

Haemophilus **b Oligosaccharide Conjugate Vaccine** *see Haemophilus b Conjugate Vaccine on previous page*

Haemophilus **b Polysaccharide Vaccine** *see Haemophilus b Conjugate Vaccine on previous page*

Halazepam (hal AZ e pam)

Brand Names Paxipam®

Therapeutic Category Benzodiazepine

Use Management of anxiety disorders; short-term relief of the symptoms of anxiety

Local Anesthetic/Vasoconstrictor Precautions No information available to require special precautions

Effects on Dental Treatment >10% of patients experience significant dry mouth; normal salivary flow occurs with cessation of drug therapy

Other Adverse Effects

>10%:

Cardiovascular: Chest pain

Central nervous system: Drowsiness, fatigue, lightheadedness, memory impairment, insomnia, anxiety, depression, headache, ataxia

Dermatologic: Rash

Endocrine & metabolic: Decreased libido

Gastrointestinal: Constipation, diarrhea, decreased salivation, nausea, vomiting, increased or decreased appetite

Neuromuscular & skeletal: Dysarthria

Miscellaneous: Sweating

1% to 10%:

Cardiovascular: Syncope, tachycardia, hypotension

Central nervous system: Confusion, nervousness, dizziness, akathisia

Dermatologic: Dermatitis

Gastrointestinal: Weight gain or loss, increased salivation

Neuromuscular & skeletal: Rigidity, tremor, muscle cramps

Ocular: Blurred vision

Otic: Tinnitus

Respiratory: Nasal congestion, hyperventilation

<1%:

Endocrine & metabolic: Menstrual irregularities

Hematologic: Blood dyscrasias

Neuromuscular & skeletal: Reflex slowing

Miscellaneous: Drug dependence

Pregnancy Risk Factor D

Generic Available No

Comments Halazepam offers no significant advantage over other benzodiazepines

Halcinonida (Mexico) *see Halcinonide on this page*

Halcinonide (hal SIN oh nide)

Related Information

Corticosteroids, Topical Comparison *on page 1140*

Brand Names Halog®; Halog®-E

Canadian/Mexican Brand Names Dermalog® Simple (Mexico)

Therapeutic Category Corticosteroid, Topical (High Potency)

Synonyms Halcinonida (Mexico)

Use Inflammation of corticosteroid-responsive dermatoses [high potency topical corticosteroid]

Usual Dosage Children and Adults: Topical: Apply sparingly 1-3 times/day, occlusive dressing may be used for severe or resistant dermatoses; a thin film of cream or ointment is effective; do not overuse

Mechanism of Action Decreases inflammation by suppression of migration of polymorphonuclear leukocytes and reversal of increased capillary permeability

Local Anesthetic/Vasoconstrictor Precautions No information available to require special precautions

Effects on Dental Treatment No effects or complications reported

Other Adverse Effects <1%:

Dermatologic: Itching, dry skin, folliculitis, hypertrichosis, acneiform eruptions, hypopigmentation, perioral dermatitis, allergic contact dermatitis, skin maceration, skin atrophy, striae

Local: Burning, irritation, miliaria

Miscellaneous: Secondary infection

Drug Interactions No data reported

Drug Uptake Absorption: Percutaneous absorption varies by location of topical application and the use of occlusive dressings

Pregnancy Risk Factor C

(Continued)

Halcinonide *(Continued)*

Dosage Forms
Cream (Halog®): 0.025% (15 g, 60 g, 240 g); 0.1% (15 g, 30 g, 60 g, 240 g)
Cream, emollient base (Halog®-E) : 0.1% (15 g, 30 g, 60 g)
Ointment, topical (Halog®): 0.1% (15 g, 30 g, 60 g, 240 g)
Solution (Halog®): 0.1% (20 mL, 60 mL)

Generic Available No

Halcion® *see Triazolam on page 957*

Haldol® *see Haloperidol on next page*

Haldol® Decanoate *see Haloperidol on next page*

Haldrone® *see Paramethasone Acetate on page 724*

Halenol® Childrens [OTC] *see Acetaminophen on page 20*

Haley's M-O® [OTC] *see Magnesium Hydroxide and Mineral Oil Emulsion on page 576*

Halfan® *see Halofantrine on this page*

Halfprin® 81® [OTC] *see Aspirin on page 90*

Halobetasol *(hal oh BAY ta sol)*

Brand Names Ultravate™

Therapeutic Category Corticosteroid, Topical (Very High Potency)

Use Relief of inflammatory and pruritic manifestations of corticosteroid-response dermatoses [very high potency topical corticosteroid]

Usual Dosage Children and Adults: Topical: Apply sparingly to skin twice daily, rub in gently and completely; treatment should not exceed 2 consecutive weeks and total dosage should not exceed 50 g/week

Mechanism of Action Corticosteroids inhibit the initial manifestations of the inflammatory process (ie, capillary dilation and edema, fibrin deposition, and migration and diapedesis of leukocytes into the inflamed site) as well as later sequelae (angiogenesis, fibroblast proliferation)

Local Anesthetic/Vasoconstrictor Precautions No information available to require special precautions

Effects on Dental Treatment No effects or complications reported

Other Adverse Effects <1%: Topical: Burning, itching, irritation, dryness, folliculitis, hypertrichosis, acneiform eruptions, hypopigmentation, perioral dermatitis, allergic contact dermatitis, skin maceration, secondary infection, skin atrophy, striae, miliaria

Drug Interactions No data reported

Drug Uptake Absorption: Percutaneous absorption varies by location of topical application and the use of occlusive dressings; ~3% of a topically applied dose of ointment enters the circulation within 96 hours

Pregnancy Risk Factor C

Dosage Forms
Cream, as propionate: 0.05% (15 g, 45 g)
Ointment, topical, as propionate: 0.05% (15 g, 45 g)

Generic Available No

Halofantrine *(ha loe FAN trin)*

Brand Names Halfan®

Therapeutic Category Antimalarial Agent

Use Treatment of mild to moderate acute malaria caused by susceptible strains of *Plasmodium falciparum* and *Plasmodium vivax*

Usual Dosage Oral:
Children <40 kg: 8 mg/kg every 6 hours for 3 doses
Adults: 500 mg every 6 hours for 3 doses

Mechanism of Action Similar to mefloquine; destruction of asexual blood forms, possible inhibition of proton pump

Local Anesthetic/Vasoconstrictor Precautions No information available to require special precautions

Effects on Dental Treatment No effects or complications reported

Other Adverse Effects
>10%: Dermatologic: Pruritus
1% to 10%:
  Cardiovascular: Edema
  Central nervous system: Malaise, headache
  Gastrointestinal: Nausea, vomiting
  Hematologic: Leukocytosis
  Hepatic: Elevated LFTs
  Local: Tenderness
  Neuromuscular & skeletal: Myalgia
  Respiratory: Cough

Miscellaneous: Lymphadenopathy

<1%:
Cardiovascular: Tachycardia, hypotension
Dermatologic: Urticaria
Endocrine & metabolic: Hypoglycemia
Local: Sterile abscesses
Respiratory: Asthma
Miscellaneous: Anaphylactic shock

Drug Interactions No data reported

Drug Uptake

Mean time to parasite clearance: 40-84 hours

Absorption: Erratic and variable; serum levels are proportional to dose up to 1000 mg; doses greater than this should be divided; may be increased 60% with high fat meals

Serum half-life: 23 hours; metabolite: 82 hours; may be increased in active disease

Pregnancy Risk Factor X

Generic Available No

Halog® *see* Halcinonide *on page 461*

Halog®-E *see* Halcinonide *on page 461*

Haloperidol (ha loe PER i dole)

Brand Names Haldol®; Haldol® Decanoate

Canadian/Mexican Brand Names Haloperil® (Mexico)

Therapeutic Category Antipsychotic Agent

Use Treatment of psychoses, Tourette's disorder, and severe behavioral problems in children; may be used for the emergency sedation of severely agitated or delirious patients

Usual Dosage

Children: 3-12 years (15-40 kg): Oral:

Initial: 0.05 mg/kg/day or 0.25-0.5 mg/day given in 2-3 divided doses; increase by 0.25-0.5 mg every 5-7 days; maximum: 0.15 mg/kg/day

Usual maintenance:

Agitation or hyperkinesia: 0.01-0.03 mg/kg/day once daily
Nonpsychotic disorders: 0.05-0.075 mg/kg/day in 2-3 divided doses
Psychotic disorders: 0.05-0.15 mg/kg/day in 2-3 divided doses

Children 6-12 years: I.M. (as lactate): 1-3 mg/dose every 4-8 hours to a maximum of 0.15 mg/kg/day; change over to oral therapy as soon as able

Adults:

Oral: 0.5-5 mg 2-3 times/day; usual maximum: 30 mg/day; some patients may require up to 100 mg/day

I.M. (as lactate): 2-5 mg every 4-8 hours as needed

I.M. (as decanoate): Initial: 10-15 times the daily oral dose administered at 3- to 4-week intervals

Sedation in the Intensive Care Unit:

I.M./IVP/IVPB: May repeat bolus doses after 30 minutes until calm achieved then administer 50% of the maximum dose every 6 hours

Mild agitation: 0.5-2 mg
Moderate agitation: 2-5 mg
Severe agitation: 10-20 mg

Continuous intravenous infusion (100 mg/100 mL D_5W): Rates of 1-40 mg/hour have been used

Elderly (nonpsychotic patients, dementia behavior):

Initial: Oral: 0.25-0.5 mg 1-2 times/day; increase dose at 4- to 7-day intervals by 0.25-0.5 mg/day; increase dosing intervals (twice daily, 3 times/day, etc) as necessary to control response or side effects

Maximum daily dose: 50 mg; gradual increases (titration) may prevent side effects or decrease their severity

Hemodialysis/peritoneal dialysis effects: Supplemental dose is not necessary

Mechanism of Action Blocks postsynaptic mesolimbic dopaminergic D_1 and D_2 receptors in the brain; exhibits a strong alpha-adrenergic blocking and anticholinergic effect, depresses the release of hypothalamic and hypophyseal hormones; believed to depress the reticular activating system thus affecting basal metabolism, body temperature, wakefulness, vasomotor tone, and emesis

Local Anesthetic/Vasoconstrictor Precautions No information available to require special precautions

Effects on Dental Treatment Orthostatic hypotension and nasal congestion possible in dental patients. Since the drug is a dopamine antagonist, extrapyramidal symptoms of the TMJ a possibility.

(Continued)

Haloperidol (Continued)

Other Adverse Effects Sedation and anticholinergic effects are more pronounced than extrapyramidal effects; EKG changes, retinal pigmentation are more common than with chlorpromazine

>10%:
Central nervous system: Sedation, drowsiness, restlessness, anxiety, extrapyramidal reactions, dystonic reactions, pseudoparkinsonian signs and symptoms, tardive dyskinesia, neuroleptic malignant syndrome, seizures, altered central temperature regulation, akathisia
Endocrine & metabolic: Swelling of breasts
Gastrointestinal: Weight gain, constipation

1% to 10%:
Cardiovascular: Hypotension (especially orthostatic), tachycardia, arrhythmias, abnormal T waves with prolonged ventricular repolarization
Central nervous system: Hallucinations, drowsiness
Gastrointestinal: Nausea, vomiting
Genitourinary: Dysuria

<1%:
Central nervous system: Tardive dystonia, heat stroke, altered central temperature regulation
Dermatologic: Hyperpigmentation, pruritus, rash, contact dermatitis, alopecia, photosensitivity (rare)
Endocrine & metabolic: Amenorrhea, galactorrhea, gynecomastia, sexual dysfunction
Gastrointestinal: Adynamic ileus, dry mouth (problem for denture user)
Genitourinary: Urinary retention, overflow incontinence, priapism
Hematologic: Agranulocytosis, leukopenia (usually inpatients with large doses for prolonged periods)
Hepatic: Cholestatic jaundice, obstructive jaundice
Ocular: Blurred vision, retinal pigmentation, decreased visual acuity (may be irreversible)
Respiratory: Laryngospasm, respiratory depression

Drug Interactions Cytochrome P-450 IID6 enzyme inhibitor
Decreased effect: Carbamazepine and phenobarbital may increase metabolism and decreased effectiveness of haloperidol
Increased toxicity: CNS depressants may increase adverse effects; epinephrine may cause hypotension; haloperidol and anticholinergic agents cause increased intraocular pressure; concurrent use with lithium has occasionally caused acute encephalopathy-like syndrome

Drug Uptake
Onset of sedation: I.V.: Within 1 hour
Duration of action: ~3 weeks for decanoate form
Serum half-life: 20 hours
Time to peak serum concentration: 20 minutes

Pregnancy Risk Factor C
Generic Available Yes

Haloprogin (ha loe PROE jin)

Brand Names Halotex®
Therapeutic Category Antifungal Agent, Topical
Use Topical treatment of tinea pedis (athlete's foot), tinea cruris (jock itch), tinea corporis (ring worm), tinea manuum caused by *Trichophyton rubrum*, *Trichophyton tonsurans*, *Trichophyton mentagrophytes*, *Microsporum canis*, or *Epidermophyton floccosum*. Topical treatment of *Malassezia furfur*.
Usual Dosage Topical: Children and Adults: Apply liberally twice daily for 2-3 weeks; intertriginous areas may require up to 4 weeks of treatment
Mechanism of Action Interferes with fungal DNA replication to inhibit yeast cell respiration and disrupt its cell membrane
Local Anesthetic/Vasoconstrictor Precautions No information available to require special precautions
Effects on Dental Treatment No effects or complications reported
Other Adverse Effects <1%: Topical: Pruritus, folliculitis, irritation, burning sensation, vesicle formation, erythema
Drug Interactions No data reported
Drug Uptake
Absorption: Poorly through the skin (~11%)
Pregnancy Risk Factor B
Generic Available No

Halotestin® *see* Fluoxymesterone *on page 420*
Halotex® *see* Haloprogin *on this page*

Halotussin® [OTC] *see* Guaifenesin *on page 452*

Halotussin® DAC *see* Guaifenesin, Pseudoephedrine, and Codeine *on page 455*

Halotussin® DM [OTC] *see* Guaifenesin and Dextromethorphan *on page 453*

Halotussin® PE [OTC] *see* Guaifenesin and Pseudoephedrine *on page 454*

Haltran® [OTC] *see* Ibuprofen *on page 495*

Havrix® *see* Hepatitis A Vaccine *on page 467*

Hayfebrol® Liquid [OTC] *see* Chlorpheniramine and Pseudoephedrine *on page 219*

HbCV *see* Haemophilus b Conjugate Vaccine *on page 460*

H-BIG® *see* Hepatitis B Immune Globulin *on page 468*

Head & Shoulders® [OTC] *see* Pyrithione Zinc *on page 826*

Healon® *see* Sodium Hyaluronate *on page 873*

Healon® GV *see* Sodium Hyaluronate *on page 873*

Helidac® *see* Bismuth Subsalicylate, Metronidazole, and Tetracycline *on page 132*

Helidac® Combination *see* Metronidazole *on page 631*

Helistat® *see* Microfibrillar Collagen Hemostat *on page 636*

Helixate® *see* Antihemophilic Factor (Recombinant) *on page 81*

Hemabate™ *see* Carboprost Tromethamine *on page 179*

Hemiacidrin *see* Citric Acid Bladder Mixture *on page 239*

Hemin (HEE min)
Brand Names Panhematin®
Therapeutic Category Blood Modifiers
Use Treatment of recurrent attacks of acute intermittent porphyria (AIP) only after an appropriate period of alternate therapy has been tried
Local Anesthetic/Vasoconstrictor Precautions No information available to require special precautions
Effects on Dental Treatment No effects or complications reported
Other Adverse Effects 1% to 10%:
Central nervous system: Mild pyrexia
Hematologic: Leukocytosis
Local: Phlebitis
Generic Available No

Hemocyte® [OTC] *see* Ferrous Fumarate *on page 400*

Hemodent® Gingival Retraction Cord *see* Aluminum Chloride *on page 47*

Hemofil® M *see* Antihemophilic Factor (Human) *on page 80*

Hemotene® *see* Microfibrillar Collagen Hemostat *on page 636*

Heparin (HEP a rin)
Brand Names Hep-Lock®
Canadian/Mexican Brand Names Dixaparine® (Mexico); Fraxiparine® (Mexico); Helberina (Mexico); Inhepar (Mexico)
Therapeutic Category Anticoagulant
Synonyms Heparin Lock Flush; Heparin Sodium, Heparin Calcium
Use Prophylaxis and treatment of thromboembolic disorders
Usual Dosage
Line flushing: When using daily flushes of heparin to maintain patency of single and double lumen central catheters, 10 units/mL is commonly used for younger infants (eg, <10 kg) while 100 units/mL is used for older infants, children, and adults. Capped PVC catheters and peripheral heparin locks require flushing more frequently (eg, every 6-8 hours). Volume of heparin flush is usually similar to volume of catheter (or slightly greater). Additional flushes should be given when stagnant blood is observed in catheter, after catheter is used for drug or blood administration, and after blood withdrawal from catheter.

Addition of heparin (0.5-1 unit/mL) to peripheral and central TPN has been shown to increase duration of line patency. The final concentration of heparin used for TPN solutions may need to be decreased to 0.5 units/mL in small infants receiving larger amounts of volume in order to avoid approaching therapeutic amounts. Arterial lines are heparinized with a final concentration of 1 unit/mL.

Children:
Intermittent I.V.: Initial: 50-100 units/kg, then 50-100 units/kg every 4 hours
I.V. infusion: Initial: 50 units/kg, then 15-25 units/kg/hour; increase dose by 2-4 units/kg/hour every 6-8 hours as required

Adults:
Prophylaxis (low-dose heparin): S.C.: 5000 units every 8-12 hours
Intermittent I.V.: Initial: 10,000 units, then 50-70 units/kg (5000-10,000 units) every 4-6 hours
(Continued)

Heparin *(Continued)*

I.V. infusion: 50 units/kg to start, then 15-25 units/kg/hour as continuous infusion; increase dose by 5 units/kg/hour every 4 hours as required according to PTT results, usual range: 10-30 units/hour

Weight-based protocol: 80 units/kg I.V. push followed by continuous infusion of 18 units/kg/hour. See table.

Standard Heparin Solution (25,000 units/500 mL D₅W)

To Administer a Dose of	Set Infusion Rate at
400 units/h	8 mL/h
500 units/h	10 mL/h
600 units/h	12 mL/h
700 units/h	14 mL/h
800 units/h	16 mL/h
900 units/h	18 mL/h
1000 units/h	20 mL/h
1100 units/h	22 mL/h
1200 units/h	24 mL/h
1300 units/h	26 mL/h
1400 units/h	28 mL/h
1500 units/h	30 mL/h
1600 units/h	32 mL/h
1700 units/h	34 mL/h
1800 units/h	36 mL/h
1900 units/h	38 mL/h
2000 units/h	40 mL/h

Mechanism of Action Potentiates the action of antithrombin III and thereby inactivates thrombin (as well as activated coagulation factors IX, X, XI, XII, and plasmin) and prevents the conversion of fibrinogen to fibrin; heparin also stimulates release of lipoprotein lipase (lipoprotein lipase hydrolyzes triglycerides to glycerol and free fatty acids)

Local Anesthetic/Vasoconstrictor Precautions No information available to require special precautions

Effects on Dental Treatment No effects or complications reported

Other Adverse Effects

>10%:
Dermatologic: Unexplained bruising
Gastrointestinal: Constipation, vomiting of blood, bleeding from gums
Hematologic: Hemorrhage, blood in urine

1% to 10%:
Cardiovascular: Chest pain
Genitourinary: Frequent or persistent erection
Neuromuscular & skeletal: Peripheral neuropathy
Miscellaneous: Allergic reactions

<1%:
Central nervous system: Fever, headache, chills
Dermatologic: Urticaria
Gastrointestinal: Nausea, vomiting
Hematologic: Thrombocytopenia (heparin-associated thrombocytopenia occurs in <1% of patients, immune thrombocytopenia occurs with progressive fall in platelet counts and, in some cases, thromboembolic complications; daily platelet counts for 5-7 days at initiation of therapy may help detect the onset of this complication)
Hepatic: Elevated liver enzymes
Local: Irritation, ulceration, cutaneous necrosis have been rarely reported with deep S.C. injections
Neuromuscular & skeletal: Osteoporosis (chronic therapy effect)

Drug Uptake

Onset of anticoagulation:
I.V.: Immediate with use
S.C.: Within 20-30 minutes
Absorption: Oral, rectal, sublingual, I.M.: Erratic
Serum half-life:
Mean: 1.5 hours

Range: 1-2 hours; affected by obesity, renal function, hepatic function, malignancy, presence of pulmonary embolism, and infections

Pregnancy Risk Factor C

Generic Available Yes

Comments Heparin does not possess fibrinolytic activity and, therefore, cannot lyse established thrombi; discontinue heparin if hemorrhage occurs; severe hemorrhage or overdosage may require protamine; monitor platelet counts, signs of bleeding, PTT.

When using daily flushes of heparin to maintain patency of single and double lumen central catheters, 10 units/mL is commonly used for younger infants (eg, <10 kg) while 100 units/mL is used for older infants and children (eg, ≥10 kg). Capped PVC catheters and peripheral heparin locks require flushing more frequently (eg, every 6-8 hours). Volume of heparin flush is usually similar to volume of catheter (or slightly greater) or may be standardized according to specific hospital's policy (eg, 2-5 mL/flush). Dose of heparin flush used should not approach therapeutic per kg dose. Additional flushes should be given when stagnant blood is observed in catheter, after catheter is used for drug or blood administration, and after blood withdrawal from catheter.

Heparin 1 unit/mL (final concentration) may be added to TPN solutions, both central and peripheral. (Addition of heparin to peripheral TPN has been shown to increase duration of line patency.) The final concentration of heparin used for TPN solutions may need to be decreased to 0.5 units/mL in small infants receiving larger amounts of volume in order to avoid approaching therapeutic amounts.

Arterial lines are heparinized with a final concentration of 1 unit/mL.

Heparin Cofactor I see Antithrombin III on page 82

Heparin Lock Flush see Heparin on page 465

Heparin Sodium, Heparin Calcium see Heparin on page 465

Hepatitis A Vaccine (hep a TYE tis aye vak SEEN)

Related Information

Systemic Viral Diseases on page 1047

Brand Names Havrix®

Therapeutic Category Vaccine, Inactivated Virus

Use For populations desiring protection against hepatitis A or for populations at high risk of exposure to hepatitis A virus (travelers to developing countries, household and sexual contacts of persons infected with hepatitis A), child day care employees, illicit drug users, male homosexuals, institutional workers (eg, institutions for the mentally and physically handicapped persons, prisons, etc), and healthcare workers who may be exposed to hepatitis A virus (eg, laboratory employees)

Usual Dosage I.M.:

Children: 0.5 mL (360 units) on days 1 and 30, with a booster dose 6-12 months later (completion of the first 2 doses [ie, the primary series] should be accomplished at least 2 weeks before anticipated exposure to hepatitis A)

Adults: 1 mL (1440 units), with a booster dose at 6-12 months

Mechanism of Action As an inactivated virus vaccine, hepatitis A vaccine offers active immunization against hepatitis A virus infection at an effective immune response rate in up to 99% of subjects

Local Anesthetic/Vasoconstrictor Precautions No information available to require special precautions

Effects on Dental Treatment No effects or complications reported

Other Adverse Effects

Central nervous system: Headache, fatigue, fever (rare)

Hepatic: Transient liver function test abnormalities

Local: Cutaneous reactions at the injection site (pain, soreness, tenderness, swelling, warmth, and redness)

Drug Interactions No interference of immunogenicity was reported when mixed with hepatitis B vaccine

Drug Uptake

Onset of action (protection): 3 weeks after a single dose

Duration: Neutralizing antibodies have persisted for >3 years; unconfirmed evidence indicates that antibody levels may persist for 5-10 years

Pregnancy Risk Factor C

Generic Available No

Hepatitis B Immune Globulin
(hep a TYE tis bee i MYUN GLOB yoo lin)

Related Information
Occupational Exposure to Bloodborne Pathogens (Universal Precautions) *on page 1151*
Systemic Viral Diseases *on page 1047*

Brand Names H-BIG®; HyperHep®

Therapeutic Category Immune Globulin

Use Provide prophylactic passive immunity to hepatitis B infection to those individuals exposed; newborns of mothers known to be hepatitis B surface antigen positive; hepatitis B immune globulin is not indicated for treatment of active hepatitis B infections and is ineffective in the treatment of chronic active hepatitis B infection

Usual Dosage I.M.:
Newborns: Hepatitis B: 0.5 mL as soon after birth as possible (within 12 hours)
Adults: Postexposure prophylaxis: 0.06 mL/kg; usual dose: 3-5 mL; repeat at 28-30 days after exposure

Mechanism of Action Hepatitis B immune globulin (HBIG) is a nonpyrogenic sterile solution containing 10% to 18% protein of which at least 80% is monomeric immunoglobulin G (IgG). HBIG differs from immune globulin in the amount of anti-HBs. Immune globulin is prepared from plasma that is not preselected for anti-HBs content. HBIG is prepared from plasma preselected for high titer anti-HBs. In the U.S., HBIG has an anti-HBs high titer of higher than 1:100,000 by IRA. There is no evidence that the causative agent of AIDS (HTLV-III/LAV) is transmitted by HBIG.

Local Anesthetic/Vasoconstrictor Precautions No information available to require special precautions

Effects on Dental Treatment No effects or complications reported

Other Adverse Effects
1% to 10%:
Central nervous system: Dizziness, malaise
Dermatologic: Urticaria, angioedema, rash, erythema
Local: Pain and tenderness at injection site
Neuromuscular & skeletal: Arthralgia
<1%: Miscellaneous: Anaphylaxis

Drug Interactions Increased toxicity: Live virus vaccines

Drug Uptake
Absorption: Slow
Time to peak serum concentration: 1-6 days

Pregnancy Risk Factor C

Generic Available No

Hepatitis B Vaccine (hep a TYE tis bee vak SEEN)
Related Information
Systemic Viral Diseases *on page 1047*

Brand Names Engerix-B®; Recombivax HB®

Therapeutic Category Vaccine, Inactivated Virus

Use Immunization against infection caused by all known subtypes of hepatitis B virus in individuals considered at high risk of potential exposure to hepatitis B virus or HB$_s$Ag-positive materials

Usual Dosage See tables.

Mechanism of Action Recombinant hepatitis B vaccine is a noninfectious subunit viral vaccine. The vaccine is derived from hepatitis B surface antigen (HB$_s$Ag) produced through recombinant DNA techniques from yeast cells. The portion of the hepatitis B gene which codes for HB$_s$Ag is cloned into yeast which is then cultured to produce hepatitis B vaccine.

Local Anesthetic/Vasoconstrictor Precautions No information available to require special precautions

Effects on Dental Treatment No effects or complications reported

Recommended Dosage for Infants Born to HB$_s$Ag Positive Mothers

Treatment	Birth	Within 7 d	1 mo	6 mo
Engerix-B® (pediatric dose 10 mcg/0.5 mL)	*	0.5 mL*	0.5 mL	0.5 mL
Recombivax HB® (pediatric dose 5 mcg/0.5 mL)	*	0.5 mL*	0.5 mL	0.5 mL
Hepatitis B immune globulin	0.5 mL	—	—	—

*The first dose may be given at birth at the same time as HBIG, but give in the opposite anterolateral thigh. This may better ensure vaccine absorption.

Immunization Regimen of Three I.M. Hepatitis B Vaccine Doses

Age	Initial		1 mo		6 mo	
	Recom-bivax HB® (mL)	Enger-ix-B® (mL)	Recom-bivax HB® (mL)	Enger-ix-B® (mL)	Recom-bivax HB® (mL)	Enger-ix-B® (mL)
Birth* - 10 y	0.25	0.5	0.25	0.5	0.25	0.5
11-19 y	0.5	1	0.5	1	0.5	1
≥20 y	1	1	1	1	1	1
Dialysis or immuno-compromised pa-tients		2†		2†		2†

*Infants born of HB$_s$Ag negative mothers.

†Two 1 mL doses given at different sites.

Other Adverse Effects
>10%:
Central nervous system: Fever, malaise, fatigue, headache
Local: Mild local tenderness, local inflammatory reaction
1% to 10%:
Gastrointestinal: Nausea, diarrhea
Respiratory: Pharyngitis
<1%:
Cardiovascular: Tachycardia, hypotension, flushing
Central nervous system: Lightheadedness, chills, somnolence, insomnia, irrita-bility, agitation
Dermatologic: Pruritus, rash, erythema, urticaria
Gastrointestinal: Vomiting, GI disturbances, constipation, abdominal cramps, dyspepsia, anorexia
Genitourinary: Dysuria
Neuromuscular & skeletal: Arthralgia, myalgia, stiffness in back/neck/arm or shoulder
Otic: Earache
Respiratory: Rhinitis, cough, epistaxis
Miscellaneous: Sweating, sensation of warmth
Drug Interactions Decreased effect: Immunosuppressive agents
Drug Uptake Duration of action: Following all 3 doses of hepatitis B vaccine, immunity will last approximately 5-7 years
Pregnancy Risk Factor C
Generic Available No

Hep-Lock® see Heparin on page 465
Heptalac® see Lactulose on page 540
Herplex® see Idoxuridine on page 498
HES see Hetastarch on this page
Hespan® see Hetastarch on this page

Hetastarch (HET a starch)
Brand Names Hespan®
Therapeutic Category Plasma Volume Expander
Synonyms HES; Hydroxyethyl Starch
Use Blood volume expander used in treatment of shock or impending shock when blood or blood products are not available; does not have oxygen-carrying capacity and is not a substitute for blood or plasma; an adjunct in leukapheresis to enhance the yield of granulocytes by centrifugal means
Usual Dosage I.V. infusion (requires an infusion pump):
Children: Safety and efficacy have not been established
Adults: 500-1000 mL (up to 1500 mL/day) or 20 mL/kg/day (up to 1500 mL/day); larger volumes (15,000 mL/24 hours) have been used safely in small numbers of patients
Mechanism of Action Produces plasma volume expansion by virtue of its highly colloidal starch structure, similar to albumin
Local Anesthetic/Vasoconstrictor Precautions No information available to require special precautions
Effects on Dental Treatment No effects or complications reported
Other Adverse Effects <1%:
Cardiovascular: Peripheral edema, heart failure, circulatory overload
Central nervous system: Fever, chills, headaches
Dermatologic: Itching, pruritus
Gastrointestinal: Vomiting
Hematologic: Bleeding, prolongation of PT, PTT, clotting time, and bleeding time
(Continued)

Hetastarch *(Continued)*

Neuromuscular & skeletal: Myalgia
Miscellaneous: Hypersensitivity

Drug Uptake
Onset of volume expansion: I.V.: Within 30 minutes
Duration: 24-36 hours

Pregnancy Risk Factor C

Generic Available No

Comments Does not have oxygen-carrying capacity and is not a substitute for blood or plasma; large volumes may interfere with platelet function and prolong PT and PTT times; safety and efficacy in children have not been established; hetastarch is a synthetic polymer derived from a waxy starch composed of amylopectin; average molecular weight = 450,000

Hexachlorophene *(heks a KLOR oh feen)*

Brand Names pHisoHex®; pHiso® Scrub; Septisol®

Therapeutic Category Antibacterial, Topical; Soap

Use Surgical scrub and as a bacteriostatic skin cleanser; control an outbreak of gram-positive infection when other procedures have been unsuccessful

Usual Dosage Children and Adults: Topical: Apply 5 mL cleanser and water to area to be cleansed; lather and rinse thoroughly under running water

Mechanism of Action Bacteriostatic polychlorinated biphenyl which inhibits membrane-bound enzymes and disrupts the cell membrane

Local Anesthetic/Vasoconstrictor Precautions No information available to require special precautions

Effects on Dental Treatment No effects or complications reported

Other Adverse Effects <1%:
Central nervous system: CNS injury, seizures, irritability
Dermatologic: Photosensitivity, dermatitis, redness, dry skin

Drug Interactions No data reported

Drug Uptake
Absorption: Percutaneously through inflamed, excoriated, and intact skin
Serum half-life: Infants: 6.1-44.2 hours

Pregnancy Risk Factor C

Dosage Forms
Foam (Septisol®): 0.23% with alcohol 56% (180 mL, 600 mL)
Liquid, topical (pHisoHex®): 3% (8 mL, 150 mL, 500 mL, 3840 mL)

Generic Available Yes

Hexadrol® *see* Dexamethasone *on page 291*

Hexalen® *see* Altretamine *on page 46*

Hexavitamin *see* Vitamins, Multiple *on page 995*

Hexobarbital *(hex oh BAR bi tal)*

Brand Names Pre-Sed®

Therapeutic Category Sedative

Use Preoperative medication; short-term sedation for diagnostic and minor surgical procedures; potentiating agent for analgesic; postoperative medication; patients suffering from mental and emotional stress that cannot fall asleep

Restrictions C-III

Usual Dosage Oral:
Children 6-12 years: One-fourth (¼) to one-half (½) tablet ~15 minutes before procedure
Children >12 years: One-half (<12)[to 1 tablet ~15 minutes before procedure
Adults: 1-2o tablets ~15 minutes before procedure

Mechanism of Action Interferes with transmission of impulses from the thalamus to the cortex of the brain resulting in an imbalance in central inhibitory and facilitatory mechanisms

Local Anesthetic/Vasoconstrictor Precautions No information available to require special precautions

Effects on Dental Treatment No effects or complications reported

Contraindications Hypersensitivity to hexobarbital or any component; pre-existing CNS depression, severe uncontrolled pain, porphyria, severe respiratory disease with dyspnea or obstruction; patients with impairment of renal function

Warnings/Precautions May be habit forming; untoward response attributable to barbiturates are particularly likely to occur in patients with fever, hyperthyroidism, diabetes mellitus, severe anemia, latent or manifest porphyria and congestive heart failure. Use with caution in patients with respiratory disease associated with dyspnea or obstruction; in patients with impaired hepatic function, the dose should be reduced.

Drug Interactions Caution should be observed when barbiturates and tranquilizers or antihistamines are administered simultaneously, as there may be a synergistic effect; smaller doses than the usual are then indicated. Barbiturate pretreatment of patients being induced with oral coumarin-type anticoagulants may prevent anticoagulation.

Drug Uptake Duration of action: ~1 hour

Dosage Forms Tablet, scored: 260 mg

Comments This tranquilizer has a rapid 10-minute onset time and ultra-short duration of 1 hour; developed exclusively for the dental industry to help reduce chair time. A comfortable patient will return and talk about the ease of his appointment.

Hexylresorcinol (heks il re ZOR si nole)
Brand Names Sucrets® Sore Throat [OTC]
Therapeutic Category Local Anesthetic
Use Minor antiseptic and local anesthetic for sore throat
Usual Dosage May be used as needed, allow to dissolve slowly in mouth
Local Anesthetic/Vasoconstrictor Precautions No information available to require special precautions
Effects on Dental Treatment No effects or complications reported
Dosage Forms Lozenge: 2.4 mg
Generic Available Yes

Hibiclens® Topical [OTC] see Chlorhexidine Gluconate on page 211

Hibistat® Topical [OTC] see Chlorhexidine Gluconate on page 211

Hib Polysaccharide Conjugate see Haemophilus b Conjugate Vaccine on page 460

HibTITER® see Haemophilus b Conjugate Vaccine on page 460

Hidralacina Clorhidrato De (Mexico) see Hydralazine on page 475

Hidroclorotiacida (Mexico) see Hydrochlorothiazide on page 476

Hidroquinona (Mexico) see Hydroquinone on page 487

Hidroxicloroquina Sulfato De (Mexico) see Hydroxychloroquine on page 488

Hidroxiprogesterona Caproato De (Mexico) see Hydroxyprogesterone Caproate on page 489

Hidroxocobalamina (Mexico) see Hydroxocobalamin on page 487

Hiprex® see Methenamine on page 610

Hismanal® see Astemizole on page 94

Histalet Forte® Tablet see Chlorpheniramine, Pyrilamine, Phenylephrine, and Phenylpropanolamine on page 223

Histalet® Syrup [OTC] see Chlorpheniramine and Pseudoephedrine on page 219

Histalet® X see Guaifenesin and Pseudoephedrine on page 454

Histatab® Plus Tablet [OTC] see Chlorpheniramine and Phenylephrine on page 218

Hista-Vadrin® Tablet see Chlorpheniramine, Phenylephrine, and Phenylpropanolamine on page 221

Histerone® Injection see Testosterone on page 910

Histolyn-CYL® Injection see Histoplasmin on this page

Histoplasmin (his toe PLAZ min)
Brand Names Histolyn-CYL® Injection
Therapeutic Category Diagnostic Agent, Skin Test
Synonyms Histoplasmosis Skin Test Antigen
Use Diagnosing histoplasmosis; to assess cell-mediated immunity
Local Anesthetic/Vasoconstrictor Precautions No information available to require special precautions
Effects on Dental Treatment No effects or complications reported
Other Adverse Effects 1% to 10%:
Dermatologic: Pruritus, urticaria
Local: Ulceration or necrosis may occur at test site
Respiratory: Dyspnea
Pregnancy Risk Factor C
Generic Available No

Histoplasmosis Skin Test Antigen see Histoplasmin on this page

Histor-D® Syrup see Chlorpheniramine and Phenylephrine on page 218

Histor-D® Timecelles® see Chlorpheniramine, Phenylephrine, and Methscopolamine on page 220

Histrelin (his TREL in)
Brand Names Supprelin™
Therapeutic Category Gonadotropin Releasing Hormone Analog
(Continued)

Histrelin *(Continued)*

Use Treatment of central idiopathic precocious puberty; treatment of estrogen-associated gynecological disorders such as acute intermittent porphyria, endometriosis, leiomyomata uteri, and premenstrual syndrome

Usual Dosage
Central idiopathic precocious puberty: S.C.: Usual dose is 10 mcg/kg/day given as a single daily dose at the same time each day
Acute intermittent porphyria in women: S.C.: 5 mcg/day
Endometriosis: S.C.: 100 mcg/day
Leiomyomata uteri: S.C.: 20-50 mcg/day or 4 mcg/kg/day

Mechanism of Action Histrelin is a synthetic long-acting gonadotropin-releasing hormone analog; with daily administration, it desensitizes the pituitary to endogenous gonadotropin-releasing hormone (ie, suppresses gonadotropin release by causing down regulation of the pituitary); this results in a decrease in gonadal sex steroid production which stops the secondary sexual development

Local Anesthetic/Vasoconstrictor Precautions No information available to require special precautions

Effects on Dental Treatment No effects or complications reported

Other Adverse Effects
>10%:
Cardiovascular: Vasodilation
Central nervous system: Headache
Gastrointestinal: Abdominal pain
Genitourinary: Vaginal bleeding, vaginal dryness
Local: Skin reaction at injection site
1% to 10%:
Central nervous system: Mood swings
Dermatologic: Skin rashes, urticaria
Endocrine & metabolic: Breast tenderness, hot flashes
Gastrointestinal: Nausea, vomiting
Neuromuscular & skeletal: Joint stiffness, pain
Renal: Increased urinary calcium excretion

Drug Interactions No data reported

Drug Uptake
Precocious puberty: Onset of hormonal responses: Within 3 months of initiation of therapy
Acute intermittent porphyria associated with menses: Amelioration of symptoms: After 1-2 months of therapy
Treatment of endometriosis or leiomyomata uteri: Onset of responses: After 3-6 months of treatment

Pregnancy Risk Factor X
Generic Available No

Hi-Vegi-Lip® *see* Pancreatin *on page 721*
Hivid® *see* Zalcitabine *on page 1001*
HIV Infection and AIDS *see page 1024*
HMS Liquifilm® *see* Medrysone *on page 587*
Hold® DM [OTC] *see* Dextromethorphan *on page 298*

Homatropine *(hoe MA troe peen)*

Brand Names AK-Homatropine® Ophthalmic; Isopto® Homatropine Ophthalmic
Therapeutic Category Anticholinergic Agent, Ophthalmic; Ophthalmic Agent, Mydriatic
Use Producing cycloplegia and mydriasis for refraction; treatment of acute inflammatory conditions of the uveal tract

Usual Dosage
Children:
Mydriasis and cycloplegia for refraction: Instill 1 drop of 2% solution immediately before the procedure; repeat at 10-minute intervals as needed
Uveitis: Instill 1 drop of 2% solution 2-3 times/day

Adults:
Mydriasis and cycloplegia for refraction: Instill 1-2 drops of 2% solution or 1 drop of 5% solution before the procedure; repeat at 5- to 10-minute intervals as needed
Uveitis: Instill 1-2 drops of 2% or 5% 2-3 times/day up to every 3-4 hours as needed

Mechanism of Action Blocks response of iris sphincter muscle and the accommodative muscle of the ciliary body to cholinergic stimulation resulting in dilation and loss of accommodation

Local Anesthetic/Vasoconstrictor Precautions No information available to require special precautions

Effects on Dental Treatment No effects or complications reported
Other Adverse Effects
>10%: Ocular: Blurred vision, photophobia
1% to 10%:
　Local: Stinging, local irritation
　Ocular: Increased intraocular pressure
　Respiratory: Congestion
<1%:
　Cardiovascular: Vascular congestion, edema
　Central nervous system: Drowsiness
　Dermatologic: Exudate, eczematoid dermatitis
　Ocular: Follicular conjunctivitis
Drug Uptake
Onset of accommodation and pupil effect: Ophthalmic:
　Maximum mydriatic effect: Within 10-30 minutes
　Maximum cycloplegic effect: Within 30-90 minutes
Duration:
　Mydriasis: 6 hours to 4 days
　Cycloplegia: 10-48 hours
Pregnancy Risk Factor C
Generic Available Yes

Homatropine and Hydrocodone *see* Hydrocodone and Homatropine *on page 481*

Horse Anti-human Thymocyte Gamma Globulin *see* Lymphocyte Immune Globulin *on page 572*

H.P. Acthar® Gel *see* Corticotropin *on page 262*

Humalog® *see* Insulin Preparations *on page 509*

Human Growth Hormone (HYU man grothe HOR mone)

Brand Names Genotropin® Injection; Humatrope® Injection; Norditropin® Injection; Nutropin® AQ Injection; Nutropin® Injection; Protropin® Injection; Serostim® Injection

Therapeutic Category Growth Hormone
Use
Long-term treatment of growth failure from lack of adequate endogenous growth hormone secretion
Nutropin®: Treatment of children who have growth failure associated with chronic renal insufficiency up until the time of renal transplantation
Usual Dosage Children (individualize dose):
Somatrem (Protropin®): I.M., S.C.: Up to 0.1 mg (0.26 units)/kg/dose 3 times/week
Somatropin (Humatrope®): I.M., S.C.: Up to 0.06 mg (0.16 units)/kg/dose 3 times/week
Somatropin (Nutropin®): S.C.:
　Growth hormone inadequacy: Weekly dosage of 0.3 mg/kg (0.78 units/kg) administered daily
　Chronic renal insufficiency: Weekly dosage of 0.35 mg/kg (0.91 units/kg) administered daily
　Therapy should be discontinued when patient has reached satisfactory adult height, when epiphyses have fused, or when the patient ceases to respond
　Growth of 5 cm/year or more is expected, if growth rate does not exceed 2.5 cm in a 6-month period, double the dose for the next 6 months, if there is still no satisfactory response, discontinue therapy
Mechanism of Action Somatrem and somatropin are purified polypeptide hormones of recombinant DNA origin; somatrem contains the identical sequence of amino acids found in human growth hormone while somatropin's amino acid sequence is identical plus an additional amino acid, methionine; human growth hormone stimulates growth of linear bone, skeletal muscle, and organs; stimulates erythropoietin which increases red blood cell mass; exerts both insulin-like and diabetogenic effects
Local Anesthetic/Vasoconstrictor Precautions No information available to require special precautions
Effects on Dental Treatment No effects or complications reported
Other Adverse Effects S.C. administration can cause local lipoatrophy or lipodystrophy and may enhance the development of neutralizing antibodies
1% to 10%: Endocrine & metabolism: Hypothyroidism
<1%:
　Dermatologic: Skin rash, itching
　Endocrine & metabolic: Hypoglycemia
　Local: Pain at injection site
　Neuromuscular & skeletal: Pain in hip/knee
(Continued)

Human Growth Hormone (Continued)

Miscellaneous: Small risk for developing leukemia

Drug Interactions Decreased effect: Glucocorticoid therapy may inhibit growth-promoting effects.

Drug Uptake Somatrem and somatropin have equivalent pharmacokinetic properties

Duration of action: Maintains supraphysiologic levels for 18-20 hours

Absorption: I.M.: Well absorbed

Serum half-life: 15-50 minutes

Pregnancy Risk Factor C

Generic Available No

Humate-P® see Antihemophilic Factor (Human) on page 80

Humatin® see Paromomycin on page 725

Humatrope® Injection see Human Growth Hormone on previous page

Humegon™ see Menotropins on page 591

Humibid® DM [OTC] see Guaifenesin and Dextromethorphan on page 453

Humibid® L.A. see Guaifenesin on page 452

Humibid® Sprinkle see Guaifenesin on page 452

HuMist® Nasal Mist [OTC] see Sodium Chloride on page 870

Humorsol® see Demecarium on page 286

Humulin® 50/50 see Insulin Preparations on page 509

Humulin® 70/30 see Insulin Preparations on page 509

Humulin® L see Insulin Preparations on page 509

Humulin® N see Insulin Preparations on page 509

Humulin® R see Insulin Preparations on page 509

Humulin® U see Insulin Preparations on page 509

Hurricaine® see Benzocaine on page 118

Hyaluronic Acid see Sodium Hyaluronate on page 873

Hyaluronidase (hye al yoor ON i dase)

Brand Names Wydase® Injection

Therapeutic Category Antidote, Extravasation

Use Increase the dispersion and absorption of other drugs; increase rate of absorption of parenteral fluids administered by hypodermoclysis; management of I.V. extravasations

Usual Dosage

Children:

Management of I.V. extravasation: Reconstitute the 150 unit vial of lyophilized powder with 1 mL normal saline; take 0.1 mL of this solution and dilute with 0.9 mL normal saline to yield 15 units/mL; using a 25- or 26-gauge needle, five 0.2 mL injections are made subcutaneously or intradermally into the extravasation site at the leading edge, changing the needle after each injection

Hypodermoclysis:

S.C.: 1 mL (150 units) is added to 1000 mL of infusion fluid and 0.5 mL (75 units) in injected into each clysis site at the initiation of the infusion

I.V.: 15 units is added to each 100 mL of I.V. fluid to be administered

Adults: Absorption and dispersion of drugs: 150 units are added to the vehicle containing the drug

Mechanism of Action Modifies the permeability of connective tissue through hydrolysis of hyaluronic acid, one of the chief ingredients of tissue cement which offers resistance to diffusion of liquids through tissues

Local Anesthetic/Vasoconstrictor Precautions No information available to require special precautions

Effects on Dental Treatment No effects or complications reported

Other Adverse Effects <1%:

Cardiovascular: Tachycardia, hypotension

Central nervous system: Dizziness, chills

Dermatologic: Urticaria, erythema

Gastrointestinal: Nausea, vomiting

Drug Uptake

Onset of action: Immediate by the subcutaneous or intradermal routes for the treatment of extravasation

Duration: 24-48 hours

Pregnancy Risk Factor C

Generic Available No

Comments The USP hyaluronidase unit is equivalent to the turbidity-reducing (TR) unit and the International Unit; each unit is defined as being the activity contained in 100 mcg of the International Standard Preparation

Hyate®:C see Antihemophilic Factor (Porcine) on page 81

Hybolin™ Decanoate Injection see Nandrolone on page 663

Hybolin™ Improved Injection see Nandrolone on page 663

Hycamptamine see Topotecan on page 945

Hycamtin® see Topotecan on page 945

HycoClear Tuss® see Hydrocodone and Guaifenesin on page 481

Hycodan® see Hydrocodone and Homatropine on page 481

Hycomine® see Hydrocodone and Phenylpropanolamine on page 483

Hycomine® Compound see Hydrocodone, Chlorpheniramine, Phenylephrine, Acetaminophen and Caffeine on page 483

Hycomine® Pediatric see Hydrocodone and Phenylpropanolamine on page 483

Hycotuss® Expectorant Liquid see Hydrocodone and Guaifenesin on page 481

Hydergine® see Ergoloid Mesylates on page 358

Hydergine® LC see Ergoloid Mesylates on page 358

Hydralazine (hye DRAL a zeen)

Related Information
Cardiovascular Diseases on page 1010

Brand Names Apresoline®

Canadian/Mexican Brand Names Apo®-Hydralazine (Canada); Apresolina® (Mexico); Novo-Hylazin® (Canada); Nu-Hydral® (Canada)

Therapeutic Category Vasodilator

Synonyms Hidralacina Clorhidrato De (Mexico)

Use Management of moderate to severe hypertension, congestive heart failure, hypertension secondary to pre-eclampsia/eclampsia; also used to treat primary pulmonary hypertension

Usual Dosage
Children:
Oral: Initial: 0.75-1 mg/kg/day in 2-4 divided doses, not to exceed 25 mg/dose; increase over 3-4 weeks to maximum of 7.5 mg/kg/day in 2-4 divided doses; maximum daily dose: 200 mg/day
I.M., I.V.: 0.1-0.2 mg/kg/dose (not to exceed 20 mg) every 4-6 hours as needed, up to 1.7-3.5 mg/kg/day in 4-6 divided doses

Adults:
Oral: Hypertension:
Initial dose: 10 mg 4 times/day
Increase by 10-25 mg/dose every 2-5 days
Maximum dose: 300 mg/day
Oral: Congestive heart failure:
Initial dose: 10-25 mg TID
Target dose: 75 mg TID
Maximum dose: 100 mg TID
I.M., I.V.:
Hypertensive Initial: 10-20 mg/dose every 4-6 hours as needed, may increase to 40 mg/dose; change to oral therapy as soon as possible
Pre-eclampsia/eclampsia: 5 mg/dose then 5-10 mg every 20-30 minutes as needed

Elderly: Oral: Initial: 10 mg 2-3 times/day; increase by 10-25 mg/day every 2-5 days

Mechanism of Action Direct vasodilation of arterioles (with little effect on veins) with decreased systemic resistance

Local Anesthetic/Vasoconstrictor Precautions No information available to require special precautions

Effects on Dental Treatment No effects or complications reported

Other Adverse Effects
>10%:
Cardiovascular: Palpitations, flushing, tachycardia, angina pectoris
Central nervous system: Headache
Gastrointestinal: Nausea, vomiting, diarrhea, anorexia

1% to 10%:
Cardiovascular: Hypotension, redness or flushing of face
Gastrointestinal: Constipation
Ocular: Lacrimation
Respiratory: Dyspnea, nasal congestion

<1%:
Cardiovascular: Edema
Central nervous system: Malaise, fever, dizziness
Dermatologic: Rash
Neuromuscular & skeletal: Arthralgias, peripheral neuritis, weakness

(Continued)

Hydralazine *(Continued)*

Drug Interactions Increased toxicity: Concomitant administration of MAO inhibitors causes significant decrease in blood pressure; indomethacin leads to decreased hypotensive effects

Drug Uptake
Onset of action:
Oral: 20-30 minutes
I.V.: 5-20 minutes
Duration:
Oral: 2-4 hours
I.V.: 2-6 hours
Serum half-life:
Normal renal function: 2-8 hours
End stage renal disease: 7-16 hours

Pregnancy Risk Factor C
Generic Available Yes

Hydralazine and Hydrochlorothiazide
(hye DRAL a zeen & hye droe klor oh THYE a zide)

Brand Names Apresazide®
Therapeutic Category Antihypertensive Agent, Combination
Synonyms Hydrochlorothiazide and Hydralazine
Use Management of moderate to severe hypertension and treatment of congestive heart failure
Local Anesthetic/Vasoconstrictor Precautions No information available to require special precautions
Effects on Dental Treatment No effects or complications reported
Pregnancy Risk Factor C
Generic Available Yes

Hydralazine, Hydrochlorothiazide, and Reserpine
(hye DRAL a zeen, hye droe klor oh THYE a zide, & re SER peen)

Brand Names Hydrap-ES®; Marpres®; Ser-Ap-Es®
Therapeutic Category Antihypertensive Agent, Combination
Use Hypertensive disorders
Local Anesthetic/Vasoconstrictor Precautions No information available to require special precautions
Effects on Dental Treatment No effects or complications reported
Pregnancy Risk Factor C
Generic Available Yes

Hydramyn® Syrup [OTC] *see* Diphenhydramine *on page 323*
Hydrap-ES® *see* Hydralazine, Hydrochlorothiazide, and Reserpine *on this page*
Hydrate® Injection *see* Dimenhydrinate *on page 320*
Hydrea® *see* Hydroxyurea *on page 490*
Hydrobexan® *see* Hydroxocobalamin *on page 487*
Hydrocet® [5/500] *see* Hydrocodone and Acetaminophen *on page 478*

Hydrochlorothiazide (hye droe klor oh THYE a zide)

Related Information
Cardiovascular Diseases *on page 1010*
Moexipril and Hydrochlorothiazide *on page 645*

Brand Names Esidrix®; Ezide®; HydroDIURIL®; Hydro-Par®; Oretic®
Canadian/Mexican Brand Names Apo®-Hydro (Canada); Diclotride® (Mexico); Diuchlor® (Canada); Neo-Codema® (Canada); Novo-Hydrazide® (Canada); Urozide® (Canada)
Therapeutic Category Diuretic, Thiazide
Synonyms Hidroclorotiacida (Mexico)
Use Management of mild to moderate hypertension; treatment of edema in congestive heart failure and nephrotic syndrome
Usual Dosage Oral (effect of drug may be decreased when used every day):
Children (In pediatric patients, chlorothiazide may be preferred over hydrochlorothiazide as there are more dosage formulations (eg, suspension) available):
<6 months: 2-3 mg/kg/day in 2 divided doses
>6 months: 2 mg/kg/day in 2 divided doses
Adults: 25-100 mg/day in 1-2 doses
Maximum: 200 mg/day
Elderly: 12.5-25 mg once daily
Minimal increase in response and more electrolyte disturbances are seen with doses >50 mg/day

Mechanism of Action Inhibits sodium reabsorption in the distal tubules causing increased excretion of sodium and water as well as potassium and hydrogen ions

Local Anesthetic/Vasoconstrictor Precautions No information available to require special precautions

Effects on Dental Treatment No effects or complications reported

Other Adverse Effects
1% to 10%: Endocrine & metabolic: Hypokalemia
<1%:
Cardiovascular: Hypotension
Dermatologic: Photosensitivity
Endocrine & metabolic: Fluid and electrolyte imbalances (hypocalcemia, hypomagnesemia, hyponatremia), hyperglycemia
Hematologic: Rarely blood dyscrasias
Renal: Prerenal azotemia

Drug Interactions
Decreased effect: Decreased antidiabetic drug efficacy
Increased toxicity:
Hypotensive agents cause increased hypotensive potential
Increased digoxin related arrhythmias when given with digoxin
Increased lithium levels due to reduced lithium clearance

Drug Uptake
Onset of diuretic action: Oral: Within 2 hours
Peak effect: 4 hours
Duration: 6-12 hours
Absorption: Oral: ~60% to 80%

Pregnancy Risk Factor D

Generic Available Yes: Tablet

Hydrochlorothiazide and Amiloride *see* Amiloride and Hydrochlorothiazide *on page 54*

Hydrochlorothiazide and Hydralazine *see* Hydralazine and Hydrochlorothiazide *on previous page*

Hydrochlorothiazide and Methyldopa *see* Methyldopa and Hydrochlorothiazide *on page 622*

Hydrochlorothiazide and Reserpine
(hye droe klor oh THYE a zide & re SER peen)

Brand Names Hydropres®; Hydro-Serp®; Hydroserpine®

Therapeutic Category Antihypertensive Agent, Combination

Synonyms Reserpine and Hydrochlorothiazide

Use Management of mild to moderate hypertension; treatment of edema in congestive heart failure and nephrotic syndrome

Local Anesthetic/Vasoconstrictor Precautions No information available to require special precautions

Effects on Dental Treatment No effects or complications reported

Pregnancy Risk Factor C

Generic Available Yes

Hydrochlorothiazide and Spironolactone
(hye droe klor oh THYE a zide & speer on oh LAK tone)

Related Information
Cardiovascular Diseases *on page 1010*

Brand Names Alazide®; Aldactazide®; Spironazide®; Spirozide®

Therapeutic Category Antihypertensive Agent, Combination; Diuretic, Combination

Synonyms Spironolactone and Hydrochlorothiazide

Use Management of mild to moderate hypertension; treatment of edema in congestive heart failure and nephrotic syndrome

Usual Dosage Oral:
Children: 1.66-3.3 mg/kg/day (of spironolactone) in 2-4 divided doses

Adults: 1-8 tablets in 1-2 divided doses

Local Anesthetic/Vasoconstrictor Precautions No information available to require special precautions

Effects on Dental Treatment No effects or complications reported

Other Adverse Effects 1% to 10%:
Central nervous system: Headache, lethargy
Dermatology: Rash
Endocrine & metabolic: Hyperkalemia, gynecomastia, hyperchloremic metabolic acidosis (in decompensated hepatic cirrhosis), dehydration, hyponatremia
Gastrointestinal: Anorexia, nausea, vomiting, diarrhea

Contraindications Anuria, hyperkalemia, renal or hepatic failure, hypersensitivity to hydrochlorothiazide, spironolactone, or any component

(Continued)

477

Hydrochlorothiazide and Spironolactone *(Continued)*

Pregnancy Risk Factor C

Dosage Forms Tablet:
25/25: Hydrochlorothiazide 25 mg and spironolactone 25 mg
50/50: Hydrochlorothiazide 50 mg and spironolactone 50 mg

Generic Available Yes

Hydrochlorothiazide and Triamterene

(hye droe klor oh THYE a zide & trye AM ter een)

Related Information
Cardiovascular Diseases *on page 1010*

Brand Names Dyazide®; Maxzide®

Canadian/Mexican Brand Names Apo®-Triazide (Canada); Novo-Triamzide® (Canada); Nu-Triazide® (Canada)

Therapeutic Category Diuretic, Combination

Synonyms Triamtereno Hidroclorotiacida (Mexico)

Use Management of mild to moderate hypertension; treatment of edema in congestive heart failure and nephrotic syndrome

Usual Dosage Oral:
Adults: 1-2 capsules twice daily after meals
Elderly: Initial: 1 capsule/day or every other day

Mechanism of Action Competes with aldosterone for receptor sites in the distal renal tubules, increasing sodium, chloride, and water excretion while conserving potassium and hydrogen ions; may block the effect of aldosterone on arteriolar smooth muscle as well

Inhibits sodium reabsorption in the distal tubules causing increased excretion of sodium and water as well as potassium and hydrogen ions

Local Anesthetic/Vasoconstrictor Precautions No information available to require special precautions

Effects on Dental Treatment No effects or complications reported

Other Adverse Effects
1% to 10%: Gastrointestinal: Loss of appetite, nausea, vomiting, stomach cramps, diarrhea, upset stomach
<1%:
Central nervous system: Dizziness, fatigue
Dermatologic: Purpura, cracked corners of mouth
Endocrine & metabolic: Electrolyte disturbances
Gastrointestinal: Bright orange tongue, burning of tongue
Hematologic: Aplastic anemia, agranulocytosis, hemolytic anemia, leukopenia, thrombocytopenia, megaloblastic anemia
Neuromuscular & skeletal: Muscle cramps
Ocular: Xanthopsia, transient blurred vision
Respiratory: Allergic pneumonitis, pulmonary edema, respiratory distress

Drug Interactions
Hydrochlorothiazide:
Decreased effect of oral hypoglycemics; decreased absorption with cholestyramine and colestipol
Increased effect with furosemide and other loop diuretics
Increased toxicity/levels of lithium
Triamterene:
Increased risk of hyperkalemia if given together with amiloride, spironolactone, angiotensin-converting enzyme (ACE) inhibitors
Increased toxicity of amantadine (possibly by decreasing its renal excretion)

Pregnancy Risk Factor C

Generic Available Yes (Dyazide® strength only)

Hydrocil® [OTC] *see* Psyllium *on page 822*

Hydro Cobex® *see* Hydroxocobalamin *on page 487*

Hydrocodone and Acetaminophen

(hye droe KOE done & a seet a MIN oh fen)

Related Information
Acetaminophen *on page 20*
Dental Drug Interactions: Update on Drug Combinations Requiring Special Considerations *on page 1144*
Narcotic Agonists *on page 1141*
Oral Pain *on page 1053*

Brand Names Anexsia® 5/500; Anexsia® 7.5/650; Anexsia® 10/660; Anodynos-DHC® [5/500]; Bancap HC® [5/500]; Co-Gesic® [5/500]; Dolacet® [5/500]; DuoCet™ [5/500]; Duradyne DHC® [5/500]; Hydrocet® [5/500]; Hydrogesic® [5/500]; Hy-Phen® [5/500]; Lorcet® [5/500]; Lorcet®-HD [5/500]; Lorcet® Plus [7.5/

650]; Lortab® 2.5/500; Lortab® 5/500; Lortab® 7.5/500; Lortab® 10/500; Lortab® 10/650; Lortab® Elixir; Lortab® Solution; Margesic® H [5/500]; Norcet® [5/500]; Stagesic® [5/500]; T-Gesic® [5/500]; Vicodin® [5/500]; Vicodin® ES [7.5/750]; Zydone® [5/500]

Canadian/Mexican Brand Names Vapocet® (Canada)

Therapeutic Category Analgesic, Narcotic

Use

Dental: Treatment of postoperative pain

Medical: Relief of pain

Restrictions C-III; Refillable up to 5 times in 6 months

Usual Dosage Oral:

Children: Not recommended in pediatric dental patients

Adults: Analgesic: 1-2 tablets or capsules every 4-6 hours or 5-10 mL solution every 4-6 hours as needed for pain; maximum dose: 12 tablets or capsules/day

Mechanism of Action

Hydrocodone, as with other narcotic (opiate) analgesics, blocks pain perception in the cerebral cortex by binding to specific receptor molecules (opiate receptors) within the neuronal membranes of synapses. This binding results in a decreased synaptic chemical transmission throughout the CNS thus inhibiting the flow of pain sensations into the higher centers. Mu and kappa are the two subtypes of the opiate receptor which hydrocodone binds to to cause analgesia.

Acetaminophen inhibits the synthesis of prostaglandins in the CNS and peripherally blocks pain impulse generation; produces antipyresis from inhibition of hypothalamic heat-regulating center.

Local Anesthetic/Vasoconstrictor Precautions No information available to require special precautions

Effects on Dental Treatment <1% of patients experience dry mouth

Other Adverse Effects

>10%:

Cardiovascular: Hypotension

Central nervous system: Lightheadedness, dizziness, sedation

1% to 10%: Gastrointestinal: Nausea

Contraindications Patients with known G-6-PD deficiency; hypersensitivity to acetaminophen; hypersensitivity to hydrocodone

Warnings/Precautions Use with caution in patients with hypersensitivity reactions to other phenanthrene derivative opioid agonists (morphine, codeine, levorphanol, oxycodone, oxymorphone); respiratory diseases including asthma, emphysema, COPD, or severe liver or renal insufficiency; some preparations contain sulfites which may cause allergic reactions; may be habit-forming

Drug Interactions The use of MAO inhibitors or tricyclic antidepressants with hydrocodone may **increase** the effect of either the antidepressant or hydrocodone; concurrent use of hydrocodone with anticholinergics may cause paralytic ileus; patients taking other narcotic agents, antipsychotics, antianxiety agents or other CNS depressants (including alcohol) with hydrocodone may experience an additive CNS depression; with acetaminophen component, refer to Acetaminophen monograph

Drug Uptake

Onset of effect: Narcotic analgesia: Within 10-20 minutes

Duration of effect: 3-6 hours

Serum half-life: 3.8 hours

Pregnancy Risk Factor C

Breast-feeding Considerations

Hydrocodone: No data reported

Acetaminophen: May be taken while breast-feeding

Dosage Forms

Capsule:

Bancap HC®, Dolacet®, Hydrocet®, Hydrogesic®, Lorcet®-HD, Margesic® H, Medipain 5®, Norcet®, Stagesic®, T-Gesic®, Zydone®: Hydrocodone bitartrate 5 mg and acetaminophen 500 mg

Elixir (tropical fruit punch flavor) (Lortab®): Hydrocodone bitartrate 2.5 mg and acetaminophen 167 mg per 5 mL with alcohol 7% (480 mL)

Solution, oral (tropical fruit punch flavor) (Lortab®): Hydrocodone bitartrate 2.5 mg and acetaminophen 167 mg per 5 mL with alcohol 7% (480 mL)

Tablet:

Lortab® 2.5/500: Hydrocodone bitartrate 2.5 mg and acetaminophen 500 mg

Anexsia® 5/500, Anodynos-DHC®, Co-Gesic®, DuoCet™, Duradyne DHC®, Hy-Phen®, Lorcet®, Lortab®® 5/500, Vicodin®: Hydrocodone bitartrate 5 mg and acetaminophen 500 mg

Lortab® 7.5/500: Hydrocodone bitartrate 7.5 mg and acetaminophen 500 mg

Anexsia® 7.5/650, Lorcet® Plus: Hydrocodone bitartrate 7.5 mg and acetaminophen 650 mg

(Continued)

Hydrocodone and Acetaminophen *(Continued)*

Vicodin® ES: Hydrocodone bitartrate 7.5 mg and acetaminophen 750 mg

Lortab® 10/500: Hydrocodone bitartrate 10 mg and acetaminophen 500 mg

Lortab® 10/650: Hydrocodone bitartrate 10 mg and acetaminophen 650 mg

Anexsia® 10/660, Vicodin® HP: Hydrocodone bitartrate 10 mg and acetaminophen 660 mg

Dietary Considerations No data reported

Generic Available Yes

Comments Neither hydrocodone nor acetaminophen elicit anti-inflammatory effects. Because of addiction liability of opiate analgesics, the use of hydrocodone should be limited to 2-3 days postoperatively for treatment of dental pain. Nausea is the most common adverse effect seen after use in dental patients; sedation and constipation are second. Nausea elicited by narcotic analgesics is centrally mediated and the presence or absence of food will not affect the degree nor incidence of nausea.

Selected Readings

Dionne RA, "New Approaches to Preventing and Treating Postoperative Pain," *J Am Dent Assoc*, 1992, 123(6):26-34.

Gobetti JP, "Controlling Dental Pain," *J Am Dent Assoc*, 1992, 123(6):47-52.

Hydrocodone and Aspirin *(hye droe KOE done & AS pir in)*

Related Information

Dental Drug Interactions: Update on Drug Combinations Requiring Special Considerations *on page 1144*

Narcotic Agonists *on page 1141*

Brand Names Alor® 5/500; Azdone®; Damason-P®; Lortab® ASA; Panasal® 5/500

Therapeutic Category Analgesic, Narcotic

Use

Dental: Treatment of postoperative pain

Medical: Relief of pain

Restrictions C-III; Refillable up to 5 times in 6 months

Usual Dosage Oral:

Children: Not recommended in pediatric dental patients

Adults: 1-2 tablets every 4-6 hours as needed for pain

Mechanism of Action Hydrocodone, as with other narcotic (opiate) analgesics, blocks pain perception in the cerebral cortex by binding to specific receptor molecules (opiate receptors) within the neuronal membranes of synapsis. This binding results in a decreased synaptic chemical transmission throughout the CNS thus inhibiting the flow of pain sensations into the higher centers. Mu and kappa are the two subtypes of the opiate receptor which hydrocodone binds to to cause analgesia.

Aspirin inhibits prostaglandin synthesis by decreasing the activity of the enzyme, cyclo-oxygenase, which results in decreased formation of prostaglandin precursors, acts on the hypothalamic heat-regulating center to reduce fever, blocks thromboxane synthetase action which prevents formation of the platelet-aggregating substance thromboxane A_2

Local Anesthetic/Vasoconstrictor Precautions No information available to require special precautions

Effects on Dental Treatment <1% of patients experience dry mouth; use with caution in patients with platelet and bleeding disorders, renal dysfunction, erosive gastritis, or peptic ulcer disease, previous nonreaction does not guarantee future safe taking of medication; do not use aspirin in children <16 years of age for chickenpox or flu symptoms due to the association with Reye's syndrome

Avoid aspirin if possible, for 1 week prior to surgery because of the possibility of postoperative bleeding; use with caution in impaired hepatic function

Elderly are a high-risk population for adverse effects from nonsteroidal anti-inflammatory agents. As much as 60% of elderly with GI complications to NSAIDs can develop peptic ulceration and/or hemorrhage asymptomatically. Also, concomitant disease and drug use contribute to the risk for GI adverse effects. Use lowest effective dose for shortest period possible. Consider renal function decline with age. Use with caution in patients with history of asthma.

Other Adverse Effects

>10%:

Central nervous system: Lightheadedness, dizziness, sedation

Gastrointestinal: Nausea, heartburn, stomach pains, dyspepsia

1% to 10%: Gastrointestinal: Gastrointestinal ulceration

Warnings/Precautions Because of aspirin component, use with caution in patients with impaired renal function, erosive gastritis, or peptic ulcer disease;

children and teenagers should not use for chickenpox or flu symptoms before a physician is consulted about Reye's syndrome

Drug Interactions The use of MAO inhibitors or tricyclic antidepressants with hydrocodone may **increase** the effect of either the antidepressant or hydrocodone; concurrent use of hydrocodone with anticholinergics may cause paralytic ileus; patients taking other narcotic agents, antipsychotic, antianxiety agents or other CNS depressants (including alcohol) with hydrocodone and aspirin may experience an additive CNS depression; aspirin interacts with warfarin to cause bleeding

Drug Uptake
Onset of effect: Onset of narcotic analgesia: Within 10-20 minutes
Duration of effect: 3-6 hours
Serum half-life: 3.8 hours

Pregnancy Risk Factor D

Breast-feeding Considerations
Hydrocodone: No data reported
Aspirin: Cautious use due to potential adverse effects in nursing infants

Dosage Forms Tablet: Hydrocodone bitartrate 5 mg and aspirin 500 mg

Dietary Considerations May be taken with food or milk to minimize GI distress

Generic Available Yes

Comments Because of addiction liability of opiate analgesics, the use of hydrocodone should be limited to 2-3 days postoperatively for treatment of dental pain; nausea is the most common adverse effect seen after use in dental patients; sedation and constipation are second; aspirin component affects bleeding times and could influence time of wound healing

Selected Readings
Dionne RA, "New Approaches to Preventing and Treating Postoperative Pain," *J Am Dent Assoc*, 1992, 123(6):26-34.
Gobetti JP, "Controlling Dental Pain," *J Am Dent Assoc*, 1992, 123(6):47-52.

Hydrocodone and Chlorpheniramine
(hye droe KOE done & klor fen IR a meen)
Brand Names Tussionex®
Therapeutic Category Antitussive; Cough Preparation
Use Symptomatic relief of cough
Local Anesthetic/Vasoconstrictor Precautions No information available to require special precautions
Effects on Dental Treatment Prolonged use will cause significant xerostomia
Pregnancy Risk Factor C
Generic Available Yes

Hydrocodone and Guaifenesin
(hye droe KOE done & gwye FEN e sin)
Brand Names Codiclear® DH; HycoClear Tuss®; Hycotuss® Expectorant Liquid; Kwelcof®
Therapeutic Category Antitussive; Cough Preparation
Synonyms Guaifenesin and Hydrocodone
Use Symptomatic relief of nonproductive coughs associated with upper and lower respiratory tract congestion
Local Anesthetic/Vasoconstrictor Precautions No information available to require special precautions
Effects on Dental Treatment No effects or complications reported
Pregnancy Risk Factor C
Generic Available Yes

Hydrocodone and Homatropine
(hye droe KOE done & hoe MA troe peen)
Brand Names Hycodan®; Hydromet®; Oncet®; Tussigon®
Therapeutic Category Antitussive; Cough Preparation
Synonyms Homatropine and Hydrocodone
Use Symptomatic relief of cough
Usual Dosage Oral (based on hydrocodone component):
Children: 0.6 mg/kg/day in 3-4 divided doses; do not administer more frequently than every 4 hours
A single dose should not exceed 1.25 mg in children <2 years of age, 5 mg in children 2-12 years, and 10 mg in children >12 years
Adults: 5-10 mg every 4-6 hours, a single dose should not exceed 15 mg; do not administer more frequently than every 4 hours
Local Anesthetic/Vasoconstrictor Precautions No information available to require special precautions
Effects on Dental Treatment Dry mouth
(Continued)

Hydrocodone and Homatropine *(Continued)*

Other Adverse Effects

>10%:
  Cardiovascular: Hypotension
  Central nervous system: Lightheadedness, dizziness, sedation, drowsiness, fatigue
  Neuromuscular & skeletal: Weakness

1% to 10%:
  Cardiovascular: Bradycardia, tachycardia
  Central nervous system: Confusion
  Gastrointestinal: Nausea, vomiting
  Renal: Decreased urination
  Respiratory: Dyspnea

<1%:
  Cardiovascular: Hypertension
  Central nervous system: Hallucinations
  Dermatologic: Dry hot skin
  Gastrointestinal: Dry mouth, anorexia, biliary spasm, impaired GI motility
  Genitourinary: Urinary tract spasm
  Ocular: Miosis, mydriasis, blurred vision, diplopia
  Miscellaneous: Histamine release, physical and psychological dependence with prolonged use

Pregnancy Risk Factor C
Generic Available Yes

Hydrocodone and Ibuprofen

(hye droe KOE done & eye byoo PROE fen)

Brand Names Vicoprofen®

Therapeutic Category Analgesic, Narcotic

Use Relief of moderate to moderately severe pain

Usual Dosage Adults: Oral: 1-2 tablets every 4-6 hours as needed for pain

Mechanism of Action Refer to individual agents

Local Anesthetic/Vasoconstrictor Precautions No information available to require special precautions

Effects on Dental Treatment Use with caution in patients taking anticoagulants (ibuprofen)

Other Adverse Effects

>10%:
  Cardiovascular: Hypotension
  Central nervous system: Lightheadedness, dizziness, sedation, drowsiness, fatigue
  Dermatologic: Rash, urticaria
  Gastrointestinal: Abdominal cramps, heartburn, indigestion, nausea
  Neuromuscular & skeletal: Weakness

1% to 10%:
  Cardiovascular: Bradycardia
  Central nervous system: Headache, nervousness, confusion
  Dermatologic: Itching
  Endocrine & metabolic: Fluid retention
  Gastrointestinal: Dyspepsia, vomiting, abdominal pain, peptic ulcer, GI bleed, GI perforation, nausea
  Genitourinary: Decreased urination
  Otic: Tinnitus
  Respiratory: Shortness of breath, dyspnea

<1%:
  Cardiovascular: Edema, congestive heart failure, arrhythmias, tachycardia, hypertension
  Central nervous system: Confusion, hallucinations, mental depression, drowsiness, insomnia, aseptic meningitis
  Dermatologic: Urticaria, erythema multiforme, toxic epidermal necrolysis, Stevens-Johnson syndrome
  Endocrine & metabolic: Polydipsia, hot flashes
  Gastrointestinal: Gastritis, GI ulceration, xerostomia, anorexia, biliary tract spasm
  Genitourinary: Cystitis, urinary tract spasm
  Hematologic: Neutropenia, anemia, agranulocytosis, inhibition of platelet aggregation, hemolytic anemia, bone marrow suppression, leukopenia, thrombocytopenia
  Hepatic: Hepatitis
  Neuromuscular & skeletal: Peripheral neuropathy

Ocular: Vision changes, blurred vision, conjunctivitis, dry eyes, toxic amblyopia, diplopia, miosis

Otic: Decreased hearing

Renal: Acute renal failure, polyuria

Respiratory: Allergic rhinitis, shortness of breath, epistaxis

Miscellaneous: Histamine release, physical and psychological dependence with prolonged use

Dosage Forms Tablet: Hydrocodone bitartrate 7.5 mg and ibuprofen 200 mg

Generic Available No

Comments The combination of 15 mg hydrocodone bitartrate with 400 mg ibuprofen was compared to 400 mg ibuprofen alone and placebo for the ability to diminish postoperative pain (pain after cesarean section or gynecologic surgery, 120 patients). Analgesia was measured during a 6-hour period after dosing based on onset of relief, hourly and summary variables, and duration of effect. A significantly greater proportion of patients treated with the hydrocodone/ibuprofen combination reported onset of relief compared with ibuprofen or placebo. Time to onset of relief did not differ among treatments. Hydrocodone with ibuprofen and ibuprofen alone were significantly more effective than placebo for all measures. The combination of hydrocodone with ibuprofen was significantly superior to ibuprofen for all hourly analgesic evaluations, weighted sum of pain intensity differences, total pain relief, and global rating of study medications. This report demonstrated an analgesic superiority of 15 mg hydrocodone bitartrate combined with 400 mg ibuprofen compared to 400 mg ibuprofen alone.

Selected Readings

Sunshine A, Olson NZ, O'Neill E, et al, "Analgesic Efficacy of a Hydrocodone With Ibuprofen Combination Compared With Ibuprofen Alone for the Treatment of Acute Postoperative Pain," *J Clin Pharmacol*, 1997, 37:908-15.

Hydrocodone and Phenylpropanolamine

(hye droe KOE done & fen il proe pa NOLE a meen)

Brand Names Codamine®; Codamine® Pediatric; Hycomine®; Hycomine® Pediatric; Hydrocodone PA® Syrup

Therapeutic Category Cough Preparation; Decongestant

Synonyms Phenylpropanolamine and Hydrocodone

Use Symptomatic relief of cough and nasal congestion

Local Anesthetic/Vasoconstrictor Precautions Use with caution since phenylpropanolamine is a sympathomimetic amine which could interact with epinephrine to cause a pressor response

Effects on Dental Treatment Up to 10% of patients could experience tachycardia, palpitations, and dry mouth; use vasoconstrictor with caution

Pregnancy Risk Factor C

Generic Available Yes

Hydrocodone, Chlorpheniramine, Phenylephrine, Acetaminophen and Caffeine

(hye droe KOE done, klor fen IR a meen, fen il EF rin, a seet a MIN oh fen, & KAF een)

Brand Names Hycomine® Compound

Therapeutic Category Antitussive; Cough Preparation

Use Symptomatic relief of cough and symptoms of upper respiratory infections

Local Anesthetic/Vasoconstrictor Precautions Use with caution since phenylephrine is a sympathomimetic amine which could interact with epinephrine to cause a pressor response

Effects on Dental Treatment

Acetaminophen: No effects or complications reported

Chlorpheniramine: Prolonged use will cause significant xerostomia

Phenylephrine: Up to 10% of patients could experience tachycardia, palpitations, and dry mouth; use vasoconstrictor with caution

Pregnancy Risk Factor C

Generic Available Yes

Selected Readings

Barker JD Jr, de Carle DJ, and Anuras S, "Chronic Excessive Acetaminophen Use in Liver Damage," *Ann Intern Med*, 1977, 87(3):299-301.

Dionne RA, Campbell RA, Cooper SA, et al, "Suppression of Postoperative Pain by Preoperative Administration of Ibuprofen in Comparison to Placebo, Acetaminophen, and Acetaminophen Plus Codeine," *J Clin Pharmacol*, 1983, 23(1):37-43.

Licht H, Seeff LB, and Zimmerman HJ, "Apparent Potentiation of Acetaminophen Hepatotoxicity by Alcohol," *Ann Intern Med*, 1980, 92(4):511.

Hydrocodone PA® Syrup *see* Hydrocodone and Phenylpropanolamine *on this page*

Hydrocodone, Phenylephrine, Pyrilamine, Phenindamine, Chlorpheniramine, and Ammonium Chloride

(hye droe KOE done, fen il EF rin, peer IL a meen, fen IN da meen, klor fen IR a meen, & a MOE nee um KLOR ide)

Brand Names P-V-Tussin®

Therapeutic Category Antihistamine/Decongestant Combination; Cough Preparation

Use Symptomatic relief of cough and nasal congestion

Local Anesthetic/Vasoconstrictor Precautions Use with caution since phenylephrine is a sympathomimetic amine which could interact with epinephrine to cause a pressor response

Effects on Dental Treatment

Chlorpheniramine: Prolonged use will cause significant xerostomia

Phenylephrine: Up to 10% of patients could experience tachycardia, palpitations, and dry mouth; use vasoconstrictor with caution

Generic Available Yes

Hydrocodone, Pseudoephedrine, and Guaifenesin

(hye droe KOE done, soo doe e FED rin & gwye FEN e sin)

Brand Names Cophene XP®; Detussin® Expectorant; SRC® Expectorant; Tussafin® Expectorant

Therapeutic Category Cough Preparation; Decongestant; Expectorant

Use Symptomatic relief of irritating, nonproductive cough associated with respiratory conditions such as bronchitis, bronchial asthma, tracheobronchitis, and the common cold

Local Anesthetic/Vasoconstrictor Precautions Use with caution since pseudoephedrine is a sympathomimetic amine which could interact with epinephrine to cause a pressor response

Effects on Dental Treatment

Guaifenesin: No effects or complications reported

Pseudoephedrine: Up to 10% of patients could experience tachycardia, palpitations, and dry mouth; use vasoconstrictor with caution

Generic Available Yes

Hydrocortisone (hye droe KOR ti sone)

Related Information

Corticosteroid Equivalencies Comparison *on page 1139*

Corticosteroids, Topical Comparison *on page 1140*

Brand Names Cortef®; Hydrocortone® Acetate; Hydrocortone® Phosphate; Orabase® HCA; Solu-Cortef®

Canadian/Mexican Brand Names Flebocortid® [Sodium Succinate] (Mexico); Nositrol® [Sodium Succinate] (Mexico)

Therapeutic Category Anti-inflammatory Agent; Corticosteroid, Systemic; Corticosteroid, Topical (Low Potency)

Use

Dental: Treatment of a variety of oral diseases of allergic, inflammatory or auto-immune origin

Medical: Management of adrenocortical insufficiency; relief of inflammation of corticosteroid-responsive dermatoses (low and medium potency topical corticosteroid); adjunctive treatment of ulcerative colitis

Usual Dosage Adults: Anti-inflammatory or immunosuppressive:

Oral: 20-240 mg/day in 2-4 divided doses;

I.M., I.V.: Succinate: 100-500 mg every 2-10 hours

I.M., I.V., S.C.: Sodium phosphate: Initially 15-240 mg/day (approximately 1/3 to 1/2 of the oral dose) in divided doses every 12 hours. In acute diseases, doses higher than 240 mg may be required.

Mechanism of Action Decreases inflammation by suppression of migration of polymorphonuclear leukocytes and reversal of increased capillary permeability

Local Anesthetic/Vasoconstrictor Precautions No information available to require special precautions

Effects on Dental Treatment No effects or complications reported

Other Adverse Effects >10%:

Central nervous system: Insomnia, nervousness

Gastrointestinal: Increased appetite, indigestion

Contraindications Serious infections, except septic shock or tuberculous meningitis; known hypersensitivity to hydrocortisone; viral, fungal, or tubercular skin lesions

Warnings/Precautions
Use with caution in patients with hyperthyroidism, cirrhosis, nonspecific ulcerative colitis, hypertension, osteoporosis, thromboembolic tendencies, CHF, convulsive disorders, myasthenia gravis, thrombophlebitis, peptic ulcer, diabetes

Acute adrenal insufficiency may occur with abrupt withdrawal after long-term therapy or with stress; young pediatric patients may be more susceptible to adrenal axis suppression from topical therapy

Because of the risk of adverse effects, systemic corticosteroids should be used cautiously in the elderly, in the smallest possible dose, and for the shortest possible time

Drug Interactions Insulin decreases hypoglycemic effect; phenytoin, phenobarbital, ephedrine, and rifampin have caused increased metabolism of hydrocortisone and decreased steroid blood level; oral anticoagulants change prothrombin time; potassium- depleting diuretics increase risk of hypokalemia; cardiac glucosides increase risk of arrhythmias or digitalis toxicity secondary to hypokalemia

Drug Uptake
Hydrocortisone acetate salt has a slow onset but long duration of action when compared with more soluble preparations
Hydrocortisone sodium phosphate salt is a water soluble salt with a rapid onset but short duration of action
Hydrocortisone sodium succinate salt is a water soluble salt with is rapidly active
Absorption: Rapid by all routes, except rectally
Serum half-life, biologic: 8-12 hours

Pregnancy Risk Factor C

Breast-feeding Considerations No data reported

Dosage Forms
Hydrocortisone acetate: Injection, suspension: 25 mg/mL (5 mL, 10 mL); 50 mg/mL (5 mL, 10 mL)
Hydrocortisone base: Tablet, oral: 5 mg, 10 mg, 20 mg
Hydrocortisone cypionate: Suspension, oral: 10 mg/5 mL (120 mL)
Hydrocortisone sodium phosphate: Injection, IM/IV/SC: 50 mg/mL (2 mL, 10 mL)
Hydrocortisone sodium succinate: Injection, IM/IV: 100 mg, 250 mg, 500 mg, 1000 mg

Dietary Considerations May be taken with meals to decrease GI upset; limit caffeine; need diet rich in pyridoxine, vitamin C, vitamin D, folate, calcium, and phosphorus

Generic Available Yes

Hydrocortisone and Clioquinol *see* Clioquinol and Hydrocortisone *on page 245*

Hydrocortisone and Dibucaine *see* Dibucaine and Hydrocortisone *on page 303*

Hydrocortisone and Pramoxine *see* Pramoxine and Hydrocortisone *on page 784*

Hydrocortisone and Urea *see* Urea and Hydrocortisone *on page 978*

Hydrocortone® Acetate *see* Hydrocortisone *on previous page*

Hydrocortone® Phosphate *see* Hydrocortisone *on previous page*

Hydro-Crysti-12® *see* Hydroxocobalamin *on page 487*

HydroDIURIL® *see* Hydrochlorothiazide *on page 476*

Hydroflumethiazide (hye droe floo meth EYE a zide)
Related Information
Cardiovascular Diseases *on page 1010*
Brand Names Diucardin®; Saluron®
Therapeutic Category Diuretic, Thiazide
Use Management of mild to moderate hypertension; treatment of edema in congestive heart failure and nephrotic syndrome
Usual Dosage Oral:
Children: 1 mg/kg/24 hours
Adults: 50-200 mg/day
Mechanism of Action The diuretic mechanism of action is primarily inhibition of sodium, chloride, and water reabsorption in the renal distal tubules, thereby producing diuresis with a resultant reduction in plasma volume
Local Anesthetic/Vasoconstrictor Precautions No information available to require special precautions
Effects on Dental Treatment No effects or complications reported
Other Adverse Effects
1% to 10%: Endocrine & metabolic: Hypokalemia
<1%:
Cardiovascular: Hypotension
Central nervous system: Drowsiness
(Continued)

Hydroflumethiazide *(Continued)*

Dermatologic: Photosensitivity, rash

Endocrine & metabolic: Fluid and electrolyte imbalances (hypocalcemia, hypomagnesemia, hyponatremia), hyperglycemia

Gastrointestinal: Anorexia

Hematologic: Aplastic anemia, hemolytic anemia, leukopenia, agranulocytosis, thrombocytopenia, rarely blood dyscrasias

Hepatic: Hepatitis

Neuromuscular & skeletal: Paresthesia

Renal: Polyuria, prerenal azotemia, uremia

Drug Interactions

Decreased effect of oral hypoglycemics; decreased absorption with cholestyramine and colestipol

Increased effect with furosemide and other loop diuretics

Increased toxicity/levels of lithium

Drug Uptake

Onset of diuretic effect: Within ~2 hours

Peak effect: Within ~4 hours

Duration of action: 12-24 hours

Pregnancy Risk Factor D

Generic Available Yes

Hydroflumethiazide and Reserpine

(hye droe floo meth EYE a zide & re SER peen)

Brand Names Salutensin®

Therapeutic Category Antihypertensive Agent, Combination

Use Management of hypertension

Local Anesthetic/Vasoconstrictor Precautions No information available to require special precautions

Effects on Dental Treatment No effects or complications reported

Pregnancy Risk Factor C

Generic Available Yes

Hydrogesic® [5/500] *see* Hydrocodone and Acetaminophen *on page 478*

Hydromagnesium Aluminate *see* Magaldrate *on page 574*

Hydromet® *see* Hydrocodone and Homatropine *on page 481*

Hydromorphone (hye droe MOR fone)

Related Information

Narcotic Agonists *on page 1141*

Brand Names Dilaudid®; Dilaudid-5®; Dilaudid-HP®; HydroStat IR®

Canadian/Mexican Brand Names PMS-Hydromorphone® (Canada)

Therapeutic Category Analgesic, Narcotic; Antitussive

Use Management of moderate to severe pain; antitussive at lower doses

Usual Dosage

Doses should be titrated to appropriate analgesic effects; when changing routes of administration, note that oral doses are less than half as effective as parenteral doses (may be only one-fifth as effective)

Pain: Older Children and Adults:

Oral, I.M., I.V., S.C.: 1-4 mg/dose every 4-6 hours as needed; usual adult dose: 2 mg/dose

Rectal: 3 mg every 6-8 hours

Antitussive: Oral:

Children 6-12 years: 0.5 mg every 3-4 hours as needed

Children >12 years and Adults: 1 mg every 3-4 hours as needed

Mechanism of Action Binds to opiate receptors in the CNS, causing inhibition of ascending pain pathways, altering the perception of and response to pain; causes cough supression by direct central action in the medulla; produces generalized CNS depression

Local Anesthetic/Vasoconstrictor Precautions No information available to require special precautions

Effects on Dental Treatment Dry mouth and nausea in 10% of patients

Other Adverse Effects

Endocrine & metabolic: Antidiuretic hormone release

Gastrointestinal: Biliary spasm

Genitourinary: Urinary tract spasm

Ocular: Miosis

Miscellaneous: Physical and psychological dependence, histamine release

>10%:

Cardiovascular: Palpitations, hypotension, peripheral vasodilation

Central nervous system: Dizziness, lightheadedness, drowsiness
Gastrointestinal: Anorexia
1% to 10%:
  Cardiovascular: Tachycardia, bradycardia, flushing of face
  Central nervous system: CNS depression, increased intracranial pressure, fatigue, headache, nervousness, restlessness
  Gastrointestinal: Nausea, vomiting, constipation, stomach cramps, dry mouth
  Genitourinary: Ureteral spasm
  Neuromuscular & skeletal: Trembling, weakness
  Renal: Decreased urination
  Respiratory: Respiratory depression, dyspnea
<1%:
  Central nervous system: Hallucinations, mental depression, paralytic ileus
  Dermatologic: Pruritus, skin rash, urticaria

Drug Interactions Increased toxicity: CNS depressants, phenothiazines, tricyclic antidepressants may potentiate the adverse effects of hydromorphone

Drug Uptake
Onset of analgesic effect: Within 15-30 minutes
Duration: 4-5 hours
Serum half-life: 1-3 hours

Pregnancy Risk Factor B (D if used for prolonged periods or in high doses at term)

Generic Available Yes

Hydromox® *see* Quinethazone *on page 829*

Hydro-Par® *see* Hydrochlorothiazide *on page 476*

Hydrophed® *see* Theophylline, Ephedrine, and Hydroxyzine *on page 922*

Hydropres® *see* Hydrochlorothiazide and Reserpine *on page 477*

Hydroquinone (HYE droe kwin one)

Brand Names Ambi® Skin Tone [OTC]; Eldopaque® [OTC]; Eldopaque Forte®; Eldoquin® [OTC]; Eldoquin® Forte®; Esoterica® Facial [OTC]; Esoterica® Regular [OTC]; Esoterica® Sensitive Skin Formula [OTC]; Esoterica® Sunscreen [OTC]; Melanex®; Porcelana® [OTC]; Porcelana® Sunscreen [OTC]; Solaquin® [OTC]; Solaquin Forte®

Canadian/Mexican Brand Names Crema Blanca Bustillos (Mexico); Neostrata® HQ (Canada); Ultraquin® (Canada)

Therapeutic Category Depigmenting Agent

Synonyms Hidroquinona (Mexico)

Use Gradual bleaching of hyperpigmented skin conditions

Usual Dosage Children >12 years and Adults: Topical: Apply thin layer and rub in twice daily

Mechanism of Action Produces reversible depigmentation of the skin by suppression of melanocyte metabolic processes, in particular the inhibition of the enzymatic oxidation of tyrosine to DOPA (3,4-dihydroxyphenylalanine); sun exposure reverses this effect and will cause repigmentation.

Local Anesthetic/Vasoconstrictor Precautions No information available to require special precautions

Effects on Dental Treatment No effects or complications reported

Other Adverse Effects 1% to 10%: Dermatologic: Dermatitis, dryness, erythema, stinging, irritation, inflammatory reaction, sensitization

Drug Interactions No data reported

Drug Uptake Onset and duration of depigmentation produced by hydroquinone varies among individuals

Pregnancy Risk Factor C

Generic Available No

Hydro-Serp® *see* Hydrochlorothiazide and Reserpine *on page 477*

Hydroserpine® *see* Hydrochlorothiazide and Reserpine *on page 477*

HydroStat IR® *see* Hydromorphone *on previous page*

Hydroxacen® *see* Hydroxyzine *on page 491*

Hydroxocobalamin (hye droks oh koe BAL a min)

Brand Names Hydrobexan®; Hydro Cobex®; Hydro-Crysti-12®; LA-12®

Canadian/Mexican Brand Names Acti-B$_{12}$® (Canada); Duradoce® (Mexico)

Therapeutic Category Vitamin, Water Soluble

Synonyms Hidroxocobalamina (Mexico)

Use Treatment of pernicious anemia, vitamin B$_{12}$ deficiency, increased B$_{12}$ requirements due to pregnancy, thyrotoxicosis, hemorrhage, malignancy, liver or kidney disease

(Continued)

Hydroxocobalamin *(Continued)*

Usual Dosage Vitamin B₁₂ deficiency: I.M.:
Children: 1-5 mg given in single doses of 100 mcg over 2 or more weeks, followed by 30-50 mcg/month
Adults: 30 mcg/day for 5-10 days, followed by 100-200 mcg/month

Mechanism of Action Coenzyme for various metabolic functions, including fat and carbohydrate metabolism and protein synthesis, used in cell replication and hematopoiesis

Local Anesthetic/Vasoconstrictor Precautions No information available to require special precautions

Effects on Dental Treatment No effects or complications reported

Other Adverse Effects
1% to 10%:
Dermatologic: Itching
Gastrointestinal: Diarrhea
<1%:
Cardiovascular: Peripheral vascular thrombosis
Dermatologic: Urticaria
Miscellaneous: Anaphylaxis

Drug Interactions No data reported

Pregnancy Risk Factor C

Generic Available Yes

Hydroxyamphetamine *(hye droks ee am FET a meen)*

Brand Names Paredrine®

Therapeutic Category Ophthalmic Agent, Mydriatic

Use Produce mydriasis in diagnostic eye examination

Local Anesthetic/Vasoconstrictor Precautions No information available to require special precautions

Effects on Dental Treatment No effects or complications reported

Generic Available No

Hydroxyamphetamine and Tropicamide
(hye droks ee am FET a meen & troe PIK a mide)

Brand Names Paremyd® Ophthalmic

Therapeutic Category Ophthalmic Agent, Mydriatic

Use Mydriasis with cycloplegia

Local Anesthetic/Vasoconstrictor Precautions No information available to require special precautions

Effects on Dental Treatment No effects or complications reported

Generic Available No

Hydroxycarbamide *see* Hydroxyurea *on page 490*

Hydroxychloroquine *(hye droks ee KLOR oh kwin)*

Related Information
Rheumatoid Arthritis and Osteoarthritis *on page 1030*

Brand Names Plaquenil®

Therapeutic Category Antimalarial Agent

Synonyms Hidroxicloroquina Sulfato De (Mexico)

Use Suppresses and treats acute attacks of malaria; treatment of systemic lupus erythematosus and rheumatoid arthritis

Usual Dosage Oral:
Children:
Chemoprophylaxis of malaria: 5 mg/kg (base) once weekly; should not exceed the recommended adult dose; begin 2 weeks before exposure; continue for 4-6 weeks after leaving endemic area
Acute attack: 10 mg/kg (base) initial dose; followed by 5 mg/kg at 6, 24, and 48 hours
JRA or SLE: 3-5 mg/kg/day divided 1-2 times/day to a maximum of 400 mg/day; not to exceed 7 mg/kg/day
Adults:
Chemoprophylaxis of malaria: 2 tablets weekly on same day each week; begin 2 weeks before exposure; continue for 4-6 weeks after leaving endemic area
Acute attack: 4 tablets first dose day 1; 2 tablets in 6 hours day 1; 2 tablets in 1 dose day 2; and 2 tablets in 1 dose on day 3
Rheumatoid arthritis: 2-3 tablets/day to start taken with food or milk; increase dose until optimum response level is reached; usually after 4-12 weeks dose should be reduced by ½ and a maintenance dose of 1-2 tablets/day given
Lupus erythematosus: 2 tablets every day or twice daily for several weeks depending on response; 1-2 tablets/day for prolonged maintenance therapy

Mechanism of Action Interferes with digestive vacuole function within sensitive malarial parasites by increasing the pH and interfering with lysosomal degradation of hemoglobin; inhibits locomotion of neutrophils and chemotaxis of eosinophils; impairs complement-dependent antigen-antibody reactions

Local Anesthetic/Vasoconstrictor Precautions No information available to require special precautions

Effects on Dental Treatment No effects or complications reported

Other Adverse Effects

>10%:

Central nervous system: Headache

Dermatologic: Itching

Gastrointestinal: Diarrhea, loss of appetite, nausea, stomach cramps, vomiting

Ocular: Ciliary muscle dysfunction

1% to 10%:

Central nervous system: Dizziness, lightheadedness, nervousness, restlessness

Dermatologic: Bleaching of hair, skin rash blue-black discoloration of skin

Ocular: Ocular toxicity, keratopathy, retinopathy

<1%:

Central nervous system: Emotional changes, seizures

Hematologic: Agranulocytosis, aplastic anemia, neutropenia, thrombocytopenia

Neuromuscular & skeletal: Neuromyopathy

Otic: Ototoxicity

Drug Interactions No data reported

Drug Uptake

Absorption: Oral: Complete

Pregnancy Risk Factor C

Generic Available Yes

Hydroxydaunomycin Hydrochloride *see* Doxorubicin *on page 336*

Hydroxyethylcellulose *see* Artificial Tears *on page 87*

Hydroxyethyl Starch *see* Hetastarch *on page 469*

Hydroxyprogesterone Caproate

(hye droks ee proe JES te rone KAP roe ate)

Brand Names Hylutin® Injection; Hyprogest® 250 Injection

Canadian/Mexican Brand Names Primolut® Depot (Mexico)

Therapeutic Category Progestin

Synonyms Hidroxiprogesterona Caproato De (Mexico)

Use Treatment of amenorrhea, abnormal uterine bleeding, endometriosis, uterine carcinoma

Usual Dosage Adults: Female: I.M.:

Amenorrhea: 375 mg; if no bleeding, begin cyclic treatment with estradiol valerate

Production of secretory endometrium and desquamation: (Medical D and C): 125-250 mg administered on day 10 of cycle; repeat every 7 days until supression is no longer desired.

Uterine carcinoma: 1 g one or more times/day (1-7 g/week) for up to 12 weeks

Mechanism of Action Natural steroid hormone that induces secretory changes in the endometrium, promotes mammary gland development, relaxes uterine smooth muscle, blocks follicular maturation and ovulation and maintains pregnancy

Local Anesthetic/Vasoconstrictor Precautions No information available to require special precautions

Effects on Dental Treatment No effects or complications reported

Other Adverse Effects

>10%:

Cardiovascular: Edema

Endocrine & metabolic: Breakthrough bleeding, spotting, changes in menstrual flow, amenorrhea

Gastrointestinal: Anorexia

Local: Pain at injection site

Neuromuscular & skeletal: Weakness

1% to 10%:

Central nervous system: Mental depression, insomnia, fever

Dermatologic: Melasma or chloasma, allergic rash with or without pruritus

Gastrointestinal: Weight gain or loss

Genitourinary: Changes in cervical erosion and secretions, increased breast tenderness

Hepatic: Cholestatic jaundice

(Continued)

Hydroxyprogesterone Caproate *(Continued)*

Drug Interactions Decreased effect: Rifampin causes an increased clearance of hydroxyprogesterone

Drug Uptake
Peak serum concentration: I.M.: 3-7 days; concentrations are measurable for 3-4 weeks after injection

Pregnancy Risk Factor D

Generic Available Yes

Hydroxypropyl Cellulose (hye droks ee PROE pil SEL yoo lose)

Brand Names Lacrisert®

Therapeutic Category Ophthalmic Agent, Miscellaneous

Use Dry eyes

Local Anesthetic/Vasoconstrictor Precautions No information available to require special precautions

Effects on Dental Treatment No effects or complications reported

Other Adverse Effects 1% to 10%: Local irritation

Generic Available Yes

Hydroxypropyl Methylcellulose
(hye droks ee PROE pil meth il SEL yoo lose)

Brand Names Gonak™ [OTC]; Goniosol® [OTC]

Therapeutic Category Ophthalmic Agent, Miscellaneous

Synonyms Gonioscopic Ophthalmic Solution

Use Ophthalmic surgical aid in cataract extraction and intraocular implantation; gonioscopic examinations

Local Anesthetic/Vasoconstrictor Precautions No information available to require special precautions

Effects on Dental Treatment No effects or complications reported

Other Adverse Effects 1% to 10%: Local irritation

Pregnancy Risk Factor C

Generic Available No

Hydroxyurea (hye droks ee yoor EE a)

Brand Names Droxia®; Hydrea®

Therapeutic Category Antineoplastic Agent, Miscellaneous

Synonyms Hydroxycarbamide

Use Treatment of chronic myelocytic leukemia (CML), melanoma, and ovarian carcinomas; also used with radiation in treatment of tumors of the head and neck; adjunct in the management of sickle cell patients

Usual Dosage Oral (**refer to individual protocols**):

Children:
No FDA-approved dosage regimens have been established. Dosages of 1500-3000 mg/m^2 as a single dose in combination with other agents every 4-6 weeks have been used in the treatment of pediatric astrocytoma, medulloblastoma and primitive neuroectodermal tumors.

CML: Initial: 10-20 mg/kg/day once daily; adjust dose according to hematologic response

Adults: Dose should always be titrated to patient response and WBC counts; usual oral doses range from 10-30 mg/kg/day or 500-3000 mg/day; if WBC count falls <2500 cells/mm^3, or the platelet count <100,000/mm^3, therapy should be stopped for at least 3 days and resumed when values rise toward normal

Solid tumors:
Intermittent therapy: 80 mg/kg as a single dose every third day
Continuous therapy: 20-30 mg/kg/day given as a single dose/day

Concomitant therapy with irradiation: 80 mg/kg as a single dose every third day starting at least 7 days before initiation of irradiation

Resistant chronic myelocytic leukemia: 20-30 mg/kg/day divided daily

Sickle cell anemia (moderate/severe disease): Hydroxyurea administration in adults (age range: 22-42 years) has produced beneficial effects in several small studies

Initial: 15 mg/kg/day, increased by 5 mg/kg every 12 weeks unless toxicity is observed or the maximum tolerated dose of 35 mg/kg/day is achieved.

Monitor for toxicity every 2 weeks. If toxicity occurs, stop treatment until the bone marrow recovers. Restart at 2.5 mg/kg/day less than the dose at which toxicity occurs. If no toxicity occurs over the next 12 weeks, then the subsequent dose should be increased by 2.5 mg/kg/day. Reduced dosage of hydroxyurea alternating with erythropoietin may decrease myelotoxicity and increase levels of fetal hemoglobin in patients who have not been helped by hydroxyurea alone

Mechanism of Action Interferes with synthesis of DNA, during the S phase of cell division, without interfering with RNA synthesis; inhibits ribonucleoside diphosphate reductase, preventing conversion of ribonucleotides to deoxyribonucleotides; cell-cycle specific for the S phase and may hold other cells in the G_1 phase of the cell cycle.

Local Anesthetic/Vasoconstrictor Precautions No information available to require special precautions

Effects on Dental Treatment No effects or complications reported

Other Adverse Effects

>10%:

Central nervous system: Drowsiness

Gastrointestinal: Mild to moderate nausea and vomiting may occur, as well as diarrhea, constipation, mucositis, ulceration of the GI tract, anorexia, and stomatitis

Hematologic: Myelosuppression: Dose-limiting toxicity, causes a rapid drop in leukocyte count (seen in 4-5 days in nonhematologic malignancy and more rapidly in leukemia). Thrombocytopenia and anemia occur less often; reversal of WBC count occurs rapidly, but the platelet count may take 7-10 days to recover.

1% to 10%:

Dermatologic: Dermatologic changes (hyperpigmentation, erythema of the hands and face, maculopapular rash, or dry skin), alopecia

Hepatic: Abnormal LFTs and hepatitis

Renal: Elevated BUN/creatinine

Miscellaneous: Carcinogenic potential

<1%:

Central nervous system: Neurotoxicity, renal tubular function impairment, dizziness, disorientation, hallucination, seizures, headache

Endocrine & metabolic: Hyperuricemia

Genitourinary: Dysuria

Hepatic: Elevation of hepatic enzymes

Drug Uptake

Absorption: Readily absorbed from GI tract (≥80%)

Serum half-life: 3-4 hours

Time to peak serum concentration: Within 2 hours

Pregnancy Risk Factor D

Generic Available Yes

Hydroxyzine (hye DROKS i zeen)

Related Information

Patients Requiring Sedation *on page 1081*

Brand Names Anxanil®; Atarax®; E-Vista®; Hydroxacen®; Hyzine-50®; QYS®; Vistacon®; Vistaject-25®; Vistaject-50®; Vistaquel®; Vistaril®; Vistazine®

Canadian/Mexican Brand Names Apo®-Hydroxyzine (Canada); Multipax® (Canada); Novo-Hydroxyzin (Canada); PMS-Hydroxyzine (Canada)

Therapeutic Category Antianxiety Agent; Antiemetic; Antihistamine; Sedative; Tranquilizer, Minor

Use

Dental: Treatment of anxiety, as a preoperative sedative in pediatric dentistry

Medical: Antipruritic, antiemetic, and in alcohol withdrawal symptoms

Usual Dosage

Children:

>6 years:

Oral: 25-50 mg 1 hour before procedure or 0.6 mg/kg/dose every 6 hours

I.M.: 0.5-1 mg/kg/dose every 4-6 hours as needed

<6 years: Oral: 12.5-25 mg 1 hours before procedure

Adults: Very rarely used in adults as preoperative sedative

Oral: 50-100 mg 1 hour before procedure

I.M.: 25-100 mg 1 hour before procedure

Mechanism of Action Competes with histamine for H_1-receptor sites on effector cells in the gastrointestinal tract, blood vessels, and respiratory tract

Local Anesthetic/Vasoconstrictor Precautions No information available to require special precautions

Effects on Dental Treatment 1% to 10% of patients experience dry mouth

Other Adverse Effects

>10%:

Central nervous system: Slight to moderate drowsiness

Respiratory: Thickening of bronchial secretions

1% to 10%:

Central nervous system: Headache, fatigue, nervousness, dizziness

(Continued)

Hydroxyzine *(Continued)*

Gastrointestinal: Appetite increase, weight gain, nausea, diarrhea, abdominal pain

Neuromuscular & skeletal: Arthralgia

Respiratory: Pharyngitis

Contraindications Hypersensitivity to hydroxyzine or any component

Warnings/Precautions S.C., intra-arterial and I.V. administration **not** recommended since thrombosis and digital gangrene can occur; extravasation can result in sterile abscess and marked tissue induration; should be used with caution in patients with narrow-angle glaucoma, prostatic hypertrophy, and bladder neck obstruction; should also be used with caution in patients with asthma or COPD

Anticholinergic effects are not well tolerated in the elderly. Hydroxyzine may be useful as a short-term antipruritic, but it is not recommended for use as a sedative or anxiolytic in the elderly.

Drug Interactions Increased toxicity with CNS depressants, anticholinergics

Drug Uptake

Absorption: Oral: Rapid

Onset of effect: Within 15-30 minutes

Duration: 4-6 hours

Serum half-life: 3-7 hours

Pregnancy Risk Factor C

Breast-feeding Considerations No data reported

Dosage Forms

Hydroxyzine hydrochloride:

Injection: 25 mg/mL (1 mL, 2 mL, 10 mL); 50 mg/mL (1 mL, 2 mL, 10 mL)

Syrup: 10 mg/5 mL (120 mL, 480 mL, 4000 mL)

Tablet: 10 mg, 25 mg, 50 mg, 100 mg

Hydroxyzine pamoate:

Capsule: 25 mg, 50 mg, 100 mg

Suspension, oral: 25 mg/5 mL (120 mL, 480 mL)

Dietary Considerations No data reported

Generic Available Yes

Hygroton® see Chlorthalidone on page 227

Hylorel® see Guanadrel on page 457

Hylutin® Injection see Hydroxyprogesterone Caproate on page 489

Hyoscyamine *(hye oh SYE a meen)*

Brand Names Anaspaz®; A-Spas® S/L; Cystospaz®; Cystospaz-M®; Donnamar®; ED-SPAZ®; Gastrosed™; Levbid®; Levsin®; Levsinex®; Levsin/SL®

Therapeutic Category Anticholinergic Agent; Antispasmodic Agent, Gastrointestinal

Use Treatment of GI tract disorders caused by spasm, adjunctive therapy for peptic ulcers

Usual Dosage

Children: Oral, S.L.: Dose as per table repeated every 4 hours as needed

Hyoscyamine

Weight (kg)	Dose (mcg)	Maximum 24-Hour Dose (mcg)
Children <2 y		
2.3	12.5	75
3.4	16.7	100
5	20.8	125
7	25	150
10	31.3-33.3	200
15	45.8	275
Children 2-10 y		
10	31.3-33.3	
20	62.5	Do not exceed
40	93.8	0.75 mg
50	125	

Adults:

Oral or S.L.: 0.125-0.25 mg 3-4 times/day before meals or food and at bedtime

Oral: 0.375-0.75 mg (timed release) every 12 hours

I.M., I.V., S.C.: 0.25-0.5 mg every 6 hours

Mechanism of Action Blocks the action of acetylcholine at parasympathetic sites in smooth muscle, secretory glands and the CNS; increases cardiac output, dries secretions, antagonizes histamine and serotonin

Local Anesthetic/Vasoconstrictor Precautions No information available to require special precautions

Effects on Dental Treatment >10% of patients experience dry mouth (normal salivary flow returns with cessation of drug therapy)

Other Adverse Effects

>10%:
  Dermatologic: Dry skin
  Local: Irritation at injection site
  Respiratory: Dry nose, throat
  Miscellaneous: Decreased sweating

1% to 10%:
  Dermatologic: Photosensitivity
  Gastrointestinal: Constipation, dysphagia
  Ocular: Blurred vision, mydriasis

<1%:
  Cardiovascular: Palpitations, orthostatic hypotension
  Central nervous system: Headache, lightheadedness, memory loss, fatigue, delirium, restlessness, ataxia
  Dermatologic: Skin rash
  Genitourinary: Dysuria
  Neuromuscular & skeletal: Tremor
  Ocular: Increased intraocular pressure

Drug Interactions

Decreased effect with antacids

Increased toxicity with amantadine, antimuscarinics, haloperidol, phenothiazines, TCAs, MAO inhibitors

Drug Uptake

Onset of effect: 2-3 minutes
Duration: 4-6 hours
Absorption: Oral: Absorbed well
Serum half-life: 13% to 38%

Pregnancy Risk Factor C

Generic Available Yes

Hyoscyamine, Atropine, Scopolamine, and Phenobarbital

(hye oh SYE a meen, A troe peen, skoe POL a meen & fee noe BAR bi tal)

Brand Names Barbidonna®; Donnatal®; Hyosophen®; Malatal®; Spasmolin®

Therapeutic Category Anticholinergic Agent; Antispasmodic Agent, Gastrointestinal

Use Adjunct in treatment of peptic ulcer disease, irritable bowel, spastic colitis, spastic bladder, and renal colic

Usual Dosage Oral:

Children 2-12 years: Kinesed® dose: ½ to 1 tablet 3-4 times/day

Children: Donnatal® elixir: 0.1 mL/kg/dose every 4 hours; maximum dose: 5 mL **or** see table for alternative.

Weight (kg)	Dose (mL)	
	q4h	q6h
4.5	0.5	0.75
10	1	1.5
14	1.5	2
23	2.5	3.8
34	3.8	5
≥45	5	7.5

Adults: 1-2 capsules or tablets 3-4 times/day; or 1 Donnatal® Extentab® in sustained release form every 12 hours; or 5-10 mL elixir 3-4 times/day or every 8 hours

Mechanism of Action Refer to individual agents

Local Anesthetic/Vasoconstrictor Precautions No information available to require special precautions

Effects on Dental Treatment >10% of patients experience dry mouth (normal salivary flow returns with cessation of drug therapy)

(Continued)

Hyoscyamine, Atropine, Scopolamine, and Phenobarbital *(Continued)*

Other Adverse Effects
>10%:
Dermatologic: Dry skin
Gastrointestinal: Constipation
Local: Irritation at injection site
Respiratory: Dry nose, throat
Miscellaneous: Decreased sweating

1% to 10%:
Dermatologic: Photosensitivity
Endocrine & metabolic: Decreased flow of breast milk
Gastrointestinal: Dysphagia

<1%:
Cardiovascular: Orthostatic hypotension, ventricular fibrillation, tachycardia, palpitations
Central nervous system: Confusion, drowsiness, headache, loss of memory, fatigue, ataxia
Dermatologic: Skin rash
Gastrointestinal: Bloated feeling, nausea, vomiting
Genitourinary: Dysuria
Ocular: Increased intraocular pain, blurred vision

Drug Interactions The following drugs may cause enhanced effects of this preparation: CNS depressants, amantadine, antihistamine, phenothiazines, corticosteroids, digitalis, griseofulvin, anticonvulsants, MAO inhibitors, tricyclic antidepressants

Drug Uptake Absorption: Well absorbed from GI tract

Pregnancy Risk Factor C

Generic Available Yes

Hyoscyamine, Atropine, Scopolamine, Kaolin, and Pectin
(hye oh SYE a meen, A troe peen, skoe POL a meen, KAY oh lin & PEK tin)

Therapeutic Category Antidiarrheal

Use Antidiarrheal; also used in gastritis, enteritis, colitis, and acute gastrointestinal upsets, and nausea which may accompany any of these conditions

Local Anesthetic/Vasoconstrictor Precautions No information available to require special precautions

Effects on Dental Treatment Dry mouth in >10% of patients (normal salivary flow returns with cessation of drug therapy)

Pregnancy Risk Factor C

Generic Available Yes

Hyoscyamine, Atropine, Scopolamine, Kaolin, Pectin, and Opium
(hye oh SYE a meen, A troe peen, skoe POL a meen, KAY oh lin, PEK tin, & OH pee um)

Brand Names Donnapectolin-PG®; Kapectolin PG®

Therapeutic Category Antidiarrheal

Use Treatment of diarrhea

Local Anesthetic/Vasoconstrictor Precautions No information available to require special precautions

Effects on Dental Treatment Dry mouth in >10% of patients (normal salivary flow returns with cessation of drug therapy)

Pregnancy Risk Factor C

Generic Available Yes

Comments Hyoscyamine is dialyzable

Hyosophen® *see* Hyoscyamine, Atropine, Scopolamine, and Phenobarbital *on previous page*

Hyperab® *see* Rabies Immune Globulin (Human) *on page 832*

HyperHep® *see* Hepatitis B Immune Globulin *on page 468*

Hyperstat® I.V. *see* Diazoxide *on page 301*

Hyper-Tet® *see* Tetanus Immune Globulin (Human) *on page 911*

Hy-Phen® [5/500] *see* Hydrocodone and Acetaminophen *on page 478*

HypoTears PF Solution [OTC] *see* Artificial Tears *on page 87*

HypoTears Solution [OTC] *see* Artificial Tears *on page 87*

HypRho®-D *see* Rh₀(D) Immune Globulin *on page 840*

HypRho®-D Mini-Dose *see* Rh₀(D) Immune Globulin *on page 840*

Hyprogest® 250 Injection *see* Hydroxyprogesterone Caproate *on page 489*

Hyrexin-50® Injection *see* Diphenhydramine *on page 323*

Hytakerol® *see* Dihydrotachysterol *on page 317*

Hytinic® [OTC] *see* Polysaccharide-Iron Complex *on page 773*

Hytrin® *see* Terazosin *on page 906*

Hytuss® [OTC] *see* Guaifenesin *on page 452*

Hytuss-2X® [OTC] *see* Guaifenesin *on page 452*

Hyzaar® *see* Losartan and Hydrochlorothiazide *on page 570*

Hyzine-50® *see* Hydroxyzine *on page 491*

Iberet-Folic-500® *see* Ferrous Sulfate, Ascorbic Acid, Vitamin B-Complex, and Folic Acid *on page 403*

Iberet®-Liquid [OTC] *see* Ferrous Sulfate, Ascorbic Acid, and Vitamin B-Complex *on page 402*

IBU® *see* Ibuprofen *on this page*

Ibuprin® [OTC] *see* Ibuprofen *on this page*

Ibuprofen (eye byoo PROE fen)

Related Information

Dental Drug Interactions: Update on Drug Combinations Requiring Special Considerations *on page 1144*

Nonsteroidal Anti-Inflammatory Agents, Comparative Dosages, and Pharmacokinetics *on page 1143*

Oral Pain *on page 1053*

Rheumatoid Arthritis and Osteoarthritis *on page 1030*

Temporomandibular Dysfunction (TMD) *on page 1078*

Brand Names Advil® [OTC]; Bayer® Select® Pain Relief Formula [OTC]; Children's Advil® Oral Suspension [OTC]; Children's Motrin® Oral Suspension [OTC]; Genpril® [OTC]; Haltran® [OTC]; IBU®; Ibuprin® [OTC]; Ibuprohm® [OTC]; Junior Strength Motrin® [OTC]; Menadol® [OTC]; Midol® IB [OTC]; Motrin®; Motrin® IB [OTC]; Nuprin® [OTC]; Pediatric Advil® [OTC]; Saleto-200® [OTC]; Saleto-400®; Saleto-600®; Saleto-800®

Canadian/Mexican Brand Names Actiprofen™ (Canada); Apo®-Ibuprofen (Canada); Butacortelone® (Mexico); Dibufen® (Mexico); Kedvil® (Mexico); Novo-Profen® (Canada); Nu-Ibuprofen (Canada); proartinal® (Mexico); Quadrax® (Mexico); Tabalon® (Mexico)

Therapeutic Category Analgesic, Non-narcotic; Anti-inflammatory Agent; Nonsteroidal Anti-inflammatory Agent (NSAID), Oral

Use

Dental: Management of pain and swelling

Medical: Inflammatory diseases and rheumatoid disorders including juvenile rheumatoid arthritis, mild to moderate pain, fever, dysmenorrhea, gout, ankylosing spondylitis, acute migraine headache

Usual Dosage Oral:

Children: Analgesic: 4-10 mg/kg/dose every 6-8 hours

Adults: 400-800 mg/dose 3-4 times/day; maximum daily dose: 3.2 (3200 mg) g/day

Mechanism of Action Inhibits prostaglandin synthesis by decreasing the activity of the enzyme, cyclo-oxygenase, which results in decreased formation of prostaglandin precursors

Local Anesthetic/Vasoconstrictor Precautions No information available to require special precautions

Effects on Dental Treatment <1% of patients experience dry mouth; use with caution in patients taking anticoagulants

Other Adverse Effects

>10%: Gastrointestinal: Indigestion, nausea

1% to 10%: Gastrointestinal: Abdominal pain

Contraindications Hypersensitivity to ibuprofen, any component, aspirin, or other nonsteroidal anti-inflammatory drugs (NSAIDs)

Warnings/Precautions Do not exceed 3200 mg/day; use with caution in patients with congestive heart failure, hypertension, decreased renal or hepatic function, history of GI disease (bleeding or ulcers), or those receiving anticoagulants; safety and efficacy in children <6 months of age have not yet been established; elderly are a high-risk population for adverse effects from nonsteroidal anti-inflammatory agents. As much as 60% of elderly can develop peptic ulceration and/or hemorrhage asymptomatically.

Use lowest effective dose for shortest period possible. CNS adverse effects such as confusion, agitation, and hallucination are generally seen in overdose or high dose situations; but elderly may demonstrate these adverse effects at lower doses than younger adults.

(Continued)

Ibuprofen *(Continued)*

Drug Interactions

Warfarin (Coumadin®): Ibuprofen can cause a decrease in platelet aggregation which may result in enhancement of the anticoagulant effect of coumarins

Lithium: Ibuprofen may inhibit prostaglandin-induced renal secretion of lithium, which increases lithium plasma levels and produces symptoms of lithium toxicity

Methotrexate: Ibuprofen has been reported to increase the serum levels of methotrexate resulting in possible methotrexate toxicity

Aspirin: Aspirin may decrease ibuprofen serum levels thereby reducing the effectiveness of ibuprofen

Drug Uptake

Absorption: Rapid

Onset of effect: 30-60 minutes

Time to peak serum concentration: Within 1-2 hours

Duration of effect: 4-6 hours

Serum half-life: 2-4 hours

Pregnancy Risk Factor B (D if used in the 3rd trimester)

Breast-feeding Considerations May be taken while breast-feeding

Dosage Forms

Caplet: 100 mg

Drops, oral (berry flavor): 40 mg/mL (15 mL)

Suppository, rectal: 80 mg

Suspension, oral: 100 mg/5 mL [OTC] (60 mL, 120 mL, 480 mL)

Suspension, oral, drops: 40 mg/mL [OTC]

Tablet: 100 mg [OTC], 200 mg [OTC], 300 mg, 400 mg, 600 mg, 800 mg

Tablet, chewable: 50 mg, 100 mg

Dietary Considerations May be taken with food or milk to decrease GI adverse effects; food decreases rate of absorption but extent remains the same

Generic Available Yes: Tablet

Comments Preoperative use of ibuprofen at a dose of 400-600 mg every 6 hours 24 hours before the appointment decreases postoperative edema and hastens healing time

Selected Readings

Brooks PM and Day RO, "Nonsteroidal Anti-inflammatory Drugs-Differences and Similarities," *N Engl J Med,* 1991, 324(24):1716-25.

Dionne RA, "New Approaches to Preventing and Treating Postoperative Pain," *J Am Dent Assoc,* 1992, 123(6):26-34.

Gobetti JP, "Controlling Dental Pain," *J Am Dent Assoc,* 1992, 123(6):47-52.

Pearlman B, Boyatzis S, Daly C, et al, "The Analgesic Efficacy of Ibuprofen in Periodontal Surgery: A Multicentre Study," *Aust Dent J,* 1997, 42(5):328-34.

Winter L Jr, Bass E, Recant B, et al, "Analgesic Activity of Ibuprofen (Motrin®) in Postoperative Oral Surgical Pain," *Oral Surg Oral Med Oral Pathol,* 1978, 45(2):159-66.

Ibuprohm® [OTC] *see* Ibuprofen *on previous page*

Ibutilide *(i BYOO ti lide)*

Brand Names Corvert®

Therapeutic Category Antiarrhythmic Agent, Class III

Synonyms Ibutilide Fumarate

Use Acute termination of atrial fibrillation or flutter of recent onset; the effectiveness of ibutilide has not been determined in patients with arrhythmias of >90 days in duration

Usual Dosage I.V.: Initial:

<60 kg: 0.01 mg/kg over 10 minutes

≥60 kg: 1 mg over 10 minutes

If the arrhythmia does not terminate within 10 minutes after the end of the initial infusion, a second infusion of equal strength may be infused over a 10-minute period

Mechanism of Action Exact mechanism of action is unknown; prolongs the action potential in cardiac tissue

Local Anesthetic/Vasoconstrictor Precautions No information available to require special precautions

Effects on Dental Treatment No effects or complications reported

Other Adverse Effects

1% to 10%:

Cardiovascular: Sustained polymorphic ventricular tachycardia (ie, torsade de pointes) (1.7%), often requiring cardioversion, nonsustained polymorphic ventricular tachycardia (2.7%), nonsustained monomorphic ventricular extrasystoles (5.1%), nonsustained monomorphic VT (4.9%), tachycardia/supraventricular tachycardia, hypotension (2%), bundle branch block (1.9%), A-V block (1.5%), bradycardia, Q-T segment prolongation, hypertension (1.2%), palpitations (1%)

Central nervous system: Headache (3.6%)
Gastrointestinal: Nausea (>1%)
<1%:
Cardiovascular: Supraventricular extrasystoles (0.9%), nodal arrhythmia (0.7%), congestive heart failure (0.5%), syncope, idioventricular rhythm, sustained monomorphic VT (0.2%)
Renal: Renal failure: (0.3%)

Warnings/Precautions Potentially fatal arrhythmias (eg, polymorphic ventricular tachycardia) can occur with ibutilide, **usually** in association with torsade de pointes (Q-T prolongation). Studies indicate a 1.7% incidence of arrhythmias in treated patients. The drug should be given in a setting of continuous EKG monitoring and by personnel trained in treating arrhythmias particularly polymorphic ventricular tachycardia. Patients with chronic atrial fibrillation may not be the best candidates for ibutilide since they often revert after conversion and the risks of treatment may not be justified when compared to alternative management. Dosing adjustments in patients with renal or hepatic dysfunction since a maximum of only two 10-minute infusions are indicated and drug distribution is one of the primary mechanisms responsible for termination of the pharmacologic effect; safety and efficacy in children have not been established.

Drug Interactions
Increased toxicity: Class Ia antiarrhythmic drugs (disopyramide, quinidine, and procainamide) and other class III drugs such as amiodarone and sotalol, should not be given concomitantly with ibutilide due to their potential to prolong refractoriness; the potential for prolongation of the Q-T interval may occur if ibutilide is given concurrently with phenothiazines, tricyclic and tetracyclic antidepressants, and the nonsedating antihistamines (terfenadine and astemizole); signs of digoxin toxicity may be masked when coadministered with ibutilide

Drug Uptake
Absorption: Onset: Within 90 minutes after start of infusion (½ of conversions to sinus rhythm occur during infusion)
Serum half-life: 2-12 hours (average: 6 hours)

Pregnancy Risk Factor C
Generic Available No

Ibutilide Fumarate see Ibutilide on previous page
Idamycin® see Idarubicin on this page

Idarubicin (eye da ROO bi sin)

Brand Names Idamycin®
Therapeutic Category Antineoplastic Agent, Antibiotic
Synonyms 4-demethoxydaunorubicin; IDR
Use In combination with other antineoplastic agents for treatment of acute myelogenous leukemia (AML) in adults and acute lymphocytic leukemia (ALL) in children

Usual Dosage I.V.:
Children:
Leukemia: 10-12 mg/m² once daily for 3 days and repeat every 3 weeks
Solid tumors: 5 mg/m² once daily for 3 days and repeat every 3 weeks
Adults: 12 mg/m²/day for 3 days by slow I.V. injection (10-15 minutes) in combination with Ara-C. The Ara-C may be given as 100 mg/m²/day by continuous infusion for 7 days or 25 mg/m² bolus followed by Ara-C 200 mg/m²/day for 5 days continuous infusion

Mechanism of Action Similar to daunorubicin, idarubicin exhibits inhibitory effects on DNA and RNA polymerase *in vitro*. Idarubicin has an affinity for DNA similar to daunorubicin and somewhat higher efficacy in stabilizing the DNA double helix against heat denaturation. Idarubicin has been as active or more active than daunorubicin in inhibiting 3H-TdR uptake by DNA or RNA of mouse embryo fibroblasts.

Local Anesthetic/Vasoconstrictor Precautions No information available to require special precautions
Effects on Dental Treatment No effects or complications reported
Other Adverse Effects
>10%:
Central nervous system: Headache, fever
Dermatologic: Alopecia, rash, urticaria
Gastrointestinal: Mucositis, nausea, vomiting, diarrhea, stomatitis
Genitourinary: Discoloration of urine (red)
Hematologic: Hemorrhage, anemia
Leukopenia (nadir: 8-29 days)
Thrombocytopenia (nadir: 10-15 days)
Local: Tissue necrosis upon extravasation, erythematous streaking
Vesicant chemotherapy
(Continued)

Idarubicin (Continued)

Miscellaneous: Infection
1% to 10%:
  Central nervous system: Seizures
  Neuromuscular & skeletal: Peripheral neuropathy
  Respiratory: Pulmonary allergy
<1%:
  Cardiovascular: Arrhythmias, EKG changes, cardiomyopathy, congestive heart
    failure, myocardial toxicity, acute life-threatening arrhythmias
  Endocrine & metabolic: Hyperuricemia
  Hepatic: Elevations in liver enzymes or bilirubin

Drug Uptake
  Absorption: Oral: Rapid but erratic (20% to 30%) from GI tract
  Serum half-life, elimination:
    Oral: 14-35 hours
    I.V.: 12-27 hours
  Time to peak serum concentration: Within 2-4 hours and varies considerably

Pregnancy Risk Factor D

Generic Available No

Comments Discoloration of urine may persist for 48 hours

Idoxuridina (Mexico) see Idoxuridine on this page

Idoxuridine (eye doks YOOR i deen)

Brand Names Herplex®

Therapeutic Category Antiviral Agent, Ophthalmic

Synonyms Idoxuridina (Mexico)

Use Treatment of herpes simplex keratitis

Usual Dosage Adults: Ophthalmic:
  Ointment: Instill 5 times/day (every 4 hours) in the conjunctival sac with last dose
    at bedtime; continue therapy for 5-7 days after healing appears complete
  Solution: Instill 1 drop in eye(s) every hour during day and every 2 hours at night,
    continue until definite improvement is noted, then reduce daytime dose to 1
    drop every 2 hours and every 4 hours at night; continue for 5-7 days after
    healing appears complete
  Alternative dosing schedule: Instill 1 drop every minute for 5 minutes; repeat
    every 4 hours day and night

Mechanism of Action Incorporated into viral DNA in place of thymidine resulting
  in mutations and inhibition of viral replication

Local Anesthetic/Vasoconstrictor Precautions No information available to
  require special precautions

Effects on Dental Treatment No effects or complications reported

Other Adverse Effects
  1% to 10%:
    Dermatologic: Pruritus, follicular conjunctivitis
    Local: Irritation, pain, inflammation, mild edema of the eyelids and cornea
    Ocular: Visual haze, corneal clouding, photophobia, small punctate defects on
      the corneal epithelium
  <1%: Ocular: Small punctate defects on the corneal epithelium

Drug Interactions Increased toxicity: Do not coadminister with boric acid
  containing solutions

Drug Uptake
  Absorption: Ophthalmic: Poorly absorbed following instillation; tissue uptake is a
    function of cellular metabolism, which is inhibited by high concentrations of the
    drug (absorption decreases as the concentration of drug increases)

Pregnancy Risk Factor C

Generic Available No

IDR see Idarubicin on previous page

Ifex® Injection see Ifosfamide on this page

Ifosfamide (eye FOSS fa mide)

Brand Names Ifex® Injection

Canadian/Mexican Brand Names Ifoxan® (Mexico)

Therapeutic Category Antineoplastic Agent, Alkylating Agent

Use In combination with other antineoplastics in treatment of lung cancer,
  Hodgkin's and non-Hodgkin's lymphoma, breast cancer, acute and chronic
  lymphocytic leukemia, ovarian cancer, testicular cancer, and sarcomas

Usual Dosage I.V. (refer to individual protocols):
  Children: 1200-1800 mg/m^2/day for 3-5 days every 21-28 days or 5 g/m^2 as a
    single 24-hour infusion or 3 g/m^2/day for 2 days

Adults:
  Doses may be given as 50 mg/kg/day **or** 700-2000 mg/m²/day for 5 days
  Alternatives include 2400 mg/m²/day for 3 days **or** 5000 mg/m² as a single dose
  Doses of 700-900 mg/m²/day for 5 days may be given IVP; courses may be repeated every 3-4 weeks

To prevent bladder toxicity, ifosfamide should be given with extensive hydration consisting of at least 2 L of oral or I.V. fluid per day. A protector, such as mesna, should also be used to prevent hemorrhagic cystitis. The dose-limiting toxicity is hemorrhagic cystitis and ifosfamide should be used in conjunction with a uroprotective agent.

Mechanism of Action Causes cross-linking of strands of DNA by binding with nucleic acids and other intracellular structures; inhibits protein synthesis and DNA synthesis; an analogue of cyclophosphamide, and like cyclophosphamide, it undergoes activation by microsomal enzymes in the liver. Ifosfamide is metabolized to active compounds, ifosfamide mustard, and acrolein

Local Anesthetic/Vasoconstrictor Precautions No information available to require special precautions

Effects on Dental Treatment No effects or complications reported

Other Adverse Effects
>10%:
  Dermatologic: Alopecia occurs in 50% to 83% of patients 2-4 weeks after initiation of therapy; may be as high as 100% in combination therapy patients.
  Endocrine & metabolic: Metabolic acidosis may occur in up to 31% of
  Gastrointestinal: Nausea and vomiting in 58% of patients is dose and schedule related (more common with higher doses and after bolus regimens); nausea and vomiting can persist up to 3 days after therapy; also anorexia, diarrhea, constipation, and stomatitis noted.
  Emetic potential: Moderate (58%)
  Genitourinary toxicity: Hemorrhagic cystitis has been frequently associated with the use of ifosfamide. A urinalysis prior to each dose should be obtained. **Ifosfamide should never be administered without a uroprotective agent (MESNA).**
  Hepatic: Transient elevation in LFTS
  Renal: Hematuria has been reported in 6% to 92% of patients. Renal toxicity occurs in 6% of patients and is manifested as an elevation in BUN or serum creatinine and is most likely related to tubular damage.
1% to 10%:
  Cardiovascular: Cardiotoxicity
  Central nervous system: Polyneuropathy, somnolence, confusion, hallucinations in 12% and coma (rare) have occurred and are usually reversible; usually occur with higher doses; depressive psychoses
  Dermatologic: Skin hyperpigmentation, dermatitis
  Endocrine & metabolic: SIADH
  Gastrointestinal: Stomatitis
  Hematologic: Leukopenia is mild to moderate, thrombocytopenia and anemia are rare
    Myelosuppression: Less of a problem than with cyclophosphamide if used alone. However, myelosuppression can be severe when used with other chemotherapeutic agents. Be cautious with patients with compromised bone marrow reserve. WBC: Moderate; Platelets: Mild; Onset (days): 7; Nadir (days): 10-14; Recovery (days): 21
  Hepatic: Elevated liver enzymes
  Local: Phlebitis
  Respiratory: Nasal congestion, pulmonary fibrosis
  Miscellaneous: Immunosuppression, sterility, nail ridging, possible secondary malignancy, impaired wound healing, and allergic reactions

Drug Uptake Pharmacokinetics are dose-dependent
  Absorption: Oral: Peak plasma levels occur within 1 hour
  Serum half-life: Beta phase: 11-15 hours with high-dose (3800-5000 mg/m²) or 4-7 hours with lower doses (1800 mg/m²)

Pregnancy Risk Factor D

Generic Available No

Comments Usually used in combination with mesna, a prophylactic agent for hemorrhagic cystitis

Ilozyme® *see* Pancrelipase *on page 722*
Imdur™ *see* Isosorbide Mononitrate *on page 526*
I-Methasone® *see* Dexamethasone *on page 291*
Imidazole Carboxamide *see* Dacarbazine *on page 276*

Imiglucerase (imi GLOO ser ase)
Brand Names Cerezyme®
Therapeutic Category Enzyme, Glucocerebrosidase
Use Long-term enzyme replacement therapy for patients with Type 1 Gaucher's disease
Local Anesthetic/Vasoconstrictor Precautions No information available to require special precautions
Effects on Dental Treatment No effects or complications reported
Pregnancy Risk Factor C
Generic Available No

Imipenem and Cilastatin (i mi PEN em & sye la STAT in)
Related Information
Animal and Human Bites Guidelines *on page 1093*
Brand Names Primaxin®
Canadian/Mexican Brand Names Tienam® (Mexico)
Therapeutic Category Antibiotic, Miscellaneous
Use Treatment of documented multidrug resistant gram-negative infection due to organisms proven or suspected to be susceptible to imipenem/cilastatin; treatment of multiple organism infection in which other agents have an insufficient spectrum of activity or are contraindicated due to toxic potential; Antibacterial activity includes resistant gram-negative bacilli (*Pseudomonas aeruginosa* and *Enterococcus* sp.), gram-positive bacteria (methicillin-sensitive *Staphylococcus aureus* and *Enterococcus* sp.) and anaerobes
Usual Dosage I.M. and I.V. (dosing based on imipenem component):
Children: I.V.: 60-100 mg/kg/24 hours divided every 6 hours (maximum: 4 g/day)
Adults: I.V.: 500 mg every 6-8 hours (1 g every 6-8 hours for severe *Pseudomonas* infection); infuse each 250-500 mg dose over 20-30 minutes; infuse each 1 g dose over 40-60 minutes
Mild to moderate infection **only**: I.M.: 500-750 mg every 12 hours (**Note:** 750 mg is recommended for intra-abdominal and more severe respiratory, dermatologic, or gynecologic infections; total daily I.M. dosages >1500 mg are not recommended; deep I.M. injection should be carefully made into a large muscle mass only)
Mechanism of Action
A carbapenem with broad-spectrum antibacterial activity including resistant gram-negative bacilli (*Pseudomonas aeruginosa* and *Enterococcus* sp.), gram-positive bacteria (methicillin-sensitive *Staphylococcus aureus* and *Enterococcus* sp.) and anaerobes
Inhibits cell wall synthesis by binding to penicillin-binding proteins on the bacterial outer membrane; cilastatin prevents renal metabolism of imipenem by competitive inhibition of dehydropeptidase along the brush border of the proximal renal tubules
Local Anesthetic/Vasoconstrictor Precautions No information available to require special precautions
Effects on Dental Treatment No effects or complications reported
Other Adverse Effects
1% to 10%:
Gastrointestinal: Nausea, diarrhea, vomiting
Local: Phlebitis
<1%:
Cardiovascular: Hypotension, palpitations
Central nervous system: Seizures
Dermatologic: Rash
Gastrointestinal: Pseudomembranous colitis
Hematologic: Neutropenia, eosinophilia
Local: Pain at injection site
Miscellaneous: Emergence of resistant strains of *P. aeruginosa*
Drug Interactions Increased toxicity: Probenecid causes increased toxic potential
Drug Uptake
Imipenem: Serum half-life: 1 hour, extended with renal insufficiency
Cilastatin: Serum half-life: 1 hour, extended with renal insufficiency
Pregnancy Risk Factor C
Generic Available No

Imipramine (im IP ra meen)

Brand Names Janimine®; Tofranil®; Tofranil-PM®

Canadian/Mexican Brand Names Apo®-Imipramine (Canada); Novo-Pramine® (Canada); PMS-Imipramine® (Canada); Talpramin® (Mexico)

Therapeutic Category Antidepressant, Tricyclic

Use Treatment of various forms of depression, often in conjunction with psychotherapy; enuresis in children; analgesic for certain chronic and neuropathic pain

Usual Dosage Maximum antidepressant effect may not be seen for 2 or more weeks after initiation of therapy.

Children: Oral:

Depression: 1.5 mg/kg/day with dosage increments of 1 mg/kg every 3-4 days to a maximum dose of 5 mg/kg/day in 1-4 divided doses; monitor carefully especially with doses ≥3.5 mg/kg/day

Enuresis: ≥6 years: Initial: 10-25 mg at bedtime, if inadequate response still seen after 1 week of therapy, increase by 25 mg/day; dose should not exceed 2.5 mg/kg/day or 50 mg at bedtime if 6-12 years of age or 75 mg at bedtime if ≥12 years of age

Adjunct in the treatment of cancer pain: Initial: 0.2-0.4 mg/kg at bedtime; dose may be increased by 50% every 2-3 days up to 1-3 mg/kg/dose at bedtime

Adolescents: Oral: Initial: 25-50 mg/day; increase gradually; maximum: 100 mg/day in single or divided doses

Adults:

Oral: Initial: 25 mg 3-4 times/day, increase dose gradually, total dose may be given at bedtime; maximum: 300 mg/day

I.M.: Initial: Up to 100 mg/day in divided doses; change to oral as soon as possible

Elderly: Initial: 10-25 mg at bedtime; increase by 10-25 mg every 3 days for inpatients and weekly for outpatients if tolerated; average daily dose to achieve a therapeutic concentration: 100 mg/day; range: 50-150 mg/day

Mechanism of Action Traditionally believed to increase the synaptic concentration of serotonin and/or norepinephrine in the central nervous system by inhibition of their reuptake by the presynaptic neuronal membrane. However, additional receptor effects have been found including desensitization of adenyl cyclase, down regulation of beta-adrenergic receptors, and down regulation of serotonin receptors.

Local Anesthetic/Vasoconstrictor Precautions Use with caution; epinephrine, norepinephrine and levonordefrin have been shown to have an increased pressor response in combination with TCAs

Effects on Dental Treatment >10% of patients experience dry mouth; long-term treatment with TCAs such as imipramine increases the risk of caries by reducing salivation and salivary buffer capacity. In a study by Rundergren, et al, pathological alterations were observed in the oral mucosa of 72% of 58 patients; 55% had new carious lesions after taking TCAs for a median of 5½ years. Current research is investigating the use of the salivary stimulant pilocarpine to overcome the xerostomia from imipramine.

Other Adverse Effects Less sedation and anticholinergic effects than amitriptyline

>10%:

Central nervous system: Dizziness, drowsiness, headache

Gastrointestinal: Increased appetite, nausea, unpleasant taste, weight gain, constipation

Genitourinary: Urinary retention

Neuromuscular & skeletal: Weakness

1% to 10%:

Cardiovascular: Postural hypotension, arrhythmias, tachycardia, sudden death

Central nervous system: Confusion, delirium, hallucinations, nervousness, restlessness, parkinsonian syndrome, insomnia

Endocrine & metabolic: Sexual dysfunction

Gastrointestinal: Diarrhea, heartburn

Genitourinary: Dysuria

Neuromuscular & skeletal: Fine muscle tremors

Ocular: Blurred vision, eye pain

Miscellaneous: Excessive sweating

<1%:

Central nervous system: Anxiety, seizures

Dermatologic: Alopecia, photosensitivity

Endocrine & metabolic: Breast enlargement, galactorrhea, SIADH

Genitourinary: Testicular swelling

Hematologic: Leukopenia, eosinophilia, rarely agranulocytosis

Hepatic: Elevated liver enzymes, cholestatic jaundice

(Continued)

Imipramine *(Continued)*

Ocular: Increased intraocular pressure

Otic: Tinnitus

Miscellaneous: Allergic reactions, trouble with gums, decreased lower esophageal sphincter tone may cause GE reflux, allergic reactions, has been associated with falls

Drug Interactions

Decreased effect: Phenobarbital may increase the metabolism of imipramine; imipramine blocks the uptake of guanethidine and thus prevents the hypotensive effect of guanethidine

Increased toxicity: Clonidine may increase hypertensive crisis; imipramine may be additive with or may potentiate the action of other CNS depressants such as sedatives or hypnotics; with MAO inhibitors, hyperpyrexia, hypertension, tachycardia, confusion, and seizures. Imipramine may increase the prothrombin time in patients stabilized on warfarin; imipramine potentiates the pressor and cardiac effects of sympathomimetic agents such as isoproterenol, epinephrine, etc; cimetidine and methylphenidate may decrease the metabolism of imipramine

Additive anticholinergic effects seen with other anticholinergic agents

Drug Uptake

Peak antidepressant effect: Usually after ≥2 weeks

Absorption: Oral: Well absorbed

Serum half-life: 6-18 hours

Pregnancy Risk Factor D

Generic Available Yes: Tablet

Selected Readings

Boakes AJ, Laurence DR, Teoh PC, et al, "Interactions Between Sympathomimetic Amines and Antidepressant Agents in Man," *Br Med J,* 1973, 1(849):311-5.

Jastak JT and Yagiela JA, "Vasoconstrictors and Local Anesthesia: A Review and Rationale for Use," *J Am Dent Assoc,* 1983, 107(4):623-30.

Larochelle P, Hamet P, and Enjalbert M, "Responses to Tyramine and Norepinephrine After Imipramine and Trazodone," *Clin Pharmacol Ther,* 1979, 26(1):24-30.

Mitchell JR, "Guanethidine and Related Agents. III Antagonism by Drugs Which Inhibit the Norepinephrine Pump in Man," *J Clin Invest,* 1970, 49(8):1596-604.

Rundegren J, van Dijken J, Mörnstad H, et al, "Oral Conditions in Patients Receiving Long-Term Treatment With Cyclic Antidepressant Drugs," *Swed Dent J,* 1985, 9(2):55-64.

Svedmyr N, "The Influence of a Tricyclic Antidepressive Agent (Protriptyline) on Some of the Circulatory Effects of Noradrenaline and Adrenalin in Man," *Life Sci,* 1968, 7(1):77-84.

Wynn RL, "New Antidepressant Medications," *Gen Dent,* 1997, 45(1):24-8.

Imiquimod *(i mi KWI mod)*

Brand Names Aldara®

Therapeutic Category Immune Response Modifier

Use Genital and perianal warts (condyloma acuminata)

Usual Dosage Adults: Topical: Apply three times/week, prior to bedtime, leave on for 6-10 hours, remove cream by washing area with mild soap and water

Local Anesthetic/Vasoconstrictor Precautions No information available to require special precautions

Effects on Dental Treatment No effects or complications reported

Pregnancy Risk Factor B

Imitrex® *see* Sumatriptan Succinate *on page 899*

Immune Globulin, Intramuscular

(i MYUN GLOB yoo lin, IN tra MUS kyoo ler)

Related Information

Systemic Viral Diseases *on page 1047*

Brand Names Gamastan®; Gammar®

Canadian/Mexican Brand Names Gammabulin Immuno (Canada); Iveegam® (Canada)

Therapeutic Category Immune Globulin

Use Household and sexual contacts of persons with hepatitis A, measles, varicella, and possibly rubella; travelers to high-risk areas outside tourist routes; staff, attendees, and patients of diapered attendees in day-care center outbreaks

For travelers, IG is not an alternative to careful selection of foods and water; immune globulin can interfere with the antibody response to parenterally administered live virus vaccines. Frequent travelers should be tested for hepatitis A antibody, immune hemolytic anemia, and neutropenia (with ITP, I.V. route is usually used).

Usual Dosage I.M.:

Hepatitis A:

Pre-exposure prophylaxis upon travel into endemic areas:

0.02 mL/kg for anticipated risk 1-3 months

0.06 mL/kg for anticipated risk >3 months
Repeat approximate dose every 4-6 months if exposure continues
Postexposure prophylaxis: 0.02 mL/kg given within 2 weeks of exposure
Measles:
Prophylaxis: 0.25 mL/kg/dose (maximum dose: 15 mL) given within 6 days of exposure followed by live attenuated measles vaccine in 3 months or at 15 months of age (whichever is later)
For patients with leukemia, lymphoma, immunodeficiency disorders, generalized malignancy, or receiving immunosuppressive therapy: 0.5 mL/kg (maximum dose: 15 mL)
Poliomyelitis: Prophylaxis: 0.3 mL/kg/dose as a single dose
Rubella: Prophylaxis: 0.55 mL/kg/dose within 72 hours of exposure
Varicella:: Prophylaxis: 0.6-1.2 mL/kg (varicella zoster immune globulin preferred) within 72 hours of exposure
IgG deficiency: 1.3 mL/kg, then 0.66 mL/kg in 3-4 weeks
Hepatitis B: Prophylaxis: 0.06 mL/kg/dose (HBIG preferred)

Mechanism of Action Provides passive immunity by increasing the antibody titer and antigen-antibody reaction potential

Local Anesthetic/Vasoconstrictor Precautions No information available to require special precautions

Effects on Dental Treatment No effects or complications reported

Other Adverse Effects
>10%: Local: Pain, tenderness, muscle stiffness at I.M. site
1% to 10%:
Cardiovascular: Flushing
Central nervous system: Chills
Gastrointestinal: Nausea
<1%:
Central nervous system: Lethargy, fever
Dermatologic: Urticaria, angioedema, erythema
Gastrointestinal: Vomiting
Neuromuscular & skeletal: Myalgia
Miscellaneous: Hypersensitivity reactions

Drug Interactions Increased toxicity: Live virus, vaccines (measles, mumps, rubella); do not administer within 3 months after administration of these vaccines

Drug Uptake
Duration of immune effect: Usually 3-4 weeks
Serum half-life: 23 days
Time to peak serum concentration: I.M.: Within 24-48 hours

Pregnancy Risk Factor C

Generic Available Yes

Immune Globulin, Intravenous
(i MYUN GLOB yoo lin, IN tra VEE nus)

Related Information
Systemic Viral Diseases on page 1047

Brand Names Gamimune® N; Gammagard®; Gammagard® S/D; Gammar®-P I.V.; Polygam®; Polygam® S/D; Sandoglobulin®; Venoglobulin®-I; Venoglobulin®-S

Canadian/Mexican Brand Names Citax (Mexico); Intacglobin® (Mexico); Sandoglubolina® (Mexico)

Therapeutic Category Immune Globulin

Synonyms IVIG

Use Immunodeficiency syndrome, idiopathic thrombocytopenic purpura (ITP) and B-cell chronic lymphocytic leukemia (CLL); used in conjunction with appropriate anti-infective therapy to prevent or modify acute bacterial or viral infections in patients with iatrogenically-induced or disease-associated immunodepression; autoimmune neutropenia, bone marrow transplantation patients, Kawasaki disease, Guillain-Barré syndrome, demyelinating polyneuropathies

Usual Dosage Children and Adults: I.V.:
Dosages should be based on ideal body weight and not actual body weight in morbidly obese patients
Primary immunodeficiency disorders: 200-400 mg/kg every 4 weeks or as per monitored serum IgG concentrations
Chronic lymphocytic leukemia (CLL): 400 mg/kg/dose every 3 weeks
Idiopathic thrombocytopenic purpura (ITP): Maintenance dose:
400 mg/kg/day for 5 consecutive days
800 mg/kg/day for 2 consecutive days
Chronic ITP: 400-1000 mg/kg/dose every 7 or 14 days
Kawasaki disease:
400 mg/kg/day for 4 days within 10 days of onset of fever
800 mg/kg/day for 1-2 days within 10 days of onset of fever
(Continued)

Immune Globulin, Intravenous *(Continued)*

2 g/kg for one dose only

Acquired immunodeficiency syndrome (patients must be symptomatic):
200-250 mg/kg/dose every 2 weeks
400-500 mg/kg/dose every month or every 4 weeks

Autoimmune hemolytic anemia and neutropenia: 1000 mg/kg/dose for 2-3 days

Autoimmune diseases: 400 mg/kg/day for 4 days

Post allogeneic bone marrow transplant: 500 mg/kg/week for 4 months post-transplant

Adjuvant to severe cytomegalovirus infections: 500 mg/kg/dose every other day for 7 doses

Severe systemic viral and bacterial infections:
Children: 500-1000 mg/kg/week

Prevention of gastroenteritis: Children: Oral: 50 mg/kg/day divided every 6 hours

Guillain-Barré syndrome:
400 mg/kg/day for 4 days
1000 mg/kg/day for 2 days
2000 mg/kg/day for one day

Refractory dermatomyositis: 2 g/kg/dose every month x 3-4 doses

Refractory polymyositis: 1 g/kg/day x 2 days every month x 4 doses

Chronic inflammatory demyelinating polyneuropathy:
400 mg/kg/day for 5 doses once each month
800 mg/kg/day for 3 doses once each month
1000 mg/kg/day for 2 days once each month

Mechanism of Action Replacement therapy for primary and secondary immunodeficiencies; interference with F_c receptors on the cells of the reticuloendothelial system for autoimmune cytopenias and ITP; possible role of contained antiviral-type antibodies

Local Anesthetic/Vasoconstrictor Precautions No information available to require special precautions

Effects on Dental Treatment No effects or complications reported

Other Adverse Effects

1% to 10%:
Cardiovascular: Flushing of the face, tachycardia
Central nervous system: Chills
Gastrointestinal: Nausea
Respiratory: Dyspnea

<1%:
Cardiovascular: Hypotension, tightness in the chest
Central nervous system: Dizziness, fever, headache
Miscellaneous: Sweating, hypersensitivity reactions

Drug Uptake I.V. provides immediate antibody levels
Half-life: 21-24 days

Pregnancy Risk Factor C

Generic Available No

Comments Gammagard®, Polygam®, or Iveegam® have low titers of IgA and may be used in patients with IgA deficiency

Imodium® *see Loperamide on page 565*

Imodium® A-D [OTC] *see Loperamide on page 565*

Imogam® *see Rabies Immune Globulin (Human) on page 832*

Imovax® Rabies I.D. Vaccine *see Rabies Virus Vaccine on page 832*

Imovax® Rabies Vaccine *see Rabies Virus Vaccine on page 832*

Imuran® *see Azathioprine on page 102*

I-Naphline® Ophthalmic *see Naphazoline on page 664*

Inapsine® *see Droperidol on page 340*

Indapamide *(in DAP a mide)*

Related Information
Cardiovascular Diseases *on page 1010*

Brand Names Lozol®

Canadian/Mexican Brand Names Lozide® (Canada)

Therapeutic Category Diuretic, Thiazide

Use Management of mild to moderate hypertension; treatment of edema in congestive heart failure and nephrotic syndrome

Usual Dosage Adults: Oral: 2.5-5 mg/day. **Note:** There is little therapeutic benefit to increasing the dose >5 mg/day; there is, however, an increased risk of electrolyte disturbances.

Mechanism of Action Diuretic effect is localized at the proximal segment of the distal tubule of the nephron; it does not appear to have significant effect on glomerular filtration rate nor renal blood flow; like other diuretics, it enhances sodium, chloride, and water excretion by interfering with the transport of sodium ions across the renal tubular epithelium

Local Anesthetic/Vasoconstrictor Precautions No information available to require special precautions

Effects on Dental Treatment No effects or complications reported

Other Adverse Effects

1% to 10%: Endocrine & metabolic: Hypokalemia

<1%:

Cardiovascular: Arrhythmia, weak pulse, hypotension

Central nervous system: Mood changes

Dermatologic: Photosensitivity

Endocrine & metabolic: Fluid and electrolyte imbalances (hypocalcemia, hypomagnesemia, hyponatremia), hyperglycemia

Gastrointestinal: Dry mouth, increased thirst

Hematologic: Rarely blood dyscrasias

Neuromuscular & skeletal: Numbness in hands, feet, or lips; paresthesia, muscle cramps or pain, weakness (unusual)

Renal: Prerenal azotemia

Respiratory: Dyspnea

Drug Interactions

Decreased effect of oral hypoglycemics; decreased absorption with cholestyramine and colestipol

Increased effect with furosemide and other loop diuretics

Increased toxicity/levels of lithium; when given with digoxin, diuretic-induced hypokalemia increases the risk of digoxin toxicity

Drug Uptake

Absorption: Completely from GI tract

Serum half-life: 14-18 hours

Time to peak serum concentration: 2-2.5 hours

Pregnancy Risk Factor D

Generic Available Yes

Inderal® *see* Propranolol *on page 814*

Inderal® LA *see* Propranolol *on page 814*

Inderide® *see* Propranolol and Hydrochlorothiazide *on page 816*

Indinavir (in DIN a veer)

Related Information

HIV Infection and AIDS *on page 1024*

Systemic Viral Diseases *on page 1047*

Brand Names Crixivan®

Therapeutic Category Antiviral Agent, Oral; Protease Inhibitor

Use Treatment of HIV infection, especially advanced disease; usually administered as part of a three-drug regimen (two nucleosides plus a protease inhibitor) or double therapy (one nucleoside plus a protease inhibitor)

Usual Dosage Adults: Oral: 800 mg every 8 hours

Dosage adjustment in hepatic impairment: 600 mg every 8 hours with mild/medium impairment due to cirrhosis or with ketoconazole coadministration

Mechanism of Action Indinavir is a protease inhibitor which prevents cleavage of protein precursors essential for HIV infection of new cells and viral replication. Some patients with advanced HIV infection have significantly improved clinically with the use of a protease inhibitor; resistant strains are cross-resistant to ritonavir and saquinavir.

Local Anesthetic/Vasoconstrictor Precautions No information available to require special precautions

Effects on Dental Treatment No effects or complications reported

Other Adverse Effects 1% to 10%:

Hepatic: Mild elevation of indirect bilirubin (10%)

Renal: Kidney stones (2% to 3%)

Contraindications Hypersensitivity to the drug or its components; avoid use with terfenadine, astemizole, cisapride, or benzodiazepines

Warnings/Precautions Use caution in patients with hepatic insufficiency; dosage reduction may be needed; nephrolithiasis may occur with use; if signs and symptoms of nephrolithiasis occur, interrupt therapy for 1-3 days; ensure adequate hydration

Drug Interactions

Decreased effect: Concurrent use of rifampin and rifabutin may decrease the effectiveness of indinavir; dosage decreases of rifampin/rifabutin is recommended

Increase toxicity: Gastric pH is lowered and absorption may be decreased when didanosine and indinavir are taken <1 hour apart; a reduction of dose is often required when coadministered with ketoconazole; terfenadine, astemizole, (Continued)

Indinavir *(Continued)*

cisapride, and benzodiazepines should be avoided with indinavir due to a potentially serious toxicity

Drug Uptake
Bioavailability: Oral: Good; T_{max}: 0.8 ± 0.3 hour
Half-life: 1.8 ± 0.4 hour

Pregnancy Risk Factor C

Dosage Forms Capsule: 400 mg

Generic Available No

Comments One study of previously untreated patients with a mean CD4-cell count of 250 cell/mm^3 found that indinavir plus zidovudine lowered serum HIV below detectable levels in 56% of 52 patients treated for 24 weeks. Other studies show similar results. Indinavir alone has suppressed serum HIV below detectable levels in 40% to 60% of patients treated up to 48 weeks.

Indochron E-R® *see* Indomethacin *on this page*

Indocin® *see* Indomethacin *on this page*

Indocin® **I.V.** *see* Indomethacin *on this page*

Indocin® **SR** *see* Indomethacin *on this page*

Indocyanine Green *(in doe SYE a neen green)*

Brand Names Cardio-Green®

Therapeutic Category Diagnostic Agent, Cardiac Function

Use Determining hepatic function, cardiac output and liver blood flow and for ophthalmic angiography

Local Anesthetic/Vasoconstrictor Precautions No information available to require special precautions

Effects on Dental Treatment No effects or complications reported

Other Adverse Effects 1% to 10%:
Central nervous system: Headache
Dermatologic: Pruritus, skin discoloration
Miscellaneous: Sweating, anaphylactoid reactions

Pregnancy Risk Factor C

Generic Available Yes

Indometacina (Mexico) *see* Indomethacin *on this page*

Indomethacin *(in doe METH a sin)*

Related Information
Nonsteroidal Anti-Inflammatory Agents, Comparative Dosages, and Pharmacokinetics *on page 1143*
Rheumatoid Arthritis and Osteoarthritis *on page 1030*

Brand Names Indochron E-R®; Indocin®; Indocin® I.V.; Indocin® SR

Canadian/Mexican Brand Names Antalgin® Dialicels (Mexico); Apo®-Indomethacin (Canada); Indocid® (Canada); Indocid® (Mexico); Indocid-SR® (Canada); Malival® y Malival® AP (Mexico); Novo-Methacin® (Canada); Nu-Indo® (Canada); Pro-Indo® (Canada)

Therapeutic Category Analgesic, Non-narcotic; Anti-inflammatory Agent; Nonsteroidal Anti-inflammatory Agent (NSAID), Oral; Nonsteroidal Anti-inflammatory Agent (NSAID), Parenteral

Synonyms Indometacina (Mexico)

Use Management of inflammatory diseases and rheumatoid disorders; moderate pain; acute gouty arthritis; I.V. form used as alternative to surgery for closure of patent ductus arteriosus in neonates

Usual Dosage
Patent ductus arteriosus:
Neonates: I.V.: Initial: 0.2 mg/kg; followed with: 2 doses of 0.1 mg/kg at 12- to 24-hour intervals if age <48 hours at time of first dose; 0.2 mg/kg 2 times if 2-7 days old at time of first dose; or 0.25 mg/kg 2 times if over 7 days at time of first dose; discontinue if significant adverse effects occur. Dose should be withheld if patient has anuria or oliguria.
Analgesia:
Children: Oral: Initial: 1-2 mg/kg/day in 2-4 divided doses; maximum: 4 mg/kg/day; not to exceed 150-200 mg/day
Adults: Oral, rectal: 25-50 mg/dose 2-3 times/day; maximum dose: 200 mg/day; extended release capsule should be given on a 1-2 times/day schedule

Mechanism of Action Inhibits prostaglandin synthesis by decreasing the activity of the enzyme, cyclo-oxygenase, which results in decreased formation of prostaglandin precursors

Local Anesthetic/Vasoconstrictor Precautions No information available to require special precautions

Effects on Dental Treatment No effects or complications reported
Other Adverse Effects
>10%:
Central nervous system: Dizziness
Dermatologic: Rash
Gastrointestinal: Nausea, epigastric pain, abdominal pain, anorexia, GI bleeding, ulcers, perforation, abdominal cramps, heartburn, indigestion
1% to 10%:
Central nervous system: Headache, nervousness
Dermatologic: Itching
Endocrine & metabolic: Fluid retention
Gastrointestinal: Vomiting
Otic: Tinnitus
<1%:
Cardiovascular: Hypertension, congestive heart failure, arrhythmias, tachycardia
Central nervous system: Somnolence, fatigue, depression, confusion, hallucinations
Dermatologic: Urticaria, erythema multiforme, toxic epidermal necrolysis, Stevens-Johnson syndrome, angioedema
Endocrine & metabolic: Hyperkalemia, dilutional hyponatremia (I.V.), oliguria, hypoglycemia (I.V.), hot flashes, polydipsia
Gastrointestinal: Gastritis
Genitourinary: Cystitis
Hematologic: Hemolytic anemia, bone marrow suppression, agranulocytosis, thrombocytopenia, inhibition of platelet aggregation, anemia, leukopenia
Hepatic: Hepatitis
Neuromuscular & skeletal: Peripheral neuropathy
Ocular: Corneal opacities, blurred vision, conjunctivitis, dry eyes, toxic amblyopia
Otic: Decreased hearing
Renal: Polyuria, renal failure
Respiratory: Dyspnea, allergic rhinitis, epistaxis
Miscellaneous: Aseptic meningitis, hypersensitivity reactions

Drug Interactions
Decreased effect: May decrease antihypertensive effects of beta-blockers, hydralazine and captopril
Increased toxicity: May increase serum potassium with potassium-sparing diuretics; probenecid may increase indomethacin serum concentrations; other NSAIDs may increase GI adverse effects; may increase nephrotoxicity of cyclosporin
Indomethacin may increase serum concentrations of digoxin, methotrexate, lithium, and aminoglycosides (reported with I.V. use in neonates)

Drug Uptake
Onset of action: Within 30 minutes
Duration: 4-6 hours
Absorption: Prompt and extensive
Serum half-life: 4.5 hours
Time to peak serum concentration: Oral: Within 3-4 hours

Pregnancy Risk Factor B (D if used longer than 48 hours or after 34-week gestation)

Generic Available Yes (capsule and oral suspension)

Infants Feverall™ [OTC] see Acetaminophen on page 20

Infants' Silapap® [OTC] see Acetaminophen on page 20

Infectious Disease - Antimicrobial Activity Against Selected Organisms see page 1155

InFeD™ Injection see Iron Dextran Complex on page 519

Inflamase® see Prednisolone on page 788

Inflamase® Mild see Prednisolone on page 788

Influenza Virus Vaccine (in floo EN za VYE rus vak SEEN)
Brand Names Fluogen®; Fluzone®
Canadian/Mexican Brand Names Fluviral® (Canada)
Therapeutic Category Vaccine, Inactivated Virus
Use Provide active immunity to influenza virus strains contained in the vaccine; for high risk persons, previous year vaccines should not be to prevent present year influenza

Those at risk for influenza injection:
Persons ≥65 years of age
Institutionalized patients
(Continued)

Influenza Virus Vaccine *(Continued)*

Persons of any age with chronic disorders of pulmonary and/or cardiovascular system

Persons who have required medical follow-up following hospitalization for other chronic diseases such as diabetes, renal disease, immunodepressive disorders, etc

Travelers, especially those at·risk (above)

Usual Dosage Adults: I.M.: 0.5 mL each year of appropriate vaccine for the year, one dose is all that is necessary; administer in late fall to allow maximum titers to develop by peak epidemic periods usually occurring in early December

Local Anesthetic/Vasoconstrictor Precautions No information available to require special precautions

Effects on Dental Treatment No effects or complications reported

Other Adverse Effects

1% to 10%:

Central nervous system: Fever, malaise

Local: Tenderness, redness, or induration at the site of injection

<1%:

Central nervous system: Guillain-Barré syndrome

Dermatologic: Urticaria, angioedema

Neuromuscular & skeletal: Myalgia

Respiratory: Asthma

Miscellaneous: Anaphylactoid reactions (most likely to residual egg protein), allergic reactions

Drug Interactions

Decreased effect with immunosuppressive agents; do not administer within 7 days after administration of diphtheria and tetanus toxoids and pertussis vaccine adsorbed (DTP)

Increased effect/toxicity of theophylline and warfarin

Pregnancy Risk Factor C

Generic Available No

Infumorph™ Injection *see Morphine Sulfate on page 648*

INH™ *see Isoniazid on page 522*

Inhalant, crushable glass perles: 0.18 mL, 0.3 mL Amyl Nitrite *(AM il NYE trite)*

Therapeutic Category Vasodilator, Coronary

Use Coronary vasodilator in angina pectoris; adjunct in treatment of cyanide poisoning; used to produce changes in the intensity of heart murmurs

Usual Dosage Adults: 1-6 inhalations from one capsule are usually sufficient to produce the desired effect

Local Anesthetic/Vasoconstrictor Precautions No information available to require special precautions

Effects on Dental Treatment No effects or complications reported

Other Adverse Effects

1% to 10%:

Cardiovascular: Postural hypotension, cutaneous flushing of head, neck, and clavicular area

Central nervous system: Headache

<1%:

Dermatologic: Skin rash

Hematologic: Hemolytic anemia

Drug Interactions Increased toxicity: Alcohol

Drug Uptake

Onset of action: Angina relieved within 30 seconds

Duration: 3-15 minutes

Pregnancy Risk Factor X

Generic Available Yes

Inocor® *see Amrinone on page 76*

Insect Sting Kit *(IN sekt sting kit)*

Brand Names Ana-Kit®

Therapeutic Category Antidote, Insect Sting

Use Anaphylaxis emergency treatment of insect bites or stings by the sensitive patient that may occur within minutes of insect sting or exposure to an allergic substance

Local Anesthetic/Vasoconstrictor Precautions No information available to require special precautions

Effects on Dental Treatment No effects or complications reported

Generic Available No

Comments Not intended for I.V. use (I.M. or S.C. only)

Insta-Char® [OTC] *see Charcoal on page 206*

Insta-Glucose® [OTC] *see Glucose on page 444*

Insulina (Mexico) *see Insulin Preparations on this page*

Insulin Preparations (IN su lin prep a RAY shuns)

Related Information
Endocrine Disorders & Pregnancy *on page 1021*

Brand Names Humalog®; Humulin® 50/50; Humulin® 70/30; Humulin® L; Humulin® N; Humulin® R; Humulin® U; Lente® Iletin® I; Lente® Iletin® II; Lente® Insulin; Lente® L; Novolin® 70/30; Novolin® L; Novolin® N; Novolin® R; NPH Iletin® I; NPH Insulin; NPH-N; Pork NPH Iletin® II; Pork Regular Iletin® II; Regular (Concentrated) Iletin® II U-500; Regular Iletin® I; Regular Insulin; Regular Purified Pork Insulin; Velosulin® Human

Canadian/Mexican Brand Names Insulina Lenta® (Mexico); Insulina NPH® (Mexico); Insulina Regular® (Mexico)

Therapeutic Category Antidiabetic Agent

Synonyms Insulina (Mexico)

Use Treatment of insulin-dependent diabetes mellitus, also noninsulin-dependent diabetes mellitus unresponsive to treatment with diet and/or oral hypoglycemics; to assure proper utilization of glucose and reduce glucosuria in nondiabetic patients receiving parenteral nutrition whose glucosuria cannot be adequately controlled with infusion rate adjustments or those who require assistance in achieving optimal caloric intakes; hyperkalemia (use with glucose to shift potassium into cells to lower serum potassium levels)

Usual Dosage Dose requires continuous medical supervision; may administer I.V. (regular), I.M., S.C.

Diabetes mellitus:
  Children and Adults: 0.5-1 unit/kg/day in divided doses
  Adolescents (growth spurts): 0.8-1.2 units/kg/day in divided doses
  Adjust dose to maintain premeal and bedtime blood glucose of 80-140 mg/dL (children <5 years: 100-200 mg/dL)

Hyperkalemia: Give calcium gluconate and $NaHCO_3$ first then 50% dextrose at 0.5-1 mL/kg and insulin 1 unit for every 4-5 g dextrose given

Diabetic ketoacidosis: Children and Adults: I.V. loading dose: 0.1 unit/kg, then maintenance continuous infusion: 0.1 unit/kg/hour (range: 0.05-0.2 units/kg/hour depending upon the rate of decrease of serum glucose - too rapid decrease of serum glucose may lead to cerebral edema).
  Optimum rate of decrease (serum glucose): 80-100 mg/dL/hour

  Note: Newly diagnosed patients with IDDM presenting in DKA and patients with blood sugars <800 mg/dL may be relatively "sensitive" to insulin and should receive loading and initial maintenance doses approximately $1/2$ of those indicated above.

Mechanism of Action Replacement therapy for persons unable to produce the hormone naturally or in insufficient amounts to maintain glycemic control

Drug Interactions With Insulin Injection

Decrease Hypoglycemic Effect of Insulin	Increase Hypoglycemic Effect of Insulin
Contraceptives, oral	Alcohol
Corticosteroids	Alpha blockers
Dextrothyroxine	Anabolic steroids
Diltiazem	Beta-blockers*
Dobutamine	Clofibrate
Epinephrine	Fenfluramine
Smoking	Guanethidine
Thiazide diuretics	MAO inhibitors
Thyroid hormone	Pentamidine
Niacin	Phenylbutazone
	Salicylates
	Sulfinpyrazone
	Tetracyclines

*Nonselective beta-blockers may delay recovery from hypoglycemic episodes and mask signs/symptoms of hypoglycemia. Cardioselective agents may be alternatives.

(Continued)

Insulin Preparations (Continued)

Local Anesthetic/Vasoconstrictor Precautions No information available to require special precautions

Effects on Dental Treatment Insulin-dependent diabetics (juvenile onset, type I) should be appointed for dental treatment in the morning in order to minimize chance of stress-induced hypoglycemia

Other Adverse Effects 1% to 10%:
Cardiovascular: Palpitation, tachycardia, pallor
Central nervous system: Fatigue, mental confusion, loss of consciousness, headache, hypothermia
Dermatologic: Urticaria
Endocrine & metabolic: Hypoglycemia
Gastrointestinal: Hunger, nausea, numbness of mouth
Local: Itching, redness, swelling, stinging, or warmth at injection site, atrophy or hypertrophy of S.C. fat tissue
Neuromuscular & skeletal: Muscle weakness, tremor, paresthesia
Ocular: Transient presbyopia, blurred vision
Miscellaneous: Perspiration, anaphylaxis

Drug Interactions See table.

Drug Uptake
Onset and duration of hypoglycemic effects depend upon preparation administered. See table.

Pharmacokinetics/Pharmacodynamics: Onset and Duration of Hypoglycemic Effects Depend Upon Preparation Administered

	Onset (h)	Peak (h)	Duration (h)
Insulin, regular (Novolin® R)	0.5–1	2-3	5–7
Prompt insulin zinc suspension (Semilente®)	0.5–1	4–7	18–24
Insulin zinc suspension (NPH) (Novolin® N)	1–1.5	4–12	18–24
Isophane insulin suspension (Lente®)	1–2.5	8–12	18–24
Isophane insulin suspension and regular insulin injection (Novolin® 70/30)	0.5	4–8	24
Prompt zinc insulin suspension (PZI)	4-8	14-24	36
Extended insulin zinc suspension (Ultralente®)	4-8	16–18	>36

Onset and duration: Biosynthetic NPH human insulin shows a more rapid onset and shorter duration of action than corresponding porcine insulins; human insulin and purified porcine regular insulin are similarly efficacious following S.C. administration. The duration of action of highly purified porcine insulins is shorter than that of conventional insulin equivalents. Duration depends on type of preparation and route of administration as well as patient related variables. In general, the larger the dose of insulin, the longer the duration of activity.

Absorption: Biosynthetic regular human insulin is absorbed from the S.C. injection site more rapidly than insulins of animal origin (60-90 minutes peak vs 120-150 minutes peak respectively) and lowers the initial blood glucose much faster. Human Ultralente® insulin is absorbed about twice as quickly as its bovine equivalent, and bioavailability is also improved. Human Lente® insulin preparations are also absorbed more quickly than their animal equivalents.

Pregnancy Risk Factor B

Generic Available Yes

Intal® *see* Cromolyn Sodium *on page 264*

Interferon Alfa-2a (in ter FEER on AL fa too aye)

Related Information
Systemic Viral Diseases *on page 1047*

Brand Names Roferon-A®

Therapeutic Category Antineoplastic Agent, Miscellaneous; Interferon

Use FDA approved: Patients >18 years of age: Hairy cell leukemia, AIDS related Kaposi's sarcoma; multiple **unlabeled uses**; indications and dosage regimens are specific for a particular brand of interferon

Usual Dosage Refer to individual protocols
Children: Hemangiomas of infancy, pulmonary hemangiomatosis: S.C.: 1-3 million units/m²/day once daily

Adults >18 years: I.M., S.C.:
Hairy cell leukemia:
Induction: 3 million units/day for 16-24 weeks.
Maintenance: 3 million units 3 times/week (may be treated for up to 20 consecutive weeks)
AIDS-related Kaposi's sarcoma:
Induction: 36 million units/day for 10-12 weeks
Maintenance: 36 million units 3 times/week (may begin with dose escalation from 3-9-18 million units each day over 3 consecutive days followed by 36 million units/day for the remainder of the 10-12 weeks of induction)
If severe adverse reactions occur, modify dosage (50% reduction) or temporarily discontinue therapy until adverse reactions abate

Local Anesthetic/Vasoconstrictor Precautions No information available to require special precautions

Effects on Dental Treatment >10% of patients experience significant dry mouth and metallic taste

Other Adverse Effects
>10%:
Central nervous system: Dizziness, fatigue, malaise, fever (usually within 4-6 hours), chills
Dermatologic: Skin rash
Gastrointestinal: Nausea, vomiting, diarrhea, abdominal cramps, weight loss
Hematologic: Mildly myelosuppressive and well tolerated if used without adjunct antineoplastic agents; thrombocytosis has been reported, leukopenia (mainly neutropenia), anemia, thrombocytopenia, decreased hemoglobin, hematocrit, platelets
Neuromuscular & skeletal: Rigors, arthralgia
Miscellaneous: Flu-like syndrome, sweating
1% to 10%:
Central nervous system: Headache, delirium, somnolence, neurotoxicity
Dermatologic: alopecia, dry skin
Gastrointestinal: Anorexia, stomatitis
Hepatic: Hepatotoxicity
Neuromuscular & skeletal: Peripheral neuropathy, leg cramps
Ocular: Blurred vision
<1%:
Cardiovascular: Tachycardia, arrhythmias, chest pain, hypotension, SVT, edema
Central nervous system: Confusion, sensory neuropathy, psychiatric effects, EEG abnormalities, depression
Dermatologic: Partial alopecia
Endocrine & metabolic: Hypothyroidism, hyperuricemia
Gastrointestinal: Change in taste
Hepatic: Elevated hepatic transaminase
Local: Sensitivity to injection
Neuromuscular & skeletal: Myalgia
Ocular: Visual disturbances
Renal: Proteinuria, elevated Cr, elevated BUN
Respiratory: Coughing, chest pain, dyspnea, nasal congestion
Miscellaneous: Neutralizing antibodies; usually patient can build up a tolerance to side effects

Drug Interactions
Increased effect:
Cimetidine: May augment the antitumor effects of interferon in melanoma
Theophylline: Clearance has been reported to be decreased in hepatitis patients receiving interferon
Increased toxicity: Vinblastine: Enhances interferon toxicity in several patients; increased incidence of paresthesia has also been noted

Drug Uptake
Absorption: Filtered and absorbed at the renal tubule
Serum half-life: Elimination:
I.M., I.V.: 2 hours after administration
S.C.: 3 hours
Time to peak serum concentration: I.M., S.C.: ~6-8 hours

Pregnancy Risk Factor C
Generic Available No

Interferon Alfa-2b (in ter FEER on AL fa too bee)
Related Information
Systemic Viral Diseases on page 1047
Brand Names Intron® A
(Continued)

Interferon Alfa-2b (Continued)

Therapeutic Category Antineoplastic Agent, Miscellaneous; Biological Response Modulator; Interferon

Use FDA approved: Patients >18 years of age: Hairy cell leukemia, condylomata acuminata, AIDS-related Kaposi's sarcoma, chronic hepatitis non-A, non-B(C), chronic hepatitis B; indications and dosage regimens are specific for a particular brand of interferon

Usual Dosage Adults (**refer to individual protocols**):

Hairy cell leukemia: I.M., S.C.: 2 million units/m^2 3 times/week for 2 to ≥6 months of therapy

AIDS-related Kaposi's sarcoma: I.M., S.C. (use 50 million unit vial): 30 million units/m^2 3 times/week

Condylomata acuminata: Intralesionally (use 10 million unit vial): 1 million units/lesion 3 times/week for 4-8 weeks; not to exceed 5 million units per treatment (maximum: 5 lesions at one time)

Chronic hepatitis C (non-A/non-B): I.M., S.C.: 3 million units 3 times/week for approximately a 6-month course

Chronic hepatitis B: I.M., S.C.: 5 million units/day or 10 million units 3 times/week for 16 weeks; if severe adverse reactions occur, reduce dosage 50% or temporarily discontinue therapy until adverse reactions abate; when platelet/granulocyte count returns to normal, reinstitute therapy

Mechanism of Action Alpha interferons are a family of proteins, produced by nucleated cells, that have antiviral, antiproliferative, and immune-regulating activity. There are 16 known subtypes of alpha interferons. Interferons interact with cells through high affinity cell surface receptors. Following activation, multiple effects can be detected including induction of gene transcription. Inhibits cellular growth, alters the state of cellular differentiation, interferes with oncogene expression, alters cell surface antigen expression, increases phagocytic activity of macrophages, and augments cytotoxicity of lymphocytes for target cells

Local Anesthetic/Vasoconstrictor Precautions No information available to require special precautions

Effects on Dental Treatment >10% of patients experience dry mouth and metallic taste

Other Adverse Effects

>10%:

Central nervous system: Dizziness, fatigue, malaise, fever (usually within 4-6 hours)

Dermatologic: Skin rash

Gastrointestinal: Nausea, vomiting, diarrhea, abdominal cramps, weight loss, anorexia

Hematologic: Mildly myelosuppressive and well tolerated if used without adjunct antineoplastic agents; thrombocytosis has been reported, leukopenia (mainly neutropenia), anemia, thrombocytopenia, decreased hemoglobin, hematocrit, platelets

Neuromuscular & skeletal: Rigors, arthralgia

Miscellaneous: Flu-like syndrome, sweating

1% to 10%:

Central nervous system: Neurotoxicity

Dermatologic: Dry skin, alopecia

Gastrointestinal: Stomatitis

Hepatic: Hepatotoxicity

Neuromuscular & skeletal: Peripheral neuropathy, leg cramps

Ocular: Blurred vision

<1%:

Cardiovascular: Cardiotoxicity, tachycardia, arrhythmias, hypotension, SVT, arrhythmias, chest pain, edema

Central nervous system: EEG abnormalities, confusion, sensory neuropathy, headache, psychiatric effects, delirium, somnolence

Dermatologic: Partial alopecia

Endocrine & metabolic: Hypothyroidism, hyperuricemia

Gastrointestinal: Change in taste

Hepatic: Elevated hepatic transaminase, elevated ALT and AST

Local: Sensitivity to injection

Neuromuscular & skeletal: Myalgia

Ocular: Visual disturbances

Renal: Proteinuria, elevated creatinine, elevated BUN

Respiratory: Coughing, dyspnea, nasal congestion

Miscellaneous: Neutralizing antibodies; usually patient can build up a tolerance to side effects

Drug Interactions
Increased effect: Cimetidine: May augment the antitumor effects of interferon in melanoma

Increased toxicity:

Theophylline: Clearance has been reported to be decreased in hepatitis patients receiving interferon

Vinblastine: Enhances interferon toxicity in several patients; increased incidence of paresthesia has also been noted

Drug Uptake
Absorption: Filtered and absorbed at the renal tubule

Serum half-life: Elimination:

I.M., I.V.: 2 hours

S.C.: 3 hours

Time to peak serum concentration: I.M., S.C.: ~6-8 hours

Pregnancy Risk Factor C

Generic Available No

Interferon Alfa-n3 (in ter FEER on AL fa en three)

Related Information
Systemic Viral Diseases *on page 1047*

Brand Names Alferon® N

Therapeutic Category Antineoplastic Agent, Miscellaneous; Interferon

Use FDA approved: Patients ≥18 years of age: Condylomata acuminata, intralesional treatment of refractory or recurring genital or venereal warts; useful in patients who do not respond or are not candidates for usual treatments; indications and dosage regimens are specific for a particular brand of interferon

Usual Dosage Adults: Inject 250,000 units (0.05 mL) in each wart twice weekly for a maximum of 8 weeks; therapy should not be repeated for at least 3 months after the initial 8-week course of therapy

Mechanism of Action Interferons interact with cells through high affinity cell surface receptors. Following activation, multiple effects can be detected including induction of gene transcription. Inhibits cellular growth, alters the state of cellular differentiation, interferes with oncogene expression, alters cell surface antigen expression, increases phagocytic activity of macrophages, and augments cytotoxicity of lymphocytes for target cells

Local Anesthetic/Vasoconstrictor Precautions No information available to require special precautions

Effects on Dental Treatment >10% of patients experience dry mouth and metallic taste

Other Adverse Effects
>10%:

Central nervous system: Fatigue, malaise, fever (usually within 4-6 hours), chills, dizziness

Dermatologic: Skin rash

Gastrointestinal: Nausea, vomiting, diarrhea, abdominal cramps, weight loss, anorexia

Hematologic: Mildly myelosuppressive and well tolerated if used without adjunct antineoplastic agents; thrombocytosis has been reported, leukopenia (mainly neutropenia), anemia, thrombocytopenia, decreased hemoglobin, hematocrit, platelets

Neuromuscular & skeletal: Arthralgia, rigors

Miscellaneous: Flu-like syndrome, sweating

1% to 10%:

Central nervous system: Headache, delirium, somnolence, neurotoxicity

Dermatologic: Alopecia, dry skin

Gastrointestinal: Stomatitis

Hepatic: Hepatotoxicity

Neuromuscular & skeletal: Peripheral neuropathy, leg cramps

Ocular: Blurred vision

<1%:

Cardiovascular: Tachycardia, arrhythmias, chest pain, hypotension, SVT, edema

Central nervous system: EEG abnormalities, confusion, sensory neuropathy, confusion, psychiatric effects, depression

Dermatologic: Rash, partial alopecia, local sensitivity to injection

Endocrine & metabolic: Hypothyroidism, hyperuricemia

Gastrointestinal: Change in taste

Hepatic: Elevated hepatic transaminase, elevated ALT and AST

Neuromuscular & skeletal: Myalgia

Ocular: Visual disturbances

Renal: Proteinuria, elevated Cr, elevated BUN

Respiratory: Coughing, chest pain, dyspnea, cough, nasal congestion

(Continued)

Interferon Alfa-n3 (Continued)

Miscellaneous: Neutralizing antibodies, usually patient can build up a tolerance to side effects

Drug Interactions
Increased effect: Cimetidine: May augment the antitumor effects of interferon in melanoma
Increased toxicity:
Vinblastine: Enhances interferon toxicity in several patients; increased incidence of paresthesia has also been noted
Theophylline: Clearance has been reported to be decreased in hepatitis patients receiving interferon

Pregnancy Risk Factor C
Generic Available No

Interferon Beta-1a (in ter FEER on BAY ta won aye)

Brand Names Avonex®
Therapeutic Category Biological Response Modulator
Use Treatment of relapsing forms of multiple sclerosis (MS); to slow the accumulation of physical disability and decrease the frequency of clinical exacerbations
Usual Dosage Adults >18 years: I.M.: 30 mcg once weekly
Mechanism of Action Interferon beta differs from naturally occurring human protein by a single amino acid substitution and the lack of carbohydrate side chains; alters the expression and response to surface antigens and can enhance immune cell activities. Properties of interferon beta that modify biologic responses are mediated by cell surface receptor interactions; mechanism in the treatment of MS is unknown.
Local Anesthetic/Vasoconstrictor Precautions No information available to require special precautions
Effects on Dental Treatment No effects or complications reported
Other Adverse Effects 1% to 10%:
Cardiovascular: CHF (rare), tachycardia, syncope
Central nervous system: Headache, lethargy, depression, emotional lability, anxiety, suicidal ideations, somnolence, agitation, confusion
Dermatologic: Alopecia (rare)
Endocrine & metabolic: Hypocalcemia
Gastrointestinal: Nausea, anorexia, vomiting, diarrhea, chronic weight loss
Hematologic: Leukopenia, thrombocytopenia, anemia (frequent, dose-related, but not usually severe)
Hepatic: Elevated liver enzymes (mild, transient)
Local: Pain/redness at injection site (80%)
Neuromuscular & skeletal: Weakness
Ocular: Retinal toxicity/visual changes
Renal: Elevated BUN and S_{cr}
Miscellaneous: Flu-like syndrome (fever, nausea, malaise, myalgia) occurs in most patients, but is usually controlled by acetaminophen or NSAIDs; dose related abortifacient activity was reported in rhesus monkeys
Warnings/Precautions Interferon beta-1a should be used with caution in patients with a history of depression, seizures, or cardiac disease; because its use has not been evaluated during lactation, its use in breast-feeding mothers may not be safe and should be warned against
Drug Interactions Decreases clearance of zidovudine thus increasing zidovudine toxicity
Drug Uptake Limited data due to small doses used
Serum half-life: 10 hours
Time to peak serum concentration: 3-15 hours
Pregnancy Risk Factor C
Generic Available No

Interferon Beta-1b (in ter FEER on BAY ta won bee)

Brand Names Betaseron®
Therapeutic Category Interferon
Use Reduces the frequency of clinical exacerbations in ambulatory patients with relapsing-remitting multiple sclerosis (MS)
Usual Dosage S.C.:
Children <18 years: Not recommended
Adults >18 years: 0.25 mg (8 million units) every other day
Mechanism of Action Interferon beta-1b differs from naturally occurring human protein by a single amino acid substitution and the lack of carbohydrate side chains; alters the expression and response to surface antigens and can enhance immune cell activities. Properties of interferon beta-1b that modify biologic

responses are mediated by cell surface receptor interactions; mechanism in the treatment of MS is unknown.

Local Anesthetic/Vasoconstrictor Precautions No information available to require special precautions

Effects on Dental Treatment No effects or complications reported

Other Adverse Effects Due to the pivotal position of interferon in the immune system, toxicities can affect nearly every organ system. Injection site reactions, injection site necrosis, flu-like symptoms, menstrual disorders, depression (with suicidal ideations), somnolence, palpitations, peripheral vascular disorders, hypertension, blood dyscrasias, dyspnea, laryngitis, cystitis, gastrointestinal complaints.

Drug Interactions No data reported

Pregnancy Risk Factor C

Generic Available No

Interferon Gamma-1b (in ter FEER on GAM ah won bee)

Brand Names Actimmune®

Therapeutic Category Biological Response Modulator; Interferon

Use Reduce the frequency and severity of serious infections associated with chronic granulomatous disease

Local Anesthetic/Vasoconstrictor Precautions No information available to require special precautions

Effects on Dental Treatment No effects or complications reported

Other Adverse Effects

>10%:
  Central nervous system: Fever, headache, chills, fatigue
  Dermatologic: Rash
  Gastrointestinal: Diarrhea, vomiting, nausea

1% to 10%:
  Central nervous system: Depression
  Gastrointestinal: Abdominal pain, weight loss, anorexia
  Neuromuscular & skeletal: Arthralgia, back pain, myalgia

Pregnancy Risk Factor C

Generic Available No

Comments More heat- and acid-labile than alfa interferons

Interleukin-2 *see* Aldesleukin *on page 37*

Intralipid® *see* Fat Emulsion *on page 393*

Intravenous Fat Emulsion *see* Fat Emulsion *on page 393*

Intron® A *see* Interferon Alfa-2b *on page 511*

Inversine® *see* Mecamylamine *on page 584*

Invirase® *see* Saquinavir *on page 856*

Iobid DM® *see* Guaifenesin and Dextromethorphan *on page 453*

Iodex® Regular *see* Povidone-Iodine *on page 783*

Iodinated Glycerol (EYE oh di nay ted GLI ser ole)

Brand Names Iophen®; Organidin®; Par Glycerol®; R-Gen®

Therapeutic Category Expectorant

Use Mucolytic expectorant in adjunctive treatment of bronchitis, bronchial asthma, pulmonary emphysema, cystic fibrosis, or chronic sinusitis

Usual Dosage Oral:
  Children: Up to 30 mg 4 times/day
  Adults: 60 mg 4 times/day

Mechanism of Action Increases respiratory tract secretions by decreasing surface tension and thereby decreases the viscosity of mucus, which aids in removal of the mucus

Local Anesthetic/Vasoconstrictor Precautions No information available to require special precautions

Effects on Dental Treatment No effects or complications reported

Other Adverse Effects

1% to 10%: Gastrointestinal: Diarrhea, nausea, vomiting
<1%:
  Central nervous system: Headache
  Dermatologic: Acne, dermatitis
  Endocrine & metabolic: Acute parotitis, thyroid gland enlargement
  Gastrointestinal: GI irritation
  Ocular: Swelling of the eyelids
  Respiratory: Pulmonary edema
  Miscellaneous: Hypersensitivity

Drug Interactions Increased toxicity: Disulfiram, metronidazole, procarbazine, MAO inhibitors, CNS depressants, lithium

(Continued)

515

Iodinated Glycerol *(Continued)*

Drug Uptake Absorption: From GI tract

Pregnancy Risk Factor X

Dosage Forms Organically bound iodine in brackets

Elixir: 60 mg/5 mL [30 mg/5 mL] (120 mL, 480 mL)

Solution: 50 mg/mL [25 mg/mL] (30 mL)

Tablet: 30 mg [15 mg]

Iodine (EYE oh dyne)

Therapeutic Category Topical Skin Product

Use Used topically as an antiseptic in the management of minor, superficial skin wounds and has been used to disinfect the skin preoperatively

Local Anesthetic/Vasoconstrictor Precautions No information available to require special precautions

Effects on Dental Treatment No effects or complications reported

Other Adverse Effects 1% to 10%:

Central nervous system: Fever, headache

Dermatologic: Skin rash, angioedema, urticaria, acne

Gastrointestinal: Metallic taste, diarrhea

Endocrine & metabolic: Hypothyroidism

Hematologic: Eosinophilia, hemorrhage (mucosal)

Neuromuscular & skeletal: Arthralgia

Ocular: Swelling of eyelids

Respiratory: Pulmonary edema

Miscellaneous: Lymph node enlargement

Pregnancy Risk Factor D

Generic Available Yes

Comments Sodium thiosulfate inactivates iodine and is an effective chemical antidote for codeine poisoning; solutions of sodium thiosulfate may be used to remove iodine stains from skin and clothing

Iodine *see* Trace Metals *on page 948*

Iodochlorhydroxyquin and Hydrocortisone *see* Clioquinol and Hydrocortisone *on page 245*

Iodopen® *see* Trace Metals *on page 948*

Iodoquinol (eye oh doe KWIN ole)

Brand Names Yodoxin®

Canadian/Mexican Brand Names Diodoquin® (Canada)

Therapeutic Category Amebicide

Use Treatment of acute and chronic intestinal amebiasis; asymptomatic cyst passers; *Blastocystis hominis* infections; ineffective for amebic hepatitis or hepatic abscess

Usual Dosage Oral:

Children: 30-40 mg/kg/day (maximum: 650 mg/dose) in 3 divided doses for 20 days; not to exceed 1.95 g/day

Adults: 650 mg 3 times/day after meals for 20 days; not to exceed 2 g/day

Mechanism of Action Contact amebicide that works in the lumen of the intestine by an unknown mechanism

Local Anesthetic/Vasoconstrictor Precautions No information available to require special precautions

Effects on Dental Treatment No effects or complications reported

Other Adverse Effects

>10%: Gastrointestinal: Diarrhea, nausea, vomiting, stomach pain

1% to 10%:

Central nervous system: Fever, chills, agitation, retrograde amnesia, headache

Dermatologic: Skin rash, urticaria

Endocrine & metabolic: Thyroid gland enlargement

Gastrointestinal: Itching of rectal area

Neuromuscular & skeletal: Peripheral neuropathy, weakness

Ocular: Optic neuritis, optic atrophy, visual impairment

Drug Interactions No data reported

Drug Uptake

Absorption: Oral: Poor and irregular

Pregnancy Risk Factor C

Generic Available No

Iodoquinol and Hydrocortisone
(eye oh doe KWIN ole & hye droe KOR ti sone)

Brand Names Vytone® Topical

Therapeutic Category Antifungal Agent, Topical; Corticosteroid, Topical (Low Potency)

Use Treatment of eczema; infectious dermatitis; chronic eczematoid otitis externa; mycotic dermatoses

Local Anesthetic/Vasoconstrictor Precautions No information available to require special precautions

Effects on Dental Treatment No effects or complications reported

Pregnancy Risk Factor C

Generic Available No

Iofed® *see* Brompheniramine and Pseudoephedrine *on page 144*

Iofed® PD *see* Brompheniramine and Pseudoephedrine *on page 144*

Ionamin® *see* Phentermine *on page 750*

Iophen® *see* Iodinated Glycerol *on page 515*

Iopidine® *see* Apraclonidine *on page 83*

I-Paracaine® *see* Proparacaine *on page 808*

Ipecac Syrup (IP e kak SIR up)

Therapeutic Category Antidote, Emetic

Use Treatment of acute oral drug overdosage and certain poisonings

Usual Dosage Oral:

Children:

6-12 months: 5-10 mL followed by 10-20 mL/kg of water; repeat dose one time if vomiting does not occur within 20 minutes

1-12 years: 15 mL followed by 10-20 mL/kg of water; repeat dose one time if vomiting does not occur within 20 minutes

If emesis does not occur within 30 minutes after second dose, ipecac must be removed from stomach by gastric lavage

Adults: 15-30 mL followed by 200-300 mL of water; repeat dose one time if vomiting does not occur within 20 minutes

Mechanism of Action Irritates the gastric mucosa and stimulates the medullary chemoreceptor trigger zone to induce vomiting

Local Anesthetic/Vasoconstrictor Precautions No information available to require special precautions

Effects on Dental Treatment No effects or complications reported

Other Adverse Effects 1% to 10%:

Cardiovascular: Cardiotoxicity

Central nervous system: Lethargy

Gastrointestinal: Protracted vomiting, diarrhea

Ocular: Myopathy

Drug Uptake

Onset of action: Within 15-30 minutes

Duration: 20-25 minutes; can last longer, 60 minutes in some cases

Absorption: Significant amounts, mainly when it does not produce emesis

Pregnancy Risk Factor C

Generic Available Yes

I-Pentolate® *see* Cyclopentolate *on page 269*

I-Phrine® Ophthalmic Solution *see* Phenylephrine *on page 752*

IPOL™ *see* Poliovirus Vaccine, Inactivated *on page 770*

Ipratropium (i pra TROE pee um)

Related Information

Ipratropium and Albuterol *on next page*
Respiratory Diseases *on page 1018*

Brand Names Atrovent®

Therapeutic Category Anticholinergic Agent; Bronchodilator

Use Anticholinergic bronchodilator in bronchospasm associated with COPD, bronchitis, and emphysema

Usual Dosage

Children:

<2 years: Nebulization: 250 mcg 3 times/day

3-14 years: Metered dose inhaler: 1-2 inhalations 3 times/day, up to 6 inhalations/24 hours

Children >12 years and Adults: Nebulization: 500 mcg (1 unit-dose vial) administered 3-4 times/day by oral nebulization, with doses 6-8 hours apart

Children >14 years and Adults: Metered dose inhaler: 2 inhalations 4 times/day every 4-6 hours up to 12 inhalations in 24 hours

(Continued)

517

Ipratropium (Continued)

Mechanism of Action Blocks the action of acetylcholine at parasympathetic sites in bronchial smooth muscle causing bronchodilation

Local Anesthetic/Vasoconstrictor Precautions No information available to require special precautions

Effects on Dental Treatment >10% of patients experience dry mouth

Other Adverse Effects Note: Ipratropium is poorly absorbed from the lung, so systemic effects are rare

>10%:
Central nervous system: Nervousness, dizziness, fatigue, headache
Gastrointestinal: Nausea, stomach upset
Respiratory: Cough

1% to 10%:
Cardiovascular: Palpitations, hypotension
Central nervous system: Insomnia
Genitourinary: Urinary retention
Neuromuscular & skeletal: Trembling
Ocular: Blurred vision
Respiratory: Nasal congestion

<1%:
Dermatologic: Skin rash, urticaria
Gastrointestinal: Stomatitis

Drug Interactions
Increased effect with albuterol
Increased toxicity with anticholinergics or drugs with anticholinergic properties, dronabinol

Drug Uptake
Onset of bronchodilation: 1-3 minutes after administration
Duration: Up to 4-6 hours
Absorption: Not readily absorbed into the systemic circulation from the surface of the lung or from the GI tract

Pregnancy Risk Factor B
Generic Available Yes

Ipratropium and Albuterol (i pra TROE pee um & al BYOO ter ole)

Brand Names Combivent®
Therapeutic Category Bronchodilator
Use Treatment of chronic obstructive pulmonary disease (COPD) in those patients that are currently on a regular bronchodilator who continue to have bronchospasms and require a second bronchodilator
Usual Dosage Adults: 2 inhalations 4 times/day, maximum of 12 inhalations/24 hours
Mechanism of Action See individual agents
Local Anesthetic/Vasoconstrictor Precautions No information available to require special precautions
Effects on Dental Treatment >10% of patients experience dry mouth
Other Adverse Effects See individual agents
Drug Interactions See individual agents
Dosage Forms Aerosol: Ipratropium bromide 21 mcg and albuterol sulfate 120 mcg per actuation [200 doses] (14.7 g)
Generic Available No

IPV see Poliovirus Vaccine, Inactivated on page 770

Irbesartan (ir be SAR tan)

Brand Names Avapro®
Therapeutic Category Angiotensin II Antagonists
Use Treatment of hypertension alone or in combination with other antihypertensives
Usual Dosage Adults: Oral: 150 mg once daily with or without food; patients may be titrated to 300 mg once daily
Local Anesthetic/Vasoconstrictor Precautions No information available to require special precautions
Effects on Dental Treatment No effects or complications reported
Dosage Forms Tablet: 75 mg, 150 mg, 300 mg

Ircon® [OTC] see Ferrous Fumarate on page 400

Irinotecan (eye rye no TEE kan)

Brand Names Camptosar®
Therapeutic Category Antineoplastic Agent, Miscellaneous

Use Treatment of metastatic carcinoma of the colon or rectum which has recurred or progressed following 5-FU fluorouracil-based therapy

Mechanism of Action Irinotecan and its active metabolite (SN-38) bind reversibly to topoisomerase I and stabilize the cleavable complex so that religation of the cleaved DNA strand cannot occur. This results in the accumulation of cleavable complexes and single-strand DNA breaks. This interaction results in double-stranded DNA breaks and cell death consistent with S-phase cell cycle specificity.

Local Anesthetic/Vasoconstrictor Precautions No information available to require special precautions

Effects on Dental Treatment No effects or complications reported

Other Adverse Effects

>10%:

Cardiovascular: Vasodilation

Central nervous system: Insomnia, dizziness, fever (45.4%)

Dermatologic: Alopecia (60.5%), rash

Gastrointestinal: Irinotecan therapy may induce two different forms of diarrhea. Onset, symptoms, proposed mechanisms and treatment are different. Overall, 56.9% of patients treated experience abdominal pain and/or cramping during therapy. Anorexia, constipation, flatulence, stomatitis, and dyspepsia have also been reported.

Diarrhea: Dose-limiting toxicity with weekly dosing regimen

Early diarrhea (50.7% incidence) usually occurs during or within 24 hours of administration. May be accompanied by symptoms of cramping, vomiting, flushing, and diaphoresis. It is thought to be mediated by cholinergic effects which can be successfully managed with atropine (refer to Warnings/Precautions).

Late diarrhea (87.8% incidence) usually occurs >24 hours after treatment. National Cancer Institute (NCI) grade 3 or 4 diarrhea occurs in 30.6% of patients. Late diarrhea generally occurs with a median of 11 days after therapy and lasts approximately 3 days. Patients experiencing grade 3 or 4 diarrhea were noted to have symptoms a total of 7 days. Correlated with irinotecan or SN-38 levels in plasma and bile. Due to the duration, dehydration and electrolyte imbalances are significant clinical concerns. Loperamide therapy is recommended. The incidence of grade 3 or 4 late diarrhea is significantly higher in patients ≥ 65 years of age: close monitoring and prompt initiation of high-dose loperamide therapy is prudent (refer to Warnings/Precautions).

Emetic potential: Moderately high (86.2% incidence, however, only 12.5% grade 3 or 4 vomiting)

Hematologic: Myelosuppressive: Dose-limiting toxicity with 3 week dosing regimen

Grade 1-4 neutropenia occurred in 53.9% of patients. Patients who had previously received pelvic or abdominal radiation therapy were noted to have a significantly increased incidence of grade 3 or 4 neutropenia. White blood cell count nadir is 15 days after administration and is more frequent than thrombocytopenia. Recovery is usually within 24-28 days and cumulative toxicity has not been observed.

WBC: Mild to severe

Platelets: Mild

Onset (days): 10

Nadir (days): 14-16

Recovery (days): 21-28

Neuromuscular & skeletal: Weakness (75.7%)

Respiratory: Dyspnea (22%), coughing, rhinitis

Miscellaneous: Diaphoresis

1% to 10%: **Irritant chemotherapy**; thrombophlebitis has been reported

Drug Interactions Increased toxicity: Prochlorperazine: Increased incidence of akathisia

Drug Uptake Serum half-life: Terminal: Irinotecan = 10 hours; SN-38 = 10 hours

Pregnancy Risk Factor D

Dosage Forms Injection: 20 mg/mL (5 mL)

Generic Available No

Iron Dextran Complex (EYE ern DEKS tran KOM pleks)

Brand Names Dexferrum® Injection; InFeD™ Injection

Canadian/Mexican Brand Names Driken® (Mexico)

Therapeutic Category Iron Salt

Use Treatment of microcytic, hypochromic anemia resulting from iron deficiency when oral iron administration is infeasible or ineffective

(Continued)

Iron Dextran Complex *(Continued)*

Usual Dosage I.M. (Z-track method should be used for I.M. injection), I.V.:

A 0.5 mL test dose (0.25 mL in infants) should be given prior to starting iron dextran therapy; total dose should be divided into a daily schedule for I.M., total dose may be given as a single continuous infusion

Iron deficiency anemia: Dose (mL) = 0.0476 x wt (kg) x (normal hemoglobin - observed hemoglobin) + (1 mL/5 kg) to maximum of 14 mL for iron stores

Iron replacement therapy for blood loss: Replacement iron (mg) = blood loss (mL) x hematocrit

Maximum daily dose (can give total dose at one time I.V.):
Children:
5-10 kg: 50 mg iron (1 mL)
10-50 kg: 100 mg iron (2 mL)
Adults >50 kg: 100 mg iron (2 mL)

Mechanism of Action The released iron, from the plasma, eventually replenishes the depleted iron stores in the bone marrow where it is incorporated into hemoglobin

Local Anesthetic/Vasoconstrictor Precautions No information available to require special precautions

Effects on Dental Treatment No effects or complications reported

Other Adverse Effects
>10%:
Central nervous system: Chills, fever, headache
Gastrointestinal: Metallic taste, nausea, vomiting
Local: Pain at injection site, staining of skin at the site of I.M. injection
Miscellaneous: Sweating
1% to 10%:
Gastrointestinal: Diarrhea
Genitourinary: Discolored urine
<1%:
Cardiovascular: Flushing
Local: Phlebitis
Neuromuscular & skeletal: Arthralgia
Respiratory: Respiratory difficulty
Miscellaneous: Lymphadenopathy

Drug Uptake
Absorption:
I.M.: 50% to 90% is promptly absorbed, the balance is slowly absorbed over month
I.V.: Uptake of iron by the reticuloendothelial system appears to be constant at about 10-20 mg/hour

Pregnancy Risk Factor C

Generic Available Yes

Comments 2 mL of undiluted iron dextran is the maximum recommended daily dose; epinephrine should be immediately available in the event of acute hypersensitivity reaction

Ismelin® *see* Guanethidine *on page 458*

ISMO™ *see* Isosorbide Mononitrate *on page 526*

Ismotic® *see* Isosorbide *on page 524*

Isobamate *see* Carisoprodol, Aspirin, and Codeine *on page 181*

Isocaine® HCl *see* Mepivacaine *on page 595*

Isocaine® HCl 2% *see* Mepivacaine and Levonordefrin *on page 596*

Isocaine® HCl 3% *see* Mepivacaine Dental Anesthetic *on page 597*

Isocal® [OTC] *see* Enteral Nutritional Products *on page 350*

Isocarboxazid *(eye soe kar BOKS a zid)*

Brand Names Marplan®

Therapeutic Category Antidepressant, Monoamine Oxidase Inhibitor

Use Symptomatic treatment of atypical, nonendogenous or neurotic depression

Usual Dosage Adults: Oral: 10 mg 3 times/day; reduce to 10-20 mg/day in divided doses when condition improves

Mechanism of Action Thought to act by increasing endogenous concentrations of epinephrine, norepinephrine, dopamine, and serotonin through inhibition of the enzyme (monoamine oxidase) responsible for the breakdown of these neurotransmitters

Local Anesthetic/Vasoconstrictor Precautions Attempts should be made to avoid use of vasoconstrictor due to possibility of hypertensive episodes with monoamine oxidase inhibitors

Effects on Dental Treatment Orthostatic hypotension in >10% of patients; meperidine should be avoided as an analgesic due to toxic reactions with MAO inhibitors

Other Adverse Effects

>10%:

Cardiovascular: Orthostatic hypotension

Central nervous system: Drowsiness

Endocrine & metabolic: Decreased sexual ability

Neuromuscular & skeletal: Trembling, weakness

Ocular: Blurred vision

1% to 10%:

Cardiovascular: Tachycardia, peripheral edema

Central nervous system: Nervousness, chills

Gastrointestinal: Diarrhea, anorexia, dry mouth, constipation

<1%:

Central nervous system: Parkinsonian syndrome

Hematologic: Leukopenia

Hepatic: Hepatitis

Drug Interactions

Decreased effect of antihypertensives

Increased toxicity with disulfiram (possible seizures), fluoxetine (and other serotonin active agents), TCAs (cardiovascular instability), meperidine (cardiovascular instability), phenothiazines (hyperpyretic crisis), levodopa, sympathomimetics (hypertensive crisis), barbiturates, rauwolfia alkaloids (eg, reserpine), dextroamphetamine (psychoses), foods containing tyramine

Pregnancy Risk Factor C

Generic Available No

Isoclor® Expectorant *see* Guaifenesin, Pseudoephedrine, and Codeine *on page 455*

Isocom® *see* Acetaminophen, Isometheptene, and Dichloralphenazone *on page 25*

Isodine® [OTC] *see* Povidone-Iodine *on page 783*

Isoetharine (eye soe ETH a reen)

Related Information

Respiratory Diseases *on page 1018*

Brand Names Arm-a-Med® Isoetharine; Beta-2®; Bronkometer®; Bronkosol®; Dey-Lute® Isoetharine

Therapeutic Category Adrenergic Agonist Agent; Antiasthmatic; Bronchodilator

Use Bronchodilator in bronchial asthma and for reversible bronchospasm occurring with bronchitis and emphysema

Usual Dosage Treatments are usually not repeated more often than every 4 hours, except in severe cases

Nebulizer: Children: 0.01 mL/kg; minimum dose 0.1 mL; maximum dose: 0.5 mL diluted in 2-3 mL normal saline

Inhalation: Oral: Adults: 1-2 inhalations every 4 hours as needed

Mechanism of Action Relaxes bronchial smooth muscle by action on beta$_2$-receptors with very little effect on heart rate

Local Anesthetic/Vasoconstrictor Precautions Isoetharine is selective for beta-adrenergic receptors and not alpha receptors; therefore, there is no precaution in the use of vasoconstrictor

Effects on Dental Treatment Dry mouth in 1% to 10% of patients

Other Adverse Effects

1% to 10%:

Cardiovascular: Tachycardia, hypertension, pounding heartbeat

Central nervous system: Dizziness, lightheadedness, headache, nervousness, insomnia

Gastrointestinal: Dry mouth, nausea, vomiting

Neuromuscular & skeletal: Trembling, weakness

<1%: Respiratory: Paradoxical bronchospasm

Drug Interactions

Decreased effect with beta-blockers

Increased toxicity with other sympathomimetics (eg, epinephrine)

Drug Uptake Duration: 1-4 hours

Pregnancy Risk Factor C

Generic Available Yes

Isoflurophate (eye soe FLURE oh fate)

Brand Names Floropryl®

Therapeutic Category Antiglaucoma Agent; Cholinergic Agent, Ophthalmic; Ophthalmic Agent, Miotic

Use Treat primary open-angle glaucoma and conditions that obstruct aqueous outflow and to treat accommodative convergent strabismus

Usual Dosage Adults: Ophthalmic:

Glaucoma: Instill 0.25" strip in eye every 8-72 hours

Strabismus: Instill 0.25" strip to each eye every night for 2 weeks then reduce to 0.25" every other night to once weekly for 2 months

Mechanism of Action Cholinesterase inhibitor that causes contraction of the iris and ciliary muscles producing miosis, reduced intraocular pressure, and increased aqueous humor outflow

Local Anesthetic/Vasoconstrictor Precautions No information available to require special precautions

Effects on Dental Treatment No effects or complications reported

Other Adverse Effects

1% to 10%: Ocular: Stinging, burning, myopia, visual blurring

<1%:

Cardiovascular: Bradycardia, hypotension, flushing

Gastrointestinal: Nausea, vomiting, diarrhea

Neuromuscular & skeletal: Muscle weakness

Ocular: Retinal detachment, browache, miosis, twitching eyelids, watering eyes

Respiratory: Dyspnea

Miscellaneous: Sweating

Drug Interactions Increased toxicity: Succinylcholine, systemic anticholinesterases, carbamate or organic phosphate insecticides, cause decrease in cholinesterase levels

Drug Uptake

Peak IOP reduction: 24 hours

Duration: 1 week

Onset of miosis: Within 5-10 minutes

Duration: Up to 4 weeks

Pregnancy Risk Factor X

Generic Available No

Isollyl Improved® see Butalbital Compound on page 154

Isollyl® Improved see Butalbital Compound and Aspirin on page 156

Isomeprobamate (Canada) see Carisoprodol on page 180

Isoniazid (eye soe NYE a zid)

Related Information

Nonviral Infectious Diseases on page 1032

Brand Names INH™; Laniazid® Oral; Nydrazid® Injection

Canadian/Mexican Brand Names PMS-Isoniazid® (Canada)

Therapeutic Category Antitubercular Agent

Use Treatment of susceptible tuberculosis infections and prophylactically to those individuals exposed to tuberculosis

Usual Dosage Oral, I.M. (recommendations often change due to resistant strains and newly developed information; consult *MMWR* for current CDC recommendations):

Children: 10-20 mg/kg/day in 1-2 divided doses (maximum: 300 mg total dose)

Prophylaxis: 10 mg/kg/day given daily (up to 300 mg total dose) for 6 months

Adults: 5 mg/kg/day given daily (usual dose is 300 mg)

Disseminated disease: 10 mg/kg/day in 1-2 divided doses

Treatment should be continued for 9 months with rifampin or for 6 months with rifampin and pyrazinamide

Prophylaxis: 300 mg/day given daily for 6 months

American Thoracic Society and CDC currently recommend twice weekly therapy as part of a short-course regimen which follows 1-2 months of daily treatment for uncomplicated pulmonary tuberculosis in compliant patients

Children: 20-40 mg/kg/dose (up to 900 mg) twice weekly

Adults: 15 mg/kg/dose (up to 900 mg) twice weekly

Mechanism of Action Unknown, but may include the inhibition of myocolic acid synthesis resulting in disruption of the bacterial cell wall

Local Anesthetic/Vasoconstrictor Precautions No information available to require special precautions

Effects on Dental Treatment No effects or complications reported

Other Adverse Effects

>10%:
  Gastrointestinal: Loss of appetite, nausea, vomiting, stomach pain
  Hepatic: Hepatitis
  Neuromuscular & skeletal: Peripheral neuritis, weakness
1% to 10%:
  Central nervous system: Dizziness, slurred speech, lethargy
  Neuromuscular & skeletal: Hyper-reflexia
<1%:
  Central nervous system: Fever, seizures, mental depression, psychosis
  Dermatologic: Skin rash
  Hematologic: Blood dyscrasias
  Neuromuscular & skeletal: Arthralgia
  Ocular: Blurred vision, loss of vision

Drug Interactions

Decreased effect/levels of isoniazid with aluminum salts
Increased toxicity/levels of oral anticoagulants, carbamazepines, cycloserine, hydantoins, hepatically metabolized benzodiazepines; reaction with disulfiram

Drug Uptake

Absorption: Oral, I.M.: Rapid and complete; rate can be slowed when orally administered with food
Serum half-life:
  Fast acetylators: 30-100 minutes
  Slow acetylators: 2-5 hours; half-life may be prolonged in patients with impaired hepatic function or severe renal impairment
Time to peak serum concentration: Within 1-2 hours

Pregnancy Risk Factor C

Generic Available Yes

Isonipecaine (Canada) *see* Meperidine *on page 592*

Isopap® *see* Acetaminophen, Isometheptene, and Dichloralphenazone *on page 25*

Isoproterenol (eye soe proe TER e nole)

Related Information

Cardiovascular Diseases *on page 1010*

Brand Names Arm-a-Med® Isoproterenol; Dey-Dose® Isoproterenol; Isuprel®; Medihaler-Iso®

Therapeutic Category Adrenergic Agonist Agent; Bronchodilator

Use Treatment of reversible airway obstruction as in asthma or COPD; used parenterally in ventricular arrhythmias due to A-V nodal block; hemodynamically compromised bradyarrhythmias or atropine-resistant bradyarrhythmias; temporary use in third degree A-V block until pacemaker insertion; low cardiac output; vasoconstrictive shock states

Usual Dosage

Children:
  Bronchodilation: Inhalation: Metered dose inhaler: 1-2 metered doses up to 5 times/day
  Bronchodilation (using 1:200 inhalation solution) 0.01 mL/kg/dose every 4 hours as needed (maximum: 0.05 mL/dose) diluted with NS to 2 mL
  Sublingual: 5-10 mg every 3-4 hours, not to exceed 30 mg/day
  Cardiac arrhythmias: I.V.: Start 0.1 mcg/kg/minute (usual effective dose 0.2-2 mcg/kg/minute)

Adults:
  Bronchodilation: Inhalation: Metered dose inhaler: 1-2 metered doses 4-6 times/day
  Bronchodilation: 1-2 inhalations of a 0.25% solution, no more than 2 inhalations at any one time (1-5 minutes between inhalations); no more than 6 inhalations in any hour during a 24-hour period; maintenance therapy: 1-2 inhalations 4-6 times/day. Alternatively: 0.5% solution via hand bulb nebulizer is 5-15 deep inhalations repeated once in 5-10 minutes if necessary; treatments may be repeated up to 5 times/day.
  Sublingual: 10-20 mg every 3-4 hours; not to exceed 60 mg/day
  Cardiac arrhythmias: I.V.: 5 mcg/minute initially, titrate to patient response (2-20 mcg/minute)
  Shock: I.V.: 0.5-5 mcg/minute; adjust according to response

Mechanism of Action Stimulates beta$_1$- and beta$_2$-receptors resulting in relaxation of bronchial, GI, and uterine smooth muscle, increased heart rate and contractility, vasodilation of peripheral vasculature

Local Anesthetic/Vasoconstrictor Precautions Isoproterenol is selective for beta-adrenergic receptors and not alpha receptors; therefore, there is no precaution in the use of vasoconstrictor such as epinephrine

(Continued)

Isoproterenol *(Continued)*

Effects on Dental Treatment >10% of patients experience dry mouth

Other Adverse Effects

>10%:

Central nervous system: Insomnia, restlessness

Gastrointestinal: Dry throat, discoloration of saliva (pinkish-red)

1% to 10%:

Cardiovascular: Flushing of the face or skin, ventricular arrhythmias, tachycardias, profound hypotension, hyperfension

Central nervous system: Nervousness, anxiety, dizziness, headache, lightheadedness

Gastrointestinal: Vomiting, nausea

Neuromuscular & skeletal: Trembling, tremor, weakness

Miscellaneous: Sweating

<1%:

Cardiovascular: Arrhythmias, chest pain

Respiratory: Paradoxical bronchospasm

Drug Interactions Increased toxicity: Sympathomimetic agents lead to headaches; general anesthetics lead to arrhythmias

Drug Uptake

Onset of bronchodilation: Oral inhalation: Immediately

Duration:

Oral inhalation: 1 hour

S.C.: Up to 2 hours

Serum half-life: 2.5-5 minutes

Time to peak serum concentration: Oral: Within 1-2 hours

Pregnancy Risk Factor C

Generic Available Yes

Isoproterenol and Phenylephrine

(eye soe proe TER e nole & fen il EF rin)

Brand Names Duo-Medihaler® Aerosol

Therapeutic Category Adrenergic Agonist Agent

Use Treatment of bronchospasm associated with acute and chronic bronchial asthma, bronchitis, pulmonary emphysema, and bronchiectasis

Local Anesthetic/Vasoconstrictor Precautions No information available to require special precautions

Effects on Dental Treatment No effects or complications reported

Generic Available No

Isoptin® *see* Verapamil *on page 987*

Isoptin® SR *see* Verapamil *on page 987*

Isopto® Atropine *see* Atropine *on page 98*

Isopto® Carbachol Ophthalmic *see* Carbachol *on page 173*

Isopto® Carpine® *see* Pilocarpine *on page 759*

Isopto® Cetamide® Ophthalmic *see* Sulfacetamide Sodium *on page 890*

Isopto® Cetapred® Ophthalmic *see* Sulfacetamide Sodium and Prednisolone *on page 891*

Isopto® Eserine® *see* Physostigmine *on page 758*

Isopto® Homatropine Ophthalmic *see* Homatropine *on page 472*

Isopto® Hyoscine Ophthalmic *see* Scopolamine *on page 858*

Isopto® Plain Solution [OTC] *see* Artificial Tears *on page 87*

Isopto® Tears Solution [OTC] *see* Artificial Tears *on page 87*

Isordil® *see* Isosorbide Dinitrate *on next page*

Isosorbide *(eye soe SOR bide)*

Brand Names Ismotic®

Therapeutic Category Antiglaucoma Agent; Diuretic, Osmotic; Ophthalmic Agent, Osmotic

Use Short-term emergency treatment of acute angle-closure glaucoma and short-term reduction of intraocular pressure prior to and following intraocular surgery; may be used to interrupt an acute glaucoma attack; preferred agent when need to avoid nausea and vomiting

Usual Dosage Adults: Oral: Initial: 1.5 g/kg with a usual range of 1-3 g/kg 2-4 times/day as needed

Mechanism of Action Elevates osmolarity of glomerular filtrate to hinder the tubular resorption of water and increase excretion of sodium and chloride to result in diuresis; creates an osmotic gradient between plasma and ocular fluids

Local Anesthetic/Vasoconstrictor Precautions No information available to require special precautions

Effects on Dental Treatment No effects or complications reported
Other Adverse Effects
1% to 10%:
Central nervous system: Headache, confusion, disorientation
Gastrointestinal: Vomiting
<1%:
Cardiovascular: Syncope
Central nervous system: Lethargy, vertigo, dizziness, lightheadedness, irritability
Dermatologic: Rash
Endocrine & metabolic: Hypernatremia, hyperosmolarity
Gastrointestinal: Nausea, abdominal/gastric discomfort (infrequently), anorexia, thirst
Miscellaneous: Hiccups
Drug Interactions No data reported
Drug Uptake
Onset of action: Within 10-30 minutes
Peak action: 1-1.5 hours
Duration: 5-6 hours
Serum half-life: 5-9.5 hours
Pregnancy Risk Factor B
Generic Available No

Isosorbide Dinitrate (eye soe SOR bide dye NYE trate)
Related Information
Cardiovascular Diseases *on page 1010*
Brand Names Dilatrate®-SR; Isordil®; Sorbitrate®
Canadian/Mexican Brand Names Apo®-ISDN (Canada); Cedocard-SR® (Canada); Coradur® (Canada); Isoket® (Mexico); Isorbid® (Mexico)
Therapeutic Category Antianginal Agent; Nitrate; Vasodilator, Coronary
Use Prevention and treatment of angina pectoris; for congestive heart failure; to relieve pain, dysphagia, and spasm in esophageal spasm with GE reflux
Usual Dosage Adults (elderly should be given lowest recommended daily doses initially and titrate upward):
Oral: Angina: 5-40 mg 4 times/day or 40 mg every 8-12 hours in sustained released dosage form
Oral: Congestive heart failure:
Initial dose: 10 mg 3 times/day
Target dose: 40 mg 3 times/day
Maximum dose: 80 mg 3 times/day
Sublingual: 2.5-10 mg every 4-6 hours
Chew: 5-10 mg every 2-3 hours
Tolerance to nitrate effects develops with chronic exposure
Dose escalation does not overcome this effect. Tolerance can only be overcome by short periods of nitrate absence from the body. Short periods (10-12 hours) or nitrate withdrawal help minimize tolerance.

Hemodialysis: During hemodialysis, administer dose postdialysis or administer supplemental 10-20 mg dose; during peritoneal dialysis, supplemental dose is not necessary
Mechanism of Action Stimulation of intracellular cyclic-GMP results in vascular smooth muscle relaxation of both arterial and venous vasculature. Increased venous pooling decreases left ventricular pressure (preload) and arterial dilation decreases arterial resistance (afterload). Therefore, this reduces cardiac oxygen demand by decreasing left ventricular pressure and systemic vascular resistance by dilating arteries. Additionally, coronary artery dilation improves collateral flow to ischemic regions; esophageal smooth muscle is relaxed via the same mechanism.
Local Anesthetic/Vasoconstrictor Precautions No information available to require special precautions
Effects on Dental Treatment No effects or complications reported
Other Adverse Effects
>10%:
Cardiovascular: Flushing, postural hypotension
Central nervous system: Headache, lightheadedness, dizziness
Neuromuscular & skeletal: Weakness
1% to 10%: Dermatologic: Drug rash, exfoliative dermatitis
<1%:
Gastrointestinal: Nausea, vomiting
Hematologic: Methemoglobinemia (overdose)
Drug Interactions No data reported
(Continued)

Isosorbide Dinitrate *(Continued)*

Drug Uptake
Serum half-life:
Parent drug: 1-4 hours
Metabolite (5-mononitrate): 4 hours

Pregnancy Risk Factor C
Generic Available Yes

Isosorbide Mononitrate *(eye soe SOR bide mon oh NYE trate)*

Related Information
Cardiovascular Diseases *on page 1010*

Brand Names Imdur™; ISMO™; Monoket®
Canadian/Mexican Brand Names Elantan® (Mexico); Mono-Mack® (Mexico)
Therapeutic Category Antianginal Agent; Vasodilator, Coronary
Use Long-acting metabolite of the vasodilator isosorbide dinitrate used for the prophylactic treatment of angina pectoris

Usual Dosage Adults: Oral:
Regular tablet: 20 mg twice daily separated by 7 hours

Extended release tablet (Imdur™): Initial: 30-60 mg once daily; after several days the dosage may be increased to 120 mg/day (given as two 60 mg tablets); daily dose should be taken in the morning upon arising; maximum: 240 mg/day

Asymmetrical dosing regimen of 7 AM and 3 PM or 9 AM and 5 PM to allow for a nitrate-free dosing interval to minimize nitrate tolerance

Mechanism of Action Prevailing mechanism of action for nitroglycerin (and other nitrates) is systemic venodilation, decreasing preload as measured by pulmonary capillary wedge pressure and left ventricular end diastolic volume and pressure; the average reduction in LVEDV is 25% at rest, with a corresponding increase in ejection fractions of 50% to 60%. This effect improves congestive symptoms in heart failure and improves the myocardial perfusion gradient in patients with coronary artery disease.

Local Anesthetic/Vasoconstrictor Precautions No information available to require special precautions
Effects on Dental Treatment No effects or complications reported
Other Adverse Effects
>10%: Central nervous system: Headache, dizziness

1% to 10%: Gastrointestinal: Nausea, vomiting

<1%:
Cardiovascular: Angina pectoris, arrhythmias, atrial fibrillation, hypotension, palpitations, postural hypotension, premature ventricular contractions, supraventricular tachycardia, syncope, edema

Central nervous system: Malaise, agitation, anxiety, confusion, hypoesthesia, insomnia, nervousness, nightmares

Dermatologic: Pruritus, rash

Gastrointestinal: Abdominal pain, diarrhea, dyspepsia, tenesmus, increased appetite

Genitourinary: Impotence, dysuria

Hematologic: Methemoglobinemia (rarely)

Neuromuscular & skeletal: Neck stiffness, rigors, arthralgia, dyscoordination, weakness

Ocular: Blurred vision, diplopia

Renal: Polyuria

Respiratory: Bronchitis, pneumonia, upper respiratory tract infection

Miscellaneous: Tooth disorder, cold sweat

Drug Interactions No data reported
Drug Uptake
Absorption: Oral: Nearly complete and low intersubject variability in its pharmacokinetic parameters and plasma concentrations

Pregnancy Risk Factor C
Generic Available No

Isotretinoin *(eye soe TRET i noyn)*

Brand Names Accutane®
Canadian/Mexican Brand Names Isotrex® (Canada)
Therapeutic Category Acne Products; Retinoic Acid Derivative; Vitamin A Derivative
Use Treatment of severe recalcitrant cystic and/or conglobate acne unresponsive to conventional therapy; used investigationally for the treatment of children with metastatic neuroblastoma or leukemia that does not respond to conventional therapy

Usual Dosage Oral:

Children: Maintenance therapy for neuroblastoma: 100-250 mg/m²/day in 2 divided doses has been used investigationally

Children and Adults: 0.5-2 mg/kg/day in 2 divided doses (dosages as low as 0.05 mg/kg/day have been reported to be beneficial) for 15-20 weeks or until the total cyst count decreases by 70%, whichever is sooner

Mechanism of Action Reduces sebaceous gland size and reduces sebum production; regulates cell proliferation and differentiation

Local Anesthetic/Vasoconstrictor Precautions No information available to require special precautions

Effects on Dental Treatment >10% of patients experience dry mouth

Other Adverse Effects

>10%:

Dermatologic: Cheilitis, inflammation of lips, dry skin, pruritus, photosensitivity

Endocrine/metabolic: Elevated serum concentration of triglycerides

Local: Burning, redness

Neuromuscular & skeletal: Bone pain, arthralgia, myalgia

Ocular: Itching of eye

Respiratory: Dry nose, epistaxis

1% to 10%:

Central nervous system: Fatigue, headache, mental depression

Dermatologic: Skin peeling on hands or soles of feet, skin rash

Gastrointestinal: Stomach upset

Ocular: Dry eyes, photophobia

<1%:

Central nervous system: Mood changes, pseudomotor cerebri

Dermatologic: Alopecia

Endocrine & metabolic: Hyperuricemia

Gastrointestinal: Anorexia, nausea, vomiting, inflammatory bowel syndrome, bleeding of gums

Hematologic: Elevated erythrocyte sedimentation rate, decrease in hemoglobin and hematocrit

Hepatic: Hepatitis

Ocular: Conjunctivitis, corneal opacities, optic neuritis, cataracts

Note: Not to be used in women of childbearing potential unless woman is capable of complying with effective contraceptive measures; therapy is normally begun on the second or third day of next normal menstrual period; effective contraception must be used for at least 1 month before beginning therapy, during therapy, and for 1 month after discontinuation of therapy. Because of the high likelihood of teratogenic effects (~20%), physicians do not prescribe isotretinoin for women who are or who are likely to become pregnant while using the drug.

Drug Interactions

Increased effect: Increased clearance of carbamazepine

Increased toxicity: Avoid other vitamin A products; may interfere with medications used to treat hypertriglyceridemia

Drug Uptake

Absorption: Oral: Demonstrates biphasic absorption

Serum half-life, terminal:

Parent drug: 10-20 hours

Time to peak serum concentration: Within 3 hours

Pregnancy Risk Factor X

Generic Available No

Isovex® see Ethaverine on page 374

Isoxsuprine (eye SOKS syoo preen)

Brand Names Vasodilan®

Canadian/Mexican Brand Names Vadosilan® 20 (Mexico); Vadosilan® (Mexico)

Therapeutic Category Vasodilator

Use Treatment of peripheral vascular diseases, such as arteriosclerosis obliterans and Raynaud's disease

Usual Dosage Adults: 10-20 mg 3-4 times/day; start with lower dose in elderly due to potential hypotension

Mechanism of Action In studies on normal human subjects, isoxsuprine increases muscle blood flow, but skin blood flow is usually unaffected. Rather than increasing muscle blood flow by beta-receptor stimulation, isoxsuprine probably has a direct action on vascular smooth muscle. The generally accepted mechanism of action of isoxsuprine on the uterus is beta-adrenergic stimulation. Isoxsuprine was shown to inhibit prostaglandin synthetase at high serum concentrations, with low concentrations there was an increase in the P-G synthesis.
(Continued)

Isoxsuprine (Continued)

Local Anesthetic/Vasoconstrictor Precautions No information available to require special precautions

Effects on Dental Treatment No effects or complications reported

Other Adverse Effects

1% to 10%: Gastrointestinal: Nausea, vomiting

<1%:

Cardiovascular: Chest pain, hypotension

Dermatologic: Rash

Respiratory: Pulmonary edema

Drug Interactions No data reported

Drug Uptake

Absorption: Nearly complete

Serum half-life, serum: 1.25 hours mean

Time to peak serum concentration: Oral, I.M.: Within 1 hour

Pregnancy Risk Factor C

Generic Available Yes

Isradipine (iz RA di peen)

Related Information

Calcium Channel Blockers & Gingival Hyperplasia on page 1132

Cardiovascular Diseases on page 1010

Brand Names DynaCirc®

Canadian/Mexican Brand Names DynaCirc SRO® (Mexico)

Therapeutic Category Calcium Channel Blocker

Use Treatment of hypertension, congestive heart failure, migraine prophylaxis

Usual Dosage Adults: 2.5 mg twice daily; antihypertensive response seen in 2-3 hours; maximal response in 2-4 weeks; increase dose at 2- to 4-week intervals at 2.5-5 mg increments; usual dose range: 5-20 mg/day. **Note:** Most patients show no improvement with doses >10 mg/day except adverse reaction rate increases; therefore, maximal dose in elderly should be 10 mg/day.

Mechanism of Action Inhibits calcium ion from entering the "slow channels" or select voltage-sensitive areas of vascular smooth muscle and myocardium during depolarization, producing a relaxation of coronary vascular smooth muscle and coronary vasodilation; increases myocardial oxygen delivery in patients with vasospastic angina

Local Anesthetic/Vasoconstrictor Precautions No information available to require special precautions

Effects on Dental Treatment Other drugs of this class can cause gingival hyperplasia (ie, nifedipine) but there have been no reports for isradipine

Other Adverse Effects

>10%: Central nervous system: Headache

1% to 10%:

Cardiovascular: Edema, palpitations, flushing, chest pain, tachycardia, hypotension

Central nervous system: Dizziness, fatigue

Dermatologic: Rash

Gastrointestinal: Nausea, abdominal discomfort, vomiting, diarrhea

Neuromuscular & skeletal: Weakness

Respiratory: Dyspnea

<1%:

Cardiovascular: Heart failure, atrial and ventricular fibrillation, TIAs, A-V block, myocardial infarction, abnormal EKG

Central nervous system: Disturbed sleep

Dermatologic: Pruritus, urticaria

Gastrointestinal: Dry mouth

Genitourinary: Nocturia

Hematologic: Leukopenia

Neuromuscular & skeletal: Foot cramps, paresthesia

Ocular: Visual disturbance

Respiratory: Cough

Drug Interactions Increased toxicity/effect/levels: H_2-blockers cause increased bioavailability of isradipine

Severe hypotension has been reported during fentanyl anesthesia with concomitant use of beta-blockers and calcium channel blockers; even though such interactions have not been seen specifically with isradipine, caution is suggested in using isradipine with fentanyl

Drug Uptake

Absorption: Oral: 90% to 95%

Serum half-life: 8 hours

Time to peak: Serum concentration: 1-1.5 hours

Pregnancy Risk Factor C
Generic Available No
Selected Readings
Westbrook P, Bednarczyk EM, Carlson M, et al, "Regression of Nifedipine-Induced Gingival Hyperplasia Following Switch to a Same Class Calcium Channel Blocker, Isradipine," *J Periodontol*, 1997, 68(7):645-50.

Isuprel® *see* Isoproterenol *on page 523*
Itch-X® [OTC] *see* Pramoxine *on page 784*

Itraconazole (i tra KOE na zole)

Related Information
Oral Fungal Infections *on page 1063*
Brand Names Sporanox®
Canadian/Mexican Brand Names Isox® (Mexico); Itranax® (Mexico)
Therapeutic Category Antifungal Agent, Systemic
Use

Dental: Treatment of susceptible fungal infections in immunocompromised and immunocompetent patients including blastomycosis and histoplasmosis; also has activity against *Aspergillus, Candida, Coccidioides, Cryptococcus, Sporothrix* and chromomycosis

Medical: Treatment of susceptible fungal infection as described for dental use

Usual Dosage Oral (absorption is best if taken with food, therefore, it is best to administer itraconazole after meals):

Children: Efficacy and safety have not been established; a small number of patients 3-16 years of age have been treated with 100 mg/day for systemic fungal infections with no serious adverse effects reported

Adults: 200 mg once daily, if obvious improvement or there is evidence of progressive fungal disease, increase the dose in 100 mg increments to a maximum of 400 mg/day; doses >200 mg/day are given in 2 divided doses

Mechanism of Action Inhibits fungal cytochrome P-450-dependent enzymes (cytochrome P-450 3A4 and cytochrome P-450 2C); this blocks the synthesis of ergosterol which is the vital component in the fungal cell membrane. Triazoles contain three nitrogen atoms in the five-membered azole ring; the triazole ring increases tissue penetration, prolongs half-life, and enhances efficacy while decreasing toxicity compared with the imidazoles.

Local Anesthetic/Vasoconstrictor Precautions No information available to require special precautions

Effects on Dental Treatment No effects or complications reported

Other Adverse Effects

>10%: Gastrointestinal: Nausea
1% to 10%:
Central nervous system: Headache
Dermatologic: Rash
Gastrointestinal: Abdominal pain, vomiting

Contraindications Known hypersensitivity to itraconazole or other azoles; terfenadine

Warnings/Precautions Rare cases of serious cardiovascular adverse event, including death, ventricular tachycardia and torsade de pointes have been observed due to increased terfenadine concentrations induced by itraconazole; patients who develop abnormal liver function tests during fluconazole therapy should be monitored and therapy discontinued if symptoms of liver disease develop

Drug Interactions Decreased serum levels with isoniazid and phenytoin; decreased/undetectable serum levels with rifampin - **should not be administered concomitantly with rifampin**; absorption requires gastric acidity, therefore, antacids, H_2 antagonists (cimetidine and ranitidine), omeprazole, and sucralfate significantly reduce bioavailability resulting in treatment failures and should not be administered concomitantly; amphotericin B or fluconazole should be used instead. May increase cyclosporine levels (by 50%) when high doses are used; may increase phenytoin serum concentration; may inhibit warfarins metabolism; may increase digoxin serum levels; may increase terfenadine levels - **concomitant administration is not recommended**. If used concomitantly with an HMG-CoA reductase inhibitor (atorvastatin, lovastatin, pravastatin, simvastatin) itraconazole can increase HMG-CoA levels significantly (possibly 20-fold). This is probably due to hepatic enzyme inhibition or competition. In order to decrease the risk of myositis or myopathy, it may be necessary to temporarily stop HMG-CoA reductase inhibitors if systemic azole antifungals are needed.

Drug Uptake
Absorption: Oral: ~55%
Serum half-life: After single 200 mg dose: 21±5 hours
Time to peak serum concentration: 1-2 hours

Pregnancy Risk Factor C

(Continued)

Itraconazole *(Continued)*
Breast-feeding Considerations No data reported
Dosage Forms
Capsule: 100 mg
Solution, oral: 100 mg/10 mL (150 mL)
Dietary Considerations Absorption enhanced by food and requires gastric acidity
Generic Available No

I-Tropine® *see* Atropine *on page 98*

Ivermectin *(eye ver MEK tin)*
Brand Names Stromectol®
Therapeutic Category Antibiotic, Miscellaneous
Use Treatment of the following infections: Strongyloidiasis of the intestinal tract due the nematode parasite *Strongyloides stercoralis*. Onchocerciasis due to the nematode parasite *Onchocerca volvulus*. Note: Ivermectin is ineffective against adult *Onchocerca volvulus* parasites because they reside in subcutaneous nodules which are infrequently palpable. Surgical excision of these nodules may be considered in the management of patients with onchocerciasis.
Usual Dosage Oral:
Children >5 years: 150 mcg/kg as a single dose once every 12 months
Adults: 150 mcg/kg as a single dose; may be repeated every 6-12 **months**
Local Anesthetic/Vasoconstrictor Precautions No information available to require special precautions
Effects on Dental Treatment No effects or complications reported
Pregnancy Risk Factor C
Dosage Forms Tablet: 6 mg
Generic Available No

IVIG *see* Immune Globulin, Intravenous *on page 503*
IvyBlock® *see* Bentoquatam *on page 117*
Janimine® *see* Imipramine *on page 501*

Japanese Encephalitis Virus Vaccine, Inactivated
(jap a NEESE en sef a LYE tis VYE rus vak SEEN, in ak ti VAY ted)
Brand Names JE-VAX®
Therapeutic Category Vaccine, Live Virus
Use Active immunization against Japanese encephalitis for persons spending a month or longer in endemic areas, especially if travel will include rural areas
Local Anesthetic/Vasoconstrictor Precautions No information available to require special precautions
Effects on Dental Treatment No effects or complications reported
Other Adverse Effects
1% to 10%:
Cardiovascular: Hypotension
Central nervous system: Fever, headache, malaise, chills, dizziness
Dermatologic: Rash, urticaria, itching with or without accompanying rash
Gastrointestinal: Nausea, vomiting, abdominal pain
Local: Tenderness, redness, and swelling at injection site
Neuromuscular & skeletal: Myalgia
<1%:
Central nervous system: Encephalitis, encephalopathy, seizure
Dermatologic: Erythema multiforme, erythema nodosum, angioedema
Neuromuscular & skeletal: Peripheral neuropathy, joint swelling
Respiratory: Dyspnea
Miscellaneous: Anaphylactic reaction
Report allergic or unusual adverse reactions to the Vaccine Adverse Event Reporting System (VAERS 1-800-822-7967)
Pregnancy Risk Factor C
Generic Available No
Comments Japanese encephalitis vaccine is currently available only from the Centers for Disease Control. Contact Centers for Disease Control at (404) 639-6370 (Mon-Fri) or (404) 639-2888 (nights, weekends, or holidays).

Jenest-28™ *see* Ethinyl Estradiol and Norethindrone *on page 379*
JE-VAX® *see* Japanese Encephalitis Virus Vaccine, Inactivated *on this page*
Junior Strength Motrin® [OTC] *see* Ibuprofen *on page 495*
Junior Strength Panadol® [OTC] *see* Acetaminophen *on page 20*
Just Tears® Solution [OTC] *see* Artificial Tears *on page 87*
K+ 10® *see* Potassium Chloride *on page 778*

Kabikinase® see Streptokinase on page 884
Kadian® Capsule see Morphine Sulfate on page 648
Kalcinate® see Calcium Gluconate on page 166

Kanamycin (kan a MYE sin)
Related Information
Nonviral Infectious Diseases on page 1032
Brand Names Kantrex®
Canadian/Mexican Brand Names Randikan® (Mexico)
Therapeutic Category Antibiotic, Aminoglycoside
Use
Oral: Preoperative bowel preparation in the prophylaxis of infections and adjunctive treatment of hepatic coma (oral kanamycin is not indicated in the treatment of systemic infections); treatment of susceptible bacterial infection including gram-negative aerobes, gram-positive *Bacillus* as well as some mycobacteria
Parenteral: Rarely used in antibiotic irrigations during surgery
Usual Dosage
Children:
Infections: I.M., I.V.: 15-30 mg/kg/day in divided doses every 8 hours
Suppression of bowel flora: Oral: 150-250 mg/kg/day in divided doses administered every 1-6 hours
Adults:
Infections: I.M., I.V.: 5-7.5 mg/kg/dose in divided doses every 8-12 hours
Preoperative intestinal antisepsis: Oral: 1 g every 4-6 hours for 36-72 hours
Hepatic coma: Oral: 8-12 g/day in divided doses
Mechanism of Action Interferes with protein synthesis in bacterial cell by binding to ribosomal subunit
Local Anesthetic/Vasoconstrictor Precautions No information available to require special precautions
Effects on Dental Treatment No effects or complications reported
Other Adverse Effects
>10%: Renal: Nephrotoxicity
1% to 10%:
Cardiovascular: Swelling
Central nervous system: Neurotoxicity
Dermatologic: Skin itching, redness, rash
Otic: Ototoxicity (auditory), ototoxicity (vestibular)
<1%:
Central nervous system: Drowsiness, headache, pseudomotor cerebri
Dermatologic: Photosensitivity, erythema
Gastrointestinal: Anorexia, nausea, vomiting, weight loss, increased salivation, enterocolitis
Hematologic: Granulocytopenia, agranulocytosis, thrombocytopenia
Local: Burning, stinging
Neuromuscular & skeletal: Tremors, muscle cramps, weakness
Respiratory: Dyspnea
Drug Interactions
Increased toxicity:
Penicillins, cephalosporins, amphotericin B, diuretics cause increased nephrotoxicity of kanamycin
Neuromuscular blocking agents cause increased neuromuscular blockade of kanamycin
Drug Uptake
Absorption: Oral: Not absorbed following administration
Serum half-life: 2-4 hours, increases in anuria to 80 hours
End stage renal disease: 40-96 hours
Time to peak serum concentration: I.M.: 1-2 hours
Pregnancy Risk Factor D
Generic Available Yes

Kantrex® see Kanamycin on this page
Kaochlor® see Potassium Chloride on page 778
Kaochlor-Eff® see Potassium Bicarbonate, Potassium Chloride, and Potassium Citrate on page 778
Kaochlor® SF see Potassium Chloride on page 778
Kaodene® [OTC] see Kaolin and Pectin on this page

Kaolin and Pectin (KAY oh lin & PEK tin)
Brand Names Kaodene® [OTC]; Kao-Spen® [OTC]; Kapectolin® [OTC]
Therapeutic Category Antidiarrheal
Synonyms Pectin and Kaolin
Use Treatment of uncomplicated diarrhea
(Continued)

Kaolin and Pectin *(Continued)*

Local Anesthetic/Vasoconstrictor Precautions No information available to require special precautions
Effects on Dental Treatment No effects or complications reported
Other Adverse Effects 1% to 10%: Gastrointestinal: Constipation, fecal impaction
Pregnancy Risk Factor C
Generic Available Yes

Kaolin and Pectin With Opium

(KAY oh lin & PEK tin with OH pee um)
Brand Names Parepectolin®
Therapeutic Category Antidiarrheal
Use Symptomatic relief of diarrhea
Local Anesthetic/Vasoconstrictor Precautions No information available to require special precautions
Effects on Dental Treatment No effects or complications reported
Pregnancy Risk Factor C
Generic Available Yes

Kaon® *see Potassium Gluconate on page 780*
Kaon-Cl® *see Potassium Chloride on page 778*
Kaon-Cl-10® *see Potassium Chloride on page 778*
Kaopectate® Advanced Formula [OTC] *see Attapulgite on page 99*
Kaopectate® II [OTC] *see Loperamide on page 565*
Kaopectate® Maximum Strength Caplets *see Attapulgite on page 99*
Kao-Spen® [OTC] *see Kaolin and Pectin on previous page*
Kapectolin® [OTC] *see Kaolin and Pectin on previous page*
Kapectolin PG® *see Hyoscyamine, Atropine, Scopolamine, Kaolin, Pectin, and Opium on page 494*
Karidium® *see Fluoride on page 415*
Karigel® *see Fluoride on page 415*
Karigel®-N *see Fluoride on page 415*
Kasof® [OTC] *see Docusate on page 331*
Kay Ciel® *see Potassium Chloride on page 778*
K+ Care® *see Potassium Chloride on page 778*
K+ Care® Effervescent *see Potassium Bicarbonate on page 777*
K-Dur® 10 *see Potassium Chloride on page 778*
K-Dur® 20 *see Potassium Chloride on page 778*
Keflex® *see Cephalexin on page 201*
Keflin® *see Cephalothin on page 202*
Keftab® *see Cephalexin on page 201*
Kefurox® *see Cefuroxime on page 199*
Kefzol® *see Cefazolin on page 188*
K-Electrolyte® Effervescent *see Potassium Bicarbonate on page 777*
Kemadrin® *see Procyclidine on page 801*
Kenacort® *see Triamcinolone on page 954*
Kenaject-40® *see Triamcinolone on page 954*
Kenalog® *see Triamcinolone on page 954*
Kenalog-10® *see Triamcinolone on page 954*
Kenalog-40® *see Triamcinolone on page 954*
Kenalog® H *see Triamcinolone on page 954*
Kenalog® in Orabase® *see Triamcinolone on page 954*
Kenalog® in Orabase® *see Triamcinolone Acetonide Dental Paste on page 955*
Kenonel® *see Triamcinolone on page 954*
Keoxifene Hydrochloride *see Raloxifene on page 833*
Keralyt® Gel *see Salicylic Acid and Propylene Glycol on page 854*
Kerlone® *see Betaxolol on page 127*
Kestrone® *see Estrone on page 369*
Ketalar® *see Ketamine on this page*

Ketamine (KEET a meen)

Brand Names Ketalar®
Canadian/Mexican Brand Names Ketalin® (Mexico)
Therapeutic Category General Anesthetic, Intravenous
Use Induction of anesthesia; short surgical procedures; dressing changes

Usual Dosage Used in combination with anticholinergic agents to ↓ hypersalivation

Children: Initial induction:

    Oral: 6-10 mg/kg for 1 dose (mixed in 0.2-0.3 mL/kg of cola or other beverage) given 30 minutes before the procedure

    I.M.: 3-7 mg/kg

    I.V.: Range: 0.5-2 mg/kg, use smaller doses (0.5-1 mg/kg) for sedation for minor procedures; usual induction dosage: 1-2 mg/kg

    Continuous I.V. infusion: Sedation: 5-20 mcg/kg/minute

Adults: Initial induction:

    I.M.: 3-8 mg/kg

    I.V.: Range: 1-4.5 mg/kg; usual induction dosage: 1-2 mg/kg

Children and Adults: Maintenance: Supplemental doses of ½ to the full induction dose; repeat as needed

Mechanism of Action Produces dissociative anesthesia by direct action on the cortex and limbic system

Local Anesthetic/Vasoconstrictor Precautions No information available to require special precautions

Effects on Dental Treatment No effects or complications reported

Other Adverse Effects

>10%:

    Cardiovascular: Hypertension, tachycardia, increased cardiac output, paradoxical direct myocardial depression

    Central nervous system: Increased intracranial pressure, vivid dreams, visual hallucinations

    Neuromuscular & skeletal: Tonic-clonic movements, tremors

    Miscellaneous: Emergence reactions, vocalization

1% to 10%:

    Cardiovascular: Bradycardia, hypotension

    Dermatologic: Skin rash

    Gastrointestinal: Vomiting, anorexia, nausea

    Local: Pain at injection site

    Ocular: Nystagmus, diplopia

    Respiratory: Respiratory depression

<1%:

    Cardiovascular: Cardiac arrhythmias, myocardial depression, increases in cerebral blood

    Endocrine & metabolic: Increased metabolic rate

    Gastrointestinal: Hypersalivation

    Neuromuscular & skeletal: Increased skeletal muscle tone, fasciculations

    Ocular: Increased intraocular pressure

    Respiratory: Increased airway resistance, cough reflex may be depressed, decreased bronchospasm, respiratory depression or apnea with large doses or rapid infusions, laryngospasm

Drug Interactions

Increased toxicity:

    Barbiturates, narcotics, hydroxyzine increase prolonged recovery from ketamine

    Muscle relaxants, thyroid hormones cause increased blood pressure and heart rate in combination with ketamine

    Halothane causes decreased blood pressure in combination with ketamine

Drug Uptake Duration of action (following a single dose):

Unconsciousness: 10-15 minutes

Analgesia: 30-40 minutes

Amnesia: May persist for 1-2 hours

Pregnancy Risk Factor D

Generic Available No

Ketoconazole (kee toe KOE na zole)

Related Information

Dental Drug Interactions: Update on Drug Combinations Requiring Special Considerations *on page 1144*

Oral Fungal Infections *on page 1063*

Respiratory Diseases *on page 1018*

Brand Names Nizoral®

Canadian/Mexican Brand Names Akorazol® (Mexico)

Therapeutic Category Antifungal Agent, Systemic; Antifungal Agent, Topical

Use

Dental: Treatment of susceptible fungal infections in the oral cavity including candidiasis, oral thrush, and chronic mucocutaneous candidiasis

(Continued)

Ketoconazole *(Continued)*

Medical: Treatment of susceptible fungal infections including blastomycosis, histoplasmosis, paracoccidioidomycosis, as well as certain recalcitrant cutaneous dermatophytosis; used topically for treatment of tinea corporis, tinea cruris, tinea versicolor, and cutaneous candidiasis, seborrheic dermatitis

Usual Dosage

Children >2 years:

Oral: 5-10 mg/kg/day divided every 12-24 hours for 2-4 weeks

Topical: Rub gently to affected area 1-2 times/day

Adults:

Oral: 200-400 mg/day as a single daily dose

Topical: Rub gently to affected area 1-2 times/day

Mechanism of Action Alters the permeability of the cell wall; inhibits biosynthesis of triglycerides and phospholipids by fungi; inhibits several fungal enzymes that results in a build-up of toxic concentrations of hydrogen peroxide

Local Anesthetic/Vasoconstrictor Precautions No information available to require special precautions

Effects on Dental Treatment No effects or complications reported

Other Adverse Effects

Oral: 1% to 10%:

Dermatologic: Pruritus

Gastrointestinal: Nausea, vomiting, abdominal pain, diarrhea

Cream: Dermatologic: Severe irritation, pruritus, stinging (~5%)

Shampoo: Increases in normal hair loss, irritation (<1%), abnormal hair texture, scalp pustules, mild dryness of skin, itching, oiliness/dryness of hair

Contraindications Hypersensitivity to ketoconazole or any component; CNS fungal infections (due to poor CNS penetration); coadministration with terfenadine is contraindicated

Warnings/Precautions Rare cases of serious cardiovascular adverse event, including death, ventricular tachycardia and torsade de pointes have been observed due to increased terfenadine concentrations induced by ketoconazole. Use with caution in patients with impaired hepatic function; has been associated with hepatotoxicity, including some fatalities; perform periodic liver function tests; high doses of ketoconazole may depress adrenocortical function.

Drug Interactions Decreased serum levels with isoniazid and phenytoin; decreased/undetectable serum levels with rifampin - **should not be administered concomitantly with rifampin**; absorption requires gastric acidity, therefore, antacids, H_2 antagonists (cimetidine and ranitidine), omeprazole, and sucralfate significantly reduce bioavailability resulting in treatment failures and should not be administered concomitantly; amphotericin B or fluconazole should be used instead. May increase cyclosporine levels (by 50%) when high doses are used; may increase phenytoin serum concentration; may inhibit warfarins metabolism; may increase digoxin serum levels; may increase terfenadine levels - **concomitant administration is not recommended**.

Drug Uptake

Serum half-life: Biphasic: Initial: 2 hours; terminal: 8 hours

Time to peak serum concentration: 1-2 hours

Pregnancy Risk Factor C

Breast-feeding Considerations No data reported

Dosage Forms

Cream: 2% (15 g, 30 g, 60 g)

Shampoo: 2% (120 mL)

Tablet: 200 mg

Dietary Considerations May be taken with food or milk to decrease GI adverse effects

Generic Available No

Selected Readings

Wynn RL, "Erythromycin and Ketoconazole (Nizoral®) Associated With Terfenadine (Seldane®)-Induced Ventricular Arrhythmias," *Gen Dent*, 1993, 41(1):27-9.

Ketoprofen *(kee toe PROE fen)*

Related Information

Nonsteroidal Anti-Inflammatory Agents, Comparative Dosages, and Pharmacokinetics *on page 1143*

Oral Pain *on page 1053*

Rheumatoid Arthritis and Osteoarthritis *on page 1030*

Brand Names Actron® [OTC]; Orudis®; Orudis® KT [OTC]; Oruvail®

Canadian/Mexican Brand Names Apo®-Keto (Canada); Apo®-Keto-E (Canada); Keduril® (Mexico); K-Profen® (Mexico); Novo-Keto-EC (Canada); Nu-Ketoprofen (Canada); Nu-Ketoprofen-E (Canada); PMS-Ketoprofen (Canada);

Profenid® 200 (Mexico); Profenid-IM® (Mexico); Pro-Fenid® (Mexico); Rhodis™ (Canada); Rhodis-EC™ (Canada)

Therapeutic Category Analgesic, Non-narcotic; Anti-inflammatory Agent; Nonsteroidal Anti-inflammatory Agent (NSAID), Oral

Synonyms Ketoprofeno (Mexico)

Use

Dental: Management of pain and swelling

Medical: Acute and long-term treatment of rheumatoid arthritis and osteoarthritis; primary dysmenorrhea; mild to moderate pain

Usual Dosage Oral:

Children: Not recommended

Adults: 25-50 mg every 6-8 hours as necessary; daily doses >300 mg are not recommended

Mechanism of Action Inhibits prostaglandin synthesis by decreasing the activity of the enzyme, cyclo-oxygenase, which results in decreased formation of prostaglandin precursors

Local Anesthetic/Vasoconstrictor Precautions No information available to require special precautions

Effects on Dental Treatment Use with caution in patients taking anticoagulants

Other Adverse Effects >10%:

Central nervous system: Dizziness

Dermatologic: Skin rash

Gastrointestinal: Cramps, heartburn, nausea

Contraindications Ketoprofen is contraindicated in patients who have known hypersensitivity to it; should not be given to patients in whom aspirin or other nonsteroidal anti-inflammatory drugs induce asthma, urticaria, or other allergic-type reactions because severe, rarely fatal, anaphylactic reactions to ketoprofen have been reported in such patients

Warnings/Precautions Use lowest effective dose for shortest period possible; use with caution in patients with a history of GI disease (bleeding or ulcers)

Drug Interactions Probenecid increases both free and bound ketoprofen by reducing the plasma clearance of ketoprofen to about one-third, as well as decreasing its protein-binding; the combination of ketoprofen and probenecid is not recommended; coadministration of ketoprofen and methotrexate should be avoided because increased toxicity due to displacement of protein-bound methotrexate has been reported to occur

Drug Uptake

Absorption: Rapid and complete

Onset of effect: 30-60 minutes

Serum half-life: 2-4 hours

Time to peak serum concentration: 0.5-2 hours

Pregnancy Risk Factor B (D if used in the 3rd trimester or near delivery)

Breast-feeding Considerations May be taken while breast-feeding

Dosage Forms

Capsule (Orudis®): 25 mg, 50 mg, 75 mg

Actron®, Orudis® KT [OTC]: 12.5 mg

Capsule, extended release (Oruvail®): 100 mg, 200 mg

Dietary Considerations In order to minimize gastrointestinal effects, ketoprofen can be prescribed to be taken with food or milk; although food affects the bioavailability of ketoprofen, analgesic efficacy is not significantly diminished; food slows rate of absorption resulting in delayed and reduced peak serum concentrations

Generic Available Yes

Selected Readings

Balevi B, "Ketorolac Versus Ibuprofen: A Simple Cost-Efficacy Comparison for Dental Use," *J Can Dent Assoc*, 1994, 60(1):31-2.

Brooks PM and Day RO, "Nonsteroidal Anti-Inflammatory Drugs - Differences and Similarities," *N Engl J Med*, 1991, 324(24):1716-25.

Cooper SA, "Ketoprofen in Oral Surgery Pain: A Review," *J Clin Pharmacol*, 1988, 28(12 Suppl):S40-6.

Hersh EV, "The Efficacy and Safety of Ketoprofen in Postsurgical Dental Pain," *Compendium*, 1991, 12(4):234.

Ketoprofeno (Mexico) *see Ketoprofen on previous page*

Ketorolac Tromethamine (KEE toe role ak troe METH a meen)

Related Information

Dental Drug Interactions: Update on Drug Combinations Requiring Special Considerations *on page 1144*

Nonsteroidal Anti-Inflammatory Agents, Comparative Dosages, and Pharmacokinetics *on page 1143*

Brand Names Acular® Ophthalmic; Toradol® Injection; Toradol® Oral

(Continued)

Ketorolac Tromethamine *(Continued)*

Canadian/Mexican Brand Names Dolac® Inyectable (Mexico); Dolac® Oral (Mexico)

Therapeutic Category Analgesic, Non-narcotic; Anti-inflammatory Agent; Nonsteroidal Anti-inflammatory Agent (NSAID), Oral

Use

Dental: Short-term (<5 days) management of pain

Medical: First parenteral NSAID for analgesia; 30 mg I.M. provides the analgesia comparable to 12 mg of morphine or 100 mg of meperidine

Usual Dosage Adults: Treatment of acute postsurgical pain:

Manufacturer recommendation: I.M.: 30 mg followed by an oral dose (10 mg) as needed, then 10 mg every 4-6 hours as needed thereafter; total time for drug administration should be no longer than 5 days; maximum oral daily dose: 40 mg (or 120 mg combined oral and I.M.)

I.M.: Initial: 30-60 mg, then 15-30 mg every 6 hours as needed for up to 5 days maximum; maximum dose in the first 24 hours: 150 mg with 120 mg/24 hours for up to 5 days total

Mechanism of Action Inhibits prostaglandin synthesis by decreasing the activity of the enzyme, cyclo-oxygenase, which results in decreased formation of prostaglandin precursors

Local Anesthetic/Vasoconstrictor Precautions No information available to require special precautions

Effects on Dental Treatment No effects or complications reported

Other Adverse Effects 1% to 10%: Gastrointestinal: Abdominal pain, nausea, gastric ulcers

Contraindications In patients who have developed nasal polyps, angioedema, or bronchospastic reactions to other NSAIDs, active peptic ulcer disease, recent GI bleeding or perforation, patients with advanced renal disease or risk of renal failure, labor and delivery, nursing mothers, patients with hypersensitivity to ketorolac, aspirin, or other NSAIDs, **prophylaxis before major surgery**, suspected or confirmed cerebrovascular bleeding, hemorrhagic diathesis, concurrent aspirin or other NSAIDs, epidural or intrathecal administration, concomitant probenecid

Warnings/Precautions Use extra caution and reduce dosages in the elderly because it is cleared renally somewhat slower, and the elderly are also more sensitive to the renal effects of NSAIDs; use with caution in patients with congestive heart failure, hypertension, decreased renal or hepatic function, history of GI disease (bleeding or ulcers), or those receiving anticoagulants

Drug Interactions High dose salicylates may increase plasma levels of ketorolac by displacing from plasma proteins; coadministration with probenecid reduces renal excretion of ketorolac causing increased plasma levels; ketorolac reduces diuretic effect of furosemide; some NSAIDs may prevent renal excretion of lithium; effect of ketorolac on lithium is unknown

Drug Uptake

Absorption: Oral: Rapid and complete

Onset of effect: I.M.: Within 10 minutes

Duration of effect: 6-8 hours

Serum half-life: 2-8 hours

Time to peak serum concentration: I.M.: 30-60 minutes

Pregnancy Risk Factor B (D if used in the 3rd trimester)

Breast-feeding Considerations No data reported

Dosage Forms

Injection: 15 mg/mL (1 mL); 30 mg/mL (1 mL, 2 mL)

Solution, ophthalmic: 0.5% (5 mL)

Tablet: 10 mg

Dietary Considerations May be taken with food to decrease GI distress; food decreases rate of absorption but extent remains the same

Generic Available Yes (tablet)

Comments According to the manufacturer, ketorolac has been used inappropriately by physicians in the past. The drug had been prescribed to NSAID-sensitive patients, patients with GI bleeding, and for long-term use; a warning has been issued regarding increased incidence and severity of GI complications with increasing doses and duration of use. Labeling now includes the statement that ketorolac inhibits platelet function and is indicated for up to 5 days use only.

Selected Readings

Brown CR, Moodie JE, Evans SE, et al, "Efficacy of Intramuscular (I.M.) Ketorolac and Meperidine in Pain Following Major Oral Surgery," *Clin Pharmacol Ther*, 1988, 43:161 (abstract).

Forbes JA, Butterworth GA, Burchfield WH, et al, "Evaluation of Ketorolac, Aspirin, and an Acetaminophen-Codeine Combination in Postoperative Oral Surgery Pain," *Pharmacotherapy*, 1990, 10(6 Pt 2): 77S-93S.

Forbes JA, Kehm CJ, Grodin CD, et al, "Evaluation of Ketorolac, Ibuprofen, Acetaminophen, and an Acetaminophen-Codeine Combination in Postoperative Oral Surgery Pain," *Pharmacotherapy*, 1990, 10(6 Pt 2):94S-105S.

Fricke J and Angelocci D, "The Analgesic Efficacy of I.M. Ketorolac and Meperidine for the Control of Postoperative Dental Pain," *Clin Pharmacol Ther*, 1987, 41:181.

Fricke JR Jr, Angelocci D, Fox K, et al, "Comparison of the Efficacy and Safety of Ketorolac and Meperidine in the Relief of Dental Pain," *J Clin Pharmacol*, 1992, 32(4):376-84.

Gannon R, "Focus on Ketorolac: A Nonsteroidal, Anti-inflammatory Agent for the Treatment of Moderate to Severe Pain," *Hosp Formul*, 1989, 24:695-702.

Wynn RL, "Ketorolac (Toradol®) for Dental Pain," *Gen Dent*, 1992, 40(6):476-9.

Key-Pred® *see* Prednisolone *on page 788*

Key-Pred-SP® *see* Prednisolone *on page 788*

K-G® *see* Potassium Gluconate *on page 780*

K-Gen® Effervescent *see* Potassium Bicarbonate *on page 777*

K-Ide® *see* Potassium Bicarbonate and Potassium Citrate, Effervescent *on page 777*

Kinevac® *see* Sincalide *on page 866*

Klaron® Lotion *see* Sulfacetamide Sodium *on page 890*

K-Lease® *see* Potassium Chloride *on page 778*

Klerist-D® Tablet [OTC] *see* Chlorpheniramine and Pseudoephedrine *on page 219*

Klonopin™ *see* Clonazepam *on page 249*

K-Lor™ *see* Potassium Chloride *on page 778*

Klor-Con® *see* Potassium Chloride *on page 778*

Klor-Con® 8 *see* Potassium Chloride *on page 778*

Klor-Con® 10 *see* Potassium Chloride *on page 778*

Klor-Con/25® *see* Potassium Chloride *on page 778*

Klor-con®/EF *see* Potassium Bicarbonate and Potassium Citrate, Effervescent *on page 777*

Klorvess® *see* Potassium Chloride *on page 778*

Klorvess® Effervescent *see* Potassium Bicarbonate and Potassium Chloride, Effervescent *on page 777*

Klotrix® *see* Potassium Chloride *on page 778*

K-Lyte® *see* Potassium Bicarbonate and Potassium Citrate, Effervescent *on page 777*

K/Lyte/CL® *see* Potassium Bicarbonate and Potassium Chloride, Effervescent *on page 777*

K-Lyte®/Cl *see* Potassium Chloride *on page 778*

K-Lyte® Effervescent *see* Potassium Bicarbonate *on page 777*

K-Norm® *see* Potassium Chloride *on page 778*

Koāte®-HP *see* Antihemophilic Factor (Human) *on page 80*

Koāte®-HS *see* Antihemophilic Factor (Human) *on page 80*

Kogenate® *see* Antihemophilic Factor (Recombinant) *on page 81*

Kolephrin® GG/DM [OTC] *see* Guaifenesin and Dextromethorphan *on page 453*

Kolyum® *see* Potassium Chloride and Potassium Gluconate *on page 779*

Konakion® *see* Phytonadione *on page 758*

Kondon's Nasal® [OTC] *see* Ephedrine *on page 351*

Konsyl® [OTC] *see* Psyllium *on page 822*

Konsyl-D® [OTC] *see* Psyllium *on page 822*

Konȳne® 80 *see* Factor IX Complex (Human) *on page 391*

Koromex® [OTC] *see* Nonoxynol 9 *on page 689*

K-Phos® Neutral *see* Potassium Phosphate and Sodium Phosphate *on page 783*

K-Phos® Original *see* Potassium Acid Phosphate *on page 776*

K-Tab® *see* Potassium Chloride *on page 778*

Ku-Zyme® HP *see* Pancrelipase *on page 722*

K-Vescent® *see* Potassium Bicarbonate and Potassium Citrate, Effervescent *on page 777*

Kwelcof® *see* Hydrocodone and Guaifenesin *on page 481*

Kytril® *see* Granisetron *on page 449*

LA-12® *see* Hydroxocobalamin *on page 487*

Labetalol (la BET a lole)

Related Information

Cardiovascular Diseases *on page 1010*

Brand Names Normodyne®; Trandate®

Canadian/Mexican Brand Names Midotens® (Mexico)

Therapeutic Category Alpha-/Beta- Adrenergic Blocker

Use Treatment of mild to severe hypertension; I.V. for hypertensive emergencies

(Continued)

Labetalol *(Continued)*

Usual Dosage Due to limited documentation of its use, labetalol should be initiated cautiously in pediatric patients with careful dosage adjustment and blood pressure monitoring

Children:

Oral: Limited information regarding labetalol use in pediatric patients is currently available in literature. Some centers recommend initial oral doses of 4 mg/kg/day in 2 divided doses. Reported oral doses have started at 3 mg/kg/day and 20 mg/kg/day and have increased up to 40 mg/kg/day.

I.V., intermittent bolus doses of 0.3-1 mg/kg/dose have been reported

For treatment of pediatric hypertensive emergencies, initial continuous infusions of 0.4-1 mg/kg/hour with a maximum of 3 mg/kg/hour have been used; administration requires the use of an infusion pump

Adults:

Oral: Initial: 100 mg twice daily, may increase as needed every 2-3 days by 100 mg until desired response is obtained; usual dose: 200-400 mg twice daily; not to exceed 2.4 g/day

I.V.: 20 mg or 1-2 mg/kg whichever is lower, IVP over 2 minutes, may give 40-80 mg at 10-minute intervals, up to 300 mg total dose

I.V. infusion: Initial: 2 mg/minute; titrate to response up to 300 mg total dose; administration requires the use of an infusion pump

I.V. infusion (500 mg/250 mL D$_5$) rates:

1 mg/minute: 30 mL/hour
2 mg/minute: 60 mL/hour
3 mg/minute: 90 mL/hour
4 mg/minute: 120 mL/hour
5 mg/minute: 150 mL/hour
6 mg/minute: 180 mL/hour

Not removed by hemo- or peritoneal dialysis; supplemental dose is not necessary

Mechanism of Action Blocks alpha-, beta$_1$-, and beta$_2$-adrenergic receptor sites; elevated renins are reduced

Local Anesthetic/Vasoconstrictor Precautions Use with caution; epinephrine has interacted with nonselective beta-blockers to result in initial hypertensive episode followed by bradycardia

Effects on Dental Treatment Noncardioselective beta-blockers (ie, propranolol, nadolol) enhance the pressor response to epinephrine, resulting in hypertension and bradycardia. Many nonsteroidal anti-inflammatory drugs such as ibuprofen and indomethacin can reduce the hypotensive effect of beta-blockers after 3 or more weeks of therapy with the NSAID. Short-term NSAID use (ie, 3 days) requires no special precautions in patients taking beta-blockers.

Other Adverse Effects

1% to 10%:

Cardiovascular: Congestive heart failure, arrhythmia, reduced peripheral circulation, orthostatic hypotension

Central nervous system: Mental depression, dizziness, drowsiness

Dermatologic: Itching, numbness of skin

Endocrine & metabolic: Decreased sexual ability

Gastrointestinal: Nausea, vomiting, stomach discomfort, changes in taste

Neuromuscular & skeletal: Weakness

Respiratory: Dyspnea, nasal congestion

<1%:

Cardiovascular: Bradycardia, chest pain

Dermatologic: Skin rash

Gastrointestinal: Diarrhea

Hepatic: Hepatotoxicity

Neuromuscular & skeletal: Arthralgia

Ocular: Dry eyes

Drug Interactions

Decreased effect of beta-blockers:

Barbiturates (increased liver metabolism of beta-blockers to result in lower serum levels)

NSAIDs (attenuate the hypotensive therapeutic effects of beta-blockers)

Rifampin (increased liver metabolism of beta-blockers to result in lower serum levels)

Increased effects of beta-blockers:

Calcium channel blockers (increase serum levels of beta-blockers by unknown mechanism to enhance hypotension)

Beta-blockers increase the effects of:
   Epinephrine (vasoconstrictor; initial hypertensive episode followed by brady-cardia) only from noncardioselective type beta-blockers
   Phenylephrine (Neosynephrine®; enhanced pressor response)
   Theophylline (inhibit theophylline metabolism causing increase in serum concentrations)
Drug Uptake
   Onset of action:
      Oral: 20 minutes to 2 hours
      I.V.: 2-5 minutes
   Peak effect:
      Oral: 1-4 hours
      I.V.: 5-15 minutes
   Duration:
      Oral: 8-24 hours (dose-dependent)
      I.V.: 2-4 hours
   Serum half-life, normal renal function: 6-8 hours
Pregnancy Risk Factor C
Generic Available No

Lac-Hydrin® see Lactic Acid With Ammonium Hydroxide on this page

Lacril® Ophthalmic Solution [OTC] see Artificial Tears on page 87

Lacrisert® see Hydroxypropyl Cellulose on page 490

LactAid® [OTC] see Lactase on this page

Lactase (LAK tase)
Brand Names Dairy Ease® [OTC]; LactAid® [OTC]; Lactrase® [OTC]
Therapeutic Category Nutritional Supplement
Use Help digest lactose in milk for patients with lactose intolerance
Local Anesthetic/Vasoconstrictor Precautions No information available to require special precautions
Effects on Dental Treatment No effects or complications reported
Generic Available No

Lactic Acid and Salicylic Acid see Salicylic Acid and Lactic Acid on page 853

Lactic Acid and Sodium-PCA
(LAK tik AS id & SOW dee um-pee see aye)
Brand Names LactiCare® [OTC]
Therapeutic Category Topical Skin Product
Synonyms Sodium-PCA and Lactic Acid
Use Lubricate and moisturize the skin counteracting dryness and itching
Local Anesthetic/Vasoconstrictor Precautions No information available to require special precautions
Effects on Dental Treatment No effects or complications reported
Generic Available No

Lactic Acid With Ammonium Hydroxide
(LAK tik AS id with a MOE nee um hye DROKS ide)
Brand Names Lac-Hydrin®
Therapeutic Category Topical Skin Product
Synonyms Ammonium Lactate
Use Treatment of moderate to severe xerosis and ichthyosis vulgaris
Local Anesthetic/Vasoconstrictor Precautions No information available to require special precautions
Effects on Dental Treatment No effects or complications reported
Generic Available No

LactiCare® [OTC] see Lactic Acid and Sodium-PCA on this page

Lactinex® [OTC] see Lactobacillus acidophilus and Lactobacillus bulgaricus on this page

Lactobacillus acidophilus and Lactobacillus bulgaricus
(lak toe ba SIL us as i DOF il us & lak toe ba SIL us bul GAR i cus)
Related Information
   Oral Nonviral Soft Tissue Ulcerations or Erosions on page 1070
Brand Names Bacid® [OTC]; Lactinex® [OTC]; More-Dophilus® [OTC]
Canadian/Mexican Brand Names Fermalac® (Canada); Lacteol® Fort (Mexico); Sinuberase® (Mexico)
Therapeutic Category Antidiarrheal
Use Treatment of uncomplicated diarrhea particularly that caused by antibiotic therapy; re-establish normal physiologic and bacterial flora of the intestinal tract
Usual Dosage Children >3 years and Adults: Oral:
   (Continued)

Lactobacillus acidophilus and *Lactobacillus bulgaricus* (Continued)

Capsules: 2 capsules 2-4 times/day

Granules: 1 packet added to or taken with cereal, food, milk, fruit juice, or water, 3-4 times/day

Powder: 1 teaspoonful daily with liquid

Tablet, chewable: 4 tablets 3-4 times/day; may follow each dose with a small amount of milk, fruit juice, or water

Mechanism of Action Creates an environment unfavorable to potentially pathogenic fungi or bacteria through the production of lactic acid, and favors establishment of an aciduric flora, thereby suppressing the growth of pathogenic microorganisms; helps re-establish normal intestinal flora

Local Anesthetic/Vasoconstrictor Precautions No information available to require special precautions

Effects on Dental Treatment No effects or complications reported

Other Adverse Effects 1% to 10%: Gastrointestinal: Flatulence

Drug Interactions No data reported

Drug Uptake Absorption: Oral: Not absorbed

Pregnancy Risk Factor No rating

Dosage Forms

Capsule: 50s, 100s

Granules: 1 g/packet (12 packets/box)

Powder: 12 oz

Tablet, chewable: 50s

Generic Available No

Lactrase® [OTC] *see Lactase on previous page*

Lactulose (LAK tyoo lose)

Brand Names Cephulac®; Cholac®; Chronulac®; Constilac®; Constulose®; Duphalac®; Enulose®; Evalose®; Heptalac®; Lactulose PSE®

Therapeutic Category Ammonia Detoxicant; Laxative, Miscellaneous

Use Adjunct in the prevention and treatment of portal-systemic encephalopathy (PSE); treatment of chronic constipation

Usual Dosage Diarrhea may indicate overdosage and responds to dose reduction

Prevention of portal systemic encephalopathy (PSE): Oral:

Older Children: Daily dose of 40-90 mL divided 3-4 times/day; if initial dose causes diarrhea, then reduce it immediately; adjust dosage to produce 2-3 stools/day

Constipation:

Children: 5 g/day (7.5 mL) after breakfast

Adults:

Acute PSE:

Oral: 20-30 g (30-45 mL) every 1-2 hours to induce rapid laxation; adjust dosage daily to produce 2-3 soft stools; doses of 30-45 mL may be given hourly to cause rapid laxation, then reduce to recommended dose; usual daily dose: 60-100 g or 20-30 g (30-45 mL), 3-4 times/day

Rectal administration: 200 g (300 mL) diluted with 700 mL of H_2O or NS; administer rectally via rectal balloon catheter and retain 30-60 minutes every 4-6 hours

Constipation: Oral: 15-30 mL/day increased to 60 mL/day if necessary

Mechanism of Action The bacterial degradation of lactulose resulting in an acidic pH inhibits the diffusion of NH_3 into the blood by causing the conversion of NH_3 to NH_4+; also enhances the diffusion of NH_3 from the blood into the gut where conversion to NH_4+ occurs; produces an osmotic effect in the colon with resultant distention promoting peristalsis

Local Anesthetic/Vasoconstrictor Precautions No information available to require special precautions

Effects on Dental Treatment No effects or complications reported

Other Adverse Effects

>10%: Gastrointestinal: Flatulence, diarrhea (excessive dose)

1% to 10%: Gastrointestinal: Abdominal discomfort, nausea, vomiting

Drug Interactions

Absorption: Oral: Not absorbed appreciably following administration; this is desirable since the intended site of action is within the colon

Pregnancy Risk Factor B

Generic Available Yes

Lactulose PSE® *see Lactulose on this page*

Ladakamycin *see Azacitidine on page 101*

Lamictal® see Lamotrigine on this page
Lamisil® see Terbinafine on page 907
Lamisil® Oral see Terbinafine, Oral on page 908

Lamivudine (la MI vyoo deen)

Related Information

HIV Infection and AIDS on page 1024
Systemic Viral Diseases on page 1047
Zidovudine and Lamivudine on page 1003

Brand Names Epivir®

Therapeutic Category Antiviral Agent, Oral

Synonyms 3TC

Use In combination with zidovudine (or other nucleoside) and often a protease inhibitor for treatment of HIV infection when therapy is warranted based on clinical and/or immunological evidence of disease progression; recommended with zidovudine for prophylaxis of HIV following needle sticks; has also demonstrated positive effects in the treatment of hepatitis B

Mechanism of Action In vitro, lamivudine is phosphorylated to its active 5'-triphosphate metabolite (L-TP), which inhibits HIV reverse transcription via viral DNA chain termination; L-TP also inhibits the RNA- and DNA-dependent DNA polymerase activities of reverse transcriptase

Local Anesthetic/Vasoconstrictor Precautions No information available to require special precautions

Effects on Dental Treatment No effects or complications reported

Other Adverse Effects

>10%:
  Central nervous system: Headache, insomnia, malaise, fatigue, pain
  Gastrointestinal: Nausea, diarrhea, vomiting
  Neuromuscular & skeletal: Peripheral neuropathy, paresthesia
  Respiratory: Nasal signs and symptoms, cough

1% to 10%:
  Central nervous system: Dizziness, depression, fever, chills
  Dermatologic: Rashes
  Gastrointestinal: Anorexia, abdominal pain, dyspepsia, elevated amylase
  Hematologic: Neutropenia, anemia
  Hepatic: Elevated AST, ALT
  Neuromuscular & skeletal: Myalgia, arthralgia

<1%:
  Gastrointestinal: Pancreatitis
  Hematologic: Thrombocytopenia
  Hepatic: Hyperbilirubinemia

Drug Interactions Increased effect: Zidovudine concentrations increase significantly (~39%) with coadministration with lamivudine; trimethoprim/sulfamethoxazole increases lamivudine's AUC and decreases its renal clearance by 44% and 29%, respectively; although the AUC was not significantly affected, absorption of lamivudine was slowed and C_{max} was 40% lower when administered to patients in the fed versus the fasted state

Drug Uptake
  Absorption: Oral: Rapid in HIV-infected patients
  Serum half-life:
    Children: 2 hours
    Adults: 5-7 hours

Pregnancy Risk Factor C

Dosage Forms
  Solution, oral: 10 mg/mL (240 mL)
  Tablet: 150 mg

Generic Available No

Lamotrigina (Mexico) see Lamotrigine on this page

Lamotrigine (la MOE tri jeen)

Brand Names Lamictal®

Therapeutic Category Anticonvulsant, Miscellaneous

Synonyms Lamotrigina (Mexico)

Use Partial/secondary generalized seizures in adults; childhood epilepsy (not approved for use in children <16 years of age)

Usual Dosage Oral:
  Children: 2-15 mg/kg/day in 2 divided doses
  Adults: Initial dose: 50-100 mg/day then titrate to daily maintenance dose of 100-400 mg/day in 1-2 divided daily doses
    With concomitant valproic acid therapy: Start initial dose at 25 mg/day then titrate to maintenance dose of 50-200 mg/day in 1-2 divided daily doses

(Continued)

Lamotrigine *(Continued)*

Mechanism of Action A triazine derivative which inhibits release of glutamate (an excitatory amino acid) and inhibits voltage-sensitive sodium channels, which stabilizes neuronal membranes

Local Anesthetic/Vasoconstrictor Precautions No information available to require special precautions

Effects on Dental Treatment No effects or complications reported

Other Adverse Effects 1% to 10%:
Central nervous system: Dizziness, sedation, ataxia
Dermatologic: Hypersensitivity rash, Stevens-Johnson syndrome, angioedema
Ocular: Nystagmus, diplopia
Renal: Hematuria

Drug Interactions
Decreased effect: Acetaminophen (increases renal clearance); carbamazepine, phenobarbital, and phenytoin (increases metabolic clearance)
Increased effect: Valproic acid increases half-life of lamotrigine (decreased metabolic clearance)

Drug Uptake
Serum half-life: 24 hours; increases to 59 hours with concomitant valproic acid therapy; decreases with concomitant phenytoin or carbamazepine therapy to 15 hours

Pregnancy Risk Factor C

Generic Available No

Lamprene® *see* Clofazimine *on page 246*

Lanacane® [OTC] *see* Benzocaine *on page 118*

Laniazid® Oral *see* Isoniazid *on page 522*

Lanolin, Cetyl Alcohol, Glycerin, and Petrolatum

(LAN oh lin, SEE til AL koe hol, GLIS er in, & pe troe LAY tum)

Brand Names Lubriderm® [OTC]

Therapeutic Category Topical Skin Product

Use Treatment of dry skin

Local Anesthetic/Vasoconstrictor Precautions No information available to require special precautions

Effects on Dental Treatment No effects or complications reported

Other Adverse Effects 1% to 10%: Local irritation

Pregnancy Risk Factor C

Generic Available Yes

Lanorinal® *see* Butalbital Compound *on page 154*

Lanorinal® *see* Butalbital Compound and Aspirin *on page 156*

Lanoxicaps® *see* Digoxin *on page 313*

Lanoxin® *see* Digoxin *on page 313*

Lansoprazole (lan SOE pra zole)

Brand Names Prevacid®

Therapeutic Category Gastric Acid Secretion Inhibitor

Use Short-term treatment (up to 4 weeks) for healing and symptom relief of active duodenal ulcers (should not be used for maintenance therapy of duodenal ulcers); up to 8 weeks of treatment for all grades of erosive esophagitis (8 additional weeks can be given for incompletely healed esophageal erosions or for recurrence); and long-term treatment of pathological hypersecretory conditions, including Zollinger-Ellison syndrome

Usual Dosage
Duodenal or gastric ulcer: 30 mg once daily for 4-8 weeks
Erosive esophagitis: 30 mg once daily for 4-8 weeks
Hypersecretory conditions: 30-180 mg once daily, titrated to reduce acid secretion to <10 mEq/hour (5 mEq/hour in patients with prior gastric surgery)

Local Anesthetic/Vasoconstrictor Precautions No information available to require special precautions

Effects on Dental Treatment No effects or complications reported

Other Adverse Effects
1% to 10%:
Central nervous system: Fatigue, dizziness, headache
Gastrointestinal: Abdominal pain, diarrhea, nausea, increased appetite, hypergastrinoma
<1%:
Dermatologic: Rash
Otic: Tinnitus
Renal: Proteinuria

Pregnancy Risk Factor B
Dosage Forms Capsule, delayed release: 15 mg, 30 mg
Generic Available No

Largon® Injection *see* Propiomazine *on page 809*
Lariam® *see* Mefloquine *on page 589*
Larodopa® *see* Levodopa *on page 547*
Larotid® *see* Amoxicillin *on page 68*
Lasix® *see* Furosemide *on page 434*
L-asparaginase *see* Asparaginase *on page 89*
Lassar's Zinc Paste *see* Zinc Oxide *on page 1004*

Latanoprost (la TAN oh prost)

Brand Names Xalatan®
Therapeutic Category Ophthalmic Agent, Miscellaneous
Use Reduction of elevated intraocular pressure in patients with open-angle glaucoma and ocular hypertension who are intolerant of the other IOP lowering medications or insufficiently responsive (failed to achieve target IOP determined after multiple measurements over time) to another IOP lowering medication
Mechanism of Action Latanoprost is a prostaglandin F_2-alpha analog believed to reduce intraocular pressure by increasing the outflow of the aqueous humor
Local Anesthetic/Vasoconstrictor Precautions No information available to require special precautions
Effects on Dental Treatment No effects or complications reported
Other Adverse Effects
  >10%: Ocular: Blurred vision, burning and stinging, conjunctival hyperemia, foreign body sensation, itching, increased pigmentation of the iris, and punctate epithelial keratopathy
  1% to 10%:
    Cardiovascular: Chest pain, angina pectoris
    Dermatologic: Rash, allergic skin reaction
    Neuromuscular & skeletal: Myalgia, arthralgia, back pain
    Ocular: Dry eye, excessive tearing, eye pain, lid crusting, lid edema, lid erythema, lid discomfort/pain, photophobia
    Respiratory: Upper respiratory tract infection, cold, flu
  <1%: Ocular: Conjunctivitis, diplopia, discharge from the eye, retinal artery embolus, retinal detachment, vitreous hemorrhage from diabetic retinopathy
Drug Interactions Decreased effect: *In vitro* studies have shown that precipitation occurs when eye drops containing thimerosal are mixed with latanoprost. If such drugs are used, administer with an interval of at least 5 minutes between applications
Drug Uptake
  Onset of effect: 3-4 hours
  Maximum effect: 8-12 hours
  Absorption: Through the cornea where the isopropyl ester prodrug is hydrolyzed by esterases to the biologically active acid. Peak concentration is reached in 2 hours after topical administration in the aqueous humor.
  Serum half-life: 17 minutes
Pregnancy Risk Factor C
Dosage Forms Solution, ophthalmic: 0.005% (2.5 mL)
Generic Available No

L-Carnitine *see* Levocarnitine *on page 547*
LCD *see* Coal Tar *on page 254*
LCR *see* Vincristine *on page 990*
Lederplex® [OTC] *see* Vitamin B Complex *on page 993*
Legatrin® [OTC] *see* Quinine *on page 831*
Lente® Iletin® I *see* Insulin Preparations *on page 509*
Lente® Iletin® II *see* Insulin Preparations *on page 509*
Lente® Insulin *see* Insulin Preparations *on page 509*
Lente® L *see* Insulin Preparations *on page 509*
Lescol® *see* Fluvastatin *on page 425*

Letrozole (LET roe zole)

Brand Names Femara®
Therapeutic Category Antineoplastic Agent, Hormone (Antiestrogen)
Use Treatment of advanced breast cancer in postmenopausal women with disease progression following tamoxifen therapy. Patients with ER-negative disease and patients who did not respond to tamoxifen therapy rarely responded to anastrozole.
Usual Dosage Adults: Oral: 2.5 mg once/day, without regard to meals
(Continued)

Letrozole *(Continued)*

Local Anesthetic/Vasoconstrictor Precautions No information available to require special precautions

Effects on Dental Treatment No effects or complications reported

Dosage Forms Tablet: 2.5 mg

Leucovorin (loo koe VOR in)

Brand Names Wellcovorin®

Canadian/Mexican Brand Names Dalisol (Mexico); Medasavorin (Mexico)

Therapeutic Category Antidote, Methotrexate; Folic Acid Derivative

Synonyms Calcium Leucovorin; Citrovorum Factor; Folinic Acid; 5-Formyl Tetra-hydrofolate; Leucovorin Calcium

Use Antidote for folic acid antagonists; treatment of folate deficient megaloblastic anemias of infancy, sprue, pregnancy; nutritional deficiency when oral folate therapy is not possible

Usual Dosage Children and Adults:

Treatment of folic acid antagonist overdosage (eg, pyrimethamine or trimethoprim): Oral: 2-15 mg/day for 3 days or until blood counts are normal or 5 mg every 3 days; doses of 6 mg/day are needed for patients with platelet counts <100,000/mm³

Folate-deficient megaloblastic anemia: I.M.: 1 mg/day

Megaloblastic anemia secondary to congenital deficiency of dihydrofolate reductase: I.M.: 3-6 mg/day

Rescue dose (rescue therapy should start within 24 hours of MTX therapy): I.V.: 10 mg/m² to start, then 10 mg/m² every 6 hours orally for 72 hours until serum MTX concentration is <10⁻⁸ molar; if serum creatinine 24 hours after methotrexate is elevated 50% or more above the pre-MTX serum creatinine **or** the serum MTX concentration is >5 x 10⁻⁶ molar (see graph), increase dose to 100 mg/m²/dose every 3 hours until serum methotrexate level is <1 x 10⁻⁸ molar

Investigational: Post I.T. methotrexate: Oral, I.V.: 12 mg/m² as a single dose; post high-dose methotrexate: 100-1000 mg/m²/dose until the serum methotrexate level is less than 1 x 10⁻⁷ molar

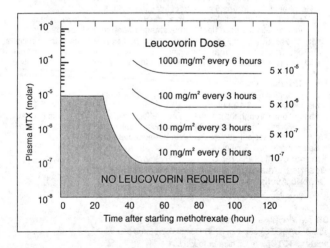

The drug should be given parenterally instead of orally in patients with GI toxicity, nausea, vomiting, and when individual doses are >25 mg

Mechanism of Action A reduced form of folic acid, but does not require a reduction reaction by an enzyme for activation, allows for purine and thymidine synthesis, a necessity for normal erythropoiesis; leucovorin supplies the necessary cofactor blocked by MTX, enters the cells via the same active transport system as MTX

Local Anesthetic/Vasoconstrictor Precautions No information available to require special precautions

Effects on Dental Treatment No effects or complications reported

Other Adverse Effects <1%:

Dermatologic: Rash, pruritus, erythema, urticaria

Hematologic: Thrombocytosis

Respiratory: Wheezing
Drug Uptake
  Onset of activity:
    Oral: Within 30 minutes
    I.V.: Within 5 minutes
  Absorption: Oral, I.M.: Rapid
  Serum half-life:
    Leucovorin: 15 minutes
    5MTHF: 33-35 minutes
Pregnancy Risk Factor C
Generic Available Yes
Comments Drug should be given parenterally instead of orally in patients with GI toxicity, nausea, vomiting, and when individual doses are >25 mg

Leucovorin Calcium *see Leucovorin on previous page*

Leukeran® *see Chlorambucil on page 208*

Leukine™ *see Sargramostim on page 857*

Leuprolide Acetate (loo PROE lide AS e tate)
Brand Names Lupron®; Lupron® Depot; Lupron® Depot-Ped
Canadian/Mexican Brand Names Lucrin Depot (Mexico); Lucrin (Mexico)
Therapeutic Category Antineoplastic Agent, Hormone (Gonadotropin Hormone-Releasing Antigen); Gonadotropin Releasing Hormone Analog
Synonyms Leuprorelin Acetate
Use Treatment of precocious puberty; palliative treatment of advanced prostate carcinoma
Usual Dosage Requires parenteral administration
  Children: Precocious puberty:
    S.C.: 20-45 mcg/kg/day
    I.M. (Depot®) formulation: 0.3 mg/kg/dose given every 28 days
      ≤25 kg: 7.5 mg
      >25-37.5 kg: 11.25 mg
      >37.5 kg: 15 mg
  Adults:
    Male: Advanced prostatic carcinoma:
      S.C.: 1 mg/day **or**
      I.M., Depot® (suspension): 7.5 mg/dose given monthly (every 28-33 days)
    Female: Endometriosis: I.M., Depot® (suspension): 3.75 mg monthly for up to 6 months
Mechanism of Action Continuous daily administration results in suppression of ovarian and testicular steroidogenesis due to decreased levels of LH and FSH with subsequent decrease in testosterone (male) and estrogen (female) levels
Local Anesthetic/Vasoconstrictor Precautions No information available to require special precautions
Effects on Dental Treatment No effects or complications reported
Other Adverse Effects
  >10%:
    Central nervous system: Depression, pain
    Endocrine & metabolic: Hot flashes
    Gastrointestinal: Weight gain, nausea, vomiting
  1% to 10%:
    Cardiovascular: Cardiac arrhythmias, edema
    Central nervous system: Dizziness, lethargy, insomnia, headache
    Dermatologic: Rash
    Endocrine & metabolic: Estrogenic effects (gynecomastia, breast tenderness)
    Gastrointestinal: Diarrhea, GI bleed
    Hematologic: Decreased hemoglobin and hematocrit
    Neuromuscular & skeletal: Paresthesia, myalgia
    Ocular: Blurred vision
  <1%:
    Cardiovascular: Myocardial infarction
    Local: Thrombophlebitis
    Respiratory: Pulmonary embolism
Drug Uptake
  Onset of action: Serum testosterone levels first increase within 3 days of therapy
  Duration: Levels decrease after 2-4 weeks with continued therapy
  Serum half-life: 3-4.25 hours
Pregnancy Risk Factor X
Generic Available No
Comments Has the advantage of not increasing risk of atherosclerotic vascular disease, causing swelling of breasts, fluid retention, and thromboembolism as compared to estrogen therapy

Leuprorelin Acetate *see* Leuprolide Acetate *on previous page*

Leurocristine *see* Vincristine *on page 990*

Leustatin™ *see* Cladribine *on page 239*

Levamisole (lee VAM i sole)

Brand Names Ergamisol®

Therapeutic Category Immune Modulator

Use Adjuvant treatment with fluorouracil in Dukes stage C colon cancer

Usual Dosage Adults: Oral: Initial: 50 mg every 8 hours for 3 days, then 50 mg every 8 hours for 3 days every 2 weeks (fluorouracil is always given concomitantly)

Mechanism of Action Clinically, combined therapy with levamisole and 5-fluorouracil has been effective in treating colon cancer patients, whereas demonstrable activity has been. Due to the broad range of pharmacologic activities of levamisole, it has been suggested that the drug may act as a biochemical modulator (of fluorouracil, for example, in colon cancer), an effect entirely independent of immune modulation. Further studies are needed to evaluate the mechanisms of action of the drug in cancer patients.

Local Anesthetic/Vasoconstrictor Precautions No information available to require special precautions

Effects on Dental Treatment No effects or complications reported

Other Adverse Effects

>10%: Gastrointestinal: Nausea, diarrhea

1% to 10%:

Cardiovascular: Edema

Central nervous system: Fatigue, fever, dizziness, headache, somnolence, depression, nervousness, insomnia

Dermatologic: Dermatitis, alopecia

Gastrointestinal: Stomatitis, vomiting, anorexia, abdominal pain, constipation, taste perversion

Hematologic: Leukopenia

Neuromuscular & skeletal: Rigors, arthralgia, myalgia, paresthesia

Miscellaneous: Infection

<1%:

Cardiovascular: Chest pain

Central nervous system: Anxiety

Dermatologic: Pruritus, urticaria

Gastrointestinal: Flatulence, dyspepsia

Hematologic: Thrombocytopenia, anemia, granulocytopenia

Ocular: Abnormal tearing, blurred vision, conjunctivitis

Respiratory: Epistaxis

Miscellaneous: Altered sense of smell

Drug Uptake

Absorption: Well absorbed

Half-life, elimination: 2-6 hours

Time to peak serum concentration: 1-2 hours

Pregnancy Risk Factor C

Generic Available No

Comments Should not be used at dose exceeding the recommended dose or frequency due to increasing adverse reactions

Levaquin® *see* Levofloxacin *on page 549*

Levarterenol Bitartrate *see* Norepinephrine *on page 689*

Levatol® *see* Penbutolol *on page 729*

Levbid® *see* Hyoscyamine *on page 492*

Levlen® *see* Ethinyl Estradiol and Levonorgestrel *on page 377*

Levobunolol (lee voe BYOO noe lole)

Brand Names AKBeta®; Betagan®

Therapeutic Category Antiglaucoma Agent; Beta-Adrenergic Blocker, Ophthalmic

Use To lower intraocular pressure in chronic open-angle glaucoma or ocular hypertension

Usual Dosage Adults: Instill 1 drop in the affected eye(s) 1-2 times/day

Mechanism of Action A nonselective beta-adrenergic blocking agent that lowers intraocular pressure by reducing aqueous humor production and possibly increases the outflow of aqueous humor

Local Anesthetic/Vasoconstrictor Precautions No information available to require special precautions

Effects on Dental Treatment No effects or complications reported

Other Adverse Effects
>10%: Ocular: Stinging/burning of eye
1% to 10%:
Cardiovascular: Bradycardia, arrhythmia, hypotension
Central nervous system: Dizziness, headache
Dermatologic: Alopecia, erythema
Local: Stinging, burning
Ocular: Blepharoconjunctivitis, conjunctivitis
Respiratory: Bronchospasm
<1%:
Dermatologic: Skin rash
Local: Itching
Ocular: Visual disturbances, keratitis, decreased visual acuity

Drug Interactions
Increased toxicity:
Systemic beta-adrenergic blocking agents
Ophthalmic epinephrine (increased blood pressure/loss of IOP effect)
Quinidine (sinus bradycardia)
Verapamil (bradycardia and asystole have been reported)

Drug Uptake
Onset of action: Decreases in intraocular pressure (IOP) can be noted within 1 hour
Peak effect: 2-6 hours
Duration: 1-7 days

Pregnancy Risk Factor C
Generic Available Yes

Levocabastine (LEE voe kab as teen)

Brand Names Livostin®
Canadian/Mexican Brand Names Livostin® Nasal (Mexico); Livostin® Oftalmico (Mexico)
Therapeutic Category Ophthalmic Agent, Miscellaneous
Use Treatment of allergic conjunctivitis
Usual Dosage Children >12 years and Adults: Instill 1 drop in affected eye(s) 4 times/day for up to 2 weeks
Mechanism of Action Potent, selective histamine H_1-receptor antagonist for topical ophthalmic use
Local Anesthetic/Vasoconstrictor Precautions No information available to require special precautions
Effects on Dental Treatment No effects or complications reported
Other Adverse Effects
>10%: Local: Transient burning, stinging, discomfort
1% to 10%:
Central nervous system: Headache, somnolence, fatigue
Dermatologic: Rash
Gastrointestinal: Dry mouth
Ocular: Blurred vision, eye pain, red eyes, eyelid edema
Respiratory: Dyspnea
Drug Interactions No data reported
Drug Uptake Absorption: Topical: Systemically absorbed
Pregnancy Risk Factor B
Dosage Forms Suspension, ophthalmic, as hydrochloride: 0.05% (2.5 mL, 5 mL, 10 mL)
Generic Available No

Levocarnitine (lee voe KAR ni teen)

Brand Names Carnitor® Injection; Carnitor® Oral; VitaCarn® Oral
Therapeutic Category Dietary Supplement
Synonyms L-Carnitine
Use Treatment of primary or secondary carnitine deficiency
Local Anesthetic/Vasoconstrictor Precautions No information available to require special precautions
Effects on Dental Treatment No effects or complications reported
Pregnancy Risk Factor B
Generic Available Yes
Comments Tolerance may be improved by mixing the product with liquids or food and spacing doses evenly throughout the day with meals

Levodopa (lee voe DOE pa)

Brand Names Dopar®; Larodopa®
Therapeutic Category Anti-Parkinson's Agent
(Continued)

Levodopa *(Continued)*

Use Treatment of Parkinson's disease; used as a diagnostic agent for growth hormone deficiency

Usual Dosage Oral:

Children (give as a single dose to evaluate growth hormone deficiency):

0.5 g/m^2 **or**

<30 lb: 125 mg

30-70 lb: 250 mg

>70 lb: 500 mg

Adults: 500-1000 mg/day in divided doses every 6-12 hours; increase by 100-750 mg/day every 3-7 days until response or total dose of 8,000 mg is reached

A significant therapeutic response may not be obtained for 6 months

Mechanism of Action Increases dopamine levels in the brain, then stimulates dopaminergic receptors in the basal ganglia to improve the balance between cholinergic and dopaminergic activity

Local Anesthetic/Vasoconstrictor Precautions No information available to require special precautions

Effects on Dental Treatment No effects or complications reported

Other Adverse Effects

>10%:

Cardiovascular: Orthostatic hypotension, arrhythmias

Central nervous system: Dizziness, anxiety, confusion, nightmares

Gastrointestinal: Anorexia, nausea, vomiting, constipation

Genitourinary: Dysuria

Neuromuscular & skeletal: Choreiform and involuntary movements

Ocular: Blepharospasm

1% to 10%:

Central nervous system: Headache

Gastrointestinal: Diarrhea, dry mouth

Genitourinary: Discoloration of urine

Neuromuscular & skeletal: Muscle twitching

Ocular: Eyelid spasms

Miscellaneous: Discoloration of sweat

<1%:

Cardiovascular: Hypertension

Gastrointestinal: Duodenal ulcer, GI bleeding

Hematologic: Hemolytic anemia

Ocular: Blurred vision

Drug Interactions

Decreased effect:

Hydantoins cause decreased effectiveness of levodopa

Phenothiazines and hypotensive agents cause decreased effect of levodopa

Pyridoxine causes increased peripheral conversion, causing decreased levodopa effectiveness

Increased toxicity:

Monoamine oxidase inhibitors may increase hypertensive reactions

Antacids cause increased levodopa

Drug Uptake

Time to peak serum concentration: Oral: 1-2 hours

Serum half-life: 1.2-2.3 hours

Pregnancy Risk Factor C

Generic Available No

Levodopa and Carbidopa *(lee voe DOE pa & kar bi DOE pa)*

Brand Names Sinemet®

Canadian/Mexican Brand Names Racovel® (Mexico)

Therapeutic Category Anti-Parkinson's Agent

Use Treatment of parkinsonian syndrome; 50-100 mg/day of carbidopa is needed to block the peripheral conversion of levodopa to dopamine. "On-off" can be managed by giving smaller, more frequent doses of Sinemet® or adding a dopamine agonist or selegiline; when adding a new agent, doses of Sinemet® should usually be decreased.

Usual Dosage Oral:

Adults: Initial: 25/100 2-4 times/day, increase as necessary to a maximum of 200/2000 mg/day

Elderly: Initial: 25/100 twice daily, increase as necessary

Conversion from Sinemet® to Sinemet® CR (50/200): (Sinemet® [total daily dose of levodopa] / Sinemet® CR)

300-400 mg / 1 tablet twice daily

500-600 mg / 1½ tablets twice daily or one 3 times/day

700-800 mg / 4 tablets in 3 or more divided doses
900-1000 mg / 5 tablets in 3 or more divided doses
Intervals between doses of Sinemet® CR should be 4-8 hours while awake

Mechanism of Action Parkinson's symptoms are due to a lack of striatal dopamine; levodopa circulates in the plasma to the blood-brain-barrier (BBB), where it crosses, to be converted by striatal enzymes to dopamine; carbidopa inhibits the peripheral plasma breakdown of levodopa by inhibiting its decarboxylation, and thereby increases available levodopa at the BBB

Local Anesthetic/Vasoconstrictor Precautions No information available to require special precautions

Effects on Dental Treatment No effects or complications reported

Other Adverse Effects

>10%:
Cardiovascular: Orthostatic hypotension, palpitations, cardiac arrhythmias
Central nervous system: Confusion, nightmares, dizziness, anxiety
Gastrointestinal: Nausea, vomiting, anorexia, constipation
Genitourinary: Dysuria
Neuromuscular & skeletal: Dystonic movements, "on-off", choreiform and involuntary movements
Ocular: Blepharospasm

1% to 10%:
Central nervous system: Headache
Gastrointestinal: Diarrhea, dry mouth
Genitourinary: Discoloration of urine
Neuromuscular & skeletal: Muscle twitching
Ocular: Eyelid spasms
Miscellaneous: Discoloration of sweat

<1%:
Cardiovascular: Hypertension
Central nervous system: Memory loss, nervousness, insomnia, fatigue, hallucinations, ataxia
Gastrointestinal: Duodenal ulcer, GI bleeding
Hematologic: Hemolytic anemia
Ocular: Blurred vision

Drug Interactions

Decreased effect:
Hydantoins cause decreased effectiveness
Phenothiazines and hypotensive agents cause decreased effect of levodopa
Increased toxicity: Monoamine oxidase inhibitors may increase hypertensive reactions

Drug Uptake

Carbidopa:
Absorption: Oral: 40% to 70%
Serum half-life: 1-2 hours

Levodopa:
Absorption: May be decreased if given with a high protein meal
Serum half-life: 1.2-2.3 hours

Pregnancy Risk Factor C

Generic Available Yes

Levo-Dromoran® *see* Levorphanol *on page 551*

Levofloxacin (lee voe FLOKS a sin)

Brand Names Levaquin®

Therapeutic Category Antibiotic, Quinolone

Use Treatment of bacterial respiratory tract infections

Usual Dosage Adults: Oral, I.V. (infuse I.V. solution over 60 minutes):
Acute bacterial exacerbation of chronic bronchitis: 500 mg every 24 hours for at least 7 days
Community acquired pneumonia: 500 mg every 24 hours for 7-14 days
Acute maxillary sinusitis: 500 mg every 24 hours for 10-14 days
Uncomplicated skin infections: 500 mg every 24 hours for 7-10 days
Complicated urinary tract infections include acute pyelonephritis: 250 mg every 24 hours for 10 days

Mechanism of Action As the S (-) enantiomer of the fluoroquinolone, ofloxacin, levofloxacin, inhibits DNA-gyrase in susceptible organisms; inhibits relaxation of supercoiled DNA and promotes breakage of double-stranded DNA

Local Anesthetic/Vasoconstrictor Precautions No information available to require special precautions

Effects on Dental Treatment No effects or complications reported
(Continued)

Levofloxacin (Continued)

Other Adverse Effects
>1%:
Central nervous system: Dizziness, headache, insomnia
Dermatologic: Rash
Gastrointestinal: Nausea, vomiting, increased transaminases
Hematologic: Leukopenia, thrombocytopenia
Neuromuscular & skeletal: Tremor, arthralgia

Warnings/Precautions Not recommended in children <18 years of age; other quinolones have caused transient arthropathy in children; CNS stimulation may occur (tremor, restlessness, confusion, and very rarely hallucinations or seizures); use with caution in patients with known or suspected CNS disorders or renal dysfunction; prolonged use may result in superinfection; if an allergic reaction (itching, urticaria, dyspnea, pharyngeal or facial edema, loss of consciousness, tingling, cardiovascular collapse) occurs, discontinue the drug immediately; use caution to avoid possible photosensitivity reactions during and for several days following fluoroquinolone therapy; pseudomembranous colitis may occur and should be considered in patients who present with diarrhea

Drug Interactions
Decreased effect: Decreased absorption with antacids containing aluminum, magnesium, and/or calcium (by up to 98% if given at the same time); phenytoin serum levels may be reduced by quinolones; antineoplastic agents may also decrease serum levels of fluoroquinolones
Increased toxicity/serum levels: Quinolones cause increased levels of caffeine, warfarin, azlocillin, cyclosporine, and theophylline (one study indicates no effect on theophylline metabolism); azlocillin, cimetidine, and probenecid increases quinolone levels; an increased incidence of seizures may occur with foscarnet

Drug Uptake
Absorption: Well absorbed
Serum half-life: 6 hours
Time to peak serum concentration: 1 hour

Pregnancy Risk Factor C

Generic Available No

Levomepromazine see Methotrimeprazine on page 617

Levomethadyl Acetate Hydrochloride
(lee voe METH a dil AS e tate hye droe KLOR ide)

Brand Names ORLAAM®

Therapeutic Category Analgesic, Narcotic

Use Management of opiate dependence

Usual Dosage Adults: Oral: 20-40 mg 3 times/week, with ranges of 10 mg to as high as 140 mg 3 times/week; always dilute before administration and mix with diluent prior to dispensing

Local Anesthetic/Vasoconstrictor Precautions No information available to require special precautions

Effects on Dental Treatment No effects or complications reported

Other Adverse Effects
>10%:
Cardiovascular: Bradycardia, hypotension
Central nervous system: Drowsiness
Gastrointestinal: Nausea, vomiting
Respiratory: Respiratory depression
1% to 10%:
Cardiovascular: Peripheral vasodilation, orthostatic hypotension
Central nervous system: Dizziness/vertigo, CNS depression, confusion, sedation, increased intracranial pressure
Endocrine & metabolic: Antidiuretic hormone release
Gastrointestinal: Constipation, biliary spasm
Genitourinary: Urinary tract spasm
Ocular: Miosis, blurred vision

Drug Interactions Decreased effect/levels with phenobarbital

Pregnancy Risk Factor C

Dosage Forms Solution, oral: 10 mg/mL (474 mL)

Generic Available No

Levonorgestrel (LEE voe nor jes trel)

Related Information
Endocrine Disorders & Pregnancy on page 1021

Brand Names Norplant® Implant

Canadian/Mexican Brand Names Microlut® (Mexico)

Therapeutic Category Contraceptive, Implant; Contraceptive, Progestin Only; Progestin

Use Prevention of pregnancy. The net cumulative 5 year pregnancy rate for levonorgestrel implant use has been reported to be from 1.5-3.9 pregnancies/100 users. Norplant® is a very efficient, yet reversible, method of contraception. The long duration of action may be particularly advantageous in women who desire an extended period of contraceptive protection without sacrificing the possibility of future fertility.

Usual Dosage Total administration doses (implanted): 216 mg in 6 capsules which should be implanted during the first 7 days of onset of menses subdermally in the upper arm; each Norplant® silastic capsule releases 80 mcg of drug/day for 6-18 months, following which a rate of release of 25-30 mcg/day is maintained for ≤5 years; capsules should be removed by end of 5th year

Mechanism of Action Ovulation is inhibited in about 50% to 60% of implant users from a negative feedback mechanism on the hypothalamus, leading to reduced secretion of follicle stimulating hormone (FSH) and luteinizing hormone (LH). An insufficient luteal phase has also been demonstrated with levonorgestrel administration and may result from defective gonadotropin stimulation of the ovary or from a direct effect of the drug on progesterone synthesis by the corpora lutea.

Local Anesthetic/Vasoconstrictor Precautions No information available to require special precautions

Effects on Dental Treatment Progestins may predispose the patient to gingival bleeding

Other Adverse Effects
>10%: Endocrine & metabolic: Prolonged menstrual flow, spotting
1% to 10%:
  Central nervous system: Headache, nervousness, dizziness
  Dermatologic: Dermatitis, acne
  Endocrine & metabolic: Amenorrhea, irregular menstrual cycles, scanty bleeding, breast discharge
  Gastrointestinal: Nausea, change in appetite, weight gain
  Genitourinary: Vaginitis, leukorrhea
  Local: Pain or itching at implant site
  Neuromuscular & skeletal: Myalgia
<1%: Miscellaneous: Infection at implant site

Drug Interactions Decreased effect: Carbamazepine/phenytoin

Drug Uptake
Serum half-life, terminal: 11-45 hours

Pregnancy Risk Factor X

Generic Available No

Levophed® Injection see Norepinephrine on page 689

Levoprome® see Methotrimeprazine on page 617

Levora® see Ethinyl Estradiol and Levonorgestrel on page 377

Levorphanol (lee VOR fa nole)

Related Information
Narcotic Agonists on page 1141

Brand Names Levo-Dromoran®

Therapeutic Category Analgesic, Narcotic

Use Relief of moderate to severe pain; also used parenterally for preoperative sedation and an adjunct to nitrous oxide/oxygen anesthesia; 2 mg levorphanol produces analgesia comparable to that produced by 10 mg of morphine

Usual Dosage Adults:
Oral: 2 mg every 6-24 hours as needed
S.C.: 2 mg, up to 3 mg if necessary, every 6-8 hours

Mechanism of Action Levorphanol tartrate is a synthetic opioid agonist that is classified as a morphinan derivative. Opioids interact with stereospecific opioid receptors in various parts of the central nervous system and other tissues. Analgesic potency parallels the affinity for these binding sites. These drugs do not alter the threshold or responsiveness to pain, but the perception of pain.

Local Anesthetic/Vasoconstrictor Precautions No information available to require special precautions

Effects on Dental Treatment ~10% of patients experience dry mouth (will disappear with cessation of therapy)

Other Adverse Effects
>10%:
  Cardiovascular: Palpitations, hypotension, bradycardia, peripheral vasodilation
  Central nervous system: CNS depression, fatigue, drowsiness, dizziness
  Dermatologic: Pruritus
  Gastrointestinal: Nausea, vomiting
(Continued)

Levorphanol (Continued)

Neuromuscular & skeletal: Weakness

1% to 10%:

Central nervous system: Nervousness, headache, restlessness, anorexia, malaise, confusion

Endocrine & metabolic: Antidiuretic hormone release

Gastrointestinal: Stomach cramps, constipation, biliary spasm

Genitourinary: Decreased urination, urinary tract spasm

Local: Pain at injection site

Ocular: Miosis

Respiratory: Respiratory depression

<1%:

Central nervous system: Mental depression, hallucinations, paradoxical CNS stimulation, increased intracranial pressure

Dermatologic: Skin rash, urticaria

Gastrointestinal: Paralytic ileus

Miscellaneous: Physical and psychological dependence, histamine release

Drug Interactions Increased toxicity: CNS depressants increased CNS depression

Pregnancy Risk Factor B (D if used for prolonged periods or in high doses at term)

Generic Available No

Levo-T™ see Levothyroxine on this page

Levothroid® see Levothyroxine on this page

Levothyroxine (lee voe thye ROKS een)

Related Information

Endocrine Disorders & Pregnancy on page 1021

Brand Names Eltroxin™; Levo-T™; Levothroid®; Levoxyl™; Synthroid®

Canadian/Mexican Brand Names Eltroxin® (Canada); Eutirox® (Mexico); PMS-Levothyroxine® Sodium (Canada); Tiroidine® (Mexico)

Therapeutic Category Thyroid Product

Synonyms Levotiroxina (Mexico)

Use Replacement or supplemental therapy in hypothyroidism; some clinicians suggest levothyroxine is the drug of choice for replacement therapy

Usual Dosage

Children:

Oral:

0-6 months: 8-10 mcg/kg/day **or** 25-50 mcg/day

6-12 months: 6-8 mcg/kg/day **or** 50-75 mcg/day

1-5 years: 5-6 mcg/kg/day **or** 75-100 mcg/day

6-12 years: 4-5 mcg/kg/day **or** 100-150 mcg/day

>12 years: 2-3 mcg/kg/day **or** ≥150 mcg/day

I.M., I.V.: 50% to 75% of the oral dose

Adults:

Oral: 12.5-50 mcg/day to start, then increase by 25-50 mcg/day at intervals of 2-4 weeks; average adult dose: 100-200 mcg/day

I.M., I.V.: 50% of the oral dose

Myxedema coma or stupor: I.V.: 200-500 mcg one time, then 100-300 mcg the next day if necessary

Thyroid suppression therapy: Oral: 2-6 mcg/kg/day for 7-10 days

Mechanism of Action Exact mechanism of action is unknown; however, it is believed the thyroid hormone exerts its many metabolic effects through control of DNA transcription and protein synthesis; involved in normal metabolism, growth, and development; promotes gluconeogenesis, increases utilization and mobilization of glycogen stores, and stimulates protein synthesis, increases basal metabolic rate

Local Anesthetic/Vasoconstrictor Precautions No precautions with vasoconstrictor are necessary if patient is well controlled with levothyroxine

Effects on Dental Treatment No effects or complications reported

Other Adverse Effects <1%:

Cardiovascular: Palpitations, cardiac arrhythmias, tachycardia, chest pain

Central nervous system: Nervousness, headache, insomnia, fever, clumsiness

Dermatologic: Alopecia

Endocrine: Changes in menstrual cycle

Gastrointestinal: Weight loss, increased appetite, diarrhea, abdominal cramps, constipation

Neuromuscular & skeletal: Myalgia, hand tremors, tremor

Respiratory: Dyspnea

Miscellaneous: Sweating

Drug Interactions
Decreased effect:
Phenytoin may decreased levothyroxine levels
Cholestyramine may decreased absorption of levothyroxine
Increases oral hypoglycemic requirements
Increased effect: Increased effects of oral anticoagulants
Increased toxicity: Tricyclic antidepressants cause increased toxic potential of both drugs

Drug Uptake
Onset of therapeutic effect:
Oral: 3-5 days
I.V. Within 6-8 hours
Peak effect: I.V.: Within 24 hours
Absorption: Oral: Erratic
Time to peak serum concentration: 2-4 hours

Pregnancy Risk Factor A
Generic Available Yes

Levotiroxina (Mexico) see Levothyroxine on previous page

Levoxyl™ see Levothyroxine on previous page

Levsin® see Hyoscyamine on page 492

Levsinex® see Hyoscyamine on page 492

Levsin/SL® see Hyoscyamine on page 492

Levulose, Dextrose and Phosphoric Acid see Phosphorated Carbohydrate Solution on page 757

Lexxel® see Enalapril and Felodipine on page 348

Librax® see Clidinium and Chlordiazepoxide on page 243

Libritabs® see Chlordiazepoxide on page 210

Librium® see Chlordiazepoxide on page 210

Lice-Enz® Shampoo [OTC] see Pyrethrins on page 824

Lida-Mantle HC® Topical see Lidocaine and Hydrocortisone on page 555

Lidex® see Fluocinonide on page 415

Lidex-E® see Fluocinonide on page 415

Lidocaine (LYE doe kane)

Related Information
Cardiovascular Diseases on page 1010
Oral Pain on page 1053
Oral Viral Infections on page 1066
Patients Undergoing Cancer Therapy on page 1083

Brand Names Dilocaine®; Duo-Trach®; Nervocaine®; Octocaine®; Xylocaine®

Canadian/Mexican Brand Names Pisacina® (Mexico); PMS-Lidocaine Viscous (Canada); Xylocaina® (Mexico); Xylocard® (Canada)

Therapeutic Category Antiarrhythmic Agent (Supraventricular & Ventricular); Dental/Local Anesthetics; Local Anesthetic, Injectable

Use
Dental: Amide-type injectable local anesthetic and topical local anesthetic; Patch: Production of mild topical anesthesia of accessible mucous membranes of the mouth prior to superficial dental procedures
Medical: Drug of choice for ventricular ectopy, ventricular tachycardia, ventricular fibrillation; for pulseless VT or VF preferably give **after** defibrillation and epinephrine; control of premature ventricular contractions, wide-complex PSVT

Usual Dosage Dental anesthetic, infiltration, or conduction block: Do not exceed 6.6 mg/kg of body weight or 300 mg/dental appointment. A 2% solution of lidocaine hydrochloride provides 20 mg of anesthetic per mL. The effective anesthetic dose varies with procedure, intensity of anesthesia needed, duration of anesthesia required, and physical condition of the patient. Always use the lowest effective dose along with careful aspiration.

Note: Maximum dose for lidocaine hydrochloride cited from USP Dispensing Information (USP DI) 17th ed, The United Pharmacopeial Convention, Inc, Rockville, MD, 1997, 137.

Mechanism of Action Class IB antiarrhythmic; local anesthetics bind selectively to the intracellular surface of sodium channels to block influx of sodium into the axon. As a result, depolarization necessary for action potential propagation and subsequent nerve function is prevented. The block at the sodium channel is reversible. When drug diffuses away from the axon, sodium channel function is restored and nerve propagation returns.

Local Anesthetic/Vasoconstrictor Precautions No information available to require special precautions

Effects on Dental Treatment No effects or complications reported
(Continued)

Lidocaine *(Continued)*

Other Adverse Effects No data reported

Contraindications Known hypersensitivity to amide-type local anesthetics; patients with Adams-Stokes syndrome or with severe degree of S-A, A-V, or intraventricular heart block (without a pacemaker)

Drug Interactions No data reported

Pregnancy Risk Factor C

Breast-feeding Considerations May be taken while breast-feeding

Dosage Forms
Injection: 0.5% [5 mg/mL] (50 mL); 1% [10 mg/mL] (2 mL, 5 mL, 10 mL, 20 mL, 30 mL, 50 mL); 1.5% [15 mg/mL] (20 mL); 2% [20 mg/mL] (2 mL, 5 mL, 10 mL, 20 mL, 30 mL, 50 mL); 4% [40 mg/mL] (5 mL)
Liquid, viscous: 2% (20 mL, 100 mL)

Generic Available Yes

Comments Lidocaine without epinephrine is not marketed as a dental 1.8 mL carpule and as such is not used as a dental local anesthetic

Lidocaine and Epinephrine (LYE doe kane & ep i NEF rin)

Related Information
Oral Pain *on page 1053*

Brand Names Octocaine® 50; Octocaine® 100; Xylocaine® With Epinephrine

Canadian/Mexican Brand Names Pisacaina® (Mexico); Uvega® (Mexico); Xylocaina® (Mexico)

Therapeutic Category Dental/Local Anesthetics; Local Anesthetic, Injectable

Use Dental: Amide-type anesthetic used for local infiltration anesthesia; injection near nerve trunks to produce nerve block

Usual Dosage
Children <10 years: Dental anesthesia, infiltration, or conduction block: 20-30 mg (1-1.5 mL) of lidocaine hydrochloride as a 2% solution with epinephrine 1:100,000; maximum: 4-5 mg of lidocaine hydrochloride/kg of body weight or 100-150 mg as a single dose

Children >10 years and Adults: Dental anesthesia, infiltration, or conduction block: Do not exceed 6.6 mg/kg body weight or 300 mg of lidocaine hydrochloride and 3 mcg (0.003 mg) of epinephrine/kg of body weight or 0.2 mg epinephrine per dental appointment. The effective anesthetic dose varies with procedure, intensity of anesthesia needed, duration of anesthesia required, and physical condition of the patient. Always use the lowest effective dose along with careful aspiration. The following numbers of dental carpules (1.8 mL) provide the indicated amounts of lidocaine hydrochloride 2% and epinephrine 1:100,000.

For most routine dental procedures, lidocaine hydrochloride 2% with epinephrine 1:100,000 is preferred. When a more pronounced hemostasis is required, a 1:50,000 epinephrine concentration should be used. The following numbers of dental carpules (1.8 mL) provide the indicated amounts of lidocaine hydrochloride 2% and epinephrine 1:50,000.

# of Cartridges	Mg Lidocaine (2%)	Mg Vasoconstrictor (Epinephrine 1:50,000)
1	36	0.036
2	72	0.072
3	108	0.108
4	144	0.144
5	180	0.180
6	216	0.216

Note: Adult and children doses of lidocaine hydrochloride and epinephrine cited from USP Dispensing Information (USP DI) 17th ed, The United States Pharmacopeial Convention, Inc, Rockville, MD, 1997, 138-9.

Mechanism of Action Local anesthetics bind selectively to the intracellular surface of sodium channels to block influx of sodium into the axon. As a result, depolarization necessary for action potential propagation and subsequent nerve function is prevented. The block at the sodium channel is reversible. When drug diffuses away from the axon, sodium channel function is restored and nerve propagation returns.

Epinephrine prolongs the duration of the anesthetic actions of lidocaine by causing vasoconstriction (alpha adrenergic receptor agonist) of the vasculature surrounding the nerve axons. This prevents the diffusion of lidocaine away from the nerves resulting in a longer retention in the axon.

Local Anesthetic/Vasoconstrictor Precautions No information available to require special precautions

Effects on Dental Treatment No effects or complications reported

Other Adverse Effects Degree of adverse effects in the central nervous system and cardiovascular system are directly related to the blood levels of lidocaine. The effects below are more likely to occur after systemic administration rather than infiltration.

Cardiovascular: Myocardial effects include a decrease in contraction force as well as a decrease in electrical excitability and myocardial conduction rate resulting in bradycardia and reduction in cardiac output.

Central nervous system: High blood levels result in anxiety, restlessness, disorientation, confusion, dizziness, tremors and seizures. This is followed by depression of CNS resulting in somnolence, unconsciousness and possible respiratory arrest. In some cases, symptoms of CNS stimulation may be absent and the primary CNS effects are somnolence and unconsciousness.

Gastrointestinal: Nausea and vomiting may occur

Hypersensitivity reactions: Extremely rare, but may be manifest as dermatologic reactions and edema at injection site. Asthmatic syndromes have occurred. Patients may exhibit hypersensitivity to bisulfites contained in local anesthetic solution to prevent oxidation of epinephrine. In general, patients reacting to bisulfites have a history of asthma and their airways are hyper-reactive to asthmatic syndrome.

Psychogenic reactions: It is common to misinterpret psychogenic responses to local anesthetic injection as an allergic reaction. Intraoral injections are perceived by many patients as a stressful procedure in dentistry. Common symptoms to this stress are sweating, palpitations, hyperventilation, generalized pallor and a fainting feeling

Contraindications Hypersensitivity to local anesthetics of the amide-type

Warnings/Precautions Should be avoided in patients with uncontrolled hyperthyroidism. Should be used in minimal amounts in patients with significant cardiovascular problems (because of epinephrine component). Aspirate the syringe after tissue penetration and before injection to minimize chance of direct vascular injection.

Drug Interactions Due to epinephrine component, use with tricyclic antidepressants or MAO inhibitors could result in increased pressor response; use with nonselective beta-blockers (ie, propranolol) could result in serious hypertension and reflex bradycardia

Drug Uptake

Onset of action: Infiltration less than 2 minutes; nerve block 2-4 minutes

Duration after infiltration: Soft tissue anesthesia ~2.5 hours; pulp anesthesia <60 minutes

Duration after nerve block: Soft tissue anesthesia ~3.25 hours; pulp anesthesia at least 90 minutes

Pregnancy Risk Factor B

Breast-feeding Considerations Usual infiltration doses of lidocaine with epinephrine given to nursing mothers has not been shown to affect the health of the nursing infant

Dosage Forms Injection:

Lidocaine Hydrochloride 2% with epinephrine 1:100,000 (Octocaine® 100, Xylocaine®): (1.8 mL dental cartridges)

Lidocaine Hydrochloride 2% with epinephrine 1:50,000 (Octocaine® 50, Xylocaine®): (1.8 mL dental cartridges)

Dietary Considerations No data reported

Generic Available Yes

Selected Readings
Jastak JT and Yagiela JA, "Vasoconstrictors and Local Anesthesia: A Review and Rationale for Use," J Am Dent Assoc, 1983, 107(4):623-30.
MacKenzie TA and Young ER, "Local Anesthetic Update," Anesth Prog, 1993, 40(2):29-34.
Wynn RL, "Epinephrine Interactions With Beta-Blockers," Gen Dent, 1994, 42(1):16, 18.
Wynn RL, "Recent Research on Mechanisms of Local Anesthetics," Gen Dent, 1995, 43(4):316-8.
Yagiela JA, "Local Anesthetics," Anesth Prog, 1991, 38(4-5):128-41.

Lidocaine and Hydrocortisone

(LYE doe kane & hye droe KOR ti sone)

Brand Names Lida-Mantle HC® Topical

Therapeutic Category Corticosteroid, Topical (Low Potency); Local Anesthetic, Topical

Use Topical anti-inflammatory and anesthetic for skin disorders

Local Anesthetic/Vasoconstrictor Precautions No information available to require special precautions

Effects on Dental Treatment No effects or complications reported

Generic Available No

Lidocaine and Prilocaine (LYE doe kane & PRIL oh kane)

Brand Names EMLA® Cream; EMLA® Disc

Therapeutic Category Analgesic, Topical; Antipruritic, Topical; Local Anesthetic, Topical

Use

Dental: Amide-type topical anesthetic for use on normal intact skin to provide local analgesia for minor procedures such as I.V. cannulation or venipuncture

Medical: Has also been used for painful procedures such as lumbar puncture and skin graft harvesting; topical anesthetic for local anesthesia on normal skin

Mechanism of Action Local anesthetics bind selectively to the intracellular surface of sodium channels to block influx of sodium into the axon. As a result, depolarization necessary for action potential propagation and subsequent nerve function is prevented. The block at the sodium channel is reversible. When drug diffuses away from the axon, sodium channel function is restored and nerve propagation returns.

Local Anesthetic/Vasoconstrictor Precautions No information available to require special precautions

Effects on Dental Treatment No effects or complications reported

Other Adverse Effects 1% to 10%:

Dermatologic: Angioedema, contact dermatitis

Local: Burning, stinging

Contraindications Known hypersensitivity to lidocaine, prilocaine, any component or local anesthetics of the amide type; patients with congenital or idiopathic methemoglobinemia, infants <1 month of age, infants <12 months of age who are receiving concurrent treatment with methemoglobin-inducing agents (ie, sulfas, acetaminophen, benzocaine, chloroquine, dapsone, nitrofurantoin, nitroglycerin, nitroprusside, phenobarbital, phenytoin)

Warnings/Precautions Use with caution in patients receiving class I antiarrhythmic drugs, since systemic absorption occurs and synergistic toxicity is possible

Drug Interactions Increased toxicity with Class I antiarrhythmic drugs (tocainide, mexiletine) - effects are additive and potentially synergistic and with drugs known to induce methemoglobinemia

Drug Uptake

Absorption: Related to the duration of application and to the area over which it is applied

3-hour application: 3.6% lidocaine and 6.1% prilocaine were absorbed

24-hour application: 16.2% lidocaine and 33.5% prilocaine were absorbed

Onset of action: 1 hour for sufficient dermal analgesia

Peak effect: 2-3 hours

Duration: 1-2 hours after removal of the cream

Serum half-life:

Lidocaine: 65-150 minutes, prolonged with cardiac or hepatic dysfunction

Prilocaine: 10-150 minutes, prolonged in hepatic or renal dysfunction

Pregnancy Risk Factor B

Breast-feeding Considerations Usual infiltration doses of lidocaine and prilocaine given to nursing mothers has not been shown to affect the health of the nursing infant

Dosage Forms

Cream: Lidocaine 2.5% and prilocaine 2.5% [2 Tegaderm® dressings] (5 g, 30 g)

Disc:

Generic Available No

Selected Readings

Vickers ER, Mazbani N, Gerzina TM, et al, "Pharmacokinetics of EMLA Cream 5% Application to Oral Mucosa," *Anesth Prog*, 1997, 44:32-7.

Lidocaine Transoral (LYE doe kane)

Related Information

Oral Pain on page 1053

Brand Names Dentipatch®

Therapeutic Category Local Anesthetic, Transoral

Use Local anesthesia of the oral mucosa prior to oral injections and soft-tissure dental procedures

Usual Dosage One patch on selected area of oral mucosa

Mechanism of Action Blocks both the initiation and conduction of nerve impulses by decreasing the neuronal membrane's permeability to sodium ions, which results in inhibition of depolarization with resultant blockade of conduction

Local Anesthetic/Vasoconstrictor Precautions No information available to require special precautions

Effects on Dental Treatment No effects or complications reported

Other Adverse Effects No data reported

Contraindications Known hypersensitivity to any of its components

Drug Uptake

Onset of action: 2 minutes

Duration of anesthesia after patch application: 45 minutes

Dosage Forms Patch: 23 mg/2 cm², 46.1 mg/2 cm² (50s, 100s)

Generic Available No

Comments The manufacturer· claims Dentipatch® is safe, with "negligible systemic absorption" of lidocaine. The agent is "clinically proven to prevent injection pain from 25-gauge needles that are inserted to the level of the bone."

Selected Readings

Hersh EV, Houpt MI, Cooper SA, et al, "Analgesic Efficacy and Safety of an Intraoral Lidocaine Patch," *J Am Dent Assoc*, 1996, 127(11):1626-34.

Houpt MI, Heins P, Lamster I, et al, "An Evaluation of Intraoral Lidocaine Patches in Reducing Needle-Insertion Pain," *Compendium*, 1997, 4:309-16.

Limbitrol® DS 10-25 *see* Amitriptyline and Chlordiazepoxide *on page 61*

Lincocin® *see* Lincomycin *on this page*

Lincomicina (Mexico) *see* Lincomycin *on this page*

Lincomycin (lin koe MYE sin)

Brand Names Lincocin®

Canadian/Mexican Brand Names Princol® (Mexico)

Therapeutic Category Antibiotic, Macrolide

Synonyms Lincomicina (Mexico)

Use Treatment of susceptible bacterial infections, mainly those caused by streptococci and staphylococci resistant to other agents

Usual Dosage

Children >1 month:

Oral: 30-60 mg/kg/day in divided doses every 8 hours

I.M.: 10 mg/kg every 8-12 hours

I.V.: 10-20 mg/kg/day in divided doses every 8-12 hours

Adults:

Oral: 500 mg every 6-8 hours

I.M.: 600 mg every 12-24 hours

I.V.: 600-1 g every 8-12 hours up to 8 g/day

Mechanism of Action Lincosamide antibiotic which was isolated from a strain of *Streptomyces lincolnensis*; lincomycin, like clindamycin, inhibits bacterial protein synthesis by specifically binding on the 50S subunit and affecting the process of peptide chain initiation. Other macrolide antibiotics (erythromycin) also bind to the 50S subunit. Since only one molecule of antibiotic can bind to a single ribosome, the concomitant use of erythromycin and lincomycin is not recommended.

Local Anesthetic/Vasoconstrictor Precautions No information available to require special precautions

Effects on Dental Treatment No effects or complications reported

Other Adverse Effects

1% to 10%: Gastrointestinal: Nausea, vomiting, diarrhea

<1%:

Cardiovascular: Hypotension

Central nervous system: Vertigo

Dermatologic: Urticaria, rash, Stevens-Johnson syndrome

Gastrointestinal: Pseudomembranous colitis, glossitis, stomatitis, pruritus ani

Genitourinary: Vaginitis

Hematologic: Granulocytopenia, thrombocytopenia, pancytopenia

Hepatic: Elevation of liver enzymes

Local: Sterile abscess at I.M. injection site, thrombophlebitis

Otic: Tinnitus

Drug Interactions

Decreased effect with erythromycin

Increased activity/toxicity of neuromuscular blocking agents

Drug Uptake

Absorption: Oral: ~20% to 30%

Serum half-life, elimination: 2-11.5 hours

Time to peak serum concentration:

Oral: 2-4 hours

I.M.: 1 hour

Pregnancy Risk Factor B

Generic Available No

Lindane (LIN dane)
Brand Names G-well®; Scabene®
Canadian/Mexican Brand Names Herklin® (Mexico); Hexit® (Canada); Kwellada® (Canada); PMS-Lindane® (Canada); Scabisan® Shampoo (Mexico)
Therapeutic Category Antiparasitic Agent, Topical; Pediculocide; Scabicidal Agent; Shampoos
Synonyms Lindano (Mexico)
Use Treatment of scabies (*Sarcoptes scabiei*), *Pediculus capitis* (head lice), and *Pediculus pubis* (crab lice)
Usual Dosage Children and Adults: Topical:

Scabies: Apply a thin layer of lotion or cream and massage it on skin from the neck to the toes (head to toe in infants). For adults, bathe and remove the drug after 8-12 hours; for children, wash off 6-8 hours after application (for infants, wash off 6 hours after application); repeat treatment in 7 days if lice or nits are still present

Pediculosis, capitis and pubis: 15-30 mL of shampoo is applied and lathered for 4-5 minutes; rinse hair thoroughly and comb with a fine tooth comb to remove nits; repeat treatment in 7 days if lice or nits are still present

Mechanism of Action Directly absorbed by parasites and ova through the exoskeleton; stimulates the nervous system resulting in seizures and death of parasitic arthropods
Local Anesthetic/Vasoconstrictor Precautions No information available to require special precautions
Effects on Dental Treatment No effects or complications reported
Other Adverse Effects <1%:
Cardiovascular: Cardiac arrhythmia
Central nervous system: Dizziness, restlessness, seizures, headache, ataxia
Dermatologic: Eczematous eruptions, contact dermatitis, skin and adipose tissue may act as repositories
Gastrointestinal: Nausea, vomiting
Hematologic: Aplastic anemia
Hepatic: Hepatitis
Local: Burning and stinging
Renal: Hematuria
Respiratory: Pulmonary edema
Drug Interactions Increased toxicity: Oil-based hair dressing may increase toxic potential
Drug Uptake
Absorption: Systemic absorption of up to 13% may occur
Serum half-life: Children: 17-22 hours
Time to peak serum concentration: Topical: Children: 6 hours
Pregnancy Risk Factor B
Generic Available Yes

Lindano (Mexico) see Lindane on this page
Lioresal® see Baclofen on page 109

Liothyronine (lye oh THYE roe neen)
Related Information
Endocrine Disorders & Pregnancy on page 1021
Brand Names Cytomel®; Triostat™
Therapeutic Category Thyroid Product
Use Replacement or supplemental therapy in hypothyroidism, management of nontoxic goiter, chronic lymphocytic thyroiditis, as an adjunct in thyrotoxicosis and as a diagnostic aid; **levothyroxine is recommended for chronic therapy**
Usual Dosage
Congenital hypothyroidism: Children: Oral: 5 mcg/day increase by 5 mcg every 3 days to 20 mcg/day for infants, 50 mcg/day for children 1-3 years of age, and give adult dose for children >3 years.

Hypothyroidism: Oral:
Adults: 25 mcg/day increase by 12.5-25 mcg/day every 1-2 weeks to a maximum of 100 mcg/day
Elderly: Initial: 5 mcg/day, increase by 5 mcg/day every 1-2 weeks; usual maintenance dose: 25-75 mcg/day

T_3 suppression test: Oral: 75-100 mcg/day for 7 days; use lowest dose for elderly

Myxedema coma: I.V.: 25-50 mcg
Patients with known or suspected cardiovascular disease: 10-20 mcg
Note: Normally, at least 4 hours should be allowed between doses to adequately assess therapeutic response and no more than 12 hours should elapse between doses to avoid fluctuations in hormone levels. Oral therapy

should be resumed as soon as the clinical situation has been stabilized and the patient is able to take oral medication. If levothyroxine rather than liothyronine sodium is used in initiating oral therapy, the physician should bear in mind that there is a delay of several days in the onset of levothyroxine activity and that I.V. therapy should be discontinued gradually.

Mechanism of Action Primary active compound is T_3 (triiodothyronine), which may be converted from T_4 (thyroxine) and then circulates throughout the body to influence growth and maturation of various tissues; exact mechanism of action is unknown; however, it is believed the thyroid hormone exerts its many metabolic effects through control of DNA transcription and protein synthesis; involved in normal metabolism, growth, and development; promotes gluconeogenesis, increases utilization and mobilization of glycogen stores, and stimulates protein synthesis, increases basal metabolic rate

Local Anesthetic/Vasoconstrictor Precautions No precautions with vasoconstrictor are necessary if patient is well controlled with liothyronine

Effects on Dental Treatment No effects or complications reported

Other Adverse Effects <1%:
Cardiovascular: Palpitations, tachycardia, cardiac arrhythmias, chest pain
Central nervous system: Nervousness, fever, headache, insomnia, clumsiness
Dermatologic: Alopecia
Endocrine & metabolic: Changes in menstrual cycle
Gastrointestinal: Weight loss, increased appetite, diarrhea, abdominal cramps, constipation
Neuromuscular & skeletal: Myalgia, hand tremors, tremor
Respiratory: Dyspnea
Miscellaneous: Sweating

Drug Interactions
Decreased effect:
Cholestyramine resin causes decreased absorption of liothyronine
Antidiabetic drug requirements are increased
Estrogens cause increased thyroid requirements
Increased effect: Increased oral anticoagulant effects

Drug Uptake
Onset of effect: Within 24-72 hours
Duration: Up to 72 hours
Absorption: Oral: Well absorbed (~85% to 90%)
Serum half-life: 16-49 hours

Pregnancy Risk Factor A

Generic Available Yes

Liotrix (LYE oh triks)

Related Information
Endocrine Disorders & Pregnancy *on page 1021*

Brand Names Thyrolar®

Therapeutic Category Thyroid Product

Use Replacement or supplemental therapy in hypothyroidism (uniform mixture of T_4:T_3 in 4:1 ratio by weight); little advantage to this product exists and cost is not justified

Usual Dosage Oral:
Congenital hypothyroidism:
Children (dose of T_4 or levothyroxine/day):
0-6 months: 8-10 mcg/kg or 25-50 mcg/day
6-12 months: 6-8 mcg/kg or 50-75 mcg/day
1-5 years: 5-6 mcg/kg or 75-100 mcg/day
6-12 years: 4-5 mcg/kg or 100-150 mcg/day
>12 years: 2-3 mcg/kg or >150 mcg/day
Hypothyroidism (dose of thyroid equivalent):
Adults: 30 mg/day, increasing by 15 mg/day at 2- to 3-week intervals to a maximum of 180 mg/day (usual maintenance dose: 60-120 mg/day)
Elderly: Initial: 15 mg, adjust dose at 2- to 4-week intervals by increments of 15 mg

Mechanism of Action The primary active compound is T_3 (triiodothyronine), which may be converted from T_4 (thyroxine) and then circulates throughout the body to influence growth and maturation of various tissues. Liotrix is uniform mixture of synthetic T_4 and T_3 in 4:1 ratio; exact mechanism of action is unknown; however, it is believed the thyroid hormone exerts its many metabolic effects through control of DNA transcription and protein synthesis; involved in normal metabolism, growth, and development; promotes gluconeogenesis, increases utilization and mobilization of glycogen stores and stimulates protein synthesis, increases basal metabolic rate

Local Anesthetic/Vasoconstrictor Precautions No precautions with vasoconstrictor are necessary if patient is well controlled with liotrix
(Continued)

Liotrix *(Continued)*

Effects on Dental Treatment No effects or complications reported

Other Adverse Effects <1%:
    Cardiovascular: Palpitations, tachycardia, cardiac arrhythmias, chest pain
    Central nervous system: Nervousness, headache, insomnia, fever, clumsiness
    Dermatologic: Alopecia
    Endocrine & metabolic: Excessive bone loss with overtreatment (excess thyroid
        replacement), heat intolerance, changes in menstrual cycle
    Gastrointestinal: Weight loss, increased appetite, diarrhea, abdominal cramps,
        vomiting, constipation
    Neuromuscular & skeletal: Tremor, myalgia, hand tremors
    Respiratory: Dyspnea
    Miscellaneous: Sweating

Drug Interactions
    Decreased effect:
        Thyroid hormones increase hypoglycemic drug requirements
        Phenytoin may decrease clinical lymphothyroidism
        Cholestyramine causes decreased drug absorption of liotrix
    Increased effect: Increased oral anticoagulant effect
    Increased toxicity: Tricyclic antidepressants cause increased potential of both
        drugs

Drug Uptake
    Absorption: 50% to 95% from GI tract
    Serum half-life: 6-7 days
    Time to peak serum concentration: 12-48 hours

Pregnancy Risk Factor A

Generic Available No

Lipancreatin *see* Pancrelipase *on page 722*

Lipidil® *see* Fenofibrate *on page 396*

Lipitor® *see* Atorvastatin *on page 97*

Liposyn® *see* Fat Emulsion *on page 393*

Lipovite® [OTC] *see* Vitamin B Complex *on page 993*

Liquibid® *see* Guaifenesin *on page 452*

Liqui-Char® [OTC] *see* Charcoal *on page 206*

Liquid Pred® *see* Prednisone *on page 789*

Liqui-E® *see* Tocophersolan *on page 940*

Liquifilm® Forte Solution [OTC] *see* Artificial Tears *on page 87*

Liquifilm® Tears Solution [OTC] *see* Artificial Tears *on page 87*

Liquiprin® [OTC] *see* Acetaminophen *on page 20*

Lisinopril *(lyse IN oh pril)*

Related Information
    Cardiovascular Diseases *on page 1010*

Brand Names Prinivil®; Zestril®

Therapeutic Category Angiotensin-Converting Enzyme (ACE) Inhibitors

Use Treatment of hypertension, either alone or in combination with other antihypertensive agents; adjunctive therapy in treatment of CHF (afterload reduction)

Usual Dosage
    Adults: Initial: 10 mg/day; increase doses 5-10 mg/day at 1- to 2-week intervals;
        maximum daily dose: 40 mg
    Elderly: Initial: 2.5-5 mg/day; increase doses 2.5-5 mg/day at 1- to 2-week inter-
        vals; maximum daily dose: 40 mg
    Patients taking diuretics should have them discontinued 2-3 days prior to initia-
        ting lisinopril if possible; restart diuretic after blood pressure is stable if needed;
        in patients with hyponatremia (<130 mEq/L), start dose at 2.5 mg/day

    Acute myocardial infarction (within 24 hours in hemodynamically stable patients):
        Oral: 5 mg immediately, then 5 mg at 24 hours, 10 mg at 48 hours, and 10 mg
        every day thereafter for 6 weeks; patients should continue to receive standard
        treatments such as thrombolytics, aspirin, and beta-blockers

Mechanism of Action Competitive inhibitor of angiotensin-converting enzyme
(ACE); prevents conversion of angiotensin I to angiotensin II, a potent vasoconstrictor; results in lower levels of angiotensin II which causes an increase in
plasma renin activity and a reduction in aldosterone secretion; a CNS mechanism may also be involved in hypotensive effect as angiotensin II increases
adrenergic outflow from CNS; vasoactive kallikreins may be decreased in
conversion to active hormones by ACE inhibitors, thus reducing blood pressure

Local Anesthetic/Vasoconstrictor Precautions No information available to
require special precautions

Effects on Dental Treatment No effects or complications reported

Other Adverse Effects

1% to 10%:

Cardiovascular: Hypotension

Central nervous system: Dizziness, headache, fatigue

Gastrointestinal: Diarrhea

Renal: Elevated BUN and serum creatinine

Respiratory: Upper respiratory symptoms, cough

<1%:

Cardiovascular: Chest discomfort, flushing, myocardial infarction, angina pectoris, orthostatic hypotension, rhythm disturbances, tachycardia, peripheral edema, vasculitis, palpitations, syncope

Central nervous system: Fever, malaise, depression, somnolence, insomnia

Dermatologic: Urticaria, pruritus, angioedema

Endocrine & metabolic: Gout

Gastrointestinal: Pancreatitis, abdominal pain, anorexia, constipation, flatulence, dry mouth

Hematologic: Neutropenia, bone marrow suppression

Hepatic: Hepatitis

Neuromuscular & skeletal: Arthralgia, shoulder pain

Ocular: Blurred vision

Respiratory: Bronchitis, sinusitis, pharyngeal pain

Miscellaneous: Sweating

Drug Interactions See table.

Drug-Drug Interactions With ACEIs

Precipitant Drug	Drug (Category) and Effect	Description
Antacids	ACE Inhibitors: decreased	Decreased bioavailability of ACEIs. May be more likely with captopril. Separate administration times by 1-2 hours.
NSAIDs (indomethacin)	ACEIs: decreased	Reduced hypotensive effects of ACEIs. More prominent in low renin or volume dependent hypertensive patients.
Phenothiazines	ACEIs: increased	Pharmacologic effects of ACEIs may be increased.
ACEIs	Allopurinol: increased	Higher risk of hypersensitivity reaction possible when given concurrently. Three case reports of Stevens-Johnson syndrome with captopril.
ACEIs	Digoxin: increased	Increased plasma digoxin levels.
ACEIs	Lithium: increased	Increased serum lithium levels and symptoms of toxicity may occur.
ACEIs	Potassium preps/ potassium sparing diuretics increased	Coadministration may result in elevated potassium levels.

Increased toxicity: Lisinopril and diuretics have additive hypotensive effects

Drug Uptake

Peak hypotensive effect: Oral: Within 6 hours

Absorption: Well absorbed; unaffected by food

Serum half-life: 11-12 hours

Pregnancy Risk Factor C (first trimester); D (second and third trimesters)

Generic Available No

Lisinopril and Hydrochlorothiazide

(lyse IN oh pril & hye droe klor oh THYE a zide)

Related Information

Cardiovascular Diseases *on page 1010*

Brand Names Prinzide®; Zestoretic®

Therapeutic Category Antihypertensive Agent, Combination

Use Treatment of hypertension

Local Anesthetic/Vasoconstrictor Precautions No information available to require special precautions

Effects on Dental Treatment No effects or complications reported

Generic Available No

Listerine® Antiseptic [OTC] *see Mouthwash, Antiseptic on page 650*

Listermint® with Fluoride [OTC] *see Fluoride on page 415*

Lithane® *see Lithium on next page*

Lithium (LITH ee um)
Related Information
Dental Drug Interactions: Update on Drug Combinations Requiring Special Considerations *on page 1144*

Brand Names Eskalith®; Lithane®; Lithobid®; Lithonate®; Lithotabs®

Canadian/Mexican Brand Names Carbolit® (Mexico); Lithellm® 300 (Mexico)

Therapeutic Category Antimanic Agent

Synonyms Lito Carbonato De (Mexico)

Use Management of acute manic episodes, bipolar disorders, and depression

Usual Dosage Oral: Monitor serum concentrations and clinical response (efficacy and toxicity) to determine proper dose

Children 6-12 years: 15-60 mg/kg/day in 3-4 divided doses; dose not to exceed usual adult dosage

Adults: 300-600 mg 3-4 times/day; usual maximum maintenance dose: 2.4 g/day or 450-900 mg of sustained release twice daily

Elderly: Initial dose: 300 mg twice daily; increase weekly in increments of 300 mg/day, monitoring levels; rarely need to go >900-1200 mg/day

Mechanism of Action Alters cation transport across cell membrane in nerve and muscle cells and influences reuptake of serotonin and/or norepinephrine

Local Anesthetic/Vasoconstrictor Precautions No information available to require special precautions

Effects on Dental Treatment Avoid NSAIDs if analgesics are required since lithium toxicity has been reported with concomitant administration; acetaminophen products (ie, singly or with narcotics) are recommended

Other Adverse Effects
>10%:
Endocrine & metabolic: Polydipsia, stress
Gastrointestinal: Nausea, diarrhea, impaired taste
Neuromuscular & skeletal: Trembling

1% to 10%:
Central nervous system: Fatigue
Dermatologic: Skin rash
Gastrointestinal: Bloated feeling, weight gain
Neuromuscular: Muscle twitching, weakness

<1%:
Central nervous system: Lethargy, dizziness, vertigo, pseudotumor cerebri
Dermatologic: Eruptions, discoloration of fingers and toes
Endocrine & metabolic: Hypothyroidism, goiter, acneiform, diabetes insipidus
Gastrointestinal: Anorexia, dry mouth
Hematologic: Leukocytosis
Neuromuscular & skeletal: Muscle weakness, cogwheel rigidity, chronic movements of the limbs, tremor
Ocular: Vision problems
Renal: Nonspecific nephron atrophy, renal tubular acidosis

Drug Interactions
Decreased effect with xanthines (eg, theophylline, caffeine)

Increased effect/toxicity of CNS depressants, alfentanil, iodide salts increased hypothyroid effect

Increased toxicity with thiazide diuretics (dose may need to be reduced by 30%), NSAIDs, haloperidol, phenothiazines (neurotoxicity), neuromuscular blockers, carbamazepine, fluoxetine, ACE inhibitors

Drug Uptake
Serum half-life: 18-24 hours; can increase to more than 36 hours in elderly or patients with renal impairment

Time to peak serum concentration (nonsustained release product): Within 0.5-2 hours following oral absorption

Pregnancy Risk Factor D

Generic Available Yes

Lithobid® *see* Lithium *on this page*

Lithonate® *see* Lithium *on this page*

Lithostat® *see* Acetohydroxamic Acid *on page 28*

Lithotabs® *see* Lithium *on this page*

Lito Carbonato De (Mexico) *see* Lithium *on this page*

Livostin® *see* Levocabastine *on page 547*

LKV-Drops® [OTC] *see* Vitamins, Multiple *on page 995*

L-Lysine (el LYE seen)
Brand Names Enisyl® [OTC]; Lycolan® Elixir [OTC]

Therapeutic Category Dietary Supplement

Use Improves utilization of vegetable proteins

Local Anesthetic/Vasoconstrictor Precautions No information available to require special precautions
Effects on Dental Treatment No effects or complications reported
Pregnancy Risk Factor C
Generic Available Yes

LMD® *see* Dextran *on page 295*
Lodine® *see* Etodolac *on page 387* ·
Lodine® XL *see* Etodolac *on page 387*
Lodosyn® *see* Carbidopa *on page 176*

Lodoxamide Tromethamine (loe DOKS a mide troe METH a meen)
Brand Names Alomide®
Therapeutic Category Ophthalmic Agent, Miscellaneous
Use Treatment of vernal keratoconjunctivitis, vernal conjunctivitis, and vernal keratitis
Usual Dosage Children >2 years and Adults: Instill 1-2 drops in eye(s) 4 times/day for up to 3 months
Mechanism of Action Mast cell stabilizer that inhibits the *in vivo* type I immediate hypersensitivity reaction to increase cutaneous vascular permeability associated with IgE and antigen-mediated reactions
Local Anesthetic/Vasoconstrictor Precautions No information available to require special precautions
Effects on Dental Treatment No effects or complications reported
Other Adverse Effects
>10%: Local: Transient burning, stinging, discomfort
1% to 10%:
Central nervous system: Headache
Ocular: Blurred vision, corneal erosion/ulcer, eye pain, corneal abrasion, blepharitis
<1%:
Central nervous system: Dizziness, somnolence
Dermatologic: Rash
Gastrointestinal: Nausea, stomach discomfort
Ocular: Blepharitis
Respiratory: Sneezing, dry nose
Drug Interactions No data reported
Drug Uptake Absorption: Topical: Very small and undetectable
Pregnancy Risk Factor B
Dosage Forms Solution, ophthalmic: 0.1% (10 mL)
Generic Available No

Loestrin® *see* Ethinyl Estradiol and Norethindrone *on page 379*
Logen® *see* Diphenoxylate and Atropine *on page 324*
Lomanate® *see* Diphenoxylate and Atropine *on page 324*

Lomefloxacin (loe me FLOKS a sin)
Brand Names Maxaquin®
Therapeutic Category Antibiotic, Quinolone
Synonyms Lomefloxacino Clorhidato De (Mexico)
Use Quinolone antibiotic for skin and skin structure, lower respiratory and urinary tract infections, and sexually transmitted diseases
Usual Dosage Oral: Adults: 400 mg once daily for 10-14 days
Mechanism of Action Inhibits DNA-gyrase in susceptible organisms thereby inhibits relaxation of supercoiled DNA and promotes breakage of DNA strands. DNA gyrase (topoisomerase II), is an essential bacterial enzyme that maintains the superhelical structure of DNA and is required for DNA replication and transcription, DNA repair, recombination, and transposition.
Local Anesthetic/Vasoconstrictor Precautions No information available to require special precautions
Effects on Dental Treatment No effects or complications reported
Other Adverse Effects
1% to 10%:
Central nervous system: Headache, dizziness
Dermatologic: Photosensitivity
Gastrointestinal: Nausea
<1%:
Cardiovascular: Flushing, chest pain, hypotension, hypertension, edema, syncope, tachycardia, bradycardia, arrhythmia, extrasystoles, cyanosis, cardiac failure, angina pectoris, myocardial infarction, face edema
Central nervous system: Fatigue, malaise, chills, convulsions, vertigo, coma
Dermatologic: Purpura, rash
(Continued)

Lomefloxacin (Continued)

Endocrine & metabolic: Gout, hypoglycemia

Gastrointestinal: Abdominal pain, vomiting, flatulence, constipation, dry mouth, thirst, taste perversion, tongue discoloration

Genitourinary: Micturition disorder, dysuria

Hematologic: Thrombocytopenia

Neuromuscular & skeletal: Back pain, hyperkinesia, tremor, paresthesias, leg cramps, myalgia, weakness

Otic: Earache

Renal: Hematuria, anuria

Respiratory: Dyspnea, cough, epistaxis

Miscellaneous: Increased sweating, allergic reaction, flu-like symptoms, decreased heat tolerance, increased fibrinolysis

Drug Interactions

Decreased effect: Decreased absorption with antacids containing aluminum, magnesium, and/or calcium (by up to 98% if given at the same time)

Increased toxicity/serum levels: Quinolones cause increased levels of caffeine, warfarin, cyclosporine, and theophylline; azlocillin, cimetidine, probenecid increase quinolone levels

Drug Uptake

Absorption: Well absorbed

Serum half-life, elimination: 5-7.5 hours

Pregnancy Risk Factor C

Generic Available No

Lomefloxacino Clorhidato De (Mexico) *see* Lomefloxacin *on previous page*

Lomotil® *see* Diphenoxylate and Atropine *on page 324*

Lomustine (loe MUS teen)

Brand Names CeeNU® Oral

Therapeutic Category Antineoplastic Agent, Alkylating Agent (Nitrosourea)

Synonyms CCNU

Use Treatment of brain tumors, Hodgkin's and non-Hodgkin's lymphomas, melanoma, renal carcinoma, lung cancer, colon cancer

Usual Dosage Oral (**refer to individual protocols**):

Children: 75-150 mg/m² as a single dose every 6 weeks. Subsequent doses are readjusted after initial treatment according to platelet and leukocyte counts.

Adults: 100-130 mg/m² as a single dose every 6 weeks; readjust after initial treatment according to platelet and leukocyte counts

With compromised marrow function: Initial dose: 100 mg/m² as a single dose every 6 weeks

Subsequent dosing adjustment based on nadir:

Leukocytes 2000-2900/mm³, platelets 25,000-74,999/mm³: Administer 70% of prior dose

Leukocytes <2000/mm³, platelets <25,000/mm³: Administer 50% of prior dose

Mechanism of Action Inhibits DNA and RNA synthesis via carbamylation of DNA polymerase, alkylation of DNA, and alteration of RNA, proteins, and enzymes

Local Anesthetic/Vasoconstrictor Precautions No information available to require special precautions

Effects on Dental Treatment No effects or complications reported

Other Adverse Effects

>10%:

Gastrointestinal: Nausea and vomiting occur 3-6 hours after oral administration; this is due to a centrally mediated mechanism, not a direct effect on the GI lining; if vomiting occurs, it is not necessary to replace the dose unless it occurs immediately after drug administration

Hematologic: Anemia; myelosuppressive effects occur 4-6 weeks after a dose and may persist for 1-2 weeks

1% to 10%:

Central nervous system: Neurotoxicity

Dermatologic: Rash

Gastrointestinal: Stomatitis, diarrhea

Hematologic: Anemia

<1%:

Central nervous system: Disorientation, lethargy, ataxia

Dermatologic: Alopecia

Hepatic: Hepatotoxicity

Neuromuscular & skeletal: Dysarthria

Renal: Renal failure

Respiratory: Pulmonary fibrosis with cumulative doses >600 mg

Drug Uptake
Absorption: Complete from GI tract; appears in plasma within 3 minutes after administration
Serum half-life: Parent drug: 16-72 hours
Active metabolite: Terminal half-life: 1.3-2 days
Time to peak serum concentration: Active metabolite: Within 3 hours

Pregnancy Risk Factor D

Generic Available No

Comments Myelosuppression is delayed about 4-6 weeks after a dose

Loniten® see Minoxidil on page 640

Lonox® see Diphenoxylate and Atropine on page 324

Lo/Ovral® see Ethinyl Estradiol and Norgestrel on page 381

Loperamide (loe PER a mide)

Brand Names Diar-aid® [OTC]; Imodium®; Imodium® A-D [OTC]; Kaopectate® II [OTC]; Pepto® Diarrhea Control [OTC]

Canadian/Mexican Brand Names Acanol® (Mexico); PMS-Loperamine® (Canada); Pramidal® (Mexico); Raxedin® (Mexico)

Therapeutic Category Antidiarrheal

Use Treatment of acute diarrhea and chronic diarrhea associated with inflammatory bowel disease; chronic functional diarrhea (idiopathic), chronic diarrhea caused by bowel resection or organic lesions; to decrease the volume of ileostomy discharge

Unlabeled use: Treatment of traveler's diarrhea in combination with trimethoprim-sulfamethoxazole (co-trimoxazole) (3 days therapy)

Usual Dosage Oral:
Children:
Acute diarrhea: Initial doses (in first 24 hours):
2-6 years: 1 mg three times/day
6-8 years: 2 mg twice daily
8-12 years: 2 mg three times/day
Maintenance: After initial dosing, 0.1 mg/kg doses after each loose stool, but not exceeding initial dosage
Chronic diarrhea: 0.08-0.24 mg/kg/day divided 2-3 times/day, maximum: 2 mg/dose
Adults: Initial: 4 mg (2 capsules), followed by 2 mg after each loose stool, up to 16 mg/day (8 capsules)

Mechanism of Action Acts directly on intestinal muscles to inhibit peristalsis and prolongs transit time enhancing fluid and electrolyte movement through intestinal mucosa; reduces fecal volume, increases viscosity, and diminishes fluid and electrolyte loss; demonstrates antisecretory activity; exhibits peripheral action

Local Anesthetic/Vasoconstrictor Precautions No information available to require special precautions

Effects on Dental Treatment No effects or complications reported

Other Adverse Effects
Central nervous system: Sedation, fatigue, dizziness, drowsiness
Dermatologic: Rash
Gastrointestinal: Nausea, vomiting, constipation, abdominal cramping, dry mouth, abdominal distention

Drug Interactions Increased toxicity: CNS depressants, phenothiazines, tricyclic antidepressants may potentiate the adverse effects of loperamide

Drug Uptake
Onset of action: Oral: Within 0.5-1 hour
Absorption: Oral: <40%; levels in breast milk expected to be very low
Serum half-life: 7-14 hours

Pregnancy Risk Factor B

Generic Available Yes

Lopid® see Gemfibrozil on page 439

Lopremone see Protirelin on page 818

Lopressor® [Tartrate] see Metoprolol on page 629

Loprox® see Ciclopirox on page 233

Lorabid™ see Loracarbef on this page

Loracarbef (lor a KAR bef)

Brand Names Lorabid™

Canadian/Mexican Brand Names Carbac® (Mexico)

Therapeutic Category Antibiotic, Carbacephem
(Continued)

Loracarbef *(Continued)*

Use Infections caused by susceptible organisms involving the respiratory tract, acute otitis media, sinusitis, skin and skin structure, bone and joint, and urinary tract and gynecologic

Usual Dosage Oral:

Children:

Acute otitis media: 15 mg/kg twice daily for 10 days

Pharyngitis: 7.5-15 mg/kg twice daily for 10 days

Adults: Women:

Uncomplicated urinary tract infections: 200 mg once daily for 7 days

Skin and soft tissue: 200-400 mg every 12-24 hours

Uncomplicated pyelonephritis: 400 mg every 12 hours for 14 days

Mechanism of Action Inhibits bacterial cell wall synthesis by binding to one or more of the penicillin binding proteins (PBPs); inhibits the final transpeptidation step of peptidoglycan synthesis in bacterial cell walls, thus inhibiting cell wall biosynthesis. It is thought that beta-lactam antibiotics inactivate transpeptidase via acylation of the enzyme with cleavage of the CO-N bond of the beta-lactam ring. Upon exposure to beta-lactam antibiotics, bacteria eventually lyse due to ongoing activity of cell wall autolytic enzymes (autolysins and murein hydrolases) while cell wall assembly is arrested.

Local Anesthetic/Vasoconstrictor Precautions No information available to require special precautions

Effects on Dental Treatment No effects or complications reported

Other Adverse Effects

1% to 10%:

Central nervous system: Headache

Dermatologic: Skin rashes

Gastrointestinal: Diarrhea, nausea, vomiting, abdominal pain, anorexia

Genitourinary: Vaginitis, vaginal moniliasis

<1%:

Cardiovascular: Vasodilation

Central nervous system: Somnolence, nervousness, dizziness

Hematologic: Transient thrombocytopenia, leukopenia, and eosinophilia

Hepatic: Transient elevations of ALT, AST, alkaline phosphatase

Renal: Transient elevations of BUN and creatinine

Drug Interactions Increased serum levels with probenecid

Drug Uptake

Absorption: Oral: Rapid

Serum half-life, elimination: ~1 hour

Time to peak serum concentration: Oral: Within 1 hour

Pregnancy Risk Factor B

Generic Available No

Loracepam (Mexico) *see* Lorazepam *on next page*
Loratadina (Mexico) *see* Loratadine *on this page*

Loratadine (lor AT a deen)

Brand Names Claritin®

Canadian/Mexican Brand Names Clarityne® (Mexico); Lertamine® (Mexico); Lowadina® (Mexico)

Therapeutic Category Antihistamine

Synonyms Loratadina (Mexico)

Use Relief of nasal and non-nasal symptoms of seasonal allergic rhinitis

Usual Dosage Children >12 years and Adults: Oral: 10 mg/day on an empty stomach

Mechanism of Action Long-acting tricyclic antihistamine with selective peripheral histamine H_1 receptor antagonistic properties

Local Anesthetic/Vasoconstrictor Precautions No information available to require special precautions

Effects on Dental Treatment >10% of patients experience dry mouth which will disappear with cessation of drug therapy

Other Adverse Effects

>10%: Central nervous system: Headache, somnolence, fatigue

1% to 10%:

Cardiovascular: Hypotension, hypertension, palpitations, tachycardia

Central nervous system: Anxiety, depression

Endocrine & metabolic: Breast pain

Neuromuscular & skeletal: Hyperkinesia, arthralgias

Respiratory: Nasal dryness, pharyngitis, dyspnea

Miscellaneous: Sweating

Drug Interactions
Increased plasma concentrations of loratadine and its active metabolite with ketoconazole; erythromycin increases the AUC of loratadine and its active metabolite; no change in Q-T$_c$ interval was seen
Increased toxicity: Procarbazine, other antihistamines, alcohol

Drug Uptake
Onset of action: Within 1-3 hours
Peak effect: 8-12 hours
Duration: >24 hours
Absorption: Rapid
Serum half-life: 12-15 hours

Pregnancy Risk Factor B

Dosage Forms
Syrup: 1 mg/mL (480 mL)
Tablet: 10 mg
Rapid-disintegrating tablets: 10 mg (RediTabs®)

Generic Available No

Loratadine and Pseudoephedrine
(lor AT a deen & soo doe e FED rin)

Related Information
Oral Bacterial Infections on page 1059

Brand Names Claritin-D®; Claritin-D 24-Hour®

Therapeutic Category Antihistamine/Decongestant Combination

Use Temporary relief of symptoms of seasonal and perennial allergic rhinitis, and vasomotor rhinitis, including nasal obstruction

Local Anesthetic/Vasoconstrictor Precautions Use with caution since pseudoephedrine is a sympathomimetic amine which could interact with epinephrine to cause a pressor response

Effects on Dental Treatment Up to 10% of patients could experience tachycardia, palpitations, and dry mouth; use vasoconstrictor with caution; over 10% of patients may experience dry mouth which will disappear with cessation of drug therapy

Other Adverse Effects
>10%:
Cardiovascular: Tachycardia
Central nervous system: Slight to moderate drowsiness, nervousness, transient stimulation, insomnia
Respiratory: Thickening of bronchial secretions

1% to 10%:
Central nervous system: Headache, fatigue, dizziness
Gastrointestinal: Appetite increase, weight gain, nausea, diarrhea, abdominal pain, dry mouth
Genitourinary: Dysuria
Neuromuscular & skeletal: Arthralgia, weakness
Respiratory: Pharyngitis
Miscellaneous: Sweating

<1%:
Cardiovascular: Edema, palpitations, hypotension
Central nervous system: Depression, sedation, paradoxical excitement, convulsions, hallucinations
Dermatologic: Angioedema, rash, photosensitivity
Genitourinary: Urinary retention
Hepatic: Hepatitis
Neuromuscular & skeletal: Myalgia, paresthesia, tremor
Ocular: Blurred vision
Respiratory: Bronchospasm, epistaxis, dyspnea

Generic Available No

Lorazepam (lor A ze pam)

Related Information
Patients Requiring Sedation on page 1081
Temporomandibular Dysfunction (TMD) on page 1078

Brand Names Ativan®

Canadian/Mexican Brand Names Apo®-Lorazepam (Canada); Novo-Lorazepam® (Canada); Nu-Loraz® (Canada); PMS-Lorazepam® (Canada); Pro-Lorazepam® (Canada)

Therapeutic Category Antianxiety Agent; Benzodiazepine; Hypnotic; Sedative; Tranquilizer, Minor

Synonyms Loracepam (Mexico)

Use Management of anxiety, status epilepticus, preoperative sedation, for desired amnesia, and as an antiemetic adjunct
(Continued)

Lorazepam (Continued)

Unapproved uses: Alcohol detoxification, insomnia, psychogenic catatonia, partial complex seizures

Usual Dosage

Antiemetic:
Children 2-15 years: I.V.: 0.05 mg/kg (up to 2 mg/dose) prior to chemotherapy
Adults: Oral, I.V.: 0.5-2 mg every 4-6 hours as needed

Anxiety and sedation:
Children: Oral, I.V.: Usual: 0.05 mg/kg/dose (range: 0.02-0.09 mg/kg) every 4-8 hours
Adults: Oral: 1-10 mg/day in 2-3 divided doses; usual dose: 2-6 mg/day in divided doses

Insomnia: Adults: Oral: 2-4 mg at bedtime

Preoperative: Adults:
I.M.: 0.05 mg/kg administered 2 hours before surgery; maximum: 4 mg/dose
I.V.: 0.044 mg/kg 15-20 minutes before surgery; usual maximum: 2 mg/dose

Operative amnesia: Adults: I.V.: up to 0.05 mg/kg; maximum: 4 mg/dose

Status epilepticus: I.V.:
Children: 0.1 mg/kg slow I.V. over 2-5 minutes, do not exceed 4 mg/single dose; may repeat second dose of 0.05 mg/kg slow I.V. in 10-15 minutes if needed
Adolescents: 0.07 mg/kg slow I.V. over 2-5 minutes; maximum: 4 mg/dose; may repeat in 10-15 minutes
Adults: 4 mg/dose given slowly over 2-5 minutes; may repeat in 10-15 minutes; usual maximum dose: 8 mg

Mechanism of Action Depresses all levels of the CNS, including the limbic and reticular formation, probably through the increased action of gamma-aminobutyric acid (GABA), which is a major inhibitory neurotransmitter in the brain

Local Anesthetic/Vasoconstrictor Precautions No information available to require special precautions

Effects on Dental Treatment >10% of patients experience dry mouth; normal salivary flow occurs with cessation of drug therapy

Other Adverse Effects

>10%: Central nervous system: Sedation
1% to 10%:
Central nervous system: Dizziness, unsteadiness
Neuromuscular & skeletal: Weakness
<1%:
Cardiovascular: Hypotension
Central nervous system: Disorientation, fatigue, depression, headache, sleep disturbance
Gastrointestinal: Nausea, appetite changes

Drug Interactions

Decreased effect with oral contraceptives (combination products), cigarette smoking; decreased effect of levodopa
Increased effect with morphine
Increased toxicity with alcohol, CNS depressants, MAO inhibitors, loxapine, tricyclic antidepressants

Drug Uptake

Onset of hypnosis: I.M.: 20-30 minutes
Duration: 6-8 hours
Absorption: Oral, I.M.: Prompt following administration
Serum half-life:
Older Children: 10.5 hours
Adults: 12.9 hours
Elderly: 15.9 hours
End stage renal disease: 32-70 hours

Pregnancy Risk Factor D

Dosage Forms

Injection: 2 mg/mL (1 mL, 10 mL); 4 mg/mL (1 mL, 10 mL)
Solution, oral concentrated, alcohol and dye free: 2 mg/mL (30 mL)
Tablet: 0.5 mg, 1 mg, 2 mg

Generic Available Yes

Lorcet® [5/500] see Hydrocodone and Acetaminophen on page 478

Lorcet®-HD [5/500] see Hydrocodone and Acetaminophen on page 478

Lorcet® Plus [7.5/650] see Hydrocodone and Acetaminophen on page 478

Lorelco® see Probucol on page 796

Loroxide® [OTC] see Benzoyl Peroxide on page 120

Lortab® 2.5/500 *see* Hydrocodone and Acetaminophen *on page 478*

Lortab® 5/500 *see* Hydrocodone and Acetaminophen *on page 478*

Lortab® 7.5/500 *see* Hydrocodone and Acetaminophen *on page 478*

Lortab® 10/500 *see* Hydrocodone and Acetaminophen *on page 478*

Lortab® 10/650 *see* Hydrocodone and Acetaminophen *on page 478*

Lortab® ASA *see* Hydrocodone and Aspirin *on page 480*

Lortab® Elixir *see* Hydrocodone and Acetaminophen *on page 478*

Lortab® Solution *see* Hydrocodone and Acetaminophen *on page 478*

Losartan (loe SAR tan)

Related Information
Cardiovascular Diseases *on page 1010*

Brand Names Cozaar®

Therapeutic Category Angiotensin II Antagonists

Synonyms DuP 753; Losartan Potassium; MK594

Use Treatment of hypertension alone or in combination with other antihypertensives; in considering the use of monotherapy with Cozaar®, it should be noted that in controlled trials Cozaar® had an effect on blood pressure that was notably less in black patients than in nonblacks, a finding similar to the small effect of ACE inhibitors in blacks

Usual Dosage
Oral: 25-100 mg once or twice daily (adjust dosage at weekly intervals; maximum effect may not be apparent for 3-6 weeks)
Usual initial doses in patients receiving diuretics or those with intravascular volume depletion: 25 mg
Patients not receiving diuretics: 50 mg

Mechanism of Action As a selective and competitive, nonpeptide angiotensin II receptor antagonist, losartan blocks the vasoconstrictor and aldosterone-secreting effects of angiotensin II; losartan interacts reversibly at the AT1 and AT2 receptors of many tissues and has slow dissociation kinetics; its affinity for the AT1 receptor is 1000 times greater than the AT2 receptor. Angiotensin II receptor antagonists may induce a more complete inhibition of the renin-angiotensin system than ACE inhibitors, they do not affect the response to bradykinin, and are less likely to be associated with nonrenin-angiotensin effects (eg, cough and angioedema). Losartan increases urinary flow rate and in addition to being natriuretic and kaliuretic, increases excretion of chloride, magnesium, uric acid, calcium, and phosphate.

Local Anesthetic/Vasoconstrictor Precautions No information available to require special precautions

Effects on Dental Treatment No effects or complications reported

Other Adverse Effects
1% to 10%:
Cardiovascular: Hypotension without reflex tachycardia
Central nervous system: Dizziness, insomnia
Endocrine & metabolic: Hyperkalemia
Gastrointestinal: Diarrhea, dyspepsia
Hematologic: Slight decreases in hemoglobin and hematocrit
Neuromuscular & skeletal: Back and leg pain, myalgia
Renal: Hypouricemia (with large doses)
Respiratory: Cough (less than ACE inhibitors), nasal congestion, sinus disorders, sinusitis
<1%:
Cardiovascular: Orthostatic effects, angina, second degree A-V block, CVA, palpitations, sinus bradycardia, tachycardia, flushing, facial edema
Central nervous system: Anxiety, ataxia, confusion, depression, dream abnormality, migraine headache, sleep disorders, vertigo, fever
Dermatologic: Alopecia, dermatitis, dry skin, bruising, erythema, photosensitivity, pruritus, rash, urticaria
Endocrine & metabolic: Gout, decreased libido
Gastrointestinal: Anorexia, constipation, flatulence, vomiting, taste alteration, gastritis
Genitourinary: Impotence, nocturia, urinary tract infection
Hepatic: Slight elevations of LFTs and bilirubin
Neuromuscular & skeletal: Paresthesia; tremor; arm, hip, shoulder, and knee pain; joint swelling; fibromyalgia; muscle weakness
Ocular: Blurred vision, burning and stinging eyes, conjunctivitis, decreased visual acuity
Otic: Tinnitus
Renal: Mild elevation in BUN/creatinine, polyuria
Respiratory: Dyspnea, bronchitis, pharyngeal discomfort, epistaxis, rhinitis, respiratory congestion
(Continued)

Losartan *(Continued)*

Miscellaneous: Sweating

Drug Uptake
Onset of effect: 6 hours
Serum half-life:
Losartan: 1.5-2 hours
E-3174: 6-9 hours
Time to peak: Peak serum levels of losartan: 1 hour; metabolite, E-3174: 3-4 hours

Pregnancy Risk Factor C (first trimester); D (second & third trimester)
Generic Available No
Comments Cozaar® may be administered with other antihypertensive agents

Losartan and Hydrochlorothiazide
(loe SAR tan & hye droe klor oh THYE a zide)

Brand Names Hyzaar®
Therapeutic Category Angiotensin II Antagonists; Diuretic, Thiazide
Use Treatment of hypertension
Local Anesthetic/Vasoconstrictor Precautions No information available to require special precautions
Effects on Dental Treatment No effects or complications reported
Pregnancy Risk Factor C (1st trimester); D (2nd and 3rd trimesters)
Generic Available No

Losartan Potassium *see Losartan on previous page*

Lotensin® *see Benazepril on page 115*

Lotensin HCT® *see Benazepril and Hydrochlorothiazide on page 116*

Lotrel™ *see Amlodipine and Benazepril on page 64*

Lotrimin® AF Powder [OTC] *see Miconazole on page 635*

Lotrimin® AF Spray Liquid [OTC] *see Miconazole on page 635*

Lotrimin® AF Spray Powder [OTC] *see Miconazole on page 635*

Lotrisone® *see Betamethasone and Clotrimazole on page 127*

Lovastatin (LOE va sta tin)

Related Information
Cardiovascular Diseases *on page 1010*
Brand Names Mevacor®
Therapeutic Category HMG-CoA Reductase Inhibitor; Lipid Lowering Drugs
Synonyms Lovastatina (Mexico)
Use Adjunct to dietary therapy to decrease elevated serum total and LDL cholesterol concentrations in primary hypercholesterolemia
Usual Dosage Adults: Oral: Initial: 20 mg with evening meal, then adjust at 4-week intervals; maximum dose: 80 mg/day; before initiation of therapy, patients should be placed on a standard cholesterol-lowering diet for 3-6 months and the diet should be continued during drug therapy
Mechanism of Action Lovastatin acts by competitively inhibiting 3-hydroxyl-3-methylglutaryl-coenzyme A (HMG-CoA) reductase, the enzyme that catalyzes the rate-limiting step in cholesterol biosynthesis
Local Anesthetic/Vasoconstrictor Precautions No information available to require special precautions
Effects on Dental Treatment No effects or complications reported
Other Adverse Effects
Endocrine & metabolic: Gynecomastia

1% to 10%: Elevated creatine phosphokinase (CPK)
Central nervous system: Headache, dizziness
Dermatologic: Rash, pruritus
Gastrointestinal: Flatulence, abdominal pain, cramps, diarrhea, pancreatitis, constipation, nausea, dyspepsia, heartburn
Neuromuscular & skeletal: Myalgia
<1%:
Gastrointestinal: Dysgeusia
Ocular: Blurred vision, myositis, lenticular opacities

Drug Interactions
Increased toxicity: Gemfibrozil (musculoskeletal effects such as myopathy, myalgia and/or muscle weakness accompanied by markedly elevated CK concentrations, rash and/or pruritus); clofibrate, niacin (myopathy), erythromycin, cyclosporine, oral anticoagulants (elevated PT)
Increased effect/toxicity of levothyroxine
Concurrent use of erythromycin and lovastatin may result in rhabdomyolysis

Drug Uptake
Onset of effect: 3 days of therapy required for LDL cholesterol concentration reductions
Absorption: Oral: 30%
Serum half-life: 1.1-1.7 hours
Time to peak serum concentration: Oral: 2-4 hours

Pregnancy Risk Factor X

Generic Available No

Lovastatina (Mexico) *see* Lovastatin *on previous page*

Lovenox® *see* Enoxaparin *on page 349*

Loxapine (LOKS a peen)

Brand Names Loxitane®

Canadian/Mexican Brand Names Loxapac® (Canada)

Therapeutic Category Antiemetic; Antipsychotic Agent; Phenothiazine Derivative

Use Treatment of psychoses, nausea and vomiting; Tourette's syndrome; mania; intractable hiccups (adults); behavioral problems (children)

Usual Dosage Adults:
Oral: 10 mg twice daily, increase dose until psychotic symptoms are controlled; usual dose range: 60-100 mg/day in divided doses 2-4 times/day; dosages >250 mg/day are not recommended
I.M.: 12.5-50 mg every 4-6 hours or longer as needed and change to oral therapy as soon as possible

Mechanism of Action Blocks postsynaptic mesolimbic dopaminergic receptors in the brain; exhibits a strong alpha-adrenergic blocking effect and depresses the release of hypothalamic and hypophyseal hormones; believed to depress the reticular-activating system, thus affecting basal metabolism, body temperatures, wakefulness, vasomotor tone, and emesis

Local Anesthetic/Vasoconstrictor Precautions No information available to require special precautions

Effects on Dental Treatment >10% of patients experience dry mouth. Significant hypotension may occur, especially when the drug is administered parenterally; orthostatic hypotension is due to alpha-receptor blockade, the elderly are at greater risk for orthostatic hypotension

Tardive dyskinesia: Prevalence rate may be 40% in elderly; development of the syndrome and the irreversible nature are proportional to duration and total cumulative dose over time

Extrapyramidal reactions are more common in elderly with up to 50% developing these reactions after 60 years of age; drug-induced **Parkinson's syndrome** occurs often; **Akathisia** is the most common extrapyramidal reaction in elderly

Increased confusion, memory loss, psychotic behavior, and agitation frequently occur as a consequence of anticholinergic effects

Antipsychotic associated sedation in nonpsychotic patients is extremely unpleasant due to feelings of depersonalization, derealization, and dysphoria

Other Adverse Effects
>10%:
Cardiovascular: Orthostatic hypotension
Central nervous system: Drowsiness, extrapyramidal effects (parkinsonian), confusion, persistent tardive dyskinesia
Ocular: Blurred vision
1% to 10%:
Dermatologic: Skin rash
Endocrine & metabolic: Enlargement of breasts
Gastrointestinal: Constipation, nausea, vomiting
<1%:
Cardiovascular: Tachycardia, arrhythmias, abnormal T-waves with prolonged ventricular repolarization
Central nervous system: Neuroleptic malignant syndrome (NMS), sedation, restlessness, anxiety, seizures, altered central temperature regulation
Dermatologic: Hyperpigmentation, pruritus, rash, photosensitivity
Endocrine & metabolic: Galactorrhea, amenorrhea, gynecomastia, sexual dysfunction
Gastrointestinal: Weight gain, adynamic ileus
Genitourinary: Urinary retention, overflow incontinence, priapism
Hematologic: Agranulocytosis (more often in women between fourth and tenth week of therapy), leukopenia (usually in patients with large doses for prolonged periods)
Hepatic: Cholestatic jaundice
Ocular: Retinal pigmentation
(Continued)

Loxapine *(Continued)*

Drug Interactions
Decreased effect of guanethidine, phenytoin
Increased toxicity with CNS depressants, metrizamide (increased seizure potential), guanabenz, MAO inhibitors

Drug Uptake
Onset of neuroleptic effect: Oral: Within 20-30 minutes
Peak effect: 1.5-3 hours
Duration: ~12 hours
Serum half-life, biphasic:
  Initial: 5 hours
  Terminal: 12-19 hours

Pregnancy Risk Factor C
Generic Available Yes

Loxitane® see Loxapine on previous page

Lozol® see Indapamide on page 504

L-PAM see Melphalan on page 590

L-Sarcolysin see Melphalan on page 590

Lubriderm® [OTC] see Lanolin, Cetyl Alcohol, Glycerin, and Petrolatum on page 542

LubriTears® Solution [OTC] see Artificial Tears on page 87

Ludiomil® see Maprotiline on page 579

Lufyllin® see Dyphylline on page 342

Luminal® see Phenobarbital on page 747

Lupron® see Leuprolide Acetate on page 545

Lupron® Depot see Leuprolide Acetate on page 545

Lupron® Depot-Ped see Leuprolide Acetate on page 545

Luride® see Fluoride on page 415

Luride® Lozi-Tab® see Fluoride on page 415

Luride®-SF Lozi-Tab® see Fluoride on page 415

Luvox® see Fluvoxamine on page 426

Lycolan® Elixir [OTC] see L-Lysine on page 562

Lymphocyte Immune Globulin (LIM foe site i MYUN GLOB yoo lin)

Brand Names Atgam®

Therapeutic Category Immunosuppressant Agent

Synonyms Antithymocyte Globulin (Equine); Antithymocyte Immunoglobulin; ATG; Horse Anti-human Thymocyte Gamma Globulin

Use Prevention and treatment of acute allograft rejection; treatment of moderate to severe aplastic anemia in patients not considered suitable candidates for bone marrow transplantation; prevention of graft-vs-host disease following bone marrow transplantation

Usual Dosage An intradermal skin test is recommended prior to administration of the initial dose of ATG; use 0.1 mL of a 1:1000 dilution of ATG in normal saline

Children: I.V.:
  Aplastic anemia protocol: 10-20 mg/kg/day for 8-14 days, then give every other day for 7 more doses
  Cardiac allograft: 10 mg/kg/day for 7 days
  Renal allograft: 5-25 mg/kg/day

Adults: I.V.:
  Aplastic anemia protocol: 10-20 mg/kg/day for 8-14 days, then give every other day for 7 more doses **or** 40 mg/kg/day for 4 days
  Rejection prevention: 15 mg/kg/day for 14 days, then give every other day for 7 more doses for a total of 21 doses in 28 days; initial dose should be administered within 24 hours before or after transplantation
  Rejection treatment: 10-15 mg/kg/day for 14 days, then give every other day for 7 more doses

Mechanism of Action May involve elimination of antigen-reactive T-lymphocytes (killer cells) in peripheral blood or alteration of T-cell function

Local Anesthetic/Vasoconstrictor Precautions No information available to require special precautions

Effects on Dental Treatment No effects or complications reported

Other Adverse Effects
>10%:
  Central nervous system: Fever, chills
  Dermatologic: Rash
  Hematologic: Leukopenia, thrombocytopenia
  Miscellaneous: Systemic infection

1% to 10%:
Cardiovascular: Hypotension, hypertension, tachycardia, edema, chest pain
Central nervous system: Headache, malaise
Gastrointestinal: Diarrhea, nausea, stomatitis, GI bleeding
Respiratory: Dyspnea
Local: Pain, swelling or redness at injection site, thrombophlebitis
Neuromuscular & skeletal: Myalgia, back pain
Renal: Abnormal renal function tests
Miscellaneous: Viral infection, anaphylaxis may be indicated by hypotension, respiratory distress, serum sickness

<1%:
Central nervous system: Seizures
Dermatologic: Pruritus, urticaria
Hematologic: Hemolysis, anemia
Neuromuscular & skeletal: Arthralgia, weakness
Renal: Acute renal failure
Miscellaneous: Lymphadenopathy

Drug Uptake
Serum half-life: 1.5-12 days
Pregnancy Risk Factor C
Generic Available No
Comments Do not dilute with D_5W (may cause precipitation). The use of highly acidic infusion solutions is not recommended because of possible physical instability. When the dose of corticosteroids and other immunosuppressants is being reduced, some previously masked reaction to Atgam® may appear.

Lyphocin® *see* Vancomycin *on page 983*

Lypressin (lye PRES in)
Brand Names Diapid®
Therapeutic Category Antidiuretic Hormone Analog
Use Controls or prevents signs and complications of neurogenic diabetes insipidus
Usual Dosage Children and Adults: Instill 1-2 sprays into one or both nostrils whenever frequency of urination increases or significant thirst develops; usual dosage is 1-2 sprays 4 times/day; range: 1 spray/day at bedtime to 10 sprays each nostril every 3-4 hours
Mechanism of Action Increases cyclic adenosine monophosphate (cAMP) which increases water permeability at the renal tubule resulting in decreased urine volume and increased osmolality; causes peristalsis by directly stimulating the smooth muscle in the GI tract
Local Anesthetic/Vasoconstrictor Precautions No information available to require special precautions
Effects on Dental Treatment No effects or complications reported
Other Adverse Effects
1% to 10%:
Central nervous system: Dizziness, headache
Gastrointestinal: Abdominal cramping, increased bowel movements
Respiratory: Chest tightness, coughing, dyspnea, rhinorrhea, nasal congestion, irritation or burning
<1%:
Endocrine & metabolic: Water intoxication
Respiratory: Inadvertent inhalation
Drug Interactions Increased effect: Chlorpropamide, clofibrate, carbamazepine causes prolongation of antidiuretic effects
Drug Uptake
Onset of antidiuretic effect: Intranasal spray: Within 0.5-2 hours
Duration: 3-8 hours
Serum half-life: 15-20 minutes
Pregnancy Risk Factor C
Generic Available No

Lysodren® *see* Mitotane *on page 643*
Maalox® [OTC] *see* Aluminum Hydroxide and Magnesium Hydroxide *on page 48*
Maalox Anti-Gas® [OTC] *see* Simethicone *on page 865*
Maalox® Plus [OTC] *see* Aluminum Hydroxide, Magnesium Hydroxide, and Simethicone *on page 49*
Maalox® Therapeutic Concentrate [OTC] *see* Aluminum Hydroxide and Magnesium Hydroxide *on page 48*
Macrobid® *see* Nitrofurantoin *on page 684*
Macrodantin® *see* Nitrofurantoin *on page 684*
Macrodex® *see* Dextran *on page 295*

Mafenide (MA fe nide)
Brand Names Sulfamylon®

Therapeutic Category Antibacterial, Topical; Antibiotic, Topical

Use Adjunct in the treatment of second and third degree burns to prevent septicemia caused by susceptible organisms such as *Pseudomonas aeruginosa*; prevention of graft loss of meshed autografts on excised burn wounds

Usual Dosage Children and Adults: Topical: Apply once or twice daily with a sterile gloved hand; apply to a thickness of approximately 16 mm; the burned area should be covered with cream at all times

Mechanism of Action Interferes with bacterial folic acid synthesis through competitive inhibition of para-aminobenzoic acid

Local Anesthetic/Vasoconstrictor Precautions No information available to require special precautions

Effects on Dental Treatment No effects or complications reported

Other Adverse Effects
>10%: Local: Burning sensation, excoriation, pain

1% to 10%:
  Cardiovascular: Swelling of face
  Dermatologic: Skin rash
  Respiratory: Dyspnea

<1%:
  Dermatologic: Erythema
  Endocrine & metabolic: Hyperchloremia, metabolic acidosis
  Hematologic: Bone marrow suppression, hemolytic anemia, bleeding, porphyria
  Respiratory: Hyperventilation, tachypnea
  Miscellaneous: Hypersensitivity

Drug Interactions No data reported

Drug Uptake
Absorption: Diffuses through devascularized areas and is rapidly absorbed from burned surface

Time to peak serum concentration: Topical: 2-4 hours

Pregnancy Risk Factor C

Generic Available No

Magaldrate (MAG al drate)
Brand Names Riopan® [OTC]

Therapeutic Category Antacid

Synonyms Hydromagnesium Aluminate

Use Symptomatic relief of hyperacidity associated with peptic ulcer, gastritis, peptic esophagitis and hiatal hernia

Local Anesthetic/Vasoconstrictor Precautions No information available to require special precautions

Effects on Dental Treatment No effects or complications reported

Other Adverse Effects
>10%: Gastrointestinal: Constipation, chalky taste, stomach cramps, fecal impaction

1% to 10%: Gastrointestinal: Nausea, vomiting, discoloration of feces (white speckles)

<1%: Endocrine & metabolic: Hypophosphatemia, hypomagnesemia

Pregnancy Risk Factor C

Generic Available Yes

Comments Chemical entity known as hydroxy magnesium aluminate equivalent to magnesium oxide and aluminum oxide; unlike other magnesium-containing antacids, Riopan® is safe to use in renal patients

Magaldrate and Simethicone (MAG al drate & sye METH i kone)
Brand Names Riopan Plus® [OTC]

Therapeutic Category Antacid; Antiflatulent

Synonyms Simethicone and Magaldrate

Use Relief of hyperacidity associated with peptic ulcer, gastritis, peptic esophagitis and hiatal hernia which are accompanied by symptoms of gas

Local Anesthetic/Vasoconstrictor Precautions No information available to require special precautions

Effects on Dental Treatment No effects or complications reported

Pregnancy Risk Factor C

Generic Available Yes

Comments Chemical entity known as hydroxy magnesium aluminate equivalent to magnesium oxide and aluminum oxide; unlike other magnesium containing antacids, Riopan® is safe to use in renal patients if used cautiously

Magalox Plus® [OTC] *see* Aluminum Hydroxide, Magnesium Hydroxide, and Simethicone *on page 49*

Magan® *see* Magnesium Salicylate *on page 577*

Magnacal® [OTC] *see* Enteral Nutritional Products *on page 350*

Magnesio, Hidroxido De (Mexico) *see* Magnesium Hydroxide *on next page*

Magnesio, Oxide De (Mexico) *see* Magnesium Oxide *on page 577*

Magnesium Chloride (mag NEE zhum KLOR ide)
Brand Names Slow-Mag® [OTC]

Therapeutic Category Magnesium Salt

Use Correct or prevent hypomagnesemia

Local Anesthetic/Vasoconstrictor Precautions No information available to require special precautions

Effects on Dental Treatment Magnesium products may prevent gastrointestinal absorption of tetracyclines by forming a large ionized chelated molecule with the tetracyclines in the stomach. Tetracyclines should be given at least 1 hour before magnesium.

Other Adverse Effects 1% to 10%:
Cardiovascular: Flushing
Central nervous system: Depressed CNS, somnolence
Gastrointestinal: Diarrhea
Neuromuscular & skeletal: Blocked peripheral neuromuscular transmission, deep tendon reflexes
Respiratory: Respiratory paralysis

Pregnancy Risk Factor D

Generic Available Yes

Magnesium Citrate (mag NEE zhum SIT rate)
Brand Names Evac-Q-Mag® [OTC]

Therapeutic Category Laxative, Saline

Synonyms Citrate of Magnesia

Use To evacuate bowel prior to certain surgical and diagnostic procedures

Mechanism of Action Promotes bowel evacuation by causing osmotic retention of fluid which distends the colon with increased peristaltic activity

Local Anesthetic/Vasoconstrictor Precautions No information available to require special precautions

Effects on Dental Treatment Magnesium products may prevent gastrointestinal absorption of tetracyclines by forming a large ionized chelated molecule with the tetracyclines in the stomach. Tetracyclines should be given at least 1 hour before magnesium.

Other Adverse Effects 1% to 10%:
Cardiovascular: Hypotension
Endocrine & metabolic: Hypermagnesemia
Gastrointestinal: Abdominal cramps, diarrhea, gas formation
Respiratory: Respiratory depression

Drug Uptake Absorption: Oral: 15% to 30%

Pregnancy Risk Factor B

Generic Available Yes

Comments Magnesium content of 5 mL: 3.85-4.71 mEq

Magnesium Gluconate (mag NEE zhum GLOO koe nate)
Brand Names Magonate® [OTC]

Therapeutic Category Magnesium Salt

Use Dietary supplement for treatment of magnesium deficiencies

Usual Dosage The recommended dietary allowance (RDA) of magnesium is 4.5 mg/kg which is a total daily allowance of 350-400 mg for adult men and 280-300 mg for adult women. During pregnancy the RDA is 300 mg and during lactation the RDA is 355 mg. Average daily intakes of dietary magnesium have declined in recent years due to processing of food. The latest estimate of the average American dietary intake was 349 mg/day.

Dietary supplement: Oral:
Children: 3-6 mg/kg/day in divided doses 3-4 times/day; maximum: 400 mg/day
Adults: 27-54 mg 2-3 times/day or 100 mg 4 times/day

Mechanism of Action Magnesium is important as a cofactor in many enzymatic reactions in the body involving protein synthesis and carbohydrate metabolism, (at least 300 enzymatic reactions require magnesium). Actions on lipoprotein lipase have been found to be important in reducing serum cholesterol and on sodium/potassium ATPase in promoting polarization (ie, neuromuscular functioning).
(Continued)

Magnesium Gluconate *(Continued)*

Local Anesthetic/Vasoconstrictor Precautions No information available to require special precautions

Effects on Dental Treatment Magnesium products may prevent gastrointestinal absorption of tetracyclines by forming a large ionized chelated molecule with the tetracyclines in the stomach. Tetracyclines should be given at least 1 hour before magnesium.

Other Adverse Effects ˙

1% to 10%: Gastrointestinal: Diarrhea (excessive dose)

<1%:

Endocrine & metabolic: Hypotension, hypermagnesemia

Gastrointestinal: Abdominal cramps

Neuromuscular & skeletal: Muscle weakness

Respiratory: Respiratory depression

Drug Uptake

Absorption: Oral: 15% to 30%

Generic Available Yes

Comments Magnesium content of 500 mg: 27 mg

Magnesium Hydroxide *(mag NEE zhum hye DROKS ide)*

Brand Names Phillips'® Milk of Magnesia [OTC]

Canadian/Mexican Brand Names Leche De Magnesia Normex (Mexico)

Therapeutic Category Antacid; Laxative, Saline; Magnesium Salt

Synonyms Magnesio, Hidroxido De (Mexico)

Use Short-term treatment of occasional constipation and symptoms of hyperacidity, magnesium replacement therapy

Usual Dosage Oral:

Laxative:

<2 years: 0.5 mL/kg/dose

2-5 years: 5-15 mL/day or in divided doses

6-12 years: 15-30 mL/day or in divided doses

≥12 years: 30-60 mL/day or in divided doses

Antacid:

Children: 2.5-5 mL as needed up to 4 times/day

Adults: 5-15 mL or 650 mg to 1.3 g tablets up to 4 times/day as needed

Mechanism of Action Promotes bowel evacuation by causing osmotic retention of fluid which distends the colon with increased peristaltic activity; reacts with hydrochloric acid in stomach to form magnesium chloride

Local Anesthetic/Vasoconstrictor Precautions No information available to require special precautions

Effects on Dental Treatment Magnesium products may prevent gastrointestinal absorption of tetracyclines by forming a large ionized chelated molecule with the tetracyclines in the stomach. Tetracyclines should be given at least 1 hour before magnesium.

Other Adverse Effects

>10%: Diarrhea

1% to 10%:

Cardiovascular: Hypotension

Endocrine & metabolic: Hypermagnesemia

Gastrointestinal: Abdominal cramps

Neuromuscular & skeletal: Muscle weakness

Respiratory: Respiratory depression

Drug Interactions Decreased effect: Decreased absorption of tetracyclines, digoxin, indomethacin, or iron salts

Drug Uptake Onset of laxative action: 4-8 hours

Pregnancy Risk Factor B

Generic Available Yes

Magnesium Hydroxide and Aluminum Hydroxide *see* Aluminum Hydroxide and Magnesium Hydroxide *on page 48*

Magnesium Hydroxide and Mineral Oil Emulsion

(mag NEE zhum hye DROKS ide & MIN er al oyl e MUL shun)

Brand Names Haley's M-O® [OTC]

Therapeutic Category Laxative, Lubricant; Laxative, Saline

Synonyms MOM/Mineral Oil Emulsion

Use Short-term treatment of occasional constipation

Local Anesthetic/Vasoconstrictor Precautions No information available to require special precautions

Effects on Dental Treatment Magnesium products may prevent gastrointestinal absorption of tetracyclines by forming a large ionized chelated molecule with the tetracyclines in the stomach. Tetracyclines should be given at least 1 hour before magnesium.

Pregnancy Risk Factor B
Generic Available Yes

Magnesium Oxide (mag NEE zhum OKS ide)

Brand Names Maox®
Therapeutic Category Antacid
Synonyms Magnesio, Oxide De (Mexico)
Use Short-term treatment of occasional constipation and symptoms of hyperacidity
Usual Dosage Magnesium RDA: 4.5 mg/kg, which is a total daily allowance of 350 mg for adult men and 280-300 mg for adult women. During pregnancy, the RDA is 200 mg and during lactation it is 355 mg. Average daily intakes of dietary magnesium have declined in recent years due to processing in food. The latest estimate of the average American dietary intake was 349 mg/day.

Adults: Oral:
  Dietary supplement: 27-54 mEq (1-2 tablets) 2-3 times
  Antacid: 1/2 to 3 tablets (0.21-1.68 g) with water or milk 4 times/day after meals and at bedtime
  Laxative: 2-4 g at bedtime with full glass of water

Mechanism of Action Promotes bowel evacuation by causing osmotic retention of fluid which distends the colon with increased peristaltic activity
Local Anesthetic/Vasoconstrictor Precautions No information available to require special precautions
Effects on Dental Treatment Magnesium products may prevent gastrointestinal absorption of tetracyclines by forming a large ionized chelated molecule with the tetracyclines in the stomach. Tetracyclines should be given at least 1 hour before magnesium.
Other Adverse Effects
  >10%: Diarrhea
  1% to 10%:
    Cardiovascular: Hypotension, EKG changes
    Central nervous system: Mental depression, coma
    Gastrointestinal: Nausea, vomiting
    Respiratory: Respiratory depression
Drug Interactions Decreased effect: Tetracyclines, digoxin, indomethacin, iron salts, isoniazid, quinolones
Drug Uptake Onset of laxative action: 4-8 hours
Pregnancy Risk Factor B
Generic Available Yes

Magnesium Salicylate (mag NEE zhum sa LIS i late)

Brand Names Doan's®, Original [OTC]; Extra Strength Doan's® [OTC]; Magan®; Mobidin®
Therapeutic Category Nonsteroidal Anti-inflammatory Agent (NSAID), Oral
Use Mild to moderate pain, fever, various inflammatory conditions
Usual Dosage Oral: Adults: 650 mg 4 times daily or 1090 mg 3 times daily; may increase to 3.6-4.8 mg/day in 3 or 4 divided doses
Local Anesthetic/Vasoconstrictor Precautions No information available to require special precautions
Effects on Dental Treatment No effects or complications reported
Dosage Forms
  Caplet:
    Doan's®, Original: 325 mg
    Extra Strength Doan's®: 500 mg
  Tablet:
    Magan®: 545 mg
    Mobidin®: 600 mg
Generic Available Yes

Magnesium Sulfate (mag NEE zhum SUL fate)

Therapeutic Category Anticonvulsant, Miscellaneous; Electrolyte Supplement, Parenteral; Laxative, Saline; Magnesium Salt
Synonyms Epsom Salts
Use Treatment and prevention of hypomagnesemia; hypertension; encephalopathy and seizures associated with acute nephritis in children; also used as a cathartic
Usual Dosage The recommended dietary allowance (RDA) of magnesium is 4.5 mg/kg which is a total daily allowance of 350-400 mg for adult men and 280-300 mg for adult women. During pregnancy the RDA is 300 mg and during lactation the RDA is 355 mg. Average daily intakes of dietary magnesium have declined in
(Continued)

Magnesium Sulfate *(Continued)*

recent years due to processing of food. The latest estimate of the average American dietary intake was 349 mg/day. Dose represented as $MgSO_4$ unless stated otherwise.

Note: Serum magnesium is poor reflection of repletional status as the majority of magnesium is intracellular; serum levels may be transiently normal for a few hours after a dose is given, therefore, aim for consistently high normal serum levels in patients with normal renal function for most efficient repletion

Hypomagnesemia:
Children: I.M., I.V.: 25-50 mg/kg/dose (0.2-0.4 mEq/kg/dose) every 4-6 hours for 3-4 doses, maximum single dose: 2000 mg (16 mEq), may repeat if hypomagnesemia persists (higher dosage up to 100 mg/kg/dose $MgSO_4$ I.V. has been used); maintenance: I.V.: 30-60 mg/kg/day (0.25-0.5 mEq/kg/day)

Management of seizures and hypertension:
Children:
Oral: 100-200 mg/kg/dose 4 times/day
I.M., I.V.: 20-100 mg/kg/dose every 4-6 hours as needed; in severe cases doses as high as 200 mg/kg/dose have been used
Adults:
Oral: 3 g every 6 hours for 4 doses as needed
I.M., I.V.: 1 g every 6 hours for 4 doses; for severe hypomagnesemia: 8-12 g $MgSO_4$/day in divided doses has been used

Eclampsia, pre-eclampsia: Adults:
I.M.: 1-4 g every 4 hours
I.V.: Initial: 4 g, then switch to I.M. or 1-4 g/hour by continuous infusion

Maximum dose should not exceed 30-40 g/day; maximum rate of infusion: 1-2 g/hour

Maintenance electrolyte requirements:
Daily requirements: 0.2-0.5 mEq/kg/24 hours or 3-10 mEq/1000 kcal/24 hours
Maximum: 8-16 mEq/24 hours

Cathartic: Oral:
Children: 0.25 g/kg every 4-6 hours
Adults: 10-15 g in a glass of water

Mechanism of Action Promotes bowel evacuation by causing osmotic retention of fluid which distends the colon with increased peristaltic activity when taken orally; parenterally, decreases acetylcholine in motor nerve terminals and acts on myocardium by slowing rate of S-A node impulse formation and prolonging conduction time

Local Anesthetic/Vasoconstrictor Precautions No information available to require special precautions

Effects on Dental Treatment Magnesium products may prevent gastrointestinal absorption of tetracyclines by forming a large ionized chelated molecule with the tetracyclines in the stomach. Tetracyclines should be given at least 1 hour before magnesium.

Other Adverse Effects
1% to 10%:
Serum magnesium levels >3 mg/dL:
Central nervous system: Depressed CNS
Gastrointestinal: Diarrhea
Neuromuscular & skeletal: Blocked peripheral neuromuscular transmission leading to anticonvulsant effects
Serum magnesium levels >5 mg/dL:
Cardiovascular: Flushing
Central nervous system: Somnolence
Serum magnesium levels >12.5 mg/dL:
Cardiovascular: Complete heart block
Respiratory: Respiratory paralysis

Drug Uptake
Oral: Onset of cathartic action: Within 1-2 hours
I.M.:
Onset of action: 1 hour
Duration: 3-4 hours
I.V.:
Onset of action: Immediate
Duration: 30 minutes

Pregnancy Risk Factor B

Generic Available Yes

Comments $MgSO_4$ 500 mg = magnesium 4.06 mEq = elemental magnesium 49.3 mg

Magonate® [OTC] *see* Magnesium Gluconate *on page 575*

Malatal® *see* Hyoscyamine, Atropine, Scopolamine, and Phenobarbital *on page 493*

Mallamint® [OTC] *see* Calcium Carbonate *on page 162*

Mallazine® Eye Drops [OTC] *see* Tetrahydrozoline *on page 916*

Malt Soup Extract (malt soop EKS trakt)
Brand Names Maltsupex® [OTC]
Therapeutic Category Laxative, Bulk-Producing
Use Short-term treatment of constipation
Local Anesthetic/Vasoconstrictor Precautions No information available to require special precautions
Effects on Dental Treatment No effects or complications reported
Other Adverse Effects 1% to 10%: Gastrointestinal: Abdominal cramps, diarrhea, rectal obstruction
Generic Available No

Maltsupex® [OTC] *see* Malt Soup Extract *on this page*

Mandelamine® *see* Methenamine *on page 610*

Mandol® *see* Cefamandole *on page 187*

Manganese *see* Trace Metals *on page 948*

Mantoux *see* Tuberculin Purified Protein Derivative *on page 975*

Maolate® *see* Chlorphenesin *on page 217*

Maox® *see* Magnesium Oxide *on page 577*

Mapap® [OTC] *see* Acetaminophen *on page 20*

Maprotilina, Clorhidrato De (Mexico) *see* Maprotiline *on this page*

Maprotiline (ma PROE ti leen)
Related Information
Vasoconstrictor Interactions With Antidepressants *on page 1226*
Brand Names Ludiomil®
Therapeutic Category Antidepressant, Tetracyclic
Synonyms Maprotilina, Clorhidrato De (Mexico)
Use Treatment of depression and anxiety associated with depression
Usual Dosage Oral:
Children 6-14 years: 10 mg/day, increase to a maximum daily dose of 75 mg
Adults: 75 mg/day to start, increase by 25 mg every 2 weeks up to 150-225 mg/day; given in 3 divided doses or in a single daily dose
Elderly: Initial: 25 mg at bedtime, increase by 25 mg every 3 days for inpatients and weekly for outpatients if tolerated; usual maintenance dose: 50-75 mg/day, higher doses may be necessary in nonresponders
Mechanism of Action Traditionally believed to increase the synaptic concentration of norepinephrine in the central nervous system by inhibition of their reuptake by the presynaptic neuronal membrane. However, additional receptor effects have been found including desensitization of adenyl cyclase, down regulation of beta-adrenergic receptors, and down regulation of serotonin receptors.
Local Anesthetic/Vasoconstrictor Precautions Use with caution; epinephrine, norepinephrine and levonordefrin have been shown to have an increased pressor response in combination with TCAs
Effects on Dental Treatment >10% of patients experience dry mouth; long-term treatment with TCAs such as amoxapine increases the risk of caries by reducing salivation and salivary buffer capacity
Other Adverse Effects
>10%:
Cardiovascular: Orthostatic hypotension
Central nervous system: Drowsiness
Dermatologic: Skin rash
Genitourinary: Urinary retention
Neuromuscular & skeletal: Weakness
1% to 10%:
Central nervous system: Insomnia
Gastrointestinal: Constipation, nausea, vomiting, increased appetite and weight gain, weight loss
Neuromuscular & skeletal: Trembling
<1%:
Central nervous system: Confusion
Endocrine & metabolic: Breast enlargement
Genitourinary: Swelling of testicles
Hepatic: Cholestatic hepatitis
Ocular: Blurred vision, increased intraocular pressure
Otic: Tinnitus
(Continued)

Maprotiline *(Continued)*

Drug Interactions

Decreased effect: Phenobarbital may increase the metabolism of maprotiline; maprotiline blocks the uptake of guanethidine and thus prevents the hypotensive effect of guanethidine

Increased toxicity: Clonidine causes hypertensive crisis; maprotiline may be additive with or may potentiate the action of other CNS depressants such as sedatives or hypnotics; with MAO inhibitors, hyperpyrexia, hypertension, tachycardia, confusion, and seizures. Maprotiline may increase the prothrombin time in patients stabilized on warfarin; maprotiline potentiate the pressor and cardiac effects of sympathomimetic agents such as isoproterenol, epinephrine, etc; cimetidine and methylphenidate may decrease the metabolism of maprotiline

Additive anticholinergic effects seen with other anticholinergic agents

Drug Uptake

Absorption: Slow

Serum half-life: 27-58 hours (mean, 43 hours)

Time to peak serum concentration: Within 12 hours

Pregnancy Risk Factor B

Generic Available Yes

Selected Readings

Boakes AJ, Laurence DR, Teoh PC, et al, "Interactions Between Sympathomimetic Amines and Antidepressant Agents in Man," *Br Med J*, 1973, 1(849):311-5.

Jastak JT and Yagiela JA, "Vasoconstrictors and Local Anesthesia: A Review and Rationale for Use," *J Am Dent Assoc*, 1983, 107(4):623-30.

Larochelle P, Hamet P, and Enjalbert M, "Responses to Tyramine and Norepinephrine After Imipramine and Trazodone," *Clin Pharmacol Ther*, 1979, 26(1):24-30.

Mitchell JR, "Guanethidine and Related Agents. III Antagonism by Drugs Which Inhibit the Norepinephrine Pump in Man," *J Clin Invest*, 1970, 49(8):1596-604.

Rundegren J, van Dijken J, Mörnstad H, et al, "Oral Conditions in Patients Receiving Long-Term Treatment With Cyclic Antidepressant Drugs," *Swed Dent J*, 1985, 9(2):55-64.

Svedmyr N, "The Influence of a Tricyclic Antidepressive Agent (Protriptyline) on Some of the Circulatory Effects of Noradrenaline and Adrenalin in Man," *Life Sci*, 1968, 7(1):77-84.

Wynn RL, "New Antidepressant Medications," *Gen Dent*, 1997, 45(1):24-8.

Maranox® [OTC] *see* Acetaminophen *on page 20*

Marax® *see* Theophylline, Ephedrine, and Hydroxyzine *on page 922*

Marcaine® *see* Bupivacaine *on page 148*

Marcaine® With Epinephrine *see* Bupivacaine and Epinephrine *on page 149*

Marcillin® *see* Ampicillin *on page 73*

Marezine® [OTC] *see* Cyclizine *on page 267*

Marezine® *see* Meclizine *on page 584*

Margesic® H [5/500] *see* Hydrocodone and Acetaminophen *on page 478*

Marinol® *see* Dronabinol *on page 340*

Marnal® *see* Butalbital Compound *on page 154*

Marplan® *see* Isocarboxazid *on page 520*

Marpres® *see* Hydralazine, Hydrochlorothiazide, and Reserpine *on page 476*

Marthritic® *see* Salsalate *on page 855*

Masoprocol *(ma SOE pro kole)*

Brand Names Actinex®

Therapeutic Category Topical Skin Product

Use Treatment of actinic keratosis

Usual Dosage Adults: Topical: Wash and dry area; gently massage into affected area every morning and evening for 28 days

Mechanism of Action Antiproliferative activity against keratinocytes

Local Anesthetic/Vasoconstrictor Precautions No information available to require special precautions

Effects on Dental Treatment No effects or complications reported

Other Adverse Effects

>10%:

Dermatologic: Erythema, flaking, dryness, itching

Local: Burning

1% to 10%:

Dermatologic: Soreness, rash

Neuromuscular & skeletal: Paresthesia

Ocular: Eye irritation

<1%: Dermatologic: Blistering, excoriation, skin roughness, wrinkling

Drug Interactions No data reported

Drug Uptake Absorption: Topical: <1% to 2%

Pregnancy Risk Factor B

Dosage Forms Cream: 10% (30 g)

Generic Available Yes

Massé® Breast Cream [OTC] *see* Glycerin, Lanolin, and Peanut Oil *on page 447*

Matulane® *see* Procarbazine *on page 798*

Mavik® *see* Trandolapril *on page 949*

Maxair™ *see* Pirbuterol *on page 766*

Maxaquin® *see* Lomefloxacin *on page 563*

Max-Caro® [OTC] *see* Beta-Carotene *on page 125*

Maxiflor® *see* Diflorasone *on page 311*

Maximum Strength Anbesol® [OTC] *see* Benzocaine *on page 118*

Maximum Strength Desenex® Antifungal Cream [OTC] *see* Miconazole *on page 635*

Maximum Strength Dex-A-Diet® [OTC] *see* Phenylpropanolamine *on page 754*

Maximum Strength Dexatrim® [OTC] *see* Phenylpropanolamine *on page 754*

Maximum Strength Nytol® [OTC] *see* Diphenhydramine *on page 323*

Maximum Strength Orajel® [OTC] *see* Benzocaine *on page 118*

Maxipime® *see* Cefepime *on page 189*

Maxitrol® *see* Neomycin, Polymyxin B, and Dexamethasone *on page 672*

Maxivate® *see* Betamethasone *on page 126*

Maxolon® *see* Metoclopramide *on page 627*

Maxzide® *see* Hydrochlorothiazide and Triamterene *on page 478*

Mazanor® *see* Mazindol *on this page*

Mazindol (MAY zin dole)
Brand Names Mazanor®; Sanorex®
Therapeutic Category Anorexiant
Use Short-term adjunct in exogenous obesity
Local Anesthetic/Vasoconstrictor Precautions No information available to require special precautions
Effects on Dental Treatment No effects or complications reported
Other Adverse Effects
>10%:
  Cardiovascular: Hypertension
  Central nervous system: Euphoria, nervousness, insomnia
1% to 10%:
  Central nervous system: Confusion, mental depression, restlessness
  Endocrine & metabolic: Changes in libido
  Gastrointestinal: Nausea, vomiting, constipation
  Hematologic: Blood dyscrasias
  Neuromuscular & skeletal: Tremor
  Ocular: Blurred vision
<1%:
  Cardiovascular: Tachycardia, arrhythmias
  Central nervous system: Headache
  Dermatologic: Alopecia
  Gastrointestinal: Diarrhea, abdominal cramps
  Genitourinary: Dysuria, testicular pain
  Neuromuscular & skeletal: Myalgia
  Renal: Polyuria
  Respiratory: Dyspnea
  Miscellaneous: Increased sweating
Pregnancy Risk Factor C
Generic Available No

m-Cresyl Acetate (em-KREE sil AS e tate)
Brand Names Cresylate®
Therapeutic Category Otic Agent, Anti-infective
Use Provides an acid medium; for external otitis infections caused by susceptible bacteria or fungus
Local Anesthetic/Vasoconstrictor Precautions No information available to require special precautions
Effects on Dental Treatment No effects or complications reported
Generic Available No

MCT Oil® [OTC] *see* Medium Chain Triglycerides *on page 586*

Measles and Rubella Vaccines, Combined
(MEE zels & roo BEL a vak SEENS, kom BINED)
Brand Names M-R-VAX® II
Therapeutic Category Vaccine, Live Virus
(Continued)

Measles and Rubella Vaccines, Combined *(Continued)*

Synonyms Rubella and Measles Vaccines, Combined

Use Simultaneous immunization against measles and rubella

Usual Dosage Children at 15 months and Adults: S.C.: Inject 0.5 mL into outer aspect of upper arm; no routine booster for rubella

Local Anesthetic/Vasoconstrictor Precautions No information available to require special precautions

Effects on Dental Treatment No effects or complications reported

Other Adverse Effects All serious adverse reactions must be reported to the FDA

>10%:

Central nervous system: Fever <100°F

Dermatologic: Urticaria, rash, local erythema

Local: Burning at injection site, local tenderness

Neuromuscular & skeletal: Arthralgias

1% to 10%:

Central nervous system: Fever between 100°F and 103°F, malaise, headache

Gastrointestinal: Sore throat

Miscellaneous: Allergic reaction (delayed type), lymphadenopathy

<1%:

Central nervous system: Fatigue, convulsions, encephalitis, confusion, severe headache, fever >103°F (prolonged)

Dermatologic: Itching, reddening of skin (especially around ears and eyes)

Gastrointestinal: Vomiting

Hematologic: Thrombocytopenic purpura

Neuromuscular & skeletal: Stiff neck

Ocular: Diplopia, optic neuritis

Respiratory: Dyspnea

Miscellaneous: Hypersensitivity

The chance of a child having a convulsion after receiving the measles vaccine is small. The risk is up to 5 times greater if the child has ever had a convulsion before or if the child's brother, sister, or parent has ever had a convulsion.

Pregnancy Risk Factor X

Generic Available No

Comments Federal law requires that the date of administration, the vaccine manufacturer, lot number of vaccine, and the administering person's name, title and address be entered into the patient's permanent medical record

Measles, Mumps, and Rubella Vaccines, Combined

(MEE zels, mumpz & roo BEL a vak SEENS, kom BINED)

Brand Names M-M-R® II

Therapeutic Category Vaccine, Live Virus

Synonyms MMR; Mumps, Measles and Rubella Vaccines, Combined; Rubella, Measles and Mumps Vaccines, Combined

Use Measles, mumps, and rubella prophylaxis

Usual Dosage

Infants <12 months: If there is risk of exposure to measles, single-antigen measles vaccine should be administered at 6-11 months of age with a second dose (of MMR) at >12 months of age

Give S.C. in outer aspect of the upper arm to children ≥15 months of age:

0.5 mL at 15 months of age and then repeated at 4-6 years* of age

In some areas, MMR vaccine may be given at 12 months

*Many experts recommend that this dose of MMR be given at entry to middle school or junior high school

Local Anesthetic/Vasoconstrictor Precautions No information available to require special precautions

Effects on Dental Treatment No effects or complications reported

Other Adverse Effects All serious adverse reactions must be reported to the FDA

1% to 10%:

Dermatologic: Transient rash, tenderness erythema and swelling

Gastrointestinal: Sore throat

Miscellaneous: Allergic reactions

<1%: Central nervous system: Seizures, malaise, fever

The chance of a child having a convulsion after receiving the measles vaccine is small. The risk is up to 5 times greater if the child has ever had a convulsion before or if the child's brother, sister, or parent has ever had a convulsion.

Pregnancy Risk Factor X

Generic Available No

Comments Federal law requires that the date of administration, the vaccine manufacturer, lot number of vaccine, and the administering person's name, title and address be entered into the patient's permanent medical record

Measles Virus Vaccine, Live (MEE zels VYE rus vak SEEN, live)
Brand Names Attenuvax®
Canadian/Mexican Brand Names Ervevax (Mexico)
Therapeutic Category Vaccine, Live Virus
Synonyms More Attenuated Enders Strain; Rubeola Vaccine
Use Immunization against measles (rubeola) in persons ≥15 months of age
Usual Dosage Children >15 months and Adults: S.C.: 0.5 mL in outer aspect of the upper arm, no routine boosters
Local Anesthetic/Vasoconstrictor Precautions No information available to require special precautions
Effects on Dental Treatment No effects or complications reported
Other Adverse Effects All serious adverse reactions must be reported to the FDA
Dermatologic: Rarely urticaria, erythema

>10%:
  Cardiovascular: Swelling
  Central nervous system: Fever <100°F
  Local: Burning or stinging, induration
1% to 10%:
  Central nervous system: Fever between 100°F and 103°F
  Miscellaneous: Allergic reaction (delayed type)
<1%:
  Central nervous system: Fatigue, convulsions, confusion, severe headache, fever >103°F (prolonged)
  Dermatologic: Itching, reddening of skin (especially around ears and eyes)
  Gastrointestinal: Vomiting, sore throat
  Hematologic: Thrombocytopenic purpura
  Ocular: Diplopia
  Neuromuscular & skeletal: Stiff neck
  Respiratory: Dyspnea, coryza
  Miscellaneous: Lymphadenopathy
Pregnancy Risk Factor X
Generic Available No
Comments Federal law requires that the date of administration, the vaccine manufacturer, lot number of vaccine, and the administering person's name, title and address be entered into the patient's permanent medical record

Mebaral® *see* Mephobarbital *on page 594*

Mebendazole (me BEN da zole)
Brand Names Vermox®
Canadian/Mexican Brand Names Helminzole® (Mexico); Mebensole® (Mexico); Revapol® (Mexico); Soltric® (Mexico); Vermicol® (Mexico)
Therapeutic Category Anthelmintic
Use Treatment of pinworms, whipworms, roundworms, and hookworms
Usual Dosage Children and Adults: Oral:
  Pinworms: 100 mg as a single dose; may need to repeat after 2 weeks; treatment should include family members in close contact with patient
  Whipworms, roundworms, hookworms: One tablet twice daily, morning and evening on 3 consecutive days; if patient is not cured within 3-4 weeks, a second course of treatment may be administered
  Capillariasis: 200 mg twice daily for 20 days
Mechanism of Action Selectively and irreversibly blocks glucose uptake and other nutrients in susceptible adult intestine-dwelling helminths
Local Anesthetic/Vasoconstrictor Precautions No information available to require special precautions
Effects on Dental Treatment No effects or complications reported
Other Adverse Effects
1% to 10%: Gastrointestinal: Abdominal pain, diarrhea, nausea, vomiting
<1%:
  Central nervous system: Fever, dizziness, headache, fatigue
  Dermatologic: Skin rash, itching, alopecia (with high dose)
  Gastrointestinal: Sore throat
  Hematologic: Neutropenia
  Neuromuscular & skeletal: Weakness
Drug Interactions Decreased effect: Anticonvulsants such as carbamazepine and phenytoin may increase metabolism of mebendazole
(Continued)

583

Mebendazole *(Continued)*

Drug Uptake
Absorption: Only 2% to 10%
Serum half-life: 1-11.5 hours
Time to peak serum concentration: Within 2-4 hours
Pregnancy Risk Factor C
Generic Available Yes

Mecamylamine *(mek a MIL a meén)*

Brand Names Inversine®
Therapeutic Category Ganglionic Blocking Agent
Use Treatment of moderately severe to severe hypertension and in uncomplicated malignant hypertension
Usual Dosage Adults: Oral: 2.5 mg twice daily after meals for 2 days; increased by increments of 2.5 mg at intervals ≥2 days until desired blood pressure response is achieved; average daily dose: 25 mg
Mechanism of Action Mecamylamine is a ganglion blocker. This agent inhibits acetylcholine at the autonomic ganglia, causing a decrease in blood pressure. Mecamylamine also blocks central nicotinic cholinergic receptors, which inhibits the effects of nicotine and may suppress the desire to smoke.
Local Anesthetic/Vasoconstrictor Precautions No information available to require special precautions
Effects on Dental Treatment >10% of patients experience dry mouth
Other Adverse Effects
>10%:
Cardiovascular: Postural hypotension
Central nervous system: Drowsiness
Endocrine & metabolic: Decreased sexual ability
Ocular: Blurred vision, enlarged pupils
1% to 10%:
Gastrointestinal: Loss of appetite, nausea, vomiting
Genitourinary: Dysuria
<1%:
Central nervous system: Convulsions, confusion, mental depression
Gastrointestinal: Bloating, frequent stools, followed by severe constipation
Neuromuscular & skeletal: Uncontrolled movements of hands, arms, legs, or face, trembling
Respiratory: Dyspnea
Pregnancy Risk Factor C
Generic Available No

Meclan® *see* Meclocycline *on next page*

Meclizine *(MEK li zeen)*

Brand Names Antivert®; Antrizine®; Bonine® [OTC]; Dizmiss® [OTC]; Dramamine® II [OTC]; Marezine®; Meni-D®; Ru-Vert-M®; Vergon® [OTC]
Therapeutic Category Antiemetic; Antihistamine
Synonyms Meclozina, Clorhidrato De (Mexico)
Use Prevention and treatment of symptoms of motion sickness; management of vertigo with diseases affecting the vestibular system
Usual Dosage Children >12 years and Adults: Oral:
Motion sickness: 12.5-25 mg 1 hour before travel, repeat dose every 12-24 hours if needed; doses up to 50 mg may be needed
Vertigo: 25-100 mg/day in divided doses
Mechanism of Action Has central anticholinergic action by blocking chemoreceptor trigger zone; decreases excitability of the middle ear labyrinth and blocks conduction in the middle ear vestibular-cerebellar pathways
Local Anesthetic/Vasoconstrictor Precautions No information available to require special precautions
Effects on Dental Treatment Up to 10% of patients will have significant dry mouth which will disappear with cessation of drug therapy
Other Adverse Effects
>10%:
Central nervous system: Slight to moderate drowsiness
Respiratory: Thickening of bronchial secretions
1% to 10%:
Central nervous system: Headache, fatigue, nervousness, dizziness
Gastrointestinal: Appetite increase, weight gain, nausea, diarrhea, abdominal pain, dry mouth
Neuromuscular & skeletal: Arthralgia
Respiratory: Pharyngitis

<1%:
  Cardiovascular: Palpitations, hypotension
  Central nervous system: Depression, sedation
  Dermatologic: Photosensitivity, rash, angioedema
  Genitourinary: Urinary retention
  Hepatic: Hepatitis
  Neuromuscular & skeletal: Myalgia, tremor, paresthesia
  Ocular: Blurred vision
  Respiratory: Bronchospasm, epistaxis
Drug Interactions Increased toxicity: CNS depressants, neuroleptics, anticholinergics
Drug Uptake
  Onset of action: Oral: Within 1 hour
  Duration: 8-24 hours
  Serum half-life: 6 hours
Pregnancy Risk Factor B
Generic Available Yes

Meclocycline (me kloe SYE kleen)
Brand Names Meclan®
Therapeutic Category Antibiotic, Topical; Topical Skin Product, Acne
Use Topical treatment of inflammatory acne vulgaris
Usual Dosage Children >11 years and Adults: Topical: Apply generously to affected areas twice daily
Mechanism of Action Inhibits bacterial protein synthesis by binding with the 30S and possibly the 50S ribosomal subunit(s) of susceptible bacteria; may also cause alterations in the cytoplasmic membrane
Local Anesthetic/Vasoconstrictor Precautions No information available to require special precautions
Effects on Dental Treatment No effects or complications reported
Other Adverse Effects
  >10%: Topical: Follicular staining, yellowing of the skin, burning/stinging feeling
  1% to 10%: Topical: Pain, redness, skin irritation, dermatitis
Drug Interactions No data reported
Drug Uptake Absorption: Topical: Very little
Pregnancy Risk Factor B
Dosage Forms Cream, topical, as sulfosalicylate: 1% (20 g, 45 g)
Generic Available No

Meclofenamate (me kloe fen AM ate)
Related Information
  Nonsteroidal Anti-Inflammatory Agents, Comparative Dosages, and Pharmacokinetics *on page 1143*
  Rheumatoid Arthritis and Osteoarthritis *on page 1030*
Brand Names Meclomen®
Therapeutic Category Analgesic, Non-narcotic; Anti-inflammatory Agent; Nonsteroidal Anti-inflammatory Agent (NSAID), Oral
Use Treatment of inflammatory disorders
Usual Dosage Children >14 years and Adults: Oral:
  Mild to moderate pain: 50 mg every 4-6 hours, not to exceed 400 mg/day
  Rheumatoid arthritis/osteoarthritis: 200-400 mg/day in 3-4 equal doses
Mechanism of Action Inhibits prostaglandin synthesis by decreasing the activity of the enzyme, cyclo-oxygenase, which results in decreased formation of prostaglandin precursors
Local Anesthetic/Vasoconstrictor Precautions No information available to require special precautions
Effects on Dental Treatment Caution is recommended in dental patients requiring surgery since most NSAIDs inhibit platelet aggregation and prolong bleeding time. Recovery of platelet function usually occurs 1-2 days after discontinuation of NSAIDs.
Other Adverse Effects
  >10%:
    Central nervous system: Dizziness
    Dermatologic: Skin rash
    Gastrointestinal: Abdominal cramps, heartburn, indigestion, nausea
  1% to 10%:
    Cardiovascular: Fluid retention
    Central nervous system: Headache, nervousness
    Dermatologic: Itching
    Gastrointestinal: Vomiting
    Otic: Tinnitus
(Continued)

Meclofenamate *(Continued)*

<1%:
Cardiovascular: Congestive heart failure, hypertension, arrhythmia, tachy-cardia
Central nervous system: Confusion, hallucinations, aseptic meningitis, mental depression, drowsiness, insomnia
Dermatologic: Urticaria, erythema multiforme, toxic epidermal necrolysis, Stevens-Johnson syndrome, angioedema
Endocrine & metabolic: Polydipsia, hot flashes
Gastrointestinal: Gastritis, GI ulceration
Genitourinary: Cystitis
Hematologic: Agranulocytosis, anemia, hemolytic anemia, bone marrow suppression, leukopenia, thrombocytopenia
Hepatic: Hepatitis
Neuromuscular & skeletal: Peripheral neuropathy
Ocular: Toxic amblyopia, blurred vision, conjunctivitis, dry eyes
Otic: Decreased hearing
Renal: Polyuria, acute renal failure
Respiratory: Allergic rhinitis, dyspnea, epistaxis

Drug Interactions
Decreased effect with aspirin; decreased effect of diuretics, antihypertensives
Increased effect/toxicity of warfarin, methotrexate

Drug Uptake
Duration of action: 2-4 hours
Serum half-life: 2-3.3 hours
Time to peak serum concentration: Within 0.5-1.5 hours

Pregnancy Risk Factor B (D if used in the 3rd trimester)
Generic Available Yes

Meclomen® *see* Meclofenamate *on previous page*

Meclozina, Clorhidrato De (Mexico) *see* Meclizine *on page 584*

Medigesic® *see* Butalbital Compound *on page 154*

Medigesic® *see* Butalbital Compound and Acetaminophen *on page 155*

Medihaler-Iso® *see* Isoproterenol *on page 523*

Mediplast® Plaster [OTC] *see* Salicylic Acid *on page 853*

Medi-Quick® Topical Ointment [OTC] *see* Bacitracin, Neomycin, and Polymyxin B *on page 108*

Medi-Tuss® [OTC] *see* Guaifenesin *on page 452*

Medium Chain Triglycerides

(mee DEE um chane trye GLIS er ides)
Brand Names MCT Oil® [OTC]
Therapeutic Category Nutritional Supplement
Synonyms Triglycerides, Medium Chain
Use Dietary supplement for those who cannot digest long chain fats; malabsorption associated with disorders such as pancreatic insufficiency, bile salt deficiency, and bacterial overgrowth of the small bowel; induce ketosis as a prevention for seizures (akinetic, clonic, and petit mal)
Local Anesthetic/Vasoconstrictor Precautions No information available to require special precautions
Effects on Dental Treatment No effects or complications reported
Other Adverse Effects
Central nervous system: May result in **narcosis** and **coma** in cirrhotic patients due to high levels of medium chain fatty acids in the serum which then enter the cerebral spinal fluid; electroencephalogram effects include slowing of the alpha wave (can occur during infusion of fatty acids of 2-6 carbon lengths)
Endocrine & metabolic:
MCT therapy does not produce recognized metabolic side effects of any clinical importance, nor do they interfere with the metabolism of other food stuffs or with the absorption of drugs; when administered in the form of a mixed diet with carbohydrates and protein, there is no clinical evidence of **hyperketonemia**; hyperketonemia may occur in normal or diabetic subjects in the absence of carbohydrates; has been reported that MCT may increase hepatic free fatty acid synthesis and reduce ketone clearance
Fecal water, sodium and potassium excretion are decreased in patients with steatorrhea who are treated with MCT; enhanced calcium absorption has been demonstrated in patients with steatorrhea who are given MCT
Gastrointestinal: Nausea, occasional vomiting, gastritis and distention, diarrhea, and borborygmi are common adverse reactions occurring in about 10% of the patients receiving supplements or diets containing MCT; these symptoms may be related to rapid hydrolysis of MCT, high concentrations of free fatty acids in

the stomach and small intestine, hyperosmolarity causing influx of large amounts of fluid, and lactose intolerance; abdominal cramps, nausea and vomiting occurred despite cautionary administration of MCT in small sips throughout meals, but subsided with continued administration

Pregnancy Risk Factor C

Generic Available No

Comments Does not provide any essential fatty acids; only saturated fats are contained; supplementation with safflower, corn oil, or other polyunsaturated vegetable oil must be given to provide the patient with the essential fatty acids. The minimum daily requirement has not been established for oral intake, but 10-15 mL of safflower oil (60% to 70% linoleic acid) appears to be satisfactory. Contains 7.7 kcal/mL

Medralone® see Methylprednisolone on page 624

Medrol® see Methylprednisolone on page 624

Medroxyprogesterone Acetate

(me DROKS ee proe JES te rone AS e tate)

Related Information

Endocrine Disorders & Pregnancy on page 1021

Brand Names Amen®; Curretab®; Cycrin®; Depo-Provera®; Provera®

Therapeutic Category Contraceptive, Progestin Only; Progestin

Use Endometrial carcinoma or renal carcinoma as well as secondary amenorrhea or abnormal uterine bleeding due to hormonal imbalance; prevention of pregnancy

Usual Dosage

Adolescents and Adults: Oral:

Amenorrhea: 5-10 mg/day for 5-10 days or 2.5 mg/day

Abnormal uterine bleeding: 5-10 mg for 5-10 days starting on day 16 or 21 of cycle

Accompanying cyclic estrogen therapy, postmenopausal: 2.5-10 mg the last 10-13 days of estrogen dosing each month

Adults: I.M.:

Endometrial or renal carcinoma: 400-1000 mg/week

Contraception: 150 mg every 3 months or 450 mg every 6 months

Mechanism of Action Inhibits secretion of pituitary gonadotropins, which prevents follicular maturation and ovulation, stimulates growth of mammary tissue

Local Anesthetic/Vasoconstrictor Precautions No information available to require special precautions

Effects on Dental Treatment Progestins may predispose the patient to gingival bleeding

Other Adverse Effects

>10%:

Cardiovascular: Edema

Endocrine & metabolic: Breakthrough bleeding, spotting, changes in menstrual flow, amenorrhea

Gastrointestinal: Anorexia

Local: Pain at injection site

Neuromuscular & skeletal: Weakness

1% to 10%:

Cardiovascular: Embolism, central thrombosis

Central nervous system: Mental depression, fever, insomnia

Dermatologic: Melasma or chloasma, allergic rash with or without pruritus

Endocrine & metabolic: Changes in cervical erosion and secretions, increased breast tenderness

Gastrointestinal: Weight gain or loss

Hepatic: Cholestatic jaundice

Local: Thrombophlebitis

Drug Interactions Decreased effect: Aminoglutethimide may decrease effects by increasing hepatic metabolism

Drug Uptake

Absorption: I.M.: Slow

Pregnancy Risk Factor X

Generic Available Yes

Medrysone (ME dri sone)

Brand Names HMS Liquifilm®

Therapeutic Category Anti-inflammatory Agent, Ophthalmic; Corticosteroid, Ophthalmic

Use Treatment of allergic conjunctivitis, vernal conjunctivitis, episcleritis, ophthalmic epinephrine sensitivity reaction

(Continued)

Medrysone *(Continued)*

Usual Dosage Children and Adults: Ophthalmic: Instill 1 drop in conjunctival sac 2-4 times/day up to every 4 hours; may use every 1-2 hours during first 1-2 days

Mechanism of Action Decreases inflammation by suppression of migration of polymorphonuclear leukocytes and reversal of increased capillary permeability

Local Anesthetic/Vasoconstrictor Precautions No information available to require special precautions

Effects on Dental Treatment No effects or complications reported

Other Adverse Effects

1% to 10%: Ocular: Temporary mild blurred vision

<1%: Ocular: Stinging, burning eyes, corneal thinning, increased intraocular pressure, glaucoma, damage to the optic nerve, defects in visual activity, cataracts, secondary ocular infection

Drug Uptake Absorption: Through aqueous humor

Pregnancy Risk Factor C

Dosage Forms Solution, ophthalmic: 1% (5 mL, 10 mL)

Generic Available No

Comments Medrysone is a synthetic corticosteroid; structurally related to progesterone; if no improvement after several days of treatment, discontinue medrysone and institute other therapy; duration of therapy: 3-4 days to several weeks dependent on type and severity of disease; taper dose to avoid disease exacerbation

Mefenamic Acid *(me fe NAM ik AS id)*

Related Information

Nonsteroidal Anti-Inflammatory Agents, Comparative Dosages, and Pharmacokinetics *on page 1143*

Brand Names Ponstel®

Canadian/Mexican Brand Names Ponstan-500® (Mexico); Ponstan® (Canada)

Therapeutic Category Analgesic, Non-narcotic; Nonsteroidal Anti-inflammatory Agent (NSAID), Oral

Synonyms Mefenamico, Acido (Mexico)

Use Short-term relief of mild to moderate pain including primary dysmenorrhea

Usual Dosage Children >14 years and Adults: Oral: 500 mg to start then 250 mg every 4 hours as needed; maximum therapy: 1 week

Mechanism of Action Inhibits prostaglandin synthesis by decreasing the activity of the enzyme, cyclo-oxygenase, which results in decreased formation of prostaglandin precursors

Local Anesthetic/Vasoconstrictor Precautions No information available to require special precautions

Effects on Dental Treatment Caution is recommended in dental patients requiring surgery since most NSAIDs inhibit platelet aggregation and prolong bleeding time. Recovery of platelet function usually occurs 1-2 days after discontinuation of NSAIDs.

Other Adverse Effects

>10%:

Central nervous system: Dizziness

Dermatologic: Skin rash

Gastrointestinal: Abdominal cramps, heartburn, indigestion, nausea

1% to 10%:

Central nervous system: Headache, nervousness

Dermatologic: Itching

Endocrine & metabolic: Fluid retention

Gastrointestinal: Vomiting

Otic: Tinnitus

<1%:

Cardiovascular: Congestive heart failure, hypertension, arrhythmias, tachycardia

Central nervous system: Confusion, hallucinations, aseptic meningitis, mental depression, drowsiness, insomnia

Dermatologic: Urticaria, erythema multiforme, toxic epidermal necrolysis, Stevens-Johnson syndrome, angioedema

Endocrine & metabolic: Polydipsia, hot flashes

Gastrointestinal: Gastritis, GI ulceration

Genitourinary: Cystitis

Hematologic: Agranulocytosis, anemia, hemolytic anemia, bone marrow suppression, leukopenia, thrombocytopenia

Hepatic: Hepatitis

Neuromuscular & skeletal: Peripheral neuropathy

Ocular: Toxic amblyopia, blurred vision, conjunctivitis, dry eyes

Otic: Decreased hearing

Renal: Polyuria, acute renal failure
Respiratory: Dyspnea, allergic rhinitis, epistaxis
Drug Interactions
Decreased effect of diuretics, antihypertensives; decreased effect with aspirin
Increased effect/toxicity with oral anticoagulants, methotrexate
Drug Uptake
Duration of action: Up to 6 hours
Serum half-life: 3.5 hours.
Pregnancy Risk Factor C
Generic Available No

Mefenamico, Acido (Mexico) see Mefenamic Acid on previous page

Mefloquine (ME floe kwin)
Brand Names Lariam®
Therapeutic Category Antimalarial Agent
Use Treatment of acute malarial infections and prevention of malaria
Usual Dosage Oral:
Children: Malaria prophylaxis:
15-19 kg: ¼ tablet
20-30 kg: ½ tablet
31-45 kg: ¾ tablet
>45 kg: 1 tablet
Administer weekly starting 1 week before travel, continuing weekly during travel and for 4 weeks after leaving endemic area

Adults:
Treatment of mild to moderate malaria infection: 5 tablets (1250 mg) as a single dose with at least 8 oz of water
Malaria prophylaxis: 1 tablet (250 mg) weekly starting 1 week before travel, continuing weekly during travel and for 4 weeks after leaving endemic area
Mechanism of Action Mefloquine is a quinoline-methanol compound structurally similar to quinine; mefloquine's effectiveness in the treatment and prophylaxis of malaria is due to the destruction of the asexual blood forms of the malarial pathogens that affect humans, Plasmodium falciparum, P. vivax, P. malariae, P. ovale
Local Anesthetic/Vasoconstrictor Precautions No information available to require special precautions
Effects on Dental Treatment No effects or complications reported
Other Adverse Effects
1% to 10%:
Central nervous system: Difficulty concentrating, headache, insomnia, light-headedness, vertigo
Gastrointestinal: Vomiting, diarrhea, stomach pain, nausea
Ocular: Visual disturbances
Otic: Tinnitus
<1%:
Cardiovascular: Bradycardia, extrasystoles, syncope
Central nervous system: Anxiety, dizziness, confusion, seizures, hallucinations, mental depression, psychosis
Drug Uptake
Absorption: Oral: Well absorbed
Serum half-life: 21-22 days
Pregnancy Risk Factor C
Generic Available No
Comments To avoid relapse after initial treatment with mefloquine, patients should subsequently be treated with an 8-aminoquinolone (eg, primaquine)

Mefoxin® see Cefoxitin on page 193
Mega B® [OTC] see Vitamin B Complex on page 993
Megace® see Megestrol Acetate on this page
Megaton™ [OTC] see Vitamin B Complex on page 993

Megestrol Acetate (me JES trole AS e tate)
Brand Names Megace®
Therapeutic Category Antineoplastic Agent, Hormone; Progestin
Use Palliative treatment of breast and endometrial carcinomas, appetite stimulation, and promotion of weight gain in cachexia
Usual Dosage Adults: Oral (refer to individual protocols):
Female:
Breast carcinoma: 40 mg 4 times/day
Endometrial: 40-320 mg/day in divided doses; use for 2 months to determine efficacy; maximum doses used have been up to 800 mg/day
(Continued)

Megestrol Acetate *(Continued)*

Uterine bleeding: 40 mg 2-4 times/day

Male and Female: HIV-related cachexia: Initial dose: 800 mg/day; daily doses of 400 and 800 mg/day were found to be clinically effective

Mechanism of Action Megestrol is an antineoplastic progestin thought to act through an antileutenizing effect mediated via the pituitary

Local Anesthetic/Vasoconstrictor Precautions No information available to require special precautions

Effects on Dental Treatment No effects or complications reported

Other Adverse Effects

>10%:

Cardiovascular: Edema

Endocrine & metabolic: Breakthrough bleeding and amenorrhea, spotting, changes in menstrual flow

Neuromuscular & skeletal: Weakness

1% to 10%:

Central nervous system: Insomnia, depression, fever, headache

Dermatologic: Allergic rash with or without pruritus, melasma or chloasma, skin rash, and rarely alopecia

Endocrine & metabolic: Changes in cervical erosion and secretions, increased breast tenderness, changes in vaginal bleeding pattern, fluid retention, hyperglycemia

Gastrointestinal: Weight gain (not attributed to edema or fluid retention), nausea, vomiting, stomach cramps

Hepatic: Cholestatic jaundice, hepatotoxicity

Hematologic: Myelosuppressive: WBC: None; Platelets: None

Local: Thrombophlebitis

Neuromuscular & skeletal: Carpal tunnel syndrome

Respiratory: Hyperpnea

Drug Interactions No data reported

Drug Uptake

Onset of action: At least 2 months of continuous therapy is necessary

Absorption: Oral: Well absorbed

Serum half-life, elimination: 15-20 hours

Time to peak serum concentration: Oral: Within 1-3 hours

Pregnancy Risk Factor X

Generic Available Yes

Melanex® *see* Hydroquinone *on page 487*

Mellaril® *see* Thioridazine *on page 927*

Mellaril-S® *see* Thioridazine *on page 927*

Melphalan (MEL fa lan)

Brand Names Alkeran®

Therapeutic Category Antineoplastic Agent, Alkylating Agent (Nitrogen Mustard)

Synonyms L-PAM; L-Sarcolysin; Phenylalanine Mustard

Use Palliative treatment of multiple myeloma and nonresectable epithelial ovarian carcinoma; neuroblastoma, rhabdomyosarcoma, breast cancer, sarcoma; I.V. formulation: Use in patients in whom oral therapy is not appropriate

Usual Dosage

Oral (refer to individual protocols); dose should always be adjusted to patient response and weekly blood counts:

Children: 4-20 mg/m²/day for 1-21 days

Adults:

Multiple myeloma: 6 mg/day initially adjusted as indicated **or** 0.15 mg/kg/day for 7 days **or** 0.25 mg/kg/day for 4 days; repeat at 4- to 6-week intervals

Ovarian carcinoma: 0.2 mg/kg/day for 5 days, repeat every 4-5 weeks

I.V. (refer to individual protocols):

Children:

Pediatric rhabdomyosarcoma: 10-35 mg/m²/dose every 21-28 days

High-dose melphalan with bone marrow transplantation for neuroblastoma: 70-100 mg/m²/day on day 7 and 6 before BMT; **or** 140-220 mg/m² single dose before BMT **or** 50 mg/m²/day for 4 days; **or** 70 mg/m²/day for 3 days

Adults: Multiple myeloma: 16 mg/m² administered at 2-week intervals for 4 doses, then repeat monthly as per protocol for multiple myeloma

Mechanism of Action Alkylating agent which is a derivative of mechlorethamine that inhibits DNA and RNA synthesis via formation of carbonium ions; cross-links strands of DNA

Local Anesthetic/Vasoconstrictor Precautions No information available to require special precautions

Effects on Dental Treatment No effects or complications reported

Other Adverse Effects

>10%:

Dermatologic: Alopecia, pruritus, rash

Endocrine & metabolic: SIADH, amenorrhea

Hematologic: Leukopenia and thrombocytopenia are the most common effects of melphalan; anemia, agranulocytosis, hemolytic anemia; irreversible bone marrow failure has been reported

Myelosuppression: WBC: Moderate; Platelets: Moderate; Onset (days): 7; Nadir (days): 8-10 and 27-32; Recovery (days): 42-50

Second malignancies: Reported are melphalan more frequently

Respiratory: Pulmonary fibrosis, interstitial pneumonitis

Miscellaneous: Sterility, hypersensitivity

1% to 10%:

Cardiovascular: Vasculitis

Dermatologic: Vesiculation of skin

Gastrointestinal: Nausea and vomiting are mild; stomatitis and diarrhea are infrequent

Genitourinary: Bladder irritation, hemorrhagic cystitis

Drug Uptake

Absorption: Oral: Variable and incomplete from the GI tract; food interferes with absorption

Serum half-life, terminal: 1.5 hours

Time to peak serum concentration: Reportedly within 2 hours

Pregnancy Risk Factor D

Generic Available No

Menadol® [OTC] see Ibuprofen on page 495

Menest® see Estrogens, Esterified on page 369

Meni-D® see Meclizine on page 584

Meningococcal Polysaccharide Vaccine, Groups A, C, Y, and W-135

(me NIN joe kok al pol i SAK a ride vak SEEN groops aye, see, why & dubl yoo won thur tee fyve)

Brand Names Menomune®-A/C/Y/W-135

Therapeutic Category Vaccine, Live Bacteria

Use Immunization against infection caused by *Neisseria meningitidis* groups A,C,Y, and W-135 in persons ≥2 years

Usual Dosage One dose I.M. (0.5 mL); the need for booster is unknown

Mechanism of Action Induces the formation of bactericidal antibodies to meningococcal antigens; the presence of these antibodies is strongly correlated with immunity to meningococcal disease caused by *Neisseria meningitidis* groups A, C, Y and W-135.

Local Anesthetic/Vasoconstrictor Precautions No information available to require special precautions

Effects on Dental Treatment No effects or complications reported

Other Adverse Effects

>10%:

Central nervous system: Pain

Dermatologic: Erythema and induration

Local: Tenderness

1% to 10%: Central nervous system: Headache, malaise, fever, chills

Drug Uptake

Onset: Antibody levels are achieved within 10-14 days after administration

Duration: Antibodies against group A and C polysaccharides decline markedly (to prevaccination levels) over the first 3 years following a single dose of vaccine, especially in children <4 years of age

Pregnancy Risk Factor C

Generic Available No

Menomune®-A/C/Y/W-135 see Meningococcal Polysaccharide Vaccine, Groups A, C, Y, and W-135 on this page

Menotropins (men oh TROE pins)

Brand Names Humegon™; Pergonal®

Therapeutic Category Gonadotropin; Ovulation Stimulator

Use Sequentially with hCG to induce ovulation and pregnancy in the infertile woman with functional anovulation; used with hCG in men to stimulate spermatogenesis in those with primary hypogonadotropic hypogonadism

(Continued)

Menotropins *(Continued)*

Mechanism of Action Actions occur as a result of both follicle stimulating hormone (FSH) effects and luteinizing hormone (LH) effects; menotropins stimulate the development and maturation of the ovarian follicle (FSH), cause ovulation (LH), and stimulate the development of the corpus luteum (LH); in males it stimulates spermatogenesis (LH)

Local Anesthetic/Vasoconstrictor Precautions No information available to require special precautions

Effects on Dental Treatment No effects or complications reported

Other Adverse Effects

Male:

>10%: Endocrine & metabolic: Gynecomastia

1% to 10%: Erythrocytosis (shortness of breath, dizziness, anorexia, syncope, epistaxis)

Female:

>10%:

Endocrine & metabolic: Ovarian enlargement

Gastrointestinal: Abdominal distention

Local: Pain/rash at injection site

1% to 10%: Ovarian hyperstimulation syndrome

<1%:

Cardiovascular: Thromboembolism,

Central nervous system: Pain, febrile reactions

Drug Interactions No data reported

Pregnancy Risk Factor X

Dosage Forms Injection:

Follicle stimulating hormone activity 75 units and luteinizing hormone activity 75 units per 2 mL ampul

Follicle stimulating hormone activity 150 units and luteinizing hormone activity 150 units per 2 mL ampul

Generic Available Yes

Mentax® *see Butenafine on page 157*

Mepenzolate Bromide *(me PEN zoe late)*

Brand Names Cantil®

Therapeutic Category Anticholinergic Agent; Antispasmodic Agent, Gastrointestinal

Use Management of peptic ulcer disease; inhibit salivation and excessive secretions in respiratory tract preoperatively

Local Anesthetic/Vasoconstrictor Precautions No information available to require special precautions

Effects on Dental Treatment >10% of patients experience dry mouth

Other Adverse Effects

>10%:

Dermatologic: Dry skin

Gastrointestinal: Constipation

Respiratory: Dry nose, throat

Miscellaneous: Decreased sweating

1% to 10%: Gastrointestinal: Dysphagia

<1%:

Cardiovascular: Tachycardia

Central nervous system: Confusion, headache, loss of memory, fatigue, drowsiness, nervousness, insomnia

Dermatologic: Rash

Gastrointestinal: Bloated feeling, nausea, vomiting

Genitourinary: Urinary retention

Neuromuscular & skeletal: Weakness

Ocular: Increased intraocular pressure, blurred vision

Pregnancy Risk Factor C

Generic Available No

Mepergan® *see Meperidine and Promethazine on page 594*

Meperidine *(me PER i deen)*

Related Information

Dental Drug Interactions: Update on Drug Combinations Requiring Special Considerations *on page 1144*

Narcotic Agonists *on page 1141*

Oral Pain *on page 1053*

Brand Names Demerol®

Therapeutic Category Analgesic, Narcotic

Synonyms Isonipecaine (Canada); Pethidine Hydrochloride (Canada)

Use

Dental: Adjunct in preoperative intravenous conscious sedation in patients under-going dental surgery; alternate oral narcotic in patients allergic to codeine to treat moderate to moderate-severe pain

Medical: Management of moderate to severe pain

Restrictions C-II; Nonrefillable .

Usual Dosage

Children: Oral: 25-50 mg every 4-6 hours as needed for pain

Adults:

I.V.: 50-100 mg titrated as a single dose to produce sedation

Oral: 50-100 mg every 4-6 hours as needed for pain

Mechanism of Action Binds to opiate receptors in the CNS, causing inhibition of ascending pain pathways, altering the perception of and response to pain; produces generalized CNS depression

Local Anesthetic/Vasoconstrictor Precautions No information available to require special precautions

Effects on Dental Treatment 1% to 10% of patients experience dry mouth

Other Adverse Effects >10%:

Cardiovascular: Hypotension

Central nervous system: Fatigue, drowsiness, dizziness

Gastrointestinal: Nausea, vomiting, constipation

Neuromuscular & skeletal: Weakness

Miscellaneous: Histamine release

Contraindications Hypersensitivity to meperidine or any component; patients receiving MAO inhibitors presently or in the past 14 days

Warnings/Precautions Use with caution in patients with pulmonary, hepatic, renal disorders, or increased intracranial pressure; use with caution in patients with renal failure or seizure disorders or those receiving high-dose meperidine; normeperidine (an active metabolite and CNS stimulant) may accumulate and precipitate twitches, tremors, or seizures; some preparations contain sulfites which may cause allergic reaction

Enhanced analgesia has been seen in elderly patients on therapeutic doses of narcotics; duration of action may be increased in the elderly; the elderly may be particularly susceptible to the CNS depressant and constipating effects of narcotics

Drug Interactions Phenytoin may decrease the analgesic effects of meperidine; meperidine may aggravate the adverse effects of isoniazid; MAO inhibitors, fluoxetine, and other serotonin uptake inhibitors greatly potentiate the effects of meperidine; acute opioid overdosage symptoms can be seen, including severe toxic reactions; CNS depressants, tricyclic antidepressants, phenothiazines may potentiate the effects of meperidine

Drug Uptake

Onset of effect: I.V.: Within 5 minutes

Duration: 4-6 hours

Serum half-life:

Parent drug, terminal phase:

Adults: 2.5-4 hours

Adults with liver disease: 7-11 hours

Normeperidine (active metabolite): 15-30 hours; dependent on renal function and can accumulate with higher doses or in patients with decreased renal function

Time to peak serum concentration: Oral: 90-120 minutes

Pregnancy Risk Factor B (D if used for prolonged periods or in high doses at term)

Breast-feeding Considerations Considered compatible by AAO in 1983 state-ment; however, not included in the 1989 statement

Dosage Forms

Syrup: 50 mg/5 mL (500 mL)

Tablet: 50 mg, 100 mg

Dietary Considerations No data reported

Generic Available Yes

Comments Meperidine is not to be used as the narcotic drug of first choice. It is recommended only to be used in codeine-allergic patients when a narcotic anal-gesic is indicated. Meperidine is not an anti-inflammatory agent. Meperidine, as with other narcotic analgesics, is recommended only for limited acute dosing (ie, 3 days or less); common adverse effects in the dental patient are nausea, sedation, and constipation. Meperidine has a significant addiction liability, espe-cially when given long term.

Meperidine and Promethazine
(me PER i deen & proe METH a zeen)
Brand Names Mepergan®
Therapeutic Category Analgesic, Narcotic
Use Management of moderate to severe pain
Local Anesthetic/Vasoconstrictor Precautions No information available to require special precautions
Effects on Dental Treatment 1% to 10% of patients experience dry mouth
Pregnancy Risk Factor B
Generic Available No

Mephenytoin (me FEN i toyn)
Brand Names Mesantoin®
Therapeutic Category Anticonvulsant, Hydantoin
Use Treatment of tonic-clonic and partial seizures in patients who are uncontrolled with less toxic anticonvulsants
Mechanism of Action Stabilizes neuronal membranes and decreases seizure activity by increasing efflux or decreasing influx of sodium ions across cell membranes in the motor cortex during generation of nerve impulses; prolongs effective refractory period and suppresses ventricular pacemaker automaticity, shortens action potential in the heart
Local Anesthetic/Vasoconstrictor Precautions No information available to require special precautions
Effects on Dental Treatment Mephenytoin, like phenytoin, causes gingival hyperplasia. Usually starts during the first 6 months of dental treatment as gingivitis. The incidence is higher in patients under 20 years of age. To minimize severity and growth rate of gingival tissue begin a program of professional cleaning and patient plaque control within 10 days of starting anticonvulsant therapy. GH induced by mephenytoin disappears with cessation of drug therapy.
Other Adverse Effects
>10%:
Central nervous system: Psychiatric changes, slurred speech, dizziness, somnolence
Gastrointestinal: Constipation, nausea, vomiting
Neuromuscular & skeletal: Trembling
1% to 10%:
Central nervous system: Headache, insomnia
Dermatologic: Skin rash
Gastrointestinal: Anorexia, weight loss
Hematologic: Leukopenia
Hepatic: Hepatitis
Renal: Elevated serum creatinine
<1%:
Cardiovascular: Hypotension, bradycardia, cardiac arrhythmias, cardiovascular collapse
Central nervous system: Confusion, fever, ataxia
Dermatologic: Stevens-Johnson syndrome or SLE-like syndrome
Gastrointestinal: Gingival hyperplasia
Hematologic: Blood dyscrasias, Hodgkin's disease-like syndrome
Local: Venous irritation and pain, thrombophlebitis
Neuromuscular & skeletal: Paresthesia, peripheral neuropathy
Ocular: Diplopia, nystagmus, blurred vision, photophobia
Miscellaneous: Lymphadenopathy, serum sickness
Drug Interactions
Decreased effect with carbamazepine, TCAs, calcium antacids; decreased effect of oral anticoagulants, oral contraceptives, steroids, quinidine, vitamin D, vitamin K, doxycycline, furosemide, TCAs
Increased effect/toxicity with alcohol, sulfonamides, chloramphenicol, cimetidine, isoniazid, disulfiram, phenothiazines, benzodiazepines
Pregnancy Risk Factor C
Generic Available No

Mephobarbital (me foe BAR bi tal)
Brand Names Mebaral®
Therapeutic Category Anticonvulsant, Barbiturate
Use Sedative; treatment of grand mal and petit mal epilepsy
Usual Dosage Oral:
Epilepsy:
Children: 6-12 mg/kg/day in 2-4 divided doses
Adults: 200-600 mg/day in 2-4 divided doses

Sedation:

Children:

<5 years: 16-32 mg 3-4 times/day

>5 years: 32-64 mg 3-4 times/day

Adults: 32-100 mg 3-4 times/day

Mechanism of Action Increases seizure threshold in the motor cortex; depresses monosynaptic and polysynaptic transmission in the CNS

Local Anesthetic/Vasoconstrictor Precautions No information available to require special precautions

Effects on Dental Treatment No effects or complications reported

Other Adverse Effects

>10%: Central nervous system: Dizziness, lightheadedness, drowsiness, "hangover" effect

1% to 10%:

Central nervous system: Confusion, mental depression, unusual excitement, nervousness, faint feeling, headache, insomnia, nightmares

Gastrointestinal: Constipation, nausea, vomiting

<1%:

Cardiovascular: Hypotension

Central nervous system: Hallucinations

Dermatologic: Skin rash, exfoliative dermatitis, Stevens-Johnson syndrome, angioedema

Hematologic: Agranulocytosis, megaloblastic anemia, thrombocytopenia

Local: Thrombophlebitis

Respiratory: Respiratory depression

Miscellaneous: Dependence

Drug Interactions

Mephobarbital causes decreased effects of the following drugs: Phenothiazines, haloperidol, quinidine, cyclosporine, TCAs, corticosteroids, theophylline, ethosuximide, warfarin, oral contraceptives, chloramphenicol, griseofulvin, doxycycline, beta-blockers

The following drugs enhance the CNS effects of mephobarbital: Propoxyphene, benzodiazepines, CNS depressants, valproic acid, methylphenidate, chloramphenicol

Drug Uptake

Onset of action: 20-60 minutes

Duration: 6-8 hours

Absorption: Oral: ~50%

Serum half-life: 34 hours

Pregnancy Risk Factor D

Generic Available No

Mephyton® *see* Phytonadione *on page 758*

Mepivacaine (me PIV a kane)

Brand Names Carbocaine®; Isocaine® HCl; Polocaine®

Therapeutic Category Local Anesthetic

Synonyms Mepivacaine Hydrochloride

Use Local anesthesia by nerve block; infiltration in dental procedures

Usual Dosage Children and Adults: Injectable local anesthetic: Varies with procedure, degree of anesthesia needed, vascularity of tissue, duration of anesthesia required, and physical condition of patient

Mechanism of Action Mepivacaine is an amino amide local anesthetic similar to lidocaine; like all local anesthetics, mepivacaine acts by preventing the generation and conduction of nerve impulses

Local Anesthetic/Vasoconstrictor Precautions No information available to require special precautions

Effects on Dental Treatment No effects or complications reported

Other Adverse Effects

<1%:

Cardiovascular: Bradycardia, myocardial depression, hypotension, cardiovascular collapse, edema

Central nervous system: Anxiety, restlessness, disorientation, confusion, seizures, drowsiness, unconsciousness, chills

Dermatologic: Urticaria

Gastrointestinal: Nausea, vomiting

Local: Transient stinging or burning at injection site

Neuromuscular & skeletal: Tremors

Ocular: Blurred vision

Otic: Tinnitus

Respiratory: Respiratory arrest

Miscellaneous: Anaphylactoid reactions, shivering

(Continued)

Mepivacaine *(Continued)*

Warnings/Precautions Use with caution in patients with cardiac disease, renal disease, and hyperthyroidism; convulsions due to systemic toxicity leading to cardiac arrest have been reported presumably due to intravascular injection

Drug Uptake

Onset of action: Epidural: Within 7-15 minutes

Duration: 2-2.5 hours; similar onset and duration is seen following infiltration

Protein binding: 70% to 85%

Metabolism: Chiefly in the liver by N-demethylation, hydroxylation, and glucuronidation

Half-life: 1.9 hours

Elimination: Urinary excretion (95% as metabolites)

Pregnancy Risk Factor C

Dosage Forms Injection, as hydrochloride: 1% [10 mg/mL] (30 mL, 50 mL); 1.5% [15 mg/mL] (30 mL); 2% [20 mg/mL] (20 mL, 50 mL); 3% [30 mg/mL] (1.8 mL)

Generic Available Yes

Selected Readings

Dodson WE, Hillman RE, and Hillman LS, "Brain Tissue Levels in a Fatal Case of Neonatal Mepivacaine (Carbocaine®) Poisoning," *J Pediatr*, 1975, 86(4):624-7.

Torres MJ, Garcia JJ, del Cano Moratinos AM, et al, "Fixed Drug Eruption Induced by Mepivacaine," *J Allergy Clin Immunol*, 1995, 96(1):130-1.

Mepivacaine and Levonordefrin

(me PIV a kane & lee voe nor DEF rin)

Related Information

Oral Pain *on page 1053*

Brand Names Carbocaine® 2% With Neo-Cobefrin®; Isocaine® HCl 2%; Polocaine® 2%

Canadian/Mexican Brand Names Polocaine® and Levonordefrin (Canada)

Therapeutic Category Dental/Local Anesthetics; Local Anesthetic, Injectable

Use Dental: Amide-type anesthetic used for local infiltration anesthesia; injection near nerve trunks to produce nerve block

Usual Dosage

Children <10 years: Maximum pediatric dosage must be carefully calculated on the basis of patient's weight but should not exceed 6.6 mg/kg of body weight or 180 mg of mepivacaine hydrochloride as a 2% solution with levonordefrin 1:20,000

Children >10 years and Adults:

Dental infiltration and nerve block, single site: 36 mg (1.8 mL) of mepivacaine hydrochloride as a 2% solution with levonordefrin 1:20,000

Entire oral cavity: 180 mg (9 mL) of mepivacaine hydrochloride as a 2% solution with levonordefrin 1:20,000; up to a maximum of 6.6 mg/kg of body weight but not to exceed 400 mg of mepivacaine hydrochloride per appointment. The effective anesthetic dose varies with procedure, intensity of anesthesia needed, duration of anesthesia required, and physical condition of the patient. Always use the lowest effective dose along with careful aspiration.

The following numbers of dental carpules (1.8 mL) provide the indicated amounts of mepivacaine hydrochloride 2% and levonordefrin 1:20,000.

# of Cartridges	Mg Mepivacaine (2%)	Mg Vasoconstrictor (Levonordefrin 1:20,000)
1	36	0.090
2	72	0.180
3	108	0.270
4	144	0.360
5	180	0.450
6	216	0.540
7	252	0.630
8	288	0.720
9	324	0.810
10	360	0.900

Note: Adult and children doses of mepivacaine hydrochloride with levonordefrin cited from USP Dispensing Information (USP DI), 17th ed, The United States Pharmacopeial Convention, Inc, Rockville, MD, 1997, 139.

Mechanism of Action Local anesthetics bind selectively to the intracellular surface of sodium channels to block influx of sodium into the axon. As a result, depolarization necessary for action potential propagation and subsequent nerve function is prevented. The block at the sodium channel is reversible. When drug diffuses away from the axon, sodium channel function is restored and nerve propagation returns.

Levonordefrin prolongs the duration of the anesthetic actions of mepivacaine by causing vasoconstriction (alpha adrenergic receptor agonist) of the vasculature surrounding the nerve axons. This prevents the diffusion of mepivacaine away from the nerves resulting in a longer retention in the axon.

Local Anesthetic/Vasoconstrictor Precautions No information available to require special precautions

Effects on Dental Treatment No effects or complications reported

Other Adverse Effects Degree of adverse effects in the CNS and cardiovascular system are directly related to the blood levels of mepivacaine. The effects below are more likely to occur after systemic administration rather than infiltration.

Central nervous system: High blood levels result in anxiety, restlessness, disorientation, confusion, dizziness, and seizures. This is followed by depression of CNS resulting in somnolence, unconsciousness and possible respiratory arrest. In some cases, symptoms of CNS stimulation may be absent and the primary CNS effects are somnolence and unconsciousness.

Cardiovascular: Myocardial effects include a decrease in contraction force as well as a decrease in electrical excitability and myocardial conduction rate resulting in bradycardia and reduction in cardiac output.

Gastrointestinal: Nausea and vomiting may occur

Hypersensitivity reactions: Extremely rare, but may be manifest as dermatologic reactions and edema at injection site. Asthmatic syndromes have occurred. Patients may exhibit hypersensitivity to bisulfites contained in local anesthetic solution to prevent oxidation of levonordefrin. In general, patients reacting to bisulfites have a history of asthma and their airways are hyper-reactive to asthmatic syndrome.

Neuromuscular & skeletal: Tremors

Psychogenic reactions: It is common to misinterpret psychogenic responses to local anesthetic injection as an allergic reaction. Intraoral injections are perceived by many patients as a stressful procedure in dentistry. Common symptoms to this stress are sweating, palpitations, hyperventilation, generalized pallor and a fainting feeling.

Contraindications Hypersensitivity to local anesthetics of the amide-type

Warnings/Precautions Should be avoided in patients with uncontrolled hyperthyroidism. Should be used in minimal amounts in patients with significant cardiovascular problems (because of levonordefrin component). Aspirate the syringe after tissue penetration and before injection to minimize chance of direct vascular injection.

Drug Interactions Due to levonordefrin component, use with tricyclic antidepressants or MAO inhibitors could result in increased pressor response; use with nonselective beta-blockers (ie, propranolol) could result in serious hypertension and reflex bradycardia

Drug Uptake
Duration: 1-2.5 hours in upper jaw and 2.5-5.5 hours in lower jaw
Infiltration: 50 minutes
Inferior alveolar block: 60-75 minutes

Pregnancy Risk Factor C

Breast-feeding Considerations Usual infiltration doses of mepivacaine with levonordefrin given to nursing mothers has not been shown to affect the health of the nursing infant

Dosage Forms Injection: Mepivacaine hydrochloride 2% with levonordefrin 1:20,000 (1.8 mL dental cartridges)

Dietary Considerations No data reported

Generic Available No

Selected Readings
Jastak JT and Yagiela JA, "Vasoconstrictors and Local Anesthesia: A Review and Rationale for Use," *J Am Dent Assoc*, 1983, 107(4):623-30.
MacKenzie TA and Young ER, "Local Anesthetic Update," *Anesth Prog*, 1993, 40(2):29-34.
Wynn RL, "Epinephrine Interactions With Beta-Blockers," *Gen Dent*, 1994, 42(1):16, 18.
Wynn RL, "Recent Research on Mechanisms of Local Anesthetics," *Gen Dent*, 1995, 43(4):316-8.
Yagiela JA, "Local Anesthetics," *Anesth Prog*, 1991, 38(4-5):128-41.

Mepivacaine Dental Anesthetic

(me PIV a kane DEN tal an es THE tik)

Related Information
Oral Pain *on page 1053*

Brand Names Carbocaine® 3%; Isocaine® HCl 3%; Polocaine® 3%

Canadian/Mexican Brand Names Polocaine® (Canada)

Therapeutic Category Dental/Local Anesthetics; Local Anesthetic, Injectable

(Continued)

Mepivacaine Dental Anesthetic *(Continued)*

Use Dental: Amide-type anesthetic used for local infiltration anesthesia; injection near nerve trunks to produce nerve block

Usual Dosage

Children <10 years: Up to 5-6 mg/kg of body weight; maximum pediatric dosage must be carefully calculated on the basis of patient's weight but must not exceed 270 mg (9 mL) of the 3% solution

Children >10 years and Adults:

Dental anesthesia, single site in upper or lower jaw: 54 mg (1.8 mL) as a 3% solution

Infiltration and nerve block of entire oral cavity: 270 mg (9 mL) as a 3% solution; up to a maximum of 6.6 mg/kg of body weight but not to exceed 300 mg per appointment. Manufacturer's maximum recommended dose is not more than 400 mg to normal healthy adults. The effective anesthetic dose varies with procedure, intensity of anesthesia needed, duration of anesthesia required, and physical condition of the patient. Always use the lowest effective dose along with careful aspiration.

The following number of dental carpules (1.8 mL) provide the indicated amounts of mepivacaine dental anesthetic 3%.

# of Cartridges	Mg Mepivacaine (3%)
1	54
2	108
3	162
4	216
5	270
6	324
7	378
8	432

Note: Adult and children doses of mepivacaine dental anesthetic cited from USP Dispensing Information (USP DI), 17th ed, The United States Pharmacopeial Convention, Inc, Rockville, MD, 1997, 138-9.

Mechanism of Action Local anesthetics bind selectively to the intracellular surface of sodium channels to block influx of sodium into the axon. As a result, depolarization necessary for action potential propagation and subsequent nerve function is prevented. The block at the sodium channel is reversible. When drug diffuses away from the axon, sodium channel function is restored and nerve propagation returns.

Local Anesthetic/Vasoconstrictor Precautions No information available to require special precautions

Effects on Dental Treatment No effects or complications reported

Other Adverse Effects Degree of adverse effects in the CNS and cardiovascular system are directly related to the blood levels of local anesthetic.

Cardiovascular: Myocardial effects include a decrease in contraction force as well as a decrease in electrical excitability and myocardial conduction rate resulting in bradycardia and reduction in cardiac output

Central nervous system: High blood levels result in anxiety, restlessness, disorientation, confusion, dizziness, and seizures. This is followed by depression of CNS resulting in somnolence, unconsciousness and possible respiratory arrest. In some cases, symptoms of CNS stimulation may be absent and the primary CNS effects are somnolence and unconsciousness.

Gastrointestinal: Nausea and vomiting may occur

Hypersensitivity reactions: May manifest as dermatologic reactions and edema at injection site. Asthmatic syndromes have occurred.

Neuromuscular & skeletal: Tremors

Psychogenic reactions: It is common to misinterpret psychogenic responses to local anesthetic injection as an allergic reaction. Intraoral injections is perceived by many patients as a stressful procedure in dentistry. Common symptoms to this stress are sweating, palpitations, hyperventilation, generalized pallor and a fainting feeling.

Contraindications Hypersensitivity to local anesthetics of the amide type

Warnings/Precautions Aspirate the syringe after tissue penetration and before injection to minimize chance of direct vascular injection

Drug Interactions No data reported

Drug Uptake

Onset of action: 30-120 seconds in upper jaw; 1-4 minutes in lower jaw

Duration: 20 minutes in upper jaw; 40 minutes in lower jaw

Serum half-life: 1.9 hours

Pregnancy Risk Factor C

Breast-feeding Considerations Usual infiltration doses of mepivacaine dental anesthetic given to nursing mothers has not been shown to affect the health of the nursing infant

Dosage Forms Injection: Mepivacaine hydrochloride 3% (1.8 mL dental cartridges)

Dietary Considerations No data reported

Generic Available Yes

Selected Readings

Wynn RL, "Recent Research on Mechanisms of Local Anesthetics," *Gen Dent*, 1995, 43(4):316-8.

Mepivacaine Hydrochloride *see* Mepivacaine *on page 595*

Meprobamate (me proe BA mate)

Brand Names Equanil®; Miltown®; Neuramate®

Canadian/Mexican Brand Names Apo®-Meprobamate (Canada); Meditran® (Canada); Novo-Mepro® (Canada)

Therapeutic Category Antianxiety Agent; Muscle Relaxant; Skeletal Muscle Relaxant; Tranquilizer, Minor

Use

Dental: Treatment of muscle spasm associated with acute temporomandibular joint pain; management of dental anxiety disorders

Medical: Management of anxiety disorders

Unlabeled use: Demonstrated value for muscle contraction, headache, premenstrual tension, external sphincter spasticity, muscle rigidity, opisthotonos-associated with tetanus

Restrictions C-IV; Refillable up to 5 times in 6 months

Usual Dosage Oral:

Children 6-12 years: 100-200 mg 2-3 times/day

Sustained release: 200 mg twice daily

Adults: 400 mg 3-4 times/day, up to 2400 mg/day

Sustained release: 400-800 mg twice daily

Mechanism of Action Precise mechanism is not yet clear, but many effects have been ascribed to its central depressant actions

Local Anesthetic/Vasoconstrictor Precautions No information available to require special precautions

Effects on Dental Treatment <1% of patients experience stomatitis

Other Adverse Effects

>10%: Central nervous system: Drowsiness, clumsiness, ataxia, loss of motor coordination

1% to 10%: Central nervous system: Dizziness

Contraindications Acute intermittent porphyria; hypersensitivity to meprobamate or any component; do not use in patients with pre-existing CNS depression, narrow-angle glaucoma, or severe uncontrolled pain

Warnings/Precautions Physical and psychological dependence and abuse may occur; not recommended in children <6 years of age; allergic reaction may occur in patients with history of dermatological condition (usually by fourth dose); use with caution in patients with renal or hepatic impairment, or with a history of seizures

Drug Interactions CNS depressants cause increased CNS depression

Drug Uptake

Absorption: Oral: Rapid and nearly complete

Onset of sedation: Oral: Within 1 hour

Serum half-life: 10 hours

Pregnancy Risk Factor D

Breast-feeding Considerations Milk concentrations are higher then plasma; effects unknown; not recommended

Dosage Forms

Capsule, sustained release: 200 mg, 400 mg

Tablet: 200 mg, 400 mg, 600 mg

Dietary Considerations No data reported

Generic Available Yes

Meprobamate and Aspirin *see* Aspirin and Meprobamate *on page 94*

Mepron™ *see* Atovaquone *on page 97*

Merbromin (mer BROE min)

Brand Names Mercurochrome®

Therapeutic Category Topical Skin Product

Use Topical antiseptic

(Continued)

Merbromin (Continued)

Local Anesthetic/Vasoconstrictor Precautions No information available to require special precautions

Effects on Dental Treatment No effects or complications reported

Generic Available Yes

Mercaptopurine (mer kap toe PYOOR een)

Brand Names Purinethol®

Therapeutic Category Antineoplastic Agent, Antimetabolite; Antineoplastic Agent, Purine

Synonyms 6-Mercaptopurine; 6-MP

Use Treatment of acute leukemias (ALL, CML)

Usual Dosage Oral (**refer to individual protocols**):

Children:

Induction: 2.5-5 mg/kg/day given once daily

Maintenance: 1.5-2.5 mg/kg/day given once daily **or** 70-100 mg/m^2/day once daily

Adults:

Induction: 2.5-5 mg/kg/day (100-200 mg)

Maintenance: 1.5-2.5 mg/kg/day **or** 80-100 mg/m^2/day given once daily

Elderly: Due to renal decline with age, start with lower recommended doses for adults

Mechanism of Action Purine antagonist which inhibits DNA and RNA synthesis; acts as false metabolite and is incorporated into DNA and RNA, eventually inhibiting their synthesis. 6-MP is substituted for hypoxanthine; must be metabolized to active nucleotides once inside the cell.

Local Anesthetic/Vasoconstrictor Precautions No information available to require special precautions

Effects on Dental Treatment No effects or complications reported

Other Adverse Effects

>10%: Hepatic: 6-MP can cause an intrahepatic cholestasis and focal centralobular necrosis manifested as hyperbilirubinemia, elevated alkaline phosphatase, and elevated AST. This may be dose related, occurring more frequently at doses >2.5 mg/kg/day; jaundice is noted 1-2 months into therapy, but has ranged from 1 week to 8 years.

1% to 10%:

Central nervous system: Drug fever

Dermatologic: Hyperpigmentation, rash

Endocrine & metabolic: Hyperuricemia

Gastrointestinal: Nausea, vomiting, diarrhea, stomatitis, anorexia, stomach pain, and mucositis may require parenteral nutrition and dose reduction; 6-TG is less GI toxic than 6-MP

Hematologic: Leukopenia, thrombocytopenia, anemia may occur at high doses

Myelosuppressive: WBC: Moderate; Platelets: Moderate; Onset (days): 7-10; Nadir (days): 14; Recovery (days): 21

Neuromuscular & skeletal: Weakness

Renal: Renal toxicity

<1%:

Dermatologic: Dry, scaling rash

Gastrointestinal: Glossitis, tarry stools

Hematologic: Eosinophilia

Drug Uptake

Absorption: Variable and incomplete (16% to 50%)

Serum half-life (age-dependent):

Children: 21 minutes

Adults: 47 minutes

Time to peak serum concentration: Within 2 hours

Pregnancy Risk Factor D

Generic Available No

6-Mercaptopurine see Mercaptopurine on this page

Mercuric Oxide (mer KYOOR ik OKS ide)

Therapeutic Category Antibiotic, Ophthalmic

Synonyms Yellow Mercuric Oxide

Use Treatment of irritation and minor infections of the eyelids

Local Anesthetic/Vasoconstrictor Precautions No information available to require special precautions

Effects on Dental Treatment No effects or complications reported

Generic Available Yes

Mercurochrome® *see* Merbromin *on page 599*
Meridia™ *see* Sibutramine *on page 864*

Meropenem (mer oh PEN em)
Brand Names Merrem® I.V.
Therapeutic Category Antibiotic, Carbacephem
Use Meropenem is indicated as single agent therapy for the treatment of intra-abdominal infections including complicated appendicitis and peritonitis in adults and bacterial meningitis in pediatric patients >3 months of age caused by *S. pneumoniae, H. influenzae,* and *N. meningitidis* (penicillin-resistant pneumococci have not been studied in clinical trials); it is better tolerated than imipenem and highly effective against a broad range of bacteria
Usual Dosage
Children:
Intra-abdominal infections: 20 mg/kg every 8 hours (maximum dose: 1 g every 8 hours)
Meningitis: 40 mg/kg every 8 hours (maximum dose: 2 g every 8 hours)
Adults: 1 g every 8 hours (see Administration)

Dosing adjustment in renal impairment: Adults:
Cl_{cr} 26-50 mL/minute: Administer 1 g every 12 hours
Cl_{cr} 10-25 mL/minute: Administer 500 mg every 12 hours
Cl_{cr} <10 mL/minute: Administer 500 mg every 24 hours
Meropenem and its metabolites are readily dialyzable
Mechanism of Action Inhibits bacterial cell wall synthesis by binding to several of the penicillin-binding proteins, which in turn inhibit the final transpeptidation step of peptidoglycan synthesis in bacterial cell walls, thus inhibiting cell wall biosynthesis; bacteria eventually lyse due to ongoing activity of cell wall autolytic enzymes (autolysins and murein hydrolases) while cell wall assembly is arrested
Local Anesthetic/Vasoconstrictor Precautions No information available to require special precautions
Effects on Dental Treatment 1% to 10% of patients will experience oral moniliasis and glossitis
Other Adverse Effects
1% to 10%:
Central nervous system: Headache
Dermatologic: Rash, pruritus
Gastrointestinal: Diarrhea, nausea/vomiting, constipation, glossitis
Local: Injection site reaction/thrombophlebitis
Respiratory: Apnea
Miscellaneous: Oral moniliasis
<1%:
Cardiovascular: Heart failure, other cardiac symptoms including myocardial infarction and arrhythmias, edema
Central nervous system: Pain, fever, agitation/delirium, dizziness, seizure, hallucinations
Dermatologic: Urticaria
Gastrointestinal: Anorexia, flatulence
Hematologic: Bleeding event, anemia, hematologic effects both increase and decrease in cell counts
Hepatic: Hepatic failure, hepatic effects, elevated LFTs
Renal: Kidney failure
Respiratory: Dyspnea
Miscellaneous: Sweating
Warnings/Precautions Do not administer to patients with serious hypersensitivity reactions to beta-lactam agents. Seizures and other CNS events have been reported during treatment with meropenem; these experiences have occurred most commonly in patients with pre-existing CNS disorders, with bacterial meningitis, and/or decreased renal function; may cause pseudomembranous colitis
Drug Interactions Probenecid interferes with renal excretion of meropenem
Drug Uptake
Serum half-life: ~1 hours
Pregnancy Risk Factor B
Generic Available No
Comments 1 g of meropenem contains 90.2 mg of sodium as sodium carbonate (3.92 mEq)
Selected Readings
Wiseman LR, Wagstaff AJ, Brogden RN, et al, "Meropenem: A Review of Its Antibacterial Activity, Pharmacokinetic Properties, and Clinical Efficacy," *Drugs,* 1995, 50(1):73-101.

Merrem® I.V. *see* Meropenem *on this page*
Mersol® [OTC] *see* Thimerosal *on page 925*
Merthiolate® [OTC] *see* Thimerosal *on page 925*

Meruvax® II *see* Rubella Virus Vaccine, Live *on page 851*

Mesalamine (me SAL a meen)
Brand Names Asacol®; Pentasa®; Rowasa®
Therapeutic Category 5-Aminosalicylic Acid Derivative; Anti-inflammatory Agent, Rectal
Use Treatment of ulcerative colitis, proctosigmoiditis, and proctitis
Usual Dosage Adults (usual course of therapy is 3-6 weeks):
  Oral:
    Capsule: 1 g 4 times/day
    Tablet: 800 mg 3 times/day
  Retention enema: 60 mL (4 g) at bedtime, retained overnight, approximately 8 hours
  Rectal suppository: Insert 1 suppository in rectum twice daily
  Some patients may require rectal and oral therapy concurrently
Mechanism of Action Mesalamine (5-aminosalicylic acid) is the active component of sulfasalazine; the specific mechanism of action of mesalamine is unknown; however, it is thought that it modulates local chemical mediators of the inflammatory response, especially leukotrienes; action appears topical rather than systemic
Local Anesthetic/Vasoconstrictor Precautions No information available to require special precautions
Effects on Dental Treatment No effects or complications reported
Other Adverse Effects
  >10%:
    Central nervous system: Headache, malaise
    Gastrointestinal: Abdominal pain, cramps, flatulence, gas
  1% to 10%: Dermatologic: Alopecia, rash
  <1%: Anal irritation, acute intolerance syndrome (bloody diarrhea, severe abdominal cramps, severe headache)
Drug Interactions Decreased effect: Decreased digoxin bioavailability
Drug Uptake
  Absorption: Rectal: ~15%; variable and dependent upon retention time, underlying GI disease, and colonic pH
  Serum half-life:
    5-ASA: 0.5-1.5 hours
    Acetyl 5-ASA: 5-10 hours
  Time to peak serum concentration: Within 4-7 hours
Pregnancy Risk Factor B
Generic Available No

Mesantoin® *see* Mephenytoin *on page 594*

Mesoridazine (mez oh RID a zeen)
Brand Names Serentil®
Therapeutic Category Antipsychotic Agent; Phenothiazine Derivative
Use Symptomatic management of psychotic disorders, including schizophrenia, behavioral problems, alcoholism as well as reducing anxiety and tension occurring in neurosis
Usual Dosage Concentrate may be diluted just prior to administration with distilled water, acidified tap water, orange or grape juice; do not prepare and store bulk dilutions

  Adults:
    Oral: 25-50 mg 3 times/day; maximum: 100-400 mg/day
    I.M.: 25 mg initially, repeat in 30-60 minutes as needed; optimal dosage range: 25-200 mg/day

  Not dialyzable (0% to 5%)
Mechanism of Action Blockade of postsynaptic CNS dopamine receptors
Local Anesthetic/Vasoconstrictor Precautions No information available to require special precautions
Effects on Dental Treatment No effects or complications reported
Other Adverse Effects
  >10%:
    Cardiovascular: Hypotension, orthostatic hypotension
    Central nervous system: Pseudoparkinsonism, akathisia, dystonias, tardive dyskinesia (persistent), dizziness
    Gastrointestinal: Constipation
    Ocular: Pigmentary retinopathy
    Respiratory: Nasal congestion
    Miscellaneous: Decreased sweating

1% to 10%:
  Dermatologic: Photosensitivity, skin rash
  Endocrine & metabolic: Changes in menstrual cycle, changes in libido, pain in breasts
  Gastrointestinal: Weight gain, nausea, vomiting, stomach pain
  Genitourinary: Dysuria, ejaculatory disturbances
  Neuromuscular & skeletal: Trembling of fingers
<1%:
  Central nervous system: Neuroleptic malignant syndrome (NMS), impairment of temperature regulation, lowering of seizures threshold
  Dermatologic: Discoloration of skin (blue-gray)
  Endocrine & metabolic: Galactorrhea
  Genitourinary: Priapism
  Hematologic: Agranulocytosis, leukopenia
  Hepatic: Cholestatic jaundice, hepatotoxicity
  Ocular: Cornea and lens changes, pigmentary retinopathy

Drug Interactions
  Decreased effect with anticonvulsants, anticholinergics
  Increased toxicity with CNS depressants, metrizamide (increased seizures), propranolol

Drug Uptake
  Duration of action: 4-6 hours
  Absorption: Very erratic with oral tablet; oral liquids much more dependable
  Serum half-life: 24-48 hours
  Time to peak serum concentration: 2-4 hours

Pregnancy Risk Factor C
Generic Available No

Mestranol and Norethindrone (MES tra nole & nor eth IN drone)
Related Information
  Endocrine Disorders & Pregnancy *on page 1021*

Brand Names Genora® 1/50; Nelova™ 1/50M; Norethin™ 1/50M; Norinyl® 1+50; Ortho-Novum™ 1/50

Therapeutic Category Contraceptive, Oral; Progestin

Use Prevention of pregnancy; treatment of hypermenorrhea, endometriosis, female hypogonadism [monophasic oral contraceptive]

Usual Dosage Adults: Female: Oral:
  Contraception: 1 tablet daily, beginning on day 5 of menstrual cycle (first day of menstrual flow is day 1). With 20-tablet and 21-tablet packages, new dosing cycle begins 7 days after last tablet taken. With 28-tablet packages, dosage is 1 tablet daily without interruption; extra tablets are placebos or contain iron. If next menstrual period does not begin on schedule, rule out pregnancy before starting new dosing cycle. If menstrual period begins, start new dosing cycle 7 days after last tablet was taken. If all doses have been taken on schedule and one menstrual period is missed, continue dosing cycle. If two consecutive menstrual periods are missed, pregnancy test is required before new dosing cycle is started.
  One dose missed: Take as soon as remembered or take 2 tablets next day
  Two doses missed: Take 2 tablets as soon as remembered or 2 tablets next 2 days
  Three doses missed: Begin new compact of tablets starting on day 1 of next cycle

Mechanism of Action Inhibits ovulation via a negative feedback mechanism on the hypothalamus, which alters the normal pattern of gonadotropin secretion of a follicle-stimulating hormone (FSH) and luteinizing hormone by the anterior pituitary. Follicular phase FSH and midcycle surge of gonadotropins are inhibited. Produces alterations in the genital tract, including changes in the cervical mucus, rendering it unfavorable for sperm penetration even if ovulation occurs. Changes in the endometrium may also occur, producing an unfavorable environment for nidation. May alter the tubal transport of the ova through the fallopian tubes. Progestational agents may also alter sperm fertility.

Local Anesthetic/Vasoconstrictor Precautions No information available to require special precautions

Effects on Dental Treatment When prescribing antibiotics, patients must be advised to use additional methods of birth control when taking oral contraceptives

Other Adverse Effects
  >10%:
  Cardiovascular: Peripheral edema
  Central nervous system: Headache
  Endocrine: Enlargement of breasts, breast tenderness, increased libido
  Gastrointestinal: Nausea, anorexia, bloating

(Continued)

Mestranol and Norethindrone *(Continued)*

1% to 10%: Gastrointestinal: Vomiting, diarrhea

<1%:

Cardiovascular: Hypertension, thromboembolism, edema, myocardial infarction

Central nervous system: Depression, dizziness, anxiety, stroke

Dermatologic: Chloasma, melasma, rash

Endocrine: Decreased glucose tolerance, breast tumors, amenorrhea, alterations in frequency and flow of menses, elevated triglycerides and LDL

Gastrointestinal: GI distress

Hepatic: Cholestatic jaundice

Ocular: Intolerance to contact lenses

Miscellaneous: Increased susceptibility to *Candida* infection

See tables.

Achieving Proper Hormonal Balance in an Oral Contraceptive

Estrogen		Progestin	
Excess	**Deficiency**	**Excess**	**Deficiency**
Nausea, bloating	Early or midcycle	Increased appetite	Late breakthrough
Cervical mucorrhea,	breakthrough	Weight gain	bleeding
polyposis	bleeding	Tiredness, fatigue	Amenorrhea
Melasma	Increased spotting	Hypomenorrhea	Hypermenorrhea
Migraine headache	Hypomenorrhea	Acne, oily scalp*	
Breast fullness or		Hair loss, hirsutism*	
tenderness		Depression	
Edema		Monilial vaginitis	
Hypertension		Breast regression	

*Result of androgenic activity of progestins.

Pharmacological Effects of Progestins Used in Oral Contraceptives

	Progestin	Estrogen	Antiestrogen	Androgen
Norgestrel/levonorgestrel	+++	0	++	+++
Ethynodiol diacetate	++	+*	+*	+
Norethindrone acetate	+	+	+++	+
Norethindrone	+	+*	+*	+
Norethynodrel	+	+++	0	0

*Has estrogenic effect at low doses; may have antiestrogenic effect at higher doses.

+++ = pronounced effect

++ = moderate effect

+ = slight effect

0 = no effect

Drug Interactions

Decreased effect of oral contraceptives with barbiturates, hydantoins - phenytoin, rifampin, antibiotics - penicillins, tetracyclines, erythromycins, clindamycin, griseofulvin

Increased toxicity of acetaminophen, anticoagulants, benzodiazepines, caffeine, corticosteroids, metoprolol, theophylline, tricyclic antidepressants

Pregnancy Risk Factor X

Generic Available Yes

Mestranol and Norethynodrel

(MES tra nole & nor e THYE noe drel)

Related Information

Endocrine Disorders & Pregnancy *on page 1021*

Brand Names Enovid®

Therapeutic Category Contraceptive, Oral

Use Treatment of hypermenorrhea, endometriosis, female hypogonadism

Usual Dosage Adults: Female: Oral:

Endometriosis: 5-10 mg/day for 2 weeks beginning on day 5 of menstrual cycle; increase by 5-10 mg increments at 2-week intervals up to 20 mg/day for 6-9 months

Hypermenorrhea: 20-30 mg/day until bleeding is controlled, then reduce to 10 mg/day and continue through day 24 of cycle; administer 5-10 mg/day from day 5 through day 24 of next 2-3 cycles

Mechanism of Action Inhibits ovulation via a negative feedback mechanism on the hypothalamus, which alters the normal pattern of gonadotropin secretion of a follicle-stimulating hormone (FSH) and luteinizing hormone by the anterior pituitary. The follicular phase FSH and midcycle surge of gonadotropins are inhibited. Oral contraceptives produce alterations in the genital tract, including changes in the cervical mucus, rendering it unfavorable for sperm penetration even if ovulation occurs. Changes in the endometrium may also occur, producing an unfavorable environment for nidation. May alter the tubal transport of the ova through the fallopian tubes. Progestational agents may also alter sperm fertility.

Local Anesthetic/Vasoconstrictor Precautions No information available to require special precautions

Effects on Dental Treatment When prescribing antibiotics, patients must be advised to use additional methods of birth control when taking oral contraceptives

Other Adverse Effects
>10%:
  Cardiovascular: Peripheral edema
  Endocrine & metabolic: Enlargement of breasts, breast tenderness
  Gastrointestinal: Nausea, anorexia, bloating

1% to 10%:
  Central nervous system: Headache
  Endocrine & metabolic: Increased libido
  Gastrointestinal: Vomiting, diarrhea

<1%:
  Cardiovascular: Hypertension, thromboembolism, myocardial infarction, edema
  Central nervous system: Depression, dizziness, anxiety, stroke
  Dermatologic: Chloasma, melasma, rash
  Endocrine & metabolic: Decreased glucose tolerance, breast tumors, amenorrhea, alterations in frequency and flow of menses, elevated triglycerides and LDL
  Gastrointestinal: GI distress
  Hepatic: Cholestatic jaundice
  Ocular: Intolerance to contact lenses
  Miscellaneous: Increased susceptibility to *Candida* infection

Drug Interactions
  Decreased effect with barbiturates, hydantoins - phenytoin, rifampin, antibiotics - penicillins, tetracyclines, erythromycins, clindamycin, griseofulvin
  Increased toxicity of acetaminophen, anticoagulants, benzodiazepines, caffeine, corticosteroids, metoprolol, theophylline, tricyclic antidepressants

Drug Uptake
  Mestranol:
    Demethylated to ethinyl estradiol
    Serum half-life: 6-20 hours
  Norethynodrel:
    Serum half-life, terminal: 5-14 hours

Pregnancy Risk Factor X
Generic Available Yes

Metahydrin® *see* Trichlormethiazide *on page 958*
Metamucil® [OTC] *see* Psyllium *on page 822*
Metamucil® Instant Mix [OTC] *see* Psyllium *on page 822*
Metaprel® *see* Metaproterenol *on this page*

Metaproterenol (met a proe TER e nol)

Related Information
  Respiratory Diseases *on page 1018*

Brand Names Alupent®; Arm-a-Med® Metaproterenol; Dey-Dose® Metaproterenol; Metaprel®; Prometa®

Therapeutic Category Adrenergic Agonist Agent; Antiasthmatic; Beta$_2$-Adrenergic Agonist Agent; Bronchodilator

Use Bronchodilator in reversible airway obstruction due to asthma or COPD; because of its delayed onset of action (one hour) and prolonged effect (4 or more hours), this may not be the drug of choice for assessing response to a bronchodilator

Usual Dosage
  Oral:
    Children:
      <2 years: 0.4 mg/kg/dose given 3-4 times/day; in infants, the dose can be given every 8-12 hours
      2-6 years: 1-2.6 mg/kg/day divided every 6 hours
      6-9 years: 10 mg/dose 3-4 times/day

(Continued)

605

Metaproterenol *(Continued)*

Children >9 years and Adults: 20 mg 3-4 times/day
Elderly: Initial: 10 mg 3-4 times/day, increasing as necessary up to 20 mg 3-4 times/day
Inhalation: Children >12 years and Adults: 2-3 inhalations every 3-4 hours, up to 12 inhalations in 24 hours
Nebulizer:
Children: 0.01-0.02 mL/kg of 5% solution; minimum dose: 0.1 mL; maximum dose: 0.3 mL diluted in 2-3 mL normal saline every 4-6 hours (may be given more frequently according to need)
Adolescents and Adults: 5-20 breaths of full strength 5% metaproterenol **or** 0.2 to 0.3 mL 5% metaproterenol in 2.5-3 mL normal saline until nebulized every 4-6 hours (can be given more frequently according to need)

Mechanism of Action Relaxes bronchial smooth muscle by action on beta$_2$-receptors with very little effect on heart rate

Local Anesthetic/Vasoconstrictor Precautions No information available to require special precautions

Effects on Dental Treatment No effects or complications reported

Other Adverse Effects
>10%:
Central nervous system: Nervousness
Neuromuscular & skeletal: Tremor
1% to 10%:
Cardiovascular: Tachycardia, palpitations, hypertension
Central nervous system: Headache, dizziness
Gastrointestinal: Nausea, vomiting, bad taste
Neuromuscular & skeletal: Trembling, muscle cramps, weakness
Respiratory: Coughing
Miscellaneous: Increased sweating
<1%: Respiratory: Paradoxical bronchospasm

Drug Interactions
Decreased effect: Beta-blockers
Increased toxicity: Sympathomimetics, TCAs, MAO inhibitors

Drug Uptake
Oral:
Onset of bronchodilation: Within 15 minutes
Peak effect: Within 1 hour
Duration of action: ~1-5 hours
Inhalation:
Onset of effects: Within 60 seconds
Duration of action: Similar (~1-5 hours) regardless of route administered

Pregnancy Risk Factor C

Generic Available Yes (except inhaler)

Metasep® [OTC] *see* Parachlorometaxylenol *on page 723*

Metaxalone *(me TAKS a lone)*

Brand Names Skelaxin®
Therapeutic Category Muscle Relaxant; Skeletal Muscle Relaxant
Use Relief of discomfort associated with acute, painful musculoskeletal conditions
Usual Dosage Children >12 years and Adults: Oral: 800 mg 3-4 times/day
Mechanism of Action Does not have a direct effect on skeletal muscle; most of its therapeutic effect comes from actions on the central nervous system
Local Anesthetic/Vasoconstrictor Precautions No information available to require special precautions
Effects on Dental Treatment No effects or complications reported
Other Adverse Effects
>10%:
Central nervous system: Paradoxical stimulation, headache, somnolence, dizziness
Gastrointestinal: Nausea, vomiting, stomach cramps
<1%:
Dermatologic: Allergic dermatitis
Hematologic: Leukopenia, hemolytic anemia
Hepatic: Hepatotoxicity
Miscellaneous: Anaphylaxis
Drug Interactions Increased effect of alcohol, CNS depressants
Drug Uptake
Onset of action: ~1 hour
Duration: ~4-6 hours
Serum half-life: 2-3 hours

Pregnancy Risk Factor C
Generic Available No

Metforma (Mexico) *see* Metformin *on this page*

Metformin (met FOR min)
Related Information
Endocrine Disorders & Pregnancy *on page 1021*
Brand Names Glucophage®
Canadian/Mexican Brand Names Glucophage® Forte (Mexico); Novo-Metformin® (Canada)
Therapeutic Category Hypoglycemic Agent, Oral
Synonyms Metforma (Mexico)
Use Management of noninsulin-dependent diabetes mellitus (type II) as monotherapy when hyperglycemia cannot be managed on diet alone. May be used concomitantly with a sulfonylurea when diet and metformin or sulfonylurea alone do not result in adequate glycemic control.
Usual Dosage Oral (allow 1-2 weeks between dose titrations):
Adults:
> 500 mg tablets: Initial: 500 mg twice daily (given with the morning and evening meals). Dosage increases should be made in increments of one tablet every week, given in divided doses, up to a maximum of 2,500 mg/day. Doses of up to 2000 mg/day may be given twice daily. If a dose of 2,500 mg/day is required, it may be better tolerated 3 times/day (with meals).

> 850 mg tablets: Initial: 850 mg once daily (given with the morning meal). Dosage increases should be made in increments of one tablet every OTHER week, given in divided doses, up to a maximum of 2550 mg/day. The usual maintenance dose is 850 mg twice daily (with the morning and evening meals). Some patients may be given 850 mg 3 times/day (with meals).

Elderly patients: The initial and maintenance dosing should be conservative, due to the potential for decreased renal function. Generally, elderly patients should not be titrated to the maximum dose of metformin.

Transfer from other antidiabetic agents: No transition period is generally necessary except when transferring from chlorpropamide. When transferring from chlorpropamide, care should be exercised during the first 2 weeks because of the prolonged retention of chlorpropamide in the body, leading to overlapping drug effects and possible hypoglycemia.

Concomitant metformin and oral sulfonylurea therapy: If patients have not responded to 4 weeks of the maximum dose of metformin monotherapy, consideration to a gradually addition of an oral sulfonylurea while continuing metformin at the maximum dose, even if prior primary or secondary failure to a sulfonylurea has occurred.

Mechanism of Action Decreases hepatic glucose production, decreasing intestinal absorption of glucose and improves insulin sensitivity (increases peripheral glucose uptake and utilization)
Local Anesthetic/Vasoconstrictor Precautions No information available to require special precautions
Effects on Dental Treatment Metformin-dependent diabetics (noninsulin dependent, Type II) should be appointed for dental treatment in morning in order to minimize chance of stress-induced hypoglycemia
Other Adverse Effects
> \>10%: Gastrointestinal: Anorexia, nausea, vomiting, diarrhea, epigastric fullness, constipation, heartburn

> 1% to 10%:
> Dermatologic: Rash, urticaria, photosensitivity
> Endocrine & metabolic: Decreased vitamin B_{12} levels

> <1%: Hematologic: Blood dyscrasias, aplastic anemia, hemolytic anemia, bone marrow suppression, thrombocytopenia, agranulocytosis

Drug Interactions
> Decreased effects: Drugs which tend to produce hyperglycemia (eg, diuretics, corticosteroids, phenothiazines, thyroid products, estrogens, oral contraceptives, phenytoin, nicotinic acid, sympathomimetics, calcium channel blocking drugs, isoniazid) may lead to a loss of glycemic control

> Increased toxicity:
> Cationic drugs (eg, amiloride, digoxin, morphine, procainamide, quinidine, quinine, ranitidine, triamterene, trimethoprim, and vancomycin) which are eliminated by renal tubular secretion could have the potential for interaction with metformin by competing for common renal tubular transport systems
> Cimetidine increases (by 60%) peak metformin plasma and whole blood concentrations

Drug Uptake
> Serum half-life, plasma elimination: 6.2 hours

(Continued)

Metformin *(Continued)*
Pregnancy Risk Factor B
Generic Available No

Methadone (METH a done)
Related Information
Narcotic Agonists *on page 1141·*
Brand Names Dolophine®
Canadian/Mexican Brand Names Methadose® (Canada)
Therapeutic Category Analgesic, Narcotic
Use Management of severe pain, used in narcotic detoxification maintenance programs
Usual Dosage Doses should be titrated to appropriate effects
Children: Analgesia:
Oral, I.M., S.C.: 0.7 mg/kg/24 hours divided every 4-6 hours as needed or 0.1-0.2 mg/kg every 4-12 hours as needed; maximum: 10 mg/dose
I.V.: 0.1 mg/kg every 4 hours initially for 2-3 doses, then every 6-12 hours as needed; maximum: 10 mg/dose
Adults:
Analgesia: Oral, I.M., I.V., S.C.: 2.5-10 mg every 3-8 hours as needed, up to 5-20 mg every 6-8 hours
Detoxification: Oral: 15-40 mg/day; should not exceed 21 days and may not be repeated earlier than 4 weeks after completion of preceding course
Maintenance of opiate dependence: Oral: 20-120 mg/day
Mechanism of Action Binds to opiate receptors in the CNS, causing inhibition of ascending pain pathways, altering the perception of and response to pain; produces generalized CNS depression
Local Anesthetic/Vasoconstrictor Precautions No information available to require special precautions
Effects on Dental Treatment 1% to 10% of patients experience significant dry mouth which will disappear with cessation of drug therapy
Other Adverse Effects
Central nervous system: CNS depression
Endocrine & metabolic: Antidiuretic hormone release
Ocular: Miosis
Respiratory: Respiratory depression

>10%:
Cardiovascular: Palpitations, hypotension, bradycardia, peripheral vasodilation
Central nervous system: Fatigue, drowsiness, dizziness
Gastrointestinal: Nausea, vomiting, constipation
Neuromuscular & skeletal: Weakness
Miscellaneous: Histamine release
1% to 10%:
Central nervous system: Nervousness, headache, restlessness, anorexia, malaise, confusion, increased intracranial pressure
Gastrointestinal: Stomach cramps, dry mouth, biliary spasm
Genitourinary: Decreased urination, urinary tract spasm
Local: Pain at injection site
Respiratory: Dyspnea
<1%:
Central nervous system: Mental depression, hallucinations, paradoxical CNS stimulation
Dermatologic: Pruritus, skin rash, urticaria
Gastrointestinal: Paralytic ileus
Miscellaneous: Physical and psychological dependence
Drug Interactions
Decreased effect: Phenytoin, pentazocine and rifampin may increase the metabolism of methadone and may precipitate withdrawal
Increased toxicity: CNS depressants, phenothiazines, tricyclic antidepressants, MAO inhibitors may potentiate the adverse effects of methadone
Drug Uptake
Oral:
Onset of analgesia: Within 0.5-1 hour
Duration: 6-8 hours, increases to 22-48 hours with repeated doses
Parenteral:
Onset of effect: Within 10-20 minutes
Peak effect: Within 1-2 hours
Serum half-life: 15-29 hours, may be prolonged with alkaline pH
Pregnancy Risk Factor B (D if used for prolonged periods or in high doses at term)
Generic Available Yes

Methamphetamine (meth am FET a meen)
Brand Names Desoxyn®
Therapeutic Category Amphetamine; Central Nervous System Stimulant, Amphetamine
Use Treatment of narcolepsy, exogenous obesity, abnormal behavioral syndrome in children (minimal brain dysfunction)
Usual Dosage
Attention deficit disorder: Children >6 years: 2.5-5 mg 1-2 times/day, may increase by 5 mg increments weekly until optimum response is achieved, usually 20-25 mg/day

Exogenous obesity: Children >12 years and Adults: 5 mg, 30 minutes before each meal; long-acting formulation: 10-15 mg in morning; treatment duration should not exceed a few weeks
Local Anesthetic/Vasoconstrictor Precautions Use vasoconstriction with caution in patients taking methamphetamine. Amphetamines enhance the sympathomimetic response of epinephrine and norepinephrine leading to potential hypertension and cardiotoxicity.
Effects on Dental Treatment Up to 10% of patients taking dextroamphetamines may present with hypertension. The use of local anesthetic without vasoconstrictor is recommended in these patients.
Other Adverse Effects
>10%:
Cardiovascular: Arrhythmia
Central nervous system: False feeling of well being, nervousness, restlessness, insomnia
1% to 10%:
Cardiovascular: Hypertension
Central nervous system: Mood or mental changes, dizziness, lightheadedness, headache
Endocrine & metabolic: Changes in libido
Gastrointestinal: Diarrhea, nausea, vomiting, stomach cramps, constipation, anorexia, weight loss, dry mouth
Ocular: Blurred vision
Miscellaneous: Increased sweating
<1%:
Cardiovascular: Chest pain
Central nervous system: CNS stimulation (severe), Tourette's syndrome, hyperthermia, seizures, paranoia
Dermatologic: Skin rash, urticaria
Miscellaneous: Tolerance and withdrawal with prolonged use
Drug Interactions Increased toxicity with MAO inhibitors (hypertensive crisis)
Pregnancy Risk Factor C
Generic Available No

Methantheline (meth AN tha leen)
Brand Names Banthine®
Therapeutic Category Anticholinergic Agent; Antispasmodic Agent, Gastrointestinal
Synonyms Methanthelinium Bromide
Use Adjunctive treatment of peptic ulcer, irritable bowel syndrome, pancreatitis, ureteral and urinary bladder spasm; to reduce duodenal motility during diagnostic radiologic procedures and treatment of an uninhibited neurogenic bladder
Local Anesthetic/Vasoconstrictor Precautions No information available to require special precautions
Effects on Dental Treatment >10% of patients experience dry mouth
Other Adverse Effects
>10%:
Dermatologic: Dry skin
Gastrointestinal: Constipation
Respiratory: Dry nose, throat
Miscellaneous: Decreased sweating
1% to 10%: Gastrointestinal: Dysphagia
<1%:
Cardiovascular: Tachycardia
Central nervous system: Confusion, headache, loss of memory, fatigue, drowsiness, nervousness, insomnia
Dermatologic: Rash
Gastrointestinal: Bloated feeling, nausea, vomiting
Genitourinary: Urinary retention
Neuromuscular & skeletal: Weakness
Ocular: Increased intraocular pressure, blurred vision
(Continued)

Methantheline *(Continued)*
Pregnancy Risk Factor C
Generic Available No

Methanthelinium Bromide *see* Methantheline *on previous page*

Methazolamide *(meth a ZOE la mide)*
Brand Names GlaucTabs®; Neptazane®
Therapeutic Category Antiglaucoma Agent; Carbonic Anhydrase Inhibitor; Diuretic, Carbonic Anhydrase Inhibitor
Use Adjunctive treatment of open-angle or secondary glaucoma; short-term therapy of narrow-angle glaucoma when delay of surgery is desired
Usual Dosage Adults: Oral: 50-100 mg 2-3 times/day
Mechanism of Action Noncompetitive inhibition of the enzyme carbonic anhydrase; thought that carbonic anhydrase is located at the luminal border of cells of the proximal tubule. When the enzyme is inhibited, there is an increase in urine volume and a change to an alkaline pH with a subsequent decrease in the excretion of titratable acid and ammonia.
Local Anesthetic/Vasoconstrictor Precautions No information available to require special precautions
Effects on Dental Treatment No effects or complications reported
Other Adverse Effects
>10%:
Central nervous system: Malaise
Gastrointestinal: Metallic taste, anorexia
Neuromuscular & skeletal: Weakness
Renal: Polyuria
1% to 10%:
Central nervous system: Mental depression, drowsiness, dizziness
Renal: Crystalluria
<1%:
Central nervous system: Fever, headache, seizures, unsteadiness, fatigue
Dermatologic: Rash, sulfonamide rash, Stevens-Johnson syndrome
Endocrine & metabolic: Hyperchloremic metabolic acidosis, hypokalemia, hyperglycemia
Gastrointestinal: GI irritation, constipation, anorexia, dry mouth, black tarry stools
Genitourinary: Dysuria
Hematologic: Bone marrow suppression
Neuromuscular & skeletal: Paresthesia, trembling
Ocular: Myopia
Otic: Tinnitus
Miscellaneous: Loss of smell, hypersensitivity
Drug Interactions
Increased toxicity:
May induce hypokalemia which would sensitize a patient to digitalis toxicity
May increase the potential for salicylate toxicity
Hypokalemia may be compounded with concurrent diuretic use or steroids
Primidone absorption may be delayed
Decreased effect: Increased lithium excretion and altered excretion of other drugs by alkalinization of the urine, such as amphetamines, quinidine, procainamide, methenamine, phenobarbital, salicylates
Drug Uptake
Onset of action: Slow in comparison with acetazolamide (2-4 hours)
Peak effect: 6-8 hours
Duration: 10-18 hours
Absorption: Slowly from GI tract
Serum half-life: ~14 hours
Pregnancy Risk Factor C
Generic Available Yes

Methenamine *(meth EN a meen)*
Brand Names Hiprex®; Mandelamine®; Urex®; Urised®
Canadian/Mexican Brand Names Dehydral® (Canada); Hip-Rex® (Canada); Urasal® (Canada)
Therapeutic Category Antibiotic, Miscellaneous
Use Prophylaxis or suppression of recurrent urinary tract infections; urinary tract discomfort secondary to hypermotility; should not be used to treat infections outside of urinary tract
Usual Dosage Oral:
Children: 6-12 years:
Hippurate: 25-50 mg/kg/day divided every 12 hours

Mandelate: 50-75 mg/kg/day divided every 6 hours

Children >12 years and Adults:
Hippurate: 1 g twice daily
Mandelate: 1 g 4 times/day after meals and at bedtime

Mechanism of Action Methenamine is hydrolyzed to formaldehyde and ammonia in acidic urine; formaldehyde has nonspecific bactericidal action

Local Anesthetic/Vasoconstrictor Precautions No information available to require special precautions

Effects on Dental Treatment No effects or complications reported

Other Adverse Effects
1% to 10%:
Dermatologic: Skin rash
Gastrointestinal: Nausea, vomiting, diarrhea, anorexia, abdominal cramping
<1%:
Central nervous system: Headache
Genitourinary: Bladder irritation, dysuria
Hepatic: Elevation in AST and ALT
Renal: Hematuria, crystalluria

Drug Interactions
Decreased effect: Sodium bicarbonate and acetazolamide will decrease effect secondary to alkalinization of urine
Increased toxicity: Sulfonamides (may precipitate)

Drug Uptake
Absorption: Readily absorbed from GI tract
Serum half-life: 3-6 hours

Pregnancy Risk Factor C

Generic Available Yes

Methergine® *see Methylergonovine* *on page 623*

Methicillin (meth i SIL in)

Brand Names Staphcillin®

Therapeutic Category Antibiotic, Penicillin

Use Treatment of susceptible bacterial infections such as osteomyelitis, septicemia, endocarditis, and CNS infections due to penicillinase-producing strains of *Staphylococcus*; other antistaphylococcal penicillins are usually preferred

Usual Dosage I.M., I.V.:
Children: 150-200 mg/kg/day divided every 6 hours; 200-400 mg/kg/day divided every 4-6 hours has been used for treatment of severe infections; maximum dose: 12 g/day
Adults: 4-12 g/day in divided doses every 4-6 hours

Mechanism of Action Inhibits bacterial cell wall synthesis by binding to one or more of the penicillin binding proteins (PBPs); which in turn inhibits the final transpeptidation step of peptidoglycan synthesis in bacterial cell walls, thus inhibiting cell wall biosynthesis. Bacteria eventually lyse due to ongoing activity of cell wall autolytic enzymes (autolysins and murein hydrolases) while cell wall assembly is arrested.

Local Anesthetic/Vasoconstrictor Precautions No information available to require special precautions

Effects on Dental Treatment Prolonged use of penicillins may lead to development of oral candidiasis

Other Adverse Effects
1% to 10%:
Dermatologic: Skin rash
Renal: Acute interstitial nephritis
<1%:
Central nervous system: Fever
Dermatologic: Rash
Genitourinary: Hemorrhagic cystitis
Hematologic: Eosinophilia, anemia, leukopenia, neutropenia, thrombocytopenia
Local: Phlebitis
Miscellaneous: Serum sickness-like reactions

Drug Interactions
Decreased effect: Efficacy of oral contraceptives may be reduced
Increased effect: Disulfiram, probenecid may increase penicillin levels, increased effect of anticoagulants

Drug Uptake
Serum half-life (with normal renal function):
Children 2-16 years: 0.8 hour
Adults: 0.4-0.5 hour
(Continued)

Methicillin *(Continued)*

Time to peak serum concentration:
I.M.: 0.5-1 hour
I.V. infusion: Within 5 minutes
Pregnancy Risk Factor B
Generic Available No

Methimazole *(meth IM'a zole)*

Related Information
Endocrine Disorders & Pregnancy *on page 1021*

Brand Names Tapazole®

Therapeutic Category Antithyroid Agent

Use Palliative treatment of hyperthyroidism, return the hyperthyroid patient to a normal metabolic state prior to thyroidectomy, and to control thyrotoxic crisis that may accompany thyroidectomy. The use of antithyroid thioamides is as effective in elderly as they are in younger adults; however, the expense, potential adverse effects, and inconvenience (compliance, monitoring) make them undesirable. The use of radioiodine due to ease of administration and less concern for long-term side effects and reproduction problems (some older males) makes it a more appropriate therapy.

Usual Dosage Oral: Administer in 3 equally divided doses at approximately 8-hour intervals
Children: Initial: 0.4 mg/kg/day in 3 divided doses; maintenance: 0.2 mg/kg/day in 3 divided doses up to 30 mg/24 hours maximum
Adults: Initial: 5 mg every 8 hours; maintenance dose: 5-15 mg/day up to 60 mg/day for severe hyperthyroidism
Adjust dosage as required to achieve and maintain serum T_3, T_4, and TSH levels in the normal range. An elevated T_3 may be the sole indicator of inadequate treatment. An elevated TSH indicates excessive antithyroid treatment.

Mechanism of Action Inhibits the synthesis of thyroid hormones by blocking the oxidation of iodine in the thyroid gland, blocking iodine's ability to combine with tyrosine to form thyroxine and triiodothyronine (T_3), does not inactivate circulating T_4 and T_3

Local Anesthetic/Vasoconstrictor Precautions No information available to require special precautions

Effects on Dental Treatment No effects or complications reported

Other Adverse Effects
>10%:
Central nervous system: Fever
Dermatologic: Skin rash
Hematologic: Leukopenia
1% to 10%:
Central nervous system: Dizziness
Gastrointestinal: Nausea, vomiting, stomach pain, dysgeusia
Hematologic: Agranulocytosis
Miscellaneous: SLE-like syndrome
<1%:
Cardiovascular: Edema
Central nervous system: Drowsiness, vertigo, headache
Dermatologic: Rash, urticaria, pruritus, alopecia
Endocrine & metabolic: Goiter
Gastrointestinal: Constipation, weight gain, swollen salivary glands
Hematologic: Thrombocytopenia, aplastic anemia
Hepatic: Cholestatic jaundice
Neuromuscular & skeletal: Arthralgia, paresthesia
Renal: Nephrotic syndrome

Drug Interactions Increased toxicity: Iodinated glycerol, lithium, potassium iodide; anticoagulant activity increased

Drug Uptake
Onset of antithyroid effect: Oral: Within 30-40 minutes
Duration: 2-4 hours
Serum half-life: 4-13 hours

Pregnancy Risk Factor D
Generic Available No

Methionine *(me THYE oh neen)*

Brand Names Pedameth®

Therapeutic Category Dietary Supplement

Use Treatment of diaper rash and control of odor, dermatitis and ulceration caused by ammoniacal urine

Local Anesthetic/Vasoconstrictor Precautions No information available to require special precautions
Effects on Dental Treatment No effects or complications reported
Generic Available Yes

Methocarbamol (meth oh KAR ba mole)

Related Information
Temporomandibular Dysfunction (TMD) *on page 1078*
Brand Names Robaxin®
Therapeutic Category Muscle Relaxant; Skeletal Muscle Relaxant
Use
Dental: Treatment of muscle spasm associated with acute temporomandibular joint pain
Medical: Treatment of muscle spasm associated with acute painful musculoskeletal conditions, supportive therapy in tetanus
Usual Dosage Adults: Muscle spasm: Oral: 1.5 g 4 times/day for 2-3 days, then decrease to 4-4.5 g/day in 3-6 divided doses
Mechanism of Action Causes skeletal muscle relaxation by reducing the transmission of impulses from the spinal cord to skeletal muscle
Local Anesthetic/Vasoconstrictor Precautions No information available to require special precautions
Effects on Dental Treatment No effects or complications reported
Other Adverse Effects >10%: Central nervous system: Drowsiness, dizziness, lightheadedness
Contraindications Renal impairment, hypersensitivity to methocarbamol or any component
Warnings/Precautions Rate of injection should not exceed 3 mL/minute; solution is hypertonic; avoid extravasation; use with caution in patients with a history of seizures
Drug Interactions Increased effect/toxicity with CNS depressants
Drug Uptake
Absorption: Rapid
Onset of muscle relaxation: Oral: Within 30 minutes
Serum half-life: 1-2 hours
Time to peak serum concentration: Oral: ~2 hours
Pregnancy Risk Factor C
Breast-feeding Considerations May be taken while breast-feeding
Dosage Forms
Injection: 100 mg/mL in polyethylene glycol 50% (10 mL)
Tablet: 500 mg, 750 mg
Dietary Considerations Tablets may be crushed and mixed with food or liquid if needed
Generic Available Yes

Methocarbamol and Aspirin (meth oh KAR ba mole & AS pir in)

Brand Names Robaxisal®
Therapeutic Category Muscle Relaxant; Skeletal Muscle Relaxant
Use
Dental: Treatment of muscle spasm associated with acute temporomandibular joint pain
Medical: Treatment of muscle spasm associated with acute painful musculoskeletal conditions, supportive therapy in tetanus
Usual Dosage Children >12 years and Adults: Oral: 2 tablets 4 times/day
Mechanism of Action Causes skeletal muscle relaxation by reducing the transmission of impulses from the spinal cord to skeletal muscle
Local Anesthetic/Vasoconstrictor Precautions No information available to require special precautions
Effects on Dental Treatment Use with caution in patients with platelet and bleeding disorders, renal dysfunction, erosive gastritis, or peptic ulcer disease, previous nonreaction does not guarantee future safe taking of medication; do not use aspirin in children <16 years of age for chickenpox or flu symptoms due to the association with Reye's syndrome

Avoid aspirin if possible, for 1 week prior to surgery because of the possibility of postoperative bleeding; use with caution in impaired hepatic function

Elderly are a high-risk population for adverse effects from nonsteroidal anti-inflammatory agents. As much as 60% of elderly with GI complications to NSAIDs can develop peptic ulceration and/or hemorrhage asymptomatically. Also, concomitant disease and drug use contribute to the risk for GI adverse effects. Use lowest effective dose for shortest period possible. Consider renal function decline with age. Use with caution in patients with history of asthma
(Continued)

Methocarbamol and Aspirin *(Continued)*

Other Adverse Effects
Methocarbamol: >10%: Central nervous system: Drowsiness, dizziness, light-headedness

Aspirin:
>10%: Gastrointestinal: Nausea, vomiting, dyspepsia, epigastric discomfort, heartburn, stomach pains
1% to 10%: Gastrointestinal: Ulceration

Contraindications
Methocarbamol: Renal impairment, hypersensitivity to methocarbamol or any component
Aspirin: Bleeding disorders (factor VII or IX deficiencies), hypersensitivity to salicylates or other NSAIDs, tartrazine dye and asthma

Warnings/Precautions
Use aspirin with caution in patients with platelet and bleeding disorders, renal dysfunction, erosive gastritis, or peptic ulcer disease, previous nonreaction does not guarantee future safe taking of medication; do not use aspirin in children <16 years of age for chickenpox or flu symptoms due to the association with Reye's syndrome

Avoid aspirin if possible, for 1 week prior to surgery because of the possibility of postoperative bleeding; use with caution in impaired hepatic function

Elderly are a high-risk population for adverse effects from nonsteroidal anti-inflammatory agents. As much as 60% of elderly with GI complications to NSAIDs can develop peptic ulceration and/or hemorrhage asymptomatically. Also, concomitant disease and drug use contribute to the risk for GI adverse effects. Use lowest effective dose for shortest period possible. Consider renal function decline with age. Use with caution in patients with history of asthma

Drug Interactions
Methocarbamol: Increased effect/toxicity with CNS depressants
Aspirin: Concomitant use of aspirin may result in possible decreased serum concentration of NSAIDs; aspirin may antagonize effects of probenecid; aspirin may increase methotrexate serum levels. Aspirin may displace valproic acid from binding sites which can result in toxicity; warfarin and aspirin result in increased bleeding; NSAIDs and aspirin result in increased GI adverse effects.

Drug Uptake
Methocarbamol:
Absorption: Rapid
Onset of muscle relaxation: Oral: Within 30 minutes
Time to peak serum concentration: Oral: ~2 hours
Serum half-life: 1-2 hours
Aspirin:
Absorption: Rapid
Time to peak serum concentration: ~1-2 hours
Serum half-life:
Parent drug: 15-20 minutes
Salicylates (dose-dependent): From 3 hours at lower doses (300-600 mg), to 5-6 hours (after 1 g) to 10 hours with higher doses

Pregnancy Risk Factor
C (D if full-dose aspirin in 3rd trimester)

Breast-feeding Considerations
Use cautiously due to potential adverse effects in nursing infants

Dosage Forms
Tablet: Methocarbamol 400 mg and aspirin 325 mg

Dietary Considerations
Food decreases rate but not extent of absorption (oral)

Generic Available
Yes

Methohexital *(meth oh HEKS i tal)*

Brand Names
Brevital® Sodium

Canadian/Mexican Brand Names
Brietal Sodium® (Canada)

Therapeutic Category
Barbiturate; General Anesthetic, Intravenous; Sedative

Use
Dental: I.V. induction and maintenance of general anesthesia for short periods
Medical: None

Restrictions
C-IV

Usual Dosage
I.V.:
Children: 1-2 mg/kg/dose
Adults: 50-120 mg to start; 20-40 mg every 4-7 minutes

Mechanism of Action
Ultrashort-acting I.V. barbiturate anesthetic; acts as agonist within the multisubunit $GABA_A$ receptor ion chloride-channel complex in central nervous system neurons; this leads to inhibition of many brain functions resulting in loss of consciousness. May also dissolve in neuronal membranes to cause stabilization and eventual loss of action potentials which also leads to inhibition of brain function.

Local Anesthetic/Vasoconstrictor Precautions No information available to require special precautions

Effects on Dental Treatment No effects or complications reported

Other Adverse Effects >10%: Local: Pain on I.M. injection

Contraindications Porphyria, hypersensitivity to methohexital or any component

Warnings/Precautions Use with extreme caution in patients with liver impairment, asthma, cardiovascular instability

Drug Interactions CNS depressants worsen CNS depression

Drug Uptake
Onset of effect: Immediately after I.V. injection
Duration: 10-20 minutes after a single dose

Pregnancy Risk Factor C

Breast-feeding Considerations No data reported

Dosage Forms Injection, as sodium: 500 mg, 2.5 g, 5 g

Dietary Considerations Should not be given to patients with food in stomach because of danger of vomiting during anesthesia

Generic Available No

Methotrexate (meth oh TREKS ate)

Related Information
Rheumatoid Arthritis and Osteoarthritis *on page 1030*

Brand Names Folex® PFS; Rheumatrex®

Canadian/Mexican Brand Names Ledertrexate® (Mexico)

Therapeutic Category Antineoplastic Agent, Antimetabolite

Synonyms Metotrexato (Mexico)

Use Treatment of trophoblastic neoplasms; leukemias; psoriasis; rheumatoid arthritis; breast, head, and lung carcinomas; osteosarcoma; sarcomas; carcinoma of gastric, esophagus, testes; lymphomas

Usual Dosage Refer to individual protocols. May be administered orally, I.M., intra-arterially, intrathecally, I.V., or S.C.

Leucovorin may be administered concomitantly or within 24 hours of methotrexate

Children:
Juvenile rheumatoid arthritis: Oral, I.M.: 5-15 mg/m^2/week as a single dose **or** as 3 divided doses given 12 hours apart
Antineoplastic dosage range:
Oral, I.M.: 7.5-30 mg/m^2/week **or** every 2 weeks
I.V.: 10-12,000 mg/m^2 bolus dosing **or** continuous infusion over 6-42 hours

Methotrexate Dosing Schedules

	Dose	Route	Frequency
Conventional dose	15-20 mg/m^2 30-50 mg/m^2 15 mg/day for 5 days	Oral Oral, I.V. Oral, I.M.	Twice weekly Weekly Every 2-3 weeks
Intermediate dose	50-150 mg/m^2 240 mg/m^{2*} 0.5-1 g/m^{2*}	I.V. push I.V. infusion I.V. infusion	Every 2-3 weeks Every 4-7 days Every 2-3 weeks
High dose	1-12 g/m^{2*}	I.V. infusion	Every 1-3 weeks

Pediatric solid tumors: I.V.:
<12 years: 12 g/m^2 (dosage range: 12-18 g)
≥ 12 years: 8 g/m^2 (maximum: 18 g)
Meningeal leukemia: I.V.: Loading dose: 6 g/m^2 followed by I.V. continuous infusion of 1.2 g/m^2/hour for 23 hours
Acute lymphocytic leukemia (high dose): I.V.: Loading: 200 mg/m^2 followed by a 24-hour infusion of 1200 mg/m^2/day
ANLL: I.V.: 7.5 mg/m^2/day on days 1-5
Resistant ANLL: I.V.: 100 mg/m^2/dose on day 1
Hodgkin's lymphoma: I.V.: 200-500 mg/m^2; repeat every 28 days
Induction of remission in acute lymphoblastic leukemias: Oral: 3.3 mg/m^2/day for 4-6 weeks; remission maintenance: Oral, I.M.: 20-30 mg/m^2 twice weekly

Meningeal leukemia: I.T.: 10-15 mg/m^2 (maximum dose: 15 mg)
or
≤3 months: 3 mg/dose
4-11 months: 6 mg/dose
1 year: 8 mg/dose
2 years: 10 mg/dose
≥3 years: 12 mg/dose
(Continued)

Methotrexate *(Continued)*

I.T. doses are prepared with preservative-free MTX **only**. Hydrocortisone may be added to the I.T. preparation; total volume should range from 3-6 mL. Doses should be repeated at 2- to 5-day intervals until CSF counts return to normal followed by a dose once weekly for 2 weeks then monthly thereafter.

Adults: I.V.: Range is wide from 30-40 mg/m²/week to 100-7500 mg/m² with leucovorin rescue

Doses not requiring leucovorin rescue range from 30-40 mg/m² I.V. or I.M. repeated weekly, or oral regimens of 10 mg/m² twice weekly

High-dose MTX is considered to be >100 mg/m² and can be as high as 1500-7500 mg/m². These doses require leucovorin rescue. Patients receiving doses ≥1000 mg/m² should have their urine alkalinized with bicarbonate or Bicitra® prior to and following MTX therapy.

Trophoblastic neoplasms: Oral, I.M.: 15-30 mg/day for 5 days; repeat in 7 days for 3-5 courses

Head and neck cancer: Oral, I.M., I.V.: 25-50 mg/m² once weekly

Rheumatoid arthritis: Oral: 7.5 mg once weekly **or** 2.5 mg every 12 hours for 3 doses/week; not to exceed 20 mg/week

Psoriasis: Oral: 2.5-5 mg/dose every 12 hours for 3 doses given once weekly **or**
Oral, I.M.: 10-25 mg/dose given once weekly

Elderly: Rheumatoid arthritis/psoriasis: Oral:
Initial: 5 mg once weekly
If nausea occurs, split dose to 2.5 mg every 12 hours for the day of administration
Dose may be increased to 7.5 mg/week based on response, not to exceed 20 mg/week

Ectopic pregnancy: I.M./I.V.: 50 mg/m² single-dose without leucovorin rescue

Mechanism of Action Antimetabolite that inhibits DNA synthesis and cell reproduction in cancerous cells

Folates must be in the reduced form (FH_4) to be active
Folates are activated by dihydrofolate reductase (DHFR)
DHFR is inhibited by MTX (by binding irreversibly), causing an increase in the intracellular dihydrofolate pool (the inactive cofactor) and inhibition of both purine and thymidylate synthesis (TS)
MTX enters the cell through an energy-dependent and temperature-dependent process which is mediated by an intramembrane protein; this carrier mechanism is also used by naturally occurring reduced folates, including folinic acid (leucovorin), making this a competitive process
At high drug concentrations (>20 μM), MTX enters the cell by a second mechanism which is not shared by reduced folates; the process may be passive diffusion or a specific, saturable process, and provides a rationale for high-dose MTX
A small fraction of MTX is converted intracellularly to polyglutamates, which leads to a prolonged inhibition of DHFR

Local Anesthetic/Vasoconstrictor Precautions No information available to require special precautions

Effects on Dental Treatment Methotrexate commonly causes ulceration stomatitis, gingivitis, and pharyngitis associated with oral discomfort

Other Adverse Effects

>10%:
Gastrointestinal: Mucositis is dose-dependent; appears in 3-7 days after therapy, resolving within 2 weeks
Cardiovascular: Vasculitis
Central nervous system (with I.T. administration only):
Arachnoiditis: Acute reaction manifested as severe headache, nuchal rigidity, vomiting, and fever; may be alleviated by reducing the dose
Subacute toxicity: 10% of patients treated with 12-15 mg/m² of I.T. MTX may develop this in the second or third week of therapy; consists of motor paralysis of extremities, cranial nerve palsy, seizures, or coma. This has also been seen in pediatric cases receiving very high-dose MTX (when enough MTX can get across into the CSF).
Demyelinating encephalopathy: Seen months or years after receiving MTX; usually in association with cranial irradiation or other systemic chemotherapy
Dermatologic: Reddening of skin
Gastrointestinal: Ulcerative stomatitis, pharyngitis, glossitis, gingivitis, nausea, vomiting, diarrhea, anorexia, intestinal perforation
Emetic potential: <100 mg: Moderately low (10% to 30%); ≥100 mg or <250 mg: Moderate (30% to 60%); ≥250 mg: Moderately high (60% to 90%)

Endocrine & metabolic: Hyperuricemia
Hematologic: Leukopenia, thrombocytopenia
Renal: Renal failure, azotemia, nephropathy

1% to 10%:

Central nervous system: Dizziness, malaise, encephalopathy, seizures, fever, chills

Dermatologic: Alopecia, rash, photosensitivity, depigmentation or hyperpigmentation of skin

Endocrine & metabolic: Diabetes

Genitourinary: Cystitis

Hematologic: Hemorrhage

Myelosuppressive: This is the primary dose-limiting factor (along with mucositis) of MTX; occurs about 5-7 days after MTX therapy, and should resolve within 2 weeks; WBC: Mild; Platelets: Moderate; Onset (days): 7; Nadir (days): 10; Recovery (days): 21

Hepatic abnormalities: Cirrhosis and portal fibrosis have been associated with chronic MTX therapy; acute elevation of liver enzymes are common after high-dose MTX, and usually resolve within 10 days

Neuromuscular & skeletal: Arthralgia

Ocular: Blurred vision

Respiratory: Pneumonitis associated with fever, cough, and interstitial pulmonary infiltrates; treatment is to withhold MTX during the acute reaction

Renal dysfunction: Manifested by an abrupt rise in serum creatinine and BUN and a fall in urine output; more common with high-dose MTX, and may be due to precipitation of the drug. The best treatment is prevention: Aggressively hydrate with 3 L/m^2/day starting 12 hours before therapy and continue for 24-36 hours; alkalinize the urine by adding 50 mEq of bicarbonate to each liter of fluid; keep urine flow >100 mL/hour and urine pH >7.

Renal: Vasculitis

Miscellaneous: Anaphylaxis, decreased resistance to infection

Drug Interactions

Decreased effect: Decreased phenytoin, 5-FU, nonsteroidal anti-inflammatory drugs (NSAIDs)

Corticosteroids: Reported to decrease uptake of MTX into leukemia cells. Administration of these drugs should be separated by 12 hours. Dexamethasone has been reported to not affect methotrexate influx into cells.

Increased toxicity:

Live virus vaccines cause vaccinia infections

Vincristine: Inhibits MTX efflux from the cell, leading to increased and prolonged MTX levels in the cell; the dose of VCR needed to produce this effect is not achieved clinically

Organic acids: Salicylates, sulfonamides, probenecid, and high doses of penicillins compete with MTX for transport and reduce renal tubular secretion. Salicylates and sulfonamides may also displace MTX from plasma proteins, increasing MTX levels.

Ara-C: Increased formation of the Ara-C nucleotide can occur when MTX precedes Ara-C, thus promoting the action of Ara-C

Cyclosporine: CSA and MTX interfere with each others renal elimination, which may result in increased toxicity

Drug Uptake

Absorption:

Oral: Rapid; well absorbed orally at low doses (<30 mg/m^2), incomplete absorption after large doses

I.M. injection: Completely absorbed

Serum half-life: 8-12 hours with high doses and 3-10 hours with low doses

Time to peak serum concentration:

Oral: 1-2 hours

Parenteral: 30-60 minutes

Pregnancy Risk Factor D

Generic Available Yes

Methotrimeprazine (meth oh trye MEP ra zeen)

Brand Names Levoprome®

Therapeutic Category Analgesic, Non-narcotic; Phenothiazine Derivative; Sedative

Synonyms Levomepromazine; Methotrimeprazine Hydrochloride

Use Relief of moderate to severe pain in nonambulatory patients; for analgesia and sedation when respiratory depression is to be avoided, as in obstetrics; preanesthetic for producing sedation, somnolence and relief of apprehension and anxiety

Usual Dosage Adults: I.M.:

Sedation analgesia: 10-20 mg every 4-6 hours as needed

(Continued)

Methotrimeprazine *(Continued)*

Preoperative medication: 2-20 mg, 45 minutes to 3 hours before surgery
Postoperative analgesia: 2.5-7.5 mg every 4-6 hours is suggested as necessary since residual effects of anesthetic may be present
Pre- and postoperative hypotension: I.M.: 5-10 mg

Mechanism of Action Methotrimeprazine is a phenothiazine with sites of action thought to be in the thalamus, hypothalamus, reticular and limbic systems, producing suppression of sensory impulses. This results with sedation, an elevated pain threshold, and induction of amnesia. The analgesic effect of methotrimeprazine is comparable to meperidine and morphine without the respiratory suppression. This agent also has antihistamine, anticholinergic, and antiepinephrine effects.

Local Anesthetic/Vasoconstrictor Precautions No information available to require special precautions

Effects on Dental Treatment Anticholinergic side effects can cause a reduction of saliva production or secretion contributes to discomfort and dental disease (ie, caries, oral candidiasis and periodontal disease); phenothiazines can cause extrapyramidal reactions which may appear as muscle twitching or increased motor activity of the face, neck or head

Other Adverse Effects

>10%:
Cardiovascular: Hypotension, orthostatic hypotension
Central nervous system: Pseudoparkinsonism, akathisia, dystonias, tardive dyskinesia (persistent), dizziness
Gastrointestinal: Constipation
Ocular: Pigmentary retinopathy
Respiratory: Nasal congestion
Miscellaneous: Decreased sweating

1% to 10%:
Dermatologic: Photosensitivity, skin rash
Endocrine & metabolic: Changes in menstrual cycle, changes in libido, pain in breasts
Gastrointestinal: Weight gain, nausea, vomiting, stomach pain
Genitourinary: Dysuria, ejaculatory disturbances
Neuromuscular & skeletal: Trembling of fingers

<1%:
Central nervous system: Neuroleptic malignant syndrome (NMS), impairment of temperature regulation, lowering of seizures threshold
Dermatologic: Discoloration of skin (blue-gray)
Endocrine & metabolic: Galactorrhea
Genitourinary: Priapism
Hematologic: Agranulocytosis, leukopenia
Hepatic: Cholestatic jaundice, hepatotoxicity
Ocular: Cornea and lens changes, pigmentary retinopathy

Drug Interactions Increased toxicity: Additive effects with other CNS-depressants

Drug Uptake
Peak effect: Within 20-40 minutes
Duration: 4 hours
Serum half-life, elimination: 20 hours
Time to peak serum concentration: Within 0.5-1.5 hours

Pregnancy Risk Factor C

Generic Available No

Methotrimeprazine Hydrochloride *see* Methotrimeprazine *on previous page*

Methoxsalen *(meth OKS a len)*

Brand Names Oxsoralen® Topical; Oxsoralen-Ultra® Oral

Therapeutic Category Psoralen

Synonyms Methoxypsoralen; 8-Methoxypsoralen; 8-MOP

Use Symptomatic control of severe, recalcitrant, disabling psoriasis in conjunction with long wave ultraviolet radiation; induce repigmentation in vitiligo topical repigmenting agent in conjunction with controlled doses of ultraviolet A (UVA) or sunlight

Usual Dosage

Psoriasis: Adults: Oral: 10-70 mg 1½-2 hours before exposure to ultraviolet light, 2-3 times at least 48 hours apart; dosage is based upon patient's body weight and skin type

Vitiligo: Children >12 years and Adults:
Oral: 20 mg 2-4 hours before exposure to UVA light or sunlight; limit exposure to 15-40 minutes based on skin basic color and exposure

Topical: Apply lotion 1-2 hours before exposure to UVA light, no more than once weekly

Mechanism of Action Bonds covalently to pyrimidine bases in DNA, inhibits the synthesis of DNA, and suppresses cell division. The augmented sunburn reaction involves excitation of the methoxsalen molecule by radiation in the long-wave ultraviolet light (UVA), resulting in transference of energy to the methoxsalen molecule producing an excited state ("triplet electronic state"). The molecule, in this "triplet state", then reacts with cutaneous DNA.

Local Anesthetic/Vasoconstrictor Precautions No information available to require special precautions

Effects on Dental Treatment No effects or complications reported

Other Adverse Effects
>10%:
Dermatologic: Itching
Gastrointestinal: Nausea
1% to 10%:
Cardiovascular: Severe edema, hypotension
Central nervous system: Nervousness, vertigo, depression
Dermatologic: Pruritus, freckling, hypopigmentation, rash, cheilitis, erythema; painful blistering, burning, and peeling of skin
Neuromuscular & skeletal: Loss of muscle coordination

Drug Uptake
Time to peak serum concentration: Oral: 2-4 hours

Pregnancy Risk Factor C

Generic Available No

Comments Absorption is increased with food; peak levels occur in 30 minutes to 1 hour after ingestion; plasma half-life is approximately 2 hours

Methoxycinnamate and Oxybenzone
(meth OKS ee SIN a mate & oks i BEN zone)

Brand Names PreSun® 29 [OTC]; Ti-Screen® [OTC]

Therapeutic Category Sunscreen

Synonyms Sunscreen, PABA-Free

Use Reduce the chance of premature aging of the skin and skin cancer from overexposure to the sun

Local Anesthetic/Vasoconstrictor Precautions No information available to require special precautions

Effects on Dental Treatment No effects or complications reported

Generic Available Yes

Methoxypsoralen *see* Methoxsalen *on previous page*

8-Methoxypsoralen *see* Methoxsalen *on previous page*

Methscopolamine (meth skoe POL a meen)

Brand Names Pamine®

Therapeutic Category Anticholinergic Agent; Antispasmodic Agent, Gastrointestinal

Use Adjunctive therapy in the treatment of peptic ulcer

Usual Dosage Adults: Oral: 2.5 mg 30 minutes before meals or food and 2.5-5 mg at bedtime

Mechanism of Action Methscopolamine is a peripheral anticholinergic agent that does not cross the blood-brain barrier and provides a peripheral blockade of muscarinic receptors. This agent reduces the volume and the total acid content of gastric secretions, inhibits salivation, and reduces gastrointestinal motility.

Local Anesthetic/Vasoconstrictor Precautions No information available to require special precautions

Effects on Dental Treatment >10% of patients experience dry mouth; anticholinergic side effects can cause a reduction of saliva production or secretion contributes to discomfort and dental disease (ie, caries, oral candidiasis and periodontal disease)

Other Adverse Effects
>10%:
Dermatologic: Dry skin
Gastrointestinal: Constipation
Respiratory: Dry nose, throat
Miscellaneous: Decreased sweating
1% to 10%: Gastrointestinal: Dysphagia
<1%:
Cardiovascular: Tachycardia
Central nervous system: Confusion, drowsiness, nervousness, insomnia, headache, loss of memory, fatigue
Dermatologic: Rash
(Continued)

Methscopolamine *(Continued)*

Gastrointestinal: Bloated feeling, nausea, vomiting
Genitourinary: Urinary retention
Neuromuscular & skeletal: Weakness
Ocular: Increased intraocular pressure, blurred vision
Drug Interactions No data reported
Pregnancy Risk Factor C
Generic Available No

Methsuximide (meth SUKS i mide)
Brand Names Celontin®
Canadian/Mexican Brand Names Celontin® (Canada)
Therapeutic Category Anticonvulsant, Succinimide
Use Control of absence (petit mal) seizures; useful adjunct in refractory, partial complex (psychomotor) seizures
Usual Dosage Oral:
Children: Initial: 10-15 mg/kg/day in 3-4 divided doses; increase weekly up to maximum of 30 mg/kg/day

Adults: 300 mg/day for the first week; may increase by 300 mg/day at weekly intervals up to 1.2 g/day in 2-4 divided doses/day
Mechanism of Action Increases the seizure threshold and suppresses paroxysmal spike-and-wave pattern in absence seizures; depresses nerve transmission in the motor cortex
Local Anesthetic/Vasoconstrictor Precautions No information available to require special precautions
Effects on Dental Treatment No effects or complications reported
Other Adverse Effects
>10%:
Central nervous system: Ataxia, dizziness, drowsiness, headache
Dermatologic: Stevens-Johnson syndrome
Gastrointestinal: Anorexia, nausea, vomiting, weight loss
Miscellaneous: Hiccups, SLE
1% to 10%:
Central nervous system: Aggressiveness, mental depression, nightmares, fatigue
Neuromuscular & skeletal: Weakness
<1%:
Central nervous system: Paranoid psychosis
Dermatologic: Urticaria, exfoliative dermatitis
Hematologic: Agranulocytosis, leukopenia, aplastic anemia, thrombocytopenia, pancytopenia
Drug Interactions No data reported
Drug Uptake
Serum half-life: 2-4 hours
Time to peak serum concentration: Oral: Within 1-3 hours
Pregnancy Risk Factor C
Generic Available No

Methyclothiazide (meth i kloe THYE a zide)
Related Information
Cardiovascular Diseases *on page 1010*
Brand Names Aquatensen®; Enduron®
Therapeutic Category Diuretic, Thiazide
Use Management of mild to moderate hypertension; treatment of edema in congestive heart failure and nephrotic syndrome
Usual Dosage Oral:
Children: 0.05-0.2 mg/kg/day

Adults:
Edema: 2.5-10 mg/day
Hypertension: 2.5-5 mg/day
Mechanism of Action Inhibits sodium reabsorption in the distal tubules causing increased excretion of sodium and water, as well as, potassium and hydrogen ions
Local Anesthetic/Vasoconstrictor Precautions No information available to require special precautions
Effects on Dental Treatment No effects or complications reported
Other Adverse Effects
1% to 10%: Endocrine & metabolic: Hypokalemia
<1%:
Cardiovascular: Hypotension

Central nervous system: Drowsiness
Dermatologic: Photosensitivity, rash
Endocrine & metabolic: Fluid and electrolyte imbalances (hypocalcemia, hypomagnesemia, hyponatremia), hyperglycemia
Gastrointestinal: Nausea, vomiting, anorexia
Hematologic: Rarely blood dyscrasias, aplastic anemia, hemolytic anemia, leukopenia, agranulocytosis, thrombocytopenia
Hepatic: Hepatitis
Neuromuscular & skeletal: Paresthesia
Renal: Polyuria, prerenal azotemia, uremia
Drug Interactions Increased toxicity/levels of lithium
Drug Uptake
Onset of diuresis: Oral: 2 hours
Peak effect: 6 hours
Duration: ~1 day
Pregnancy Risk Factor D
Generic Available Yes

Methyclothiazide and Deserpidine
(meth i kloe THYE a zide & de SER pi deen)
Brand Names Enduronyl®; Enduronyl® Forte
Therapeutic Category Antihypertensive Agent, Combination
Use Management of mild to moderately severe hypertension
Local Anesthetic/Vasoconstrictor Precautions No information available to require special precautions
Effects on Dental Treatment No effects or complications reported
Pregnancy Risk Factor C
Generic Available No

Methyclothiazide and Pargyline
(meth i kloe THYE a zide & PAR gi leen)
Brand Names Eutron®
Therapeutic Category Antihypertensive Agent, Combination
Synonyms Pargyline and Methyclothiazide
Use Management of hypertension
Local Anesthetic/Vasoconstrictor Precautions No information available to require special precautions
Effects on Dental Treatment No effects or complications reported
Pregnancy Risk Factor C
Generic Available No

Methylbenzethonium Chloride
(meth il ben ze THOE nee um KLOR ide)
Brand Names Diaparene® [OTC]; Puri-Clens™ [OTC]; Sween® Cream [OTC]
Therapeutic Category Topical Skin Product
Use Diaper rash and ammonia dermatitis
Local Anesthetic/Vasoconstrictor Precautions No information available to require special precautions
Effects on Dental Treatment No effects or complications reported
Generic Available No

Methylcellulose (meth il SEL yoo lose)
Brand Names Citrucel® [OTC]
Therapeutic Category Ophthalmic Agent, Miscellaneous
Use Adjunct in treatment of constipation
Local Anesthetic/Vasoconstrictor Precautions No information available to require special precautions
Effects on Dental Treatment No effects or complications reported
Pregnancy Risk Factor C
Generic Available Yes
Comments Each dose contains sodium 3 mg, potassium 105 mg, and 60 calories from sucrose

Methyldopa (meth il DOE pa)
Related Information
Cardiovascular Diseases *on page 1010*
Brand Names Aldomet®
Canadian/Mexican Brand Names Apo®-Methyldopa (Canada); Dopamet® (Canada); Medimet® (Canada); Novo-Medopa® (Canada); Nu-Medopa® (Canada)
(Continued)

Methyldopa *(Continued)*

Therapeutic Category Alpha-Adrenergic Blockers - Peripheral-Acting (Alpha$_1$-Blockers)

Synonyms Metildopa (Mexico)

Use Management of moderate to severe hypertension

Usual Dosage

Children:

Oral: Initial: 10 mg/kg/day in 2-4 divided doses; increase every 2 days as needed to maximum dose of 65 mg/kg/day; do not exceed 3 g/day

I.V.: 5-10 mg/kg/dose every 6-8 hours up to a total dose of 65 mg/kg/24 hours or 3 g/24 hours

Adults:

Oral: Initial: 250 mg 2-3 times/day; increase every 2 days as needed; usual dose 1-1.5 g/day in 2-4 divided doses; maximum dose: 3 g/day

I.V.: 250-1000 mg every 6-8 hours; maximum dose: 1 g every 6 hours

Mechanism of Action Stimulation of central alpha-adrenergic receptors by a false transmitter that results in a decreased sympathetic outflow to the heart, kidneys, and peripheral vasculature

Local Anesthetic/Vasoconstrictor Precautions No information available to require special precautions

Effects on Dental Treatment Anticholinergic side effects can cause a reduction of saliva production or secretion. This may result in discomfort and dental disease (ie, caries, oral candidiasis and periodontal disease)

Other Adverse Effects

>10%: Cardiovascular: Peripheral edema

1% to 10%:

Central nervous system: Drug fever, mental depression, anxiety, nightmares, drowsiness, headache

Gastrointestinal: Dry mouth

<1%:

Cardiovascular: Orthostatic hypotension, bradycardia (sinus)

Central nervous system: Fever, chills, sedation, vertigo, depression, memory lapse

Dermatologic: Rash

Endocrine & metabolic: Sodium retention, sexual dysfunction, gynecomastia, hyperprolactinemia

Gastrointestinal: Colitis, pancreatitis, diarrhea, nausea, vomiting, "black" tongue

Genitourinary: Decreased libido

Hematologic: Thrombocytopenia, hemolytic anemia, positive Coombs' test, leukopenia, transient leukopenia or granulocytopenia

Hepatic: Cholestasis or hepatitis and heptocellular injury, elevated liver enzymes, jaundice, cirrhosis

Neuromuscular & skeletal: Paresthesias, weakness

Respiratory: Dyspnea

Miscellaneous: SLE-like syndrome

Drug Interactions

Decreased effect: Iron supplements can interact and cause a significant **increase** in blood pressure

Increased toxicity: Lithium causes increased lithium toxicity; tolbutamide and levodopa effects/toxicity increased

Drug Uptake

Peak hypotensive effect: Oral, parenteral: Within 3-6 hours

Duration: 12-24 hours

Serum half-life: 75-80 minutes

End stage renal disease: 6-16 hours

Pregnancy Risk Factor C

Generic Available Yes

Methyldopa and Chlorothiazide *see* Chlorothiazide and Methyldopa *on* page 216

Methyldopa and Hydrochlorothiazide

(meth il DOE pa & hye droe klor oh THYE a zide)

Brand Names Aldoril®

Therapeutic Category Antihypertensive Agent, Combination

Synonyms Hydrochlorothiazide and Methyldopa

Use Management of moderate to severe hypertension

Local Anesthetic/Vasoconstrictor Precautions No information available to require special precautions

Effects on Dental Treatment Anticholinergic side effects can cause a reduction of saliva production or secretion. This may result in discomfort and dental disease (ie, caries, oral candidiasis and periodontal disease)

Pregnancy Risk Factor C

Generic Available Yes

Methylergonovine (meth il er goe NOE veen)

Brand Names Methergine®

Therapeutic Category Ergot Alkaloid

Synonyms Metilergometrina, Maleato De (Mexico)

Use Prevention and treatment of postpartum and postabortion hemorrhage caused by uterine atony or subinvolution

Usual Dosage Adults:

Oral: 0.2 mg 3-4 times/day for 2-7 days

I.M.: 0.2 mg after delivery of anterior shoulder, after delivery of placenta, or during puerperium; may be repeated as required at intervals of 2-4 hours

I.V.: Same dose as I.M., but should not be routinely administered I.V. because of possibility of inducing sudden hypertension and cerebrovascular accident

Mechanism of Action Similar smooth muscle actions as seen with ergotamine; however, it affects primarily uterine smooth muscles producing sustained contractions and thereby shortens the third stage of labor

Local Anesthetic/Vasoconstrictor Precautions No information available to require special precautions

Effects on Dental Treatment No effects or complications reported

Other Adverse Effects

>10%:
Cardiovascular: Hypertension
Central nervous system: Headache, seizures

1% to 10%: Gastrointestinal: Nausea, vomiting

<1%:
Cardiovascular: Temporary chest pain, palpitations
Central nervous system: Hallucinations, dizziness
Endocrine & metabolic: Water intoxication
Gastrointestinal: Diarrhea, foul taste
Local: Thrombophlebitis
Neuromuscular & skeletal: Leg cramps
Otic: Tinnitus
Renal: Hematuria
Respiratory: Dyspnea, nasal congestion
Miscellaneous: Sweating

Drug Interactions No data reported

Drug Uptake

Onset of oxytocic effect:
Oral: 5-10 minutes
I.M.: 2-5 minutes
I.V.: Immediately

Duration of action:
Oral: ~3 hours
I.M.: ~3 hours
I.V.: 45 minutes

Absorption: Rapid

Serum half-life (biphasic):
Initial: 1-5 minutes
Terminal: 30 minutes to 2 hours

Time to peak serum concentration: Within 30 minutes to 3 hours

Pregnancy Risk Factor C

Generic Available No

Methylmorphine (Canada) *see* Codeine *on page 256*

Methylone® *see* Methylprednisolone *on next page*

Methylphenidate (meth il FEN i date)

Brand Names Ritalin®; Ritalin-SR®

Canadian/Mexican Brand Names PMS-Methylphenidate® (Canada)

Therapeutic Category Central Nervous System Stimulant, Nonamphetamine

Synonyms Metifenidato, Clorhidrato De (Mexico)

Use Treatment of attention deficit disorder and symptomatic management of narcolepsy; many **unlabeled uses**

Usual Dosage Oral: (Discontinue periodically to re-evaluate or if no improvement occurs within 1 month)

Children ≥6 years: Attention deficit disorder: Initial: 0.3 mg/kg/dose or 2.5-5 mg/dose given before breakfast and lunch; increase by 0.1 mg/kg/dose or by 5-10 (Continued)

Methylphenidate *(Continued)*

mg/day at weekly intervals; usual dose: 0.5-1 mg/kg/day; maximum dose: 2 mg/kg/day or 60 mg/day

Adults:

Narcolepsy: 10 mg 2-3 times/day, up to 60 mg/day

Depression: Initial: 2.5 mg every morning before 9 AM; dosage may be increased by 2.5-5 mg every 2-3 days as tolerated to a maximum of 20 mg/ day; may be divided (ie, 7 AM and 12 noon), but should not be given after noon; do not use sustained release product

Mechanism of Action Blocks the reuptake mechanism of dopaminergic neurons; appears to stimulate the cerebral cortex and subcortical structures similar to amphetamines

Local Anesthetic/Vasoconstrictor Precautions No information available to require special precautions

Effects on Dental Treatment Up to 10% of patients taking dextroamphetamines may present with hypertension. The use of local anesthetic without vasoconstrictor is recommended in these patients.

Other Adverse Effects

>10%:

Cardiovascular: Tachycardia

Central nervous system: Nervousness, insomnia

Gastrointestinal: Anorexia

1% to 10%:

Central nervous system: Dizziness, drowsiness

Gastrointestinal: Stomach pain

Miscellaneous: Hypersensitivity reactions

<1%:

Cardiovascular: Hypertension, hypotension, palpitations, cardiac arrhythmias

Central nervous system: Movement disorders, precipitation of Tourette's syndrome, and toxic psychosis (rare), fever, headache, convulsions

Dermatologic: Rash

Gastrointestinal: Nausea, weight loss, vomiting

Endocrine & metabolic: Growth retardation

Hematologic: Thrombocytopenia, anemia, leukopenia

Ocular: Blurred vision

Drug Interactions

Decreased effect: Effects of guanethidine, bretylium may be antagonized by methylphenidate

Increased toxicity: May increase serum concentrations of tricyclic antidepressants, warfarin, phenytoin, phenobarbital, and primidone; MAO inhibitors may potentiate effects of methylphenidate

Drug Uptake

Immediate release tablet:

Duration: 3-6 hours

Sustained release tablet:

Peak effect: Within 4-7 hours

Duration: 8 hours

Absorption: Slow and incomplete from GI tract

Serum half-life: 2-4 hours

Pregnancy Risk Factor C

Generic Available Yes

Methylprednisolone (meth il pred NIS oh lone)

Related Information

Corticosteroid Equivalencies Comparison *on page 1139*

Corticosteroids, Topical Comparison *on page 1140*

Respiratory Diseases *on page 1018*

Brand Names Adlone®; A-Methapred®; depMedalone®; Depoject®; Depo-Medrol®; Depopred®; Duralone®; Medralone®; Medrol®; Methylone®; Solu-Medrol®

Canadian/Mexican Brand Names Cryosolona® (Mexico)

Therapeutic Category Adrenal Corticosteroid; Anti-inflammatory Agent; Corticosteroid, Systemic; Corticosteroid, Topical (Low Potency)

Use

Dental: Treatment of a variety of oral diseases of allergic, inflammatory or autoimmune origin

Medical: Primarily as an anti-inflammatory or immunosuppressant agent in the treatment of a variety of diseases including those of hematologic, allergic, inflammatory, neoplastic, and autoimmune origin

Usual Dosage Only sodium succinate salt may be given I.V.. Methylprednisolone sodium succinate is highly soluble and has a rapid effect by I.M. and I.V.

routes. Methylprednisolone acetate has a low solubility and has a sustained I.M. effect.

Children:
Anti-inflammatory or immunosuppressive: Oral, I.M., I.V. (sodium succinate): 0.12-1.7 mg/kg/day or 5-25 mg/m²/day in divided doses every 6-12 hours

Adults:
Anti-inflammatory or immunosuppressive: Oral: 2-60 mg/day in 1-4 divided doses to start, followed by gradual reduction in dosage to the lowest possible level consistent with maintaining an adequate clinical response

I.M. (sodium succinate): 10-80 mg/day once daily

I.M. (acetate): 40-120 mg every 1-2 weeks

I.V. (sodium succinate): 10-40 mg over a period of several minutes and repeated I.V. or I.M. at intervals depending on clinical response; when high dosages are needed, give 30 mg/kg over a period of 10-20 minutes and may be repeated every 4-6 hours for 48 hours

Mechanism of Action Decreases inflammation by suppression of migration of polymorphonuclear leukocytes and reversal of increased capillary permeability

Local Anesthetic/Vasoconstrictor Precautions No information available to require special precautions

Effects on Dental Treatment No effects or complications reported

Other Adverse Effects >10%:
Central nervous system: Insomnia, nervousness
Gastrointestinal: Increased appetite, indigestion

Contraindications Serious infections, except septic shock or tuberculous meningitis; known hypersensitivity to methylprednisolone; viral, fungal, or tubercular skin lesions; administration of live virus vaccines

Warnings/Precautions

Use with caution in patients with hyperthyroidism, cirrhosis, nonspecific ulcerative colitis, hypertension, osteoporosis, thromboembolic tendencies, CHF, convulsive disorders, myasthenia gravis, thrombophlebitis, peptic ulcer, diabetes

Acute adrenal insufficiency may occur with abrupt withdrawal after long-term therapy or with stress; young pediatric patients may be more susceptible to adrenal axis suppression from topical therapy

Because of the risk of adverse effects, systemic corticosteroids should be used cautiously in the elderly, in the smallest possible dose, and for the shortest possible time.

Drug Interactions Phenytoin, phenobarbital, rifampin increases clearance of methylprednisolone; potassium depleting diuretics enhance potassium depletion; skin test antigens, immunizations increase response and increase potential infections; methylprednisolone may increase circulating glucose levels → may need adjustments of insulin or oral hypoglycemics

Drug Uptake Methylprednisolone sodium succinate is highly soluble and has a rapid effect by I.M. and I.V. routes; methylprednisolone acetate has a low solubility and has a sustained I.M. effect

Serum half-life: 3-3.5 hours

Time to obtain peak effect and the duration of these effects is dependent upon the route of administration. See table.

Route	Peak Effect	Duration
Oral	1-2 h	30-36 h
I.M.	4-8 d	1-4 wk
Intra-articular	1 wk	1-5 wk

Pregnancy Risk Factor C

Breast-feeding Considerations No data reported

Dosage Forms

Injection, as sodium succinate: 40 mg (1 mL, 3 mL); 125 mg (2 mL, 5 mL); 500 mg (1 mL, 4 mL, 8 mL, 20 mL); 1,000 mg (1 mL, 8 mL, 50 mL); 2,000 mg (30.6 mL)

Injection, as acetate: 20 mg/mL (5 mL, 10 mL); 40 mg/mL (1 mL, 5 mL, 10 mL); 80 mg/mL (1 mL, 5 mL)

Tablet: 2 mg, 4 mg, 8 mg, 16 mg, 24 mg, 32 mg

Tablet, dose pack: 4 mg (21s)

Dietary Considerations Should be taken after meals or with food or milk; limit caffeine; need diet rich in pyridoxine, vitamin C, vitamin D, folate, calcium, phosphorus, and protein

Generic Available Yes

4-Methylpyrazole see Fomepizole on page 428

Methyltestosterone (meth il tes TOS te rone)

Brand Names Android-25®; Oreton® Methyl; Testred®; Virilon®
Therapeutic Category Androgen
Use
  Male: Hypogonadism; delayed puberty; impotence and climacteric symptoms
  Female: Palliative treatment of metastatic breast cancer; postpartum breast pain and/or engorgement

Usual Dosage Adults (buccal absorption produces twice the androgenic activity of oral tablets):
  Male:
    Oral: 10-40 mg/day
    Buccal: 5-25 mg/day

  Female:
    Breast pain/engorgement:
      Oral: 80 mg/day for 3-5 days
      Buccal: 40 mg/day for 3-5 days
    Breast cancer:
      Oral: 50-200 mg/day
      Buccal: 25-100 mg/day

Mechanism of Action Stimulates receptors in organs and tissues to promote growth and development of male sex organs and maintains secondary sex characteristics in androgen-deficient males

Local Anesthetic/Vasoconstrictor Precautions No information available to require special precautions

Effects on Dental Treatment No effects or complications reported

Other Adverse Effects
  >10%:
    Male: Virilism, priapism
    Female: Virilism, menstrual problems (amenorrhea), breast soreness
    Cardiovascular: Edema
    Dermatologic: Acne
  1% to 10%:
    Females: Hirsutism (increase in pubic hair growth)
    Men: Prostatic hypertrophy, prostatic carcinoma, impotence, testicular atrophy
    Gastrointestinal: GI irritation, nausea, vomiting
    Hepatic: Hepatic dysfunction
  <1%:
    Endocrine & metabolic: Gynecomastia, amenorrhea, hypercalcemia
    Hematologic: Leukopenia, polycythemia
    Hepatic: Hepatic necrosis, cholestatic hepatitis
    Miscellaneous: Hypersensitivity reactions

Drug Interactions Decreased effect: Oral anticoagulant effect or insulin requirements may be increased

Drug Uptake
  Absorption: From GI tract and oral mucosa
Pregnancy Risk Factor X
Generic Available Yes

Methysergide (meth i SER jide)

Brand Names Sansert®
Therapeutic Category Ergot Alkaloid
Use Prophylaxis of vascular headache
Usual Dosage Adults: Oral: 4-8 mg/day with meals; if no improvement is noted after 3 weeks, drug is unlikely to be beneficial; must not be given continuously for longer than 6 months, and a drug-free interval of 3-4 weeks must follow each 6-month course

Mechanism of Action Ergotamine congener, however actions appear to differ; methysergide has minimal ergotamine-like oxytocic or vasoconstrictive properties, and has significantly greater serotonin-like properties

Local Anesthetic/Vasoconstrictor Precautions No information available to require special precautions

Effects on Dental Treatment No effects or complications reported

Other Adverse Effects
  >10%:
    Cardiovascular: Postural hypotension, peripheral ischemia
    Central nervous system: Insomnia
    Gastrointestinal: Nausea, vomiting, abdominal pain, diarrhea
  1% to 10%:
    Cardiovascular: Peripheral edema, tachycardia, bradycardia
    Dermatologic: Skin rash
    Gastrointestinal: Heartburn

<1%:
  Central nervous system: Overstimulation, drowsiness, mild euphoria, lethargy, mental depression, vertigo, unsteadiness, confusion, hyperesthesia; rebound headache may occur if methysergide is discontinued abruptly
  Ocular: Visual disturbances
  Respiratory: Fibrosis
Drug Interactions No data reported
Drug Uptake
  Serum half-life, plasma elimination: ~10 hours
Pregnancy Risk Factor X
Generic Available No

Meticorten® *see* Prednisone *on page 789*

Metifenidato, Clorhidrato De (Mexico) *see* Methylphenidate *on page 623*

Metildopa (Mexico) *see* Methyldopa *on page 621*

Metilergometrina, Maleato De (Mexico) *see* Methylergonovine *on page 623*

Metimyd® Ophthalmic *see* Sulfacetamide Sodium and Prednisolone *on page 891*

Metipranolol (met i PRAN oh lol)
Brand Names OptiPranolol®
Therapeutic Category Antiglaucoma Agent; Beta-Adrenergic Blocker, Ophthalmic
Use Agent for lowering intraocular pressure in patients with chronic open-angle glaucoma
Usual Dosage Ophthalmic: Adults: Instill 1 drop in the affected eye(s) twice daily
Mechanism of Action Beta-adrenoceptor-blocking agent; lacks intrinsic sympathomimetic activity and membrane-stabilizing effects and possesses only slight local anesthetic activity; mechanism of action of metipranolol in reducing intraocular pressure appears to be via reduced production of aqueous humor. This effect may be related to a reduction in blood flow to the iris root-ciliary body. It remains unclear if the reduction in intraocular pressure observed with beta-blockers is actually secondary to beta-adrenoceptor blockade.
Local Anesthetic/Vasoconstrictor Precautions No information available to require special precautions
Effects on Dental Treatment No effects or complications reported
Other Adverse Effects
  >10%: Ocular: Mild ocular stinging and discomfort, eye irritation
  1% to 10%: Ocular: Blurred vision, browache
  <1%:
    Cardiovascular: Bradycardia, A-V block, congestive heart failure
    Neuromuscular & skeletal: Weakness
    Ocular: Conjunctivitis, blepharitis, tearing, erythema, itching, keratitis, photophobia, decreased corneal sensitivity
    Respiratory: Bronchospasm
Drug Interactions No data reported
Drug Uptake
  Onset of action: ≤30 minutes
  Maximum effects: ~2 hours
  Duration of action: Intraocular pressure reduction has persisted for 24 hours following ocular instillation
  Serum half-life, elimination: ~3 hours
Pregnancy Risk Factor C
Generic Available No

Metoclopramida (Mexico) *see* Metoclopramide *on this page*

Metoclopramide (met oh kloe PRA mide)
Related Information
  Endocrine Disorders & Pregnancy *on page 1021*
Brand Names Clopra®; Maxolon®; Octamide® PFS; Reglan®
Canadian/Mexican Brand Names Apo®-Metoclop (Canada); Carnotprim Primperan® (Mexico); Carnotprim Primperan® Retard (Mexico); Maxeran® (Canada); Meclomid® (Mexico); Plasil® (Mexico); Pramotil® (Mexico)
Therapeutic Category Antiemetic
Synonyms Metoclopramida (Mexico)
Use Symptomatic treatment of diabetic gastric stasis, gastroesophageal reflux; prevention of nausea associated with chemotherapy or postsurgery and facilitates intubation of the small intestine
(Continued)

Metoclopramide *(Continued)*

Usual Dosage

Children:

Gastroesophageal reflux: Oral: 0.1-0.2 mg/kg/dose up to 4 times/day; efficacy of continuing metoclopramide beyond 12 weeks in reflux has not been determined; total daily dose should not exceed 0.5 mg/kg/day

Gastrointestinal hypomotility (gastroparesis): Oral, I.M., I.V.: 0.1 mg/kg/dose up to 4 times/day, not to exceed 0.5 mg/kg/day

Antiemetic (chemotherapy-induced emesis): I.V.: 1-2 mg/kg 30 minutes before chemotherapy and every 2-4 hours

Facilitate intubation: I.V.:
<6 years: 0.1 mg/kg
6-14 years: 2.5-5 mg

Adults:

Gastroesophageal reflux: Oral: 10-15 mg/dose up to 4 times/day 30 minutes before meals or food and at bedtime; single doses of 20 mg are occasionally needed for provoking situations; efficacy of continuing metoclopramide beyond 12 weeks in reflux has not been determined

Gastrointestinal hypomotility (gastroparesis):
Oral: 10 mg 30 minutes before each meal and at bedtime for 2-8 weeks
I.V. (for severe symptoms): 10 mg over 1-2 minutes; 10 days of I.V. therapy may be necessary for best response

Antiemetic (chemotherapy-induced emesis): I.V.: 1-2 mg/kg 30 minutes before chemotherapy and every 2-4 hours to every 4-6 hours (and usually given with diphenhydramine 25-50 mg I.V./oral)

Postoperative nausea and vomiting: I.M.: 10 mg near end of surgery; 20 mg doses may be used

Facilitate intubation: I.V.: 10 mg

Elderly:

Gastroesophageal reflux: Oral: 5 mg 4 times/day (30 minutes before meals and at bedtime); increase dose to 10 mg 4 times/day if no response at lower dose

Gastrointestinal hypomotility:
Oral: Initial: 5 mg 30 minutes before meals and at bedtime for 2-8 weeks; increase if necessary to 10 mg doses
I.V.: Initiate at 5 mg over 1-2 minutes; increase to 10 mg if necessary

Postoperative nausea and vomiting: I.M.: 5 mg near end of surgery; may repeat dose if necessary

Mechanism of Action
Blocks dopamine receptors in chemoreceptor trigger zone of the CNS; enhances the response to acetylcholine of tissue in upper GI tract causing enhanced motility and accelerated gastric emptying without stimulating gastric, biliary, or pancreatic secretions

Local Anesthetic/Vasoconstrictor Precautions
No information available to require special precautions

Effects on Dental Treatment
No effects or complications reported

Other Adverse Effects

>10%:
Central nervous system: Restlessness, drowsiness
Gastrointestinal: Diarrhea
Neuromuscular & skeletal: Weakness

1% to 10%:
Central nervous system: Insomnia, depression
Dermatologic: Skin rash
Endocrine & metabolic: Breast tenderness, prolactin stimulation
Gastrointestinal: Nausea, dry mouth

<1%:
Cardiovascular: Tachycardia, hypertension or hypotension
Central nervous system: Extrapyramidal reactions*, tardive dyskinesia, fatigue, anxiety, agitation
Gastrointestinal: Constipation
Hematologic: Methemoglobinemia

*Note: A recent study suggests the incidence of extrapyramidal reactions due to metoclopramide may be as high as 34% and the incidence appears more often in the elderly

Drug Interactions
Decreased effect: Anticholinergic agents antagonize metoclopramide's actions
Increased toxicity: Opiate analgesics causes increased CNS depression

Drug Uptake
Onset of effect:
Oral: Within 0.5-1 hour
I.V.: Within 1-3 minutes
Duration of therapeutic effect: 1-2 hours, regardless of route administered

Serum half-life, normal renal function: 4-7 hours (may be dose-dependent)
Pregnancy Risk Factor B
Generic Available Yes

Metolazone (me TOLE a zone)
Related Information
Cardiovascular Diseases *on page 1010*
Brand Names Mykrox®; Zaroxolyn®
Therapeutic Category Diuretic, Thiazide
Use Management of mild to moderate hypertension; treatment of edema in congestive heart failure and nephrotic syndrome, impaired renal function
Usual Dosage Oral:
Children: 0.2-0.4 mg/kg/day divided every 12-24 hours
Adults:
Edema: 5-20 mg/dose every 24 hours
Hypertension: 2.5-5 mg/dose every 24 hours
Hypertension (Mykrox®): 0.5 mg/day; if response is not adequate, increase dose to maximum of 1 mg/day

Not dialyzable (0% to 5%) via hemo- or peritoneal dialysis; supplemental dose is not necessary
Mechanism of Action Inhibits sodium reabsorption in the distal tubules causing increased excretion of sodium and water, as well as, potassium and hydrogen ions
Local Anesthetic/Vasoconstrictor Precautions No information available to require special precautions
Effects on Dental Treatment No effects or complications reported
Other Adverse Effects
1% to 10%: Endocrine & metabolic: Hypokalemia
<1%:
Cardiovascular: Hypotension
Central nervous system: Drowsiness
Dermatologic: Photosensitivity, rash
Endocrine & metabolic: Fluid and electrolyte imbalances (hypocalcemia, hypomagnesemia, hyponatremia), hyperglycemia
Gastrointestinal: Nausea, vomiting, anorexia
Hematologic: Rarely blood dyscrasias, aplastic anemia, hemolytic anemia, leukopenia, agranulocytosis, thrombocytopenia
Hepatic: Hepatitis
Neuromuscular & skeletal: Paresthesia
Renal: Prerenal azotemia, polyuria, uremia
Drug Interactions
Increased toxicity:
Concurrent administration with furosemide may cause excessive volume and electrolyte depletion
Increased digitalis glycosides toxicity
Increased lithium toxicity
Drug Uptake Same for all routes:
Onset of diuresis: Within 60 minutes
Duration: 12-24 hours
Absorption: Oral: Incomplete
Serum half-life: 6-20 hours, renal function dependent
Pregnancy Risk Factor D
Generic Available No

Metoprolol (me toe PROE lole)
Related Information
Cardiovascular Diseases *on page 1010*
Brand Names Lopressor® [Tartrate]; Toprol XL® [Succinate]
Canadian/Mexican Brand Names Apo®-Metoprolol (Type L) (Canada); Betaloc® (Canada); Betaloc Durules® (Canada); Kenaprol® (Mexico); Lopresor® (Mexico); Novo-Metoprolol® (Canada); Nu-Metop® (Canada); Proken® M (Mexico); Prolaken® (Mexico); Ritmolol® (Mexico); Seloken® (Mexico); Selopres® (Mexico)
Therapeutic Category Beta-adrenergic Blocker, Cardioselective
Use Treatment of hypertension and angina pectoris; prevention of myocardial infarction, atrial fibrillation, flutter, symptomatic treatment of hypertrophic subaortic stenosis

Unlabeled use: Treatment of ventricular arrhythmias, atrial ectopy, migraine prophylaxis, essential tremor, aggressive behavior
(Continued)

Metoprolol *(Continued)*

Usual Dosage

Children: Oral: 1-5 mg/kg/24 hours divided twice daily; allow 3 days between dose adjustments

Adults:

Oral: 100-450 mg/day in 2-3 divided doses, begin with 50 mg twice daily and increase doses at weekly intervals to desired effect

I.V.: 5 mg every 2 minutes for 3 doses in early treatment of myocardial infarction; thereafter give 50 mg orally every 6 hours 15 minutes after last I.V. dose and continue for 48 hours; then administer a maintenance dose of 100 mg twice daily

Elderly: Oral: Initial: 25 mg/day; usual range: 25-300 mg/day

Hemodialysis: Administer dose posthemodialysis or administer 50 mg supplemental dose supplemental dose is not necessary following peritoneal dialysis

Mechanism of Action

Selective inhibitor of beta$_1$-adrenergic receptors; competitively blocks beta$_1$-receptors, with little or no effect on beta$_2$-receptors at doses <100 mg; does not exhibit any membrane stabilizing or intrinsic sympathomimetic activity

Local Anesthetic/Vasoconstrictor Precautions

No information available to require special precautions

Effects on Dental Treatment

Noncardioselective beta-blockers (ie, propranolol, nadolol) enhance the pressor response to epinephrine, resulting in hypertension and bradycardia. This has not been reported for metoprolol, a cardioselective beta-blocker. Therefore, local anesthetic with vasoconstrictor can be safely used in patients medicated with metoprolol. Many nonsteroidal anti-inflammatory drugs such as ibuprofen and indomethacin can reduce the hypotensive effect of beta-blockers after 3 or more weeks of therapy with the NSAID. Short-term NSAID use (ie, 3 days) requires no special precautions in patients taking beta-blockers.

Other Adverse Effects

>10%:

Central nervous system: Mental depression, fatigue, dizziness

Neuromuscular & skeletal: Weakness

1% to 10%:

Cardiovascular: Bradycardia, arrhythmia, reduced peripheral circulation

Gastrointestinal: Heartburn

Respiratory: Wheezing

<1%:

Cardiovascular: Chest pain, heart failure, Raynaud's phenomenon

Central nervous system: Insomnia, nightmares, confusion, headache

Dermatologic: Rash, itching

Endocrine & metabolic: Decreased sexual activity

Gastrointestinal: Constipation, nausea, vomiting, stomach discomfort

Genitourinary: Impotence

Miscellaneous: Cold extremities

Drug Interactions

Decreased effect of beta-blockers:

Barbiturates (increased liver metabolism of beta-blockers to result in lower serum levels)

NSAIDs (attenuate the hypotensive therapeutic effects of beta-blockers)

Rifampin (increased liver metabolism of beta-blockers to result in lower serum levels)

Increased effects of beta-blockers:

Calcium channel blockers (increase serum levels of beta-blockers by unknown mechanism to enhance hypotension)

Beta-blockers increase the effects of:

Epinephrine (vasoconstrictor; initial hypertensive episode followed by bradycardia) only from noncardioselective type beta-blockers

Phenylephrine (Neosynephrine®; enhanced pressor response)

Theophylline (inhibit theophylline metabolism causing increase in serum concentrations)

Drug Uptake

Peak antihypertensive effect: Oral: Within 1.5-4 hours

Duration: 10-20 hours

Absorption: 95%

Serum half-life: 3-4 hours

End stage renal disease: 2.5-4.5 hours

Pregnancy Risk Factor B

Generic Available Yes

Selected Readings

Foster CA and Aston SJ, "Propranolol-Epinephrine Interaction: A Potential Disaster," *Plast Reconstr Surg*, 1983, 72(1):74-8.

Wong DG, Spence JD, Lamki L, et al, "Effect of Nonsteroidal Anti-inflammatory Drugs on Control of Hypertension of Beta-Blockers and Diuretics," *Lancet*, 1986, 1(8488):997-1001.

Wynn RL, "Dental Nonsteroidal Anti-inflammatory Drugs and Prostaglandin-Based Drug Interactions, Part Two," *Gen Dent*, 1992, 40(2):104, 106, 108.

Wynn RL, "Epinephrine Interactions With Beta-Blockers," *Gen Dent*, 1994, 42(1):16, 18.

Metotrexato (Mexico) *see* Methotrexate *on page 615*

Metreton® *see* Prednisolone *on page 788*

Metrodin® Injection *see* Urofollitropin *on page 978*

MetroGel® *see* Metronidazole *on this page*

Metro I.V.® *see* Metronidazole *on this page*

Metronidazole (me troe NI da zole)

Related Information
Oral Bacterial Infections *on page 1059*
Oral Nonviral Soft Tissue Ulcerations or Erosions *on page 1070*

Brand Names Flagyl®; Helidac® Combination; MetroGel®; Metro I.V.®; Noritate® Cream; Protostat®

Canadian/Mexican Brand Names Ameblin® (Mexico); Apo®-Metronidazole (Canada); Flagenase® (Mexico); Milezzol® (Mexico); Novo-Nidazol (Canada); Otrozol® (Mexico); Vatrix-S® (Mexico); Vertisal® (Mexico)

Therapeutic Category Amebicide; Antibiotic, Anaerobic; Antibiotic, Topical; Antiprotozoal

Use

Dental: Treatment of oral soft tissue infections due to anaerobic bacteria including all anaerobic cocci, anaerobic gram-negative bacilli (*Bacteroides*), and gram-positive spore-forming bacilli (*Clostridium*). Useful as single agent or in combination with amoxicillin, Augmentin®, or ciprofloxacin in the treatment of periodontitis associated with the presence of *Actinobacillus actinomycetem-comitans*, (AA).

Medical: Treatment of susceptible anaerobic bacterial and protozoal infections in the following conditions: amebiasis, symptomatic and asymptomatic trichomoniasis; skin and skin structure infections; CNS infections; intra-abdominal infections; systemic anaerobic infections; topically for the treatment of acne rosacea; treatment of antibiotic-associated pseudomembranous colitis (AAPC); Helidac® in combination with an H_2 antagonist for the treatment active duodenal ulcer associated with *H. pylori* infection; topical cream is indicated for topical application in the treatment of inflammatory papules, pustules and erythema of rosacea

Usual Dosage Adults: Oral:

Anaerobic infections: 500 mg every 6-8 hours, not to exceed 4 g/day

Treatment of periodontitis associated with AA:

Oral, singly: 200-400 mg 3 times/day for 7-10 days;

In combination: metronidazole plus Augmentin® 250 mg 3 times/day of each for 7 days; metronidazole 250 mg plus amoxicillin 250 mg each 3 times/day for 7 days; metronidazole plus ciprofloxacin 500 mg each twice daily for 8 days

Helidac®: Take metronidazole 250 mg tablet, bismuth subsalicylate 262.4 mg tablet x2, and tetracycline 500 mg capsule plus an H_2 antagonist four times daily at meals and bedtime for 14 days; chew and swallow the bismuth subsalicylate tablets, swallow the metronidazole tablet and tetracycline capsule with a full glass of water

Mechanism of Action Reduced to a product which interacts with DNA to cause a loss of helical DNA structure and strand breakage resulting in inhibition of protein synthesis and cell death in susceptible organisms

Local Anesthetic/Vasoconstrictor Precautions No information available to require special precautions

Effects on Dental Treatment <1% of patients may experience dry mouth and metallic taste

Other Adverse Effects

>10%:
Central nervous system: Dizziness, headache
Gastrointestinal: Nausea, diarrhea, loss of appetite, vomiting

<1%: Endocrine & metabolic: Disulfiram-type reaction with alcohol

Contraindications Hypersensitivity to metronidazole or any component, 1st trimester of pregnancy

Warnings/Precautions Use with caution in patients with liver impairment, blood dyscrasias; history of seizures, congestive heart failure, or other sodium retaining states; reduce dosage in patients with severe liver impairment, CNS disease, and severe renal failure. Has been shown to be carcinogenic in rodents.

(Continued)

Metronidazole *(Continued)*

Drug Interactions Phenytoin, phenobarbital cause decreased metronidazole half-life; alcohol, disulfiram cause disulfiram-like reactions which includes flushing, headache, nausea, and in some patients, vomiting and chest and/or abdominal pain, therefore, absolutely contraindicated with alcohol; warfarin increases PT prolongation

Drug Uptake

Absorption: Oral: ~80%

Serum half-life: 6-8 hours, increases with hepatic impairment

Time to peak serum concentration: Within 1-2 hours

Pregnancy Risk Factor B

Breast-feeding Considerations Not compatible; resume breast-feeding 12-24 hours after last dose

Dosage Forms

Gel, topical: 0.75% [7.5 mg/mL] (30 g)

Injection, ready to use: 5 mg/mL (100 mL)

Powder for injection, as hydrochloride: 500 mg

Tablet: 250 mg, 500 mg

Helidac® (One day supply): Contains metronidazole 250 mg tablet (#4), bismuth subsalicylate 262.4 mg tablet [Pepto-Bismol®] (#8), and tetracycline 500 mg capsule (#4)

Dietary Considerations Food has no effect on extent of absorption, but delays rate and decreases maximum concentration; however, may be taken with food if gastric irritation

Generic Available Yes

Selected Readings

Eisenberg L, Suchow R, Coles RS, et al, "The Effects of Metronidazole Administration on Clinical and Microbiologic Parameters of Periodontal Disease," *Clin Prev Dent*, 1991, 13(1):28-34.

Jenkins WM, MacFarlane TW, Gilmour WH, et al, "Systemic Metronidazole in the Treatment of Periodontitis," *J Clin Periodontol*, 1989, 16(7):433-50.

Loesche WJ, Giordano JR, Hujoel P, et al, "Metronidazole in Periodontitis: Reduced Need for Surgery," *J Clin Periodontol*, 1992, 19(2):103-12.

Loesche WJ, Schmidt E, Smith BA, et al, "Effects of Metronidazole on Periodontal Treatment Needs," *J Periodontol*, 1991, 62(4):247-57.

Soder PO, Frithiof L, Wikner S, et al, "The Effect of Systemic Metronidazole After Nonsurgical Treatment in Moderate and Advanced Periodontitis in Young Adults," *J Periodontol*, 1990, 61(5):281-8.

Metyrosine *(me TYE roe seen)*

Brand Names Demser®

Therapeutic Category Tyrosine Hydroxylase Inhibitor

Synonyms AMPT; OGMT

Use Short-term management of pheochromocytoma before surgery, long-term management when surgery is contraindicated or when malignant

Usual Dosage Children >12 years and Adults: Oral: Initial: 250 mg 4 times/day, increased by 250-500 mg/day up to 4 g/day; maintenance: 2-3 g/day in 4 divided doses; for preoperative preparation, administer optimum effective dosage for 5-7 days

Dosing adjustment in renal impairment: Adjustment should be considered

Mechanism of Action Blocks the rate-limiting step in the biosynthetic pathway of catecholamines. It is a tyrosine hydroxylase inhibitor, blocking the conversion of tyrosine to dihydroxyphenylalanine. This inhibition results in decreased levels of endogenous catecholamines. Catecholamine biosynthesis is reduced by 35% to 80% in patients treated with metyrosine 1-4 g/day.

Local Anesthetic/Vasoconstrictor Precautions No information available to require special precautions

Effects on Dental Treatment No effects or complications reported

Other Adverse Effects

>10%:

Central nervous system: Drowsiness, extrapyramidal symptoms

Gastrointestinal: Diarrhea

1% to 10%:

Endocrine & metabolic: Galactorrhea, edema of the breasts

Gastrointestinal: Nausea, vomiting, xerostomia

Genitourinary: Impotence

Respiratory: Nasal congestion

<1%:

Cardiovascular: Lower extremity edema

Central nervous system: Depression, hallucinations, disorientation, parkinsonism

Dermatologic: Urticaria

Genitourinary: Urinary problems

Hematologic: Anemia, eosinophilia
Renal: Hematuria
Miscellaneous: Hyperstimulation after withdrawal
Contraindications Hypertension of unknown etiology, known hypersensitivity to metyrosine
Warnings/Precautions Maintain fluid volume during and after surgery; use with caution in patients with impaired renal or hepatic function
Drug Uptake
Serum half-life: 7.2 hours
Pregnancy Risk Factor C
Dosage Forms Capsule: 250 mg
Dietary Considerations Alcohol: Additive CNS effect, avoid use
Generic Available No

Mevacor® *see* Lovastatin *on page 570*

Mexiletina (Mexico) *see* Mexiletine *on this page*

Mexiletine (MEKS i le teen)
Related Information
Cardiovascular Diseases *on page 1010*
Brand Names Mexitil®
Therapeutic Category Antiarrhythmic Agent, Class I-B; Antiarrhythmic Agent (Supraventricular & Ventricular)
Synonyms Mexiletina (Mexico)
Use Management of serious ventricular arrhythmias; suppression of PVCs

Unlabeled use: Diabetic neuropathy
Usual Dosage Adults: Oral: Initial: 200 mg every 8 hours (may load with 400 mg if necessary); adjust dose every 2-3 days; usual dose: 200-300 mg every 8 hours; maximum dose: 1.2 g/day (some patients respond to every 12-hour dosing); patients with hepatic impairment or CHF may require dose reduction; when switching from another antiarrhythmic, initiate a 200 mg dose 6-12 hours after stopping former agents, 3-6 hours after stopping procainamide
Mechanism of Action Class IB antiarrhythmic, structurally related to lidocaine, which may cause increase in systemic vascular resistance and decrease in cardiac output; no significant negative inotropic effect; inhibits inward sodium current, decreases rate of rise of phase 0, increases effective refractory period/action potential duration ratio
Local Anesthetic/Vasoconstrictor Precautions No information available to require special precautions
Effects on Dental Treatment No effects or complications reported
Other Adverse Effects
>10%:
Central nervous system: Lightheadedness, dizziness, nervousness
Neuromuscular & skeletal: Trembling, unsteady gait
1% to 10%:
Cardiovascular: Chest pain, premature ventricular contractions
Central nervous system: Confusion, headache, insomnia
Dermatologic: Rash
Gastrointestinal: Constipation or diarrhea
Hepatic: Elevated LFTs
Neuromuscular & skeletal: Numbness of fingers/toes, weakness
Ocular: Blurred vision
Otic: Tinnitus
Respiratory: Dyspnea
<1%:
Hematologic: Leukopenia, agranulocytosis, thrombocytopenia, positive antinuclear antibody
Ocular: Diplopia
Drug Interactions
Decreased plasma levels: Phenobarbital, phenytoin, rifampin, and other hepatic enzyme inducers, cimetidine and drugs which make the urine acidic
Increased effect: Allopurinol
Increased toxicity/levels of caffeine and theophylline
Drug Uptake
Absorption: Elderly have a slightly slower rate of absorption but extent of absorption is the same as young adults
Serum half-life: Adults: 10-14 hours (average: 14.4 hours elderly, 12 hours in younger adults); increase in half-life with hepatic or heart failure
Time to peak: Peak levels attained in 2-3 hours
Pregnancy Risk Factor C
Generic Available Yes

Mexitil® *see* Mexiletine *on previous page*
Mezlin® *see* Mezlocillin *on this page*

Mezlocillin (mez loe SIL in)
Brand Names Mezlin®
Therapeutic Category Antibiotic, Penicillin
Use Treatment of infections caused by susceptible gram-negative aerobic bacilli (*Klebsiella, Proteus, Escherichia coli, Enterobacter, Pseudomonas aeruginosa, Serratia*) involving the skin and skin structure, bone and joint, respiratory tract, urinary tract, gastrointestinal tract, as well as, septicemia
Usual Dosage I.M., I.V.:
Children: 200-300 mg/kg/day divided every 4-6 hours; maximum: 24 g/day
Adults:
Uncomplicated urinary tract infection: 1.5-2 g every 6 hours
Serious infections: 3-4 g every 4-6 hours
Mechanism of Action Interferes with bacterial cell wall synthesis during active multiplication causing cell death and resultant bactericidal activity against susceptible bacteria
Local Anesthetic/Vasoconstrictor Precautions No information available to require special precautions
Effects on Dental Treatment Prolonged use of penicillins may lead to development of oral candidiasis
Other Adverse Effects
1% to 10%: Gastrointestinal: Nausea, diarrhea
<1%:
Central nervous system: Fever, seizures, dizziness, headache
Dermatologic: Rash, exfoliative dermatitis
Endocrine & metabolic: Hypokalemia, hypernatremia
Gastrointestinal: Vomiting
Hematologic: Eosinophilia, leukopenia, neutropenia, thrombocytopenia, agranulocytosis, hemolytic anemia, prolonged bleeding time, positive Coombs' [direct]
Hepatic: Hepatotoxicity, elevated liver enzymes
Renal: Hematuria, elevated serum creatinine and BUN, interstitial nephritis
Miscellaneous: Serum sickness-like reactions
Drug Interactions Aminoglycosides (synergy), probenecid (decreased clearance), vecuronium (increased duration of neuromuscular blockade), heparin (increased risk of bleeding)
Drug Uptake
Absorption: I.M.: 63%
Serum half-life: Dose dependent:
Children 2-19 years: 0.9 hour
Adults: 50-70 minutes, increased in renal impairment
Time to peak serum concentration:
I.M.: 45-90 minutes after administration
I.V. infusion: Within 5 minutes
Pregnancy Risk Factor B
Generic Available No

Miacalcin® Injection *see* Calcitonin *on page 160*
Miacalcin® Nasal Spray *see* Calcitonin *on page 160*

Mibefradil (mi be FRA dil)
Brand Names Posicor®
Therapeutic Category Calcium Channel Blocker; Vasodilator
Synonyms Mibefradil Dihydrochloride; Mibefradilum
Use Treatment of hypertension, alone or in combination with other antihypertensive agents; chronic stable angina pectoris, alone or in combination with other antianginal drugs
Usual Dosage Oral: 50-100 mg/day; larger dose is, on average, more effective; doses >100 mg offer little or no additional benefit and induce a great rate of adverse reactions; can be taken with or without food

Hypertension: 50 mg once daily; titrate to 100 mg once daily based on blood pressure response; full effect of given dose level is generally seen after 1-2 weeks
Chronic stable angina pectoris: 50 mg once daily
Mechanism of Action At therapeutic concentrations, mibefradil blocks both the T-type (low-voltage) and L-type (high-voltage) calcium channels, with greater selectivity for T-type channels, in contrast to benzothiazepine, dihydropyridine, and phenylalkylamine calcium antagonists, which at therapeutic concentrations block only the L-type channels. The binding site of mibefradil is different from that of the dihydropyridines. The contractile processes of cardiac muscle and

vascular smooth muscle are dependent upon the movement of extracellular calcium ions into these cells through specific ion channels. In vitro, mibefradil selectively inhibits calcium ion influx across cell membranes of cardiac and vascular smooth muscle with a pronounced dependence on membrane potential.

Local Anesthetic/Vasoconstrictor Precautions No information available to require special precautions

Effects on Dental Treatment No effects or complications reported

Other Adverse Effects Most side effects (adverse reactions) were transient and of only mild or moderate intensity. The most common side effects included headache and runny nose.

Pregnancy Risk Factor C

Dosage Forms Tablet, as dihydrochloride: 50 mg, 100 mg

Mibefradil Dihydrochloride see Mibefradil on previous page

Mibefradilum see Mibefradil on previous page

Micanol® Cream see Anthralin on page 79

Micatin® Topical [OTC] see Miconazole on this page

Miconazole (mi KON a zole)

Brand Names Absorbine® Antifungal Foot Powder [OTC]; Breezee® Mist Antifungal [OTC]; Femizol-M® [OTC]; Fungoid® Creme; Fungoid® Tincture; Lotrimin® AF Powder [OTC]; Lotrimin® AF Spray Liquid [OTC]; Lotrimin® AF Spray Powder [OTC]; Maximum Strength Desenex® Antifungal Cream [OTC]; Micatin® Topical [OTC]; Monistat-Derm™ Topical; Monistat i.v.™ Injection; Monistat™ Vaginal; Ony-Clear® Spray; Prescription Strength Desenex® [OTC]; Zeasorb-AF® Powder [OTC]

Canadian/Mexican Brand Names Aloid® (Mexico); Daktarin® (Mexico); Dermifun® (Mexico); Fungiquim® (Mexico); Gyno-Daktarin® (Mexico); Gyno-Daktarin® V (Mexico); Neomicol® (Mexico)

Therapeutic Category Antifungal Agent, Topical; Antifungal Agent, Vaginal

Use
I.V.: Treatment of severe systemic fungal infections and fungal meningitis that are refractory to standard treatment
Topical: Treatment of vulvovaginal candidiasis and a variety of skin and mucous membrane fungal infections

Usual Dosage
Children:
I.V.: 20-40 mg/kg/day divided every 8 hours
Topical: Apply twice daily for up to 1 month
Adults:
Topical: Apply twice daily for up to 1 month
I.T.: 20 mg every 1-2 days
I.V.: Initial: 200 mg, then 1.2-3.6 g/day divided every 8 hours for up to 20 weeks
Bladder candidal infections: 200 mg diluted solution instilled in the bladder
Vaginal: Insert contents of 1 applicator of vaginal cream (100 mg) or 100 mg suppository at bedtime for 7 days, or 200 mg suppository at bedtime for 3 days

Not dialyzable (0% to 5%)

Mechanism of Action Inhibits biosynthesis of ergosterol, damaging the fungal cell wall membrane, which increases permeability causing leaking of nutrients

Local Anesthetic/Vasoconstrictor Precautions No information available to require special precautions

Effects on Dental Treatment No effects or complications reported

Other Adverse Effects
>10%:
Central nervous system: Fever, chills
Dermatologic: Skin rash, itching
Local: Pain at injection site
Gastrointestinal: Anorexia, diarrhea, nausea, vomiting
1% to 10%: Hematologic: Anemia, thrombocytopenia
<1%:
Cardiovascular: Flushing of face or skin
Central nervous system: Drowsiness

Drug Interactions Warfarin (increased anticoagulant effect), oral sulfonylureas, amphotericin B (decreased antifungal effect of both agents), phenytoin (levels may be increased)

Drug Uptake
Serum half-life, multiphasic:
Initial: 40 minutes
Secondary: 126 minutes
Terminal phase: 24 hours
(Continued)

Miconazole *(Continued)*

Pregnancy Risk Factor C
Dosage Forms
Cream:
Topical, as nitrate: 2% (15 g, 30 g, 56.7 g, 85 g)
Vaginal, as nitrate: 2% (45 g is equivalent to 7 doses)
Injection: 1% [10 mg/mL] (20 mL)
Lotion, as nitrate: 2% (30 mL, 60 mL)
Powder, topical: 2% (45 g, 90 g, 113 g)
Spray, topical: 2% (105 mL)
Suppository, vaginal, as nitrate: 100 mg (7s); 200 mg (3s)
Tincture: 2% with alcohol (7.39 mL, 29.57 mL)
Generic Available Yes

MICRhoGAM™ *see* Rh₀(D) Immune Globulin *on page 840*

Microfibrillar Collagen Hemostat

(mye kro FI bri lar KOL la jen HEE moe stat)
Brand Names Avitene®; Helistat®; Hemotene®
Therapeutic Category Hemostatic Agent
Use
Dental & Medical: Adjunct to hemostasis when control of bleeding by ligature is
ineffective or impractical
Usual Dosage Apply dry directly to source of bleeding
Mechanism of Action Microfibrillar collagen hemostat (MCH) is an absorbable
topical hemostatic agent prepared from purified bovine corium collagen and
shredded into fibrils. Physically, microfibrillar collagen hemostat yields a large
surface area. Chemically, it is collagen with hydrochloric acid noncovalently
bound to some of the available amino groups in the collagen molecules. When in
contact with a bleeding surface, microfibrillar collagen hemostat attracts platelets
which adhere to its fibrils and undergo the release phenomenon. This triggers
aggregation of the platelets into thrombi in the interstices of the fibrous mass,
initiating the formation of a physiologic platelet plug.
Local Anesthetic/Vasoconstrictor Precautions No information available to
require special precautions
Effects on Dental Treatment No effects or complications reported
Other Adverse Effects 1% to 10%:
Local: Adhesion formation
Miscellaneous: Potentiation of infection, allergic reaction
Contraindications Closure of skin incisions, contaminated wounds
Warnings/Precautions Fragments of MCH may pass through filters of blood
scavenging systems, avoid reintroduction of blood from operative sites treated
with MCH; after several minutes remove excess material
Drug Interactions No data reported
Drug Uptake Resorption: By animal tissue in 3 months
Pregnancy Risk Factor C
Breast-feeding Considerations No data reported
Dosage Forms
Fibrous: 1 g, 5 g
Nonwoven web: 70 mm x 70 mm x 1 mm; 70 mm x 35 mm x 1 mm
Generic Available No

Micro-K® 10 *see* Potassium Chloride *on page 778*
Micro-K Extencaps® *see* Potassium Chloride *on page 778*
Micro-K® LS *see* Potassium Chloride *on page 778*
Microlipid™ [OTC] *see* Enteral Nutritional Products *on page 350*
Micronase® *see* Glyburide *on page 445*
microNefrin® *see* Epinephrine, Racemic *on page 354*
Micronor® *see* Norethindrone *on page 690*
Microsulfon® *see* Sulfadiazine *on page 892*
Midamor® *see* Amiloride *on page 53*

Midazolam (MID aye zoe lam)

Brand Names Versed®
Canadian/Mexican Brand Names Dormicum® (Mexico)
Therapeutic Category Benzodiazepine; Hypnotic; Sedative
Use
Dental: Sedation component in I.V. conscious sedation in oral surgery patients
Medical: In medicine, preoperative sedation and provides conscious sedation
prior to diagnostic or radiographic procedures
Restrictions C-IV

Usual Dosage

Children:

Preoperative sedation:

I.M.: 0.07-0.08 mg/kg 30-60 minutes presurgery

I.V.: 0.035 mg/kg/dose, repeat over several minutes as required to achieve the desired sedative effect up to a total dose of 0.1-0.2 mg/kg

Conscious sedation for procedures:

Oral, Intranasal: 0.2-0.4 mg/kg (maximum: 15 mg) 30-45 minutes before the procedure

I.V.: 0.05 mg/kg 3 minutes before procedure

Adults: Conscious sedation: I.V.: Initial: 0.5-2 mg slow I.V. over at least 2 minutes; slowly titrate to effect by repeating doses every 2-3 minutes if needed; usual total dose: 2.5-5 mg; use decreased doses in elderly

Healthy Adults <60 years: I.V.: Some patients respond to doses as low as 1 mg; no more than 2.5 mg should be administered over a period of 2 minutes. Additional doses of midazolam may be administered after a 2-minute waiting period and evaluation of sedation after each dose increment. A total dose >5 mg is generally not needed. If narcotics or other CNS depressants are administered concomitantly, the midazolam dose should be reduced by 30%.

Mechanism of Action Depresses all levels of the CNS, including the limbic and reticular formation, probably through the increased action of gamma-aminobutyric acid (GABA), which is a major inhibitory neurotransmitter in the brain

Local Anesthetic/Vasoconstrictor Precautions No information available to require special precautions

Effects on Dental Treatment No effects or complications reported

Other Adverse Effects

>10%: Miscellaneous: Hiccups

1% to 10%:

Central nervous system: Drowsiness, ataxia, amnesia, dizziness, sedation

Respiratory: Respiratory depression, apnea, laryngospasm, bronchospasm

Contraindications Hypersensitivity to midazolam or any component (cross-sensitivity with other benzodiazepines may occur); uncontrolled pain; existing CNS depression; shock; narrow-angle glaucoma

Warnings/Precautions Use with caution in patients with congestive heart failure, renal impairment, pulmonary disease, hepatic dysfunction, the elderly, and those receiving concomitant narcotics; midazolam may cause respiratory depression/arrest; deaths and hypoxic encephalopathy have resulted when these were not promptly recognized and treated appropriately

Drug Interactions Theophylline may antagonize the sedative effects of midazolam; CNS depressants cause increased sedation and respiratory depression; doses of general anesthetic agents should be reduced when used in conjunction with midazolam; cimetidine may increase midazolam serum concentrations

Note: If narcotics or other CNS depressants are administered concomitantly, the midazolam dose should be reduced by 30%, if <65 years of age or by at least 50%, if >65 years of age.

Drug Uptake

Onset of action:

I.M.: Within 15-60 minutes

I.V.: Within 1-5 minutes

Serum half-life: 1-4 hours, increased with cirrhosis, CHF, obesity, elderly

Time to recovery: Usually within 2 hours, but may take up to 6 hours

Pregnancy Risk Factor D

Breast-feeding Considerations No data reported

Dosage Forms Injection, as hydrochloride: 1 mg/mL (2 mL, 5 mL, 10 mL); 5 mg/mL (1 mL, 2 mL, 5 mL, 10 mL)

Dietary Considerations No data reported

Generic Available No

Midchlor® see Acetaminophen, Isometheptene, and Dichloralphenazone on page 25

Midodrine (MI doe dreen)

Brand Names ProAmatine™

Therapeutic Category Alpha-Adrenergic Agonist

Synonyms Midodrine Hydrochloride

Use Treatment of symptomatic orthostatic hypotension in patients whose lives are considerably impaired despite standard clinical care.

Usual Dosage Adults: Oral: 10 mg 3 times/day during daytime hours (every 3-4 hours) when patient is upright (maximum: 40 mg/day)

Mechanism of Action Midodrine forms an active metabolite, desglymidodrine, that is an alpha$_1$-agonist. This agent increases arteriolar and venous tone (Continued)

Midodrine *(Continued)*

resulting in a rise in standing, sitting, and supine systolic and diastolic blood pressure in patients with orthostatic hypotension.

Local Anesthetic/Vasoconstrictor Precautions No information available to require special precautions

Effects on Dental Treatment 1% to 10% of patients experience significant dry mouth

Other Adverse Effects
>10%:
Dermatologic: Piloerection, pruritus
Genitourinary: Urinary urgency, retention, or polyuria
Neuromuscular & skeletal: Paresthesia
1% to 10%:
Cardiovascular: Supine hypertension, facial flushing
Central nervous system: Confusion, anxiety, dizziness, chills
Dermatologic: Rash, dry skin
Gastrointestinal: Xerostomia, nausea, abdominal pain
Genitourinary: Dysuria
Neuromuscular & skeletal: Pain
<1%:
Cardiovascular: Flushing
Central nervous system: Headache, insomnia
Gastrointestinal: Flatulence
Neuromuscular & skeletal: Leg cramps
Ocular: Visual changes

Warnings/Precautions Only indicated for patients for whom orthostatic hypotension significantly impairs their daily life. Use is not recommended with supine hypertension and caution should be exercised in patients with diabetes, visual problems, urinary retention (reduce initial dose) or hepatic dysfunction; monitor renal and hepatic function prior to and periodically during therapy; safety and efficacy has not been established in children; discontinue and re-evaluate therapy if signs of bradycardia occur.

Drug Interactions Increased effect: Concomitant fludrocortisone results in hypernatremia or an increase in intraocular pressure and glaucoma; bradycardia may be accentuated with concomitant administration of cardiac glycosides, psychotherapeutics, and beta-blockers; alpha-agonists may increase the pressure effects and alpha-antagonists may negate the effects of midodrine

Drug Uptake
Absorption: Rapid
Serum half-life: ~3-4 hours (active drug); 25 minutes (prodrug)
Time to peak serum concentration: 1-2 hours (active drug); 30 minutes (prodrug)

Pregnancy Risk Factor C

Generic Available No

Midodrine Hydrochloride *see Midodrine on previous page*

Midol® IB [OTC] *see Ibuprofen on page 495*

Midol® PM [OTC] *see Acetaminophen and Diphenhydramine on page 23*

Midrin® *see Acetaminophen, Isometheptene, and Dichloralphenazone on page 25*

Miglitol

Brand Names Glyset®

Therapeutic Category Antidiabetic Agent; Hypoglycemic Agent, Oral

Use As an adjunct to diet to lower blood glucose in patients with noninsulin-dependent diabetes mellitus (NIDDM)

Usual Dosage Oral: Adults: 25 mg three times/day with the first bite of food at each meal; the dose may be increased to 50 mg three times/day after 4-8 weeks; maximum recommended dose is 100 mg three times/day

Mechanism of Action In contrast to sulfonylureas, miglitol does not enhance insulin secretion; the antihyperglycemic action of miglitol results from a reversible inhibition of membrane-bound intestinal a-glucosidases hydrolyze oligosaccharides and disaccharides to glucose and other monosaccharides in the brush border of the small intestine; in diabetic patients, this enzyme inhibition results in delayed glucose absorption and lowering of postprandial hyperglycemia

Local Anesthetic/Vasoconstrictor Precautions No information available to require special precautions

Effects on Dental Treatment No effects or complications reported

Dosage Forms Tablet: 25 mg, 50 mg, 100 mg

Migranal® Nasal Spray *see Dihydroergotamine on page 317*

Migratine® *see Acetaminophen, Isometheptene, and Dichloralphenazone on page 25*

Miles Nervine® Caplets [OTC] see Diphenhydramine on page 323
Milontin® see Phensuximide on page 750
Milophene® see Clomiphene on page 247

Milrinone (MIL ri none)

Brand Names Primacor®

Therapeutic Category Cardiovascular Agent, Other

Use Short-term I.V. therapy of congestive heart failure; used for calcium antagonist intoxication

Usual Dosage Adults: I.V.: Loading dose: 50 mcg/kg administered over 10 minutes followed by a maintenance dose titrated according to the hemodynamic and clinical response

Mechanism of Action Phosphodiesterase inhibitor resulting in vasodilation

Local Anesthetic/Vasoconstrictor Precautions No information available to require special precautions

Effects on Dental Treatment No effects or complications reported

Other Adverse Effects
>10%: Cardiovascular: Ventricular arrhythmias
1% to 10%:
Cardiovascular: Supraventricular arrhythmias, hypotension, angina, chest pain
Central nervous system: Headache
<1%:
Cardiovascular: Ventricular fibrillation
Endocrine & metabolic: Hypokalemia
Hematologic: Thrombocytopenia
Neuromuscular & skeletal: Tremor

Drug Interactions No data reported

Drug Uptake
Serum level: I.V.: Following a 125 mcg/kg dose, peak plasma concentrations of ~1000 ng/mL were observed at 2 minutes postinjection, decreasing to <100 ng/mL in 2 hours
Therapeutic effect: Oral: Following doses of 7.5-15 mg, peak hemodynamic effects occurred at 90 minutes
Serum half-life, elimination: I.V.: 136 minutes in patients with CHF; patients with severe CHF have a more prolonged half-life, with values ranging from 1.7-2.7 hours. Patients with CHF have a reduction in the systemic clearance of milrinone, resulting in a prolonged elimination half-life. Alternatively, one study reported that 1 month of therapy with milrinone did not change the pharmacokinetic parameters for patients with CHF despite improvement in cardiac function.

Pregnancy Risk Factor C
Generic Available No

Miltown® see Meprobamate on page 599
Mini-Gamulin® Rh see Rh₀(D) Immune Globulin on page 840
Minipress® see Prazosin on page 787
Minitran® see Nitroglycerin on page 685
Minizide® see Prazosin and Polythiazide on page 787
Minociclina (Mexico) see Minocycline on this page
Minocin® IV Injection see Minocycline on this page
Minocin® Oral see Minocycline on this page

Minocycline (mi noe SYE kleen)

Brand Names Dynacin® Oral; Minocin® IV Injection; Minocin® Oral

Canadian/Mexican Brand Names Apo®-Minocycline (Canada); Syn-Minocycline (Canada)

Therapeutic Category Antibiotic, Tetracycline Derivative

Synonyms Minociclina (Mexico)

Use
Dental: Treatment of periodontitis associated with presence of *Actinobacillus actinomycetemocomitams* (AA); as adjunctive therapy in recurrent aphthous ulcers
Medical: Treatment of susceptible bacterial infections of both gram-negative and gram-positive organisms; acne, meningococcal carrier state

Usual Dosage Infection: Oral, I.V.:
Children >8 years: Initial: 4 mg/kg followed by 2 mg/kg/dose every 12 hours
Adults: 200 mg stat, 100 mg every 12 hours not to exceed 400 mg/24 hours

Mechanism of Action Inhibits bacterial protein synthesis by binding with the 30S and possibly the 50S ribosomal subunit(s) of susceptible bacteria; cell wall synthesis is not affected
(Continued)

Minocycline (Continued)

Local Anesthetic/Vasoconstrictor Precautions No information available to require special precautions

Effects on Dental Treatment Opportunistic "superinfection" with *Candida albicans*; tetracycline's are not recommended for use during pregnancy or in children ≤8 years of age since they have been reported to cause enamel hypoplasia and permanent teeth discoloration. The use of tetracycline's should only be used in these patients if other agents are contraindicated or alternative antimicrobials will not eradicate the organism. Long-term use associated with oral candidiasis.

Other Adverse Effects
>10%: Miscellaneous: Discoloration of teeth in children

1% to 10%:
  Dermatologic: Photosensitivity
  Gastrointestinal: Nausea, diarrhea

Warnings/Precautions Use of tetracyclines during tooth development may cause permanent discoloration of the teeth and enamel, hypoplasia and retardation of skeletal development and bone growth with risk being the greatest for children <4 years of age and those receiving high doses; use with caution in patients with renal or hepatic impairment and in pregnancy; dosage modification required in patients with renal impairment; pseudotumor cerebri has been reported with tetracycline use; outdated drug can cause nephropathy.

Drug Interactions Decreased effect with antacids (aluminum, calcium, zinc, or magnesium), bismuth salts, barbiturates, carbamazepine, hydantoins; decreased effect of oral contraceptives; increased effect of warfarin

Drug Uptake Serum half-life: 15 hours

Pregnancy Risk Factor D

Breast-feeding Considerations No data reported

Dosage Forms
Capsule, as hydrochloride: 50 mg, 100 mg
Capsule, as hydrochloride (Dynacin®): 50 mg, 100 mg
Capsule, pellet-filled, as hydrochloride (Minocin®): 50 mg, 100 mg
Injection, as hydrochloride (Minocin® IV): 100 mg
Suspension, oral, as hydrochloride (Minocin®)50 mg/5 mL (60 mL)

Dietary Considerations No data reported

Generic Available Yes

Minoxidil (mi NOKS i dil)

Related Information
Cardiovascular Diseases on page 1010

Brand Names Loniten®; Rogaine® Extra Strength for Men [OTC]; Rogaine® for Men [OTC]; Rogaine® for Women [OTC]

Canadian/Mexican Brand Names Apo®-Gain (Canada); Gen-Minoxidil® (Canada); Regaine® (Mexico)

Therapeutic Category Vasodilator

Use Management of severe hypertension (usually in combination with a diuretic and beta-blocker); treatment of male pattern baldness (alopecia androgenetica)

Usual Dosage
Children <12 years: Hypertension: Oral: Initial: 0.1-0.2 mg/kg once daily; maximum: 5 mg/day; increase gradually every 3 days; usual dosage: 0.25-1 mg/kg/day in 1-2 divided doses; maximum: 50 mg/day

Children >12 years and Adults:
  Hypertension: Oral: Initial: 5 mg once daily, increase gradually every 3 days; usual dose: 10-40 mg/day in 1-2 divided doses; maximum: 100 mg/day
  Alopecia: Topical: Apply twice daily; 4 months of therapy may be necessary for hair growth

Elderly: Initial: 2.5 mg once daily; increase gradually

Supplemental dose is not necessary via hemo- or peritoneal dialysis

Mechanism of Action Produces vasodilation by directly relaxing arteriolar smooth muscle, with little effect on veins; effects may be mediated by cyclic AMP; stimulation of hair growth is secondary to vasodilation, increased cutaneous blood flow and stimulation of resting hair follicles

Local Anesthetic/Vasoconstrictor Precautions No information available to require special precautions

Effects on Dental Treatment No effects or complications reported

Other Adverse Effects
>10%:
  Cardiovascular: EKG changes, tachycardia, congestive heart failure, edema
  Dermatologic: Hypertrichosis (commonly occurs within 1-2 months of therapy)

1% to 10%: Endocrine & metabolic: Fluid and electrolyte imbalance

<1%:
  Cardiovascular: Angina, pericardial effusion tamponade
  Central nervous system: Dizziness, headache
  Dermatologic: Rashes, coarsening facial features, dermatologic reactions, Stevens-Johnson syndrome, sunburn
  Endocrine & metabolic: Breast tenderness
  Gastrointestinal: Weight gain
  Hematologic: Thrombocytopenia, leukopenia
Drug Interactions Increased toxicity: .
  Concurrent administration with guanethidine may cause profound orthostatic hypotensive effects
  Additive hypotensive effects with other hypotensive agents or diuretics
Drug Uptake
  Onset of hypotensive effect: Oral: Within 30 minutes
  Peak effect: Within 2-8 hours
  Duration: Up to 2-5 days
  Serum half-life: Adults: 3.5-4.2 hours
Pregnancy Risk Factor C
Generic Available Yes

Mintezol® see Thiabendazole on page 923

Minute-Gel® see Fluoride on page 415

Miochol-E® see Acetylcholine on page 29

Miostat® Intraocular see Carbachol on page 173

Mirapex® see Pramipexole on page 784

Mirtazapine (mir TAZ a peen)
  Brand Names Remeron®
  Therapeutic Category Antidepressant, Tetracyclic
  Use Treatment of depression
  Usual Dosage Adults: Oral: Starting dose is 15 mg/day, usually given in the evening
  Local Anesthetic/Vasoconstrictor Precautions No information available to require special precautions
  Effects on Dental Treatment Significant xerostomia occurs in up to 25% of patients
  Other Adverse Effects >10%:
    Central nervous system: Somnolence, insomnia
    Gastrointestinal: Constipation, weight gain
  Warnings/Precautions Use with caution in patients with cardiac conduction disturbances, history of hyperthyroid, renal, or hepatic dysfunction; safe use of tricyclic antidepressants in children <12 years of age has not been established; to avoid cholinergic crisis do not discontinue abruptly in patients receiving high doses chronically
  Drug Interactions
    Decreased effect: Barbiturates, phenytoin, carbamazepine
    Increased toxicity: CNS depressants, MAO inhibitors (hyperpyretic crisis), anticholinergics, sympathomimetics, thyroid increases cardiotoxicity, phenothiazines (seizures), benzodiazepines
  Pregnancy Risk Factor C
  Generic Available No

Misoprostol (mye soe PROST ole)
  Brand Names Cytotec®
  Therapeutic Category Prostaglandin
  Use Prevention of NSAID-induced gastric ulcers
  Usual Dosage Adults: Oral: 200 mcg 4 times/day with food; if not tolerated, may decrease dose to 100 mcg 4 times/day with food or 200 mcg twice daily with food
  Mechanism of Action Misoprostol is a synthetic prostaglandin E_1 analog that replaces the protective prostaglandins consumed with prostaglandin-inhibiting therapies eg, nonsteroidal anti-inflammatory drugs
  Local Anesthetic/Vasoconstrictor Precautions No information available to require special precautions
  Effects on Dental Treatment No effects or complications reported
  Other Adverse Effects
    >10%: Gastrointestinal: Diarrhea, abdominal pain
    1% to 10%:
      Central nervous system: Headache
      Gastrointestinal: Constipation, flatulence
    <1%:
      Gastrointestinal: Nausea, vomiting
  (Continued)

Misoprostol *(Continued)*

Genitourinary: Uterine stimulation, vaginal bleeding

Drug Interactions No data reported

Drug Uptake

Absorption: Oral: Rapid

Serum half-life (parent and metabolite combined): 1.5 hours

Time to peak serum concentration (active metabolite): Within 15-30 minutes

Pregnancy Risk Factor X

Dosage Forms Tablet: 100 mcg, 200 mcg

Generic Available No

Mithracin® *see Plicamycin on page 768*

Mitomycin *(mye toe MYE sin)*

Brand Names Mutamycin®

Therapeutic Category Antineoplastic Agent, Antibiotic

Synonyms Mitomycin-C; MTC

Use Therapy of disseminated adenocarcinoma of stomach, colon, or pancreas in combination with other approved chemotherapeutic agents; bladder cancer, breast cancer

Usual Dosage Refer to individual protocols.

Children and Adults: I.V.:

Single agent therapy: 20 mg/m² every 6-8 weeks

Combination therapy: 10 mg/m² every 6-8 weeks

Bone marrow transplant:

40-50 mg/m²

2-40 mg/m²/day for 3 days

Total cumulative dose should not exceed 50 mg/m²; see table.

Nadir After Prior Dose/mm³		% of Prior Dose to Be Given
Leukocytes	Platelets	
4000	>100,000	100
3000-3999	75,000-99,999	100
2000-2999	25,000-74,999	70
2000	<25,000	50

Mechanism of Action Isolated from *Streptomyces caespitosus*; acts primarily as an alkylating agent and produces DNA cross-linking (primarily with guanine and cytosine pairs); cell-cycle nonspecific; inhibits DNA and RNA synthesis by alkylation and cross-linking the strands of DNA

Local Anesthetic/Vasoconstrictor Precautions No information available to require special precautions

Effects on Dental Treatment No effects or complications reported

Other Adverse Effects

>10%:

Extravasation: May cause severe tissue irritation if infiltrated; can progress to cellulitis, ulceration, and sloughing of tissue

Gastrointestinal: **Emetic potential:** Moderately high (60% to 90%); **nausea and vomiting (mild to moderate) seen in almost 100% of patients;** usually begins 1-2 hours after treatment and persists for 3 hours to 4 days; other toxicities include stomatitis, hepatic toxicity, diarrhea, anorexia

Hematologic: Myelosuppressive: Dose-related toxicity and may be cumulative; related to both total dose (incidence higher at doses >50 mg) and schedule

1% to 10%:

Dermatologic: Discolored fingernails (violet), alopecia

Gastrointestinal: Mouth ulcers

Neuromuscular & skeletal: Paresthesia

Respiratory: Interstitial pneumonitis or pulmonary fibrosis have been noticed in 7% of patients, and it occurs independent of dosing. Manifested as dry cough and progressive dyspnea; usually is responsive to steroid therapy.

Renal: Elevation of creatinine seen in 2% of patients; hemolytic uremic syndrome observed in <10% of patients and is dose-dependent (doses >30 mg have higher risk)

<1%:

Cardiovascular: Cardiac failure (in patients treated with doses >30 mg)

Central nervous system: Malaise, fever

Dermatologic: Pruritus, rash

Hematologic: Bone marrow suppression (leukopenia, thrombocytopenia), microangiopathic hemolytic anemia

Local: Thrombophlebitis

Neuromuscular & skeletal: Weakness
Drug Uptake
Absorption: Fairly well from the GI tract
Serum half-life: 23-78 minutes
Terminal: 50 minutes
Pregnancy Risk Factor C
Generic Available No

Mitomycin-C *see* Mitomycin *on previous page*

Mitotane (MYE toe tane)
Brand Names Lysodren®
Therapeutic Category Antiadrenal Agent; Antineoplastic Agent, Miscellaneous
Synonyms o,p'-DDD
Use Treatment of inoperable adrenal cortical carcinoma
Usual Dosage Oral:
Children: 0.1-0.5 mg/kg or 1-2 g/day in divided doses increasing gradually to a maximum of 5-7 g/day
Adults: Start at 1-6 g/day in divided doses, then increase incrementally to 8-10 g/day in 3-4 divided doses; dose is changed on basis of side effect with aim of giving as high a dose as tolerated; maximum daily dose: 18 g
Mechanism of Action Causes adrenal cortical atrophy; drug affects mitochondria in adrenal cortical cells and decreases production of cortisol; also alters the peripheral metabolism of steroids
Local Anesthetic/Vasoconstrictor Precautions No information available to require special precautions
Effects on Dental Treatment No effects or complications reported
Other Adverse Effects
>10%:
Central nervous system: Vertigo, mental depression, dizziness; all are reversible with discontinuation of the drug and can occur in 15% to 26% of patients
Dermatologic: Rash (15%) which may subside without discontinuation of therapy, hyperpigmentation
Gastrointestinal: 75% to 80% will experience nausea, vomiting, and anorexia; diarrhea can occur in 20% of patients
Ocular: Visual disturbances, diplopia, blurred vision; all are reversible with discontinuation of drug
1% to 10%:
Cardiovascular: Orthostatic hypotension, flushing of skin
Central nervous system: Fever
Genitourinary: Hemorrhagic cystitis
Neuromuscular & skeletal: Myalgia
<1%:
Cardiovascular: Hypertension
Central nervous system: Lethargy, somnolence, mental depression, irritability, confusion, fatigue, headache
Endocrine & metabolic: Hypercholesterolemia, adrenal insufficiency may develop and may require steroid replacement
Genitourinary: Hemorrhagic cystitis, hypouricemia
Hematologic: Myelosuppressive: WBC: None; Platelets: None
Neuromuscular & skeletal: Tremor, weakness
Ocular: Lens opacities, toxic retinopathy
Renal: Hematuria, albuminuria
Respiratory: Dyspnea, wheezing
Drug Uptake
Absorption: Oral: ~35% to 40%
Serum half-life: 18-159 days
Time to peak serum concentration: Within 3-5 hours
Pregnancy Risk Factor C
Generic Available No
Comments Myelosuppressive effects:
WBC: None
Platelets: None

Mitoxantrone (mye toe ZAN trone)
Brand Names Novantrone®
Canadian/Mexican Brand Names Misostol (Mexico); Novantrone® (Mexico)
Therapeutic Category Antineoplastic Agent, Anthracycline; Antineoplastic Agent, Antibiotic
Synonyms DHAD; Mitoxantrone Hydrochloride
(Continued)

643

Mitoxantrone *(Continued)*

Use FDA approved for remission-induction therapy of acute nonlymphocytic leukemia (ANLL); mitoxantrone is also active against other various leukemias, lymphoma, and breast cancer, and moderately active against pediatric sarcoma

Usual Dosage

Refer to individual protocols. I.V. (may dilute in D_5W or NS):

ANLL leukemias:

Children ≤2 years: 0.4 mg/kg/day once daily for 3-5 days

Children >2 years and Adults: 12 mg/m²/day once daily for 3 days; acute leukemia in relapse: 8-12 mg/m²/day once daily for 4-5 days

Solid tumors:

Children: 18-20 mg/m² every 3-4 weeks **OR** 5-8 mg/m² every week

Adults: 12-14 mg/m² every 3-4 weeks **OR** 2-4 mg/m²/day for 5 days

Maximum total dose: 80-120 mg/m² in patients with predisposing factor and <160 mg in patients with no predisposing factor

Mechanism of Action Analogue of the anthracyclines, but different in mechanism of action, cardiac toxicity, and potential for tissue necrosis; mitoxantrone does intercalate DNA; binds to nucleic acids and inhibits DNA and RNA synthesis by template disordering and steric obstruction; replication is decreased by binding to DNA topoisomerase II (enzyme responsible for DNA helix supercoiling); active throughout entire cell cycle; does not appear to produce free radicals

Local Anesthetic/Vasoconstrictor Precautions No information available to require special precautions

Effects on Dental Treatment No effects or complications reported

Other Adverse Effects

>10%:

Central nervous system: Headache

Dermatologic: Alopecia

Gastrointestinal: Nausea, vomiting, diarrhea, abdominal pain, mucositis, stomatitis, GI bleeding

Emetic potential: Moderate (31% to 72%)

Genitourinary: Discoloration of urine (blue-green)

Hepatic: Abnormal LFTs

Respiratory: Coughing, dyspnea

1% to 10%:

Cardiac toxicity: Much reduced compared to doxorubicin and has been reported primarily in patients who have received prior anthracycline therapy, congestive heart failure, hypotension

Central nervous system: Seizures, fever

Dermatologic: Pruritus, skin desquamation

Hepatic: Transient elevation of liver enzymes, jaundice

Ocular: Conjunctivitis

Renal: Renal failure

<1%: Local: Pain or redness at injection site

Drug Uptake

Absorption: Oral: Poor

Serum half-life: Terminal: 37 hours; may be prolonged with liver impairment

Pregnancy Risk Factor D

Generic Available No

Mitoxantrone Hydrochloride *see* Mitoxantrone *on previous page*

Mitran® *see* Chlordiazepoxide *on page 210*

Mitrolan® Chewable Tablet [OTC] *see* Calcium Polycarbophil *on page 168*

MK594 *see* Losartan *on page 569*

M-KYA® [OTC] *see* Quinine *on page 831*

MMR *see* Measles, Mumps, and Rubella Vaccines, Combined *on page 582*

M-M-R® II *see* Measles, Mumps, and Rubella Vaccines, Combined *on page 582*

Moban® *see* Molindone *on page 646*

Mobidin® *see* Magnesium Salicylate *on page 577*

Modane® Bulk [OTC] *see* Psyllium *on page 822*

Modane® Soft [OTC] *see* Docusate *on page 331*

Modicon™ *see* Ethinyl Estradiol and Norethindrone *on page 379*

Modified Dakin's Solution *see* Sodium Hypochlorite Solution *on page 873*

Modified Shohl's Solution *see* Sodium Citrate and Citric Acid *on page 872*

Moducal® [OTC] *see* Glucose Polymers *on page 444*

Moduretic® *see* Amiloride and Hydrochlorothiazide *on page 54*

Moexipril (mo EKS i pril)
Related Information
Cardiovascular Diseases *on page 1010*
Moexipril and Hydrochlorothiazide *on this page*
Brand Names Univasc®
Therapeutic Category Angiotensin-Converting Enzyme (ACE) Inhibitors
Use Treatment of hypertension, alone or in combination with thiazide diuretics
Usual Dosage Adults: Oral: Initial: 7.5 mg once daily (in patients **not** receiving diuretics), one hour prior to a meal **or** 3.75 mg once daily (when combined with thiazide diuretics); maintenance dose: 7.5-30 mg/day in 1 or 2 divided doses one hour before meals
Mechanism of Action Competitive inhibitor of angiotensin-converting enzyme (ACE); prevents conversion of angiotensin I to angiotensin II, a potent vasoconstrictor; results in lower levels of angiotensin II which causes an increase in plasma renin activity and a reduction in aldosterone secretion
Local Anesthetic/Vasoconstrictor Precautions No information available to require special precautions
Effects on Dental Treatment No effects or complications reported
Other Adverse Effects
1% to 10%:
Cardiovascular: Flushing
Central nervous system: Headache, dizziness, fatigue
Dermatologic: Rash, pruritus, alopecia, rash
Endocrine & metabolic: Hyperkalemia
Gastrointestinal: Diarrhea
Renal: Oliguria, reversible elevations in creatinine or BUN, polyuria
Respiratory: Nonproductive cough (6%), pharyngitis, upper respiratory infections, rhinitis
Miscellaneous: Flu-like symptoms
<1%:
Cardiovascular: Symptomatic hypotension, chest pain, angina, peripheral edema, myocardial infarction, palpitations, arrhythmias
Central nervous system: Sleep disturbances, anxiety, mood changes
Dermatologic: Angioedema, photosensitivity, pemphigus
Endocrine & metabolic: Hypercholesterolemia
Gastrointestinal: Abdominal pain, taste disturbance, constipation, vomiting, changes in appetite, pancreatitis, dysgeusia
Hematologic: Neutropenia
Hepatic: Elevated LFTs
Neuromuscular & skeletal: Myalgia, arthralgia
Renal: Proteinuria
Respiratory: Bronchospasm, dyspnea
Drug Uptake
Absorption: Food decreases bioavailability (AUC decreased by ~40%)
Serum half-life:
Moexipril: 1 hour
Moexiprilat: 2-10 hours
Time to peak: 1.5 hours
Pregnancy Risk Factor D
Generic Available No

Moexipril and Hydrochlorothiazide
(mo EKS i pril & hye droe klor oh THYE a zide)
Brand Names Uniretic®
Therapeutic Category Angiotensin-Converting Enzyme (ACE) Inhibitors; Diuretic, Thiazide
Use Treatment of hypertension
Usual Dosage Adults: Oral: 7.5-30 mg of moexipril, taken either in a single or divided dose one hour before meals
Mechanism of Action See individual agents
Local Anesthetic/Vasoconstrictor Precautions No information available to require special precautions
Effects on Dental Treatment No effects or complications reported
Other Adverse Effects See individual agents
Drug Interactions See individual agents
Dosage Forms Tablet: Moexipril hydrochloride 7.5 mg and hydrochlorothiazide 12.5 mg; moexipril hydrochloride 15 mg and hydrochlorothiazide 25 mg
Generic Available No

Moi-Stir® Solution [OTC] *see* Saliva Substitute *on page 854*
Moi-Stir® Swabsticks [OTC] *see* Saliva Substitute *on page 854*

Moisture® Ophthalmic Drops [OTC] *see* Artificial Tears *on page 87*

Molindone (moe LIN done)
Brand Names Moban®
Therapeutic Category Antipsychotic Agent
Use Management of psychotic disorder
Usual Dosage Oral:
  Children:
    3-5 years: 1-2.5 mg/day divided into 4 doses
    5-12 years: 0.5-1 mg/kg/day in 4 divided doses

  Adults: 50-75 mg/day increase at 3- to 4-day intervals up to 225 mg/day
Mechanism of Action Mechanism of action mimics that of chlorpromazine; however, it produces more extrapyramidal effects and less sedation than chlorpromazine
Local Anesthetic/Vasoconstrictor Precautions No information available to require special precautions
Effects on Dental Treatment >10% of patients experience dry mouth; anticholinergic side effects can cause a reduction of saliva production or secretion. This may result in discomfort and dental disease (ie, caries, oral candidiasis and periodontal disease); molindone can cause extrapyramidal reactions which may appear as muscle twitching or increased motor activity of the face, neck or head
Other Adverse Effects
  >10%:
    Cardiovascular: Orthostatic hypotension
    Central nervous system: Akathisia, extrapyramidal effects, persistent tardive dyskinesia
    Gastrointestinal: Constipation
    Ocular: Blurred vision
    Miscellaneous: Decreased sweating
  1% to 10%:
    Central nervous system: Mental depression
    Endocrine & metabolic: Change in menstrual periods, swelling of breasts
  <1%:
    Cardiovascular: Tachycardia, arrhythmias
    Central nervous system: Sedation, drowsiness, restlessness, anxiety, seizures, neuroleptic malignant syndrome (NMS), altered central temperature regulation
    Dermatologic: Hyperpigmentation, pruritus, rash, photosensitivity
    Endocrine & metabolic: Galactorrhea, gynecomastia
    Gastrointestinal: Weight gain
    Genitourinary: Urinary retention
    Hematologic: Agranulocytosis (more often in women between fourth and tenth weeks of therapy), leukopenia (usually in patients with large doses for prolonged periods)
    Ocular: Retinal pigmentation
Drug Interactions Increased toxicity: CNS depressants, antihypertensives, anticonvulsants
Drug Uptake
  Serum half-life: 1.5 hours
  Time to peak serum concentration: Oral: Within 1.5 hours
Pregnancy Risk Factor C
Generic Available No

Mol-Iron® [OTC] *see* Ferrous Sulfate *on page 401*

Mollifene® Ear Wax Removing Formula [OTC] *see* Carbamide Peroxide *on page 175*

Molybdenum *see* Trace Metals *on page 948*

Molypen® *see* Trace Metals *on page 948*

Mometasona, Furoata De (Mexico) *see* Mometasone Furoate *on this page*

Mometasone Furoate (moe MET a sone FYOOR oh ate)
Brand Names Elocon®; Nasonex®
Canadian/Mexican Brand Names Elocom® (Canada); Elomet® (Mexico)
Therapeutic Category Corticosteroid, Topical (Medium Potency)
Synonyms Mometasona, Furoata De (Mexico)
Use Relief of the inflammatory and pruritic manifestations of corticosteroid-responsive dermatoses (medium potency topical corticosteroid)
Usual Dosage Adults: Topical: Apply sparingly to area once daily, do not use occlusive dressings
Mechanism of Action May depress the formation, release, and activity of endogenous chemical mediators of inflammation (kinins, histamine, liposomal

enzymes, prostaglandins). Leukocytes and macrophages may have to be present for the initiation of responses mediated by the above substances. Inhibits the margination and subsequent cell migration to the area of injury, and also reverses the dilatation and increased vessel permeability in the area resulting in decreased access of cells to the sites of injury.

Local Anesthetic/Vasoconstrictor Precautions No information available to require special precautions

Effects on Dental Treatment No effects or complications reported

Other Adverse Effects <1%:
  Dermatologic: Acne, hypopigmentation, allergic dermatitis, maceration of the skin, skin atrophy, striae, miliaria, folliculitis, hypertrichosis
  Endocrine & metabolic: HPA suppression, Cushing's syndrome, growth retardation
  Local: Burning, itching, irritation, dryness
  Miscellaneous: Secondary infection

Drug Interactions No data reported

Pregnancy Risk Factor C

Generic Available No

MOM/Mineral Oil Emulsion *see* Magnesium Hydroxide and Mineral Oil Emulsion *on page 576*

Monafed® *see* Guaifenesin *on page 452*

Monafed® DM *see* Guaifenesin and Dextromethorphan *on page 453*

Monistat-Derm™ Topical *see* Miconazole *on page 635*

Monistat i.v.™ Injection *see* Miconazole *on page 635*

Monistat™ Vaginal *see* Miconazole *on page 635*

Monobenzone (mon oh BEN zone)
Brand Names Benoquin®

Therapeutic Category Topical Skin Product

Use Final depigmentation in extensive vitiligo

Local Anesthetic/Vasoconstrictor Precautions No information available to require special precautions

Effects on Dental Treatment No effects or complications reported

Other Adverse Effects 1% to 10%: Irritation, burning sensation, dermatitis

Pregnancy Risk Factor C

Generic Available No

Monocid® *see* Cefonicid *on page 191*

Monoclate-P® *see* Antihemophilic Factor (Human) *on page 80*

Monoclonal Antibody *see* Muromonab-CD3 *on page 652*

Monoethanolamine (Canada) *see* Ethanolamine Oleate *on page 373*

Mono-Gesic® *see* Salsalate *on page 855*

Monoket® *see* Isosorbide Mononitrate *on page 526*

Mononine® *see* Factor IX Complex (Human) *on page 391*

Monopril® *see* Fosinopril *on page 431*

Montelukast (mon te LOO kast)
Brand Names Singulair®

Therapeutic Category Leukotriene Receptor Antagonist

Synonyms Montelukast Sodium

Use Prophylaxis and chronic treatment of asthma in adults and children ≥6 years of age

Usual Dosage Oral:
  Children 6-14 years: 5 mg once daily
  Children >14 years and Adults: 10 mg once daily

Local Anesthetic/Vasoconstrictor Precautions No information available to require special precautions

Effects on Dental Treatment No effects or complications reported

Dosage Forms
  Tablet, as sodium: 10 mg
  Tablet, chewable (cherry), as sodium: 5 mg

Montelukast Sodium *see* Montelukast *on this page*

Monurol™ *see* Fosfomycin *on page 430*

8-MOP *see* Methoxsalen *on page 618*

More Attenuated Enders Strain *see* Measles Virus Vaccine, Live *on page 583*

More-Dophilus® [OTC] *see* Lactobacillus acidophilus and Lactobacillus bulgaricus *on page 539*

Morfina (Mexico) *see* Morphine Sulfate *on next page*

Moricizine (mor I siz een)

Related Information
Cardiovascular Diseases *on page 1010*

Brand Names Ethmozine®

Therapeutic Category Antiarrhythmic Agent, Class I; Antiarrhythmic Agent (Supraventricular & Ventricular)

Use For treatment of ventricular tachycardia and life-threatening ventricular arrhythmias

Unlabeled use: PVCs, complete and nonsustained ventricular tachycardia

Usual Dosage Adults: Oral: 200-300 mg every 8 hours, adjust dosage at 150 mg/day at 3-day intervals. See table for dosage recommendations of transferring from other antiarrhythmic agents to Ethmozine®.

Moricizine

Transferred From	Start Ethmozine®
Encainide, propafenone, tocainide, or mexiletine	8-12 hours after last dose
Flecainide	12-24 hours after last dose
Procainamide	3-6 hours after last dose
Quinidine, disopyramide	6-12 hours after last dose

Mechanism of Action Class I antiarrhythmic agent; reduces the fast inward current carried by sodium ions, shortens Phase I and Phase II repolarization, resulting in decreased action potential duration and effective refractory period

Local Anesthetic/Vasoconstrictor Precautions No information available to require special precautions

Effects on Dental Treatment No effects or complications reported

Other Adverse Effects
>10%: Central nervous system: Dizziness
1% to 10%:
   Cardiovascular: Proarrhythmia, palpitations, cardiac death, EKG abnormalities, congestive heart failure
   Central nervous system: Headache, fatigue, insomnia
   Endocrine & metabolic: Decreased libido
   Gastrointestinal: Nausea, diarrhea, ileus
   Ocular: Blurred vision, periorbital edema
   Respiratory: Dyspnea
<1%:
   Cardiovascular: Ventricular tachycardia, cardiac chest pain, hypotension or hypertension, syncope, supraventricular arrhythmias, myocardial infarction
   Central nervous system: Anxiety, drug fever, confusion, loss of memory, vertigo, anorexia
   Dermatologic: Rash, dry skin
   Gastrointestinal: GI upset, vomiting, dyspepsia, flatulence, bitter taste
   Genitourinary: Urinary retention, urinary incontinence, impotence
   Neuromuscular & skeletal: Tremor
   Otic: Tinnitus
   Respiratory: Apnea
   Miscellaneous: Sweating

Drug Interactions
Decreased levels of theophylline (50%)
Increased levels with cimetidine (50%)

Drug Uptake
Serum half-life:
   Normal patients: 3-4 hours
   Cardiac disease patients: 6-13 hours

Pregnancy Risk Factor B

Generic Available No

Morphine Sulfate (MOR feen SUL fate)

Related Information
Narcotic Agonists *on page 1141*

Brand Names Astramorph™ PF Injection; Duramorph® Injection; Infumorph™ Injection; Kadian® Capsule; MS Contin® Oral; MSIR® Oral; MS/L®; MS/S®; OMS® Oral; Oramorph SR™ Oral; RMS® Rectal; Roxanol™ Oral; Roxanol Rescudose®; Roxanol SR™ Oral

Canadian/Mexican Brand Names Epimorph® (Canada); Morphine-HP® (Canada); MS-IR® (Canada); MST-Continus® (Mexico); Statex® (Canada)

Therapeutic Category Analgesic, Narcotic

Synonyms Morfina (Mexico)

Use Relief of moderate to severe acute and chronic pain; pain of myocardial infarction; relieves dyspnea of acute left ventricular failure and pulmonary edema; preanesthetic medication

Usual Dosage Doses should be titrated to appropriate effect; when changing routes of administration in chronically treated patients, please note that oral doses are approximately one-half as effective as parenteral dose

Children:
    Oral: Tablet and solution (prompt release): 0.2-0.5 mg/kg/dose every 4-6 hours as needed; tablet (controlled release): 0.3-0.6 mg/kg/dose every 12 hours
    I.M., I.V., S.C.: 0.1-0.2 mg/kg/dose every 2-4 hours as needed; usual maximum: 15 mg/dose; may initiate at 0.05 mg/kg/dose
    I.V., S.C. continuous infusion: Sickle cell or cancer pain: 0.025-2 mg/kg/hour; postoperative pain: 0.01-0.04 mg/kg/hour
    Sedation/analgesia for procedures: I.V.: 0.05-0.1 mg/kg 5 minutes before the procedure

Adolescents >12 years: Sedation/analgesia for procedures: I.V.: 3-4 mg and repeat in 5 minutes if necessary

Adults:
    Oral: Prompt release: 10-30 mg every 4 hours as needed; controlled release: 15-30 mg every 8-12 hours
    I.M., I.V., S.C.: 2.5-20 mg/dose every 2-6 hours as needed; usual: 10 mg/dose every 4 hours as needed
    I.V., S.C. continuous infusion: 0.8-10 mg/hour; may increase depending on pain relief/adverse effects; usual range: up to 80 mg/hour
    Epidural: Initial: 5 mg in lumbar region; if inadequate pain relief within 1 hour, give 1-2 mg, maximum dose: 10 mg/24 hours
    Intrathecal ($\frac{1}{10}$ of epidural dose): 0.2-1 mg/dose; repeat doses **not** recommended
    Rectal: 10-20 mg every 4 hours

Mechanism of Action Binds to opiate receptors in the CNS, causing inhibition of ascending pain pathways, altering the perception of and response to pain; produces generalized CNS depression

Local Anesthetic/Vasoconstrictor Precautions No information available to require special precautions

Effects on Dental Treatment >10% of patients experience dry mouth; anticholinergic side effects can cause a reduction of saliva production or secretion contributes to discomfort and dental disease (ie, caries, oral candidiasis and periodontal disease)

Other Adverse Effects
Cardiovascular: Flushing
Central nervous system: CNS depression, drowsiness, sedation
Endocrine & metabolic: Antidiuretic hormone release
Miscellaneous: Physical and psychological dependence

>10%:
    Cardiovascular: Palpitations, hypotension, bradycardia
    Central nervous system: Dizziness
    Gastrointestinal: Nausea, vomiting, constipation
    Local: Pain at injection site
    Neuromuscular & skeletal: Weakness
    Miscellaneous: Histamine release, sweating

1% to 10%:
    Central nervous system: Restlessness, headache, false feeling of well being, confusion
    Gastrointestinal: Anorexia, GI irritation, dry mouth, paralytic ileus
    Genitourinary: Decreased urination
    Neuromuscular & skeletal: Trembling
    Ocular: Vision problems
    Respiratory: Respiratory depression, dyspnea

<1%:
    Cardiovascular: Peripheral vasodilation
    Central nervous system: Insomnia, mental depression, hallucinations, paradoxical CNS stimulation
    Dermatologic: Pruritus
    Gastrointestinal: Biliary spasm
    Genitourinary: Urinary tract spasm
    Neuromuscular & skeletal: Muscle rigidity
    Ocular: Miosis

Drug Interactions
Decreased effect: Phenothiazines may antagonize the analgesic effect of morphine and other opiate agonists
(Continued)

Morphine Sulfate *(Continued)*

Increased toxicity: CNS depressants, tricyclic antidepressants may potentiate the effects of morphine and other opiate agonists; dextroamphetamine may enhance the analgesic effect of morphine and other opiate agonists

Drug Uptake
Absorption: Oral: Variable
Serum half-life: Adults: 2-4 hours

Pregnancy Risk Factor B (D if used for prolonged periods or in high doses at term)

Generic Available Yes

Morrhuate Sodium *(MOR yoo ate SOW dee um)*

Brand Names Scleromate™

Therapeutic Category Sclerosing Agent

Use Treatment of small, uncomplicated varicose veins of the lower extremities

Usual Dosage I.V.:
Children 1-18 years: Esophageal hemorrhage: 2, 3, or 4 mL of 5% repeated every 3-4 days until bleeding is controlled, then every 6 weeks until varices obliterated

Adults: 50-250 mg, repeated at 5- to 7-day intervals (50-100 mg for small veins, 150-250 mg for large veins)

Mechanism of Action Both varicose veins and esophageal varices are treated by the thrombotic action of morrhuate sodium. By causing inflammation of the vein's intima, a thrombus is formed. Occlusion secondary to the fibrous tissue and the thrombus results in the obliteration of the vein.

Local Anesthetic/Vasoconstrictor Precautions No information available to require special precautions

Effects on Dental Treatment No effects or complications reported

Other Adverse Effects
>10%:
Cardiovascular: Thrombosis, valvular incompetency
Dermatologic: Urticaria
Local: Burning at the site of injection, severe extravasation effects
<1%:
Cardiovascular: Vascular collapse
Central nervous system: Drowsiness, headache, dizziness
Gastrointestinal: Nausea, vomiting
Neuromuscular & skeletal: Weakness
Respiratory: Asthma
Miscellaneous: Anaphylaxis

Drug Interactions No data reported

Drug Uptake
Onset of action: ~5 minutes
Absorption: Most of the dose stays at the site of injection

Pregnancy Risk Factor C

Generic Available No

Mosco® Liquid [OTC] *see* Salicylic Acid *on page 853*

Motofen® *see* Difenoxin and Atropine *on page 311*

Motrin® *see* Ibuprofen *on page 495*

Motrin® IB [OTC] *see* Ibuprofen *on page 495*

Motrin® IB Sinus [OTC] *see* Pseudoephedrine and Ibuprofen *on page 821*

Mouthkote® Solution [OTC] *see* Saliva Substitute *on page 854*

Mouth Pain, Cold Sore, Canker Sore Products *see page 1183*

Mouthwash, Antiseptic

Related Information
Oral Bacterial Infections *on page 1059*
Oral Nonviral Soft Tissue Ulcerations or Erosions *on page 1070*
Oral Rinse Products *on page 1187*

Brand Names Cool Mint Listerine® Antiseptic [OTC]; Fresh Burst Listerine® Antiseptic [OTC]; Listerine® Antiseptic [OTC]

Therapeutic Category Antimicrobial Mouth Rinse; Antiplaque Agent; Mouthwash

Use Help prevent and reduce plaque and gingivitis; bad breath

Usual Dosage Rinse full strength for 30 seconds with 20 mL (2/3 fluid ounce or 4 teaspoonfuls) morning and night

Local Anesthetic/Vasoconstrictor Precautions No information available to require special precautions

Effects on Dental Treatment No effects or complications reported

Other Adverse Effects No data reported
Contraindications Known hypersensitivity to any of its components
Dosage Forms Rinse: 250 mL, 500 mL, 1000 mL
Comments
Active ingredients:
Listerine® Antiseptic: Thymol 0.064%, eucalyptus 0.092%, methyl salicylate 0.060%, menthol 0.042%, alcohol 26.9%, water, benzoic acid, poloxamer 407, sodium benzoate, caramel
Fresh Burst Listerine® Antiseptic: Thymol 0.064%, eucalyptus 0.092%, methyl salicylate 0.060%, menthol 0.042%, alcohol 26.9%, water, benzoic acid, poloxamer 407, sodium benzoate, flavoring, sodium, saccharin, sodium citrate, citric acid, D&C yellow #10, FD&C green #3
Cool Mint Listerine® Antiseptic: Thymol 0.064%, eucalyptus 0.092%, methyl salicylate 0.060%, menthol 0.042%, alcohol 26.9%, water, benzoic acid, poloxamer 407, sodium benzoate, flavoring, sodium, saccharin, sodium citrate, citric acid, FD&C green #3
The following information is endorsed on the label of the Listerine® products by the Council on Scientific Affairs, American Dental Association: "Listerine Antiseptic has been shown to help prevent and reduce supragingival plaque accumulation and gingivitis when used in a conscientiously applied program of oral hygiene and regular professional care. Its effect on periodontitis has not been determined."

4-MP *see* Fomepizole *on page 428*
6-MP *see* Mercaptopurine *on page 600*
M-R-VAX® II *see* Measles and Rubella Vaccines, Combined *on page 581*
MS Contin® Oral *see* Morphine Sulfate *on page 648*
MSIR® Oral *see* Morphine Sulfate *on page 648*
MS/L® *see* Morphine Sulfate *on page 648*
MS/S® *see* Morphine Sulfate *on page 648*
MTC *see* Mitomycin *on page 642*
M.T.E.-4® *see* Trace Metals *on page 948*
M.T.E.-5® *see* Trace Metals *on page 948*
M.T.E.-6® *see* Trace Metals *on page 948*
Muco-Fen-DM® *see* Guaifenesin and Dextromethorphan *on page 453*
Muco-Fen-LA® *see* Guaifenesin *on page 452*
Mucomyst® *see* Acetylcysteine *on page 29*
Mucoplex® [OTC] *see* Vitamin B Complex *on page 993*
Mucosil™ *see* Acetylcysteine *on page 29*
MulTE-PAK-4® *see* Trace Metals *on page 948*
MulTE-PAK-5® *see* Trace Metals *on page 948*
Multiple Sulfonamides *see* Sulfadiazine, Sulfamethazine, and Sulfamerazine *on page 892*
Multiple Vitamins *see* Vitamins, Multiple *on page 995*
Multitest CMI® *see* Skin Test Antigens, Multiple *on page 867*
Multivitamins/Fluoride *see* Vitamins, Multiple *on page 995*
Multi Vit® Drops [OTC] *see* Vitamins, Multiple *on page 995*
Mumps, Measles and Rubella Vaccines, Combined *see* Measles, Mumps, and Rubella Vaccines, Combined *on page 582*
Mumpsvax® *see* Mumps Virus Vaccine, Live, Attenuated *on this page*

Mumps Virus Vaccine, Live, Attenuated
(mumpz VYE rus vak SEEN, live, a ten YOO ate ed)
Brand Names Mumpsvax®
Therapeutic Category Vaccine, Live Virus
Use Mumps prophylaxis by promoting active immunity
Usual Dosage 1 vial (5000 units) S.C. in outer aspect of the upper arm, no booster
Local Anesthetic/Vasoconstrictor Precautions No information available to require special precautions
Effects on Dental Treatment No effects or complications reported
Other Adverse Effects
>10%: Local: Burning or stinging at injection site
1% to 10%:
Central nervous system: Fever ≤100°F
Dermatologic: Rash
Endocrine & metabolic: Parotitis
<1%:
Central nervous system: Convulsions, confusion, severe or continuing headache, fever >103°F
(Continued)

Mumps Virus Vaccine, Live, Attenuated *(Continued)*

Genitourinary: Orchitis in postpubescent and adult males
Hematologic: Thrombocytopenic purpura
Miscellaneous: Anaphylactic reactions

Drug Interactions Decreased effect with concurrent infection, immunoglobulin with in 1 month, other live vaccines with the exception of attenuated measles, rubella, or polio

Pregnancy Risk Factor X

Dosage Forms Injection: Single dose

Generic Available No

Comments Federal law requires that the date of administration, the vaccine manufacturer, lot number of vaccine, and the administering person's name, title and address be entered into the patient's permanent medical record

Mupirocin (myoo PEER oh sin)

Brand Names Bactroban®; Bactroban® Nasal

Canadian/Mexican Brand Names Mupiban® (Mexico)

Therapeutic Category Antibiotic, Topical

Use Topical treatment of impetigo due to *Staphylococcus aureus*, beta-hemolytic *Streptococcus* and *S. pyogenes*; intranasally for the eradication of nasal colonization with methicillin-resistant *Streptococcus aureus* in adult patients and healthcare workers during institutional outbreaks; eradication of nasal colonization with methicillin-resistant Staphylococcus aureus in adult patients and health care workers; use as part of a comprehensive infection control program to reduce the risk of infection among patients at high risk of methicillin-resistant S. aureus infection during institutional outbreaks of infections with this pathogen

Usual Dosage Children and Adults: Topical: Apply small amount to affected area 2-5 times/day for 5-14 days

Mechanism of Action Binds to bacterial isoleucyl transfer-RNA synthetase resulting in the inhibition of protein and RNA synthesis

Local Anesthetic/Vasoconstrictor Precautions No information available to require special precautions

Effects on Dental Treatment No effects or complications reported

Other Adverse Effects 1% to 10%:
Dermatologic: Pruritus, rash, erythema, dry skin
Local: Burning, stinging, pain, tenderness, swelling

Drug Interactions No data reported

Drug Uptake
Absorption: Topical: Penetrates the outer layers of the skin; systemic absorption minimal through intact skin
Serum half-life: 17-36 minutes

Pregnancy Risk Factor B

Generic Available No

Murine® Ear Drops [OTC] *see* Carbamide Peroxide *on page 175*

Murine® Plus Ophthalmic [OTC] *see* Tetrahydrozoline *on page 916*

Murine® Solution [OTC] *see* Artificial Tears *on page 87*

Muro 128® Ophthalmic [OTC] *see* Sodium Chloride *on page 870*

Murocel® Ophthalmic Solution [OTC] *see* Artificial Tears *on page 87*

Murocoll-2® Ophthalmic *see* Phenylephrine and Scopolamine *on page 754*

Muromonab-CD3 (myoo roe MOE nab see dee three)

Brand Names Orthoclone® OKT3

Canadian/Mexican Brand Names Orthoclone® OKT3 (Mexico)

Therapeutic Category Immunosuppressant Agent

Synonyms Monoclonal Antibody; OKT3

Use Treatment of acute allograft rejection in renal transplant patients; effective in reversing acute hepatic, cardiac, and bone marrow transplant rejection episodes resistant to conventional treatment

Usual Dosage I.V. (refer to individual protocols):
Children <30 kg: 2.5 mg/day once daily for 7-14 days
Children >30 kg: 5 mg/day once daily for 7-14 days
or
Children <12 years: 0.1 mg/kg/day once daily for 10-14 days
Children ≥12 years and Adults: 5 mg/day once daily for 10-14 days

Removal by dialysis: Molecular size of OKT_3 is 150,000 daltons; not dialyzed by most standard dialyzers; however, may be dialyzed by high flux dialysis; OKT_3 will be removed by plasmapheresis; administer following dialysis treatments

Mechanism of Action Reverses graft rejection by binding to T-cells and interfering with their function

Local Anesthetic/Vasoconstrictor Precautions No information available to require special precautions

Effects on Dental Treatment No effects or complications reported

Other Adverse Effects

>10%:
    Cardiovascular: Tachycardia, faintness
    Central nervous system: Dizziness
    Gastrointestinal: Diarrhea, nausea, vomiting
    Neuromuscular & skeletal: Trembling
    Respiratory: Dyspnea

1% to 10%:
    Central nervous system: Headache
    Neuromuscular & skeletal: Stiff neck
    Ocular: Photophobia
    Respiratory: Pulmonary edema

<1%:
    Cardiovascular: Hypertension, hypotension, chest pain, tightness in chest
    Central nervous system: Aseptic meningitis, seizures, fatigue, confusion, coma, hallucinations, pyrexia
    Dermatologic: Pruritus, rash
    Neuromuscular & skeletal: Arthralgia, tremor
    Renal: Elevated BUN/creatinine
    Respiratory: Wheezing
    Miscellaneous: Flu-like symptoms (ie, fever, chills), infection, anaphylactic-type reactions

Drug Uptake

Absorption: I.V.: Immediate
Time to steady-state: Trough level: 3-14 days; pretreatment levels are restored within 7 days after treatment is terminated

Pregnancy Risk Factor C

Generic Available No

Comments Recommend decreasing dose of prednisone to 0.5 mg/kg, azathioprine to 0.5 mg/kg (approximate 50% decrease in dose), and discontinuing cyclosporine while patient is receiving OKT_3

Muroptic-5® [OTC] see Sodium Chloride on page 870

Muse® Pellet see Alprostadil on page 44

Mutamycin® see Mitomycin on page 642

M.V.I.® see Vitamins, Multiple on page 995

M.V.I.®-12 see Vitamins, Multiple on page 995

M.V.I.® Concentrate see Vitamins, Multiple on page 995

M.V.I.® Pediatric see Vitamins, Multiple on page 995

Myambutol® see Ethambutol on page 372

Mycelex® Troche see Clotrimazole on page 252

Mycifradin® Sulfate see Neomycin on page 670

Mycinettes® [OTC] see Benzocaine on page 118

Mycitracin® Topical [OTC] see Bacitracin, Neomycin, and Polymyxin B on page 108

Mycobutin® see Rifabutin on page 842

Mycogen II Topical see Nystatin and Triamcinolone on page 695

Mycolog®-II Topical see Nystatin and Triamcinolone on page 695

Myconel® Topical see Nystatin and Triamcinolone on page 695

Mycophenolate (mye koe FEN oh late)

Brand Names CellCept®

Therapeutic Category Immunosuppressant Agent

Use Immunosuppressant used with corticosteroids and cyclosporine to prevent organ rejection in patients receiving allogenic renal transplants

Usual Dosage Oral:
    Children: Doses of 15-23 mg/kg given twice daily have been used, further studies are necessary
    Adults: 1 g twice daily within 72 hours of transplant (although 3 g/day has been given in some clinical trials, there was decreased tolerability and no efficacy advantage)

Mechanism of Action Inhibition of purine synthesis of human lymphocytes and proliferation of human lymphocytes

Local Anesthetic/Vasoconstrictor Precautions No information available to require special precautions

Effects on Dental Treatment No effects or complications reported

Other Adverse Effects See table.

(Continued)

653

Mycophenolate *(Continued)*

Adverse Reactions Reported in >10%

Adverse Reaction	MM 2 g/day	MM 3 g/day
Body as a Whole		
Pain	33	31.2
Abdominal pain	12.1-24.7	11.9-27.6
Fever	20.4	23.3
Headache	20.1	16.1
Infection	12.7-18.2	15.6-20.9
Sepsis	17.6-20.8	17.5-19.7
Asthenia	13.7	16.1
Chest pain	13.4	13.3
Back pain	11.6	12.1
Hypertension	17.6-32.4	16.9-28.2
Central Nervous System		
Tremor	11	11.8
Insomnia	8.9	11.8
Dizziness	5.7	11.2
Dermatologic		
Acne	10.1	9.7
Rash	7.7	6.4
Gastrointestinal		
Diarrhea	16.4-31	18.8-36.1
Constipation	21.9	18.5
Nausea	19.9	23.6
Dyspepsia	17.6	13.6
Vomiting	12.5	13.6
Nausea & vomiting	10.4	9.7
Oral monoliasis	10.1	12.1
Hemic/Lymphatic		
Anemia	25.6	25.8
Leukopenia	11.5-23.2	16.3-34.5
Thrombocytopenia	10.1	8.2
Hypochromic anemia	7.4	11.5
Leukocytosis	7.1	10.9
Metabolic/Nutritional		
Peripheral edema	28.6	27
Hypercholesterolemia	12.8	8.5
Hypophosphatemia	12.5	15.8
Edema	12.2	11.8
Hypokalemia	10.1	10
Hyperkalemia	8.9	10.3
Hyperglycemia	8.6	12.4
Respiratory		
Infection	15.8-21	13.1-23.9
Dyspnea	15.5	17.3
Cough increase	15.5	13.3
Pharyngitis	9.5	11.2
Bronchitis	8.5	11.9
Pneumonia	3.6	10.6
Urogenital		
UTI	37.2-45.5	37-44.4
Hematuria	14	12.1
Kidney tubular necrosis	6.3	10
Urinary tract disorder	6.7	10.6

Drug Interactions
Decreased effect: Antacids and cholestyramine decrease serum levels of mycophenolate

Increased toxicity: Acyclovir and ganciclovir levels may elevate due to competition for tubular secretion of these drugs; probenecid may elevate mycophenolate levels due to inhibition of tubular secretion; salicylates: high doses may increase free fraction of mycophenolic acid

Drug Uptake
Absorption: Mycophenolate mofetil is hydrolyzed to mycophenolic acid in the liver and gastrointestinal tract; food does not alter the extent of absorption, but the maximum concentration is decreased
Serum half-life: 18 hours
Serum concentrations: Correlation of toxicity or efficacy is still being developed, however, one study indicated that 12-hour AUCs of >40 mcg/mL/hour were correlated with efficacy and decreased episodes of rejection

Pregnancy Risk Factor C
Dosage Forms Capsule, as mofetil: 250 mg
Generic Available No

Mycostatin® see Nystatin on page 695

Myco-Triacet® II see Nystatin and Triamcinolone on page 695

Mydfrin® Ophthalmic Solution see Phenylephrine on page 752

Mydriacyl® see Tropicamide on page 973

Mykrox® see Metolazone on page 629

Mylanta® [OTC] see Aluminum Hydroxide, Magnesium Hydroxide, and Simethicone on page 49

Mylanta Gas® [OTC] see Simethicone on page 865

Mylanta® Gelcaps® see Calcium Carbonate and Magnesium Carbonate on page 163

Mylanta®-II [OTC] see Aluminum Hydroxide, Magnesium Hydroxide, and Simethicone on page 49

Myleran® see Busulfan on page 152

Mylicon® [OTC] see Simethicone on page 865

Mylosar® see Azacitidine on page 101

Myminic® Expectorant [OTC] see Guaifenesin and Phenylpropanolamine on page 454

Myoflex® [OTC] see Triethanolamine Salicylate on page 960

Myotonachol™ see Bethanechol on page 128

Myphetane DC® see Brompheniramine, Phenylpropanolamine, and Codeine on page 145

Mysoline® see Primidone on page 794

Mytelase® Caplets® see Ambenonium on page 51

Mytrex® F Topical see Nystatin and Triamcinolone on page 695

Mytussin® [OTC] see Guaifenesin on page 452

Mytussin® AC see Guaifenesin and Codeine on page 452

Mytussin® DAC see Guaifenesin, Pseudoephedrine, and Codeine on page 455

Mytussin® DM [OTC] see Guaifenesin and Dextromethorphan on page 453

Nabilone (NA bi lone)
Brand Names Cesamet®
Therapeutic Category Antiemetic
Use Treatment of nausea and vomiting associated with cancer chemotherapy
Usual Dosage Oral:
Children >4 years:
<18 kg: 0.5 mg twice daily
18-30 kg: 1 mg twice daily
>30 kg: 1 mg 3 times/day

Adults: 1-2 mg twice daily beginning 1-3 hours before chemotherapy is administered and continuing around-the-clock until 1 dose after chemotherapy is completed; maximum daily dose: 6 mg divided in 3 doses

Mechanism of Action Nabilone is a synthetic cannabinoid utilized as an antiemetic drug in the control of nausea and vomiting in patients receiving cancer chemotherapy; like delta-9-tetrahydrocannabinol (the active principal of marijuana), nabilone is a dibenzo(b,d)pyrans

Local Anesthetic/Vasoconstrictor Precautions No information available to require special precautions

Effects on Dental Treatment >10% of patients experience dry mouth
Other Adverse Effects
>10%: Central nervous system: Dizziness, drowsiness, vertigo, euphoria, clumsiness
1% to 10%:
Cardiovascular: Orthostatic hypotension
Central nervous system: Depression
(Continued)

Nabilone *(Continued)*

Ocular: Blurred vision

<1%:

Central nervous system: Changes of mood, confusion, hallucinations, headache

Gastrointestinal: Loss of appetite

Respiratory: Dyspnea

Drug Interactions No data reported

Drug Uptake

Absorption: Rapid

Serum half-life: 35 hours

Pregnancy Risk Factor C

Generic Available No

Nabumetone (na BYOO me tone)

Related Information

Nonsteroidal Anti-Inflammatory Agents, Comparative Dosages, and Pharmacokinetics *on page 1143*

Rheumatoid Arthritis and Osteoarthritis *on page 1030*

Brand Names Relafen®

Therapeutic Category Nonsteroidal Anti-inflammatory Agent (NSAID), Oral

Use Management of osteoarthritis and rheumatoid arthritis

Unlabeled use: Sunburn, mild to moderate pain

Usual Dosage Adults: Oral: 1000 mg/day; an additional 500-1000 mg may be needed in some patients to obtain more symptomatic relief; may be administered once or twice daily

Mechanism of Action Nabumetone is a nonacidic, nonsteroidal anti-inflammatory drug that is rapidly metabolized after absorption to a major active metabolite, 6-methoxy-2-naphthylacetic acid. As found with previous nonsteroidal anti-inflammatory drugs, nabumetone's active metabolite inhibits the cyclooxygenase enzyme which is indirectly responsible for the production of inflammation and pain during arthritis by way of enhancing the production of endoperoxides and prostaglandins E_2 and I_2 (prostacyclin). The active metabolite of nabumetone is felt to be the compound primarily responsible for therapeutic effect. Comparatively, the parent drug is a poor inhibitor of prostaglandin synthesis.

Local Anesthetic/Vasoconstrictor Precautions No information available to require special precautions

Effects on Dental Treatment No effects or complications reported

Other Adverse Effects

>10%:

Central nervous system: Dizziness

Dermatologic: Skin rash

Gastrointestinal: Abdominal cramps, heartburn, indigestion, nausea

1% to 10%:

Central nervous system: Headache, nervousness

Dermatologic: Itching

Endocrine & metabolic: Fluid retention

Gastrointestinal: Vomiting

Otic: Tinnitus

<1%:

Cardiovascular: Congestive heart failure, hypertension, arrhythmia, tachycardia

Central nervous system: Confusion, hallucinations, aseptic meningitis, mental depression, drowsiness, insomnia

Dermatologic: Angioedema, urticaria, erythema multiforme, toxic epidermal necrolysis, Stevens-Johnson syndrome

Endocrine & metabolic: Polydipsia, hot flashes

Gastrointestinal: Gastritis, GI ulceration

Genitourinary: Cystitis

Hematologic: Agranulocytosis, anemia, hemolytic anemia, bone marrow suppression, leukopenia, thrombocytopenia

Hepatic: Hepatitis

Neuromuscular & skeletal: Peripheral neuropathy

Ocular: Toxic amblyopia, blurred vision, conjunctivitis, dry eyes

Otic: Decreased hearing

Renal: Polyuria, acute renal failure

Respiratory: Allergic rhinitis, dyspnea, epistaxis

Drug Interactions No data reported

Drug Uptake

Serum half-life, elimination: Major metabolite: 24 hours

Time to peak serum concentration: Metabolite: Oral: Within 3-6 hours
Pregnancy Risk Factor C
Generic Available No

NaCl *see* Sodium Chloride *on page 870*

Nadolol (nay DOE lole)

Related Information
Cardiovascular Diseases *on page 1010*

Brand Names Corgard®

Canadian/Mexican Brand Names Apo®-Nadol (Canada); Syn-Nadolol® (Canada)

Therapeutic Category Antianginal Agent; Beta-adrenergic Blocker, Noncardioselective

Use Treatment of hypertension and angina pectoris; prevention of myocardial infarction; prophylaxis of migraine headaches

Usual Dosage Oral:

Children: No information regarding pediatric dosage is currently available in the literature

Adults: Initial: 40-80 mg/day, increase dosage gradually by 40-80 mg increments at 3- to 7-day intervals until optimum clinical response is obtained with profound slowing of heart rate; doses up to 160-240 mg/day in angina and 240-320 mg/day in hypertension may be necessary; doses as high as 640 mg/day have been used

Elderly: Initial: 20 mg/day; increase doses by 20 mg increments at 3- to 7-day intervals; usual dosage range: 20-240 mg/day

Mechanism of Action Competitively blocks response to beta$_1$- and beta$_2$-adrenergic stimulation; does not exhibit any membrane stabilizing or intrinsic sympathomimetic activity

Local Anesthetic/Vasoconstrictor Precautions Use with caution; epinephrine has interacted with nonselective beta-blockers to result in initial hypertensive episode followed by bradycardia

Effects on Dental Treatment Noncardioselective beta-blockers (ie, propranolol, nadolol) may enhance the pressor response to epinephrine, resulting in hypertension and bradycardia. Many nonsteroidal anti-inflammatory drugs such as ibuprofen and indomethacin can reduce the hypotensive effect of beta-blockers after 3 or more weeks of therapy with the NSAID. Short-term NSAID use (ie, 3 days) requires no special precautions in patients taking beta-blockers.

Other Adverse Effects
>10%: Cardiovascular: Bradycardia
1% to 10%:
Cardiovascular: Reduced peripheral circulation
Central nervous system: Mental depression, dizziness
Endocrine & metabolic: Decreased sexual ability
Gastrointestinal: Constipation
Neuromuscular & skeletal: Weakness
Respiratory: Dyspnea, wheezing
<1%:
Cardiovascular: Congestive heart failure, chest pain, orthostatic hypotension, edema, Raynaud's phenomenon
Central nervous system: Drowsiness, nightmares, vivid dreams, insomnia, lethargy, fatigue, confusion, headache
Dermatologic: Itching, rash
Gastrointestinal: Vomiting, stomach discomfort, diarrhea, nausea
Genitourinary: Impotence
Hematologic: Thrombocytopenia
Neuromuscular & skeletal: Paresthesia
Ocular: Dry eyes
Respiratory: Nasal congestion
Miscellaneous: Cold extremities

Drug Interactions
Decreased effect of beta-blockers:
Barbiturates (increased liver metabolism of beta-blockers to result in lower serum levels)
NSAIDs (attenuate the hypotensive therapeutic effects of beta-blockers)
Rifampin (increased liver metabolism of beta-blockers to result in lower serum levels)
Increased effects of beta-blockers:
Calcium channel blockers (increase serum levels of beta-blockers by unknown mechanism to enhance hypotension)
(Continued)

Nadolol *(Continued)*

Beta-blockers increase the effects of:
Epinephrine (vasoconstrictor; initial hypertensive episode followed by brady-cardia) only from noncardioselective type beta-blockers
Phenylephrine (Neosynephrine®; enhanced pressor response)
Theophylline (inhibit theophylline metabolism causing increase in serum concentrations)

Drug Uptake
Duration of effect: 24 hours
Absorption: Oral: 30% to 40%
Time to peak serum concentration: Within 2-4 hours persisting for 17-24 hours
Serum half-life: Adults: 10-24 hours; increased half-life with decreased renal function
End stage renal disease: 45 hours
Pregnancy Risk Factor C
Generic Available Yes

Nafarelin *(NAF a re lin)*

Brand Names Synarel®
Therapeutic Category Hormone, Posterior Pituitary; Luteinizing Hormone-Releasing Hormone Analog
Use Treatment of endometriosis, including pain and reduction of lesions; treatment of central precocious puberty (gonadotropin-dependent precocious puberty) in children of both sexes
Usual Dosage
Endometriosis: Adults: Female: 1 spray (200 mcg) in 1 nostril each morning and the other nostril each evening starting on days 2-4 of menstrual cycle for 6 months
Central precocious puberty: Children: Males/Females: 2 sprays (400 mcg) into each nostril in the morning 2 sprays (400 mcg) into each nostril in the evening. If inadequate suppression, may increase dose to 3 sprays (600 mcg) into alternating nostrils 3 times/day.
Mechanism of Action Potent synthetic decapeptide analogue of gonadotropin-releasing hormone (GnRH; LHRH) which is approximately 200 times more potent than GnRH in terms of pituitary release of luteinizing hormone (LH) and follicle-stimulating hormone (FSH). Effects on the pituitary gland and sex hormones are dependent upon its length of administration. After acute administration, an initial stimulation of the release of LH and FSH from the pituitary is observed; an increase in androgens and estrogens subsequently follows. Continued administration of nafarelin, however, suppresses gonadotrope responsiveness to endogenous GnRH resulting in reduced secretion of LH and FSH and, secondarily, decreased ovarian and testicular steroid production.
Local Anesthetic/Vasoconstrictor Precautions No information available to require special precautions
Effects on Dental Treatment No effects or complications reported
Other Adverse Effects
>10%:
Central nervous system: Headache, emotional lability
Dermatologic: Acne
Endocrine & metabolic: Hot flashes, decreased libido, decreased breast size
Genitourinary: Vaginal dryness
Neuromuscular & skeletal: Myalgia
Respiratory: Nasal irritation
1% to 10%:
Cardiovascular: Edema
Central nervous system: Insomnia
Dermatologic: Urticaria, rash, pruritus, seborrhea
Respiratory: Dyspnea, chest pain
<1%:
Endocrine & metabolic: Increased libido
Gastrointestinal: Weight loss
Drug Interactions No data reported
Drug Uptake
Absorption: Not absorbed from GI tract
Maximum serum concentration: 10-45 minutes
Pregnancy Risk Factor X
Generic Available No

Nafazair® Ophthalmic *see* Naphazoline *on page 664*
Nafazolina, Clorhidrato De (Mexico) *see* Naphazoline *on page 664*
Nafcil™ *see* Nafcillin *on next page*

Nafcillin (naf SIL in)

Brand Names Nafcil™; Nallpen®; Unipen®

Therapeutic Category Antibiotic, Penicillin

Use Treatment of susceptible bacterial infections such as osteomyelitis, septicemia, endocarditis, and CNS infections due to penicillinase-producing strains of *Staphylococcus*

Usual Dosage
Children: I.M., I.V.:
Mild to moderate infections: 50-100 mg/kg/day in divided doses every 6 hours
Severe infections: 100-200 mg/kg/day in divided doses every 4-6 hours
Maximum dose: 12 g/day
Adults:
I.M.: 500 mg every 4-6 hours
I.V.: 500-2000 mg every 4-6 hours

Mechanism of Action Interferes with bacterial cell wall synthesis during active multiplication, causing cell wall death and resultant bactericidal activity against susceptible bacteria

Local Anesthetic/Vasoconstrictor Precautions No information available to require special precautions

Effects on Dental Treatment Prolonged use of penicillins may lead to the development of oral candidiasis

Other Adverse Effects <1%:
Central nervous system: Fever, pain
Dermatologic: Skin rash
Gastrointestinal: Nausea, diarrhea
Hematologic: Neutropenia
Local: Thrombophlebitis; oxacillin (less likely to cause phlebitis) is often preferred in pediatric patients
Renal: Acute interstitial nephritis
Miscellaneous: Hypersensitivity reactions

Drug Interactions
Decreased effect: Chloramphenicol may decrease nafcillin levels; oral contraceptive may have a decreased effectiveness
Increased effect: Probenecid may increase nafcillin levels
Increased toxicity: Oral anticoagulants, heparin increase risk of bleeding

Drug Uptake
Absorption: Oral: Poor and erratic
Serum half-life:
Adults: 0.5-1.5 hours, with normal hepatic function
End stage renal disease: 1.2 hours
Time to peak serum concentration:
Oral: Within 2 hours
I.M.: Within 0.5-1 hour

Pregnancy Risk Factor B

Generic Available Yes

Naftifine (NAF ti feen)

Brand Names Naftin®

Therapeutic Category Antifungal Agent, Topical

Use Topical treatment of tinea cruris (jock itch), tinea corporis (ring worm), and tinea pedis (athlete's foot)

Usual Dosage Adults: Topical: Apply cream once daily and gel twice daily (morning and evening) for up to 4 weeks

Mechanism of Action Synthetic, broad-spectrum antifungal agent in the allylamine class; appears to have both fungistatic and fungicidal activity. Exhibits antifungal activity by selectively inhibiting the enzyme squalene epoxidase in a dose-dependent manner which results in the primary sterol, ergosterol, within the fungal membrane not being synthesized.

Local Anesthetic/Vasoconstrictor Precautions No information available to require special precautions

Effects on Dental Treatment No effects or complications reported

Other Adverse Effects
>10%: Local: Burning, stinging
1% to 10%: Local: Dryness, erythema, itching, irritation

Drug Interactions No data reported

Drug Uptake
Absorption: Systemic, 6% for cream, ≤4% for gel
Serum half-life: 2-3 days

Pregnancy Risk Factor B

Generic Available No

Naftin® see Naftifine on previous page
NaHCO₃ see Sodium Bicarbonate on page 869
Nalbufina, Clorhidrato De (Mexico) see Nalbuphine on this page

Nalbuphine (NAL byoo feen)
Related Information
Narcotic Agonists on page 1141.
Brand Names Nubain®
Therapeutic Category Analgesic, Narcotic
Synonyms Nalbufina, Clorhidrato De (Mexico)
Use Relief of moderate to severe pain; preoperative analgesia, postoperative and surgical anesthesia, and obstetrical analgesia during labor and delivery
Usual Dosage I.M., I.V., S.C.:
Children 10 months to 14 years: Premedication: 0.2 mg/kg; maximum: 20 mg/dose

Adults: 10 mg/70 kg every 3-6 hours; maximum single dose: 20 mg; maximum daily dose: 160 mg
Mechanism of Action Binds to opiate receptors in the CNS, causing inhibition of ascending pain pathways, altering the perception of and response to pain; produces generalized CNS depression
Local Anesthetic/Vasoconstrictor Precautions No information available to require special precautions
Effects on Dental Treatment Anticholinergic side effects can cause a reduction of saliva production or secretion contributes to discomfort and dental disease (ie, caries, oral candidiasis and periodontal disease)
Other Adverse Effects
>10%:
Central nervous system: Drowsiness, CNS depression
Miscellaneous: Histamine release, narcotic withdrawal
1% to 10%:
Cardiovascular: Hypotension, flushing
Central nervous system: Dry mouth, dizziness, headache
Dermatologic: Urticaria, skin rash
Gastrointestinal: Nausea, vomiting, anorexia
Local: Pain at injection site
Neuromuscular & skeletal: Weakness
Respiratory: Pulmonary edema
<1%:
Cardiovascular: Hypertension, tachycardia
Central nervous system: Mental depression, hallucinations, confusion, paradoxical CNS stimulation, nervousness, restlessness, nightmares, insomnia
Gastrointestinal: GI irritation, ureteral spasm, biliary spasm, toxic megacolon
Genitourinary: Decreased urination
Ocular: Blurred vision
Respiratory: Dyspnea, respiratory depression
Drug Interactions Increased toxicity: Barbiturate anesthetics cause increased CNS depression
Drug Uptake Serum half-life: 3.5-5 hours
Pregnancy Risk Factor B (D if used for prolonged periods or in high doses at term)
Generic Available Yes

Naldecon® see Chlorpheniramine, Phenyltoloxamine, Phenylpropanolamine, and Phenylephrine on page 222
Naldecon® DX Adult Liquid [OTC] see Guaifenesin, Phenylpropanolamine, and Dextromethorphan on page 455
Naldecon-EX® Children's Syrup [OTC] see Guaifenesin and Phenylpropanolamine on page 454
Naldecon® Senior DX [OTC] see Guaifenesin and Dextromethorphan on page 453
Naldecon® Senior EX [OTC] see Guaifenesin on page 452
Naldelate® see Chlorpheniramine, Phenyltoloxamine, Phenylpropanolamine, and Phenylephrine on page 222
Nalfon® see Fenoprofen on page 398
Nalgest® see Chlorpheniramine, Phenyltoloxamine, Phenylpropanolamine, and Phenylephrine on page 222

Nalidixic Acid (nal i DIKS ik AS id)
Brand Names NegGram®
Therapeutic Category Antibiotic, Quinolone
Synonyms Nalidixio Acido (Mexico)

Use Treatment of urinary tract infections

Usual Dosage Oral:

Children 3 months to 12 years: 55 mg/kg/day divided every 6 hours; suppressive therapy is 33 mg/kg/day divided every 6 hours

Adults: 1 g 4 times/day for 2 weeks; then suppressive therapy of 500 mg 4 times/day

Mechanism of Action Inhibits. DNA polymerization in late stages of chromosomal replication　·

Local Anesthetic/Vasoconstrictor Precautions No information available to require special precautions

Effects on Dental Treatment No effects or complications reported

Other Adverse Effects

>10%: Central nervous system: Dizziness, drowsiness, headache

1% to 10%: Gastrointestinal: Nausea, vomiting

<1%:

Central nervous system: Increased intracranial pressure, malaise, vertigo, confusion, toxic psychosis, convulsions, fever, chills

Dermatologic: Rash, urticaria, photosensitivity reactions

Endocrine & metabolic: Metabolic acidosis

Hematologic: Leukopenia, thrombocytopenia

Hepatic: Hepatotoxicity

Ocular: Visual disturbances

Drug Interactions

Decreased effect with antacids

Increased effect of warfarin

Drug Uptake

Serum half-life: 6-7 hours; increases significantly with renal impairment

Time to peak serum concentration: Oral: Within 1-2 hours

Pregnancy Risk Factor B

Generic Available Yes

Nalidixio Acido (Mexico) *see* Nalidixic Acid *on previous page*

Nallpen® *see* Nafcillin *on page 659*

Nalmefene (NAL me feen)

Brand Names Revex®

Therapeutic Category Antidote for Narcotic Agonists

Use Complete or partial of opioid drug effects; management of known or suspected opioid overdose

Usual Dosage

Reversal of postoperative opioid depression: Blue labeled product (100 mcg/mL): Titrate to reverse the undesired effects of opioids; initial dose for nonopioid dependent patients: 0.25 mcg/kg followed by 0.25 mcg/kg incremental doses at 2- to 5-minute intervals; after a total dose of >1 mcg/kg, further therapeutic response is unlikely

Management of known/suspected opioid overdose: Green labeled product (1000 mcg/mL): Initial dose: 0.5 mg/70 kg; may repeat with 1 mg/70 kg in 2-5 minutes; further increase beyond a total dose of 1.5 mg/70 kg will not likely result in improved response and may result in cardiovascular stress and precipitated withdrawal syndrome. (If opioid dependency is suspected, administer a challenge dose of 0.1 mg/70 kg; if no withdrawal symptoms are observed in 2 minutes, the recommended doses can be administered.)

Local Anesthetic/Vasoconstrictor Precautions No information available to require special precautions

Effects on Dental Treatment No effects or complications reported

Other Adverse Effects

>10%: Gastrointestinal: Nausea

1% to 10%:

Cardiovascular: Tachycardia, hypertension

Central nervous system: Postoperative pain, fever, dizziness

Gastrointestinal: Vomiting

<1%:

Cardiovascular: Hypotension, vasodilation, arrhythmia

Central nervous system: Headache, chills, nervousness, confusion

Gastrointestinal: Diarrhea, dry mouth

Genitourinary: Urinary retention

Neuromuscular & skeletal: Tremor

Miscellaneous: Withdrawal syndrome

Drug Uptake

Onset of action: I.M., S.C.: 5-15 minutes

Serum half-life: 10.8 hours

(Continued)

Nalmefene *(Continued)*

Time to peak serum concentration: 2.3 hours

Pregnancy Risk Factor B

Generic Available No

Comments Nalmefene is supplied in two concentrations 100 mcg/mL has a blue label, 1000 mcg/mL has a green label; proper steps should be used to prevent use of the incorrect dosage strength; duration of action of nalmefene is as long as most opioid analgesics; may cause acute withdrawal symptoms in individuals who have some degree of tolerance to and dependence on opioids

Naloxone *(nal OKS one)*

Related Information

Narcotic Agonists *on page 1141*

Brand Names Narcan®

Therapeutic Category Narcotic Antagonist

Use

Dental: Reverses CNS and respiratory depressant effects of fentanyl and meperidine during I.V. conscious state

Medical: Reverses CNS and respiratory depression in suspected narcotic overdose; neonatal opiate depression; coma of unknown etiology

Usual Dosage Adults: Narcotic overdose: I.V.: 0.4-2 mg every 2-3 minutes as needed; may need to repeat doses every 20-60 minutes, if no response is observed after 10 mg, question the diagnosis. **Note:** Use 0.1-0.2 mg increments in patients who are opioid-dependent and in postoperative patients to avoid large cardiovascular changes.

Mechanism of Action Competes and displaces narcotics at narcotic receptor sites (mu, kappa, delta, and sigma subtypes)

Local Anesthetic/Vasoconstrictor Precautions No information available to require special precautions

Effects on Dental Treatment No effects or complications reported

Other Adverse Effects 1% to 10%:

Cardiovascular: Hypertension, hypotension, tachycardia, ventricular arrhythmias

Central nervous system: Insomnia, irritability, anxiety

Dermatologic: Rash

Gastrointestinal: Nausea, vomiting

Ocular: Blurred vision

Miscellaneous: Narcotic withdrawal, sweating

Contraindications Hypersensitivity to naloxone or any component

Warnings/Precautions Use with caution in patients with cardiovascular disease; excessive dosages should be avoided after use of opiates in surgery, because naloxone may cause an increase in blood pressure and reversal of anesthesia; may precipitate withdrawal symptoms in patients addicted to opiates, including pain, hypertension, sweating, agitation, irritability, shrill cry, failure to feed

Drug Interactions Decreased effect of narcotic analgesics

Drug Uptake

Onset of effect: I.V.: Within 2 minutes

Duration of effect: 20-60 minutes; since shorter than that of most opioids, repeated doses are usually needed

Time to peak serum concentration: 5-15 minutes

Serum half-life: 1-1.5 hours

Pregnancy Risk Factor B

Breast-feeding Considerations No data reported

Dosage Forms Injection: 0.02 mg/mL (2 mL); 0.4 mg/mL (1 mL, 2 mL, 10 mL); 1 mg/mL (2 mL, 10 mL)

Dietary Considerations No data reported

Generic Available Yes

Comments Naloxone is an antagonist to all narcotic analgesics. Its use in dental practice is to reverse overdose effects of the two narcotic agents fentanyl and meperidine, used in the technique of I.V. conscious sedation.

Nalspan® *see* Chlorpheniramine, Phenyltoloxamine, Phenylpropanolamine, and Phenylephrine *on page 222*

Naltrexone *(nal TREKS one)*

Brand Names ReVia™ Oral

Therapeutic Category Narcotic Antagonist

Use Adjunct to the maintenance of an opioid-free state in detoxified individual

Usual Dosage Do not give until patient is opioid-free for 7-10 days as required by urine analysis

Adults: Oral: 25 mg; if no withdrawal signs within 1 hour give another 25 mg; maintenance regimen is flexible, variable and individualized (50 mg/day to 100-150 mg 3 times/week)

Mechanism of Action Naltrexone is a cyclopropyl derivative of oxymorphone similar in structure to naloxone and nalorphine (a morphine derivative); it acts as a competitive antagonist at opioid receptor sites

Local Anesthetic/Vasoconstrictor Precautions No information available to require special precautions

Effects on Dental Treatment No effects or complications reported

Other Adverse Effects

>10%:

Central nervous system: Insomnia, nervousness, headache

Gastrointestinal: Abdominal cramping, nausea, vomiting

Neuromuscular & skeletal: Arthralgia

1% to 10%:

Central nervous system: Dizziness

Dermatologic: Skin rash

Gastrointestinal: Anorexia

Endocrine & metabolic: Polydipsia

Respiratory: Sneezing

<1%:

Central nervous system: Irritability, anxiety

Hematologic: Thrombocytopenia, agranulocytosis, hemolytic anemia

Ocular: Blurred vision

Miscellaneous: Narcotic withdrawal

Drug Interactions No data reported

Drug Uptake

Duration of action:

50 mg: 24 hours

100 mg: 48 hours

150 mg: 72 hours

Absorption: Oral: Almost completely

Serum half-life: 4 hours; 6-β-naltrexol: 13 hours

Time to peak serum concentration: Within 60 minutes

Pregnancy Risk Factor C

Generic Available No

Nandrolone (NAN droe lone)

Brand Names Anabolin® Injection; Androlone®-D Injection; Androlone® Injection; Deca-Durabolin® Injection; Hybolin™ Decanoate Injection; Hybolin™ Improved Injection; Neo-Durabolic Injection

Therapeutic Category Androgen

Use Control of metastatic breast cancer; management of anemia of renal insufficiency

Usual Dosage Deep I.M. (into gluteal muscle):

Children 2-13 years: (decanoate): 25-50 mg every 3-4 weeks

Adults:

Male:

Breast cancer (phenpropionate): 50-100 mg/week

Anemia of renal insufficiency (decanoate): 100-200 mg/week

Female: 50-100 mg/week

Breast cancer (phenproprionate): 50-100 mg/week

Anemia of renal insufficiency (decanoate): 50-100 mg/week

Mechanism of Action Promotes tissue-building processes, increases production of erythropoietin, causes protein anabolism; increases hemoglobin and red blood cell volume

Local Anesthetic/Vasoconstrictor Precautions No information available to require special precautions

Effects on Dental Treatment No effects or complications reported

Other Adverse Effects

Male:

Postpubertal:

>10%:

Dermatologic: Acne

Endocrine & metabolic: Gynecomastia

Genitourinary: Bladder irritability, priapism

1% to 10%:

Central nervous system: Insomnia, chills

Endocrine & metabolic: Decreased libido

Gastrointestinal: Nausea, diarrhea

Genitourinary: Prostatic hypertrophy (elderly)

Hematologic: Iron deficiency anemia, suppression of clotting factors

(Continued)

Nandrolone *(Continued)*

  Hepatic: Hepatic dysfunction
  <1%:
  Hepatic: Hepatic necrosis, hepatocellular carcinoma
 Prepubertal:
  >10%:
   Dermatologic: Acne
   Endocrine & metabolic: Virilism
  1% to 10%:
   Central nervous system: Chills, insomnia
   Dermatologic: Hyperpigmentation
   Gastrointestinal: Diarrhea, nausea
   Hematologic: Iron deficiency anemia, suppression of clotting
  <1%: Hepatic: necrosis, hepatocellular carcinoma

 Female:
  >10%: Endocrine & metabolic: Virilism
  1% to 10%:
   Central nervous system: Chills, insomnia
   Endocrine & metabolic: Hypercalcemia
   Gastrointestinal: Nausea, diarrhea
   Hematologic: Iron deficiency anemia, suppression of clotting factors
   Hepatic: Hepatic dysfunction
  <1%: Hepatic: Hepatic necrosis, hepatocellular carcinoma
Drug Interactions Increased toxicity: Oral anticoagulants, insulin, oral hypoglycemic agents, adrenal steroids, ACTH
Pregnancy Risk Factor X
Generic Available Yes

Naphazoline *(naf AZ oh leen)*

Brand Names AK-Con® Ophthalmic; Albalon® Liquifilm® Ophthalmic; Allerest® Eye Drops [OTC]; Clear Eyes® [OTC]; Comfort® Ophthalmic [OTC]; Degest® 2 Ophthalmic [OTC]; Estivin® II Ophthalmic [OTC]; I-Naphline® Ophthalmic; Nafazair® Ophthalmic; Naphcon Forte® Ophthalmic; Naphcon® Ophthalmic [OTC]; Opcon® Ophthalmic; Privine® Nasal [OTC]; VasoClear® Ophthalmic [OTC]; Vasocon Regular® Ophthalmic
Canadian/Mexican Brand Names Nazil® Ofteno (Mexico)
Therapeutic Category Adrenergic Agonist Agent, Ophthalmic; Decongestant, Nasal; Nasal Agent, Vasoconstrictor; Ophthalmic Agent, Vasoconstrictor
Synonyms Nafazolina, Clorhidrato De (Mexico)
Use Topical ocular vasoconstrictor; will temporarily relieve congestion, itching, and minor irritation, and to control hyperemia in patients with superficial corneal vascularity
Usual Dosage
 Nasal:
  Children:
   <6 years: Intranasal: Not recommended (especially infants) due to CNS depression
   6-12 years: 1 spray of 0.05% into each nostril every 6 hours if necessary; therapy should not exceed 3-5 days
  Children >12 years and Adults: 0.05%, instill 1-2 drops or sprays every 6 hours if needed; therapy should not exceed 3-5 days

 Ophthalmic:
  Children <6 years: Not recommended for use due to CNS depression (especially in infants)
  Children >6 years and Adults: Instill 1-2 drops into conjunctival sac of affected eye(s) every 3-4 hours; therapy generally should not exceed 3-4 days
Mechanism of Action Stimulates alpha-adrenergic receptors in the arterioles of the conjunctiva and the nasal mucosa to produce vasoconstriction
Local Anesthetic/Vasoconstrictor Precautions No information available to require special precautions
Effects on Dental Treatment No effects or complications reported
Other Adverse Effects 1% to 10%:
 Cardiovascular: Systemic cardiovascular stimulation
 Central nervous system: Dizziness, headache, nervousness
 Gastrointestinal: Nausea
 Local: Transient stinging, nasal mucosa irritation, dryness
 Ocular: Mydriasis, increased intraocular pressure, blurring of vision
 Respiratory: Sneezing, rebound congestion

Drug Interactions Increased toxicity: Anesthetics (discontinue mydriatic prior to use of anesthetics that sensitize the myocardium to sympathomimetics, ie, cyclo-propane, halothane), MAO inhibitors, tricyclic antidepressants causes hyperten-sive reactions

Drug Uptake
Onset of decongestant action: Topical: Within 10 minutes
Duration: 2-6 hours

Pregnancy Risk Factor C

Generic Available Yes

Naphazoline and Antazoline (naf AZ oh leen & an TAZ oh leen)

Brand Names Albalon-A® Ophthalmic; Antazoline-V® Ophthalmic; Vasocon-A® [OTC] Ophthalmic

Therapeutic Category Ophthalmic Agent, Vasoconstrictor

Use Topical ocular congestion, irritation and itching

Local Anesthetic/Vasoconstrictor Precautions No information available to require special precautions

Effects on Dental Treatment No effects or complications reported

Other Adverse Effects 1% to 10%:
Cardiovascular: Systemic cardiovascular stimulation, hypertension
Central nervous system: Nervousness, dizziness, headache
Gastrointestinal: Nausea
Local: Transient stinging
Neuromuscular & skeletal: Weakness
Ocular: Mydriasis, increased intraocular pressure, blurring of vision
Respiratory: Nasal mucosa irritation, dryness, rebound congestion
Miscellaneous: Sweating

Pregnancy Risk Factor C

Generic Available No

Comments Discontinue drug and consult physician if ocular pain or visual changes occur, ocular redness or irritation, or condition worsens or persists for more than 72 hours

Naphazoline and Pheniramine (naf AZ oh leen & fen NIR a meen)

Brand Names Naphcon-A® Ophthalmic [OTC]

Therapeutic Category Ophthalmic Agent, Vasoconstrictor

Synonyms Pheniramine and Naphazoline

Use Topical ocular vasoconstrictor

Local Anesthetic/Vasoconstrictor Precautions No information available to require special precautions

Effects on Dental Treatment No effects or complications reported

Other Adverse Effects 1% to 10%:
Cardiovascular: Systemic effects due to absorption (hypertension, cardiac irregu-larities, hyperglycemia)
Ocular: Pupillary dilation, increase in intraocular pressure

Pregnancy Risk Factor C

Generic Available No

Naphcon-A® Ophthalmic [OTC] see Naphazoline and Pheniramine on this page

Naphcon Forte® Ophthalmic see Naphazoline on previous page

Naphcon® Ophthalmic [OTC] see Naphazoline on previous page

Naprosyn® (Naproxen Base) see Naproxen on this page

Naproxen (na PROKS en)

Related Information
Dental Drug Interactions: Update on Drug Combinations Requiring Special Considerations on page 1144
Nonsteroidal Anti-Inflammatory Agents, Comparative Dosages, and Pharmacoki-netics on page 1143
Oral Pain on page 1053
Rheumatoid Arthritis and Osteoarthritis on page 1030
Temporomandibular Dysfunction (TMD) on page 1078

Brand Names Aleve® (Naproxen Sodium) (OTC); Anaprox® (Naproxen Sodium); Naprosyn® (Naproxen Base)

Canadian/Mexican Brand Names Apo®-Naproxen (Canada); Atiflan® (Mexico); Atiquim® (Mexico); Dafloxen® (Mexico); Faraxen® (Mexico); Flanax® (Mexico); Flexen® (Mexico); Flogen® (Mexico); Fuxen® (Mexico); Naprodil® (Mexico); Naxen® (Canada); Naxen® (Mexico); Naxil® (Mexico); Novo-Naprox (Canada); Nu-Naprox (Canada); Pactens® (Mexico); Pronaxil® (Mexico); Supradol® (Mexico); Velsay® (Mexico)
(Continued)

Naproxen *(Continued)*

Therapeutic Category Analgesic, Non-narcotic; Anti-inflammatory Agent; Nonsteroidal Anti-inflammatory Agent (NSAID), Oral

Use

Dental: Management of pain and swelling

Medical: Management of inflammatory disease and rheumatoid disorders (including juvenile rheumatoid arthritis); acute gout; mild to moderate pain; dysmenorrhea; fever, migraine headache

Usual Dosage Adults: Oral:

Naproxen base: Initial: 500 mg, then 250 mg every 6-8 hours

Naproxen sodium: Initial: 550 mg, then 275 mg every 6-8 hours

Maximum daily dose: 1250 mg/day naproxen base and 1375 mg naproxen sodium

Mechanism of Action Inhibits prostaglandin synthesis by decreasing the activity of the enzyme, cyclo-oxygenase, which results in decreased formation of prostaglandin precursors

Local Anesthetic/Vasoconstrictor Precautions No information available to require special precautions

Effects on Dental Treatment Use with caution in patients taking anticoagulants

Other Adverse Effects >10%: Gastrointestinal: Nausea, heartburn, ulcers, indigestion

Contraindications Hypersensitivity to naproxen, aspirin, or other nonsteroidal anti-inflammatory drugs (NSAIDs)

Warnings/Precautions Use with caution in patients with GI disease (bleeding or ulcers), cardiovascular disease (CHF, hypertension), renal or hepatic impairment, and patients receiving anticoagulants; perform ophthalmologic evaluation for those who develop eye complaints during therapy (blurred vision, diminished vision, changes in color vision, retinal changes); NSAIDs may mask signs/symptoms of infections; photosensitivity reported; elderly are at especially high-risk for adverse effects

Drug Interactions Decreased effect of furosemide; naproxen could displace other highly protein bound drugs, such as oral anticoagulants, hydantoins, salicylates, sulfonamides, and sulfonylureas; naproxen and warfarin may result in slight increase in free warfarin; naproxen and probenecid may result in increased plasma half-life of naproxen; naproxen and methotrexate may result in significantly increased and prolonged blood methotrexate concentration, which may be severe or fatal

Drug Uptake

Onset of effect: 1 hour

Duration of effect: Up to 7 hours

Serum half-life: 12-15 hours

Time to peak serum concentration: Within 1-2 hours and persisting for up to 12 hours

Pregnancy Risk Factor B (D if used in the 3rd trimester or near delivery)

Breast-feeding Considerations May be taken while breast-feeding

Dosage Forms

Suspension, oral: 125 mg/5 mL (15 mL, 30 mL, 480 mL)

Tablet, as sodium:

220 mg (200 mg base)

Anaprox®: 220 mg (200 mg base); 275 mg (250 mg base); 550 mg (500 mg base)

Tablet:

Aleve®: 200 mg

Naprosyn®: 250 mg, 375 mg, 500 mg

Tablet, controlled release (Naprelan®): 375 mg, 500 mg

Dietary Considerations May be taken with food, milk, or antacids to decrease GI adverse effects

Generic Available Yes

Comments The sodium salt of naproxen provides better effects because of better oral absorption; the sodium salt also provides a faster onset and a longer duration of action

Selected Readings

Brooks PM and Day RO, "Nonsteroidal Anti-inflammatory Drugs-Differences and Similarities," *N Engl J Med*, 1991, 324(24):1716-25.

Forbes JA, Keller CK, Smith JW, et al, "Analgesic Effect of Naproxen Sodium, Codeine, a Naproxen-Codeine Combination and Aspirin on the Postoperative Pain of Oral Surgery," *Pharmacotherapy*, 1986, 6(5):211-8.

Naqua® *see* Trichlormethiazide *on page 958*

Naratriptan (NAR a trip tan)
Brand Names Amerge®
Therapeutic Category Antimigraine Agent; Serotonin Agonist
Synonyms Naratriptan Hydrochloride
Use Acute treatment of migraine with or without aura
Local Anesthetic/Vasoconstrictor Precautions No information available to require special precautions
Effects on Dental Treatment No effects or complications reported
Dosage Forms Tablet: 1 mg, 2.5 mg

Naratriptan Hydrochloride *see* Naratriptan *on this page*
Narcan® *see* Naloxone *on page 662*
Narcotic Agonists *see page 1141*
Nardil® *see* Phenelzine *on page 746*
Naropin® *see* Ropivacaine *on page 850*
Nasabid™ *see* Guaifenesin and Pseudoephedrine *on page 454*
Nasacort® *see* Triamcinolone *on page 954*
Nasacort® AQ *see* Triamcinolone *on page 954*
Nasahist B® *see* Brompheniramine *on page 142*
NãSal™ [OTC] *see* Sodium Chloride *on page 870*
Nasalcrom® *see* Cromolyn Sodium *on page 264*
Nasalide® Nasal Aerosol *see* Flunisolide *on page 413*
Nasal Moist® [OTC] *see* Sodium Chloride *on page 870*
Nasarel® Nasal Spray *see* Flunisolide *on page 413*
Nasonex® *see* Mometasone Furoate *on page 646*
Natabec® [OTC] *see* Vitamins, Multiple *on page 995*
Natabec® FA [OTC] *see* Vitamins, Multiple *on page 995*
Natabec® Rx *see* Vitamins, Multiple *on page 995*
Natacyn® *see* Natamycin *on this page*
Natalins® [OTC] *see* Vitamins, Multiple *on page 995*
Natalins® Rx *see* Vitamins, Multiple *on page 995*

Natamycin (na ta MYE sin)
Brand Names Natacyn®
Therapeutic Category Antifungal Agent, Ophthalmic
Use Treatment of blepharitis, conjunctivitis, and keratitis caused by susceptible fungi (*Aspergillus*, *Candida*), *Cephalosporium*, *Curvularia*, *Fusarium*, *Penicillium*, *Microsporum*, *Epidermophyton*, *Blastomyces dermatitidis*, *Coccidioides immitis*, *Cryptococcus neoformans*, *Histoplasma capsulatum*, *Sporothrix schenckii*, *Trichomonas vaginalis*
Usual Dosage Adults: Ophthalmic: Instill 1 drop in conjunctival sac every 1-2 hours, after 3-4 days reduce to 1 drop 6-8 times/day; usual course of therapy is 2-3 weeks
Mechanism of Action Increases cell membrane permeability in susceptible fungi
Local Anesthetic/Vasoconstrictor Precautions No information available to require special precautions
Effects on Dental Treatment No effects or complications reported
Other Adverse Effects <1%: Ocular: Blurred vision, photophobia, eye pain, eye irritation not present before therapy
Drug Interactions Increased toxicity: Topical corticosteroids (concomitant use contraindicated)
Drug Uptake Absorption: Ophthalmic: <2% systemically absorbed
Pregnancy Risk Factor C
Dosage Forms Suspension, ophthalmic: 5% (15 mL)
Generic Available No

Natural Products, Herbals, and Dietary Supplements *see page 1096*
Nature's Tears® Solution [OTC] *see* Artificial Tears *on page 87*
Naturetin® *see* Bendroflumethiazide *on page 116*
Naus-A-Way® [OTC] *see* Phosphorated Carbohydrate Solution *on page 757*
Nausetrol® [OTC] *see* Phosphorated Carbohydrate Solution *on page 757*
Navane® *see* Thiothixene *on page 928*
Navelbine® *see* Vinorelbine *on page 991*
ND-Stat® *see* Brompheniramine *on page 142*
Nebcin® Injection *see* Tobramycin *on page 937*
NebuPent™ Inhalation *see* Pentamidine *on page 736*

Nedocromil Sodium (ne doe KROE mil SOW dee um)

Related Information
Respiratory Diseases *on page 1018*

Brand Names Tilade® Inhalation Aerosol

Therapeutic Category Antiasthmatic; Antihistamine, Inhalation

Use Maintenance therapy in patients with mild to moderate bronchial asthma

Usual Dosage Children >12 years and Adults: Inhalation: 2 inhalations 4 times/day; may reduce dosage to 2-3 times/day once desired clinical response to initial dose is observed

Local Anesthetic/Vasoconstrictor Precautions No information available to require special precautions

Effects on Dental Treatment No effects or complications reported

Other Adverse Effects 1% to 10%:
Cardiovascular: Chest pain
Central nervous system: Dizziness, headache, fatigue
Gastrointestinal: Nausea, vomiting, dry mouth, diarrhea, unpleasant taste
Respiratory: Coughing, pharyngitis, rhinitis, bronchitis, dyspnea, bronchospasm

Drug Uptake
Duration of therapeutic effect: 2 hours
Serum half-life: 1.5-2 hours

Pregnancy Risk Factor B

Generic Available No

Comments Not a bronchodilator and, therefore, should not be used for reversal of acute bronchospasm; has no known therapeutic systemic activity when delivered by inhalation

N.E.E.® 1/35 *see* Ethinyl Estradiol and Norethindrone *on page 379*

Nefazodone (nef AY zoe done)

Brand Names Serzone®

Therapeutic Category Antidepressant, Miscellaneous

Use Treatment of depression

Usual Dosage Adults: Oral: 200 mg/day, administered in two divided doses initially, with a range of 300-600 mg/day in two divided doses thereafter

Mechanism of Action Inhibits reuptake of serotonin and norepinephrine by the presynaptic neuronal membrane and desensitization of adenyl cyclase, down regulation of beta-adrenergic receptors, and down regulation of serotonin receptors

Local Anesthetic/Vasoconstrictor Precautions No information available to require special precautions

Effects on Dental Treatment >10% of patients experience significant dry mouth which will disappear with cessation of drug therapy

Other Adverse Effects
>10%:
Central nervous system: Headache, drowsiness, insomnia, agitation, dizziness, confusion
Gastrointestinal: Nausea
Neuromuscular & skeletal: Tremor
1% to 10%:
Cardiovascular: Postural hypotension
Gastrointestinal: Constipation, vomiting
Neuromuscular & skeletal: Weakness
Ocular: Blurred vision, amblyopia
<1%:
Gastrointestinal: Diarrhea
Genitourinary: Prolonged priapism

Drug Interactions
Alprazolam and triazolam: Coadministration with nefazodone has resulted in significant increased blood levels of these two benzodiazepines. A 50% reduction in alprazolam dosage is recommended; a 75% reduction in triazolam dosage is recommended
Digoxin: Coadministration with nefazodone has resulted in increased blood levels of digoxin; because of the narrow margin of safety of digoxin, caution is advised in administration with nefazodone
Monoamine oxidase inhibitors: In patients taking antidepressants similar to nefazodone, concomitant administration of monoamine oxidase inhibitors has resulted in serious, sometimes fatal, reactions. It is recommended that nefazodone not be given in combination with monoamine oxidase inhibitors.

Drug Uptake
Onset of action: Therapeutic effects take at least 2 weeks to appear
Serum half-life: 2-4 hours (parent compound), active metabolites persist longer

Time to peak serum concentration: 30 minutes, prolonged in presence of food
Pregnancy Risk Factor C
Generic Available No

NegGram® *see* Nalidixic Acid *on page 660*

Nelfinavir (nel FIN a veer)
Related Information
HIV Infection and AIDS *on page 1024*
Brand Names Viracept®
Therapeutic Category Protease Inhibitor
Use As monotherapy or preferably in combination with nucleoside analogs in the treatment of HIV infection when antiretroviral therapy is warranted
Usual Dosage Oral:
Children 2-13 years: 20-30 mg/kg 3 times/day with a meal or light snack; if tablets are unable to be taken, use oral powder in small amount of water, milk, formula, or dietary supplements; do not use acidic food/juice or store for >6 hours
Adults: 750 mg 3 times/day with meals
Mechanism of Action Inhibits the HIV-1 protease; inhibition of the viral protease prevents cleavage of the gag-pol polyprotein resulting in the production of immature, noninfectious virus; cross-resistance with other protease inhibitors is possible although, as yet, unknown
Local Anesthetic/Vasoconstrictor Precautions No information available to require special precautions
Effects on Dental Treatment <1% of patients experience mouth ulcers
Other Adverse Effects
>10%: Gastrointestinal: Diarrhea
1% to 10%:
Central nervous system: Decreased concentration
Dermatologic: Rash
Gastrointestinal: Nausea, flatulence, abdominal pain
Neuromuscular & skeletal: Weakness
<1%:
Central nervous system: Anxiety, depression, dizziness, emotional lability, hyperkinesia, insomnia, migraine, seizures, sleep disorder, somnolence, suicide ideation, fever, headache, malaise
Dermatologic: Dermatitis, pruritus, urticaria
Endocrine & metabolic: Increased LFTs, hyperlipemia, hyperuricemia, hypoglycemia
Gastrointestinal: Anorexia, dyspepsia, epigastric pain, mouth ulceration, GI bleeding, pancreatitis, vomiting
Genitourinary: Kidney calculus, sexual dysfunction
Hematologic: Anemia, leukopenia, thrombocytopenia
Hepatic: Hepatitis
Neuromuscular & skeletal: Arthralgia, arthritis, cramps, myalgia, myasthenia, myopathy, paresthesia, back pain
Respiratory: Dyspnea, pharyngitis, rhinitis, sinusitis
Miscellaneous: Diaphoresis, allergy
Warnings/Precautions Avoid use of powder in phenylketonurics since contains phenylalanine; use extreme caution when administered to patients with hepatic insufficiency since nelfinavir is metabolized in the liver and excreted predominantly in the feces; avoid use, if possible, with terfenadine, astemizole, cisapride, triazolam, or midazolam. Concurrent use with some anticonvulsants may significantly limit nelfinavir's effectiveness.
Drug Interactions Unlike other protease inhibitors, nelfinavir may be administered with dapsone, trimethoprim/sulfamethoxazole, clarithromycin, azithromycin, erythromycin, itraconazole, and fluconazole

Increased effect: Nelfinavir inhibits the metabolism of cisapride and astemizole and should, therefore, not be administered concurrently due to risk of cardiac arrhythmias. A 20% increase in rifabutin plasma AUC has been observed when coadministered with nelfinavir (decrease rifabutin's dose by 50%). An increase in midazolam and triazolam serum levels may occur resulting in significant oversedation when administered with nelfinavir. These drugs should not be administered together. Indinavir and ritonavir may increase nelfinavir plasma concentrations resulting in potential increases in side effects (the safety of these combinations have not been established).
Decreased effect: Rifampin decreases nelfinavir's plasma AUC by ~82%; the two drugs should not be administered together. Serum levels of the hormones in oral contraceptives may decrease significantly with administration of nelfinavir. Patients should use alternative methods of contraceptives during
(Continued)

669

Nelfinavir *(Continued)*

nelfinavir therapy. Phenobarbital, phenytoin, and carbamazepine may decrease serum levels and consequently effectiveness of nelfinavir.

Drug Uptake
Serum half-life: 3.5-5 hours
Time to peak serum concentration: 2-4 hours

Pregnancy Risk Factor B

Nelova™ 0.5/35E *see* Ethinyl Estradiol and Norethindrone *on page 379*

Nelova™ 1/50M *see* Mestranol and Norethindrone *on page 603*

Nelova™ 10/11 *see* Ethinyl Estradiol and Norethindrone *on page 379*

Nembutal® *see* Pentobarbital *on page 738*

Neo-Calglucon® [OTC] *see* Calcium Glubionate *on page 165*

Neo-Cortef® *see* Neomycin and Hydrocortisone *on next page*

NeoDecadron® Ophthalmic *see* Neomycin and Dexamethasone *on next page*

NeoDecadron® Topical *see* Neomycin and Dexamethasone *on next page*

Neo-Dexameth® Ophthalmic *see* Neomycin and Dexamethasone *on next page*

Neo-Durabolic Injection *see* Nandrolone *on page 663*

Neo-fradin® *see* Neomycin *on this page*

Neoloid® [OTC] *see* Castor Oil *on page 184*

Neomixin® Topical [OTC] *see* Bacitracin, Neomycin, and Polymyxin B *on page 108*

Neomycin *(nee oh MYE sin)*

Related Information
Antimicrobial Prophylaxis in Surgical Patients *on page 1163*
Neomycin and Polymyxin B *on next page*
Neomycin, Polymyxin B, and Dexamethasone *on page 672*
Neomycin, Polymyxin B, and Prednisolone *on page 673*

Brand Names Mycifradin® Sulfate; Neo-fradin®; Neo-Tabs®

Therapeutic Category Ammonia Detoxicant; Antibiotic, Aminoglycoside; Antibiotic, Topical

Use Prepares GI tract for surgery; treat minor skin infections; treat diarrhea caused by *E. coli*; adjunct in the treatment of hepatic encephalopathy, as irrigant during surgery

Usual Dosage
Children: Oral:
Preoperative intestinal antisepsis: 90 mg/kg/day divided every 4 hours for 2 days; or 25 mg/kg at 1 PM, 2 PM, and 11 PM on the day preceding surgery as an adjunct to mechanical cleansing of the intestine and in combination with erythromycin base
Hepatic coma: 50-100 mg/kg/day in divided doses every 6-8 hours or 2.5-7 g/m^2/day divided every 4-6 hours for 5-6 days not to exceed 12 g/day

Children and Adults: Topical: Apply ointment 1-4 times/day; topical solutions containing 0.1% to 1% neomycin have been used for irrigation

Adults: Oral:
Preoperative intestinal antisepsis: 1 g each hour for 4 doses then 1 g every 4 hours for 5 doses; or 1 g at 1 PM, 2 PM, and 11 PM on day preceding surgery as an adjunct to mechanical cleansing of the bowel and oral erythromycin; or 6 g/day divided every 4 hours for 2-3 days
Hepatic coma: 500-2000 mg every 6-8 hours or 4-12 g/day divided every 4-6 hours for 5-6 days
Chronic hepatic insufficiency: 4 g/day for an indefinite period

Dialyzable (50% to 100%)

Mechanism of Action Interferes with bacterial protein synthesis by binding to 30S ribosomal subunits

Local Anesthetic/Vasoconstrictor Precautions No information available to require special precautions

Effects on Dental Treatment No effects or complications reported

Other Adverse Effects
1% to 10%:
Dermatologic: Dermatitis, rash, urticaria, erythema
Local: Burning
Ocular: Contact conjunctivitis
<1%:
Gastrointestinal: Nausea, vomiting, diarrhea
Neuromuscular & skeletal: Neuromuscular blockade
Otic: Ototoxicity
Renal: Nephrotoxicity

Drug Interactions
Decreased effect: May decrease GI absorption of digoxin and methotrexate
Increased effect: Synergistic effects with penicillins
Increased toxicity:
Oral neomycin may potentiate the effects of oral anticoagulants
Increased adverse effects with other neurotoxic, ototoxic, or nephrotoxic drugs
Drug Uptake
Absorption: Oral, percutaneous: Poor (3%)
Serum half-life: 3 hours (age and renal function dependent)
Time to peak serum concentration:
Oral: 1-4 hours
I.M.: Within 2 hours
Pregnancy Risk Factor C
Generic Available Yes

Neomycin and Dexamethasone
(nee oh MYE sin & deks a METH a sone)
Brand Names AK-Neo-Dex® Ophthalmic; NeoDecadron® Ophthalmic; NeoDecadron® Topical; Neo-Dexameth® Ophthalmic
Therapeutic Category Antibiotic, Ophthalmic; Corticosteroid, Ophthalmic
Synonyms Dexamethasone and Neomycin
Use Treatment of steroid responsive inflammatory conditions of the palpebral and bulbar conjunctiva, lid, cornea, and anterior segment of the globe
Local Anesthetic/Vasoconstrictor Precautions No information available to require special precautions
Effects on Dental Treatment No effects or complications reported
Other Adverse Effects <1%:
Local: Transient stinging, burning, or local irritation
Ocular: Increased intraocular pressure, mydriasis, ptosis, epithelial punctate keratitis, and possible corneal or scleral malacia can occur
Pregnancy Risk Factor C
Generic Available No

Neomycin and Hydrocortisone
(nee oh MYE sin & hye droe KOR ti sone)
Brand Names Neo-Cortef®
Therapeutic Category Antibiotic, Topical; Corticosteroid, Topical (Low Potency)
Use Treatment of susceptible topical bacterial infections with associated swelling
Local Anesthetic/Vasoconstrictor Precautions No information available to require special precautions
Effects on Dental Treatment No effects or complications reported
Generic Available No

Neomycin and Polymyxin B (nee oh MYE sin & pol i MIKS in bee)
Brand Names Neosporin® Cream [OTC]; Neosporin® G.U. Irrigant
Therapeutic Category Antibiotic, Topical; Antibiotic, Urinary Irrigation
Use Short-term as a continuous irrigant or rinse in the urinary bladder to prevent bacteriuria and gram-negative rod septicemia associated with the use of indwelling catheters; to help prevent infection in minor cuts, scrapes, and burns; treatment of superficial ocular infections involving the conjunctiva or cornea
Usual Dosage Children and Adults:
Bladder irrigation: **Not for injection;** add 1 mL irrigant to 1 liter isotonic saline solution and connect container to the inflow of lumen of 3-way catheter. Continuous irrigant or rinse in the urinary bladder for up to a maximum of 10 days with administration rate adjusted to patient's urine output; usually no more than 1 L of irrigant is used per day.
Ophthalmic:
Ointment: Instill ½" ribbon into the conjunctival sac every 3-4 hours for acute infections or 2-3 times/day for mild to moderate infections for 7-10 days
Solution: Instill 1-2 drops every 15-30 minutes for acute infections; 1-2 drops every 3-6 hours for mild-moderate infections.
Topical: Apply cream 1-4 times/day to affected area
Mechanism of Action Refer to individual monographs
Local Anesthetic/Vasoconstrictor Precautions No information available to require special precautions
Effects on Dental Treatment No effects or complications reported
Other Adverse Effects 1% to 10%:
Dermatologic: Contact dermatitis, erythema, rash, urticaria
Genitourinary: Bladder irritation
Local: Burning
(Continued)

Neomycin and Polymyxin B *(Continued)*

Neuromuscular & skeletal: Neuromuscular blockade
Otic: Ototoxicity
Renal: Nephrotoxicity
Drug Interactions No data reported
Drug Uptake Absorption: Topical: Not absorbed following application to intact skin; absorbed through denuded or abraded skin, peritoneum, wounds, or ulcers
Pregnancy Risk Factor C (D - G.U. irrigant)
Dosage Forms
Cream: Neomycin sulfate 3.5 mg and polymyxin B sulfate 10,000 units per g (0.94 g, 15 g)
Solution, irrigant: Neomycin sulfate 40 mg and polymyxin B sulfate 200,000 units per mL (1 mL, 20 mL)
Generic Available Yes

Neomycin, Polymyxin B, and Dexamethasone

(nee oh MYE sin, pol i MIKS in bee, & deks a METH a sone)
Brand Names AK-Trol®; Dexacidin®; Dexasporin®; Maxitrol®
Therapeutic Category Antibiotic, Ophthalmic
Use Steroid-responsive inflammatory ocular conditions in which a corticosteroid is indicated and where bacterial infection or a risk of bacterial infection exists
Mechanism of Action Refer to individual monographs
Local Anesthetic/Vasoconstrictor Precautions No information available to require special precautions
Effects on Dental Treatment No effects or complications reported
Other Adverse Effects
1% to 10%:
Dermatologic: Contact dermatitis, delayed wound healing
Ocular: Cutaneous sensitization, eye pain, development of glaucoma, cataract, increased intraocular pressure, optic nerve damage
Drug Interactions No data reported
Drug Uptake Refer to individual monographs
Pregnancy Risk Factor C
Generic Available Yes

Neomycin, Polymyxin B, and Gramicidin

(nee oh MYE sin, pol i MIKS in bee, & gram i SYE din)
Related Information
Antimicrobial Prophylaxis in Surgical Patients *on page 1163*
Brand Names AK-Spore® Ophthalmic Solution; Neosporin® Ophthalmic Solution
Canadian/Mexican Brand Names Neosporin® Oftalmico (Mexico)
Therapeutic Category Antibiotic, Ophthalmic
Use Treatment of superficial ocular infection, infection prophylaxis in minor skin abrasions
Mechanism of Action Interferes with bacterial protein synthesis by binding to 30S ribosomal subunits; binds to phospholipids, alters permeability, and damages the bacterial cytoplasmic membrane permitting leakage of intracellular constituents
Local Anesthetic/Vasoconstrictor Precautions No information available to require special precautions
Effects on Dental Treatment No effects or complications reported
Other Adverse Effects 1% to 10%:
Cardiovascular: Edema
Dermatologic: Itching
Local: Reddening, failure to heal
Ocular: Low grade conjunctivitis
Drug Interactions No data reported
Pregnancy Risk Factor C
Generic Available Yes

Neomycin, Polymyxin B, and Hydrocortisone

(nee oh MYE sin, pol i MIKS in bee, & hye droe KOR ti sone)
Brand Names AK-Spore H.C.® Ophthalmic Suspension; AK-Spore H.C.® Otic; AntibiOtic® Otic; Cortatrigen® Otic; Cortisporin® Ophthalmic Suspension; Cortisporin® Otic; Cortisporin® Topical Cream; Octicair® Otic; Otic-Care® Otic; Otocort® Otic; Otosporin® Otic; Pediotic® Otic; UAD Otic®
Therapeutic Category Antibiotic, Ophthalmic; Antibiotic, Otic; Antibiotic, Topical; Corticosteroid, Ophthalmic; Corticosteroid, Otic; Corticosteroid, Topical (Low Potency)

Use Steroid-responsive inflammatory condition for which a corticosteroid is indicated and where bacterial infection or a risk of bacterial infection exists

Usual Dosage Duration of use should be limited to 10 days unless otherwise directed by the physician

Otic solution is used **only** for swimmer's ear (infections of external auditory canal)

Otic:

Children: Instill 3 drops jnto affected ear 3-4 times/day

Adults: Instill 4 drops 3-4 times/day; otic suspension is the preferred otic preparation

Children and Adults:

Ophthalmic: Drops: Instill 1-2 drops 2-4 times/day, or more frequently as required for severe infections; in acute infections, instill 1-2 drops every 15-30 minutes gradually reducing the frequency of administration as the infection is controlled

Topical: Apply a thin layer 1-4 times/day

Mechanism of Action Refer to individual monographs for neomycin, Polymyxin B, and Hydrocortisone

Local Anesthetic/Vasoconstrictor Precautions No information available to require special precautions

Effects on Dental Treatment No effects or complications reported

Other Adverse Effects

>10%: Miscellaneous: Hypersensitivity

1% to 10%:

Dermatologic: Contact dermatitis, erythema, rash, urticaria

Genitourinary: Bladder irritation

Local: Burning, itching, swelling, pain, stinging

Neuromuscular & skeletal: Neuromuscular blockade

Ocular: Increased intraocular pressure, glaucoma, cataracts, conjunctival erythema

Otic: Ototoxicity

Renal: Nephrotoxicity

Miscellaneous: Sensitization to neomycin, secondary infections

Drug Interactions No data reported

Pregnancy Risk Factor C

Generic Available Yes

Neomycin, Polymyxin B, and Prednisolone

(nee oh MYE sin, pol i MIKS in bee, & pred NIS oh lone)

Brand Names Poly-Pred®

Therapeutic Category Antibiotic, Ophthalmic; Corticosteroid, Ophthalmic

Use Steroid-responsive inflammatory ocular condition in which bacterial infection or a risk of bacterial ocular infection exists

Mechanism of Action Refer to individual monographs

Local Anesthetic/Vasoconstrictor Precautions No information available to require special precautions

Effects on Dental Treatment No effects or complications reported

Other Adverse Effects 1% to 10%:

Dermatologic: Cutaneous sensitization, skin rash, delayed wound healing

Ocular: Increased intraocular pressure, glaucoma, optic nerve damage, cataracts, conjunctival sensitization

Drug Interactions No data reported

Drug Uptake Refer to individual monographs

Pregnancy Risk Factor C

Generic Available Yes

Netilmicin (ne til MYE sin)

Brand Names Netromycin®

Canadian/Mexican Brand Names Netromicina® (Mexico)

Therapeutic Category Antibiotic, Aminoglycoside

Synonyms Netilmicina Sulfato De (Mexico)

Use Short-term treatment of serious or life-threatening infections including septicemia, peritonitis, intra-abdominal abscess, lower respiratory tract infections, urinary tract infections; skin, bone, and joint infections caused by sensitive *Pseudomonas aeruginosa*, *Escherichia coli*, *Proteus*, *Klebsiella*, *Serratia*, *Enterobacter*, *Citrobacter*, and *Staphylococcus*

Usual Dosage Individualization is critical because of the low therapeutic index. Use of ideal body weight (IBW) for determining the mg/kg/dose appears to be more accurate than dosing on the basis of total body weight (TBW). In morbid obesity, dosage requirement may best be estimated using a dosing weight of IBW + 0.4 (TBW - IBW). Peak and trough plasma drug levels should be determined, particularly in critically ill patients with serious infections or in disease states known to significantly alter aminoglycoside pharmacokinetics (eg, cystic fibrosis, burns, or major surgery).

Once daily dosing: Higher peak serum drug concentration to MIC ratios, demonstrated aminoglycoside postantibiotic effect, decreased renal cortex drug uptake, and improved cost-time efficiency are supportive reasons for the use of once daily dosing regimens for aminoglycosides. Current research indicates these regimens to be as effective for nonlife-threatening infections, with no higher incidence of nephrotoxicity, than those requiring multiple daily doses. Doses are determined by calculating the entire day's dose via usual multiple dose calculation techniques and administering this quantity as a single dose. Doses are then adjusted to maintain mean serum concentrations above the MIC(s) of the causative organism(s). (Example: 4.5-6.5 mg/kg as a single dose; expected Cp_{max}: 10-20 mcg/mL, and Cp_{min}: <1 mcg/mL). Further research is needed for universal recommendation in all patient populations and gram-negative disease; exceptions may include those with known high clearance (eg, children, patients with cystic fibrosis, or burns who may require shorter dosage intervals) and patients with renal function impairment for whom longer than conventional dosage intervals are usually required.

I.M., I.V.:
  Children 6 weeks to 12 years: 1-2.5 mg/kg/dose every 8 hours
  Children >12 years and Adults: 1.5-2 mg/kg/dose every 8-12 hours
  Some clinicians suggest a daily dose of 4-7 mg/kg for all patients with normal renal function. This dose is at least as efficacious with similar, if not less, toxicity than conventional dosing.

Mechanism of Action Interferes with protein synthesis in bacterial cell by binding to ribosomal subunit

Local Anesthetic/Vasoconstrictor Precautions No information available to require special precautions

Effects on Dental Treatment No effects or complications reported

Other Adverse Effects
>10%:
  Central nervous system: Neurotoxicity
  Otic: Ototoxicity (auditory), ototoxicity (vestibular)
  Renal: Decreased creatinine clearance, nephrotoxicity

1% to 10%:
  Cardiovascular: Swelling
  Dermatologic: Skin itching, redness, rash
<1%:
  Central nervous system: Drowsiness, headache, pseudomotor cerebri
  Dermatologic: Photosensitivity, erythema
  Gastrointestinal: Anorexia, nausea, vomiting, weight loss, increased salivation,
    enterocolitis
  Hematologic: Granulocytopenia, agranulocytosis, thrombocytopenia
  Local: Burning, stinging
  Neuromuscular & skeletal: Tremors, muscle cramps, weakness
  Respiratory: Dyspnea
Drug Interactions Increased toxicity:
  Penicillins, cephalosporins, amphotericin B, loop diuretics, vancomycin cause
    increased nephrotoxic potential
  Neuromuscular blocking agents cause increased neuromuscular blockade
Drug Uptake
  Absorption: I.M.: Well absorbed
  Serum half-life: 2-3 hours (age and renal function dependent)
  Time to peak serum concentration: I.M.: Within 0.5-1 hour
Pregnancy Risk Factor D
Generic Available No

Netilmicina Sulfato De (Mexico) see Netilmicin on previous page

Netromycin® see Netilmicin on previous page

Neupogen® Injection see Filgrastim on page 404

Neuramate® see Meprobamate on page 599

Neurontin® see Gabapentin on page 436

Neut® Injection see Sodium Bicarbonate on page 869

Neutra-Phos® see Potassium Phosphate and Sodium Phosphate on page 783

Neutra-Phos®-K see Potassium Phosphate on page 781

Neutrexin™ see Trimetrexate Glucuronate on page 966

Neutrogena® Acne Mask [OTC] see Benzoyl Peroxide on page 120

Neutrogena® T/Derm see Coal Tar on page 254

Nevirapine (ne VYE ra peen)
  Brand Names Viramune®
  Therapeutic Category Antiviral Agent, Parenteral
  Use In combination therapy with nucleoside antiretroviral agents in HIV-1 infected
    adults previously treated for whom current therapy is deemed inadequate
  Usual Dosage Adults: Oral: 200 mg once daily for 2 weeks followed by 200 mg
    twice daily
  Mechanism of Action Nevirapine is a non-nucleoside reverse transcriptase
    inhibitor specific for HIV-1; nevirapine does not require intracellular phosphoryla-
    tion for antiviral activity
  Local Anesthetic/Vasoconstrictor Precautions No information available to
    require special precautions
  Effects on Dental Treatment No effects or complications reported
  Other Adverse Effects >10%:
    Central nervous system: Headache, drowsiness, drug fever
    Dermatologic: Rash
    Gastrointestinal: Diarrhea, nausea
    Hepatic: LFTs (elevated)
  Contraindications Previous hypersensitivity to nevirapine
  Drug Interactions Decreased effect: Rifampin and rifabutin may decrease
    nevirapine trough concentrations due to induction of CYP3A; since nevirapine
    may decrease concentrations of protease inhibitors, they should not be adminis-
    tered concomitantly; nevirapine may decrease the effectiveness of oral contra-
    ceptives - suggest alternate method of birth control
  Drug Uptake
    Absorption: Rapidly absorbed with peak levels occurring within 2 hours of admin-
      istration
    Serum half-life: 22-84 hours
  Pregnancy Risk Factor C
  Generic Available No

New Decongestant® see Chlorpheniramine, Phenyltoloxamine, Phenylpropanolamine,
and Phenylephrine on page 222

N.G.T.® Topical see Nystatin and Triamcinolone on page 695

Niacin (NYE a sin)

Related Information
Cardiovascular Diseases *on page 1010*

Brand Names Nicobid® [OTC]; Nicolar® [OTC]; Nicotinex [OTC]; Slo-Niacin® [OTC]

Therapeutic Category Lipid Lowering Drugs; Vitamin, Water Soluble

Use Adjunctive treatment of hyperlipidemias; peripheral vascular disease and circulatory disorders; treatment of pellagra; dietary supplement

Usual Dosage Give I.M., I.V., or S.C. only if oral route is unavailable and use only for vitamin deficiencies (not for hyperlipidemia)

Children: Pellagra: Oral: 50-100 mg/dose 3 times/day
Oral: Recommended daily allowances:
0-0.5 years: 5 mg/day
0.5-1 year: 6 mg/day
1-3 years: 9 mg/day
4-6 years: 12 mg/day
7-10 years: 13 mg/day
Males:
11-14 years: 17 mg/day
15-18 years: 20 mg/day
19-24 years: 19 mg/day
Females: 11-24 years: 15 mg/day

Adults: Oral:
Recommended daily allowances:
Males: 25-50 years: 19 mg/day; >51 years: 15 mg/day
Females: 25-50 years: 15 mg/day; >51 years: 13 mg/day
Hyperlipidemia: 1.5-6 g/day in 3 divided doses with or after meals
Pellagra: 50-100 mg 3-4 times/day, maximum: 500 mg/day
Niacin deficiency: 10-20 mg/day, maximum: 100 mg/day

Mechanism of Action Component of two coenzymes which is necessary for tissue respiration, lipid metabolism, and glycogenolysis; inhibits the synthesis of very low density lipoproteins

Local Anesthetic/Vasoconstrictor Precautions No information available to require special precautions

Effects on Dental Treatment No effects or complications reported

Other Adverse Effects
1% to 10%:
Cardiovascular: Generalized flushing with sensation of warmth
Central nervous system: Headache
Gastrointestinal: Bloating, flatulence, nausea
Hepatic: Abnormalities of hepatic function tests, jaundice
Neuromuscular & skeletal: Paresthesia
Miscellaneous: Increased sebaceous gland activity
<1%:
Cardiovascular: Tachycardia, syncope, vasovagal attacks
Central nervous system: Dizziness
Dermatologic: Skin rash
Hepatic: Chronic liver damage
Ocular: Blurred vision
Respiratory: Wheezing

Drug Interactions
Decreased effect of oral hypoglycemics; may inhibit uricosuric effects of sulfinpyrazone and probenecid
Decreased toxicity (flush) with aspirin
Increased toxicity with lovastatin (myopathy) and possibly with other HMG-CoA reductase inhibitors; adrenergic blocking agents → additive vasodilating effect and postural hypotension

Drug Uptake
Serum half-life: 45 minutes
Peak serum concentrations: Oral: Within 45 minutes

Pregnancy Risk Factor A (C if used in doses greater than RDA suggested doses)

Generic Available Yes

Niacinamide (nye a SIN a mide)

Therapeutic Category Vitamin, Water Soluble

Use Prophylaxis and treatment of pellagra

Usual Dosage Oral:
Children: Pellagra: 100-300 mg/day in divided doses

Adults: 50 mg 3-10 times/day

Pellagra: 300-500 mg/day

Recommended daily allowance: 13-19 mg/day

Mechanism of Action Used by the body as a source of niacin; is a component of two coenzymes which is necessary for tissue respiration, lipid metabolism, and glycogenolysis; inhibits the synthesis of very low density lipoproteins

Local Anesthetic/Vasoconstrictor Precautions No information available to require special precautions

Effects on Dental Treatment No effects or complications reported

Other Adverse Effects

1% to 10%:

Gastrointestinal: Bloating, flatulence, nausea

Neuromuscular & skeletal: Paresthesia

Miscellaneous: Increased sebaceous gland activity

<1%:

Cardiovascular: Tachycardia

Dermatologic: Skin rash

Ocular: Blurred vision

Respiratory: Wheezing

Drug Interactions No data reported

Drug Uptake

Absorption: Rapid from GI tract

Serum half-life: 45 minutes

Time to peak serum concentration: 20-70 minutes

Pregnancy Risk Factor A (C if used in doses greater than RDA suggested doses)

Generic Available Yes

Nicardipina (Mexico) *see* Nicardipine *on this page*

Nicardipine (nye KAR de peen)

Related Information

Calcium Channel Blockers & Gingival Hyperplasia *on page 1132*

Cardiovascular Diseases *on page 1010*

Brand Names Cardene®; Cardene® SR

Canadian/Mexican Brand Names Ridene® (Mexico)

Therapeutic Category Antianginal Agent; Calcium Channel Blocker

Synonyms Nicardipina (Mexico)

Use Chronic stable angina; management of essential hypertension, migraine prophylaxis

Unlabeled use: CHF

Usual Dosage Adults:

Oral: 40 mg 3 times/day (allow 3 days between dose increases)

Oral, sustained release: Initial: 30 mg twice daily, titrate up to 60 mg twice daily

I.V. (dilute to 0.1 mg/mL): Initial: 5 mg/hour increased by 2.5 mg/hour every 15 minutes to a maximum of 15 mg/hour

Mechanism of Action Inhibits calcium ion from entering the "slow channels" or select voltage-sensitive areas of vascular smooth muscle and myocardium during depolarization, producing a relaxation of coronary vascular smooth muscle and coronary vasodilation; increases myocardial oxygen delivery in patients with vasospastic angina

Local Anesthetic/Vasoconstrictor Precautions No information available to require special precautions

Effects on Dental Treatment Other drugs of this class can cause gingival hyperplasia (ie, nifedipine). The first case of nicardipine-induced gingival hyperplasia has been reported in a child taking 40-50 mg daily for 20 months

Other Adverse Effects

1% to 10%:

Cardiovascular: Flushing, palpitations, tachycardia, pedal edema

Central nervous system: Headache, dizziness, somnolence

Gastrointestinal: Nausea

Neuromuscular & skeletal: Weakness

<1%:

Cardiovascular: Edema, syncope, abnormal EKG

Central nervous system: Insomnia, malaise, abnormal dreams

Dermatologic: Rash

Gastrointestinal: Vomiting, constipation, dyspepsia, dry mouth

Genitourinary: Nocturia

Neuromuscular & skeletal: Tremor

Drug Interactions

Increased toxicity/effect/levels:

Calcium channel blockers (CCB) and H_2-blockers cause increased bioavailability CCB

(Continued)

Nicardipine *(Continued)*

CCB and beta-blockers cause increased cardiac depressant effects on A-V conduction

H_2-blockers cause increased bioavailability of nicardipine

Severe hypotension has been reported during fentanyl anesthesia with concomitant use of beta-blockers and calcium channel blockers; even though such interactions have not been ·seen specifically with nicardipine, caution is suggested in using nicardipine with fentanyl

Drug Uptake

Absorption: Oral: Well absorbed, ~100%

Serum half-life: 2-4 hours

Time to peak: Peak serum levels occur within 20-120 minutes and an onset of hypotension occurs within 20 minutes

Pregnancy Risk Factor C

Generic Available Yes: Capsule

Selected Readings

Pascual-Castroviejo I and Pascual Pascual SI, "Nicardipine-Induced Gingival Hyperplasia," *Neurologia*, 1997, 12(1):37-9.

N'ice® Vitamin C Drops [OTC] *see Ascorbic Acid on page 88*

Niclocide® *see Niclosamide on this page*

Niclosamide *(ni KLOE sa mide)*

Brand Names Niclocide®

Therapeutic Category Anthelmintic

Use Treatment of intestinal beef and fish tapeworm infections and dwarf tapeworm infections

Usual Dosage Oral:

Beef and fish tapeworm:

Children:

11-34 kg: 1 g (2 tablets) as a single dose

>34 kg: 1.5 g (3 tablets) as a single dose

Adults: 2 g (4 tablets) in a single dose

May require a second course of treatment 7 days later

Dwarf tapeworm:

Children:

11-34 g: 1 g (2 tablets) chewed thoroughly in a single dose the first day, then 500 mg/day (1 tablet) for next 6 days

>34 g: 1.5 g (3 tablets) in a single dose the first day, then 1 g/day for 6 days

Adults: 2 g (4 tablets) in a single daily dose for 7 days

Mechanism of Action Inhibits the synthesis of ATP through inhibition of oxidative phosphorylation in the mitochondria of cestodes

Local Anesthetic/Vasoconstrictor Precautions No information available to require special precautions

Effects on Dental Treatment No effects or complications reported

Other Adverse Effects

1% to 10%:

Central nervous system: Drowsiness, dizziness, headache

Gastrointestinal: Nausea, vomiting, loss of appetite, diarrhea

<1%:

Cardiovascular: Palpitations, edema in the arm

Central nervous system: Fever

Dermatologic: Rash, pruritus ani, alopecia

Gastrointestinal: Constipation, oral irritation, bad taste in mouth, rectal bleeding

Neuromuscular & skeletal: Backache, weakness

Miscellaneous: Sweating

Drug Interactions No data reported

Drug Uptake

Absorption: Oral: Not significant

Pregnancy Risk Factor B

Generic Available No

Nicobid® [OTC] *see Niacin on page 676*

Nicoderm® *see Nicotine on this page*

Nicolar® [OTC] *see Niacin on page 676*

Nicorette® *see Nicotine on this page*

Nicotine *(nik oh TEEN)*

Brand Names Habitrol™; Nicoderm®; Nicorette®; Nicotrol®; ProStep®

Canadian/Mexican Brand Names Nicolan® (Mexico); Nicorette™ Plus (Canada); Nicotinell®-TTS (Mexico)

Therapeutic Category Smoking Deterrent

Use

Dental: Treatment aid to smoking cessation while participating in a behavioral modification program under dental or medical supervision

Medical: None

Usual Dosage

Gum: Chew 1 piece of gum when urge to smoke, up to 30 pieces/day; most patients require 10-12 pieces of gum/day

Transdermal patch (patients should be advised to completely stop smoking upon initiation of therapy): Apply new patch every 24 hours to nonhairy, clean, dry skin on the upper body or upper outer arm; each patch should be applied to a different site

Initial starting dose: 21 mg/day for 4-8 weeks for most patients

First weaning dose: 14 mg/day for 2-4 weeks

Second weaning dose: 7 mg/day for 2-4 weeks

Initial starting dose for patients <100 pounds, smoke <10 cigarettes/day, have a history of cardiovascular disease: 14 mg/day for 4-8 weeks followed by 7 mg/day for 2-4 weeks

In patients who are receiving >600 mg/day of cimetidine: Decrease to the next lower patch size

Benefits of use of nicotine transdermal patches beyond 3 months have not been demonstrated

Mechanism of Action Nicotine is one of two naturally-occurring alkaloids which exhibit their primary effects via autonomic ganglia stimulation. The other alkaloid is lobeline which has many actions similar to those of nicotine but is less potent. Nicotine is a potent ganglionic and central nervous system stimulant, the actions of which are mediated via nicotine-specific receptors. Biphasic actions are observed depending upon the dose administered. The main effect of nicotine in small doses is stimulation of all autonomic ganglia; with larger doses, initial stimulation is followed by blockade of transmission. Biphasic effects are also evident in the adrenal medulla; discharge of catecholamines occurs with small doses, whereas prevention of catecholamines release is seen with higher doses as a response to splanchnic nerve stimulation. Stimulation of the central nervous system (CNS) is characterized by tremors and respiratory excitation. However, convulsions may occur with higher doses, along with respiratory failure secondary to both central paralysis and peripheral blockade to respiratory muscles.

Local Anesthetic/Vasoconstrictor Precautions No information available to require special precautions

Effects on Dental Treatment >10% of patients using chewing gum form of product experience excessive salivation, mouth, or throat soreness

Other Adverse Effects

Chewing gum:

>10%:

Cardiovascular: Tachycardia

Central nervous system: Headache (mild)

Gastrointestinal: Nausea, vomiting, indigestion, excessive salivation, belching, increased appetite, mouth or throat soreness

Neuromuscular & skeletal: Jaw muscle ache

Miscellaneous: Hiccups

1% to 10%:

Central nervous system: Insomnia, dizziness, nervousness

Endocrine & metabolic: Dysmenorrhea

Gastrointestinal: GI distress, eructation

Neuromuscular & skeletal: Myalgia

Respiratory: Hoarseness

Miscellaneous: Hiccups

<1%:

Cardiovascular: Atrial fibrillation

Dermatologic: Erythema, itching, hypersensitivity reactions

Transdermal systems:

>10%:

Cardiovascular: Tachycardia

Central nervous system: Headache (mild)

Dermatologic: Pruritus, erythema

Gastrointestinal: Increased appetite

1% to 10%:

Central nervous system: Insomnia, nervousness

Endocrine & metabolic: Dysmenorrhea

<1%:

Cardiovascular: Atrial fibrillation

Dermatologic: Itching

Miscellaneous: Hypersensitivity reactions

(Continued)

Nicotine *(Continued)*

Contraindications Nonsmokers, patients with a history of hypersensitivity or allergy to nicotine or any components used in the transdermal system, pregnant or nursing women, patients who are smoking during the postmyocardial infarction period, patients with life-threatening arrhythmias, or severe or worsening angina pectoris, active temporomandibular joint disease (gum)

Warnings/Precautions Use with caution in oropharyngeal inflammation and in patients with history of esòphagitis, peptic ulcer, coronary artery disease, vasospastic disease, angina, hypertension; hyperthyroidism, diabetes, and hepatic dysfunction; nicotine is known to be one of the most toxic of all poisons; while the gum is being used to help the patient overcome a health hazard, it also must be considered a hazardous drug vehicle

Drug Interactions

Smoking cessation may alter response to concomitant medications:
    Decreased effect of caffeine, imipramine, oxazepam, pentazocine, propranolol, theophylline, glutethimide
    Increased effect of furosemide, insulin, propoxyphene
Smoking and nicotine can increase circulating cortisol and catecholamines; therapy with adrenergic agonists or adrenergic blockers may need to be adjusted
Decrease dose of patch in patients taking lithium

Drug Uptake

Gum: 15-30 minutes
Transdermal: 8-9 hours
Duration of effect: Transdermal: 24 hours
Serum half-life:
    Nicotine: 1-2 hours
    Cotinine: 15-20 hours
Time to peak serum concentration:

Pregnancy Risk Factor D (transdermal)/X (chewing gum)

Breast-feeding Considerations No data reported

Dosage Forms

Patch, transdermal:
    Habitrol™: 21 mg/day; 14 mg/day; 7 mg/day (30 systems/box)
    Nicoderm®: 21 mg/day; 14 mg/day; 7 mg/day (14 systems/box)
    Nicotrol® [OTC]: 15 mg/day (gradually released over 16 hours)
    ProStep®: 22 mg/day; 11 mg/day (7 systems/box)
Pieces, chewing gum, as polacrilex: 2 mg/square [OTC] (96 pieces/box); 4 mg/ square (96 pieces/box)
Spray, nasal: 0.5 mg/actuation [10 mg/mL-200 actuations] (10 mL)

Dietary Considerations No data reported

Generic Available No

Comments At least 10 reported studies have documented the effectiveness of nicotine patches in smoking cessation. Approximately 45% of treated patients quit smoking after 6 weeks of patch therapy. Control patients given placebo patches accounted for about a 20% success rate. At 52 weeks, approximately ½ of the 45% 6-week successful patients continued to abstain. Control placebo patients accounted for an approximate 11% success rate after 52 weeks.

Selected Readings

Li Wan Po A, "Transdermal Nicotine in Smoking Cessation. A Meta-Analysis," *Eur J Clin Pharmacol,* 1993, 45(6):519-28.

Transdermal Nicotine Study Group, "Transdermal Nicotine for Smoking Cessation. Six-month Results from Two Multicenter Controlled Clinical Trials," *JAMA,* 1991, 266(22):3133-8.

Westman EC, Levin ED, and Rose JE, "The Nicotine Patch in Smoking Cessation," *Arch Intern Med,* 1993, 153(16):1917-23.

Wynn RL, "Nicotine Patches in Smoking Cessation," *AGD Impact,* 1994, 22:14.

Nicotinex [OTC] *see* Niacin *on page 676*

Nicotrol® *see* Nicotine *on page 678*

Nifedipine *(nye FED i peen)*

Related Information

Calcium Channel Blockers & Gingival Hyperplasia *on page 1132*
Cardiovascular Diseases *on page 1010*

Brand Names Adalat®; Adalat® CC; Procardia®; Procardia XL®

Canadian/Mexican Brand Names Adalat® Oros (Mexico); Adalat PA® (Canada); Adalat® Retard (Mexico); Apo®-Nifed (Canada); Corogal® (Mexico); Corotrend® (Mexico); Corotrend® Retard (Mexico); Gen-Nifedipine® (Canada); Nifedipres® (Mexico); Noviken-N® (Mexico); Novo-Nifedin® (Canada); Nu-Nifedin® (Canada)

Therapeutic Category Antianginal Agent; Calcium Channel Blocker

Synonyms Nifedipino (Mexico)

Use Angina, hypertrophic cardiomyopathy, hypertension (sustained release only), pulmonary hypertension

Usual Dosage Capsule may be punctured and drug solution administered sublingually to reduce blood pressure

Children: Oral, S.L.:
Hypertensive emergencies: 0.25-0.5 mg/kg/dose
Hypertrophic cardiomyopathy: 0.6-0.9 mg/kg/24 hours in 3-4 divided doses

Adults:
Initial: 10 mg 3 times/day as capsules or 30 mg once daily as sustained release
Usual dose: 10-30 mg 3 times/day as capsules or 30-60 mg once daily as sustained release
Maximum dose: 120-180 mg/day
Increase sustained release at 7- to 14-day intervals

Not removed by hemo- or peritoneal dialysis; supplemental dose is not necessary

Mechanism of Action Inhibits calcium ion from entering the "slow channels" or select voltage-sensitive areas of vascular smooth muscle and myocardium during depolarization, producing a relaxation of coronary vascular smooth muscle and coronary vasodilation; increases myocardial oxygen delivery in patients with vasospastic angina

Local Anesthetic/Vasoconstrictor Precautions No information available to require special precautions

Effects on Dental Treatment Nifedipine has the greatest incidence in causing gingival hyperplasia than any other calcium channel blocker. Effects from the use of nifedipine (30-100 mg/day) have appeared after 1-9 months. Discontinuance of the drug results in complete disappearance or marked regression of symptoms; symptoms will reappear upon remediation. Marked regression occurs after 1 week and complete disappearance of symptoms has occurred within 15 days. If a gingivectomy is performed and use of the drug is continued or resumed, hyperplasia usually will reoccur. The success of the gingivectomy usually requires that the medication be discontinued or that a switch to a noncalcium channel blocker be made. If for some reason, nifedipine cannot be discontinued, hyperplasia has not reoccurred after gingivectomy when extensive plaque control was performed. If nifedipine is changed to another class of cardiovascular agent, the gingival hyperplasia will probably regress and disappear. A switch to another calcium channel blocker probably may result in continued hyperplasia.

Other Adverse Effects
>10%:
Cardiovascular: Flushing
Central nervous system: Dizziness, lightheadedness, giddiness, headache
Gastrointestinal: Nausea, heartburn
Neuromuscular & skeletal: Weakness
Miscellaneous: Heat sensation
1% to 10%:
Cardiovascular: Peripheral edema, palpitations, hypotension
Central nervous system: Nervousness, mood changes
Gastrointestinal: Sore throat
Neuromuscular & skeletal: Muscle cramps, tremor
Respiratory: Dyspnea, cough, nasal congestion
<1%:
Cardiovascular: Tachycardia, syncope
Central nervous system: Fever, chills
Dermatologic: Dermatitis, urticaria, purpura
Gastrointestinal: Diarrhea, constipation, gingival hyperplasia
Hematologic: Thrombocytopenia, leukopenia, anemia
Neuromuscular & skeletal: Joint stiffness, arthritis with increased ANA
Ocular: Blurred vision, transient blindness
Miscellaneous: Sweating

Drug Interactions
Increased toxicity/effect/levels:
H_2-blockers cause increased bioavailability of nifedipine
Beta-blockers cause increased cardiac depressant effects on A-V conduction
Severe hypotension has been reported during fentanyl anesthesia with concomitant use of beta-blockers and calcium channel blockers; even though such interactions have not been seen specifically with nifedipine, caution is suggested in using nifedipine with fentanyl

Drug Uptake
Onset of action:
Oral: Within 20 minutes
S.L.: Within 1-5 minutes
(Continued)

Nifedipine *(Continued)*

Serum half-life:
    Adults, normal: 2-5 hours
    Adults with cirrhosis: 7 hours
Pregnancy Risk Factor C
Generic Available Yes: Capsule
Selected Readings

Deen-Duggins L, Fry HR, Clay JR, et al, "Nifedipine-Associated Gingival Overgrowth: A Survey of the Literature and Report of Four Cases," *Quintessence Int*, 1996, 27(3):163-70.

Harel-Raviv M, Eckler M, Lalani K, et al, "Nifedipine-Induced Gingival Hyperplasia. A Comprehensive Review and Analysis," *Oral Surg Oral Med Oral Pathol Oral Radiol Endod*, 1995, 79(6):715-22.

Lederman D, Lumerman H, Reuben S, et al, "Gingival Hyperplasia Associated With Nifedipine Therapy," *Oral Surg Oral Med Oral Pathol*, 1984, 57(6):620-2.

Lucas RM, Howell LP, and Wall BA, "Nifedipine-Induced Gingival Hyperplasia: A Histochemical and Ultrastructural Study," *J Periodontol*, 1985, 56(4):211-5.

Nery EB, Edson RG, Lee KK, et al, "Prevalence of Nifedipine-Induced Gingival Hyperplasia," *J Periodontol*, 1995, 66(7):572-8.

Nishikawa SJ, Tada H, Hamasaki A, et al, "Nifedipine-Induced Gingival Hyperplasia: A Clinical and In Vitro Study," *J Periodontol*, 1991, 62(1):30-5.

Saito K, Mori S, Iwakura M, et al, "Immunohistochemical Localization of Transforming Growth Factor Beta, Basic Fibroblast Growth Factor and Heparin Sulphate Glycosaminoglycan in Gingival Hyperplasia Induced by Nifedipine and Phenytoin," *J Periodontal Res*, 1996, 31(8):545-5.

Silverstein LH, Koch JP, Lefkove MD, et al, "Nifedipine-Induced Gingival Enlargement Around Dental Implants: A Clinical Report," *J Oral Implantol*, 1995, 21(2):116-20.

Westbrook P, Bednarczyk EM, Carlson M, et al, "Regression of Nifedipine-Induced Gingival Hyperplasia Following Switch to a Same Class Calcium Channel Blocker, Isradipine," *J Periodontol*, 1997, 68(7):645-50.

Wynn RL, "Calcium Channel Blockers and Gingival Hyperplasia," *Gen Dent*, 1991, 39(4):240-3.

Wynn RL, "Update on Calcium Channel Blocker-Induced Gingival Hyperplasia," *Gen Dent*, 1995, 43(3):218-22.

Nifedipino (Mexico) *see* Nifedipine *on page 680*

Niferex® [OTC] *see* Polysaccharide-Iron Complex *on page 773*

Niferex®-PN *see* Vitamins, Multiple *on page 995*

Nilandron® *see* Nilutamide *on this page*

Nilstat® *see* Nystatin *on page 695*

Nilutamide *(ni LU ta mide)*

Brand Names Nilandron®
Canadian/Mexican Brand Names Anandron® (Can)
Therapeutic Category Antineoplastic Agent, Miscellaneous
Use In combination with surgical castration in treatment of metastatic prostatic carcinoma (Stage D_2); for maximum benefit, nilutamide treatment must begin on the same day as or on the day after surgical castration
Usual Dosage Adults: Oral: 300 mg (6-50 mg tablets) once daily for 30 days, then 150 mg (3-50 mg tablets) once daily; starting on the same day or day after surgical castration
Mechanism of Action Nonsteroidal antiandrogen that inhibits androgen uptake or inhibits binding of androgen in target tissues
Local Anesthetic/Vasoconstrictor Precautions No information available to require special precautions
Effects on Dental Treatment No effects or complications reported
Other Adverse Effects
>10%:
    Central nervous system: Pain, headache, insomnia
    Gastrointestinal: Nausea, constipation, anorexia
    Genitourinary: Impotence, testicular atrophy, gynecomastia
    Endocrine & metabolic: Loss of libido, hot flashes
    Neuromuscular & skeletal: Weakness
    Ocular: Impaired adaption to dark
1% to 10%:
    Cardiovascular: Hypertension
    Central nervous system: Flu syndrome, fever, dizziness, depression, hypesthesia
    Dermatologic: Alopecia, dry skin, rash
    Gastrointestinal: Dyspepsia, vomiting, abdominal pain
    Genitourinary: Urinary tract infection, hematuria, urinary tract disorder, nocturia
    Respiratory: Dyspnea, upper respiratory infection, pneumonia
    Ocular: Chromatopsia, impaired adaption to light, abnormal vision
    Miscellaneous: Diaphoresis
Drug Uptake
Absorption: Rapid and complete
Serum half-life: 38-59 hours
Pregnancy Risk Factor C
Dosage Forms Tablet: 50 mg

NIM *see* Bleomycin *on page 135*

Nimodipina (Mexico) *see* Nimodipine *on this page*

Nimodipine (nye MOE di peen)
Related Information
Calcium Channel Blockers & Gingival Hyperplasia *on page 1132*
Cardiovascular Diseases *on page 1010*
Brand Names Nimotop® .
Therapeutic Category Calcium Channel Blocker
Synonyms Nimodipina (Mexico)
Use Improvement of neurological deficits due to spasm following subarachnoid hemorrhage from ruptured congenital intracranial aneurysms in patients who are in good neurological condition postictus

Usual Dosage Adults: Oral: 60 mg every 4 hours for 21 days, start therapy within 96 hours after subarachnoid hemorrhage

Not removed by hemo- or peritoneal dialysis; supplemental dose is not necessary

Mechanism of Action Nimodipine shares the pharmacology of other calcium channel blockers; animal studies indicate that nimodipine has a greater effect on cerebral arterials than other arterials; this increased specificity may be due to the drug's increased lipophilicity and cerebral distribution as compared to nifedipine; inhibits calcium ion from entering the "slow channels" or select voltage sensitive areas of vascular smooth muscle and myocardium during depolarization

Local Anesthetic/Vasoconstrictor Precautions No information available to require special precautions

Effects on Dental Treatment Other drugs of this class can cause gingival hyperplasia (ie, nifedipine) but there have been no reports for nimodipine

Other Adverse Effects
1% to 10%: Cardiovascular: Reductions in systemic blood pressure

<1%:
Cardiovascular: Edema, EKG abnormalities, tachycardia, bradycardia
Central nervous system: Headache, depression
Dermatologic: Rash, acne
Gastrointestinal: Diarrhea, nausea
Hematologic: Hemorrhage
Hepatic: Hepatitis
Neuromuscular & skeletal: Muscle cramps
Respiratory: Dyspnea

Drug Interactions
Increased toxicity/effect/levels:
H_2 blockers cause increased bioavailability of nimodipine
Beta-blockers cause increased cardiac depressant effects on A-V conduction
Severe hypotension has been reported during fentanyl anesthesia with concomitant use of beta-blockers and calcium channel blockers; even though such interactions have not been seen specifically with nimodipine, caution is suggested in using nimodipine with fentanyl

Drug Uptake
Serum half-life: 3 hours, increases with reduced renal function
Time to peak serum concentration: Oral: Within 1 hour
Pregnancy Risk Factor C
Generic Available No

Nimotop® *see* Nimodipine *on this page*

Nipent™ Injection *see* Pentostatin *on page 740*

Nipride® *see* Nitroprusside *on page 686*

Nisoldipine (NYE sole di peen)
Related Information
Cardiovascular Diseases *on page 1010*
Brand Names Sular™
Therapeutic Category Calcium Channel Blocker
Use Management of hypertension, may be used alone or in combination with other antihypertensive agents

Usual Dosage Adults: Oral: Initial: 20 mg once daily, then increase by 10 mg/week (or longer intervals) to attain adequate control of blood pressure; doses >60 mg once daily are not recommended. A starting dose not exceeding 10 mg/day is recommended for the elderly and those with hepatic impairment.

Mechanism of Action As a dihydropyridine calcium channel blocker, structurally similar to nifedipine, nisoldipine impedes the movement of calcium ions into vascular smooth muscle and cardiac muscle. Dihydropyridines are potent vasodilators and are not as likely to suppress cardiac contractility and slow cardiac
(Continued)

Nisoldipine *(Continued)*

conduction as other calcium antagonists such as verapamil and diltiazem; nisoldipine is 5-10 times as potent a vasodilator as nifedipine.

Local Anesthetic/Vasoconstrictor Precautions No information available to require special precautions

Effects on Dental Treatment Other drugs in this class can cause gingival hyperplasia, but there have been no reports for nisoldipine

Other Adverse Effects
Cardiovascular: Peripheral edema, tachycardia
Central nervous system: Dizziness, headache

Warnings/Precautions Increased angina and/or myocardial infarction in patients with coronary artery disease

Drug Interactions Increased toxicity:
Nisoldipine and digoxin may increase digoxin effect
Nisoldipine and propranolol may increase cardiovascular adverse effects
Nisoldipine and H_2-antagonists increase bioavailability and may increase nisoldipine serum concentration
Nisoldipine and omeprazole increase bioavailability and may increase nisoldipine serum concentration

Drug Uptake
Absorption: Well absorbed
Serum half-life: 7-12 hours

Pregnancy Risk Factor C

Dosage Forms Tablet, extended release: 10 mg, 20 mg, 30 mg, 40 mg

Generic Available No

Nitro-Bid® *see* Nitroglycerin *on next page*
Nitrocine® *see* Nitroglycerin *on next page*
Nitrodisc® *see* Nitroglycerin *on next page*
Nitro-Dur® *see* Nitroglycerin *on next page*

Nitrofurantoin *(nye troe fyoor AN toyn)*

Brand Names Furadantin®; Macrobid®; Macrodantin®

Canadian/Mexican Brand Names Apo®-Nitrofurantoin (Canada); Furadantina® (Mexico); Macrodantina® (Mexico); Nephronex® (Canada); Novo-Furan® (Canada)

Therapeutic Category Antibiotic, Miscellaneous

Synonyms Nitrofurantoina (Mexico)

Use Prevention and treatment of urinary tract infections caused by susceptible gram-negative and some gram-positive organisms; *Pseudomonas, Serratia,* and most species of *Proteus* are generally resistant to nitrofurantoin

Usual Dosage Oral:
Children >1 month: 5-7 mg/kg/day in divided doses every 6 hours; maximum: 400 mg/day
Chronic therapy: 1-2 mg/kg/day in divided doses every 24 hours; maximum dose: 400 mg/day
Adults: 50-100 mg/dose every 6 hours (not to exceed 400 mg/24 hours)
Prophylaxis: 50-100 mg/dose at at bedtime

Mechanism of Action Inhibits several bacterial enzyme systems including acetyl coenzyme A interfering with metabolism and possibly cell wall synthesis

Local Anesthetic/Vasoconstrictor Precautions No information available to require special precautions

Effects on Dental Treatment No effects or complications reported

Other Adverse Effects
>10%:
Cardiovascular: Chest pains
Central nervous system: Chills, fever
Gastrointestinal: Stomach upset, diarrhea, loss of appetite, vomiting
Respiratory: Cough, dyspnea
1% to 10%:
Central nervous system: Fatigue, drowsiness, headache, dizziness
Gastrointestinal: Sore throat
Neuromuscular & skeletal: Paresthesia, weakness
<1%:
Dermatologic: Skin rash, itching
Hematologic: Hemolytic anemia
Hepatic: Hepatitis
Neuromuscular & skeletal: Arthralgia

Drug Interactions
Decreased effect: Antacids (decreases absorption of nitrofurantoin)
Increased toxicity: Probenecid (decreases renal excretion of nitrofurantoin)

Drug Uptake
Absorption: Well absorbed from GI tract; the macrocrystalline form is absorbed more slowly due to slower dissolution, but causes less GI distress
Serum half-life: 20-60 minutes; prolonged with renal impairment
Pregnancy Risk Factor B
Generic Available Yes: Tablet and suspension

Nitrofurantoina (Mexico) *see* Nitrofurantoin *on previous page*
Nitrofurazona (Mexico) *see* Nitrofurazone *on this page*

Nitrofurazone (nye troe FYOOR a zone)
Brand Names Furacin®
Therapeutic Category Antibacterial, Topical
Synonyms Nitrofurazona (Mexico)
Use Antibacterial agent in second and third degree burns and skin grafting
Usual Dosage Children and Adults: Topical: Apply once daily or every few days to lesion or place on gauze
Mechanism of Action A broad antibacterial spectrum; it acts by inhibiting bacterial enzymes involved in carbohydrate metabolism; effective against a wide range of gram-negative and gram-positive organisms; bactericidal against most bacteria commonly causing surface infections including *Staphylococcus aureus*, *Streptococcus*, *Escherichia coli*, *Enterobacter cloacae*, *Clostridium perfringens*, *Aerobacter aerogenes*, and *Proteus* sp; not particularly active against most *Pseudomonas aeruginosa* strains and does not inhibit viruses or fungi. Topical preparations of nitrofurazone are readily soluble in blood, pus, and serum and are nonmacerating.
Local Anesthetic/Vasoconstrictor Precautions No information available to require special precautions
Effects on Dental Treatment No effects or complications reported
Other Adverse Effects Women should inform their physicians if signs or symptoms of any of the following occur thromboembolic or thrombotic disorders including sudden severe headache or vomiting, disturbance of vision or speech, loss of vision, numbness or weakness in an extremity, sharp or crushing chest pain, calf pain, dyspnea, severe abdominal pain or mass, mental depression or unusual bleeding

Women should discontinue taking the medication if they suspect they are pregnant or become pregnant. Notify physician if area under dermal patch becomes irritated or a rash develops.
Drug Interactions Decreased effect: Sutilains decrease activity of nitrofurazone
Pregnancy Risk Factor C
Generic Available Yes

Nitrogard® *see* Nitroglycerin *on this page*
Nitroglicerina (Mexico) *see* Nitroglycerin *on this page*

Nitroglycerin (nye troe GLI ser in)
Related Information
Cardiovascular Diseases *on page 1010*
Brand Names Deponit®; Minitran®; Nitro-Bid®; Nitrocine®; Nitrodisc®; Nitro-Dur®; Nitrogard®; Nitroglyn®; Nitrol®; Nitrolingual®; Nitrong®; Nitrostat®; Transdermal-NTG®; Transderm-Nitro®; Tridil®
Canadian/Mexican Brand Names Cardinit® (Mexico); Nitradisc® (Mexico); Nitroderm-TTS® (Mexico)
Therapeutic Category Antianginal Agent; Nitrate; Vasodilator, Coronary
Synonyms Nitroglicerina (Mexico)
Use Treatment of angina pectoris; I.V. for congestive heart failure (especially when associated with acute myocardial infarction); pulmonary hypertension; hypertensive emergencies occurring perioperatively (especially during cardiovascular surgery)
Usual Dosage Note: Hemodynamic and antianginal tolerance often develop within 24-48 hours of continuous nitrate administration

Children: Pulmonary hypertension: Continuous infusion: Start 0.25-0.5 mcg/kg/minute and titrate by 1 mcg/kg/minute at 20- to 60-minute intervals to desired effect; usual dose: 1-3 mcg/kg/minute; maximum: 5 mcg/kg/minute

Adults:
Buccal: Initial: 1 mg every 3-5 hours while awake (3 times/day); titrate dosage upward if angina occurs with tablet in place
Oral: 2.5-9 mg 2-4 times/day (up to 26 mg 4 times/day)
I.V.: 5 mcg/minute, increase by 5 mcg/minute every 3-5 minutes to 20 mcg/minute; if no response at 20 mcg/minute increase by 10 mcg/minute every 3-5 minutes, up to 200 mcg/minute
(Continued)

Nitroglycerin *(Continued)*

Ointment: 1" to 2" every 8 hours up to 4" to 5" every 4 hours

Patch, transdermal: 0.2-0.4 mg/hour initially and titrate to doses of 0.4-0.8 mg/hour; tolerance is minimized by using a patch-on period of 12-14 hours and patch-off period of 10-12 hours

Sublingual: 0.2-0.6 mg every 5 minutes for maximum of 3 doses in 15 minutes; may also use prophylactically 5-10 minutes prior to activities which may provoke an attack

Translingual: 1-2 sprays into mouth under tongue every 3-5 minutes for maximum of 3 doses in 15 minutes, may also be used 5-10 minutes prior to activities which may provoke an attack prophylactically

May need to use nitrate-free interval (10-12 hours/day) to avoid tolerance development; tolerance may possibly be reversed with acetylcysteine; gradually decrease dose in patients receiving NTG for prolonged period to avoid withdrawal reaction

Mechanism of Action Reduces cardiac oxygen demand by decreasing left ventricular pressure and systemic vascular resistance; dilates coronary arteries and improves collateral flow to ischemic regions

Local Anesthetic/Vasoconstrictor Precautions No information available to require special precautions

Effects on Dental Treatment No effects or complications reported

Other Adverse Effects

>10%:

Cardiovascular: Postural hypotension, flushing

Central nervous system: Headache, lightheadedness, dizziness

Neuromuscular & skeletal: Weakness

1% to 10%: Dermatologic: Drug rash, exfoliative dermatitis

<1%:

Cardiovascular: Reflex tachycardia, bradycardia, coronary vascular insufficiency, arrhythmias

Dermatologic: Allergic contact dermatitis, exfoliative dermatitis

Gastrointestinal: Nausea, vomiting

Hematologic: Methemoglobinemia (overdose)

Miscellaneous: Perspiration, collapse, alcohol intoxication

Drug Interactions

Decreased effect: I.V. nitroglycerin may antagonize the anticoagulant effect of heparin, monitor closely; may need to decrease heparin dosage when nitroglycerin is discontinued

Increased toxicity: Alcohol, beta-blockers, calcium channel blockers may enhance nitroglycerin's hypotensive effect

Drug Uptake

Onset and duration of action is dependent upon dosage form administered

Serum half-life: 1-4 minutes

Pregnancy Risk Factor C

Generic Available Yes

Nitroglyn® *see* Nitroglycerin *on previous page*

Nitrol® *see* Nitroglycerin *on previous page*

Nitrolingual® *see* Nitroglycerin *on previous page*

Nitrong® *see* Nitroglycerin *on previous page*

Nitropress® *see* Nitroprusside *on this page*

Nitroprusside *(nye troe PRUS ide)*

Brand Names Nipride®; Nitropress®

Therapeutic Category Vasodilator

Use Management of hypertensive crises; congestive heart failure; used for controlled hypotension to reduce bleeding during surgery

Usual Dosage Administration requires the use of an infusion pump. Average dose: 5 mcg/kg/minute

Children: Pulmonary hypertension: I.V.: Initial: 1 mcg/kg/minute by continuous I.V. infusion; increase in increments of 1 mcg/kg/minute at intervals of 20-60 minutes; titrating to the desired response; usual dose: 3 mcg/kg/minute, rarely need >4 mcg/kg/minute; maximum: 5 mcg/kg/minute.

Adults: I.V. Initial: 0.3-0.5 mcg/kg/minute; increase in increments of 0.5 mcg/kg/minute, titrating to the desired hemodynamic effect or the appearance of headache or nausea; usual dose: 3 mcg/kg/minute; rarely need >4 mcg/kg/minute; maximum: 10 mcg/kg/minute. When >500 mcg/kg is administered by prolonged infusion of faster than 2 mcg/kg/minute, cyanide is generated faster than an unaided patient can handle.

Mechanism of Action Causes peripheral vasodilation by direct action on venous and arteriolar smooth muscle, thus reducing peripheral resistance; will increase cardiac output by decreasing afterload; reduces aortal and left ventricular impedance

Local Anesthetic/Vasoconstrictor Precautions No information available to require special precautions

Effects on Dental Treatment No effects or complications reported

Other Adverse Effects 1% to 10%:

Cardiovascular: Excessive hypotensive response, palpitations, substernal distress

Central nervous system: Disorientation, psychosis, headache, restlessness

Endocrine & metabolic: Thyroid suppression

Gastrointestinal: Nausea, vomiting

Neuromuscular & skeletal: Muscle spasm, weakness

Otic: Tinnitus

Respiratory: Hypoxia

Miscellaneous: Sweating, thiocyanate toxicity

Drug Interactions No data reported

Drug Uptake

Onset of hypotensive effect: <2 minutes

Duration: Within 1-10 minutes following discontinuation of therapy, effects cease

Serum half-life:

Parent drug: <10 minutes

Thiocyanate: 2.7-7 days

Pregnancy Risk Factor C

Generic Available Yes

Nitrostat® see Nitroglycerin on page 685

Nitrous Oxide (NYE trus OKS ide)

Related Information

Patients Requiring Sedation on page 1081

Therapeutic Category Dental Gases

Use

Dental: To induce sedation and analgesia in anxious dental patients

Medical: A principal adjunct to inhalation and intravenous general anesthesia in medical patients undergoing surgery; prehospital relief of pain of differing etiologies (ie, burns, fractures, back injury, abrasions, lacerations)

Usual Dosage Children and Adults: For sedation and analgesia: Concentrations of 25% to 50% nitrous oxide with oxygen inhaled through the nose via a nasal mask

Mechanism of Action General CNS depressant action; may act similarly as inhalant general anesthetics by mildly stabilizing axonal membranes to partially inhibit action potentials leading to sedation; may partially act on opiate receptor systems to cause mild analgesia

Local Anesthetic/Vasoconstrictor Precautions No information available to require special precautions

Effects on Dental Treatment No effects or complications reported

Other Adverse Effects

An increased risk of renal and hepatic diseases and peripheral neuropathy similar to that of vitamin B_{12} deficiency have been reported in dental personnel who work in areas where nitrous oxide is used

Methionine synthase, a vitamin B_{12} dependent enzyme, is inactivated following very prolonged administration of nitrous oxide, and the subsequent interference with DNA synthesis prevents production of both leukocytes and red blood cells by bone marrow. These effects do not occur within the time frame of clinical sedation.

Female dental personnel who were exposed to unscavenged nitrous oxide for more than 5 hours/week were significantly less fertile than women who were not exposed, or who were exposed to lower levels of scavenged or unscavenged nitrous oxide. Fertility was measured by the number of menstrual cycles, without use of contraception, required to become pregnant. Women who were exposed to nitrous oxide for more than 5 hours/week were only 41% as likely as unexposed women to conceive during each monthly cycle.

Contraindications Nitrous oxide should not be administered without oxygen. Nitrous oxide should not be given to patients after a full meal

Warnings/Precautions Nausea and vomiting occurs postoperatively in ~15% of patients. Prolonged use may produce bone marrow suppression and/or neurologic dysfunction. Oxygen should be briefly administered during emergence from prolonged anesthesia with nitrous oxide to prevent diffusion hypoxia. Patients with vitamin B_{12} deficiency (pernicious anemia) and those with other nutritional (Continued)

Nitrous Oxide *(Continued)*

deficiencies (alcoholics) are at increased risk of developing neurologic disease and bone marrow suppression with exposure to nitrous oxide. May be addictive

Drug Interactions No data reported

Drug Uptake Nitrous oxide is rapidly absorbed via inhalation. The blood/gas partition coefficient is 0.5. The gas is rapidly eliminated via the lungs, with minimal amounts eliminated through the skin.

Onset time: Inhalation: 5-10 minutes

Pregnancy Risk Factor No data reported

Breast-feeding Considerations No data reported

Dosage Forms Supplied in blue cylinders

Dietary Considerations No data reported

Generic Available Yes

Comments Results of a mail survey of more than 30,000 dentists and 30,000 chairside assistants, who were exposed to trace anesthetics in dental operatories were published in 1980 (Cohen et al, 1980). This study suggested that long-term exposure to nitrous oxide and to nitrous oxide/halogenated anesthetics was associated with an increase in general health problems and reproductive difficulties in these dental personnel. Schuyt et al (1986) observed that 4 female dental personnel who were exposed to inhalation sedation with 35% nitrous oxide reported 6 spontaneous abortions among 7 pregnancies over 17 months

Selected Readings

Babich S and Burakoff RP, "Occupational Hazards of Dentistry. A Review of Literature From 1990," *N Y State Dent J*, 1997, 63(8):26-31.

Baird PA, "Occupational Exposure to Nitrous Oxide - Not a Laughing Matter," *N Engl J Med*, 1992, 327(14):1026-7.

Cohen EN, Gift HC, Brown BW, et al, "Occupational Disease in Dentistry and Chronic Exposure to Trace Anesthetic Gases," *J Am Dent Assoc*, 1980, 101(1):21-31.

Dunning DG, McFarland K, and Safarik M, "Nitrous-Oxide Use. II. Risks, Compliance, and Exposure Levels Among Nebraska Dentists and Dental Assistants," *Gen Dent*, 1997, 45(1):82-6.

Howard WR, "Nitrous Oxide in the Dental Environment: Assessing the Risk, Reducing the Exposure," *J Am Dent Assoc*, 1997, 128(3):356-60.

Johnsen KG, "Nitrous Oxide Safety," *J Am Dent Assoc*, 1997, 128(8):1066-7.

"Nitrous Oxide in the Dental Office. ADA Council on Scientific Affairs; ADA Council on Dental Practice," *J Am Dent Assoc*, 1997, 128(3):364-5.

Petersen JK, "Nitrous Oxide Analgesia in Dental Practice," *Acta Anaesthesiol Scand*, 1994, 38(8):773-4.

Quarnstrom F, "Nitrous Oxide," *J Am Dent Assoc*, 1997, 128(6):690, 692.

Rowland AS, Baird DD, Weinberg CR, et al, "Reduced Fertility Among Women Employed as Female Dental Assistants Exposed to High Levels of Nitrous Oxide," *N Engl J Med*, 1992, 327(14):993-7.

Schuyt HC, Brakel K, Oostendorp SG, et al, "Abortions Among Dental Personnel Exposed to Nitrous Oxide," *Anaesthesia*, 1986, 41(1):82-3.

Wynn RL, "Nitrous Oxide and Fertility, Part I," *Gen Dent*, 1993, 41(2):122-3.

Wynn RL, "Nitrous Oxide and Fertility, Part II," *Gen Dent*, 1993, 41(3):212, 214.

Nix™ [OTC] *see* Permethrin *on page 744*

Nizatidina (Mexico) *see* Nizatidine *on this page*

Nizatidine *(ni ZA ti deen)*

Brand Names Axid®; Axid® AR [OTC]

Therapeutic Category Histamine H_2 Antagonist

Synonyms Nizatidina (Mexico)

Use Treatment and maintenance of duodenal ulcer; treatment of gastroesophageal reflux disease (GERD)

Usual Dosage Adults: Active duodenal ulcer: Oral:

Treatment: 300 mg at bedtime or 150 mg twice daily

Maintenance: 150 mg/day

Mechanism of Action Nizatidine is an H_2-receptor antagonist. In healthy volunteers, nizatidine has been effective in suppressing gastric acid secretion induced by pentagastrin infusion or food. Nizatidine reduces gastric acid secretion by 29.4% to 78.4%. This compares with a 60.3% reduction by cimetidine. Nizatidine 100 mg is reported to provide equivalent acid suppression as cimetidine 300 mg.

Local Anesthetic/Vasoconstrictor Precautions No information available to require special precautions

Effects on Dental Treatment No effects or complications reported

Other Adverse Effects

1% to 10%:

Central nervous system: Dizziness, headache

Gastrointestinal: Constipation, diarrhea

<1%:

Cardiovascular: Bradycardia, tachycardia, palpitations, hypertension

Central nervous system: Fever, fatigue, seizures, insomnia, drowsiness

Dermatologic: Acne, pruritus, urticaria, dry skin

Gastrointestinal: Abdominal discomfort, flatulence, belching, anorexia

Hematologic: Agranulocytosis, neutropenia, thrombocytopenia

Hepatic: Elevated AST, ALT
Neuromuscular & skeletal: Paresthesia, weakness
Renal: Elevated BUN and creatinine, proteinuria
Respiratory: Bronchospasm
Miscellaneous: Allergic reaction
Drug Interactions No data reported
Pregnancy Risk Factor C
Generic Available No

Nizoral® see Ketoconazole on page 533

N-Methylhydrazine see Procarbazine on page 798

Nolahist® [OTC] see Phenindamine on page 747

Nolamine® see Chlorpheniramine, Phenindamine, and Phenylpropanolamine on page 220

Nolex® LA see Guaifenesin and Phenylpropanolamine on page 454

Nolvadex® see Tamoxifen on page 903

Nonoxynol 9 (non OKS i nole nine)

Brand Names Because® [OTC]; Delfen® [OTC]; Emko® [OTC]; Encare® [OTC]; Gynol II® [OTC]; Koromex® [OTC]; Ramses® [OTC]; Semicid® [OTC]; Shur-Seal® [OTC]

Therapeutic Category Spermicide

Use Spermatocide in contraception

Local Anesthetic/Vasoconstrictor Precautions No information available to require special precautions

Effects on Dental Treatment No effects or complications reported

Pregnancy Risk Factor C

Generic Available Yes

Nonsteroidal Anti-Inflammatory Agents, Comparative Dosages, and Pharmacokinetics see page 1143

Nonviral Infectious Diseases see page 1032

No Pain-HP® [OTC] see Capsaicin on page 170

Noradrenaline see Norepinephrine on this page

Noradrenaline Acid Tartrate see Norepinephrine on this page

Norcet® [5/500] see Hydrocodone and Acetaminophen on page 478

Nordette® see Ethinyl Estradiol and Levonorgestrel on page 377

Norditropin® Injection see Human Growth Hormone on page 473

Norepinephrine (nor ep i NEF rin)

Brand Names Levophed® Injection

Therapeutic Category Adrenergic Agonist Agent

Synonyms Levarterenol Bitartrate; Noradrenaline; Noradrenaline Acid Tartrate; Norepinephrine Bitartrate

Use Treatment of shock which persists after adequate fluid volume replacement; severe hypotension; cardiogenic shock

Usual Dosage Note: Norepinephrine dosage is stated in terms of norepinephrine base and intravenous formulation is norepinephrine bitartrate

Norepinephrine bitartrate 2 mg = norepinephrine base 1 mg

Continuous I.V. infusion:
Children:
Initial: 0.05-0.1 mcg/kg/minute; titrate to desired effect
Maximum dose: 1-2 mcg/kg/minute
Adults: Initiate at 4 mcg/minute and titrate to desired response; 8-12 mcg/minute is usual range
ACLS dosing range: 0.5-30 mcg/minute
Rate of infusion: 4 mg in 500 mL D$_5$W
2 mcg/minute = 15 mL/hour
4 mcg/minute = 30 mL/hour
6 mcg/minute = 45 mL/hour
8 mcg/minute = 60 mL/hour
10 mcg/minute = 75 mL/hour
12 mcg/minute = 90 mL/hour
14 mcg/minute = 105 mL/hour
16 mcg/minute = 120 mL/hour
18 mcg/minute = 135 mL/hour
20 mcg/minute = 150 mL/hour
Mechanism of Action Stimulates beta$_1$-adrenergic receptors and alpha-adrenergic receptors causing increased contractility and heart rate as well as vasoconstriction, thereby increasing systemic blood pressure and coronary blood flow;
(Continued)

Norepinephrine *(Continued)*

clinically alpha effects (vasoconstriction) are greater than beta effects (inotropic and chronotropic effects)

Local Anesthetic/Vasoconstrictor Precautions No information available to require special precautions

Effects on Dental Treatment No effects or complications reported

Other Adverse Effects

1% to 10%:

Central nervous system: Dizziness, anxiety, headache, insomnia

Endocrine & metabolic: Thyroid gland enlargement

Neuromuscular & skeletal: Trembling

<1%:

Cardiovascular: Cardiac arrhythmias, palpitations, bradycardia, tachycardia, hypertension, chest pain, pallor, gangrene of extremities

Gastrointestinal: Vomiting

Genitourinary: Uterine contractions

Local: Sloughing at the infusion site

Ocular: Photophobia

Respiratory: Respiratory distress

Miscellaneous: Diaphoresis

Warnings/Precautions Blood/volume depletion should be corrected, if possible, before norepinephrine therapy; extravasation may cause severe tissue necrosis, administer into a large vein. The drug should not be given to patients with peripheral or mesenteric vascular thrombosis because ischemia may be increased and the area of infarct extended; use with caution during cyclopropane and halothane anesthesia; use with caution in patients with occlusive vascular disease; some products may contain sulfites

Drug Interactions

Increased effect with tricyclic antidepressants, MAO inhibitors, antihistamines (diphenhydramine, tripelennamine), guanethidine, ergot alkaloids, and methyldopa

Atropine sulfate may block the reflex bradycardia caused by norepinephrine and enhances the pressor response

Drug Uptake

Onset of action: I.V.: Very rapid-acting

Duration: Limited

Metabolism: By catechol-o-methyltransferase (COMT) and monoamine oxidase (MAO)

Elimination: In urine (84% to 96% as inactive metabolites)

Pregnancy Risk Factor D

Dosage Forms Injection, as bitartrate: 1 mg/mL (4 mL)

Generic Available No

Selected Readings

Martin C, Papazian L, Perrin G, et al, "Norepinephrine or Dopamine for the Treatment of Hyperdynamic Septic Shock?" *Chest*, 1993, 103(6):1826-31.

Norepinephrine Bitartrate *see* Norepinephrine *on previous page*

Norethin™ 1/35E *see* Ethinyl Estradiol and Norethindrone *on page 379*

Norethin™ 1/50M *see* Mestranol and Norethindrone *on page 603*

Norethindrone *(nor eth IN drone)*

Related Information

Endocrine Disorders & Pregnancy *on page 1021*

Brand Names Aygestin®; Micronor®; NOR-Q.D.®

Canadian/Mexican Brand Names Syngestal® (Mexico)

Therapeutic Category Contraceptive, Oral; Contraceptive, Progestin Only; Progestin

Synonyms Noretindrona (Mexico)

Use Treatment of amenorrhea; abnormal uterine bleeding; endometriosis, oral contraceptive; **higher rate of failure with progestin only contraceptives**

Mechanism of Action Inhibits secretion of pituitary gonadotropin (LH) which prevents follicular maturation and ovulation

Local Anesthetic/Vasoconstrictor Precautions No information available to require special precautions

Effects on Dental Treatment Until we know more about the mechanism of interaction, caution is required in prescribing antibiotics to female dental patients taking progestin-only oral contraceptives

Other Adverse Effects

>10%:

Cardiovascular: Edema

Endocrine & metabolic: Breakthrough bleeding, spotting, changes in menstrual flow, amenorrhea

Gastrointestinal: Anorexia

Neuromuscular & skeletal: Weakness

1% to 10%:

Cardiovascular: Embolism, central thrombosis

Central nervous system: Mental depression, fever, insomnia

Dermatologic: Melasma.or chloasma, allergic rash with or without pruritus

Endocrine & metabolic: Changes in cervical erosion and secretions, weight gain or loss, increased breast tenderness

Hepatic: Cholestatic jaundice

Local: Thrombophlebitis

Drug Interactions Decreased effect: Aminoglutethimide may decrease effects by increasing hepatic metabolism

Pregnancy Risk Factor X

Generic Available No

Noretindrona (Mexico) *see* Norethindrone *on previous page*

Norflex™ *see* Orphenadrine *on page 704*

Norfloxacin (nor FLOKS a sin)

Brand Names Chibroxin™; Noroxin®

Canadian/Mexican Brand Names Floxacin® (Mexico); Oranor® (Mexico)

Therapeutic Category Antibiotic, Quinolone

Synonyms Norfloxacina (Mexico)

Use Complicated and uncomplicated urinary tract infections caused by susceptible gram-negative and gram-positive bacteria; ophthalmic solution for conjunctivitis

Usual Dosage

Ophthalmic: Children >1 year and Adults: Instill 1-2 drops in affected eye(s) 4 times/day for up to 7 days

Oral: Adults:

Urinary tract infections: 400 mg twice daily for 3-21 days depending on severity of infection or organism sensitivity; maximum: 800 mg/day

Uncomplicated gonorrhea: 800 mg as a single dose (CDC recommends as an alternative regimen to ciprofloxacin or ofloxacin)

Prostatitis: 400 mg every 12 hours for 4 weeks

Mechanism of Action Norfloxacin is a DNA gyrase inhibitor. DNA gyrase is an essential bacterial enzyme that maintains the superhelical structure of DNA. DNA gyrase is required for DNA replication and transcription, DNA repair, recombination, and transposition; bactericidal

Local Anesthetic/Vasoconstrictor Precautions No information available to require special precautions

Effects on Dental Treatment No effects or complications reported

Other Adverse Effects

1% to 10%:

Central nervous system: Headache, dizziness, fatigue

Gastrointestinal: Nausea

<1%:

Central nervous system: Somnolence, depression, insomnia, fever

Dermatologic: Pruritus, hyperhidrosis, erythema, rash

Gastrointestinal: Abdominal pain, dyspepsia, constipation, flatulence, heartburn, dry mouth, diarrhea, vomiting, loose stools, anorexia, bitter taste, GI bleeding

Hepatic: Elevated liver enzymes

Neuromuscular & skeletal: Back pain, weakness

Renal: Elevated serum creatinine and BUN, acute renal failure

Drug Interactions

Decreased effect: Decreased absorption with antacids containing aluminum, magnesium, and/or calcium (by up to 98% if given at the same time)

Increased toxicity/serum levels: Quinolones cause increased levels of caffeine, warfarin, cyclosporine, and theophylline; azlocillin, cimetidine, probenecid increase quinolone levels

Drug Uptake

Absorption: Oral: Rapid, up to 40%

Serum half-life: 4.8 hours (can be higher with reduced glomerular filtration rates)

Time to peak serum concentration: Within 1-2 hours

Pregnancy Risk Factor C

Generic Available No

Norfloxacina (Mexico) *see* Norfloxacin *on this page*

Norgesic™ *see* Orphenadrine, Aspirin, and Caffeine *on page 704*

Norgesic™ Forte *see* Orphenadrine, Aspirin, and Caffeine *on page 704*

Norgestimate and Ethinyl Estradiol *see* Ethinyl Estradiol and Norgestimate *on page 381*

Norgestrel (nor JES trel)
Related Information
Endocrine Disorders & Pregnancy *on page 1021*
Brand Names Ovrette®
Therapeutic Category Contraceptive, Oral; Progestin
Use Prevention of pregnancy; **progestin only products have higher risk of failure in contraceptive use**
Usual Dosage Administer daily, starting the first day of menstruation, take 1 tablet at the same time each day, every day of the year. If 1 dose is missed, take as soon as remembered, then next tablet at regular time; if 2 doses are missed, take 1 tablet and discard the other, then take daily at usual time; if 3 doses are missed, use an additional form of birth control until menses or pregnancy is ruled out.
Mechanism of Action Inhibits secretion of pituitary gonadotropin (LH) which prevents follicular maturation and ovulation
Local Anesthetic/Vasoconstrictor Precautions No information available to require special precautions
Effects on Dental Treatment Until we know more about the mechanism of interaction, caution is required in prescribing antibiotics to female dental patients taking progestin-only oral contraceptives
Other Adverse Effects
>10%:
Cardiovascular: Edema
Endocrine & metabolic: Breakthrough bleeding, spotting, changes in menstrual flow, amenorrhea
Gastrointestinal: Anorexia
Neuromuscular & skeletal: Weakness
1% to 10%:
Cardiovascular: Embolism, central thrombosis
Central nervous system: Mental depression, fever, insomnia
Dermatologic: Melasma or chloasma, allergic rash with or without pruritus
Endocrine & metabolic: Changes in cervical erosion and secretions, weight gain or loss, increased breast tenderness
Hepatic: Cholestatic jaundice
Local: Thrombophlebitis
Drug Interactions Decreased effect: Aminoglutethimide may decrease effects by increasing hepatic metabolism
Pregnancy Risk Factor X
Generic Available No

Norinyl® 1+35 *see* Ethinyl Estradiol and Norethindrone *on page 379*
Norinyl® 1+50 *see* Mestranol and Norethindrone *on page 603*
Noritate® Cream *see* Metronidazole *on page 631*
Normal Saline *see* Sodium Chloride *on page 870*
Normiflo® *see* Ardeparin *on page 85*
Normodyne® *see* Labetalol *on page 537*
Noroxin® *see* Norfloxacin *on previous page*
Norpace® *see* Disopyramide *on page 327*
Norplant® Implant *see* Levonorgestrel *on page 550*
Norpramin® *see* Desipramine *on page 288*
NOR-Q.D.® *see* Norethindrone *on page 690*
Nortriptilina Clorhidrato De (Mexico) *see* Nortriptyline *on this page*

Nortriptyline (nor TRIP ti leen)
Brand Names Aventyl® Hydrochloride; Pamelor®
Therapeutic Category Antidepressant, Tricyclic
Synonyms Nortriptilina Clorhidrato De (Mexico)
Use Treatment of various forms of depression, often in conjunction with psychotherapy. Maximum antidepressant effect may not be seen for 2 or more weeks after initiation of therapy; has also demonstrated effectiveness for chronic pain.
Usual Dosage Oral:
Nocturnal enuresis:
Children:
6-7 years (20-25 kg): 10 mg/day
8-11 years (25-35 kg): 10-20 mg/day
>11 years (35-54 kg): 25-35 mg/day
Depression:
Adolescents: 30-50 mg/day in divided doses

Adults: 25 mg 3-4 times/day up to 150 mg/day

Elderly:

Initial: 10-25 mg at bedtime

Dosage can be increased by 25 mg every 3 days for inpatients and weekly for outpatients if tolerated

Usual maintenance dose: 75 mg as a single bedtime dose, however, lower or higher doses may be required to stay within the therapeutic window

Mechanism of Action Traditionally believed to increase the synaptic concentration of serotonin and/or norepinephrine in the central nervous system by inhibition of their reuptake by the presynaptic neuronal membrane. However, additional receptor effects have been found including desensitization of adenyl cyclase, down regulation of beta-adrenergic receptors, and down regulation of serotonin receptors.

Local Anesthetic/Vasoconstrictor Precautions Use with caution; epinephrine, norepinephrine and levonordefrin have been shown to have an increased pressor response in combination with TCAs

Effects on Dental Treatment >10% of patients experience dry mouth; long-term treatment with TCAs such as amoxapine increases the risk of caries by reducing salivation and salivary buffer capacity

Other Adverse Effects

>10%:

Central nervous system: Dizziness, drowsiness, headache

Gastrointestinal: Constipation, increased appetite, nausea, unpleasant taste, weight gain

Neuromuscular & skeletal: Weakness

1% to 10%:

Cardiovascular: Postural hypotension, arrhythmias, tachycardia, sudden death

Central nervous system: Confusion, delirium, hallucinations, nervousness, restlessness, parkinsonian syndrome, insomnia

Endocrine & metabolic: Sexual dysfunction

Gastrointestinal: Diarrhea, heartburn

Genitourinary: Dysuria

Ocular: Blurred vision, eye pain

Neuromuscular & skeletal: Fine muscle tremors

Miscellaneous: Excessive sweating

<1%:

Central nervous system: Anxiety, seizures

Dermatologic: Alopecia, photosensitivity

Endocrine & metabolic: Breast enlargement, galactorrhea, SIADH

Gastrointestinal: Trouble with gums, decreased lower esophageal sphincter tone may cause GE reflux

Genitourinary: Testicular swelling

Hematologic: Leukopenia, rarely agranulocytosis, eosinophilia

Hepatic: Elevated liver enzymes, cholestatic jaundice

Otic: Tinnitus

Miscellaneous: Allergic reactions

Drug Interactions Blocks the uptake of guanethidine and thus prevents the hypotensive effect of guanethidine; may be additive with or may potentiate the action of other CNS depressants such as sedatives or hypnotics; potentiates the pressor and cardiac effects of sympathomimetic agents such as isoproterenol, epinephrine, etc; with MAO inhibitors, hyperpyrexia, hypertension, tachycardia, confusion, seizures, and death have been reported; anticholinergic effect seen with other anticholinergic agents; cimetidine reduces the metabolism of nortriptyline; may increase the prothrombin time in patients stabilized on warfarin

Drug Uptake

Onset of action: 1-3 weeks before therapeutic effects are seen

Serum half-life: 28-31 hours

Time to peak serum concentration: Oral: Within 7-8.5 hours

Pregnancy Risk Factor D

Generic Available Yes

Selected Readings

Boakes AJ, Laurence DR, Teoh PC, et al, "Interactions Between Sympathomimetic Amines and Antidepressant Agents in Man," *Br Med J*, 1973, 1(849):311-5.

Jastak JT and Yagiela JA, "Vasoconstrictors and Local Anesthesia: A Review and Rationale for Use," *J Am Dent Assoc*, 1983, 107(4):623-30.

Larochelle P, Hamet P, and Enjalbert M, "Responses to Tyramine and Norepinephrine After Imipramine and Trazodone," *Clin Pharmacol Ther*, 1979, 26(1):24-30.

Mitchell JR, "Guanethidine and Related Agents. III Antagonism by Drugs Which Inhibit the Norepinephrine Pump in Man," *J Clin Invest*, 1970, 49(8):1596-604.

Rundegren J, van Dijken J, Mörnstad H, et al, "Oral Conditions in Patients Receiving Long-Term Treatment With Cyclic Antidepressant Drugs," *Swed Dent J*, 1985, 9(2):55-64.

Svedmyr N, "The Influence of a Tricyclic Antidepressive Agent (Protriptyline) on Some of the Circulatory Effects of Noradrenaline and Adrenalin in Man," *Life Sci*, 1968, 7(1):77-84.

Norvasc® see Amlodipine on page 63

Norvir® see Ritonavir on page 847

Norzine® see Thiethylperazine on page 924

Nõstrilla® [OTC] see Oxymetazoline on page 714

Nostril® Nasal Solution [OTC] see Phenylephrine on page 752

Novacet® Topical see Sulfur and Sulfacetamide Sodium on page 898

Novahistine® DMX Liquid [OTC] See Guaifenesin, Pseudoephedrine, and Dextromethorphan on page 456

Novantrone® see Mitoxantrone on page 643

Novocain® see Procaine on page 798

Novolin® 70/30 see Insulin Preparations on page 509

Novolin® L see Insulin Preparations on page 509

Novolin® N see Insulin Preparations on page 509

Novolin® R see Insulin Preparations on page 509

NP-27® [OTC] see Tolnaftate on page 943

NPH lletin® I see Insulin Preparations on page 509

NPH Insulin see Insulin Preparations on page 509

NPH-N see Insulin Preparations on page 509

NSC-102816 see Azacitidine on page 101

NSC-106977 see Erwinia Asparaginase on page 360

NTZ® Long Acting Nasal Solution [OTC] see Oxymetazoline on page 714

Nubain® see Nalbuphine on page 660

Nucofed® see Guaifenesin, Pseudoephedrine, and Codeine on page 455

Nucofed® Pediatric Expectorant see Guaifenesin, Pseudoephedrine, and Codeine on page 455

Nucotuss® see Guaifenesin, Pseudoephedrine, and Codeine on page 455

Nu-Iron® [OTC] see Polysaccharide-Iron Complex on page 773

Nullo® [OTC] see Chlorophyll on page 212

NuLytely® see Polyethylene Glycol-Electrolyte Solution on page 771

Numorphan® see Oxymorphone on page 715

Numzitdent® [OTC] see Benzocaine on page 118

Numzit Teething® [OTC] see Benzocaine on page 118

Nupercainal® [OTC] see Dibucaine on page 302

Nuprin® [OTC] see Ibuprofen on page 495

Nu-Tears® II Solution [OTC] see Artificial Tears on page 87

Nu-Tears® Solution [OTC] see Artificial Tears on page 87

Nutraplus® [OTC] see Urea on page 977

Nutrilipid® see Fat Emulsion on page 393

Nutropin® AQ Injection see Human Growth Hormone on page 473

Nutropin® Injection see Human Growth Hormone on page 473

Nydrazid® Injection see Isoniazid on page 522

Nylidrin (NYE li drin)

Brand Names Arlidin®

Canadian/Mexican Brand Names PMS-Nylidrin® (Canada)

Therapeutic Category Vasodilator, Peripheral

Use Considered "possibly effective" for increasing blood supply to treat peripheral disease (arteriosclerosis obliterans, diabetic vascular disease, nocturnal leg cramps, Raynaud's disease, frost bite, ischemic ulcer, thrombophlebitis) and circulatory disturbances of the inner ear (cochlear ischemia, macular or ampullar ischemia, etc)

Mechanism of Action Nylidrin is a peripheral vasodilator; this results from direct relaxation of vascular smooth muscle and beta agonist action. Nylidrin does not appear to affect cutaneous blood flow; it reportedly increases heart rate and cardiac output; cutaneous blood flow is not enhanced to any appreciable extent.

Local Anesthetic/Vasoconstrictor Precautions No information available to require special precautions

Effects on Dental Treatment No effects or complications reported

Other Adverse Effects

1% to 10%:

Central nervous system: Nervousness

Neuromuscular & skeletal: Trembling

<1%:

Cardiovascular: Palpitations, postural hypotension

Central nervous system: Dizziness

Gastrointestinal: Nausea, vomiting

Neuromuscular & skeletal: Weakness

Drug Interactions No data reported
Pregnancy Risk Factor C

Nystatin (nye STAT in)
Related Information
Oral Fungal Infections *on page 1063*
Patients Undergoing Cancer Therapy *on page 1083*
Brand Names Mycostatin®; Nilstat®; Nystex®
Canadian/Mexican Brand Names Mestatin® (Canada); Micostatin® (Mexico); Nadostine® (Canada); Nistaquim® (Mexico); Nyaderm (Canada); PMS-Nystatin (Canada)
Therapeutic Category Antifungal Agent, Oral Nonabsorbed; Antifungal Agent, Topical; Antifungal Agent, Vaginal
Use
Dental: Treatment of susceptible cutaneous, mucocutaneous, and oral cavity fungal infections normally caused by the *Candida* species
Medical: None
Usual Dosage Oral candidiasis: Suspension (swish and swallow orally):
Children and Adults: 400,000-600,000 units 4 times/day; troche: 200,000-400,000 units 4-5 times/day
Adults: 400,000-600,000 units 4 times/day; pastilles: 200,000-400,000 units 4-5 times/day
Mechanism of Action Binds to sterols in fungal cell membrane, changing the cell wall permeability allowing for leakage of cellular contents
Local Anesthetic/Vasoconstrictor Precautions No information available to require special precautions
Effects on Dental Treatment No effects or complications reported
Other Adverse Effects
1% to 10%: Gastrointestinal: Nausea, vomiting, diarrhea, abdominal pain
<1%:
Dermatologic: Contact dermatitis, Stevens-Johnson syndrome
Miscellaneous: Hypersensitivity reactions
Contraindications Hypersensitivity to nystatin or any component
Drug Interactions No data reported
Drug Uptake
Onset of symptomatic relief from candidiasis: Within 24-72 hours
Absorption: Not absorbed through mucous membranes or intact skin; poorly absorbed from GI tract
Pregnancy Risk Factor B/C (oral)
Breast-feeding Considerations Compatible (not absorbed orally)
Dosage Forms
Cream: 100,000 units/g (15 g, 30 g)
Ointment, topical: 100,000 units/g (15 g, 30 g)
Powder, for preparation of oral suspension: 50 million units, 1 billion units, 2 billion units, 5 billion units
Powder, topical: 100,000 units/g (15 g)
Suspension, oral: 100,000 units/mL (5 mL, 60 mL, 480 mL)
Tablet:
Oral: 500,000 units
Vaginal: 100,000 units (15 and 30/box with applicator)
Troche: 200,000 units
Dietary Considerations No data reported
Generic Available Yes

Nystatin and Triamcinolone (nye STAT in & trye am SIN oh lone)
Related Information
Oral Fungal Infections *on page 1063*
Brand Names Mycogen II Topical; Mycolog®-II Topical; Myconel® Topical; Myco-Triacet® II; Mytrex® F Topical; N.G.T.® Topical; Tri-Statin® II Topical
Therapeutic Category Antifungal Agent, Topical; Corticosteroid, Topical (Medium Potency)
Use Treatment of cutaneous candidiasis
Usual Dosage Children and Adults: Topical: Apply sparingly 2-4 times/day
Mechanism of Action Nystatin is an antifungal agent that binds to sterols in fungal cell membrane, changing the cell wall permeability allowing for leakage of cellular contents. Triamcinolone is a synthetic corticosteroid; it decreases inflammation by suppression of migration of polymorphonuclear leukocytes and reversal of increased capillary permeability. It suppresses the immune system reducing activity and volume of the lymphatic system. It suppresses adrenal function at high doses.
(Continued)

Nystatin and Triamcinolone *(Continued)*

Local Anesthetic/Vasoconstrictor Precautions No information available to require special precautions

Effects on Dental Treatment No effects or complications reported

Other Adverse Effects 1% to 10%:

Dermatologic: Dryness, folliculitis, hypertrichosis, acne, hypopigmentation, allergic dermatitis, maceration of the skin, skin atrophy

Local: Burning, itching, irritation

Miscellaneous: Increased incidence of secondary infection

Contraindications Known hypersensitivity to nystatin or triamcinolone

Warnings/Precautions Avoid use of occlusive dressings; limit therapy to least amount necessary for effective therapy, pediatric patients may be more susceptible to HPA axis suppression due to larger BSA to weight ratio

Drug Interactions No data reported

Pregnancy Risk Factor C

Breast-feeding Considerations

Nystatin: Compatible

Triamcinolone: No data reported

Dosage Forms

Cream: Nystatin 100,000 units and triamcinolone acetonide 0.1% (15 g, 30 g, 45 g, 60 g, 240 g)

Ointment, topical: Nystatin 100,000 units and triamcinolone acetonide 0.1% (15 g, 30 g, 60 g, 120 g)

Generic Available Yes

Nystex® *see* Nystatin *on previous page*

Nytol® Oral [OTC] *see* Diphenhydramine *on page 323*

Occlusal-HP Liquid *see* Salicylic Acid *on page 853*

Occupational Exposure to Bloodborne Pathogens (Universal Precautions) *see page 1151*

Ocean Nasal Mist [OTC] *see* Sodium Chloride *on page 870*

OCL® *see* Polyethylene Glycol-Electrolyte Solution *on page 771*

Octamide® PFS *see* Metoclopramide *on page 627*

Octicair® Otic *see* Neomycin, Polymyxin B, and Hydrocortisone *on page 672*

Octocaine® *see* Lidocaine *on page 553*

Octocaine® 50 *see* Lidocaine and Epinephrine *on page 554*

Octocaine® 100 *see* Lidocaine and Epinephrine *on page 554*

Octreotide Acetate *(ok TREE oh tide AS e tate)*

Brand Names Sandostatin®

Canadian/Mexican Brand Names Sandostatina® (Mexico)

Therapeutic Category Antisecretory Agent; Somatostatin Analog

Use Control of symptoms in patients with metastatic carcinoid, vasoactive intestinal peptide-secreting tumors (VIPomas), and secretory diarrhea

Usual Dosage Adults: S.C.: Initial: 50 mcg 1-2 times/day and titrate dose based on patient tolerance and response

Carcinoid: 100-600 mcg/day in 2-4 divided doses

VIPomas: 200-300 mcg/day in 2-4 divided doses

Diarrhea: Initial: I.V.: 50-100 mcg every 8 hours; increase by 100 mcg/dose at 48-hour intervals; maximum dose: 500 mcg every 8 hours

Esophageal varices bleeding: I.V. bolus: 25-50 mcg followed by continuous I.V. infusion of 25-50 mcg/hour

Mechanism of Action Mimics natural somatostatin by inhibiting serotonin release, and the secretion of gastrin, VIP, insulin, glucagon, secretin, motilin, and pancreatic polypeptide

Local Anesthetic/Vasoconstrictor Precautions No information available to require special precautions

Effects on Dental Treatment No effects or complications reported

Other Adverse Effects

1% to 10%:

Cardiovascular: Flushing, edema

Central nervous system: Headache, dizziness, fatigue

Endocrine & metabolic: Hyperglycemia, hypoglycemia

Gastrointestinal: Nausea, diarrhea, abdominal pain, vomiting, fat malabsorption

Local: Pain at injection site

Neuromuscular & skeletal: Weakness

<1%:
Cardiovascular: Chest pain
Central nervous system: Anxiety, fever
Dermatologic: Erythema, alopecia, rash
Endocrine & metabolic: Galactorrhea
Gastrointestinal: Constipation, flatulence, throat discomfort
Hepatic: Hepatitis
Respiratory: Dyspnea, rhinorrhea
Ocular: Burning eyes
Neuromuscular & skeletal: Leg cramps, Bell's palsy

Drug Uptake
Duration of action: 6-12 hours
Absorption:
Oral: Absorbed but still under study
S.C.: Rapid
Serum half-life: 60-110 minutes

Pregnancy Risk Factor B

Generic Available No

Comments Doses of 1-10 mcg/kg every 12 hours have been used in children beginning at the low end of the range and increasing by 0.3 mcg/kg/dose at 3-day intervals; suppression of growth hormone (animal data) is of concern when used as long-term therapy

Ocu-Carpine® see Pilocarpine on page 759

OcuClear® Ophthalmic [OTC] see Oxymetazoline on page 714

OcuCoat® Ophthalmic Solution [OTC] see Artificial Tears on page 87

OcuCoat® PF Ophthalmic Solution [OTC] see Artificial Tears on page 87

Ocuflox™ see Ofloxacin on this page

Ocupress® see Carteolol on page 182

Ocusert® Pilo see Pilocarpine on page 759

Ocusert Pilo-20® see Pilocarpine on page 759

Ocusert Pilo-40® see Pilocarpine on page 759

Ocusulf-10® Ophthalmic see Sulfacetamide Sodium on page 890

Ocutricin® Topical Ointment see Bacitracin, Neomycin, and Polymyxin B on page 108

Off-Ezy® Wart Remover [OTC] see Salicylic Acid on page 853

Ofloxacin (oh FLOKS a sin)

Related Information
Nonviral Infectious Diseases on page 1032

Brand Names Floxin® Oral; Floxin® Otic; Ocuflox™

Canadian/Mexican Brand Names Bactocin® (Mexico); Floxil® (Mexico); Flox-stat® (Mexico)

Therapeutic Category Antibiotic, Quinolone

Synonyms Ofloxacina (Mexico)

Use Quinolone antibiotic for skin and skin structure, lower respiratory and urinary tract infections, and sexually transmitted diseases, bacterial conjunctivitis caused by susceptible organisms; for the ear, otitis externa; acute otitis media in children aged 1 to 12 years of age with tympanostomy tubes; chronic suppurative otitis media in children aged 12 years or older with perforated tympanic membranes

Usual Dosage
Children >1 year and Adults: Ophthalmic: Instill 1-2 drops in affected eye(s) every 2-4 hours for the first 2 days, then use 4 times/day for an additional 5 days

Adults: Oral, I.V.: 200-400 mg every 12 hours for 7-10 days for most infections or for 6 weeks for prostatitis

Children 1 to 12 years and older: Otic: Five (5) or ten (10) drops, respectively, twice daily

Mechanism of Action Ofloxacin, a fluorinated quinolone, is a pyridine carboxylic acid derivative which exerts a broad spectrum bactericidal effect. It inhibits DNA gyrase, an essential bacterial enzyme that maintains the superhelical structure of DNA. DNA gyrase is required for DNA replication and transcription, DNA repair, recombination, and transposition within the bacteria.

Local Anesthetic/Vasoconstrictor Precautions No information available to require special precautions

Effects on Dental Treatment No effects or complications reported

Other Adverse Effects
>10%: Gastrointestinal: Nausea
1% to 10%:
Cardiovascular: Chest pain
(Continued)

697

Ofloxacin *(Continued)*

Central nervous system: Headache, insomnia, dizziness, fatigue, somnolence, sleep disorders, nervousness, pyrexia

Dermatologic: External genital pruritus in women, rash, pruritus

Gastrointestinal: Diarrhea, vomiting, GI distress, pain and cramps, flatulence, dysgeusia, dry mouth, decreased appetite

Genitourinary: Vaginitis

Neuromuscular & skeletal: Trunk pain

Ocular: Superinfection (ophthalmic), photophobia, lacrimation, dry eyes, stinging, visual disturbances

<1%:

Cardiovascular: Syncope, edema, hypertension, palpitations, vasodilation

Central nervous system: Anxiety, cognitive change, depression, dream abnormality, euphoria, hallucinations, vertigo, chills, malaise, extremity pain

Gastrointestinal: Thirst, weight loss

Neuromuscular & skeletal: Paresthesia, weakness

Ocular: Photophobia

Otic: Decreased hearing acuity, tinnitus

Respiratory: Cough

Drug Interactions

Decreased effect: decreased absorption with antacids containing aluminum, magnesium, and/or calcium (by up to 98% if given at the same time)

Increased toxicity/serum levels: Quinolones cause increased caffeine, warfarin, cyclosporine, and theophylline levels; azlocillin, cimetidine, probenecid increase quinolone levels

Drug Uptake

Absorption: Well absorbed; administration with food causes only minor alterations in absorption

Serum half-life, elimination 5-7.5 hours

Pregnancy Risk Factor C

Generic Available No

Ofloxacina (Mexico) *see* Ofloxacin *on previous page*

Ogen® *see* Estropipate *on page 370*

OGMT *see* Metyrosine *on page 632*

OKT3 *see* Muromonab-CD3 *on page 652*

Olanzapine *(oh LAN za peen)*

Brand Names Zyprexa®

Therapeutic Category Antipsychotic Agent

Use Treatment of manifestations of psychotic disorders

Usual Dosage Adults: Oral: Usual starting dose: 5-10 mg/day, given in a once-a-day dosing schedule; up to a maximum of 20 mg/day

Mechanism of Action Olanzapine is a thienobenzodiazepine neuroleptic; thought to work by antagonizing dopamine and serotonin activities. It is a selective monoaminergic antagonist with high affinity binding to serotonin $5HT2_A$ and $5HT2_C$, dopamine D_{1-4}, muscarinic M_{1-5}, histamine H_1 and alpha$_1$-adrenergic receptor sites.

Local Anesthetic/Vasoconstrictor Precautions No information available to require special precautions

Effects on Dental Treatment No effects or complications reported

Other Adverse Effects

>10%: Central nervous system: Headache, somnolence, insomnia, agitation, nervousness, hostility, dizziness

1% to 10%:

Central nervous system: Dystonic reactions, Parkinsonian events, akathisia, anxiety, personality changes, fever

Gastrointestinal: Xerostomia, constipation, abdominal pain, weight gain

Neuromuscular & skeletal: Arthralgia

Ocular: Amblyopia

Respiratory: Rhinitis, cough, pharyngitis

<1%:

Cardiovascular: Peripheral edema

Central nervous system: Tardive dyskinesia, neuroleptic malignant syndrome

Drug Interactions

Decreased effect: Cigarette smoking, levodopa, pergolide, bromocriptine, charcoal, and reduction of effects may be seen with cytochrome P-450 enzyme inducers such as rifampin, omeprazole, carbamazepine

Increased effect: Effects may be potentiated with cytochrome P-450 $1A_2$ inhibitors such as fluvoxamine

Increased toxicity: Increased sedation with alcohol or other CNS depressants, increased risk of hypotension and orthostatic hypotension with antihypertensives

Pregnancy Risk Factor C

Dosage Forms Tablet: 5 mg, 7.5 mg, 10 mg

Comments Olanzapine (Zyprexa®) is chemically similar to clozapine (Clozaril®), but without as many side effects. Also, olanzapine (Zyprexa®) does not produce side effects such as Parkinson's disease-like tremors which are associated with other antipsychotics such as haloperidol.

Olopatadine (oh LOP ah tah deen)

Brand Names Patanol®

Therapeutic Category Antihistamine

Use Allergic conjunctivitis

Usual Dosage Adults: Ophthalmic: One drop in affected eye(s) every 6-8 hours (2 times daily)

Local Anesthetic/Vasoconstrictor Precautions No information available to require special precautions

Effects on Dental Treatment No effects or complications reported

Pregnancy Risk Factor C

Dosage Forms Solution, ophthalmic: 0.1% (5 mL)

Olsalazine (ole SAL a zeen)

Brand Names Dipentum®

Therapeutic Category 5-Aminosalicylic Acid Derivative; Anti-inflammatory Agent

Use Maintenance of remission of ulcerative colitis in patients intolerant to sulfasalazine

Usual Dosage Adults: Oral: 1 g/day in 2 divided doses

Mechanism of Action The mechanism of action appears to be topical rather than systemic

Local Anesthetic/Vasoconstrictor Precautions No information available to require special precautions

Effects on Dental Treatment No effects or complications reported

Other Adverse Effects

>10%: Gastrointestinal: Diarrhea, cramps, abdominal pain

1% to 10%:
Central nervous system: Headache, fatigue, depression
Dermatologic: Rash, itching
Gastrointestinal: Nausea, dyspepsia, bloating, anorexia
Neuromuscular & skeletal: Arthralgia

<1%:
Central nervous system: Fever
Gastrointestinal: Bloody diarrhea
Hematologic: Blood dyscrasias
Hepatic: Hepatitis

Drug Interactions No data reported

Drug Uptake

Absorption: <3%; very little intact olsalazine is systemically absorbed

Serum half-life, elimination: 56 minutes or 55 hours depending on the analysis used

Pregnancy Risk Factor C

Dosage Forms Capsule, as sodium: 250 mg

Generic Available No

Omeprazole (oh ME pray zol)

Brand Names Prilosec™

Canadian/Mexican Brand Names Inhibitron® (Mexico); Losec® (Canada); Ozoken® (Mexico); Prazidec® (Mexico); Ulsen® (Mexico)

Therapeutic Category Gastric Acid Secretion Inhibitor

Synonyms Omeprazol (Mexico)

Use Short-term (4-8 weeks) treatment of severe erosive esophagitis (grade 2 or above), diagnosed by endoscopy and short-term treatment of symptomatic gastroesophageal reflux disease (GERD) poorly responsive to customary medical treatment; pathological hypersecretory conditions; peptic ulcer disease

Unlabeled use: Gastric ulcer therapy and healing NSAID-induced ulcers

Usual Dosage Adults: Oral:

Active duodenal ulcer: 20 mg/day for 4-8 weeks

GERD or severe erosive esophagitis: 20 mg/day for 4-8 weeks

(Continued)

Omeprazole *(Continued)*

Pathological hypersecretory conditions: 60 mg once daily to start; doses up to 120 mg 3 times/day have been administered; administer daily doses >80 mg in divided doses

Helicobacter pylori: Combination therapy with bismuth subsalicylate, tetracycline, clarithromycin, and H$_2$ antagonist; or clarithromycin and omeprazole. Adult dose: Oral: 20 mg twice daily

Gastric ulcers: 40 mg/day for 4-8 weeks

Mechanism of Action Suppresses gastric acid secretion by inhibiting the parietal cell H+/K+ ATP pump

Local Anesthetic/Vasoconstrictor Precautions No information available to require special precautions

Effects on Dental Treatment No effects or complications reported

Other Adverse Effects

1% to 10%:

Cardiovascular: Angina, tachycardia, bradycardia, edema

Central nervous system: Headache (7%), dizziness

Dermatologic: Rash, urticaria, pruritus, dry skin

Gastrointestinal: Diarrhea, nausea, abdominal pain, vomiting, constipation, anorexia, irritable colon, fecal discoloration, esophageal candidiasis, dry mouth, taste alterations

Genitourinary: Testicular pain, urinary tract infection

Neuromuscular & skeletal: Back pain, muscle cramps, myalgia, arthralgia, leg pain, weakness

Renal: Pyuria, proteinuria, hematuria, glycosuria, polyuria

Respiratory: Cough

<1%:

Cardiovascular: Chest pain

Central nervous system: Fever, fatigue, malaise, apathy, somnolence, nervousness, anxiety, pain

Gastrointestinal: Abdominal swelling

Drug Interactions

Cytochrome P-450 1A2 enzyme inducer and cytochrome P-450 IIC enzyme inhibitor

Decreased effect: Decreased ketoconazole; decreased itraconazole because of reduced absorption from gastrointestinal tract

Increased toxicity: Diazepam causes increased half-life; increased digoxin, increased phenytoin, increased warfarin

Drug Uptake

Onset of antisecretory action: Oral: Within 1 hour

Duration: 72 hours

Serum half-life: 30-90 minutes

Pregnancy Risk Factor C

Dosage Forms Capsule, delayed release: 10 mg, 20 mg, 40 mg

Generic Available No

Omeprazol (Mexico) *see* Omeprazole *on previous page*

OmniHIB® *see* Haemophilus b Conjugate Vaccine *on page 460*

Omnipen® *see* Ampicillin *on page 73*

Omnipen®-N *see* Ampicillin *on page 73*

OMS® Oral *see* Morphine Sulfate *on page 648*

Oncaspar® *see* Pegaspargase *on page 727*

Oncet® *see* Hydrocodone and Homatropine *on page 481*

Oncovin® Injection *see* Vincristine *on page 990*

Ondansetron *(on DAN se tron)*

Brand Names Zofran®

Therapeutic Category Antiemetic; Serotonin Antagonist

Use May be prescribed for patients who are refractory to or have severe adverse reactions to standard antiemetic therapy. Ondansetron may be prescribed for young patients (ie, <45 years of age who are more likely to develop extrapyramidal reactions to high-dose metoclopramide) who are to receive highly emetogenic chemotherapeutic agents as listed:

Agents with high emetogenic potential (>90%) (dose/m^2):

Carmustine ≥200 mg

Cisplatin ≥75 mg

Cyclophosphamide ≥1000 mg

Cytarabine ≥1000 mg

Dacarbazine ≥500 mg

Ifosfamide ≥1000 mg

Lomustine ≥60 mg
Mechlorethamine
Pentostatin
Streptozocin

or two agents classified as having high or moderately high emetogenic potential as listed:

Agents with moderately high emetogenic potential (60% to 90%) (dose/m²):
Carmustine <200 mg
Cisplatin <75 mg
Cyclophosphamide 1000 mg
Cytarabine 250-1000 mg
Dacarbazine <500 mg
Doxorubicin ≥75 mg
Ifosfamide
Lomustine <60 mg
Methotrexate ≥250 mg
Mitomycin
Mitoxantrone
Procarbazine

Ondansetron should not be prescribed for chemotherapeutic agents with a low emetogenic potential (eg, bleomycin, busulfan, cyclophosphamide <1000 mg, etoposide, 5-fluorouracil, vinblastine, vincristine)

Usual Dosage
Oral:
Children 4-11 years: 4 mg 30 minutes before chemotherapy; repeat 4 and 8 hours after initial dose
Children >11 years and Adults: 8 mg 30 minutes before chemotherapy; repeat 4 and 8 hours after initial dose or every 8 hours for a maximum of 48 hours

I.V.: Administer either three 0.15 mg/kg doses or a single 32 mg dose; with the 3-dose regimen, the initial dose is given 30 minutes prior to chemotherapy with subsequent doses administered 4 and 8 hours after the first dose. With the single-dose regimen 32 mg is infused over 15 minutes beginning 30 minutes before the start of emetogenic chemotherapy. Dosage should be calculated based on weight:
Children: Pediatric dosing should follow the manufacturer's guidelines for 0.15 mg/kg/dose administered 30 minutes prior to chemotherapy, 4 and 8 hours after the first dose. While not as yet FDA-approved, literature supports the day's total dose administered as a single dose 30 minutes prior to chemotherapy.
Adults:
>80 kg: 12 mg IVPB
45-80 kg: 8 mg IVPB
<45 kg: 0.15 mg/kg/dose IVPB

Mechanism of Action Selective 5-HT₃ receptor antagonist, blocking serotonin, both peripherally on vagal nerve terminals and centrally in the chemoreceptor trigger zone

Local Anesthetic/Vasoconstrictor Precautions No information available to require special precautions

Effects on Dental Treatment No effects or complications reported

Other Adverse Effects
>10%:
Central nervous system: Headache, fever
Gastrointestinal: Constipation, diarrhea
1% to 10%:
Central nervous system: Dizziness
Gastrointestinal: Abdominal cramps, dry mouth
Neuromuscular & skeletal: Weakness
<1%:
Cardiovascular: Tachycardia
Central nervous system: Lightheadedness, seizures
Dermatologic: Rash
Endocrine & metabolic: Hypokalemia
Hepatic: Transient elevations in serum levels of aminotransferases and bilirubin
Respiratory: Bronchospasm, dyspnea, wheezing

Drug Interactions
Decreased effect: Metabolized by the hepatic cytochrome P-450 enzymes; therefore, the drug's clearance and half-life may be changed with concomitant use of cytochrome P-450 inducers (eg, barbiturates, carbamazepine, rifampin, phenytoin, and phenylbutazone)
Increased toxicity: Inhibitors (eg, cimetidine, allopurinol, and disulfiram)
(Continued)

Ondansetron *(Continued)*

Drug Uptake
Serum half-life:
Children <15 years: 2-3 hours
Adults: 4 hours
Pregnancy Risk Factor B
Generic Available No

Ony-Clear® Nail *see* Triacetin *on page 954*

Ony-Clear® Spray *see* Miconazole *on page 635*

OP-CCK *see* Sincalide *on page 866*

Opcon® Ophthalmic *see* Naphazoline *on page 664*

o,p'-DDD *see* Mitotane *on page 643*

Ophthalgan® Ophthalmic *see* Glycerin *on page 446*

Ophthetic® *see* Proparacaine *on page 808*

Ophthochlor® *see* Chloramphenicol *on page 209*

Ophthocort® Ophthalmic *see* Chloramphenicol, Polymyxin B, and Hydrocortisone *on page 210*

Opium Alkaloids (OH pee um AL ka loyds)

Brand Names Pantopon®
Therapeutic Category Analgesic, Narcotic
Use For relief of severe pain
Local Anesthetic/Vasoconstrictor Precautions No information available to require special precautions
Effects on Dental Treatment 1% to 10% of patients will experience significant dry mouth
Other Adverse Effects
>10%:
Cardiovascular: Hypotension
Central nervous system: Fatigue, drowsiness, dizziness
Gastrointestinal: Nausea, vomiting
Neuromuscular & skeletal: Weakness
1% to 10%:
Central nervous system: Nervousness, headache, confusion restlessness, malaise
Gastrointestinal: Anorexia, stomach cramps, dry mouth, constipation, biliary tract spasm
Genitourinary: Ureteral spasms, decreased urination
Local: Pain at injection site
Respiratory: Dyspnea
<1%:
Central nervous system: Mental depression, paradoxical CNS stimulation, hallucinations, increased intracranial pressure
Dermatologic: Skin rash, urticaria
Gastrointestinal: Paralytic ileus
Miscellaneous: Histamine release, physical and psychological dependence
Pregnancy Risk Factor B (D if used for prolonged periods or in high doses at term)
Generic Available Yes
Comments Abrupt discontinuation after sustained use (generally >10 days) may cause withdrawal symptoms

Opium Tincture (OH pee um TING chur)

Therapeutic Category Analgesic, Narcotic; Antidiarrheal
Use Treatment of diarrhea or relief of pain
Usual Dosage Oral:
Children:
Diarrhea: 0.005-0.01 mL/kg/dose every 3-4 hours for a maximum of 6 doses/24 hours
Analgesia: 0.01-0.02 mL/kg/dose every 3-4 hours

Adults:
Diarrhea: 0.3-1 mL/dose every 2-6 hours to maximum of 6 mL/24 hours
Analgesia: 0.6-1.5 mL/dose every 3-4 hours
Mechanism of Action Contains many narcotic alkaloids including morphine; its mechanism for gastric motility inhibition is primarily due to this morphine content; it results in a decrease in digestive secretions, an increase in GI muscle tone, and therefore a reduction in GI propulsion
Local Anesthetic/Vasoconstrictor Precautions No information available to require special precautions

Effects on Dental Treatment No effects or complications reported
Other Adverse Effects
>10%:
Cardiovascular: Palpitations, hypotension, bradycardia
Central nervous system: Drowsiness, dizziness
Neuromuscular & skeletal: Weakness
1% to 10%:
Central nervous system; Restlessness, headache, malaise
Genitourinary: Decreased urination
Miscellaneous: Histamine release
<1%:
Cardiovascular: Peripheral vasodilation
Central nervous system: CNS depression, increased intracranial pressure, insomnia, mental depression
Gastrointestinal: Nausea, vomiting, constipation, anorexia, stomach cramps, biliary spasm
Genitourinary: Urinary tract spasm
Ocular: Miosis
Respiratory: Respiratory depression
Miscellaneous: Physical and psychological dependence
Drug Interactions
Decreased effect: Phenothiazines may antagonize the analgesic effect of opiate agonists
Increased toxicity: CNS depressants, MAO inhibitors, tricyclic antidepressants may potentiate the effects of opiate agonists; dextroamphetamine may enhance the analgesic effect of opiate agonists
Drug Uptake
Duration of effect: 4-5 hours
Absorption: Variable from GI tract
Pregnancy Risk Factor B (D if used for prolonged periods or in high doses at term)
Generic Available No

Opticyl® *see* Tropicamide *on page 973*
Optigene® Ophthalmic [OTC] *see* Tetrahydrozoline *on page 916*
Optimine® *see* Azatadine *on page 101*
Optimoist® Solution [OTC] *see* Saliva Substitute *on page 854*
OptiPranolol® *see* Metipranolol *on page 627*
OPV *see* Poliovirus Vaccine, Live, Trivalent, Oral *on page 770*
Orabase®-B [OTC] *see* Benzocaine *on page 118*
Orabase® HCA *see* Hydrocortisone *on page 484*
Orabase®-O [OTC] *see* Benzocaine *on page 118*
Orabase® Plain [OTC] *see* Gelatin, Pectin, and Methylcellulose *on page 438*
Orabase® With Benzocaine [OTC] *see* Benzocaine, Gelatin, Pectin, and Sodium Carboxymethylcellulose *on page 119*
Oracit® *see* Sodium Citrate and Citric Acid *on page 872*
Orajel® Brace-Aid Oral Anesthetic [OTC] *see* Benzocaine *on page 118*
Orajel® Maximum Strength [OTC] *see* Benzocaine *on page 118*
Orajel® Mouth-Aid [OTC] *see* Benzocaine *on page 118*
Orajel® Perioseptic [OTC] *see* Carbamide Peroxide *on page 175*
Oral Bacterial Infections *see page 1059*
Oral Fungal Infections *see page 1063*
Oral Nonviral Soft Tissue Ulcerations or Erosions *see page 1070*
Oral Pain *see page 1053*
Oral Rinse Products *see page 1187*
Oral Viral Infections *see page 1066*
Oramorph SR™ Oral *see* Morphine Sulfate *on page 648*
Orap™ *see* Pimozide *on page 762*
Orasept® [OTC] *see* Benzocaine *on page 118*
Orasol® [OTC] *see* Benzocaine *on page 118*
Orasone® *see* Prednisone *on page 789*
Orazinc® [OTC] *see* Zinc Supplements *on page 1005*
Orazinc® Oral [OTC] *see* Zinc Sulfate *on page 1005*
Ordrine AT® Extended Release Capsule *see* Caramiphen and Phenylpropanolamine *on page 173*
Oretic® *see* Hydrochlorothiazide *on page 476*
Oreton® Methyl *see* Methyltestosterone *on page 626*
Orexin® [OTC] *see* Vitamin B Complex *on page 993*
Orfenadrina (Mexico) *see* Orphenadrine *on next page*

Organidin® *see* Iodinated Glycerol *on page 515*
Organidin® NR *see* Guaifenesin *on page 452*
Orgaran® *see* Danaparoid *on page 279*
Orimune® *see* Poliovirus Vaccine, Live, Trivalent, Oral *on page 770*
Orinase® *see* Tolbutamide *on page 941*
ORLAAM® *see* Levomethadyl Acetate Hydrochloride *on page 550*
Ormazine *see* Chlorpromazine *on page 223*
Ornade® Spansule® *see* Chlorpheniramine and Phenylpropanolamine *on page 219*
Ornex® No Drowsiness [OTC] *see* Acetaminophen and Pseudoephedrine *on page 24*

Orphenadrine (or FEN a dreen)

Related Information
Temporomandibular Dysfunction (TMD) *on page 1078*
Brand Names Norflex™
Therapeutic Category Muscle Relaxant; Skeletal Muscle Relaxant
Synonyms Orfenadrina (Mexico)
Use Treatment of muscle spasm associated with acute painful musculoskeletal conditions; supportive therapy in tetanus
Usual Dosage Adults:
Oral: 100 mg twice daily
I.M., I.V.: 60 mg every 12 hours
Mechanism of Action Indirect skeletal muscle relaxant thought to work by central atropine-like effects; has some euphorgenic and analgesic properties
Local Anesthetic/Vasoconstrictor Precautions No information available to require special precautions
Effects on Dental Treatment The peripheral anticholinergic effects of orphenadrine may decrease or inhibit salivary flow; normal salivation will return with cessation of drug therapy
Other Adverse Effects
>10%:
Central nervous system: Drowsiness, dizziness
Ocular: Blurred vision
1% to 10%:
Cardiovascular: Flushing of face, tachycardia, syncope
Dermatologic: Skin rash
Gastrointestinal: Nausea, vomiting, constipation
Genitourinary: Decreased urination
Neuromuscular & skeletal: Weakness
Ocular: Nystagmus, increased intraocular pressure
Respiratory: Nasal congestion
<1%:
Central nervous system: Hallucinations
Hematologic: Aplastic anemia
Drug Interactions No data reported
Drug Uptake
Duration: 4-6 hours
Serum half-life: 14-16 hours
Pregnancy Risk Factor C
Generic Available Yes

Orphenadrine, Aspirin, and Caffeine

(or FEN a dreen, AS pir in, & KAF een)
Brand Names Norgesic™; Norgesic™ Forte
Therapeutic Category Analgesic, Non-narcotic; Muscle Relaxant; Skeletal Muscle Relaxant
Use Relief of discomfort associated with skeletal muscular conditions
Local Anesthetic/Vasoconstrictor Precautions No information available to require special precautions
Effects on Dental Treatment The peripheral anticholinergic effects of orphenadrine may decrease or inhibit salivary flow; normal salivation will return with cessation of drug therapy
Pregnancy Risk Factor D
Generic Available Yes

Ortho-Cept® *see* Ethinyl Estradiol and Desogestrel *on page 375*
Orthoclone® OKT3 *see* Muromonab-CD3 *on page 652*
Ortho-Cyclen® *see* Ethinyl Estradiol and Norgestimate *on page 381*
Ortho-Dienestrol® Vaginal *see* Dienestrol *on page 309*
Ortho-Est® *see* Estropipate *on page 370*

Ortho-Novum® 1/35 *see* Ethinyl Estradiol and Norethindrone *on page 379*
Ortho-Novum™ 1/50 *see* Mestranol and Norethindrone *on page 603*
Ortho-Novum® 7/7/7 *see* Ethinyl Estradiol and Norethindrone *on page 379*
Ortho-Novum® 10/11 *see* Ethinyl Estradiol and Norethindrone *on page 379*
Ortho Tri-Cyclen® *see* Ethinyl Estradiol and Norgestimate *on page 381*
Or-Tyl® Injection *see* Dicyclomine *on page 307*
Orudis® *see* Ketoprofen *on page 534*
Orudis® KT [OTC] *see* Ketoprofen *on page 534*
Oruvail® *see* Ketoprofen *on page 534*
Os-Cal® 500 [OTC] *see* Calcium Carbonate *on page 162*
Osmoglyn® Ophthalmic *see* Glycerin *on page 446*
Osmolite® HN [OTC] *see* Enteral Nutritional Products *on page 350*
Osteocalcin® Injection *see* Calcitonin *on page 160*
Otic-Care® Otic *see* Neomycin, Polymyxin B, and Hydrocortisone *on page 672*
Otic Domeboro® *see* Aluminum Acetate and Acetic Acid *on page 47*
Otobiotic® Otic *see* Polymyxin B and Hydrocortisone *on page 773*
Otocalm® Ear *see* Antipyrine and Benzocaine *on page 82*
Otocort® Otic *see* Neomycin, Polymyxin B, and Hydrocortisone *on page 672*
Otosporin® Otic *see* Neomycin, Polymyxin B, and Hydrocortisone *on page 672*
Otrivin® [OTC] *see* Xylometazoline *on page 999*
Ovcon® 35 *see* Ethinyl Estradiol and Norethindrone *on page 379*
Ovcon® 50 *see* Ethinyl Estradiol and Norethindrone *on page 379*
Ovral® *see* Ethinyl Estradiol and Norgestrel *on page 381*
Ovrette® *see* Norgestrel *on page 692*

Oxacillin (oks a SIL in)

Brand Names Bactocill®; Prostaphlin®
Therapeutic Category Antibiotic, Penicillin
Use Treatment of susceptible bacterial infections such as osteomyelitis, septicemia, endocarditis, and CNS infections due to penicillinase-producing strains of *Staphylococcus*
Usual Dosage
  Children:
    Oral: 50-100 mg/kg/day divided every 6 hours
    I.M., I.V.: 150-200 mg/kg/day in divided doses every 6 hours; maximum dose: 12 g/day

  Adults:
    Oral: 500-1000 mg every 4-6 hours for at least 5 days
    I.M., I.V.: 250 mg to 2 g/dose every 4-6 hours
Mechanism of Action Inhibits bacterial cell wall synthesis by binding to one or more of the penicillin binding proteins (PBPs); which in turn inhibits the final transpeptidation step of peptidoglycan synthesis in bacterial cell walls, thus inhibiting cell wall biosynthesis. Bacteria eventually lyse due to ongoing activity of cell wall autolytic enzymes (autolysins and murein hydrolases) while cell wall assembly is arrested.
Local Anesthetic/Vasoconstrictor Precautions No information available to require special precautions
Effects on Dental Treatment Prolonged use of penicillins may lead to development of oral candidiasis
Other Adverse Effects
  1% to 10%: Gastrointestinal: Nausea, diarrhea
  <1%:
    Central nervous system: Fever
    Dermatologic: Rash
    Gastrointestinal: Vomiting
    Hematologic: Eosinophilia, leukopenia, neutropenia, thrombocytopenia, agranulocytosis
    Hepatic: Hepatotoxicity, elevated AST
    Renal: Hematuria, acute interstitial nephritis
    Miscellaneous: Serum sickness-like reactions
Drug Interactions
  Decreased effect: Efficacy of oral contraceptives may be reduced
  Increased effect: Disulfiram, probenecid causes increased penicillin levels
Drug Uptake
  Absorption: Oral: 35% to 67%
  Serum half-life:
    Children 1 week to 2 years: 0.9-1.8 hours
    Adults: 23-60 minutes (prolonged with reduced renal function and in neonates)
(Continued)

Oxacillin *(Continued)*

Time to peak serum concentration:
Oral: Within 2 hours
I.M.: Within 30-60 minutes
Pregnancy Risk Factor B
Generic Available Yes

Oxamniquine (oks AM'ni kwin)
Brand Names Vansil™
Therapeutic Category Anthelmintic
Use Treat all stages of *Schistosoma mansoni* infection
Local Anesthetic/Vasoconstrictor Precautions No information available to require special precautions
Effects on Dental Treatment No effects or complications reported
Other Adverse Effects
>10%: Central nervous system: Dizziness, drowsiness, headache
<10%:
Central nervous system: Insomnia, malaise, hallucinations, behavior changes
Dermatologic: Rash, urticaria, pruritus
Gastrointestinal: GI effects
Genitourinary: Urine discoloration (orange/red)
Hepatic: Elevated LFTs
Renal: Proteinuria
Pregnancy Risk Factor C
Generic Available No
Comments Strains other than from the western hemisphere may require higher doses

Oxandrin® *see* Oxandrolone *on this page*

Oxandrolone (oks AN droe lone)
Brand Names Oxandrin®
Therapeutic Category Androgen
Use Treatment of catabolic or tissue-depleting processes
Local Anesthetic/Vasoconstrictor Precautions No information available to require special precautions
Effects on Dental Treatment No effects or complications reported
Other Adverse Effects
Male:
Postpubertal:
>10%: Bladder irritability, priapism, gynecomastia, acne
1% to 10%: Decreased libido, hepatic dysfunction, chills, nausea, diarrhea, insomnia, iron deficiency anemia, suppression of clotting factors, prostatic hypertrophy (geriatric)
<1%: Hepatic necrosis, hepatocellular carcinoma
Prepubertal: Virilism
>10%: Acne, virilism
1% to 10%: Hyperpigmentation, chills, diarrhea, nausea, insomnia, iron deficiency anemia, suppression of clotting factors
<1%: Hepatic necrosis, hepatocellular carcinoma

Female:
>10%: Virilism
1% to 10%: Hypercalcemia, hepatic dysfunction, nausea, chills, diarrhea, insomnia, iron deficiency anemia, suppression of clotting factors
<1%: Hepatic necrosis, hepatocellular carcinoma
Pregnancy Risk Factor X
Generic Available No
Comments This medication is currently on the market as an Orphan Drug. It is distributed by Gynex Pharmaceuticals, Inc. to physicians who document their expertise in endocrinology and agree to participate in a study to gather data for the FDA.

Oxaprozin (oks a PROE zin)
Related Information
Rheumatoid Arthritis and Osteoarthritis *on page 1030*
Brand Names Daypro™
Therapeutic Category Nonsteroidal Anti-inflammatory Agent (NSAID), Oral
Use Acute and long-term use in the management of signs and symptoms of osteoarthritis and rheumatoid arthritis
Usual Dosage Adults: Oral (individualize dosage to lowest effective dose to minimize adverse effects):

Osteoarthritis: 600-1200 mg once daily
Rheumatoid arthritis: 1200 mg once daily
Maximum dose: 1800 mg/day or 26 mg/kg (whichever is lower) in divided doses

Mechanism of Action Inhibits prostaglandin synthesis by decreasing the activity of the enzyme, cyclo-oxygenase, which results in decreased formation of prostaglandin precursors

Local Anesthetic/Vasoconstrictor Precautions No information available to require special precautions

Effects on Dental Treatment No effects or complications reported

Other Adverse Effects
>10%:
    Central nervous system: Dizziness
    Dermatologic: Skin rash
    Gastrointestinal: Abdominal cramps, heartburn, indigestion, nausea
1% to 10%:
    Cardiovascular: Angina pectoris, arrhythmia
    Central nervous system: Nervousness
    Dermatologic: Itching
    Gastrointestinal: GI ulceration, vomiting
    Genitourinary: Vaginal bleeding
    Otic: Tinnitus
<1%:
    Cardiovascular: Chest pain, congestive heart failure, hypertension, tachycardia
    Central nervous system: Convulsions, forgetfulness, mental depression, drowsiness, insomnia
    Dermatologic: Urticaria, exfoliative dermatitis, erythema multiforme, Stevens-Johnson syndrome, angioedema
    Gastrointestinal: Stomatitis
    Genitourinary: Cystitis
    Hematologic: Agranulocytosis, anemia, pancytopenia, leukopenia, thrombocytopenia
    Hepatic: Hepatitis
    Neuromuscular & skeletal: Peripheral neuropathy, trembling, weakness
    Ocular: Blurred vision, change in vision
    Otic: Decreased hearing
    Renal: Interstitial nephritis, nephrotic syndrome, renal impairment
    Respiratory: Dyspnea, wheezing, laryngeal edema, epistaxis
    Miscellaneous: Anaphylaxis, increased sweating

Drug Interactions Oxaprozin, like other NSAIDs, may cause increased toxicity of aspirin, oral anticoagulants, diuretics

Drug Uptake
    Absorption: Almost completely
    Serum half-life: 40-50 hours
    Time to peak: 2-4 hours

Pregnancy Risk Factor C

Generic Available No

Oxazepam (oks A ze pam)
Related Information
    Patients Requiring Sedation *on page 1081*

Brand Names Serax®

Canadian/Mexican Brand Names Apo®-Oxazepam (Canada); Novo-Oxazepam® (Canada); Oxpam® (Canada); PMS-Oxazepam® (Canada); Zapex® (Canada)

Therapeutic Category Benzodiazepine

Use Treatment of anxiety and management of alcohol withdrawal; may also be used as an anticonvulsant in management of simple partial seizures

Usual Dosage Oral:
    Children: 1 mg/kg/day has been administered

    Adults:
        Anxiety: 10-30 mg 3-4 times/day
        Alcohol withdrawal: 15-30 mg 3-4 times/day
        Hypnotic: 15-30 mg
        Not dialyzable (0% to 5%)

Mechanism of Action Benzodiazepine anxiolytic sedative that produces CNS depression at the subcortical level, except at high doses, whereby it works at the cortical level

Local Anesthetic/Vasoconstrictor Precautions No information available to require special precautions

Effects on Dental Treatment >10% of patients experience dry mouth which disappears with cessation of drug therapy
(Continued)

Oxazepam *(Continued)*

Other Adverse Effects
>10%: Central nervous system: Drowsiness
1% to 10%: Central nervous system: Dizziness, vertigo, headache
<1%:
  Cardiovascular: Syncope
  Central nervous system: Slurred speech, lethargy, ataxia
  Dermatologic: Rash
  Endocrine & metabolic: Altered libido
  Gastrointestinal: Nausea
  Hematologic: Leukopenia
  Hepatic: Jaundice
  Neuromuscular & skeletal: Tremor
Drug Interactions Increased toxicity (CNS depression): Alcohol, tricyclic antidepressants, sedative-hypnotics, MAO inhibitors
Drug Uptake
Absorption: Oral: Almost completely
Serum half-life: 2.8-5.7 hours
Time to peak serum concentration: Within 2-4 hours
Pregnancy Risk Factor D
Generic Available Yes

Oxiconazole (oks i KON a zole)
Brand Names Oxistat®
Canadian/Mexican Brand Names Myfungar® (Mexico)
Therapeutic Category Antifungal Agent, Topical
Synonyms Oxiconazol, Nitrato De (Mexico)
Use Treatment of tinea pedis (athlete's foot), tinea cruris (jock itch), and tinea corporis (ring worm)
Usual Dosage Children and Adults: Topical: Apply once to twice daily to affected areas for 2 weeks (tinea corporis/tinea cruris) to 1 month (tinea pedis)
Mechanism of Action Inhibition of ergosterol synthesis. Effective for treatment of tinea pedis, tinea cruris, and tinea corporis. Active against *Trichophyton rubrum, Trichophyton mentagrophytes, Trichophyton violaceum, Microsporum canis, Microsporum audouini, Microsporum gypseum, Epidermophyton floccosum, Candida albicans,* and *Malassezia furfur.*
Local Anesthetic/Vasoconstrictor Precautions No information available to require special precautions
Effects on Dental Treatment No effects or complications reported
Other Adverse Effects 1% to 10%: Local: Itching, transient burning, local irritation, stinging, erythema, dryness
Drug Interactions No data reported
Drug Uptake
Absorption: In each layer of the dermis; very little is absorbed systemically after one topical dose
Pregnancy Risk Factor B
Generic Available No

Oxiconazol, Nitrato De (Mexico) *see* Oxiconazole *on this page*
Oxipor® VHC [OTC] *see* Coal Tar *on page 254*
Oxistat® *see* Oxiconazole *on this page*
Oxitetraciclina (Mexico) *see* Oxytetracycline *on page 717*
Oxitocina (Mexico) *see* Oxytocin *on page 719*
Oxsoralen® Topical *see* Methoxsalen *on page 618*
Oxsoralen-Ultra® Oral *see* Methoxsalen *on page 618*

Oxtriphylline (oks TRYE fi lin)
Related Information
Respiratory Diseases *on page 1018*
Brand Names Choledyl®
Therapeutic Category Antiasthmatic; Bronchodilator; Theophylline Derivative
Synonyms Choline Theophyllinate
Use Bronchodilator in symptomatic treatment of asthma and reversible bronchospasm
Local Anesthetic/Vasoconstrictor Precautions No information available to require special precautions
Effects on Dental Treatment Do not prescribe any erythromycin product to patients taking theophylline products. Erythromycin will delay the normal metabolic inactivation of theophyllines leading to increased blood levels; this has resulted in nausea, vomiting and CNS restlessness

Other Adverse Effects Uncommon with theophylline levels <20 mcg/mL

1% to 10%:

Cardiovascular: Tachycardia

Central nervous system: Nervousness, restlessness

Gastrointestinal: Nausea, vomiting

<1%:

Central nervous system: Insomnia, irritability, seizures

Dermatologic: Skin rash

Gastrointestinal: Gastric irritation

Neuromuscular & skeletal: Tremor

Miscellaneous: Allergic reactions

Pregnancy Risk Factor C

Generic Available Yes

Comments Oxtriphylline is 64% theophylline

Oxy-5® Advanced Formula for Sensitive Skin [OTC] *see* Benzoyl Peroxide *on page 120*

Oxy-5® Tinted [OTC] *see* Benzoyl Peroxide *on page 120*

Oxy-10® Advanced Formula for Sensitive Skin [OTC] *see* Benzoyl Peroxide *on page 120*

Oxy 10® Wash [OTC] *see* Benzoyl Peroxide *on page 120*

Oxybutynin (oks i BYOO ti nin)

Brand Names Ditropan®

Therapeutic Category Antispasmodic Agent, Urinary

Use Antispasmodic for neurogenic bladder (urgency, frequency, urge incontinence) and uninhibited bladder

Usual Dosage Oral:

Children:

1-5 years: 0.2 mg/kg/dose 2-4 times/day

>5 years: 5 mg twice daily, up to 5 mg 4 times/day maximum

Adults: 5 mg 2-3 times/day up to 5 mg 4 times/day maximum

Elderly: 2.5-5 mg twice daily; increase by 2.5 mg increments every 1-2 days

Note: Should be discontinued periodically to determine whether the patient can manage without the drug and to minimize resistance to the drug

Mechanism of Action Direct antispasmodic effect on smooth muscle, also inhibits the action of acetylcholine on smooth muscle (exhibits $\frac{1}{5}$ the anticholinergic activity of atropine, but is 4-10 times the antispasmodic activity); does not block effects at skeletal muscle or at autonomic ganglia; increases bladder capacity, decreases uninhibited contractions, and delays desire to void; therefore, decreases urgency and frequency

Local Anesthetic/Vasoconstrictor Precautions No information available to require special precautions

Effects on Dental Treatment >10% of patients experience dry mouth; prolonged use of oxybutynin may decrease or inhibit salivary flow; normal salivation returns with cessation of drug therapy

Other Adverse Effects

>10%:

Central nervous system: Drowsiness

Gastrointestinal: Constipation

Miscellaneous: Decreased sweating

1% to 10%:

Cardiovascular: Tachycardia, palpitations

Central nervous system: Dizziness, insomnia, fever, headache

Dermatologic: Rash

Endocrine & metabolic: Hot flashes, decreased flow of breast milk

Gastrointestinal: Nausea, vomiting

Genitourinary: Urinary hesitancy or retention, decreased sexual ability

Neuromuscular & skeletal: Weakness

Ocular: Blurred vision, mydriatic effect

<1%:

Ocular: Increased intraocular pressure

Miscellaneous: Allergic reaction

Drug Interactions

Increased toxicity:

Additive sedation with CNS depressants and alcohol

Additive anticholinergic effects with antihistamines and anticholinergic agents

Drug Uptake

Onset of effect: Oral: 30-60 minutes

Peak effect: 3-6 hours

Duration: 6-10 hours

Absorption: Oral: Rapid and well absorbed

(Continued)

Oxybutynin *(Continued)*

Serum half-life: 1-2.3 hours
Time to peak serum concentration: Within 60 minutes
Pregnancy Risk Factor B
Generic Available Yes

Oxycel® *see* Cellulose, Oxidized *on page 200*

Oxychlorosene (oks i KLOR oh seen)

Brand Names Clorpactin® WCS-90
Therapeutic Category Antibiotic, Topical
Use Treating localized infections
Local Anesthetic/Vasoconstrictor Precautions No information available to require special precautions
Effects on Dental Treatment No effects or complications reported
Generic Available No
Comments Product is available as powder which must be diluted with sterile water or isotonic saline

Oxycodone (oks i KOE done)

Brand Names OxyContin®; OxyIR®; Roxicodone™
Canadian/Mexican Brand Names Supeudol® (Canada)
Therapeutic Category Analgesic, Narcotic
Synonyms Dihydrohydroxycodeinone; Oxycodone Hydrochloride
Use
Dental: Treatment of postoperative pain
Medical: Management of moderate to severe pain, normally used in combination with non-narcotic analgesics
Restrictions C-II
Usual Dosage Oral:
Immediate release:
Children:
6-12 years: 1.25 mg every 6 hours as needed
>12 years: 2.5 mg every 6 hours as needed
Adults: 5 mg every 6 hours as needed
Controlled release: Adults: 10 mg every 12 hours around-the-clock

Dosing adjustment in hepatic impairment: Reduce dosage in patients with severe liver disease
Mechanism of Action Oxycodone, as with other narcotic (opiate) analgesics, blocks pain perception in the cerebral cortex by binding to specific receptor molecules (opiate receptors) within the neuronal membranes of synapses. This binding results in a decreased synaptic chemical transmission throughout the CNS thus inhibiting the flow of pain sensations into the higher centers. Mu and kappa are the two subtypes of the opiate receptor which oxycodone binds to to cause analgesia.
Local Anesthetic/Vasoconstrictor Precautions No information available to require special precautions
Effects on Dental Treatment 1% to 10% of patients experience dry mouth
Other Adverse Effects
>10%:
Central nervous system: Fatigue, drowsiness, dizziness
Gastrointestinal: Nausea, vomiting
1% to 10%:
Gastrointestinal: Anorexia, stomach cramps, xerostomia, constipation, biliary spasm
Contraindications Patients with known hypersensitivity to oxycodone
Warnings/Precautions Use with caution in patients with hypersensitivity reactions to other phenanthrene derivative opioid agonists (morphine, hydrocodone, hydromorphone, levorphanol, oxycodone, oxymorphone); respiratory diseases including asthma, emphysema, COPD, or severe liver or renal insufficiency; some preparations contain sulfites which may cause allergic reactions; may be habit-forming
Drug Interactions The use of MAO inhibitors or tricyclic antidepressants with oxycodone may **increase** the effect of either the antidepressant or oxycodone; concurrent use of oxycodone with anticholinergics may cause paralytic ileus; patients taking other narcotic agents, antipsychotics, antianxiety agents or other CNS depressants (including alcohol) with oxycodone may experience an additive CNS depression
Drug Uptake
Onset of effect: Narcotic analgesia: 0.5-1 hour
Duration of effect: 4-6 hours

Serum half-life: 2-3 hours

Pregnancy Risk Factor B (D if used for prolonged periods or in high doses at term)

Dosage Forms

Capsule, as hydrochloride, immediate release (OxyIR®): 5 mg

Liquid, oral, as hydrochloride: 5 mg/5 mL (500 mL)

Solution, oral concentrate, as hydrochloride: 20 mg/mL (30 mL)

Tablet, as hydrochloride: 5 mg

Tablet, controlled release, as hydrochloride (OxyContin®): 10 mg, 20 mg, 40 mg, 80 mg

Dietary Considerations No data reported

Generic Available No

Comments Prophylactic use of a laxative should be considered; oxycodone, as with other narcotic analgesics, is recommended only for limited acute dosing (ie, 3 days or less). The most common adverse effect is nausea, followed by sedation and constipation. Oxycodone has an addictive liability, especially when given long term.

Oxycodone and Acetaminophen
(oks i KOE done & a seet a MIN oh fen)

Related Information

Acetaminophen *on page 20*

Dental Drug Interactions: Update on Drug Combinations Requiring Special Considerations *on page 1144*

Narcotic Agonists *on page 1141*

Oral Pain *on page 1053*

Brand Names Percocet®; Roxicet® 5/500; Roxilox®; Tylox®

Canadian/Mexican Brand Names Endocet® (Canada); Oxycocet (Canada); Percocet®-Demi (Canada)

Therapeutic Category Analgesic, Narcotic

Use

Dental: Treatment of postoperative pain

Medical: Relief of pain

Restrictions C-II; Nonrefillable

Usual Dosage Oral:

Children: Not recommended in pediatric dental patients

Adults: 1-2 tablets every 4-6 hours as needed for pain; maximum dose: 12 tablets/day

Mechanism of Action

Oxycodone, as with other narcotic (opiate) analgesics, blocks pain perception in the cerebral cortex by binding to specific receptor molecules (opiate receptors) within the neuronal membranes of synapses. This binding results in a decreased synaptic chemical transmission throughout the CNS thus inhibiting the flow of pain sensations into the higher centers. Mu and kappa are the two subtypes of the opiate receptor which oxycodone binds to to cause analgesia.

Acetaminophen inhibits the synthesis of prostaglandins in the CNS and peripherally blocks pain impulse generation; produces antipyresis from inhibition of hypothalamic heat-regulating center

Local Anesthetic/Vasoconstrictor Precautions No information available to require special precautions

Effects on Dental Treatment 1% to 10% of patients experience dry mouth

Other Adverse Effects

>10%:

Central nervous system: Drowsiness, dizziness, sedation

Gastrointestinal: Nausea

1% to 10%: Gastrointestinal: Constipation

Contraindications Patients with known G-6-PD deficiency; hypersensitivity to acetaminophen; hypersensitivity to oxycodone

Warnings/Precautions Use with caution in patients with hypersensitivity reactions to other phenanthrene derivative opioid agonists (morphine, codeine, hydrocodone, hydromorphone, levorphanol, oxymorphone); respiratory diseases including asthma, emphysema, COPD, or severe liver or renal insufficiency; some preparations contain sulfites which may cause allergic reactions; may be habit-forming

Enhanced analgesia has been seen in elderly patients on therapeutic doses of narcotics; duration of action may be increased in the elderly; the elderly may be particularly susceptible to the CNS depressant and constipating effects of narcotics

Drug Interactions The use of MAO inhibitors or tricyclic antidepressants with oxycodone may **increase** the effect of either the antidepressant or oxycodone; concurrent use of oxycodone with anticholinergics may cause paralytic ileus; (Continued)

Oxycodone and Acetaminophen *(Continued)*

patients taking other narcotic agents, antipsychotics, antianxiety agents or other CNS depressants (including alcohol) with oxycodone may experience an additive CNS depression; with acetaminophen component, refer to Acetaminophen monograph

Drug Uptake

Onset of effect: Narcotic analgesia: 0.5-1 hour

Duration of effect: 4-6 hours

Serum half-life: Oxycodone: 2-3 hours

Pregnancy Risk Factor C

Breast-feeding Considerations

Oxycodone: No data reported

Acetaminophen: May be taken while breast-feeding

Dosage Forms

Caplet: Oxycodone hydrochloride 5 mg and acetaminophen 500 mg

Capsule: Oxycodone hydrochloride 5 mg and acetaminophen 500 mg

Solution, oral: Oxycodone hydrochloride 5 mg and acetaminophen 325 mg per 5 mL (5 mL, 500 mL)

Tablet: Oxycodone hydrochloride 5 mg and acetaminophen 325 mg

Dietary Considerations No data reported

Generic Available Yes

Comments Oxycodone, as with other narcotic analgesics, is recommended only for limited acute dosing (ie, 3 days or less). The most common adverse effect is nausea, followed by sedation and constipation. Oxycodone has an addictive liability, especially when given long term. The acetaminophen component requires use with caution in patients with alcoholic liver disease.

Selected Readings

Cooper SA, Precheur H, Rauch D, et al, "Evaluation of Oxycodone and Acetaminophen in Treatment of Postoperative Pain," *Oral Surg Oral Med Oral Pathol*, 1980, 50(6):496-501.

Dionne RA, "New Approaches to Preventing and Treating Postoperative Pain," *J Am Dent Assoc*, 1992, 123(6):26-34.

Gobetti JP, "Controlling Dental Pain," *J Am Dent Assoc*, 1992, 123(6):47-52.

Oxycodone and Aspirin (oks i KOE done & AS pir in)

Related Information

Dental Drug Interactions: Update on Drug Combinations Requiring Special Considerations *on page 1144*

Narcotic Agonists *on page 1141*

Oral Pain *on page 1053*

Brand Names Codoxy®; Percodan®; Percodan®-Demi; Roxiprin®

Canadian/Mexican Brand Names Endodan® (Canada); Oxycodan (Canada)

Therapeutic Category Analgesic, Narcotic

Use

Dental: Treatment of postoperative pain

Medical: Relief of pain

Restrictions C-II; Nonrefillable

Usual Dosage Oral:

Children: Not recommended in pediatric dental patients

Adults: Percodan®: 1 tablet every 6 hours as needed for pain or Percodan®-Demi: 1-2 tablets every 6 hours as needed for pain

Mechanism of Action

Oxycodone, as with other narcotic (opiate) analgesics, blocks pain perception in the cerebral cortex by binding to specific receptor molecules (opiate receptors) within the neuronal membranes of synapses. This binding results in a decreased synaptic chemical transmission throughout the CNS thus inhibiting the flow of pain sensations into the higher centers. Mu and kappa are the two subtypes of the opiate receptor which oxycodone binds to to cause analgesia.

Aspirin inhibits prostaglandin synthesis by decreasing the activity of the enzyme, cyclo-oxygenase, which results in decreased formation of prostaglandin precursors, acts on the hypothalamic heat-regulating center to reduce fever, blocks thromboxane synthetase action which prevents formation of the platelet-aggregating substance thromboxane A_2

Local Anesthetic/Vasoconstrictor Precautions No information available to require special precautions

Effects on Dental Treatment 1% to 10% of patients experience dry mouth; use with caution in patients with platelet and bleeding disorders, renal dysfunction, erosive gastritis, or peptic ulcer disease, previous nonreaction does not guarantee future safe taking of medication; do not use aspirin in children <16 years of age for chickenpox or flu symptoms due to the association with Reye's syndrome

Avoid aspirin if possible, for 1 week prior to surgery because of the possibility of postoperative bleeding; use with caution in impaired hepatic function

Elderly are a high-risk population for adverse effects from nonsteroidal anti-inflammatory agents. As much as 60% of elderly with GI complications to NSAIDs can develop peptic ulceration and/or hemorrhage asymptomatically. Also, concomitant disease and drug use contribute to the risk for GI adverse effects. Use lowest effective dose for shortest period possible. Consider renal function decline with age. Use with caution in patients with history of asthma.

Other Adverse Effects

>10%:
  Central nervous system: Drowsiness, dizziness, sedation
  Gastrointestinal: Nausea, heartburn, stomach pains, dyspepsia
1% to 10%: Gastrointestinal: Constipation

Contraindications Known hypersensitivity to oxycodone or aspirin; severe respiratory depression

Warnings/Precautions Use with caution in patients with hypersensitivity to other phenanthrene derivative opioid agonists (morphine, codeine, hydrocodone, hydromorphone, oxymorphone, levorphanol); children and teenagers should not be given aspirin products if chickenpox or flu symptoms are present; aspirin use has been associated with Reye's syndrome; severe liver or renal insufficiency, pre-existing CNS and depression

Enhanced analgesia has been seen in elderly patients on therapeutic doses of narcotics; duration of action may be increased in the elderly; the elderly may be particularly susceptible to the CNS depressant and constipating effects of narcotics

Drug Interactions The use of MAO inhibitors or tricyclic antidepressants with oxycodone may **increase** effect of either the antidepressant or oxycodone; concurrent use of oxycodone with anticholinergics may cause paralytic ileus; patients taking other narcotic agents, antipsychotics, antianxiety agents or other CNS depressants (including alcohol) with oxycodone and aspirin may experience an additive CNS depression; aspirin interacts with warfarin to cause bleeding

Drug Uptake

Onset of effect: Narcotic analgesia: 0.5-1 hour
Duration of effect 4-6 hours
Serum half-life: Oxycodone: 2-3 hours

Pregnancy Risk Factor D

Breast-feeding Considerations

Aspirin: Caution is suggested due to potential adverse effects in nursing infants
Oxycodone: No data reported

Dosage Forms Tablet:
Percodan®: Oxycodone hydrochloride 4.5 mg, oxycodone terephthalate 0.38 mg, and aspirin 325 mg
Percodan®-Demi: Oxycodone hydrochloride 2.25 mg, oxycodone terephthalate 0.19 mg, and aspirin 325 mg

Dietary Considerations May be taken with food or water

Generic Available Yes

Comments Oxycodone, as with other narcotic analgesics, is recommended only for limited acute dosing (ie, 3 days or less). The most common adverse effect is nausea, followed by sedation and constipation. Oxycodone has an addictive liability, especially when given long term. The oxycodone with aspirin could have anticoagulant effects and could possibly affect bleeding times.

Selected Readings
Dionne RA, "New Approaches to Preventing and Treating Postoperative Pain," *J Am Dent Assoc,* 1992, 123(6):26-34.
Gobetti JP, "Controlling Dental Pain," *J Am Dent Assoc,* 1992, 123(6):47-52.

Oxycodone Hydrochloride *see* Oxycodone *on page 710*

OxyContin® *see* Oxycodone *on page 710*

Oxygen (OKS i jen)

Therapeutic Category Dental Gases

Use

Dental: Administered as a supplement with nitrous oxide to ensure adequate ventilation during sedation; a resuscitative agent for medical emergencies in dental office

Medical: To treat various clinical disorders, both respiratory and nonrespiratory; relief of arterial hypoxia and secondary complications; treatment of pulmonary hypertension, polycythemia secondary to hypoxemia, chronic disease states complicated by anemia, cancer, migraine headaches, coronary artery disease, seizure disorders, sickle-cell crisis and sleep apnea

Usual Dosage Children and Adults: Average rate of 2 L/minute

Mechanism of Action Increased oxygen in tidal volume and oxygenation of tissues at molecular level

(Continued)

Oxygen *(Continued)*

Local Anesthetic/Vasoconstrictor Precautions No information available to require special precautions

Effects on Dental Treatment No effects or complications reported

Other Adverse Effects No data reported

Contraindications No data reported

Warnings/Precautions Oxygen-induced hypoventilation is the greatest potential hazard of oxygen therapy. In patients with severe chronic obstructive pulmonary disease (COPD), the respiratory drive results from hypoxic stimulation of the carotid chemoreceptors. If this hypoxic drive is diminished by excessive oxygen therapy, hypoventilation may occur and further carbon dioxide retention with possible cessation of ventilation could result.

Drug Interactions No data reported

Pregnancy Risk Factor No data reported

Breast-feeding Considerations No data reported

Dosage Forms Liquid system with large reservoir holding 75-100 lb of liquid oxygen; compressed gas system consisting of high-pressure tank; tank sizes are "H" (6900 L of oxygen), "E" (622 L of oxygen) and "D" (356 L of oxygen)

Dietary Considerations No data reported

Generic Available Yes

OxyIR® *see* Oxycodone *on page 710*

Oxymetazoline *(oks i met AZ oh leen)*

Related Information

Oral Bacterial Infections *on page 1059*

Brand Names Afrin® Children's Nose Drops [OTC]; Afrin® Sinus [OTC]; Allerest® 12 Hour Nasal Solution [OTC]; Chlorphed®-LA Nasal Solution [OTC]; Dristan® Long Lasting Nasal Solution [OTC]; Duramist® Plus [OTC]; Duration® Nasal Solution [OTC]; Neo-Synephrine® 12 Hour Nasal Solution [OTC]; Nōstrilla® [OTC]; NTZ® Long Acting Nasal Solution [OTC]; OcuClear® Ophthalmic [OTC]; Sinarest® 12 Hour Nasal Solution; Sinex® Long-Acting [OTC]; Twice-A-Day® Nasal [OTC]; Visine® L.R. Ophthalmic [OTC]; 4-Way® Long Acting Nasal Solution [OTC]

Canadian/Mexican Brand Names Drixoral® Nasal (Canada)

Therapeutic Category Adrenergic Agonist Agent; Decongestant, Nasal; Nasal Agent, Vasoconstrictor

Use

Dental: Symptomatic relief of nasal mucosal congestion

Medical:

Adjunctive therapy of middle ear infections, associated with acute or chronic rhinitis, the common cold, sinusitis, hay fever, or other allergies

Ophthalmic: Relief of redness of eye due to minor eye irritations

Usual Dosage Intranasal (therapy should not exceed 3-5 days):

Children 2-5 years: 0.025% solution: Instill 2-3 drops in each nostril twice daily

Children ≥6 years and Adults: 0.05% solution: Instill 2-3 drops or 2-3 sprays into each nostril twice daily

Mechanism of Action Stimulates alpha-adrenergic receptors in the arterioles of the nasal mucosa to produce vasoconstriction

Local Anesthetic/Vasoconstrictor Precautions No information available to require special precautions

Effects on Dental Treatment No effects or complications reported

Other Adverse Effects

>10%:

Local: Transient burning, stinging

Respiratory: Dryness of the nasal mucosa, sneezing

1% to 10%:

Cardiovascular: Hypertension, palpitations

Respiratory: Rebound congestion with prolonged use

Contraindications Hypersensitivity to oxymetazoline or any component

Warnings/Precautions Rebound congestion may occur with extended use (>3 days); use with caution in the presence of hypertension, diabetes, hyperthyroidism, heart disease, coronary artery disease, cerebral arteriosclerosis, or long-standing bronchial asthma

Drug Interactions Increased toxicity with MAO inhibitors

Drug Uptake

Onset of effect: Intranasal: Within 5-10 minutes

Duration: 5-6 hours

Pregnancy Risk Factor C

Breast-feeding Considerations No data reported

Dosage Forms Solution, nasal:
  Drops: 0.05% drops (15 mL, 20 mL)
  Drops, pediatric: 0.025% (20 mL)
  Spray: 0.05% (15 mL, 30 mL)
Dietary Considerations No data reported
Generic Available Yes

Oxymetholone (oks i METH oh lone)
Brand Names Anadrol®
Canadian/Mexican Brand Names Anapolon® (Canada)
Therapeutic Category Anabolic Steroid
Use Anemias caused by the administration of myelotoxic drugs
Usual Dosage Adults: Erythropoietic effects: Oral: 1-5 mg/kg/day in 1 daily dose; maximum: 100 mg/day; give for a minimum trial of 3-6 months because response may be delayed
Mechanism of Action Stimulates receptors in organs and tissues to promote growth and development of male sex organs and maintains secondary sex characteristics in androgen-deficient males
Local Anesthetic/Vasoconstrictor Precautions No information available to require special precautions
Effects on Dental Treatment No effects or complications reported
Other Adverse Effects
  Male:
  Postpubertal:
    >10%:
      Dermatologic: Acne
      Endocrine & metabolic: Gynecomastia
      Genitourinary: Bladder irritability, priapism
    1% to 10%:
      Central nervous system: Insomnia, chills
      Endocrine & metabolic: Decreased libido
      Gastrointestinal: Nausea, diarrhea
      Genitourinary: Prostatic hypertrophy (elderly)
      Hematologic: Iron deficiency anemia, suppression of clotting factors
    Hepatic: Hepatic dysfunction
    <1%:
      Hepatic: Hepatic necrosis, hepatocellular carcinoma
  Prepubertal:
    >10%:
      Dermatologic: Acne
      Endocrine & metabolic: Virilism
    1% to 10%:
      Central nervous system: Chills, insomnia
      Dermatologic: Hyperpigmentation
      Gastrointestinal: Diarrhea, nausea
      Hematologic: Iron deficiency anemia, suppression of clotting factors
    <1%: Hepatic: Hepatic necrosis, hepatocellular carcinoma

  Female:
    >10%: Endocrine & metabolic: Virilism
    1% to 10%:
      Central nervous system: Chills, insomnia
      Endocrine & metabolic: Hypercalcemia
      Gastrointestinal: Nausea, diarrhea
      Hematologic: Iron deficiency anemia, suppression of clotting factors
      Hepatic: Hepatic dysfunction
    <1%: Hepatic: Hepatic necrosis, hepatocellular carcinoma
Drug Interactions Increased toxicity: Increased oral anticoagulants, insulin requirements may be decreased
Drug Uptake
  Serum half-life: 9 hours
Pregnancy Risk Factor X
Generic Available No

Oxymorphone (oks i MOR fone)
Related Information
  Narcotic Agonists *on page 1141*
Brand Names Numorphan®
Therapeutic Category Analgesic, Narcotic
Use Management of moderate to severe pain and preoperatively as a sedative and a supplement to anesthesia
  (Continued)

Oxymorphone *(Continued)*

Usual Dosage Adults:
    I.M., S.C.: 0.5 mg initially, 1-1.5 mg every 4-6 hours as needed
    I.V.: 0.5 mg initially
    Rectal: 5 mg every 4-6 hours

Mechanism of Action Oxymorphone hydrochloride (Numorphan®) is a potent narcotic analgesic with uses similar to those of morphine. The drug is a semisynthetic derivative of morphine (phenanthrene derivative) and is closely related to hydromorphone chemically (Dilaudid®).

Local Anesthetic/Vasoconstrictor Precautions No information available to require special precautions

Effects on Dental Treatment Anticholinergic side effects can cause a reduction of saliva production or secretion contributes to discomfort and dental disease (ie, caries, oral candidiasis and periodontal disease)

Other Adverse Effects
>10%:
    Cardiovascular: Hypotension
    Central nervous system: Fatigue, drowsiness, dizziness
    Gastrointestinal: Nausea, vomiting, constipation
    Neuromuscular & skeletal: Weakness
    Miscellaneous: Histamine release

1% to 10%:
    Central nervous system: Nervousness, headache, restlessness, malaise, confusion
    Gastrointestinal: Anorexia, stomach cramps, dry mouth, biliary spasm
    Genitourinary: Decreased urination, ureteral spasms
    Local: Pain at injection site
    Respiratory: Dyspnea

<1%:
    Central nervous system: Mental depression, hallucinations, paradoxical CNS stimulation, increased intracranial pressure
    Dermatologic: Skin rash, urticaria
    Gastrointestinal: Paralytic ileus
    Miscellaneous: Histamine release, physical and psychological dependence

Drug Interactions
Decreased effect with phenothiazines
Increased effect/toxicity with CNS depressants, TCAs, dextroamphetamine

Drug Uptake
Onset of analgesia:
    I.V., I.M., S.C.: Within 5-10 minutes
    Rectal: Within 15-30 minutes
Duration of analgesia: Parenteral, rectal: 3-4 hours

Pregnancy Risk Factor B (D if used for prolonged periods or in high doses at term)

Generic Available No

Oxyphenbutazone *(oks i fen BYOO ta zone)*

Therapeutic Category Analgesic, Non-narcotic; Nonsteroidal Anti-inflammatory Agent (NSAID), Oral

Use Management of inflammatory disorders, as an analgesic in the treatment of mild to moderate pain and as an antipyretic; I.V. form used as an alternate to surgery in management of patent ductus arteriosus in premature neonates; acute gouty arthritis

Local Anesthetic/Vasoconstrictor Precautions No information available to require special precautions

Effects on Dental Treatment No effects or complications reported

Other Adverse Effects
>10%:
    Central nervous system: Dizziness
    Dermatologic: Skin rash
    Gastrointestinal: Abdominal cramps, heartburn, indigestion, nausea

1% to 10%:
    Central nervous system: Headache, nervousness
    Dermatologic: Itching
    Endocrine & metabolic: Fluid retention
    Gastrointestinal: Vomiting
    Otic: Tinnitus

<1%:
    Cardiovascular: Congestive heart failure, hypertension, arrhythmia, tachycardia

Central nervous system: Confusion, hallucinations, aseptic meningitis, mental depression, drowsiness, insomnia

Dermatologic: Urticaria, erythema multiforme, toxic epidermal necrolysis, Stevens-Johnson syndrome, angioedema

Endocrine & metabolic: Polydipsia, hot flashes

Gastrointestinal: Gastritis, GI ulceration

Genitourinary: Cystitis

Hematologic: Agranulocytosis, anemia, hemolytic anemia, bone marrow suppression, leukopenia, thrombocytopenia

Hepatic: Hepatitis

Neuromuscular & skeletal: Peripheral neuropathy

Ocular: Toxic amblyopia, blurred vision, conjunctivitis, dry eyes

Otic: Decreased hearing

Renal: Polyuria, acute renal failure

Respiratory: Allergic rhinitis, dyspnea, epistaxis

Pregnancy Risk Factor D

Generic Available Yes

Oxyphencyclimine (oks i fen SYE kli meen)

Brand Names Daricon®

Therapeutic Category Anticholinergic Agent; Antispasmodic Agent, Gastrointestinal

Use Adjunctive treatment of peptic ulcer

Local Anesthetic/Vasoconstrictor Precautions No information available to require special precautions

Effects on Dental Treatment >10% of patients experience dry mouth

Other Adverse Effects

>10%:

Dermatologic: Dry skin

Gastrointestinal: Constipation, dry throat

Respiratory: Dry nose

Miscellaneous: Decreased sweating

1% to 10%:

Gastrointestinal: Dysphagia

Ocular: Photosensitivity

<1%:

Cardiovascular: Tachycardia

Central nervous system: Confusion, headache, loss of memory, fatigue, drowsiness, nervousness, insomnia

Dermatologic: Rash

Gastrointestinal: Bloated feeling, nausea, vomiting

Genitourinary: Urinary retention

Neuromuscular & skeletal: Weakness

Ocular: Increased intraocular pressure, blurred vision

Pregnancy Risk Factor C

Generic Available No

Oxytetracycline (oks i tet ra SYE kleen)

Brand Names Terramycin® I.M. Injection; Terramycin® Oral

Canadian/Mexican Brand Names Oxitraklin® (Mexico); Terramicina® (Mexico)

Therapeutic Category Antibiotic, Tetracycline Derivative

Synonyms Oxitetraciclina (Mexico)

Use Treatment of susceptible bacterial infections; both gram-positive and gram-negative, as well as, *Rickettsia* and *Mycoplasma* organisms

Usual Dosage

Oral:

Children: 40-50 mg/kg/day in divided doses every 6 hours (maximum: 2 g/24 hours)

Adults: 250-500 mg/dose every 6 hours

I.M.:

Children >8 years: 15-25 mg/kg/day (maximum: 250 mg/dose) in divided doses every 8-12 hours

Adults: 250-500 mg every 24 hours or 300 mg/day divided every 8-12 hours

Mechanism of Action Inhibits bacterial protein synthesis by binding with the 30S and possibly the 50S ribosomal subunit(s) of susceptible bacteria, cell wall synthesis is not affected

Local Anesthetic/Vasoconstrictor Precautions No information available to require special precautions

Effects on Dental Treatment Tetracycline's are not recommended for use during pregnancy or in children ≤8 years of age since they have been reported to (Continued)

Oxytetracycline *(Continued)*

cause enamel hypoplasia and permanent teeth discoloration. The use of tetracycline's should only be used in these patients if other agents are contraindicated or alternative antimicrobials will not eradicate the organism. Long-term use associated with oral candidiasis.

Other Adverse Effects
>10%: Miscellaneous: Discoloration of teeth and enamel hypoplasia (infants)
1% to 10%:
 Dermatologic: Photosensitivity
 Gastrointestinal: Nausea, diarrhea
<1%:
 Cardiovascular: Pericarditis
 Central nervous system: Increased intracranial pressure, bulging fontanels in infants, pseudotumor cerebri
 Dermatologic: Pruritus, exfoliative dermatitis, dermatologic effects
 Endocrine & metabolic: Diabetes insipidus syndrome
 Gastrointestinal: Vomiting, esophagitis, anorexia, abdominal cramps, antibiotic-associated pseudomembranous colitis, staphylococcal enterocolitis
 Hepatic: Hepatotoxicity
 Local: Thrombophlebitis,
 Neuromuscular & skeletal: Paresthesia
 Renal: Renal damage, acute renal failure, azotemia
 Miscellaneous: Superinfections, anaphylaxis, pigmentation of nails, hypersensitivity reactions, candidal superinfection

Drug Interactions
Decreased effect with antacids containing aluminum, calcium or magnesium
Iron and bismuth subsalicylate may decrease oxytetracycline bioavailability
Barbiturates, phenytoin, and carbamazepine decrease oxytetracycline's half-life
Increased effect of warfarin

Drug Uptake
Absorption:
 Oral: Adequate (~75%)
 I.M.: Poor
Serum half-life: 8.5-9.6 hours (increases with renal impairment)
Time to peak serum concentration: Within 2-4 hours

Pregnancy Risk Factor D
Dosage Forms
Capsule, as hydrochloride: 250 mg
Injection, as hydrochloride, with lidocaine 2%: 5% [50 mg/mL] (2 mL, 10 mL); 12.5% [125 mg/mL] (2 mL)

Generic Available Yes

Oxytetracycline and Hydrocortisone
(oks i tet ra SYE kleen & hye droe KOR ti sone)
Brand Names Terra-Cortril® Ophthalmic Suspension
Therapeutic Category Antibiotic, Ophthalmic
Use Treatment of susceptible ophthalmic bacterial infections with associated swelling
Local Anesthetic/Vasoconstrictor Precautions No information available to require special precautions
Effects on Dental Treatment No effects or complications reported
Pregnancy Risk Factor C
Generic Available Yes

Oxytetracycline and Polymyxin B
(oks i tet ra SYE kleen & pol i MIKS in bee)
Brand Names Terak® Ophthalmic Ointment; Terramycin® Ophthalmic Ointment; Terramycin® w/Polymyxin B Ophthalmic Ointment
Therapeutic Category Antibiotic, Ophthalmic
Synonyms Polymyxin B and Oxytetracycline
Use Treatment of superficial ocular infections involving the conjunctiva and/or cornea
Local Anesthetic/Vasoconstrictor Precautions No information available to require special precautions
Effects on Dental Treatment No effects or complications reported
Pregnancy Risk Factor D
Generic Available No

Oxytocin (oks i TOE sin)

Brand Names Pitocin®; Syntocinon®

Canadian/Mexican Brand Names Oxitopisa® (Mexico); Syntocinon® (Mexico); Toesen® (Canada); Xitocin® (Mexico)

Therapeutic Category Oxytocic Agent

Synonyms Oxitocina (Mexico)

Use Induces labor at term; controls postpartum bleeding; nasal preparation used to promote milk letdown in lactating females

Usual Dosage I.V. administration requires the use of an infusion pump

Adults:

Induction of labor: I.V.: 0.001-0.002 units/minute; increase by 0.001-0.002 units every 15-30 minutes until contraction pattern has been established; maximum dose should not exceed 20 milliunits/minute

Postpartum bleeding:

I.M.: Total dose of 10 units after delivery

I.V.: 10-40 units by I.V. infusion in 1000 mL of intravenous fluid at a rate sufficient to control uterine atony

Promotion of milk letdown: Intranasal: 1 spray or 3 drops in one or both nostrils 2-3 minutes before breast-feeding

Mechanism of Action Produces the rhythmic uterine contractions characteristic to delivery and stimulates breast milk flow during nursing

Local Anesthetic/Vasoconstrictor Precautions No information available to require special precautions

Effects on Dental Treatment No effects or complications reported

Other Adverse Effects

Fetal: <1%:

Cardiovascular: Bradycardia, arrhythmias

Central nervous system: Brain damage, intracranial hemorrhage

Hepatic: Neonatal jaundice

Respiratory: Hypoxia

Miscellaneous: Death

Maternal: <1%:

Cardiovascular: Cardiac arrhythmias, premature ventricular contractions, hypotension, tachycardia, arrhythmias

Central nervous system: Seizures, coma

Endocrine & metabolic: SIADH with hyponatremia

Gastrointestinal: Nausea, vomiting

Genitourinary: Increased uterine motility, pelvic hematoma

Hematologic: Postpartum hemorrhage, fatal afibrinogenemia, increased blood loss

Miscellaneous: Death, anaphylactic reactions

Drug Interactions No data reported

Drug Uptake

Onset of uterine contractions: I.V.: Within 1 minute

Duration: <30 minutes

Serum half-life: 1-5 minutes

Pregnancy Risk Factor X (nasal solution)

Generic Available Yes

Oyst-Cal 500 [OTC] see Calcium Carbonate on page 162

Oystercal® 500 see Calcium Carbonate on page 162

P-071 see Cetirizine on page 205

Paclitaxel (PAK li taks el)

Brand Names Taxol®

Therapeutic Category Antineoplastic Agent, Antimicrotubular

Use Treatment of metastatic carcinoma of the ovary after failure of first-line or subsequent chemotherapy; treatment of metastatic breast cancer

Usual Dosage Corticosteroids (dexamethasone), H_1 antagonists (diphenhydramine), and H_2 antagonists (cimetidine or ranitidine), should be administered prior to paclitaxel administration to minimize potential for anaphylaxis

Adults: I.V. infusion: **Refer to individual protocol**

Ovarian carcinoma: 135-175 mg/m² over 1-24 hours administered every 3 weeks

Metastatic breast cancer: Treatment is still undergoing investigation; most protocols have used doses of 175-250 mg/m² over 1-24 hours every 3 weeks

Local Anesthetic/Vasoconstrictor Precautions No information available to require special precautions

Effects on Dental Treatment No effects or complications reported

(Continued)

Paclitaxel (Continued)

Other Adverse Effects

>10%:

Bone marrow suppression: Major dose-limiting (ie, more severe at doses of 200-250 mg/m^2) toxicity

Dermatologic: Alopecia has been observed in almost all patients; loss of scalp hair occurs suddenly between day 14 and 21 and is reversible. Some patients experience a loss of all body hair. Local venous effects include erythema, tenderness, and discomfort during infusion and areas of extravasation include erythema, swelling, and induration. Necrotic changes and ulcers have not been reported even after extravasation of large volumes of infusate.

Hypersensitivity: Based on observations during early clinical trials, reactions were principally nonimmunologically mediated by the direct release of histamine or other vasoactive substances from mast cells and basophils

Neurotoxicity: Typically cumulative, with symptoms progressing after each treatment at both high and low doses. Patients with pre-existing neuropathies due to previous chemotherapy or coexisting medical illness (diabetes mellitus, alcoholism) appear to be predisposed to neurotoxicity. Neurotoxic effects such as sensory neuropathy, motor neuropathy, autonomic neuropathy, myopathy or myopathic effects, and central nervous system toxicity have been reported. Sensory neuropathy occurs invariably when the paclitaxel dose approaches 250 mg/m^2. Symptoms include numbness, tingling, and/or burning pain in the distal lower extremities, toes and/or fingers and begin as early as 24-72 hours after treatment with high single doses. Motor neuropathy occurs primarily at relatively high doses (250-275 mg/m^2) and in those patients with diabetes mellitus who may be more predisposed to toxic neuropathies. Myopathy effects are commonly observed after treatment with moderate to high doses (ie, >200 mg/m^2) administered over 6-24 hours. These symptoms generally occur 2-3 days after treatment and resolve within 5-6 days.

Miscellaneous: Hypersensitivity reactions, myalgia, abnormal liver function tests

1% to 10%:

Cardiovascular: Bradycardia, severe cardiovascular events

Gastrointestinal: Nausea and vomiting are not severe at any dose level

Irritant chemotherapy

Drug Interactions Increased toxicity:

In phase I trials, myelosuppression was more profound when given after cisplatin than with alternative sequence; pharmacokinetic data demonstrates a decrease in clearance of -33% when administered following cisplatin

Possibility of an inhibition of metabolism in patients treated with ketoconazole

Drug Uptake Administered by I.V. infusion and exhibits a biphasic decline in plasma concentrations

Serum half-life, mean, terminal: 5.3-17.4 hours after 1- and 6-hour infusions at dosing levels of 15-275 mg/m^2

Pregnancy Risk Factor D

Generic Available No

PALS® [OTC] see Chlorophyll on page 212

Pamelor® see Nortriptyline on page 692

Pamidronate (pa mi DROE nate)

Brand Names Aredia™

Therapeutic Category Antidote, Hypercalcemia; Bisphosphonate Derivative

Use FDA-approved: Treatment of hypercalcemia associated with malignancy; treatment of osteolytic bone lesions associated with multiple myeloma; treatment of osteolytic bone metastases of breast cancer; moderate to severe Paget's disease of bone

Usual Dosage Drug must be diluted properly before administration and infused slowly (over at least 1 hour)

Adults: I.V.:

Moderate cancer-related hypercalcemia (corrected serum calcium: 12-13 mg/dL): 60-90 mg given as a slow infusion over 2-24 hours

Severe cancer-related hypercalcemia (corrected serum calcium: >13.5 mg/dL): 90 mg as a slow infusion over 2-24 hours

A period of 7 days should elapse before the use of second course; repeat infusions every 2-3 weeks have been suggested, however, could be administered every 2-3 months according to the degree and of severity of hypercalcemia and/or the type of malignancy

Osteolytic bone lesions with multiple myeloma: 90 mg in 500 mL D$_5$W, 0.45% NaCl or 0.9% NaCl administered over 4 hours on a monthly basis

Paget's disease: 30 mg in 500 mL 0.45% NaCl, 0.9% NaCl or D$_5$W administered over 4 hours for 3 consecutive days

Mechanism of Action A biphosphonate which inhibits bone resorption via actions on osteoclasts or on osteoclast precursors. Does not appear to produce any significant effects on renal tubular calcium handling and is poorly absorbed following oral administration (high oral doses have been reported effective); therefore, I.V. therapy is preferred.

Local Anesthetic/Vasoconstrictor Precautions No information available to require special precautions

Effects on Dental Treatment No effects or complications reported

Other Adverse Effects
1% to 10%:
Central nervous system: Malaise, fever, convulsions
Endocrine & metabolic: Hypomagnesemia, hypocalcemia, hypokalemia, hypophosphatemia, fluid overload
Gastrointestinal: GI symptoms, nausea, diarrhea, constipation, anorexia
Hepatic: Abnormal hepatic function
Neuromuscular & skeletal: Bone pain
Respiratory: Dyspnea
<1%:
Central nervous system: Pain
Dermatologic: Skin rash, angioedema
Gastrointestinal: Dysgeusia, occult blood in stools
Hematologic: Leukopenia
Neuromuscular & skeletal: Increased risk of fractures
Renal: Nephrotoxicity
Miscellaneous: Hypersensitivity reactions

Drug Interactions No data reported

Drug Uptake
Onset of effect: 24-48 hours
Maximum effect: 5-7 days
Absorption: Poorly from the GI tract; pharmacokinetic studies are lacking
Serum half-life, unmetabolized: 2.5 hours

Pregnancy Risk Factor C

Generic Available No

Pamine® *see* Methscopolamine *on page 619*

p-Aminoclonidine *see* Apraclonidine *on page 83*

Panadol® [OTC] *see* Acetaminophen *on page 20*

Panasal® 5/500 *see* Hydrocodone and Aspirin *on page 480*

Pancrease® *see* Pancrelipase *on next page*

Pancrease® MT 4 *see* Pancrelipase *on next page*

Pancrease® MT 10 *see* Pancrelipase *on next page*

Pancrease® MT 16 *see* Pancrelipase *on next page*

Pancrease® MT 20 *see* Pancrelipase *on next page*

Pancreatin (PAN kree a tin)

Brand Names Creon®; Digepepsin®; Donnazyme®; Hi-Vegi-Lip®

Therapeutic Category Pancreatic Enzyme

Use Replacement therapy in symptomatic treatment of malabsorption syndrome caused by pancreatic insufficiency

Local Anesthetic/Vasoconstrictor Precautions No information available to require special precautions

Effects on Dental Treatment No effects or complications reported

Other Adverse Effects
1% to 10%: High doses:
Endocrine & metabolic: Hyperuricemia
Gastrointestinal: Nausea, cramps, constipation, diarrhea
Ocular: Lacrimation
Renal: Hyperuricosuria
Respiratory: Sneezing
<1%:
Dermatologic: Rash
Gastrointestinal: Irritation of the mouth
Respiratory: Dyspnea, bronchospasm

Pregnancy Risk Factor C

Generic Available No

Comments On a weight basis, pancreatin has $^1/_{12}$ the lipolytic activity of pancrelipase

Pancrelipase (pan kre LI pase)

Brand Names Cotazym®; Cotazym-S®; Creon® 10; Creon® 20; Ilozyme®; Ku-Zyme® HP; Pancrease®; Pancrease® MT 4; Pancrease® MT 10; Pancrease® MT 16; Pancrease® MT 20; Protilase®; Ultrase® MT12; Ultrase® MT20; Viokase®; Zymase®

Therapeutic Category Pancreatic Enzyme

Synonyms Lipancreatin

Use Replacement therapy in symptomatic treatment of malabsorption syndrome caused by pancreatic insufficiency

Usual Dosage Oral:

Powder: Actual dose depends on the digestive requirements of the patient

Children <1 year: Start with 1/8 teaspoonful with feedings

Adults: 0.7 g with meals

Enteric coated microspheres and microtablets: The following dosage recommendations are only an approximation for initial dosages. The actual dosage will depend on the digestive requirements of the individual patient.

Children:

<1 year: 2000 units of lipase with meals

1-6 years: 4000-8000 units of lipase with meals and 4000 units with snacks

7-12 years: 4000-12,000 units of lipase with meals and snacks

Adults: 4000-16,000 units of lipase with meals and with snacks or 1-3 tablets/capsules before or with meals and snacks; in severe deficiencies, dose may be increased to 8 tablets/capsules

Occluded feeding tubes: One tablet of Viokase® crushed with one 325 mg tablet of sodium bicarbonate (to activate the Viokase®) in 5 mL of water can be instilled into the nasogastric tube and clamped for 5 minutes; then, flushed with 50 mL of tap water

Mechanism of Action Replaces endogenous pancreatic enzymes to assist in digestion of protein, starch and fats

Local Anesthetic/Vasoconstrictor Precautions No information available to require special precautions

Effects on Dental Treatment No effects or complications reported

Other Adverse Effects

1% to 10%: High doses:

Endocrine & metabolic: Hyperuricemia

Gastrointestinal: Nausea, cramps, constipation, diarrhea

Ocular: Lacrimation

Renal: Hyperuricosuria

Respiratory: Sneezing

<1%:

Dermatologic: Rash

Gastrointestinal: Irritation of the mouth

Respiratory: Dyspnea, bronchospasm

Drug Uptake

Absorption: Not absorbed, acts locally in GI tract

Pregnancy Risk Factor C

Generic Available Yes

Comments Concomitant administration of conventional pancreatin enzymes with an H_2-receptor antagonist has been used to decrease the inactivation of enzyme activity

Panhematin® see Hemin on page 465

PanOxyl®-AQ see Benzoyl Peroxide on page 120

PanOxyl® Bar [OTC] see Benzoyl Peroxide on page 120

Panscol® [OTC] see Salicylic Acid on page 853

Panthoderm® [OTC] see Dexpanthenol on page 294

Pantopon® see Opium Alkaloids on page 702

Pantothenic Acid (pan toe THEN ik AS id)

Therapeutic Category Vitamin, Water Soluble

Synonyms Calcium Pantothenate; Vitamin B_5

Use Pantothenic acid deficiency

Local Anesthetic/Vasoconstrictor Precautions No information available to require special precautions

Effects on Dental Treatment No effects or complications reported

Pregnancy Risk Factor A (C if used in doses above RDA recommendations)

Generic Available Yes

Papaverine (pa PAV er een)

Brand Names Genabid®; Pavabid®; Pavatine®

Therapeutic Category Vasodilator

Use
Oral: Relief of peripheral and cerebral ischemia associated with arterial spasm; smooth muscle relaxant
Parenteral: Various vascular spasms associated with muscle spasms as in myocardial infarction, angina, peripheral and pulmonary embolism, peripheral vascular disease, angiospastic states, and visceral spasm (ureteral, biliary, and GI colic); testing for impotence

Usual Dosage
Children: I.M., I.V.: 1.5 mg/kg 4 times/day
Adults:
Oral: 100-300 mg 3-5 times/day
Oral, sustained release: 150-300 mg every 12 hours
I.M., I.V.: 30-120 mg every 3 hours as needed; for cardiac extrasystoles, give 2 doses 10 minutes apart I.V. or I.M.

Mechanism of Action Smooth muscle spasmolytic producing a generalized smooth muscle relaxation including: vasodilatation, gastrointestinal sphincter relaxation, bronchiolar muscle relaxation, and potentially a depressed myocardium (with large doses); muscle relaxation may occur due to inhibition or cyclic nucleotide phosphodiesterase, increasing cyclic AMP; muscle relaxation is unrelated to nerve innervation; papaverine increases cerebral blood flow in normal subjects; oxygen uptake is unaltered

Local Anesthetic/Vasoconstrictor Precautions No information available to require special precautions

Effects on Dental Treatment No effects or complications reported

Other Adverse Effects <1%:
Cardiovascular: Flushing of the face, tachycardia, hypotension, arrhythmias with rapid I.V. use
Central nervous system: Depression, dizziness, vertigo, drowsiness, sedation, lethargy, headache
Dermatologic: Pruritus
Gastrointestinal: Dry mouth, nausea, constipation
Hepatic: Hepatic hypersensitivity
Local: Thrombosis at the I.V. administration site
Respiratory: Apnea with rapid I.V. use
Miscellaneous: Sweating

Drug Interactions
Decreased effect: Papaverine decreases the effects of levodopa
Increased toxicity: Additive effects with CNS depressants or morphine

Drug Uptake
Onset of action: Oral: Rapid
Serum half-life: 0.5-1.5 hours

Pregnancy Risk Factor C
Generic Available Yes

Para-Aminosalicylate Sodium
(PAIR a-a MEE noe sa LIS i late SOW dee um)
Related Information
Nonviral Infectious Diseases *on page 1032*
Therapeutic Category Analgesic, Non-narcotic; Salicylate
Synonyms Aminosalicylate Sodium; PAS
Use Adjunctive treatment of tuberculosis
Local Anesthetic/Vasoconstrictor Precautions No information available to require special precautions
Effects on Dental Treatment No effects or complications reported
Other Adverse Effects 1% to 10%:
Endocrine & metabolic: Hypokalemia
Gastrointestinal: Nausea, vomiting, diarrhea
Hepatic: Hepatitis, jaundice
Miscellaneous: Allergy reactions
Pregnancy Risk Factor C
Generic Available No
Comments Capsules contain bentonite which may decrease absorption of concomitantly ingested drugs

Paracetamol (Mexico) *see Acetaminophen on page 20*

Parachlorometaxylenol (PAIR a klor oh met a ZYE le nol)
Brand Names Metasep® [OTC]
Therapeutic Category Antiseborrheic Agent, Topical
Synonyms PCMX
Use Aid in relief of dandruff and associated conditions
(Continued)

Parachlorometaxylenol *(Continued)*

Local Anesthetic/Vasoconstrictor Precautions No information available to require special precautions

Effects on Dental Treatment No effects or complications reported

Generic Available No

Paraflex® *see* Chlorzoxazone *on page 228*

Parafon Forte™ DSC *see* Chlorzoxazone *on page 228*

Para-Hist AT® *see* Promethazine, Phenylephrine, and Codeine *on page 806*

Paramethasone Acetate (par a METH a sone AS e tate)

Brand Names Haldrone®; Stemex®

Therapeutic Category Adrenal Corticosteroid

Use Treatment of variety of diseases including those of hematologic, allergic, inflammatory, neoplastic, and autoimmune in origin

Local Anesthetic/Vasoconstrictor Precautions No information available to require special precautions

Effects on Dental Treatment No effects or complications reported

Pregnancy Risk Factor C

Generic Available No

Comments Likely to inhibit maturation and growth in adolescents; at high doses (>15 mg/d) increased urinary excretion of nitrogen and calcium will occur

Paraplatin® *see* Carboplatin *on page 178*

Par Decon® *see* Chlorpheniramine, Phenyltoloxamine, Phenylpropanolamine, and Phenylephrine *on page 222*

Paredrine® *see* Hydroxyamphetamine *on page 488*

Paregoric (par e GOR ik)

Therapeutic Category Analgesic, Narcotic; Antidiarrheal

Use Treatment of diarrhea or relief of pain; neonatal opiate withdrawal

Usual Dosage Oral:

Neonatal opiate withdrawal: Instill 3-6 drops every 3-6 hours as needed, or initially 0.2 mL every 3 hours; increase dosage by approximately 0.05 mL every 3 hours until withdrawal symptoms are controlled; it is rare to exceed 0.7 mL/ dose. Stabilize withdrawal symptoms for 3-5 days, then gradually decrease dosage over a 2- to 4-week period.

Children: 0.25-0.5 mL/kg 1-4 times/day

Adults: 5-10 mL 1-4 times/day

Mechanism of Action Increases smooth muscle tone in GI tract, decreases motility and peristalsis, diminishes digestive secretions

Local Anesthetic/Vasoconstrictor Precautions No information available to require special precautions

Effects on Dental Treatment No effects or complications reported

Other Adverse Effects

>10%:

Cardiovascular: Hypotension

Central nervous system: Drowsiness, dizziness

Gastrointestinal: Constipation

Neuromuscular & skeletal: Weakness

1% to 10%:

Central nervous system: Restlessness, headache, malaise

Genitourinary: Ureteral spasms, decreased urination

Miscellaneous: Histamine release

<1%:

Cardiovascular: Peripheral vasodilation

Central nervous system: Insomnia, CNS depression, mental depression, increased intracranial pressure

Gastrointestinal: Anorexia, stomach cramps, nausea, vomiting, biliary spasm

Genitourinary: Urinary tract spasm

Ocular: Miosis

Respiratory: Respiratory depression

Miscellaneous: Physical and psychological dependence

Drug Interactions Increased effect/toxicity with CNS depressants (eg, alcohol, narcotics, benzodiazepines, TCAs, MAO inhibitors, phenothiazine)

Pregnancy Risk Factor B (D when used long-term or in high doses)

Generic Available Yes

Paremyd® Ophthalmic *see* Hydroxyamphetamine and Tropicamide *on page 488*

Parenteral Multiple Vitamin *see* Vitamins, Multiple *on page 995*

Parepectolin® *see* Kaolin and Pectin With Opium *on page 532*

Par Glycerol® *see* Iodinated Glycerol *on page 515*

Pargyline and Methyclothiazide *see* Methyclothiazide and Pargyline *on page 621*

Parlodel® *see* Bromocriptine *on page 141*

Parnate® *see* Tranylcypromine *on page 951*

Paromomycin (par oh moe MYE sin)
Brand Names Humatin®
Therapeutic Category Amebicide
Use Treatment of acute and chronic intestinal amebiasis due to susceptible *Entamoeba histolytica* (not effective in the treatment of extraintestinal amebiasis); tapeworm infestations; adjunctive management of hepatic coma; treatment of cryptosporidial diarrhea
Usual Dosage Oral:
Intestinal amebiasis: Children and Adults: 25-35 mg/kg/day in 3 divided doses for 5-10 days
Dientamoeba fragilis: Children and Adults: 25-30 mg/kg/day in 3 divided doses for 7 days
Cryptosporidium: Adults with AIDS: 1.5-2.25 g/day in 3-6 divided doses for 10-14 days (occasionally courses of up to 4-8 weeks may be needed)
Tapeworm (fish, dog, bovine, porcine):
Children: 11 mg/kg every 15 minutes for 4 doses
Adults: 1 g every 15 minutes for 4 doses
Hepatic coma: Adults: 4 g/day in 2-4 divided doses for 5-6 days
Dwarf tapeworm: Children and Adults: 45 mg/kg/dose every day for 5-7 days
Mechanism of Action Acts directly on ameba; has antibacterial activity against normal and pathogenic organisms in the GI tract; interferes with bacterial protein synthesis by binding to 30S ribosomal subunits
Local Anesthetic/Vasoconstrictor Precautions No information available to require special precautions
Effects on Dental Treatment No effects or complications reported
Other Adverse Effects
1% to 10%: Gastrointestinal: Diarrhea, abdominal cramps, nausea, vomiting, heartburn
<1%:
Central nervous system: Headache, vertigo
Dermatologic: Rash, pruritus, exanthema
Gastrointestinal: Steatorrhea, secondary enterocolitis
Hematologic: Eosinophilia
Otic: Ototoxicity
Drug Uptake
Absorption: Not absorbed via oral route
Pregnancy Risk Factor C
Generic Available No

Paroxetina (Mexico) *see* Paroxetine *on this page*

Paroxetine (pa ROKS e teen)
Related Information
Vasoconstrictor Interactions With Antidepressants *on page 1226*
Brand Names Paxil™
Therapeutic Category Antidepressant, Selective Serotonin Reuptake Inhibitor
Synonyms Paroxetina (Mexico)
Use Treatment of depression; indicated for treatment of obsessions and compulsions in patients with obsessive-compulsive disorder (OCD) as defined in the DSM-IV
Usual Dosage Adults: Oral:
Depression: 20 mg once daily (maximum: 60 mg/day), preferably in the morning; in elderly, debilitated, or patients with hepatic or renal impairment, start with 10 mg/day (maximum: 40 mg/day); adjust doses at 7-day intervals
Panic disorder and obsessive compulsive disorder: Recommended average daily dose: 40 mg, this dosage should be given after an adequate trial on 20 mg/day and then titrating upward
Mechanism of Action Paroxetine is a selective serotonin reuptake inhibitor, chemically unrelated to tricyclic, tetracyclic, or other antidepressants; presumably, the inhibition of serotonin reuptake from brain synapse stimulated serotonin activity in the brain
Local Anesthetic/Vasoconstrictor Precautions Although caution should be used in patients taking tricyclic antidepressants, no interactions have been reported with vasoconstrictor and paroxetine, a nontricyclic antidepressant which acts to increase serotonin
(Continued)

Paroxetine *(Continued)*

Effects on Dental Treatment >10% of patients experience dry mouth; prolonged use of paroxetine may decrease or inhibit salivary flow; normal salivary flow will resume with cessation of drug therapy

Other Adverse Effects
>10%:
  Central nervous system: Headache, somnolence, dizziness, insomnia
  Gastrointestinal: Nausea, constipation, diarrhea
  Genitourinary: Ejaculatory disturbances
  Neuromuscular & skeletal: Weakness
  Miscellaneous: Sweating
1% to 10%:
  Cardiovascular: Palpitations, vasodilation, postural hypotension
  Central nervous system: Nervousness, anxiety
  Endocrine & metabolic: Decreased libido
  Gastrointestinal: Anorexia, flatulence, vomiting
  Neuromuscular & skeletal: Tremor, paresthesia
<1%:
  Cardiovascular: Bradycardia, hypotension
  Central nervous system: Migraine, akinesia
  Dermatologic: Alopecia
  Endocrine & metabolic: Amenorrhea
  Gastrointestinal: Gastritis, thirst
  Hematologic: Anemia, leukopenia
  Neuromuscular & skeletal: Arthritis
  Otic: Ear pain
  Ocular: Eye pain
  Respiratory: Asthma
  Miscellaneous: Bruxism

Drug Interactions
Decreased effect of paroxetine when taken with phenobarbital, phenytoin
Increased toxicity: Alcohol, cimetidine, MAO inhibitors (hyperpyrexic crisis); increased effect/toxicity of tricyclic antidepressants, fluoxetine, sertraline, phenothiazines, class 1C antiarrhythmics, warfarin

Drug Uptake Serum half-life: 21 hours
Pregnancy Risk Factor B
Generic Available No

PedTE-PAK-4® *see* Trace Metals *on page 948*

Pedtrace-4® *see* Trace Metals *on page 948*

PedvaxHIB™ *see* Haemophilus b Conjugate Vaccine *on page 460*

Pegademase Bovine (peg A de mase BOE vine)

Brand Names Adagen™

Therapeutic Category Enzyme, Replacement Therapy

Use Enzyme replacement therapy for adenosine deaminase (ADA) deficiency in patients with severe combined immunodeficiency disease (SCID) who cannot benefit from bone marrow transplant; not a cure for SCID, unlike bone marrow transplants, injections must be used the rest of the child's life, therefore, is not really an alternative

Usual Dosage Children: I.M.: Dose given every 7 days, 10 units/kg the first dose, 15 units/kg the second dose, and 20 units/kg the third dose; maintenance dose: 20 units/kg/week is recommended depending on patient's ADA level; maximum single dose: 30 units/kg

Mechanism of Action Adenosine deaminase is an enzyme that catalyzes the deamination of both adenosine and deoxyadenosine. Hereditary lack of adenosine deaminase activity results in severe combined immunodeficiency disease, a fatal disorder of infancy characterized by profound defects of both cellular and humoral immunity. It is estimated that 25% of patients with the autosomal recessive form of severe combined immunodeficiency lack adenosine deaminase.

Local Anesthetic/Vasoconstrictor Precautions No information available to require special precautions

Effects on Dental Treatment No effects or complications reported

Other Adverse Effects <1%:
Central nervous system: Headache
Local: Pain at injection site

Drug Interactions Decreased effect: Vidarabine

Drug Uptake
Plasma adenosine deaminase activity generally normalizes after 2-3 weeks of weekly I.M. injections
Absorption: Rapid
Serum half-life: 48-72 hours

Pregnancy Risk Factor C

Generic Available No

Peganone® *see* Ethotoin *on page 383*

Pegaspargase (peg AS par jase)

Brand Names Oncaspar®

Therapeutic Category Antineoplastic Agent, Miscellaneous

Synonyms PEG-L-asparaginase

Use Induction treatment of acute lymphoblastic leukemia in combination with other chemotherapeutic agents in patients who have developed hypersensitivity to native forms of asparaginase derived from *E. coli* and/or *Erwinia chrysanthemia*, treatment of lymphoma

Usual Dosage
Dose must be individualized based upon clinical response and tolerance of the patient (refer to individual protocols)
I.M. administration is **preferred** over I.V. administration; I.M. administration may decrease the incidence of hepatotoxicity, coagulopathy, and GI and renal disorders

Children: I.M., I.V.:
Body surface area ≤0.6 m²: 82.5 units/kg every 14 days
Body surface area ≥0.6 m²: 2500 units/m² every 14 days
Adults: I.M., I.V.: 2,500 units/m² every 14 days

Mechanism of Action
Pegaspargase is a modified version of the enzyme asparaginase. The asparaginase used in the manufacture of pegaspargase is derived from *Escherichia coli*.
Some malignant cells (ie, lymphoblastic leukemia cells and those of lymphocyte derivation) must acquire the amino acid asparagine from surrounding fluid such as blood, whereas normal cells can synthesize their own asparagine. asparaginase is an enzyme that deaminates asparagine to aspartic acid and ammonia in the plasma and extracellular fluid and therefore deprives tumor cells of the amino acid for protein synthesis.

Local Anesthetic/Vasoconstrictor Precautions No information available to require special precautions

Effects on Dental Treatment No effects or complications reported

(Continued)

Pegaspargase *(Continued)*

Other Adverse Effects Overall, the adult patients had a somewhat higher incidence of asparaginase toxicities, except for hypersensitivity reactions, than the pediatric patients

>10%:
Cardiovascular: Edema
Central nervous system: Pain
Dermatologic: Urticaria, erythema
Gastrointestinal: Pancreatitis, (sometimes fulminant and fatal); elevated serum amylase and lipase, swelling lip
Hepatic: Elevations of AST, ALT, and bilirubin (direct and indirect); jaundice, ascites and hypoalbuminemia, fatty changes in the liver; liver failure
Local: Induration, tenderness
Neuromuscular: Arthralgia
Respiratory: Bronchospasm, dyspnea
Miscellaneous: Hypersensitivity (acute or delayed), acute anaphylaxis,

>5%:
Allergic reactions: Rash, erythema, edema, pain, fever, chills, dyspnea or bronchospasm
Central nervous system: Malaise
Gastrointestinal: **Emetic potential:** Mild (>5%)

1% to 5%:
Cardiovascular: Hypotension, tachycardia, thrombosis
Central nervous system: Chills
Dermatologic: Lip edema
Gastrointestinal: Abdominal pain
Hematologic: Decreased anticoagulant effect, disseminated intravascular coagulation, decreased fibrinogen, hemolytic anemia, leukopenia, pancytopenia, thrombocytopenia, increased thromboplastin.
Myelosuppressive effects: WBC: Mild; Platelets: Mild; Onset (days): 7; Nadir (days): 14; Recovery (days): 21
Local: Injection site hypersensitivity
Respiratory: Dyspnea

Drug Uptake
Serum half-life: 5.73 days
Pregnancy Risk Factor C
Generic Available No

PEG-L-asparaginase *see Pegaspargase on previous page*

Pemoline *(PEM oh leen)*
Brand Names Cylert®
Therapeutic Category Central Nervous System Stimulant, Nonamphetamine
Use Treatment of attention deficit disorder with hyperactivity (ADDH); narcolepsy
Usual Dosage Children ≥6 years: Oral: Initial: 37.5 mg given once daily in the morning, increase by 18.75 mg/day at weekly intervals; usual effective dose range: 56.25-75 mg/day; maximum: 112.5 mg/day; dosage range: 0.5-3 mg/kg/24 hours; significant benefit may not be evident until third or fourth week of administration
Mechanism of Action Blocks the reuptake mechanism of dopaminergic neurons, appears to act at the cerebral cortex and subcortical structures; CNS and respiratory stimulant with weak sympathomimetic effects; actions may be mediated via increase in CNS dopamine
Local Anesthetic/Vasoconstrictor Precautions Pemoline has minimal sympathomimetic effects; there are no precautions in using vasoconstrictors
Effects on Dental Treatment No effects or complications reported
Other Adverse Effects
>10%:
Central nervous system: Insomnia
Gastrointestinal: Anorexia, weight loss
1% to 10%:
Central nervous system: Dizziness, drowsiness, mental depression
Dermatologic: Skin rash
Gastrointestinal: Stomach pain, nausea
<1%:
Central nervous system: Seizures, precipitation of Tourette's syndrome, hallucination, headache, movement disorders
Endocrine & metabolic: Growth reaction
Gastrointestinal: Diarrhea
Hepatic: Elevated liver enzymes (usually reversible upon discontinuation), hepatitis, jaundice

Drug Interactions Decreased effect of insulin

Drug Uptake
Duration: 8 hours
Serum half-life:
Children: 7-8.6 hours
Adults: 12 hours
Time to peak serum concentration: Oral: Within 2-4 hours

Pregnancy Risk Factor B

Generic Available No

Penbutolol (pen BYOO toe lole)

Related Information
Cardiovascular Diseases on page 1010

Brand Names Levatol®

Therapeutic Category Beta-adrenergic Blocker, Noncardioselective

Use Treatment of mild to moderate arterial hypertension

Mechanism of Action Blocks both beta$_1$- and beta$_2$-receptors and has mild intrinsic sympathomimetic activity; has negative inotropic and chronotropic effects and can significantly slow A-V nodal conduction

Local Anesthetic/Vasoconstrictor Precautions No information available to require special precautions

Effects on Dental Treatment No effects or complications reported

Other Adverse Effects
1% to 10%:
Cardiovascular: Congestive heart failure, arrhythmia
Central nervous system: Mental depression, headache, dizziness
Neuromuscular & skeletal: Back pain, arthralgia
<1%:
Cardiovascular: Bradycardia, chest pain, mesenteric arterial thrombosis, A-V block, persistent bradycardia, hypotension, chest pain, edema, Raynaud's phenomenon
Central nervous system: Fatigue, insomnia, lethargy, nightmares, depression, confusion
Dermatologic: Purpura
Endocrine & metabolic: Hyperglycemia
Gastrointestinal: Ischemic colitis, constipation, nausea, diarrhea
Genitourinary: Impotence
Hematologic: Thrombocytopenia
Respiratory: Bronchospasm
Miscellaneous: Cold extremities

Pregnancy Risk Factor C

Generic Available No

Penciclovir (pen SYE kloe veer)

Related Information
Oral Viral Infections on page 1066

Brand Names Denavir®

Therapeutic Category Antiviral Agent, Topical

Use Antiviral cream for the treatment of recurrent herpes labialis (cold sores) in adults

Usual Dosage Apply cream at the first sign or symptom of cold sore (eg, tingling, swelling); apply every 2 hours during waking hours for 4 days

Mechanism of Action In cells infected with HSV-1 or HSV-2, viral thymidine kinase phosphorylates penciclovir to a monophosphate form which, in turn, is converted to penciclovir triphosphate by cellular kinases. Penciclovir triphosphate inhibits HSV polymerase competitively with deoxyguanosine triphosphate. Consequently, herpes viral DNA synthesis and, therefore, replication are selectively inhibited

Local Anesthetic/Vasoconstrictor Precautions No information available to require special precautions

Effects on Dental Treatment No effects or complications reported

Other Adverse Effects 1% to 10%:
Central nervous system: Headache
Local: Application site reaction

Contraindications Patients with known hypersensitivity to the product or any of its components

Warnings/Precautions Penciclovir should only be used on herpes labialis on the lips and face; because no data are available, application to mucous membranes is not recommended. Avoid application in or near eyes since it may cause irritation. The effect of penciclovir has not been established in immuno-compromised patients.
(Continued)

Penciclovir *(Continued)*

Drug Interactions No data reported

Drug Uptake Measurable penciclovir concentrations were not detected in plasma or urine of health male volunteers following single or repeat application of the 1% cream at a dose of 180 mg penciclovir daily (approximately 67 times the usual clinical dose)

Pregnancy Risk Factor B

Dosage Forms Cream: 1% [10 mg/g] (2 g)

Generic Available No

Penetrex™ *see* Enoxacin *on page 349*

Penicilina G Procainica (Mexico) *see* Penicillin G Procaine *on page 733*

Penicillamine *(pen i SIL a meen)*

Brand Names Cuprimine®; Depen®

Canadian/Mexican Brand Names Sufortan® (Mex)

Therapeutic Category Chelating Agent

Synonyms D-3-Mercaptovaline; β,β-Dimethylcysteine; D-Penicillamine

Use Treatment of Wilson's disease, cystinuria, adjunct in the treatment of severe rheumatoid arthritis; lead poisoning, primary biliary cirrhosis

Usual Dosage Oral:

Rheumatoid arthritis:

Children: Initial: 3 mg/kg/day (≤250 mg/day) for 3 months, then 6 mg/kg/day (≤500 mg/day) in divided doses twice daily for 3 months to a maximum of 10 mg/kg/day in 3-4 divided doses

Adults: 125-250 mg/day, may increase dose at 1- to 3-month intervals up to 1-1.5 g/day

Wilson's disease (doses titrated to maintain urinary copper excretion >1 mg/day):

Infants <6 months: 250 mg/dose once daily

Children <12 years: 250 mg/dose 2-3 times/day

Adults: 250 mg 4 times/day

Cystinuria:

Children: 30 mg/kg/day in 4 divided doses

Adults: 1-4 g/day in divided doses every 6 hours

Lead poisoning (continue until blood lead level is <60 µg/dL): Children and Adults: 25-35 mg/kg/d, administered in 3-4 divided doses; initiating treatment at 25% of this dose and gradually increasing to the full dose over 2-3 weeks may minimize adverse reactions

Primary biliary cirrhosis: 250 mg/day to start, increase by 250 mg every 2 weeks up to a maintenance dose of 1 g/day, usually given 250 mg 4 times/day

Arsenic poisoning: Children: 100 mg/kg/day in divided doses every 6 hours for 5 days; maximum: 1 g/day

Mechanism of Action Chelates with lead, copper, mercury and other heavy metals to form stable, soluble complexes that are excreted in urine; depresses circulating IgM rheumatoid factor, depresses T-cell but not B-cell activity; combines with cystine to form a compound which is more soluble, thus cystine calculi are prevented

Local Anesthetic/Vasoconstrictor Precautions No information available to require special precautions

Effects on Dental Treatment No effects or complications reported

Other Adverse Effects

>10%:

Central nervous system: Fever

Dermatologic: Rash, urticaria, itching

Gastrointestinal: Hypogeusia

Neuromuscular & skeletal: Arthralgia

1% to 10%:

Cardiovascular: Edema of the face, feet, or lower legs

Central nervous system: Fever, chills

Gastrointestinal: Weight gain, sore throat

Genitourinary: Bloody or cloudy urine

Hematologic: Aplastic or hemolytic anemia, leukopenia, thrombocytopenia

Miscellaneous: White spots on lips or mouth

<1%:

Central nervous system: Fatigue

Dermatologic: Toxic epidermal necrolysis, pemphigus, increased friability of the skin

Endocrine & metabolic: Iron deficiency

Gastrointestinal: Nausea, vomiting, anorexia, pancreatitis

Hepatic: Cholestatic jaundice, hepatitis

Neuromuscular & skeletal: Myasthenia gravis syndrome, weakness
Ocular: Optic neuritis
Otic: Tinnitus
Renal: Nephrotic syndrome
Respiratory: Coughing, wheezing
Miscellaneous: SLE-like syndrome, spitting of blood allergic reactions, lymph-adenopathy

Warnings/Precautions Cross-sensitivity with penicillin is possible; therefore, should be used cautiously in patients with a history of penicillin allergy. Patients on penicillamine for Wilson's disease or cystinuria should receive pyridoxine supplementation 25 mg/day; once instituted for Wilson's disease or cystinuria, continue treatment on a daily basis; interruptions of even a few days have been followed by hypersensitivity with reinstitution of therapy. Penicillamine has been associated with fatalities due to agranulocytosis, aplastic anemia, thrombocytopenia, Goodpasture's syndrome, and myasthenia gravis; patients should be warned to report promptly any symptoms suggesting toxicity; approximately 33% of patients will experience an allergic reaction; since toxicity may be dose related, it is recommended not to exceed 750 mg/day in elderly.

Drug Interactions
Decreased effect with iron and zinc salts, antacids (magnesium, calcium, aluminum) and food
Decreased effect/levels of digoxin
Increased effect of gold, antimalarials, immunosuppressants, phenylbutazone (hematologic, renal toxicity)

Drug Uptake
Absorption: Oral: 40% to 70%
Serum half-life: 1.7-3.2 hours
Time to peak serum concentration: Within 2 hours

Pregnancy Risk Factor D

Dosage Forms
Capsule: 125 mg, 250 mg
Tablet: 250 mg

Dietary Considerations Should be administered at least 1 hour before a meal on an empty stomach; do not administer with milk; iron and zinc may decrease drug action; increase dietary intake of pyridoxine; for Wilson's disease, decrease copper in diet and omit chocolate, nuts, shellfish, mushrooms, liver, raisins, broccoli, and molasses; for lead poisoning, decrease calcium in diet
Patients unable to swallow capsules may mix contents of capsule with fruit juice or chilled pureed fruit; limit alcohol

Generic Available No

Selected Readings
Aronow R and Fleschmann LE, "Mercury Poisoning in Children," *Clin Pediatr*, 1976, 15(10):936-45.
Hryhorczuk DO, Meyers L, and Chen G, "Treatment of Mercury Intoxication in a Dentist With N-Acetyl-D,L-Penicillamine," *J Toxicol Clin Toxicol*, 1982, 19(4):401-8.
Lyle WH, "Penicillamine in Metal Poisoning," *J Rheumatol Suppl*, 1981, 7:96-9.
Rosa FW, "Teratogen Update. Penicillamine," *Teratology*, 1986, 33(1):127-31.

Penicillin G Benzathine (pen i SIL in jee BENZ a theen)

Related Information
Dental Drug Interactions: Update on Drug Combinations Requiring Special Considerations *on page 1144*
Nonviral Infectious Diseases *on page 1032*

Brand Names Bicillin® L-A; Permapen®

Canadian/Mexican Brand Names Benzetacil® (Mexico); Benzilfan® (Mexico); Megacillin® Susp (Canada)

Therapeutic Category Antibiotic, Penicillin

Use Active against some gram-positive organisms, few gram-negative organisms such as *Neisseria gonorrhoeae*, and some anaerobes and spirochetes; used only for the treatment of mild to moderately severe infections caused by organisms susceptible to low concentrations of penicillin G or for prophylaxis of infections caused by these organisms; used when patient cannot be kept in a hospital environment and neurosyphilis has been ruled out

The CDC and AAP do not currently recommend the use of penicillin G benzathine to treat congenital syphilis or neurosyphilis due to reported treatment failures and lack of published clinical data on its efficacy

Usual Dosage I.M.: Give undiluted injection; higher doses result in more sustained rather than higher levels. Use a penicillin G benzathine-penicillin G procaine combination to achieve early peak levels in acute infections.
Children:
Group A streptococcal upper respiratory infection: 25,000-50,000 units/kg as a single dose; maximum: 1.2 million units

(Continued)

Penicillin G Benzathine *(Continued)*

Prophylaxis of recurrent rheumatic fever: 25,000-50,000 units/kg every 3-4 weeks; maximum: 1.2 million units/dose

Early syphilis: 50,000 units/kg as a single injection; maximum: 2.4 million units

Syphilis of more than 1-year duration: 50,000 units/kg every week for 3 doses; maximum: 2.4 million units/dose

Adults:

Group A streptococcal upper respiratory infection: 1.2 million units as a single dose

Prophylaxis of recurrent rheumatic fever: 1.2 million units every 3-4 weeks or 600,000 units twice monthly

Early syphilis: 2.4 million units as a single dose in 2 injection sites

Syphilis of more than 1-year duration: 2.4 million units in 2 injection sites once weekly for 3 doses

Not indicated as single drug therapy for neurosyphilis, but may be given 1 time/week for 3 weeks following I.V. treatment (refer to Penicillin G monograph for dosing)

Mechanism of Action Interferes with bacterial cell wall synthesis during active multiplication, causing cell wall death and resultant bactericidal activity against susceptible bacteria

Local Anesthetic/Vasoconstrictor Precautions No information available to require special precautions

Effects on Dental Treatment No effects or complications reported

Other Adverse Effects

1% to 10%: Local: Pain

<1%:

Central nervous system: Convulsions, confusion, drowsiness, fever

Dermatologic: Rash

Endocrine & metabolic: Electrolyte imbalance

Hematologic: Hemolytic anemia, positive Coombs' reaction

Local: Thrombophlebitis

Neuromuscular & skeletal: Myoclonus

Renal: Acute interstitial nephritis

Miscellaneous: Hypersensitivity reactions, anaphylaxis, Jarisch-Herxheimer reaction

Drug Interactions

Decreased effect: Tetracyclines cause decreased penicillin effectiveness

Increased effect:

Probenecid causes increased penicillin levels

Drug Uptake

Absorption: I.M.: Slow

Time to peak serum concentration: Within 12-24 hours; serum levels are usually detectable for 1-4 weeks depending on the dose; larger doses result in more sustained levels rather than higher levels

Pregnancy Risk Factor B

Generic Available No

Penicillin G Benzathine and Procaine Combined

(pen i SIL in jee BENZ a theen & PROE kane KOM bined)

Brand Names Bicillin® C-R 900/300 Injection; Bicillin® C-R Injection

Therapeutic Category Antibiotic, Penicillin

Synonyms Penicillin G Procaine and Benzathine Combined

Use Active against most gram-positive organisms, mostly streptococcal and pneumococcal

Local Anesthetic/Vasoconstrictor Precautions No information available to require special precautions

Effects on Dental Treatment No effects or complications reported

Other Adverse Effects 1% to 10%:

Central nervous system: CNS toxicity (convulsions, confusion, drowsiness, myoclonus)

Hematologic: Positive Coombs' reaction, hemolytic anemia

Renal: Interstitial nephritis

Miscellaneous: Hypersensitivity reactions, Jarisch-Herxheimer reaction

Pregnancy Risk Factor B

Generic Available No

Penicillin G, Parenteral, Aqueous

(pen i SIL in jee, pa REN ter al, AYE kwee us)

Related Information

Antimicrobial Prophylaxis in Surgical Patients *on page 1163*

Dental Drug Interactions: Update on Drug Combinations Requiring Special Considerations *on page 1144*
Nonviral Infectious Diseases *on page 1032*

Brand Names Pfizerpen®

Canadian/Mexican Brand Names Benzanil® (Mexico); Lentopenil® (Mexico)

Therapeutic Category Antibiotic, Penicillin

Use Active against some gram-positive organisms, generally not *Staphylococcus aureus*; some gram-negative such as *Neisseria gonorrhoeae*, and some anaerobes and spirochetes; although ceftriaxone is now the drug of choice for Lyme disease and gonorrhea

Usual Dosage I.M., I.V.:

Children (sodium salt is preferred in children): 100,000-250,000 units/kg/day in divided doses every 4 hours; maximum: 4.8 million units/24 hours

Severe infections: Up to 400,000 units/kg/day in divided doses every 4 hours; maximum dose: 24 million units/day

Adults: 2-24 million units/day in divided doses every 4 hours

Congenital syphilis:

Disseminated gonococcal infections or gonococcus ophthalmia (if organism proven sensitive): 100,000 units/kg/day in 2 equal doses (4 equal doses/day for infants >1 week)

Gonococcal meningitis: 150,000 units/kg in 2 equal doses (4 doses/day for infants >1 week)

Mechanism of Action Interferes with bacterial cell wall synthesis during active multiplication, causing cell wall death and resultant bactericidal activity against susceptible bacteria

Local Anesthetic/Vasoconstrictor Precautions No information available to require special precautions

Effects on Dental Treatment No effects or complications reported

Other Adverse Effects <1%:

Central nervous system: Convulsions, confusion, drowsiness, fever

Dermatologic: Rash

Endocrine & metabolic: Electrolyte imbalance

Hematologic: Hemolytic anemia, positive Coombs' reaction

Local: Thrombophlebitis

Neuromuscular & skeletal: Myoclonus

Renal: Acute interstitial nephritis

Miscellaneous: Hypersensitivity reactions, anaphylaxis, Jarisch-Herxheimer reaction

Drug Interactions

Decreased effect: Tetracyclines cause decreased penicillin effectiveness

Increased effect: Probenecid causes increased penicillin levels

Drug Uptake

Serum half-life:

Children and adults with normal renal function: 20-50 minutes

End stage renal disease: 3.3-5.1 hours

Time to peak serum concentration:

I.M.: Within 30 minutes

I.V. Within 1 hour

Pregnancy Risk Factor B

Generic Available Yes

Penicillin G Procaine (pen i SIL in jee PROE kane)

Related Information

Dental Drug Interactions: Update on Drug Combinations Requiring Special Considerations *on page 1144*

Brand Names Crysticillin® A.S.; Pfizerpen®-AS; Wycillin®

Canadian/Mexican Brand Names Ayercillin® (Canada); Penicil® (Mexico); Penipot® (Mexico); Penprocilina® (Mexico)

Therapeutic Category Antibiotic, Penicillin

Synonyms Penicilina G Procainica (Mexico)

Use Moderately severe infections due to *Neisseria gonorrhoeae*, *Treponema pallidum* and other penicillin G-sensitive microorganisms that are susceptible to low but prolonged serum penicillin concentrations

Usual Dosage I.M.:

Children: 25,000-50,000 units/kg/day in divided doses 1-2 times/day; not to exceed 4.8 million units/24 hours

Gonorrhea: 100,000 units/kg (maximum 4.8 million units) one time (in 2 injection sites) along with probenecid 25 mg/kg (maximum: 1 g orally) 30 minutes prior to procaine penicillin

Congenital syphilis: 50,000 units/kg/day for 10-14 days

(Continued)

Penicillin G Procaine *(Continued)*

Adults: 0.6-4.8 million units/day in divided doses every 12-24 hours

Uncomplicated gonorrhea: 1 g probenecid orally, then 4.8 million units procaine penicillin divided into 2 injection sites 30 minutes later

Endocarditis caused by susceptible viridans *Streptococcus* (when used in conjunction with an aminoglycoside): 1.2 million units every 6 hours for 2-4 weeks

Neurosyphilis: I.M.: 2-4 million units/day with 500 mg probenecid by mouth 4 times/day for 10-14 days; **penicillin G aqueous I.V. is the preferred agent**

Moderately dialyzable (20% to 50%)

Mechanism of Action Inhibits bacterial cell wall synthesis by binding to one or more of the penicillin binding proteins (PBPs); which in turn inhibits the final transpeptidation step of peptidoglycan synthesis in bacterial cell walls, thus inhibiting cell wall biosynthesis. Bacteria eventually lyse due to ongoing activity of cell wall autolytic enzymes (autolysins and murein hydrolases) while cell wall assembly is arrested.

Local Anesthetic/Vasoconstrictor Precautions No information available to require special precautions

Effects on Dental Treatment No effects or complications reported

Other Adverse Effects

>10%: Local: Pain at injection site

<1%:

Cardiovascular: Myocardial depression, vasodilation, conduction disturbances

Central nervous system: CNS stimulation, seizures, confusion, drowsiness

Hematologic: Hemolytic anemia, positive Coombs' reaction

Local: Sterile abscess at injection site

Neuromuscular & skeletal: Myoclonus

Renal: Interstitial nephritis

Miscellaneous: Pseudoanaphylactic reactions, hypersensitivity reactions, Jarisch-Herxheimer reaction

Drug Interactions

Decreased effect: Tetracyclines cause decreased penicillin effectiveness

Increased effect: Probenecid causes increased penicillin levels

Drug Uptake

Absorption: I.M.: Slowly absorbed

Time to peak serum concentration: Within 1-4 hours; can persist within the therapeutic range for 15-24 hours

Pregnancy Risk Factor B

Generic Available Yes

Penicillin G Procaine and Benzathine Combined *see* Penicillin G Benzathine and Procaine Combined *on page 732*

Penicillin V Potassium *(pen i SIL in vee poe TASS ee um)*

Related Information

Dental Drug Interactions: Update on Drug Combinations Requiring Special Considerations *on page 1144*

Oral Bacterial Infections *on page 1059*

Oral Viral Infections *on page 1066*

Brand Names Beepen-VK®; Betapen®-VK; Pen.Vee® K; Robicillin® VK; V-Cillin K®; Veetids®

Canadian/Mexican Brand Names Anapenil® (Mexico); Apo®-Pen VK (Canada); Nadopen-V® (Canada); Novo-Pen-VK® (Canada); Nu-Pen-VK (Canada); Pen-Vi-K® (Mexico); PVF® K (Canada)

Therapeutic Category Antibiotic, Penicillin

Use

Dental: Antibiotic of first choice in treating common orofacial infections caused by aerobic gram-positive cocci and anaerobes. These orofacial infections include cellulitis, periapical abscess, periodontal abscess, acute suppurative pulpitis, oronasal fistula, pericoronitis, osteitis, osteomyelitis, postsurgical and post-traumatic infection. It is no longer recommended for dental procedure prophylaxis.

Medical: Treatment of moderate to severe susceptible bacterial infections involving the respiratory tract, otitis media, sinusitis, skin, and and urinary tract

Usual Dosage

Children <12 years: Daily dose: 25-50 mg/kg in divided doses every 6-8 hours for 7 days; maximum daily dose: 3 g

Children >12 years and Adults: 250-500 mg every 6 hours for at least 7 days

Mechanism of Action Inhibits bacterial cell wall synthesis by binding to one or more of the penicillin binding proteins (PBPs); which in turn inhibits the final transpeptidation step of peptidoglycan synthesis in bacterial cell walls, thus inhibiting cell wall biosynthesis. Bacteria eventually lyse due to ongoing activity of cell wall autolytic enzymes (autolysins and murein hydrolases) while cell wall assembly is arrested.

Local Anesthetic/Vasoconstrictor Precautions No information available to require special precautions

Effects on Dental Treatment Prolonged use of penicillins may lead to development of oral candidiasis

Other Adverse Effects
>10%: Gastrointestinal: Mild diarrhea, vomiting, nausea
1% to 10%: Miscellaneous: Hypersensitivity reactions

Contraindications Known hypersensitivity to penicillin or any component

Warnings/Precautions Use with caution in patients with severe renal impairment (modify dosage), history of seizures, or hypersensitivity to cephalosporins

Drug Interactions Tetracyclines may decrease penicillin effectiveness; probenecid may increase penicillin levels; aminoglycosides cause synergistic efficacy

Drug Uptake
Absorption: Oral: 60% to 73% from GI tract
Time to peak serum concentration: Oral: Within 0.5-1 hour
Serum half-life: 0.5 hours

Pregnancy Risk Factor B

Breast-feeding Considerations No data reported; however, other penicillins may be taken while breast-feeding

Dosage Forms
Powder for oral solution: 125 mg/5 mL (3 mL, 100 mL, 150 mL, 200 mL); 250 mg/5 mL (100 mL, 150 mL, 200 mL)
Tablet: 125 mg, 250 mg, 500 mg

Dietary Considerations Peak concentration may be delayed with food; may be taken with water on an empty stomach 1 hour before or 2 hours after meals or may be taken with food

Generic Available Yes

Selected Readings
Wynn RL and Bergman SA, "Antibiotics and Their Use in the Treatment of Orofacial Infections, Part I and Part II," *Gen Dent*, 1994, 42(5):398-402, 498-502.

Pentacarinat® Injection *see* Pentamidine *on next page*

Pentaerythritol Tetranitrate (pen ta er ITH ri tole te tra NYE trate)
Related Information
Cardiovascular Diseases *on page 1010*

Brand Names Duotrate®; Peritrate®; Peritrate® SA

Therapeutic Category Antianginal Agent; Nitrate; Vasodilator, Coronary

Use Possibly effective for the prophylactic long-term management of angina pectoris. **Note:** Not indicated to abort acute anginal episodes

Usual Dosage Adults: Oral: 10-20 mg 4 times/day up to 40 mg 4 times/day before or after meals and at bedtime; sustained release preparation 80 mg twice daily; use lowest recommended doses in elderly initially; titrations up to 240 mg/day are tolerated, however, headache may occur with increasing doses (reduce dose for a few days; if headache returns or is persistent, an analgesic can be used to treat symptoms)

Mechanism of Action Stimulation of intracellular cyclic-GMP results in vascular smooth muscle relaxation of both arterial and venous vasculature. Increased venous pooling decreases left ventricular pressure (preload) and arterial dilatation decreases arterial resistance (afterload). Therefore, this reduces cardiac oxygen demand by decreasing left ventricular pressure and systemic vascular resistance by dilating arteries. Additionally, coronary artery dilation improves collateral flow to ischemic regions; esophageal smooth muscle is relaxed via the same mechanism.

Local Anesthetic/Vasoconstrictor Precautions No information available to require special precautions

Effects on Dental Treatment No effects or complications reported

Other Adverse Effects
>10%:
Cardiovascular: Flushing, postural hypotension
Central nervous system: Headache, lightheadedness, dizziness
Neuromuscular & skeletal: Weakness
1% to 10%: Dermatologic: Drug rash, exfoliative dermatitis
<1%:
Gastrointestinal: Nausea, vomiting
Hematologic: Methemoglobinemia (overdose)

Drug Interactions No data reported
(Continued)

Pentaerythritol Tetranitrate *(Continued)*

Drug Uptake
Onset of hemodynamic effect: Oral: Within 20-60 minutes
Duration: 4-5 hours, or up to 12 hours with the sustained release formulations
Serum half-life: 10 minutes

Pregnancy Risk Factor C

Generic Available Yes

Pentagastrin *(pen ta GAS trin)*

Brand Names Peptavlon®

Therapeutic Category Diagnostic Agent, Gastric Acid Secretory Function

Use Evaluate gastric acid secretory function in pernicious anemia, gastric carcinoma; in suspected duodenal ulcer or Zollinger-Ellison tumor

Usual Dosage Adults:
I.M., S.C.: 6 mcg/kg
I.V. infusion: 0.1-12 mcg/kg/hour in 0.9% sodium chloride

Mechanism of Action Excites the oxyntic cells of the stomach to secrete to their maximum capacity similar to the naturally occurring hormone, gastrin

Local Anesthetic/Vasoconstrictor Precautions No information available to require special precautions

Effects on Dental Treatment No effects or complications reported

Other Adverse Effects
>10%: Gastrointestinal: Abdominal pain, desire to defecate, nausea, vomiting
1% to 10%:
Cardiovascular: Flushing, tachycardia, palpitations, hypotension, faintness
Central nervous system: Dizziness, headache
Respiratory: Dyspnea
<1%: Miscellaneous: Allergic reactions

Drug Uptake
Absorption: I.M., S.C.: Well absorbed
Serum half-life: 1 minute

Pregnancy Risk Factor C

Generic Available No

Pentam-300® Injection *see* Pentamidine *on this page*

Pentamidina (Mexico) *see* Pentamidine *on this page*

Pentamidine *(pen TAM i deen)*

Brand Names NebuPent™ Inhalation; Pentacarinat® Injection; Pentam-300® Injection

Canadian/Mexican Brand Names Pentacarinat® (Mexico)

Therapeutic Category Antibiotic, Miscellaneous

Synonyms Pentamidina (Mexico)

Use Treatment and prevention of pneumonia caused by *Pneumocystis carinii*; treatment of trypanosomiasis

Usual Dosage
Children:
Treatment: I.M., I.V. (I.V. preferred): 4 mg/kg/day once daily for 10-14 days
Prevention:
I.M., I.V.: 4 mg/kg monthly or every 2 weeks
Inhalation (aerosolized pentamidine in children ≥5 years): 300 mg/dose given every 3-4 weeks via Respirgard® II inhaler (8 mg/kg dose has also been used in children <5 years)
Treatment of trypanosomiasis: I.V.: 4 mg/kg/day once daily for 10 days

Adults:
Treatment: I.M., I.V. (I.V. preferred): 4 mg/kg/day once daily for 14 days
Prevention: Inhalation: 300 mg every 4 weeks via Respirgard® II nebulizer

Not removed by hemo or peritoneal dialysis or continuous arterio-venous or veno-venous hemofiltration (CAVH/CAVHD); supplemental dosage is not necessary

Mechanism of Action Interferes with RNA/DNA, phospholipids and protein synthesis, through inhibition of oxidative phosphorylation and/or interference with incorporation of nucleotides and nucleic acids into RNA and DNA, in protozoa

Local Anesthetic/Vasoconstrictor Precautions No information available to require special precautions

Effects on Dental Treatment No effects or complications reported

Other Adverse Effects
>10%:
Cardiovascular: Chest pain
Dermatologic: Skin rash

Endocrine & metabolic: Hyperkalemia
Local: Local reactions at injection site
Respiratory: Wheezing, dyspnea, coughing, pharyngitis
1% to 10%: Gastrointestinal: Bitter or metallic taste
<1%:
Cardiovascular: Hypotension, tachycardia
Central nervous system: Dizziness, fever, fatigue
Endocrine & metabolic: Hyperglycemia or hypoglycemia, hypocalcemia
Gastrointestinal: Pancreatitis, vomiting
Hematologic: Megaloblastic anemia, granulocytopenia, leukopenia, thrombocytopenia
Hepatic: Mild hepatic injury
Renal: Renal insufficiency, mild renal injury
Respiratory: Extrapulmonary pneumocystosis, irritation of the airway, pneumothorax
Miscellaneous: Jarisch-Herxheimer-like reaction
Drug Interactions No data reported
Drug Uptake
Absorption: I.M.: Well absorbed
Serum half-life, terminal: 6.4-9.4 hours; may be prolonged in patients with severe renal impairment
Pregnancy Risk Factor C
Generic Available Yes

Pentasa® *see* Mesalamine *on page 602*

Pentaspan® *see* Pentastarch *on this page*

Pentastarch (PEN ta starch)
Brand Names Pentaspan®
Therapeutic Category Blood Modifiers
Use Adjunct in leukapheresis to improve the harvesting and increase the yield of leukocytes by centrifugal means
Local Anesthetic/Vasoconstrictor Precautions No information available to require special precautions
Effects on Dental Treatment No effects or complications reported
Generic Available No

Pentazocine (pen TAZ oh seen)
Related Information
Narcotic Agonists *on page 1141*
Brand Names Talwin®; Talwin® NX
Therapeutic Category Analgesic, Narcotic
Use Relief of moderate to severe pain; has also been used as a sedative prior to surgery and as a supplement to surgical anesthesia
Usual Dosage
Children: I.M., S.C.:
5-8 years: 15 mg
8-14 years: 30 mg

Children >12 years and Adults: Oral: 50 mg every 3-4 hours; may increase to 100 mg/dose if needed, but should not exceed 600 mg/day

Adults:
I.M., S.C.: 30-60 mg every 3-4 hours, not to exceed total daily dose of 360 mg
I.V.: 30 mg every 3-4 hours
Mechanism of Action Binds to opiate receptors in the CNS, causing inhibition of ascending pain pathways, altering the perception of and response to pain; produces generalized CNS depression; partial agonist-antagonist
Local Anesthetic/Vasoconstrictor Precautions No information available to require special precautions
Effects on Dental Treatment No effects or complications reported
Other Adverse Effects
>10%:
Central nervous system: Euphoria, drowsiness
Gastrointestinal: Nausea, vomiting
Neuromuscular & skeletal: Weakness
1% to 10%:
Cardiovascular: Hypotension
Central nervous system: Malaise, headache, restlessness, nightmares
Dermatologic: Skin rash
Gastrointestinal: Dry mouth
Genitourinary: Ureteral spasm
Ocular: Blurred vision
(Continued)

Pentazocine *(Continued)*

Respiratory: Dyspnea

<1%:

Cardiovascular: Palpitations, bradycardia, peripheral vasodilation

Central nervous system: Insomnia, CNS depression, sedation, hallucinations, confusion, disorientation, seizures may occur in seizure-prone patients, increased intracranial pressure

Dermatologic: Pruritus

Endocrine & metabolic: Antidiuretic hormone release

Gastrointestinal: GI irritation, constipation, biliary spasm

Genitourinary: Urinary tract spasm

Local: Tissue damage and irritation with I.M./S.C. use

Ocular: Miosis

Miscellaneous: Histamine release physical and psychological dependence

Drug Interactions May potentiate or reduce analgesic effect of opiate agonist, (eg, morphine) depending on patients tolerance to opiates can precipitate withdrawal in narcotic addicts

Increased effect/toxicity with tripelennamine (can be lethal), CNS depressants (phenothiazines, tranquilizers, anxiolytics, sedatives, hypnotics, or alcohol)

Drug Uptake

Onset of action:

Oral, I.M., S.C.: Within 15-30 minutes

I.V.: Within 2-3 minutes

Duration:

Oral: 4-5 hours

Parenteral: 2-3 hours

Serum half-life: 2-3 hours; increased with decreased hepatic function

Pregnancy Risk Factor B (D if used for prolonged periods or in high doses at term)

Dosage Forms

Injection, as lactate: 30 mg/mL (1 mL, 1.5 mL, 2 mL, 10 mL)

Tablet: Pentazocine hydrochloride 50 mg and naloxone hydrochloride 0.5 mg

Generic Available Yes

Pentazocine Compound (pen TAZ oh seen KOM pownd)

Brand Names Talacen®; Talwin® Compound

Therapeutic Category Analgesic, Narcotic

Use Relief of moderate to severe pain; has also been used as a sedative prior to surgery and as a supplement to surgical anesthesia

Local Anesthetic/Vasoconstrictor Precautions No information available to require special precautions

Effects on Dental Treatment No effects or complications reported

Pregnancy Risk Factor D

Generic Available No

Comments Abrupt discontinuation after sustained use (generally >10 days) may cause withdrawal symptoms

Pentobarbital (pen toe BAR bi tal)

Brand Names Nembutal®

Therapeutic Category Barbiturate; Sedative

Use Short-term treatment of insomnia; preoperative sedation; high-dose barbiturate coma for treatment of increased intracranial pressure or status epilepticus unresponsive to other therapy

Usual Dosage

Children:

Sedative: Oral: 2-6 mg/kg/day divided in 3 doses; maximum: 100 mg/day

Hypnotic: I.M.: 2-6 mg/kg; maximum: 100 mg/dose

Rectal:

2 months to 1 year (10-20 lb): 30 mg

1-4 years (20-40 lb): 30-60 mg

5-12 years (40-80 lb): 60 mg

12-14 years (80-110 lb): 60-120 mg

or

<4 years: 3-6 mg/kg/dose

>4 years: 1.5-3 mg/kg/dose

Preoperative/preprocedure sedation: ≥6 months:

Oral, I.M., rectal: 2-6 mg/kg; maximum: 100 mg/dose

I.V.: 1-3 mg/kg to a maximum of 100 mg until asleep

Children 5-12 years: Conscious sedation prior to a procedure: I.V.: 2 mg/kg 5-10 minutes before procedures, may repeat one time

Adolescents: Conscious sedation: Oral, I.V.: 100 mg prior to a procedure

Adults:
Hypnotic:
Oral: 100-200 mg at bedtime or 20 mg 3-4 times/day for daytime sedation
I.M.: 150-200 mg
I.V.: Initial: 100 mg, may repeat every 1-3 minutes up to 200-500 mg total dose
Rectal: 120-200 mg at bedtime
Preoperative sedation: I.M.: 150-200 mg

Children and Adults: Barbiturate coma in head injury patients: I.V.: Loading dose: 5-10 mg/kg given slowly over 1-2 hours; monitor blood pressure and respiratory rate; Maintenance infusion: Initial: 1 mg/kg/hour; may increase to 2-3 mg/kg/hour; maintain burst suppression on EEG

Mechanism of Action Short-acting barbiturate with sedative, hypnotic, and anticonvulsant properties

Local Anesthetic/Vasoconstrictor Precautions No information available to require special precautions

Effects on Dental Treatment No effects or complications reported

Other Adverse Effects
Renal: Oliguria
>10%:
Cardiovascular: Cardiac arrhythmias, bradycardia, hypotension, arterial spasm, and gangrene with inadvertent intra-arterial injection
Central nervous system: Drowsiness, lethargy, CNS excitation or depression, impaired judgment, "hangover" effect
Local: Pain at injection site, thrombophlebitis with I.V. use
1% to 10%:
Central nervous system: Confusion, mental depression, unusual excitement, nervousness, faint feeling, headache, insomnia, nightmares
Gastrointestinal: Nausea, vomiting, constipation
<1%:
Cardiovascular: Hypotension
Central nervous system: Hallucinations, hypothermia
Dermatologic: Rash, exfoliative dermatitis, Stevens-Johnson syndrome
Hematologic: Agranulocytosis, thrombocytopenia, megaloblastic anemia
Local: Thrombophlebitis
Respiratory: Laryngospasm, respiratory depression, apnea (especially with rapid I.V. use)

Drug Interactions
Decreased effect: Decreased chloramphenicol; decreased doxycycline effects
Increased toxicity: Increased CNS depressants, cimetidine; causes increase effect of pentobarbital

Drug Uptake
Onset of action:
Oral, rectal: 15-60 minutes
I.M.: Within 10-15 minutes
I.V.: Within 1 minute
Duration:
Oral, rectal: 1-4 hours
I.V.: 15 minutes
Serum half-life, terminal:
Children: 25 hours
Adults, normal: 22 hours; range: 35-50 hours

Pregnancy Risk Factor D

Generic Available Yes

Pentosan Polysulfate Sodium
(PEN toe san pol i SUL fate SOW dee um)

Brand Names Elmiron®

Therapeutic Category Analgesic, Urinary

Synonyms PPS

Use Bladder pain relief or discomfort associated with interstitial cystitis

Usual Dosage Adults: Oral: 100 mg 3 times/day taken with water 1 hour before or 2 hours after meals

Patients should be evaluated at 3 months and may be continued an additional 3 months if there has been no improvement and if there are no therapy-limiting side effects. **The risks and benefits of continued use beyond 6 months in patients who have not responded is not yet known.**

Mechanism of Action Although pentosan polysulfate sodium is a low-molecular weight heparinoid, it is not known whether these properties play a role in its mechanism of action in treating interstitial cystitis; the drug appears to adhere to
(Continued)

Pentosan Polysulfate Sodium *(Continued)*

the bladder wall mucosa where it may act as a buffer to protect the tissues from irritating substances in the urine.

Local Anesthetic/Vasoconstrictor Precautions No information available to require special precautions

Effects on Dental Treatment <1% of patients experience gum bleeding, mouth ulcers

Other Adverse Effects

1% to 10%:

Central nervous system: Headache, dizziness

Dermatologic: Alopecia, rash

Gastrointestinal: Diarrhea, nausea, dyspepsia, abdominal pain

Hepatic: Liver function test abnormalities

<1%:

Dermatologic: Pruritus, urticaria, photosensitivity, bruising

Gastrointestinal: Vomiting, mouth ulcer, colitis, esophagitis, gastritis, flatulence, constipation, anorexia, gum bleeding

Hematologic: Anemia, increased prothrombin time, increased partial thromboplastin time, leukopenia, thrombocytopenia

Ocular: Conjunctivitis, optic neuritis, amblyopia, retinal hemorrhage

Otic: Tinnitus

Respiratory: Pharyngitis, rhinitis, epistaxis, dyspnea

Miscellaneous: Allergic reactions

Warnings/Precautions Pentosan polysulfate is a low-molecular weight heparin-like compound with anticoagulant and fibrinolytic effects, therefore, bleeding complications such as ecchymosis, epistaxis and gum bleeding, may occur; patients with the following diseases should be carefully evaluated before initiating therapy: aneurysm, thrombocytopenia, hemophilia, gastrointestinal ulcerations, polyps, diverticula, or hepatic insufficiency; patients undergoing invasive procedures or having signs or symptoms of underlying coagulopathies or other increased risk of bleeding (eg, receiving heparin, warfarin, thrombolytics, or high dose aspirin) should be evaluated for hemorrhage; elevations in transaminases and alopecia can occur

Drug Interactions Although there is no information about potential drug interactions, it is expected that pentosan polysulfate sodium would have at least additive anticoagulant effects when administered with anticoagulant drugs such as warfarin or heparin, and possible similar effects when administered with aspirin or thrombolytics

Drug Uptake

Absorption: ~3%

Serum half-life: 4-8 hours

Pregnancy Risk Factor B

Generic Available No

Pentostatin *(PEN toe stat in)*

Brand Names Nipent™ Injection

Therapeutic Category Antineoplastic Agent, Antimetabolite; Antineoplastic Agent, Nonirritant

Synonyms DCF; Deoxycoformycin; 2′-deoxycoformycin

Use Treatment of adult patients with alpha-interferon-refractory hairy cell leukemia; significant antitumor activity in various lymphoid neoplasms has been demonstrated; pentostatin also is known as 2′-deoxycoformycin; it is a purine analogue capable of inhibiting adenosine deaminase

Usual Dosage Refractory hairy cell leukemia: Adults (refer to individual protocols): 4 mg/m^2 every other week; I.V. bolus over ≥3-5 minutes in D$_5$W or NS at concentrations ≥2 mg/mL

Mechanism of Action An antimetabolite inhibiting adenosine deaminase (ADA), prevents ADA from controlling intracellular adenosine levels through the irreversible deamination of adenosine and deoxyadenosine. ADA is found to exhibit the highest activity in lymphoid tissue. Patients receiving pentostatin accumulate deoxyadenosine (dAdo) and deoxyadenosine 5′-triphosphate (dATP); accumulation of dATP results in cell death, probably through inhibiting DNA or RNA synthesis. Following a single dose, pentostatin has the ability to inhibit ADA for periods exceeding 1 week.

Local Anesthetic/Vasoconstrictor Precautions No information available to require special precautions

Effects on Dental Treatment No effects or complications reported

Other Adverse Effects

>10%:

Central nervous system: Headache, neurologic disorder, fever, fatigue, chills, pain

Dermatologic: Rash
Gastrointestinal: Vomiting, nausea, anorexia, diarrhea
Hematologic: Leukopenia, anemia, thrombocytopenia
Hepatic: Hepatic disorder, liver function tests (abnormal)
Neuromuscular & skeletal: Myalgia
Respiratory: Coughing
Miscellaneous: Allergic reaction
1% to 10%:
Cardiovascular: Chest pain, arrhythmia, peripheral edema
Central nervous system: Anxiety, confusion, depression, dizziness, insomnia, lethargy, coma, seizures, malaise
Dermatologic: Dry skin, eczema, pruritus
Gastrointestinal: Constipation, flatulence, stomatitis, weight loss
Genitourinary: Dysuria
Hematologic: Myelosuppression
Hepatic: Liver dysfunction
Local: Thrombophlebitis
Neuromuscular & skeletal: Arthralgia, paresthesia, back pain, weakness
Ocular: Abnormal vision, eye pain, keratoconjunctivitis
Otic: Ear pain
Renal: Renal failure, hematuria
Respiratory: Bronchitis, dyspnea, lung edema, pneumonia
Miscellaneous: Death, opportunistic infections, sweating
Drug Uptake
Serum half-life, terminal: 5-15 hours
Pregnancy Risk Factor D
Generic Available No

Pentothal® Sodium *see* Thiopental *on page 925*
Pentoxifilina (Mexico) *see* Pentoxifylline *on this page*

Pentoxifylline (pen toks I fi leen)
Brand Names Trental®
Canadian/Mexican Brand Names Peridane® (Mexico)
Therapeutic Category Blood Viscosity Reducer Agent
Synonyms Pentoxifilina (Mexico)
Use Symptomatic management of peripheral vascular disease, mainly intermittent claudication

Unapproved use: AIDS patients with increased TNF, CVA, cerebrovascular diseases, diabetic atherosclerosis, diabetic neuropathy, gangrene, hemodialysis shunt thrombosis, vascular impotence, cerebral malaria, septic shock, sickle cell syndromes, and vasculitis
Usual Dosage Adults: Oral: 400 mg 3 times/day with meals; may reduce to 400 mg twice daily if GI or CNS side effects occur
Mechanism of Action Mechanism of action remains unclear; is thought to reduce blood viscosity and improve blood flow by altering the rheology of red blood cells
Local Anesthetic/Vasoconstrictor Precautions No information available to require special precautions
Effects on Dental Treatment No effects or complications reported
Other Adverse Effects
1% to 10%:
Central nervous system: Dizziness, headache
Gastrointestinal: Dyspepsia, nausea, vomiting
<1%:
Cardiovascular: Mild hypotension, angina
Central nervous system: Agitation
Ocular: Blurred vision
Otic: Earache
Drug Interactions Increased effect/toxic potential with cimetidine (increased levels) and other H_2 antagonists, warfarin; increased effect of antihypertensives
Drug Uptake
Absorption: Oral: Well absorbed
Serum half-life:
Parent drug: 24-48 minutes
Metabolites: 60-96 minutes
Time to peak serum concentration: Within 2-4 hours
Pregnancy Risk Factor C
Generic Available Yes

Pentrax® [OTC] *see* Coal Tar *on page 254*
Pen.Vee® K *see* Penicillin V Potassium *on page 734*

Pepcid® *see* Famotidine *on page 393*

Pepcid® AC Acid Controller [OTC] *see* Famotidine *on page 393*

Peptavlon® *see* Pentagastrin *on page 736*

Pepto-Bismol® (subsalicylate) [OTC] *see* Bismuth *on page 131*

Pepto® Diarrhea Control [OTC] *see* Loperamide *on page 565*

Percocet® *see* Oxycodone and Acetaminophen *on page 711*

Percodan® *see* Oxycodone and Aspirin *on page 712*

Percodan®-Demi *see* Oxycodone and Aspirin *on page 712*

Percogesic® [OTC] *see* Acetaminophen and Phenyltoloxamine *on page 23*

Perdiem® Plain [OTC] *see* Psyllium *on page 822*

Perfectoderm® Gel [OTC] *see* Benzoyl Peroxide *on page 120*

Perfenacina (Mexico) *see* Perphenazine *on page 744*

Pergolida, Mesilato De (Mexico) *see* Pergolide Mesylate *on this page*

Pergolide Mesylate (PER go lide)

Brand Names Permax®

Therapeutic Category Anti-Parkinson's Agent; Ergot Alkaloid

Synonyms Pergolida, Mesilato De (Mexico)

Use Adjunctive treatment to levodopa/carbidopa in the management of Parkinson's Disease

Usual Dosage When adding pergolide to levodopa/carbidopa, the dose of the latter can usually and should be decreased. Patients no longer responsive to bromocriptine may benefit by being switched to pergolide.

Adults: Oral: Start with 0.05 mg/day for 2 days, then increase dosage by 0.1 or 0.15 mg/day every 3 days over next 12 days, increase dose by 0.25 mg/day every 3 days until optimal therapeutic dose is achieved, up to 5 mg/day maximum; usual dosage range: 2-3 mg/day in 3 divided doses

Mechanism of Action Pergolide is a semisynthetic ergot alkaloid similar to bromocriptine but stated to be more potent and longer acting; it is a centrally-active dopamine agonist stimulating both D_1 and D_2 receptors

Local Anesthetic/Vasoconstrictor Precautions No information available to require special precautions

Effects on Dental Treatment Pergolide may decrease or inhibit salivary flow; normal salivary flow will resume with cessation of drug therapy; prolonged salivary reduction could enhance development of periodontal disease, oral candidiasis and discomfort

Other Adverse Effects

>10%:

Central nervous system: Dizziness, somnolence, insomnia, confusion, hallucinations, anxiety, dystonia

Gastrointestinal: Nausea, constipation

Neuromuscular & skeletal: Dyskinesias

Respiratory: Rhinitis

1% to 10%:

Cardiovascular: Myocardial infarction, postural hypotension, syncope, arrhythmias, peripheral edema, vasodilation, palpitations, chest pain

Central nervous system: Chills

Gastrointestinal: Diarrhea, abdominal pain, vomiting, dry mouth, anorexia, weight gain

Neuromuscular & skeletal: Weakness

Ocular: Abnormal vision

Respiratory: Dyspnea

Miscellaneous: Flu syndrome

Drug Interactions Decreased effect: Dopamine antagonists, metoclopramide

Drug Uptake

Absorption: Oral: Well absorbed

Pregnancy Risk Factor B

Generic Available No

Pergonal® *see* Menotropins *on page 591*

Periactin® *see* Cyproheptadine *on page 273*

Peri-Colace® [OTC] *see* Docusate and Casanthranol *on page 331*

Peridex® Oral Rinse *see* Chlorhexidine Gluconate *on page 211*

Perindopril Erbumine (per IN doe pril er BYOO meen)

Brand Names Aceon®

Therapeutic Category Antihypertensive

Use Treatment of stage I or II hypertension and congestive heart failure

Usual Dosage Adults: Oral:

Congestive heart failure: 4 mg once daily

Hypertension: Initial: 4 mg/day but may be titrated to response; usual range: 4-8 mg/day, maximum: 16 mg/day

Mechanism of Action Competitive inhibitor of angiotensin-converting enzyme (ACE); prevents conversion of angiotensin I to angiotensin II, a potent vasoconstrictor; results in lower levels of angiotensin II which, in turn, causes an increase in plasma renin activity and a reduction in aldosterone secretion

Local Anesthetic/Vasoconstrictor Precautions No information available to require special precautions

Effects on Dental Treatment <1%: Taste disturbances

Other Adverse Effects

1% to 10%

Central nervous system: Headache, dizziness, mood and sleep disorders, fatigue

Dermatologic: Rash, pruritus

Gastrointestinal: Nausea, epigastric pain, diarrhea, vomiting

Neuromuscular & skeletal: Muscle cramps

Respiratory: Cough (incidence is greater in women, 3:1)

<1%:

Cardiovascular: Hypotension

Dermatologic: Angioedema, psoriasis

Endocrine & metabolic: Hyperkalemia

Genitourinary: Impotence

Hematologic: Agranulocytosis for all ACE inhibitors (especially in patients with renal impairment or collagen vascular disease), possibly neutropenia

Ocular: Dry eyes, blurred vision, optic phosphenes

Renal: Decreases in creatinine clearance in some elderly hypertensive patients or those with chronic renal failure, worsening of renal function in patients with bilateral renal artery stenosis, or furosemide therapy; proteinuria

Drug Interactions See table.

Drug-Drug Interactions With ACEIs

Precipitant Drug	Drug (Category) and Effect	Description
Antacids	ACE Inhibitors: decreased	Decreased bioavailability of ACEIs. May be more likely with captopril. Separate administration times by 1-2 hours.
NSAIDs (indomethacin)	ACEIs: decreased	Reduced hypotensive effects of ACEIs. More prominent in low renin or volume dependent hypertensive patients.
Phenothiazines	ACEIs: increased	Pharmacologic effects of ACEIs may be increased.
ACEIs	Allopurinol: increased	Higher risk of hypersensitivity reaction possible when given concurrently. Three case reports of Stevens-Johnson syndrome with captopril.
ACEIs	Digoxin: increased	Increased plasma digoxin levels.
ACEIs	Lithium: increased	Increased serum lithium levels and symptoms of toxicity may occur.
ACEIs	Potassium preps/ potassium sparing diuretics increased	Coadministration may result in elevated potassium levels.

Drug Uptake

Serum half-life:

Parent drug: 1.5-3 hours

Metabolite: 25-30 hours

Time to peak: Occurs in 1 and 3-4 hours for perindopril and perindoprilat, respectively after chronic therapy; (maximum perindoprilat serum levels are 2-3 times higher and T_{max} is shorter following chronic therapy); in CHF, the peak of perindoprilat is prolonged to 6 hours

Pregnancy Risk Factor D (especially during 2nd and 3rd trimester)

Generic Available No

PerioGard® *see* Chlorhexidine Gluconate *on page 211*

Peritrate® *see* Pentaerythritol Tetranitrate *on page 735*

Peritrate® SA *see* Pentaerythritol Tetranitrate *on page 735*

Permapen® *see* Penicillin G Benzathine *on page 731*

Permax® *see* Pergolide Mesylate *on previous page*

Permethrin (per METH rin)
Brand Names Elimite™; Nix™ [OTC]
Therapeutic Category Antiparasitic Agent, Topical; Scabicidal Agent
Use Single application treatment of infestation with *Pediculus humanus capitis* (head louse) and its nits or *Sarcoptes scabiei* (scabies)
Usual Dosage Topical: Children >2 months and Adults:
Head lice: After hair has been washed with shampoo, rinsed with water, and towel dried, apply a sufficient volume of topical liquid to saturate the hair and scalp. Leave on hair for 10 minutes before rinsing off with water; remove remaining nits; may repeat in 1 week if lice or nits still present.
Scabies: Apply cream from head to toe; leave on for 8-14 hours before washing off with water; for infants, also apply on the hairline, neck, scalp, temple, and forehead; may reapply in 1 week if live mites appear
Permethrin 5% cream was shown to be safe and effective when applied to an infant <1 month of age with neonatal scabies; time of application was limited to 6 hours before rinsing with soap and water
Mechanism of Action Inhibits sodium ion influx through nerve cell membrane channels in parasites resulting in delayed repolarization and thus paralysis and death of the pest
Local Anesthetic/Vasoconstrictor Precautions No information available to require special precautions
Effects on Dental Treatment No effects or complications reported
Other Adverse Effects 1% to 10%:
Cardiovascular: Local edema
Dermatologic: Pruritus, erythema, rash of the scalp, numbness or scalp discomfort
Local: Burning, stinging, tingling
Drug Interactions No data reported
Drug Uptake
Absorption: Topical: Minimal (<2%)
Pregnancy Risk Factor B
Generic Available No

Permitil® *see* Fluphenazine *on page 420*

Pernox® [OTC] *see* Sulfur and Salicylic Acid *on page 898*

Peroxin A5® *see* Benzoyl Peroxide *on page 120*

Peroxin A10® *see* Benzoyl Peroxide *on page 120*

Perphenazine (per FEN a zeen)
Brand Names Trilafon®
Canadian/Mexican Brand Names Apo®-Perphenazine (Canada); Leptopsique® (Mexico); PMS-Perphenazine® (Canada)
Therapeutic Category Antiemetic; Antipsychotic Agent; Phenothiazine Derivative
Synonyms Perfenacina (Mexico)
Use Management of manifestations of psychotic disorders, depressive neurosis, alcohol withdrawal, nausea and vomiting, nonpsychotic symptoms associated with dementia in elderly, Tourette's syndrome, Huntington's chorea, spasmodic torticollis and Reye's syndrome
Usual Dosage
Children:
Psychoses: Oral:
1-6 years: 4-6 mg/day in divided doses
6-12 years: 6 mg/day in divided doses
>12 years: 4-16 mg 2-4 times/day
I.M.: 5 mg every 6 hours
Nausea/vomiting: I.M.: 5 mg every 6 hours

Adults:
Psychoses:
Oral: 4-16 mg 2-4 times/day not to exceed 64 mg/day
I.M.: 5 mg every 6 hours up to 15 mg/day in ambulatory patients and 30 mg/day in hospitalized patients
Nausea/vomiting:
Oral: 8-16 mg/day in divided doses up to 24 mg/day
I.M.: 5-10 mg every 6 hours as necessary up to 15 mg/day in ambulatory patients and 30 mg/day in hospitalized patients
I.V. (severe): 1 mg at 1- to 2-minute intervals up to a total of 5 mg

Not dialyzable (0% to 5%)
Mechanism of Action Blocks postsynaptic mesolimbic dopaminergic receptors in the brain; exhibits a strong alpha-adrenergic blocking effect and depresses the release of hypothalamic and hypophyseal hormones

Local Anesthetic/Vasoconstrictor Precautions No information available to require special precautions

Effects on Dental Treatment Significant hypotension may occur, especially when the drug is administered parenterally; orthostatic hypotension is due to alpha-receptor blockade, the elderly are at greater risk for orthostatic hypotension

Tardive dyskinesia: Prevalence rate may be 40% in elderly; development of the syndrome and the irreversible nature are proportional to duration and total cumulative dose over time

Extrapyramidal reactions are more common in elderly with up to 50% developing these reactions after 60 years of age; drug-induced **Parkinson's syndrome** occurs often; **Akathisia** is the most common extrapyramidal reaction in elderly

Increased confusion, memory loss, psychotic behavior, and agitation frequently occur as a consequence of anticholinergic effects

Antipsychotic associated sedation in nonpsychotic patients is extremely unpleasant due to feelings of depersonalization, derealization, and dysphoria

Other Adverse Effects
>10%:
    Cardiovascular: Hypotension, orthostatic hypotension
    Central nervous system: Pseudoparkinsonism, akathisia, dystonias, tardive dyskinesia (persistent), dizziness
    Gastrointestinal: Constipation
    Ocular: Pigmentary retinopathy
    Respiratory: Nasal congestion
    Miscellaneous: Decreased sweating
1% to 10%:
    Dermatologic: Photosensitivity, skin rash
    Endocrine & metabolic: Changes in menstrual cycle, changes in libido, pain in breasts
    Gastrointestinal: Weight gain, vomiting, stomach pain, nausea
    Genitourinary: Dysuria, ejaculatory disturbances
    Neuromuscular & skeletal: Trembling of fingers
<1%:
    Central nervous system: Neuroleptic malignant syndrome (NMS), impairment of temperature regulation, lowering of seizures threshold
    Dermatologic: Discoloration of skin (blue-gray)
    Endocrine & metabolic: Galactorrhea
    Genitourinary: Priapism
    Hematologic: Agranulocytosis, leukopenia
    Hepatic: Cholestatic jaundice, hepatotoxicity
    Ocular: Cornea and lens changes, pigmentary retinopathy

Drug Interactions Increased toxicity: Additive effects with other CNS depressants

Drug Uptake
    Absorption: Oral: Well absorbed
    Serum half-life: 9 hours
    Time to peak serum concentration: Within 4-8 hours

Pregnancy Risk Factor C
Generic Available Yes

Perphenazine and Amitriptyline see Amitriptyline and Perphenazine on page 62

Persa-Gel® see Benzoyl Peroxide on page 120

Persantine® see Dipyridamole on page 326

Pertofrane® see Desipramine on page 288

Pertussin® CS [OTC] see Dextromethorphan on page 298

Pertussin® ES [OTC] see Dextromethorphan on page 298

Pethidine Hydrochloride (Canada) see Meperidine on page 592

Pfizerpen® see Penicillin G, Parenteral, Aqueous on page 732

Pfizerpen®-AS see Penicillin G Procaine on page 733

PGE$_1$ see Alprostadil on page 44

PGE$_2$ see Dinoprostone on page 322

PGF$_{2\alpha}$ see Dinoprost Tromethamine on page 322

Phanatuss® Cough Syrup [OTC] see Guaifenesin and Dextromethorphan on page 453

Pharmacology of Drug Metabolism and Interactions see page 11

Pharmaflur® see Fluoride on page 415

Phazyme® [OTC] see Simethicone on page 865

Phenadex® Senior [OTC] see Guaifenesin and Dextromethorphan on page 453

Phenahist-TR® *see* Chlorpheniramine, Phenylephrine, Phenylpropanolamine, and Belladonna Alkaloids *on page 221*

Phenameth® DM *see* Promethazine and Dextromethorphan *on page 805*

Phenaphen® With Codeine *see* Acetaminophen and Codeine *on page 21*

Phenazine® *see* Promethazine *on page 804*

Phenazopyridine (fen az oh PEER i deen)

Brand Names Azo-Standard® [OTC]; Baridium® [OTC]; Prodium® [OTC]; Pyridiate®; Pyridium®; Urodine®; Urogesic®

Canadian/Mexican Brand Names Azo Wintomylon® (Mexico); Madel® (Mexico); Phenazo® (Canada); Pyronium® (Canada); Urovalidin® (Mexico); Vito Reins® (Canada)

Therapeutic Category Analgesic, Urinary; Local Anesthetic, Urinary

Synonyms Fenazopiridina (Mexico)

Use Symptomatic relief of urinary burning, itching, frequency and urgency in association with urinary tract infection or following urologic procedures

Usual Dosage Oral:

Children: 12 mg/kg/day in 3 divided doses administered after meals for 2 days

Adults: 100-200 mg 3 times/day after meals for 2 days when used concomitantly with an antibacterial agent

Mechanism of Action An azo dye which exerts local anesthetic or analgesic action on urinary tract mucosa through an unknown mechanism

Local Anesthetic/Vasoconstrictor Precautions No information available to require special precautions

Effects on Dental Treatment No effects or complications reported

Other Adverse Effects

1% to 10%:
Central nervous system: Headache, dizziness
Gastrointestinal: Stomach cramps

<1%:
Central nervous system: Vertigo
Dermatologic: Skin pigmentation, rash
Hematologic: Methemoglobinemia, hemolytic anemia
Hepatic: Hepatitis
Renal: Acute renal failure

Drug Interactions No data reported

Pregnancy Risk Factor B

Generic Available Yes

Phenchlor® S.H.A. *see* Chlorpheniramine, Phenylephrine, Phenylpropanolamine, and Belladonna Alkaloids *on page 221*

Phendry® Oral [OTC] *see* Diphenhydramine *on page 323*

Phenelzine (FEN el zeen)

Brand Names Nardil®

Therapeutic Category Antidepressant, Monoamine Oxidase Inhibitor

Use Symptomatic treatment of atypical, nonendogenous or neurotic depression

The MAO inhibitors are usually reserved for patients who do not tolerate or respond to the traditional "cyclic" or "second generation" antidepressants. The brain activity of monoamine oxidase increases with age and even more so in patients with Alzheimer's disease. Therefore, the MAO inhibitors may have an increased role in patients with Alzheimer's disease who are depressed. Phenelzine is less stimulating than tranylcypromine.

Usual Dosage Oral:

Adults: 15 mg 3 times/day; may increase to 60-90 mg/day during early phase of treatment, then reduce to dose for maintenance therapy slowly after maximum benefit is obtained; takes 2-4 weeks for a significant response to occur

Elderly: Initial: 7.5 mg/day; increase by 7.5-15 mg/day every 3-4 days as tolerated; usual therapeutic dose: 15-60 mg/day in 3-4 divided doses

Mechanism of Action Thought to act by increasing endogenous concentrations of epinephrine, norepinephrine, dopamine and serotonin through inhibition of the enzyme (monoamine oxidase) responsible for the breakdown of these neurotransmitters

Local Anesthetic/Vasoconstrictor Precautions Attempts should be made to avoid use of vasoconstrictor due to possibility of hypertensive episodes with monoamine oxidase inhibitors

Effects on Dental Treatment Orthostatic hypotension in >10% of patients; meperidine should be avoided as an analgesic due to toxic reactions with MAO inhibitors

Other Adverse Effects
>10%:
Cardiovascular: Orthostatic hypotension
Central nervous system: Drowsiness
Endocrine & metabolic: Decreased sexual ability
Neuromuscular & skeletal: Trembling, weakness
Ocular: Blurred vision
1% to 10%:
Cardiovascular; Tachycardia, peripheral edema
Central nervous system: Nervousness, chills
Gastrointestinal: Diarrhea, anorexia, dry mouth, constipation
<1%:
Central nervous system: Parkinsonism syndrome
Hematologic: Leukopenia
Hepatic: Hepatitis

Drug Interactions
Decreased effect of antihypertensives
Increased toxicity with disulfiram (possible seizures), fluoxetine (and other serotonin active agents), tricyclic antidepressants (cardiovascular instability),
meperidine (cardiovascular instability), phenothiazines (hyperpyretic crisis),
levodopa, sympathomimetics (hypertensive crisis), barbiturates, rauwolfia alkaloids (eg, reserpine), dextroamphetamine (psychoses), foods containing tyramine

Drug Uptake
Onset of action: Within 2-4 weeks
Duration: May continue to have a therapeutic effect and interactions 2 weeks
after discontinuing therapy
Absorption: Oral: Well absorbed

Pregnancy Risk Factor C
Generic Available No

Phenerbel-S® see Belladonna, Phenobarbital, and Ergotamine Tartrate *on page 114*

Phenergan® *see Promethazine on page 804*

Phenergan® VC Syrup *see Promethazine and Phenylephrine on page 805*

Phenergan® VC With Codeine *see Promethazine, Phenylephrine, and Codeine on page 806*

Phenergan® With Codeine *see Promethazine and Codeine on page 805*

Phenergan® with Dextromethorphan *see Promethazine and Dextromethorphan on page 805*

Phenetron® *see Chlorpheniramine on page 217*

Phenhist® Expectorant *see Guaifenesin, Pseudoephedrine, and Codeine on page 455*

Phenindamine (fen IN dah meen)
Brand Names Nolahist® [OTC]
Therapeutic Category Decongestant, Nasal
Use Treatment of perennial and seasonal allergic rhinitis and chronic urticaria
Local Anesthetic/Vasoconstrictor Precautions No information available to
require special precautions
Effects on Dental Treatment No effects or complications reported
Generic Available Yes

Pheniramine and Naphazoline *see Naphazoline and Pheniramine on page 665*

Pheniramine, Phenylpropanolamine, and Pyrilamine
(fen EER a meen, fen il proe pa NOLE a meen, & peer IL a meen)
Brand Names Triaminic® Oral Infant Drops
Therapeutic Category Antihistamine/Decongestant Combination
Use Symptomatic relief of nasal congestion and postnasal drip as well as allergic
rhinitis
Local Anesthetic/Vasoconstrictor Precautions No information available to
require special precautions
Effects on Dental Treatment No effects or complications reported
Pregnancy Risk Factor C
Generic Available Yes

Phenobarbital (fee noe BAR bi tal)
Brand Names Barbita®; Luminal®; Solfoton®
Canadian/Mexican Brand Names Alepsal® (Mexico); Barbilixir® (Canada)
Therapeutic Category Anticonvulsant, Barbiturate; Barbiturate; Hypnotic;
Sedative
(Continued)

Phenobarbital *(Continued)*

Synonyms Fenobarbital (Mexico)

Use Management of generalized tonic-clonic (grand mal) and partial seizures; neonatal seizures; febrile seizures in children; sedation; may also be used for prevention and treatment of neonatal hyperbilirubinemia and lowering of bilirubin in chronic cholestasis

Usual Dosage

Children:

Sedation: Oral: 2 mg/kg 3 times/day

Hypnotic: I.M., I.V., S.C.: 3-5 mg/kg at bedtime

Preoperative sedation: Oral, I.M., I.V.: 1-3 mg/kg 1-1.5 hours before procedure

Anticonvulsant: Status epilepticus **Loading dose:** I.V.:

Children: 10-20 mg/kg in a single or divided dose; in select patients may give additional 5 mg/kg/dose every 15-30 minutes until seizure is controlled or a total dose of 40 mg/kg is reached

Adults: 300-800 mg initially followed by 120-240 mg/dose at 20-minute intervals until seizures are controlled or a total dose of 1-2 g

Anticonvulsant maintenance dose: Oral, I.V.:

Children:

1-5 years: 6-8 mg/kg/day in 1-2 divided doses

5-12 years: 4-6 mg/kg/day in 1-2 divided doses

Children >12 years and Adults: 1-3 mg/kg/day in divided doses or 50-100 mg 2-3 times/day

Adults:

Sedation: Oral, I.M.: 30-120 mg/day in 2-3 divided doses

Hypnotic: Oral, I.M., I.V., S.C.: 100-320 mg at bedtime

Preoperative sedation: I.M.: 100-200 mg 1-1.5 hours before procedure

Mechanism of Action Interferes with transmission of impulses from the thalamus to the cortex of the brain resulting in an imbalance in central inhibitory and facilitatory mechanisms

Local Anesthetic/Vasoconstrictor Precautions No information available to require special precautions

Effects on Dental Treatment No effects or complications reported

Other Adverse Effects

>10%:

Cardiovascular: Hypotension, cardiac arrhythmias, bradycardia, arterial spasm, and gangrene with inadvertent intra-arterial injection

Central nervous system: Dizziness, lightheadedness, "hangover" effect, drowsiness, lethargy, CNS excitation or depression, impaired judgment

Local: Pain at injection site, thrombophlebitis with I.V. use

1% to 10%:

Central nervous system: Confusion, mental depression, unusual excitement, nervousness, faint feeling, headache, insomnia, nightmares

Gastrointestinal: Nausea, vomiting, constipation

<1%:

Central nervous system: Hallucinations, hypothermia

Dermatologic: Exfoliative dermatitis, Stevens-Johnson syndrome, rash

Hematologic: Agranulocytosis, megaloblastic anemia, thrombocytopenia

Respiratory: Laryngospasm, respiratory depression, apnea (especially with rapid I.V. use)

Drug Interactions

Decreased effect: Phenobarbital appears to increase the metabolism of the following drugs to cause a decrease in their actions: Phenothiazines, haloperidol, quinidine, cyclosporine, tricyclic antidepressants, corticosteroids, theophylline, ethosuximide, warfarin, oral contraceptives, chloramphenicol, griseofulvin, doxycycline, beta-blockers

Increased toxicity: Phenobarbital enhances the sedative effects of propoxyphene, benzodiazepines, CNS depressants, valproic acid, methylphenidate, chloramphenicol

Drug Uptake

Oral:

Onset of hypnosis: Within 20-60 minutes

Duration: 6-10 hours

I.V.:

Onset of action: Within 5 minutes

Duration: 4-10 hours

Absorption: Oral: 70% to 90%

Serum half-life:

Children: 37-73 hours

Adults: 53-140 hours

Time to peak serum concentration: Oral: Within 1-6 hours
Pregnancy Risk Factor D
Generic Available Yes

Phenol (FEE nol)
Related Information
Mouth Pain, Cold Sore, Canker Sore Products *on page 1183*
Brand Names Baker's P&S Topical [OTC]; Cēpastat® [OTC]; Chloraseptic® Oral [OTC]
Therapeutic Category Pharmaceutical Aid
Synonyms Carbolic Acid
Use Relief of sore throat pain, mouth, gum, and throat irritations
Local Anesthetic/Vasoconstrictor Precautions No information available to require special precautions
Effects on Dental Treatment No effects or complications reported
Other Adverse Effects In overdose situation:
1% to 10%:
Cardiovascular: Hypotension, cardiovascular collapse, tachycardia, atrial and ventricular arrhythmias, edema
Central nervous system: slurred speech, CNS depression, agitation, confusion, seizures, coma
Dermatologic: White, red, or brown skin discoloration
Gastrointestinal: Nausea, vomiting, oral burns GI ulceration, GI bleeding
Genitourinary: Urine discoloration (green)
Hematologic: Hemorrhage
Local: Irritation, burns
Renal: Nephritis
Respiratory: Bronchospasm/wheezing, coughing, dyspnea, pneumonia, pulmonary

When used for spinal neurolysis/motor point blocks: 1% to 10%:
Cardiovascular: Dysrhythmias
Central nervous system: Headache, hyperesthesia, dysesthesia
Gastrointestinal: Bowel incontinence
Genitourinary: Urinary incontinence
Local: Tissue necrosis, pain at injection site
Neuromuscular & skeletal: Motor weakness, nerve damage
Respiratory: Pleural irritation
Pregnancy Risk Factor C
Generic Available Yes
Comments Cepastat® contains 8 calories/lozenge (2 g sorbitol)

Phenoxine® [OTC] *see* Phenylpropanolamine *on page 754*

Phenoxybenzamine (fen oks ee BEN za meen)
Brand Names Dibenzyline®
Therapeutic Category Alpha-Adrenergic Blocking Agent, Oral; Antihypertensive; Vasodilator, Coronary
Use Symptomatic management of pheochromocytoma; treatment of hypertensive crisis caused by sympathomimetic amines

Unlabeled use: Micturition problems associated with neurogenic bladder, functional outlet obstruction, and partial prostate obstruction
Usual Dosage Oral:
Children: Initial: 0.2 mg/kg (maximum: 10 mg) once daily, increase by 0.2 mg/kg increments; usual maintenance dose: 0.4-1.2 mg/kg/day every 6-8 hours, higher doses may be necessary
Adults: Initial: 10 mg twice daily, increase by 10 mg every other day until optimum dose is achieved; usual range: 20-40 mg 2-3 times/day
Mechanism of Action Produces long-lasting noncompetitive alpha-adrenergic blockade of postganglionic synapses in exocrine glands and smooth muscle; relaxes urethra and increases opening of the bladder
Local Anesthetic/Vasoconstrictor Precautions No information available to require special precautions
Effects on Dental Treatment No effects or complications reported
Other Adverse Effects
>10%:
Cardiovascular: Postural hypotension, tachycardia, syncope
Ocular: Miosis
Respiratory: Nasal congestion
1% to 10%:
Cardiovascular: Shock
Central nervous system: Lethargy, headache, confusion, fatigue
(Continued)

Phenoxybenzamine *(Continued)*

Gastrointestinal: Vomiting, nausea, diarrhea, dry mouth
Genitourinary: Inhibition of ejaculation
Neuromuscular & skeletal: Weakness

Drug Interactions
Decreased effect: Alpha agonists
Increased toxicity: Beta-blockers (hypotension, tachycardia)

Drug Uptake
Onset of action: Oral: Within 2 hours
Duration: Can continue for 4 or more days
Serum half-life: 24 hours

Pregnancy Risk Factor C
Generic Available No

Phensuximide (fen SUKS i mide)

Brand Names Milontin®
Therapeutic Category Anticonvulsant, Succinimide
Use Control of absence (petit mal) seizures
Local Anesthetic/Vasoconstrictor Precautions No information available to require special precautions
Effects on Dental Treatment No effects or complications reported
Other Adverse Effects
>10%:
Central nervous system: Ataxia, dizziness, drowsiness, headache
Dermatologic: Stevens-Johnson syndrome
Gastrointestinal: Anorexia, nausea, vomiting, weight loss
Miscellaneous: Systemic lupus erythematosus (SLE), hiccups
1% to 10%:
Central nervous system: Mental depression, nightmares, fatigue, aggressiveness
Neuromuscular & skeletal: Weakness
<1%:
Central nervous system: Paranoid psychosis
Dermatologic: Urticaria, exfoliative dermatitis
Hematologic: Agranulocytosis, leukopenia, aplastic anemia, thrombocytopenia, pancytopenia

Pregnancy Risk Factor D
Generic Available No

Phentermine (FEN ter meen)

Brand Names Adipex-P®; Fastin®; Ionamin®; Zantryl®
Canadian/Mexican Brand Names Diminex® (Mexico)
Therapeutic Category Anorexiant
Synonyms Fentermina (Mexico)
Use Short-term adjunct in exogenous obesity
Usual Dosage Oral:
Children 3-15 years: 5-15 mg/day for 4 weeks

Adults: 8 mg 3 times/day 30 minutes before meals or food or 15-37.5 mg/day before breakfast or 10-14 hours before retiring

Mechanism of Action Phentermine is structurally similar to dextroamphetamine and is comparable to dextroamphetamine as an appetite suppressant, but is generally associated with a lower incidence and severity of CNS side effects. Phentermine, like other anorexiants, stimulates the hypothalamus to result in decreased appetite; anorexiant effects are most likely mediated via norepinephrine and dopamine metabolism. However, other CNS effects or metabolic effects may be involved.

Local Anesthetic/Vasoconstrictor Precautions Use vasoconstriction with caution in patients taking phentermine. Amphetamines enhance the sympathomimetic response of epinephrine and norepinephrine leading to potential hypertension and cardiotoxicity.

Effects on Dental Treatment Up to 10% of patients may present with hypertension. The use of local anesthetic without vasoconstrictor is recommended in these patients.

Other Adverse Effects
>10%:
Cardiovascular: Hypertension
Central nervous system: Euphoria, nervousness, insomnia
1% to 10%:
Central nervous system: Confusion, mental depression, restlessness
Gastrointestinal: Nausea, vomiting, constipation

Endocrine & metabolic: Changes in libido
Hematologic: Blood dyscrasias
Neuromuscular & skeletal: Tremor
Ocular: Blurred vision
<1%:
Cardiovascular: Tachycardia, arrhythmias
Central nervous system: Headache
Dermatologic: Alopecia
Gastrointestinal: Diarrhea, abdominal cramps
Genitourinary: Dysuria
Neuromuscular & skeletal: Myalgia
Renal: Polyuria
Respiratory: Dyspnea
Miscellaneous: Increased sweating

Drug Interactions
Adrenergic blockers are inhibited by amphetamines
Amphetamines enhance the activity of tricyclic or sympathomimetic agents
MAO inhibitors slow the metabolism of amphetamines
Amphetamines will counteract the sedative effects of antihistamines
Amphetamines potentiate the analgesic effects of meperidine

Drug Uptake
Absorption: Well absorbed; resin absorbed slower and produces more prolonged clinical effects
Serum half-life: 20 hours

Pregnancy Risk Factor C

Generic Available Yes

Comments Many diet doctors have prescribed fenfluramine ("fen") and phentermine ("phen"). When taken together the combination is known as "fen-phen". The diet drug dexfenfluramine (Redux®) is chemically similar to fenfluramine (Pondimin®) and was also used in combination with phentermine called "Redux-phen". While each of the three drugs alone had approval from the FDA for sale in the treatment of obesity, neither combination had an official approval. The use of the combinations in the treatment of obesity was considered an "off-label" use. Reports in medical literature have been accumulating for some years about significant side effects associated with fenfluramine and dexfenfluramine. In 1997, the manufacturers, at the urging of the FDA, agreed to voluntarily withdraw the drugs from the market. The action was based on findings from physicians who evaluated patients taking fenfluramine and dexfenfluramine with echocardiograms. The findings indicated that approximately 30% of patients had abnormal echocardiograms, even though they had no symptoms. This was a much higher than expected percentage of abnormal test results. This conclusion was based on a sample of 291 patients examined by five different physicians. Under normal conditions, fewer than 1% of patients would be expected to show signs of heart valve disease. The findings suggested that fenfluramine and dexfenfluramine were the likely cause of heart valve problems of the type that promoted FDA's earlier warnings concerning "fen-phen". The earlier warning included the following: The mitral valve and other valves in the heart are damaged by a strange white coating and allow blood to flow back, causing heart muscle damage. In several cases, valve replacement surgery has been done. As a rule, the person must, thereafter for life, be on a blood thinner to prevent clots from the mechanical valve. This type of valve damage had only been seen before in persons who were exposed to large amounts of serotonin. The fenfluramine increases the availability of serotonin.

Phentolamine (fen TOLE a meen)

Brand Names Regitine®

Canadian/Mexican Brand Names Rogitine® (Canada)

Therapeutic Category Alpha-Adrenergic Blocking Agent, Parenteral; Alpha-Adrenergic Inhibitors, Central; Antidote, Extravasation; Antihypertensive; Diagnostic Agent, Pheochromocytoma; Vasodilator, Coronary

Use Diagnosis of pheochromocytoma and treatment of hypertension associated with pheochromocytoma or other caused by excess sympathomimetic amines; as treatment of dermal necrosis after extravasation of drugs with alpha-adrenergic effects (norepinephrine, dopamine, epinephrine, dobutamine)

Usual Dosage
Treatment of alpha-adrenergic drug extravasation: S.C.:
Children: 0.1-0.2 mg/kg diluted in 10 mL 0.9% sodium chloride infiltrated into area of extravasation within 12 hours
Adults: Infiltrate area with small amount of solution made by diluting 5-10 mg in 10 mL 0.9% sodium chloride within 12 hours of extravasation
If dose is effective, normal skin color should return to the blanched area within 1 hour

(Continued)

Phentolamine *(Continued)*

Diagnosis of pheochromocytoma: I.M., I.V.:
  Children: 0.05-0.1 mg/kg/dose, maximum single dose: 5 mg
  Adults: 5 mg

Surgery for pheochromocytoma: Hypertension: I.M., I.V.:
  Children: 0.05-0.1 mg/kg/dose given 1-2 hours before procedure; repeat as
    needed every 2-4 hours until hypertension is controlled; maximum single
    dose: 5 mg
  Adults: 5 mg given 1-2 hours before procedure and repeated as needed every
    2-4 hours

Hypertensive crisis: Adults: 5-20 mg

Mechanism of Action Competitively blocks alpha-adrenergic receptors to produce brief antagonism of circulating epinephrine and norepinephrine to reduce hypertension caused by alpha effects of these catecholamines; also has a positive inotropic and chronotropic effect on the heart

Local Anesthetic/Vasoconstrictor Precautions No information available to require special precautions

Effects on Dental Treatment No effects or complications reported

Other Adverse Effects

>10%:
  Cardiovascular: Hypotension, tachycardia, arrhythmias, reflex tachycardia,
    anginal pain, orthostatic hypotension
  Gastrointestinal: Nausea, vomiting, diarrhea, exacerbation of peptic ulcer,
    abdominal pain
  Respiratory: Nasal congestion

1% to 10%:
  Cardiovascular: Flushing of face, syncope
  Central nervous system: Dizziness
  Neuromuscular & skeletal: Weakness

<1%:
  Cardiovascular: Myocardial infarction
  Central nervous system: Severe headache

Drug Interactions
Decreased effect: Epinephrine, ephedrine
Increased toxicity: Ethanol (disulfiram reaction)

Drug Uptake
Onset of action:
  I.M.: Within 15-20 minutes
  I.V.: Immediate
Duration:
  I.M.: 30-45 minutes
  I.V.: 15-30 minutes
Serum half-life: 19 minutes

Pregnancy Risk Factor C

Generic Available No

Phenylalanine Mustard *see* Melphalan *on page 590*

Phenyldrine® [OTC] *see* Phenylpropanolamine *on page 754*

Phenylephrine *(fen il EF rin)*

Related Information
Dentin Hypersensitivity; High Caries Index; Xerostomia *on page 1074*
Guaifenesin and Phenylephrine *on page 454*

Brand Names AK-Dilate® Ophthalmic Solution; AK-Nefrin® Ophthalmic Solution; Alconefrin® Nasal Solution [OTC]; I-Phrine® Ophthalmic Solution; Mydfrin® Ophthalmic Solution; Neo-Synephrine® Nasal Solution [OTC]; Neo-Synephrine® Ophthalmic Solution; Nostril® Nasal Solution [OTC]; Prefrin™ Ophthalmic Solution; Relief® Ophthalmic Solution; Rhinall® Nasal Solution [OTC]; Sinarest® Nasal Solution [OTC]; St. Joseph® Measured Dose Nasal Solution [OTC]; Vicks Sinex® Nasal Solution [OTC]

Canadian/Mexican Brand Names Dionephrine® (Canada)

Therapeutic Category Adrenergic Agonist Agent; Adrenergic Agonist Agent, Ophthalmic; Antiglaucoma Agent; Nasal Agent, Vasoconstrictor; Ophthalmic Agent, Mydriatic

Synonyms Fenilefrina (Mexico)

Use Treatment of hypotension, vascular failure in shock; as a vasoconstrictor in regional analgesia; symptomatic relief of nasal and nasopharyngeal mucosal congestion; as a mydriatic in ophthalmic procedures and treatment of wide-angle glaucoma; supraventricular tachycardia

Usual Dosage

Ophthalmic procedures:

Children and Adults: Instill 1 drop of 2.5% or 10% solution, may repeat in 10-60 minutes as needed

Nasal decongestant: (therapy should not exceed 5 continuous days)

Children:

2-6 years: Instill 1 drop every 2-4 hours of 0.125% solution as needed

6-12 years: Instill 1-2 sprays or instill 1-2 drops every 4 hours of 0.25% solution as needed

Children >12 years and Adults: Instill 1-2 sprays or instill 1-2 drops every 4 hours of 0.25% to 0.5% solution as needed; 1% solution may be used in adult in cases of extreme nasal congestion; do not use nasal solutions more than 3 days

Hypotension/shock:

Children:

I.M., S.C.: 0.1 mg/kg/dose every 1-2 hours as needed (maximum: 5 mg)

I.V. bolus: 5-20 mcg/kg/dose every 10-15 minutes as needed

I.V. infusion: 0.1-0.5 mcg/kg/minute

Adults:

I.M., S.C.: 2-5 mg/dose every 1-2 hours as needed (initial dose should not exceed 5 mg)

I.V. bolus: 0.1-0.5 mg/dose every 10-15 minutes as needed (initial dose should not exceed 0.5 mg)

I.V. infusion: 10 mg in 250 mL D_5W or NS (1:25,000 dilution) (40 mcg/mL); start at 100-180 mcg/minute (2-5 mL/minute; 50-90 drops/minute) initially; when blood pressure is stabilized, maintenance rate: 40-60 mcg/minute (20-30 drops/minute)

Paroxysmal supraventricular tachycardia: I.V.:

Children: 5-10 mcg/kg/dose over 20-30 seconds

Adults: 0.25-0.5 mg/dose over 20-30 seconds

Mechanism of Action Potent, direct-acting alpha-adrenergic stimulator with weak beta-adrenergic activity; causes vasoconstriction of the arterioles of the nasal mucosa and conjunctiva; activates the dilator muscle of the pupil to cause contraction; produces vasoconstriction of arterioles in the body; produces systemic arterial vasoconstriction

Local Anesthetic/Vasoconstrictor Precautions Use with caution since phenylephrine is a sympathomimetic amine which could interact with epinephrine to cause a pressor response

Effects on Dental Treatment Up to 10% of patients could experience tachycardia, palpitations, and dry mouth; use vasoconstrictor with caution

Other Adverse Effects

Nasal:

>10%: Respiratory: Burning, rebound congestion, sneezing

1% to 10%: Respiratory: Stinging, dryness

Ophthalmic:

>10%: Ocular: Transient stinging

1% to 10%:

Central nervous system: Headache, browache

Ocular: Blurred vision, photophobia, lacrimation

Systemic:

>10%: Neuromuscular & skeletal: Tremor

1% to 10%:

Cardiovascular: Peripheral vasoconstriction hypertension, angina, reflex bradycardia, arrhythmias

Central nervous system: Restlessness, excitability

Drug Interactions

Decreased effect of phenylephrine with alpha- and beta-adrenergic blocking agents

Increased effect of phenylephrine with oxytocic drugs

Increased toxicity: With sympathomimetics, tachycardia or arrhythmias may occur; with MAO inhibitors, actions may be potentiated

Drug Uptake

Onset of effect:

I.M., S.C.: Within 10-15 minutes

I.V.: Immediate

Duration:

I.M.: 30 minutes to 2 hours

I.V.: 15-30 minutes

S.C.: 1 hour

Serum half-life: 2.5 hours

Pregnancy Risk Factor C

(Continued)

Phenylephrine *(Continued)*

Generic Available Yes

Phenylephrine and Chlorpheniramine *see* Chlorpheniramine and Phenylephrine *on page 218*

Phenylephrine and Cyclopentolate *see* Cyclopentolate and Phenylephrine *on page 269*

Phenylephrine and Guaifenesin *see* Guaifenesin and Phenylephrine *on page 454*

Phenylephrine and Scopolamine

(fen il EF rin & skoe POL a meen)

Brand Names Murocoll-2® Ophthalmic

Therapeutic Category Ophthalmic Agent, Mydriatic

Synonyms Scopolamine and Phenylephrine

Use Mydriasis, cycloplegia, and to break posterior synechiae in iritis

Local Anesthetic/Vasoconstrictor Precautions Use with caution since phenylephrine is a sympathomimetic amine which could interact with epinephrine to cause a pressor response

Effects on Dental Treatment This form of phenylephrine will have no effect on dental treatment when given as eye drops

Pregnancy Risk Factor C

Generic Available Yes

Phenylephrine and Zinc Sulfate (fen il EF rin & zingk SUL fate)

Brand Names Zincfrin® Ophthalmic [OTC]

Therapeutic Category Ophthalmic Agent, Miscellaneous

Use Soothe, moisturize, and remove redness due to minor eye irritation

Local Anesthetic/Vasoconstrictor Precautions No information available to require special precautions

Effects on Dental Treatment No effects or complications reported

Generic Available Yes

Phenylephrine, Chlorpheniramine, Phenylpropanolamine, and Belladonna Alkaloids *see* Chlorpheniramine, Phenylephrine, Phenylpropanolamine, and Belladonna Alkaloids *on page 221*

Phenylfenesin® L.A. *see* Guaifenesin and Phenylpropanolamine *on page 454*

Phenylpropanolamine (fen il proe pa NOLE a meen)

Related Information

Phenyltoloxamine, Phenylpropanolamine, Pyrilamine, and Pheniramine *on next page*

Brand Names Acutrim® 16 Hours [OTC]; Acutrim® II, Maximum Strength [OTC]; Acutrim® Late Day [OTC]; Control® [OTC]; Dexatrim® Pre-Meal [OTC]; Maximum Strength Dex-A-Diet® [OTC]; Maximum Strength Dexatrim® [OTC]; Phenoxine® [OTC]; Phenyldrine® [OTC]; Prolamine® [OTC]; Propagest® [OTC]; Rhindecon®; Unitrol® [OTC]

Therapeutic Category Adrenergic Agonist Agent; Anorexiant; Decongestant; Nasal Agent, Vasoconstrictor

Synonyms Fenilpropanolamina (Mexico)

Use Anorexiant; nasal decongestant

Usual Dosage Oral:

Children: Decongestant:

2-6 years: 6.25 mg every 4 hours

6-12 years: 12.5 mg every 4 hours not to exceed 75 mg/day

Adults:

Decongestant: 25 mg every 4 hours or 50 mg every 8 hours, not to exceed 150 mg/day

Anorexic: 25 mg 3 times/day 30 minutes before meals or 75 mg (timed release) once daily in the morning

Precision release: 75 mg after breakfast

Mechanism of Action Releases tissue stores of epinephrine and thereby produces an alpha- and beta-adrenergic stimulation; this causes vasoconstriction and nasal mucosa blanching; also appears to depress central appetite centers

Local Anesthetic/Vasoconstrictor Precautions Use with caution since phenylpropanolamine is a sympathomimetic amine which could interact with epinephrine to cause a pressor response

Effects on Dental Treatment Up to 10% of patients could experience tachycardia, palpitations, and dry mouth; use vasoconstrictor with caution

Other Adverse Effects

>10%: Cardiovascular: Hypertension, palpitations

1% to 10%:
  Central nervous system: Insomnia, restlessness, dizziness
  Gastrointestinal: Dry mouth, nausea
<1%:
  Cardiovascular: Tightness in chest, bradycardia, arrhythmias, angina
  Central nervous system: Severe headache, anxiety, nervousness
  Genitourinary: Dysuria
Drug Interactions
  Decreased effect of antihypertensives
  Increased effect/toxicity with MAO inhibitors (hypertensive crisis), beta-blockers
  (increased pressor effects)
Drug Uptake
  Absorption: Oral: Well absorbed
  Serum half-life: 4.6-6.6 hours
Pregnancy Risk Factor C
Generic Available Yes

Phenylpropanolamine and Brompheniramine see Brompheniramine and Phenyl-propanolamine *on page 143*

Phenylpropanolamine and Caramiphen see Caramiphen and Phenylpropanolamine *on page 173*

Phenylpropanolamine and Chlorpheniramine see Chlorpheniramine and Phenyl-propanolamine *on page 219*

Phenylpropanolamine and Guaifenesin see Guaifenesin and Phenylpropanolamine *on page 454*

Phenylpropanolamine and Hydrocodone see Hydrocodone and Phenylpropanola-mine *on page 483*

Phenylpropanolamine, Chlorpheniramine, Phenylephrine, and Belladonna Alkaloids see Chlorpheniramine, Phenylephrine, Phenylpropanolamine, and Bella-donna Alkaloids *on page 221*

Phenyltoloxamine, Phenylpropanolamine, and Acetaminophen

(fen il tol OKS a meen, fen il proe pa NOLE a meen, & a seet a MIN oh fen)
Brand Names Sinubid®
Therapeutic Category Analgesic, Non-narcotic; Antihistamine/Decongestant Combination
Use Intermittent symptomatic treatment of nasal congestion in sinus or other frontal headache; allergic rhinitis, vasomotor rhinitis, coryza; facial pain and pressure of acute and chronic sinusitis
Local Anesthetic/Vasoconstrictor Precautions Use with caution since phenylpropanolamine is a sympathomimetic amine which could interact with epinephrine to cause a pressor response
Effects on Dental Treatment
  Acetaminophen: No effects or complications reported
  Phenylpropanolamine: Up to 10% of patients could experience tachycardia, palpitations, and dry mouth; use vasoconstrictor with caution
Pregnancy Risk Factor C
Generic Available Yes
Selected Readings
  Barker JD Jr, de Carle DJ, and Anuras S, "Chronic Excessive Acetaminophen Use in Liver Damage," *Ann Intern Med*, 1977, 87(3):299-301.
  Dionne RA, Campbell RA, Cooper SA, et al, "Suppression of Postoperative Pain by Preoperative Administration of Ibuprofen in Comparison to Placebo, Acetaminophen, and Acetaminophen Plus Codeine," *J Clin Pharmacol*, 1983, 23(1):37-43.
  Licht H, Seeff LB, and Zimmerman HJ, "Apparent Potentiation of Acetaminophen Hepatotoxicity by Alcohol," *Ann Intern Med*, 1980, 92(4):511.

Phenyltoloxamine, Phenylpropanolamine, Pyrilamine, and Pheniramine

(fen il tol OKS a meen, fen il proe pa NOLE a meen, peer IL a meen, & fen IR a meen)
Brand Names Poly-Histine-D® Capsule
Therapeutic Category Cold Preparation
Use Treatment of nasal congestion
Usual Dosage Oral: Adults: One capsule every 8-12 hours
Local Anesthetic/Vasoconstrictor Precautions Use with caution since phenylpropanolamine is a sympathomimetic amine which could interact with epinephrine to cause a pressor response
Effects on Dental Treatment
  Phenylpropanolamine: Up to 10% of patients could experience tachycardia, palpitations, and dry mouth; use vasoconstrictor with caution
  Pyrilamine: No effects or complications reported
(Continued)

Phenyltoloxamine, Phenylpropanolamine, Pyrilamine, and Pheniramine *(Continued)*

Pheniramine: No effects or complications reported

Other Adverse Effects See individual agents

Drug Interactions See individual agents

Dosage Forms Capsule: Phenyltoloxamine citrate 16 mg, phenylpropanolamine hydrochloride 50 mg, pyrilamine maleate 16 mg, and pheniramine maleate 16 mg

Generic Available Yes

Phenytoin (FEN i toyn)

Related Information

Cardiovascular Diseases *on page 1010*

Brand Names Dilantin®; Diphenylan Sodium®

Canadian/Mexican Brand Names Tremytoine® (Canada)

Therapeutic Category Antiarrhythmic Agent, Class I-B; Antiarrhythmic Agent (Supraventricular & Ventricular); Anticonvulsant, Hydantoin

Use Management of generalized tonic-clonic (grand mal), simple partial and complex partial seizures; prevention of seizures following head trauma/neurosurgery; ventricular arrhythmias, including those associated with digitalis intoxication, prolonged Q-T interval and surgical repair of congenital heart diseases in children; also used for epidermolysis bullosa

Usual Dosage

Status epilepticus: I.V.:

Children: Loading dose: 15-20 mg/kg in a single or divided dose; maintenance dose: Initial: 5 mg/kg/day in 2 divided doses, usual doses:

6 months to 3 years: 8-10 mg/kg/day

4-6 years: 7.5-9 mg/kg/day

7-9 years: 7-8 mg/kg/day

10-16 years: 6-7 mg/kg/day, some patients may require every 8 hours dosing

Adults: Loading dose: 15-20 mg/kg in a single or divided dose, followed by 100-150 mg/dose at 30-minute intervals up to a maximum of 1500 mg/24 hours; maintenance dose: 300 mg/day or 5-6 mg/kg/day in 3 divided doses or 1-2 divided doses using extended release

Anticonvulsant: Children and Adults: Oral:

Loading dose: 15-20 mg/kg; based on phenytoin serum concentrations and recent dosing history; administer oral loading dose in 3 divided doses given every 2-4 hours to decrease GI adverse effects and to ensure complete oral absorption; maintenance dose: same as I.V.

Mechanism of Action Stabilizes neuronal membranes and decreases seizure activity by increasing efflux or decreasing influx of sodium ions across cell membranes in the motor cortex during generation of nerve impulses; prolongs effective refractory period and suppresses ventricular pacemaker automaticity, shortens action potential in the heart

Local Anesthetic/Vasoconstrictor Precautions No information available to require special precautions

Effects on Dental Treatment Gingival hyperplasia is a common problem observed during the first 6 months of phenytoin therapy appearing as gingivitis or gum inflammation. To minimize severity and growth rate of gingival tissue begin a program of professional cleaning and patient plaque control within 10 days of starting anticonvulsant therapy.

Other Adverse Effects

>10%:

Central nervous system: Psychiatric changes, slurred speech, dizziness, drowsiness

Gastrointestinal: Constipation, nausea, vomiting, gingival hyperplasia

Neuromuscular & skeletal: Trembling

1% to 10%:

Central nervous system: Headache, insomnia

Dermatologic: Skin rash

Gastrointestinal: Anorexia, weight loss

Hematologic: Leukopenia, elevated serum creatinine

Hepatic: Hepatitis

<1%:

Cardiovascular: Hypotension, bradycardia, cardiac arrhythmias, cardiovascular collapse

Central nervous system: Confusion, fever, ataxia

Local: Thrombophlebitis, venous irritation and pain

Neuromuscular & skeletal: Peripheral neuropathy, paresthesia

Ocular: Diplopia, nystagmus, blurred vision

Rarely seen effects: SLE-like syndrome, lymphadenopathy, hepatitis, Stevens-Johnson syndrome, blood dyscrasias, dyskinesias, pseudolymphoma, lymphoma

Drug Interactions Phenytoin is an inducer of cytochrome P-450 IIIA enzymes and is associated with many drug interactions

Decreased effect: Rifampin, cisplatin, vinblastine, bleomycin, folic acid, continuous NG feedings

Increased toxicity: Amiodarone decreases metabolism of phenytoin; disulfiram decreases metabolism of phenytoin; fluconazole, itraconazole decreases phenytoin serum concentrations; isoniazid may increase phenytoin serum concentrations

Increased effect/toxicity of valproic acid, ethosuximide, primidone, warfarin, oral contraceptives, corticosteroids, cyclosporine, theophylline, chloramphenicol, rifampin, doxycycline, quinidine, mexiletine, disopyramide, dopamine, nondepolarizing skeletal muscle relaxants

Drug Uptake

Absorption: Oral: Slow

Time to peak serum concentration (dependent upon formulation administered): Oral:

Extended-release capsule: Within 4-12 hours

Immediate release preparation: Within 2-3 hours

Pregnancy Risk Factor D

Generic Available Yes

Selected Readings

Dooley G and Vasan N, "Dilantin Hyperplasia: A Review of the Literature," *J N Z Soc Periodontol*, 1989, 68:19-22.

Iacopino AM, Doxey D, Cutler CW, et al, "Phenytoin and Cyclosporine A Specifically Regulate Macrophage Phenotype and Expression of Platelet-Derived Growth Factor and Interleukin-1 In Vitro and In Vivo: Possible Molecular Mechanism of Drug-Induced Gingival Hyperplasia," *J Periodontol*, 1997, 68(1):73-83.

Pihlstrom BL, "Prevention and Treatment of Dilantin-Associated Gingival Enlargement," *Compendium*, 1990, 14:S506-10.

Saito K, Mori S, Iwakura M, et al, "Immunohistochemical Localization of Transforming Growth Factor Beta, Basic Fibroblast Growth Factor and Heparin Sulphate Glycosaminoglycan in Gingival Hyperplasia Induced by Nifedipine and Phenytoin," *J Periodontal Res*, 1996, 31(8):545-5.

Zhou LX, Pihlstrom B, Hardwick JP, et al, "Metabolism of Phenytoin by the Gingiva of Normal Humans: The Possible Role of Reactive Metabolites of Phenytoin in the Initiation of Gingival Hyperplasia," *Clin Pharmacol Ther*, 1996, 60(2):191-8.

Phenytoin With Phenobarbital (FEN i toyn with fee noe BAR bi tal)

Brand Names Dilantin® With Phenobarbital

Therapeutic Category Anticonvulsant, Barbiturate; Anticonvulsant, Hydantoin

Use Management of generalized tonic-clonic (grand mal), simple partial and complex partial seizures

Local Anesthetic/Vasoconstrictor Precautions No information available to require special precautions

Effects on Dental Treatment Gingival hyperplasia is a common problem observed during the first 6 months of phenytoin therapy appearing as gingivitis or gum inflammation. To minimize severity and growth rate of gingival tissue begin a program of professional cleaning and patient plaque control within 10 days of starting anticonvulsant therapy.

Pregnancy Risk Factor D

Generic Available No

Pherazine® VC w/ Codeine see Promethazine, Phenylephrine, and Codeine *on page 806*

Pherazine® w/DM see Promethazine and Dextromethorphan *on page 805*

Pherazine® With Codeine see Promethazine and Codeine *on page 805*

Phicon® [OTC] see Pramoxine *on page 784*

Phillips'® Milk of Magnesia [OTC] see Magnesium Hydroxide *on page 576*

pHisoHex® see Hexachlorophene *on page 470*

pHiso® Scrub see Hexachlorophene *on page 470*

Phos-Flur® see Fluoride *on page 415*

PhosLo® see Calcium Acetate *on page 162*

Phospholine Iodide® see Echothiophate Iodide *on page 343*

Phosphorated Carbohydrate Solution

(FOS for ate ed kar boe HYE drate soe LOO shun)

Brand Names Emecheck® [OTC]; Emetrol® [OTC]; Naus-A-Way® [OTC]; Nausetrol® [OTC]

Therapeutic Category Antiemetic

Synonyms Dextrose, Levulose and Phosphoric Acid; Levulose, Dextrose and Phosphoric Acid; Phosphoric Acid, Levulose and Dextrose

(Continued)

Phosphorated Carbohydrate Solution *(Continued)*

Use Relief of nausea associated with upset stomach that occurs with intestinal flu, pregnancy, food indiscretions, and emotional upsets

Local Anesthetic/Vasoconstrictor Precautions No information available to require special precautions

Effects on Dental Treatment No effects or complications reported

Other Adverse Effects 1% to 10%: Gastrointestinal: Abdominal pain, diarrhea

Generic Available Yes

Phosphoric Acid, Levulose and Dextrose *see* Phosphorated Carbohydrate Solution *on previous page*

Photofrin® *see* Porfimer *on page 774*

Phrenilin® *see* Butalbital Compound *on page 154*

Phrenilin® *see* Butalbital Compound and Acetaminophen *on page 155*

Phrenilin® Forte® *see* Butalbital Compound *on page 154*

Phrenilin Forte® *see* Butalbital Compound and Acetaminophen *on page 155*

Phyllocontin® *see* Aminophylline *on page 56*

Phylloquinone (Canada) *see* Phytonadione *on this page*

Physostigmine *(fye zoe STIG meen)*

Brand Names Antilirium®; Isopto® Eserine®

Therapeutic Category Antidote, Anticholinergic Agent; Antiglaucoma Agent; Cholinergic Agent; Cholinergic Agent, Ophthalmic

Use Reverse toxic CNS effects caused by anticholinergic drugs; used as miotic in treatment of glaucoma

Usual Dosage

Children: Anticholinergic drug overdose: Reserve for life-threatening situations only: I.V.: 0.01-0.03 mg/kg/dose, (maximum: 0.5 mg/minute); may repeat after 5-10 minutes to a maximum total dose of 2 mg or until response occurs or adverse cholinergic effects occur

Adults: Anticholinergic drug overdose:

I.M., I.V., S.C.: 0.5-2 mg to start, repeat every 20 minutes until response occurs or adverse effect occurs

Repeat 1-4 mg every 30-60 minutes as life-threatening signs (arrhythmias, seizures, deep coma) recur; maximum I.V. rate: 1 mg/minute

Ophthalmic:

Ointment: Instill a small quantity to lower fornix up to 3 times/day

Solution: Instill 1-2 drops into eye(s) up to 4 times/day

Mechanism of Action Inhibits destruction of acetylcholine by acetylcholinesterase which facilitates transmission of impulses across myoneural junction and prolongs the central and peripheral effects of acetylcholine

Local Anesthetic/Vasoconstrictor Precautions No information available to require special precautions

Effects on Dental Treatment No effects or complications reported

Other Adverse Effects Ophthalmic:

>10%:

Ocular: Lacrimation, marked miosis, blurred vision, eye pain

Miscellaneous: Sweating

1% to 10%:

Central nervous system: Headache, browache

Dermatologic: Burning, redness

Drug Interactions No data reported with ophthalmic use

Drug Uptake

Onset of action:

Ophthalmic instillation: Within 2 minutes

Parenteral: Within 5 minutes

Absorption: I.M., ophthalmic, S.C.: Readily absorbed

Serum half-life: 15-40 minutes

Pregnancy Risk Factor C

Generic Available Yes: Ophthalmic

Phytomenadione (Canada) *see* Phytonadione *on this page*

Phytonadione *(fye toe na DYE one)*

Brand Names AquaMEPHYTON®; Konakion®; Mephyton®

Therapeutic Category Vitamin, Fat Soluble

Synonyms Phylloquinone (Canada); Phytomenadione (Canada)

Use Prevention and treatment of hypoprothrombinemia caused by drug-induced or anticoagulant-induced vitamin K deficiency, hemorrhagic disease of the newborn; phytonadione is more effective and is preferred to other vitamin K preparations in the presence of impending hemorrhage; oral absorption depends on the presence of bile salts

Usual Dosage I.V. route should be restricted for emergency use only

Minimum daily requirement: Not well established

Adults: 0.03 mcg/kg/day

Hemorrhagic disease of the newborn:

Prophylaxis: I.M., S.C.: 0.5-1 mg within 1 hour of birth

Treatment: I.M., S.C.: 1-2 mg/dose/day

Oral anticoagulant overdose:

Children and Adults: Oral, I.M., I.V., S.C.: 2.5-10 mg/dose; rarely up to 25-50 mg has been used; may repeat in 6-8 hours if given by I.M., I.V., S.C. route; may repeat 12-48 hours after oral route

Vitamin K deficiency: Due to drugs, malabsorption or decreased synthesis of vitamin K

Children:

Oral: 2.5-5 mg/24 hours

I.M., I.V.: 1-2 mg/dose as a single dose

Adults:

Oral: 5-25 mg/24 hours

I.M., I.V.: 10 mg

Mechanism of Action Promotes liver synthesis of clotting factors (II, VII, IX, X); however, the exact mechanism as to this stimulation is unknown. Menadiol is a water soluble form of vitamin K; phytonadione has a more rapid and prolonged effect than menadione; menadiol sodium diphosphate (K_4) is half as potent as menadione (K_3).

Local Anesthetic/Vasoconstrictor Precautions No information available to require special precautions

Effects on Dental Treatment No effects or complications reported

Other Adverse Effects <1%:

Cardiovascular: Transient flushing reaction, rarely hypotension, cyanosis

Central nervous system: Rarely dizziness, pain

Gastrointestinal: Dysgeusia, GI upset (oral)

Hematologic: Hemolysis in neonates and in patients with G-6-PD deficiency

Local: Tenderness at injection site

Respiratory: Dyspnea

Miscellaneous: Sweating, anaphylaxis, hypersensitivity reactions

Drug Interactions Warfarin sodium, dicumarol, and anisindione effects antagonized by phytonadione

Drug Uptake

Onset of increased coagulation factors:

Oral: Within 6-12 hours

Parenteral: Within 1-2 hours; patient may become normal after 12-14 hours

Absorption: Oral: Absorbed from the intestines in the presence of bile

Pregnancy Risk Factor C

Generic Available Yes

Pilagan® see Pilocarpine *on this page*

Pilocar® see Pilocarpine *on this page*

Pilocarpine (pye loe KAR peen)

Related Information

Dentin Hypersensitivity; High Caries Index; Xerostomia *on page 1074*

Patients Undergoing Cancer Therapy *on page 1083*

Brand Names Adsorbocarpine®; Akarpine®; Isopto® Carpine®; Ocu-Carpine®; Ocusert® Pilo; Ocusert Pilo-20®; Ocusert Pilo-40®; Pilagan®; Pilocar®; Pilopine HS®; Piloptic®; Pilostat®

Canadian/Mexican Brand Names Minims® Pilocarpine (Canada)

Therapeutic Category Antiglaucoma Agent; Cholinergic Agent, Ophthalmic; Ophthalmic Agent, Miotic

Use Management of chronic simple glaucoma, chronic and acute angle-closure glaucoma; counter effects of cycloplegics

Usual Dosage Adults:

Ophthalmic:

Nitrate solution: Shake well before using; instill 1-2 drops 2-4 times/day

Hydrochloride solution:

Instill 1-2 drops up to 6 times/day; adjust the concentration and frequency as required to control elevated intraocular pressure

To counteract the mydriatic effects of sympathomimetic agents: Instill 1 drop of a 1% solution in the affected eye

Gel: Instill 0.5" ribbon into lower conjunctival sac once daily at bedtime

(Continued)

Pilocarpine *(Continued)*

Ocular systems: Systems are labeled in terms of mean rate of release of pilocarpine over 7 days; begin with 20 mcg/hour at night and adjust based on response

Oral: 5 mg 3 times/day, titration up to 10 mg 3 times/day may be considered for patients who have not responded adequately

Mechanism of Action Directly stimulates cholinergic receptors in the eye causing miosis (by contraction of the iris sphincter), loss of accommodation (by constriction of ciliary muscle), and lowering of intraocular pressure (with decreased resistance to aqueous humor outflow)

Local Anesthetic/Vasoconstrictor Precautions No information available to require special precautions

Effects on Dental Treatment No effects or complications reported

Other Adverse Effects

>10%: Ocular: Blurred vision, miosis

1% to 10%:

Central nervous system: Headache, browache

Genitourinary: Frequent urination

Local: Stinging, burning, lacrimation

Ocular: Ciliary spasm, retinal detachment, photophobia, acute iritis, conjunctival and ciliary congestion early in therapy

Miscellaneous: Hypersensitivity reactions

<1%:

Cardiovascular: Hypertension, tachycardia

Gastrointestinal: Nausea, vomiting, diarrhea, salivation

Miscellaneous: Sweating

Drug Interactions Concurrent use with beta-blockers may cause conduction disturbances; pilocarpine may antagonize the effects of anticholinergic drugs

Drug Uptake

Ophthalmic instillation:

Miosis:

Onset of effect: Within 10-30 minutes

Duration: 4-8 hours

Intraocular pressure reduction:

Onset of effect: 1 hour required

Duration: 4-12 hours

Ocusert® Pilo application:

Miosis: Onset of effect: 1.5-2 hours

Reduced intraocular pressure:

Onset: Within 1.5-2 hours; miosis within 10-30 minutes

Duration: ~1 week

Pregnancy Risk Factor C

Dosage Forms See table.

Pilocarpine

Dosage Form	Strength %	1 mL	2 mL	15 mL	30 mL	3.5 g
Gel	4					x
Solution as hydrochloride	0.25			x		
	0.5			x	x	
	1	x	x	x	x	
	2	x	x	x	x	
	3			x	x	
	4	x	x	x	x	
	6			x	x	
	8		x			
	10			x		
Solution as nitrate	1			x		
	2			x		
	4			x		
Ocusert® Pilo-20: Releases 20 mcg/hour for 1 week						
Ocusert® Pilo-40: Releases 40 mcg/hour for 1 week						

Generic Available Yes: Hydrochloride Solution

Pilocarpine and Epinephrine (pye loe KAR peen & ep i NEF rin)

Brand Names E-Pilo-x® Ophthalmic; P₁E₁® Ophthalmic

Therapeutic Category Antiglaucoma Agent; Ophthalmic Agent, Miotic

Use Treatment of glaucoma; counter effect of cycloplegics

Local Anesthetic/Vasoconstrictor Precautions No information available to require special precautions

Effects on Dental Treatment No effects or complications reported

Other Adverse Effects 1% to 10%:

Cardiovascular: Tachycardia, hypertension

Central nervous system: Headache

Gastrointestinal: Salivation

Ocular: Miosis, ciliary spasm, blurred vision, retinal detachment, stinging, lacrimation, itching, vitreous hemorrhages, photophobia, acute iritis

Miscellaneous: Hypersensitivity reactions

Pregnancy Risk Factor C

Generic Available No

Pilocarpine (Dental) (pye loe KAR peen)

Brand Names Salagen®

Therapeutic Category Cholinergic Agent

Use

Dental: Treatment of xerostomia caused by radiation therapy in patients with head and neck cancer and from Sjögren's syndrome

Medical: No data reported

Usual Dosage Adults: 1-2 tablets 3-4 times/day not to exceed 30 mg/day; patients should be treated for a minimum of 90 days for optimum effects

Mechanism of Action Pilocarpine stimulates the muscarinic-type acetylcholine receptors in the salivary glands within the parasympathetic division of the autonomic nervous system to cause an increase in serous-type saliva

Local Anesthetic/Vasoconstrictor Precautions No information available to require special precautions

Effects on Dental Treatment Salivation - therapeutic effect

Other Adverse Effects

>10%: Miscellaneous: Sweating

1% to 10%:

Central nervous system: Chills, headache, dizziness

Gastrointestinal: Nausea

Ocular: Lacrimation

Renal: Polyuria

Respiratory: Rhinitis, pharyngitis

Contraindications In patients with uncontrolled asthma, known hypersensitivity to pilocarpine and when miosis is undesirable (eg, narrow-angle glaucoma)

Warnings/Precautions In patients with chronic obstructive pulmonary disease, pilocarpine may stimulate the mucous cells of the respiratory tract and may increase airway resistance. Patients with cardiovascular disease may be unable to compensate for changes in heart rhythm that could be induced by pilocarpine.

Drug Interactions Concurrent use with anticholinergics may cause antagonism of pilocarpine's cholinergic effect; medications with cholinergic actions may result in additive cholinergic effects; beta-adrenergic receptor blocking drugs when used with pilocarpine may increase the possibility of myocardial conduction disturbances

Drug Uptake

Onset of action after single dose: 20 minutes

Duration: 3-5 hours

Serum half-life: 0.76 hours

Time to peak serum concentration: 1.25 hours

Pregnancy Risk Factor C

Breast-feeding Considerations May be taken while breast-feeding

Dosage Forms Tablet: 5 mg

Dietary Considerations No data reported

Generic Available Yes: Hydrochloride Solution

Comments Pilocarpine may have potential as a salivary stimulant in individuals suffering from xerostomia induced by antidepressants and other medications. At the present time however, the FDA has not approved pilocarpine for use in drug-induced xerostomia. Clinical studies are needed to evaluate pilocarpine for this type of indication. In an attempt to discern the efficacy of pilocarpine as a salivary stimulant in patients suffering from Sjögren's syndrome (SS), Rhodus and Schuh studied 9 patients with SS given daily doses of pilocarpine over a 6-week period. A dose of 5 mg daily produced a significant overall increase in both whole unstimulated salivary flow and parotid stimulated salivary flow. These results support the use of pilocarpine to increase salivary flow in patients with SS.

(Continued)

Pilocarpine (Dental) *(Continued)*

Selected Readings

Davies AN and Singer J, "A Comparison of Artificial Saliva and Pilocarpine in Radiation-Induced Xerostomia," *J Laryngol Otol*, 1994, 108(8):663-5.

Fox PC, "Management of Dry Mouth," *Dent Clin North Am*, 1997, 41(4):863-75.

Fox PC, Atkinson JC, Macynski AA, et al, " Pilocarpine Treatment of Salivary Gland Hypofunction and Dry Mouth (Xerostomia)," *Arch Intern Med*, 1991, 151(6):1149-52.

Garg AK and Malo M, "Manifestations and Treatment of Xerostomia and Associated Oral Effects Secondary to Head and Neck Radiation Therapy," *J Am Dent Assoc*, 1997, 128(8):1128-33.

Greenspan D and Daniels TE, "The Use of Pilocarpine in Postradiation Xerostomia," *J Dent Res*, 1979, 58:420.

Johnson JT, Ferretti GA, Nethery WJ, et al, "Oral Pilocarpine for Post-Irradiation Xerostomia in Patients With Head and Neck Cancer," *N Engl J Med*, 1993, 329(6):390-5.

Rhodus NL and Schuh MJ, "Effects of Pilocarpine on Salivary Flow in Patients With Sjögren's Syndrome," *Oral Surg Oral Med Oral Pathol*, 1991, 72:545-9.

Rieke JW, Hafermann MD, Johnson JT, et al, "Oral Pilocarpine for Radiation-Induced Xerostomia: Integrated Efficacy and Safety Results From Two Prospective Randomized Clinical Trials," *Int J Radiat Oncol Biol Phys*, 1995, 31(3):661-9.

Rousseau P, "Pilocarpine in Radiation-Induced Xerostomia," *Am J Hosp Palliat Care*, 1995, 12(2):38-9.

Schuller DE, Stevens P, Clausen KP, et al, "Treatment of Radiation Side Effects With Pilocarpine," *J Surg Oncol*, 1989, 42(4):272-6.

Singhal S, Mehta J, Rattenbury H, et al, "Oral Pilocarpine Hydrochloride for the Treatment of Refractory Xerostomia Associated With Chronic Graft-Versus-Host Disease," *Blood*, 1995, 85(4):1147-8.

Valdez IH, Wolff A, Atkinson JC, et al, "Use of Pilocarpine During Head and Neck Radiation Therapy to Reduce Xerostomia Salivary Dysfunction," *Cancer*, 1993, 71(5):1848-51.

Wiseman LR and Faulds D, "Oral Pilocarpine: A Review of Its Pharmacological Properties and Clinical Potential in Xerostomia," *Drugs*, 1995, 49(1):143-55.

Wynn RL, "Oral Pilocarpine (Salagen®) - A Recently Approved Salivary Stimulant," *Gen Dent*, 1996, 44(1):26,29-30.

Zimmerman RP, Mark RJ, Tran LM, et al, "Concomitant Pilocarpine During Head and Neck Irradiation Is Associated With Decreased Post-Treatment Xerostomia," *Int J Radiat Oncol Biol Phys*, 1997, 37(3):571-5.

Pilopine HS® *see Pilocarpine on page 759*

Piloptic® *see Pilocarpine on page 759*

Pilostat® *see Pilocarpine on page 759*

Pima® *see Potassium Iodide on page 781*

Pimozide *(PI moe zide)*

Brand Names Orap™

Therapeutic Category Neuroleptic Agent

Use Suppression of severe motor and phonic tics in patients with Tourette's disorder

Usual Dosage Children >12 years and Adults: Oral: Initial: 1-2 mg/day, then increase dosage as needed every other day; range is usually 7-16 mg/day, maximum dose: 20 mg/day or 0.3 mg/kg/day should not be exceeded

Mechanism of Action A potent centrally acting dopamine receptor antagonist resulting in its characteristic neuroleptic effects

Local Anesthetic/Vasoconstrictor Precautions No information available to require special precautions

Effects on Dental Treatment >10% of patients experience dry mouth

Other Adverse Effects

>10%:

    Cardiovascular: Tachycardia, orthostatic hypotension

    Central nervous system: Akathisia, akinesia, extrapyramidal effects, drowsiness

    Dermatologic: Skin rash

    Endocrine & metabolic: Swelling of breasts

    Gastrointestinal: Constipation

1% to 10%:

    Cardiovascular: Swelling of face

    Central nervous system: Tardive dyskinesia, mental depression

    Gastrointestinal: Diarrhea, anorexia

<1%:

    Central nervous system: Neuroleptic malignant syndrome (NMS)

    Hematologic: Blood dyscrasias

    Hepatic: Jaundice

Contraindications Simple tics other than Tourette's, history of cardiac dysrhythmias, known hypersensitivity to pimozide; use in patients receiving macrolide antibiotics such as clarithromycin, erythromycin, azithromycin, and dirithromycin

Drug Interactions Increased effect/toxicity of alfentanil, CNS depressants, guanabenz (increased sedation), MAO inhibitors

Drug Uptake

    Absorption: Oral: 50%

    Serum half-life: 50 hours

Time to peak serum concentration: Within 6-8 hours

Pregnancy Risk Factor C

Generic Available No

Selected Readings

"Pimozide (Orap) Contraindicated With Clarithromycin (Biaxin) and Other Macrolide Antibiotics," *FDA Medical Bulletin*, October 1996, 3.

Pindolol (PIN doe lole)

Related Information

Cardiovascular Diseases *on page 1010*

Brand Names Visken®

Canadian/Mexican Brand Names Apo®-Pindol (Canada); Gen-Pindolol® (Canada); Novo-Pindol® (Canada); Nu-Pindol® (Canada); Syn-Pindol® (Canada)

Therapeutic Category Beta-adrenergic Blocker, Noncardioselective

Use Management of hypertension

Unlabeled use: Ventricular arrhythmias/tachycardia, antipsychotic-induced akathisia, situational anxiety; aggressive behavior associated with dementia

Usual Dosage

Adults: Initial: 5 mg twice daily, increase as necessary by 10 mg/day every 3-4 weeks; maximum daily dose: 60 mg

Elderly: Initial: 5 mg once daily, increase as necessary by 5 mg/day every 3-4 weeks

Mechanism of Action Blocks both $beta_1$- and $beta_2$-receptors and has mild intrinsic sympathomimetic activity; pindolol has negative inotropic and chronotropic effects and can significantly slow A-V nodal conduction

Local Anesthetic/Vasoconstrictor Precautions Use with caution; epinephrine has interacted with nonselective beta-blockers to result in initial hypertensive episode followed by bradycardia

Effects on Dental Treatment Noncardioselective beta-blockers (ie, propranolol, nadolol, pindolol) enhance the pressor response to epinephrine, resulting in hypertension and bradycardia. Many nonsteroidal anti-inflammatory drugs such as ibuprofen and indomethacin can reduce the hypotensive effect of beta-blockers after 3 or more weeks of therapy with the NSAID. Short-term NSAID use (ie, 3 days) requires no special precautions in patients taking beta-blockers.

Other Adverse Effects

>10%:

Central nervous system: Anxiety, dizziness, insomnia, fatigue

Endocrine & metabolic: Decreased sexual ability

Neuromuscular & skeletal: Arthralgia, back pain, weakness

1% to 10%:

Cardiovascular: Congestive heart failure, arrhythmia, reduced peripheral circulation

Central nervous system: Hallucinations, nightmares, vivid dreams

Dermatologic: Skin rash, itching

Gastrointestinal: Diarrhea, nausea, vomiting, stomach discomfort

Neuromuscular & skeletal: Numbness of extremities

Respiratory: Dyspnea

<1%:

Cardiovascular: Bradycardia, chest pain

Central nervous system: Confusion, mental depression

Hematologic: Thrombocytopenia

Ocular: Dry eyes

Drug Interactions

Decreased effect of beta-blockers:

Barbiturates (increased liver metabolism of beta-blockers to result in lower serum levels)

NSAIDs (attenuate the hypotensive therapeutic effects of beta-blockers)

Rifampin (increased liver metabolism of beta-blockers to result in lower serum levels)

Increased effects of beta-blockers:

Calcium channel blockers (increase serum levels of beta-blockers by unknown mechanism to enhance hypotension)

Beta-Blockers increase the effects of:

Epinephrine (vasoconstrictor; initial hypertensive episode followed by bradycardia) only from noncardioselective type beta-blockers

Drug Uptake

Absorption: Oral: Rapid, 50% to 95%

Serum half-life: 2.5-4 hours; increased with renal insufficiency, age, and cirrhosis

Time to peak serum concentration: Within 1-2 hours

Pregnancy Risk Factor B

Generic Available Yes

(Continued)

Pindolol *(Continued)*

Selected Readings

Foster CA and Aston SJ, "Propranolol-Epinephrine Interaction: A Potential Disaster," *Plast Reconstr Surg*, 1983, 72(1):74-8.

Wong DG, Spence JD, Lamki L, et al, "Effect of Nonsteroidal Anti-inflammatory Drugs on Control of Hypertension of Beta-Blockers and Diuretics," *Lancet*, 1986, 1(8488):997-1001.

Wynn RL, "Dental Nonsteroidal Anti-inflammatory Drugs and Prostaglandin-Based Drug Interactions, Part Two," *Gen Dent*, 1992, 40(2):104, 106, 108.

Wynn RL, "Epinephrine Interactions With Beta-Blockers," *Gen Dent*, 1994, 42(1):16, 18.

Pink Bismuth® (subsalicylate) [OTC] *see* Bismuth *on page 131*

Pin-Rid® [OTC] *see* Pyrantel Pamoate *on page 822*

Pin-X® [OTC] *see* Pyrantel Pamoate *on page 822*

Piperacilina (Mexico) *see* Piperacillin *on this page*

Piperacillin *(pi PER a sil in)*

Brand Names Pipracil®

Therapeutic Category Antibiotic, Penicillin

Synonyms Piperacilina (Mexico)

Use Treatment of susceptible infections such as septicemia, acute and chronic respiratory tract infections, skin and soft tissue infections, and urinary tract infections due to susceptible strains of *Pseudomonas*, *Proteus*, and *Escherichia coli* and *Enterobacter*; normally used with other antibiotics (ie, aminoglycosides)

Usual Dosage

Children: I.M., I.V.: 200-300 mg/kg/day in divided doses every 4-6 hours; maximum dose: 24 g/day

Higher doses have been used in cystic fibrosis: 350-500 mg/kg/day in divided doses every 4 hours

Adults:

I.M.: 2-3 g/dose every 6-12 hours; maximum: 24 g/24 hours

I.V.: 3-4 g/dose every 4-6 hours; maximum: 24 g/24 hours

Mechanism of Action Inhibits bacterial cell wall synthesis by binding to one or more of the penicillin binding proteins (PBPs); which in turn inhibits the final transpeptidation step of peptidoglycan synthesis in bacterial cell walls, thus inhibiting cell wall biosynthesis. Bacteria eventually lyse due to ongoing activity of cell wall autolytic enzymes (autolysins and murein hydrolases) while cell wall assembly is arrested.

Local Anesthetic/Vasoconstrictor Precautions No information available to require special precautions

Effects on Dental Treatment Prolonged use of penicillins may lead to development of oral candidiasis

Other Adverse Effects <1%:

Central nervous system: Convulsions, confusion, drowsiness, fever

Dermatologic: Rash

Endocrine & metabolic: Electrolyte imbalance

Hematologic: Hemolytic anemia, positive Coombs' reaction, abnormal platelet aggregation and prolonged prothrombin time (high doses)

Local: Thrombophlebitis

Neuromuscular: Myoclonus

Renal: Acute interstitial nephritis

Miscellaneous: Hypersensitivity reactions, anaphylaxis, Jarisch-Herxheimer reaction

Drug Interactions

Decreased effect: Tetracyclines cause decreased penicillin effectiveness

Increased effect: Probenecid causes increased penicillin levels

Drug Uptake

Absorption: I.M.: 70% to 80%

Serum half-life: Dose-dependent; prolonged with moderately severe renal or hepatic impairment:

Adults: 36-80 minutes

Time to peak serum concentration: I.M.: Within 30-50 minutes

Pregnancy Risk Factor B

Generic Available No

Piperacillin and Tazobactam Sodium

(pi PER a sil in & ta zoe BAK tam SOW dee um)

Brand Names Zosyn™

Therapeutic Category Antibiotic, Penicillin

Use

Treatment of infections of lower respiratory tract, urinary tract, skin and skin structures, gynecologic, bone and joint infections, and septicemia caused by susceptible organisms. Tazobactam expands activity of piperacillin to include beta-lactamase producing strains of *S. aureus, H. influenzae, Enterobacteriaceae, Pseudomonas, Klebsiella, Citrobacter, Serratia, Bacteroides,* and other gram-negative anaerobes.

Application to nosocomial infections may be limited by restricted activity against gram-negative organisms producing class I beta-lactamases and inactivity against methicillin-resistant *Staphylococcus aureus*

Usual Dosage

Children <12 years: Not recommended due to lack of data

Children >12 years and Adults:

Severe infections: I.V.: Piperacillin/tazobactam 4/0.5 g every 8 hours or 3/0.375 g every 6 hours

Moderate infections: I.M.: Piperacillin/tazobactam 2/0.25 g every 6-1 hours; treatment should be continued for ≥7-10 days depending on severity of disease

Mechanism of Action Piperacillin interferes with bacterial cell wall synthesis during active multiplication, causing cell wall death and resultant bactericidal activity against susceptible bacteria; tazobactam prevents degradation of piperacillin by binding to the active side on beta-lactamase; tazobactam inhibits many beta-lactamases, including staphylococcal penicillinase and Richmond and Sykes types II, III, IV, and V, including extended spectrum enzymes; it has only limited activity against class I beta-lactamases other than class Ic types

Local Anesthetic/Vasoconstrictor Precautions No information available to require special precautions

Effects on Dental Treatment Prolonged use of penicillins may lead to development of oral candidiasis

Other Adverse Effects

>10%: Gastrointestinal: Diarrhea

1% to 10%:

Central nervous system: Insomnia, headache

Dermatologic: Rash, pruritus

Gastrointestinal: Constipation, nausea, vomiting, dyspepsia

Hematologic: Leukopenia

Miscellaneous: Serum sickness-like reaction

<1%:

Cardiovascular: Hypertension, hypotension, edema

Central nervous system: Dizziness, agitation, confusion

Gastrointestinal: Pseudomembranous colitis

Respiratory: Bronchospasm

Several laboratory abnormalities have rarely been associated with piperacillin/tazobactam including reversible eosinophilia, and neutropenia (associated most often with prolonged therapy), positive direct Coombs' test, prolonged PT and PTT, transient elevations of LFT, elevated creatinine

Drug Interactions

Decreased effect: Tetracyclines cause decreased penicillin effectiveness

Increased effect: Probenecid causes increased penicillin levels

Drug Uptake Both AUC and peak concentrations are dose proportional

Serum half-life:

Piperacillin: 1 hour

Metabolite: 1-1.5 hours

Tazobactam: 0.7-0.9 hour

Pregnancy Risk Factor B

Generic Available No

Piperazine (PI per a zeen)

Brand Names Vermizine®

Therapeutic Category Anthelmintic

Use Treatment of pinworm and roundworm infections (used as an alternative to first-line agents, mebendazole, or pyrantel pamoate)

Usual Dosage Oral:

Pinworms: Children and Adults: 65 mg/kg/day (not to exceed 2.5 g/day) as a single daily dose for 7 days; in severe infections, repeat course after a 1-week interval

Roundworms:

Children: 75 mg/kg/day as a single daily dose for 2 days; maximum: 3.5 g/day

Adults: 3.5 g/day for 2 days (in severe infections, repeat course, after a 1-week interval)

Mechanism of Action Causes muscle paralysis of the roundworm by blocking the effects of acetylcholine at the neuromuscular junction

Local Anesthetic/Vasoconstrictor Precautions No information available to require special precautions

Effects on Dental Treatment No effects or complications reported

(Continued)

Piperazine *(Continued)*

Other Adverse Effects <1%:
Central nervous system: Dizziness, seizures, EEG changes, headache, vertigo
Gastrointestinal: Nausea, vomiting, diarrhea
Hematologic: Hemolytic anemia
Neuromuscular & skeletal: Weakness
Ocular: Visual impairment
Respiratory: Bronchospasms
Miscellaneous: Hypersensitivity reactions
Drug Interactions None reported
Drug Uptake
Absorption: Well absorbed from GI tract
Time to peak serum concentration: 1 hour
Pregnancy Risk Factor B
Generic Available Yes

Pipobroman (pi poe BROE man)

Brand Names Vercyte®
Therapeutic Category Antineoplastic Agent, Alkylating Agent
Use Treat polycythemia vera; chronic myelocytic leukemia
Usual Dosage Children >15 years and Adults: Oral:
Polycythemia: 1 mg/kg/day for 30 days; may increase to 1.5-3 mg/kg until hematocrit reduced to 50% to 55%; maintenance: 0.1-0.2 mg/kg/day
Myelocytic leukemia: 1.5-2.5 mg/kg/day until WBC drops to 10,000/mm^3 then start maintenance 7-175 mg/day; stop if WBC falls to <3000/mm^3 or platelets fall to <150,000/mm^3
Mechanism of Action An alkylating agent considered to be cell-cycle nonspecific and capable of killing tumor cells in any phase of the cell cycle. Alkylating agents form covalent cross-links with DNA thereby resulting in cytotoxic, mutagenic, and carcinogenic effects. The end result of the alkylation process results in the misreading of the DNA code and the inhibition of DNA, RNA, and protein synthesis in rapidly proliferating tumor cells.
Local Anesthetic/Vasoconstrictor Precautions No information available to require special precautions
Effects on Dental Treatment No effects or complications reported
Other Adverse Effects 1% to 10%:
Dermatologic: Rash
Gastrointestinal: Vomiting, diarrhea, nausea, abdominal cramps
Hematologic: Leukopenia, thrombocytopenia, anemia
Pregnancy Risk Factor D
Generic Available No

Pipracil® *see* Piperacillin *on page 764*
Pirazinamida (Mexico) *see* Pyrazinamide *on page 823*

Pirbuterol (peer BYOO ter ole)

Related Information
Respiratory Diseases *on page 1018*
Brand Names Maxair™
Therapeutic Category Antiasthmatic; Beta$_2$-Adrenergic Agonist Agent; Bronchodilator
Use Prevention and treatment of reversible bronchospasm including asthma
Usual Dosage Children >12 years and Adults: 2 inhalations every 4-6 hours for prevention; two inhalations at an interval of at least 1-3 minutes, followed by a third inhalation in treatment of bronchospasm, not to exceed 12 inhalations/day
Mechanism of Action Pirbuterol is a beta$_2$-adrenergic agonist with a similar structure to albuterol, specifically a pyridine ring has been substituted for the benzene ring in albuterol. The increased beta$_2$ selectivity of pirbuterol results from the substitution of a tertiary butyl group on the nitrogen of the side chain, which additionally imparts resistance of pirbuterol to degradation by monoamine oxidase and provides a lengthened duration of action in comparison to the less selective previous beta-agonist agents.
Local Anesthetic/Vasoconstrictor Precautions No information available to require special precautions
Effects on Dental Treatment No effects or complications reported
Other Adverse Effects
>10%:
Central nervous system: Nervousness, restlessness
Neuromuscular & skeletal: Trembling
1% to 10%:
Central nervous system: Headache, dizziness

Gastrointestinal: Taste changes, vomiting, nausea
<1%:
Cardiovascular: Hypertension, arrhythmias, chest pain
Central nervous system: Insomnia
Dermatologic: Bruising
Gastrointestinal: Anorexia
Neuromuscular & skeletal: Numbness in hands, weakness
Respiratory: Paradoxical bronchospasm
Drug Interactions Increased toxicity: Cardiovascular effects are potentiated in patients also receiving MAO inhibitors, tricyclic antidepressants, sympathomimetic agents (eg, amphetamine, dopamine, dobutamine), inhaled anesthetics (eg, enflurane)
Drug Uptake
Peak therapeutic effect:
Oral: 2-3 hours with peak serum concentration of 6.2-9.8 mcg/L
Inhalation: 0.5-1 hour
Serum half-life: 2-3 hours
Pregnancy Risk Factor C
Generic Available No

Piridoxina (Mexico) *see* Pyridoxine *on page 824*

Pirimetamina (Mexico) *see* Pyrimethamine *on page 825*

Piroxicam (peer OKS i kam)
Related Information
Nonsteroidal Anti-Inflammatory Agents, Comparative Dosages, and Pharmacokinetics *on page 1143*
Rheumatoid Arthritis and Osteoarthritis *on page 1030*
Brand Names Feldene®
Canadian/Mexican Brand Names Apo®-Piroxicam (Canada); Artyflam® (Mexico); Citoken® (Mexico); Facicam® (Mexico); Flogosan® (Mexico); Novo-Piroxicam® (Canada); Nu-Pirox® (Canada); Oxicanol® (Mexico); Piroxan® (Mexico); Piroxen® (Mexico); Pro-Piroxicam® (Canada); Rogal® (Mexico)
Therapeutic Category Analgesic, Non-narcotic; Anti-inflammatory Agent; Nonsteroidal Anti-inflammatory Agent (NSAID), Oral
Use Management of inflammatory disorders; symptomatic treatment of acute and chronic rheumatoid arthritis, osteoarthritis, and ankylosing spondylitis; also used to treat sunburn
Usual Dosage Oral:
Children: 0.2-0.3 mg/kg/day once daily; maximum dose: 15 mg/day
Adults: 10-20 mg/day once daily; although associated with increase in GI adverse effects, doses >20 mg/day have been used (ie, 30-40 mg/day)
Mechanism of Action Inhibits prostaglandin synthesis, acts on the hypothalamus heat-regulating center to reduce fever, blocks prostaglandin synthetase action which prevents formation of the platelet-aggregating substance thromboxane A_2; decreases pain receptor sensitivity. Other proposed mechanisms of action for salicylate anti-inflammatory action are lysosomal stabilization, kinin and leukotriene production, alteration of chemotactic factors, and inhibition of neutrophil activation. This latter mechanism may be the most significant pharmacologic action to reduce inflammation.
Local Anesthetic/Vasoconstrictor Precautions No information available to require special precautions
Effects on Dental Treatment No effects or complications reported
Other Adverse Effects
>10%:
Central nervous system: Dizziness
Dermatologic: Skin rash
Gastrointestinal: Abdominal cramps, heartburn, indigestion, nausea
1% to 10%:
Central nervous system: Headache, nervousness
Dermatologic: Itching
Endocrine & metabolic: Fluid retention
Gastrointestinal: Vomiting
Otic: Tinnitus
<1%:
Cardiovascular: Congestive heart failure, hypertension, arrhythmias, tachycardia
Central nervous system: Confusion, hallucinations, aseptic meningitis, mental depression, drowsiness, insomnia
Dermatologic: Urticaria, erythema multiforme, toxic epidermal necrolysis, Stevens-Johnson syndrome, angioedema
Endocrine & metabolic: Polydipsia, hot flashes
(Continued)

Piroxicam (Continued)

Gastrointestinal: Gastritis, GI ulceration
Genitourinary: Cystitis
Hematologic: Agranulocytosis, anemia, hemolytic anemia, bone marrow suppression, leukopenia, thrombocytopenia
Hepatic: Hepatitis
Neuromuscular & skeletal: Peripheral neuropathy
Ocular: Toxic amblyopia, blurred vision, conjunctivitis, dry eyes
Otic: Decreased hearing
Renal: Polyuria, acute renal failure
Respiratory: Allergic rhinitis, dyspnea, epistaxis

Drug Interactions
Decreased effect of diuretics, beta-blockers; decreased effect with aspirin, antacids, cholestyramine
Increased effect/toxicity of lithium, warfarin, methotrexate (controversial)

Drug Uptake
Onset of analgesia: Oral: Within 1 hour
Serum half-life: 45-50 hours

Pregnancy Risk Factor B (D if used in the 3rd trimester or near delivery)

Generic Available Yes

Pitocin® *see* Oxytocin *on page 719*

Pitressin® *see* Vasopressin *on page 985*

Pix Carbonis *see* Coal Tar *on page 254*

Placidyl® *see* Ethchlorvynol *on page 374*

Plaquenil® *see* Hydroxychloroquine *on page 488*

Platinol® *see* Cisplatin *on page 237*

Platinol®-AQ *see* Cisplatin *on page 237*

Plavix® *see* Clopidogrel *on page 251*

Plendil® *see* Felodipine *on page 395*

Plicamycin (plye kay MYE sin)

Brand Names Mithracin®

Therapeutic Category Antidote, Hypercalcemia; Antineoplastic Agent, Antibiotic

Use Malignant testicular tumors, in the treatment of hypercalcemia and hypercalciuria of malignancy not responsive to conventional treatment; Paget's disease

Usual Dosage Refer to individual protocols. Dose should be diluted in 1 L of D₅W or NS and administered over 4-6 hours

Dosage should be based on the patient's body weight. If a patient has abnormal fluid retention (ie, edema, hydrothorax or ascites), the patient's ideal weight rather than actual body weight should be used to calculate the dose.

Adults: I.V.:
Testicular cancer: 25-30 mcg/kg/day for 8-10 days
Blastic chronic granulocytic leukemia: 25 mcg/kg over 2-4 hours every other day for 3 weeks
Paget's disease: 15 mcg/kg/day once daily for 10 days
Hypercalcemia:
25 mcg/kg single dose which may be repeated in 48 hours if no response occurs
or 25 mcg/kg for 3-4 days
or 25-50 mcg/kg every other day for 3-8 doses

Mechanism of Action Potent osteoclast inhibitor; may inhibit parathyroid hormone effect on osteoclasts; inhibits bone resorption; forms a complex with DNA in the presence of magnesium or other divalent cations inhibiting DNA-directed RNA synthesis

Local Anesthetic/Vasoconstrictor Precautions No information available to require special precautions

Effects on Dental Treatment No effects or complications reported

Other Adverse Effects
>10%: Gastrointestinal: Nausea and vomiting occur in almost 100% of patients within the first 6 hours after treatment; incidence increases with rapid injection; stomatitis has also occurred; anorexia, diarrhea
1% to 10%:
Cardiovascular: Facial flushing
Central nervous system: Headache, fever, mental depression, drowsiness
Endocrine & metabolic: Hypocalcemia
Hematologic: Hemorrhagic diathesis, mild leukopenia and thrombocytopenia

Clotting disorders: May also depress hepatic synthesis of clotting factors, leading to a form of coagulopathy; petechiae, increased prothrombin time, epistaxis, and thrombocytopenia may be seen and may require discontinuation of the drug

Hepatic: Elevation in liver enzymes, hepatotoxicity

Local: Extravasation: Irritant; may produce local tissue irritation or cellulitis if infiltrated; if extravasation occurs, follow hospital procedure, discontinue I.V., and apply ice for 24 hours

Irritant chemotherapy

Neuromuscular & skeletal: Weakness

Renal: Nephrotoxicity, azotemia

Drug Interactions Increased toxicity: Calcitonin, etidronate, glucagon, causes additive hypoglycemic effects

Drug Uptake

Decreasing calcium levels:

Onset of action: Within 24 hours

Peak effect: 48-72 hours

Duration: 5-15 days

Serum half-life, plasma: 1 hour

Pregnancy Risk Factor D

Generic Available No

Pneumomist® see Guaifenesin *on page 452*

Podocon-25® see Podophyllum Resin *on this page*

Podofilox (po do FIL oks)

Brand Names Condylox®

Therapeutic Category Keratolytic Agent

Use Treatment of external genital warts

Local Anesthetic/Vasoconstrictor Precautions No information available to require special precautions

Effects on Dental Treatment No effects or complications reported

Pregnancy Risk Factor C

Generic Available No

Podofin® see Podophyllum Resin *on this page*

Podophyllin and Salicylic Acid (po DOF fil um & sal i SIL ik AS id)

Brand Names Verrex-C&M®

Therapeutic Category Keratolytic Agent

Synonyms Salicylic Acid and Podophyllin

Use Topical treatment of benign growths including external genital and perianal warts, papillomas, fibroids

Local Anesthetic/Vasoconstrictor Precautions No information available to require special precautions

Effects on Dental Treatment No effects or complications reported

Generic Available No

Podophyllum Resin (po DOF fil um REZ in)

Brand Names Podocon-25®; Podofin®

Canadian/Mexican Brand Names Podofilm® (Canada)

Therapeutic Category Keratolytic Agent

Use Topical treatment of benign growths including external genital and perianal warts, papillomas, fibroids; compound benzoin tincture generally is used as the medium for topical application

Usual Dosage Topical:

Children and Adults: 10% to 25% solution in compound benzoin tincture; apply drug to dry surface, use 1 drop at a time allowing drying between drops until area is covered; total volume should be limited to <0.5 mL per treatment session

Condylomata acuminatum: 25% solution is applied daily; use a 10% solution when applied to or near mucous membranes

Verrucae: 25% solution is applied 3-5 times/day directly to the wart

Mechanism of Action Directly affects epithelial cell metabolism by arresting mitosis through binding to a protein subunit of spindle microtubules (tubulin)

Local Anesthetic/Vasoconstrictor Precautions No information available to require special precautions

Effects on Dental Treatment No effects or complications reported

Other Adverse Effects Local: Pain, swelling

1% to 10%:

Dermatologic: Pruritus

(Continued)

Podophyllum Resin *(Continued)*

Gastrointestinal: Nausea, vomiting, abdominal pain, diarrhea

<1%:

Central nervous system: Confusion, lethargy, hallucinations
Hematologic: Leukopenia, thrombocytopenia
Hepatic: Hepatotoxicity
Neuromuscular & skeletal: Peripheral neuropathy
Renal: Renal failure

Drug Interactions No data reported

Pregnancy Risk Factor X

Generic Available Yes

Point-Two® *see* Fluoride *on page 415*

Poison Information Centers *see page 1206*

Poladex® *see* Dexchlorpheniramine *on page 293*

Polaramine® *see* Dexchlorpheniramine *on page 293*

Poliovirus Vaccine, Inactivated

(POE lee oh VYE rus vak SEEN, in ak ti VAY ted)

Brand Names IPOL™

Therapeutic Category Vaccine, Live Virus and Inactivated Virus

Synonyms Enhanced-potency Inactivated Poliovirus Vaccine; IPV; Salk Vaccine

Use Although a protective immune response to E-IPV cannot be assured in the immunocompromised individual, E-IPV is recommended because the vaccine is safe and some protection may result from its administration.

Usual Dosage Subcutaneous: **Enhanced-potency inactivated poliovirus vaccine (E-IPV) is preferred for primary vaccination of adults**, 2 doses S.C. 4-8 weeks apart, a third dose 6-12 months after the second. For adults with a completed primary series and for whom a booster is indicated, either OPV or E-IPV can be given. If immediate protection is needed, either OPV or E-IPV is recommended.

Local Anesthetic/Vasoconstrictor Precautions No information available to require special precautions

Effects on Dental Treatment No effects or complications reported

Other Adverse Effects All serious adverse reactions must be reported to the FDA

1% to 10%:

Central nervous system: Fever >101.3°F
Dermatologic: Skin rash
Local: Tenderness or pain at injection site

<1%:

Central nervous system: Fatigue, fussiness, sleepiness, crying, Guillain-Barré
Dermatologic: Reddening of skin, erythema
Gastrointestinal: Decreased appetite
Neuromuscular & skeletal: Weakness
Respiratory: Dyspnea

Drug Interactions Decreased effect with immunosuppressive agents, immune globulin, other live vaccines within 1 month; may temporarily suppress tuberculin skin test sensitivity (4-6 weeks)

Pregnancy Risk Factor C

Generic Available No

Poliovirus Vaccine, Live, Trivalent, Oral

(POE lee oh VYE rus vak SEEN, live, try VAY lent, OR al)

Brand Names Orimune®

Therapeutic Category Vaccine, Live Virus

Synonyms OPV; Sabin Vaccine; TOPV

Use Poliovirus immunization

Local Anesthetic/Vasoconstrictor Precautions No information available to require special precautions

Effects on Dental Treatment No effects or complications reported

Other Adverse Effects All serious adverse reactions must be reported to the Vaccine Adverse Event Reporting System (1-800-822-7967)

Pregnancy Risk Factor C

Generic Available No

Comments

Oral vaccine: Live, attenuated vaccine

Federal law requires that the date of administration, the vaccine manufacturer, lot number of vaccine, and the administering person's name, title and address be entered into the patient's permanent medical record; live virus vaccine

Polyestradiol (pol i es tra DYE ole)

Brand Names Estradurin®

Therapeutic Category Estrogen Derivative

Use Palliative treatment of advanced, inoperable carcinoma of the prostate

Usual Dosage Adults: Deep I.M.: 40 mg every 2-4 weeks or less frequently; maximum dose: 80 mg

Mechanism of Action Estrogens exert their primary effects on the interphase DNA-protein complex (chromatin) by binding to a receptor (usually located in the cytoplasm of a target cell) and initiating translocation of the hormone-receptor complex to the nucleus

Local Anesthetic/Vasoconstrictor Precautions No information available to require special precautions

Effects on Dental Treatment No effects or complications reported

Other Adverse Effects

>10%:

Cardiovascular: Peripheral edema

Endocrine & metabolic: Enlargement of breasts (female and male), breast tenderness

Gastrointestinal: Nausea, anorexia, bloating

1% to 10%:

Central nervous system: Headache

Endocrine & metabolic: Increased libido (female), decrease libido (male)

Gastrointestinal: Vomiting, diarrhea

<1%:

Cardiovascular: Hypertension, thromboembolism, myocardial infarction, edema

Central nervous system: Depression, dizziness, anxiety, stroke

Dermatologic: Chloasma, melasma, rash

Endocrine & metabolic: Breast tumors, amenorrhea, alterations in frequency and flow of menses, decreased glucose tolerance, elevated triglycerides and LDL

Gastrointestinal: GI distress

Hepatic: Cholestatic jaundice

Ocular: Intolerance to contact lenses

Miscellaneous: Increased susceptibility to *Candida* infection

Drug Interactions No data reported

Drug Uptake

90% of injected dose leaves blood stream within 24 hours

Passive storage in reticuloendothelial system

Increasing the dose prolongs duration of action

Pregnancy Risk Factor X

Generic Available No

Polyethylene Glycol-Electrolyte Solution

(pol i ETH i leen GLY kol ee LEK troe lite soe LOO shun)

Brand Names Colovage®; CoLyte®; GoLYTELY®; NuLytely®; OCL®

Therapeutic Category Laxative, Bowel Evacuant

Synonyms Electrolyte Lavage Solution

Use For bowel cleansing prior to GI examination

Usual Dosage The recommended dose for adults is 4 L of solution prior to gastrointestinal examination, as ingestion of this dose produces a satisfactory preparation in >95% of patients. Ideally the patient should fast for approximately 3-4 hours prior to administration, but in no case should solid food be given for at least 2 hours before the solution is given. The solution is usually administered orally, but may be given via nasogastric tube to patients who are unwilling or unable to drink the solution.

Children: Oral: 25-40 mL/kg/hour for 4-10 hours

(Continued)

Polyethylene Glycol-Electrolyte Solution *(Continued)*

Adults:

Oral: At a rate of 240 mL (8 oz) every 10 minutes, until 4 liters are consumed or the rectal effluent is clear; rapid drinking of each portion is preferred to drinking small amounts continuously

Nasogastric tube: At a rate of 20-30 mL/minute (1.2-1.8 L/hour); the first bowel movement should occur approximately 1 hour after the start of administration

Mechanism of Action Induces catharsis by strong electrolyte and osmotic effects

Local Anesthetic/Vasoconstrictor Precautions No information available to require special precautions

Effects on Dental Treatment No effects or complications reported

Other Adverse Effects GI side effect may be reduced by premedication with single doses of simethicone and metoclopramide, given 30 minutes to 1 hour prior to beginning prep

>10%: Gastrointestinal: Nausea, abdominal fullness, bloating

1% to 10%: Gastrointestinal: Abdominal cramps, vomiting, anal irritation

<1%: Dermatologic: Skin rash

Drug Uptake Onset of effect: Oral: Within 1-2 hours

Pregnancy Risk Factor C

Generic Available No

Comments Do not add flavorings as additional ingredients before use

Polygam® *see* Immune Globulin, Intravenous *on page 503*

Polygam® S/D *see* Immune Globulin, Intravenous *on page 503*

Poly-Histine CS® *see* Brompheniramine, Phenylpropanolamine, and Codeine *on page 145*

Poly-Histine-D® Capsule *see* Phenyltoloxamine, Phenylpropanolamine, Pyrilamine, and Pheniramine *on page 755*

Polymox® *see* Amoxicillin *on page 68*

Polymyxin B *(pol i MIKS in bee)*

Related Information

Neomycin and Polymyxin B *on page 671*

Neomycin, Polymyxin B, and Dexamethasone *on page 672*

Neomycin, Polymyxin B, and Prednisolone *on page 673*

Brand Names Aerosporin®

Therapeutic Category Antibiotic, Ophthalmic; Antibiotic, Topical

Use

Topical: Wound irrigation and bladder irrigation against *Pseudomonas aeruginosa*; used occasionally for gut decontamination

Parenteral use of polymyxin B has mainly been replaced by less toxic antibiotics; it is reserved for life-threatening infections caused by organisms resistant to the preferred drugs

Usual Dosage

Otic: 1-2 drops, 3-4 times/day; should be used sparingly to avoid accumulation of excess debris

Children ≥2 years and Adults:

I.M.: 25,000-30,000 units/kg/day divided every 4-6 hours

I.V.: 15,000-25,000 units/kg/day divided every 12 hours or by continuous infusion

Intrathecal: 50,000 units/day for 3-4 days, then every other day for at least 2 weeks

Total daily dose should not exceed 2,000,000 units/day

Bladder irrigation: Continuous irrigant or rinse in the urinary bladder for up to 10 days using 20 mg (equal to 200,000 units) added to 1 L of normal saline; usually no more than 1 L of irrigant is used per day unless urine flow rate is high; administration rate is adjusted to patient's urine output

Topical irrigation or topical solution: 500,000 units/L of normal saline; topical irrigation should not exceed 2 million units/day in adults

Gut sterilization: Oral: 15,000-25,000 units/kg/day in divided doses every 6 hours

Clostridium difficile enteritis: Oral: 25,000 units every 6 hours for 10 days

Ophthalmic: A concentration of 0.1% to 0.25% is administered as 1-3 drops every hour, then increasing the interval as response indicates to 1-2 drops 4-6 times/day

Mechanism of Action Binds to phospholipids, alters permeability, and damages the bacterial cytoplasmic membrane permitting leakage of intracellular constituents

Local Anesthetic/Vasoconstrictor Precautions No information available to require special precautions

Effects on Dental Treatment No effects or complications reported
Other Adverse Effects <1%:
Cardiovascular: Facial flushing
Central nervous system: Neurotoxicity, irritability, drowsiness, ataxia, drug fever
Dermatologic: Urticarial rash
Endocrine & metabolic: Hypocalcemia, hyponatremia, hypokalemia, hypochloremia
Neuromuscular & skeletal: Neuromuscular blockade, perioral paresthesia, weakness
Ocular: Blurring of vision
Renal: Nephrotoxicity
Respiratory: Respiratory arrest
Miscellaneous: Anaphylactoid reaction, meningeal irritation with intrathecal administration
Drug Interactions Increased/prolonged effect of neuromuscular blocking agents
Drug Uptake
Absorption: Well absorbed from the peritoneum; minimal absorption from the GI tract (except in neonates) from mucous membranes or intact skin
Serum half-life: 4.5-6 hours, increased with reduced renal function
Time to peak serum concentration: I.M.: Within 2 hours
Pregnancy Risk Factor B
Generic Available Yes

Polymyxin B and Hydrocortisone
(pol i MIKS in bee & hye droe KOR ti sone)
Brand Names Otobiotic® Otic
Therapeutic Category Antibacterial, Otic; Corticosteroid, Otic
Use Treatment of superficial bacterial infections of external ear canal
Local Anesthetic/Vasoconstrictor Precautions No information available to require special precautions
Effects on Dental Treatment No effects or complications reported
Pregnancy Risk Factor C
Generic Available No

Polymyxin B and Oxytetracycline *see* Oxytetracycline and Polymyxin B *on page 718*
Polymyxin B and Trimethoprim *see* Trimethoprim and Polymyxin B *on page 965*
Polymyxin E *see* Colistin *on page 259*
Poly-Pred® *see* Neomycin, Polymyxin B, and Prednisolone *on page 673*

Polysaccharide-Iron Complex
(pol i SAK a ride-EYE ern KOM pleks)
Brand Names Hytinic® [OTC]; Niferex® [OTC]; Nu-Iron® [OTC]
Therapeutic Category Iron Salt
Use Prevention and treatment of iron deficiency anemias
Local Anesthetic/Vasoconstrictor Precautions No information available to require special precautions
Effects on Dental Treatment No effects or complications reported
Other Adverse Effects
>10%: Gastrointestinal: Stomach cramping, constipation, nausea, vomiting, dark stools, GI irritation, epigastric pain, nausea
1% to 10%:
Gastrointestinal: Heartburn, diarrhea
Genitourinary: Discolored urine
Miscellaneous: Staining of teeth
<1%: Dermatologic: Contact irritation
Pregnancy Risk Factor A
Generic Available Yes
Comments 100% elemental iron

Polysporin® Ophthalmic *see* Bacitracin and Polymyxin B *on page 108*
Polysporin® Topical *see* Bacitracin and Polymyxin B *on page 108*
Polytar® [OTC] *see* Coal Tar *on page 254*

Polythiazide (pol i THYE a zide)
Related Information
Cardiovascular Diseases *on page 1010*
Brand Names Renese®
Therapeutic Category Diuretic, Thiazide
Use Adjunctive therapy in treatment of edema and hypertension
Usual Dosage Adults: Oral: 1-4 mg/day
(Continued)

Polythiazide *(Continued)*

Mechanism of Action The diuretic mechanism of action of the thiazides is primarily inhibition of sodium, chloride, and water reabsorption in the renal distal tubules, thereby producing diuresis with a resultant reduction in plasma volume. The antihypertensive mechanism of action of the thiazides is unknown. It is known that doses of thiazides produce greater reductions in blood pressure than equivalent diuretic doses of loop diuretics (eg, furosemide). There has been speculation that the thiazides may have some influence on vascular tone mediated through sodium depletion, but this remains to be proven.

Local Anesthetic/Vasoconstrictor Precautions No information available to require special precautions

Effects on Dental Treatment No effects or complications reported

Other Adverse Effects

1% to 10%: Endocrine & metabolic: Hypokalemia

<1%:
Cardiovascular: Hypotension
Central nervous system: Drowsiness
Dermatologic: Photosensitivity, rash
Endocrine & metabolic: Fluid and electrolyte imbalances (hypocalcemia, hypomagnesemia, hyponatremia), hyperglycemia
Gastrointestinal: Nausea, vomiting, anorexia
Hematologic: Rarely blood dyscrasias
Hepatic: Hepatitis
Renal: Prerenal azotemia, polyuria, uremia

Drug Interactions Increased toxicity/levels of lithium

Drug Uptake
Onset of diuretic effect: Within ~2 hours
Duration: 24-48 hours

Pregnancy Risk Factor D

Generic Available No

Polytrim® Ophthalmic *see* Trimethoprim and Polymyxin B *on page 965*

Poly-Vi-Flor® *see* Vitamins, Multiple *on page 995*

Polyvinyl Alcohol *see* Artificial Tears *on page 87*

Poly-Vi-Sol® [OTC] *see* Vitamins, Multiple *on page 995*

Pondimin® *see* Fenfluramine *Withdrawn from Market 1997* *on page 396*

Ponstel® *see* Mefenamic Acid *on page 588*

Pontocaine® *see* Tetracaine *on page 913*

Pontocaine® With Dextrose Injection *see* Tetracaine and Dextrose *on page 914*

Porcelana® [OTC] *see* Hydroquinone *on page 487*

Porcelana® Sunscreen [OTC] *see* Hydroquinone *on page 487*

Porfimer *(POR fi mer)*

Brand Names Photofrin®

Therapeutic Category Antineoplastic Agent, Miscellaneous

Synonyms Porfimer Sodium

Use Esophageal cancer: Photodynamic therapy (PDT) with porfimer for palliation of patients with completely obstructing esophageal cancer, or of patients with partially obstructing esophageal cancer who cannot be satisfactorily treated with Nd:YAG laser therapy

Usual Dosage I.V. (refer to individual protocols):
Children: Safety and efficacy have not been established
Adults: I.V.: 2 mg/kg over 3-5 minutes
Photodynamic therapy is a two-stage process requiring administration of both drug and light. The first stage of PDT is the I.V. injection of porfimer. Illumination with laser light 40-50 hours following the injection with porfimer constitutes the second stage of therapy. A second laser light application may be given 90-120 hours after injection, preceded by gentle debridement of residual tumor.
Patients may receive a second course of PDT a minimum of 30 days after the initial therapy; up to three courses of PDT (each separated by a minimum of 30 days) can be given. Before each course of treatment, evaluate patients for the presence of a tracheoesophageal or bronchoesophageal fistula.

Mechanism of Action Photosensitizing agent used in the photodynamic therapy (PDT) of tumors: cytotoxic and antitumor actions of porfimer are light and oxygen dependent. Cellular damage caused by porfimer PDT is a consequence of the propagation of radical reactions.

Local Anesthetic/Vasoconstrictor Precautions No information available to require special precautions

Effects on Dental Treatment No effects or complications reported

Other Adverse Effects

>10%:

Cardiovascular: Atrial fibrillation, chest pain

Central nervous system: Fever, pain, insomnia

Dermatologic: Photosensitivity reaction

Gastrointestinal: abdominal pain, constipation, dysphagia, nausea, vomiting

Hematologic: Anemia

Neuromuscular & skeletal: Back pain

Respiratory: Dyspnea, pharyngitis, pleural effusion, pneumonia, respiratory insufficiency

1% to 10%:

Cardiovascular: Hypertension, hypotension, edema, cardiac failure, tachycardia, chest pain (substernal)

Central nervous system: Anxiety, confusion

Endocrine & metabolic: Dehydration

Gastrointestinal: Diarrhea, dyspepsia, eructation, esophageal edema, esophageal tumor bleeding, esophageal stricture, esophagitis, hematemesis, melena, weight loss, anorexia

Genitourinary: Urinary tract infection

Neuromuscular & skeletal: Weakness

Respiratory: Coughing, tracheoesophageal fistula

Miscellaneous: Moniliasis, surgical complication

Warnings/Precautions The U.S. Food and Drug Administration (FDA) currently recommends that procedures for proper handling and disposal of antineoplastic agents be considered. If the esophageal tumor is eroding into the trachea or bronchial tree, the likelihood of tracheoesophageal or bronchoesophageal fistula resulting from treatment is sufficiently high that PDT is not recommended. All patients who receive porfimer sodium will be photosensitive and must observe precautions to avoid exposure of skin and eyes to direct sunlight or bright indoor light for 30 days. The photosensitivity is due to residual drug which will be present in all parts of the skin. Exposure of the skin to ambient indoor light is, however, beneficial because the remaining drug will be inactivated gradually and safely through a photobleaching reaction. Patients should not stay in a darkened room during this period and should be encouraged to expose their skin to ambient indoor light. Ocular discomfort has been reported; for 30 days, when outdoors, patients should wear dark sunglasses which have an average white light transmittance of <4%.

Drug Interactions

Decreased effect: Compounds that quench active oxygen species or scavenge radicals (eg, dimethyl sulfoxide, beta-carotene, ethanol, mannitol) would be expected to decrease PDT activity; allopurinol, calcium channel blockers and some prostaglandin synthesis inhibitors could interfere with porfimer; drugs that decrease clotting, vasoconstriction or platelet aggregation could decrease the efficacy of PDT; glucocorticoid hormones may decrease the efficacy of the treatment

Increased toxicity: Concomitant administration of other photosensitizing agents (eg, tetracyclines, sulfonamides, phenothiazines, sulfonylureas, thiazide diuretics, griseofulvin) could increase the photosensitivity reaction

Drug Uptake

Serum half-life: 250 hours

Time to peak serum concentration: Within 2 hours

Pregnancy Risk Factor C

Generic Available No

Porfimer Sodium *see* Porfimer *on previous page*

Pork NPH Iletin® II *see* Insulin Preparations *on page 509*

Pork Regular Iletin® II *see* Insulin Preparations *on page 509*

Portagen® [OTC] *see* Enteral Nutritional Products *on page 350*

Porton Asparaginase *see* Erwinia Asparaginase *on page 360*

Posicor® *see* Mibefradil *on page 634*

Posture® [OTC] *see* Calcium Phosphate, Tribasic *on page 168*

Potasalan® *see* Potassium Chloride *on page 778*

Potassium Acetate (poe TASS ee um AS e tate)

Therapeutic Category Electrolyte Supplement, Parenteral; Potassium Salt

Use Potassium deficiency; to avoid chloride when high concentration of potassium is needed, source of bicarbonate

Usual Dosage I.V. doses should be incorporated into the patient's maintenance I.V. fluids, intermittent I.V. potassium administration should be reserved for severe depletion situations and requires EKG monitoring; doses listed as mEq of potassium

(Continued)

Potassium Acetate *(Continued)*

Treatment of hypokalemia: I.V.:
Children: 2-5 mEq/kg/day
Adults: 40-100 mEq/day
I.V. intermittent infusion (must be diluted prior to administration):
Children: 0.5-1 mEq/kg/dose (maximum: 30 mEq) to infuse at 0.3-0.5 mEq/kg/hour (maximum: 1 mEq/kg/hour)
Adults: 10-20 mEq/dose (maximum: 40 mEq/dose) to infuse over 2-3 hours (maximum: 40 mEq over 1 hour)

Mechanism of Action Potassium is the major cation of intracellular fluid and is essential for the conduction of nerve impulses in heart, brain, and skeletal muscle; contraction of cardiac, skeletal and smooth muscles; maintenance of normal renal function, acid-base balance, carbohydrate metabolism, and gastric secretion

Local Anesthetic/Vasoconstrictor Precautions No information available to require special precautions

Effects on Dental Treatment No effects or complications reported

Other Adverse Effects
>10%: Gastrointestinal: Diarrhea, nausea, stomach pain, flatulence, vomiting (oral)
1% to 10%:
Cardiovascular: Bradycardia
Endocrine & metabolic: Hyperkalemia
Local: Local tissue necrosis with extravasation
Neuromuscular & skeletal: Weakness
Respiratory: Dyspnea
<1%:
Cardiovascular: Chest pain
Central nervous system: Mental confusion
Endocrine & metabolic: Alkalosis
Gastrointestinal: Abdominal pain, throat pain
Local: Phlebitis
Neuromuscular & skeletal: Paresthesias, paralysis

Drug Interactions Increased effect/levels with potassium-sparing diuretics, salt substitutes, ACE inhibitors

Drug Uptake
Absorption: Absorbed well from upper GI tract

Pregnancy Risk Factor C

Generic Available Yes

Potassium Acetate, Potassium Bicarbonate, and Potassium Citrate

(poe TASS ee um AS e tate, poe TASS ee um bye KAR bun ate, & poe TASS ee um SIT rate)

Brand Names Tri-K®

Therapeutic Category Electrolyte Supplement, Oral; Potassium Salt

Use Treatment or prevention of hypokalemia

Local Anesthetic/Vasoconstrictor Precautions No information available to require special precautions

Effects on Dental Treatment No effects or complications reported

Pregnancy Risk Factor C

Generic Available Yes

Potassium Acid Phosphate (poe TASS ee um AS id FOS fate)

Brand Names K-Phos® Original

Therapeutic Category Electrolyte Supplement, Oral; Potassium Salt; Urinary Acidifying Agent

Use Acidifies urine and lowers urinary calcium concentration; reduces odor and rash caused by ammoniacal urine; increases the antibacterial activity of methenamine

Usual Dosage Adults: Oral: 1000 mg dissolved in 6-8 oz of water 4 times/day with meals and at bedtime; for best results, soak tablets in water for 2-5 minutes, then stir and swallow

Mechanism of Action The principal intracellular cation; involved in transmission of nerve impulses, muscle contractions, enzyme activity, and glucose utilization

Local Anesthetic/Vasoconstrictor Precautions No information available to require special precautions

Effects on Dental Treatment No effects or complications reported

Other Adverse Effects
>10%: Gastrointestinal: Diarrhea, nausea, stomach pain, flatulence, vomiting

1% to 10%:
  Cardiovascular: Bradycardia
  Endocrine & metabolic: Hyperkalemia
  Local: Local tissue necrosis with extravasation
  Neuromuscular & skeletal: Weakness
  Respiratory: Dyspnea
<1%:
  Cardiovascular: Chest pain, arrhythmia, edema
  Central nervous system: Mental confusion, tetany
  Endocrine & metabolic: Hyperphosphatemia, hypocalcemia, alkalosis
  Gastrointestinal: Abdominal pain, weight gain, thirst, throat pain
  Genitourinary: Decreased urine output
  Local: Phlebitis
  Neuromuscular & skeletal: Paresthesias, paralysis, bone pain, arthralgia, pain/
    weakness of extremities
Drug Interactions
  Increased effect/levels with potassium-sparing diuretics, salt substitutes, salicy-
  lates, ACE inhibitors
Drug Uptake
  Absorption: Absorbed well from upper GI tract
Pregnancy Risk Factor C
Generic Available No

Potassium Bicarbonate (poe TASS ee um bye KAR bun ate)

Brand Names K+ Care® Effervescent; K-Electrolyte® Effervescent; K-Gen® Effer-
vescent; K-Lyte® Effervescent
Therapeutic Category Electrolyte Supplement, Oral; Potassium Salt
Use Potassium deficiency, hypokalemia
Local Anesthetic/Vasoconstrictor Precautions No information available to
require special precautions
Effects on Dental Treatment No effects or complications reported
Pregnancy Risk Factor C
Generic Available No

Potassium Bicarbonate and Potassium Chloride, Effervescent

(poe TASS ee um bye KAR bun ate & poe TASS ee um KLOR ide, ef er VES
ent)
Brand Names Klorvess® Effervescent; K/Lyte/CL®
Therapeutic Category Electrolyte Supplement, Oral; Potassium Salt
Use Treatment or prevention of hypokalemia
Local Anesthetic/Vasoconstrictor Precautions No information available to
require special precautions
Effects on Dental Treatment No effects or complications reported
Pregnancy Risk Factor C
Generic Available Yes

Potassium Bicarbonate and Potassium Citrate, Effervescent

(poe TASS ee um bye KAR bun ate & poe TASS ee um SIT rate, ef er VES
ent)
Brand Names Effer-K™; K-Ide®; Klor-con®/EF; K-Lyte®; K-Vescent®
Therapeutic Category Electrolyte Supplement, Oral; Potassium Salt
Use Treatment or prevention of hypokalemia
Usual Dosage Oral:
  Children: 1-4 mEq/kg/24 hours in divided doses as required to maintain normal
    serum potassium

  Adults:
    Prevention: 16-24 mEq/day in 2-4 divided doses
    Treatment: 40-100 mEq/day in 2-4 divided doses
Mechanism of Action Needed for the conduction of nerve impulses in heart,
brain, and skeletal muscle; contraction of cardiac, skeletal and smooth muscles;
maintenance of normal renal function
Local Anesthetic/Vasoconstrictor Precautions No information available to
require special precautions
Effects on Dental Treatment No effects or complications reported
Other Adverse Effects
  >10%: Gastrointestinal: Diarrhea, nausea, stomach pain, flatulence, vomiting
  1% to 10%:
    Cardiovascular: Bradycardia
(Continued)

Potassium Bicarbonate and Potassium Citrate, Effervescent *(Continued)*

Endocrine & metabolic: Hyperkalemia
Local: Local tissue necrosis with extravasation
Neuromuscular & skeletal: Weakness
Respiratory: Dyspnea

<1%:
Cardiovascular: Chest pain
Central nervous system: Mental confusion
Endocrine & metabolic: Alkalosis
Gastrointestinal: Abdominal pain, throat pain
Local: Phlebitis
Neuromuscular & skeletal: Paresthesias, paralysis

Drug Interactions Increased effect/levels with potassium-sparing diuretics, salt substitutes, ACE inhibitors

Drug Uptake
Absorption: Absorbed well from upper GI tract

Pregnancy Risk Factor C

Generic Available No

Potassium Bicarbonate, Potassium Chloride, and Potassium Citrate

(poe TASS ee um bye KAR bun ate, poe TASS ee um KLOR ide & poe TASS ee um SIT rate)

Brand Names Kaochlor-Eff®

Therapeutic Category Electrolyte Supplement, Oral; Potassium Salt

Use Treatment or prevention of hypokalemia

Local Anesthetic/Vasoconstrictor Precautions No information available to require special precautions

Effects on Dental Treatment No effects or complications reported

Pregnancy Risk Factor C

Generic Available Yes

Potassium Chloride (poe TASS ee um KLOR ide)

Brand Names Cena-K®; Gen-K®; K+ 10®; Kaochlor®; Kaochlor® SF; Kaon-Cl®; Kaon-Cl-10®; Kay Ciel®; K+ Care®; K-Dur® 10; K-Dur® 20; K-Lease®; K-Lor™; Klor-Con®; Klor-Con® 8; Klor-Con® 10; Klor-Con/25®; Klorvess®; Klotrix®; K-Lyte®/Cl; K-Norm®; K-Tab®; Micro-K® 10; Micro-K Extencaps®; Micro-K® LS; Potasalan®; Rum-K®; Slow-K®; Ten-K®

Canadian/Mexican Brand Names Celek® 20 (Mexico); Clor-K-Zaf® (Mexico); Cloruro® De Potasio (Mexico); Kaliolite® (Mexico)

Therapeutic Category Electrolyte Supplement, Oral; Electrolyte Supplement, Parenteral; Potassium Salt

Use Treatment or prevention of hypokalemia

Usual Dosage I.V. doses should be incorporated into the patient's maintenance I.V. fluids; intermittent I.V. potassium administration should be reserved for severe depletion situations in patients undergoing EKG monitoring.

Normal daily requirements: Oral, I.V.:
Children: 2-3 mEq/kg/day
Adults: 40-80 mEq/day

Prevention during diuretic therapy: Oral:
Children: 1-2 mEq/kg/day in 1-2 divided doses
Adults: 20-40 mEq/day in 1-2 divided doses

Treatment of hypokalemia: Children:
Oral: 1-2 mEq/kg initially, then as needed based on frequently obtained lab values. If deficits are severe or ongoing losses are great, I.V. route should be considered.
I.V.: 1 mEq/kg over 1-2 hours initially, then repeated as needed based on frequently obtained lab values; severe depletion or ongoing losses may require >200% of normal limit needs

Potassium Dosage/Rate of Infusion Guidelines

Serum Potassium*	Maximum Infusion Rate	Maximum Concentration	Maximum 24-Hour Dose
>2.5 mEq/L	10 mEq/h	40 mEq/L	200 mEq
<2.5 mEq/L	40 mEq/h	80 mEq/L	400 mEq

I.V. intermittent infusion: Dose should not exceed 1 mEq/kg/hour, or 40 mEq/hour; if it exceeds 0.5 mEq/kg/hour, physician should be at bedside and patient should have continuous EKG monitoring

Treatment of hypokalemia: Adults:
I.V. intermittent infusion: 10-20 mEq/hour, not to exceed 40 mEq/hour and 150 mEq/day. See table.
Potassium >2.5 mEq/L:
Oral: 60-80 mEq/day plus additional amounts if needed
I.V.: 10 mEq over 1 hour with additional doses if needed
Potassium <2.5 mEq/L:
Oral: Up to 40-60 mEq initial dose, followed by further doses based on lab values; deficits at a plasma level of 2 mEq/L may be as high as 400-800 mEq of potassium
I.V.: Up to 40 mEq over 1 hour, with doses based on frequent lab monitoring; deficits at a plasma level of 2 mEq/L may be as high as 400-800 mEq of potassium

Mechanism of Action Potassium is the major cation of intracellular fluid and is essential for the conduction of nerve impulses in heart, brain, and skeletal muscle; contraction of cardiac, skeletal and smooth muscles; maintenance of normal renal function, acid-base balance, carbohydrate metabolism, and gastric secretion

Local Anesthetic/Vasoconstrictor Precautions No information available to require special precautions

Effects on Dental Treatment No effects or complications reported

Other Adverse Effects
>10%: Gastrointestinal: Diarrhea, nausea, stomach pain, flatulence, vomiting (oral)
1% to 10%:
Cardiovascular: Bradycardia
Endocrine & metabolic: Hyperkalemia
Local: Local tissue necrosis with extravasation, pain at the site of injection
Neuromuscular & skeletal: Weakness
Respiratory: Dyspnea
<1%:
Cardiovascular: Chest pain, arrhythmias, heart block, hypotension
Central nervous system: Mental confusion
Endocrine & metabolic: Alkalosis
Gastrointestinal: Abdominal pain, throat pain
Local: Phlebitis
Neuromuscular & skeletal: Paresthesias, paralysis

Drug Interactions No data reported

Drug Uptake
Absorption: Absorbed well from upper GI tract

Pregnancy Risk Factor A

Generic Available Yes

Potassium Chloride and Potassium Gluconate
(poe TASS ee um KLOR ide & poe TASS ee um GLOO coe nate)
Brand Names Kolyum®
Therapeutic Category Electrolyte Supplement, Oral; Potassium Salt
Use Treatment or prevention of hypokalemia
Local Anesthetic/Vasoconstrictor Precautions No information available to require special precautions
Effects on Dental Treatment No effects or complications reported
Generic Available Yes

Potassium Citrate (poe TASS ee um SIT rate)
Brand Names Urocit®-K
Therapeutic Category Alkalinizing Agent, Oral
Use Prevention of uric acid nephrolithiasis; prevention of calcium renal stones in patients with hypocitraturia; urinary alkalinizer when sodium citrate is contraindicated
Local Anesthetic/Vasoconstrictor Precautions No information available to require special precautions
Effects on Dental Treatment No effects or complications reported
Pregnancy Risk Factor A
Generic Available Yes
Comments Parenteral K_3PO_4 contains 3 mmol of phosphorous/mL and 4.4 mEq of potassium/mL. If ordering by phosphorous content, use mmol instead of mEq since the mEq value for phosphorous varies with the pH of the solution due to valence changes of the phosphorus ion. (1 mmol of phosphorous = 31 mg)

Potassium Citrate and Citric Acid
(poe TASS ee um SIT rate & SI trik AS id)

Brand Names Polycitra®-K

Therapeutic Category Electrolyte Supplement, Oral; Potassium Salt

Use Treatment of metabolic acidosis; alkalinizing agent in conditions where long-term maintenance of an alkaline urine is desirable

Local Anesthetic/Vasoconstrictor Precautions No information available to require special precautions

Effects on Dental Treatment No effects or complications reported

Pregnancy Risk Factor C

Generic Available No

Comments Potassium citrate 3.4 mmol/5 mL and citric acid 1.6 mmol/5 mL = total of 5.0 mmol/5 mL citrate content

Potassium Citrate and Potassium Gluconate
(poe TASS ee um SIT rate & poe TASS ee um GLOO coe nate)

Brand Names Twin-K®

Therapeutic Category Electrolyte Supplement, Oral; Potassium Salt

Use Treatment or prevention of hypokalemia

Local Anesthetic/Vasoconstrictor Precautions No information available to require special precautions

Effects on Dental Treatment No effects or complications reported

Pregnancy Risk Factor C

Generic Available Yes

Potassium Gluconate (poe TASS ee um GLOO coe nate)

Brand Names Kaon®; K-G®

Therapeutic Category Electrolyte Supplement, Oral; Potassium Salt

Use Treatment or prevention of hypokalemia

Usual Dosage Oral (doses listed as mEq of potassium):
Normal daily requirement:
Children: 2-3 mEq/kg/day
Adults: 40-80 mEq/day
Prevention of hypokalemia during diuretic therapy:
Children: 1-2 mEq/kg/day in 1-2 divided doses
Adults: 20-40 mEq/day in 1-2 divided doses
Treatment of hypokalemia:
Children: 2-5 mEq/kg/day in 2-4 divided doses
Adults: 40-100 mEq/day in 2-4 divided doses

Mechanism of Action Potassium is the major cation of intracellular fluid and is essential for the conduction of nerve impulses in heart, brain, and skeletal muscle; contraction of cardiac, skeletal and smooth muscles; maintenance of normal renal function, acid-base balance, carbohydrate metabolism, and gastric secretion

Local Anesthetic/Vasoconstrictor Precautions No information available to require special precautions

Effects on Dental Treatment No effects or complications reported

Other Adverse Effects
>10%: Gastrointestinal: Diarrhea, nausea, stomach pain, flatulence, vomiting (oral)
1% to 10%:
Cardiovascular: Bradycardia
Endocrine & metabolic: Hyperkalemia
Neuromuscular & skeletal: Weakness
Respiratory: Dyspnea
<1%:
Cardiovascular: Chest pain
Central nervous system: Mental confusion
Endocrine & metabolic: Alkalosis
Gastrointestinal: Throat pain
Local: Phlebitis
Neuromuscular & skeletal: Paresthesias, paralysis

Drug Interactions
Increased effect/levels with potassium-sparing diuretics, salt substitutes, ACE inhibitors
Increased effect of digitalis

Drug Uptake
Absorption: Absorbed well from upper GI tract

Pregnancy Risk Factor A

Generic Available Yes

Potassium Iodide (poe TASS ee um EYE oh dide)
Related Information
Endocrine Disorders & Pregnancy *on page 1021*
Brand Names Pima®; SSKI®; Thyro-Block®
Therapeutic Category Antithyroid Agent; Expectorant
Use Facilitate bronchial drainage and cough; reduce thyroid vascularity prior to thyroidectomy and management of thyrotoxic crisis; block thyroidal uptake of radioactive isotopes of iodine in a radiation emergency
Usual Dosage Oral:
Adults: RDA: 130 mcg

Expectorant:
Children: 60-250 mg every 6-8 hours; maximum single dose: 500 mg
Adults: 300-650 mg 2-3 times/day
Preoperative thyroidectomy: Children and Adults: 50-250 mg (1-5 drops SSKI®) 3 times/day **or** 0.1-0.3 mL (3-5 drops) of strong iodine (Lugol's solution) 3 times/day; give for 10 days before surgery
Thyrotoxic crisis:
Children and Adults: 300-500 mg (6-10 drops SSKI®) 3 times/day or 1 mL strong iodine (Lugol's solution) 3 times/day
Graves' disease in neonates: 1 drop of strong iodine (Lugol's solution) 3 times/day
Sporotrichosis:
Initial:
Preschool: 50 mg/dose 3 times/day
Children: 250 mg/dose 3 times/day
Adults: 500 mg/dose 3 times/day
Oral increase 50 mg/dose daily
Maximum dose:
Preschool: 500 mg/dose 3 times/day
Children and Adults: 1-2 g/dose 3 times/day
Continue treatment for 4-6 weeks after lesions have completely healed
Mechanism of Action Reduces viscosity of mucus by increasing respiratory tract secretions; inhibits secretion of thyroid hormone, fosters colloid accumulation in thyroid follicles
Local Anesthetic/Vasoconstrictor Precautions No information available to require special precautions
Effects on Dental Treatment No effects or complications reported
Other Adverse Effects 1% to 10%:
Central nervous system: Fever, headache
Dermatologic: Urticaria, acne, angioedema
Endocrine & metabolic: Goiter with hypothyroidism
Gastrointestinal: Metallic taste, GI upset, soreness of teeth and gums
Hematologic: Cutaneous and mucosal hemorrhage, eosinophilia
Neuromuscular & skeletal: Arthralgia
Respiratory: Rhinitis
Miscellaneous: Lymph node enlargement
Drug Interactions Increased toxicity: Lithium causes additive hypothyroid effects
Drug Uptake
Onset of action: 24-48 hours
Peak effect: 10-15 days after continuous therapy
Pregnancy Risk Factor D
Generic Available Yes

Potassium Phosphate (poe TASS ee um FOS fate)
Brand Names Neutra-Phos®-K
Therapeutic Category Electrolyte Supplement, Parenteral; Phosphate Salt; Potassium Salt
Use Treatment and prevention of hypophosphatemia or hypokalemia
Usual Dosage I.V. doses should be incorporated into the patient's maintenance I.V. fluids; intermittent I.V. infusion should be reserved for severe depletion situations in patients undergoing continuous EKG monitoring. It is difficult to determine total body phosphorus deficit; the following dosages are empiric guidelines:

Normal requirements elemental phosphorus: Oral:
0-6 months: 240 mg
6-12 months: 360 mg
1-10 years: 800 mg
>10 years: 1200 mg
Pregnancy lactation: Additional 400 mg/day

Adults RDA: 800 mg
(Continued)

Potassium Phosphate (Continued)

Treatment: It is difficult to provide concrete guidelines for the treatment of severe hypophosphatemia because the extent of total body deficits and response to therapy are difficult to predict. Aggressive doses of phosphate may result in a transient serum elevation followed by redistribution into intracellular compartments or bone tissue. It is recommended that repletion of severe hypophosphatemia (<1 mg/dL in adults) be done I.V. because large doses of oral phosphate may cause diarrhea and intestinal absorption may be unreliable

Pediatric I.V. phosphate repletion: Children: 0.25-0.5 mmol/kg **administer over 4-6 hours and repeat if symptomatic hypophosphatemia persists;** to assess the need for further phosphate administration, obtain serum inorganic phosphate after administration of the first dose and base further doses on serum levels and clinical status

Adult I.V. phosphate repletion:

Initial dose: 0.08 mmol/kg if recent uncomplicated hypophosphatemia

Initial dose: 0.16 mmol/kg if prolonged hypophosphatemia with presumed total body deficits; increase dose by 25% to 50% if patient symptomatic with severe hypophosphatemia

Do not exceed 0.24 mmol/kg/day; administer over 6 hours by I.V. infusion

With orders for I.V. phosphate, there is considerable confusion associated with the use of millimoles (mmol) versus milliequivalents (mEq) to express the phosphate requirement. Because inorganic phosphate exists as monobasic and dibasic anions, with the mixture of valences dependent on pH, ordering by mEq amounts is unreliable and may lead to large dosing errors. In addition, I.V. phosphate is available in the sodium and potassium salt; therefore, the content of these cations must be considered when ordering phosphate. The most reliable method of ordering I.V. phosphate is by millimoles, then specifying the potassium or sodium salt. For example, an order for 15 mmol of phosphate as potassium phosphate in one liter of normal saline would also provide 22 mEq of potassium.

Phosphate maintenance electrolyte requirement in parenteral nutrition: 2 mmol/kg/24 hours or 35 mmol/kcal/24 hours; maximum: 15-30 mmol/24 hours

Maintenance:

I.V. solutions:

Children: 0.5-1.5 mmol/kg/24 hours I.V. or 2-3 mmol/kg/24 hours orally in divided doses

Adults: 15-30 mmol/24 hours I.V. or 50-150 mmol/24 hours orally in divided doses

Oral:

Children <4 years: 1 capsule (250 mg phosphorus/8 mmol) 4 times/day; dilute as instructed

Children >4 years and Adults: 1-2 capsules (250-500 mg phosphorus/8-16 mmol) 4 times/day; dilute as instructed

Fleet® Phospho®-Soda: Laxative: Oral: Single dose

Children: 5-15 mL

Adults: 20-30 mL mixed with 120 mL cold water

Local Anesthetic/Vasoconstrictor Precautions No information available to require special precautions

Effects on Dental Treatment No effects or complications reported

Other Adverse Effects

>10%: Gastrointestinal: Diarrhea, nausea, stomach pain, flatulence, vomiting

1% to 10%:

Cardiovascular: Bradycardia

Endocrine & metabolic: Hyperkalemia

Neuromuscular & skeletal: Weakness

Respiratory: Dyspnea

<1%:

Cardiovascular: Chest pain

Central nervous system: Mental confusion

Endocrine & metabolic: Alkalosis

Gastrointestinal: Abdominal pain, throat pain

Local: Phlebitis

Neuromuscular & skeletal: Paresthesias, paralysis

Renal: Acute renal failure

Drug Interactions

Decreased effect/levels with aluminum and magnesium-containing antacids or sucralfate which can act as phosphate binders

Increased effect/levels with potassium-sparing diuretics, salt substitutes, or ACE-inhibitors

Increased effect of digitalis
Pregnancy Risk Factor C
Generic Available Yes

Potassium Phosphate and Sodium Phosphate
(poe TASS ee um FOS fate & SOW dee um FOS fate)

Brand Names K-Phos® Neutral; Neutra-Phos®; Uro-KP-Neutral®

Therapeutic Category Electrolyte Supplement, Oral; Phosphate Salt; Potassium Salt

Use Treatment of conditions associated with excessive renal phosphate loss or inadequate GI absorption of phosphate; to acidify the urine to lower calcium concentrations; to increase the antibacterial activity of methenamine; reduce odor and rash caused by ammonia in urine

Usual Dosage All dosage forms to be mixed in 6-8 oz of water prior to administration

Children: 2-3 mmol phosphate/kg/24 hours given 4 times/day **or** 1 capsule 4 times/day

Adults: 1-2 capsules (250-500 mg phosphorus/8-16 mmol) 4 times/day after meals and at bedtime

Local Anesthetic/Vasoconstrictor Precautions No information available to require special precautions

Effects on Dental Treatment No effects or complications reported

Other Adverse Effects

>10%: Gastrointestinal: Diarrhea, nausea, stomach pain, flatulence, vomiting

1% to 10%:

Cardiovascular: Bradycardia
Endocrine & metabolic: Hyperkalemia
Neuromuscular & skeletal: Weakness
Respiratory: Dyspnea

<1%:

Cardiovascular: Arrhythmia, chest pain, edema
Central nervous system: Mental confusion, tetany
Endocrine & metabolic: Alkalosis
Gastrointestinal: Weight gain, thirst, throat pain
Genitourinary: Decreased urine output
Local: Phlebitis
Neuromuscular & skeletal: Paresthesias, paralysis, pain/weakness of extremities, bone pain, arthralgia
Renal: Acute renal failure

Drug Interactions

Decreased effect/levels with aluminum and magnesium-containing antacids or sucralfate which can act as phosphate binders
Increased effect/levels with potassium-sparing diuretics or ACE-inhibitors
Increased effect/levels of digitalis, salicylates

Pregnancy Risk Factor C
Generic Available Yes

Povidone-Iodine (POE vi done EYE oh dyne)

Related Information

Patients Undergoing Cancer Therapy *on page 1083*

Brand Names Betadine® [OTC]; Efodine® [OTC]; Iodex® Regular; Isodine® [OTC]

Therapeutic Category Antibacterial, Topical

Use External antiseptic with broad microbicidal spectrum against bacteria, fungi, viruses, protozoa, and yeasts

Usual Dosage

Shampoo: Apply 2 tsp to hair and scalp, lather and rinse; repeat application 2 times/week until improvement is noted, then shampoo weekly
Topical: Apply as needed for treatment and prevention of susceptible microbial infections

Mechanism of Action Povidone-iodine is known to be a powerful broad spectrum germicidal agent effective against a wide range of bacteria, viruses, fungi, protozoa, and spores.

Local Anesthetic/Vasoconstrictor Precautions No information available to require special precautions

Effects on Dental Treatment No effects or complications reported

Other Adverse Effects

1% to 10%:

Cardiovascular: Local edema
Dermatologic: Rash, pruritus

<1%:

Endocrine & metabolic: Metabolic acidosis

(Continued)

783

Povidone-Iodine *(Continued)*

    Local: Systemic absorption in extensive burns causing iododerma
    Renal: Renal impairment
Drug Interactions No data reported
Drug Uptake Absorption: In normal individuals, topical application results in very little systemic absorption; with vaginal administration, however, absorption is rapid and serum concentrations of total iodine and inorganic iodide are increased significantly
Pregnancy Risk Factor D
Generic Available Yes

PPD *see* Tuberculin Purified Protein Derivative *on page 975*

PPS *see* Pentosan Polysulfate Sodium *on page 739*

PrameGel® [OTC] *see* Pramoxine *on this page*

Pramet® FA *see* Vitamins, Multiple *on page 995*

Pramilet® FA *see* Vitamins, Multiple *on page 995*

Pramipexole *(pra mi PEX ole)*

Brand Names Mirapex®
Therapeutic Category Anti-Parkinson's Agent
Use Treatment of the signs and symptoms of idiopathic Parkinson's Disease
Usual Dosage Adults: Oral: Initial: 0.375 mg/day given in 3 divided doses, increase gradually by 0.125 mg/dose every 5-7 days; range: 1.5-4.5 mg/day
Local Anesthetic/Vasoconstrictor Precautions No information available to require special precautions
Effects on Dental Treatment No effects or complications reported
Pregnancy Risk Factor C
Dosage Forms Tablet: 0.125 mg, 0.25 mg, 1 mg, 1.5 mg

Pramosone® *see* Pramoxine and Hydrocortisone *on this page*

Pramoxine *(pra MOKS een)*

Brand Names Anusol® Ointment [OTC]; Fleet® Pain Relief [OTC]; Itch-X® [OTC]; Phicon® [OTC]; PrameGel® [OTC]; Prax® [OTC]; ProctoFoam® NS [OTC]; Tronolane® [OTC]
Therapeutic Category Local Anesthetic, Topical
Use Temporary relief of pain and itching associated with anogenital pruritus or irritation; dermatosis, minor burns, or hemorrhoids
Usual Dosage Adults: Topical: Apply as directed, usually every 3-4 hours to affected area (maximum adult dose: 200 mg)
Mechanism of Action Pramoxine, like other anesthetics, decreases the neuronal membrane's permeability to sodium ions; both initiation and conduction of nerve impulses are blocked, thus depolarization of the neuron is inhibited
Local Anesthetic/Vasoconstrictor Precautions No information available to require special precautions
Effects on Dental Treatment No effects or complications reported
Other Adverse Effects
    1% to 10%:
        Dermatologic: Angioedema
        Local: Contact dermatitis, burning, stinging
    <1%:
        Cardiovascular: Edema
        Dermatologic: Urticaria
        Genitourinary: Urethritis
        Hematologic: Methemoglobinemia in infants
        Local: Tenderness
Drug Interactions No data reported
Drug Uptake
    Onset of therapeutic effect: Within 2-5 minutes
    Peak effect: 3-5 minutes
    Duration: May last for several days
Pregnancy Risk Factor C
Generic Available No

Pramoxine and Hydrocortisone
    (pra MOKS een & hye droe KOR ti sone)
Brand Names Enzone®; Pramosone®; Proctofoam®-HC; Zone-A Forte®
Therapeutic Category Anti-inflammatory Agent; Corticosteroid, Topical (Low Potency); Local Anesthetic, Topical
Synonyms Hydrocortisone and Pramoxine
Use Treatment of severe anorectal or perianal swelling

Local Anesthetic/Vasoconstrictor Precautions No information available to require special precautions

Effects on Dental Treatment No effects or complications reported

Pregnancy Risk Factor C

Generic Available No

Prandin™ see Repaglinide on page 838

Pravachol® see Pravastatin on this page

Pravastatin (PRA va stat in)

Related Information

Cardiovascular Diseases on page 1010

Brand Names Pravachol®

Therapeutic Category HMG-CoA Reductase Inhibitor; Lipid Lowering Drugs

Use Adjunct to diet for the reduction of elevated total and LDL cholesterol levels in patients with hypercholesterolemia (type IIa, IIb, and IIc); used in hypercholesterolemic patients without clinically evident heart disease to reduce the risk of myocardial infarction, to reduce the risk for revascularization, and reduce the risk of death due to cardiovascular causes with no increase in death from noncardiovascular diseases

Usual Dosage Adults: Oral: 10-20 mg once daily at bedtime, may increase to 40 mg/day at bedtime

Mechanism of Action Pravastatin is a competitive inhibitor of 3-hydroxy-3-methylglutaryl coenzyme A (HMG-CoA) reductase, which is the rate-limiting enzyme involved in de novo cholesterol synthesis.

Local Anesthetic/Vasoconstrictor Precautions No information available to require special precautions

Effects on Dental Treatment No effects of complications reported

Other Adverse Effects

1% to 10%:
Central nervous system: Headache, dizziness
Dermatologic: Rash
Gastrointestinal: flatulence, abdominal cramps, diarrhea, constipation, nausea, dyspepsia, heartburn
Neuromuscular & skeletal: Myalgia, elevated creatine phosphokinase (CPK)
<1%:
Gastrointestinal: Dysgeusia
Ocular: Lenticular opacities, blurred vision

Drug Interactions

Increased effect with cholestyramine
Increased effect/toxicity of oral anticoagulants
Increased toxicity with gemfibrozil, clofibrate
Concurrent use of erythromycin and HMG-CoA reductase inhibitors may result in rhabdomyolysis

Drug Uptake

Absorption: Poor
Serum half-life, elimination: ~2-3 hours
Time to peak serum concentration: 1-1.5 hours

Pregnancy Risk Factor X

Generic Available No

Prax® [OTC] see Pramoxine on previous page

Prazepam (PRA ze pam)

Brand Names Centrax®

Therapeutic Category Antianxiety Agent; Anticonvulsant, Benzodiazepine; Benzodiazepine; Tranquilizer, Minor

Use Treatment of anxiety and management of alcohol withdrawal; may also be used as an anticonvulsant in management of simple partial seizures

Usual Dosage Adults: Oral: 30 mg/day in divided doses, may increase gradually to a maximum of 60 mg/day

Mechanism of Action Benzodiazepine anxiolytic sedative that produces CNS depression at the subcortical level, except at high doses, whereby it works at the cortical level

Local Anesthetic/Vasoconstrictor Precautions No information available to require special precautions

Effects on Dental Treatment >10% of patients experience dry mouth which disappears with cessation of drug therapy

Other Adverse Effects

>10%:
Cardiovascular Tachycardia, chest pain
(Continued)

Prazepam *(Continued)*

Central nervous system: Drowsiness, fatigue, lightheadedness, memory impairment, insomnia, anxiety, depression, headache, impaired coordination

Dermatologic: Rash

Endocrine & metabolic: Decreased libido

Gastrointestinal: Constipation, diarrhea, decreased salivation, nausea, vomiting, increased or decreased appetite

Neuromuscular & skeletal: Dysarthria

Ocular: Blurred vision

Miscellaneous: Sweating

1% to 10%:

Cardiovascular: Syncope, hypotension

Central nervous system: Confusion, nervousness, dizziness, akathisia

Dermatologic: Dermatitis

Gastrointestinal: Weight gain or loss, increased salivation

Neuromuscular & skeletal: Muscle cramps, rigidity, tremor

Ocular: Blurred vision

Otic: Tinnitus

Respiratory: Hyperventilation, nasal congestion

<1%:

Endocrine & metabolic: Menstrual irregularities

Hematologic: Blood dyscrasias

Neuromuscular & skeletal: Reflex slowing

Miscellaneous: Drug dependence

Drug Interactions Increased toxicity (CNS depression): Alcohol, tricyclic antidepressants, sedative-hypnotics, MAO inhibitors

Drug Uptake

Duration: 48 hours

Serum half-life:

Parent drug: 78 minutes

Desmethyldiazepam: 30-100 hours

Pregnancy Risk Factor D

Generic Available Yes

Praziquantel *(pray zi KWON tel)*

Brand Names Biltricide®

Canadian/Mexican Brand Names Cisticid® (Mexico); Tecprazin (Mexico)

Therapeutic Category Anthelmintic

Use Treatment of all stages of schistosomiasis caused by *Schistosoma* species pathogenic to humans; also active in the treatment of clonorchiasis, opisthorchiasis, cysticercosis, and many intestinal tapeworm infections and trematode

Usual Dosage Children >4 years and Adults: Oral:

Schistosomiasis: 20 mg/kg/dose 2-3 times/day for 1 day at 4- to 6-hour intervals

Flukes: 25 mg/kg/dose every 8 hours for 1-2 days

Cysticercosis: 50 mg/kg/day divided every 8 hours for 14 days

Tapeworms: 10-20 mg/kg as a single dose (25 mg/kg for *Hymenolepis nana*)

Mechanism of Action Increases the cell permeability to calcium in schistosomes, causing strong contractions and paralysis of worm musculature leading to detachment of suckers from the blood vessel walls and to dislodgment

Local Anesthetic/Vasoconstrictor Precautions No information available to require special precautions

Effects on Dental Treatment No effects or complications reported

Other Adverse Effects

1% to 10%:

Central nervous system: Dizziness, drowsiness, headache, malaise

Gastrointestinal: Abdominal pain, loss of appetite, nausea, vomiting

Miscellaneous: Sweating

<1%:

Central nervous system: Fever

Dermatologic: Skin rash, urticaria, itching

Gastrointestinal: Diarrhea

Miscellaneous: CSF reaction syndrome in patients being treated for neurocysticercosis

Drug Uptake

Absorption: Oral: ~80%; CSF concentration is 14% to 20% of plasma concentration

Serum half-life:

Parent drug: 0.8-1.5 hours

Metabolites: 4.5 hours

Time to peak serum concentration: Within 1-3 hours

Pregnancy Risk Factor B

Generic Available No

Prazosin (PRA zoe sin)
Related Information
Cardiovascular Diseases *on page 1010*
Brand Names Minipress®
Canadian/Mexican Brand Names Apo®-Prazo (Canada); Novo-Prazin® (Canada); Nu-Prazo® (Canada)
Therapeutic Category Alpha-Adrenergic Blockers - Peripheral-Acting (Alpha$_1$-Blockers); Antihypertensive; Vasodilator, Coronary
Use Treatment of hypertension, severe congestive heart failure (in conjunction with diuretics and cardiac glycosides); reduce mortality in stable postmyocardial patients with left ventricular dysfunction (ejection fraction ≤40%)

Unlabeled use: Symptoms of benign prostatic hypertrophy
Usual Dosage Oral:
Children: Initial: 5 mcg/kg/dose (to assess hypotensive effects); usual dosing interval: every 6 hours; increase dosage gradually up to maximum of 25 mcg/kg/dose every 6 hours
Adults: Initial: 1 mg/dose 2-3 times/day; usual maintenance dose: 3-15 mg/day in divided doses 2-4 times/day; maximum daily dose: 20 mg
Mechanism of Action Competitively inhibits postsynaptic alpha-adrenergic receptors which results in vasodilation of veins and arterioles and a decrease in total peripheral resistance and blood pressure
Local Anesthetic/Vasoconstrictor Precautions No information available to require special precautions
Effects on Dental Treatment Significant orthostatic hypotension a possibility; monitor patient when getting out of dental chair; significant dry mouth in up to 10% of patients
Other Adverse Effects
>10%:
Cardiovascular: Orthostatic hypotension
Central nervous system: Dizziness, lightheadedness, drowsiness, headache, malaise
1% to 10%:
Cardiovascular: Edema, palpitations
Central nervous system: Fatigue, nervousness
Gastrointestinal: Dry mouth
Genitourinary: Urinary incontinence
<1%:
Cardiovascular: Angina
Central nervous system: Nightmares, hypothermia
Dermatologic: Rash
Endocrine & metabolic: Sexual dysfunction
Gastrointestinal: Nausea
Genitourinary: Priapism
Renal: Polyuria
Respiratory: Dyspnea, nasal congestion
Drug Interactions
Decreased effect in combination with NSAIDs: Indomethacin pretreatment has been reported to inhibit the hypotensive effect of a single dose of prazosin. The effect of chronic therapy with both drugs is not known. It is suggested however that, as a general rule, indomethacin may inhibit the antihypertensive response to prazosin. The effect of other NSAIDs is not known and the use of NSAIDs such as ibuprofen for treatment of acute postoperative pain in patients taking prazosin is not contraindicated. Inhibition of prostaglandin synthesis by NSAIDs is probably responsible for the decreased effect of prazosin.
Increased effect (hypotensive) with diuretics and antihypertensive medications (especially beta-blockers)
Drug Uptake
Onset of hypotensive effect: Within 2 hours
Maximum decrease: 2-4 hours
Duration: 10-24 hours
Serum half-life: 2-4 hours; increased with congestive heart failure
Pregnancy Risk Factor C
Generic Available Yes

Prazosin and Polythiazide (PRA zoe sin & pol i THYE a zide)
Brand Names Minizide®
Therapeutic Category Antihypertensive Agent, Combination
Use Management of mild to moderate hypertension
(Continued)

Prazosin and Polythiazide *(Continued)*

Local Anesthetic/Vasoconstrictor Precautions No information available to require special precautions

Effects on Dental Treatment No effects or complications reported

Pregnancy Risk Factor C

Generic Available No

Precose® *see Acarbose on page 18*

Predair® *see Prednisolone on this page*

Predaject® *see Prednisolone on this page*

Predalone T.B.A.® *see Prednisolone on this page*

Predcor® *see Prednisolone on this page*

Predcor-TBA® *see Prednisolone on this page*

Pred Forte® *see Prednisolone on this page*

Pred-G® Ophthalmic *see Prednisolone and Gentamicin on next page*

Pred Mild® *see Prednisolone on this page*

Prednicarbate (PRED ni kar bate)

Brand Names Dermatop®

Therapeutic Category Corticosteroid, Topical (Medium Potency)

Use Relief of the inflammatory and pruritic manifestations of corticosteroid-responsive dermatoses (medium potency topical corticosteroid)

Usual Dosage Adults: Topical: Apply a thin film to affected area twice daily

Mechanism of Action Topical corticosteroids have anti-inflammatory, antipruritic, vasoconstrictive, and antiproliferative actions

Local Anesthetic/Vasoconstrictor Precautions No information available to require special precautions

Effects on Dental Treatment No effects or complications reported

Other Adverse Effects <10%:

Dermatologic: Acne, hypopigmentation, allergic dermatitis, maceration of the skin, skin atrophy, folliculitis, hypertrichosis

Endocrine & metabolic: HPA suppression, Cushing's syndrome, growth retardation

Local: Burning, itching, irritation, dryness

Miscellaneous: Secondary infection

Drug Interactions No data reported

Pregnancy Risk Factor C

Dosage Forms Cream: 0.1% (15 g, 60 g)

Generic Available No

Prednicen-M® *see Prednisone on next page*

Prednisolone (pred NIS oh lone)

Related Information

Corticosteroid Equivalencies Comparison *on page 1139*

Corticosteroids, Topical Comparison *on page 1140*

Neomycin, Polymyxin B, and Prednisolone *on page 673*

Respiratory Diseases *on page 1018*

Brand Names AK-Pred®; Articulose-50®; Delta-Cortef®; Econopred®; Econopred® Plus; Inflamase®; Inflamase® Mild; Key-Pred®; Key-Pred-SP®; Metreton®; Pediapred®; Predair®; Predaject®; Predalone T.B.A.®; Predcor®; Predcor-TBA®; Pred Forte®; Pred Mild®; Prelone®

Canadian/Mexican Brand Names Fisopred® (Mexico); Novo-Prednisolone® (Canada); Sophipren® Ofteno (Mexico)

Therapeutic Category Adrenal Corticosteroid; Anti-inflammatory Agent; Corticosteroid, Ophthalmic; Corticosteroid, Systemic

Use

Dental: Treatment of a variety of oral diseases of allergic, inflammatory or autoimmune origin

Medical: Treatment of palpebral and bulbar conjunctivitis; corneal injury from chemical, radiation, thermal burns, or foreign body penetration; endocrine disorders, rheumatic disorders, collagen diseases, dermatologic diseases, allergic states, ophthalmic diseases, respiratory diseases, hematologic disorders, neoplastic diseases, edematous states, and gastrointestinal diseases; useful in patients with inability to activate prednisone (liver disease)

Usual Dosage Dose depends upon condition being treated and response of patient; dosage for infants and children should be based on severity of the disease and response of the patient rather than on strict adherence to dosage indicated by age, weight, or body surface area. Consider alternate day therapy for long-term therapy. Discontinuation of long-term therapy requires gradual withdrawal by tapering the dose.

Children: Anti-inflammatory or immunosuppressive dose: Oral, I.V., I.M. (sodium phosphate salt): 0.1-2 mg/kg/day in divided doses 1-4 times/day

Adults: Oral, I.V., I.M. (sodium phosphate salt): 5-60 mg/day

Elderly: Use lowest effective adult dose

Mechanism of Action Decreases inflammation by suppression of migration of polymorphonuclear leukocytes and reversal of increased capillary permeability; suppresses the immune system by reducing activity and volume of the lymphatic system

Local Anesthetic/Vasoconstrictor Precautions No information available to require special precautions

Effects on Dental Treatment No effects or complications reported

Other Adverse Effects >10%:

Central nervous system: Insomnia, nervousness

Gastrointestinal: Increased appetite, indigestion

Contraindications Acute superficial herpes simplex keratitis; systemic fungal infections; varicella; hypersensitivity to prednisolone or any component

Warnings/Precautions Use with caution in patients with hyperthyroidism, cirrhosis, nonspecific ulcerative colitis, hypertension, osteoporosis, thromboembolic tendencies, CHF, convulsive disorders, myasthenia gravis, thrombophlebitis, peptic ulcer, diabetes; acute adrenal insufficiency may occur with abrupt withdrawal after long-term therapy or with stress; young pediatric patients may be more susceptible to adrenal axis suppression from topical therapy. Because of the risk of adverse effects, systemic corticosteroids should be used cautiously in the elderly, in the smallest possible dose, and for the shortest possible time.

Drug Interactions Decreased effect with barbiturates, phenytoin, rifampin; decreased effect of salicylates, vaccines, toxoids

Drug Uptake

Absorption: Rapid and nearly complete

Serum half-life: 3.6 hours; biological: 18-36 hours

Pregnancy Risk Factor C

Breast-feeding Considerations May be taken while breast-feeding

Dosage Forms

Injection, as acetate (for I.M., intralesional, intra-articular, or soft tissue administration only): 25 mg/mL (10 mL, 30 mL); 50 mg/mL (30 mL)

Injection, as sodium phosphate (for I.M., I.V., intra-articular, intralesional, or soft tissue administration): 20 mg/mL (2 mL, 5 mL, 10 mL)

Injection, as tebutate (for intra-articular, intralesional, soft tissue administration only): 20 mg/mL (1 mL, 5 mL, 10 mL)

Liquid, oral, as sodium phosphate: 5 mg/5 mL (120 mL)

Solution, ophthalmic, as sodium phosphate: 0.125% (5 mL, 10 mL, 15 mL); 1% (5 mL, 10 mL, 15 mL)

Syrup: 15 mg/5 mL (240 mL)

Tablet: 5 mg

Dietary Considerations Should be taken after meals or with food or milk to decrease GI effects; limit caffeine; increase dietary intake of pyridoxine, vitamin C, vitamin D, folate, calcium, and phosphorus

Generic Available Yes

Prednisolone and Gentamicin (pred NIS oh lone & jen ta MYE sin)

Brand Names Pred-G® Ophthalmic

Therapeutic Category Antibiotic, Ophthalmic; Corticosteroid, Ophthalmic

Synonyms Gentamicin and Prednisolone

Use Treatment of steroid responsive inflammatory conditions and superficial ocular infections due to strains of microorganisms susceptible to gentamicin such as *Staphylococcus, E. coli, H. influenzae, Klebsiella, Neisseria, Pseudomonas, Proteus,* and *Serratia* species

Local Anesthetic/Vasoconstrictor Precautions No information available to require special precautions

Effects on Dental Treatment No effects or complications reported

Other Adverse Effects 1% to 10%:

Dermatologic: Delayed wound healing

Local: Burning, stinging

Ocular: Increased intraocular pressure, glaucoma, superficial punctate keratitis, infrequent optic nerve damage, posterior subcapsular cataract formation

Miscellaneous: Development of secondary infection, allergic sensitization

Pregnancy Risk Factor C

Generic Available Yes

Prednisone (PRED ni sone)

Related Information

Corticosteroid Equivalencies Comparison *on page 1139*

(Continued)

Prednisone *(Continued)*

Oral Nonviral Soft Tissue Ulcerations or Erosions *on page 1070*
Respiratory Diseases *on page 1018*
Rheumatoid Arthritis and Osteoarthritis *on page 1030*

Brand Names Deltasone®; Liquid Pred®; Meticorten®; Orasone®; Prednicen-M®; Sterapred®

Canadian/Mexican Brand Names Apo®-Prednisone (Canada); Jaa-Prednisone® (Canada); Novo-Prednisone® (Canada); Winpred (Canada)

Therapeutic Category Adrenal Corticosteroid; Anti-inflammatory Agent; Corticosteroid, Systemic

Use

Dental: Treatment of a variety of oral diseases of allergic, inflammatory or autoimmune origin

Medical: Treatment of a variety of diseases including adrenocortical insufficiency, hypercalcemia, rheumatic and collagen disorders; dermatologic, ocular, respiratory, gastrointestinal, and neoplastic diseases; organ transplantation; not available in injectable form, prednisolone must be used

Usual Dosage Dose depends upon condition being treated and response of patient; dosage for infants and children should be based on severity of the disease and response of the patient rather than on strict adherence to dosage indicated by age, weight, or body surface area. Consider alternate day therapy for long-term therapy. Discontinuation of long-term therapy requires gradual withdrawal by tapering the dose.

Children: Oral: Anti-inflammatory or immunosuppressive dose: 0.05-2 mg/kg/day divided 1-4 times/day

Adults: 5-60 mg/day in divided doses 1-4 times/day

Elderly: Use the lowest effective dose

Mechanism of Action Decreases inflammation by suppression of migration of polymorphonuclear leukocytes and reversal of increased capillary permeability; suppresses the immune system by reducing activity and volume of the lymphatic system; suppresses adrenal function at high doses

Local Anesthetic/Vasoconstrictor Precautions No information available to require special precautions

Effects on Dental Treatment No effects or complications reported

Other Adverse Effects >10%:

Central nervous system: Insomnia, nervousness

Gastrointestinal: Increased appetite, indigestion

Contraindications Serious infections, except septic shock or tuberculous meningitis; systemic fungal infections; hypersensitivity to prednisone or any component; varicella

Warnings/Precautions Use with caution in patients with hypothyroidism, cirrhosis, hypertension, congestive heart failure, ulcerative colitis, thromboembolic disorders, and patients with an increased risk for peptic ulcer disease; may retard bone growth; gradually taper dose to withdraw therapy. Because of the risk of adverse effects, systemic corticosteroids should be used cautiously in the elderly, in the smallest possible dose, and for the shortest possible time.

Drug Interactions Decreased effect with barbiturates, phenytoin, rifampin; decreased effect of salicylates, vaccines, toxoids

Drug Uptake Prednisone is inactive and must be metabolized to prednisolone which may be impaired in patients with impaired liver function

Absorption: Rapid and nearly complete

Serum half-life: Normal renal function: 2.5-3.5 hours

Pregnancy Risk Factor B

Breast-feeding Considerations May be taken while breast-feeding

Dosage Forms

Solution, oral: Concentrate (30% alcohol): 5 mg/mL (30 mL); Nonconcentrate (5% alcohol): 5 mg/5 mL (5 mL, 500 mL)

Syrup: 5 mg/5 mL (120 mL, 240 mL)

Tablet: 1 mg, 2.5 mg, 5 mg, 10 mg, 20 mg, 50 mg

Dietary Considerations Should be taken after meals or with food or milk; limit caffeine; increase dietary intake of pyridoxine, vitamin C, vitamin D, folate, calcium, and phosphorus

Generic Available Yes

Predominant Cultivable Microorganisms From Various Sites of the Oral Cavity *see page 1166*

Prefrin™ Ophthalmic Solution *see Phenylephrine on page 752*

Pregestimil® [OTC] *see Enteral Nutritional Products on page 350*

Pregnyl® *see Chorionic Gonadotropin on page 231*

Prelone® *see Prednisolone on page 788*

Premarin® *see* Estrogens, Conjugated *on page 368*

Premarin® With Methyltestosterone Oral *see* Estrogens and Methyltestosterone *on page 368*

Premphase™ *see* Estrogens and Medroxyprogesterone *on page 367*

Prempro™ *see* Estrogens and Medroxyprogesterone *on page 367*

Prenatal Vitamins *see* Vitamins, Multiple *on page 995*

Prenavite® [OTC] *see* Vitamins, Multiple *on page 995*

Pre-Pen® *see* Benzylpenicilloyl-polylysine *on page 123*

Prepidil® Vaginal Gel *see* Dinoprostone *on page 322*

Prescription Strength Desenex® [OTC] *see* Miconazole *on page 635*

Prescription Writing *see page 1218*

Pre-Sed® *see* Hexobarbital *on page 470*

PreSun® 29 [OTC] *see* Methoxycinnamate and Oxybenzone *on page 619*

Pretz® [OTC] *see* Sodium Chloride *on page 870*

Pretz-D® [OTC] *see* Ephedrine *on page 351*

Prevacid® *see* Lansoprazole *on page 542*

Prevalite® *see* Cholestyramine Resin *on page 229*

PreviDent® *see* Fluoride *on page 415*

Prilocaine (PRIL oh kane)

Related Information
Oral Pain *on page 1053*

Brand Names
Citanest Plain 4% Injection

Therapeutic Category
Dental/Local Anesthetics; Local Anesthetic, Injectable

Use
Dental: Amide-type anesthetic used for local infiltration anesthesia; injection near nerve trunks to produce nerve block

Usual Dosage
Children <10 years: Doses >40 mg (1 mL) as a 4% solution per procedure rarely needed

Children >10 years and Adults: Dental anesthesia, infiltration, or conduction block: Initial: 40-80 mg (1-2 mL) as a 4% solution; up to a maximum of 400 mg (10 mL) as a 4% solution within a 2-hour period. Manufacturer's maximum recommended dose is not more than 600 mg to normal healthy adults. The effective anesthetic dose varies with procedure, intensity of anesthesia needed, duration of anesthesia required and physical condition of the patient. Always use the lowest effective dose along with careful aspiration.

The following numbers of dental carpules (1.8 mL) provide the indicated amounts of prilocaine hydrochloride 4%.

# of Cartridges	Mg Prilocaine (4%)
1	72
2	144
3	216
4	288
5	360
6	432
7	504
8	576

Note: Adult and children doses of prilocaine hydrochloride cited from USP Dispensing Information (USP DI), 17th ed, The United States Pharmacopeial Convention, Inc, Rockville, MD, 1997, 139.

Mechanism of Action
Local anesthetics bind selectively to the intracellular surface of sodium channels to block influx of sodium into the axon. As a result, depolarization necessary for action potential propagation and subsequent nerve function is prevented. The block at the sodium channel is reversible. When drug diffuses away from the axon, sodium channel function is restored and nerve propagation returns.

Local Anesthetic/Vasoconstrictor Precautions
No information available to require special precautions

Effects on Dental Treatment
No effects or complications reported

Other Adverse Effects
Degree of adverse effects in the central nervous system and cardiovascular system are directly related to the blood levels of local anesthetic. The effects below are more likely to occur after systemic administration rather than infiltration.

Cardiovascular: Myocardial effects include a decrease in contraction force as well as a decrease in electrical excitability and myocardial conduction rate
(Continued)

Prilocaine *(Continued)*

resulting in bradycardia and reduction in cardiac output.

Central nervous system: High blood levels result in anxiety, restlessness, disorientation, confusion, dizziness, tremors and seizures. This is followed by depression of CNS resulting in somnolence, unconsciousness and possible respiratory arrest. Nausea and vomiting may also occur. In some cases, symptoms of CNS stimulation may be absent and the primary CNS effects are somnolence and unconsciousness.

Hypersensitivity reactions: May be manifest as dermatologic reactions and edema at injection site. Asthmatic syndromes have occurred.

Psychogenic reactions: It is common to misinterpret psychogenic responses to local anesthetic injection as an allergic reaction. Intraoral injections are perceived by many patients as a stressful procedure in dentistry. Common symptoms to this stress are sweating, palpitations, hyperventilation, generalized pallor and a fainting feeling

Contraindications Hypersensitivity to local anesthetics of the amide type

Warnings/Precautions Aspirate the syringe after tissue penetration and before injection to minimize chance of direct vascular injection

Drug Interactions No data reported

Drug Uptake
Infiltration
Onset: ~2 minutes
Duration: Complete anesthesia for procedures lasting 20 minutes
Inferior alveolar nerve block
Onset: ~3 minutes
Duration: ~2.5 hours

Pregnancy Risk Factor B

Breast-feeding Considerations Usual infiltration doses of prilocaine given to nursing mothers has not been shown to affect the health of the nursing infant

Dosage Forms Prilocaine hydrochloride 4%, 1.8 mL cartridges, containers of 100

Dietary Considerations No data reported

Generic Available No

Selected Readings
Jastak JT and Yagiela JA, "Vasoconstrictors and Local Anesthesia: A Review and Rationale for Use," *J Am Dent Assoc*, 1983, 107(4):623-30.
MacKenzie TA and Young ER, "Local Anesthetic Update," *Anesth Prog*, 1993, 40(2):29-34.
Wynn RL, "Epinephrine Interactions With Beta-Blockers," *Gen Dent*, 1994, 42(1):16, 18.
Yagiela JA, "Local Anesthetics," *Anesth Prog*, 1991, 38(4-5):128-41.

Prilocaine With Epinephrine *(PRIL oh kane with ep i NEF rin)*

Related Information
Oral Pain *on page 1053*

Brand Names Citanest Forte® With Epinephrine

Canadian/Mexican Brand Names Citanest® Forte (Canada); Citanest® Octapresin (Mexico)

Therapeutic Category Dental/Local Anesthetics; Local Anesthetic, Injectable

Use Dental: Amide-type anesthetic used for local infiltration anesthesia; injection near nerve trunks to produce nerve block

Usual Dosage

Children <10 years: Doses >40 mg (1 mL) of prilocaine hydrochloride as a 4% solution with epinephrine 1:200,000 are rarely needed

Children >10 years and Adults: Dental anesthesia, infiltration, or conduction block: Initial: 40-80 mg (1-2 mL) of prilocaine hydrochloride as a 4% solution with epinephrine 1:200,000; up to a maximum of 400 mg (10 mL) of prilocaine hydrochloride within a 2-hour period. The effective anesthetic dose varies with procedure, intensity of anesthesia needed, duration of anesthesia required, and physical condition of the patient. Always use the lowest effective dose along with careful aspiration.

The following numbers of dental carpules (1.8 mL) provide the indicated amounts of prilocaine hydrochloride 4% and epinephrine 1:200,000.

# of Cartridges	Mg Prilocaine (4%)	Mg Vasoconstrictor (Epinephrine 1:200,000)
1	72	0.009
2	144	0.018
3	216	0.027
4	288	0.036
5	360	0.045
6	432	0.054
7	504	0.063
8	576	0.072

Note: Adult and children doses of prilocaine hydrochloride with epinephrine cited from USP Dispensing Information (USP DI), 17th ed, The United States Pharmacopeial Convention, Inc, Rockville, MD, 1997, 140.

Mechanism of Action Local anesthetics bind selectively to the intracellular surface of sodium channels to block influx of sodium into the axon. As a result, depolarization necessary for action potential propagation and subsequent nerve function is prevented. The block at the sodium channel is reversible. When drug diffuses away from the axon, sodium channel function is restored and nerve propagation returns.

Epinephrine prolongs the duration of the anesthetic actions of prilocaine by causing vasoconstriction (alpha adrenergic receptor agonist) of the vasculature surrounding the nerve axons. This prevents the diffusion of prilocaine away from the nerves resulting in a longer retention in the axon.

Local Anesthetic/Vasoconstrictor Precautions No information available to require special precautions

Effects on Dental Treatment No effects or complications reported

Other Adverse Effects Degree of adverse effects in the CNS and cardiovascular system are directly related to the blood levels of prilocaine. The effects below are more likely to occur after systemic administration rather than infiltration.

Cardiovascular: Myocardial effects include a decrease in contraction force as well as a decrease in electrical excitability and myocardial conduction rate resulting in bradycardia and reduction in cardiac output.

Central nervous system: High blood levels result in anxiety, restlessness, disorientation, confusion, dizziness, tremors and seizures. This is followed by depression of CNS resulting in somnolence, unconsciousness and possible respiratory arrest. Nausea and vomiting may also occur. In some cases, symptoms of CNS stimulation may be absent and the primary CNS effects are somnolence and unconsciousness.

Hypersensitivity reactions: Extremely rare, but may be manifest as dermatologic reactions and edema at injection site. Asthmatic syndromes have occurred. Patients may exhibit hypersensitivity to bisulfites contained in local anesthetic solution to prevent oxidation of epinephrine. In general, patients reacting to bisulfites have a history of asthma and their airways are hyper-reactive to asthmatic syndrome.

Psychogenic reactions: It is common to misinterpret psychogenic responses to local anesthetic injection as an allergic reaction. Intraoral injections are perceived by many patients as a stressful procedure in dentistry. Common symptoms to this stress are sweating, palpitations, hyperventilation, generalized pallor, and a fainting feeling.

Contraindications Hypersensitivity to local anesthetics of the amide-type

Warnings/Precautions Should be avoided in patients with uncontrolled hyperthyroidism. Should be used in minimal amounts in patients with significant cardiovascular problems (because of epinephrine component). Aspirate the syringe after tissue penetration and before injection to minimize chance of direct vascular injection

Drug Interactions Due to epinephrine component, use with tricyclic antidepressants or MAO inhibitors could result in increased pressor response; use with nonselective beta-blockers (ie, propranolol) could result in serious hypertension and reflex bradycardia

Drug Uptake
Onset of action:
Infiltration <2 minutes
Inferior alveolar nerve block: <3 minutes
Duration:
Infiltration 2.25 hours
Inferior alveolar nerve block: 3 hours

Pregnancy Risk Factor C

Breast-feeding Considerations Usual infiltration doses of prilocaine with epinephrine given to nursing mothers has not been shown to affect the health of the nursing infant

Dosage Forms Injection: Prilocaine hydrochloride 4% with epinephrine 1:200,000 (1.8 mL cartridges, in boxes of 100)

Dietary Considerations No data reported

Generic Available No
(Continued)

Prilocaine With Epinephrine *(Continued)*

Selected Readings
Blanton PL and Roda RS, "The Anatomy of Local Anesthesia," *J Calif Dent Assoc*, 1995, 23(4):55-65.

Jastak JT and Yagiela JA, "Vasoconstrictors and Local Anesthesia: A Review and Rationale for Use," *J Am Dent Assoc*, 1983, 107(4):623-30.

MacKenzie TA and Young ER, "Local Anesthetic Update," *Anesth Prog*, 1993, 40(2):29-34.

Wynn RL, "Epinephrine Interactions With Beta-Blockers," *Gen Dent*, 1994, 42(1):16, 18.

Yagiela JA, "Local Anesthetics," *Anesth Prog*, 1991, 38(4-5):128-41.

Yagiela JA, "Vasoconstrictor Agents for Local Anesthesia," *Anesth Prog*, 1995, 42(3-4):116-20.

Prilosec™ *see* Omeprazole *on page 699*

Primacor® *see* Milrinone *on page 639*

Primaquine Phosphate (PRIM a kween FOS fate)

Therapeutic Category Antimalarial Agent

Use Provides radical cure of *P. vivax* or *P. ovale* malaria after a clinical attack has been confirmed by blood smear or serologic titer and postexposure prophylaxis

Usual Dosage Oral:

Children: 0.3 mg base/kg/day once daily for 14 days (not to exceed 15 mg/day) or 0.9 mg base/kg once weekly for 8 weeks not to exceed 45 mg base/week

Adults: 15 mg/day (base) once daily for 14 days or 45 mg base once weekly for 8 weeks

Mechanism of Action Eliminates the primary tissue exoerythrocytic forms of *P. falciparum*; disrupts mitochondria and binds to DNA

Local Anesthetic/Vasoconstrictor Precautions No information available to require special precautions

Effects on Dental Treatment No effects or complications reported

Other Adverse Effects

>10%:

Gastrointestinal: Abdominal pain, nausea, vomiting

Hematologic: Hemolytic anemia

1% to 10%: Hematologic: Methemoglobinemia

<1%:

Cardiovascular: Arrhythmias

Central nervous system: Headache

Dermatologic: Pruritus

Hematologic: Leukopenia, agranulocytosis, leukocytosis

Ocular: Interference with visual accommodation

Drug Interactions Increased toxicity/levels with quinacrine

Drug Uptake

Absorption: Oral: Well absorbed

Serum half-life: 3.7-9.6 hours

Time to peak serum concentration: Within 1-2 hours

Pregnancy Risk Factor C

Generic Available Yes

Primaxin® *see* Imipenem and Cilastatin *on page 500*

Primidone (PRI mi done)

Brand Names Mysoline®

Canadian/Mexican Brand Names Apo®-Primidone (Canada); Sertan® (Canada)

Therapeutic Category Anticonvulsant, Barbiturate

Use Management of grand mal, complex partial, and focal seizures

Unlabeled use: Benign familial tremor (essential tremor)

Usual Dosage Oral:

Children <8 years: Initial: 50-125 mg/day given at bedtime; increase by 50-125 mg/day increments every 3-7 days; usual dose: 10-25 mg/kg/day in divided doses 3-4 times/day

Children >8 years and Adults: Initial: 125-250 mg/day at bedtime; increase by 125-250 mg/day every 3-7 days; usual dose: 750-1500 mg/day in divided doses 3-4 times/day with maximum dosage of 2 g/day

Mechanism of Action Decreases neuron excitability, raises seizure threshold similar to phenobarbital; primidone has two active metabolites, phenobarbital and phenylethylmalonamide (PEMA); PEMA may enhance the activity of phenobarbital

Local Anesthetic/Vasoconstrictor Precautions No information available to require special precautions

Effects on Dental Treatment No effects or complications reported

Other Adverse Effects

>10%: Central nervous system: Drowsiness, vertigo, ataxia, lethargy, behavior change, sedation, headache

1% to 10%:
  Gastrointestinal: Nausea, vomiting, anorexia
  Genitourinary: Impotence
<1%:
  Dermatologic: Rash
  Hematologic: Leukopenia, malignant lymphoma-like syndrome, megaloblastic anemia
  Ocular: Diplopia, nystagmus
  Miscellaneous: Systemic lupus-like syndrome

Drug Interactions
  Decreased effect: Primidone may decrease serum concentrations of ethosuximide, valproic acid, griseofulvin; phenytoin may decrease primidone serum concentrations
  Increased toxicity: Methylphenidate may increase primidone serum concentrations; valproic acid may increase phenobarbital concentrations derived from primidone

Drug Uptake
  Serum half-life (age dependent):
    Primidone: 10-12 hours
    PEMA: 16 hours
    Phenobarbital: 52-118 hours
  Time to peak serum concentration: Oral: Within 4 hours

Pregnancy Risk Factor D
Generic Available Yes: Tablet

Principen® see Ampicillin on page 73
Prinivil® see Lisinopril on page 560
Prinzide® see Lisinopril and Hydrochlorothiazide on page 561
Priscoline® see Tolazoline on page 941
Privine® Nasal [OTC] see Naphazoline on page 664
ProAmatine™ see Midodrine on page 637
Probalan® see Probenecid on this page
Probampacin® see Ampicillin and Probenecid on page 74
Pro-Banthine® see Propantheline on page 807

Probenecid (proe BEN e sid)
  Related Information
    Dental Drug Interactions: Update on Drug Combinations Requiring Special Considerations on page 1144
  Brand Names Benemid®; Probalan®
  Canadian/Mexican Brand Names Benecid® Probenecida Valdecasas (Mexico); Benuryl® (Canada)
  Therapeutic Category Adjuvant Therapy, Penicillin Level Prolongation; Uric Acid Lowering Agent
  Use Prevention of gouty arthritis; hyperuricemia; prolongation of beta-lactam effect (ie, serum levels)
  Usual Dosage Oral:
    Children:
      <2 years: Not recommended
      2-14 years: Prolong penicillin serum levels: 25 mg/kg starting dose, then 40 mg/kg/day given 4 times/day
      Gonorrhea: <45 kg: 25 mg/kg x 1 (maximum: 1 g/dose) 30 minutes before penicillin, ampicillin or amoxicillin
    Adults:
      Hyperuricemia with gout: 250 mg twice daily for one week; increase to 250-500 mg/day; may increase by 500 mg/month, if needed, to maximum of 2-3 g/day (dosages may be increased by 500 mg every 6 months if serum urate concentrations are controlled)
      Prolong penicillin serum levels: 500 mg 4 times/day
      Gonorrhea: 1 g 30 minutes before penicillin, ampicillin or amoxicillin
  Mechanism of Action Competitively inhibits the reabsorption of uric acid at the proximal convoluted tubule, thereby promoting its excretion and reducing serum uric acid levels; increases plasma levels of weak organic acids (penicillins, cephalosporins, or other beta-lactam antibiotics) by competitively inhibiting their renal tubular secretion
  Local Anesthetic/Vasoconstrictor Precautions No information available to require special precautions
  Effects on Dental Treatment No effects or complications reported
  Other Adverse Effects
    >10%:
      Central nervous system: Headache
  (Continued)

Probenecid *(Continued)*

Gastrointestinal: Anorexia, nausea, vomiting
Neuromuscular & skeletal: Gouty arthritis (acute)

1% to 10%:
Central nervous system: Dizziness
Cardiovascular: Flushing of face
Dermatologic: Skin rash, itching
Gastrointestinal: Sore gums
Genitourinary: Painful urination
Renal: Renal calculi

<1%:
Hematologic: Leukopenia, hemolytic anemia, aplastic anemia
Hepatic: Hepatic necrosis
Renal: Urate nephropathy, nephrotic syndrome
Miscellaneous: Anaphylaxis

Drug Interactions
Decreased effect:
Salicylates (high dose) cause decreased uricosuria
Decreased urinary levels of nitrofurantoin cause decreased efficacy
Increased toxicity:
Increased methotrexate toxic potential
Increased penicillin and cephalosporin (beta-lactam) serum levels
Increased toxicity of acyclovir, thiopental, benzodiazepines, dapsone, sulfonyl-ureas, zidovudine

Drug Uptake
Onset of action: Effect on penicillin levels reached in about 2 hours
Absorption: Rapid and complete from GI tract
Serum half-life: Normal renal function: 6-12 hours and is dose dependent
Time to peak serum concentration: 2-4 hours

Pregnancy Risk Factor B
Generic Available Yes

Probenecid and Colchicine *see* Colchicine and Probenecid *on page 258*

Probucol *(PROE byoo kole)*

Related Information
Cardiovascular Diseases *on page 1010*

Brand Names Lorelco®

Canadian/Mexican Brand Names Lesterol® (Mexico)

Therapeutic Category Lipid Lowering Drugs

Use Adjunct to dietary therapy to decrease elevated serum total and LDL cholesterol concentrations in primary hypercholesterolemia

Mechanism of Action Increases the fecal loss of bile acid-bound low density lipoprotein cholesterol, decreases the synthesis of cholesterol and inhibits enteral cholesterol absorption

Local Anesthetic/Vasoconstrictor Precautions No information available to require special precautions

Effects on Dental Treatment No effects or complications reported

Other Adverse Effects
>10%:
Cardiovascular: Q-T prolongation, serious arrhythmias
Gastrointestinal: Bloating, diarrhea, stomach pain, nausea, vomiting

1% to 10%:
Central nervous system: Dizziness, headache
Neuromuscular & skeletal: Paresthesia

<1%:
Cardiovascular: Tachycardia
Hematologic: Anemia, thrombocytopenia

Drug Interactions Increased toxicity: Drugs that prolong the Q-T interval (eg, tricyclic antidepressants, some antiarrhythmic agents, phenothiazines) or with drugs that affect the atrial rate (eg, beta-adrenergic blocking agents) or that can cause A-V block (eg, digoxin)

Pregnancy Risk Factor B
Generic Available No

Procainamide *(proe kane A mide)*

Related Information
Cardiovascular Diseases *on page 1010*

Brand Names Procanbid®; Pronestyl®

Canadian/Mexican Brand Names Apo®-Procainamide (Canada)

Therapeutic Category Antiarrhythmic Agent, Class I-A; Antiarrhythmic Agent (Supraventricular & Ventricular)

Use Treatment of ventricular tachycardia, premature ventricular contractions, paroxysmal atrial tachycardia, and atrial fibrillation; to prevent recurrence of ventricular tachycardia, paroxysmal supraventricular tachycardia, atrial fibrillation or flutter

Usual Dosage Must be titrated to patient's response

Children:

Oral: 15-50 mg/kg/24 hours divided every 3-6 hours; maximum: 4 g/24 hours

I.M.: 20-30 mg/kg/24 hours divided every 4-6 hours in divided doses; maximum: 4 g/24 hours

I.V. (infusion requires use of an infusion pump):

Load: 3-6 mg/kg/dose over 5 minutes not to exceed 100 mg/dose; may repeat every 5-10 minutes to maximum of 15 mg/kg/load

Maintenance as continuous I.V. infusion: 20-80 mcg/kg/minute; maximum: 2 g/24 hours

Adults:

Oral: 250-500 mg/dose every 3-6 hours or 500 mg to 1 g every 6 hours sustained release; usual dose: 50 mg/kg/24 hours; maximum: 4 g/24 hours

I.M.: 0.5-1 g every 4-8 hours until oral therapy is possible

I.V. (infusion requires use of an infusion pump): Loading dose: 15-18 mg/kg administered as slow infusion over 25-30 minutes or 100-200 mg/dose repeated every 5 minutes as needed to a total dose of 1 g; maintenance dose: 1-6 mg/minute by continuous infusion

Infusion rate: 2 g/250 mL D_5W/NS (I.V. infusion requires use of an infusion pump):

1 mg/minute: 7 mL/hour

2 mg/minute: 15 mL/hour

3 mg/minute: 21 mL/hour

4 mg/minute: 30 mL/hour

5 mg/minute: 38 mL/hour

6 mg/minute: 45 mL/hour

Refractory ventricular fibrillation: 30 mg/minute, up to a total of 17 mg/kg; I.V. maintenance infusion: 1-4 mg/minute; monitor levels and do not exceed 3 mg/minute for >24 hours in adults with renal failure

ACLS guidelines: I.V.: Infuse 20 mg/minute until arrhythmia is controlled, hypotension occurs, QRS complex widens by 50% of its original width, or total of 17 mg/kg is given

Mechanism of Action Decreases myocardial excitability and conduction velocity and may depress myocardial contractility, by increasing the electrical stimulation threshold of ventricle, HIS-Purkinje system and through direct cardiac effects

Local Anesthetic/Vasoconstrictor Precautions No information available to require special precautions

Effects on Dental Treatment No effects or complications reported

Other Adverse Effects

>10%: Miscellaneous: SLE-like syndrome

1% to 10%:

Cardiovascular: Tachycardia, arrhythmias, A-V block, Q-T prolongation, widening QRS complex

Central nervous system: Dizziness, lightheadedness

Gastrointestinal: Diarrhea

<1%:

Cardiovascular: Hypotension

Central nervous system: Confusion, hallucinations, mental depression, confusion, disorientation, drug fever

Dermatologic: Rash

Gastrointestinal: Nausea, vomiting, GI complaints

Hematologic: Hemolytic anemia, agranulocytosis, neutropenia, thrombocytopenia, positive Coombs' test

Neuromuscular & skeletal: Arthralgia, myalgia

Respiratory: Pleural effusion

Drug Interactions

Increased plasma procainamide and procainamide metabolite concentrations with cimetidine, ranitidine, beta-blockers, and amiodarone

Increased effect of skeletal muscle relaxants, quinidine and lidocaine and neuromuscular blockers (succinylcholine)

Increased procainamide metabolite levels/toxicity with trimethoprim

Drug Uptake

Onset of action: I.M. 10-30 minutes

(Continued)

Procainamide *(Continued)*

Serum half-life:
Procainamide: (Dependent upon hepatic acetylator, phenotype, cardiac function, and renal function):
Adults: 2.5-4.7 hours
Anephric: 11 hours
NAPA: (Dependent upon renal function):
Children: 6 hours
Adults: 6-8 hours
Anephric: 42 hours
Time to peak serum concentration:
Capsule: Within 45 minutes to 2.5 hours
I.M.: 15-60 minutes
Pregnancy Risk Factor C
Generic Available Yes

Procaine *(PROE kane)*

Related Information
Oral Pain *on page 1053*
Brand Names Novocain®
Therapeutic Category Dental/Local Anesthetics; Local Anesthetic, Injectable
Use Produces spinal anesthesia and epidural and peripheral nerve block by injection and infiltration methods
Usual Dosage Dose varies with procedure, desired depth, and duration of anesthesia, desired muscle relaxation, vascularity of tissues, physical condition, and age of patient
Mechanism of Action Blocks both the initiation and conduction of nerve impulses by decreasing the neuronal membrane's permeability to sodium ions, which results in inhibition of depolarization with resultant blockade of conduction
Local Anesthetic/Vasoconstrictor Precautions No information available to require special precautions
Effects on Dental Treatment This is no longer a useful anesthetic in dentistry because of high incidence of allergic reactions
Other Adverse Effects
1% to 10%: Local: Burning sensation at site of injection, pain, tissue irritation
<1%:
Central nervous system: Aseptic meningitis resulting in paralysis can occur, CNS stimulation followed by CNS depression, chills
Dermatologic: Skin discoloration
Gastrointestinal: Nausea, vomiting
Ocular: Miosis
Otic: Tinnitus
Miscellaneous: Anaphylactoid reaction
Drug Interactions
Decreased effect of sulfonamides with the PABA metabolite of procaine, chloroprocaine, and tetracaine
Decreased/increased effect of vasopressors, ergot alkaloids, and MAO inhibitors on blood pressure when using anesthetic solutions with a vasoconstrictor
Drug Uptake
Onset of effect: Injection: Within 2-5 minutes
Duration: 0.5-1.5 hours (dependent upon patient, type of block, concentration, and method of anesthesia)
Serum half-life: 7.7 minutes
Pregnancy Risk Factor C
Dosage Forms Injection, as hydrochloride: 1% [10 mg/mL] (2 mL, 6 mL, 30 mL, 100 mL); 2% [20 mg/mL] (30 mL, 100 mL); 10% (2 mL)
Generic Available Yes

Pro-Cal-Sof® [OTC] *see Docusate on page 331*
Procanbid® *see Procainamide on page 796*

Procarbazine *(proe KAR ba zeen)*

Brand Names Matulane®
Canadian/Mexican Brand Names Natulan® (Mexico)
Therapeutic Category Antineoplastic Agent, Miscellaneous
Synonyms Benzmethyzin; N-Methylhydrazine; Procarbazine Hydrochloride
Use Treatment of Hodgkin's disease, non-Hodgkin's lymphoma, brain tumor, bronchogenic carcinoma
Usual Dosage Refer to individual protocols

Oral (dose based on patients ideal weight if the patients has abnormal fluid retention):

Children:

BMT aplastic anemia conditioning regimen: 12.5 mg/kg/dose every other day for 4 doses

Hodgkin's disease: MOPP/IC-MOPP regimens: 100 mg/m²/day for 14 days and repeated every 4 weeks

Neuroblastoma and medulloblastoma: Doses as high as 100-200 mg/m²/day once daily have been used

Adults: Initial: 2-4 mg/kg/day in single or divided doses for 7 days then increase dose to 4-6 mg/kg/day until response is obtained or leukocyte count decreased <4000/mm³ or the platelet count decreased <100,000/mm³; maintenance: 1-2 mg/kg/day

In MOPP, 100 mg/m²/day on days 1-14 of a 28-day cycle

Mechanism of Action Mechanism of action is not clear, methylating of nucleic acids; inhibits DNA, RNA, and protein synthesis; may damage DNA directly and suppresses mitosis; metabolic activation required by host

Local Anesthetic/Vasoconstrictor Precautions No information available to require special precautions

Effects on Dental Treatment No effects or complications reported

Other Adverse Effects

>10%:

Central nervous system: Mental depression, manic reactions, hallucinations, dizziness, headache, nervousness, insomnia, nightmares, ataxia, foot drop, confusion, and seizures

Endocrine & metabolic: Amenorrhea

Gastrointestinal: Severe nausea and vomiting occur frequently and may be dose-limiting; anorexia, abdominal pain, stomatitis, dysphagia, diarrhea, and constipation; use a nonphenothiazine antiemetic, when possible

Emetic potential: Moderately high (60% to 90%)

Hematologic: May be dose-limiting toxicity; procarbazine should be discontinued if leukocyte count is <4000/mm³ or platelet count <100,000/mm³

Neuromuscular & skeletal: Paresthesia, neuropathies, disorientation, decreased reflexes, tremors

Ocular: Nystagmus

Respiratory: Pleural effusion, cough

1% to 10%:

Dermatologic: Alopecia, hyperpigmentation

Hepatic: Hepatotoxicity

<1%:

Cardiovascular: Hypotension (orthostatic), hypertensive crisis

Central nervous system: Irritability, somnolence

Dermatologic: Dermatitis, hypersensitivity rash, pruritus

Endocrine & metabolic: Cessation of menses, disulfiram-like reaction of alcohol

Hepatic: Jaundice

Neuromuscular & skeletal: Arthralgia, myalgia

Ocular: Diplopia, photophobia

Respiratory: Pneumonitis, hoarseness

Miscellaneous: Flu-like syndrome, secondary malignancy, allergic reactions

Drug Uptake

Absorption: Oral: Rapid and complete

Serum half-life: 1 hour

Pregnancy Risk Factor D

Generic Available No

Procarbazine Hydrochloride *see* Procarbazine *on previous page*

Procardia® *see* Nifedipine *on page 680*

Procardia XL® *see* Nifedipine *on page 680*

Prochlorperazine (proe klor PER a zeen)

Brand Names Compazine®

Canadian/Mexican Brand Names Nu-Prochlor® (Canada); PMS-Prochlorperazine® (Canada); Prorazin® (Canada)

Therapeutic Category Antiemetic; Antipsychotic Agent; Phenothiazine Derivative

Use Management of nausea and vomiting; acute and chronic psychosis

Usual Dosage

Antiemetic: Children:

Oral, rectal:

>10 kg: 0.4 mg/kg/24 hours in 3-4 divided doses; **or**

9-14 kg: 2.5 mg every 12-24 hours as needed; maximum: 7.5 mg/day

14-18 kg: 2.5 mg every 8-12 hours as needed; maximum: 10 mg/day

(Continued)

Prochlorperazine *(Continued)*

18-39 kg: 2.5 mg every 8 hours or 5 mg every 12 hours as needed; maximum: 15 mg/day

I.M.: 0.1-0.15 mg/kg/dose; usual: 0.13 mg/kg/dose; change to oral as soon as possible

I.V.: Not recommended in children <10 kg or <2 years

Antiemetic: Adults:

Oral: 5-10 mg 3-4 times/day; usual maximum: 40 mg/day

I.M.: 5-10 mg every 3-4 hours; usual maximum: 40 mg/day

I.V.: 2.5-10 mg; maximum 10 mg/dose or 40 mg/day; may repeat dose every 3-4 hours as needed

Rectal: 25 mg twice daily

Antipsychotic:

Children 2-12 years:

Oral, rectal: 2.5 mg 2-3 times/day; increase dosage as needed to maximum daily dose of 20 mg for 2-5 years and 25 mg for 6-12 years

I.M.: 0.13 mg/kg/dose; change to oral as soon as possible

Adults:

Oral: 5-10 mg 3-4 times/day; doses up to 150 mg/day may be required in some patients for treatment of severe disturbances

I.M.: 10-20 mg every 4-6 hours may be required in some patients for treatment of severe disturbances; change to oral as soon as possible

Dementia behavior (nonpsychotic): Elderly: Initial: 2.5-5 mg 1-2 times/day; increase dose at 4- to 7-day intervals by 2.5-5 mg/day; increase dosing intervals (twice daily, 3 times/day, etc) as necessary to control response or side effects; maximum daily dose should probably not exceed 75 mg in elderly; gradual increases (titration) may prevent some side effects or decrease their severity

Not dialyzable (0% to 5%)

Mechanism of Action Blocks postsynaptic mesolimbic dopaminergic D_1 and D_2 receptors in the brain, including the medullary chemoreceptor trigger zone; exhibits a strong alpha-adrenergic and anticholinergic blocking effect and depresses the release of hypothalamic and hypophyseal hormones; believed to depress the reticular activating system, thus affecting basal metabolism, body temperature, wakefulness, vasomotor tone and emesis

Local Anesthetic/Vasoconstrictor Precautions No information available to require special precautions

Effects on Dental Treatment >10% of patients experience dry mouth

Significant hypotension may occur especially when the drug is administered parenterally; orthostatic hypotension is due to alpha-receptor blockade, the elderly are at greater risk for orthostatic hypotension

Tardive dyskinesia: Prevalence rate may be 40% in elderly; development of the syndrome and the irreversible nature are proportional to duration and total cumulative dose over time

Extrapyramidal reactions are more common in elderly with up to 50% developing these reactions after 60 years of age; drug-induced **Parkinson's syndrome** occurs often; **Akathisia** is the most common extrapyramidal reaction in elderly

Increased confusion, memory loss, psychotic behavior, and agitation frequently occur as a consequence of anticholinergic effects

Antipsychotic associated sedation in nonpsychotic patients is extremely unpleasant due to feelings of depersonalization, derealization, and dysphoria

Other Adverse Effects Incidence of extrapyramidal reactions are higher with prochlorperazine than chlorpromazine

Central nervous system: Sedation, drowsiness, restlessness, anxiety, extrapyramidal reactions, parkinsonian signs and symptoms, seizures, altered central temperature regulation

Dermatologic: Photosensitivity, hyperpigmentation, pruritus, rash

Endocrine & metabolic: Amenorrhea, gynecomastia

Miscellaneous: Anaphylactoid reactions

>10%:

Cardiovascular: Hypotension (especially with I.V. use), orthostatic hypotension, tachycardia, arrhythmias

Central nervous system: Pseudoparkinsonism, akathisia, tardive dyskinesia (persistent), dizziness, dystonias

Gastrointestinal: Constipation

Genitourinary: Urinary retention

Ocular: Pigmentary retinopathy, blurred vision

Respiratory: Nasal congestion

Miscellaneous: Decreased sweating
1% to 10%:
Dermatologic: Skin rash
Endocrine & metabolic: Changes in menstrual cycle pain in breasts, changes in libido
Gastrointestinal: Weight gain, nausea, vomiting, stomach pain
Genitourinary: Dysuria, ejaculatory disturbances
Neuromuscular & skeletal: Trembling of fingers
<1%:
Central nervous system: Neuroleptic malignant syndrome (NMS), impairment of temperature regulation lowering of seizures threshold
Dermatologic: Discoloration of skin (blue-gray)
Endocrine & metabolic: Galactorrhea
Genitourinary: Priapism
Hematologic: Agranulocytosis, leukopenia, thrombocytopenia
Hepatic: Cholestatic jaundice, hepatotoxicity
Ocular: Cornea and lens changes, pigmentary retinopathy
Drug Interactions Increased toxicity: Additive effects with other CNS depressants
Drug Uptake
Onset of effect:
Oral: Within 30-40 minutes
I.M.: Within 10-20 minutes
Rectal: Within 60 minutes
Duration: Persists longest with I.M. and oral extended-release doses (12 hours); shortest following rectal and immediate release oral administration (3-4 hours)
Serum half-life: 23 hours
Pregnancy Risk Factor C
Generic Available Yes

Procrit® see Epoetin Alfa on page 355

Proctofoam®-HC see Pramoxine and Hydrocortisone on page 784

ProctoFoam® NS [OTC] see Pramoxine on page 784

Procyclidine (proe SYE kli deen)
Brand Names Kemadrin®
Canadian/Mexican Brand Names PMS-Procyclidine® (Canada); Procyclid® (Canada)
Therapeutic Category Anticholinergic Agent; Anti-Parkinson's Agent
Use Relieves symptoms of parkinsonian syndrome and drug-induced extrapyramidal symptoms
Usual Dosage Adults: Oral: 2.5 mg 3 times/day after meals; if tolerated, gradually increase dose, maximum of 20 mg/day if necessary
Mechanism of Action Thought to act by blocking excess acetylcholine at cerebral synapses; many of its effects are due to its pharmacologic similarities with atropine
Local Anesthetic/Vasoconstrictor Precautions No information available to require special precautions
Effects on Dental Treatment >10% of patients experience dry mouth; prolonged use of antidyskinetics may decrease or inhibit salivary flow and could contribute to development of periodontal disease, oral candidiasis or discomfort
Other Adverse Effects
>10%:
Dermatologic: Dry skin
Gastrointestinal: Constipation
Respiratory: Dry nose, throat
Miscellaneous: Decreased sweating
1% to 10%:
Dermatologic: Photosensitivity
Endocrine & metabolic: Decreased flow of breast milk
Gastrointestinal: Dysphagia
<1%:
Cardiovascular: Orthostatic hypotension, ventricular fibrillation, tachycardia, palpitations
Central nervous system: Confusion, drowsiness, headache, loss of memory, fatigue, ataxia
Dermatologic: Skin rash
Gastrointestinal: Bloated feeling, nausea, vomiting
Genitourinary: Dysuria
Neuromuscular & skeletal: Weakness
Ocular: Increased intraocular pain, blurred vision
(Continued)

Procyclidine (Continued)

Drug Interactions
Decreased effect of psychotropics
Increased toxicity with phenothiazines, meperidine, TCAs
Drug Uptake
Onset of effect: Oral: Within 30-40 minutes
Duration: 4-6 hours
Pregnancy Risk Factor C
Generic Available No

Prodium® [OTC] *see* Phenazopyridine *on page 746*
Profasi® HP *see* Chorionic Gonadotropin *on page 231*
Profenal® *see* Suprofen *on page 900*
Profen II® *see* Guaifenesin and Phenylpropanolamine *on page 454*
Profen LA® *see* Guaifenesin and Phenylpropanolamine *on page 454*
Profilate® OSD *see* Antihemophilic Factor (Human) *on page 80*
Profilate® SD *see* Antihemophilic Factor (Human) *on page 80*
Profilnine® Heat-Treated *see* Factor IX Complex (Human) *on page 391*
Progestasert® *see* Progesterone *on this page*
Progesterona (Mexico) *see* Progesterone *on this page*

Progesterone (proe JES ter one)

Brand Names Crinone® Vaginal Gel; Progestasert®
Canadian/Mexican Brand Names PMS-Progesterone® (Canada); Progesterone Oil (Canada); Utrogestan® (Mexico)
Therapeutic Category Progestin
Synonyms Progesterona (Mexico)
Use Intrauterine contraception in women who have had at least 1 child, are in a stable, mutually monogamous relationship, and have no history of pelvic inflammatory disease; amenorrhea; functional uterine bleeding
Usual Dosage Adults: Female: Insert a single system into the uterine cavity; contraceptive effectiveness is retained for 1 year and system must be replaced 1 year after insertion
Mechanism of Action Natural steroid hormone that induces secretory changes in the endometrium, promotes mammary gland development, relaxes uterine smooth muscle, blocks follicular maturation and ovulation, and maintains pregnancy
Local Anesthetic/Vasoconstrictor Precautions No information available to require special precautions
Effects on Dental Treatment Progestins may predispose the patient to gingival bleeding
Other Adverse Effects
>10%:
Cardiovascular: Edema
Endocrine & metabolic: Breakthrough bleeding, spotting, changes in menstrual flow, amenorrhea
Gastrointestinal: Anorexia
Local: Pain at injection site
Neuromuscular & skeletal: Weakness
1% to 10%:
Cardiovascular: Embolism, central thrombosis
Central nervous system: Mental depression, fever, insomnia
Dermatologic: Melasma or chloasma, allergic rash with or without pruritus
Endocrine: Changes in cervical erosion and secretions, increased breast tenderness
Gastrointestinal: Weight gain or loss
Hepatic: Cholestatic jaundice
Local: Thrombophlebitis
Drug Interactions Decreased effect: Aminoglutethimide may decrease effect by increasing hepatic metabolism
Drug Uptake
Duration of action: 24 hours
Serum half-life: 5 minutes
Pregnancy Risk Factor X
Generic Available Yes

Proglycem® *see* Diazoxide *on page 301*
Prograf® *see* Tacrolimus *on page 902*
ProHIBiT® *see* Haemophilus b Conjugate Vaccine *on page 460*
Prolamine® [OTC] *see* Phenylpropanolamine *on page 754*
Prolastin® Injection *see* Alpha₁-Proteinase Inhibitor *on page 42*

Proleukin® *see* Aldesleukin *on page 37*

Prolixin® *see* Fluphenazine *on page 420*

Prolixin Decanoate® *see* Fluphenazine *on page 420*

Prolixin Enanthate® *see* Fluphenazine *on page 420*

Proloprim® *see* Trimethoprim *on page 964*

Promazine (PROE ma zeen)

Brand Names Sparine®

Therapeutic Category Antipsychotic Agent; Phenothiazine Derivative

Use Management of manifestations of psychotic disorders; depressive neurosis; alcohol withdrawal; nausea and vomiting; nonpsychotic symptoms associated with dementia in elderly, Tourette's syndrome; Huntington's chorea; spasmodic torticollis and Reye's syndrome

Usual Dosage Oral, I.M.:

Children >12 years: Antipsychotic: 10-25 mg every 4-6 hours

Adults:
Psychosis: 10-200 mg every 4-6 hours not to exceed 1000 mg/day
Antiemetic: 25-50 mg every 4-6 hours as needed

Not dialyzable (0% to 5%)

Mechanism of Action Blocks postsynaptic mesolimbic dopaminergic D_1 and D_2 receptors in the brain; exhibits a strong alpha-adrenergic blocking and anticholinergic effect, depresses the release of hypothalamic and hypophyseal hormones; believed to depress the reticular activating system thus affecting basal metabolism, body temperature, wakefulness, vasomotor tone, and emesis

Local Anesthetic/Vasoconstrictor Precautions No information available to require special precautions

Effects on Dental Treatment Significant hypotension may occur, especially when the drug is administered parenterally; orthostatic hypotension is due to alpha-receptor blockade, the elderly are at greater risk for orthostatic hypotension

Tardive dyskinesia: Prevalence rate may be 40% in elderly; development of the syndrome and the irreversible nature are proportional to duration and total cumulative dose over time

Extrapyramidal reactions are more common in elderly with up to 50% developing these reactions after 60 years of age; drug-induced **Parkinson's syndrome** occurs often; **Akathisia** is the most common extrapyramidal reaction in elderly

Increased confusion, memory loss, psychotic behavior, and agitation frequently occur as a consequence of anticholinergic effects

Antipsychotic associated sedation in nonpsychotic patients is extremely unpleasant due to feelings of depersonalization, derealization, and dysphoria

Other Adverse Effects
>10%:
Cardiovascular: Hypotension, orthostatic hypotension
Central nervous system: Pseudoparkinsonism, akathisia, dystonias, tardive dyskinesia (persistent), dizziness
Gastrointestinal: Constipation
Ocular: Pigmentary retinopathy
Respiratory: Nasal congestion
Miscellaneous: Decreased sweating
1% to 10%:
Dermatologic: Photosensitivity, skin rash
Endocrine & metabolic: Changes in menstrual cycle, changes in libido, pain in breasts
Gastrointestinal: Weight gain, nausea, vomiting, stomach pain
Genitourinary: Dysuria, ejaculatory disturbances
Neuromuscular & skeletal: Trembling of fingers
<1%:
Central nervous system: Neuroleptic malignant syndrome (NMS), impairment of temperature regulation, lowering of seizures threshold
Dermatologic: Discoloration of skin (blue-gray)
Endocrine & metabolic: Galactorrhea
Genitourinary: Priapism
Hematologic: Agranulocytosis, leukopenia
Hepatic: Cholestatic jaundice, hepatotoxicity
Ocular: Cornea and lens changes

Drug Interactions Increased toxicity: Additive effects with other CNS depressants

Drug Uptake The specific pharmacokinetics of promazine are poorly established but probably resemble those of other phenothiazines.

(Continued)

Promazine *(Continued)*

Serum half-life: Most phenothiazines have long half-lives in the range of 24 hours or more

Pregnancy Risk Factor C

Generic Available Yes: Injection only

Prometa® *see Metaproterenol on page 605*

Promethazine *(proe METH a zeen)*

Brand Names Anergan®; Phenazine®; Phenergan®; Prorex®

Therapeutic Category Antiemetic; Antihistamine; Phenothiazine Derivative; Sedative

Use Symptomatic treatment of various allergic conditions, antiemetic, motion sickness, and as a sedative

Usual Dosage

Children:

Antihistamine: Oral, rectal: 0.1 mg/kg/dose every 6 hours during the day and 0.5 mg/kg/dose at bedtime as needed

Antiemetic: Oral, I.M., I.V., rectal: 0.25-1 mg/kg 4-6 times/day as needed

Motion sickness: Oral, rectal: 0.5 mg/kg/dose 30 minutes to 1 hour before departure, then every 12 hours as needed

Sedation: Oral, I.M., I.V., rectal: 0.5-1 mg/kg/dose every 6 hours as needed

Adults:

Antihistamine (including allergic reactions to blood or plasma):

Oral, rectal: 12.5 mg 3 times/day and 25 mg at bedtime

I.M., I.V.: 25 mg, may repeat in 2 hours when necessary; switch to oral route as soon as feasible

Antiemetic: Oral, I.M., I.V., rectal: 12.5-25 mg every 4 hours as needed

Motion sickness: Oral, rectal: 25 mg 30-60 minutes before departure, then every 12 hours as needed

Sedation: Oral, I.M., I.V., rectal: 25-50 mg/dose

Not dialyzable (0% to 5%)

Mechanism of Action Blocks postsynaptic mesolimbic dopaminergic receptors in the brain; exhibits a strong alpha-adrenergic blocking effect and depresses the release of hypothalamic and hypophyseal hormones; competes with histamine for the H_1-receptor; reduces stimuli to the brainstem reticular system

Local Anesthetic/Vasoconstrictor Precautions No information available to require special precautions

Effects on Dental Treatment Significant hypotension may occur, especially when the drug is administered parenterally; orthostatic hypotension is due to alpha-receptor blockade, the elderly are at greater risk for orthostatic hypotension

Tardive dyskinesia: Prevalence rate may be 40% in elderly; development of the syndrome and the irreversible nature are proportional to duration and total cumulative dose over time

Extrapyramidal reactions are more common in elderly with up to 50% developing these reactions after 60 years of age; drug-induced **Parkinson's syndrome** occurs often; **akathisia** is the most common extrapyramidal reaction in elderly

Increased confusion, memory loss, psychotic behavior, and agitation frequently occur as a consequence of anticholinergic effects

Antipsychotic associated sedation in nonpsychotic patients is extremely unpleasant due to feelings of depersonalization, derealization, and dysphoria

Other Adverse Effects

Hematologic: Thrombocytopenia

Hepatic: Jaundice

>10%:

Central nervous system: Slight to moderate drowsiness

Respiratory: Thickening of bronchial secretions

1% to 10%:

Central nervous system: Headache, fatigue, nervousness, dizziness

Gastrointestinal: Dry mouth, abdominal pain, nausea, diarrhea, appetite increase, weight gain

Neuromuscular & skeletal: Arthralgia

Respiratory: Pharyngitis

<1%:

Cardiovascular: Tachycardia, bradycardia, palpitations, hypotension

Central nervous system: Sedation (pronounced), confusion, excitation, extrapyramidal reactions with high doses, dystonia, faintness with I.V. administration, depression, insomnia, sedation (pronounced)

Dermatologic: Photosensitivity, rash, angioedema

Genitourinary: Urinary retention

Hepatic: Hepatitis

Neuromuscular & skeletal: Tremor, paresthesia, myalgia

Ocular: Blurred vision

Respiratory: Irregular respiration, bronchospasm, epistaxis

Miscellaneous: Allergic reactions

Drug Interactions Increased toxicity: Additive effects with other CNS depressants

Drug Uptake

Onset of effect: I.V.: Within 20 minutes (3-5 minutes with I.V. injection)

Duration: 2-6 hours

Pregnancy Risk Factor C

Generic Available Yes

Promethazine and Codeine (proe METH a zeen & KOE deen)

Brand Names Phenergan® With Codeine; Pherazine® With Codeine; Prothazine-DC®

Therapeutic Category Antihistamine; Antitussive; Cough Preparation

Use Temporary relief of coughs and upper respiratory symptoms associated with allergy or the common cold

Local Anesthetic/Vasoconstrictor Precautions No information available to require special precautions

Effects on Dental Treatment Although promethazine is a phenothiazine derivative, extrapyramidal reactions or tardive dyskinesias are not seen with the use of this drug.

Pregnancy Risk Factor C

Generic Available Yes

Promethazine and Dextromethorphan

(proe METH a zeen & deks troe meth OR fan)

Brand Names Phenameth® DM; Phenergan® with Dextromethorphan; Pherazine® w/DM

Therapeutic Category Antitussive; Cough Preparation

Use Temporary relief of coughs and upper respiratory symptoms associated with allergy or the common cold

Local Anesthetic/Vasoconstrictor Precautions No information available to require special precautions

Effects on Dental Treatment Although promethazine is a phenothiazine derivative, extrapyramidal reactions or tardive dyskinesias are not seen with the use of this drug.

Warnings/Precautions Research on chicken embryos exposed to concentrations of dextromethorphan relative to those typically taken by humans has shown to cause birth defects and fetal death; more study is needed, but it is suggested that pregnant women should be advised not to use dextromethorphan-containing medications

Pregnancy Risk Factor C (see Warnings)

Generic Available Yes

Promethazine and Phenylephrine

(proe METH a zeen & fen il EF rin)

Brand Names Phenergan® VC Syrup; Promethazine VC Plain Syrup; Promethazine VC Syrup; Prometh VC Plain Liquid

Therapeutic Category Antihistamine/Decongestant Combination

Use Temporary relief of upper respiratory symptoms associated with allergy or the common cold

Local Anesthetic/Vasoconstrictor Precautions

Phenylephrine: Use with caution since phenylephrine is a sympathomimetic amine which could interact with epinephrine to cause a pressor response

Promethazine: No information available to require special precautions

Effects on Dental Treatment

Phenylephrine: Up to 10% of patients could experience tachycardia, palpitations, and dry mouth; use vasoconstrictor with caution

Although promethazine is a phenothiazine derivative, extrapyramidal reactions or tardive dyskinesias are not seen with the use of this drug.

Pregnancy Risk Factor C

Generic Available Yes

Promethazine, Phenylephrine, and Codeine
(proe METH a zeen, fen il EF rin, & KOE deen)

Brand Names Para-Hist AT®; Phenergan® VC With Codeine; Pherazine® VC w/ Codeine; Promethist® with Codeine; Prometh® VC with Codeine

Therapeutic Category Antihistamine/Decongestant Combination; Antitussive; Cough Preparation

Use Temporary relief of coughs and upper respiratory symptoms including nasal congestion

Local Anesthetic/Vasoconstrictor Precautions
Phenylephrine: Use with caution since phenylephrine is a sympathomimetic amine which could interact with epinephrine to cause a pressor response
Promethazine: No information available to require special precautions

Effects on Dental Treatment
Phenylephrine: Up to 10% of patients could experience tachycardia, palpitations, and dry mouth; use vasoconstrictor with caution

Although promethazine is a phenothiazine derivative, extrapyramidal reactions or tardive dyskinesias are not seen with the use of this drug.

Pregnancy Risk Factor C

Generic Available Yes

Promethazine VC Plain Syrup *see* Promethazine and Phenylephrine *on previous page*

Promethazine VC Syrup *see* Promethazine and Phenylephrine *on previous page*

Promethist® with Codeine *see* Promethazine, Phenylephrine, and Codeine *on this page*

Prometh VC Plain Liquid *see* Promethazine and Phenylephrine *on previous page*

Prometh® VC with Codeine *see* Promethazine, Phenylephrine, and Codeine *on this page*

Promit® *see* Dextran 1 *on page 296*

Pronestyl® *see* Procainamide *on page 796*

Pronto® Shampoo [OTC] *see* Pyrethrins *on page 824*

Propac™ [OTC] *see* Enteral Nutritional Products *on page 350*

Propacet® *see* Propoxyphene and Acetaminophen *on page 812*

Propafenona, Clorhidrato De (Mexico) *see* Propafenone *on this page*

Propafenone (proe pa FEEN one)

Related Information
Cardiovascular Diseases *on page 1010*

Brand Names Rythmol®

Canadian/Mexican Brand Names Norfenon® (Mexico)

Therapeutic Category Antiarrhythmic Agent, Class I-C; Antiarrhythmic Agent (Supraventricular & Ventricular)

Synonyms Propafenona, Clorhidrato De (Mexico)

Use Life-threatening ventricular arrhythmias

Unlabeled use: Supraventricular tachycardias, including those patients with Wolff-Parkinson-White syndrome

Usual Dosage Adults: Oral: 150 mg every 8 hours, increase at 3- to 4-day intervals up to 300 mg every 8 hours. **Note:** Patients who exhibit significant widening of QRS complex or second or third degree A-V block may need dose reduction.

Mechanism of Action Propafenone is a 1C antiarrhythmic agent which possesses local anesthetic properties, blocks the fast inward sodium current, and slows the rate of increase of the action potential. prolongs conduction and refractoriness in all areas of the myocardium, with a slightly more pronounced effect on intraventricular conduction; it prolongs effective refractory period, reduces spontaneous automaticity and exhibits some beta-blockade activity.

Local Anesthetic/Vasoconstrictor Precautions No information available to require special precautions

Effects on Dental Treatment >10% of patients experience significant dry mouth; normal salivary flow will resume with cessation of drug therapy

Other Adverse Effects
>10%: Central nervous system: Dizziness, drowsiness
1% to 10%:
Cardiovascular: A-V block (first and second degree), cardiac conduction disturbances, palpitations, congestive heart failure, angina, bradycardia
Central nervous system: Headache, anxiety, loss of balance
Gastrointestinal: Dysgeusia, constipation, nausea, vomiting, abdominal pain, dyspepsia, anorexia, flatulence, diarrhea
Ocular: Blurred vision
Respiratory: Dyspnea

<1%:
  Cardiovascular: New or worsened arrhythmias (proarrhythmic effect), bundle branch block
  Central nervous system: Abnormal speech, vision, or dreams
  Hematologic: Leukopenia, thrombocytopenia, agranulocytosis
  Neuromuscular & skeletal: Paresthesia

Drug Interactions
  Decreased levels with rifampin
  Increased levels with cimetidine, quinidine, and beta-blockers
  Increased effect/levels of warfarin, beta-blockers metabolized by the liver, local anesthetics, cyclosporine, and digoxin (**Note:** Reduce dose of digoxin by 25%)

Drug Uptake
  Absorption: Well absorbed
  Serum half-life after a single dose (100-300 mg): 2-8 hours; half-life after chronic dosing ranges from 10-32 hours
  Time to peak: Peak levels occur in 2 hours with a 150 mg dose and 3 hours after a 300 mg dose; this agent exhibits nonlinear pharmacokinetics; when dose is increased from 300 mg to 900 mg/day, serum concentrations increase tenfold; this nonlinearity is thought to be due to saturable first-pass hepatic enzyme metabolism

Pregnancy Risk Factor C

Generic Available No

Propagest® [OTC] *see* Phenylpropanolamine *on page 754*

Propantheline (proe PAN the leen)

Brand Names Pro-Banthine®

Therapeutic Category Anticholinergic Agent; Antispasmodic Agent, Gastrointestinal

Use
  Dental: Induce dry field (xerostomia) in oral cavity
  Medical: Adjunctive treatment of peptic ulcer, irritable bowel syndrome, pancreatitis, ureteral and urinary bladder spasm; reduce duodenal motility during diagnostic radiologic procedures

Usual Dosage Adults: 15-30 mg as a single dose to induce xerostomia 1 hour before procedure

Mechanism of Action Competitively blocks the action of acetylcholine at postganglionic parasympathetic receptor sites

Local Anesthetic/Vasoconstrictor Precautions No information available to require special precautions

Effects on Dental Treatment Significant xerostomia in >10% of patients - (therapeutic effect)

Other Adverse Effects
  >10%:
    Gastrointestinal: Constipation
    Miscellaneous: Decreased sweating
  1% to 10%: Gastrointestinal: Dysphagia

Contraindications Narrow-angle glaucoma, known hypersensitivity to propantheline; ulcerative colitis; toxic megacolon; obstructive disease of the GI or urinary tract

Warnings/Precautions Use with caution in patients with hyperthyroidism, hepatic, cardiac, or renal disease, hypertension, GI infections, or other endocrine diseases

Drug Interactions Decreased effect with antacids (decreases absorption); decreased effect of sustained release dosage forms (decreases absorption); increased effect/toxicity with anticholinergics, disopyramide, narcotic analgesics, bretylium, type I antiarrhythmics, antihistamines, phenothiazines, TCAs, corticosteroids (increases intraocular pressure), CNS depressants (sedation), adenosine, amiodarone, beta-blockers, amoxapine

Drug Uptake
  Onset of effect: Oral: Within 30-45 minutes
  Duration: 4-6 hours
  Serum half-life: 1.6 hours (average)

Pregnancy Risk Factor C

Breast-feeding Considerations No data reported; however, atropine may be taken while breast-feeding

Dosage Forms Tablet, as bromide: 7.5 mg, 15 mg

Dietary Considerations Should be taken 30 minutes before meals so that the drug's peak effect occurs at the proper time

Generic Available Yes: 15 mg tablet

Proparacaine (proe PAR a kane)

Brand Names AK-Taine®; Alcaine®; I-Paracaine®; Ophthetic®

Therapeutic Category Local Anesthetic, Ophthalmic

Use Anesthesia for tonometry, gonioscopy; suture removal from cornea; removal of corneal foreign body; cataract extraction, glaucoma surgery; short operative procedure involving the cornea and conjunctiva

Usual Dosage Children and Adults:

Ophthalmic surgery: Instill 1 drop of 0.5% solution in eye every 5-10 minutes for 5-7 doses

Tonometry, gonioscopy, suture removal: Instill 1-2 drops of 0.5% solution in eye just prior to procedure

Mechanism of Action Prevents initiation and transmission of impulse at the nerve cell membrane by decreasing ion permeability through stabilizing

Local Anesthetic/Vasoconstrictor Precautions No information available to require special precautions

Effects on Dental Treatment No effects or complications reported

Other Adverse Effects

1% to 10%: Local: Burning, stinging, redness

<1%:

Cardiovascular: Arrhythmias

Central nervous system: CNS depression

Dermatologic: Allergic contact dermatitis

Local: Irritation, sensitization

Ocular: Lacrimation, keratitis, iritis, erosion of the corneal epithelium, conjunctival congestion and hemorrhage, corneal opacification, blurred vision

Miscellaneous: Increased sweating

Drug Interactions Increased effect of phenylephrine, tropicamide

Drug Uptake

Onset of action: Within 20 seconds of instillation

Duration: 15-20 minutes

Pregnancy Risk Factor C

Dosage Forms Ophthalmic, solution, as hydrochloride: 0.5% (2 mL, 15 mL)

Generic Available Yes

Proparacaine and Fluorescein

(proe PAR a kane & FLURE e seen)

Brand Names Fluoracaine® Ophthalmic

Therapeutic Category Diagnostic Agent, Ophthalmic Dye; Local Anesthetic, Ophthalmic

Use Anesthesia for tonometry, gonioscopy; suture removal from cornea; removal of corneal foreign body; cataract extraction, glaucoma surgery

Usual Dosage

Ophthalmic surgery: Children and Adults: Instill 1 drop in each eye every 5-10 minutes for 5-7 doses

Tonometry, gonioscopy, suture removal: Adults: Instill 1-2 drops in each eye just prior to procedure

Mechanism of Action Prevents initiation and transmission of impulse at the nerve cell membrane by decreasing ion permeability through stabilizing

Local Anesthetic/Vasoconstrictor Precautions No information available to require special precautions

Effects on Dental Treatment No effects or complications reported

Other Adverse Effects

1% to 10%: Local: Burning, stinging of eye

<1%:

Dermatologic: Allergic contact dermatitis

Local: Irritation, sensitization

Ocular: Keratitis, iritis, erosion of the corneal epithelium, conjunctival congestion and hemorrhage, corneal opacification

Drug Interactions No data reported

Drug Uptake

Onset of action: Within 20 seconds of instillation

Duration: 15-20 minutes

Pregnancy Risk Factor C

Generic Available Yes

Propecia® see Finasteride on page 405

Propine® Ophthalmic see Dipivefrin on page 325

Propiomazine (proe pee OH ma zeen)

Brand Names Largon® Injection

Therapeutic Category Antianxiety Agent; Antiemetic; Phenothiazine Derivative; Sedative; Tranquilizer, Minor

Use Relief of restlessness, nausea and apprehension before and during surgery or during labor

Local Anesthetic/Vasoconstrictor Precautions No information available to require special precautions

Effects on Dental Treatment >10% of patients experience dry mouth

Other Adverse Effects
>10%: Central nervous system: Dizziness, drowsiness
1% to 10%:
  Cardiovascular: Tachycardia
  Central nervous system: Confusion
  Dermatologic: Skin rash
  Gastrointestinal: Diarrhea, stomach pain
  Respiratory: Dyspnea
<1%: Central nervous system: Neuroleptic malignant syndrome

Generic Available No

Comments Do not use injection if cloudy or contains a precipitate

Proplex® SX-T see Factor IX Complex (Human) on page 391

Proplex® T see Factor IX Complex (Human) on page 391

Propofol (PROE po fole)

Brand Names Diprivan® Injection

Therapeutic Category General Anesthetic, Intravenous

Use Induction or maintenance of anesthesia; sedation

Not recommended for use in children <3 years of age; not recommended for sedation of PICU patients, especially at high doses or for prolonged periods of time; metabolic acidosis with fatal cardiac failure has occurred in several children (4 weeks to 11 years of age) who received propofol infusions at average rates of infusion of 4.5-10 mg/kg/hour for 66-115 hours (maximum rates of infusion 6.2-11.5 mg/kg/hour); see Parke, 1992; Strickland, 1995; and Bray, 1995

Usual Dosage Dosage must be individualized based on total body weight and titrated to the desired clinical effect; however, as a general guideline:

No pediatric dose has been established; however, induction for children 1-12 years 2-2.8 mg/kg has been used

Induction: I.V.:
  Adults ≤55 years, and/or ASA I or II patients: 2-2.5 mg/kg of body weight (approximately 40 mg every 10 seconds until onset of induction)
  Elderly, debilitated, hypovolemic, and/or ASA III or IV patients: 1-1.5 mg/kg of body weight (approximately 20 mg every 10 seconds until onset of induction)

Maintenance: I.V. infusion:
  Adults ≤55 years, and/or ASA I or II patients: 0.1-0.2 mg/kg of body weight/minute (6-12 mg/kg of body weight/hour)
  Elderly, debilitated, hypovolemic, and/or ASA III or IV patients: 0.05-0.1 mg/kg of body weight/minute (3-6 mg/kg of body weight/hour)

I.V. intermittent: 25-50 mg increments, as needed

ICU sedation: Rapid bolus injection should be avoided. Bolus injection can result in hypotension, oxyhemoglobin desaturation, apnea, airway obstruction, and oxygen desaturation. The preferred route of administration is slow infusion. Doses are based on individual need and titrated to response.
  Recommended starting dose: 1-3 mg/kg/hour
  Adjustments in dose can occur at 3- to 5-minute intervals. An 80% reduction in dose should be considered in elderly, debilitated, and ASA II or IV patients. Once sedation is established, the dose should be decreased for the maintenance infusion period and adjusted to response. The dose required for maintenance is 1.5-4.5 mg/kg/hour or 25-75 mcg/kg/minute. An alternative, but less preferred method of administration is intermittent slow I.V. bolus injection of 10-20 mg, administered over 3-5 minutes.

Mechanism of Action Propofol is a hindered phenolic compound with intravenous general anesthetic properties. The drug is unrelated to any of the currently used barbiturate, opioid, benzodiazepine, arylcyclohexylamine, or imidazole intravenous anesthetic agents.

Local Anesthetic/Vasoconstrictor Precautions No information available to require special precautions

Effects on Dental Treatment No effects or complications reported

(Continued)

Propofol *(Continued)*

Other Adverse Effects

>10%: Gastrointestinal: Nausea

1% to 10%:

Cardiovascular: Hypotension, bradycardia, flushing

Central nervous system: Fever

Gastrointestinal: Vomiting, abdominal cramping

Respiratory: Cough, apnea

<1%:

Cardiovascular: Chest pain, tachycardia, syncope

Central nervous system: Agitation, somnolence, confusion

Dermatologic: Pruritus

Gastrointestinal: Dry mouth, diarrhea

Neuromuscular & skeletal: Tremor, twitching

Otic: Ear pain

Respiratory: Bronchospasm, dyspnea

Drug Uptake

Onset of anesthesia: Within 9-51 seconds (average 30 seconds) after bolus infusion (dose dependent)

Duration: 3-10 minutes depending on the dose and the rate of administration

Serum half-life, elimination (biphasic):

Initial: 40 minutes

Terminal: 1-3 days

Pregnancy Risk Factor B

Generic Available No

Comments Formulated into an emulsion containing 10% w/v soybean oil, 1.2% w/v purified egg phosphatide, and 2.25% w/v glycerol; this emulsion vehicle is chemically similar to 10% Intralipid®

Propoxycaine and Procaine *Discontinued by Manufacturer* (proe POKS i kane & PROE kane)

Brand Names Ravocaine® and Novocain® With Levophed®; Ravocaine® and Novocain® With Neo-Cobefrin®

Therapeutic Category Dental/Local Anesthetics; Local Anesthetic, Injectable

Use Dental: Ester-type anesthetic used for local infiltration anesthesia; injection near nerve trunks to produce nerve block

Usual Dosage The lowest dose needed to provide effective anesthesia should be administered. The 1.8 mL cartridge contains 43.2 mg of the anesthetics (7.2 mg propoxycaine hydrochloride and 36 mg procaine hydrochloride).

Children: Based on a dose of 3 mg/lb body weight, maximum: 5 cartridges are usually adequate for any procedure

Adults: 5 cartridges (216 mg of total anesthetics) are usually adequate to affect anesthesia of the entire oral cavity. A dose of 3 mg/lb body weight may be administered for one procedure

Mechanism of Action Local anesthetics bind selectively to the intracellular surface of sodium channels to block influx of sodium into the axon. As a result, depolarization necessary for action potential propagation and subsequent nerve function is prevented. The block at the sodium channel is reversible. When drug diffuses away from the axon, sodium channel function is restored and nerve propagation is subsequently restored.

Norepinephrine (Levophed®) and levonordefrin (Neocobefrin®) prolong the duration of the anesthetic actions of propoxycaine and procaine by causing vasoconstriction (alpha adrenergic receptor agonist) of the vasculature surrounding the nerve axons. This prevents the diffusion of local anesthetic away from the nerves resulting in a longer retention in the axon.

Local Anesthetic/Vasoconstrictor Precautions No information available to require special precautions

Effects on Dental Treatment No effects or complications reported

Other Adverse Effects Degree of adverse effects in the CNS and cardiovascular system are directly related to the blood levels of local anesthetic. The effects below are more likely to occur after systemic administration rather than infiltration.

Cardiovascular: Myocardial effects include a decrease in contraction force as well as a decrease in electrical excitability and myocardial conduction rate resulting in bradycardia and reduction in cardiac output.

Central nervous system: High blood levels result in anxiety, restlessness, disorientation, confusion, dizziness, tremors and seizures. This is followed by depression of CNS resulting in somnolence, unconsciousness and possible respiratory arrest. In some cases, symptoms of CNS stimulation may be absent and the primary CNS effects are somnolence and unconsciousness.

Gastrointestinal: Nausea and vomiting may occur

Hypersensitivity reactions: May be manifest as dermatologic reactions and edema at injection site. Asthmatic syndromes have occurred. Patients may exhibit hypersensitivity to bisulfites contained in local anesthetic solution to prevent oxidation of norepinephrine or levonordefrin. In general, patients reacting to bisulfites have a history of asthma and their airways are hyper-reactive to asthmatic syndrome.

Psychogenic reactions: It is common to misinterpret psychogenic responses to local anesthetic injection as an allergic reaction. Intraoral injections are perceived by many patients as a stressful procedure in dentistry. Common symptoms to this stress are sweating, palpitations, hyperventilation, generalized pallor, and a fainting feeling.

Contraindications Hypersensitivity to local anesthetics of the ester type

Warnings/Precautions Should be avoided in patients with uncontrolled hyperthyroidism. Should be used in minimal amounts in patients with significant cardiovascular problems (because of norepinephrine or levonordefrin component). Aspirate the syringe after tissue penetration and before injection to minimize chance of direct vascular injection

Drug Interactions Due to norepinephrine or levonordefrin component, use with tricyclic antidepressants or MAO inhibitors could result in increased pressor response

Drug Uptake
Onset of action: 2-5 minutes
Duration 2-3 hours

Pregnancy Risk Factor No data reported

Breast-feeding Considerations No data reported

Dosage Forms Injection:
Ravocaine® and Novocain® with Levophed®: Propoxycaine hydrochloride 7.2 mg and procaine 36 mg with norepinephrine 0.12 mg/1.8 mL dental cartridge
Ravocaine® and Novocain® with Neo-Cobefrin®: Propoxycaine hydrochloride 7.2 mg and procaine 36 mg with levonordefrin 0.09 mg/1.8 mL dental cartridge

Dietary Considerations No data reported

Generic Available No

Selected Readings
Blanton PL and Roda RS, "The Anatomy of Local Anesthesia," *J Calif Dent Assoc*, 1995, 23(4):55-65.
Jastak JT and Yagiela JA, "Vasoconstrictors and Local Anesthesia: A Review and Rationale for Use," *J Am Dent Assoc*, 1983, 107(4):623-30.
MacKenzie TA and Young ER, "Local Anesthetic Update," *Anesth Prog*, 1993, 40(2):29-34.
Wynn RL, "Epinephrine Interactions With Beta-Blockers," *Gen Dent*, 1994, 42(1):16, 18.
Yagiela JA, "Local Anesthetics," *Anesth Prog*, 1991, 38(4-5):128-41.
Yagiela JA, "Vasoconstrictor Agents for Local Anesthetics," *Anesth Prog*, 1995, 42(3-4):116-20.

Propoxyphene (proe POKS i feen)

Related Information
Narcotic Agonists *on page 1141*

Brand Names Darvon®; Darvon-N®; Dolene®

Canadian/Mexican Brand Names Novo-Propoxyn® (Canada)

Therapeutic Category Analgesic, Narcotic

Use Management of mild to moderate pain

Usual Dosage Oral:
Children: Doses for children are not well established; doses of the hydrochloride of 2-3 mg/kg/d divided every 6 hours have been used
Adults:
Hydrochloride: 65 mg every 3-4 hours as needed for pain; maximum: 390 mg/day
Napsylate: 100 mg every 4 hours as needed for pain; maximum: 600 mg/day

Mechanism of Action Binds to opiate receptors in the CNS, causing inhibition of ascending pain pathways, altering the perception of and response to pain; produces generalized CNS depression

Local Anesthetic/Vasoconstrictor Precautions No information available to require special precautions

Effects on Dental Treatment No effects or complications reported

Other Adverse Effects Hepatic: Increased liver enzymes
>10%:
Cardiovascular: Hypotension
Central nervous system: Dizziness, lightheadedness, sedation, paradoxical excitement, insomnia, fatigue, drowsiness
Gastrointestinal: GI upset, nausea, vomiting, constipation
Neuromuscular & skeletal: Weakness
Miscellaneous: Histamine release
1% to 10%:
Central nervous system: Nervousness, headache, restlessness, malaise, confusion
(Continued)

Propoxyphene *(Continued)*

    Gastrointestinal: Anorexia, stomach cramps, dry mouth, biliary spasm
    Genitourinary: Decreased urination, ureteral spasms
    Respiratory: Dyspnea
  <1%:
    Central nervous system: Mental depression hallucinations, paradoxical CNS stimulation, increased intracranial pressure
    Dermatologic: Rash, urticaria
    Gastrointestinal: Paralytic ileus
    Miscellaneous: Psychologic and physical dependence with prolonged use

Drug Interactions
  Decreased effect with charcoal, cigarette smoking
  Increased toxicity: CNS depressants may potentiate pharmacologic effects; propoxyphene may inhibit the metabolism and increase the serum concentrations of carbamazepine, phenobarbital, MAO inhibitors, tricyclic antidepressants, and warfarin

Drug Uptake
  Onset of effect: Oral: Within 0.5-1 hour
  Duration: 4-6 hours
  Serum half-life: Adults:
    Parent drug: 8-24 hours (mean: ~15 hours)
    Norpropoxyphene: 34 hours

Pregnancy Risk Factor C (D if used for prolonged periods)

Dosage Forms
  Capsule, as hydrochloride: 65 mg
  Tablet, as napsylate: 100 mg

Dietary Considerations Should be taken with glass of water on empty stomach

Generic Available Yes: Capsule

Propoxyphene and Acetaminophen

(proe POKS i feen & a seet a MIN oh fen)

Brand Names Darvocet-N®; Darvocet-N® 100; Propacet®; Wygesic®

Therapeutic Category Analgesic, Narcotic

Use
  Dental: Management of postoperative pain
  Medical: Relief of pain

Restrictions C-IV; Refillable up to 5 times in 6 months

Usual Dosage
  Children: Not recommended in pediatric dental patients
  Adults:
    Darvocet-N®: 1-2 tablets every 4 hours as needed; maximum: 600 mg propoxyphene napsylate/day
    Darvocet-N® 100: 1 tablet every 4 hours as needed; maximum: 600 mg propoxyphene napsylate/day

Mechanism of Action
  Propoxyphene is a weak narcotic analgesic which acts through binding to opiate receptors to inhibit ascending pain pathways
  Propoxyphene, as with other narcotic (opiate) analgesics, blocks pain perception in the cerebral cortex by binding to specific receptor molecules (opiate receptors) within the neuronal membranes of synapses. This binding results in a decreased synaptic chemical transmission throughout the CNS thus inhibiting the flow of pain sensations into the higher centers. Mu and kappa are the two subtypes of the opiate receptor which propoxyphene binds to to cause analgesia.
  Acetaminophen inhibits the synthesis of prostaglandins in the CNS and peripherally blocks pain impulse generation; produces antipyresis from inhibition of hypothalamic heat-regulating center

Local Anesthetic/Vasoconstrictor Precautions No information available to require special precautions

Effects on Dental Treatment No effects or complications reported

Other Adverse Effects 1% to 10%:
  Central nervous system: Dizziness, lightheadedness, headache, sedation
  Gastrointestinal: Nausea, vomiting
  Neuromuscular & skeletal: Weakness
  Miscellaneous: Psychologic and physical dependence

Contraindications Hypersensitivity to propoxyphene, acetaminophen, or any component; patients with known G-6-PD deficiency

Warnings/Precautions When given in excessive doses, either alone or in combination with other CNS depressants, propoxyphene is a major cause of drug-related deaths; do not exceed recommended dosage; give with caution in patients dependent on opiates, substitution may result in acute opiate withdrawal symptoms

Drug Interactions Decreased effect with charcoal, cigarette smoking; increased toxicity with cimetidine, CNS depressants; increased toxicity/effect of carbamazepine, phenobarbital, TCAs, MAO inhibitors, benzodiazepines

Drug Uptake
Onset of action: 15-60 minutes
Time to peak serum concentration: 2-2.5 hours
Duration: 4-6 hours
Serum half-life:
Propoxyphene: 6-12 hours
Norpropoxyphene: 30-36 hours

Pregnancy Risk Factor C

Breast-feeding Considerations Both propoxyphene and acetaminophen may be taken while breast-feeding

Dosage Forms Tablet:
Darvocet-N®: Propoxyphene napsylate 50 mg and acetaminophen 325 mg
Darvocet-N® 100: Propoxyphene napsylate 100 mg and acetaminophen 650 mg
Genagesic®, Wygesic®: Propoxyphene hydrochloride 65 mg and acetaminophen 650 mg

Dietary Considerations Should be taken with water on an empty stomach

Generic Available Yes

Comments Propoxyphene is a narcotic analgesic and shares many properties including addiction liability. The acetaminophen component requires use with caution in patients with alcoholic liver disease.

Propoxyphene and Aspirin (proe POKS i feen & AS pir in)

Related Information
Narcotic Agonists *on page 1141*

Brand Names Bexophene®; Darvon® Compound-65 Pulvules®

Canadian/Mexican Brand Names Darvon-N® Compound (contains caffeine) (Canada); Darvon-N® with ASA (Canada); Novo-Propoxyn Compound (contains caffeine) (Canada)

Therapeutic Category Analgesic, Narcotic

Use
Dental: Management of postoperative pain
Medical: Relief of pain

Restrictions C-IV; Refillable up to 5 times in 6 months

Usual Dosage Oral:
Children: Not recommended
Adults: 1-2 capsules every 4 hours as needed

Mechanism of Action
Propoxyphene is a weak narcotic analgesic which acts through binding to opiate receptors to inhibit ascending pain pathways
Propoxyphene, as with other narcotic (opiate) analgesics, blocks pain perception in the cerebral cortex by binding to specific receptor molecules (opiate receptors) within the neuronal membranes of synapses. This binding results in a decreased synaptic chemical transmission throughout the CNS thus inhibiting the flow of pain sensations into the higher centers. Mu and kappa are the two subtypes of the opiate receptor which propoxyphene binds to to cause analgesia.
Aspirin inhibits prostaglandin synthesis by decreasing the activity of the enzyme, cyclo-oxygenase, which results in decreased formation of prostaglandin precursors, acts on the hypothalamic heat-regulating center to reduce fever, blocks thromboxane synthetase action which prevents formation of the platelet-aggregating substance thromboxane A_2

Local Anesthetic/Vasoconstrictor Precautions No effects or complications reported

Effects on Dental Treatment Use with caution in patients with platelet and bleeding disorders, renal dysfunction, erosive gastritis, or peptic ulcer disease, previous nonreaction does not guarantee future safe taking of medication; do not use aspirin in children <16 years of age for chickenpox or flu symptoms due to the association with Reye's syndrome

Avoid aspirin if possible, for 1 week prior to surgery because of the possibility of postoperative bleeding; use with caution in impaired hepatic function

Elderly are a high-risk population for adverse effects from nonsteroidal anti-inflammatory agents. As much as 60% of elderly with GI complications to NSAIDs can develop peptic ulceration and/or hemorrhage asymptomatically. Also, concomitant disease and drug use contribute to the risk for GI adverse effects. Use lowest effective dose for shortest period possible. Consider renal function decline with age. Use with caution in patients with history of asthma

(Continued)

Propoxyphene and Aspirin *(Continued)*

Other Adverse Effects 1% to 10%:

Central nervous system: Dizziness, lightheadedness, headache, sedation

Gastrointestinal: Nausea, vomiting

Neuromuscular & skeletal: Weakness

Miscellaneous: Psychologic and physical dependence

Contraindications Hypersensitivity to propoxyphene, aspirin or any component

Warnings/Precautions When given in excessive doses, either alone or in combination with other CNS depressants, propoxyphene is a major cause of drug-related deaths; do not exceed recommended dosage; because of aspirin component, children and teenagers should not use for chickenpox or flu symptoms before a physician is consulted about Reye's syndrome

Drug Interactions Decreased effect with charcoal, cigarette smoking; increased toxicity with cimetidine, CNS depressants; increased toxicity/effect of carbamazepine, phenobarbital, TCAs, warfarin, MAO inhibitors, benzodiazepines, warfarin (bleeding); see Aspirin

Drug Uptake

Onset of action: 15-60 minutes

Time to peak serum concentration: 2-2.5 hours

Duration: 4-6 hours

Serum half-life:

Propoxyphene: 6-12 hours

Norpropoxyphene: 30-36 hours

Pregnancy Risk Factor D

Breast-feeding Considerations

Propoxyphene: May be taken while breast-feeding

Aspirin: Use cautiously due to potential adverse effects in nursing infants

Dosage Forms

Capsule: Propoxyphene hydrochloride 65 mg and aspirin 389 mg with caffeine 32.4 mg

Tablet (Darvon-N® with A.S.A.): Propoxyphene napsylate 100 mg and aspirin 325 mg

Dietary Considerations No data reported

Generic Available Yes

Comments Propoxyphene is a narcotic analgesic and shares many properties including addiction liability. The aspirin component could have anticoagulant effects and could possibly affect bleeding times.

Propranolol *(proe PRAN oh lole)*

Related Information

Cardiovascular Diseases *on page 1010*

Endocrine Disorders & Pregnancy *on page 1021*

Brand Names Betachron E-R® Capsule; Inderal®; Inderal® LA

Canadian/Mexican Brand Names Apo®-Propranolol (Canada); Detensol® (Canada); Inderalici® (Mexico); Nu-Propranolol® (Canada); PMS-Propranolol® (Mexico)

Therapeutic Category Antianginal Agent; Antiarrhythmic Agent, Class I-B; Antiarrhythmic Agent, Class II; Antiarrhythmic Agent (Supraventricular & Ventricular); Beta-adrenergic Blocker, Noncardioselective

Use Management of hypertension, angina pectoris, pheochromocytoma, essential tremor, tetralogy of Fallot cyanotic spells, and arrhythmias (such as atrial fibrillation and flutter, A-V nodal re-entrant tachycardias, and catecholamine-induced arrhythmias); prevention of myocardial infarction, migraine headache; symptomatic treatment of hypertrophic subaortic stenosis

Unlabeled use: Tremor due to Parkinson's disease, alcohol withdrawal, aggressive behavior, antipsychotic-induced akathisia, esophageal varices bleeding, anxiety, schizophrenia, acute panic, and gastric bleeding in portal hypertension

Usual Dosage

Tachyarrhythmias:

Oral:

Children: Initial: 0.5-1 mg/kg/day in divided doses every 6-8 hours; titrate dosage upward every 3-7 days; usual dose: 2-4 mg/kg/day; higher doses may be needed; do not exceed 16 mg/kg/day or 60 mg/day

Adults: 10-30 mg/dose every 6-8 hours

Elderly: Initial: 10 mg twice daily; increase dosage every 3-7 days; usual dosage range: 10-320 mg given in 2 divided doses

I.V.:

Children: 0.01-0.1 mg/kg slow IVP over 10 minutes; maximum dose: 1 mg

Adults: 1 mg/dose slow IVP; repeat every 5 minutes up to a total of 5 mg

Hypertension: Oral:
   Children: Initial: 0.5-1 mg/kg/day in divided doses every 6-12 hours; increase gradually every 3-7 days; maximum: 2 mg/kg/24 hours
   Adults: Initial: 40 mg twice daily; increase dosage every 3-7 days; usual dose: ≤320 mg divided in 2-3 doses/day; maximum daily dose: 640 mg
Migraine headache prophylaxis: Oral:
   Children: 0.6-1.5 mg/kg/day **or**
      ≤35 kg: 10-20 mg 3 times/day
      >35 kg: 20-40 mg 3 times/day
   Adults: Initial: 80 mg/day divided every 6-8 hours; increase by 20-40 mg/dose every 3-4 weeks to a maximum of 160-240 mg/day given in divided doses every 6-8 hours; if satisfactory response not achieved within 6 weeks of starting therapy, drug should be withdrawn gradually over several weeks
Tetralogy spells: Children:
   Oral: 1-2 mg/kg/day every 6 hours as needed, may increase by 1 mg/kg/day to a maximum of 5 mg/kg/day, or if refractory may increase slowly to a maximum of 10-15 mg/kg/day
   I.V.: 0.15-0.25 mg/kg/dose slow IVP; may repeat in 15 minutes
Thyrotoxicosis:
   Adolescents and Adults: Oral: 10-40 mg/dose every 6 hours
   Adults: I.V.: 1-3 mg/dose slow IVP as a single dose
   Adults: Oral:
      Angina: 80-320 mg/day in doses divided 2-4 times/day
      Pheochromocytoma: 30-60 mg/day in divided doses
      Myocardial infarction prophylaxis: 180-240 mg/day in 3-4 divided doses
      Hypertrophic subaortic stenosis: 20-40 mg 3-4 times/day
      Essential tremor: 40 mg twice daily initially; maintenance doses: usually 120-320 mg/day

Mechanism of Action Nonselective beta-adrenergic blocker (class II antiarrhythmic); competitively blocks response to beta$_1$- and beta$_2$-adrenergic stimulation which results in decreases in heart rate, myocardial contractility, blood pressure, and myocardial oxygen demand

Local Anesthetic/Vasoconstrictor Precautions Use with caution; epinephrine has interacted with nonselective beta-blockers to result in initial hypertensive episode followed by bradycardia

Effects on Dental Treatment Noncardioselective beta-blockers (ie, propranolol, nadolol) enhance the pressor response to epinephrine, resulting in hypertension and bradycardia. Many nonsteroidal anti-inflammatory drugs such as ibuprofen and indomethacin can reduce the hypotensive effect of beta-blockers after 3 or more weeks of therapy with the NSAID. Short-term NSAID use (ie, 3 days) requires no special precautions in patients taking beta-blockers.

Other Adverse Effects
>10%:
   Cardiovascular: Bradycardia
   Central nervous system: Mental depression
   Endocrine & metabolic: Decreased sexual ability
1% to 10%:
   Cardiovascular: Congestive heart failure, reduced peripheral circulation
   Central nervous system: Confusion, hallucinations, dizziness, insomnia, fatigue
   Dermatologic: Skin rash
   Gastrointestinal: Diarrhea, nausea, vomiting, stomach discomfort
   Neuromuscular & skeletal: Weakness
   Respiratory: Wheezing
<1%:
   Cardiovascular: Chest pain, hypotension, impaired myocardial contractility, worsening of A-V conduction disturbances
   Central nervous system: Nightmares, vivid dreams, lethargy
   Dermatologic: Red, scaling, or crusted skin
   Endocrine & metabolic: Hypoglycemia, hyperglycemia
   Gastrointestinal: GI distress
   Hematologic: Leukopenia, thrombocytopenia, agranulocytosis
   Respiratory: Bronchospasm
   Miscellaneous: Cold extremities

Drug Interactions
   Decreased effect of beta-blockers with aluminum salts, barbiturates, calcium salts, cholestyramine, colestipol, NSAIDs, penicillins (ampicillin), rifampin, salicylates and sulfinpyrazone due to decreased bioavailability and plasma levels
   Increased effect/toxicity of beta-blockers with calcium blockers (diltiazem, felodipine, nicardipine), contraceptives, flecainide, haloperidol (propranolol, hypotensive effects), H$_2$ antagonists (metoprolol, propranolol only by cimetidine, possibly ranitidine), hydralazine (metoprolol, propranolol), loop diuretics
(Continued)

Propranolol (Continued)

(propranolol, not atenolol), MAO inhibitors (metoprolol, nadolol, bradycardia), phenothiazines (propranolol), propafenone (metoprolol, propranolol), quinidine (in extensive metabolizers), ciprofloxacin, thyroid hormones (metoprolol, propranolol, when hypothyroid patient is converted to euthyroid state)

Beta-blockers may increase the effect/toxicity* of flecainide, haloperidol (hypotensive effects), hydralazine, phenothiazines, acetaminophen, anticoagulants (propranolol, warfarin), benzodiazepines (not atenolol), clonidine (hypertensive crisis after or during withdrawal of either agent), epinephrine (initial hypertensive episode followed by bradycardia), nifedipine and verapamil lidocaine*, ergots* (peripheral ischemia), prazosin (postural hypotension)

Beta-blockers may decrease the effect of sulfonylureas

Beta-blockers may also affect the action or levels of ethanol, disopyramide, nondepolarizing muscle relaxants and theophylline although the effects are difficult to predict

Drug Uptake
Onset of beta blockade: Oral: Within 1-2 hours
Duration: ~6 hours
Serum half-life:
Children: 3.9-6.4 hours
Adults: 4-6 hours

Pregnancy Risk Factor C
Generic Available Yes
Selected Readings
Foster CA and Aston SJ, "Propranolol-Epinephrine Interaction: A Potential Disaster," *Plast Reconstr Surg*, 1983, 72(1):74-8.
Wong DG, Spence JD, Lamki L, et al, "Effect of Nonsteroidal Anti-inflammatory Drugs on Control of Hypertension of Beta-Blockers and Diuretics," *Lancet*, 1986, 1(8488):997-1001.
Wynn RL, "Dental Nonsteroidal Anti-inflammatory Drugs and Prostaglandin-Based Drug Interactions, Part Two," *Gen Dent*, 1992, 40(2):104, 106, 108.
Wynn RL, "Epinephrine Interactions With Beta-Blockers," *Gen Dent*, 1994, 42(1):16, 18.

Propranolol and Hydrochlorothiazide
(proe PRAN oh lole & hye droe klor oh THYE a zide)
Brand Names Inderide®
Therapeutic Category Antihypertensive Agent, Combination
Use Management of hypertension
Local Anesthetic/Vasoconstrictor Precautions Use with caution; epinephrine has interacted with nonselective beta-blockers to result in initial hypertensive episode followed by bradycardia
Effects on Dental Treatment Noncardioselective beta-blockers (ie, propranolol, nadolol) enhance the pressor response to epinephrine, resulting in hypertension and bradycardia. Many nonsteroidal anti-inflammatory drugs such as ibuprofen and indomethacin can reduce the hypotensive effect of beta-blockers after 3 or more weeks of therapy with the NSAID. Short-term NSAID use (ie, 3 days) requires no special precautions in patients taking beta-blockers.
Pregnancy Risk Factor C
Generic Available Immediate release: Yes

Propulsid® *see* Cisapride *on page 237*

Propylene Glycol and Salicylic Acid *see* Salicylic Acid and Propylene Glycol *on page 854*

Propylhexedrine (proe pil HEKS e dreen)
Brand Names Benzedrex® [OTC]
Therapeutic Category Decongestant
Use Topical nasal decongestant
Local Anesthetic/Vasoconstrictor Precautions No information available to require special precautions
Effects on Dental Treatment No effects or complications reported
Generic Available No
Comments Drug has been extracted from inhaler and injected I.V. as an amphetamine substitute

Propylthiouracil (proe pil thye oh YOOR a sil)
Related Information
Endocrine Disorders & Pregnancy *on page 1021*
Canadian/Mexican Brand Names Propyl-Thyracil® (Canada)
Therapeutic Category Antithyroid Agent
Use Palliative treatment of hyperthyroidism as an adjunct to ameliorate hyperthyroidism in preparation for surgical treatment or radioactive iodine therapy and in the management of thyrotoxic crisis. The use of antithyroid thioamides is as effective in elderly as they are in younger adults; however, the expense, potential

adverse effects, and inconvenience (compliance, monitoring) make them undesirable. The use of radioiodine, due to ease of administration and less concern for long-term side effects and reproduction problems, makes it a more appropriate therapy.

Usual Dosage Oral: Administer in 3 equally divided doses at approximately 8-hour intervals. Adjust dosage to maintain T_3, T_4, and TSH levels in normal range; elevated T_3 may be sole indicator of inadequate treatment. Elevated TSH indicates excessive antithyroid treatment.

Children: Initial: 5-7 mg/kg/day in divided doses every 8 hours **or**
   6-10 years: 50-150 mg/day
   >10 years: 150-300 mg/day
   Maintenance: $^1/_3$ to $^2/_3$ of the initial dose in divided doses every 8-12 hours. This usually begins after 2 months on an effective initial dose.

Adults: Initial: 300-450 mg/day in divided doses every 8 hours (severe hyperthyroidism may require 600-1200 mg/day); maintenance: 100-150 mg/day in divided doses every 8-12 hours

Elderly: Use lower dose recommendations; initial dose: 150-300 mg/day

Mechanism of Action Inhibits the synthesis of thyroid hormones by blocking the oxidation of iodine in the thyroid gland; blocks synthesis of thyroxine and triiodothyronine

Local Anesthetic/Vasoconstrictor Precautions No information available to require special precautions

Effects on Dental Treatment No effects or complications reported

Other Adverse Effects
>10%:
   Central nervous system: Fever
   Dermatologic: Skin rash
   Hematologic: Leukopenia
1% to 10%:
   Central nervous system: Dizziness
   Gastrointestinal: Nausea, vomiting, dysgeusia, stomach pain
   Hematologic: Agranulocytosis
   Miscellaneous: SLE-like syndrome
<1%:
   Cardiovascular: Edema, cutaneous vasculitis
   Central nervous system: Drowsiness, neuritis, vertigo, headache
   Dermatologic: Urticaria, pruritus, exfoliative dermatitis, alopecia
   Endocrine & metabolic: Goiter
   Gastrointestinal: Constipation, weight gain, swollen salivary glands
   Hematologic: Thrombocytopenia, bleeding, aplastic anemia
   Hepatic: Cholestatic jaundice, hepatitis
   Neuromuscular & skeletal: Arthralgia, paresthesia
   Renal: Nephritis

Drug Interactions Increased effect: Increased anticoagulant activity

Drug Uptake
Onset of action: For significant therapeutic effects 24-36 hours are required
Peak effect: Remissions of hyperthyroidism do not usually occur before 4 months of continued therapy
Serum half-life: 1.5-5 hours
End stage renal disease: 8.5 hours
Time to peak serum concentration: Oral: Within 1 hour; persists for 2-3 hours

Pregnancy Risk Factor D
Generic Available Yes

Prorex® see Promethazine on page 804

Proscar® see Finasteride on page 405

Pro-Sof® Plus [OTC] see Docusate and Casanthranol on page 331

ProSom™ see Estazolam on page 364

Prostaglandin E₁ see Alprostadil on page 44

Prostaglandin E₂ see Dinoprostone on page 322

Prostaglandin F₂ Alpha see Dinoprost Tromethamine on page 322

Prostaphlin® see Oxacillin on page 705

ProStep® see Nicotine on page 678

Prostin E₂® Vaginal Suppository see Dinoprostone on page 322

Prostin F₂ Alpha® see Dinoprost Tromethamine on page 322

Prostin VR Pediatric® Injection see Alprostadil on page 44

Protamine Sulfate (PROE ta meen SUL fate)

Therapeutic Category Antidote, Heparin

Use Treatment of heparin overdosage; neutralize heparin during surgery or dialysis procedures
(Continued)

Protamine Sulfate *(Continued)*

Usual Dosage Protamine dosage is determined by the dosage of heparin; 1 mg of protamine neutralizes 90 USP units of heparin (lung) and 115 USP units of heparin (intestinal); maximum dose: 50 mg

In the situation of heparin overdosage, since blood heparin concentrations decrease rapidly **after** administration, adjust the protamine dosage depending upon the duration of time since heparin administration as follows:

Time Elapsed	Dose of Protamine (mg) to Neutralize 100 units of Heparin
Immediate	1-1.5
30-60 min	0.5-0.75
>2 h	0.25-0.375

If heparin administered by deep S.C. injection, use 1-1.5 mg protamine per 100 units heparin; this may be done by a portion of the dose (eg, 25-50 mg) given slowly I.V. followed by the remaining portion as a continuous infusion over 8-16 hours (the expected absorption time of the S.C. heparin dose)

Mechanism of Action Combines with strongly acidic heparin to form a stable complex (salt) neutralizing the anticoagulant activity of both drugs

Local Anesthetic/Vasoconstrictor Precautions No information available to require special precautions

Effects on Dental Treatment No effects or complications reported

Other Adverse Effects

>10%:
Cardiovascular: Hypotension, bradycardia
Respiratory: Dyspnea
1% to 10%: Hematologic: Hemorrhage
<1%:
Cardiovascular: Flushing, pulmonary hypertension
Central nervous system: Lassitude
Gastrointestinal: Nausea, vomiting
Miscellaneous: Hypersensitivity reactions

Drug Uptake Onset of effect: I.V. injection: Heparin neutralization occurs within 5 minutes

Pregnancy Risk Factor C

Generic Available Yes

Comments Heparin rebound associated with anticoagulation and bleeding has been reported to occur occasionally; symptoms typically occur 8-9 hours after protamine administration, but may occur as long as 18 hours later

Prothazine-DC® *see Promethazine and Codeine on page 805*

Protilase® *see Pancrelipase on page 722*

Protirelin *(proe TYE re lin)*

Brand Names Relefact® TRH Injection; Thypinone® Injection

Therapeutic Category Diagnostic Agent, Thyroid Function

Synonyms Lopremone; Thyrotropin Releasing Hormone; TRH

Use Adjunct in the diagnostic assessment of thyroid function, and an adjunct to other diagnostic procedures in assessment of patients with pituitary or hypothalamic dysfunction; also causes release of prolactin from the pituitary and is used to detect defective control of prolactin secretion.

Usual Dosage I.V.:

Children <6 years: Experience limited, but doses of 7 mcg/kg have been administered

Children 6-16 years: 7 mcg/kg to a maximum dose of 500 mcg

Adults: 500 mcg (range 200-500 mcg)

Mechanism of Action Increase release of thyroid stimulating hormone from the anterior pituitary

Local Anesthetic/Vasoconstrictor Precautions No information available to require special precautions

Effects on Dental Treatment >10% of patients experience dry mouth

Other Adverse Effects

>10%:
Cardiovascular: Flushing of face
Central nervous system: Headache, lightheadedness
Gastrointestinal: Nausea
Genitourinary: Urge to urinate
1% to 10%:
Central nervous system: Anxiety

Endocrine & metabolic: Breast enlargement and leaking in lactating women
Gastrointestinal: Bad taste in mouth, gastritis
Neuromuscular & skeletal: Paresthesia
Miscellaneous: Sweating
<1%:
Cardiovascular: Severe hypotension
Ocular: Temporary loss of vision
Drug Uptake
Peak TSH levels: 20-30 minutes
Duration: TSH returns to baseline after ~3 hours
Serum half-life, mean plasma: 5 minutes
Pregnancy Risk Factor C
Generic Available No

Protostat® *see* Metronidazole *on page 631*

Protriptyline (proe TRIP ti leen)
Brand Names Vivactil®
Canadian/Mexican Brand Names Triptil® (Canada)
Therapeutic Category Antidepressant, Tricyclic
Use Treatment of various forms of depression, often in conjunction with psychotherapy
Usual Dosage Oral:
Adolescents: 15-20 mg/day
Adults: 15-60 mg in 3-4 divided doses
Elderly: 15-20 mg/day
Mechanism of Action Increases the synaptic concentration of serotonin and/or norepinephrine in the central nervous system by inhibition of their reuptake by the presynaptic neuronal membrane
Local Anesthetic/Vasoconstrictor Precautions No information available to require special precautions
Effects on Dental Treatment >10% of patients experience dry mouth; long-term treatment with TCAs such as protriptyline increases the risk of caries by reducing salivation and salivary buffer capacity
Other Adverse Effects
>10%:
Central nervous system: Dizziness, drowsiness, headache
Gastrointestinal: Constipation, unpleasant taste, weight gain, increased appetite, nausea
Neuromuscular & skeletal: Weakness
1% to 10%:
Cardiovascular: Arrhythmias, hypotension
Central nervous system: Confusion, delirium, hallucinations, nervousness, restlessness, parkinsonian syndrome, insomnia
Endocrine & metabolic: Sexual dysfunction
Gastrointestinal: Diarrhea, heartburn
Genitourinary: Dysuria
Neuromuscular & skeletal: Fine muscle tremors
Ocular: Blurred vision, eye pain
Miscellaneous: Excessive sweating
<1%:
Central nervous system: Anxiety, seizures
Dermatologic: Alopecia, photosensitivity
Endocrine & metabolic: Breast enlargement, galactorrhea, SIADH
Gastrointestinal: Trouble with gums, decreased lower esophageal sphincter tone may cause GE reflux
Genitourinary: Testicular swelling
Hematologic: Agranulocytosis, leukopenia, eosinophilia
Hepatic: Cholestatic jaundice, elevated liver enzymes
Ocular: Increased intraocular pressure
Otic: Tinnitus
Miscellaneous: Allergic reactions
Drug Interactions
Decreased effect: Phenobarbital may increase the metabolism of protriptyline; protriptyline blocks the uptake of guanethidine and thus prevents the hypotensive effect of guanethidine
Increased toxicity: Clonidine causes hypertensive crisis; protriptyline may be additive with or may potentiate the action of other CNS depressants such as sedatives or hypnotics; with MAO inhibitors, hyperpyrexia, hypertension, tachycardia, confusion, and seizures; protriptyline may increase the prothrombin time in patients stabilized on warfarin; protriptyline potentiates the pressor and cardiac effects of sympathomimetic agents such as isoproterenol, epinephrine,
(Continued)

Protriptyline *(Continued)*

etc; cimetidine and methylphenidate may decrease the metabolism of protriptyline

Additive anticholinergic effects seen with other anticholinergic agents

Drug Uptake

Maximum antidepressant effect: 2 weeks of continuous therapy is commonly required

Serum half-life: 54-92 hours, averaging 74 hours

Time to peak serum concentration: Oral: Within 24-30 hours

Pregnancy Risk Factor C

Generic Available No

Selected Readings

Boakes AJ, Laurence DR, Teoh PC, et al, "Interactions Between Sympathomimetic Amines and Antidepressant Agents in Man," *Br Med J*, 1973, 1(849):311-5.

Jastak JT and Yagiela JA, "Vasoconstrictors and Local Anesthesia: A Review and Rationale for Use," *J Am Dent Assoc*, 1983, 107(4):623-30.

Larochelle P, Hamet P, and Enjalbert M, "Responses to Tyramine and Norepinephrine After Imipramine and Trazodone," *Clin Pharmacol Ther*, 1979, 26(1):24-30.

Mitchell JR, "Guanethidine and Related Agents. III Antagonism by Drugs Which Inhibit the Norepinephrine Pump in Man," *J Clin Invest*, 1970, 49(8):1596-604.

Rundegren J, van Dijken J, Mörnstad H, et al, "Oral Conditions in Patients Receiving Long-Term Treatment With Cyclic Antidepressant Drugs," *Swed Dent J*, 1985, 9(2):55-64.

Svedmyr N, "The Influence of a Tricyclic Antidepressive Agent (Protriptyline) on Some of the Circulatory Effects of Noradrenaline and Adrenalin in Man," *Life Sci*, 1968, 7(1):77-84.

Protropin® Injection *see* Human Growth Hormone *on page 473*

Provatene® [OTC] *see* Beta-Carotene *on page 125*

Proventil® *see* Albuterol *on page 35*

Proventil® HFA *see* Albuterol *on page 35*

Provera® *see* Medroxyprogesterone Acetate *on page 587*

Proxigel® Oral [OTC] *see* Carbamide Peroxide *on page 175*

Prozac® *see* Fluoxetine *on page 419*

PRP-D *see* Haemophilus b Conjugate Vaccine *on page 460*

Pseudo-Car® DM *see* Carbinoxamine, Pseudoephedrine, and Dextromethorphan *on page 177*

Pseudoefedrina (Mexico) *see* Pseudoephedrine *on this page*

Pseudoephedrine *(soo doe e FED rin)*

Related Information

Acetaminophen and Pseudoephedrine *on page 24*

Acetaminophen, Dextromethorphan, and Pseudoephedrine *on page 25*

Diphenhydramine and Pseudoephedrine *on page 324*

Guaifenesin, Pseudoephedrine, and Dextromethorphan *on page 456*

Brand Names Actifed® Allergy Tablet (Day) [OTC]; Afrin® Tablet [OTC]; Cenafed® [OTC]; Children's Silfedrine® [OTC]; Decofed® Syrup [OTC]; Drixoral® Non-Drowsy [OTC]; Efidac/24® [OTC]; Pedia Care® Oral; Sudafed® [OTC]; Sudafed® 12 Hour [OTC]; Triaminic® AM Decongestant Formula [OTC]

Canadian/Mexican Brand Names Balminil® Decongestant (Canada); Eltor® (Canada); PMS-Pseudoephedrine® (Canada); Robidrine® (Canada)

Therapeutic Category Adrenergic Agonist Agent; Decongestant

Synonyms Pseudoefedrina (Mexico)

Use Temporary symptomatic relief of nasal congestion due to common cold, upper respiratory allergies, and sinusitis; also promotes nasal or sinus drainage

Usual Dosage Oral:

Children:

<2 years: 4 mg/kg/day in divided doses every 6 hours

2-5 years: 15 mg every 6 hours; maximum: 60 mg/24 hours

6-12 years: 30 mg every 6 hours; maximum: 120 mg/24 hours

Adults: 30-60 mg every 4-6 hours, sustained release: 120 mg every 12 hours; maximum: 240 mg/24 hours

Mechanism of Action Directly stimulates alpha-adrenergic receptors of respiratory mucosa causing vasoconstriction; directly stimulates beta-adrenergic receptors causing bronchial relaxation, increased heart rate and contractility

Local Anesthetic/Vasoconstrictor Precautions Use with caution since pseudoephedrine is a sympathomimetic amine which could interact with epinephrine to cause a pressor response

Effects on Dental Treatment Up to 10% of patients could experience tachycardia, palpitations, and dry mouth; use vasoconstrictor with caution

Other Adverse Effects

>10%:

Cardiovascular: Tachycardia, palpitations, arrhythmias

Central nervous system: Nervousness, transient stimulation, insomnia, excitability, dizziness, drowsiness, headache
Neuromuscular & skeletal: Tremor
1% to 10%:
Gastrointestinal: Dry mouth
Neuromuscular & skeletal: Weakness
Miscellaneous: Sweating
<1%:
Central nervous system: Convulsions, hallucinations
Gastrointestinal: Nausea, vomiting
Genitourinary: Dysuria
Respiratory: Dyspnea
Drug Interactions Increased toxicity with MAO inhibitors (hypertensive crisis) sympathomimetics, CNS depressants, alcohol (sedation)
Drug Uptake
Onset of decongestant effect: Oral: 15-30 minutes
Duration: 4-6 hours (up to 12 hours with extended release formulation administration)
Serum half-life: 9-16 hours
Pregnancy Risk Factor C
Generic Available Yes

Pseudoephedrine, Acetaminophen, and Dextromethorphan *see* Acetaminophen, Dextromethorphan, and Pseudoephedrine *on page 25*

Pseudoephedrine and Acetaminophen *see* Acetaminophen and Pseudoephedrine *on page 24*

Pseudoephedrine and Azatadine *see* Azatadine and Pseudoephedrine *on page 102*

Pseudoephedrine and Chlorpheniramine *see* Chlorpheniramine and Pseudoephedrine *on page 219*

Pseudoephedrine and Dexbrompheniramine *see* Dexbrompheniramine and Pseudoephedrine *on page 292*

Pseudoephedrine and Dextromethorphan
(soo doe e FED rin & deks troe meth OR fan)
Brand Names Drixoral® Cough & Congestion Liquid Caps [OTC]; Vicks® 44D Cough & Head Congestion; Vicks® 44 Non-Drowsy Cold & Cough Liqui-Caps [OTC]
Therapeutic Category Adrenergic Agonist Agent; Antitussive; Decongestant
Use Temporary symptomatic relief of nasal congestion due to common cold, upper respiratory allergies, and sinusitis; also promotes nasal or sinus drainage; symptomatic relief of coughs caused by minor viral upper respiratory tract infections or inhaled irritants; most effective for a chronic nonproductive cough
Local Anesthetic/Vasoconstrictor Precautions Use with caution since pseudoephedrine is a sympathomimetic amine which could interact with epinephrine to cause a pressor response
Effects on Dental Treatment Up to 10% of patients could experience tachycardia, palpitations, and dry mouth; use vasoconstrictor with caution
Warnings/Precautions Research on chicken embryos exposed to concentrations of dextromethorphan relative to those typically taken by humans has shown to cause birth defects and fetal death; more study is needed, but it is suggested that pregnant women should be advised not to use dextromethorphan-containing medications
Generic Available Yes

Pseudoephedrine and Guaifenesin *see* Guaifenesin and Pseudoephedrine *on page 454*

Pseudoephedrine and Ibuprofen
(soo doe e FED rin & eye byoo PROE fen)
Brand Names Advil® Cold & Sinus Caplets [OTC]; Dimetapp® Sinus Caplets [OTC]; Dristan® Sinus Caplets [OTC]; Motrin® IB Sinus [OTC]; Sine-Aid® IB [OTC]
Therapeutic Category Adrenergic Agonist Agent; Analgesic, Non-narcotic; Decongestant
Use Temporary symptomatic relief of nasal congestion due to common cold, upper respiratory allergies, and sinusitis; also promotes nasal or sinus drainage; sinus headaches and pains
Local Anesthetic/Vasoconstrictor Precautions Use with caution since pseudoephedrine is a sympathomimetic amine which could interact with epinephrine to cause a pressor response
Effects on Dental Treatment Up to 10% of patients could experience tachycardia, palpitations, and dry mouth; use vasoconstrictor with caution
(Continued)

Pseudoephedrine and Ibuprofen *(Continued)*

Generic Available Yes

Pseudoephedrine, Dextromethorphan, and Acetaminophen *see* Acetaminophen, Dextromethorphan, and Pseudoephedrine *on page 25*

Pseudoephedrine, Dextromethorphan, and Guaifenesin *see* Guaifenesin, Pseudoephedrine, and Dextromethorphan *on page 456*

Pseudo-Gest Plus® Tablet [OTC] *see* Chlorpheniramine and Pseudoephedrine *on page 219*

Psor-a-set® Soap [OTC] *see* Salicylic Acid *on page 853*

Psorcon™ *see* Diflorasone *on page 311*

psoriGel® [OTC] *see* Coal Tar *on page 254*

P&S® Shampoo [OTC] *see* Salicylic Acid *on page 853*

Psyllium (SIL i yum)

Brand Names Effer-Syllium® [OTC]; Fiberall® Powder [OTC]; Fiberall® Wafer [OTC]; Hydrocil® [OTC]; Konsyl® [OTC]; Konsyl-D® [OTC]; Metamucil® [OTC]; Metamucil® Instant Mix [OTC]; Modane® Bulk [OTC]; Perdiem® Plain [OTC]; Reguloid® [OTC]; Serutan® [OTC]; Syllact® [OTC]; V-Lax® [OTC]

Canadian/Mexican Brand Names Fibrepur® (Canada); Novo-Mucilax® (Canada); Prodiem® Plain (Canada)

Therapeutic Category Laxative, Bulk-Producing

Use Treatment of chronic atonic or spastic constipation and in constipation associated with rectal disorders; management of irritable bowel syndrome

Usual Dosage Oral (administer at least 3 hours before or after drugs):

Children 6-11 years: (Approximately ¹/₂ adult dosage) ¹/₂ to 1 rounded teaspoonful in 4 oz glass of liquid 1-3 times/day

Adults: 1-2 rounded teaspoonfuls or 1-2 packets or 1-2 wafers in 8 oz glass of liquid 1-3 times/day

Mechanism of Action Adsorbs water in the intestine to form a viscous liquid which promotes peristalsis and reduces transit time

Local Anesthetic/Vasoconstrictor Precautions No information available to require special precautions

Effects on Dental Treatment No effects or complications reported

Other Adverse Effects 1% to 10%:

Gastrointestinal: Esophageal or bowel obstruction, diarrhea, constipation, abdominal cramps

Respiratory: Bronchospasm, anaphylaxis upon inhalation in susceptible individuals, rhinoconjunctivitis

Drug Interactions Decreased effect of warfarin, digitalis, potassium-sparing diuretics, salicylates, tetracyclines, nitrofurantoin

Drug Uptake

Onset of action: 12-24 hour, but full effect may take 2-3 days

Absorption: Oral: Generally not absorbed following administration, small amounts of grain extracts present in the preparation have been reportedly absorbed following colonic hydrolysis

Pregnancy Risk Factor C

Generic Available Yes

P.T.E.-4® *see* Trace Metals *on page 948*

P.T.E.-5® *see* Trace Metals *on page 948*

Pulmozyme® *see* Dornase Alfa *on page 333*

Puralube® Tears Solution [OTC] *see* Artificial Tears *on page 87*

Purge® [OTC] *see* Castor Oil *on page 184*

Puri-Clens™ [OTC] *see* Methylbenzethonium Chloride *on page 621*

Purinethol® *see* Mercaptopurine *on page 600*

P-V-Tussin® *see* Hydrocodone, Phenylephrine, Pyrilamine, Phenindamine, Chlorpheniramine, and Ammonium Chloride *on page 484*

PₓEₓ® Ophthalmic *see* Pilocarpine and Epinephrine *on page 761*

Pyrantel Pamoate (pi RAN tel PAM oh ate)

Brand Names Antiminth® [OTC]; Pin-Rid® [OTC]; Pin-X® [OTC]; Reese's® Pinworm Medicine [OTC]

Canadian/Mexican Brand Names Combantrin® (Mexico)

Therapeutic Category Anthelmintic

Use Roundworm (*Ascaris lumbricoides*), pinworm (*Enterobius vermicularis*), and hookworm (*Ancylostoma duodenale* and *Necator americanus*) infestations, and trichostrongyliasis

Usual Dosage Children and Adults (purgation is not required prior to use): Oral:

Roundworm, pinworm, or trichostrongyliasis: 11 mg/kg administered as a single dose; maximum dose: 1 g. **(Note:** For pinworm infection, dosage should be repeated in 2 weeks and all family members should be treated).

Hookworm: 11 mg/kg administered once daily for 3 days

Mechanism of Action Causes the release of acetylcholine and inhibits cholinesterase; acts as a depolarizing neuromuscular blocker, paralyzing the helminths

Local Anesthetic/Vasoconstrictor Precautions No information available to require special precautions

Effects on Dental Treatment No effects or complications reported

Other Adverse Effects

1% to 10%: Gastrointestinal: Anorexia, nausea, vomiting, abdominal cramps, diarrhea

<1%:

Central nervous system: Dizziness, drowsiness, insomnia, headache

Dermatologic: Rash

Gastrointestinal: Tenesmus

Hepatic: Liver enzymes (elevated)

Neuromuscular & skeletal: Weakness

Drug Uptake

Absorption: Oral: Poor

Time to peak serum concentration: Within 1-3 hours

Pregnancy Risk Factor C

Generic Available No

Comments Purgation is not required prior to use

Pyrazinamide (peer a ZIN a mide)

Related Information

Nonviral Infectious Diseases *on page 1032*

Canadian/Mexican Brand Names Braccopril® (Mexico); PMS-Pyrazinamide® (Canada); Tebrazid® (Canada)

Therapeutic Category Antitubercular Agent

Synonyms Pirazinamida (Mexico)

Use Adjunctive treatment of tuberculosis in combination with other antituberculosis agents

Usual Dosage Oral (calculate dose on ideal body weight rather than total body weight): **Note:** A four-drug regimen (isoniazid, rifampin, pyrazinamide, and either streptomycin or ethambutol) is preferred for the initial, empiric treatment of TB. When the drug susceptibility results are available, the regimen should be altered as appropriate.

Patients with TB and without HIV infection:

OPTION 1:

Isoniazid resistance rate <4%: Administer daily isoniazid, rifampin, and pyrazinamide for 8 weeks followed by isoniazid and rifampin daily or directly observed therapy (DOT) 2-3 times/week for 16 weeks

If isoniazid resistance rate is not documented, ethambutol or streptomycin should also be administered until susceptibility to isoniazid or rifampin is demonstrated. Continue treatment for at least 6 months or 3 months beyond culture conversion.

OPTION 2: Administer daily isoniazid, rifampin, pyrazinamide, and either streptomycin or ethambutol for 2 weeks followed by DOT 2 times/week administration of the same drugs for 6 weeks, and subsequently, with isoniazid and rifampin DOT 2 times/week administration for 16 weeks

OPTION 3: Administer isoniazid, rifampin, pyrazinamide, and either ethambutol or streptomycin by DOT 3 times/week for 6 months

Patients with TB and with HIV infection:

Administer any of the above OPTIONS 1, 2 or 3, however, treatment should be continued for a total of 9 months and at least 6 months beyond culture conversion

Note: Some experts recommend that the duration of therapy should be extended to 9 months for patients with disseminated disease, miliary disease, disease involving the bones or joints, or tuberculosis lymphadenitis

Children and Adults:

Daily therapy: 15-30 mg/kg/day (maximum: 2 g/day)

Directly observed therapy (DOT): Twice weekly: 50-70 mg/kg (maximum: 4 g)

DOT: 3 times/week: 50-70 mg/kg (maximum: 3 g)

Elderly: Start with a lower daily dose (15 mg/kg) and increase as tolerated

Mechanism of Action Converted to pyrazinoic acid in susceptible strains of *Mycobacterium* which lowers the pH of the environment

Local Anesthetic/Vasoconstrictor Precautions No information available to require special precautions

(Continued)

Pyrazinamide *(Continued)*

Effects on Dental Treatment No effects or complications reported

Other Adverse Effects

1% to 10%:
Central nervous system: Malaise
Gastrointestinal: Nausea, vomiting, anorexia
Neuromuscular & skeletal: Arthralgia, myalgia
<1%:
Central nervous system: Fever
Dermatologic: Skin rash, itching, acne, photosensitivity
Endocrine & metabolic: Gout
Genitourinary: Dysuria
Hematologic: Porphyria, thrombocytopenia
Hepatic: Hepatotoxicity
Renal: Interstitial nephritis

Drug Interactions No data reported

Drug Uptake Bacteriostatic or bactericidal depending on the drug's concentration at the site of infection

Absorption: Oral: Well absorbed
Serum half-life: 9-10 hours, increased with reduced renal or hepatic function
End stage renal disease: 9 hours
Time to peak serum concentration: Within 2 hours

Pregnancy Risk Factor C

Generic Available Yes

Pyrethrins (pye RE thrins)

Brand Names A-200™ Shampoo [OTC]; Barc® Liquid [OTC]; End Lice® Liquid [OTC]; Lice-Enz® Shampoo [OTC]; Pronto® Shampoo [OTC]; Pyrinex® Pediculicide Shampoo [OTC]; Pyrinyl II® Liquid [OTC]; Pyrinyl Plus® Shampoo [OTC]; R & C® Shampoo [OTC]; RID® Shampoo [OTC]; Tisit® Blue Gel [OTC]; Tisit® Liquid [OTC]; Tisit® Shampoo [OTC]; Triple X® Liquid [OTC]

Canadian/Mexican Brand Names Lice-Enz® (Canada)

Therapeutic Category Antiparasitic Agent, Topical; Pediculocide

Use Treatment of *Pediculus humanus* infestations (head lice, body lice, pubic lice and their eggs)

Usual Dosage Application of pyrethrins: Topical:
Apply enough solution to completely wet infested area, including hair
Allow to remain on area for 10 minutes
Wash and rinse with large amounts of warm water
Use fine-toothed comb to remove lice and eggs from hair
Shampoo hair to restore body and luster
Treatment may be repeated if necessary once in a 24-hour period
Repeat treatment in 7-10 days to kill newly hatched lice

Mechanism of Action Pyrethrins are derived from flowers that belong to the chrysanthemum family. The mechanism of action on the neuronal membranes of lice is similar to that of DDT. Piperonyl butoxide is usually added to pyrethrin to enhance the product's activity by decreasing the metabolism of pyrethrins in arthropods.

Local Anesthetic/Vasoconstrictor Precautions No information available to require special precautions

Effects on Dental Treatment No effects or complications reported

Other Adverse Effects 1% to 10%: Local: Pruritus, burning, stinging, irritation with repeat use

Drug Interactions No data reported

Drug Uptake
Onset of action: ~30 minutes
Absorption: Topical into the system is minimal

Pregnancy Risk Factor C

Generic Available Yes

Pyridiate® *see* Phenazopyridine *on page 746*

Pyridium® *see* Phenazopyridine *on page 746*

Pyridoxine (peer i DOKS een)

Brand Names Nestrex®

Canadian/Mexican Brand Names Benadon® (Mexico)

Therapeutic Category Antidote, Cycloserine Toxicity; Antidote, Hydralazine Toxicity; Antidote, Isoniazid Toxicity; Vitamin, Water Soluble

Synonyms Piridoxina (Mexico)

Use Prevents and treats vitamin B_6 deficiency, pyridoxine-dependent seizures in infants, adjunct to treatment of acute toxicity from isoniazid, cycloserine, or hydralazine overdose

Usual Dosage
Recommended daily allowance (RDA):
Children:
1-3 years: 0.9 mg
4-6 years: 1.3 mg
7-10 years: 1.6 mg
Adults:
Male: 1.7-2.0 mg
Female: 1.4-1.6 mg
Dietary deficiency: Oral:
Children: 5-25 mg/24 hours for 3 weeks, then 1.5-2.5 mg/day in multiple vitamin product
Adults: 10-20 mg/day for 3 weeks
Drug-induced neuritis (eg, isoniazid, hydralazine, penicillamine, cycloserine): Oral:
Children:
Treatment: 10-50 mg/24 hours
Prophylaxis: 1-2 mg/kg/24 hours
Adults:
Treatment: 100-200 mg/24 hours
Prophylaxis: 25-100 mg/24 hours
Treatment of seizures and/or coma from acute isoniazid toxicity, a dose of pyridoxine hydrochloride equal to the amount of INH ingested can be given I.M./I.V. in divided doses together with other anticonvulsants; if the amount INH ingested is not known, administer 5 g I.V. pyridoxine
Treatment of acute hydralazine toxicity, a pyridoxine dose of 25 mg/kg in divided doses I.M./I.V. has been used

Mechanism of Action Precursor to pyridoxal, which functions in the metabolism of proteins, carbohydrates, and fats; pyridoxal also aids in the release of liver and muscle-stored glycogen and in the synthesis of GABA (within the central nervous system) and heme

Local Anesthetic/Vasoconstrictor Precautions No information available to require special precautions

Effects on Dental Treatment No effects or complications reported

Other Adverse Effects <1%:
Central nervous system: Sensory neuropathy, seizures have occurred following I.V. administration of very large doses, headache
Gastrointestinal: Nausea
Endocrine & metabolic: Decreased serum folic acid secretions
Hepatic: Elevated AST
Neuromuscular & skeletal: Paresthesia
Miscellaneous: Allergic reactions have been reported

Drug Interactions Decreased serum levels of levodopa, phenobarbital, and phenytoin

Drug Uptake
Absorption: Enteral, parenteral: Well absorbed from GI tract
Serum half-life: 15-20 days

Pregnancy Risk Factor A (C if dose exceeds RDA recommendation)

Generic Available Yes

Pyrimethamine (peer i METH a meen)

Brand Names Daraprim®
Canadian/Mexican Brand Names Daraprim® (Mexico)
Therapeutic Category Antimalarial Agent
Synonyms Pirimetamina (Mexico)
Use Prophylaxis of malaria due to susceptible strains of plasmodia; used in conjunction with quinine and sulfadiazine for the treatment of uncomplicated attacks of chloroquine-resistant *P. falciparum* malaria; used in conjunction with fast-acting schizonticide to initiate transmission control and suppression cure; synergistic combination with sulfonamide in treatment of toxoplasmosis

Usual Dosage
Malaria chemoprophylaxis (for areas where chloroquine-resistant *P. falciparum* exists): Begin prophylaxis 2 weeks before entering endemic area:
Children: 0.5 mg/kg once weekly; not to exceed 25 mg/dose
or
Children:
<4 years: 6.25 mg once weekly
4-10 years: 12.5 mg once weekly
Children >10 years and Adults: 25 mg once weekly
(Continued)

Pyrimethamine *(Continued)*

Dosage should be continued for all age groups for at least 6-10 weeks after leaving endemic areas

Chloroquine-resistant *P. falciparum* malaria (when used in conjunction with quinine and sulfadiazine):

Children:

  <10 kg: 6.25 mg/day once daily for 3 days

  10-20 kg: 12.5 mg/day once daily for 3 days

  20-40 kg: 25 mg/day once daily for 3 days

Adults: 25 mg twice daily for 3 days

Toxoplasmosis:

Infants for congenital toxoplasmosis: Oral: 1 mg/kg once daily for 6 months with sulfadiazine then every other month with sulfa, alternating with spiramycin.

Children: Loading dose: 2 mg/kg/day divided into 2 equal daily doses for 1-3 days (maximum: 100 mg/day) followed by 1 mg/kg/day divided into 2 doses for 4 weeks; maximum: 25 mg/day

With sulfadiazine or trisulfapyrimidines: 2 mg/kg/day divided every 12 hours for 3 days followed by 1 mg/kg/day once daily or divided twice daily for 4 weeks given with trisulfapyrimidines or sulfadiazine

Adults: 50-75 mg/day together with 1-4 g of a sulfonamide for 1-3 weeks depending on patient's tolerance and response, then reduce dose by 50% and continue for 4-5 weeks **or** 25-50 mg/day for 3-4 weeks

Mechanism of Action Inhibits parasitic dihydrofolate reductase, resulting in inhibition of vital tetrahydrofolic acid synthesis

Local Anesthetic/Vasoconstrictor Precautions No information available to require special precautions

Effects on Dental Treatment No effects or complications reported

Other Adverse Effects

1% to 10%:

Gastrointestinal: Anorexia, abdominal cramps, vomiting

Hematologic: Megaloblastic anemia, leukopenia, thrombocytopenia, agranulocytosis

<1%:

Central nervous system: Insomnia, lightheadedness, fever, malaise, seizures, depression

Dermatologic: Skin rash, dermatitis, abnormal skin pigmentation

Gastrointestinal: Diarrhea, dry mouth, atrophic glossitis

Hematologic: Pulmonary eosinophilia

Drug Interactions

Decreased effect: Pyrimethamine effectiveness decreased by acid

Increased effect: Sulfonamides (synergy), methotrexate, TMP/SMX

Drug Uptake

Absorption: Oral: Well absorbed

Serum half-life: 80-95 hours

Pregnancy Risk Factor C

Generic Available No

Pyrinex® Pediculicide Shampoo [OTC] *see* Pyrethrins *on page 824*

Pyrinyl II® Liquid [OTC] *see* Pyrethrins *on page 824*

Pyrinyl Plus® Shampoo [OTC] *see* Pyrethrins *on page 824*

Pyrithione Zinc *(peer i THYE one zingk)*

Brand Names DHS Zinc® [OTC]; Head & Shoulders® [OTC]; Theraplex Z® [OTC]; Zincon® Shampoo [OTC]; ZNP® Bar [OTC]

Therapeutic Category Antiseborrheic Agent, Topical

Use Relieves the itching, irritation and scalp flaking associated with dandruff and/or seborrheic dermatitis of the scalp

Local Anesthetic/Vasoconstrictor Precautions No information available to require special precautions

Effects on Dental Treatment No effects or complications reported

Generic Available No

Quazepam *(KWAY ze pam)*

Brand Names Doral®

Therapeutic Category Benzodiazepine; Hypnotic; Sedative

Use Treatment of insomnia; more likely than triazolam to cause daytime sedation and fatigue; is classified as a long-acting benzodiazepine hypnotic (like flurazepam - Dalmane®), this long duration of action may prevent withdrawal symptoms when therapy is discontinued

Usual Dosage Adults: Oral: Initial: 15 mg at bedtime, in some patients the dose may be reduced to 7.5 mg after a few nights

Mechanism of Action Depresses all levels of the CNS, including the limbic and reticular formation, probably through the increased action of gamma-aminobutyric acid (GABA), which is a major inhibitory neurotransmitter in the brain

Local Anesthetic/Vasoconstrictor Precautions No information available to require special precautions

Effects on Dental Treatment >10% of patients will experience dry mouth which disappears with cessation of drug therapy

Other Adverse Effects

>10%:
  Central nervous system: Drowsiness
1% to 10%:
  Central nervous system: Headache, fatigue, dizziness
  Gastrointestinal: Xerostomia, dyspepsia
<1%:
  Central nervous system: Slurred speech, irritability
  Endocrine & metabolic: Changes in libido
  Genitourinary: Urinary retention, incontinence
  Hematologic: Leukocytosis, thrombocytosis
  Hepatic: Jaundice, increased total bilirubin, increased alkaline phosphatase
  Neuromuscular & skeletal: Dysarthria, dystonia
  Renal: Increased BUN, increased creatinine

Drug Interactions Increased effect/toxicity with CNS depressants (narcotics, alcohol, MAO inhibitors, TCAs, anesthetics, barbiturates, phenothiazines)

Drug Uptake
  Absorption: Oral: Rapid
  Serum half-life:
    Parent drug: 25-41 hours
    Active metabolite: 40-114 hours

Pregnancy Risk Factor X
Generic Available No

Questran® see Cholestyramine Resin on page 229

Questran® Light see Cholestyramine Resin on page 229

Quetiapine (kwe TYE a peen)
Brand Names Seroquel®
Therapeutic Category Antipsychotic Agent
Synonyms Quetiapine Fumarate
Use Management of psychotic disorders; this antipsychotic drug belongs to a new chemical class, the dibenzothiazepine derivatives
Usual Dosage Adults: Oral: 25-100 mg 2-3 times/day
Local Anesthetic/Vasoconstrictor Precautions No information available to require special precautions
Effects on Dental Treatment No effects or complications reported
Dosage Forms Tablet, as fumarate: 25 mg, 100 mg, 200 mg

Quetiapine Fumarate see Quetiapine on this page

Quibron® see Theophylline and Guaifenesin on page 922

Quibron®-T see Theophylline on page 917

Quibron®-T/SR see Theophylline on page 917

Quinaglute® Dura-Tabs® see Quinidine on page 830

Quinalan® see Quinidine on page 830

Quinamm® see Quinine on page 831

Quinapril (KWIN a pril)
Related Information
  Cardiovascular Diseases on page 1010
Brand Names Accupril®
Canadian/Mexican Brand Names Acupril® (Mexico)
Therapeutic Category Angiotensin-Converting Enzyme (ACE) Inhibitors
Synonyms Quinaprilo, Clorhidrato De (Mexico)
Use Management of hypertension and treatment of congestive heart failure; increase circulation in Raynaud's phenomenon; idiopathic edema

Unlabeled use: Hypertensive crisis, diabetic nephropathy, rheumatoid arthritis, diagnosis of anatomic renal artery stenosis, hypertension secondary to scleroderma renal crisis, diagnosis of aldosteronism, idiopathic edema, Bartter's syndrome, postmyocardial infarction for prevention of ventricular failure
(Continued)

Quinapril *(Continued)*

Usual Dosage

Adults: Oral: Initial: 10 mg once daily, adjust according to blood pressure response at peak and trough blood levels; in general, the normal dosage range is 20-80 mg/day

Elderly: Initial: 2.5-5 mg/day; increase dosage at increments of 2.5-5 mg at 1- to 2-week intervals

Mechanism of Action Competitive inhibitor of angiotensin-converting enzyme (ACE); prevents conversion of angiotensin I to angiotensin II, a potent vasoconstrictor; results in lower levels of angiotensin II which causes an increase in plasma renin activity and a reduction in aldosterone secretion; a CNS mechanism may also be involved in hypotensive effect as angiotensin II increases adrenergic outflow from CNS; vasoactive kallikreins may be decreased in conversion to active hormones by ACE inhibitors, thus reducing blood pressure

Local Anesthetic/Vasoconstrictor Precautions No information available to require special precautions

Effects on Dental Treatment No effects or complications reported

Other Adverse Effects

1% to 10%:

Cardiovascular: Hypotension

Central nervous system: Dizziness, headache, fatigue

Gastrointestinal: Diarrhea

Renal: Elevated BUN and serum creatinine

Respiratory: Upper respiratory symptoms, cough

<1%:

Cardiovascular: Chest discomfort, flushing, myocardial infarction, angina pectoris, orthostatic hypotension, rhythm disturbances, tachycardia, peripheral edema, vasculitis, palpitations, syncope

Central nervous system: Fever, malaise, depression, somnolence, insomnia

Dermatologic: Urticaria, pruritus, angioedema

Endocrine & metabolic: Gout

Gastrointestinal: Pancreatitis, abdominal pain, anorexia, constipation, flatulence, dry mouth

Hematologic: Neutropenia, bone marrow suppression

Hepatic: Hepatitis

Neuromuscular & skeletal: Arthralgia, shoulder pain

Ocular: Blurred vision

Respiratory: Bronchitis, sinusitis, pharyngeal pain

Miscellaneous: Sweating

Drug Interactions See table.

Drug-Drug Interactions With ACEIs

Precipitant Drug	Drug (Category) and Effect	Description
Antacids	ACE Inhibitors: decreased	Decreased bioavailability of ACEIs. May be more likely with captopril. Separate administration times by 1-2 hours.
NSAIDs (indomethacin)	ACEIs: decreased	Reduced hypotensive effects of ACEIs. More prominent in low renin or volume dependent hypertensive patients.
Phenothiazines	ACEIs: increased	Pharmacologic effects of ACEIs may be increased.
ACEIs	Allopurinol: increased	Higher risk of hypersensitivity reaction possible when given concurrently. Three case reports of Stevens-Johnson syndrome with captopril.
ACEIs	Digoxin: increased	Increased plasma digoxin levels.
ACEIs	Lithium: increased	Increased serum lithium levels and symptoms of toxicity may occur.
ACEIs	Potassium preps/ potassium sparing diuretics increased	Coadministration may result in elevated potassium levels.

Drug Uptake

Serum half-life, elimination:

Quinapril: 0.8 hours

Quinaprilat: 2 hours

Time to peak serum concentration:

Quinapril: 1 hour

Quinaprilat: ~2 hours

Pregnancy Risk Factor C (first trimester); D (second and third trimester)
Generic Available No

Quinaprilo, Clorhidrato De (Mexico) *see* Quinapril *on page 827*

Quinestrol (kwin ES trole)
Related Information
Endocrine Disorders & Pregnancy *on page 1021*
Brand Names Estrovis®
Therapeutic Category Estrogen Derivative
Use Atrophic vaginitis; hypogonadism; primary ovarian failure; vasomotor symptoms of menopause; prostatic carcinoma; osteoporosis prophylactic
Usual Dosage Adults: Female: Oral: 100 mcg once daily for 7 days; followed by 100 mcg/week beginning 2 weeks after inception of treatment; may increase to 200 mcg/week if necessary
Mechanism of Action Increases the synthesis of DNA, RNA, and various proteins in target tissues; reduces the release of gonadotropin-releasing hormone from the hypothalamus; reduces FSH and LH release from the pituitary
Local Anesthetic/Vasoconstrictor Precautions No information available to require special precautions
Effects on Dental Treatment No effects or complications reported
Other Adverse Effects
>10%:
Cardiovascular: Peripheral edema
Endocrine & metabolic: Enlargement of breasts (female and male), breast tenderness
Gastrointestinal: Nausea, anorexia, bloating
1% to 10%:
Central nervous system: Headache
Endocrine & metabolic: Increased libido (female), decreased libido (male)
Gastrointestinal: Vomiting, diarrhea
<1%:
Cardiovascular: Hypertension, thromboembolism, myocardial infarction, edema
Central nervous system: Depression, dizziness, anxiety, stroke
Dermatologic: Chloasma, melasma, rash
Endocrine: Breast tumors, amenorrhea, alterations in frequency and flow of menses, decreased glucose tolerance, elevated triglycerides and LDL
Gastrointestinal: GI distress
Hepatic: Cholestatic jaundice
Ocular: Intolerance to contact lenses
Miscellaneous: Increased susceptibility to *Candida* infection
Drug Interactions No significant interactions reported
Drug Uptake
Onset of therapeutic effect: Commonly within 3 days of treatment
Duration: Can persist for as long as 4 months
Serum half-life: 120 hours
Pregnancy Risk Factor X
Generic Available No

Quinethazone (kwin ETH a zone)
Related Information
Cardiovascular Diseases *on page 1010*
Brand Names Hydromox®
Therapeutic Category Diuretic, Thiazide
Use Adjunctive therapy in treatment of edema and hypertension
Usual Dosage Adults: Oral: 50-100 mg once daily up to a maximum of 200 mg/day
Mechanism of Action Quinethazone is a quinazoline derivative which increases the renal excretion of sodium and chloride and an accompanying volume of water due to inhibition of the tubular mechanism of electrolyte reabsorption.
Local Anesthetic/Vasoconstrictor Precautions No information available to require special precautions
Effects on Dental Treatment No effects or complications reported
Other Adverse Effects
1% to 10%: Endocrine & metabolic: Hypokalemia
<1%:
Cardiovascular: Hypotension
Central nervous system: Drowsiness
Dermatologic: Photosensitivity, rash
Endocrine & metabolic: Fluid and electrolyte imbalances (hypocalcemia, hypomagnesemia, hyponatremia), hyperglycemia
(Continued)

Quinethazone *(Continued)*

Gastrointestinal: Nausea, vomiting, anorexia
Hematologic: Aplastic anemia, hemolytic anemia, leukopenia, agranulocytosis, thrombocytopenia
Hepatic: Hepatitis
Renal: Prerenal azotemia, polyuria, uremia

Drug Interactions
Decreased effect of oral hypoglycemics; decreased absorption with cholestyramine and colestipol
Increased effect with furosemide and other loop diuretics
Increased toxicity/levels of lithium

Drug Uptake
Onset of action: 2 hours
Duration: 18-24 hours

Pregnancy Risk Factor D
Generic Available No

Quinidex® Extentabs® *see Quinidine on this page*

Quinidina (Mexico) *see Quinidine on this page*

Quinidine *(KWIN i deen)*

Related Information
Cardiovascular Diseases *on page 1010*

Brand Names Cardioquin®; Quinaglute® Dura-Tabs®; Quinalan®; Quinidex® Extentabs®; Quinora®

Canadian/Mexican Brand Names Quini Durules® (Mexico)

Therapeutic Category Antiarrhythmic Agent, Class I-A; Antiarrhythmic Agent (Supraventricular & Ventricular)

Synonyms Quinidina (Mexico)

Use Prophylaxis after cardioversion of atrial fibrillation and/or flutter to maintain normal sinus rhythm; also used to prevent reoccurrence of paroxysmal supraventricular tachycardia, paroxysmal A-V junctional rhythm, paroxysmal ventricular tachycardia, paroxysmal atrial fibrillation, and atrial or ventricular premature contractions; also has activity against *Plasmodium falciparum* malaria

Usual Dosage Dosage expressed in terms of the salt: 267 mg of quinidine gluconate = 200 mg of quinidine sulfate

Children: Test dose for idiosyncratic reaction (sulfate, oral or gluconate, I.M.): 2 mg/kg or 60 mg/m^2
Oral (quinidine sulfate): 15-60 mg/kg/day in 4-5 divided doses or 6 mg/kg every 4-6 hours; usual 30 mg/kg/day or 900 mg/m^2/day given in 5 daily doses
I.V. **not** recommended (quinidine gluconate): 2-10 mg/kg/dose given at a rate ≤10 mg/minute every 3-6 hours as needed

Adults: Test dose: Oral, I.M.: 200 mg administered several hours before full dosage (to determine possibility of idiosyncratic reaction)
Oral:
Sulfate: 100-600 mg/dose every 4-6 hours; begin at 200 mg/dose and titrate to desired effect (maximum daily dose: 3-4 g)
Gluconate: 324-972 mg every 8-12 hours
I.M.: 400 mg/dose every 4-6 hours
I.V.: 200-400 mg/dose diluted and given at a rate ≤10 mg/minute

Mechanism of Action Class 1A antiarrhythmic agent; depresses phase O of the action potential; decreases myocardial excitability and conduction velocity, and myocardial contractility by decreasing sodium influx during depolarization and potassium efflux in repolarization; also reduces calcium transport across cell membrane

Local Anesthetic/Vasoconstrictor Precautions No information available to require special precautions

Effects on Dental Treatment When taken over a long period of time, the anticholinergic side effects from quinidine can cause a reduction of saliva production or secretion contributing to discomfort and dental disease (ie, caries, oral candidiasis and periodontal disease)

Other Adverse Effects
>10%: Gastrointestinal: Bitter taste, diarrhea, anorexia, nausea, vomiting, stomach cramping
1% to 10%:
Cardiovascular: Hypotension, syncope
Central nervous system: Lightheadedness, severe headache
Dermatologic: Skin rash
Ocular: Blurred vision
Otic: Tinnitus
Respiratory: Wheezing

<1%:
  Cardiovascular: Tachycardia, heart block, ventricular fibrillation, vascular collapse
  Central nervous system: Confusion, delirium, fever, vertigo
  Dermatologic: Angioedema
  Hematologic: Anemia, thrombocytopenic purpura, blood dyscrasias
  Otic: Impaired hearing
  Respiratory: Respiratory depression

Drug Interactions
  Decreased effect: Phenobarbital, phenytoin, and rifampin may decrease quinidine serum concentrations
  Increased toxicity:
    Verapamil, amiodarone, alkalinizing agents, and cimetidine may increase quinidine serum concentrations
    Quinidine may increase plasma concentration of digoxin, digoxin dosage may need to be reduced (by one-half) when quinidine is initiated
    Beta-blockers + quinidine may cause enhanced bradycardia
    Quinidine may enhance coumarin anticoagulants

Drug Uptake
  Serum half-life:
    Children: 2.5-6.7 hours
    Adults: 6-8 hours; increased half-life with elderly, cirrhosis, and congestive heart failure

Pregnancy Risk Factor C
Generic Available Yes

Quinine (KWYE nine)

Brand Names Formula Q® [OTC]; Legatrin® [OTC]; M-KYA® [OTC]; Quinamm®; Quiphile®; Q-vel®
Therapeutic Category Antimalarial Agent; Muscle Relaxant
Use Suppression or treatment of chloroquine-resistant *P. falciparum* malaria; treatment of *Babesia microti* infection; prevention and treatment of nocturnal recumbency leg muscle cramps
Usual Dosage Oral:
  Children:
    Treatment of chloroquine-resistant malaria: 25 mg/kg/day in divided doses every 8 hours for 3-7 days in conjunction with another agent
    Babesiosis: 25 mg/kg/day, (up to a maximum of 650 mg/dose) divided every 8 hours for 7 days
  Adults:
    Treatment of chloroquine-resistant malaria: 650 mg every 8 hours for 3-7 days in conjunction with another agent
    Suppression of malaria: 325 mg twice daily and continued for 6 weeks after exposure
    Babesiosis: 650 mg every 6-8 hours for 7 days
    Leg cramps: 200-300 mg at bedtime
Mechanism of Action Depresses oxygen uptake and carbohydrate metabolism; intercalates into DNA, disrupting the parasite's replication and transcription; affects calcium distribution within muscle fibers and decreases the excitability of the motor end-plate region; cardiovascular effects similar to quinidine
Local Anesthetic/Vasoconstrictor Precautions No information available to require special precautions
Effects on Dental Treatment No effects or complications reported
Other Adverse Effects
  >10%:
    Central nervous system: Severe headache
    Gastrointestinal: Nausea, vomiting, diarrhea
    Ocular: Blurred vision
    Otic: Tinnitus
  <1%:
    Cardiovascular: Flushing of the skin, anginal symptoms
    Central nervous system: Fever
    Dermatologic: Rash, pruritus
    Endocrine & metabolic: Hypoglycemia
    Gastrointestinal: Epigastric pain
    Hematologic: Hemolysis, thrombocytopenia
    Hepatic: Hepatitis
    Ocular: Nightblindness, diplopia, optic atrophy
    Otic: Impaired hearing
    Miscellaneous: Hypersensitivity reactions
(Continued)

Quinine *(Continued)*

Drug Interactions
Decreased effect: Phenobarbital, phenytoin, and rifampin may decrease quinine serum concentrations

Increased toxicity:

Verapamil, amiodarone, alkalizing agents, and cimetidine may increase quinidine serum concentrations

Quinidine may increase plasma concentration of digoxin, digoxin dosage may need to be reduced (by one-half) when quinidine is initiated

Beta-blockers + quinidine may cause enhanced bradycardia

Quinidine may enhance coumarin anticoagulants

Drug Uptake
Absorption: Oral: Readily absorbed mainly from the upper small intestine

Serum half-life:

Children: 6-12 hours

Adults: 8-14 hours

Time to peak serum concentration: Within 1-3 hours

Pregnancy Risk Factor D
Generic Available Yes

Quinora® *see* Quinidine *on page 830*

Quinsana Plus® [OTC] *see* Tolnaftate *on page 943*

Quiphile® *see* Quinine *on previous page*

Q-vel® *see* Quinine *on previous page*

QYS® *see* Hydroxyzine *on page 491*

Rabies Immune Globulin (Human)
(RAY beez i MYUN GLOB yoo lin, HYU man)

Related Information
Animal and Human Bites Guidelines *on page 1093*

Brand Names Hyperab®; Imogam®
Therapeutic Category Immune Globulin

Use Part of postexposure prophylaxis of persons with rabies exposure who lack a history or pre-exposure or postexposure prophylaxis with rabies vaccine or a recently documented neutralizing antibody response to previous rabies vaccination; although it is preferable to give RIG with the first dose of vaccine, it can be given up to 8 days after vaccination

Usual Dosage Children and Adults: I.M.: 20 units/kg in a single dose (RIG should always be administered in conjunction with rabies vaccine (HDCV)); infiltrate ½ of the dose locally around the wound; give the remainder I.M.

Mechanism of Action Rabies immune globulin is a solution of globulins dried from the plasma or serum of selected adult human donors who have been immunized with rabies vaccine and have developed high titers of rabies antibody. It generally contains 10% to 18% of protein of which not less than 80% is monomeric immunoglobulin G.

Local Anesthetic/Vasoconstrictor Precautions No information available to require special precautions

Effects on Dental Treatment No effects or complications reported

Other Adverse Effects
1% to 10%:

Central nervous system: Fever (mild)

Local: Soreness at injection site

<1%:

Dermatologic: Urticaria, angioedema

Neuromuscular & skeletal: Stiffness, soreness of muscles

Miscellaneous: Anaphylactic shock

Drug Interactions
Decreased effect: Live vaccines, corticosteroids, immunosuppressive agents; should not be administered within 3 months

Pregnancy Risk Factor C
Generic Available No

Rabies Virus Vaccine (RAY beez VYE rus vak SEEN)

Related Information
Animal and Human Bites Guidelines *on page 1093*

Brand Names Imovax® Rabies I.D. Vaccine; Imovax® Rabies Vaccine
Therapeutic Category Vaccine, Inactivated Virus

Use Veterinarians, animal handlers, certain laboratory workers, and persons living in or visiting countries for longer than 1 month where rabies is a constant threat.

Complete pre-exposure prophylaxis does not eliminate the need for additional therapy with rabies vaccine after a rabies exposure. The Food and Drug Administration has not approved the I.D. use of rabies vaccine for postexposure prophylaxis. Recommendations for I.D. use of HDCV are currently being discussed. The decision for postexposure rabies vaccination depends on the species of biting animal, the circumstances of biting incident, and the type of exposure (bite, saliva contamination of wound, and so on). The type of and schedule for postexposure prophylaxis depends upon the person's previous rabies vaccination status or the result of a previous or current serologic test for rabies antibody. For postexposure prophylaxis, rabies vaccine should always be administered I.M., **not** I.D.

Usual Dosage

Pre-exposure prophylaxis: Two 1 mL doses I.M. 1 week apart, third dose 3 weeks after second. If exposure continues, booster doses can be given every 2 years, or an antibody titer determined and a booster dose given if the titer is inadequate.

Postexposure prophylaxis: All postexposure treatment should begin with immediate cleansing of the wound with soap and water

Persons not previously immunized as above: Rabies immune globulin 20 units/kg body weight, half infiltrated at bite site if possible, remainder I.M.; and 5 doses of rabies vaccine, 1 mL I.M., one each on days 0, 3, 7, 14, 28

Persons who have previously received postexposure prophylaxis with rabies vaccine, received a recommended I.M. pre-exposure series of rabies vaccine or have a previously documented rabies antibody titer considered adequate: Two doses of rabies vaccine, 1 mL I.M., one each on days 0 and 3

Mechanism of Action Rabies vaccine is an inactivated virus vaccine which promotes immunity by inducing an active immune response. The production of specific antibodies requires about 7-10 days to develop. Rabies immune globulin or antirabies serum, equine (ARS) is given in conjunction with rabies vaccine to provide immune protection until an antibody response can occur.

Local Anesthetic/Vasoconstrictor Precautions No information available to require special precautions

Effects on Dental Treatment No effects or complications reported

Other Adverse Effects >10%:

Central nervous system: Dizziness, malaise, encephalomyelitis, transverse myelitis, fever, pain

Dermatologic: Itching, erythema

Gastrointestinal: Nausea, headache, abdominal pain

Local: Local discomfort, swelling

Neuromuscular & skeletal: Neuroparalytic reactions, myalgia

Drug Interactions Decreased effect with immunosuppressive agents, corticosteroids, antimalarial drugs (ie, chloroquine); persons on these drugs should receive RIG (3 doses/1 mL each) by the I.M. route

Drug Uptake

Onset of effect: I.M.: Rabies antibody appears in the serum within 7-10 days

Peak effect: Within 30-60 days and persists for at least 1 year

Pregnancy Risk Factor C

Generic Available No

Raloxifene (ral OX i feen)

Brand Names Evista®

Therapeutic Category Selective Estrogen Receptor Modulator (SERM)

Synonyms Keoxifene Hydrochloride; Raloxifene Hydrochloride

Use Prevention of osteoporosis in postmenopausal women

Mechanism of Action A selective estrogen receptor modulator, meaning that it affects some of the same receptors that estrogen does, but not all, and in some instances, it antagonizes or blocks estrogen; it acts like estrogen to prevent bone loss and improve lipid profiles, but it has the potential to block some estrogen effects such as those that lead to breast cancer and uterine cancer

Local Anesthetic/Vasoconstrictor Precautions No information available to require special precautions

Effects on Dental Treatment No effects or complications reported

Dosage Forms Tablet, as hydrochloride: 60 mg

Comments The decrease in estrogen-related adverse effects with the selective estrogen-receptor modulators in general and raloxifene in particular should improve compliance and decrease the incidence of cardiovascular events and fractures while not increasing breast cancer

Raloxifene Hydrochloride see Raloxifene on this page

Ramipril (ra MI pril)
Related Information
Cardiovascular Diseases *on page 1010*
Brand Names Altace™
Canadian/Mexican Brand Names Ramace® (Mexico); Tritace® (Mexico)
Therapeutic Category Angiotensin-Converting Enzyme (ACE) Inhibitors
Use Treatment of hypertension, alone or in combination with thiazide diuretics

Unlabeled use: Congestive heart failure

Usual Dosage Adults: Oral: 2.5-5 mg once daily, maximum: 20 mg/day

Mechanism of Action Ramipril is an angiotensin-converting enzyme (ACE) inhibitor which prevents the formation of angiotensin II from angiotensin I and exhibits pharmacologic effects that are similar to captopril. Ramipril must undergo enzymatic saponification by esterases in the liver to its biologically active metabolite, ramiprilat. The pharmacodynamic effects of ramipril result from the high-affinity, competitive, reversible binding of ramiprilat to angiotensin-converting enzyme thus preventing the formation of the potent vasoconstrictor angiotensin II. This isomerized enzyme-inhibitor complex has a slow rate of dissociation, which results in high potency and a long duration of action; a CNS mechanism may also be involved in the hypotensive effect as angiotensin II increases adrenergic outflow from CNS; vasoactive kallikreins may be decreased in conversion to active hormones by ACE inhibitors, thus reducing blood pressure

Local Anesthetic/Vasoconstrictor Precautions No information available to require special precautions

Effects on Dental Treatment No effects or complications reported

Other Adverse Effects

1% to 10%:
Cardiovascular: Tachycardia, chest pain, palpitations
Central nervous system: Insomnia, headache, dizziness, fatigue, malaise
Dermatologic: Rash, pruritus, alopecia
Gastrointestinal: Dysgeusia, abdominal pain, vomiting, nausea, diarrhea, anorexia, constipation, dysgeusia
Neuromuscular & skeletal: Paresthesia
Renal: Oliguria
Respiratory: Transient cough

<1%:
Cardiovascular: Hypotension
Dermatologic: Angioedema
Endocrine & metabolic: Hyperkalemia
Hematologic: Neutropenia, agranulocytosis
Renal: Proteinuria; elevated BUN, serum creatinine

Drug Interactions See table.

Drug-Drug Interactions With ACEIs

Precipitant Drug	Drug (Category) and Effect	Description
Antacids	ACE Inhibitors: decreased	Decreased bioavailability of ACEIs. May be more likely with captopril. Separate administration times by 1-2 hours.
NSAIDs (indomethacin)	ACEIs: decreased	Reduced hypotensive effects of ACEIs. More prominent in low renin or volume dependent hypertensive patients.
Phenothiazines	ACEIs: increased	Pharmacologic effects of ACEIs may be increased.
ACEIs	Allopurinol: increased	Higher risk of hypersensitivity reaction possible when given concurrently. Three case reports of Stevens-Johnson syndrome with captopril.
ACEIs	Digoxin: increased	Increased plasma digoxin levels.
ACEIs	Lithium: increased	Increased serum lithium levels and symptoms of toxicity may occur.
ACEIs	Potassium preps/ potassium sparing diuretics increased	Coadministration may result in elevated potassium levels.

Drug Uptake
Absorption: Well absorbed from GI tract (50% to 60%)
Serum half-life: Ramiprilat: >50 hours
Time to peak serum concentration: ~1 hour
Pregnancy Risk Factor C (first trimester); D (second and third trimesters)

Generic Available No

Ramses® [OTC] see Nonoxynol 9 on page 689

Ranitidina (Mexico) see Ranitidine Hydrochloride on this page

Ranitidine Bismuth Citrate (ra NI ti deen BIZ muth SIT rate)

Brand Names Tritec®

Therapeutic Category Histamine H$_2$ Antagonist; H. Pylori Agent

Use Used in combination with clarithromycin for the treatment of active duodenal ulcer associated with H. pylori infection; not to be used alone for the treatment of active duodenal ulcer

Usual Dosage Adults: Oral: 400 mg twice daily for 4 weeks with clarithromycin 500 mg 3 times/day for first 2 weeks

Mechanism of Action As a complex of ranitidine and bismuth citrate, gastric acid secretion is inhibited by histamine-blocking activity at the parietal cell and the structural integrity of H. pylori organisms is disrupted; additionally bismuth reduces the adherence of H. pylori to epithelial cells of the stomach and may exert a cytoprotectant effect, inhibiting pepsin, as well. Adequate eradication of Helicobacter pylori is achieved with the combination of clarithromycin.

Local Anesthetic/Vasoconstrictor Precautions No information available to require special precautions

Effects on Dental Treatment 60% to 70% of patients will have darkening of the tongue and/or stool; 11% experience taste disturbance

Other Adverse Effects

>1%:

Central nervous system: Headache (14%), dizziness (1% to 2%)

Gastrointestinal: Diarrhea (9%), nausea/vomiting (3%), constipation, abdominal pain, gastric upset (<10%)

Miscellaneous: Flu-like symptoms (2%)

<1%:

Dermatologic: Rash, pruritus

Hematologic: Anemia, thrombocytopenia

Hepatic: Elevated LFTs

Warnings/Precautions Use in children has not been established

Drug Interactions See individual monographs

Increased effect: Optimal antimicrobial effects of ranitidine bismuth citrate occur when the drug is taken with food

Drug Uptake

Absorption:

Bismuth: Minimal systemic absorption (≤1%)

Ranitidine: 50% to 60% (dose-dependent)

Serum half-life:

Complex: 5-8 days

Bismuth: 11-28 days

Ranitidine: 3 hours

Time to peak serum concentration:

Bismuth: 1-2 hours

Ranitidine: 0.5-5 hours

Time to peak effect of complex: 1 week

Pregnancy Risk Factor C

Dosage Forms Tablet: 400 mg (ranitidine 162 mg, trivalent bismuth 128 mg, and citrate 110 mg)

Ranitidine Hydrochloride (ra NI ti deen hye droe KLOR ide)

Related Information

Dental Drug Interactions: Update on Drug Combinations Requiring Special Considerations on page 1144

Ranitidine Bismuth Citrate on this page

Brand Names Zantac®; Zantac® 75 [OTC]

Canadian/Mexican Brand Names Acloral® (Mexico); Alter-H$_2$® (Mexico); Anistal® (Mexico); Apo®-Ranitidine (Canada); Azantac® (Mexico); Cauteridol® (Mexico); Credaxol® (Mexico); Galidrin® (Mexico); Gastrec® (Mexico); Microtid® (Mexico); Neugal® (Mexico); Novo-Ranidine® (Canada); Nu-Ranit® (Canada); Ranifur® (Mexico); Ranisen® (Mexico)

Therapeutic Category Histamine H$_2$ Antagonist

Synonyms Ranitidina (Mexico)

Use Short-term treatment of active duodenal ulcers and benign gastric ulcers; long-term prophylaxis of duodenal ulcer and gastric hypersecretory states, gastroesophageal reflux, recurrent postoperative ulcer, upper GI bleeding, prevention of acid-aspiration pneumonitis during surgery, and prevention of stress-induced ulcers; causes fewer interactions than cimetidine

(Continued)

Ranitidine Hydrochloride *(Continued)*

Usual Dosage Giving oral dose at 6 PM may be better than 10 PM bedtime, the highest acid production usually starts at approximately 7 PM, thus giving at 6 PM controls acid secretion better

Children:
Oral: 1.25-2.5 mg/kg/dose every 12 hours; maximum: 300 mg/day
I.M., I.V.: 0.75-1.5 mg/kg/dose every 6-8 hours, maximum daily dose: 400 mg
Continuous infusion: 0.1-0.25 mg/kg/hour (preferred for stress ulcer prophylaxis in patients with concurrent maintenance I.V.s or TPNs)

Adults:
Short-term treatment of ulceration: 150 mg/dose twice daily or 300 mg at bedtime
Prophylaxis of recurrent duodenal ulcer: Oral: 150 mg at bedtime
Gastric hypersecretory conditions:
Oral: 150 mg twice daily, up to 6 g/day
I.M., I.V.: 50 mg/dose every 6-8 hours (dose not to exceed 400 mg/day)
I.V.: 50 mg/dose IVPB every 6-8 hours (dose not to exceed 400 mg/day)
or
Continuous I.V. infusion: Initial: 50 mg IVPB, followed by 6.25 mg/hour titrated to gastric pH >4.0 for prophylaxis or >7.0 for treatment; **continuous I.V. infusion is preferred in patients with active bleeding**
Gastric hypersecretory conditions: Doses up to 2.5 mg/kg/hour (220 mg/hour) have been used

Mechanism of Action Competitive inhibition of histamine at H_2-receptors of the gastric parietal cells, which inhibits gastric acid secretion, gastric volume and hydrogen ion concentration reduced

Local Anesthetic/Vasoconstrictor Precautions No information available to require special precautions

Effects on Dental Treatment No effects or complications reported

Other Adverse Effects
Endocrine & metabolic: Gynecomastia
Hepatic: Hepatitis
Neuromuscular & skeletal: Arthralgias

1% to 10%:
Central nervous system: Dizziness, sedation, malaise, headache, drowsiness
Dermatologic: Rash
Gastrointestinal: Constipation, nausea, vomiting, diarrhea
<1%:
Cardiovascular: Bradycardia, tachycardia
Central nervous system: Fever, confusion
Hematologic: Thrombocytopenia, neutropenia, agranulocytosis
Respiratory: Bronchospasm

Drug Interactions
Decreased effect: Variable effects on warfarin; antacids may decrease absorption of ranitidine; ketoconazole and itraconazole absorptions are decreased
May produce altered serum levels of procainamide and ferrous sulfate
Decreased effect of nondepolarizing muscle relaxants, cefpodoxime, cyanocobalamin (decreased absorption), diazepam, oxaprozin
Decreased toxicity of atropine
Increased toxicity of cyclosporine (increased serum creatinine), gentamicin (neuromuscular blockade), glipizide, glyburide, midazolam (increased concentrations), metoprolol, pentoxifylline, phenytoin, quinidine

Drug Uptake
Absorption: Oral: 50% to 60%
Serum half-life:
Children 3.5-16 years: 1.8-2 hours
Adults: 2-2.5 hours
End stage renal disease: 6-9 hours
Time to peak serum concentration: Oral: Within 1-3 hours and persisting for 8 hours

Pregnancy Risk Factor B
Generic Available Yes

Raudixin® *see* Rauwolfia Serpentina *on this page*
Rauverid® *see* Rauwolfia Serpentina *on this page*

Rauwolfia Serpentina (rah WOOL fee a ser pen TEEN ah)

Brand Names Raudixin®; Rauverid®; Wolfina®
Therapeutic Category Antihypertensive; Rauwolfia Alkaloid
Synonyms Whole Root Rauwolfia
Use Mild essential hypertension; relief of agitated psychotic states

Local Anesthetic/Vasoconstrictor Precautions No information available to require special precautions

Effects on Dental Treatment No effects or complications reported

Pregnancy Risk Factor C

Generic Available Yes

Ravocaine® and Novocain® With Levophed® *see* Propoxycaine and Procaine *Discontinued by Manufacturer* on page 810

Ravocaine® and Novocain® With Neo-Cobefrin® *see* Propoxycaine and Procaine *Discontinued by Manufacturer* on page 810

Raxar® *see* Grepafloxacin on page 450

R & C® Shampoo [OTC] *see* Pyrethrins on page 824

Rea-Lo® [OTC] *see* Urea on page 977

Recombinate® *see* Antihemophilic Factor (Recombinant) on page 81

Recombivax HB® *see* Hepatitis B Vaccine on page 468

Redutemp® [OTC] *see* Acetaminophen on page 20

Redux® *see* Dexfenfluramine *Withdrawn from Market 1997* on page 293

Reese's® Pinworm Medicine [OTC] *see* Pyrantel Pamoate on page 822

Reference Values for Adults *see page 1167*

Refresh® Ophthalmic Solution [OTC] *see* Artificial Tears on page 87

Refresh® Plus Ophthalmic Solution [OTC] *see* Artificial Tears on page 87

Regitine® *see* Phentolamine on page 751

Reglan® *see* Metoclopramide on page 627

Regranex® *see* Becaplermin on page 111

Regulace® [OTC] *see* Docusate and Casanthranol on page 331

Regular (Concentrated) Iletin® II U-500 *see* Insulin Preparations on page 509

Regular Iletin® I *see* Insulin Preparations on page 509

Regular Insulin *see* Insulin Preparations on page 509

Regular Purified Pork Insulin *see* Insulin Preparations on page 509

Regular Strength Bayer® Enteric 500 Aspirin [OTC] *see* Aspirin on page 90

Regulax SS® [OTC] *see* Docusate on page 331

Reguloid® [OTC] *see* Psyllium on page 822

Relafen® *see* Nabumetone on page 656

Relefact® TRH Injection *see* Protirelin on page 818

Relief® Ophthalmic Solution *see* Phenylephrine on page 752

Remeron® *see* Mirtazapine on page 641

Remifentanil (rem i FEN ta nil)

Brand Names Ultiva®

Therapeutic Category Analgesic, Narcotic; General Anesthetic, Intravenous

Use Analgesic for use during general anesthesia for continued analgesia

Usual Dosage Adults: I.V. continuous infusion:

During induction: 0.5-1 mcg/kg/minute

During maintenance:

With nitrous oxide (66%): 0.4 mcg/kg/minute (range: 0.1-2 mcg/kg/min)

With isoflurane: 0.25 mcg/kg/minute (range: 0.05-2 mcg/kg/min)

With propofol: 0.25 mcg/kg/minute (range: 0.05-2 mcg/kg/min)

Continuation as an analgesic in immediate postoperative period: 0.1 mcg/kg/minute (range: 0.025-0.2 mcg/kg/min)

Mechanism of Action Binds with stereospecific mu-opioid receptors at many sites within the CNS, increases pain threshold, alters pain reception, inhibits ascending pain pathways

Local Anesthetic/Vasoconstrictor Precautions No information available to require special precautions

Effects on Dental Treatment No effects or complications reported

Other Adverse Effects

>10%: Gastrointestinal: Nausea, vomiting

1% to 10%:

Cardiovascular: Hypotension, bradycardia, tachycardia, hypertension

Central nervous system: Dizziness, headache, agitation, fever

Dermatologic: Pruritus

Ocular: Visual disturbances

Respiratory: Respiratory depression, apnea, hypoxia

Miscellaneous: Shivering, postoperative pain

Pregnancy Risk Factor C

Renacidin® *see* Citric Acid Bladder Mixture on page 239

Renese® *see* Polythiazide on page 773

Renoquid® *see* Sulfacytine on page 891

Renormax® *see* Spirapril *on page 881*

Rentamine® *see* Chlorpheniramine, Ephedrine, Phenylephrine, and Carbetapentane *on page 219*

ReoPro™ *see* Abciximab *on page 18*

Repaglinide (re PAG li nide)
Brand Names Prandin™

Therapeutic Category Hypoglycemic Agent, Oral

Use As an adjunct to diet and exercise to lower blood glucose on non-insulin-dependent (Type II) diabetes patients

Usual Dosage Oral: Adults: 0.5 - 4.0 mg before each meal; the starting dose in oral hypoglycemic naive individuals or in those with HbA1c levels under 8% is 0.5 mg before each meal. For other patients, the starting dose is 1-2 mg before each meal. The dose can be adjusted (by prescribers) up to 4 mg before each meal. If a meal is skipped, the patient should also skip the repaglinide dose

Mechanism of Action Stimulates insulin secretion from the beta cells of the pancreas by binding to sites on the beta cell. Prandin is minimally excreted by the kidney, which may be an advantage for patients (often elderly) who often suffer from decreased kidney function.

Local Anesthetic/Vasoconstrictor Precautions No information available to require special precautions

Effects on Dental Treatment No effects or complications reported

Dosage Forms Tablet: 0.5 mg

Comments Known as NovoNorm™ elsewhere

Repan® *see* Butalbital Compound *on page 154*

Repan® *see* Butalbital Compound and Acetaminophen *on page 155*

Reposans-10® *see* Chlordiazepoxide *on page 210*

Requip™ *see* Ropinirole *on page 849*

Resaid® *see* Chlorpheniramine and Phenylpropanolamine *on page 219*

Rescaps-D® S.R. Capsule *see* Caramiphen and Phenylpropanolamine *on page 173*

Rescon Liquid [OTC] *see* Chlorpheniramine and Phenylpropanolamine *on page 219*

Rescriptor™ *see* Delavirdine *on page 285*

Reserpina (Mexico) *see* Reserpine *on this page*

Reserpine (re SER peen)
Related Information
Cardiovascular Diseases *on page 1010*

Brand Names Serpalan®; Serpasil®

Canadian/Mexican Brand Names Novo-Reserpine® (Canada)

Therapeutic Category Alpha-Adrenergic Blockers - Peripheral-Acting (Alpha$_1$-Blockers)

Synonyms Reserpina (Mexico)

Use Management of mild to moderate hypertension

Unlabeled use: Management of tardive dyskinesia

Usual Dosage Oral (full antihypertensive effects may take as long as 3 weeks):
Children: 0.01-0.02 mg/kg/24 hours divided every 12 hours; maximum dose: 0.25 mg/day
Adults: 0.1-0.25 mg/day in 1-2 doses; initial: 0.5 mg/day for 1-2 weeks; maintenance: reduce to 0.1-0.25 mg/day
Elderly: Initial: 0.05 mg once daily, increasing by 0.05 mg every week as necessary

Mechanism of Action Reduces blood pressure via depletion of sympathetic biogenic amines (norepinephrine and dopamine); this also commonly results in sedative effects

Local Anesthetic/Vasoconstrictor Precautions No information available to require special precautions

Effects on Dental Treatment >10% of patients experience dry mouth

Other Adverse Effects
>10%:
Central nervous system: Dizziness
Gastrointestinal: Anorexia, diarrhea, nausea, vomiting
Respiratory: Nasal congestion
1% to 10%:
Cardiovascular: Peripheral edema, arrhythmias, bradycardia, chest pain
Central nervous system: Headache
Gastrointestinal: Black stools, bloody vomit
Genitourinary: Impotence

<1%:
    Cardiovascular: Hypotension
    Central nervous system: Drowsiness, fatigue, mental depression, parkinsonism
    Dermatologic: Skin rash
    Endocrine & metabolic: Sodium and water retention
    Gastrointestinal: Elevated gastric acid secretion
    Genitourinary: Dysuria
    Neuromuscular & skeletal: Trembling of hands/fingers

Drug Interactions
Decreased effect of indirect-acting sympathomimetics
Increased effect/toxicity of MAO inhibitors, direct-acting sympathomimetics, and tricyclic antidepressants

Drug Uptake
Onset of antihypertensive effect: Within 3-6 days
Duration: 2-6 weeks
Absorption: Oral: ~40%
Serum half-life: 50-100 hours

Pregnancy Risk Factor C
Generic Available Yes

Reserpine and Chlorothiazide *see* Chlorothiazide and Reserpine *on page 216*

Reserpine and Hydrochlorothiazide *see* Hydrochlorothiazide and Reserpine *on page 477*

Respa-1st® *see* Guaifenesin and Pseudoephedrine *on page 454*

Respa-DM® *see* Guaifenesin and Dextromethorphan *on page 453*

Respa-GF® *see* Guaifenesin *on page 452*

Respaire®-60 SR *see* Guaifenesin and Pseudoephedrine *on page 454*

Respaire®-120 SR *see* Guaifenesin and Pseudoephedrine *on page 454*

Respbid® *see* Theophylline *on page 917*

Respiratory Diseases *see page 1018*

Restoril® *see* Temazepam *on page 905*

Retavase® *see* Reteplase *on this page*

Reteplase (RE ta plase)
Brand Names Retavase®
Therapeutic Category Thrombolytic Agent
Use Management of acute myocardial infarction
Usual Dosage
Children: Not recommended
Adults: 10 units I.V. over 2 minutes, followed by a second dose 30 minutes later of 10 units I.V. over 2 minutes
    Withhold second dose if serious bleeding or anaphylaxis occurs
Mechanism of Action Reteplase is a nonglycosylated form of tPA produced by recombinant DNA technology using *E. coli*; it initiates local fibrinolysis by binding to fibrin in a thrombus (clot) and converts entrapped plasminogen to plasmin
Local Anesthetic/Vasoconstrictor Precautions No information available to require special precautions
Effects on Dental Treatment No effects or complications reported
Other Adverse Effects
>10%:
    Cardiovascular: Hypotension, arrhythmias, trauma arrhythmias
    Hematologic: Bleeding
1% to 10%: Hematologic: Anemia, genitourinary bleeding, gastrointestinal bleeding, injection site bleeding
<1%:
    Central nervous system: Intracranial hemorrhage
    Miscellaneous: Allergic reactions, anaphylaxis
Drug Interactions
Increased effect: Anticoagulants, aspirin, ticlopidine, dipyridamole, abciximab and heparin are at least additive
Drug Uptake
Onset: 30-90 minutes
Half-life: 13-16 minutes
Pregnancy Risk Factor C
Generic Available No

Retin-A™ Micro Topical *see* Tretinoin, Topical *on page 953*

Retin-A™ Topical *see* Tretinoin, Topical *on page 953*

Retrovir® *see* Zidovudine *on page 1002*

Revex® *see* Nalmefene *on page 661*

Rēv-Eyes™ *see* Dapiprazole *on page 281*

ReVia™ Oral *see* Naltrexone *on page 662*

Rezulin® *see* Troglitazone *on page 971*

R-Gel® [OTC] *see* Capsaicin *on page 170*

R-Gen® *see* Iodinated Glycerol *on page 515*

R-Gene® *see* Arginine *on page 85*

rGM-CSF *see* Sargramostim *on page 857*

Rheaban® [OTC] *see* Attapulgite *on page 99*

Rheomacrodex® *see* Dextran *on page 295*

Rheumatoid Arthritis and Osteoarthritis *see page 1030*

Rheumatrex® *see* Methotrexate *on page 615*

Rhinall® Nasal Solution [OTC] *see* Phenylephrine *on page 752*

Rhinatate® Tablet *see* Chlorpheniramine, Pyrilamine, and Phenylephrine *on page 223*

Rhindecon® *see* Phenylpropanolamine *on page 754*

Rhinocort™ *see* Budesonide *on page 146*

Rhinosyn-DMX® [OTC] *see* Guaifenesin and Dextromethorphan *on page 453*

Rhinosyn® Liquid [OTC] *see* Chlorpheniramine and Pseudoephedrine *on page 219*

Rhinosyn-PD® Liquid [OTC] *see* Chlorpheniramine and Pseudoephedrine *on page 219*

Rhinosyn-X® Liquid [OTC] *see* Guaifenesin, Pseudoephedrine, and Dextromethorphan *on page 456*

Rh$_o$(D) Immune Globulin (ar aych oh (dee) i MYUN GLOB yoo lin)

Brand Names Gamulin® Rh; HypRho®-D; HypRho®-D Mini-Dose; MICRhoGAM™; Mini-Gamulin® Rh; RhoGAM™

Canadian/Mexican Brand Names Anti-Rho(D)® (Mexico); Probi-Rho(D) (Mexico)

Therapeutic Category Immune Globulin

Use Prevent isoimmunization in Rh-negative individuals exposed to Rh-positive blood during delivery of an Rh-positive infant, as a result of an abortion, following amniocentesis or abdominal trauma, or following a transfusion accident; to prevent hemolytic disease of the newborn if there is a subsequent pregnancy with an Rh-positive fetus

Usual Dosage Adults (administered I.M. to mothers **not** to infant) I.M.:

Obstetrical usage: 1 vial (300 mcg) prevents maternal sensitization if fetal packed red blood cell volume that has entered the circulation is <15 mL; if it is more, give additional vials. The number of vials = RBC volume of the calculated fetomaternal hemorrhage divided by 15 mL

Postpartum prophylaxis: 300 mcg within 72 hours of delivery

Antepartum prophylaxis: 300 mcg at approximately 26-28 weeks gestation; followed by 300 mcg within 72 hours of delivery if infant is Rh-positive

Following miscarriage, abortion, or termination of ectopic pregnancy at up to 13 weeks of gestation: 50 mcg ideally within 3 hours, but may be given up to 72 hours after; if pregnancy has been terminated at 13 or more weeks of gestation, administer 300 mcg

Mechanism of Action Suppresses the immune response and antibody formation of Rh-negative individuals to Rh-positive red blood cells

Local Anesthetic/Vasoconstrictor Precautions No information available to require special precautions

Effects on Dental Treatment No effects or complications reported

Other Adverse Effects <1%:

Central nervous system: Lethargy, temperature elevation

Gastrointestinal: Splenomegaly

Hepatic: Elevated bilirubin

Local: Pain at the injection site

Neuromuscular & skeletal: Myalgia

Drug Uptake

Serum half-life: 23-26 days

Pregnancy Risk Factor C

Generic Available No

Comments Administered I.M. to mothers **not** to infant; will prevent hemolytic disease of newborn in subsequent pregnancy

RhoGAM™ *see* Rh$_o$(D) Immune Globulin *on this page*

rHuEPO-α *see* Epoetin Alfa *on page 355*

Rhulicaine® [OTC] *see* Benzocaine *on page 118*

Ribavirin (rye ba VYE rin)

Brand Names Virazole® Aerosol

Canadian/Mexican Brand Names Vilona® (Mexico); Vilona Pediatrica® (Mexico); Virazide® (Mexico)

Therapeutic Category Antiviral Agent, Inhalation Therapy

Synonyms RTCA; Tribavirin

Use Treatment of patients with respiratory syncytial virus (RSV) infections; specially indicated for treatment of severe lower respiratory tract RSV infections in patients with an underlying compromising condition (prematurity, bronchopulmonary dysplasia and other chronic lung conditions, congenital heart disease, immunodeficiency, immunosuppression), and recent transplant recipients; may also be used in other viral infections including influenza A and B and adenovirus

Usual Dosage Children and Adults:

Aerosol inhalation: Use with Viratek® small particle aerosol generator (SPAG-2) at a concentration of 20 mg/mL (6 g reconstituted with 300 mL of sterile water without preservatives)

Aerosol only: 12-18 hours/day for 3 days, up to 7 days in length

Mechanism of Action Inhibits replication of RNA and DNA viruses; inhibits influenza virus RNA polymerase activity and inhibits the initiation and elongation of RNA fragments resulting in inhibition of viral protein synthesis

Local Anesthetic/Vasoconstrictor Precautions No information available to require special precautions

Effects on Dental Treatment No effects or complications reported

Other Adverse Effects

1% to 10%:

Central nervous system: Fatigue, headache, insomnia

Gastrointestinal: Nausea, anorexia

Hematologic: Anemia

<1%:

Cardiovascular: Hypotension, cardiac arrest, digitalis toxicity

Dermatologic: Rash, skin irritation

Ocular: Conjunctivitis

Respiratory: Mild bronchospasm, worsening of respiratory function, apnea, accumulation of fluid in ventilator tubing

Drug Uptake

Absorption: Absorbed systemically from the respiratory tract following nasal and oral inhalation; absorption is dependent upon respiratory factors and method of drug delivery; maximal absorption occurs with the use of the aerosol generator via an endotracheal tube; highest concentrations are found in the respiratory tract and erythrocytes

Serum half-life, plasma:

Children: 6.5-11 hours

Adults: 24 hours, much longer in the erythrocyte (16-40 days), which can be used as a marker for intracellular metabolism

Time to peak serum concentration: Inhalation: Within 60-90 minutes

Pregnancy Risk Factor X

Generic Available No

Comments RSV season is usually December to April; viral shedding period for RSV is usually 3-8 days

Riboflavin (RYE boe flay vin)

Brand Names Riobin®

Therapeutic Category Vitamin, Water Soluble

Synonyms Riboflavina (Mexico)

Use Dental and Medical: Prevent riboflavin deficiency and treat ariboflavinosis

Usual Dosage Oral:

Riboflavin deficiency:

Children: 2.5-10 mg/day in divided doses

Adults: 5-30 mg/day in divided doses

Recommended daily allowance:

Children: 0.4-1.8 mg

Adults: 1.2-1.7 mg

Mechanism of Action Component of flavoprotein enzymes that work together, which are necessary for normal tissue respiration; also needed for activation of pyridoxine and conversion of tryptophan to niacin

Local Anesthetic/Vasoconstrictor Precautions No information available to require special precautions

Effects on Dental Treatment No effects or complications reported

Warnings/Precautions Riboflavin deficiency often occurs in the presence of other B vitamin deficiencies

Drug Interactions Decreased absorption with probenecid

(Continued)

841

Riboflavin *(Continued)*

Drug Uptake
Absorption: Readily via GI tract, however, food increases extent of GI absorption; GI absorption is decreased in patients with hepatitis, cirrhosis, or biliary obstruction

Serum half-life, biologic: 66-84 minutes

Pregnancy Risk Factor A (C if dose exceeds RDA recommendation)

Dosage Forms Tablet: 25 mg, 50 mg, 100 mg

Generic Available Yes

Riboflavina (Mexico) *see* Riboflavin *on previous page*

Rid-A-Pain® [OTC] *see* Benzocaine *on page 118*

Ridaura® *see* Auranofin *on page 99*

Ridenol® [OTC] *see* Acetaminophen *on page 20*

RID® Shampoo [OTC] *see* Pyrethrins *on page 824*

Rifabutin *(rif a BYOO tin)*

Related Information
Nonviral Infectious Diseases *on page 1032*
Systemic Viral Diseases *on page 1047*

Brand Names Mycobutin®

Therapeutic Category Antibiotic, Miscellaneous; Antitubercular Agent

Use Adjunctive therapy for the prevention of disseminated *Mycobacterium avium* complex (MAC) in patients with advanced HIV infection

Usual Dosage Oral:
Children: Efficacy and safety of rifabutin have not been established in children; a limited number of HIV-positive children with MAC have been given rifabutin for MAC prophylaxis; doses of 5 mg/kg/day have been useful

Adults: 300 mg once daily; for patients who experience gastrointestinal upset, rifabutin can be administered 150 mg twice daily with food

Mechanism of Action Inhibits DNA-dependent RNA polymerase at the beta subunit which prevents chain initiation

Local Anesthetic/Vasoconstrictor Precautions No information available to require special precautions

Effects on Dental Treatment No effects or complications reported

Other Adverse Effects
>10%:
Dermatologic: Rash
Genitourinary: Discolored urine
Hematologic: Neutropenia, leukopenia

1% to 10%:
Central nervous system: Headache
Gastrointestinal: Vomiting, nausea, abdominal pain, diarrhea, anorexia, flatulence, eructation
Hematologic: Anemia, thrombocytopenia
Neuromuscular & skeletal: Myalgia

<1%:
Cardiovascular: Chest pain
Central nervous system: Fever, insomnia
Gastrointestinal: Dyspepsia, taste perversion

Drug Interactions Decreased plasma concentration (due to induction of liver enzymes) of verapamil, methadone, digoxin, cyclosporine, corticosteroids, oral anticoagulants, theophylline, barbiturates, chloramphenicol, ketoconazole, oral contraceptives, quinidine, halothane

Drug Uptake
Absorption: Oral: Readily absorbed 53%
Serum half life, terminal: 45 hours (range: 16-69 hours)
Peak serum level: Within 2-4 hours

Pregnancy Risk Factor B

Generic Available No

Rifadin® *see* Rifampin *on this page*

Rifamate® *see* Rifampin and Isoniazid *on page 844*

Rifampicina (Mexico) *see* Rifampin *on this page*

Rifampin *(RIF am pin)*

Related Information
Nonviral Infectious Diseases *on page 1032*

Brand Names Rifadin®; Rimactane®

Canadian/Mexican Brand Names Rifadin® (Canada); Rimactane® (Canada); Rofact® (Canada)

Therapeutic Category Antibiotic, Miscellaneous; Antitubercular Agent

Synonyms Rifampicina (Mexico)

Use Management of active tuberculosis; eliminate meningococci from asymptomatic carriers; prophylaxis of *Haemophilus influenzae* type B infection; used in combination with other anti-infectives in the treatment of staphylococcal infections

Usual Dosage I.V. infusion dose is the same as for the oral route

Tuberculosis therapy: Oral:

Note: A four-drug regimen (isoniazid, rifampin, pyrazinamide, and either streptomycin or ethambutol) is preferred for the initial, empiric treatment of TB. When the drug susceptibility results are available, the regimen should be altered as appropriate.

Patients with TB and without HIV infection:

OPTION 1:

Isoniazid resistance rate <4%: Administer daily isoniazid, rifampin, and pyrazinamide for 8 weeks followed by isoniazid and rifampin daily or directly observed therapy (DOT) 2-3 times/week for 16 weeks

If isoniazid resistance rate is not documented, ethambutol or streptomycin should also be administered until susceptibility to isoniazid or rifampin is demonstrated. Continue treatment for at least 6 months or 3 months beyond culture conversion.

OPTION 2: Administer daily isoniazid, rifampin, pyrazinamide, and either streptomycin or ethambutol for 2 weeks followed by DOT 2 times/week administration of the same drugs for 6 weeks, and subsequently, with isoniazid and rifampin DOT 2 times/week administration for 16 weeks

OPTION 3: Administer isoniazid, rifampin, pyrazinamide, and either ethambutol or streptomycin by DOT 3 times/week for 6 months

Patients with TB and with HIV infection:

Administer any of the above OPTIONS 1, 2 or 3, however, treatment should be continued for a total of 9 months and at least 6 months beyond culture conversion

Note: Some experts recommend that the duration of therapy should be extended to 9 months for patients with disseminated disease, miliary disease, disease involving the bones or joints, or tuberculosis lymphadenitis

Children <12 years of age: Oral:

Daily therapy: 10-20 mg/kg/day in divided doses every 12-24 hours (maximum: 600 mg/day)

Directly observed therapy (DOT): Twice weekly: 10-20 mg/kg (maximum: 600 mg)

DOT: 3 times/week: 10-20 mg/kg (maximum: 600 mg)

Adults: Oral:

Daily therapy: 10 mg/kg/day (maximum: 600 mg/day)

Directly observed therapy (DOT): Twice weekly: 10 mg/kg (maximum: 600 mg)

DOT: 3 times/week: 10 mg/kg (maximum: 600 mg)

H. influenzae prophylaxis: Oral:

Children: 20 mg/kg/day every 24 hours for 4 days, not to exceed 600 mg/dose

Adults: 600 mg every 24 hours for 4 days

Meningococcal prophylaxis: Oral:

<1 month: 10 mg/kg/day in divided doses every 12 hours for 2 days

Children: 20 mg/kg/day in divided doses every 12 hours for 2 days

Adults: 600 mg every 12 hours for 2 days

Nasal carriers of *Staphylococcus aureus*: Oral:

Children: 15 mg/kg/day divided every 12 hours for 5-10 days in combination with other antibiotics

Adults: 600 mg/day for 5-10 days in combination with other antibiotics

Synergy for *Staphylococcus aureus* infections: Oral: Adults: 300-600 mg twice daily with other antibiotics

Mechanism of Action Inhibits bacterial RNA synthesis by binding to the beta subunit of DNA-dependent RNA polymerase, blocking RNA transcription

Local Anesthetic/Vasoconstrictor Precautions No information available to require special precautions

Effects on Dental Treatment No effects or complications reported

Other Adverse Effects

1% to 10%:

Gastrointestinal: Diarrhea, stomach cramps, discoloration of feces, saliva, sputum

Genitourinary: Discoloration of urine

Ocular: Discoloration of tears (reddish orange)

Miscellaneous: Discoloration of sweat, fungal overgrowth

(Continued)

843

Rifampin *(Continued)*

<1%:

Central nervous system: Drowsiness, fatigue, ataxia, confusion, fever, headache

Dermatologic: Rash, pruritus

Gastrointestinal: Nausea, vomiting, stomatitis

Hematologic: Eosinophilia, blood dyscrasias (leukopenia, thrombocytopenia)

Hepatic: Hepatitis

Local: Irritation at the I.V. site

Renal: Renal failure

Miscellaneous: Flu-like syndrome

Drug Interactions Inducer of both Cytochrome P-450 3A and cytochrome P-450 2D6

Decreased effect: Rifampin induces liver enzymes which may decrease the plasma concentration of verapamil, methadone, digoxin, cyclosporine, corticosteroids, oral anticoagulants, theophylline, barbiturates, chloramphenicol, ketoconazole, oral contraceptives, quinidine, halothane, ketoconazole

Drug Uptake

Absorption: Oral: Well absorbed

Serum half-life: 3-4 hours, prolonged with hepatic impairment

Time to peak serum concentration: Oral: 2-4 hours and persisting for up to 24 hours; food may delay or slightly reduce

Pregnancy Risk Factor C

Generic Available No

Rifampin and Isoniazid (RIF am pin & eye soe NYE a zid)

Brand Names Rifamate®

Therapeutic Category Antibiotic, Miscellaneous; Antitubercular Agent

Use Management of active tuberculosis; see individual monographs for additional information

Local Anesthetic/Vasoconstrictor Precautions No information available to require special precautions

Effects on Dental Treatment No effects or complications reported

Pregnancy Risk Factor C

Generic Available No

Rifampin, Isoniazid, and Pyrazinamide

(RIF am pin, eye soe NYE a zid, & peer a ZIN a mide)

Brand Names Rifater®

Therapeutic Category Antibiotic, Miscellaneous; Antitubercular Agent

Use Management of active tuberculosis

Local Anesthetic/Vasoconstrictor Precautions No information available to require special precautions

Effects on Dental Treatment No effects or complications reported

Pregnancy Risk Factor C

Generic Available No

Rifater® *see* Rifampin, Isoniazid, and Pyrazinamide *on this page*

Rilutek® *see* Riluzole *on this page*

Riluzole (RIL yoo zole)

Brand Names Rilutek®

Therapeutic Category Amyotrophic Lateral Sclerosis (ALS) Agent

Use Amyotrophic lateral sclerosis (ALS): Treatment of patients with ALS; riluzole can extend survival or time to tracheostomy

Usual Dosage Adults: Oral: 50 mg every 12 hours; no increased benefit can be expected from higher daily doses, but adverse events are increased

Mechanism of Action Inhibitory effect on glutamate release, inactivation of voltage-dependent sodium channels; and ability to interfere with intracellular events that follow transmitter binding at excitatory amino acid receptors

Local Anesthetic/Vasoconstrictor Precautions No information available to require special precautions

Effects on Dental Treatment No effects or complications reported

Other Adverse Effects

>10%:

Gastrointestinal: Nausea, abdominal pain, constipation

Hepatic: ALT (SGPT) elevations

Drug Interactions Cytochrome P-450 1A2 (CYP 1A2) substrate

Decreased effect: Drugs that induce CYP 1A2 (eg, cigarette smoke, charbroiled food, rifampin, omeprazole) could increase the rate of riluzole elimination

Increased toxicity: Inhibitors of CYP 1A2 (eg, caffeine, theophylline, amitriptyline, quinolones) could decrease the rate of riluzole elimination

Drug Uptake
Absorption: Well absorbed (90%); a high fat meal decreases absorption of riluzole (decreasing AUC by 20% and peak blood levels by 45%)
Bioavailability: Oral: Absolute (50%)

Pregnancy Risk Factor C

Dosage Forms Tablet: 50 mg

Generic Available No

Rimactane® *see* Rifampin *on page 842*

Rimantadine (ri MAN ta deen)

Related Information
Systemic Viral Diseases *on page 1047*

Brand Names Flumadine®

Therapeutic Category Antiviral Agent, Oral

Use Prophylaxis (adults and children >1 year) and treatment (adults) of influenza A viral infection

Usual Dosage Oral:
Prophylaxis:
Children <10 years: 5 mg/kg give once daily; maximum: 150 mg
Children >10 years and Adults: 100 mg twice daily; decrease to 100 mg/day in elderly or in patients with severe hepatic or renal impairment (Cl_{cr} ≤10 mL/minute)
Treatment: Adults: 100 mg twice daily; decrease to 100 mg/day in elderly or in patients with severe hepatic or renal impairment (Cl_{cr} ≤10 mL/minute)

Mechanism of Action Exerts its inhibitory effect on three antigenic subtypes of influenza A virus (H1N1, H2N2, H3N2) early in the viral replicative cycle, possibly inhibiting the uncoating process; it has no activity against influenza B virus and is 2- to 8-fold more active than amantadine

Local Anesthetic/Vasoconstrictor Precautions No information available to require special precautions

Effects on Dental Treatment No effects or complications reported

Other Adverse Effects 1% to 10%:
Cardiovascular: Orthostatic hypotension, edema
Central nervous system: Dizziness, confusion, headache, insomnia, difficulty in concentrating, anxiety, restlessness, irritability, hallucinations; incidence of CNS side effects may be less than that associated with amantadine
Gastrointestinal: Nausea, vomiting, dry mouth, abdominal pain, anorexia
Genitourinary: Urinary retention

Drug Interactions
Acetaminophen: Reduction in AUC and peak concentration of rimantadine
Aspirin: Peak plasma and AUC concentrations of rimantadine are reduced
Cimetidine: Rimantadine clearance is decreased (~16%)

Drug Uptake
Absorption: Tablet and syrup formulations are equally absorbed; T_{max}: 6 hours
Serum half-life: 25.4 hours (increased in elderly)

Pregnancy Risk Factor C

Generic Available No

Rimexolone (ri MEKS oh lone)

Brand Names Vexol®

Therapeutic Category Anti-inflammatory Agent, Ophthalmic; Corticosteroid, Ophthalmic

Use Treatment of inflammation after ocular surgery and the treatment of anterior uveitis

Usual Dosage Adults: Ophthalmic: Instill 1 drop in conjunctival sac 2-4 times/day up to every 4 hours; may use every 1-2 hours during first 1-2 days

Mechanism of Action Decreases inflammation by suppression of migration of polymorphonuclear leukocytes and reversal of increased capillary permeability

Local Anesthetic/Vasoconstrictor Precautions No information available to require special precautions

Effects on Dental Treatment No effects or complications reported

Other Adverse Effects
1% to 10%: Ocular: Temporary mild blurred vision
<1%: Ocular: Stinging, burning eyes, corneal thinning, increased intraocular pressure, glaucoma, damage to the optic nerve, defects in visual activity, cataracts, secondary ocular infection

Drug Uptake Absorption: Through aqueous humor

Pregnancy Risk Factor C

Generic Available No

Riobin® see Riboflavin on page 841

Riopan® [OTC] see Magaldrate on page 574

Riopan Plus® [OTC] see Magaldrate and Simethicone on page 574

Risperdal® see Risperidone on this page

Risperidona (Mexico) see Risperidone on this page

Risperidone (ris PER i done)

Brand Names Risperdal®

Therapeutic Category Antipsychotic Agent

Synonyms Risperidona (Mexico)

Use Management of psychotic disorders (eg, schizophrenia); nonpsychotic symptoms associated with dementia in elderly

Usual Dosage

Recommended starting dose: 1 mg twice daily; slowly increase to the optimum range of 4-8 mg/day; daily dosages >10 mg does not appear to confer any additional benefit, and the incidence of extrapyramidal reactions is higher than with lower doses

Mechanism of Action Risperidone is a benzisoxazole derivative, mixed serotonin-dopamine antagonist; binds to 5-HT$_2$ receptors in the CNS and in the periphery with a very high affinity; binds to dopamine-D$_2$ receptors with less affinity. The binding affinity to the dopamine-D$_2$ receptor is 20 times lower than the 5-HT$_2$ affinity. The addition of serotonin antagonism to dopamine antagonism (classic neuroleptic mechanism) is thought to improve negative symptoms of psychoses and reduce the incidence of extrapyramidal side effects.

Local Anesthetic/Vasoconstrictor Precautions No information available to require special precautions

Effects on Dental Treatment Up to 10% of dental patients will experience significant dry mouth and orthostatic hypotension. These effects disappear with cessation of drug therapy.

Other Adverse Effects

1% to 10%:

Cardiovascular: Hypotension (especially orthostatic), tachycardia, arrhythmias, abnormal T waves with prolonged ventricular repolarization; EKG changes, syncope

Central nervous system: Sedation (occurs at daily doses ≥20 mg/day), headache, dizziness, restlessness, anxiety, extrapyramidal reactions, dystonic reactions, pseudoparkinson signs and symptoms, tardive dyskinesia, neuroleptic malignant syndrome, altered central temperature regulation

Dermatologic: Photosensitivity (rare)

Endocrine & metabolic: Amenorrhea, galactorrhea, gynecomastia, sexual dysfunction (up to 60%)

Gastrointestinal: Constipation, adynamic ileus, GI upset, dry mouth (problem for denture user), nausea and anorexia, weight gain

Genitourinary: Urinary retention, overflow incontinence, priapism

Hematologic: Agranulocytosis, leukopenia (usually in patients with large doses for prolonged periods)

Hepatic: Cholestatic jaundice

Ocular: Blurred vision, retinal pigmentation, decreased visual acuity (may be irreversible)

<1%: Central nervous system: Seizures

Drug Interactions

May antagonize effects of levodopa; carbamazepine decreases risperidone serum concentrations; clozapine decreases clearance of risperidone

Drug Uptake

Absorption: Oral: Rapid

Serum half-life: 24 hours (risperidone and its active metabolite)

Time to peak: Peak plasma concentrations within 1 hour

Pregnancy Risk Factor C

Generic Available No

Ritalin® see Methylphenidate on page 623

Ritalin-SR® see Methylphenidate on page 623

Ritodrine (RI toe dreen)

Brand Names Yutopar®

Therapeutic Category Adrenergic Agonist Agent; Beta$_2$-Adrenergic Agonist Agent

Use Inhibits uterine contraction in preterm labor

Usual Dosage Adults:

I.V.: 50-100 mcg/minute; increase by 50 mcg/minute every 10 minutes; continue for 12 hours after contractions have stopped

Oral: Start 30 minutes before stopping I.V. infusion; 10 mg every 2 hours for 24 hours, then 10-20 mg every 4-6 hours up to 120 mg/day

Hemodialysis effects: Removed by hemodialysis

Mechanism of Action Tocolysis due to its uterine beta$_2$-adrenergic receptor stimulating effects; this agent's beta$_2$ effects can also cause bronchial relaxation and vascular smooth muscle stimulation

Local Anesthetic/Vasoconstrictor Precautions No information available to require special precautions

Effects on Dental Treatment No effects or complications reported

Other Adverse Effects

>10%:

Cardiovascular: Increases in maternal and fetal heart rates and maternal hypertension, palpitations

Endocrine & metabolic: Temporary hyperglycemia

Gastrointestinal: Nausea, vomiting

Neuromuscular & skeletal: Tremor

1% to 10%:

Cardiovascular: Chest pain

Central nervous system: Nervousness, anxiety, restlessness

<1%:

Endocrine & metabolic: Ketoacidosis

Hepatic: Impaired liver function

Miscellaneous: Anaphylactic shock

Drug Interactions

Decreased effect with beta-blockers

Increased effect/toxicity with meperidine, sympathomimetics, diazoxide, magnesium, betamethasone (pulmonary edema), potassium-depleting diuretics, general anesthetics

Drug Uptake

Absorption: Oral: Rapid

Serum half-life: 15 hours

Time to peak serum concentration: Within 0.5-1 hour

Pregnancy Risk Factor B

Generic Available No

Ritonavir (rye TON a veer)

Related Information

HIV Infection and AIDS *on page 1024*

Systemic Viral Diseases *on page 1047*

Brand Names Norvir®

Therapeutic Category Antiviral Agent, Oral; Protease Inhibitor

Use Treatment of HIV, especially advanced cases; usually is used as part of triple or double therapy with other nucleoside and protease inhibitors

Usual Dosage Adults: Oral: 600 mg twice daily with meals

Dosing adjustment in renal impairment: None necessary

Dosing adjustment in hepatic impairment: Not determined; caution advised with severe impairment

Mechanism of Action As a protease inhibitor, ritonavir prevents cleavage of protein precursors essential for HIV infection of new cells and viral replication. Saquinavir- and zidovudine-resistant HIV isolates are generally susceptible to ritonavir. Used in combination therapy, resistance to ritonavir develops slowly; strains resistant to ritonavir are cross-resistant to indinavir and saquinavir.

Local Anesthetic/Vasoconstrictor Precautions No information available to require special precautions

Effects on Dental Treatment No effects or complications reported

Other Adverse Effects

1% to 10%:

Gastrointestinal: Nausea, vomiting, diarrhea, dysgeusia

Neuromuscular & skeletal: Circumoral and peripheral paresthesias, weakness

<1%:

Central nervous system: Headache, confusion

Endocrine & metabolic: Elevated triglycerides, cholesterol

Hepatic: Elevated LFTs

Contraindications Hypersensitivity to ritonavir or any of its components; avoid use with astemizole, terfenadine, and rifabutin

Warnings/Precautions Use caution in patients with hepatic insufficiency; safety and efficacy have not been established in children <16 years of age; use caution with benzodiazepines, antiarrhythmics (flecainide, encainide, bepridil, amiodarone, quinidine) and certain analgesics (meperidine, piroxicam, propoxyphene) (Continued)

Ritonavir *(Continued)*

Drug Interactions
Decreased effect: Concurrent use of rifampin, rifabutin, dexamethasone, and many anticonvulsants lowers serum concentration of ritonavir

Increased toxicity: Ketoconazole increases ritonavir's plasma levels; ritonavir may decrease metabolism of astemizole and result in rare but serious cardiac arrhythmias; enhanced cardiac effects when administered with flecainide, encainide, quinidine, amiodarone, bepridil. Increased toxic effects also possible with coadministration with cisapride and benzodiazepines.

Drug Uptake
Absorption: Well absorbed; T_{max}: 2-4 hours

Half-life: 3-5 hours

Pregnancy Risk Factor B

Dosage Forms
Capsule: 100 mg

Solution: 80 mg/mL (240 mL)

Generic Available No

Rituxan® *see* Rituximab *on this page*

Rituximab *(ri TUK si mab)*
Brand Names Rituxan®

Therapeutic Category Antineoplastic Agent, Miscellaneous

Synonyms C2B8

Use Treatment of patients with relapsed or refractory low-grade or follicular, CD20 positive, B-cell non-Hodgkin's lymphoma

Usual Dosage Adults: I.V.: 375 mg/m² given as an I.V. infusion once weekly for 4 doses (days 1, 8, 15, and 22); may be administered in an outpatient setting; DO NOT ADMINISTER AS AN INTRAVENOUS PUSH OR BOLUS

Mechanism of Action Binds specifically to the antigen CD20 (human B-lympho-cyte-restricted differentiation antigen, Bp35), a hydrophobic transmembrane protein with a molecular weight of approximately 35 kD located on pre-B and mature B lymphocytes. The antigen is also expressed on > 90% of B-cell non-Hodgkin's lymphomas (NHL) but is not found on hematopoietic stem cells, pro-B cells, normal plasma cells or other normal tissues. CD20 regulates an early step(s) in the activation process for cell cycle initiation and differentiation, and possibly functions as a calcium ion channel. CD20 is not shed from the cell surface and does not internalize upon antibody binding. Free CD20 antigen is not found in the circulation.

Local Anesthetic/Vasoconstrictor Precautions No information available to require special precautions

Effects on Dental Treatment No effects or complications reported

Warnings/Precautions DO NOT ADMINISTER AS AN INTRAVENOUS PUSH OR BOLUS. Associated with hypersensitivity reactions which may respond to adjustments in the infusion rate. Hypotension, bronchospasm, and angioedema have occurred in association with infusion as part of an infusion-related symptom complex. Infusion should be interrupted for severe reactions and can be resumed at a 50% reduction in rate (eg, from 100 mg/hour to 50 mg/hour) when symptoms have completely resolved. Treatment of these symptoms with diphenhydramine and acetaminophen is recommended; additional treatment with bronchodilators or I.V. saline may be indicated. In most cases, patients who have experienced nonlife-threatening reactions have been able to complete the full course of therapy.

Pregnancy Risk Factor C

Dosage Forms Injection: 100 mg (10 mL); 500 mg (10 mL)

Robitussin®-DAC *see* Guaifenesin, Pseudoephedrine, and Codeine *on page 455*

Robitussin®-DM [OTC] *see* Guaifenesin and Dextromethorphan *on page 453*

Robitussin-PE® [OTC] *see* Guaifenesin and Pseudoephedrine *on page 454*

Robitussin® Pediatric [OTC] *see* Dextromethorphan *on page 298*

Robitussin® Severe Congestion Liqui-Gels [OTC] *see* Guaifenesin and Pseudoephedrine *on page 454*

Rocaltrol® *see* Calcitriol *on page 161*

Rocephin® *see* Ceftriaxone *on page 197*

Rocky Mountain Spotted Fever Vaccine
(ROK ee MOUN ten SPOT ted FEE ver vak SEEN)

Therapeutic Category Vaccine, Live Bacteria

Local Anesthetic/Vasoconstrictor Precautions No information available to require special precautions

Effects on Dental Treatment No effects or complications reported

Generic Available No

Roferon-A® *see* Interferon Alfa-2a *on page 510*

Rogaine® Extra Strength for Men [OTC] *see* Minoxidil *on page 640*

Rogaine® for Men [OTC] *see* Minoxidil *on page 640*

Rogaine® for Women [OTC] *see* Minoxidil *on page 640*

Rolaids® [OTC] *see* Dihydroxyaluminum Sodium Carbonate *on page 318*

Rolaids® Calcium Rich [OTC] *see* Calcium Carbonate *on page 162*

Rolatuss® Plain Liquid *see* Chlorpheniramine and Phenylephrine *on page 218*

Romazicon™ *see* Flumazenil *on page 412*

Rondamine®-DM Drops *see* Carbinoxamine, Pseudoephedrine, and Dextromethorphan *on page 177*

Rondec®-DM *see* Carbinoxamine, Pseudoephedrine, and Dextromethorphan *on page 177*

Rondec® Drops *see* Carbinoxamine and Pseudoephedrine *on page 177*

Rondec® Filmtab® *see* Carbinoxamine and Pseudoephedrine *on page 177*

Rondec® Syrup *see* Carbinoxamine and Pseudoephedrine *on page 177*

Rondec-TR® *see* Carbinoxamine and Pseudoephedrine *on page 177*

Ropinirole (roe PIN i role)

Brand Names Requip™

Therapeutic Category Anti-Parkinson's Agent

Synonyms Ropinirole Hydrochloride

Use Treatment of idiopathic Parkinson's disease; in patients with early Parkinson's disease who were not receiving concomitant levodopa therapy as well as in patients with advanced disease on concomitant levodopa

Usual Dosage Adults: Oral: Dosage should be increased to achieve maximum therapeutic effect, balanced against the principal side effects of nausea, dizziness, somnolence and dyskinesia

Recommended starting dose: 0.25 mg 3 times/day; based on individual patient response, dosage should be titrated with weekly increments as described below:
Week 1 = 0.25 mg 3 times/day Total daily dose= 0.75 mg
Week 2 = 0.5 mg 3 times/day Total daily dose= 1.5 mg
Week 3 = 0.75 mg 3 times/day Total daily dose= 2.25 mg
Week 4 = 1 mg 3 times/day Total daily dose= 3 mg

After week 4, if necessary, daily dosage may be increased by 1.5 mg/day on a weekly basis up to a dose of 9 mg/day, and then by up to 3 mg/day weekly to a total of 24 mg/day

Local Anesthetic/Vasoconstrictor Precautions No information available to require special precautions

Effects on Dental Treatment No effects or complications reported

Other Adverse Effects
Early Parkinson's disease:
Cardiovascular: Syncope, dependent/leg edema, orthostatic symptoms
Central nervous system: Dizziness, somnolence (40%), headache, fatigue, pain, confusion, hallucinations
Gastrointestinal: Nausea (60%), dyspepsia, constipation, abdominal pain
Genitourinary: Urinary tract infections
Neuromuscular & skeletal: Asthenia
Ocular: Abnormal vision
Respiratory: Pharyngitis
Miscellaneous: Viral infection, diaphoresis (increased)
Advanced Parkinson's disease (with levodopa):
Cardiovascular: Hypotension (2%), syncope (3%)
(Continued)

Ropinirole *(Continued)*

Central nervous system: Dizziness (26%), aggravated parkinsonism, somnolence, headache (17%), insomnia, hallucinations, confusion (9%), pain (5%), paresis (3%), amnesia (5%), anxiety (6%), abnormal dreaming (3%)

Gastrointestinal: Nausea (30%), abdominal pain (9%), vomiting (7%), constipation (6%), diarrhea (5%), dysphagia (2%), flatulence (2%), increased salivation (2%), xerostomia, weight loss (2%)

Genitourinary: Urinary tract infections

Neuromuscular & skeletal: Dyskinesias (34%), falls (10%), hypokinesia (5%), paresthesia (5%), tremor (6%), arthralgia (7%), arthritis (3%)

Respiratory: Upper respiratory tract infection

Miscellaneous: Injury, increased diaphoresis (7%), viral infection, increased drug level (7%)

Endocrine & metabolic: Hypoglycemia, increased LDH, hyperphosphatemia, hyperuricemia, diabetes mellitus, hypokalemia, hypercholesterolemia, hyperkalemia, acidosis, hyponatremia, dehydration, hypochloremia

Gastrointestinal: Weight increase

Hepatic: Increaesd alkaline phosphatase

Neuromuscular & skeletal: Increased CPK

Renal: Elevated BUN, glycosuria

Miscellaneous: Thirst, increased lactate dehydrogenase (LDH)

Drug Uptake

Absorption: Not affected by food; T_{max} increased by 2.5 hours when drug taken with a meal; absolute bioavailability was 55%, indicating first-pass effect; relative bioavailability from tablet compared to oral solution is 85%

Serum half-life, elimination: ~6 hours

Time to peak concentration: ~1-2 hours

Pregnancy Risk Factor C

Dosage Forms Tablet: 0.25 mg, 0.5 mg, 1 mg, 2 mg, 5 mg

Dietary Considerations Ropinirole can be taken with or without food

Ropinirole Hydrochloride *see Ropinirole on previous page*

Ropivacaine (roe PIV a kane)

Related Information

Oral Pain *on page 1053*

Brand Names Naropin®

Therapeutic Category Local Anesthetic, Injectable

Use Local anesthetic (injectable) for use in surgery, postoperative pain management, and obstetrical procedures when local or regional anesthesia is needed. It can be administered via local infiltration, epidural block and epidural infusion, or intermittent bolus.

Usual Dosage Dose varies with procedure, onset and depth of anesthesia desired, vascularity of tissues, duration of anesthesia, and condition of patient

Adults:

Lumbar epidural for surgery: 15-30 mL of 0.5% to 1%

Lumbar epidural block for cesarean section: 20-30 mL of 0.5%

Thoracic epidural block for postoperative pain relief: 5-15 mL of 0.5%

Major nerve block: 35-50 mL dose of 0.5% (175-250 mg)

Field block: 1-40 mL dose of 0.5% (5-200 mg)

Lumbar epidural for labor pain: Initial: 10-20 mL 0.2%; continuous infusion dose: 6-14 mL/hour of 0.2% with incremental injections of 10-15 mL/hour of 0.2% solution

Mechanism of Action Local anesthetics bind selectively to the intracellular surface of sodium channels to block influx of sodium into the axon. As a result, depolarization necessary for action potential propagation and subsequent nerve function is prevented. The block at the sodium channel is reversible. When drug diffuses away from the axon, sodium channel function is restored and nerve propagation returns.

Local Anesthetic/Vasoconstrictor Precautions No information available to require special precautions

Effects on Dental Treatment No effects or complications reported

Other Adverse Effects

>10% (dose and route related):

Cardiovascular: Hypotension, bradycardia

Gastrointestinal: Nausea, vomiting

Neuromuscular & skeletal: Back pain

Miscellaneous: Shivering

1% to 10% (dose related):

Cardiovascular: Hypertension, tachycardia, bradycardia

Central nervous system: Headache, dizziness, anxiety, lightheadedness

Gastrointestinal: Vomiting
Neuromuscular & skeletal: Hypoesthesia, paresthesia, circumoral paresthesia
Otic: Tinnitus
Respiratory: Apnea
Drug Interactions
Increased effect: Other local anesthetics or agents structurally related to the amide-type anesthetics
Increased toxicity (possible but not yet reported): Drugs that decrease cytochrome P-450 1A enzyme function
Drug Uptake
Duration of action (dependent on dose and route administered): 3-15 hours generally
Half-life:
Epidural: 5-7 hours
I.V.: 2.4 hours
Pregnancy Risk Factor B
Dosage Forms
Infusion, as hydrochloride: 2 mg/mL (100 mL, 200 mL)
Injection, as hydrochloride (single dose): 2 mg/mL (20 mL); 5 mg/mL (30 mL); 7.5 mg/mL (10 mL, 20 mL); 10 mg/mL (10 mL, 20 mL)
Generic Available No
Comments Not available with vasoconstrictor (epinephrine) and not available in dental (1-8 mL) carpules

Rowasa® see Mesalamine on page 602

Roxanol™ Oral see Morphine Sulfate on page 648

Roxanol Rescudose® see Morphine Sulfate on page 648

Roxanol SR™ Oral see Morphine Sulfate on page 648

Roxicet® 5/500 see Oxycodone and Acetaminophen on page 711

Roxicodone™ see Oxycodone on page 711

Roxilox® see Oxycodone and Acetaminophen on page 711

Roxiprin® see Oxycodone and Aspirin on page 712

R-Tannamine® Tablet see Chlorpheniramine, Pyrilamine, and Phenylephrine on page 223

R-Tannate® Tablet see Chlorpheniramine, Pyrilamine, and Phenylephrine on page 223

RTCA see Ribavirin on page 841

Rubella and Measles Vaccines, Combined see Measles and Rubella Vaccines, Combined on page 581

Rubella and Mumps Vaccines, Combined
(rue BEL a & mumpz vak SEENS, kom BINED)
Brand Names Biavax® II
Therapeutic Category Vaccine, Live Virus
Use Promote active immunity to rubella and mumps by inducing production of antibodies
Usual Dosage Children >12 months and Adults: 1 vial in outer aspect of the upper arm; children vaccinated before 12 months of age should be revaccinated
Local Anesthetic/Vasoconstrictor Precautions No information available to require special precautions
Effects on Dental Treatment No effects or complications reported
Other Adverse Effects 1% to 10%:
Central nervous system: Febrile seizures, fever
Local: Burning, stinging
Neuromuscular & skeletal: Soreness
Miscellaneous: Allergic reactions
Pregnancy Risk Factor X
Dosage Forms Injection (mixture of 2 viruses):
1. Wistar RA 27/3 strain of rubella virus
2. Jeryl Lynn (B level) mumps strain grown cell cultures of chick embryo
Generic Available No
Comments Federal law requires that the date of administration, the vaccine manufacturer, lot number of vaccine, and the administering person's name, title and address be entered into the patient's permanent medical record

Rubella, Measles and Mumps Vaccines, Combined see Measles, Mumps, and Rubella Vaccines, Combined on page 582

Rubella Virus Vaccine, Live (rue BEL a VYE rus vak SEEN, live)
Brand Names Meruvax® II
Canadian/Mexican Brand Names Rimevax (Mexico)
Therapeutic Category Vaccine, Live Virus
(Continued)

Rubella Virus Vaccine, Live *(Continued)*

Synonyms German Measles Vaccine

Use Provide vaccine-induced immunity to rubella

Usual Dosage Children ≥12 months and Adults: S.C.: 0.5 mL in outer aspect of upper arm; children vaccinated before 12 months of age should be revaccinated

Mechanism of Action Rubella vaccine is a live attenuated vaccine that contains the Wistar Institute RA 27/3 strain, which is adapted to and propagated in human diploid cell culture. It is the only strain of rubella vaccine marketed in the U.S. Antibody titers after immunization last 6 years without significant decline; 90% of those vaccinated have protection for at least 15 years.

Local Anesthetic/Vasoconstrictor Precautions No information available to require special precautions

Effects on Dental Treatment No effects or complications reported

Other Adverse Effects

>10%:

Dermatologic: Erythema, urticaria, rash

Local: Tenderness

Neuromuscular & skeletal: Arthralgias

1% to 10%:

Central nervous system: Malaise, fever, headache

Gastrointestinal: Sore throat

Miscellaneous: Lymphadenopathy

<1%:

Ocular: Optic neuritis

Miscellaneous: Hypersensitivity, allergic reactions to the vaccine

Drug Uptake

Onset of effect: Antibodies to the vaccine are detectable within 2-4 weeks following immunization

Duration: Protection against both clinical rubella and asymptomatic viremia is probably life-long. Vaccine-induced antibody levels have been shown to persist for at least 10 years without substantial decline. If the present pattern continues, it will provide a basis for the expectation that immunity following vaccination will be permanent. However, continued surveillance will be required to demonstrate this point.

Pregnancy Risk Factor X

Generic Available No

Comments Federal law requires that the date of administration, the vaccine manufacturer, lot number of vaccine, and the administering person's name, title and address be entered into the patient's permanent record

Rubeola Vaccine *see* Measles Virus Vaccine, Live *on page 583*

Rubex® *see* Doxorubicin *on page 336*

Rubidomycin Hydrochloride *see* Daunorubicin Hydrochloride *on page 283*

Rum-K® *see* Potassium Chloride *on page 778*

Ru-Tuss® *see* Chlorpheniramine, Phenylephrine, Phenylpropanolamine, and Belladonna Alkaloids *on page 221*

Ru-Tuss® DE *see* Guaifenesin and Pseudoephedrine *on page 454*

Ru-Tuss® Expectorant [OTC] *see* Guaifenesin, Pseudoephedrine, and Dextromethorphan *on page 456*

Ru-Tuss® Liquid *see* Chlorpheniramine and Phenylephrine *on page 218*

Ru-Vert-M® *see* Meclizine *on page 584*

Rymed® *see* Guaifenesin and Pseudoephedrine *on page 454*

Rymed-TR® *see* Guaifenesin and Phenylpropanolamine *on page 454*

Ryna-C® Liquid *see* Chlorpheniramine, Pseudoephedrine, and Codeine *on page 223*

Ryna-CX® *see* Guaifenesin, Pseudoephedrine, and Codeine *on page 455*

Ryna® Liquid [OTC] *see* Chlorpheniramine and Pseudoephedrine *on page 219*

Rynatan® Pediatric Suspension *see* Chlorpheniramine, Pyrilamine, and Phenylephrine *on page 223*

Rynatan® Tablet *see* Chlorpheniramine, Pyrilamine, and Phenylephrine *on page 223*

Rynatuss® Pediatric Suspension *see* Chlorpheniramine, Ephedrine, Phenylephrine, and Carbetapentane *on page 219*

Rythmol® *see* Propafenone *on page 806*

S-2® *see* Epinephrine, Racemic *on page 354*

S5614 *see* Dexfenfluramine *Withdrawn from Market 1997* *on page 293*

Sabin Vaccine *see* Poliovirus Vaccine, Live, Trivalent, Oral *on page 770*

Safe Tussin® 30 [OTC] *see* Guaifenesin and Dextromethorphan *on page 453*

Safe Writing Practices *see page 1221*

Sal-Acid® Plaster [OTC] *see* Salicylic Acid *on this page*

Salactic® Film [OTC] *see* Salicylic Acid *on this page*

Salagen® *see* Pilocarpine (Dental) *on page 761*

Salbutamol (Mexico) *see* Albuterol *on page 35*

Saleto-200® [OTC] *see* Ibuprofen *on page 495*

Saleto-400® *see* Ibuprofen *on page 495*

Saleto-600® *see* Ibuprofen *on page 495*

Saleto-800® *see* Ibuprofen *on page 495*

Salflex® *see* Salsalate *on page 855*

Salgesic® *see* Salsalate *on page 855*

Salicilico, Acido (Mexico) *see* Salicylic Acid *on this page*

Salicylic Acid (sal i SIL ik AS id)

Brand Names Clear Away® Disc [OTC]; Compound W® [OTC]; Dr Scholl's® Disk [OTC]; Dr Scholl's® Wart Remover [OTC]; DuoFilm® [OTC]; DuoPlant® Gel [OTC]; Freezone® Solution [OTC]; Gordofilm® Liquid; Mediplast® Plaster [OTC]; Mosco® Liquid [OTC]; Occlusal-HP Liquid; Off-Ezy® Wart Remover [OTC]; Panscol® [OTC]; Psor-a-set® Soap [OTC]; P&S® Shampoo [OTC]; Sal-Acid® Plaster [OTC]; Salactic® Film [OTC]; Sal-Plant® Gel [OTC]; Trans-Ver-Sal® AdultPatch [OTC]; Trans-Ver-Sal® PediaPatch [OTC]; Trans-Ver-Sal® PlantarPatch [OTC]; Wart-Off® [OTC]

Canadian/Mexican Brand Names Acnex® (Canada); Acnomel® (Canada); Trans-Planta® (Canada); Trans-Ver-Sal® (Canada)

Therapeutic Category Keratolytic Agent

Synonyms Salicilico, Acido (Mexico)

Use Topically for its keratolytic effect in controlling seborrheic dermatitis or psoriasis of body and scalp, dandruff, and other scaling dermatoses; also used to remove warts, corns, and calluses

Usual Dosage
Lotion, cream, gel: Apply a thin layer to affected area once or twice daily
Plaster: Cut to size that covers the corn or callus, apply and leave in place for 48 hours; do not exceed 5 applications over a 14-day period
Solution: Apply a thin layer directly to wart using brush applicator once daily as directed for 1 week or until wart is removed

Mechanism of Action Produces desquamation of hyperkeratotic epithelium via dissolution of the intercellular cement which causes the cornified tissue to swell, soften, macerate, and desquamate. Salicylic acid is keratolytic at concentrations of 3% to 6%; it becomes destructive to tissue at concentrations >6%. Concentrations of 6% to 60% are used to remove corns and warts and in the treatment of psoriasis and other hyperkeratotic disorders.

Local Anesthetic/Vasoconstrictor Precautions No information available to require special precautions

Effects on Dental Treatment No effects or complications reported

Other Adverse Effects
>10%: Local: Burning and irritation at site of exposure on normal tissue
1% to 10%:
Central nervous system: Dizziness, mental confusion, headache
Otic: Tinnitus
Respiratory: Hyperventilation

Drug Interactions No data reported

Drug Uptake
Absorption: Absorbed percutaneously, but systemic toxicity is unlikely with normal use
Time to peak serum concentration: Topical: Within 5 hours of application with occlusion

Pregnancy Risk Factor C

Generic Available Yes

Salicylic Acid and Benzoic Acid *see* Benzoic Acid and Salicylic Acid *on page 120*

Salicylic Acid and Lactic Acid (sal i SIL ik AS id & LAK tik AS id)

Brand Names Duofilm® Solution

Therapeutic Category Keratolytic Agent

Synonyms Lactic Acid and Salicylic Acid

Use Treatment of benign epithelial tumors such as warts

Local Anesthetic/Vasoconstrictor Precautions No information available to require special precautions

Effects on Dental Treatment No effects or complications reported

Pregnancy Risk Factor C

Generic Available Yes

(Continued)

Salicylic Acid and Lactic Acid *(Continued)*

Comments Protect normal skin tissue with a ring of petrolatum surrounding the affected area; prior to application, soak affected area in hot water for at least 5 minutes; dry thoroughly with a clean towel

Salicylic Acid and Podophyllin *see* Podophyllin and Salicylic Acid *on page 769*

Salicylic Acid and Propylene Glycol
(sal i SIL ik AS id & PROE pi leen GLYE cole)
Brand Names Keralyt® Gel
Therapeutic Category Keratolytic Agent
Synonyms Propylene Glycol and Salicylic Acid
Use Removal of excessive keratin in hyperkeratotic skin disorders, including various ichthyosis, keratosis palmaris and plantaris and psoriasis; may be used to remove excessive keratin in dorsal and plantar hyperkeratotic lesions
Local Anesthetic/Vasoconstrictor Precautions No information available to require special precautions
Effects on Dental Treatment No effects or complications reported
Pregnancy Risk Factor C
Generic Available No

Salicylic Acid and Sulfur *see* Sulfur and Salicylic Acid *on page 898*

SalineX® [OTC] *see* Sodium Chloride *on page 870*

Salivart® Solution [OTC] *see* Saliva Substitute *on this page*

Saliva Substitute (sa LYE va SUB stee tute)
Related Information
Artificial Saliva Products *on page 1171*
Patients Undergoing Cancer Therapy *on page 1083*
Brand Names Entertainer's Secret® Spray [OTC]; Moi-Stir® Solution [OTC]; Moi-Stir® Swabsticks [OTC]; Mouthkote® Solution [OTC]; Optimoist® Solution [OTC]; Salivart® Solution [OTC]; Salix® Lozenge [OTC]
Therapeutic Category Gastrointestinal Agent, Miscellaneous; Saliva Substitute
Use Relief of dry mouth and throat in xerostomia
Usual Dosage Use as needed
Local Anesthetic/Vasoconstrictor Precautions No information available to require special precautions
Effects on Dental Treatment No effects or complications reported
Dosage Forms
Lozenge: 100s
Solution: 60 mL, 75 mL, 120 mL, 180 mL, 240 mL
Swabstix: 3s
Generic Available Yes

Salix® Lozenge [OTC] *see* Saliva Substitute *on this page*

Salk Vaccine *see* Poliovirus Vaccine, Inactivated *on page 770*

Salmeterol (sal ME te role)
Related Information
Respiratory Diseases *on page 1018*
Brand Names Serevent®
Canadian/Mexican Brand Names Zantirel® (Mexico)
Therapeutic Category Adrenergic Agonist Agent; Antiasthmatic; Beta₂-Adrenergic Agonist Agent; Bronchodilator
Synonyms Salmeterol, Hidroxinaftoato De (Mexico)
Use Maintenance treatment of asthma and in prevention of bronchospasm in patients >12 years of age with reversible obstructive airway disease, including patients with symptoms of nocturnal asthma, who require regular treatment with inhaled, short-acting beta₂ agonists; prevention of exercise-induced bronchospasm
Usual Dosage
Inhalation: 42 mcg (2 puffs) twice daily (12 hours apart) for maintenance and prevention of symptoms of asthma

Prevention of exercise-induced asthma: 42 mcg (2 puffs) 30-60 minutes prior to exercise; additional doses should not be used for 12 hours
Mechanism of Action Relaxes bronchial smooth muscle by selective action on beta₂-receptors with little effect on heart rate; because salmeterol acts locally in the lung, therapeutic effect is not predicted by plasma levels
Local Anesthetic/Vasoconstrictor Precautions No information available to require special precautions
Effects on Dental Treatment No effects or complications reported

Other Adverse Effects

>10%:

Central nervous system: Headache

Respiratory: Pharyngitis

1% to 10%:

Cardiovascular: Tachycardia, palpitations, elevation or depression of blood pressure, cardiac arrhythmias

Central nervous system: Nervousness, CNS stimulation, hyperactivity, insomnia, malaise, dizziness

Gastrointestinal: GI upset, diarrhea, nausea

Neuromuscular & skeletal: Tremors (may be more common in the elderly), myalgias, back pain, arthralgia

Respiratory: Upper respiratory infection, cough, bronchitis

<1%: Miscellaneous: Immediate hypersensitivity reactions (rash, urticaria, bronchospasm)

Drug Interactions Vascular system effects of salmeterol may be potentiated by MAO inhibitors and tricyclic antidepressants

Drug Uptake

Onset of action: 5-20 minutes (average 10 minutes)

Duration: 12 hours

Serum half-life: 3-4 hours

Pregnancy Risk Factor C

Dosage Forms Aerosol, oral, as xinafoate: 21 mcg/spray [60 inhalations] (6.5 g), [120 inhalations] (13 g)

Generic Available No

Salmeterol, Hidroxinaftoato De (Mexico) *see* Salmeterol *on previous page*

Salmonine® Injection *see* Calcitonin *on page 160*

Sal-Plant® Gel [OTC] *see* Salicylic Acid *on page 853*

Salsalate (SAL sa late)

Related Information

Rheumatoid Arthritis and Osteoarthritis *on page 1030*

Brand Names Argesic®-SA; Artha-G®; Disalcid®; Marthritic®; Mono-Gesic®; Salflex®; Salgesic®; Salsitab®

Therapeutic Category Analgesic, Non-narcotic; Anti-inflammatory Agent; Antipyretic; Nonsteroidal Anti-inflammatory Agent (NSAID), Oral; Salicylate

Use Treatment of minor pain or fever; arthritis

Usual Dosage Adults: Oral: 3 g/day in 2-3 divided doses

Dosing comments in renal impairment: In patients with end stage renal disease undergoing hemodialysis: 750 mg twice daily with an additional 500 mg after dialysis

Mechanism of Action Inhibits prostaglandin synthesis, acts on the hypothalamus heat-regulating center to reduce fever, blocks prostaglandin synthetase action which prevents formation of the platelet-aggregating substance thromboxane A_2

Local Anesthetic/Vasoconstrictor Precautions No information available to require special precautions

Effects on Dental Treatment No effects or complications reported

Other Adverse Effects

>10%: Gastrointestinal: Nausea, heartburn, stomach pains, dyspepsia, epigastric discomfort

1% to 10%:

Central nervous system: Fatigue

Dermatologic: Skin rash

Gastrointestinal: Gastrointestinal ulceration

Hematologic: Hemolytic anemia

Neuromuscular & skeletal: Weakness

Respiratory: Dyspnea

Miscellaneous: Anaphylactic shock

<1%:

Central nervous system: Insomnia, nervousness, jitters

Hematologic: Leukopenia, thrombocytopenia, iron deficiency anemia, does not appear to inhibit platelet aggregation, occult bleeding

Hepatic: Hepatotoxicity

Renal: Impaired renal function

Respiratory: Bronchospasm

Drug Interactions

Decreased effect with urinary alkalinizers, antacids, corticosteroids; decreased effect of uricosurics, spironolactone

Increased effect/toxicity of oral anticoagulants, hypoglycemics, methotrexate

(Continued)

855

Salsalate *(Continued)*

Drug Uptake
Onset of action: Therapeutic effects occur within 3-4 days of continuous dosing
Absorption: Oral: Completely from the small intestine
Serum half-life: 7-8 hours

Pregnancy Risk Factor C
Generic Available Yes

Salsitab® *see* Salsalate *on previous page*

Salt *see* Sodium Chloride *on page 870*

Saluron® *see* Hydroflumethiazide *on page 485*

Salutensin® *see* Hydroflumethiazide and Reserpine *on page 486*

Sandimmune® Injection *see* Cyclosporine *on page 272*

Sandimmune® Oral *see* Cyclosporine *on page 272*

Sandoglobulin® *see* Immune Globulin, Intravenous *on page 503*

Sandostatin® *see* Octreotide Acetate *on page 696*

Sani-Supp® Suppository [OTC] *see* Glycerin *on page 446*

Sanorex® *see* Mazindol *on page 581*

Sansert® *see* Methysergide *on page 626*

Santyl® *see* Collagenase *on page 260*

Saquinavir *(sa KWIN a veer)*

Related Information
HIV Infection and AIDS *on page 1024*
Systemic Viral Diseases *on page 1047*

Brand Names Invirase®
Therapeutic Category Antiviral Agent, Oral
Use Treatment of advanced HIV infection, used in combination with older nucleoside analog medications
Usual Dosage Oral: 600 mg 3 times/day within 2 hours after a full meal; use in combination with a nucleoside analog (AZT or ddC)
Mechanism of Action As an inhibitor of HIV protease, saquinavir prevents the cleavage of viral polyprotein precursors which are needed to generate functional proteins in and maturation of HIV-infected cells
Local Anesthetic/Vasoconstrictor Precautions No information available to require special precautions
Effects on Dental Treatment No effects or complications reported
Other Adverse Effects
1% to 10%:
Dermatologic: Rash
Endocrine & metabolic: Hyperglycemia, elevated CPK
Gastrointestinal: Diarrhea, abdominal discomfort, nausea, abdominal pain, buccal mucosa, ulceration
Neuromuscular & skeletal: Paresthesia, weakness

<1%:
Central nervous system: Headache, confusion, seizures, ataxia, pain
Dermatologic: Stevens-Johnson syndrome
Endocrine & metabolic: Hypoglycemia, hyper- and hypokalemia, low serum amylase
Gastrointestinal: Upper quadrant abdominal pain
Hematologic: Acute myeloblastic leukemia, hemolytic anemia, thrombocytopenia
Hepatic: Jaundice, ascites, exacerbation of chronic liver disease, elevated LFTs, altered AST, ALT, bilirubin, Hgb
Local: Thrombophlebitis

Drug Interactions
Decreased effect: Rifampin may decrease saquinavir's plasma levels and AUC by 40% to 80%; other enzyme inducers may induce saquinavir's metabolism (eg, phenobarbital, phenytoin, dexamethasone, carbamazepine)
Increased effect: Ketoconazole significantly increases plasma levels and AUC of saquinavir; as a known, although not potent inhibitor of the cytochrome P-450 system, saquinavir may decrease the metabolism of terfenadine and astemizole (and result in rare but serious cardiac arrhythmias); other drugs which may have increased adverse effects if coadministered with saquinavir include calcium channel blockers, clindamycin, dapsone, quinidine, and triazolam

Drug Uptake Absorption: Incomplete; food, especially high fat diets, may increase the absorption and oral bioavailability of saquinavir by five-fold
Pregnancy Risk Factor B
Dosage Forms Capsule, as mesylate: 200 mg
Generic Available No

Sargramostim (sar GRAM oh stim)

Brand Names Leukine™

Canadian/Mexican Brand Names Leucomax® (Mexico)

Therapeutic Category Colony Stimulating Factor

Synonyms GM-CSF; Granulocyte-Macrophage Colony Stimulating Factor; rGM-CSF

Use Myeloid reconstitution after autologous bone marrow transplantation; to accelerate myeloid recovery in patients with non-Hodgkin's lymphoma, Hodgkin's lymphoma, and acute lymphoblastic leukemia undergoing autologous BMT; following induction chemotherapy in patients with acute myelogenous leukemia to shorten time to neutrophil recovery

Usual Dosage All orders should be scheduled between 8 AM and 10 AM daily
Children and Adults: I.V. infusion over ≥2 hours or S.C.

Bone marrow transplantation failure or engraftment delay: I.V.: 250 mcg/m^2/day for 14 days. The dose can be repeated after 7 days off therapy if engraftment has not occurred. If engraftment still has not occurred, a third course of 500 mcg/m^2/day for 14 days may be tried after another 7 days off therapy. If there is still no engraftment, it is unlikely that further dose escalation be beneficial.

Myeloid reconstitution after autologous bone marrow transplant: I.V.: 250 mcg/m^2/day to begin 2-4 hours after the marrow infusion on day 0 of autologous bone marrow transplant or ≥24 hours after chemotherapy or 12 hours after last dose of radiotherapy. If significant adverse effects or "first dose" reaction is seen at this dose, discontinue the drug until toxicity resolves, then restart at a reduced dose of 125 mcg/m^2/day.

Length of therapy: Bone marrow transplant patients: GM-CSF should be administered daily for up to 30 days or until the ANC has reached 1000/mm^3 for 3 consecutive days following the expected chemotherapy-induced neutrophil-nadir.

Cancer chemotherapy recovery: I.V.: 3-15 mcg/kg/day for 14-21 days; maximum daily dose is 15 mcg/kg/day due to dose-related adverse effects; **discontinue therapy** if the ANC count is >20,000/mm^3

Excessive blood counts return to normal or baseline levels within 3-7 days following cessation of therapy

Mechanism of Action Stimulates proliferation, differentiation and functional activity of neutrophils, eosinophils, monocytes, and macrophages; see table.

Proliferation/Differentiation	G-CSF (Filgrastim)	GM-CSF (Sargramostim)
Neutrophils	Yes	Yes
Eosinophils	No	Yes
Macrophages	No	Yes
Neutrophil migration	Enhanced	Inhibited

Local Anesthetic/Vasoconstrictor Precautions No information available to require special precautions

Effects on Dental Treatment No effects or complications reported

Other Adverse Effects

>10%:
Cardiovascular: Tachycardia
Central nervous system: Neutropenic fever
Dermatologic: Alopecia
Gastrointestinal: Nausea, vomiting, diarrhea, mucositis
Hematologic: Thrombocytopenia
Neuromuscular & skeletal: Skeletal pain

1% to 10%:
Cardiovascular: Chest pain, peripheral edema
Central nervous system: Headache
Dermatologic: Skin rash
Endocrine & metabolic: Fluid retention
Gastrointestinal: Anorexia, stomatitis, sore throat, constipation
Hematologic: Leukocytosis, capillary leak syndrome
Local: Pain at injection site
Neuromuscular & skeletal: Weakness
Respiratory: Dyspnea, cough

<1%:
Cardiovascular: Transient supraventricular arrhythmia, pericarditis
Local: Thrombophlebitis
Miscellaneous: Anaphylactic reaction

Drug Uptake

Onset of action: Increase in WBC in 7-14 days

(Continued)

Sargramostim (Continued)

Duration: WBC will return to baseline within 1 week after discontinuing drug
Serum half-life: 2 hours
Time to peak serum concentration: S.C.: Within 1-2 hours

Pregnancy Risk Factor C

Generic Available No

Comments Has been demonstrated to accelerate myeloid engraftment in autologous bone marrow transplant, decrease median duration of antibiotic administration, reduce the median duration of infectious episodes, and shorten the median duration of hospitalization, no difference in relapse rate or survival or disease response has been found in placebo-controlled trials. Safety and efficacy of GM-CSF given simultaneously with cytotoxic chemotherapy have not been established. Concurrent treatment may increase myelosuppression. Precaution should be exercised in the usage of GM-CSF in any malignancy with myeloid characteristics. GM-CSF can potentially act as a growth factor for any tumor type, particularly myeloid malignancies. Tumors of nonhematopoietic origin may have surface receptors for GM-CSF.

Sarna [OTC] see Camphor, Menthol, and Phenol on page 169

Sastid® Plain Therapeutic Shampoo and Acne Wash [OTC] see Sulfur and Salicylic Acid on page 898

Scabene® see Lindane on page 558

Scleromate™ see Morrhuate Sodium on page 650

Scopace® Tablet see Scopolamine on this page

Scopolamine (skoe POL a meen)

Brand Names Isopto® Hyoscine Ophthalmic; Scopace® Tablet; Transderm Scop® Patch

Therapeutic Category Anticholinergic Agent; Anticholinergic Agent, Ophthalmic; Anticholinergic Agent, Transdermal; Ophthalmic Agent, Mydriatic

Use Preoperative medication to produce amnesia and decrease salivation and respiratory secretions; to produce cycloplegia and mydriasis; treatment of iridocyclitis, prevention of nausea and vomiting by motion; produces more CNS depression, mydriasis, and cycloplegia but less effective in preventing reflex bradycardia and effecting the intestines than atropine

Usual Dosage
Preoperatively:
Children: I.M., S.C.: 6 mcg/kg/dose (maximum: 0.3 mg/dose) or 0.2 mg/m² may be repeated every 6-8 hours **or** alternatively:
4-7 months: 0.1 mg
7 months to 3 years: 0.15 mg
3-8 years: 0.2 mg
8-12 years: 0.3 mg
Adults: I.M., I.V., S.C.: 0.3-0.65 mg; may be repeated every 4-6 hours

Motion sickness: Transdermal: Children >12 years and Adults: Apply 1 disc behind the ear at least 4 hours prior to exposure and every 3 days as needed; effective if applied as soon as 2-3 hours before anticipated need, best if 12 hours before

Ophthalmic:
Refraction:
Children: Instill 1 drop of 0.25% to eye(s) twice daily for 2 days before procedure
Adults: Instill 1-2 drops of 0.25% to eye(s) 1 hour before procedure
Iridocyclitis:
Children: Instill 1 drop of 0.25% to eye(s) up to 3 times/day
Adults: Instill 1-2 drops of 0.25% to eye(s) up to 4 times/day

Mechanism of Action Blocks the action of acetylcholine at parasympathetic sites in smooth muscle, secretory glands and the CNS; increases cardiac output, dries secretions, antagonizes histamine and serotonin

Local Anesthetic/Vasoconstrictor Precautions No information available to require special precautions

Effects on Dental Treatment >10% of patients medicated with scopolamine patch (Transderm Scop) will experience significant dry mouth. This will disappear with cessation of drug therapy.

Other Adverse Effects
Ophthalmic:
>10%: Ocular: Blurred vision, photophobia
1% to 10%:
Ocular: Local irritation, increased intraocular pressure
Respiratory: Congestion

<1%:
　　Cardiovascular: Vascular congestion, edema
　　Central nervous system: Drowsiness
　　Dermatologic: Eczematoid dermatitis
　　Ocular: Follicular conjunctivitis
　　Miscellaneous: Exudate
Systemic:
　>10%:
　　Dermatologic: Dry skin
　　Gastrointestinal: Constipation
　　Local: Irritation at injection site
　　Respiratory: Dry nose, throat
　　Miscellaneous: Decreased sweating
　1% to 10%:
　　Dermatologic: Photosensitivity
　　Endocrine & metabolic: Decreased flow of breast milk
　　Gastrointestinal: Dysphagia
　<1%:
　　Cardiovascular: Orthostatic hypotension, ventricular fibrillation, tachycardia, palpitations
　　Central nervous system: Confusion, headache, loss of memory, ataxia, fatigue
　　Dermatologic: Skin rash
　　Gastrointestinal: Bloated feeling, nausea, vomiting
　　Genitourinary: Dysuria
　　Neuromuscular & skeletal: Weakness
　　Ocular: Increased intraocular pain, blurred vision
Note: Systemic adverse effects have been reported following ophthalmic administration

Drug Interactions
　Increased toxicity: Anticholinergics, such as scopolamine, may potentiate the CNS effects of amantadine; may potentiate the anticholinergic effects of amitriptyline and haloperidol
　Decreased effects of other drugs: Anticholinergics, such as scopolamine, slow gastric emptying. This effects has reduced the rate of GI absorption of acetaminophen, levodopa, and potassium chloride wax-matrix preparations.

Drug Uptake
　Onset of effect:
　　Oral, I.M.: 0.5-1 hour
　　I.V.: 10 minutes
　Duration of effect:
　　Oral, I.M.: 4-6 hours
　　I.V.: 2 hours
　Absorption: Well absorbed by all routes of administration

Pregnancy Risk Factor C

Generic Available Yes

Scopolamine and Phenylephrine see Phenylephrine and Scopolamine on page 754

Scot-Tussin® [OTC] see Guaifenesin on page 452

Scot-Tussin DM® Cough Chasers [OTC] see Dextromethorphan on page 298

Scot-Tussin® Senior Clear [OTC] see Guaifenesin and Dextromethorphan on page 453

SeaMist® [OTC] see Sodium Chloride on page 870

Sebizon® Topical Lotion see Sulfacetamide Sodium on page 890

Sebulex® [OTC] see Sulfur and Salicylic Acid on page 898

Secobarbital (see koe BAR bi tal)
Brand Names Seconal™
Canadian/Mexican Brand Names Novo-Secobarb® (Canada)
Therapeutic Category Barbiturate; Hypnotic; Sedative
Use Short-term treatment of insomnia and as preanesthetic agent
Usual Dosage Hypnotic:
　Children: I.M.: 3-5 mg/kg/dose; maximum: 100 mg/dose

　Adults:
　　Oral: 100 mg at bedtime
　　I.M.: 100-200 mg/dose
　　I.V.: 50-250 mg/dose
Mechanism of Action Interferes with transmission of impulses from the thalamus to the cortex of the brain resulting in an imbalance in central inhibitory and facilitatory mechanisms
(Continued)

859

Secobarbital *(Continued)*

Local Anesthetic/Vasoconstrictor Precautions No information available to require special precautions

Effects on Dental Treatment No effects or complications reported

Other Adverse Effects

>10%:

Central nervous system: Dizziness, lightheadedness, drowsiness, "hangover" effect

Local: Pain at injection site

1% to 10%:

Central nervous system: Confusion, mental depression, unusual excitement, nervousness, faint feeling, headache, insomnia, nightmares

Gastrointestinal: Constipation, nausea, vomiting

<1%:

Cardiovascular: Hypotension

Central nervous system: Hallucinations

Dermatologic: Skin rash, exfoliative dermatitis, Stevens-Johnson syndrome

Hematologic: Megaloblastic anemia, thrombocytopenia, agranulocytosis

Local: Thrombophlebitis

Respiratory: Respiratory depression

Drug Interactions

Decreased effect of betamethasone and other corticosteroids, tricyclic antidepressants (TCAs), chloramphenicol, estrogens, cyclophosphamide, oral anticoagulants, doxycycline, theophylline

Increased effect/toxicity with CNS depressants, chloramphenicol, chlorpropamide

Drug Uptake

Onset of hypnosis:

Oral: Within 1-3 minutes

I.V. injection: Within 15-30 minutes

Duration: ~15 minutes

Absorption: Oral: Well absorbed (90%)

Serum half-life: 25 hours

Time to peak serum concentration: Within 2-4 hours

Pregnancy Risk Factor D

Dosage Forms

Capsule: 100 mg

Injection, as sodium: 50 mg/mL (2 mL)

Generic Available Yes

Secobarbital and Amobarbital *see* Amobarbital and Secobarbital *on page 66*

Seconal™ *see* Secobarbital *on previous page*

Secran® *see* Vitamins, Multiple *on page 995*

Secretin *(SEE kre tin)*

Brand Names Secretin-Ferring Injection

Therapeutic Category Diagnostic Agent, Pancreatic Exocrine Insufficiency; Diagnostic Agent, Zollinger-Ellison Syndrome and Pancreatic Exocrine Disease

Use Diagnosis of Zollinger-Ellison syndrome, chronic pancreatic dysfunction, and some hepatobiliary diseases such as obstructive jaundice resulting from cancer or stones in the biliary tract

Usual Dosage Potency of secretin is expressed in terms of clinical units (CU). I.V.:

Pancreatic function: 1 CU/kg slow I.V. injection over 1 minute

Zollinger-Ellison: 2 CU/kg slow I.V. injection over 1 minute

Mechanism of Action Hormone normally secreted by duodenal mucosa and upper jejunal mucosa which increases the volume and bicarbonate content of pancreatic juice; stimulates the flow of hepatic bile with a high bicarbonate concentration, stimulates gastrin release in patients with Zollinger-Ellison syndrome

Local Anesthetic/Vasoconstrictor Precautions No information available to require special precautions

Effects on Dental Treatment No effects or complications reported

Other Adverse Effects <1%:

Cardiovascular: Venous spasm, syncope

Miscellaneous: Hypersensitivity reactions

Drug Uptake

Inactivated by proteolytic enzymes if administered orally

Peak output of pancreatic secretions: Within 30 minutes

Duration of action: At least 2 hours

Pregnancy Risk Factor Not established

Generic Available No
Comments Potency of secretin is expressed in terms of clinical units

Secretin-Ferring Injection see Secretin on previous page

Sectral® see Acebutolol on page 19

Sedapap-10® see Butalbital Compound on page 154

Sedapap-10® see Butalbital Compound and Acetaminophen on page 155

Selegiline (seh LEDGE ah leen)

Brand Names Eldepryl®
Canadian/Mexican Brand Names Novo-Selegiline® (Canada)
Therapeutic Category Anti-Parkinson's Agent
Use Adjunct in the management of parkinsonian patients in which levodopa/carbidopa therapy is deteriorating
  Unlabeled use: Early Parkinson's disease
  Investigational use: Alzheimer's disease
  Selegiline is also being studied in Alzheimer's disease. Small studies have shown some improvement in behavioral and cognitive performance in patients, however, further study is needed.
Usual Dosage Oral:
  Adults: 5 mg twice daily with breakfast and lunch or 10 mg in the morning
  Elderly: Initial: 5 mg in the morning, may increase to a total of 10 mg/day
Mechanism of Action Potent monoamine oxidase (MAO) type-B inhibitor; MAO-B plays a major role in the metabolism of dopamine; selegiline may also increase dopaminergic activity by interfering with dopamine reuptake at the synapse
Local Anesthetic/Vasoconstrictor Precautions Selegiline in doses of 10 mg a day or less does not inhibit type-A MAO. Therefore, there are no precautions with the use of vasoconstrictors.
Effects on Dental Treatment >10% of patients experience dry mouth; anticholinergic side effects can cause a reduction of saliva production or secretion contributing to discomfort and dental disease (ie, caries, oral candidiasis and periodontal disease)
Other Adverse Effects
  >10%:
    Central nervous system: Mood changes, dyskinesias, dizziness
    Gastrointestinal: Nausea, vomiting, abdominal pain
  1% to 10%:
    Cardiovascular: Orthostatic hypotension, arrhythmias, hypertension
    Central nervous system: Hallucinations, confusion, depression, insomnia, agitation, loss of balance
    Neuromuscular & skeletal: Increased involuntary movements, bradykinesia, muscle twitches
    Miscellaneous: Bruxism
Drug Interactions Meperidine in combination with selegiline has caused agitation and delirium; it may be prudent to avoid other opioids as well
Drug Uptake
  Onset of therapeutic effects: Within 1 hour
  Duration: 24-72 hours
  Serum half-life: 9 minutes
Pregnancy Risk Factor C
Dosage Forms Capsule, as hydrochloride: 5 mg
Generic Available No

Selenium see Trace Metals on page 948

Selenium Sulfide (se LEE nee um)

Brand Names Exsel®; Selsun®; Selsun Blue® [OTC]; Selsun Gold® for Women [OTC]
Canadian/Mexican Brand Names Versel® (Canada)
Therapeutic Category Shampoos
Use Treatment of itching and flaking of the scalp associated with dandruff, to control scalp seborrheic dermatitis; treatment of tinea versicolor
Usual Dosage Topical:
  Dandruff, seborrhea: Massage 5-10 mL into wet scalp, leave on scalp 2-3 minutes, rinse thoroughly, and repeat application; shampoo twice weekly for 2 weeks initially, then use once every 1-4 weeks as indicated depending upon control
  Tinea versicolor: Apply the 2.5% lotion to affected area and lather with small amounts of water; leave on skin for 10 minutes, then rinse thoroughly; apply every day for 7 days
Mechanism of Action May block the enzymes involved in growth of epithelial tissue
(Continued)

Selenium Sulfide *(Continued)*

Local Anesthetic/Vasoconstrictor Precautions No information available to require special precautions

Effects on Dental Treatment No effects or complications reported

Other Adverse Effects

>10%: Dermatologic: Unusual dryness or oiliness of scalp

1% to 10%:

Central nervous system: Lethargy

Dermatologic: Alopecia, hair discoloration

Gastrointestinal: Vomiting following long-term use on damaged skin, abdominal pain, garlic breath

Local: Irritation

Neuromuscular & skeletal: Tremors

Miscellaneous: Perspiration

Drug Interactions No data reported

Drug Uptake

Absorption: Topical: Not absorbed through intact skin, but can be absorbed through damaged skin

Pregnancy Risk Factor C

Generic Available Yes

Sele-Pak® *see* Trace Metals *on page 948*

Selepen® *see* Trace Metals *on page 948*

Selsun® *see* Selenium Sulfide *on previous page*

Selsun Blue® [OTC] *see* Selenium Sulfide *on previous page*

Selsun Gold® for Women [OTC] *see* Selenium Sulfide *on previous page*

Semicid® [OTC] *see* Nonoxynol 9 *on page 689*

Semprex-D® *see* Acrivastine and Pseudoephedrine *on page 30*

Senexon® [OTC] *see* Senna *on this page*

Senna *(SEN na)*

Brand Names Black Draught® [OTC]; Senexon® [OTC]; Senna-Gen® [OTC]; Senokot® [OTC]; Senolax® [OTC]; X-Prep® Liquid [OTC]

Therapeutic Category Laxative, Stimulant

Use Short-term treatment of constipation; evacuate the colon for bowel or rectal examinations

Local Anesthetic/Vasoconstrictor Precautions No information available to require special precautions

Effects on Dental Treatment No effects or complications reported

Other Adverse Effects 1% to 10%: Gastrointestinal: Nausea, vomiting, diarrhea, abdominal cramps

Pregnancy Risk Factor C

Generic Available Yes

Comments Some patients will experience considerable gripping

Senna-Gen® [OTC] *see* Senna *on this page*

Senokot® [OTC] *see* Senna *on this page*

Senolax® [OTC] *see* Senna *on this page*

Sensorcaine® *see* Bupivacaine *on page 148*

Sensorcaine®-MPF *see* Bupivacaine *on page 148*

Sensorcaine MPF *see* Bupivacaine and Epinephrine *on page 149*

Septa® Topical Ointment [OTC] *see* Bacitracin, Neomycin, and Polymyxin B *on page 108*

Septisol® *see* Hexachlorophene *on page 470*

Septra® *see* Trimethoprim and Sulfamethoxazole *on page 965*

Septra® DS *see* Trimethoprim and Sulfamethoxazole *on page 965*

Ser-Ap-Es® *see* Hydralazine, Hydrochlorothiazide, and Reserpine *on page 476*

Serax® *see* Oxazepam *on page 707*

Serentil® *see* Mesoridazine *on page 602*

Serevent® *see* Salmeterol *on page 854*

Sermorelin Acetate *(ser moe REL in AS e tate)*

Brand Names Geref® Injection

Therapeutic Category Diagnostic Agent, Pituitary Function

Use Evaluate ability of the somatotroph of the pituitary gland to secrete growth hormone

Local Anesthetic/Vasoconstrictor Precautions No information available to require special precautions

Effects on Dental Treatment No effects or complications reported

Other Adverse Effects 1% to 10%:
    Cardiovascular: Transient flushing of the face, tightness in the chest
    Central nervous system: Headache
    Gastrointestinal: Nausea, vomiting
    Local: Pain, redness, and/or swelling at the injection site
Pregnancy Risk Factor C
Generic Available No

Seromycin® Pulvules® *see* Cycloserine *on page 271*

Serophene® *see* Clomiphene *on page 247*

Seroquel® *see* Quetiapine *on page 827*

Serostim® Injection *see* Human Growth Hormone *on page 473*

Serpalan® *see* Reserpine *on page 838*

Serpasil® *see* Reserpine *on page 838*

Sertraline (SER tra leen)
Related Information
    Vasoconstrictor Interactions With Antidepressants *on page 1226*
Brand Names Zoloft™
Therapeutic Category Antidepressant, Selective Serotonin Reuptake Inhibitor
Use Treatment of major depression; also being studied for use in obesity and obsessive-compulsive disorder
Usual Dosage Oral:
    Adults: Start with 50 mg/day in the morning and increase by 50 mg/day increments every 2-3 days if tolerated to 100 mg/day; additional increases may be necessary; maximum dose: 200 mg/day. If somnolence is noted, give at bedtime.
    Elderly: Start treatment with 25 mg/day in the morning and increase by 25 mg/day increments every 2-3 days if tolerated to 75-100 mg/day; additional increases may be necessary; maximum dose: 200 mg/day

    Hemodialysis effects: Not removed by hemodialysis
Mechanism of Action Antidepressant with selective inhibitory effects on presynaptic serotonin (5-HT) reuptake
Local Anesthetic/Vasoconstrictor Precautions Although caution should be used in patients taking tricyclic antidepressants, no interactions have been reported with vasoconstrictor and sertraline, a nontricyclic antidepressant which acts to increase serotonin
Effects on Dental Treatment No effects or complications reported
Other Adverse Effects
    1% to 10%: In clinical trials, dizziness and nausea were two most frequent side effects that led to discontinuation of therapy
    Cardiovascular: Palpitations
    Central nervous system: Insomnia, agitation, dizziness, headache, somnolence, nervousness, fatigue, pain
    Dermatologic: Dermatological reactions, sweating
    Endocrine & metabolic: Sexual dysfunction in men
    Gastrointestinal: Dry mouth, diarrhea or loose stools, nausea, constipation
    Genitourinary: Micturition disorders
    Neuromuscular & skeletal: Tremors
    Ocular: Visual difficulty
    Otic: Tinnitus
Drug Interactions
    All serotonin reuptake inhibitors are capable of inhibiting cytochrome P-450 IID6 isoenzyme enzyme system.
    Increased/decreased effect of lithium (both increases and decreases level has been reported)
    Increased toxicity of diazepam, trazodone via decreased clearance; increased toxicity with MAO inhibitors (hyperpyrexia, tremors, seizures, delirium, coma)
Drug Uptake
    Absorption: Slow
    Serum half-life:
        Parent: 24 hours
        Metabolites: 66 hours
Pregnancy Risk Factor B
Dosage Forms Tablet, as hydrochloride: 25 mg, 50 mg, 100 mg
Generic Available No

Serutan® [OTC] *see* Psyllium *on page 822*

Serzone® *see* Nefazodone *on page 668*

Shur-Seal® [OTC] *see* Nonoxynol 9 *on page 689*

Sibutramine (si BYOO tra meen)

Brand Names Meridia™

Therapeutic Category Anorexiant

Synonyms Sibutramine Hydrochloride

Use Management of obesity, including weight loss and maintenance of weight loss, and should be used in conjunction with a reduced calorie diet

Restrictions C-IV

Mechanism of Action A monoamine uptake inhibitor antidepressant; although it has little or no action on monoamine oxidase, sibutramine blocks the neuronal uptake of norepinephrine and, to a lesser extent, serotonin and dopamine; see Additional Information

Local Anesthetic/Vasoconstrictor Precautions No information available to require special precautions

Effects on Dental Treatment No effects or complications reported

Dosage Forms Capsule: 5 mg, 10 mg, 15 mg

Comments The mechanism of action of sibutramine is thought to be different from the "fen" drugs. Sibutramine works to suppress the appetite by inhibiting the reuptake of norepinephrine and serotonin. Unlike dexfenfluramine and fenfluramine, it is not a serotonin releaser. Sibutramine is closer chemically to the widely used antidepressants such as fluoxetine (Prozac®). The FDA approved sibutramine over the objections of its own advisory panel, who called the drug too risky. FDA reported that the drug causes blood pressure to increase, generally by a small amount, though in some patients the increases were higher. It is now recommended that patients taking sibutramine have their blood pressure evaluated regularly.

Selected Readings

Colchamiro R, "FDA Clears Obesity Drug," *Am Druggist*, 1998, 12.

Sibutramine Hydrochloride *see* Sibutramine *on this page*

Silace-C® [OTC] *see* Docusate and Casanthranol *on page 331*

Siladryl® Oral [OTC] *see* Diphenhydramine *on page 323*

Silafed® Syrup [OTC] *see* Triprolidine and Pseudoephedrine *on page 969*

Silaminic® Cold Syrup [OTC] *see* Chlorpheniramine and Phenylpropanolamine *on page 219*

Silaminic® Expectorant [OTC] *see* Guaifenesin and Phenylpropanolamine *on page 454*

Sildicon-E® [OTC] *see* Guaifenesin and Phenylpropanolamine *on page 454*

Silphen® Cough [OTC] *see* Diphenhydramine *on page 323*

Silphen DM® [OTC] *see* Dextromethorphan *on page 298*

Siltussin® [OTC] *see* Guaifenesin *on page 452*

Siltussin-CF® [OTC] *see* Guaifenesin, Phenylpropanolamine, and Dextromethorphan *on page 455*

Siltussin DM® [OTC] *see* Guaifenesin and Dextromethorphan *on page 453*

Silvadene® *see* Silver Sulfadiazine *on next page*

Silver Nitrate (SIL ver NYE trate)

Therapeutic Category Ophthalmic Agent, Miscellaneous; Topical Skin Product

Synonyms AgNO$_3$

Use Prevention of gonococcal ophthalmia neonatorum; cauterization of wounds and sluggish ulcers, removal of granulation tissue and warts

Usual Dosage

Children and Adults:

Ointment: Apply in an apertured pad on affected area or lesion for approximately 5 days

Sticks: Apply to mucous membranes and other moist skin surfaces only on area to be treated 2-3 times/week for 2-3 weeks

Topical solution: Apply a cotton applicator dipped in solution on the affected area 2-3 times/week for 2-3 weeks

Mechanism of Action Free silver ions precipitate bacterial proteins by combining with chloride in tissue forming silver chloride; coagulates cellular protein to form an eschar; silver ions or salts or colloidal silver preparations can inhibit the growth of both gram-positive and gram-negative bacteria. This germicidal action is attributed to the precipitation of bacterial proteins by liberated silver ions. Silver nitrate coagulates cellular protein to form an eschar, and this mode of action is the postulated mechanism for control of benign hematuria, rhinitis, and recurrent pneumothorax.

Local Anesthetic/Vasoconstrictor Precautions No information available to require special precautions

Effects on Dental Treatment No effects or complications reported

Other Adverse Effects
>10%:
Local: Burning and skin irritation
Ocular: Chemical conjunctivitis
1% to 10%:
Dermatologic: Staining of the skin
Hematologic: Methemoglobinemia
Ocular: Cauterization of the cornea, blindness

Drug Uptake
Absorption: Because silver ions readily combine with protein, there is minimal GI and cutaneous absorption of the 0.5% and 1% preparations

Pregnancy Risk Factor C

Generic Available Yes

Comments Applicators are **not** for ophthalmic use

Silver Protein, Mild (SIL ver PRO teen mild)
Brand Names Argyrol® S.S. 20%

Therapeutic Category Antibiotic, Topical

Use Stain and coagulate mucus in eye surgery which is then removed by irrigation; eye infections

Local Anesthetic/Vasoconstrictor Precautions No information available to require special precautions

Effects on Dental Treatment No effects or complications reported

Pregnancy Risk Factor C

Generic Available No

Silver Sulfadiazine (SIL ver sul fa DYE a zeen)
Brand Names Silvadene®; SSD® AF; SSD® Cream; Thermazene®

Canadian/Mexican Brand Names Dermazin® (Canada); Flamazine® (Canada)

Therapeutic Category Antibacterial, Topical

Use Prevention and treatment of infection in second and third degree burns

Usual Dosage Children and Adults: Topical: Apply once or twice daily with a sterile-gloved hand; apply to a thickness of $^1/_{16}$"; burned area should be covered with cream at all times

Mechanism of Action Acts upon the bacterial cell wall and cell membrane. Bactericidal for many gram-negative and gram-positive bacteria and is effective against yeast. Active against *Pseudomonas aeruginosa*, *Pseudomonas maltophilia*, *Enterobacteriae* species, *Klebsiella* species, *Serratia* species, *Escherichia coli*, *Proteus mirabilis*, *Morganella morganii*, *Providencia rettgeri*, *Proteus vulgaris*, *Providencia* species, *Citrobacter* species, *Acinetobacter calcoaceticus*, *Staphylococcus aureus*, *Staphylococcus epidermidis*, *Enterococcus* species, *Candida albicans*, *Corynebacterium diphtheriae*, and *Clostridium perfringens*

Local Anesthetic/Vasoconstrictor Precautions No information available to require special precautions

Effects on Dental Treatment No effects or complications reported

Other Adverse Effects
>10%: Local: Pain, burning
1% to 10%:
Dermatologic: Itching, rash, erythema multiforme, skin discoloration
Hematologic: Hemolytic anemia, leukopenia, agranulocytosis, aplastic anemia
Hepatic: Hepatitis
Renal: Interstitial nephritis
Miscellaneous: Allergic reactions may be related to sulfa component
<1%: Dermatologic: Photosensitivity

Drug Interactions Decreased effect: Topical proteolytic enzymes are inactivated

Drug Uptake
Absorption: Significant percutaneous absorption of sulfadiazine can occur especially when applied to extensive burns
Serum half-life: 10 hours and is prolonged in patients with renal insufficiency
Time to peak serum concentration: Within 3-11 days of continuous therapy

Pregnancy Risk Factor C

Generic Available Yes

Simethicone (sye METH i kone)
Brand Names Degas® [OTC]; Flatulex® [OTC]; Gas Relief®; Gas-X® [OTC]; Maalox Anti-Gas® [OTC]; Mylanta Gas® [OTC]; Mylicon® [OTC]; Phazyme® [OTC]

Canadian/Mexican Brand Names Ovol® (Canada)

Therapeutic Category Antiflatulent

Use Relieves flatulence and functional gastric bloating, and postoperative gas pains
(Continued)

Simethicone *(Continued)*

Usual Dosage Oral:

Children <12 years: 40 mg 4 times/day

Children >12 years and Adults: 40-120 mg after meals and at bedtime as needed, not to exceed 500 mg/day

Mechanism of Action Decreases the surface tension of gas bubbles thereby disperses and prevents gas pockets in the GI system

Local Anesthetic/Vasoconstrictor Precautions No information available to require special precautions

Effects on Dental Treatment No effects or complications reported

Other Adverse Effects No data reported

Drug Interactions No data reported

Pregnancy Risk Factor C

Generic Available Yes: Tablet

Simethicone and Calcium Carbonate *see* Calcium Carbonate and Simethicone *on page 163*

Simethicone and Magaldrate *see* Magaldrate and Simethicone *on page 574*

Simron® [OTC] *see* Ferrous Gluconate *on page 401*

Simvastatin *(SIM va stat in)*

Related Information

Cardiovascular Diseases *on page 1010*

Brand Names Zocor™

Therapeutic Category HMG-CoA Reductase Inhibitor; Lipid Lowering Drugs

Use Adjunct to dietary therapy to decrease elevated serum total and LDL cholesterol concentrations in primary hypercholesterolemia

Usual Dosage Adults: Oral: Start with 5-10 mg/day as a single bedtime dose; if LDL ≤190 mg/dL start with 5 mg; if LDL >190 mg/dL, start with 10 mg/day; increase every 4 weeks as needed; maximum dose: 40 mg/day

Mechanism of Action Simvastatin is a methylated derivative of lovastatin that acts by competitively inhibiting 3 hydroxy 3 methylglutaryl coenzyme A reductase (HMG CoA reductase), the enzyme that catalyzes the rate-limiting step in cholesterol biosynthesis

Local Anesthetic/Vasoconstrictor Precautions No information available to require special precautions

Effects on Dental Treatment No effects or complications reported

Other Adverse Effects

1% to 10%:

Central nervous system: Headache, dizziness

Dermatologic: Rash

Gastrointestinal: Flatulence, abdominal cramps, diarrhea, constipation, nausea, dyspepsia, heartburn

Neuromuscular & skeletal: Myalgia, elevated creatine phosphokinase (CPK)

<1%:

Gastrointestinal: Dysgeusia

Ocular: Lenticular opacities, blurred vision

Drug Interactions

Increased effect of warfarin, erythromycin, niacin

Increased toxicity of cyclosporin, gemfibrozil

Concurrent use of erythromycin and HMG-CoA reductase inhibitors may result in rhabdomyolysis

Drug Uptake

Absorption: Oral: Although 85% is absorbed following administration, <5% reaches the general circulation due to an extensive first-pass effect

Time to peak concentrations: 1.3-2.4 hours

Pregnancy Risk Factor X

Dosage Forms Tablet: 5 mg, 10 mg, 20 mg, 40 mg

Generic Available No

Sinarest® 12 Hour Nasal Solution *see* Oxymetazoline *on page 714*

Sinarest® Nasal Solution [OTC] *see* Phenylephrine *on page 752*

Sinarest®, No Drowsiness [OTC] *see* Acetaminophen and Pseudoephedrine *on page 24*

Sincalide *(SIN ka lide)*

Brand Names Kinevac®

Therapeutic Category Diagnostic Agent, Gallbladder Function

Synonyms C8-CCK; OP-CCK

Use Postevacuation cholecystography; gallbladder bile sampling; stimulate pancreatic secretion for analysis

Usual Dosage Adults: I.V.:

Contraction of gallbladder: 0.02 mcg/kg over 30 seconds to 1 minute, may repeat in 15 minutes a 0.04 mcg/kg dose

Pancreatic function: 0.02 mcg/kg over 30 minutes administered after secretin

Mechanism of Action Stimulates contraction of the gallbladder and simultaneous relaxation of the sphincter of Oddi, inhibits gastric emptying, and increases intestinal motility. Graded doses have been shown to produce graded decreases in small intestinal transit time, thought to be mediated by acetylcholine.

Local Anesthetic/Vasoconstrictor Precautions No information available to require special precautions

Effects on Dental Treatment No effects or complications reported

Other Adverse Effects 1% to 10%:

Cardiovascular: Flushing

Central nervous system: Dizziness

Gastrointestinal: Nausea, abdominal pain, urge to defecate

Drug Uptake

Onset of action: Contraction of the gallbladder occurs within 5-15 minutes

Duration: ~1 hour

Pregnancy Risk Factor B

Generic Available No

Comments Preparation of solution: To reconstitute, add 5 mL sterile water for injection to the vial; the solution may be kept at room temperature; use within 24 hours after reconstitution; delivers 1 mcg/mL

Sine-Aid® IB [OTC] *see* Pseudoephedrine and Ibuprofen *on page 821*

Sine-Aid®, Maximum Strength [OTC] *see* Acetaminophen and Pseudoephedrine *on page 24*

Sinemet® *see* Levodopa and Carbidopa *on page 548*

Sine-Off® Maximum Strength No Drowsiness Formula [OTC] *see* Acetaminophen and Pseudoephedrine *on page 24*

Sinequan® *see* Doxepin *on page 335*

Sinex® Long-Acting [OTC] *see* Oxymetazoline *on page 714*

Singulair® *see* Montelukast *on page 647*

Sinubid® *see* Phenyltoloxamine, Phenylpropanolamine, and Acetaminophen *on page 755*

Sinufed® Timecelles® *see* Guaifenesin and Pseudoephedrine *on page 454*

Sinumist®-SR Capsulets® *see* Guaifenesin *on page 452*

Sinupan® *see* Guaifenesin and Phenylephrine *on page 454*

Sinus Excedrin® Extra Strength [OTC] *see* Acetaminophen and Pseudoephedrine *on page 24*

Sinus-Relief® [OTC] *see* Acetaminophen and Pseudoephedrine *on page 24*

Sinutab® Tablets [OTC] *see* Acetaminophen, Chlorpheniramine, and Pseudoephedrine *on page 24*

Sinutab® Without Drowsiness [OTC] *see* Acetaminophen and Pseudoephedrine *on page 24*

SK and F 104864 *see* Topotecan *on page 945*

Skelaxin® *see* Metaxalone *on page 606*

Skelid® *see* Tiludronate *on page 934*

SKF 104864 *see* Topotecan *on page 945*

SKF 104864-A *see* Topotecan *on page 945*

Skin Test Antigens, Multiple (skin test AN tee gens, MUL ti pul)

Brand Names Multitest CMI®

Therapeutic Category Diagnostic Agent, Skin Test

Use Detection of nonresponsiveness to antigens by means of delayed hypersensitivity skin testing

Usual Dosage Select only test sites that permit sufficient surface area and subcutaneous tissue to allow adequate penetration of all eight points, avoid hairy areas

Press loaded unit into the skin with sufficient pressure to puncture the skin and allow adequate penetration of all points, maintain firm contact for at least 5 seconds, during application the device should not be "rocked" back and forth and side to side without removing any of the test heads from the skin sites

If adequate pressure is applied it will be possible to observe:

1. The puncture marks of the nine tines on each of the eight test heads
2. An imprint of the circular platform surrounding each test head
3. Residual antigen and glycerin at each of the eight sites

If any of the above three criteria are not fully followed, the test results may not be reliable

(Continued)

Skin Test Antigens, Multiple (Continued)

Reading should be done in good light, read the test sites at both 24 and 48 hours, the largest reaction recorded from the two readings at each test site should be used; if two readings are not possible, a single 48 hour is recommended

A positive reaction from any of the seven delayed hypersensitivity skin test antigens is **induration ≥2 mm** providing there is no induration at the negative control site; the size of the induration reactions with this test may be smaller than those obtained with other intradermal procedures

Local Anesthetic/Vasoconstrictor Precautions No information available to require special precautions

Effects on Dental Treatment No effects or complications reported

Other Adverse Effects 1% to 10%: Local: Irritation

Pregnancy Risk Factor C

Generic Available No

Comments Contains disposable plastic applicator consisting of eight sterile test heads preloaded with the following seven delayed hypersensitivity skin test antigens and glycerin negative control for percutaneous administration

Test Head No. 1 = Tetanus toxoid antigen
Test Head No. 2 = Diphtheria toxoid antigen
Test Head No. 3 = Streptococcus antigen
Test Head No. 4 = Tuberculin, old
Test Head No. 5 = Glycerin negative control
Test Head No. 6 = Candida antigen
Test Head No. 7 = Trichophyton antigen
Test Head No. 8 = Proteus antigen

Sleep-eze 3® Oral [OTC] see Diphenhydramine on page 323

Sleepinal® [OTC] see Diphenhydramine on page 323

Sleepwell 2-nite® [OTC] see Diphenhydramine on page 323

Slim-Mint® [OTC] see Benzocaine on page 118

Slo-bid™ see Theophylline on page 917

Slo-Niacin® [OTC] see Niacin on page 676

Slo-Phyllin® see Theophylline on page 917

Slo-Phyllin GG® see Theophylline and Guaifenesin on page 922

Slow FE® [OTC] see Ferrous Sulfate on page 401

Slow-K® see Potassium Chloride on page 778

Slow-Mag® [OTC] see Magnesium Chloride on page 575

SMZ-TMP see Trimethoprim and Sulfamethoxazole on page 965

Snaplets-EX® [OTC] see Guaifenesin and Phenylpropanolamine on page 454

Sodium Acid Carbonate see Sodium Bicarbonate on next page

Sodium Ascorbate (SOW dee um a SKOR bate)

Brand Names Cenolate®

Therapeutic Category Urinary Acidifying Agent; Vitamin, Water Soluble

Use Dental and Medical: Prevention and treatment of scurvy and to acidify urine

Usual Dosage Oral, I.V.:

Children:
Scurvy: 100-300 mg/day in divided doses for at least 2 weeks
Urinary acidification: 500 mg every 6-8 hours
Dietary supplement: 35-45 mg/day

Adults:
Scurvy: 100-250 mg 1-2 times/day for at least 2 weeks
Urinary acidification: 4-12 g/day in divided doses
Dietary supplement: 50-60 mg/day
Prevention and treatment of cold: 1-3 g/day

Local Anesthetic/Vasoconstrictor Precautions No information available to require special precautions

Effects on Dental Treatment No effects or complications reported

Other Adverse Effects 1% to 10%:
Cardiovascular: Hypotension with rapid I.V. administration
Gastrointestinal: Diarrhea
Local: Soreness at injection site
Renal: Precipitation of cystine, oxalate, or urate renal stones

Contraindications Large doses during pregnancy

Warnings/Precautions Use with caution in diabetics, patients with renal calculi, and those on sodium-restricted diets

Drug Interactions No data reported

Drug Uptake
Therapeutic serum levels: 0.4-1.5 mg/dL

Time to peak serum concentration: Oral: Within 2-3 hours

Pregnancy Risk Factor C

Breast-feeding Considerations No data reported

Dosage Forms

Crystals: 1020 mg per $1/4$ teaspoonful [ascorbic acid 900 mg]

Injection: 250 mg/mL [ascorbic acid 222 mg/mL] (30 mL); 562.5 mg/mL [ascorbic acid 500 mg/mL] (1 mL, 2 mL)

Tablet: 585 mg [ascorbic acid 500 mg]

Generic Available Yes

Sodium Benzoate and Caffeine see Caffeine and Sodium Benzoate on page 159

Sodium Bicarbonate (SOW dee um bye KAR bun ate)

Brand Names Neut® Injection

Therapeutic Category Alkalinizing Agent; Antacid; Electrolyte Supplement

Synonyms Baking Soda; NaHCO$_3$; Sodium Acid Carbonate; Sodium Hydrogen Carbonate

Use Management of metabolic acidosis; antacid; alkalinize urine; stabilization of acid base status in cardiac arrest (see precautions) and treatment of life-threatening hyperkalemia

Usual Dosage

Cardiac arrest: **Routine use of NaHCO$_3$ is not recommended and should be given only after adequate alveolar ventilation has been established and effective cardiac compressions are provided**

Infants and Children: I.V.: 0.5-1 mEq/kg/dose repeated every 10 minutes or as indicated by arterial blood gases; rate of infusion should not exceed 10 mEq/minute; neonates and children <2 years of age should receive 4.2% (0.5 mEq/mL) solution

Adults: I.V.: Initial: 1 mEq/kg/dose one time; maintenance: 0.5 mEq/kg/dose every 10 minutes or as indicated by arterial blood gases

Metabolic acidosis: Dosage should be based on the following formula if blood gases and pH measurements are available:

Infants and Children:

HCO$_3^-$(mEq) = 0.3 x weight (kg) x base deficit (mEq/L) **or**

HCO$_3^-$(mEq) = 0.5 x weight (kg) x [24 - serum HCO$_3^-$ (mEq/L)]

Adults:

HCO$_3^-$(mEq) = 0.2 x weight (kg) x base deficit (mEq/L) **or**

HCO$_3^-$(mEq) = 0.5 x weight (kg) x [24 - serum HCO$_3^-$ (mEq/L)]

If acid-base status is not available: Dose for older Children and Adults: 2-5 mEq/kg I.V. infusion over 4-8 hours; subsequent doses should be based on patient's acid-base status

Chronic renal failure: Oral: Initiate when plasma HCO$_3^-$ <15 mEq/L

Children: 1-3 mEq/kg/day

Adults: Start with 20-36 mEq/day in divided doses, titrate to bicarbonate level of 18-20 mEq/L

Renal tubular acidosis: Oral:

Distal:

Children: 2-3 mEq/kg/day

Adults: 0.5-2 mEq/kg/day in 4-5 divided doses

Proximal: Children: Initial: 5-10 mEq/kg/day; maintenance: Increase as required to maintain serum bicarbonate in the normal range

Urine alkalinization: Oral:

Children: 1-10 mEq (84-840 mg)/kg/day in divided doses every 4-6 hours; dose should be titrated to desired urinary pH

Adults: Initial: 48 mEq (4 g), then 12-24 mEq (1-2 g) every 4 hours; dose should be titrated to desired urinary pH; doses up to 16 g/day (200 mEq) in patients <60 years and 8 g (100 mEq) in patients >60 years

Antacid: Adults: Oral: 325 mg to 2 g 1-4 times/day

Mechanism of Action Dissociates to provide bicarbonate ion which neutralizes hydrogen ion concentration and raises blood and urinary pH

Local Anesthetic/Vasoconstrictor Precautions No information available to require special precautions

Effects on Dental Treatment No effects or complications reported

Other Adverse Effects

>10%: Gastrointestinal: Belching, gastric distension, flatulence

1% to 10%:

Cardiovascular: Edema, cerebral hemorrhage, aggravation of congestive heart failure

Central nervous system: Tetany, intracranial acidosis

Endocrine & metabolic: Metabolic alkalosis, hypernatremia, hypokalemia, hypocalcemia, hyperosmolality

Respiratory: Pulmonary edema

(Continued)

Sodium Bicarbonate *(Continued)*

Miscellaneous: Increased affinity of hemoglobin for oxygen-reduced pH in myocardial tissue necrosis when extravasated

Warnings/Precautions Rapid administration in neonates and children <2 years of age has led to hypernatremia, decreased CSF pressure and intracranial hemorrhage. **Use of I.V. NaHCO₃ should be reserved for documented metabolic acidosis and for hyperkalemia-induced cardiac arrest.** Routine use in cardiac arrest is not recommended. Avoid extravasation, tissue necrosis can occur due to the hypertonicity of NaHCO₃. May cause sodium retention especially if renal function is impaired; not to be used in treatment of peptic ulcer; use with caution in patients with CHF, edema, cirrhosis, or renal failure. Not the antacid of choice for the elderly because of sodium content and potential for systemic alkalosis.

Drug Interactions

Decreased effect/levels of lithium, chlorpropamide, salicylates due to urinary alkalinization

Increased toxicity/levels of amphetamines, ephedrine, pseudoephedrine, flecainide, quinidine, quinine due to urinary alkalinization

Drug Uptake

Oral:

Onset of action: Rapid

Duration: 8-10 minutes

I.V.:

Onset of action: 15 minutes

Duration: 1-2 hours

Absorption: Oral: Well absorbed

Pregnancy Risk Factor C

Dosage Forms

Injection: 4% [40 mg/mL = 2.4 mEq/5 mL] (5 mL); 4.2% [42 mg/mL = 5 mEq/10 mL] (10 mL); 7.5% [75 mg/mL = 8.92 mEq/10 mL] (10 mL, 50 mL); 8.4% [84 mg/mL = 10 mEq/10 mL] (10 mL, 50 mL)

Powder: 120 g, 480 g

Tablet: 300 mg [3.6 mEq]; 325 mg [3.8 mEq]; 520 mg [6.3 mEq]; 600 mg [7.3 mEq]; 650 mg [7.6 mEq]

Dietary Considerations Oral product should be administered 1-3 hours after meals; concurrent doses with iron may decrease iron absorption

Generic Available Yes

Comments

Sodium content of injection 50 mL, 8.4% = 1150 mg = 50 mEq; each 6 mg of NaHCO₃ contains 12 mEq sodium; 1 mEq NaHCO₃ = 84 mg

Each 84 mg of sodium bicarbonate provides 1 mEq of sodium and bicarbonate ions; each gram of sodium bicarbonate provides 12 mEq of sodium and bicarbonate ions

Sodium Cellulose Phosphate *see* Cellulose Sodium Phosphate *on page 201*

Sodium Chloride (SOW dee um KLOR ide)

Brand Names Adsorbonac® Ophthalmic [OTC]; Afrin® Saline Mist [OTC]; AK-NaCl® [OTC]; Ayr® Saline [OTC]; Breathe Free® [OTC]; Dristan® Saline Spray [OTC]; HuMist® Nasal Mist [OTC]; Muro 128® Ophthalmic [OTC]; Muroptic-5® [OTC]; NāSal™ [OTC]; Nasal Moist® [OTC]; Ocean Nasal Mist [OTC]; Pretz® [OTC]; SalineX® [OTC]; SeaMist® [OTC]

Therapeutic Category Electrolyte Supplement; Lubricant, Ocular

Synonyms NaCl; Normal Saline; Salt

Use Prevention of muscle cramps and heat prostration; restoration of sodium ion in hyponatremia; restore moisture to nasal membranes; reduction of corneal edema

Usual Dosage

Newborn electrolyte requirement:

Premature: 2-8 mEq/kg/24 hours

Term:

0-48 hours: 0-2 mEq/kg/24 hours

>48 hours: 1-4 mEq/kg/24 hours

Children: I.V.: Hypertonic solutions (>0.9%) should only be used for the initial treatment of acute serious symptomatic hyponatremia; maintenance: 3-4 mEq/kg/day; maximum: 100-150 mEq/day; dosage varies widely depending on clinical condition

Replacement: Determined by laboratory determinations mEq

Sodium deficiency (mEq/kg) = [% dehydration (L/kg)/100 x 70 (mEq/L)] + [0.6 (L/kg) x (140 - serum sodium) (mEq/L)]

Nasal: Use as often as needed

Adults:

GU irrigant: 1-3 L/day by intermittent irrigation

Heat cramps: Oral: 0.5-1 g with full glass of water, up to 4.8 g/day

Replacement I.V.: Determined by laboratory determinations mEq

Sodium deficiency (mEq/kg) = [% dehydration (L/kg)/100 x 70 (mEq/L)] + [0.6 (L/kg) x (140 - serum sodium) (mEq/L)]

To correct acute, serious hyponatremia: mEq sodium = [desired sodium (mEq/L) - actual sodium (mEq/L)] x [0.6 x wt (kg)]; for acute correction use 125 mEq/L as the desired serum sodium; acutely correct serum sodium in 5 mEq/L/dose increments; more gradual correction in increments of 10 mEq/L/day is indicated in the asymptomatic patient

Chloride maintenance electrolyte requirement in parenteral nutrition: 2-4 mEq/kg/24 hours or 25-40 mEq/1000 kcals/24 hours; maximum: 100-150 mEq/24 hours

Sodium maintenance electrolyte requirement in parenteral nutrition: 3-4 mEq/kg/24 hours or 25-40 mEq/1000 kcals/24 hours; maximum: 100-150 mEq/24 hours. See table.

Approximate Deficits of Water and Electrolytes in Moderately Severe Dehydration

Condition	Water (mL/kg)	Sodium (mEq/kg)
Fasting and thirsting	100-120	5-7
Diarrhea		
isonatremic	100-120	8-10
hypernatremic	100-120	2-4
hyponatremic	100-120	10-12
Pyloric stenosis	100-120	8-10
Diabetic acidosis	100-120	9-10

*A **negative** deficit indicates total body **excess** prior to treatment.

Adapted from Behrman RE, Kleigman RM, Nelson WE, et al, eds, *Nelson Textbook of Pediatrics*, 14th ed, WB Saunders Co, 1992.

Ophthalmic:

Ointment: Apply once daily or more often

Solution: Instill 1-2 drops into affected eye(s) every 3-4 hours

Abortifacient: 20% (250 mL) administered by transabdominal intra-amniotic instillation

Mechanism of Action Principal extracellular cation; functions in fluid and electrolyte balance, osmotic pressure control, and water distribution

Local Anesthetic/Vasoconstrictor Precautions No information available to require special precautions

Effects on Dental Treatment No effects or complications reported

Other Adverse Effects

1% to 10%:

Cardiovascular: Thrombosis, hypervolemia

Endocrine & metabolic: Hypernatremia, dilution of serum electrolytes, overhydration, hypokalemia

Local: Phlebitis

Respiratory: Pulmonary edema

Miscellaneous: Congestive conditions, extravasation

Warnings/Precautions Use with caution in patients with congestive heart failure, renal insufficiency, liver cirrhosis, hypertension, edema; sodium toxicity is almost exclusively related to how fast a sodium deficit is corrected; both rate and magnitude are extremely important

Drug Interactions Decreased levels of lithium

Drug Uptake

Absorption: Oral, I.V.: Rapid

Distribution: Widely distributed

Pregnancy Risk Factor C

Dosage Forms

Drops, nasal: 0.9% with dropper

Injection: 0.2% (3 mL); 0.45% (3 mL, 5 mL, 500 mL, 1000 mL); 0.9% (1 mL, 2 mL, 3 mL, 4 mL, 5 mL, 10 mL, 20 mL, 25 mL, 30 mL, 50 mL, 100 mL, 130 mL, 150 mL, 250 mL, 500 mL, 1000 mL); 3% (500 mL); 5% (500 mL); 20% (250 mL); 23.4% (30 mL, 100 mL)

Injection:

Admixtures: 50 mEq (20 mL); 100 mEq (40 mL); 625 mEq (250 mL)

Bacteriostatic: 0.9% (30 mL)

Concentrated: 14.6% (20 mL, 40 mL, 200 mL); 23.4% (10 mL, 20 mL, 30 mL)

(Continued)

Sodium Chloride *(Continued)*

Irrigation: 0.45% (500 mL, 1000 mL, 1500 mL); 0.9% (250 mL, 500 mL, 1000 mL, 1500 mL, 2000 mL, 3000 mL, 4000 mL)

Ointment, ophthalmic (Muro 128®): 5% (3.5 g)

Solution:
Irrigation: 0.9% (1000 mL, 2000 mL)
Nasal: 0.4% (15 mL, 50 mL); 0.6% (15 mL); 0.65% (20 mL, 45 mL, 50 mL)
Ophthalmic (Adsorbonac®): 2% (15 mL); 5% (15 mL, 30 mL)

Tablet: 650 mg, 1 g, 2.25 g

Tablet:
Enteric coated: 1 g
Slow release: 600 mg

Generic Available Yes

Sodium Citrate and Citric Acid

(SOW dee um SIT rate & SI trik AS id)

Brand Names Bicitra®; Oracit®

Canadian/Mexican Brand Names PMS-Dicitrate™ (Can)

Therapeutic Category Alkalinizing Agent

Synonyms Modified Shohl's Solution

Use Treatment of chronic metabolic acidosis; alkalinizing agent in conditions where long-term maintenance of an alkaline urine is desirable

Usual Dosage Oral:
Infants and Children: 2-3 mEq/kg/day in divided doses 3-4 times/day **or** 5-15 mL with water after meals and at bedtime

Adults: 15-30 mL with water after meals and at bedtime

Local Anesthetic/Vasoconstrictor Precautions No information available to require special precautions

Effects on Dental Treatment No effects or complications reported

Other Adverse Effects
1% to 10%:
Central nervous system: Tetany
Endocrine & metabolic: Metabolic alkalosis, hyperkalemia
Gastrointestinal: Diarrhea, nausea, vomiting

Warnings/Precautions Conversion to bicarbonate may be impaired in patients with hepatic failure, in shock, or who are severely ill

Drug Interactions
Decreased effect/levels of lithium, chlorpropamide, salicylates due to urinary alkalinization
Increased toxicity/levels of amphetamines, ephedrine, pseudoephedrine, flecainide, quinidine, quinine due to urinary alkalinization

Pregnancy Risk Factor C

Dosage Forms Solution, oral:
Bicitra®: Sodium citrate 500 mg and citric acid 334 mg per 5 mL (15 mL unit dose, 480 mL)
Oracit®: Sodium citrate 490 mg and citric acid 640 mg per 5 mL
Polycitra®: Sodium citrate 500 mg and citric acid 334 mg with potassium citrate 550 mg per 5 mL

Dietary Considerations Should be administered after meals to avoid laxative effect

Generic Available No

Comments 1 mL of Bicitra® contains 1 mEq of sodium and the equivalent of 1 mEq of bicarbonate

Sodium Citrate and Potassium Citrate Mixture

(SOW dee um SIT rate & poe TASS ee um SIT rate MIKS chur)

Brand Names Polycitra®

Therapeutic Category Alkalinizing Agent

Use Conditions where long-term maintenance of an alkaline urine is desirable as in control and dissolution of uric acid and cystine calculi of the urinary tract

Usual Dosage Oral:
Children: 5-15 mL diluted in water after meals and at bedtime
Adults: 15-30 mL diluted in water after meals and at bedtime

Local Anesthetic/Vasoconstrictor Precautions No information available to require special precautions

Effects on Dental Treatment No effects or complications reported

Pregnancy Risk Factor Not established

Dosage Forms Syrup: Sodium citrate 500 mg, potassium citrate 550 mg, with citric acid 334 mg per 5 mL [sodium 1 mEq, potassium 1 mEq, bicarbonate 2 mEq]

Dietary Considerations Should be administered after meals
Generic Available Yes

Sodium Cromoglycate (Canada) *see* Cromolyn Sodium *on page 264*

Sodium Edetate *see* Edetate Disodium *on page 345*

Sodium Fluoride *see* Fluoride *on page 415*

Sodium Hyaluronate (SOW dee um hye al yoor ON nate)

Brand Names AMO Vitrax®; Amvisc®; Amvisc® Plus; Healon®; Healon® GV
Therapeutic Category Ophthalmic Agent, Viscoelastic
Synonyms Hyaluronic Acid
Use Surgical aid in cataract extraction, intraocular implantation, corneal transplant, glaucoma filtration, and retinal attachment surgery
Usual Dosage Depends upon procedure (slowly introduce a sufficient quantity into eye)
Mechanism of Action Functions as a tissue lubricant and is thought to play an important role in modulating the interactions between adjacent tissues. Sodium hyaluronate is a polysaccharide which is distributed widely in the extracellular matrix of connective tissue in man. (Vitreous and aqueous humor of the eye, synovial fluid, skin, and umbilical cord.) Sodium hyaluronate forms a viscoelastic solution in water (at physiological pH and ionic strength) which makes it suitable for aqueous and vitreous humor in ophthalmic surgery.
Local Anesthetic/Vasoconstrictor Precautions No information available to require special precautions
Effects on Dental Treatment No effects or complications reported
Other Adverse Effects 1% to 10%: Ocular: Corneal edema, corneal decompensation, transient postoperative increase in intraocular pressure, postoperative inflammatory reactions (iritis, hypopyon)
Drug Uptake
  Absorption: Following intravitreous injection, diffusion occurs slowly
Pregnancy Risk Factor C
Generic Available No
Comments Bring drug to room temperature before instillation into eye

Sodium Hyaluronate-Chrondroitin Sulfate *see* Chondroitin Sulfate-Sodium Hyaluronate *on page 231*

Sodium Hydrogen Carbonate *see* Sodium Bicarbonate *on page 869*

Sodium Hypochlorite Solution
(SOW dee um hye poe KLOR ite soe LOO shun)

Therapeutic Category Disinfectant, Antibacterial (Topical)
Synonyms Dakin's Solution; Modified Dakin's Solution
Use Treatment of athlete's foot (0.5%); wound irrigation (0.5%); disinfect utensils and equipment (5%)
Usual Dosage Topical irrigation
Local Anesthetic/Vasoconstrictor Precautions No information available to require special precautions
Effects on Dental Treatment No effects or complications reported
Other Adverse Effects 1% to 10%: Dissolves blood clots, delays clotting, irritating to skin
Contraindications Hypersensitivity
Warnings/Precautions For external use only; avoid eye or mucous membrane contact; do not use on open wounds
Pregnancy Risk Factor C
Dosage Forms
  Solution: 5% (4000 mL)
  Solution (modified Dakin's solution):
    Full strength: 0.5% (1000 mL)
    Half strength: 0.25% (1000 mL)
    Quarter strength: 0.125% (1000 mL)
Generic Available Yes

Sodium P.A.S. *see* Aminosalicylate Sodium *on page 58*

Sodium-PCA and Lactic Acid *see* Lactic Acid and Sodium-PCA *on page 539*

Sodium Phenylbutyrate (SOW dee um fen il BYOO ti rate)

Brand Names Buphenyl®
Therapeutic Category Miscellaneous Product
Synonyms Ammonapse
Use Adjunctive therapy in the chronic management of patients with urea cycle disorder involving deficiencies of carbamoylphosphate synthetase, ornithine transcarbamylase, or argininosuccinic acid synthetase
(Continued)

Sodium Phenylbutyrate *(Continued)*

Usual Dosage
Powder: Patients weighing <20 kg: 450-600 mg/kg/day or 9.9-13 g/m²/day, administered in equally divided amounts with each meal or feeding, four to six times daily; safety and efficacy of doses >20 g/day has not been established

Tablet: Children >20 kg and Adults: 450-600 mg/kg/day or 9.9-13 mg/m²/day, administered in equally divided amounts with each meal; safety and efficacy of doses >20 g/day have not been established

Mechanism of Action Sodium phenylbutyrate is a prodrug that, when given orally, is rapidly converted to phenylacetate, which is in turn conjugated with glutamine to form the active compound phenylacetyglutamine; phenylacetyglutamine serves as a substitute for urea and is excreted in the urine whereby it carries with it 2 moles of nitrogen per mole of phenylacetyglutamine and can thereby assist in the clearance of nitrogenous waste in patients with urea cycle disorders

Local Anesthetic/Vasoconstrictor Precautions No information available to require special precautions

Effects on Dental Treatment No effects or complications reported

Other Adverse Effects
>10%: Endocrine & metabolic: Amenorrhea, menstrual dysfunction

1% to 10%:
Gastrointestinal: Anorexia, abnormal taste
Miscellaneous: Offensive body odor

Warnings/Precautions Since no studies have been conducted in pregnant women, sodium phenylbutyrate should be used cautiously during pregnancy; each 1 gram of drug contains 125 mg of sodium and, therefore, should be used cautiously, if at all, in patients who must maintain a low sodium intake

Dosage Forms
Powder: 3.2 g [sodium phenylbutyrate 3 g] per teaspoon (500 mL, 950 mL); 9.1 g [sodium phenylbutyrate 8.6 g] per **tablespoon** (500 mL, 950 mL)

Tablet: 500 mg

Generic Available No

Sodium Phosphates *(SOW dee um FOS fates)*

Brand Names Fleet® Enema [OTC]; Fleet® Phospho®-Soda [OTC]

Therapeutic Category Electrolyte Supplement, Parenteral; Laxative, Saline; Phosphate Salt; Sodium Salt

Use Source of phosphate in large volume I.V. fluids; short-term treatment of constipation (oral/rectal) and to evacuate the colon for rectal and bowel exams; treatment and prevention of hypophosphatemia

Usual Dosage
Normal requirements elemental phosphorus: Oral:
0-6 months: 240 mg
6-12 months: 360 mg
1-10 years: 800 mg
>10 years: 1200 mg

Pregnancy lactation: Additional 400 mg/day

Adults RDA: 800 mg

I.V. doses should be incorporated into the patient's maintenance I.V. fluids whenever possible; intermittent I.V. infusion should be reserved for severe depletion situations and requires continuous EKG monitoring. It is difficult to determine total body phosphorus deficit due to redistribution into intracellular compartment or bone tissue; (it is recommended that repletion of severe hypophosphatemia (<1 mg/dL in adults) be done via I.V. route since large dose of oral phosphate may cause diarrhea and intestinal absorption may be unreliable). The following dosages are empiric guidelines. **Note:** Doses listed as mmol of phosphate.

Severe hypophosphatemia: I.V.:
Children:
Low dose: 0.08 mmol/kg over 6 hours; use if recent losses and uncomplicated
Intermediate dose: 0.16-0.24 mmol/kg over 4-6 hours; use if phosphorus level 0.5-1 mg/dL
High dose: 0.36 mmol/kg over 6 hours; use if serum phosphorus <0.5 mg/dL
Adults: 0.15-0.3 mmol/kg/dose over 12 hours, may repeat as needed to achieve desired serum level

Maintenance:
Children: 0.5-1.5 mmol/kg/24 hours I.V. or 2-3 mmol/kg/24 hours orally in divided doses
Adults: 50-70 mmol/24 hours I.V. or 50-150 mmol/24 hours orally in divided doses **or**

Children <4 years: Oral: 1 capsule (250 mg/8 mmol phosphorus) 4 times/day; dilute as instructed

Children >4 years and Adults: Oral: 1-2 capsules (250-500 mg/8-16 mmol phosphorus) 4 times/day; dilute as instructed

Phosphate maintenance electrolyte requirement in parenteral nutrition: 2 mmol/kg/24 hours or 35 mmol/kcal/24 hours; maximum: 15-30 mmol/24 hours

Laxative (Fleet®): Rectal:
Children 2-12 years: Contents of one 2.25 oz pediatric enema, may repeat
Children ≥12 years and Adults: Contents of one 4.5 oz enema as a single dose, may repeat

Laxative (Fleet® Phospho®-Soda): Oral:
Children 5-9 years: 5 mL as a single dose
Children 10-12 years: 10 mL as a single dose
Children ≥12 years and Adults: 20-30 mL as a single dose

Mechanism of Action As a laxative, exerts osmotic effect in the small intestine by drawing water into the lumen of the gut, producing distention and promoting peristalsis and evacuation of the bowel; phosphorous participates in bone deposition, calcium metabolism, utilization of B complex vitamins, and as a buffer in acid-base equilibrium

Local Anesthetic/Vasoconstrictor Precautions No information available to require special precautions

Effects on Dental Treatment No effects or complications reported

Other Adverse Effects 1% to 10%:
Cardiovascular: Edema, hypotension
Endocrine & metabolic: Hypocalcemia, hypernatremia, hyperphosphatemia, calcium phosphate precipitation
Gastrointestinal: Nausea, vomiting, diarrhea
Renal: Acute renal failure

Drug Interactions Do not give with magnesium- and aluminum-containing antacids or sucralfate which can bind with phosphate

Drug Uptake
Onset of action:
Cathartic: 3-6 hours
Rectal: 2-5 minutes
Absorption: Oral: ~1% to 20%

Pregnancy Risk Factor C

Generic Available Yes

Sodium Salicylate (SOW dee um sa LIS i late)

Brand Names Uracel®

Therapeutic Category Analgesic, Non-narcotic

Use Treatment of minor pain or fever; arthritis

Usual Dosage Adults: Oral: 325-650 mg every 4 hours

Mechanism of Action Inhibits prostaglandin synthesis, acts on the hypothalamus heat-regulating center to reduce fever; decreases pain receptor sensitivity. Other proposed mechanisms of action for salicylate anti-inflammatory action are lysosomal stabilization, kinin and leukotriene production, alteration of chemotactic factors, and inhibition of neutrophil activation. This latter mechanism may be the most significant pharmacologic action to reduce inflammation.

Local Anesthetic/Vasoconstrictor Precautions No information available to require special precautions

Effects on Dental Treatment No effects or complications reported

Other Adverse Effects 1% to 10%:
Dermatologic: Rash, urticaria
Gastrointestinal: Nausea, vomiting, GI distress, GI ulcers, GI bleeding
Hematologic: Platelet inhibition
Hepatic: Hepatotoxicity
Respiratory: Bronchospasm/wheezing

Drug Interactions Ammonium chloride, vitamin C (high dose), methionine, antacids, urinary alkalinizers, carbonic anhydrase inhibitors, corticosteroids, nizatidine, alcohol, ACE inhibitors, beta-blockers, loop diuretics, methotrexate, probenecid, sulfinpyrazine, spironolactone, sulfonylureas

Drug Uptake
Absorption: From the stomach and small intestine
Serum half-life, aspirin: 15-20 minutes; metabolic pathways are saturable such that salicylates half-life is dose-dependent ranging from 3 hours at lower doses (300-600 mg), 5-6 hours (after 1 g) and 15-30 hours with higher doses; in therapeutic anti-inflammatory doses, half-lives generally range from 6-12 hours

Pregnancy Risk Factor C

Dosage Forms Tablet, enteric coated: 325 mg, 650 mg

Generic Available Yes

(Continued)

Sodium Salicylate *(Continued)*

Comments Sodium content of 1 g: 6.25 mEq; less effective than an equal dose of aspirin in reducing pain or fever; patients hypersensitive to aspirin may be able to tolerate

Sodium Sulamyd® Ophthalmic *see* Sulfacetamide Sodium *on page 890*

Sodium Sulfacetamide and Sulfur *see* Sulfur and Sulfacetamide Sodium *on page 898*

Sodium Tetradecyl (SOW dee um tetra DEK il)

Brand Names Sotradecol® Injection

Therapeutic Category Sclerosing Agent

Use Treatment of small, uncomplicated varicose veins of the lower extremities; endoscopic sclerotherapy in the management of bleeding esophageal varices

Mechanism of Action Acts by irritation of the vein intimal endothelium

Local Anesthetic/Vasoconstrictor Precautions No information available to require special precautions

Effects on Dental Treatment No effects or complications reported

Other Adverse Effects

1% to 10%:
Central nervous system: Headache
Dermatologic: Urticaria
Gastrointestinal: Mucosal lesions, nausea, vomiting
Local: Discoloration at the site of injection, pain, ulceration at the site, sloughing and tissue necrosis following extravasation
Respiratory: Pulmonary edema

<1%:
Gastrointestinal: Esophageal perforation
Respiratory: Asthma

Pregnancy Risk Factor C

Dosage Forms Injection, as sulfate: 1% [10 mg/mL] (2 mL); 3% [30 mg/mL] (2 mL)

Generic Available Yes

Sodium Thiosulfate (SOW dee um thye oh SUL fate)

Brand Names Tinver® Lotion

Therapeutic Category Antidote, Cyanide; Antifungal Agent, Topical

Use

Parenteral: Used alone or with sodium nitrite or amyl nitrite in cyanide poisoning or arsenic poisoning; reduce the risk of nephrotoxicity associated with cisplatin therapy; local infiltration (in diluted form) of selected chemotherapy extravasation

Topical: Treatment of tinea versicolor

Usual Dosage

Cyanide and nitroprusside antidote: I.V.:
Children <25 kg: 50 mg/kg after receiving 4.5-10 mg/kg sodium nitrite; a half dose of each may be repeated if necessary
Children >25 kg and Adults: 12.5 g after 300 mg of sodium nitrite; a half dose of each may be repeated if necessary

Cyanide poisoning: I.V.: Dose should be based on determination as with nitrite, at rate of 2.5-5 mL/minute to maximum of 50 mL. See table.

**Variation of Sodium Nitrite and Sodium Thiosulfate
Dose With Hemoglobin Concentration***

Hemoglobin (g/dL)	Initial Dose Sodium Nitrite (mg/kg)	Initial Dose Sodium Nitrite 3% (mL/kg)	Initial Dose Sodium Thiosulfate 25% (mL/kg)
7	5.8	0.19	0.95
8	6.6	0.22	1.10
9	7.5	0.25	1.25
10	8.3	0.27	1.35
11	9.1	0.30	1.50
12	10.0	0.33	1.65
13	10.8	0.36	1.80
14	11.6	0.39	1.95

*Adapted from Berlin DM Jr, "The Treatment of Cyanide Poisoning in Children," *Pediatrics*, 1970, 46:793.

Cisplatin rescue should be given before or during cisplatin administration: I.V. infusion (in sterile water): 12 g/m² over 6 hours or 9 g/m² I.V. push followed by 1.2 g/m² continuous infusion for 6 hours

Arsenic poisoning: I.V.: 1 mL first day, 2 mL second day, 3 mL third day, 4 mL fourth day, 5 mL on alternate days thereafter

Children and Adults: Topical: 20% to 25% solution: Apply a thin layer to affected areas twice daily

Mechanism of Action

Cyanide toxicity: Increases the rate of detoxification of cyanide by the enzyme rhodanese by providing an extra sulfur

Cisplatin toxicity: Complexes with cisplatin to form a compound that is nontoxic to either normal or cancerous cells

Local Anesthetic/Vasoconstrictor Precautions No information available to require special precautions

Effects on Dental Treatment No effects or complications reported

Other Adverse Effects 1% to 10%:

Cardiovascular: Hypotension

Central nervous system: Coma, CNS depression secondary to thiocyanate intoxication, psychosis, confusion

Dermatologic: Contact dermatitis

Local: Irritation

Neuromuscular & skeletal: Weakness

Otic: Tinnitus

Drug Uptake

Serum half-life: 0.65 hour

Pregnancy Risk Factor C

Generic Available Yes

Comments White, odorless crystals or powder with a salty taste; normal body burden: 1.5 mg/kg

Solaquin® [OTC] *see* Hydroquinone *on page 487*

Solaquin Forte® *see* Hydroquinone *on page 487*

Solarcaine® [OTC] *see* Benzocaine *on page 118*

Solatene® *see* Beta-Carotene *on page 125*

Solfoton® *see* Phenobarbital *on page 747*

Solganal® *see* Aurothioglucose *on page 100*

Solu-Cortef® *see* Hydrocortisone *on page 484*

Solu-Medrol® *see* Methylprednisolone *on page 624*

Solurex L.A.® *see* Dexamethasone *on page 291*

Soma® *see* Carisoprodol *on page 180*

Soma® Compound *see* Carisoprodol *on page 180*

Soma® Compound *see* Carisoprodol and Aspirin *on page 180*

Soma® Compound w/Codeine *see* Carisoprodol, Aspirin, and Codeine *on page 181*

Sominex® Oral [OTC] *see* Diphenhydramine *on page 323*

Sorbitol (SOR bi tole)

Therapeutic Category Genitourinary Irrigant

Use Genitourinary irrigant in transurethral prostatic resection or other transurethral resection or other transurethral surgical procedures; diuretic; humectant; sweetening agent; hyperosmotic laxative; facilitate the passage of sodium polystyrene sulfonate through the intestinal tract

Usual Dosage Hyperosmotic laxative (as single dose, at infrequent intervals):

Children 2-11 years:

Oral: 2 mL/kg (as 70% solution)

Rectal enema: 30-60 mL as 25% to 30% solution

Children >12 years and Adults:

Oral: 30-150 mL (as 70% solution)

Rectal enema: 120 mL as 25% to 30% solution

Adjunct to sodium polystyrene sulfonate: 15 mL as 70% solution orally until diarrhea occurs (10-20 mL/2 hours) or 20-100 mL as an oral vehicle for the sodium polystyrene sulfonate resin

When administered with charcoal:

Oral:

Children: 4.3 mL/kg of 35% sorbitol with 1 g/kg of activated charcoal

Adults: 4.3 mL/kg of 70% sorbitol with 1 g/kg of activated charcoal every 4 hours until first stool containing charcoal is passed

Topical: 3% to 3.3% as transurethral surgical procedure irrigation

Mechanism of Action A polyalcoholic sugar with osmotic cathartic actions

(Continued)

Sorbitol *(Continued)*

Local Anesthetic/Vasoconstrictor Precautions No information available to require special precautions

Effects on Dental Treatment No effects or complications reported

Other Adverse Effects

1% to 10%:

Cardiovascular: Edema

Endocrine & metabolic: Fluid and electrolyte losses, lactic acidosis

Gastrointestinal: Diarrhea, nausea, vomiting, abdominal discomfort, xerostomia

Contraindications Anuria

Warnings/Precautions Use with caution in patients with severe cardiopulmonary or renal impairment and in patients unable to metabolize sorbitol

Drug Uptake

Onset of action: About 0.25-1 hour

Absorption: Oral, rectal: Poor

Dosage Forms

Solution: 70%

Solution, genitourinary irrigation: 3% (1500 mL, 3000 mL); 3.3% (2000 mL)

Generic Available Yes

Sorbitrate® *see* Isosorbide Dinitrate *on page 525*

Sotalol (SOE ta lole)

Related Information

Cardiovascular Diseases *on page 1010*

Brand Names Betapace®

Canadian/Mexican Brand Names Sotacor® (Canada)

Therapeutic Category Antianginal Agent; Antiarrhythmic Agent, Class II; Antiarrhythmic Agent, Class III; Antiarrhythmic Agent (Supraventricular & Ventricular); Beta-adrenergic Blocker, Cardioselective

Use Treatment of documented ventricular arrhythmias, such as sustained ventricular tachycardia, that in the judgment of the physician are life-threatening

Unlabeled use: Supraventricular arrhythmias

Usual Dosage Sotalol should be initiated and doses increased in a hospital with facilities for cardiac rhythm monitoring and assessment. Proarrhythmic events can occur after initiation of therapy and with each upward dosage adjustment.

Children (oral): The safety and efficacy of sotalol in children have not been established

Supraventricular arrhythmias: 2-4 mg/kg/24 hours was given in 2 equal doses every 12 hours to 18 infants (≤2 months of age). All infants, except one with chaotic atrial tachycardia, were successful controlled with sotalol. Ten infants discontinued therapy between the ages of 7-18 months when it was no longer necessary. Median duration of treatment was 12.8 months.

Adults (oral):

Initial: 80 mg twice daily

Dose may be increased (gradually allowing 2-3 days between dosing increments in order to attain steady-state plasma concentrations and to allow monitoring of Q-T intervals) to 240-320 mg/day

Most patients respond to a total daily dose of 160-320 mg/day in 2-3 divided doses

Some patients, with life-threatening refractory ventricular arrhythmias, may require doses as high as 480-640 mg/day; however, these doses should only be prescribed when the potential benefit outweighs the increased of adverse events

Elderly patients: Age does not significantly alter the pharmacokinetics of sotalol, but impaired renal function in elderly patients can increase the terminal half-life, resulting in increased drug accumulation

Mechanism of Action

Beta-blocker which contains both beta-adrenoreceptor-blocking (Vaughan Williams Class II) and cardiac action potential duration prolongation (Vaughan Williams Class III) properties

Class II effects: Increased sinus cycle length, slowed heart rate, decreased A-V nodal conduction, and increased A-V nodal refractoriness

Class III effects: Prolongation of the atrial and ventricular monophasic action potentials, and effective refractory prolongation of atrial muscle, ventricular muscle, and atrioventricular accessory pathways in both the antegrade and retrograde directions

Sotalol is a racemic mixture of *d*- and *L*-sotalol; both isomers have similar Class III antiarrhythmic effects while the *L*-isomer is responsible for virtually all of the beta-blocking activity

Sotalol has both beta$_1$- and beta$_2$-receptor blocking activity

The beta-blocking effect of sotalol is a noncardioselective [half maximal at about 80 mg/day and maximal at doses of 320-640 mg/day]. Significant beta blockade occurs at oral doses as low as 25 mg/day.

The Class III effects are seen only at oral doses of ≥160 mg/day

Local Anesthetic/Vasoconstrictor Precautions Use with caution; epinephrine has interacted with nonselective beta-blockers to result in initial hypertensive episode followed by bradycardia

Effects on Dental Treatment Noncardioselective beta-blockers (ie, propranolol, nadolol) enhance the pressor response to epinephrine, resulting in hypertension and bradycardia. Many nonsteroidal anti-inflammatory drugs such as ibuprofen and indomethacin can reduce the hypotensive effect of beta-blockers after 3 or more weeks of therapy with the NSAID. Short-term NSAID use (ie, 3 days) requires no special precautions in patients taking beta-blockers.

Other Adverse Effects

>10%:

Cardiovascular: Bradycardia

Central nervous system: Mental depression

Endocrine & metabolic: Decreased sexual ability

1% to 10%:

Cardiovascular: Congestive heart failure

Central nervous system: Mental confusion, hallucinations, reduced peripheral circulation, anxiety, dizziness, drowsiness, nightmares, insomnia, fatigue

Dermatologic: Itching

Gastrointestinal: Constipation, diarrhea, nausea, vomiting, stomach discomfort

Neuromuscular & skeletal: Weakness

Respiratory: Dyspnea

<1%:

Cardiovascular: Chest pain, hypotension (especially with higher doses), Raynaud's phenomenon

Dermatologic: Skin rash; red, crusted skin

Hematologic: Leukopenia

Local: Phlebitis, skin necrosis after extravasation

Miscellaneous: Sweating, cold extremities

Drug Interactions Class Ia antiarrhythmics, such as quinidine, have the potential to prolong refractoriness of sotalol; sotalol should be administered with caution with calcium-blocking drugs because of possible additional effects on A-V conduction

Drug Uptake

Onset of action: Rapid, 1-2 hours

Peak effect: 2.5-4 hours

Absorption: Decreased 20% to 30% by meals compared to fasting

Serum half-life: 12 hours

Pregnancy Risk Factor B

Dosage Forms Tablet, as hydrochloride: 80 mg, 120 mg, 160 mg, 240 mg

Generic Available No

Sotradecol® Injection *see* Sodium Tetradecyl *on page 876*

Soyacal® *see* Fat Emulsion *on page 393*

Soyalac® [OTC] *see* Enteral Nutritional Products *on page 350*

Span-FF® [OTC] *see* Ferrous Fumarate *on page 400*

Sparfloxacin (spar FLOKS a sin)

Brand Names Zagam®

Therapeutic Category Antibiotic, Quinolone

Use Treatment of adult patients with community acquired pneumonia caused by susceptible strains of *Chlamydia pneumoniae, Haemophilus influenzae, Haemophilus parainfluenzae, Moraxella catarrhalis, Mycoplasma pneumoniae,* or *Streptococcus pneumoniae* and acute bacterial exacerbations of acute bronchitis caused by susceptible strains of *Chlamydia pneumoniae, Enterobacter cloacae, Haemophilus influenzae, Haemophilus parainfluenzae, Klebsiella pneumoniae, Moraxella catarrhalis, Staphylococcus aureus,* or *Streptococcus pneumoniae*

Usual Dosage Adults: Oral:

Loading dose: 2 tablets (400 mg) on day 1

Maintenance: 1 tablet (200 mg) daily for 10 additional days (total 11 tablets)

Mechanism of Action Inhibits DNA-gyrase in susceptible organisms; inhibits relaxation of supercoiled DNA and promotes breakage of double-stranded DNA (Continued)

Sparfloxacin *(Continued)*

Local Anesthetic/Vasoconstrictor Precautions No information available to require special precautions

Effects on Dental Treatment No effects or complications reported

Other Adverse Effects

>1%:

Central nervous system: Insomnia, agitation, sleep disorders, anxiety, delirium

Gastrointestinal: Diarrhea, abdominal pain, vomiting

Hematologic: Leukopenia, eosinophilia, anemia

Hepatic: Increased LFTs

<1%:

Dermatologic: Photosensitivity, rash

Neuromuscular & skeletal: Myalgia, arthralgia

Warnings/Precautions Not recommended in children <18 years of age, other quinolones have caused transient arthropathy in children; CNS stimulation may occur (tremor, restlessness, confusion, and very rarely hallucinations or seizures); use with caution in patients with known or suspected CNS disorder or renal dysfunction; prolonged use may result in superinfection; if an allergic reaction (itching, urticaria, dyspnea, pharyngeal or facial edema, loss of consciousness, tingling, cardiovascular collapse) occurs, discontinue the drug immediately; use caution to avoid possible photosensitivity reactions during and for several days following fluoroquinolone therapy; pseudomembranous colitis may occur and should be considered in patients who present with diarrhea

Drug Interactions

Decreased effect: Decreased absorption with antacids containing aluminum, magnesium, and/or calcium (by up to 98% if given at the same time); phenytoin serum levels may be reduced by quinolones; antineoplastic agents may also decrease serum levels of fluoroquinolones

Increased toxicity/serum levels: Quinolones cause increased levels of caffeine, warfarin, azlocillin, cyclosporine, and theophylline (although one study indicates that sparfloxacin may not affect theophylline metabolism), azlocillin, cimetidine, and probenecid increase quinolone levels; an increased incidence of seizures may occur with foscarnet

Drug Uptake

Absorption: Slow and erratic

Serum half-life: 16 hours

Time to peak serum concentration: 3-5 hours

Pregnancy Risk Factor C

Dosage Forms Tablet: 200 mg

Generic Available No

Sparine® *see Promazine on page 803*

Spasmolin® *see Hyoscyamine, Atropine, Scopolamine, and Phenobarbital on page 493*

Spec-T® [OTC] *see Benzocaine on page 118*

Spectazole™ *see Econazole on page 344*

Spectinomycin *(spek ti noe MYE sin)*

Related Information

Nonviral Infectious Diseases *on page 1032*

Brand Names Trobicin®

Therapeutic Category Antibiotic, Miscellaneous

Use Treatment of uncomplicated gonorrhea (ineffective against syphilis)

Usual Dosage I.M.:

Children:

<45 kg: 40 mg/kg/dose 1 time

≥45 kg: See adult dose

Children >8 years who are allergic to PCNS/cephalosporins may be treated with oral tetracycline

Adults:

Uncomplicated urethral endocervical or rectal gonorrhea: 2 g deep I.M. or 4 g where antibiotic resistance is prevalent 1 time; 4 g (10 mL) dose should be given as two 5 mL injections, followed by doxycycline 100 mg twice daily for 7 days

Disseminated gonococcal infection: 2 g every 12 hours

Hemodialysis effects: 50% removed by hemodialysis

Mechanism of Action A bacteriostatic antibiotic that selectively binds to the 30s subunits of ribosomes, and thereby inhibiting bacterial protein synthesis

Local Anesthetic/Vasoconstrictor Precautions No information available to require special precautions

Effects on Dental Treatment No effects or complications reported

Other Adverse Effects <1%:
Central nervous system: Dizziness, headache, chills
Dermatologic: Urticaria, rash, pruritus
Gastrointestinal: Nausea, vomiting
Local: Pain at injection site
Drug Interactions No data reported
Drug Uptake
Duration of action: Up to 8 hours
Serum half-life: 1.7 hours
Time to peak serum concentration: Within 1 hour
Pregnancy Risk Factor B
Generic Available No

Spectrobid® *see* Bacampicillin *on page 106*

Spirapril (SPYE ra pril)
Related Information
Cardiovascular Diseases *on page 1010*
Brand Names Renormax®
Therapeutic Category Angiotensin-Converting Enzyme (ACE) Inhibitors
Use Management of mild to severe hypertension
Usual Dosage Adults: Oral: 12-48 mg once daily
Mechanism of Action Angiotensin-converting enzyme inhibitor; inhibits renin-angiotensin system
Local Anesthetic/Vasoconstrictor Precautions No information available to require special precautions
Effects on Dental Treatment No effects or complications reported
Other Adverse Effects
Cardiovascular: Hypotension (orthostatic)
Central nervous system: Headache, dizziness, migraine headache (exacerbation of), hypoesthesia
Dermatologic: Skin rash
Gastrointestinal: Nausea, diarrhea, vomiting
Neuromuscular & skeletal: Back pain
Ocular: Conjunctivitis
Respiratory: Cough
Warnings/Precautions Use with caution in patients with previous hypersensitivity to other ACE inhibitors, pregnancy, renal/hepatic insufficiency, hyperkalemia, autoimmune disease
Drug Uptake
Absorption: Oral: 53% to 60% (delayed by high fat meals)
Serum half-life: 1-2 hours
Pregnancy Risk Factor C (first trimester); D (second and third trimesters)
Dosage Forms Tablet: 3 mg, 6 mg, 12 mg, 24 mg
Generic Available No

Spironazide® *see* Hydrochlorothiazide and Spironolactone *on page 477*

Spironolactone (speer on oh LAK tone)
Related Information
Cardiovascular Diseases *on page 1010*
Brand Names Aldactone®
Canadian/Mexican Brand Names Novo-Spiroton® (Canada)
Therapeutic Category Diuretic, Potassium Sparing
Use Management of edema associated with excessive aldosterone excretion; hypertension; primary hyperaldosteronism; hypokalemia; treatment of hirsutism; cirrhosis of liver accompanied by edema or ascites
Usual Dosage Administration with food increases absorption. To reduce delay in onset of effect, a loading dose of 2 or 3 times the daily dose may be administered on the first day of therapy. Oral:
Children:
Diuretic, hypertension: 1.5-3.5 mg/kg/day in divided doses every 6-24 hours
Diagnosis of primary aldosteronism: 125-375 mg/m²/day in divided doses
Vaso-occlusive disease: 7.5 mg/kg/day in divided doses twice daily (not FDA approved)
Adults:
Edema, hypertension, hypokalemia: 25-200 mg/day in 1-2 divided doses
Diagnosis of primary aldosteronism: 100-400 mg/day in 1-2 divided doses
Elderly: Initial: 25-50 mg/day in 1-2 divided doses, increasing by 25-50 mg every 5 days as needed
Mechanism of Action Competes with aldosterone for receptor sites in the distal renal tubules, increasing sodium chloride and water excretion while conserving
(Continued)

Spironolactone *(Continued)*

potassium and hydrogen ions; may block the effect of aldosterone on arteriolar smooth muscle as well

Local Anesthetic/Vasoconstrictor Precautions No information available to require special precautions

Effects on Dental Treatment No effects or complications reported

Other Adverse Effects

1% to 10%:

Cardiovascular: Hypotension, edema, bradycardia, congestive heart failure

Central nervous system: Dizziness, fatigue, headache

Dermatologic: Rash

Gastrointestinal: Nausea, constipation

Respiratory: Dyspnea

<1%:

Cardiovascular: Flushing

Endocrine & metabolic: Hyperkalemia, dehydration, hyponatremia, gynecomastia, hyperchloremia, metabolic acidosis, postmenopausal bleeding

Genitourinary: Inability to achieve or maintain an erection

Drug Interactions Spironolactone potentiates the effects of other diuretics and antihypertensives; spironolactone has been shown to increase the half-life of digoxin; this may result in increased serum digoxin levels and digoxin toxicity

Drug Uptake

Serum half-life: 78-84 minutes

Time to peak serum concentration: Within 1-3 hours (primarily as the active metabolite)

Pregnancy Risk Factor D

Dosage Forms Tablet: 25 mg, 50 mg, 100 mg

Generic Available Yes

Spironolactone and Hydrochlorothiazide *see* Hydrochlorothiazide and Spironolactone *on page 477*

Spirozide® *see* Hydrochlorothiazide and Spironolactone *on page 477*

Sporanox® *see* Itraconazole *on page 529*

Sportscreme® [OTC] *see* Triethanolamine Salicylate *on page 960*

S-P-T *see* Thyroid *on page 930*

SRC® Expectorant *see* Hydrocodone, Pseudoephedrine, and Guaifenesin *on page 484*

SSD® AF *see* Silver Sulfadiazine *on page 865*

SSD® Cream *see* Silver Sulfadiazine *on page 865*

SSKI® *see* Potassium Iodide *on page 781*

Stadol® *see* Butorphanol *on page 158*

Stadol® NS *see* Butorphanol *on page 158*

Stagesic® [5/500] *see* Hydrocodone and Acetaminophen *on page 478*

Stahist® *see* Chlorpheniramine, Phenylephrine, Phenylpropanolamine, and Belladonna Alkaloids *on page 221*

Stannous Fluoride *see* Fluoride *on page 415*

Stanozolol *(stan OH zoe lole)*

Brand Names Winstrol®

Therapeutic Category Anabolic Steroid

Use Prophylactic use against hereditary angioedema

Usual Dosage

Children: Acute attacks:

<6 years: 1 mg/day

6-12 years: 2 mg/day

Adults: Oral: Initial: 2 mg 3 times/day, may then reduce to a maintenance dose of 2 mg/day or 2 mg every other day after 1-3 months

Mechanism of Action Synthetic testosterone derivative with similar androgenic and anabolic actions

Local Anesthetic/Vasoconstrictor Precautions No information available to require special precautions

Effects on Dental Treatment No effects or complications reported

Other Adverse Effects

Male:

Postpubertal:

>10%:

Dermatologic: Acne

Endocrine & metabolic: Gynecomastia

Genitourinary: Bladder irritability, priapism

1% to 10%:
  Central nervous system: Insomnia, chills
  Endocrine & metabolic: Decreased libido,
  Gastrointestinal: Nausea, diarrhea
  Genitourinary: Prostatic hypertrophy (elderly)
  Hematologic: Iron deficiency anemia, suppression of clotting factors
  Hepatic: Hepatic dysfunction
<1%: Hepatic: Hepatic necrosis, hepatocellular carcinoma
Prepubertal:
  >10%:
    Dermatologic: Acne
    Endocrine & metabolic: Virilism
  1% to 10%:
    Central nervous system: Chills, insomnia
    Dermatologic: Hyperpigmentation
    Gastrointestinal: Diarrhea, nausea
    Hematologic: Iron deficiency anemia, suppression of clotting
  <1%: Hepatic: Hepatic necrosis, hepatocellular carcinoma

Female:
  >10%: Endocrine & metabolic: Virilism
  1% to 10%:
    Central nervous system: Chills, insomnia
    Endocrine & metabolic: Hypercalcemia
    Gastrointestinal: Nausea, diarrhea
    Hematologic: Iron deficiency anemia, suppression of clotting factors
    Hepatic: Hepatic dysfunction
  <1%: Hepatic: Hepatic necrosis, hepatocellular carcinoma
Drug Interactions Stanozolol enhances the hypoprothrombinemic effects of oral anticoagulants; enhances the hypoglycemic effects of insulin and sulfonylureas (oral hypoglycemics)
Pregnancy Risk Factor X
Dosage Forms Tablet: 2 mg
Generic Available No

Staphcillin® see Methicillin on page 611
Staticin® Topical see Erythromycin, Topical on page 364

Stavudine (STAV yoo deen)
Related Information
  HIV Infection and AIDS on page 1024
  Systemic Viral Diseases on page 1047
Brand Names Zerit®
Therapeutic Category Antiviral Agent, Oral; Antiviral Agent, Parenteral
Use For the treatment of adults with advanced HIV infection who are intolerant to approved therapies with proven clinical benefit or who have experienced significant clinical or immunologic deterioration while receiving these therapies, or for whom such therapies are contraindicated
Usual Dosage
  Adults: Oral:
    ≥60 kg: 40 mg every 12 hours
    <60 kg: 30 mg every 12 hours
    Dose may be cut in half if symptoms of peripheral neuropathy occur
Mechanism of Action Inhibits reverse transcriptase of the human immunodeficiency virus (HIV)
Local Anesthetic/Vasoconstrictor Precautions No information available to require special precautions
Effects on Dental Treatment No effects or complications reported
Other Adverse Effects
  >10%: Neuromuscular & skeletal: Peripheral neuropathy
  1% to 10%:
    Central nervous system: Headache, chills/fever, malaise, insomnia, anxiety, depression
    Gastrointestinal: Nausea, vomiting, diarrhea, pancreatitis, abdominal pain
    Neuromuscular & skeletal: Myalgia, back pain, weakness
Drug Interactions No data reported
Drug Uptake
  Peak serum level: 1 hour after administration
  Serum half-life: 1-1.6 hours
Pregnancy Risk Factor C
Dosage Forms
  Capsule: 15 mg, 20 mg, 30 mg, 40 mg
  Powder for oral solution: 1 mg/mL (200 mL)
  (Continued)

Stavudine *(Continued)*

Generic Available No

Stelazine® *see* Trifluoperazine *on page 960*

Stemex® *see* Paramethasone Acetate *on page 724*

Sterapred® *see* Prednisone *on page 789*

Stilphostrol® *see* Diethylstilbestrol *on page 310*

Stimate™ *see* Desmopressin Acetate *on page 289*

St Joseph® Adult Chewable Aspirin [OTC] *see* Aspirin *on page 90*

St. Joseph® Cough Suppressant [OTC] *see* Dextromethorphan *on page 298*

St. Joseph® Measured Dose Nasal Solution [OTC] *see* Phenylephrine *on page 752*

Stop® [OTC] *see* Fluoride *on page 415*

Streptase® *see* Streptokinase *on this page*

Streptokinase *(strep toe KYE nase)*

Related Information

Cardiovascular Diseases *on page 1010*

Brand Names Kabikinase®; Streptase®

Therapeutic Category Thrombolytic Agent

Use Thrombolytic agent used in treatment of recent severe or massive deep vein thrombosis, pulmonary emboli, myocardial infarction, and occluded arteriovenous cannulas

Usual Dosage I.V.:

Children: Safety and efficacy not established; limited studies have used 3500-4000 units/kg over 30 minutes followed by 1000-1500 units/kg/hour

Clotted catheter: 25,000 units, clamp for 2 hours then aspirate contents and flush with normal saline

Adults: Antibodies to streptokinase remain for at least 3-6 months after initial dose: Administration requires the use of an infusion pump

An intradermal skin test of 100 units has been suggested to predict allergic response to streptokinase. If a positive reaction is not seen after 15-20 minutes, a therapeutic dose may be administered.

Guidelines for acute myocardial infarction (AMI): 1.5 million units over 60 minutes

Administration:

Dilute two 750,000 unit vials of streptokinase with 5 mL dextrose 5% in water (D_5W) each, gently swirl to dissolve

Add this dose of the 1.5 million units to 150 mL D_5W

This should be infused over 60 minutes; an in-line filter ≥0.45 micron should be used

Monitor for the first few hours for signs of anaphylaxis or allergic reaction. **Infusion should be slowed if lowering of 25 mm Hg in blood pressure or terminated if asthmatic symptoms appear.**

Begin heparin 5000-10,000 unit bolus followed by 1000 units/hour approximately 3-4 hours after completion of streptokinase infusion or when PTT is <100 seconds

Guidelines for acute pulmonary embolism (APE): 3 million unit dose over 24 hours

Administration:

Dilute four 750,000 unit vials of streptokinase with 5 mL dextrose 5% in water (D_5W) each, gently swirl to dissolve

Add this dose of 3 million units to 250 mL D_5W, an in-line filter ≥0.45 micron should be used

Administer 250,000 units (23 mL) over 30 minutes followed by 100,000 units/hour (9 mL/hour) for 24 hours

Monitor for the first few hours for signs of anaphylaxis or allergic reaction. **Infusion should be slowed if blood pressure is lowered by 25 mm Hg or if asthmatic symptoms appear.**

Begin heparin 1000 units/hour about 3-4 hours after completion of streptokinase infusion or when PTT is <100 seconds

Monitor PT, PTT, and fibrinogen levels during therapy

Thromboses: 250,000 units to start, then 100,000 units/hour for 24-72 hours depending on location

Cannula occlusion: 250,000 units into cannula, clamp for 2 hours, then aspirate contents and flush with normal saline

Mechanism of Action Activates the conversion of plasminogen to plasmin by forming a complex, exposing plasminogen-activating site, and cleaving a peptide bond that converts plasminogen to plasmin; plasmin degrades fibrin, fibrinogen and other procoagulant proteins into soluble fragments; effective both outside and within the formed thrombus/embolus

Local Anesthetic/Vasoconstrictor Precautions No information available to require special precautions

Effects on Dental Treatment No effects or complications reported

Other Adverse Effects

>10%:

Cardiovascular: Hypotension, arrhythmias, trauma arrhythmias, cerebral hemorrhage

Dermatologic: Angioneurotic edema

Hematologic: Surface bleeding, internal bleeding

Ocular: Periorbital swelling

Respiratory: Bronchospasm

Miscellaneous: Anaphylaxis

<1%:

Cardiovascular: Flushing

Central nervous system: Headache, chills, fever

Dermatologic: Rash, itching

Gastrointestinal: Nausea, vomiting

Hematologic: Anemia

Neuromuscular & skeletal: Musculoskeletal pain

Ocular: Eye hemorrhage

Respiratory: Epistaxis

Miscellaneous: Sweating

Drug Interactions

Antifibrinolytic agents (aminocaproic acid) cause decreased effectiveness of streptokinase

Anticoagulants, antiplatelet agents cause increased risk of bleeding of streptokinase

Drug Uptake

Onset of action: Activation of plasminogen occurs almost immediately

Duration: Fibrinolytic effects last only a few hours, while anticoagulant effects can persist for 12-24 hours

Serum half-life: 83 minutes

Pregnancy Risk Factor C

Dosage Forms Powder for injection: 250,000 units (5 mL, 6.5 mL); 600,000 units (5 mL); 750,000 units (6 mL, 6.5 mL); 1,500,000 units (6.5 mL, 10 mL, 50 mL)

Generic Available No

Streptomycin (strep toe MYE sin)

Related Information

Nonviral Infectious Diseases *on page 1032*

Therapeutic Category Antibiotic, Aminoglycoside; Antitubercular Agent

Use Combination therapy of active tuberculosis; used in combination with other agents for treatment of streptococcal or enterococcal endocarditis, mycobacterial infections, plague, tularemia, and brucellosis. Streptomycin is indicated for persons from endemic areas of drug-resistant *Mycobacterium tuberculosis* or who are HIV infected.

Usual Dosage Intramuscular (may also be given intravenous piggyback):

Tuberculosis therapy: **Note:** A four-drug regimen (isoniazid, rifampin, pyrazinamide and either streptomycin or ethambutol) is preferred for the initial, empiric treatment of TB. When the drug susceptibility results are available, the regimen should be altered as appropriate.

Patients with TB and without HIV infection:

OPTION 1:

Isoniazid resistance rate <4%: Administer daily isoniazid, rifampin, and pyrazinamide for 8 weeks followed by isoniazid and rifampin daily or directly observed therapy (DOT) 2-3 times/week for 16 weeks

If isoniazid resistance rate is not documented, ethambutol or streptomycin should also be administered until susceptibility to isoniazid or rifampin is demonstrated. Continue treatment for at least 6 months or 3 months beyond culture conversion.

OPTION 2: Administer daily isoniazid, rifampin, pyrazinamide, and either streptomycin or ethambutol for 2 weeks followed by DOT 2 times/week administration of the same drugs for 6 weeks, and subsequently, with isoniazid and rifampin DOT 2 times/week administration for 16 weeks

OPTION 3: Administer isoniazid, rifampin, pyrazinamide, and either ethambutol or streptomycin by DOT 3 times/week for 6 months

Patients with TB and with HIV infection: Administer any of the above OPTIONS 1, 2 or 3, however, treatment should be continued for a total of 9 months and at least 6 months beyond culture conversion

(Continued)

Streptomycin *(Continued)*

Note: Some experts recommend that the duration of therapy should be extended to 9 months for patients with disseminated disease, miliary disease, disease involving the bones or joints, or tuberculosis lymphadenitis

Children:
Daily therapy: 20-30 mg/kg/day (maximum: 1 g/day)
Directly observed therapy (DOT): Twice weekly: 25-30 mg/kg (maximum: 1.5 g)
DOT: 3 times/week: 25-30 mg/kg (maximum: 1 g)
Adults:
Daily therapy: 15 mg/kg/day (maximum: 1 g)
Directly observed therapy (DOT): Twice weekly: 25-30 mg/kg (maximum: 1.5 g)
DOT: 3 times/week: 25-30 mg/kg (maximum: 1 g)
Enterococcal endocarditis: 1 g every 12 hours for 2 weeks, 500 mg every 12 hours for 4 weeks in combination with penicillin
Streptococcal endocarditis: 1 g every 12 hours for 1 week, 500 mg every 12 hours for 1 week
Tularemia: 1-2 g/day in divided doses for 7-10 days or until patient is afebrile for 5-7 days
Plague: 2-4 g/day in divided doses until the patient is afebrile for at least 3 days
Elderly: 10 mg/kg/day, not to exceed 750 mg/day; dosing interval should be adjusted for renal function; some authors suggest not to give more than 5 days/week or give as 20-25 mg/dose twice weekly
Mechanism of Action Inhibits bacterial protein synthesis by binding directly to the 30S ribosomal subunits causing faulty peptide sequence to form in the protein chain
Local Anesthetic/Vasoconstrictor Precautions No information available to require special precautions
Effects on Dental Treatment No effects or complications reported
Other Adverse Effects
1% to 10%:
Neuromuscular & skeletal: Neuromuscular blockade
Otic: Ototoxicity (auditory), ototoxicity (vestibular)
Renal: Nephrotoxicity
<1%:
Cardiovascular: Hypotension
Central nervous system: Drug fever, headache, drowsiness
Dermatologic: Skin rash
Gastrointestinal: Nausea, vomiting
Hematologic: Eosinophilia, anemia
Neuromuscular & skeletal: Paresthesia, tremor, arthralgia, weakness
Respiratory: Dyspnea
Drug Interactions
Concurrent use of amphotericin, loop diuretics may increase nephrotoxicity of streptomycin
Drug Uptake
Absorption: Oral: Absorbed poorly; usually given parenterally
Serum half-life: Adults: 2-4.7 hours, prolonged with renal impairment
Time to peak serum concentration: Within 1 hour
Pregnancy Risk Factor D
Generic Available Yes

Streptozocin *(strep toe ZOE sin)*
Brand Names Zanosar®
Therapeutic Category Antineoplastic Agent, Alkylating Agent (Nitrosourea)
Use Treat metastatic islet cell carcinoma of the pancreas, carcinoid tumor and syndrome, Hodgkin's disease, palliative treatment of colorectal cancer
Usual Dosage I.V. (refer to individual protocols): Children and Adults: 500 mg/m^2 for 5 days every 4-6 weeks until optimal benefit or toxicity occurs or may be given in single dose 1000 mg/m^2 at weekly intervals for 2 doses, then increased to 1500 mg/m^2; usual course of therapy: 4-6 weeks
Mechanism of Action Interferes with the normal function of DNA by alkylation and cross-linking the strands of DNA, and by possible protein modification
Local Anesthetic/Vasoconstrictor Precautions No information available to require special precautions
Effects on Dental Treatment No effects or complications reported
Other Adverse Effects
>10%:
Endocrine & metabolic: Hypoalbuminemia, hypophosphatemia
Gastrointestinal: Nausea and vomiting in all patients usually 1-4 hours after infusion; diarrhea in 10% of patients
Emetic potential: High (>90%)

Hepatic: Elevated LFTs

Renal: Renal dysfunction occurs in 65% of patients; proteinuria, decreased Cl_{cr}, elevated BUN, renal tubular acidosis; be careful with patients on other nephrotoxic agents; nephrotoxicity (25% to 75% of patients)

1% to 10%:

Endocrine & metabolic: Hypoglycemia is seen in 6% of patients; may be prevented with the administration of nicotinamide

Gastrointestinal: Diarrhea

Local: Pain at injection site

<1%:

Central nervous system: Confusion, lethargy, depression

Hematologic: Leukopenia, thrombocytopenia

Myelosuppressive: WBC: Mild; Platelets: Mild; Onset (days): 7; Nadir (days): 14; Recovery (days): 21

Hepatic: Liver dysfunction

Secondary malignancy

Drug Interactions

Phenytoin results in negation of streptozocin cytotoxicity

Doxorubicin prolongs half-life of streptozocin and thus prolongs leukopenia and thrombocytopenia

Drug Uptake

Serum half-life: 35-40 minutes

Pregnancy Risk Factor C

Generic Available No

Stresstabs® 600 Advanced Formula Tablets [OTC] see Vitamins, Multiple on page 995

Stromectol® see Ivermectin on page 530

Stuartnatal® 1 + 1 see Vitamins, Multiple on page 995

Stuart Prenatal® [OTC] see Vitamins, Multiple on page 995

Sublimaze® see Fentanyl on page 398

Sucralfate (soo KRAL fate)

Related Information

Patients Undergoing Cancer Therapy on page 1083

Brand Names Carafate®

Canadian/Mexican Brand Names Antepsin® (Mexico); Novo-Sucralate® (Canada); Sulcrate® (Canada); Sulcrate® Suspension Plus (Canada)

Therapeutic Category Gastrointestinal Agent, Miscellaneous

Synonyms Sucralfato (Mexico)

Use Short-term management of duodenal ulcers

Unlabeled uses: Gastric ulcers; maintenance of duodenal ulcers; suspension may be used topically for treatment of stomatitis due to cancer chemotherapy and other causes of esophageal and gastric erosions; GERD, esophagitis, treatment of NSAID mucosal damage, prevention of stress ulcers, postschlerotherapy for esophageal variceal bleeding.

Usual Dosage Oral:

Children: Dose not established, doses of 40-80 mg/kg/day divided every 6 hours have been used

Stomatitis: 2.5-5 mL (1 g/15 mL suspension), swish and spit or swish and swallow 4 times/day

Adults:

Stress ulcer prophylaxis: 1 g 4 times/day

Stress ulcer treatment: 1 g every 4 hours

Duodenal ulcer:

Treatment: 1 g 4 times/day, 1 hour before meals or food and at bedtime for 4-8 weeks, or alternatively 2 g twice daily; treatment is recommended for 4-8 weeks in adults, the elderly will require 12 weeks

Maintenance: Prophylaxis: 1 g twice daily

Stomatitis: 1 g/15 mL suspension, swish and spit or swish and swallow 4 times/day

Mechanism of Action Forms a complex by binding with positively charged proteins in exudates, forming a viscous paste-like, adhesive substance, when combined with gastric acid adheres to the damaged mucosal area. This selectively forms a protective coating that protects the lining against peptic acid, pepsin, and bile salts.

Local Anesthetic/Vasoconstrictor Precautions No information available to require special precautions

Effects on Dental Treatment No effects or complications reported

Other Adverse Effects

1% to 10%: Gastrointestinal: Constipation

(Continued)

Sucralfate *(Continued)*

<1%:
Central nervous system: Dizziness, sleepiness, vertigo
Dermatologic: Rash, pruritus
Gastrointestinal: Diarrhea, nausea, gastric discomfort, indigestion, dry mouth
Neuromuscular & skeletal: Back pain

Drug Interactions Decreased effect:
Digoxin, phenytoin, theophylline, ciprofloxacin, itraconazole; because of the potential for sucralfate to alter the absorption of some drugs, separate administration (2 hours before or after) should be considered when alterations in bioavailability are believed to be critical

Antacids/cimetidine/ranitidine: Do not administer concomitantly with sucralfate; these types of drugs reduce acidity; sucralfate requires gastric acid for it's mechanism of action (ie, to form a gel in the stomach as a protective barrier)

Drug Uptake
Onset of action: Paste formation and ulcer adhesion occur within 1-2 hours
Duration: Up to 6 hours
Absorption: Oral: <5%

Pregnancy Risk Factor B

Dosage Forms
Suspension, oral: 1 g/10 mL (420 mL)
Tablet: 1 g

Generic Available Yes

Sucralfato (Mexico) *see* Sucralfate *on previous page*

Sucrets® Cough Calmers [OTC] *see* Dextromethorphan *on page 298*

Sucrets® Sore Throat [OTC] *see* Hexylresorcinol *on page 471*

Sudafed® [OTC] *see* Pseudoephedrine *on page 820*

Sudafed® 12 Hour [OTC] *see* Pseudoephedrine *on page 820*

Sudafed® Cold & Cough Liquid Caps [OTC] *see* Guaifenesin, Pseudoephedrine, and Dextromethorphan *on page 456*

Sudafed Plus® Liquid [OTC] *see* Chlorpheniramine and Pseudoephedrine *on page 219*

Sudafed Plus® Tablet [OTC] *see* Chlorpheniramine and Pseudoephedrine *on page 219*

Sudafed® Severe Cold [OTC] *see* Acetaminophen, Dextromethorphan, and Pseudoephedrine *on page 25*

Sufenta® *see* Sufentanil *on this page*

Sufentanil *(soo FEN ta nil)*

Related Information
Narcotic Agonists *on page 1141*

Brand Names Sufenta®

Therapeutic Category Analgesic, Narcotic

Use Analgesic supplement in maintenance of balanced general anesthesia

Usual Dosage
Children <12 years: 10-25 mcg/kg with 100% O_2, maintenance: 25-50 mcg as needed

Adults: Dose should be based on body weight. **Note:** In obese patients (ie, >20% above ideal body weight), use lean body weight to determine dosage.
1-2 mcg/kg with NO_2/O_2 for endotracheal intubation; maintenance: 10-25 mcg as needed
2-8 mcg/kg with NO_2/O_2 more complicated major surgical procedures; maintenance: 10-50 mcg as needed
8-30 mcg/kg with 100% O_2 and muscle relaxant produces sleep; at doses ≥8 mcg/kg maintains a deep level of anesthesia; maintenance: 10-50 mcg as needed

Mechanism of Action Binds to opiate receptors in the CNS causing inhibition of ascending pain pathways, altering the perception of and response to pain; ultra-short-acting narcotic

Local Anesthetic/Vasoconstrictor Precautions No information available to require special precautions

Effects on Dental Treatment No effects or complications reported

Other Adverse Effects
>10%:
Cardiovascular: Bradycardia, hypotension
Central nervous system: Drowsiness
Gastrointestinal: Nausea, vomiting
Respiratory: Respiratory depression
1% to 10%:
Cardiovascular: Cardiac arrhythmias, orthostatic hypotension

    Central nervous system: Confusion, CNS depression
    Gastrointestinal: Biliary spasm
    Ocular: Blurred vision
<1%:
    Cardiovascular: Circulatory depression
    Central nervous system: Convulsions, dysesthesia, paradoxical CNS excitation or delirium; mental depression, dizziness
    Dermatologic: Skin rash, urticaria, itching
    Gastrointestinal: Biliary spasm
    Genitourinary: Urinary tract spasm
    Respiratory: Laryngospasm, bronchospasm
    Miscellaneous: Cold, clammy skin; physical and psychological dependence with prolonged use
Drug Interactions Increased effect/toxicity with CNS depressants, beta-blockers
Drug Uptake
  Onset of action: 1-3 minutes
  Duration: Dose dependent
Pregnancy Risk Factor C
Dosage Forms Injection, as citrate: 50 mcg/mL (1 mL, 2 mL, 5 mL)
  Generic Available Yes

Sugar-Free Liquid Pharmaceuticals *see page 1190*

Sular™ *see Nisoldipine on page 683*

Sulconazole (sul KON a zole)
Brand Names Exelderm®
Therapeutic Category Antifungal Agent, Topical
Synonyms Sulconazol, Nitrato De (Mexico)
Use Treatment of superficial fungal infections of the skin, including tinea cruris (jock itch), tinea corporis (ringworm), tinea versicolor, and possibly tinea pedis (athlete's foot - cream only)
Usual Dosage Adults: Topical: Apply a small amount to the affected area and gently massage once or twice daily for 3 weeks (tinea cruris, tinea corporis, tinea versicolor) to 4 weeks (tinea pedis).
Mechanism of Action Substituted imidazole derivative which inhibits metabolic reactions necessary for the synthesis of ergosterol, an essential membrane component. The end result is usually fungistatic; however, sulconazole may act as a fungicide in *Candida albicans* and parapsilosis during certain growth phases.
Local Anesthetic/Vasoconstrictor Precautions No information available to require special precautions
Effects on Dental Treatment No effects or complications reported
Other Adverse Effects 1% to 10%: Local: Itching, burning, stinging, redness
Drug Interactions No data reported
Drug Uptake Absorption: Topical: About 8.7% absorbed percutaneously
Pregnancy Risk Factor C
Dosage Forms
  Cream, as nitrate: 1% (15 g, 30 g, 60 g)
  Solution, as nitrate, topical: 1% (30 mL)
  Generic Available No

Sulconazol, Nitrato De (Mexico) *see Sulconazole on this page*

Sulf-10® Ophthalmic *see Sulfacetamide Sodium on next page*

Sulfabenzamide, Sulfacetamide, and Sulfathiazole
(sul fa BENZ a mide, sul fa SEE ta mide & sul fa THYE a zole)
Brand Names Femguard®; Gyne-Sulf®; Sulfa-Gyn®; Sulfa-Trip®; Sultrin™; Trysul®; V.V.S.®
Therapeutic Category Antibiotic, Vaginal
Use Treatment of *Haemophilus vaginalis* vaginitis
Usual Dosage Adults:
  Cream: Insert one applicatorful in vagina twice daily for 4-6 days; dosage may then be decreased to ½ to ¼ of an applicatorful twice daily
  Tablet: Insert one intravaginally twice daily for 10 days
Mechanism of Action Interferes with microbial folic acid synthesis and growth via inhibition of para-aminobenzoic acid metabolism
Local Anesthetic/Vasoconstrictor Precautions No information available to require special precautions
Effects on Dental Treatment No effects or complications reported
Other Adverse Effects
  >10%:
    Dermatologic: Pruritus, urticaria
(Continued)

Sulfabenzamide, Sulfacetamide, and Sulfathiazole
(Continued)

Local: Irritation
<1%:
  Dermatologic: Stevens-Johnson syndrome
  Miscellaneous: Allergic reactions
Drug Interactions No data reported
Drug Uptake
  Absorption: Absorption from the vagina is variable and unreliable
Pregnancy Risk Factor C
Generic Available Yes

Sulfacetamide Sodium (sul fa SEE ta mide SOW dee um)
Brand Names AK-Sulf® Ophthalmic; Bleph®-10 Ophthalmic; Cetamide® Ophthalmic; Isopto® Cetamide® Ophthalmic; Klaron® Lotion; Ocusulf-10® Ophthalmic; Sebizon® Topical Lotion; Sodium Sulamyd® Ophthalmic; Sulf-10® Ophthalmic
Therapeutic Category Antibiotic, Ophthalmic
Use Treatment and prophylaxis of conjunctivitis due to susceptible organisms; corneal ulcers; adjunctive treatment with systemic sulfonamides for therapy of trachoma; topical application in scaling dermatosis (seborrheic); bacterial infections of the skin
Usual Dosage
  Children >2 months and Adults: Ophthalmic:
    Ointment: Apply to lower conjunctival sac 1-4 times/day and at bedtime
    Solution: Instill 1-3 drops several times daily up to every 2-3 hours in lower conjunctival sac during waking hours and less frequently at night
  Children >12 years and Adults: Topical:
    Seborrheic dermatitis: Apply at bedtime and allow to remain overnight; in severe cases, may apply twice daily
    Secondary cutaneous bacterial infections: Apply 2-4 times/day until infection clears
Mechanism of Action Interferes with bacterial growth by inhibiting bacterial folic acid synthesis through competitive antagonism of PABA
Local Anesthetic/Vasoconstrictor Precautions No information available to require special precautions
Effects on Dental Treatment No effects or complications reported
Other Adverse Effects
  1% to 10%: Local: Irritation, stinging, burning
  <1%:
    Central nervous system: Headache, browache
    Dermatologic: Stevens-Johnson syndrome, exfoliative dermatitis, toxic epidermal necrolysis
    Ocular: Blurred vision
    Miscellaneous: Hypersensitivity reactions
Drug Interactions Decreased effect: Silver, gentamicin (antagonism)
Drug Uptake
  Serum half-life: 7-13 hours
Pregnancy Risk Factor C
Generic Available Yes

Sulfacetamide Sodium and Fluorometholone
(sul fa SEE ta mide SOW dee um & flure oh METH oh lone)
Brand Names FML-S® Ophthalmic Suspension
Therapeutic Category Antibiotic, Ophthalmic; Anti-inflammatory Agent, Ophthalmic
Use Steroid-responsive inflammatory ocular conditions where infection is present or there is a risk of infection
Local Anesthetic/Vasoconstrictor Precautions No information available to require special precautions
Effects on Dental Treatment No effects or complications reported
Pregnancy Risk Factor C
Generic Available Yes

Sulfacetamide Sodium and Phenylephrine
(sul fa SEE ta mide SOW dee um & fen il EF rin)
Brand Names Vasosulf® Ophthalmic
Therapeutic Category Antibiotic, Ophthalmic; Ophthalmic Agent, Vasoconstrictor

Local Anesthetic/Vasoconstrictor Precautions No information available to require special precautions
Effects on Dental Treatment No effects or complications reported
Pregnancy Risk Factor C
Generic Available Yes

Sulfacetamide Sodium and Prednisolone
(sul fa SEE ta mide SOW dee um & pred NIS oh lone)
Brand Names AK-Cide® Ophthalmic; Blephamide® Ophthalmic; Cetapred® Ophthalmic; Isopto® Cetapred® Ophthalmic; Metimyd® Ophthalmic; Vasocidin® Ophthalmic
Therapeutic Category Antibiotic, Ophthalmic; Corticosteroid, Ophthalmic
Use Steroid-responsive inflammatory ocular conditions where infection is present or there is a risk of infection; ophthalmic suspension may be used as an otic preparation
Usual Dosage Children >2 months and Adults: Ophthalmic:
Ointment: Apply to lower conjunctival sac 1-4 times/day
Solution: Instill 1-3 drops every 2-3 hours while awake
Mechanism of Action Interferes with bacterial growth by inhibiting bacterial folic acid synthesis through competitive antagonism of PABA; decreases inflammation by suppression of migration of polymorphonuclear leukocytes and reversal of increased capillary permeability; suppresses the immune system by reducing activity and volume of the lymphatic system
Local Anesthetic/Vasoconstrictor Precautions No information available to require special precautions
Effects on Dental Treatment No effects or complications reported
Other Adverse Effects
1% to 10%: Local: Burning, stinging
<1%:
Central nervous system: Vertigo, seizures, psychoses, pseudotumor cerebri, headache
Dermatologic: Stevens-Johnson syndrome, skin atrophy
Endocrine & metabolic: Cushing's syndrome, pituitary-adrenal axis suppression, growth suppression
Gastrointestinal: Peptic ulcer, nausea, vomiting
Neuromuscular & skeletal: Muscle weakness, osteoporosis, fractures
Ocular: Cataracts, glaucoma
Drug Interactions Decreased effect: Silver, gentamicin, vaccines, toxoids
Pregnancy Risk Factor C
Generic Available Yes

Sulfacetamide Sodium and Sulfur see Sulfur and Sulfacetamide Sodium on page 898

Sulfacet-R® Topical see Sulfur and Sulfacetamide Sodium on page 898

Sulfacytine (sul fa SYE teen)
Brand Names Renoquid®
Therapeutic Category Antibiotic, Sulfonamide Derivative
Use Treatment of urinary tract infections
Usual Dosage Adults: Oral: Initial: 500 mg, then 250 mg every 4 hours for 10 days
Local Anesthetic/Vasoconstrictor Precautions No information available to require special precautions
Effects on Dental Treatment No effects or complications reported
Other Adverse Effects
>10%:
Central nervous system: Fever, dizziness, headache
Dermatologic: Itching, skin rash, photosensitivity
Gastrointestinal: Anorexia, nausea, vomiting, diarrhea
1% to 10%:
Dermatologic: Stevens-Johnson syndrome, Lyell's syndrome
Hematologic: Granulocytopenia, leukopenia, thrombocytopenia, aplastic anemia, hemolytic anemia
Hepatic: Hepatitis
<1%:
Endocrine & metabolic: Thyroid function disturbance
Genitourinary: Crystalluria
Hepatic: Jaundice
Renal: Hematuria, interstitial nephritis, acute nephropathy
Miscellaneous: Serum sickness-like reactions
Pregnancy Risk Factor B (D at term)
Generic Available No

Sulfadiazine (sul fa DYE a zeen)

Brand Names Microsulfon®

Canadian/Mexican Brand Names Coptin® (Canada)

Therapeutic Category Antibiotic, Sulfonamide Derivative

Use Treatment of urinary tract infections and nocardiosis, rheumatic fever prophylaxis; adjunctive treatment in toxoplasmosis; uncomplicated attack of malaria

Usual Dosage Oral:

Congenital toxoplasmosis:

Newborns and Children <2 months: 100 mg/kg/day divided every 6 hours in conjunction with pyrimethamine 1 mg/kg/day once daily and supplemental folinic acid 5 mg every 3 days for 6 months

Children >2 months: 25-50 mg/kg/dose 4 times/day

Toxoplasmosis:

Children: 120-150 mg/kg/day, maximum dose: 6 g/day; divided every 6 hours in conjunction with pyrimethamine 2 mg/kg/day divided every 12 hours for 3 days followed by 1 mg/kg/day once daily (maximum: 25 mg/day) with supplemental folinic acid

Adults: 2-8 g/day divided every 6 hours in conjunction with pyrimethamine 25 mg/day and with supplemental folinic acid

Mechanism of Action Interferes with bacterial growth by inhibiting bacterial folic acid synthesis through competitive antagonism of PABA

Local Anesthetic/Vasoconstrictor Precautions No information available to require special precautions

Effects on Dental Treatment No effects or complications reported

Other Adverse Effects

>10%:

Central nervous system: Fever, dizziness, headache

Dermatologic: Itching, skin rash, photosensitivity

Gastrointestinal: Anorexia, nausea, vomiting, diarrhea

1% to 10%:

Dermatologic: Lyell's syndrome, Stevens-Johnson syndrome

Hematologic: Granulocytopenia, leukopenia, thrombocytopenia, aplastic anemia, hemolytic anemia

Hepatic: Hepatitis

<1%:

Endocrine & metabolic: Thyroid function disturbance

Genitourinary: Crystalluria

Hepatic: Jaundice

Renal: Interstitial nephritis, acute nephropathy, hematuria

Miscellaneous: Serum sickness-like reactions

Drug Interactions Decreased effect with PABA or PABA metabolites of drugs (eg, procaine, proparacaine, tetracaine, sunscreens); decreased effect of oral anticoagulants and oral hypoglycemic agents

Drug Uptake

Absorption: Oral: Well absorbed

Serum half-life: 10 hours

Time to peak serum concentration: Within 3-6 hours

Pregnancy Risk Factor B (D at term)

Generic Available Yes

Sulfadiazine, Sulfamethazine, and Sulfamerazine

(sul fa DYE a zeen sul fa METH a zeen & sul fa MER a zeen)

Therapeutic Category Antibiotic, Sulfonamide Derivative; Antibiotic, Vaginal

Synonyms Multiple Sulfonamides; Trisulfapyrimidines

Use Treatment of toxoplasmosis

Usual Dosage Adults: Oral: 2-4 g to start, then 2-4 g/day in 3-6 divided doses

Mechanism of Action Interferes with microbial folic acid synthesis and growth via inhibition of para-aminobenzoic acid metabolism

Local Anesthetic/Vasoconstrictor Precautions No information available to require special precautions

Effects on Dental Treatment No effects or complications reported

Pregnancy Risk Factor B (D at term)

Generic Available No

Sulfadoxine and Pyrimethamine

(sul fa DOKS een & peer i METH a meen)

Brand Names Fansidar®

Therapeutic Category Antimalarial Agent

Use Treatment of *Plasmodium falciparum* malaria in patients in whom chloroquine resistance is suspected; malaria prophylaxis for travelers to areas where chloroquine-resistant malaria is endemic

Usual Dosage Children and Adults: Oral:

Treatment of acute attack of malaria: A single dose of the following number of Fansidar® tablets is used in sequence with quinine or alone:

2-11 months: $1/4$ tablet
1-3 years: $1/2$ tablet
4-8 years: 1 tablet
9-14 years: 2 tablets
>14 years: 2-3 tablets

Malaria prophylaxis:

The first dose of Fansidar® should be taken 1-2 days before departure to an endemic area (CDC recommends that therapy be initiated 1-2 weeks before such travel), administration should be continued during the stay and for 4-6 weeks after return. Dose = pyrimethamine 0.5 mg/kg/dose and sulfadoxine 10 mg/kg/dose up to a maximum of 25 mg pyrimethamine and 500 mg sulfadoxine/dose weekly.

2-11 months: $1/8$ tablet weekly **or** $1/4$ tablet once every 2 weeks
1-3 years: $1/4$ tablet once weekly **or** $1/2$ tablet once every 2 weeks
4-8 years: $1/2$ tablet once weekly **or** 1 tablet once every 2 weeks
9-14 years: $3/4$ tablet once weekly **or** $11/2$ tablets once every 2 weeks
>14 years: 1 tablet once weekly **or** 2 tablets once every 2 weeks

Mechanism of Action Sulfadoxine interferes with bacterial folic acid synthesis and growth via competitive inhibition of para-aminiobenzoic acid; pyrimethamine inhibits microbial dihydrofolate reductase, resulting in inhibition of tetrahydrofolic acid synthesis

Local Anesthetic/Vasoconstrictor Precautions No information available to require special precautions

Effects on Dental Treatment No effects or complications reported

Other Adverse Effects

>10%:
Central nervous system: Ataxia, seizures, headache
Dermatologic: Photosensitivity
Gastrointestinal: Atrophic glossitis, vomiting, gastritis
Hematologic: Megaloblastic anemia, leukopenia, thrombocytopenia, pancytopenia
Neuromuscular & skeletal: Tremors
Miscellaneous: Hypersensitivity

1% to 10%:
Dermatologic: Stevens-Johnson syndrome
Hepatic: Hepatitis

<1%:
Dermatologic: Erythema multiforme, toxic epidermal necrolysis, rash
Endocrine & metabolic: Thyroid function dysfunction
Gastrointestinal: Anorexia, glossitis
Genitourinary: Crystalluria
Hepatic: Hepatic necrosis
Respiratory: Respiratory failure

Drug Interactions
Decreased effect with PABA or PABA metabolites of local anesthetics
Increased toxicity with methotrexate, other sulfonamides, co-trimoxazole

Drug Uptake
Absorption: Oral: Well absorbed
Serum half-life:
Pyrimethamine: 80-95 hours
Sulfadoxine: 5-8 days
Time to peak serum concentration: Within 2-8 hours

Pregnancy Risk Factor C

Generic Available No

Sulfa-Gyn® see Sulfabenzamide, Sulfacetamide, and Sulfathiazole *on page 889*

Sulfalax® [OTC] *see* Docusate *on page 331*

Sulfamethoprim® *see* Trimethoprim and Sulfamethoxazole *on page 965*

Sulfamethoxazole (sul fa meth OKS a zole)

Brand Names Gantanol®; Urobak®
Canadian/Mexican Brand Names Apo®-Sulfamethoxazole (Canada)
Therapeutic Category Antibiotic, Sulfonamide Derivative
Synonyms Sulfametoxazol (Mexico)
(Continued)

Sulfamethoxazole *(Continued)*

Use Treatment of urinary tract infections, nocardiosis, toxoplasmosis, acute otitis media, and acute exacerbations of chronic bronchitis due to susceptible organisms

Usual Dosage Oral:

Children >2 months: 50-60 mg/kg as single dose followed by 50-60 mg/kg/day divided every 12 hours; maximum: 3 g/24 hours or 75 mg/kg/day

Adults: 2 g stat, 1 g 2-3 times/day; maximum: 3 g/24 hours

Mechanism of Action Interferes with bacterial growth by inhibiting bacterial folic acid synthesis through competitive antagonism of PABA

Local Anesthetic/Vasoconstrictor Precautions No information available to require special precautions

Effects on Dental Treatment No effects or complications reported

Other Adverse Effects

>10%:

Central nervous system: Fever, dizziness, headache

Dermatologic: Itching, skin rash, photosensitivity

Gastrointestinal: Anorexia, nausea, vomiting, diarrhea

1% to 10%:

Dermatologic: Lyell's syndrome, Stevens-Johnson syndrome

Hematologic: Granulocytopenia, leukopenia, thrombocytopenia, aplastic anemia, hemolytic anemia

Hepatic: Hepatitis

<1%:

Cardiovascular: Vasculitis

Endocrine & metabolic: Thyroid function disturbance

Genitourinary: Crystalluria

Hepatic: Jaundice

Renal: Hematuria, acute nephropathy, interstitial nephritis

Miscellaneous: Serum sickness-like reactions

Drug Interactions

Decreased effect with PABA or PABA metabolites of drugs (ie, procaine, proparacaine, tetracaine)

Increased effect of oral anticoagulants, oral hypoglycemic agents, and methotrexate

Drug Uptake

Absorption: Oral: 90%

Serum half-life: 9-12 hours, prolonged with renal impairment

Time to peak serum concentration: Within 3-4 hours

Pregnancy Risk Factor B (D at term)

Generic Available Yes: Tablet

Sulfamethoxazole and Phenazopyridine

(sul fa meth OKS a zole & fen az oh PEER i deen)

Brand Names Azo Gantanol®

Therapeutic Category Antibiotic, Sulfonamide Derivative

Use Treatment of urinary tract infections complicated with pain

Usual Dosage Oral: 4 tablets to start, then 2 tablets twice daily for up to 2 days, then switch to sulfamethoxazole only

Local Anesthetic/Vasoconstrictor Precautions No information available to require special precautions

Effects on Dental Treatment No effects or complications reported

Other Adverse Effects

Central nervous system: Confusion, depression, hallucinations, ataxia, seizures, fever, kernicterus in neonates

Dermatologic: Rash, erythema multiforme, Stevens-Johnson syndrome, epidermal necrolysis

Gastrointestinal: Nausea, vomiting, glossitis, stomatitis, diarrhea, pseudomembranous colitis

Hematologic: Thrombocytopenia, megaloblastic anemia, granulocytopenia, aplastic anemia, hemolysis (with G-6-PD deficiency)

Hepatic: Serum sickness, hepatitis

Renal & genitourinary: Interstitial nephritis

Drug Interactions Warfarin, methotrexate

Pregnancy Risk Factor B (D at term)

Generic Available Yes

Sulfamethoxazole and Trimethoprim *see* Trimethoprim and Sulfamethoxazole *on page 965*

Sulfametoxazol (Mexico) *see* Sulfamethoxazole *on previous page*

Sulfamylon® *see* Mafenide *on page 574*

Sulfanilamide (sul fa NIL a mide)

Brand Names AVC™ Cream; AVC™ Suppository; Vagitrol®

Therapeutic Category Antifungal Agent, Vaginal

Use Treatment of vulvovaginitis caused by *Candida albicans*

Mechanism of Action Interferes with microbial folic acid synthesis and growth via inhibition of para-aminiobenzoic acid metabolism

Local Anesthetic/Vasoconstrictor Precautions No information available to require special precautions

Effects on Dental Treatment No effects or complications reported

Other Adverse Effects

1% to 10%:
   Central nervous system: Kernicterus
   Dermatologic: Itching, skin rash, exfoliative dermatitis, Stevens-Johnson syndrome
   Gastrointestinal: Nausea, vomiting
   Hematologic: Agranulocytosis, hemolytic anemia in patients with severe G-6-PD deficiency
   Hepatic: Hepatic toxicity
   Local: Burning, irritation
   Renal: Crystalluria
<1%: Genitourinary: Irritation of penis of sexual partner

Drug Interactions No data reported

Pregnancy Risk Factor B (D at term)

Dosage Forms
   Cream, vaginal (AVC™, Vagitrol®): 15% [150 mg/g] (120 g with applicator)
   Suppository, vaginal (AVC™): 1.05 g (16s)

Generic Available No

Sulfasalazine (sul fa SAL a zeen)

Brand Names Azulfidine®; Azulfidine® EN-tabs®

Canadian/Mexican Brand Names Apo®-Sulfasalazine (Canada); PMS-Sulfasalazine® (Canada); Salazopyrin® (Canada); Salazopyrin EN-Tabs® (Canada); S.A.S® (Canada)

Therapeutic Category 5-Aminosalicylic Acid Derivative; Anti-inflammatory Agent

Use Management of ulcerative colitis

Usual Dosage Oral:
   Children >2 years: 40-60 mg/kg/day in 3-6 divided doses, not to exceed 6 g/day; maintenance dose: 20-30 mg/kg/day in 4 divided doses; not to exceed 2 g/day

   Adults: 1 g 3-4 times/day, 2 g/day maintenance in divided doses; not to exceed 6 g/day

Mechanism of Action May be related to the immunosuppressant properties that have been observed in animal and *in vitro* models, to its affinity for connective tissue, and/or to the relatively high concentration it reaches in serous fluids, the liver and intestinal walls, as demonstrated in autoradiographic studies in animals; sulfasalazine (SS) has also been described as a highly efficient vehicle for carrying its principal metabolites, 5-aminosalicylic acid (5-ASA) and sulfapyridine (SP), to the colon, where a local action for both of them has been postulated; recent clinical studies utilizing rectal administration of SS, SP and 5-ASA have indicated that the major therapeutic action may reside in the 5-ASA moiety

Local Anesthetic/Vasoconstrictor Precautions No information available to require special precautions

Effects on Dental Treatment No effects or complications reported

Other Adverse Effects

>10%:
   Central nervous system: Fever, dizziness, headache
   Dermatologic: Itching, skin rash, photosensitivity
   Gastrointestinal: Anorexia, nausea, vomiting, diarrhea
   Genitourinary: Reversible oligospermia
1% to 10%:
   Dermatologic: Lyell's syndrome, Stevens-Johnson syndrome
   Hematologic: Granulocytopenia, leukopenia, thrombocytopenia, aplastic anemia, hemolytic anemia
   Hepatic: Hepatitis
<1%:
   Endocrine & metabolic: Thyroid function disturbance
   Genitourinary: Crystalluria
   Hepatic: Jaundice
   Renal: Interstitial nephritis, acute nephropathy, hematuria
   Miscellaneous: Serum sickness-like reactions
(Continued)

Sulfasalazine *(Continued)*

Drug Interactions
Decreased effect with iron, digoxin and PABA or PABA metabolites of drugs (ie, procaine, proparacaine, tetracaine)

Decreased effect of oral anticoagulants, methotrexate, and oral hypoglycemic agents

Drug Uptake
Absorption: 10% to 15% of dose is absorbed as unchanged drug from the small intestine

Serum half-life: 5.7-10 hours

Pregnancy Risk Factor B (D at term)
Generic Available Yes

Sulfatrim® *see* Trimethoprim and Sulfamethoxazole *on page 965*

Sulfatrim® DS *see* Trimethoprim and Sulfamethoxazole *on page 965*

Sulfa-Trip® *see* Sulfabenzamide, Sulfacetamide, and Sulfathiazole *on page 889*

Sulfinpyrazone *(sul fin PEER a zone)*
Brand Names Anturane®
Canadian/Mexican Brand Names Antazone® (Canada); Anturan® (Canada); Apo®-Sulfinpyrazone (Canada); Novo-Pyrazone® (Canada); Nu-Sulfinpyrazone® (Canada)
Therapeutic Category Uric Acid Lowering Agent
Use Treatment of chronic gouty arthritis and intermittent gouty arthritis

Unlabeled use: To decrease the incidence of sudden death postmyocardial infarction

Usual Dosage Adults: Oral: 100-200 mg twice daily; maximum daily dose: 800 mg

Mechanism of Action Acts by increasing the urinary excretion of uric acid, thereby decreasing blood urate levels; this effect is therapeutically useful in treating patients with acute intermittent gout, chronic tophaceous gout, and acts to promote resorption of tophi; also has antithrombic and platelet inhibitory effects

Local Anesthetic/Vasoconstrictor Precautions No information available to require special precautions

Effects on Dental Treatment No effects or complications reported

Other Adverse Effects
>10%: Gastrointestinal: Nausea, vomiting, stomach pain

1% to 10%: Dermatologic: Dermatitis, skin rash

<1%:
Cardiovascular: Flushing
Central nervous system: Dizziness, headache
Dermatologic: Rash
Hematologic: Anemia, leukopenia, increased bleeding time (decreased platelet aggregation)
Hepatic: Hepatic necrosis
Renal: Nephrotic syndrome, polyuria, uric acid stones

Drug Interactions
Decreased effect/levels of theophylline, verapamil; decreased uricosuric activity with salicylates, niacins

Increased effect of oral hypoglycemics and anticoagulants

Risk of acetaminophen hepatotoxicity is increased, but therapeutic effects may be reduced

Drug Uptake
Absorption: Complete and rapid

Serum half-life, elimination: 2.7-6 hours

Time to peak serum concentration: 1.6 hours

Pregnancy Risk Factor C
Generic Available Yes

Sulfisoxasol (Mexico) *see* Sulfisoxazole *on this page*

Sulfisoxazole *(sul fi SOKS a zole)*
Brand Names Gantrisin®
Canadian/Mexican Brand Names Novo-Soxazole® (Canada); Sulfizole® (Canada)
Therapeutic Category Antibiotic, Sulfonamide Derivative
Synonyms Sulfisoxasol (Mexico)
Use Treatment of urinary tract infections, otitis media, *Chlamydia*; nocardiosis; treatment of acute pelvic inflammatory disease in prepubertal children; often used in combination with trimethoprim

Usual Dosage

Oral (not for use in patients <2 months of age):

Children >2 months: 75 mg/kg stat, followed by 120-150 mg/kg/day in divided doses every 4-6 hours; not to exceed 6 g/day

Pelvic inflammatory disease: 100 mg/kg/day in divided doses every 6 hours; used in combination with ceftriaxone

Chlamydia trachomatis: 100 mg/kg/day in divided doses every 6 hours

Adults: 2-4 g stat, 4-8 g/day in divided doses every 4-6 hours

Pelvic inflammatory disease: 500 mg every 6 hours for 21 days; used in combination with ceftriaxone

Chlamydia trachomatis: 500 mg every 6 hours for 10 days

Elderly: 2 g stat, then 2-8 g/day in divided doses every 6 hours

Ophthalmic: Children and Adults:

Solution: Instill 1-2 drops to affected eye every 2-3 hours

Ointment: Apply small amount to affected eye 1-3 times/day and at bedtime

Mechanism of Action Interferes with bacterial growth by inhibiting bacterial folic acid synthesis through competitive antagonism of PABA

Local Anesthetic/Vasoconstrictor Precautions No information available to require special precautions

Effects on Dental Treatment No effects or complications reported

Other Adverse Effects

>10%:

Central nervous system: Fever, dizziness, headache

Dermatologic: Itching, skin rash, photosensitivity

Gastrointestinal: Anorexia, nausea, vomiting, diarrhea

1% to 10%:

Dermatologic: Lyell's syndrome, Stevens-Johnson syndrome

Hematologic: Granulocytopenia, leukopenia, thrombocytopenia, aplastic anemia, hemolytic anemia

Hepatic: Hepatitis

<1%:

Endocrine & metabolic: Thyroid function disturbance

Genitourinary: Crystalluria

Hepatic: Jaundice

Renal: Interstitial nephritis, acute nephropathy, hematuria

Miscellaneous: Serum sickness-like reactions

Drug Interactions

Decreased effect with PABA or PABA metabolites of drugs (ie, procaine, proparacaine, tetracaine), thiopental

Increased effect of oral anticoagulants, methotrexate and oral hypoglycemic agents

Drug Uptake

Absorption: Sulfisoxazole acetyl is hydrolyzed in the GI tract to sulfisoxazole which is readily absorbed

Serum half-life: 4-7 hours, prolonged with renal impairment

Time to peak serum concentration: Within 2-3 hours

Pregnancy Risk Factor B (D at term)

Generic Available Yes

Sulfisoxazole and Phenazopyridine

(sul fi SOKS a zole & fen az oh PEER i deen)

Brand Names Azo Gantrisin®

Therapeutic Category Antibiotic, Sulfonamide Derivative; Local Anesthetic, Urinary

Use Treatment of urinary tract infections and nocardiosis

Usual Dosage Adults: Oral: 4-6 tablets to start, then 2 tablets 4 times/day for 2 days, then continue with sulfisoxazole only

Mechanism of Action Interferes with bacterial growth by inhibiting bacterial folic acid synthesis through competitive antagonism of PABA; phenazopyridine exerts local anesthetic or analgesic action on urinary tract mucosa through an unknown mechanism

Local Anesthetic/Vasoconstrictor Precautions No information available to require special precautions

Effects on Dental Treatment No effects or complications reported

Other Adverse Effects

>10%:

Central nervous system: Fever, dizziness, headache

Dermatologic: Itching, skin rash, photosensitivity

Gastrointestinal: Anorexia, nausea, vomiting, diarrhea

1% to 10%:

Dermatologic: Lyell's syndrome, Stevens-Johnson syndrome

(Continued)

Sulfisoxazole and Phenazopyridine *(Continued)*

Hematologic: Granulocytopenia, leukopenia, thrombocytopenia, aplastic anemia, hemolytic anemia
Hepatic: Hepatitis
<1%:
Endocrine & metabolic: Thyroid function disturbance
Genitourinary: Crystalluria
Hepatic: Jaundice
Renal: Hematuria, acute nephropathy, interstitial nephritis
Miscellaneous: Serum sickness-like reactions

Drug Interactions
Decreased effect with PABA or PABA metabolites of drugs (ie, procaine, proparacaine, tetracaine), thiopental
Increased effect of oral anticoagulants, methotrexate and oral hypoglycemic agents

Drug Uptake
Absorption: Sulfisoxazole acetyl is hydrolyzed in the GI tract to sulfisoxazole which is readily absorbed
Serum half-life: 4-7 hours, prolonged with renal impairment
Time to peak serum concentration: Within 2-3 hours

Pregnancy Risk Factor B (D at term)
Generic Available Yes

Sulfoxaprim® *see* Trimethoprim and Sulfamethoxazole *on page 965*
Sulfoxaprim® DS *see* Trimethoprim and Sulfamethoxazole *on page 965*

Sulfur and Salicylic Acid *(SUL fur & sal i SIL ik AS id)*

Brand Names Aveeno® Cleansing Bar [OTC]; Fostex® [OTC]; Pernox® [OTC]; Sastid® Plain Therapeutic Shampoo and Acne Wash [OTC]; Sebulex® [OTC]
Therapeutic Category Antiseborrheic Agent, Topical
Synonyms Salicylic Acid and Sulfur
Use Therapeutic shampoo for dandruff and seborrheal dermatitis; acne skin cleanser
Local Anesthetic/Vasoconstrictor Precautions No information available to require special precautions
Effects on Dental Treatment No effects or complications reported
Other Adverse Effects Local: Topical preparations containing 2% to 5% sulfur generally are well tolerated, local irritation may occur, concentration >15% is very irritating to the skin, higher concentration (eg, 10% or higher) may cause systemic toxicity (eg, headache, vomiting, muscle cramps, dizziness, collapse)
Pregnancy Risk Factor C
Generic Available Yes
Comments For external use only

Sulfur and Sulfacetamide Sodium

(SUL fur & sul fa SEE ta mide SOW dee um)
Brand Names Novacet® Topical; Sulfacet-R® Topical
Therapeutic Category Acne Products
Synonyms Sodium Sulfacetamide and Sulfur; Sulfacetamide Sodium and Sulfur
Use Aid in the treatment of acne vulgaris, acne rosacea and seborrheic dermatitis
Local Anesthetic/Vasoconstrictor Precautions No information available to require special precautions
Effects on Dental Treatment No effects or complications reported
Generic Available Yes

Sulindac *(sul IN dak)*

Related Information
Nonsteroidal Anti-Inflammatory Agents, Comparative Dosages, and Pharmacokinetics *on page 1143*
Rheumatoid Arthritis and Osteoarthritis *on page 1030*
Temporomandibular Dysfunction (TMD) *on page 1078*
Brand Names Clinoril®
Canadian/Mexican Brand Names Apo®-Sulin (Canada); Novo-Sundac® (Canada)
Therapeutic Category Analgesic, Non-narcotic; Anti-inflammatory Agent; Nonsteroidal Anti-inflammatory Agent (NSAID), Oral
Use Management of inflammatory disease, rheumatoid disorders; acute gouty arthritis; structurally similar to indomethacin but acts like aspirin; safest NSAID for use in mild renal impairment
Usual Dosage Maximum therapeutic response may not be realized for up to 3 weeks. Oral:

Children: Dose not established

Adults: 150-200 mg twice daily or 300-400 mg once daily; not to exceed 400 mg/day

Mechanism of Action Inhibits prostaglandin synthesis by decreasing the activity of the enzyme, cyclo-oxygenase, which results in decreased formation of prostaglandin precursors

Local Anesthetic/Vasoconstrictor Precautions No information available to require special precautions

Effects on Dental Treatment No effects or complications reported

Other Adverse Effects

>10%:

Central nervous system: Dizziness

Dermatologic: Skin rash

Gastrointestinal: Abdominal cramps, heartburn, indigestion, nausea

1% to 10%:

Central nervous system: Headache, nervousness

Dermatologic: Itching

Endocrine & metabolic: Fluid retention

Gastrointestinal: Vomiting

Otic: Tinnitus

<1%:

Cardiovascular: Congestive heart failure, hypertension, arrhythmias, tachycardia

Central nervous system: Confusion, hallucinations, aseptic meningitis, mental depression, drowsiness, insomnia

Dermatologic: Urticaria, erythema multiforme, toxic epidermal necrolysis, Stevens-Johnson syndrome, angioedema

Endocrine & metabolic: Polydipsia, hot flashes

Gastrointestinal: Gastritis, GI ulceration

Genitourinary: Cystitis

Hematologic: Agranulocytosis, anemia, hemolytic anemia, bone marrow suppression, leukopenia, thrombocytopenia

Hepatic: Hepatitis

Neuromuscular & skeletal: Peripheral neuropathy

Ocular: Toxic amblyopia, blurred vision, conjunctivitis, dry eyes

Otic: Decreased hearing

Renal: Polyuria, acute renal failure

Respiratory: Allergic rhinitis, dyspnea, epistaxis

Drug Interactions

Decreased effect: Aspirin may decrease sulindac serum concentrations

Increased toxicity: Sulindac may increase digoxin, methotrexate, and lithium serum concentrations; other nonsteroidal anti-inflammatories may increase adverse gastrointestinal effects of sulindac

Drug Uptake

Absorption: 90%

Serum half-life:

Parent drug: 7 hours

Active metabolite: 18 hours

Pregnancy Risk Factor B (D at term)

Dosage Forms Tablet: 150 mg, 200 mg

Generic Available Yes

Sultrin™ *see* Sulfabenzamide, Sulfacetamide, and Sulfathiazole *on page 889*

Sumacal® [OTC] *see* Glucose Polymers *on page 444*

Sumatriptan Succinate (SOO ma trip tan SUKS i nate)

Brand Names Imitrex®

Canadian/Mexican Brand Names Imigran® (Mexico)

Therapeutic Category Antimigraine Agent; Serotonin Agonist

Use Acute treatment of migraine with or without aura

Unlabeled use: Cluster headaches

Usual Dosage Adults:

Oral: 25 mg (taken with fluids); maximum recommended dose is 100 mg. If a satisfactory response has not been obtained at 2 hours, a second dose of up to 100 mg may be given. Efficacy of this second dose has not been examined. If a headache returns, additional doses may be taken at intervals of at least 2 hours up to a daily maximum of 300 mg. There is no evidence that an initial dose of 100 mg provides substantially greater relief than 25 mg.

Intranasal: Single dose of 5, 10, or 20 mg administered in one nostril; a 10 mg dose may be achieved by administration of a single 5 mg dose in each nostril; if headache returns, the dose may be repeated once after 2 hours, not to exceed a total daily dose of 40 mg

(Continued)

Sumatriptan Succinate *(Continued)*

S.C.: 6 mg; a second injection may be administered at least 1 hour after the initial dose, but not more than two injections in a 24-hour period

Mechanism of Action Selective agonist for serotonin (5HT-$_{1-D}$ receptor) in cranial arteries to cause vasoconstriction and reduces sterile inflammation associated with antidromic neuronal transmission correlating with relief of migraine

Local Anesthetic/Vasoconstrictor Precautions No information available to require special precautions

Effects on Dental Treatment No effects or complications reported

Other Adverse Effects

>10%:

Central nervous system: Dizziness

Endocrine & metabolic: Hot flashes

Local: Injection site reaction

1% to 10%:

Cardiovascular: Tightness in chest

Central nervous system: Burning sensation, drowsiness, headache

Gastrointestinal: Abdominal discomfort, mouth discomfort, jaw discomfort

Neuromuscular & skeletal: Myalgia, neck pain, weakness, numbness

Miscellaneous: Sweating

<1%:

Dermatologic: Skin rashes

Endocrine & metabolic: Polydipsia, dehydration, dysmenorrhea

Gastrointestinal: Thirst

Genitourinary: Dysuria

Renal: Renal calculus

Respiratory: Dyspnea

Miscellaneous: Hiccups

Drug Interactions Increased toxicity: Ergot-containing drugs

Drug Uptake After S.C. administration:

Serum half-life, terminal: 115 minutes

Time to peak serum concentration: 5-20 minutes

Pregnancy Risk Factor C

Dosage Forms

Injection: 12 mg/mL (0.5 mL, 2 mL)

Spray, nasal: 5 mg (100 mcL); 20 mg (100 mcL)

Tablet: 25 mg, 50 mg

Generic Available No

Sumycin® *see* Tetracycline *on page 914*

Sunscreen, PABA-Free *see* Methoxycinnamate and Oxybenzone *on page 619*

SuperChar® [OTC] *see* Charcoal *on page 206*

Supprelin™ *see* Histrelin *on page 471*

Suppress® [OTC] *see* Dextromethorphan *on page 298*

Suprax® *see* Cefixime *on page 189*

Suprofen *(soo PROE fen)*

Brand Names Profenal®

Therapeutic Category Nonsteroidal Anti-inflammatory Agent (NSAID), Ophthalmic

Use Inhibition of intraoperative miosis

Usual Dosage Adults: On day of surgery, instill 2 drops in conjunctival sac at 3, 2, and 1 hour prior to surgery; or 2 drops in sac every 4 hours, while awake, the day preceding surgery

Mechanism of Action Inhibits prostaglandin synthesis

Local Anesthetic/Vasoconstrictor Precautions No information available to require special precautions

Effects on Dental Treatment No effects or complications reported

Other Adverse Effects

1% to 10%: Topical: Transient burning or stinging, redness, iritis

<1%:

Systemic: Chemosis, photophobia

Topical: Discomfort, pain, punctate epithelial staining

Drug Interactions Decreased effect: When used concurrently with suprofen, acetylcholine chloride and carbachol ophthalmic preparations may be ineffective

Pregnancy Risk Factor C

Generic Available No

Surbex® [OTC] *see* Vitamin B Complex *on page 993*

Surbex-T® Filmtabs® [OTC] *see* Vitamin B Complex With Vitamin C *on page 994*

Surbex® with C Filmtabs® [OTC] *see* Vitamin B Complex With Vitamin C *on page 994*

Surfak® [OTC] *see* Docusate *on page 331*

Surgicel® *see* Cellulose, Oxidized *on page 200*

Surgicel® Absorbable Hemostat *see* Cellulose, Oxidized Regenerated *on page 200*

Surmontil® *see* Trimipramine *on page 967*

Survanta® *see* Beractant *on page 125*

Sus-Phrine® *see* Epinephrine (Dental) *on page 353*

Sustaire® *see* Theophylline *on page 917*

Sween® Cream [OTC] *see* Methylbenzethonium Chloride *on page 621*

Swim-Ear® Otic [OTC] *see* Boric Acid *on page 136*

Syllact® [OTC] *see* Psyllium *on page 822*

Symmetrel® *see* Amantadine *on page 50*

Synacol® CF [OTC] *see* Guaifenesin and Dextromethorphan *on page 453*

Synalar® *see* Fluocinolone *on page 414*

Synalar-HP® *see* Fluocinolone *on page 414*

Synalgos®-DC *see* Dihydrocodeine Compound *on page 315*

Synarel® *see* Nafarelin *on page 658*

Synemol® *see* Fluocinolone *on page 414*

Synthetic Lung Surfactant *see* Colfosceril Palmitate *on page 259*

Synthroid® *see* Levothyroxine *on page 552*

Syntocinon® *see* Oxytocin *on page 719*

Syracol-CF® [OTC] *see* Guaifenesin and Dextromethorphan *on page 453*

Systemic Viral Diseases *see page 1047*

Tac™-3 *see* Triamcinolone *on page 954*

Tac™-40 *see* Triamcinolone *on page 954*

TACE® *see* Chlorotrianisene *on page 216*

Tacrine (TAK reen)

Brand Names Cognex®

Therapeutic Category Cholinergic Agent

Use Treatment of mild to moderate dementia of the Alzheimer's type

Usual Dosage Adults: Initial: 10 mg 4 times/day; may increase by 40 mg/day adjusted every 6 weeks; maximum: 160 mg/day; best administered separate from meal times; see table.

Dose Adjustment Based Upon Transaminase Elevations

ALT	Regimen
≤3 x ULN*	Continue titration
>3 to ≤5 x ULN	Decrease dose by 40 mg/day, resume when ALT returns to normal
>5 x ULN	Stop treatment, may rechallenge upon return of ALT to normal

*ULN = upper limit of normal.

Patients with clinical jaundice confirmed by elevated total bilirubin (>3 mg/dL) should not be rechallenged with tacrine

Mechanism of Action A deficiency of cortical acetylcholine is believed to account for some of the clinical manifestations of mild to moderate dementia. Tacrine probably acts by elevating acetylcholine concentrations in the cortical areas by slowing the degradation of acetylcholine released by still intact cholinergic neurons.

Local Anesthetic/Vasoconstrictor Precautions No information available to require special precautions

Effects on Dental Treatment No effects or complications reported

Other Adverse Effects 1% to 10%:
Gastrointestinal: Diarrhea, nausea, abdominal discomfort, anorexia
Renal: Polyuria
Miscellaneous: Sweating, ataxia

Warnings/Precautions The use of tacrine has been associated with elevations in serum transaminases; serum transaminases (specifically ALT) must be monitored throughout therapy; use extreme caution in patients with current evidence of a history of abnormal liver function tests; use caution in patients with bladder
(Continued)

Tacrine *(Continued)*

outlet obstruction, asthma, and sick-sinus syndrome (tacrine may cause brady-cardia). Also, patients with cardiovascular disease, asthma, or peptic ulcer should use cautiously.

Drug Interactions

Cholinergic drugs: Increased cholinergic effects such as diarrhea and abdominal discomfort seen when tacrine is combined with other cholinergics such as bethanechol

Anticholinergics: Tacrine may inhibit the therapeutic effects of anticholinergics, and anticholinergics may inhibit the effects of tacrine

Cigarette smoking: Tobacco appears to significantly reduce the plasma concentrations of tacrine

Cimetidine (Tagamet®) increases tacrine plasma levels

Enoxacin (Penetrex) may be a potent inhibitor of liver metabolism of tacrine

Fluvoxamine (Luvox®) markedly increases tacrine plasma levels and may increase tacrine adverse effects

Levodopa: Tacrine may inhibit the effects of levodopa in patients with parkinsonism

Propranolol: Both tacrine and propranolol can slow heart rate; additive brady-cardia is a possibility

Theophylline: Tacrine can markedly increase theophylline plasma levels which can lead to theophylline toxicity

Drug Uptake

Peak plasma concentrations: 1-2 hours

Plasma bound: 55%

Serum half-life, elimination: 2-4 hours, steady-state achieved in 24-36 hours

Pregnancy Risk Factor C

Dosage Forms Capsule, as hydrochloride: 10 mg, 20 mg, 30 mg, 40 mg

Generic Available No

Tacrolimus *(ta KROE li mus)*

Brand Names Prograf®

Therapeutic Category Immunosuppressant Agent

Use Potent immunosuppressive drug used in liver, kidney, heart, lung, or small bowel transplant recipients

Usual Dosage

Children:

I.V. continuous infusion: 0.1 mg/kg/day

Oral: 0.3 mg/kg/day

Adults:

I.V. continuous infusion: Initial (at least 6 hours after transplantation): 0.05-0.1 mg/kg/day

Oral (within 2-3 days): 0.15-0.3 mg/kg/day in divided doses every 12 hours; give 8-12 hours after discontinuation of the I.V. infusion; may gradually adjust (decrease) maintenance dose via pharmacokinetic monitoring

Mechanism of Action Suppressed humoral immunity (inhibits T-lymphocyte activation); produced by the fungus streptomyces tsukubaensis

Local Anesthetic/Vasoconstrictor Precautions No information available to require special precautions

Effects on Dental Treatment No effects or complications reported

Other Adverse Effects

>10%:

Cardiovascular: Hypertension, peripheral edema

Central nervous system: Headache, insomnia, pain, fever

Dermatologic: Pruritus

Endocrine & metabolic: Hypo-/hyperkalemia, hyperglycemia, hypomagnesemia

Gastrointestinal: Diarrhea, nausea, anorexia, vomiting, abdominal pain

Hematologic: Anemia, leukocytosis

Hepatic: LFT abnormalities, ascites

Neuromuscular & skeletal: Tremors, paresthesias, back pain, weakness

Renal: Nephrotoxicity, elevated creatinine and BUN

Respiratory: Pleural effusion, atelectasis, dyspnea

1% to 10%:

Dermatologic: Rash

Gastrointestinal: Constipation

Genitourinary: Urinary tract infection

Hematologic: Thrombocytopenia

Renal: Oliguria

Drug Interactions

Antacids: Tacrolimus absorption impaired (separate administration by at least 2 hours)

Nephrotoxic antibiotics potentially increase tacrolimus associated nephrotoxicity; amphotericin B potentially increases tacrolimus associated nephrotoxicity

Agents which may increase tacrolimus plasma concentrations and consequently its effect and toxicity include erythromycin, clarithromycin, clotrimazole, fluconazole, itraconazole, ketoconazole, diltiazem, nicardipine, verapamil, bromocriptine, cimetidine, danazol, metoclopramide, methylprednisolone, cyclosporine (synergistic immunosuppression)

Agents which may decrease tacrolimus plasma concentrations and consequently its effect include rifampin, rifabutin, phenytoin, phenobarbital, and carbamazepine

Drug Uptake

Absorption: Better in small bowel patients with a closed stoma; unlike cyclosporine, clamping of the T-tube in liver transplant patients does not alter trough concentrations or AUC; food within 15 minutes of administration decreases absorption (27%); T_{max}: 0.5-4 hours

Serum half-life, elimination: 12 hours (range: 4-40 hours, twice as fast in children)

Pregnancy Risk Factor C; because FK-506 does cross into breast milk, breast feeding is not advised while tacrolimus therapy is ongoing

Generic Available No

Tagamet® *see* Cimetidine *on page 235*

Tagamet® HB [OTC] *see* Cimetidine *on page 235*

Talacen® *see* Pentazocine Compound *on page 738*

Talwin® *see* Pentazocine *on page 737*

Talwin® Compound *see* Pentazocine Compound *on page 738*

Talwin® NX *see* Pentazocine *on page 737*

Tambocor™ *see* Flecainide *on page 407*

Tamine® [OTC] *see* Brompheniramine and Phenylpropanolamine *on page 143*

Tamoxifen (ta MOKS i fen)

Brand Names Nolvadex®

Canadian/Mexican Brand Names Alpha-Tamoxifen® (Canada); Apo®-Tamox (Canada); Bilem® (Mexico); Cryoxifeno® (Mexico); Novo-Tamoxifen® (Canada); Tamofen® (Canada); Tamone® (Canada); Tamoxan® (Mexico); Taxus® (Mexico)

Therapeutic Category Antineoplastic Agent, Hormone (Antiestrogen)

Synonyms Tamoxifeno (Mexico)

Use Palliative or adjunctive treatment of advanced breast cancer

Unlabeled use: Treatment of mastalgia, gynecomastia, male breast cancer, and pancreatic carcinoma. Studies have shown tamoxifen to be effective in the treatment of primary breast cancer in elderly women. Comparative studies with other antineoplastic agents in elderly women with breast cancer had more favorable survival rates with tamoxifen. Initiation of hormone therapy rather than chemotherapy is justified for elderly patients with metastatic breast cancer who are responsive.

Usual Dosage Oral **(refer to individual protocols):**

Adults: 10-20 mg twice daily in the morning and evening

High-dose therapy is under investigation

Mechanism of Action Competitively binds to estrogen receptors on tumors and other tissue targets, producing a nuclear complex that decreases DNA synthesis and inhibits estrogen effects; nonsteroidal agent with potent antiestrogenic properties which compete with estrogen for binding sites in breast and other tissues; cells accumulate in the G_0 and G_1 phases; therefore, tamoxifen is cytostatic rather than cytocidal.

Local Anesthetic/Vasoconstrictor Precautions No information available to require special precautions

Effects on Dental Treatment No effects or complications reported

Other Adverse Effects

>10%:

Gastrointestinal: Little to mild nausea (10%), vomiting, weight gain

General: Flushing, increased bone and tumor pain and local disease flare shortly after starting therapy; this will subside rapidly, but patients should be aware of this since many may discontinue the drug due to the side effects; skin rash, hepatotoxicity

Hematologic: Myelosuppressive, transient thrombocytopenia occurs in ~24% of patients receiving 10-20 mg/day; platelet counts return to normal within several weeks in spite of continued administration; leukopenia has also been reported and does resolve during continued therapy; anemia has also been reported

(Continued)

Tamoxifen *(Continued)*

1% to 10%:

Cardiovascular: Thromboembolism; tamoxifen has been associated with the occurrence of venous thrombosis and pulmonary embolism; arterial thrombosis has also been described in a few case reports

Central nervous system: Lightheadedness, depression, dizziness, headache, lassitude, mental confusion

Dermatologic: Rash

Endocrine & metabolic: Hypercalcemia may occur in patients with bone metastases; galactorrhea and vitamin deficiency, menstrual irregularities

Genitourinary: Vaginal bleeding or discharge, endometriosis, priapism, possible endometrial cancer

Neuromuscular & skeletal: Weakness

Ocular: Ophthalmologic effects (visual acuity changes, cataracts, or retinopathy), corneal opacities

Drug Interactions

Increased toxicity:

Allopurinol results in exacerbation of allopurinol-induced hepatotoxicity

Cyclosporine may result in increased cyclosporine serum levels

Warfarin results in significant enhancement of the anticoagulant effects of warfarin; has been speculated that a decrease in antitumor effect of tamoxifen may also occur due to alterations in the percentage of active tamoxifen metabolites

Drug Uptake

Absorption: Well absorbed from GI tract

Serum half-life: 7 days

Time to peak serum concentration: Oral: Within 4-7 hours

Pregnancy Risk Factor D

Dosage Forms Tablet, as citrate: 10 mg, 20 mg

Generic Available Yes

Tamoxifeno (Mexico) *see* Tamoxifen *on previous page*

Tamsulosin (tam SOO loe sin)

Brand Names Flomax™

Therapeutic Category Alpha-Adrenergic Blocking Agent

Synonyms Tamsulosin Hydrochloride

Use Treatment of signs and symptoms of benign prostatic hyperplasia (BPH)

Usual Dosage Oral: Adults: 0.4 mg once daily ~30 minutes after the same meal each day

Local Anesthetic/Vasoconstrictor Precautions No information available to require special precautions

Effects on Dental Treatment No effects or complications reported

Dosage Forms Capsule, as hydrochloride: 0.4 mg

Tamsulosin Hydrochloride *see* Tamsulosin *on this page*

Tanac® [OTC] *see* Benzocaine *on page 118*

Tanoral® Tablet *see* Chlorpheniramine, Pyrilamine, and Phenylephrine *on page 223*

Tao® *see* Troleandomycin *on page 972*

Tapazole® *see* Methimazole *on page 612*

Taractan® *see* Chlorprothixene *on page 226*

Tarka® *see* Trandolapril and Verapamil *on page 950*

Tasmar® *see* Tolcapone *on page 942*

Tavist® *see* Clemastine *on page 242*

Tavist®-1 [OTC] *see* Clemastine *on page 242*

Tavist-D® *see* Clemastine and Phenylpropanolamine *on page 242*

Taxol® *see* Paclitaxel *on page 719*

Taxotere® *see* Docetaxel *on page 330*

Tazarotene (taz AR oh teen)

Brand Names Tazorac®

Therapeutic Category Keratolytic Agent

Use Topical treatment of facial acne fulgaris; topical treatment of stable plaque psoriasis of up to 20% body surface area involvement

Local Anesthetic/Vasoconstrictor Precautions No information available to require special precautions

Effects on Dental Treatment No effects or complications reported

Pregnancy Risk Factor X

Dosage Forms Gel: 0.05% (30 g, 100 g); 0.1% (30 g, 100 g)

Tazicef® *see* Ceftazidime *on page 195*

Tazidime® *see* Ceftazidime *on page 195*

Tazorac® *see* Tazarotene *on previous page*

3TC *see* Lamivudine *on page 541*

Tear Drop® Solution [OTC] *see* Artificial Tears *on page 87*

TearGard® Ophthalmic Solution [OTC] *see* Artificial Tears *on page 87*

Teargen® Ophthalmic Solution [OTC] *see* Artificial Tears *on page 87*

Tearisol® Solution [OTC] *see* Artificial Tears *on page 87*

Tears Naturale® Free Solution [OTC] *see* Artificial Tears *on page 87*

Tears Naturale® II Solution [OTC] *see* Artificial Tears *on page 87*

Tears Naturale® Solution [OTC] *see* Artificial Tears *on page 87*

Tears Plus® Solution [OTC] *see* Artificial Tears *on page 87*

Tears Renewed® Solution [OTC] *see* Artificial Tears *on page 87*

Tebamide® *see* Trimethobenzamide *on page 964*

Teczem® *see* Enalapril and Diltiazem *on page 347*

Tedral® *see* Theophylline, Ephedrine, and Phenobarbital *on page 922*

Tegison® *see* Etretinate *on page 390*

Tegopen® *see* Cloxacillin *on page 253*

Tegretol® *see* Carbamazepine *on page 174*

Tegretol-XR® *see* Carbamazepine *on page 174*

Telachlor® *see* Chlorpheniramine *on page 217*

Teladar® *see* Betamethasone *on page 126*

Teldrin® [OTC] *see* Chlorpheniramine *on page 217*

Temazepam (te MAZ e pam)

Brand Names Restoril®

Therapeutic Category Benzodiazepine; Hypnotic; Sedative

Use Treatment of anxiety and as an adjunct in the treatment of depression; also may be used in the management of panic attacks; transient insomnia and sleep latency

Usual Dosage Adults: Oral: 15-30 mg at bedtime; 15 mg in elderly or debilitated patients

Mechanism of Action Benzodiazepine anxiolytic sedative that produces CNS depression at the subcortical level, except at high doses, whereby it works at the cortical level; causes minimal change in REM sleep patterns

Local Anesthetic/Vasoconstrictor Precautions No information available to require special precautions

Effects on Dental Treatment >10% of patients will exhibit significant dry mouth; normal salivary flow returns with cessation of drug therapy

Other Adverse Effects

1% to 10%:

Central nervous system: Drowsiness, headache, fatigue, nervousness, lethargy, dizziness, "hangover" feeling, anxiety, depression, euphoria, confusion, nightmares, vertigo

Gastrointestinal: Nausea, xerostomia, diarrhea, abdominal discomfort

Neuromuscular & skeletal: Weakness

Ocular: Blurred vision

<1%:

Cardiovascular: Palpitations

Central nervous system: Ataxia, amnesia, hallucinations

Gastrointestinal: Anorexia, vomiting

Neuromuscular & skeletal: Backache, tremor

Ocular: Burning

Respiratory: Dyspnea

Miscellaneous: Diaphoresis

Warnings/Precautions Safety and efficacy in children <18 years of age have not been established; do not use in pregnant women; may cause drug dependency; avoid abrupt discontinuance in patients with prolonged therapy or seizure disorders; use with caution in patients receiving other CNS depressants, in patients with hepatic dysfunction, and the elderly

Drug Interactions Increased effect of CNS depressants; contraindicated with alcohol

Drug Uptake

Serum half-life: 9.5-12.4 hours

Time to peak serum concentration: Within 2-3 hours

Pregnancy Risk Factor X

Dosage Forms Capsule: 7.5 mg, 15 mg, 30 mg

Generic Available Yes

Temazin® Cold Syrup [OTC] *see* Chlorpheniramine and Phenylpropanolamine *on page 219*

Temovate® *see* Clobetasol *on page 245*

Temporomandibular Dysfunction (TMD) *see page 1078*

Tempra® [OTC] *see* Acetaminophen *on page 20*

Tenex® *see* Guanfacine *on page 459*

Teniposide (ten i POE side)
Brand Names Vumon Injection
Therapeutic Category Antineoplastic Agent, Miscellaneous
Synonyms EPT; VM-26
Use Treatment of Hodgkin's and non-Hodgkin's lymphomas, acute lymphocytic leukemia, bladder carcinoma and neuroblastoma
Usual Dosage I.V.:
  Children: 130 mg/m^2/week, increasing to 150 mg/m^2 after 3 weeks and up to 180 mg/m^2 after 6 weeks
  Adults: 50-180 mg/m^2 once or twice weekly for 4-6 weeks or 20-60 mg/m^2/day for 5 days
  Acute lymphoblastic leukemia (ALL): 165 mg/m^2 twice weekly for 8-9 doses **or** 250 mg/m^2 weekly for 4-8 weeks
  Small cell lung cancer: 80-90 mg/m^2/day for 5 days
Mechanism of Action Inhibits mitotic activity; inhibits cells from entering mitosis
Local Anesthetic/Vasoconstrictor Precautions No information available to require special precautions
Effects on Dental Treatment No effects or complications reported
Other Adverse Effects
  >10%:
    Gastrointestinal: Mucositis, nausea, vomiting, diarrhea
    Hematologic: Myelosuppression, leukopenia, neutropenia, thrombocytopenia
    Miscellaneous: Infection
  1% to 10%:
    Cardiovascular: Hypotension
    Central nervous system: Fever
    Dermatologic: Alopecia, rash
    Hematologic: Hemorrhage
    Miscellaneous: Hypersensitivity
  <1%:
    Endocrine & metabolic: Metabolic abnormalities
    Hepatic: Hepatic dysfunction
    Neuromuscular & skeletal: Peripheral neurotoxicity
    Renal: Renal dysfunction
Drug Interactions Increased toxicity:
  Methotrexate: Alteration of MTX transport has been found as a slow efflux of MTX and its polyglutamated form out of the cell, leading to intercellular accumulation of MTX
  Sodium salicylate, sulfamethizole, tolbutamide: displace teniposide from protein-binding sites - could cause substantial increases in free drug levels, resulting in potentiation of toxicity
Drug Uptake Serum half-life: 5 hours
Pregnancy Risk Factor D
Generic Available No

Ten-K® *see* Potassium Chloride *on page 778*

Tenoretic® *see* Atenolol and Chlorthalidone *on page 96*

Tenormin® *see* Atenolol *on page 95*

Tenuate® *see* Diethylpropion *on page 309*

Tenuate® Dospan® *see* Diethylpropion *on page 309*

Terak® Ophthalmic Ointment *see* Oxytetracycline and Polymyxin B *on page 718*

Terazol® *see* Terconazole *on page 909*

Terazosin (ter AY zoe sin)
Related Information
  Cardiovascular Diseases *on page 1010*
Brand Names Hytrin®
Therapeutic Category Alpha-Adrenergic Blockers - Peripheral-Acting (Alpha$_1$-Blockers)
Synonyms Terazosina (Mexico)
Use Management of mild to moderate hypertension; considered a step 2 drug in stepped approach to hypertension; benign prostate hypertrophy
Usual Dosage Adults: Oral:

Hypertension: Initial: 1 mg at bedtime; slowly increase dose to achieve desired blood pressure, up to 20 mg/day; usual dose: 1-5 mg/day

Dosage reduction may be needed when adding a diuretic or other antihypertensive agent; if drug is discontinued for greater than several days, consider beginning with initial dose and retitrate as needed; dosage may be given on a twice daily regimen if response is diminished at 24 hours and hypotensive is observed at 2-4 hours following a dose

Benign prostatic hypertrophy: Initial: 1 mg at bedtime, increasing as needed; most patients require 10 mg day; if no response after 4-6 weeks of 10 mg/day, may increase to 20 mg/day

Mechanism of Action Alpha$_1$-specific blocking agent with minimal alpha$_2$ effects; this allows peripheral postsynaptic blockade, with the resultant decrease in arterial tone, while preserving the negative feedback loop which is mediated by the peripheral presynaptic alpha$_2$-receptors; terazosin relaxes the smooth muscle of the bladder neck, thus reducing bladder outlet obstruction

Local Anesthetic/Vasoconstrictor Precautions No information available to require special precautions

Effects on Dental Treatment No effects or complications reported

Other Adverse Effects

>10%:
Cardiovascular: Orthostatic hypotension
Central nervous system: Dizziness, lightheadedness, drowsiness, headache, malaise

1% to 10%:
Cardiovascular: Edema, palpitations
Central nervous system: Fatigue, nervousness
Gastrointestinal: Dry mouth
Genitourinary: Urinary incontinence

<1%:
Cardiovascular: Angina
Central nervous system: Nightmares, hypothermia
Dermatologic: Rash
Endocrine & metabolic: Sexual dysfunction
Gastrointestinal: Nausea
Genitourinary: Priapism
Renal: Polyuria
Respiratory: Dyspnea, nasal congestion

Drug Interactions Increased hypotensive effect with diuretics and antihypertensive medications (especially beta-blockers)

Drug Uptake
Absorption: Oral: Rapid
Serum half-life: 9.2-12 hours
Time to peak serum concentration: Within 1 hour

Pregnancy Risk Factor C

Dosage Forms
Capsule: 1 mg, 2 mg, 5 mg, 10 mg
Tablet: 1 mg, 2 mg, 5 mg, 10 mg

Generic Available No

Terazosina (Mexico) see Terazosin on previous page

Terbenafina Clorhidrato De (Mexico) see Terbinafine on this page

Terbinafine (TER bin a feen, TOP i kal)

Brand Names Lamisil®

Therapeutic Category Antifungal Agent, Topical

Synonyms Terbenafina Clorhidrato De (Mexico)

Use Topical antifungal for the treatment of tinea pedis (athlete's foot), tinea cruris (jock itch), and tinea corporis (ring worm)

Unlabeled use: Cutaneous candidiasis and pityriasis versicolor

Usual Dosage Adults: Topical:

Athlete's foot: Apply to affected area twice daily for at least 1 week, not to exceed 4 weeks

Ringworm and jock itch: Apply to affected area once or twice daily for at least 1 week, not to exceed 4 weeks

Mechanism of Action Synthetic alkylamine derivative which inhibits squalene epoxidases which is a key enzyme in sterol biosynthesis in fungi to result in a deficiency in ergosterol within fungal cell wall and result in fungal cell death

Local Anesthetic/Vasoconstrictor Precautions No information available to require special precautions

Effects on Dental Treatment No effects or complications reported

Other Adverse Effects 1% to 10%:
Dermatologic: Pruritus, contact dermatitis
(Continued)

Terbinafine (Continued)

Local: Irritation, stinging
Drug Interactions No data reported
Drug Uptake
Absorption: Topical: Limited
Pregnancy Risk Factor B
Generic Available No

Terbinafine, Oral (TER bin a feen, OR al)

Brand Names Lamisil® Oral
Therapeutic Category Antifungal Agent
Use Treatment of onychomycosis infections of the toenail or fingernail
Usual Dosage Adults: Oral:
Fingernail onychomycosis: 250 mg once daily for 6 weeks
Toenail onychomycosis: 250 mg once daily for 12 weeks
Mechanism of Action Terbinafine is a synthetic allylamine derivative which inhibits squalene epoxidase which is a key enzyme in sterol biosynthesis in fungi. The resulting deficiency in ergosterol within the cell wall causes fungi death.
Local Anesthetic/Vasoconstrictor Precautions No information available to require special precautions
Effects on Dental Treatment No effects or complications reported
Other Adverse Effects
>10%:
Central nervous system: Headache
1% to 10%:
Dermatologic: Rash, pruritus, urticaria
Gastrointestinal: Diarrhea, dyspepsia, abdominal pain, nausea, flatulence, abnormal taste
Hepatic: Elevated liver enzyme ≥2 times upper limit of normal range
Ocular: Visual disturbance
Drug Interactions
Decreases clearance of I.V. administered caffeine
Increases clearance of cyclosporine by 15%
Terbinafine clearance increased by rifampin (100%), cimetidine (33%)
Terbinafine clearance decreased by terfenadine (16%)
Terbinafine clearance unaffected by cyclosporine
Drug Uptake
Absorption: Oral: >70%
Serum half-life: 200-400 hours
Pregnancy Risk Factor B
Dosage Forms Tablet: 250 mg
Generic Available No

Terbutalina, Sulfato De (Mexico) see Terbutaline on this page

Terbutaline (ter BYOO ta leen)

Related Information
Respiratory Diseases on page 1018
Brand Names Brethaire®; Brethine®; Bricanyl®
Therapeutic Category Adrenergic Agonist Agent; Antiasthmatic; Beta₂-Adrenergic Agonist Agent; Bronchodilator
Synonyms Terbutalina, Sulfato De (Mexico)
Use Bronchodilator in reversible airway obstruction and bronchial asthma
Usual Dosage
Children <12 years:
Oral: Initial: 0.05 mg/kg/dose 3 times/day, increased gradually as required; maximum: 0.15 mg/kg/dose 3-4 times/day or a total of 5 mg/24 hours
S.C.: 0.005-0.01 mg/kg/dose to a maximum of 0.3 mg/dose every 15-20 minutes for 3 doses
Nebulization: 0.01-0.03 mg/kg/dose every 4-6 hours
Inhalation: 1-2 inhalations every 4-6 hours

Children >12 years and Adults:
Oral:
12-15 years: 2.5 mg every 6 hours 3 times/day; not to exceed 7.5 mg in 24 hours
>15 years: 5 mg/dose every 6 hours 3 times/day; if side effects occur, reduce dose to 2.5 mg every 6 hours; not to exceed 15 mg in 24 hours
S.C.: 0.25 mg/dose repeated in 15-30 minutes for one time only; a total dose of 0.5 mg should not be exceeded within a 4-hour period
Nebulization: 0.01-0.03 mg/kg/dose every 4-6 hours
Inhalation: 2 inhalations every 4-6 hours; wait 1 minute between inhalations

Mechanism of Action Relaxes bronchial smooth muscle by action on beta$_2$-receptors with less effect on heart rate

Local Anesthetic/Vasoconstrictor Precautions No information available to require special precautions

Effects on Dental Treatment No effects or complications reported

Other Adverse Effects

>10%:

Central nervous system: Nervousness, restlessness

Neuromuscular & skeletal: Trembling

1% to 10%:

Cardiovascular: Tachycardia, hypertension

Central nervous system: Dizziness, drowsiness, headache, insomnia

Gastrointestinal: Dry mouth, nausea, vomiting, bad taste in mouth

Neuromuscular & skeletal: Muscle cramps, weakness

Miscellaneous: Sweating

<1%:

Cardiovascular: Chest pain, arrhythmias

Respiratory: Paradoxical bronchospasm

Drug Interactions

Decreased effect with beta-blockers

Increased toxicity with MAO inhibitors, tricyclic antidepressants (TCAs)

Drug Uptake

Onset of action:

Oral: 30-45 minutes

S.C.: Within 6-15 minutes

Serum half-life: 11-16 hours

Pregnancy Risk Factor B

Dosage Forms

Aerosol, oral, as sulfate: 0.2 mg/actuation (10.5 g)

Injection, as sulfate: 1 mg/mL (1 mL)

Tablet, as sulfate: 2.5 mg, 5 mg

Generic Available No

Terconazole (ter KONE a zole)

Brand Names Terazol®

Canadian/Mexican Brand Names Fungistat® Dual (Mexico); Fungistat® (Mexico)

Therapeutic Category Antifungal Agent, Vaginal

Use Local treatment of vulvovaginal candidiasis

Usual Dosage Adults: Female: Insert 1 applicatorful intravaginally at bedtime for 7 consecutive days

Mechanism of Action Triazole ketal antifungal agent; involves inhibition of fungal cytochrome P-450. Specifically, terconazole inhibits cytochrome P-450-dependent 14-alpha-demethylase which results in accumulation of membrane disturbing 14-alpha-demethylsterols and ergosterol depletion.

Local Anesthetic/Vasoconstrictor Precautions No information available to require special precautions

Effects on Dental Treatment No effects or complications reported

Other Adverse Effects 1% to 10%: Genitourinary: Vulvar/vaginal burning

Drug Interactions No data reported

Drug Uptake Absorption: Extent of systemic absorption after vaginal administration may be dependent on the presence of a uterus; 5% to 8% in women who had a hysterectomy versus 12% to 16% in nonhysterectomy women

Pregnancy Risk Factor C

Dosage Forms

Cream, vaginal: 0.4% (45 g); 0.8% (20 g)

Suppository, vaginal: 80 mg (3s)

Generic Available No

Terpin Hydrate (TER pin HYE drate)

Therapeutic Category Expectorant

Use Symptomatic relief of cough

Local Anesthetic/Vasoconstrictor Precautions No information available to require special precautions

Effects on Dental Treatment No effects or complications reported

Dosage Forms Elixir: 85 mg/5 mL (120 mL)

Generic Available Yes

Terpin Hydrate and Codeine (TER pin HYE drate & KOE deen)

Therapeutic Category Cough Preparation; Expectorant

Synonyms ETH and C

(Continued)

Terpin Hydrate and Codeine *(Continued)*

Use Symptomatic relief of cough

Local Anesthetic/Vasoconstrictor Precautions No information available to require special precautions

Effects on Dental Treatment No effects or complications reported

Pregnancy Risk Factor C

Generic Available Yes

Terra-Cortril® Ophthalmic Suspension *see* Oxytetracycline and Hydrocortisone *on page 718*

Terramycin® I.M. Injection *see* Oxytetracycline *on page 717*

Terramycin® Ophthalmic Ointment *see* Oxytetracycline and Polymyxin B *on page 718*

Terramycin® Oral *see* Oxytetracycline *on page 717*

Terramycin® w/Polymyxin B Ophthalmic Ointment *see* Oxytetracycline and Polymyxin B *on page 718*

Tesamone® Injection *see* Testosterone *on this page*

Teslac® *see* Testolactone *on this page*

TESPA *see* Thiotepa *on page 928*

Tessalon® Perles *see* Benzonatate *on page 120*

Testoderm® Transdermal System *see* Testosterone *on this page*

Testolactone *(tes toe LAK tone)*

Brand Names Teslac®

Therapeutic Category Androgen

Use Palliative treatment of advanced disseminated breast carcinoma

Usual Dosage Adults: Female: Oral: 250 mg 4 times/day for at least 3 months; desired response may take as long as 3 months

Mechanism of Action Testolactone is a synthetic testosterone derivative without significant androgen activity. The drug inhibits steroid aromatase activity, thereby blocking the production of estradiol and estrone from androgen precursors such as testosterone and androstenedione. Unfortunately, the enzymatic block provided by testolactone is transient and is usually limited to a period of 3 months.

Local Anesthetic/Vasoconstrictor Precautions No information available to require special precautions

Effects on Dental Treatment No effects or complications reported

Other Adverse Effects 1% to 10%:

Cardiovascular: Edema

Dermatologic: Maculopapular rash

Endocrine & metabolic: Hypercalcemia

Gastrointestinal: Anorexia, diarrhea, nausea, swelling of tongue

Neuromuscular & skeletal: Paresthesias, peripheral neuropathies

Drug Interactions No data reported

Drug Uptake Absorption: Oral: Absorbed well

Pregnancy Risk Factor C

Dosage Forms Tablet: 50 mg

Generic Available No

Testopel® Pellet *see* Testosterone *on this page*

Testosterona (Mexico) *see* Testosterone *on this page*

Testosterone *(tes TOS ter one)*

Brand Names Androderm® Transdermal System; Andro-L.A.® Injection; Andropository® Injection; Delatest® Injection; Delatestryl® Injection; depAndro® Injection; Depotest® Injection; Depo®-Testosterone Injection; Duratest® Injection; Durathate® Injection; Everone® Injection; Histerone® Injection; Tesamone® Injection; Testoderm® Transdermal System; Testopel® Pellet

Therapeutic Category Androgen

Synonyms Testosterona (Mexico)

Use Androgen replacement therapy in the treatment of delayed male puberty; postpartum breast pain and engorgement; inoperable breast cancer; male hypogonadism

Usual Dosage

Delayed puberty: Males: Children: I.M.: 40-50 mg/m²/dose (cypionate or enanthate) monthly for 6 months

Initiation of pubertal growth: 40-50 mg/m²/dose (cypionate or enanthate) monthly until the growth rate falls to prepubertal levels (~5 cm/year)

During terminal growth phase: 100 mg/m²/dose (cypionate or enanthate) monthly until growth ceases

Maintenance virilizing dose: 100 mg/m²/dose (cypionate or enanthate) twice monthly or 50-400 mg/dose every 2-4 weeks

Inoperable breast cancer: Adults: I.M.: 200-400 mg every 2-4 weeks

Hypogonadism: Males: Adults:

I.M.:

Testosterone or testosterone propionate: 10-25 mg 2-3 times/week

Testosterone cypionate or enanthate: 50-400 mg every 2-4 weeks

Postpubertal cryptorchism: Testosterone or testosterone propionate: 10-25 mg 2-3 times/week

Topical: Initial: 6 mg/day system applied daily applied on scrotal skin. If scrotal area is inadequate, start with a 4 mg/day system. Transdermal system should be worn for 22-24 hours. Determine total serum testosterone after 3-4 weeks of daily application. If patients have not achieved desired results after 6-8 weeks of therapy, another form of testosterone replacement therapy should be considered.

Mechanism of Action Principal endogenous androgen responsible for promoting the growth and development of the male sex organs and maintaining secondary sex characteristics in androgen-deficient males

Local Anesthetic/Vasoconstrictor Precautions No information available to require special precautions

Effects on Dental Treatment No effects or complications reported

Other Adverse Effects

>10%:

Dermatologic: Acne

Endocrine & metabolic: Menstrual problems (amenorrhea), virilism, breast soreness

Genitourinary: Epididimitis, priapism, bladder irritability

1% to 10%:

Cardiovascular: Flushing, edema

Central nervous system: Excitation, aggressive behavior, sleeplessness, anxiety, mental depression, headache

Dermatologic: Hirsutism (increase in pubic hair growth)

Gastrointestinal: Nausea, vomiting, GI irritation

Genitourinary: Prostatic hypertrophy, prostatic carcinoma, impotence, testicular atrophy

Hepatic: Hepatic dysfunction

<1%:

Endocrine & metabolic: Gynecomastia, hypercalcemia, hypoglycemia

Hematologic: Leukopenia, suppression of clotting factors, polycythemia

Hepatic: Cholestatic hepatitis, hepatic necrosis

Miscellaneous: Hypersensitivity reactions

Drug Interactions Increased toxicity: Effects of oral anticoagulants may be enhanced

Drug Uptake

Duration of effect: Based upon the route of administration and which testosterone ester is used; the cypionate and enanthate esters have the longest duration, up to 2-4 weeks after I.M. administration

Serum half-life: 10-100 minutes

Pregnancy Risk Factor X

Dosage Forms

Injection:

Aqueous suspension: 25 mg/mL (10 mL, 30 mL); 50 mg/mL (10 mL, 30 mL); 100 mg/mL (10 mL, 30 mL)

In oil, as cypionate: 100 mg/mL (1 mL, 10 mL); 200 mg/mL (1 mL, 10 mL)

In oil, as enanthate: 100 mg/mL (5 mL, 10 mL); 200 mg/mL (5 mL, 10 mL)

In oil, as propionate: 50 mg/mL (10 mL, 30 mL); 100 mg/mL (10 mL, 30 mL)

Pellet: 75 mg (1 pellet per vial)

Transdermal system:

Androderm®: 2.5 mg/day

Testoderm®: 4 mg/day; 6 mg/day

Generic Available Yes

Testosterone and Estradiol see Estradiol and Testosterone on page 366

Testred® see Methyltestosterone on page 626

Tetanus Immune Globulin (Human)

(TET a nus i MYUN GLOB yoo lin HYU man)

Related Information

Animal and Human Bites Guidelines on page 1093

Brand Names Hyper-Tet®

Canadian/Mexican Brand Names Hyper-Tet® (Mexico); Probi-Tet (Mexico); Tetanogamma® P (Mexico)

(Continued)

Tetanus Immune Globulin (Human) *(Continued)*

Therapeutic Category Immune Globulin

Synonyms TIG

Use Passive immunization against tetanus; tetanus immune globulin is preferred over tetanus antitoxin for treatment of active tetanus; part of the management of an unclean, nonminor wound in a person whose history of previous receipt of tetanus toxoid is unknown or who has received less than three doses of tetanus toxoid

Usual Dosage I.M.:

Prophylaxis of tetanus:

Children: 4 units/kg; some recommend administering 250 units to small children

Adults: 250 units

Treatment of tetanus:

Children: 500-3000 units; some should infiltrate locally around the wound

Adults: 3000-6000 units

Tetanus Prophylaxis in Wound Management

Number of Prior Tetanus Toxoid Doses	Clean, Minor Wounds		All Other Wounds	
	Td*	TIG†	Td*	TIG†
Unknown or <3	Yes	No	Yes	Yes
≥3‡	No#	No	No¶	No

Adapted from Report of the Committee on Infectious Diseases, American Academy of Pediatrics, Elk Grove Village, IL: American Academy of Pediatrics, 1986.

*Adult tetanus and diphtheria toxoids; use pediatric preparations (DT or DTP) if the patient is <7 years old.

†Tetanus immune globulin.

‡If only three doses of fluid tetanus toxoid have been received, a fourth dose of toxoid, preferably an adsorbed toxoid, should be given.

#Yes, if >10 years since last dose.

¶Yes, if >5 years since last dose.

Mechanism of Action Passive immunity toward tetanus

Local Anesthetic/Vasoconstrictor Precautions No information available to require special precautions

Effects on Dental Treatment No effects or complications reported

Other Adverse Effects

>10%: Local: Pain, tenderness, erythema at injection site

1% to 10%:

Central nervous system: Fever (mild)

Dermatologic: Urticaria, angioedema

Neuromuscular & skeletal: Muscle stiffness

Miscellaneous: Anaphylaxis reaction

<1%: Local: Sensitization to repeated injections

Drug Uptake Absorption: Well absorbed

Pregnancy Risk Factor C

Generic Available No

Comments Tetanus immune globulin is preferred over tetanus antitoxin for treatment of active tetanus

Tetanus Toxoid, Adsorbed *(TET a nus TOKS oyd, ad SORBED)*

Canadian/Mexican Brand Names Tetanol® (Mexico)

Therapeutic Category Toxoid

Use Active immunization against tetanus

Usual Dosage Adults: I.M.:

Primary immunization: 0.5 mL; repeat 0.5 mL at 4-8 weeks after first dose and at 6-12 months after second dose

Routine booster doses are recommended only every 5-10 years

Mechanism of Action Tetanus toxoid preparations contain the toxin produced by virulent tetanus bacilli (detoxified growth products of *Clostridium tetani*). The toxin has been modified by treatment with formaldehyde so that is has lost toxicity but still retains ability to act as antigen and produce active immunity.

Local Anesthetic/Vasoconstrictor Precautions No information available to require special precautions

Effects on Dental Treatment No effects or complications reported

Other Adverse Effects

>10%: Local: Induration/redness at injection site

1% to 10%:

Central nervous system: Chills, fever

Local: Sterile abscess at injection site
Miscellaneous: Allergic reaction
<1%:
Central nervous system: Fever >103°F, malaise, neurological disturbances
Local: Blistering at injection site
Miscellaneous: Arthus-type hypersensitivity reactions have occurred rarely in patients >25 years of age and who have received multiple booster doses

Drug Uptake Duration of immunization following primary immunization: ~10 years

Pregnancy Risk Factor C

Generic Available No

Comments Routine booster doses are recommended only every 10 years

Tetanus Toxoid, Fluid (TET a nus TOKS oyd FLOO id)

Canadian/Mexican Brand Names Tetinox® (Mexico); Toxoide Tetanico Myn® (Mexico)

Therapeutic Category Toxoid

Synonyms Tetanus Toxoid Plain

Use Active immunization against tetanus in adults and children

Usual Dosage

Anergy testing: Intradermal: 0.1 mL

Primary immunization (**Note:** Td, TD, DTaP/DTwP are recommended): Adults: Inject 3 doses of 0.5 mL I.M. or S.C. at 4- to 8-week intervals; give fourth dose 6-12 months after third dose

Booster doses: I.M., S.C.: 0.5 mL every 10 years

Mechanism of Action Tetanus toxoid preparations contain the toxin produced by virulent tetanus bacilli (detoxified growth products of *Clostridium tetani*). The toxin has been modified by treatment with formaldehyde so that is has lost toxicity but still retains ability to act as antigen and produce active immunity.

Local Anesthetic/Vasoconstrictor Precautions No information available to require special precautions

Effects on Dental Treatment No effects or complications reported

Other Adverse Effects

>10%: Local: Induration/redness at injection site

1% to 10%:

Central nervous system: Chills, fever

Local: Sterile abscess at injection site

Miscellaneous: Allergic reaction

<1%:

Central nervous system: Fever >103°F, malaise, neurological disturbances

Local: Blistering at injection site

Miscellaneous: Arthus-type hypersensitivity reactions

Pregnancy Risk Factor C

Generic Available No

Comments Tetanus Toxoid, Adsorbed is preferred for all basic immunizing and recall reactions because of more persistent antitoxin titer induction

Tetanus Toxoid Plain see Tetanus Toxoid, Fluid on this page

Tetracaine (TET ra kane)

Related Information

Mouth Pain, Cold Sore, Canker Sore Products on page 1183

Oral Nonviral Soft Tissue Ulcerations or Erosions on page 1070

Oral Pain on page 1053

Brand Names Pontocaine®; Viractin® [OTC]

Canadian/Mexican Brand Names Supracaine® (Canada)

Therapeutic Category Dental/Local Anesthetics; Local Anesthetic, Injectable; Local Anesthetic, Oral; Local Anesthetic, Topical

Use

Dental: Ester-type local anesthetic topically applied to nose and throat for various diagnostic procedures

Medical: Spinal anesthesia; local anesthesia in the eye for various diagnostic and examination purposes

Usual Dosage Children and Adults: Topical: Applied as a 1% or 2% cream to affected areas 3-4 times/day as needed

Mechanism of Action Local anesthetics bind selectively to the intracellular surface of sodium channels to block influx of sodium into the axon. As a result, depolarization necessary for action potential propagation and subsequent nerve function is prevented. The block at the sodium channel is reversible. When drug diffuses away from the axon, sodium channel function is restored and nerve propagation returns.
(Continued)

Tetracaine (Continued)

Local Anesthetic/Vasoconstrictor Precautions No information available to require special precautions

Effects on Dental Treatment No effects or complications reported

Other Adverse Effects 1% to 10%: Dermatologic: Contact dermatitis, burning, stinging, angioedema

Contraindications Hypersensitivity to tetracaine or any component; ophthalmic secondary bacterial infection, patients with liver disease, CNS disease, meningitis (if used for epidural or spinal anesthesia), myasthenia gravis

Warnings/Precautions No pediatric dosage recommendations

Drug Interactions No data reported

Drug Uptake
Onset: Rapid
Duration of action: Topical: 1.5-3 hours

Pregnancy Risk Factor C

Breast-feeding Considerations No data reported

Dosage Forms
Cream: 1%
Cream (Viractin®): 2% (4 g)
Gel (Viractin®): 2% (4 g)

Generic Available Yes

Tetracaine and Dextrose (TET ra kane & DEKS trose)

Related Information
Oral Pain on page 1053

Brand Names Pontocaine® With Dextrose Injection

Therapeutic Category Dental/Local Anesthetics; Local Anesthetic, Injectable

Use Spinal anesthesia (saddle block)

Local Anesthetic/Vasoconstrictor Precautions No information available to require special precautions

Effects on Dental Treatment No effects or complications reported

Pregnancy Risk Factor C

Generic Available Yes

Tetracaine Hydrochloride, Benzocaine Butyl Aminobenzoate and Benzalkonium Chloride see Benzocaine, Butyl Aminobenzoate, Tetracaine, and Benzalkonium Chloride on page 119

Tetracycline (tet ra SYE kleen)

Related Information
Dental Drug Interactions: Update on Drug Combinations Requiring Special Considerations on page 1144
Oral Bacterial Infections on page 1059
Oral Nonviral Soft Tissue Ulcerations or Erosions on page 1070

Brand Names Achromycin®; Achromycin® V; Sumycin®; Tetracyn®

Canadian/Mexican Brand Names Acromicina® (Mexico); Ambotetra® (Mexico); Apo®-Tetra (Canada); Novo-Tetra (Canada); Nu-Tetra (Canada); Quimocyclar® (Mexico); Tetra-Atlantis® (Mexico); Zorbenal-G® (Mexico)

Therapeutic Category Acne Products; Antibiotic, Ophthalmic; Antibiotic, Tetracycline Derivative; Antibiotic, Topical

Use
Dental: Treatment of periodontitis associated with presence of *Actinobacillus actinomycetemcomitans* (AA). As adjunctive therapy in recurrent aphthous ulcers
Medical: In medicine for treatment of susceptible bacterial infections of both gram-positive and gram-negative organisms; also some unusual organisms including *Mycoplasma*, *Chlamydia*, and *Rickettsia*; may also be used for acne, exacerbations of chronic bronchitis, and treatment of gonorrhea and syphilis in patients that are allergic to penicillin

Usual Dosage Adults: 250 mg every 6 hours until improvement (usually 10 days or more)

Mechanism of Action Inhibits bacterial protein synthesis by binding with the 30S and possibly the 50S ribosomal subunit(s) of susceptible bacteria; may also cause alterations in the cytoplasmic membrane

Local Anesthetic/Vasoconstrictor Precautions No information available to require special precautions

Effects on Dental Treatment Opportunistic "superinfection" with *Candida albicans*; tetracycline's are not recommended for use during pregnancy or in children ≤8 years of age since they have been reported to cause enamel hypoplasia and permanent teeth discoloration. The use of tetracycline's should only be used in these patients if other agents are contraindicated or alternative antimicrobials will not eradicate the organism. Long-term use associated with oral candidiasis.

Other Adverse Effects
>10%: Gastrointestinal: Discoloration of teeth and enamel hypoplasia (infants)
1% to 10%:
Dermatologic: Photosensitivity
Gastrointestinal: Nausea, diarrhea

Contraindications Hypersensitivity to tetracycline or any component; do not administer to children ≤8 years of age

Warnings/Precautions Use of tetracyclines during tooth development may cause permanent discoloration of the teeth and enamel, hypoplasia and retardation of skeletal development and bone growth with risk being the greatest for children <4 years of age and those receiving high doses; use with caution in patients with renal or hepatic impairment and in pregnancy; dosage modification required in patients with renal impairment; pseudotumor cerebri has been reported with tetracycline use; outdated drug can cause nephropathy.

Drug Interactions Dairy products; calcium, magnesium or aluminum-containing antacids, iron, zinc, cimetidine causes decreased tetracycline absorption; methoxyflurane anesthesia when concurrent with tetracycline may cause fatal nephrotoxicity; warfarin with tetracyclines leads to increased anticoagulation; penicillin-tetracycline combination counteracts antibiotic effects of each; decreased effect of oral contraceptives

Drug Uptake
Absorption: Oral: 75%
Serum half-life: Normal renal function: 8-11 hours
Time to peak serum concentration: Oral: Within 2-4 hours

Pregnancy Risk Factor D; B (topical)

Breast-feeding Considerations May be taken while breast-feeding

Dosage Forms
Capsule: 100 mg, 250 mg, 500 mg
Suspension, oral: 125 mg/5 mL (60 mL, 480 mL)
Tablet: 250 mg, 500 mg

Dietary Considerations Should be taken 1 hour before or 2 hours after meals with adequate amounts of fluid; food decreases absorption; avoid taking antacids, iron, dairy products, or milk formulas within 3 hours of tetracyclines; decreases absorption of magnesium, zinc, calcium, iron, and amino acids

Generic Available Yes

Comments *Helicobacter pylori*: Clinically effective treatment regimens include triple therapy with amoxicillin or tetracycline, metronidazole, and bismuth subsalicylate; amoxicillin, metronidazole, and H_2 receptor antagonist; or double therapy with amoxicillin and omeprazole. Adult dose of tetracycline against *H. pylori*: 250 mg 3 times/day to 500 mg 4 times/day

Selected Readings
Gordon JM and Walker CB, "Current Status of Systemic Antibiotic Usage in Destructive Periodontal Disease," *J Periodontol*, 1993, 64(8 Suppl): 760-71.
Rams TE and Slots J, "Antibiotics in Periodontal Therapy: An Update," *Compendium*, 1992, 13(12):1130, 1132, 1134.
Seymour RA and Heasman PA, "Tetracyclines in the Management of Periodontal Diseases. A Review," *J Clin Periodontol*, 1995, 22(1):22-35.
Seymour RA and Heasman PA, "Pharmacological Control of Periodontal Disease. II. Antimicrobial Agents," *J Dent*, 1995, 23(1):5-14

Tetracycline Periodontal Fibers
(tet ra SYE kleen per ee oh DON tal FYE bers)

Related Information
Dental Drug Interactions: Update on Drug Combinations Requiring Special Considerations *on page 1144*

Brand Names Actisite®

Therapeutic Category Antibacterial, Dental

Use
Dental: Treatment of adult periodontitis; as an adjunct to scaling and root planing for the reduction of pocket depth and bleeding on probing in selected patients with adult periodontitis
Medical: No data reported

Usual Dosage
Children: Has not been established
Adults: Insert fiber to fill the periodontal pocket; each fiber contains 12.7 mg of tetracycline in 23 cm (9 inches) and provides continuous release of drug for 10 days; fibers are to be secured in pocket with cyanoacrylate adhesive and left in place for 10 days

Mechanism of Action Tetracycline is an antibiotic which inhibits growth of susceptible microorganisms. Tetracycline binds primarily to the 30S subunits of bacterial ribosomes, and appears to prevent access of aminoacyl tRNA to the
(Continued)

Tetracycline Periodontal Fibers *(Continued)*

acceptor site on the mRNA-ribosome complex. The fiber releases tetracycline into the periodontal site at a rate of 2 mcg/cm/hour.

Local Anesthetic/Vasoconstrictor Precautions No information available to require special precautions

Effects on Dental Treatment 1% to 10% of patients experience gingival inflammation, pain in mouth, glossitis, candidiasis, staining of tongue

Other Adverse Effects 1% to 10%:
Dermatologic: Local erythema following removal
Miscellaneous: Discomfort from fiber placement

Contraindications Known hypersensitivity to tetracyclines

Warnings/Precautions Use of tetracyclines is not recommended during pregnancy because of interference with fetal bone and dental development

Drug Interactions No data reported

Drug Uptake
The fiber releases tetracycline at a rate of 2 mcg/cm/hour
Tissue fluid concentrations:
Gingival fluid: ~1590 mcg/mL of tetracycline per site over 10 days
Plasma: During fiber treatment of up to 11 teeth, the tetracycline plasma concentration was below any detectable levels (<0.1 mcg/mL)
Oral: 500 mg of tetracycline produces a peak plasma level of 3-4 mcg/mL
Saliva: ~50.7 mcg/mL of tetracycline immediately after fiber treatment of 9 teeth

Pregnancy Risk Factor C

Breast-feeding Considerations It is not known whether tetracycline from periodontal fibers is distributed into human breast milk

Dosage Forms Fibers 23 cm (9") in length; 12.7 mg of tetracycline hydrochloride per fiber

Dietary Considerations No data reported

Generic Available No

Comments A number of different facultative and obligate anaerobic bacteria have been found to be causative factors in periodontal disease. These include *Actinobacillus actinomycetemcomitans* (AA), *Fusobacterium nucleatum*, and *Porphyromonas gingivalis*. These bacteria are sensitive to tetracyclines at similar concentrations as those released from the tetracycline-impregnated fibers. Placement of tetracycline periodontal fibers into gingival pockets decreases inflammation, edema, pocket depth, and bleeding upon probing.

Selected Readings
Baer PN, "Actisite (Tetracycline Hydrochloride Periodontal Fiber): A Critique," *Periodontal Clin Investig*, 1994, 16(2):5-7.
Greenstein G, "Treating Periodontal Diseases With Tetracycline-Impregnanted Fibers: Data and Controversies," *Compend Contin Educ Dent*, 1995, 16(5):448-55.
Kerry G, "Tetracycline-Loaded Fibers as Adjunctive Treatment in Periodontal Disease," *J Am Dent Assoc*, 1994, 125(9):1199-203.
Michalowicz BS, Pihlstrom BL, Drisko CL, et al, "Evaluation of Periodontal Treatments Using Controlled-Release Tetracycline Fibers: Maintenance Response," *J Periodontol*, 1995, 66(8):708-15.
Mombelli A, Lehmann B, Tonetti M, et al, "Clinical Response to Local Delivery of Tetracycline in Relation to Overall and Local Periodontal Conditions," *J Clin Periodontol*, 1997, 24(7):470-77.
Vandekerckhove BN, Quirynen M, and van Steenberghe D, "The Use of Tetracycline-Containing Controlled-Release Fibers in the Treatment of Refractory Periodontitis," *J Periodontol*, 1997, 68(4):353-61.

Tetracyn® *see* Tetracycline *on page 914*

Tetrahydrozoline *(tet ra hye DROZ a leen)*

Brand Names Collyrium Fresh® Ophthalmic [OTC]; Eyesine® Ophthalmic [OTC]; Geneye® Ophthalmic [OTC]; Mallazine® Eye Drops [OTC]; Murine® Plus Ophthalmic [OTC]; Optigene® Ophthalmic [OTC]; Tetrasine® Extra Ophthalmic [OTC]; Tetrasine® Ophthalmic [OTC]; Tyzine® Nasal; Visine® Extra Ophthalmic [OTC]

Therapeutic Category Adrenergic Agonist Agent; Adrenergic Agonist Agent, Ophthalmic; Nasal Agent, Vasoconstrictor; Ophthalmic Agent, Vasoconstrictor

Use Symptomatic relief of nasal congestion and conjunctival congestion

Usual Dosage
Nasal congestion: Intranasal:
Children 2-6 years: Instill 2-3 drops of 0.05% solution every 4-6 hours as needed, no more frequent than every 3 hours
Children >6 years and Adults: Instill 2-4 drops or 3-4 sprays of 0.1% solution every 3-4 hours as needed, no more frequent than every 3 hours

Conjunctival congestion: Ophthalmic: Adults: Instill 1-2 drops in each eye 2-4 times/day

Mechanism of Action Stimulates alpha-adrenergic receptors in the arterioles of the conjunctiva and the nasal mucosa to produce vasoconstriction

Local Anesthetic/Vasoconstrictor Precautions No information available to require special precautions

Effects on Dental Treatment No effects or complications reported
Other Adverse Effects
>10%:
Local: Transient stinging
Respiratory: Sneezing
1% to 10%:
Cardiovascular: Tachycardia, palpitations, hypertension, heart rate
Central nervous system: Headache
Neuromuscular & skeletal: Tremor
Ocular: Blurred vision

Drug Interactions Increased toxicity: MAO inhibitors can cause an exaggerated adrenergic response if taken concurrently or within 21 days of discontinuing MAO inhibitor; beta-blockers can cause hypertensive episodes and increased risk of intracranial hemorrhage; anesthetics

Drug Uptake
Onset of decongestant effect: Intranasal: Within 4-8 hours
Duration: Ophthalmic vasoconstriction: 2-3 hours
Pregnancy Risk Factor C

Dosage Forms Solution, as hydrochloride:
Nasal: 0.05% (15 mL), 0.1% (30 mL, 473 mL)
Ophthalmic: 0.05% (15 mL)
Generic Available Yes

Tetrasine® Extra Ophthalmic [OTC] *see* Tetrahydrozoline *on previous page*
Tetrasine® Ophthalmic [OTC] *see* Tetrahydrozoline *on previous page*
Teveten® *see* Eprosartan *on page 357*

TG *see* Thioguanine *on page 925*
6-TG *see* Thioguanine *on page 925*
T/Gel® [OTC] *see* Coal Tar *on page 254*
T-Gen® *see* Trimethobenzamide *on page 964*

T-Gesic® [5/500] *see* Hydrocodone and Acetaminophen *on page 478*
Thalitone® *see* Chlorthalidone *on page 227*
THAM-E® Injection *see* Tromethamine *on page 972*
THAM® Injection *see* Tromethamine *on page 972*

Theo-24® *see* Theophylline *on this page*
Theobid® *see* Theophylline *on this page*
Theochron® *see* Theophylline *on this page*

Theoclear® L.A. *see* Theophylline *on this page*
Theo-Dur® *see* Theophylline *on this page*
Theolair™ *see* Theophylline *on this page*

Theophylline (thee OF i lin)
Related Information
Aminophylline *on page 56*
Dental Drug Interactions: Update on Drug Combinations Requiring Special Considerations *on page 1144*
Respiratory Diseases *on page 1018*

Brand Names Aerolate III®; Aerolate JR®; Aerolate SR® S; Aquaphyllin®; Asmalix®; Bronkodyl®; Elixophyllin®; Quibron®-T; Quibron®-T/SR; Respbid®; Slo-bid™; Slo-Phyllin®; Sustaire®; Theo-24®; Theobid®; Theochron®; Theoclear® L.A.; Theo-Dur®; Theolair™; Theospan®-SR; Theovent®; Theo-X®; Uni-Dur®; Uniphyl®
Canadian/Mexican Brand Names Apo®-Theo LA (Canada); Phyllocontin® (Canada); Pulmophylline® (Canada)

Therapeutic Category Antiasthmatic; Bronchodilator; Theophylline Derivative
Use Bronchodilator in reversible airway obstruction due to asthma, chronic bronchitis, and emphysema; for neonatal apnea/bradycardia

(Continued)

Theophylline (Continued)

Usual Dosage Use ideal body weight for obese patients
I.V.: Initial: Maintenance infusion rates:
  Children:
    6 weeks to 6 months: 0.5 mg/kg/hour
    6 months to 1 year: 0.6-0.7 mg/kg/hour

Children >1 year and Adults:
  Treatment of acute bronchospasm: I.V.: Loading dose (in patients not
  currently receiving aminophylline or theophylline): 6 mg/kg (based on aminophylline) given I.V. over 20-30 minutes; administration rate should not exceed
  25 mg/minute (aminophylline). See table.

Approximate I.V. Theophylline Dosage for Treatment of Acute Bronchospasm

Group	Dosage for next 12 h*	Dosage after 12 h*
Infants 6 wk to 6 mo	0.5 mg/kg/h	
Children 6 mo to 1 y	0.6-0.7 mg/kg/h	
Children 1-9 y	0.95 mg/kg/h (1.2 mg/kg/h)	0.79 mg/kg/h (1 mg/kg/h)
Children 9-16 y and young adult smokers	0.79 mg/kg/h (1 mg/kg/h)	0.63 mg/kg/h (0.8 mg/kg/h)
Healthy, nonsmoking adults	0.55 mg/kg/h (0.7 mg/kg/h)	0.39 mg/kg/h (0.5 mg/kg/h)
Older patients and patients with cor pulmonale	0.47 mg/kg/h (0.6 mg/kg/h)	0.24 mg/kg/h (0.3 mg/kg/h)
Patients with congestive heart failure or liver failure	0.39 mg/kg/h (0.5 mg/kg/h)	0.08-0.16 mg/kg/h (0.1-0.2 mg/kg/h)

*Equivalent hydrous aminophylline dosage indicated in parentheses.

Approximate I.V. maintenance dosages are based upon continuous infusions; bolus dosing (often used in children <6 months of age) may be determined by multiplying the hourly infusion rate by 24 hours and dividing by the desired number of doses/day; see table.

Maintenance Dose for Acute Symptoms

Population Group	Oral Theophylline (mg/kg/day)	I.V. Aminophylline
Premature infant or newborn - 6 wk (for apnea/bradycardia)	4	5 mg/kg/day
6 wk - 6 mo	10	12 mg/kg/day or continuous I.V. infusion*
Infants 6 mo-1 y	12-18	15 mg/kg/day or continuous I.V. infusion*
Children 1-9 y	20-24	1 mg/kg/hour
Children 9-12 y, and adolescent daily smokers of cigarettes or marijuana, and otherwise healthy adult smokers <50 y	16	0.9 mg/kg/hour
Adolescents 12-16 y (nonsmokers)	13	0.7 mg/kg/hour
Otherwise healthy nonsmoking adults (including elderly patients)	10 (not to exceed 900 mg/day)	0.5 mg/kg/hour
Cardiac decompensation, cor pulmonale and/or liver dysfunction	5 (not to exceed 400 mg/day)	0.25 mg/kg/hour

*For continuous I.V. infusion divide total daily dose by 24 = mg/kg/hour.

Dosage should be adjusted according to serum level measurements during the first 12- to 24-hour period; see table.

Dosage Adjustment After Serum Theophylline Measurement

Serum Theophylline		Guidelines
Within normal limits	10-20 mcg/mL	Maintain dosage if tolerated. Recheck serum theophylline concentration at 6- to 12-month intervals.*
Too high	20-25 mcg/mL	Decrease doses by about 10%. Recheck serum theophylline concentration at 3 days and then at 6- to 12-month intervals.*
	25-30 mcg/mL	Skip next dose and decrease subsequent doses by about 25%. Recheck serum theophylline.
	>30 mcg/mL	Skip next 2 doses and decrease subsequent doses by 50%. Recheck serum theophylline.
Too low	7.5-10 mcg/mL	Increase dose by about 25%.† Recheck serum theophylline concentration at 3 days and then at 6- to 12-month intervals.*
	5-7.5 mcg/mL	Increase dose by about 25% to the nearest dose increment† and recheck serum theophylline for guidance in further dosage adjustment (another increase will probably be needed, but this provides a safety check).

From Weinberger M and Hendeles L,"Practical Guide to Using Theophylline," *J Resp Dis*, 1981, 2:12-27.

*Finer adjustments in dosage may be needed for some patients.

†Dividing the daily dose into 3 doses administered at 8-hour intervals may be indicated if symptoms occur repeatedly at the end of a dosing interval.

Oral theophylline: Initial dosage recommendation: Loading dose (to achieve a serum level of about 10 mcg/mL; loading doses should be given using a rapidly absorbed oral product **not** a sustained release product):

Oral Theophylline Dosage for Bronchial Asthma*

Age	Initial 3 Days	Second 3 Days	Steady-State Maintenance
<1 y	0.2 x (age in weeks) + 5		0.3 x (age in weeks) + 8
1-9 y	16 up to a maximum of 400 mg/24 h	20	22
9-12 y	16 up to a maximum of 400 mg/24 h	16 up to a maximum of 600 mg/24 h	20 up to a maximum of 800 mg/24 h
12-16 y	16 up to a maximum of 400 mg/24 h	16 up to a maximum of 600 mg/24 h	18 up to a maximum of 900 mg/24 h
Adults	400 mg/24 h	600 mg/24 h	900 mg/24 h

*Dose in mg/kg/24 hours of theophylline.

If no theophylline has been administered in the previous 24 hours: 4-6 mg/kg theophylline

If theophylline has been administered in the previous 24 hours: administer ½ loading dose or 2-3 mg/kg theophylline can be given in emergencies when serum levels are not available

(Continued)

Theophylline *(Continued)*

On the average, for every 1 mg/kg theophylline given, blood levels will rise 2 mcg/mL

Ideally, defer the loading dose if a serum theophylline concentration can be obtained rapidly. However, if this is not possible, exercise clinical judgment. If the patient is not experiencing theophylline toxicity, this is unlikely to result in dangerous adverse effects.

Increasing dose: The dosage may be increased in approximately 25% increments at 2- to 3-day intervals so long as the drug is tolerated or until the maximum dose is reached

Maintenance dose: In children and healthy adults, a slow-release product can be used; the total daily dose can be divided every 8-12 hours

Mechanism of Action Causes bronchodilatation, diuresis, CNS and cardiac stimulation, and gastric acid secretion by blocking phosphodiesterase which increases tissue concentrations of cyclic adenine monophosphate (cAMP) which in turn promotes catecholamine stimulation of lipolysis, glycogenolysis, and gluconeogenesis and induces release of epinephrine from adrenal medulla cells

Local Anesthetic/Vasoconstrictor Precautions No information available to require special precautions

Effects on Dental Treatment Prescribe erythromycin products with caution to patients taking theophylline products. Erythromycin will delay the normal metabolic inactivation of theophyllines leading to increased blood levels; this has resulted in nausea, vomiting and CNS restlessness

Other Adverse Effects See table.

Theophylline Serum Levels (mcg/mL)*	Adverse Reactions
15-25	GI upset, diarrhea, N/V, abdominal pain, nervousness, headache, insomnia, agitation, dizziness, muscle cramp, tremor
25-35	Tachycardia, occasional PVC
>35	Ventricular tachycardia, frequent PVC, seizure

*Adverse effects do not necessarily occur according to serum levels. Arrhythmia and seizure can occur without seeing the other adverse effects.

Uncommon at serum theophylline concentrations ≤20 mcg/mL

1% to 10%:

Cardiovascular: Tachycardia
Central nervous system: Nervousness, restlessness
Gastrointestinal: Nausea, vomiting
<1%:
Central nervous system: Insomnia, irritability, seizures
Dermatologic: Skin rash
Gastrointestinal: Gastric irritation
Neuromuscular & skeletal: Tremor
Miscellaneous: Allergic reactions

Drug Interactions Decreased effect/increased toxicity: Changes in diet may affect the elimination of theophylline; charcoal-broiled foods may increase elimination, reducing half-life by 50%; see table for factors affecting serum levels.

Factors Reported to Affect Theophylline Serum Levels

Decreased Theophylline Level	Increased Theophylline Level
Smoking (cigarettes, marijuana)	Hepatic cirrhosis
High protein/low carbohydrate diet	Cor pulmonale
Charcoal	CHF
Phenytoin	Fever/viral illness
Phenobarbital	Propranolol
Carbamazepine	Allopurinol (>600 mg/d)
Rifampin	Erythromycin
I.V. isoproterenol	Cimetidine
Aminoglutethimide	Troleandomycin
Barbiturates	Ciprofloxacin
Hydantoins	Oral contraceptives
Ketoconazole	Beta blockers
Sulfinpyrazone	Calcium channel blockers
Isoniazid	Corticosteroids
Loop diuretics	Disulfiram
Sympathomimetics	Ephedrine
	Influenza virus vaccine
	Interferon
	Macrolides
	Mexiletine
	Quinolones
	Thiabendazole
	Thyroid hormones
	Carbamazepine
	Isoniazid
	Loop diuretics

Pregnancy Risk Factor C
Dosage Forms
  Capsule:
    Immediate release (Bronkodyl®, Elixophyllin®): 100 mg, 200 mg
    Timed release:
      8-12 hours (Aerolate®): 65 mg [III]; 130 mg [JR], 260 mg [SR]
      8-12 hours (Slo-Bid™): 50 mg, 75 mg, 100 mg, 125 mg, 200 mg, 300 mg
      8-12 hours (Slo-Phyllin® Gyrocaps®): 60 mg, 125 mg, 250 mg
      12 hours (Theobid® Duracaps®): 260 mg
      12 hours (Theoclear® L.A.): 130 mg, 260 mg
      12 hours (Theospan®-SR): 130 mg, 260 mg
      12 hours (Theovent®): 125 mg, 250 mg
      24 hours (Theo-24®): 100 mg, 200 mg, 300 mg
  Elixir (Asmalix®, Elixomin®, Elixophyllin®, Lanophyllin®): 80 mg/15 mL (15 mL, 30
    mL, 480 mL, 4000 mL)
  Infusion, in D₅W: 0.4 mg/mL (1000 mL); 0.8 mg/mL (500 mL, 1000 mL); 1.6 mg/
    mL (250 mL, 500 mL); 2 mg/mL (100 mL); 3.2 mg/mL (250 mL); 4 mg/mL (50
    mL, 100 mL);
  Solution, oral:
    Theolair™: 80 mg/15 mL (15 mL, 18.75 mL, 30 mL, 480 mL)
  Syrup:
    Aquaphyllin®, Slo-Phyllin®, Theoclear-80®, Theostat-80®: 80 mg/15 mL (15 mL,
      30 mL, 500 mL)
    Accurbron®: 150 mg/15 mL (480 mL)
  Tablet: Immediate release:
    Slo-Phyllin®: 100 mg, 200 mg
    Theolair™: 125 mg, 250 mg
    Quibron®-T: 300 mg
  Tablet:
    Controlled release (Theo-X®): 100 mg, 200 mg, 300 mg
    Timed release:
      12-24 hours: 100 mg, 200 mg, 300 mg, 450 mg
      8-12 hours (Quibron®-T/SR): 300 mg
      8-12 hours (Respbid®): 250 mg, 500 mg
      8-12 hours (Sustaire®): 100 mg, 300 mg
      8-12 hours (T-Phyl®): 200 mg
      12-24 hours (Theochron®): 100 mg, 200 mg, 300 mg
(Continued)

Theophylline *(Continued)*

8-24 hour: 100 mg, 200 mg, 300 mg
8-24 hours (Theo-Dur®): 100 mg, 200 mg, 300 mg, 450 mg
8-24 hours (Theo-Sav®): 100 mg, 200 mg, 300 mg
24 hours (Theolair™-SR): 200 mg, 250 mg, 300 mg, 500 mg
24 hours (Uni-Dur®): 400 mg, 600 mg
24 hours (Uniphyl®): 400 mg

Generic Available Yes

Theophylline and Guaifenesin (thee OF i lin & gwye FEN e sin)

Brand Names Bronchial®; Glycerol-T®; Quibron®; Slo-Phyllin GG®

Therapeutic Category Antiasthmatic; Bronchodilator; Expectorant; Theophylline Derivative

Use Symptomatic treatment of bronchospasm associated with bronchial asthma, chronic bronchitis and pulmonary emphysema

Local Anesthetic/Vasoconstrictor Precautions No information available to require special precautions

Effects on Dental Treatment Do not prescribe any erythromycin product to patients taking theophylline products. Erythromycin will delay the normal metabolic inactivation of theophyllines leading to increased blood levels; this has resulted in nausea, vomiting and CNS restlessness

Pregnancy Risk Factor C

Dosage Forms

Capsule: Theophylline 150 mg and guaifenesin 90 mg; theophylline 300 mg and guaifenesin 180 mg

Elixir: Theophylline 150 mg and guaifenesin 90 mg per 15 mL (480 mL)

Generic Available Yes

Theophylline, Ephedrine, and Hydroxyzine

(thee OF i lin, e FED rin, & hye DROKS i zeen)

Brand Names Hydrophed®; Marax®

Therapeutic Category Antiasthmatic; Bronchodilator; Theophylline Derivative

Use Possibly effective for controlling bronchospastic disorders

Local Anesthetic/Vasoconstrictor Precautions Use vasoconstrictors with caution since ephedrine may enhance cardiostimulation and vasopressor effects of sympathomimetics

Effects on Dental Treatment Prescribe erythromycin products with caution to patients taking theophylline products. Erythromycin will delay the normal metabolic inactivation of theophyllines leading to increased blood levels; this has resulted in nausea, vomiting and CNS restlessness

Pregnancy Risk Factor C

Dosage Forms

Syrup, dye free: Theophylline 32.5 mg, ephedrine 6.25 mg, and hydroxyzine 2.5 mg per 5 mL

Tablet: Theophylline 130 mg, ephedrine 25 mg, and hydroxyzine 10 mg

Generic Available Yes

Theophylline, Ephedrine, and Phenobarbital

(thee OF i lin, e FED rin, & fee noe BAR bi tal)

Brand Names Tedral®

Therapeutic Category Antiasthmatic; Bronchodilator; Theophylline Derivative

Synonyms Ephedrine, Theophylline and Phenobarbital

Use Prevention and symptomatic treatment of bronchial asthma; relief of asthmatic bronchitis and other bronchospastic disorders

Usual Dosage

Children >60 lb: 1 tablet or 5 mL every 4 hours

Adults: 1-2 tablets or 10-20 mL every 4 hours

Local Anesthetic/Vasoconstrictor Precautions Use vasoconstrictors with caution since ephedrine may enhance cardiostimulation and vasopressor effects of sympathomimetics

Effects on Dental Treatment Prescribe erythromycin products with caution to patients taking theophylline products. Erythromycin will delay the normal metabolic inactivation of theophyllines leading to increased blood levels; this has resulted in nausea, vomiting and CNS restlessness

Pregnancy Risk Factor D

Dosage Forms

Suspension: Theophylline 65 mg, ephedrine sulfate 12 mg, and phenobarbital 4 mg per 5 mL

Tablet: Theophylline 118 mg, ephedrine sulfate 25 mg, and phenobarbital 11 mg; theophylline 130 mg, ephedrine sulfate 24 mg, and phenobarbital 8 mg

Generic Available Yes

Theophylline Ethylenediamine *see Aminophylline on page 56*

Theospan®-SR *see Theophylline on page 917*

Theovent® *see Theophylline on page 917*

Theo-X® *see Theophylline on page 917*

Therabid® [OTC] *see Vitamins, Multiple on page 995*

Thera-Combex® H-P Kapseals® [OTC] *see Vitamin B Complex With Vitamin C on page 994*

TheraCys™ *see BCG Vaccine on page 111*

Theraflu® Non-Drowsy Formula Maximum Strength [OTC] *see Acetaminophen, Dextromethorphan, and Pseudoephedrine on page 25*

Thera-Flur® *see Fluoride on page 415*

Thera-Flur-N® *see Fluoride on page 415*

Theragran® [OTC] *see Vitamins, Multiple on page 995*

Theragran® Hematinic® *see Vitamins, Multiple on page 995*

Theragran® Liquid [OTC] *see Vitamins, Multiple on page 995*

Theragran-M® [OTC] *see Vitamins, Multiple on page 995*

Thera-Hist® Syrup [OTC] *see Chlorpheniramine and Phenylpropanolamine on page 219*

Theramin® Expectorant [OTC] *see Guaifenesin and Phenylpropanolamine on page 454*

Therapeutic Multivitamins *see Vitamins, Multiple on page 995*

Theraplex Z® [OTC] *see Pyrithione Zinc on page 826*

Thermazene® *see Silver Sulfadiazine on page 865*

Theroxide® Wash [OTC] *see Benzoyl Peroxide on page 120*

Thiabendazole (thye a BEN da zole)

Brand Names Mintezol®

Therapeutic Category Anthelmintic

Use Treatment of strongyloidiasis, cutaneous larva migrans, visceral larva migrans, dracunculiasis, trichinosis, and mixed helminthic infections

Usual Dosage Purgation is not required prior to use; drinking of fruit juice aids in expulsion of worms by removing the mucous to which the intestinal tapeworms attach themselves.

Children and Adults: Oral: 50 mg/kg/day divided every 12 hours; maximum dose: 3 g/day
Strongyloidiasis: For 2 consecutive days
Cutaneous larva migrans: For 2-5 consecutive days
Visceral larva migrans: For 5-7 consecutive days
Trichinosis: For 2-4 consecutive days
Dracunculosis: 50-75 mg/kg/day divided every 12 hours for 3 days

Mechanism of Action Inhibits helminth-specific mitochondrial fumarate reductase

Local Anesthetic/Vasoconstrictor Precautions No information available to require special precautions

Effects on Dental Treatment No effects or complications reported

Other Adverse Effects

>10%:
Central nervous system: Seizures, hallucinations, delirium, dizziness, drowsiness, headache
Gastrointestinal: Anorexia, diarrhea, nausea, vomiting, drying of mucous membranes
Neuromuscular & skeletal: Numbness
Otic: Tinnitus

1% to 10%: Dermatologic: Skin rash, Stevens-Johnson syndrome

<1%:
Central nervous system: Chills
Genitourinary: Malodor of urine
Hematologic: Leukopenia
Hepatic: Hepatotoxicity
Ocular: Blurred or yellow vision
Renal: Nephrotoxicity
Miscellaneous: Lymphadenopathy, hypersensitivity reactions

Drug Interactions Increased levels of theophylline and other xanthines

Drug Uptake

Absorption: Rapid and nearly complete
Time to peak serum concentration: Within 1-2 hours

Pregnancy Risk Factor C

Generic Available No

Thiamine (THYE a min)
Brand Names Betalin®S; Biamine®
Canadian/Mexican Brand Names Betaxin® (Canada); Bewon® (Canada)
Therapeutic Category Vitamin, Water Soluble
Use Treatment of thiamine deficiency including beriberi, Wernicke's encephalopathy syndrome, and peripheral neuritis associated with pellagra, alcoholic patients with altered sensorium; various genetic metabolic disorders
Usual Dosage
  Recommended daily allowance:
    <6 months: 0.3 mg
    6 months to 1 year: 0.4 mg
    1-3 years: 0.7 mg
    4-6 years: 0.9 mg
    7-10 years: 1 mg
    11-14 years: 1.1-1.3 mg
    >14 years: 1-1.5 mg
  Thiamine deficiency (beriberi):
    Children: 10-25 mg/dose I.M. or I.V. daily (if critically ill), or 10-50 mg/dose orally every day for 2 weeks, then 5-10 mg/dose orally daily for 1 month
    Adults: 5-30 mg/dose I.M. or I.V. 3 times/day (if critically ill); then orally 5-30 mg/day in single or divided doses 3 times/day for 1 month
  Wenicke's encephalopathy: Adults: Initial: 100 mg I.V., then 50-100 mg/day I.M. or I.V. until consuming a regular, balanced diet
  Dietary supplement (depends on caloric or carbohydrate content of the diet):
    Children: 0.5-1 mg/day
    Adults: 1-2 mg/day
    Note: The above doses can be found in multivitamin preparations
  Metabolic disorders: Oral: Adults: 10-20 mg/day (dosages up to 4 g/day in divided doses have been used)
Mechanism of Action An essential coenzyme in carbohydrate metabolism by combining with adenosine triphosphate to form thiamine pyrophosphate
Local Anesthetic/Vasoconstrictor Precautions No information available to require special precautions
Effects on Dental Treatment No effects or complications reported
Other Adverse Effects <1%:
  Cardiovascular: Cardiovascular collapse and death
  Dermatologic: Rash, angioedema
  Neuromuscular & skeletal: Paresthesia
  Miscellaneous: Feeling of warmth
Drug Interactions No data reported
Drug Uptake
  Absorption:
    Oral: Adequate
    I.M.: Rapid and complete
Pregnancy Risk Factor A (C if dose exceeds RDA recommendation)
Generic Available Yes

Thiethylperazine (thye eth il PER a zeen)
Brand Names Norzine®; Torecan®
Therapeutic Category Antiemetic
Use Relief of nausea and vomiting
  Unlabeled use: Treatment of vertigo
Usual Dosage Children >12 years and Adults:
  Oral, I.M., rectal: 10 mg 1-3 times/day as needed
  I.V. and S.C. routes of administration are not recommended

  Not dialyzable (0% to 5%)
  Dosing comments in hepatic impairment: Use with caution
Mechanism of Action Blocks postsynaptic mesolimbic dopaminergic receptors in the brain; exhibits a strong alpha-adrenergic blocking effect and depresses the release of hypothalamic and hypophyseal hormones; acts directly on chemoreceptor trigger zone and vomiting center
Local Anesthetic/Vasoconstrictor Precautions No information available to require special precautions
Effects on Dental Treatment >10% of patients will experience dry mouth
Other Adverse Effects
  >10%:
    Central nervous system: Drowsiness, dizziness
    Respiratory: Dry nose
  1% to 10%:
    Cardiovascular: Tachycardia, orthostatic hypotension

Central nervous system: Confusion, convulsions, extrapyramidal effects, tardive dyskinesia, fever, headache
Hematologic: Agranulocytosis
Hepatic: Cholestatic jaundice
Otic: Tinnitus

Drug Interactions Increased effect/toxicity with CNS depressants (eg, anesthetics, opiates, tranquilizers, alcohol), lithium, atropine, epinephrine, MAO inhibitors, TCAs

Drug Uptake
Onset of antiemetic effect: Within 30 minutes
Duration of action: ~4 hours

Pregnancy Risk Factor X
Generic Available No

Thimerosal (thye MER oh sal)
Brand Names Aeroaid® [OTC]; Mersol® [OTC]; Merthiolate® [OTC]
Therapeutic Category Antibacterial, Topical
Use Organomercurial antiseptic with sustained bacteriostatic and fungistatic activity
Local Anesthetic/Vasoconstrictor Precautions No information available to require special precautions
Effects on Dental Treatment No effects or complications reported
Generic Available Yes

Thioguanine (thye oh GWAH neen)
Therapeutic Category Antineoplastic Agent, Antimetabolite
Synonyms 2-Amino-6-Mercaptopurine; TG; 6-TG; 6-Thioguanine; Tioguanine
Use Remission induction in acute myelogenous (nonlymphocytic) leukemia; treatment of chronic myelogenous leukemia and acute lymphocytic leukemia
Usual Dosage Total daily dose can be given at one time; offers little advantage over mercaptopurine; is sometimes ordered as 6-thioguanine, with 6 being part of the drug name and not some kind of unit or strength

Oral (refer to individual protocols):
Children <3 years: Combination drug therapy for acute nonlymphocytic leukemia: 3.3 mg/kg/day in divided doses twice daily for 4 days
Children and Adults: 2-3 mg/kg/day calculated to nearest 20 mg or 75-200 mg/m^2/day in 1-2 divided doses for 5-7 days or until remission is attained
Dosing comments in renal or hepatic impairment: Reduce dose

Mechanism of Action Purine analog that is incorporated into DNA and RNA resulting in the blockage of synthesis and metabolism of purine nucleotides
Local Anesthetic/Vasoconstrictor Precautions No information available to require special precautions
Effects on Dental Treatment No effects or complications reported
Other Adverse Effects
1% to 10%:
Dermatologic: Skin rash
Endocrine & metabolic: Hyperuricemia
Gastrointestinal: Mild nausea or vomiting, anorexia, stomatitis, diarrhea
Emetic potential: Low (<10%)
Neuromuscular: Unsteady gait
<1%:
Central nervous system: Neurotoxicity
Dermatologic: Photosensitivity
Hepatic: Hepatitis, jaundice, veno-occlusive hepatic disease

Drug Uptake
Absorption: Oral: 30%
Serum half-life, terminal: 11 hours
Time to peak serum concentration: Within 8 hours

Pregnancy Risk Factor D
Generic Available No

6-Thioguanine see Thioguanine on this page
Thiola™ see Tiopronin on page 936

Thiopental (thye oh PEN tal)
Brand Names Pentothal® Sodium
Therapeutic Category Barbiturate; General Anesthetic, Intravenous; Sedative
Synonyms Tiopental Sodico (Mexico)
Use Induction of anesthesia; adjunct for intubation in head injury patients; control of convulsive states; treatment of elevated intracranial pressure
(Continued)

Thiopental *(Continued)*

Usual Dosage I.V.:
Induction anesthesia:
Children 1-12 years: 5-6 mg/kg
Adults: 3-5 mg/kg

Maintenance anesthesia:
Children: 1 mg/kg as needed
Adults: 25-100 mg as needed

Increased intracranial pressure: Children and Adults: 1.5-5 mg/kg/dose; repeat as needed to control intracranial pressure

Seizures:
Children: 2-3 mg/kg/dose, repeat as needed
Adults: 75-250 mg/dose, repeat as needed

Rectal administration: (Patient should be NPO for no less than 3 hours prior to administration)
Suggested initial doses of thiopental rectal suspension are:
<3 months: 15 mg/kg/dose
>3 months: 25 mg/kg/dose
Note: The age of a premature infant should be adjusted to reflect the age that the infant would have been if full-term (eg, an infant, now age 4 months, who was 2 months premature should be considered to be a 2-month old infant).
Doses should be rounded downward to the nearest 50 mg increment to allow for accurate measurement of the dose
Inactive or debilitated patients and patients recently medicated with other sedatives, (eg, chloral hydrate, meperidine, chlorpromazine, and promethazine), may require smaller doses than usual

If the patient is not sedated within 15-20 minutes, a single repeat dose of thiopental can be given. The single repeat doses are:
<3 months: <7.5 mg/kg/dose
>3 months: 15 mg/kg/dose
Adults weighing >90 kg should not receive >3 g as a total dose (initial plus repeat doses)
Children weighing >34 kg should not receive >1 g as a total dose (initial plus repeat doses)
Neither adults nor children should receive more than one course of thiopental rectal suspension (initial dose plus repeat dose) per 24-hour period

Mechanism of Action Interferes with transmission of impulses from the thalamus to the cortex of the brain resulting in an imbalance in central inhibitory and facilitatory mechanisms

Local Anesthetic/Vasoconstrictor Precautions No information available to require special precautions

Effects on Dental Treatment No effects or complications reported

Other Adverse Effects
>10%: Local: Pain on I.M. injection
1% to 10%: Gastrointestinal: Cramping, diarrhea, rectal bleeding
<1%:
Cardiovascular: Hypotension, peripheral vascular collapse, myocardial depression, cardiac arrhythmias
Central nervous system: Seizures, headache, emergence delirium, prolonged somnolence and recovery, anxiety
Dermatologic: Erythema, pruritus, urticaria
Gastrointestinal: Nausea, vomiting
Hematologic: Hemolytic anemia
Local: Thrombophlebitis
Neuromuscular & skeletal: Tremor, involuntary muscle movement, twitching, rigidity, radial nerve palsy
Respiratory: Respiratory depression, coughing, circulatory depression, rhinitis, apnea, laryngospasm, bronchospasm, sneezing, dyspnea
Miscellaneous: Hiccups, anaphylactic reactions

Drug Interactions Increased toxicity with CNS depressants (especially narcotic analgesics and phenothiazines), salicylates, sulfisoxazole

Drug Uptake
Onset of action: I.V.: Anesthesia occurs in 30-60 seconds
Duration: 5-30 minutes
Serum half-life: 3-11.5 hours, decreased in children vs adults

Pregnancy Risk Factor C

Dosage Forms
Injection, as sodium: 250 mg, 400 mg, 500 mg, 1 g, 2.5 g, 5 g
Suspension, rectal, as sodium: 400 mg/g (2 g)

Generic Available Yes

Thiophosphoramide *see* Thiotepa *on next page*

Thioridazine (thye oh RID a zeen)

Brand Names Mellaril®; Mellaril-S®

Canadian/Mexican Brand Names Apo®-Thioridazine (Canada); Novo-Ridazine® (Canada); PMS-Thioridazine® (Canada)

Therapeutic Category Antipsychotic Agent; Phenothiazine Derivative

Synonyms Tioridacina (Mexico)

Use Management of manifestations of psychotic disorders; depressive neurosis; alcohol withdrawal; dementia in elderly; behavioral problems in children

Usual Dosage Oral:

Children >2 years: Range: 0.5-3 mg/kg/day in 2-3 divided doses; usual: 1 mg/kg/day; maximum: 3 mg/kg/day

Behavior problems: Initial: 10 mg 2-3 times/day, increase gradually

Severe psychoses: Initial: 25 mg 2-3 times/day, increase gradually

Adults:

Psychoses: Initial: 50-100 mg 3 times/day with gradual increments as needed and tolerated; maximum: 800 mg/day in 2-4 divided doses; if >65 years, initial dose: 10 mg 3 times/day

Depressive disorders, dementia: Initial: 25 mg 3 times/day; maintenance dose: 20-200 mg/day

Not dialyzable (0% to 5%)

Mechanism of Action Blocks postsynaptic mesolimbic dopaminergic receptors in the brain; exhibits a strong alpha-adrenergic blocking effect and depresses the release of hypothalamic and hypophyseal hormones

Local Anesthetic/Vasoconstrictor Precautions No information available to require special precautions

Effects on Dental Treatment Significant hypotension may occur, especially when the drug is administered parenterally; orthostatic hypotension is due to alpha-receptor blockade, the elderly are at greater risk for orthostatic hypotension

Tardive dyskinesia; Prevalence rate may be 40% in elderly; development of the syndrome and the irreversible nature are proportional to duration and total cumulative dose over time

Extrapyramidal reactions are more common in elderly with up to 50% developing these reactions after 60 years of age; drug-induced **Parkinson's syndrome** occurs often; **Akathisia** is the most common extrapyramidal reaction in elderly

Increased confusion, memory loss, psychotic behavior, and agitation frequently occur as a consequence of anticholinergic effects

Antipsychotic associated sedation in nonpsychotic patients is extremely unpleasant due to feelings of depersonalization, derealization, and dysphoria

Other Adverse Effects

>10%:

Central nervous system: Pseudoparkinsonism, akathisia, dystonias, tardive dyskinesia (persistent), dizziness

Cardiovascular: Hypotension, orthostatic hypotension

Gastrointestinal: Constipation

Ocular: Pigmentary retinopathy

Respiratory: Basal congestion

Miscellaneous: Decreased sweating

1% to 10%:

Dermatologic: Photosensitivity, skin rash

Endocrine & metabolic: Changes in menstrual cycle, changes in libido, pain in breasts

Gastrointestinal: Weight gain, nausea, vomiting, stomach pain

Genitourinary: Dysuria, ejaculatory disturbances

Neuromuscular & skeletal: Trembling of fingers

<1%:

Central nervous system: Neuroleptic malignant syndrome (NMS), impairment of temperature regulation, lowering of seizures threshold

Dermatologic: Discoloration of skin (blue-gray)

Endocrine & metabolic: Galactorrhea

Genitourinary: Priapism

Hematologic: Agranulocytosis, leukopenia

Hepatic: Cholestatic jaundice, hepatotoxicity

Ocular: Cornea and lens changes

Drug Interactions

Decreased effect with anticholinergics

(Continued)

Thioridazine *(Continued)*

Decreased effect of guanethidine
Increased toxicity with CNS depressants, lithium (rare), tricyclic antidepressants (cardiotoxicity), propranolol, pindolol

Drug Uptake
Duration of action: 4-5 days
Serum half-life: 21-25 hours
Time to peak serum concentration: Within 1 hour

Pregnancy Risk Factor C
Generic Available Yes

Thiotepa (thye oh TEP a)

Therapeutic Category Antineoplastic Agent, Alkylating Agent

Synonyms TESPA; Thiophosphoramide; Triethylenethiophosphoramide; TSPA

Use Treatment of superficial tumors of the bladder; palliative treatment of adeno-carcinoma of breast or ovary; lymphomas and sarcomas; meningeal neoplasms; control pleural, pericardial or pericardial effusions caused by metastatic tumors; high-dose regimens with autologous bone marrow transplantation

Usual Dosage Refer to individual protocols. Dosing must be based on the clinical and hematologic response of the patient.

Children: Sarcomas: I.V.: 25-65 mg/m^2 as a single dose every 21 days
Adults:
  I.M., I.V., S.C.: 30-60 mg/m^2 once per week
  I.V. doses of 0.3-0.4 mg/kg by rapid I.V. administration every 1-4 weeks, or 0.2 mg/kg or 6-8 mg/m^2/day for 4-5 days every 2-4 weeks
  High-dose therapy for bone marrow transplant: I.V.: 500 mg/m^2; up to 900 mg/m^2
  I.M. doses of 15-30 mg in various schedules have been given
  Intracavitary: 0.6-0.8 mg/kg
  Intrapericardial dose: Usually 15-30 mg

Mechanism of Action Alkylating agent that reacts with DNA phosphate groups to produce cross-linking of DNA strands leading to inhibition of DNA, RNA, and protein synthesis; mechanism of action has not been explored as thoroughly as the other alkylating agents, it is presumed that the aziridine rings open and react as nitrogen mustard; reactivity is enhanced at a lower pH

Local Anesthetic/Vasoconstrictor Precautions No information available to require special precautions

Effects on Dental Treatment No effects or complications reported

Other Adverse Effects
Carcinogenesis: Like other alkylating agents, this drug is carcinogenic
>10%: Local: Pain at injection site
  Hematologic: Dose-limiting toxicity which is dose-related and cumulative; moderate to severe leukopenia and severe thrombocytopenia have occurred. Anemia and pancytopenia may become fatal, so careful hematologic monitoring is required; intravesical administration may cause bone marrow suppression as well.
    Myelosuppressive: WBC: Moderate; Platelets: Severe; Onset (days): 7-10; Nadir (days): 14; Recovery (days): 28
1% to 10%:
  Central nervous system: Dizziness, fever, headache
  Dermatologic: Alopecia, rash, pruritus
  Endocrine & metabolic: Hyperuricemia
  Gastrointestinal: Stomatitis
    Emetic potential: Low (<10%); nausea and vomiting rarely occur
  Renal: Hematuria
<1%:
  Gastrointestinal: Tightness of the throat, anorexia
  Genitourinary: Hemorrhagic cystitis
  Miscellaneous: Allergic reactions

Drug Uptake
Absorption: Following intracavitary instillation, the drug is unreliably absorbed (10% to 100%) through the bladder mucosa; variable I.M. absorption
Serum half-life, terminal: 109 minutes with dose-dependent clearance

Pregnancy Risk Factor D
Generic Available No

Thiothixene (thye oh THIKS een)

Brand Names Navane®
Therapeutic Category Antipsychotic Agent; Phenothiazine Derivative
Use Management of psychotic disorders

Usual Dosage

Children <12 years: Oral: 0.25 mg/kg/24 hours in divided doses (dose not well established)

Children >12 years and Adults: Mild to moderate psychosis:
Oral: 2 mg 3 times/day, up to 20-30 mg/day; more severe psychosis: Initial: 5 mg 2 times/day, may increase gradually, if necessary; maximum: 60 mg/day
I.M.: 4 mg 2-4 times/day, increase dose gradually; usual: 16-20 mg/day; maximum: 30 mg/day; change to oral dose as soon as able

Not dialyzable (0% to 5%)

Mechanism of Action Elicits antipsychotic activity by postsynaptic blockade of CNS dopamine receptors resulting in inhibition of dopamine-mediated effects; also has alpha-adrenergic blocking activity

Local Anesthetic/Vasoconstrictor Precautions No information available to require special precautions

Effects on Dental Treatment Significant hypotension may occur, especially when the drug is administered parenterally; orthostatic hypotension is due to alpha-receptor blockade, the elderly are at greater risk for orthostatic hypotension

Tardive dyskinesia: Prevalence rate may be 40% in elderly; development of the syndrome and the irreversible nature are proportional to duration and total cumulative dose over time

Extrapyramidal reactions are more common in elderly with up to 50% developing these reactions after 60 years of age; drug-induced **Parkinson's syndrome** occurs often; **Akathisia** is the most common extrapyramidal reaction in elderly

Increased confusion, memory loss, psychotic behavior, and agitation frequently occur as a consequence of anticholinergic effects

Antipsychotic associated sedation in nonpsychotic patients is extremely unpleasant due to feelings of depersonalization, derealization, and dysphoria

Other Adverse Effects

>10%:
Cardiovascular: Hypotension, orthostatic hypotension
Central nervous system: Pseudoparkinsonism, akathisia, dystonias, tardive dyskinesia (persistent), dizziness
Gastrointestinal: Constipation
Ocular: Pigmentary retinopathy
Respiratory: Nasal congestion
Miscellaneous: Decreased sweating

1% to 10%:
Dermatologic: Photosensitivity, skin rash
Endocrine & metabolic: Changes in menstrual cycle, changes in libido, pain in breasts
Gastrointestinal: Weight gain, nausea, vomiting, stomach pain
Genitourinary: Dysuria, ejaculatory disturbances
Neuromuscular & skeletal: Trembling of fingers

<1%:
Central nervous system: Neuroleptic malignant syndrome (NMS), impairment of temperature regulation, lowering of seizures threshold
Endocrine & metabolic: Galactorrhea
Dermatologic: Discoloration of skin (blue-gray)
Genitourinary: Priapism
Hematologic: Agranulocytosis, leukopenia
Hepatic: Cholestatic jaundice, hepatotoxicity
Ocular: Fornea and lens changes

Drug Interactions

Decreased effect of guanethidine; decreased effect with anticholinergics
Increased toxicity with CNS depressants, anticholinergics, alcohol

Drug Uptake

Serum half-life: >24 hours with chronic use

Pregnancy Risk Factor C

Generic Available Yes

Thorazine® see Chlorpromazine on page 223
Thrombate III™ see Antithrombin III on page 82
Thrombinar® see Thrombin, Topical on this page

Thrombin, Topical (THROM bin, TOP i kal)

Brand Names Thrombinar®; Thrombogen®; Thrombostat®
Therapeutic Category Hemostatic Agent
(Continued)

Thrombin, Topical *(Continued)*

Use
Dental & Medical: Hemostasis whenever minor bleeding from capillaries and small venules is accessible

Usual Dosage Use 1000-2000 units/mL of solution where bleeding is profuse; apply powder directly to the site of bleeding or on oozing surfaces; use 100 units/mL for bleeding from skin or mucosal surfaces

Mechanism of Action Catalyzes the conversion of fibrinogen to fibrin

Local Anesthetic/Vasoconstrictor Precautions No information available to require special precautions

Effects on Dental Treatment No effects or complications reported

Other Adverse Effects 1% to 10%:
Central nervous system: Fever
Miscellaneous: Allergic type reaction

Contraindications Hypersensitivity to thrombin or any component

Warnings/Precautions Do not inject, for topical use only

Drug Interactions No data reported

Pregnancy Risk Factor C

Breast-feeding Considerations No data reported

Dosage Forms Powder: 1000 units, 5000 units, 10,000 units, 20,000 units, 50,000 units

Generic Available No

Comments Topical thrombin is not to be used in conjunction with oxidized cellulose

Thrombogen® *see* Thrombin, Topical *on previous page*

Thrombostat® *see* Thrombin, Topical *on previous page*

Thypinone® Injection *see* Protirelin *on page 818*

Thyrar® *see* Thyroid *on this page*

Thyro-Block® *see* Potassium Iodide *on page 781*

Thyroid (THYE royd)

Related Information
Endocrine Disorders & Pregnancy *on page 1021*

Brand Names Armour® Thyroid; S-P-T; Thyrar®; Thyroid Strong®

Therapeutic Category Thyroid Product

Use Replacement or supplemental therapy in hypothyroidism; pituitary TSH suppressants (thyroid nodules, thyroiditis, multinodular goiter, thyroid cancer), thyrotoxicosis, diagnostic suppression tests

Usual Dosage Oral:
Children: See table.

Recommended Pediatric Dosage for Congenital Hypothyroidism

Age	Daily Dose (mg)	Daily Dose/kg (mg)
0-6 mo	15-30	4.8-6
6-12 mo	30-45	3.6-4.8
1-5 y	45-60	3-3.6
6-12 y	60-90	2.4-3
>12 y	>90	1.2-1.8

Adults: Initial: 15-30 mg; increase with 15 mg increments every 2-4 weeks; use 15 mg in patients with cardiovascular disease or myxedema. Maintenance dose: Usually 60-120 mg/day; monitor TSH and clinical symptoms.
Thyroid cancer: Requires larger amounts than replacement therapy

Mechanism of Action The primary active compound is T_3 (triiodothyronine), which may be converted from T_4 (thyroxine) and then circulates throughout the body to influence growth and maturation of various tissues; exact mechanism of action is unknown; however, it is believed the thyroid hormone exerts its many metabolic effects through control of DNA transcription and protein synthesis; involved in normal metabolism, growth, and development; promotes gluconeogenesis, increases utilization and mobilization of glycogen stores and stimulates protein synthesis, increases basal metabolic rate

Local Anesthetic/Vasoconstrictor Precautions No precautions with vasoconstrictor are necessary if patient is well controlled with thyroid preparations

Effects on Dental Treatment No effects or complications reported

Other Adverse Effects <1%:
Cardiovascular: Palpitations, tachycardia, cardiac arrhythmias, chest pain

Central nervous system: Nervousness, headache, insomnia, fever, clumsiness

Dermatologic: Alopecia

Endocrine & metabolic: Changes in menstrual cycle

Gastrointestinal: Weight loss, increased appetite, diarrhea, abdominal cramps, vomiting, constipation

Neuromuscular & skeletal: Excessive bone loss with overtreatment (excess thyroid replacement), tremor, hand tremors, myalgia

Respiratory: Dyspnea

Miscellaneous: Heat intolerance, sweating

Drug Interactions

Decreased effect:

Thyroid hormones increase the therapeutic need for oral hypoglycemics or insulin

Cholestyramine can bind thyroid and reduce its absorption

Increased toxicity: Thyroid may potentiate the hypoprothrombinemic effect of oral anticoagulants

Drug Uptake

Absorption: T_4 is 48% to 79% absorbed; T_3 is 95% absorbed; desiccated thyroid contains thyroxine, liothyronine, and iodine (primarily bound); following absorption thyroxine is largely converted to liothyronine

Serum half-life:

Liothyronine: 1-2 days

Thyroxine: 6-7 days

Pregnancy Risk Factor A

Dosage Forms

Capsule, pork source in soybean oil (S-P-T): 60 mg, 120 mg, 180 mg, 300 mg

Tablet:

Armour® Thyroid: 15 mg, 30 mg, 60 mg, 90 mg, 120 mg, 180 mg, 240 mg, 300 mg

Thyrar® (bovine source): 30 mg, 60 mg, 120 mg

Thyroid Strong® (60 mg is equivalent to 90 mg thyroid USP):

Regular: 30 mg, 60 mg, 120 mg

Sugar coated: 30 mg, 60 mg, 120 mg, 180 mg

Thyroid USP: 15 mg, 30 mg, 60 mg, 120 mg, 180 mg, 300 mg

Generic Available Yes

Thyroid Strong® *see Thyroid on previous page*

Thyrolar® *see Liotrix on page 559*

Thyrotropin (thye roe TROE pin)

Brand Names Thytropar®

Therapeutic Category Diagnostic Agent, Hypothyroidism; Diagnostic Agent, Thyroid Function

Use Diagnostic aid to differentiate thyroid failure; diagnosis of decreased thyroid reserve, to differentiate between primary and secondary hypothyroidism and between primary hypothyroidism and euthyroidism in patients receiving thyroid replacement

Usual Dosage Adults: I.M., S.C.: 10 units/day for 1-3 days; follow by a radioiodine study 24 hours past last injection, no response in thyroid failure, substantial response in pituitary failure

Mechanism of Action Stimulates formation and secretion of thyroid hormone, increases uptake of iodine by thyroid gland

Local Anesthetic/Vasoconstrictor Precautions No information available to require special precautions

Effects on Dental Treatment No effects or complications reported

Other Adverse Effects <1%:

Cardiovascular: Tachycardia

Central nervous system: Fever, headache

Endocrine & metabolic: Menstrual irregularities

Gastrointestinal: Nausea, vomiting, increased bowel motility

Miscellaneous: Anaphylaxis with repeated administration

Drug Interactions No data reported

Drug Uptake Serum half-life: 35 minutes, dependent upon thyroid state

Pregnancy Risk Factor C

Dosage Forms Injection: 10 units

Generic Available No

Thyrotropin Releasing Hormone *see Protirelin on page 818*

Thytropar® *see Thyrotropin on this page*

Tiagabine (tye AJ a bene)
Brand Names Gabitril®
Therapeutic Category Anticonvulsant, Miscellaneous
Synonyms Tiagabine Hydrochloride
Use Adjunctive therapy in adults and children 12 years and older in the treatment of partial seizures
Usual Dosage Children >12 years and Adults: Oral: Starting dose: 4 mg once daily; the total daily dose may be increased in 4 mg increments beginning the second week of therapy; thereafter, the daily dose may be increased by 4-8 mg/day until clinical response is achieved, up to a maximum of 32 mg/day; the total daily dose at higher levels should be given in divided doses 2-4 times/day
Mechanism of Action The exact mechanism by which tiagabine exerts antiseizure activity is not definitively known; however, *in vitro* experiments demonstrate that it enhances the activity of gamma aminobutyric acid (GABA), the major neuroinhibitory transmitter in the nervous system; it is thought that binding to the GABA uptake carrier inhibits the uptake of GABA into presynaptic neurons, allowing an increased amount of GABA to be available to postsynaptic neurons; based on *in vitro* studies, tiagabine does not inhibit the uptake of dopamine, norepinephrine, serotonin, glutamate or choline
Local Anesthetic/Vasoconstrictor Precautions No information available to require special precautions
Effects on Dental Treatment No effects or complications reported
Other Adverse Effects All adverse effects are dose related
Central nervous system: Dizziness, headache, somnolence, CNS depression, memory disturbance, ataxia
Neuromuscular & skeletal: Tremors, weakness
Contraindications Patients who have demonstrated hypersensitivity to the drug or any of its agreements
Warnings/Precautions Anticonvulsants should not be discontinued abruptly because of the possibility of increasing seizure frequency; clinical studies were carried out that demonstrated an increase in seizure frequency upon abrupt withdrawal; tiagabine should be withdrawn gradually to minimize the potential of increased seizure frequency, unless safety concerns require a more rapid withdrawal
Drug Interactions The clearance of tiagabine is affected by the co-administration of hepatic enzyme inducing anti-epilepsy drugs; tiagabine is cleared more rapidly in patients who have been treated with carbamazepine, phenytoin, primidone and phenobarbital than in patients who have not received these drugs
Drug Uptake
Absorption: Rapid (within 1 hour); food prolongs absorption
Serum half-life: 6.7 hours
Dosage Forms Tablet: 4 mg, 12 mg, 16 mg, 20 mg
Selected Readings
Patsalos PN and Sander JW, "Newer Antiepileptic Drugs: Towards an Improved Risk-Benefit Ratio," *Drug Saf*, 1994, 11(1):37-67.

Tiagabine Hydrochloride *see* Tiagabine *on this page*

Tiamate® *see* Diltiazem *on page 318*

Tiazac® *see* Diltiazem *on page 318*

Ticar® *see* Ticarcillin *on this page*

Ticarcilina Disodica (Mexico) *see* Ticarcillin *on this page*

Ticarcillin (tye kar SIL in)
Brand Names Ticar®
Therapeutic Category Antibiotic, Penicillin
Synonyms Ticarcilina Disodica (Mexico)
Use Treatment of susceptible infections such as septicemia, acute and chronic respiratory tract infections, skin and soft tissue infections, and urinary tract infections due to susceptible strains of *Pseudomonas, Proteus,* and *Escherichia coli* and *Enterobacter*; normally used with other antibiotics (ie, aminoglycosides)
Usual Dosage Ticarcillin is generally given I.M. only for the treatment of uncomplicated urinary tract infections
Children: I.V.: Serious Infections:200-300 mg/kg/day in divided doses every 4-6 hours; doses as high as 400 mg/kg/day divided every 4 hours have been used in acute pulmonary exacerbations of cystic fibrosis
Maximum dose: 24 g/day
Urinary tract infections: I.M., I.V.: 50-100 mg/kg/day in divided doses every 6-8 hours
Adults: I.V.: 1-4 g every 4-6 hours

Mechanism of Action Interferes with bacterial cell wall synthesis during active multiplication, causing cell wall death and resultant bactericidal activity against susceptible bacteria

Local Anesthetic/Vasoconstrictor Precautions No information available to require special precautions

Effects on Dental Treatment Prolonged use of penicillins may lead to development of oral candidiasis

Other Adverse Effects <1%:

Central nervous system: Convulsions, confusion, drowsiness, fever

Dermatologic: Rash

Endocrine & metabolic: Electrolyte imbalance

Hematologic: Hemolytic anemia, positive Coombs' reaction

Local: Thrombophlebitis

Neuromuscular & skeletal: Myoclonus

Renal: Acute interstitial nephritis

Miscellaneous: Hypersensitivity reactions, anaphylaxis, Jarisch-Herxheimer reaction

Drug Interactions

Decreased effect: Tetracyclines cause decreased ticarcillin effectiveness

Increased effect:

Probenecid causes increased ticarcillin levels

Neuromuscular blockers cause increased duration of blockade

Aminoglycosides cause synergistic efficacy

Drug Uptake

Absorption: I.M.: 86%

Serum half-life, adults: 1-1.3 hours, prolonged with renal impairment and/or hepatic impairment

Peak serum levels: I.M.: Within 30-75 minutes

Pregnancy Risk Factor B

Generic Available No

Ticarcillin and Clavulanate Potassium

(tye kar SIL in & klav yoo LAN ate poe TASS ee um)

Brand Names Timentin®

Therapeutic Category Antibiotic, Penicillin

Use Treatment of infections of lower respiratory tract, urinary tract, skin and skin structures, bone and joint, and septicemia caused by susceptible organisms. Clavulanate expands activity of ticarcillin to include beta-lactamase producing strains of *S. aureus*, *H. influenzae*, *Enterobacteriaceae*, *Klebsiella*, *Citrobacter*, and *Serratia*

Usual Dosage I.V.:

Children: 200-300 mg of ticarcillin component/kg/day in divided doses every 4-6 hours

Adults: 3.1 g (ticarcillin 3 g plus clavulanic acid 0.1 g) every 4-6 hours; maximum: 18-24 g/day

Urinary tract infections: 3.1 g every 6-8 hours

Mechanism of Action Ticarcillin interferes with bacterial cell wall synthesis during active multiplication, causing cell wall death and resultant bactericidal activity against susceptible bacteria; clavulanic acid prevents degradation of ticarcillin by binding to the active site on beta-lactamase

Local Anesthetic/Vasoconstrictor Precautions No information available to require special precautions

Effects on Dental Treatment Prolonged use of penicillins may lead to development of oral candidiasis

Other Adverse Effects <1%:

Central nervous system: Convulsions, confusion, drowsiness, fever

Dermatologic: Rash

Endocrine & metabolic: Electrolyte imbalance

Hematologic: Hemolytic anemia, positive Coombs' reaction

Local: Thrombophlebitis

Neuromuscular & skeletal: Myoclonus

Renal: Acute interstitial nephritis

Miscellaneous: Hypersensitivity reactions, anaphylaxis, Jarisch-Herxheimer reaction

Drug Interactions

Decreased effect: Tetracyclines cause decreased penicillin effectiveness; aminoglycosides cause physical inactivation of aminoglycosides in the presence of high concentrations of ticarcillin and potential toxicity in patients with mild-moderate renal dysfunction

Increased effect:

Probenecid causes increased penicillin levels

Neuromuscular blockers causes increased duration of blockade

(Continued)

933

Ticarcillin and Clavulanate Potassium *(Continued)*

Aminoglycosides cause synergistic efficacy

Drug Uptake
Serum half-life:
Clavulanate: 66-90 minutes
Ticarcillin: 66-72 minutes in patients with normal renal function; clavulanic acid does not affect the clearance of ticarcillin

Pregnancy Risk Factor B
Generic Available No

TICE® BCG *see* BCG Vaccine *on page 111*

Ticlid® *see* Ticlopidine *on this page*

Ticlopidina (Mexico) *see* Ticlopidine *on this page*

Ticlopidine *(tye KLOE pi deen)*

Brand Names Ticlid®
Therapeutic Category Antiplatelet Agent
Synonyms Ticlopidina (Mexico)
Use Platelet aggregation inhibitor that reduces the risk of thrombotic stroke in patients who have had a stroke or stroke precursors

Unlabeled use: Protection of aortocoronary bypass grafts, diabetic microangiopathy, ischemic heart disease, prevention of postoperative DVT, reduction of graft loss following renal transplant

Usual Dosage Adults: Oral: 1 tablet twice daily with food
Mechanism of Action Ticlopidine is an inhibitor of platelet function with a mechanism which is different from other antiplatelet drugs. The drug significantly increases bleeding time. This effect may not be solely related to ticlopidine's effect on platelets. The prolongation of the bleeding time caused by ticlopidine is further increased by the addition of aspirin in *ex vivo* experiments. Although many metabolites of ticlopidine have been found, none have been shown to account for *in vivo* activity.

Local Anesthetic/Vasoconstrictor Precautions No information available to require special precautions
Effects on Dental Treatment No effects or complications reported
Other Adverse Effects
1% to 10%: Dermatologic: Skin rash
<1%:
Dermatologic: Bruising
Gastrointestinal: Diarrhea, nausea, vomiting, GI pain
Hematologic: Neutropenia, thrombocytopenia
Hepatic: Elevated liver function tests
Otic: Tinnitus
Renal: Hematuria
Respiratory: Epistaxis

Drug Interactions
Decreased effect with antacids (decreased absorption), corticosteroids; decreased effect of digoxin, cyclosporine
Increased effect/toxicity of aspirin, anticoagulants, antipyrine, theophylline, cimetidine (increased levels), NSAIDs

Drug Uptake
Onset of action: Within 6 hours
Serum half-life, elimination: 24 hours
Pregnancy Risk Factor B
Generic Available No

Ticon® *see* Trimethobenzamide *on page 964*

TIG *see* Tetanus Immune Globulin (Human) *on page 911*

Tigan® *see* Trimethobenzamide *on page 964*

Tilade® Inhalation Aerosol *see* Nedocromil Sodium *on page 668*

Tiludronate *(tye LOO droe nate)*

Brand Names Skelid®
Therapeutic Category Bisphosphonate Derivative
Synonyms Tiludronate Disodium
Use Paget's disease of the bone
Usual Dosage Adults: Oral: 400 mg (2 tablets) [tiludronic acid] daily
Local Anesthetic/Vasoconstrictor Precautions No information available to require special precautions
Effects on Dental Treatment No effects or complications reported
Dosage Forms Tablet, as disodium: 240 mg [tiludronic acid 200 mg]; dosage is expressed in terms of tiludronic acid.

Tiludronate Disodium see Tiludronate *on previous page*

Timentin® see Ticarcillin and Clavulanate Potassium *on page 933*

Timolol (TYE moe lole)

Related Information

Cardiovascular Diseases *on page 1010*

Brand Names Betimol® Ophthalmic; Blocadren® Oral; Timoptic® Ophthalmic; Timoptic-XE® Ophthalmic

Canadian/Mexican Brand Names Apo®-Timol (Canada); Apo®-Timop (Canada); Gen-Timolol® (Canada); Imot® Ofteno (Mexico); Novo-Timol® (Canada); Nu-Timolol® (Canada); Timoptol® (Mexico); Timoptol® XE (Mexico)

Therapeutic Category Antianginal Agent; Antiglaucoma Agent; Beta-adrenergic Blocker, Noncardioselective; Beta-Adrenergic Blocker, Ophthalmic

Synonyms Timolol, Maleato De (Mexico)

Use Ophthalmic dosage form used to treat elevated intraocular pressure such as glaucoma or ocular hypertension; orally for treatment of hypertension and angina and reduce mortality following myocardial infarction and prophylaxis of migraine

Usual Dosage

Children and Adults: Ophthalmic: Initial: 0.25% solution, instill 1 drop twice daily; increase to 0.5% solution if response not adequate; decrease to 1 drop/day if controlled; do not exceed 1 drop twice daily of 0.5% solution

Adults: Oral:

Hypertension: Initial: 10 mg twice daily, increase gradually every 7 days, usual dosage: 20-40 mg/day in 2 divided doses; maximum: 60 mg/day

Prevention of myocardial infarction: 10 mg twice daily initiated within 1-4 weeks after infarction

Migraine headache: Initial: 10 mg twice daily, increase to maximum of 30 mg/day

Mechanism of Action Blocks both beta$_1$- and beta$_2$-adrenergic receptors, reduces intraocular pressure by reducing aqueous humor production or possibly outflow; reduces blood pressure by blocking adrenergic receptors and decreasing sympathetic outflow, produces a negative chronotropic and inotropic activity through an unknown mechanism

Local Anesthetic/Vasoconstrictor Precautions No information available to require special precautions

Effects on Dental Treatment No effects or complications reported

Other Adverse Effects

Ophthalmic:

1% to 10%:

Dermatologic: Alopecia

Ocular: Burning, stinging of eyes

<1%:

Dermatologic: Skin rash

Ocular: Blepharitis, conjunctivitis, keratitis, vision disturbances

Oral:

>10%: Endocrine & metabolic: Decreased sexual ability

1% to 10%:

Cardiovascular: Bradycardia, arrhythmia, reduced peripheral circulation

Central nervous system: Dizziness, itching, fatigue

Neuromuscular & skeletal: Weakness

Respiratory: Dyspnea

<1%:

Cardiovascular: Chest pain, congestive heart failure

Central nervous system: Hallucinations, mental depression, anxiety, nightmares

Dermatologic: Skin rashes

Gastrointestinal: Diarrhea, nausea, vomiting, stomach discomfort

Neuromuscular & skeletal: Numbness in toes and fingers

Ocular: Dry sore eyes

Drug Interactions No data reported with ophthalmic preparation

Drug Uptake

Onset of hypotensive effect: Oral: Within 15-45 minutes

Peak effect: Within 0.5-2.5 hours

Duration of action: ~4 hours; intraocular effects persist for 24 hours after ophthalmic instillation

Serum half-life: 2-2.7 hours; prolonged with reduced renal function

Pregnancy Risk Factor C

Generic Available Yes

Timolol, Maleato De (Mexico) see Timolol *on this page*

Timoptic® Ophthalmic see Timolol *on this page*

Timoptic-XE® Ophthalmic *see* Timolol *on previous page*

Tinactin® [OTC] *see* Tolnaftate *on page 943*

Tinactin® for Jock Itch [OTC] *see* Tolnaftate *on page 943*

TinBen® [OTC] *see* Benzoin *on page 120*

TinCoBen® [OTC] *see* Benzoin *on page 120*

Tindal® *see* Acetophenazine *on page 28*

Tine Test *see* Tuberculin Purified Protein Derivative *on page 975*

Tine Test PPD *see* Tuberculin Purified Protein Derivative *on page 975*

Ting® [OTC] *see* Tolnaftate *on page 943*

Tinver® Lotion *see* Sodium Thiosulfate *on page 876*

Tioconazole (tye oh KONE a zole)
Brand Names Vagistat®
Therapeutic Category Antifungal Agent, Vaginal
Synonyms Tioconazol (Mexico)
Use Local treatment of vulvovaginal candidiasis
Usual Dosage Adults: Vaginal: Insert 1 applicatorful in vagina, just prior to bedtime, as a single dose
Mechanism of Action A 1-substituted imidazole derivative with a broad antifungal spectrum against a wide variety of dermatophytes and yeasts, usually at a concentration of ≤6.25 mg/L; has been demonstrated to be at least as active *in vitro* as other imidazole antifungals. *In vitro*, tioconazole has been demonstrated 2-8 times as potent as miconazole against common dermal pathogens including *Trichophyton mentagrophytes*, *T. rubrum*, *T. erinacei*, *T. tonsurans*, *Microsporum canis*, *Microsporum gypseum*, and *Candida albicans*. Both agents appear to be similarly effective against *Epidermophyton floccosum*.
Local Anesthetic/Vasoconstrictor Precautions No information available to require special precautions
Effects on Dental Treatment No effects or complications reported
Other Adverse Effects
1% to 10%: Genitourinary: Vulvar/vaginal burning
<1%:
 Genitourinary: Vulvar itching, soreness, swelling, or discharge
 Renal: Polyuria
Drug Interactions No data reported
Drug Uptake
 Absorption: Intravaginal: Following application small amounts of drug are absorbed systemically (25%) within 2-8 hours
 Serum half-life: 21-24 hours
Pregnancy Risk Factor C
Generic Available No

Tioconazol (Mexico) *see* Tioconazole *on this page*

Tioguanine *see* Thioguanine *on page 925*

Tiopental Sodico (Mexico) *see* Thiopental *on page 925*

Tiopronin (tye oh PROE nin)
Brand Names Thiola™
Therapeutic Category Urinary Tract Product
Use Prevention of kidney stone (cystine) formation in patients with severe homozygous cystinuric who have urinary cystine >500 mg/day who are resistant to treatment with high fluid intake, alkali, and diet modification, or who have had adverse reactions to penicillamine
Local Anesthetic/Vasoconstrictor Precautions No information available to require special precautions
Effects on Dental Treatment No effects or complications reported
Pregnancy Risk Factor C
Generic Available No

Tioridacina (Mexico) *see* Thioridazine *on page 927*

Ti-Screen® [OTC] *see* Methoxycinnamate and Oxybenzone *on page 619*

Tisit® Blue Gel [OTC] *see* Pyrethrins *on page 824*

Tisit® Liquid [OTC] *see* Pyrethrins *on page 824*

Tisit® Shampoo [OTC] *see* Pyrethrins *on page 824*

Titralac® Plus Liquid [OTC] *see* Calcium Carbonate and Simethicone *on page 163*

Tizanidine (tye ZAN i deen)
Brand Names Zanaflex®
Therapeutic Category Alpha₂-Adrenergic Agonist Agent

Use Intermittent management of increased muscle tone associated with spasticity (eg, multiple sclerosis, spinal cord injury)

Usual Dosage
Adults: 2-4 mg 3 times/day
Usual initial dose: 4 mg, may increase by 2-4 mg as needed for satisfactory reduction of muscle tone every 6-8 hours to a maximum of three doses in any 24 hour period
Maximum dose: 36 mg/day

Mechanism of Action An alpha$_2$-adrenergic agonist agent which decreases excitatory input to alpha motor neurons; an imidazole derivative chemically-related to clonidine, which acts as a centrally acting muscle relaxant with alpha$_2$-adrenergic agonist properties; acts on the level of the spinal cord

Local Anesthetic/Vasoconstrictor Precautions No information available to require special precautions

Effects on Dental Treatment >10% of patients medicated with tizanidine will experience significant dry mouth; this will disappear with cessation of drug therapy

Other Adverse Effects
>10%:
Cardiovascular: Hypotension
Central nervous system: Sedation, daytime drowsiness, somnolence
Gastrointestinal: Xerostomia
1% to 10%:
Cardiovascular: Bradycardia, syncope
Central nervous system: Fatigue, dizziness, anxiety, nervousness, insomnia
Dermatologic: Pruritus, skin rash
Gastrointestinal: Nausea, vomiting, dyspepsia, constipation, diarrhea
Hepatic: Elevation of liver enzymes
Neuromuscular & skeletal: Muscle weakness, tremor
<1%:
Cardiovascular: Palpitations, ventricular extrasystoles
Central nervous system: Psychotic-like symptoms, visual hallucinations, delusions
Hepatic: Hepatic failure

Warnings/Precautions Reduce dose in patients with liver or renal disease; use with caution in patients with hypotension or cardiac disease

Drug Interactions
Increased effect: Oral contraceptives
Increased toxicity: Additive hypotensive effects may be seen with diuretics, other alpha adrenergic agonists, or antihypertensives; CNS depression with alcohol, baclofen or other CNS depressants

Drug Uptake
Duration: 3-6 hours
Serum half-life: 4-8 hours
Time to peak serum concentration: 1-5 hours

Pregnancy Risk Factor C
Generic Available No

TMP-SMZ see Trimethoprim and Sulfamethoxazole on page 965
TOBI™ Inhalation Solution see Tobramycin on this page
TobraDex® see Tobramycin and Dexamethasone on page 939
Tobramicina Sulfato De (Mexico) see Tobramycin on this page

Tobramycin (toe bra MYE sin)
Related Information
Antimicrobial Prophylaxis in Surgical Patients on page 1163
Brand Names AKTob® Ophthalmic; Nebcin® Injection; TOBI™ Inhalation Solution; Tobrex® Ophthalmic
Canadian/Mexican Brand Names Tobra® (Mexico); Trazil® Often y Trazil® Ungena (Mexico)
Therapeutic Category Antibiotic, Aminoglycoside; Antibiotic, Ophthalmic
Synonyms Tobramicina Sulfato De (Mexico)
Use Treatment of documented or suspected *Pseudomonas aeruginosa* infection; infection with a nonpseudomonal enteric bacillus which is more sensitive to tobramycin than gentamicin based on susceptibility tests; empiric therapy in cystic fibrosis and immunocompromised patients; topically used to treat superficial ophthalmic infections caused by susceptible bacteria; inhaled version used for improving lung function and controlling *Pseudomonas aeruginosa* infections in people with cystic fibrosis (CF)
Usual Dosage Individualization is critical because of the low therapeutic index
Use of ideal body weight (IBW) for determining the mg/kg/dose appears to be more accurate than dosing on the basis of total body weight (TBW)
(Continued)

Tobramycin *(Continued)*

In morbid obesity, dosage requirement may best be estimated using a dosing weight of IBW + 0.4 (TBW - IBW)

Initial and periodic peak and trough plasma drug levels should be determined, particularly in critically ill patients with serious infections or in disease states known to significantly alter aminoglycoside pharmacokinetics (eg, cystic fibrosis, burns, or major surgery); 2-3 serum level measurements should be obtained after the initial dose to measure the half-life in order to determine the frequency of subsequent doses

Once daily dosing: Higher peak serum drug concentration to MIC ratios, demonstrated aminoglycoside postantibiotic effect, decreased renal cortex drug uptake, and improved cost-time efficiency are supportive reasons for the use of once daily dosing regimens for aminoglycosides. Current research indicates these regimens to be as effective for nonlife-threatening infections, with no higher incidence of nephrotoxicity, than those requiring multiple daily doses. Doses are determined by calculating the entire day's dose via usual multiple dose calculation techniques and administering this quantity as a single dose. Doses are then adjusted to maintain mean serum concentrations above the MIC(s) of the causative organism(s). (Example: 2.5-5 mg/kg as a single dose; expected Cp_{max}: 10-20 mcg/mL and Cp_{min}: <1 mcg/mL). Further research is needed for universal recommendation in all patient populations and gram-negative disease; exceptions may include those with known high clearance (eg, children, patients with cystic fibrosis, or burns who may require shorter dosage intervals) and patients with renal function impairment for whom longer than conventional dosage intervals are usually required.

Children <5 years: I.M., I.V.: 2.5 mg/kg/dose every 8 hours

Children >5 years: 1.5-2.5 mg/kg/dose every 8 hours

Note: Some patients may require larger or more frequent doses if serum levels document the need (ie, cystic fibrosis or febrile granulocytopenic patients).

Adults: I.M., I.V.:

Severe life-threatening infections: 2-2.5 mg/kg/dose

Urinary tract infection: 1.5 mg/kg/dose

Synergy (for gram-positive infections): 1 mg/kg/dose

Children and Adults: Ophthalmic: Instill 1-2 drops of solution every 4 hours; apply ointment 2-3 times/day; for severe infections apply ointment every 3-4 hours, or solution 2 drops every 30-60 minutes initially, then reduce to less frequent intervals

Children and Adults: Inhalation: Inhaled twice daily and requires about 10-15 minutes per treatment. The TOBI treatment regimen consists of repeated cycles of 28-days on drug, followed by 28-days off drug.

Mechanism of Action Interferes with bacterial protein synthesis by binding to 30S and 50S ribosomal subunits resulting in a defective bacterial cell membrane

Local Anesthetic/Vasoconstrictor Precautions No information available to require special precautions

Effects on Dental Treatment No effects or complications reported

Other Adverse Effects

1% to 10%:

Renal: Nephrotoxicity

Neuromuscular & skeletal: Neurotoxicity (neuromuscular blockade)

Otic: Ototoxicity (auditory), ototoxicity (vestibular)

<1%:

Cardiovascular: Hypotension

Central nervous system: Drug fever, headache, drowsiness

Dermatologic: Skin rash

Gastrointestinal: Nausea, vomiting

Hematologic: Eosinophilia anemia

Neuromuscular & skeletal: Paresthesia, tremor, arthralgia, weakness

Ocular: Lacrimation, itching, edema of the eyelid, keratitis

Respiratory: Dyspnea

Drug Interactions

Increased effect: Extended spectrum penicillins (synergistic)

Increased toxicity:

Neuromuscular blockers increase neuromuscular blockade

Amphotericin B, cephalosporins, loop diuretics cause increased risk of nephrotoxicity

Drug Uptake

Absorption: I.M.: Rapid and complete

Serum half-life:

Adults: 2-3 hours, directly dependent upon glomerular filtration rate

Adults with impaired renal function: 5-70 hours

Time to peak serum concentration:
I.M.: Within 30-60 minutes
I.V.: Within 30 minutes
Pregnancy Risk Factor C
Generic Available Yes

Tobramycin and Dexamethasone
(toe bra MYE sin & deks a METH a sone)
Brand Names TobraDex®
Therapeutic Category Antibiotic, Ophthalmic; Corticosteroid, Ophthalmic
Use Treatment of external ocular infection caused by susceptible gram-negative bacteria and steroid responsive inflammatory conditions of the palpebral and bulbar conjunctiva, lid, cornea, and anterior segment of the globe
Usual Dosage Children and Adults: Ophthalmic: Instill 1-2 drops of solution every 4 hours; apply ointment 2-3 times/day; for severe infections apply ointment every 3-4 hours, or solution 2 drops every 30-60 minutes initially, then reduce to less frequent intervals
Mechanism of Action Refer to individual monographs for Dexamethasone and Tobramycin
Local Anesthetic/Vasoconstrictor Precautions No information available to require special precautions
Effects on Dental Treatment No effects or complications reported
Other Adverse Effects 1% to 10%:
Dermatologic: Allergic contact dermatitis, delayed wound healing
Ocular: Lacrimation, itching, edema of eyelid, keratitis, increased intraocular pressure, glaucoma, cataract formation
Drug Interactions Refer to individual monographs for Tobramycin and Dexamethasone
Drug Uptake
Absorption: Absorbed into the aqueous humor
Time to peak serum concentration: 1-2 hours after instillation in the cornea and aqueous humor
Pregnancy Risk Factor B
Generic Available No

Tobrex® Ophthalmic *see* Tobramycin *on page 937*

Tocainide (toe KAY nide)
Related Information
Cardiovascular Diseases *on page 1010*
Brand Names Tonocard®
Therapeutic Category Antiarrhythmic Agent, Class I-B; Antiarrhythmic Agent (Supraventricular & Ventricular)
Use Suppress and prevent symptomatic life-threatening ventricular arrhythmias

Unlabeled use: Trigeminal neuralgia
Usual Dosage Adults: Oral: 1200-1800 mg/day in 3 divided doses, up to 2400 mg/day
Mechanism of Action Class 1B antiarrhythmic agent; suppresses automaticity of conduction tissue, by increasing electrical stimulation threshold of ventricle, HIS-Purkinje system, and spontaneous depolarization of the ventricles during diastole by a direct action on the tissues; blocks both the initiation and conduction of nerve impulses by decreasing the neuronal membrane's permeability to sodium ions, which results in inhibition of depolarization with resultant blockade of conduction
Local Anesthetic/Vasoconstrictor Precautions No information available to require special precautions
Effects on Dental Treatment No effects or complications reported
Other Adverse Effects
>10%:
Central nervous system: Nervousness, confusion, ataxia, dizziness
Gastrointestinal: Nausea, anorexia
Neuromuscular & skeletal: Tremor
1% to 10%:
Cardiovascular: Hypotension, tachycardia
Dermatologic: Skin rash
Gastrointestinal: Vomiting, diarrhea
Neuromuscular & skeletal: Arthralgia, myalgia, paresthesia
Ocular: Blurred vision
<1%:
Cardiovascular: Bradycardia, palpitations
Hematologic: Agranulocytosis, anemia, leukopenia, neutropenia
Respiratory: Respiratory arrest
(Continued)

Tocainide *(Continued)*

Miscellaneous: Sweating

Drug Interactions

Decreased plasma levels: Phenobarbital, phenytoin, rifampin, and other hepatic enzyme inducers, cimetidine and drugs which make the urine acidic

Increased effect of tocainide, allopurinol

Increased toxicity/levels of caffeine and theophylline

Drug Uptake

Absorption: Oral: Extensive, 99% to 100%

Serum half-life: 11-14 hours, prolonged with renal and hepatic impairment with half-life increased to 23-27 hours

Time to peak: Peak serum levels occur within 30-160 minutes

Pregnancy Risk Factor C

Generic Available No

Tocophersolan *(toe kof er SOE lan)*

Brand Names Liqui-E®

Therapeutic Category Vitamin, Fat Soluble

Synonyms TPGS

Use Treatment of vitamin E deficiency resulting from malabsorption due to prolonged cholestatic hepatobiliary disease

Local Anesthetic/Vasoconstrictor Precautions No information available to require special precautions

Effects on Dental Treatment No effects or complications reported

Pregnancy Risk Factor A/C

Generic Available No

Comments Studies indicate that TPGS is absorbed better than fat soluble forms of vitamin E in patients with impaired digestion and absorption and when coadministered with cyclosporin to transplant recipients it improves cyclosporin absorption. Due to these findings, this product has a valuable role in the liver transplant patient population.

Tofranil® *see* Imipramine *on page 501*

Tofranil-PM® *see* Imipramine *on page 501*

Tolazamide *(tole AZ a mide)*

Related Information

Endocrine Disorders & Pregnancy *on page 1021*

Brand Names Tolinase®

Therapeutic Category Antidiabetic Agent; Hypoglycemic Agent, Oral; Sulfonylurea Agent

Use Adjunct to diet for the management of mild to moderately severe, stable, noninsulin-dependent (type II) diabetes mellitus

Usual Dosage Oral (doses >1000 mg/day normally do not improve diabetic control):

Adults: Initial: 100 mg/day, increase at 2- to 4-week intervals; maximum dose: 1000 mg; give as a single or twice daily dose

Conversion from insulin → tolazamide

10 units day = 100 mg/day

20-40 units/day = 250 mg/day

>40 units/day = 250 mg/day and 50% of insulin dose

Doses >500 mg/day should be given in 2 divided doses

Mechanism of Action Stimulates insulin release from the pancreatic beta cells; reduces glucose output from the liver; insulin sensitivity is increased at peripheral target sites

Local Anesthetic/Vasoconstrictor Precautions No information available to require special precautions

Effects on Dental Treatment Use salicylates with caution in patients taking tolazamide because of potential increased hypoglycemia; NSAIDs such as ibuprofen and naproxen may be safely used. Tolazamide-dependent diabetics (noninsulin dependent, Type II) should be appointed for dental treatment in morning in order to minimize chance of stress-induced hypoglycemia.

Other Adverse Effects

>10%:

Central nervous system: Headache, dizziness

Gastrointestinal: Anorexia, nausea, vomiting, diarrhea, constipation, heartburn, epigastric fullness

1% to 10%: Dermatologic: Rash, urticaria, photosensitivity

<1%:

Endocrine & metabolic: Hypoglycemia

Hematologic: Aplastic anemia, hemolytic anemia, bone marrow suppression, thrombocytopenia, agranulocytosis

Hepatic: Cholestatic jaundice

Renal: Diuretic effect

Drug Interactions Increased toxicity: Monitor patient closely; large number of drugs interact with sulfonylureas including salicylates, anticoagulants, H_2 antagonists, tricyclic antidepressants, MAO inhibitors, beta-blockers, thiazides

Drug Uptake

Onset of action: Oral: Within 4-6 hours

Duration: 10-24 hours

Serum half-life: 7 hours

Pregnancy Risk Factor D

Dosage Forms Tablet: 100 mg, 250 mg, 500 mg

Generic Available Yes

Tolazoline (tole AZ oh leen)

Brand Names Priscoline®

Therapeutic Category Alpha-Adrenergic Blocking Agent, Parenteral; Vasodilator, Coronary

Use Treatment of persistent pulmonary vasoconstriction and hypertension of the newborn (persistent fetal circulation), peripheral vasospastic disorders

Usual Dosage

Neonates: Initial: I.V.: 1-2 mg/kg over 10-15 minutes via scalp vein or upper extremity; maintenance: 1-2 mg/kg/hour; use lower maintenance doses in patients with decreased renal function. Also used in neonates for acute vasospasm "cath toes" at 0.25 mg/kg/hour (no load); maximum dose: 6-8 mg/kg/hour

Mechanism of Action Competitively blocks alpha-adrenergic receptors to produce brief antagonism of circulating epinephrine and norepinephrine; reduces hypertension caused by catecholamines and causes vascular smooth muscle relaxation (direct action); results in peripheral vasodilation and decreased peripheral resistance

Local Anesthetic/Vasoconstrictor Precautions No information available to require special precautions

Effects on Dental Treatment No effects or complications reported

Other Adverse Effects

>10%:

Cardiovascular: Hypotension

Endocrine & metabolic: Hypochloremic alkalosis

Gastrointestinal: GI bleeding, abdominal pain

Hematologic: Thrombocytopenia

Local: Burning at injection site

Renal: Acute renal failure, oliguria

1% to 10%:

Cardiovascular: Peripheral vasodilation, tachycardia

Gastrointestinal: Nausea, diarrhea

Neuromuscular & skeletal: Increased pilomotor activity

<1%:

Cardiovascular: Hypertension, arrhythmias

Hematologic: Increased agranulocytosis, pancytopenia

Ocular: Mydriasis

Respiratory: Pulmonary hemorrhage, increased secretions

Drug Interactions

Increased toxicity: Disulfiram reaction may possibly be seen with concomitant ethanol use

Drug Uptake

Time to peak serum concentration: Within 30 minutes

Pregnancy Risk Factor C

Generic Available No

Tolbutamida (Mexico) *see* Tolbutamide *on this page*

Tolbutamide (tole BYOO ta mide)

Related Information

Endocrine Disorders & Pregnancy *on page 1021*

Brand Names Orinase®

Canadian/Mexican Brand Names Apo®-Tolbutamide (Canada); Artosin® (Mexico); Diaval® (Mexico); Mobenol® (Canada); Novo-Butamide® (Canada); Rastinon® (Mexico)

Therapeutic Category Antidiabetic Agent; Hypoglycemic Agent, Oral; Sulfonylurea Agent

Synonyms Tolbutamida (Mexico)

(Continued)

Tolbutamide *(Continued)*

Use Adjunct to diet for the management of mild to moderately severe, stable, noninsulin-dependent (type II) diabetes mellitus

Usual Dosage Divided doses may increase gastrointestinal side effects

Adults:

Oral: Initial: 500-1000 mg 1-3 times/day; usual dose should not be more than 2 g/day

I.V. bolus: 1 g over 2-3 minutes

Elderly: Oral: Initial: 250 mg 1-3 times/day; usual: 500-2000 mg; maximum: 3 g/day

Mechanism of Action A sulfonylurea hypoglycemic agent; its ability to lower elevated blood glucose levels in patients with functional pancreatic beta cells is similar to the other sulfonylurea agents; stimulates synthesis and release of endogenous insulin from pancreatic islet tissue. The hypoglycemic effect is attributed to an increased sensitivity of insulin receptors and improved peripheral utilization of insulin. Suppression of glucagon secretion may also contribute to the hypoglycemic effects of tolbutamide.

Local Anesthetic/Vasoconstrictor Precautions No information available to require special precautions

Effects on Dental Treatment Use salicylates with caution in patients taking tolazamide because of potential increased hypoglycemia; NSAIDs such as ibuprofen and naproxen may be safely used. Tolbutamide-dependent diabetics (noninsulin dependent, Type II) should be appointed for dental treatment in morning in order to minimize chance of stress-induced hypoglycemia

Other Adverse Effects

>10%:

Central nervous system: Headache, dizziness

Gastrointestinal: Constipation, diarrhea, heartburn, anorexia, epigastric fullness

1% to 10%: Dermatologic: Skin rash, urticaria, photosensitivity

<1%:

Cardiovascular: Venospasm

Endocrine & metabolic: SIADH, hypoglycemia, disulfiram-type reactions

Hematologic: Thrombocytopenia, agranulocytosis, leukopenia, aplastic anemia, hemolytic anemia, bone marrow suppression

Hepatic: Cholestatic jaundice

Local: Thrombophlebitis

Otic: Tinnitus

Miscellaneous: Hypersensitivity reaction

Drug Interactions Increased toxicity: Monitor patient closely; large number of drugs interact with sulfonylureas including salicylates, anticoagulants, H_2 antagonists, TCA, MAO inhibitors, beta-blockers, thiazides

Drug Uptake

Peak hypoglycemic action:

Oral: 1-3 hours

I.V.: 30 minutes

Duration:

Oral: 6-24 hours

I.V.: 3 hours

Absorption: Oral: Rapid

Serum half-life: Plasma: 4-25 hours

Time to peak serum concentration: 3-5 hours

Pregnancy Risk Factor D

Dosage Forms

Injection, diagnostic, as sodium: 1 g (20 mL)

Tablet: 250 mg, 500 mg

Generic Available Yes

Tolcapone *(TOLE ka pone)*

Brand Names Tasmar®

Therapeutic Category Anti-Parkinson's Agent

Use Adjunct to levodopa and carbidopa for the treatment of signs and symptoms of idiopathic Parkinson's disease

Usual Dosage Adults: Oral: Initial 100 mg 3 times/day, may increase to 200 mg 3 times/day

Local Anesthetic/Vasoconstrictor Precautions No information available to require special precautions

Effects on Dental Treatment No effects or complications reported

Dosage Forms Tablet: 100 mg, 200 mg

Tolectin® *see* Tolmetin *on next page*

Tolectin® DS *see* Tolmetin *on this page*

Tolinase® *see* Tolazamide *on page 940*

Tolmetin (TOLE met in)

Related Information

Nonsteroidal Anti-Inflammatory Agents, Comparative Dosages, and Pharmacokinetics *on page 1143*

Rheumatoid Arthritis and Osteoarthritis *on page 1030*

Brand Names Tolectin®; Tolectin® DS

Canadian/Mexican Brand Names Novo-Tolmetin® (Canada)

Therapeutic Category Analgesic, Non-narcotic; Nonsteroidal Anti-inflammatory Agent (NSAID), Oral

Use Treatment of rheumatoid arthritis and osteoarthritis, juvenile rheumatoid arthritis

Usual Dosage Oral:

Children ≥2 years:

Anti-inflammatory: Initial: 20 mg/kg/day in 3 divided doses, then 15-30 mg/kg/day in 3 divided doses

Analgesic: 5-7 mg/kg/dose every 6-8 hours

Adults: 400 mg 3 times/day; usual dose: 600 mg to 1.8 g/day; maximum: 2 g/day

Mechanism of Action Inhibits prostaglandin synthesis by decreasing the activity of the enzyme, cyclo-oxygenase, which results in decreased formation of prostaglandin precursors

Local Anesthetic/Vasoconstrictor Precautions No information available to require special precautions

Effects on Dental Treatment No effects or complications reported

Other Adverse Effects

>10%:

Central nervous system: Dizziness

Dermatologic: Skin rash

Gastrointestinal: Abdominal cramps, heartburn, indigestion, nausea

1% to 10%:

Central nervous system: Headache, nervousness

Dermatologic: Itching

Endocrine & metabolic: Fluid retention

Gastrointestinal: Vomiting

Otic: Tinnitus

<1%:

Cardiovascular: Congestive heart failure, hypertension, arrhythmias, tachycardia

Central nervous system: Confusion, hallucinations, aseptic meningitis, mental depression, drowsiness, insomnia

Dermatologic: Urticaria, erythema multiforme, toxic epidermal necrolysis, Stevens-Johnson syndrome, angioedema

Endocrine & metabolism: Polydipsia, hot flashes

Gastrointestinal: Gastritis, GI ulceration

Genitourinary: Cystitis

Hematologic: Agranulocytosis, anemia, hemolytic anemia, bone marrow suppression, leukopenia, thrombocytopenia

Hepatic: Hepatitis

Neuromuscular & skeletal: Peripheral neuropathy

Ocular: Toxic amblyopia, blurred vision, conjunctivitis, dry eyes

Otic: Decreased hearing

Renal: Polyuria, acute renal failure

Respiratory: Allergic rhinitis, dyspnea, epistaxis

Drug Interactions

Decreased effect with aspirin; decreased effect of thiazides, furosemide

Increased toxicity of digoxin, methotrexate, cyclosporine, lithium, insulin, sulfonylureas, potassium-sparing diuretics, aspirin

Drug Uptake

Absorption: Oral: Well absorbed

Time to peak serum concentration: Within 30-60 minutes

Pregnancy Risk Factor C (D if used in the 3rd trimester or near delivery)

Dosage Forms

Capsule, as sodium (Tolectin® DS): 400 mg

Tablet, as sodium (Tolectin®): 200 mg, 600 mg

Generic Available Yes

Tolnaftate (tole NAF tate)

Brand Names Absorbine® Antifungal [OTC]; Absorbine® Jock Itch [OTC]; Absorbine Jr.® Antifungal [OTC]; Aftate® for Athlete's Foot [OTC]; Aftate® for

(Continued)

Tolnaftate *(Continued)*

Jock Itch [OTC]; Blis-To-Sol® [OTC]; Breezee® Mist Antifungal [OTC]; Dr Scholl's Athlete's Foot [OTC]; Dr Scholl's Maximum Strength Tritin [OTC]; Genaspor® [OTC]; NP-27® [OTC]; Quinsana Plus® [OTC]; Tinactin® [OTC]; Tinactin® for Jock Itch [OTC]; Ting® [OTC]; Zeasorb-AF® Powder [OTC]

Canadian/Mexican Brand Names Pitrex® (Canada); Tinaderm® (Mexico)

Therapeutic Category Antifungal Agent, Topical

Synonyms Tolnaftato (Mexico)

Use Treatment of tinea pedis, tinea cruris, tinea corporis, tinea manuum, tinea versicolor infections

Usual Dosage Children and Adults: Topical: Wash and dry affected area; apply 1-3 drops of solution or a small amount of cream or powder and rub into the affected areas 2-3 times/day for 2-4 weeks

Mechanism of Action Distorts the hyphae and stunts mycelial growth in susceptible fungi

Local Anesthetic/Vasoconstrictor Precautions No information available to require special precautions

Effects on Dental Treatment No effects or complications reported

Other Adverse Effects 1% to 10%:
Dermatologic: Pruritus, contact dermatitis
Local: Irritation, stinging

Drug Interactions No data reported

Drug Uptake Onset of action: Response may be seen 24-72 hours after initiation of therapy

Pregnancy Risk Factor C

Generic Available Yes

Tolnaftato (Mexico) *see* Tolnaftate *on previous page*

Tolu-Sed® DM [OTC] *see* Guaifenesin and Dextromethorphan *on page 453*

Tonocard® *see* Tocainide *on page 939*

Topamax® *see* Topiramate *on this page*

Topicort® *see* Desoximetasone *on page 291*

Topicort®-LP *see* Desoximetasone *on page 291*

Topiramate *(toe PYE ra mate)*

Brand Names Topamax®

Therapeutic Category Anticonvulsant, Miscellaneous

Use Adjunctive therapy for partial onset seizures in adults

Usual Dosage Adults: Initial: 50 mg/day; titrate by 50 mg/day at 1-week intervals to target dose of 200 mg twice daily; usual maximum dose: 1600 mg/day

Mechanism of Action Mechanism is not fully understood, it is thought to decrease seizure frequency by blocking sodium channels in neurons, enhancing GABA activity, and by blocking glutamate activity

Local Anesthetic/Vasoconstrictor Precautions No information available to require special precautions

Effects on Dental Treatment Up to 10% of patients may experience gingivitis and dry mouth

Other Adverse Effects
>10%:
Central nervous system: Fatigue, dizziness, ataxia, somnolence, psychomotor slowing, nervousness, memory difficulties, speech problems
Gastrointestinal: Nausea
Neuromuscular & skeletal: Paresthesia, tremor
Ocular: Nystagmus
Respiratory: Upper respiratory infections
1% to 10%:
Cardiovascular: Chest pain, edema
Central nervous system: Language problems, abnormal coordination, confusion, depression, difficulty concentrating, hypoesthesia
Endocrine & metabolic: Hot flashes
Gastrointestinal: Dyspepsia, abdominal pain, anorexia, constipation, xerostomia, gingivitis, weight loss
Neuromuscular & skeletal: Myalgia, weakness, back pain, leg pain, rigors
Otic: Decreased hearing
Renal: Nephrolithiasis
Respiratory: Pharyngitis, sinusitis, epistaxis
Miscellaneous: Flu-like symptoms

Warnings/Precautions Avoid abrupt withdrawal of topiramate therapy, withdraw slowly to minimize the potential of increased seizure frequency; the risk of kidney stones is about 2-4 times that of the untreated population; the risk of this event may be reduced by increasing fluid intake; use cautiously in patients with hepatic or renal impairment, during pregnancy, or in nursing mothers.

Drug Interactions
Decreased effect: Phenytoin can decrease topiramate levels by as much as 48%, carbamazepine reduces it by 40% and valproic acid reduces topiramate by 14%; digoxin levels and norethindrone blood levels are decreased when coadministered with topiramate
Increased toxicity: Concomitant administration with other CNS depressants will increase its sedative effects; coadministration with other carbonic anhydrase inhibitors may increase the chance of nephrolithiasis

Drug Uptake
Absorption: Good; unaffected by food
Serum half-life: Mean: 21 hours in adults
Time to peak serum concentration: ~2-4 hours

Pregnancy Risk Factor C

Dosage Forms Tablet: 25 mg, 100 mg, 200 mg

Generic Available No

TOPO see Topotecan on this page

Toposar® Injection see Etoposide on page 388

Topotecan (toe poe TEE kan)

Brand Names Hycamtin®

Therapeutic Category Antineoplastic Agent, Antibiotic

Synonyms Hycamptamine; SK and F 104864; SKF 104864; SKF 104864-A; TOPO; TPT

Use Treatment of ovarian cancer after failure of first-line chemotherapy

Usual Dosage
Children: A phase I study in pediatric patients by CCSG determined the recommended phase II dose to be 5.5 mg/mm² as a 24-hour continuous infusion
Adults: Most phase II studies currently utilize topotecan at 1.5-2.0 mg/mm²/day for 5 days, repeated every 21-28 days. Alternative dosing regimens evaluated in phase I studies have included 21-day continuous infusion (recommended phase II dose: 0.53-0.7 mg/mm²/day) and weekly 24-hour infusions (recommended phase II dose: 1.5 mg/mm²/week).
Dose modifications: Dosage modification may be required for toxicity

Mechanism of Action Topotecan (TPT), like other camptothecin (CPT) analogues, is a potent inhibitor of topoisomerase I. Structure-activity studies have revealed a direct relationship between the ability of CPT analogues to inhibit topoisomerase I catalytic activity and their potency as cytotoxic agents.

Local Anesthetic/Vasoconstrictor Precautions No information available to require special precautions

Effects on Dental Treatment No effects or complications reported

Other Adverse Effects
>10%:
Central nervous system: Headache
Dermatologic: Alopecia
Gastrointestinal: Nausea, vomiting, diarrhea
Hematologic: Neutropenia
Respiratory: Dyspnea
1% to 10%:
Central nervous system: Fatigue
Gastrointestinal: Constipation, abdominal pain
Hepatic: AST and ALT elevations, bilirubin elevation
Neuromuscular & skeletal: Paresthesia
<1%:
Gastrointestinal: Stomatitis
Neuromuscular & skeletal: Arthralgia, myalgia

Drug Interactions Concurrent administration of topotecan (TPT) and G-CSF in clinical trials results in severe myelosuppression. Concurrent in vitro exposure to TPT and the topoisomerase II inhibitor etoposide results in no altered effect; sequential exposure results in potentiation. Concurrent exposure to TPT and 5-azacytidine results in potentiation both in vitro and in vivo.

Drug Uptake
Serum half-life: 3 hours

Pregnancy Risk Factor D

Generic Available No

Comments Constituted vial: When constituted with 2 mL of sterile water for injection, USP, each mL contains topotecan 2.5 mg and mannitol 50 mg with a pH of approximately 3.5. Final infusion preparation: Topotecan constituted solution should be further diluted in 5% dextrose injection. Topotecan should NOT be diluted in buffered solutions.

Toprol XL® [Succinate] *see* Metoprolol *on page 629*

TOPV *see* Poliovirus Vaccine, Live, Trivalent, Oral *on page 770*

Toradol® Injection *see* Ketorolac Tromethamine *on page 535*

Toradol® Oral *see* Ketorolac Tromethamine *on page 535*

Torecan® *see* Thiethylperazine *on page 924*

Toremifene (TORE em i feen)

Brand Names Fareston®

Therapeutic Category Antineoplastic Agent, Miscellaneous

Synonyms 4-Chloro-1,2-Diphenyl-1(4-[2-(N,N-Dimethylamino)-Ethoxy]-Phenyl)-1-Butene; FC1157a; Toremifene Butyrate

Use Treatment of advanced breast cancer; management of desmoid tumors and endometrial carcinoma

Usual Dosage Refer to individual protocols

60-240 mg/day

200-300 mg/day

60 mg for 3 days, then 20 mg/day

Dosage adjustment in hepatic impairment: May be required, but specific guidelines have not been established

Mechanism of Action At low doses, toremifene inhibits tumor growth by depleting cytosolic estrogen receptors. At higher doses, it acts on estrogen receptors. The exact mechanism of action is not clear, but may involve effects on calcium channels, calmodulin, and/or protein kinase C.

Local Anesthetic/Vasoconstrictor Precautions No information available to require special precautions

Effects on Dental Treatment No effects or complications reported

Other Adverse Effects

>10%:

Central nervous system: Dizziness or vertigo (12%), anxiety, depression, fatigue, headache, insomnia, irritability, lethargy

Endocrine & metabolic: Hot flashes

Gastrointestinal: Nausea and vomiting (40%)

Hematologic: Decreased antithrombin III levels

Neuromuscular & skeletal: Tremors

Miscellaneous: Sweating

1% to 10%:

Dermatologic: Rash, pruritus, urticaria

Gastrointestinal: Abdominal discomfort, anorexia, constipation, diarrhea, increased appetite

Genitourinary: Vaginal bleeding and discharge (3% to 8%)

Hematologic: Anemia

Neuromuscular & skeletal: Bone pain (3%)

Ocular: Dry eyes (3%)

<1%: Endocrine & metabolic: Hypercalcemia

Contraindications Hypersensitivity to toremifene or any component

Warnings/Precautions Toremifene should be used cautiously in patients with anemia or hepatic failure

Drug Uptake

Serum half-life: Elimination:

N-desmethyltoremifene: 6 days

4-hydroxytoremifene: 5 days

Time to peak serum concentration: 1.5-4.5 hours

Dosage Forms Tablet: 10 mg, 20 mg, 60 mg, 200 mg

Generic Available No

Selected Readings

Gams R, "Phase III Trials of Toremifene vs Tamoxifen," *Oncology*, 1997, 11(5 Suppl 4): 23-8.

Hamm JT, "Phase I and II Studies of Toremifene," *Oncology*, 1997, 11(5 Suppl 4):19-22.

Holli K, "Evolving Role of Troemifene in the Adjuvant Setting," *Oncology*, 1997, 11(5 Suppl 4):48-51.

Kangas L, "Review of the Pharmacological Properties of Toremifene," *J Steroid Biochem*, 1990, 36(3):191-5.

Pyrhönen S, Valavaara R, Modig H, et al, "Comparison of Toremifene and Tamoxifen in Postmenopausal Patients With Advanced Breast Cancer: A Randomized Double-Blind, the "Nordic" Phase III Study," *Br J Cancer*, 1997, 76(2):270-7.

Williams GM and Jeffrey AM, "Safety Assessment of Tamoxifen and Toremifene," *Oncology*, 1997, 11(5 Suppl 4):41-7.

Toremifene Butyrate *see* Toremifene *on this page*

Tornalate® *see* Bitolterol *on page 134*

Torsemide (TOR se mide)

Related Information

Cardiovascular Diseases *on page 1010*

Brand Names Demadex®

Therapeutic Category Diuretic, Loop

Use Management of edema associated with congestive heart failure and hepatic or renal disease; used alone or in combination with antihypertensives in treatment of hypertension; I.V. form is indicated when rapid onset is desired

Usual Dosage Adults: Oral, I.V.:

Congestive heart failure: 10-20 mg once daily; may increase gradually for chronic treatment by doubling dose until the diuretic response is apparent (for acute treatment, I.V. dose may be repeated every 2 hours with double the dose as needed)

Chronic renal failure: 20 mg once daily; increase as described above

Hepatic cirrhosis: 5-10 mg once daily with an aldosterone antagonist or a potassium-sparing diuretic; increase as described above

Hypertension: 5 mg once daily; increase to 10 mg after 4-6 weeks if an adequate hypotensive response is not apparent; if still not effective, an additional antihypertensive agent may be added

Mechanism of Action Inhibits reabsorption of sodium and chloride in the ascending loop of Henle and distal renal tubule, interfering with the chloride-binding cotransport system, thus causing increased excretion of water, sodium, chloride, magnesium, and calcium; does not alter GFR, renal plasma flow, or acid-base balance

Local Anesthetic/Vasoconstrictor Precautions No information available to require special precautions

Effects on Dental Treatment No effects or complications reported

Other Adverse Effects

>10%: Cardiovascular: Orthostatic hypotension

1% to 10%:

Central nervous system: Headache, dizziness, vertigo

Dermatologic: Photosensitivity, urticaria

Endocrine & metabolic: Electrolyte imbalance, dehydration, hyperuricemia

Gastrointestinal: Diarrhea, loss of appetite, stomach cramps or pain, pancreatitis

Ocular: Blurred vision

<1%:

Dermatologic: Skin rash

Endocrine & metabolic: Gout

Gastrointestinal: Nausea

Hepatic: Hepatic dysfunction

Hematologic: Agranulocytosis, leukopenia, anemia, thrombocytopenia

Local: Redness at injection site

Otic: Ototoxicity

Renal: Nephrocalcinosis, prerenal azotemia, interstitial nephritis

Drug Interactions

Aminoglycosides: Ototoxicity may be increased; anticoagulant activity is enhanced

Beta-blockers: Plasma concentrations of beta-blockers may be increased

Cisplatin: Ototoxicity may be increased

Digitalis: Arrhythmias may occur with diuretic-induced electrolyte disturbances

Lithium: Plasma concentrations of lithium may be increased

NSAIDs: Torsemide efficacy may be decreased

Probenecid: Torsemide action may be reduced

Salicylates: Diuretic action may be impaired in patients with cirrhosis and ascites

Sulfonylureas: Glucose tolerance may be decreased

Thiazides: Synergistic effects may result

Drug Uptake

Onset of diuresis: 30-60 minutes

Peak effect: 1-4 hours

Duration: ~6 hours

Absorption: Oral: Rapid

Serum half-life: 2-4; 7-8 hours in cirrhosis (dose modification appears unnecessary)

Pregnancy Risk Factor B

Generic Available No

Trace Metals (trase MET als)

Brand Names Chroma-Pak®; Iodopen®; Molypen®; M.T.E.-4®; M.T.E.-5®; M.T.E.-6®; MulTE-PAK-4®; MulTE-PAK-5®; Neotrace-4®; PedTE-PAK-4®; Pedtrace-4®; P.T.E.-4®; P.T.E.-5®; Sele-Pak®; Selepen®; Trace-4®; Zinca-Pak®

Therapeutic Category Trace Element, Parenteral

Synonyms Chromium; Copper; Iodine; Manganese; Molybdenum; Neonatal Trace Metals; Selenium; Zinc

Use Prevent and correct trace metal deficiencies

Local Anesthetic/Vasoconstrictor Precautions No information available to require special precautions

Effects on Dental Treatment No effects or complications reported

Pregnancy Risk Factor C

Generic Available Yes

Comments Persistent diarrhea or excessive gastrointestinal fluid losses from ostomy sites may grossly increase zinc losses

Tramadol (TRA ma dole)

Brand Names Ultram®

Canadian/Mexican Brand Names Tradol® (Mexico)

Therapeutic Category Analgesic, Non-narcotic

Use

Dental: Relief of moderate to moderately severe dental pain

Medical: Relief of moderate to moderately severe medical pain

Usual Dosage Adults: Oral: 50-100 mg every 4-6 hours, not to exceed 400 mg/day

Mechanism of Action Binds to μ-opiate receptors in the CNS causing inhibition of ascending pain pathways, altering the perception of and response to pain; also inhibits the reuptake of norepinephrine and serotonin, which also modifies the ascending pain pathway

Local Anesthetic/Vasoconstrictor Precautions No information available to require special precautions

Effects on Dental Treatment No effects or complications reported

Other Adverse Effects >1%:

Central nervous system: Dizziness, somnolence, restlessness

Gastrointestinal: Nausea, constipation

Miscellaneous: Sweating

Contraindications Previous hypersensitivity to tramadol or any components; should not be administered in cases of acute intoxication with alcohol, hypnotics, centrally acting analgesics, opioids, or psychotropic drugs

Warnings/Precautions Elderly patients and patients with chronic respiratory disorders may be at greater risk of adverse events; liver disease; patients with myxedema, hypothyroidism, or hypoadrenalism should use tramadol with caution and at reduced dosages; not recommended during pregnancy or in nursing mothers

Drug Interactions Carbamazepine decreases half-life by 33% to 50%; increased toxicity with monoamine oxidase inhibitors (seizures); quinidine inhibits cytochrome P450IID6, thereby increasing tramadol serum concentrations; cimetidine increases tramadol half-life by 20% to 25%

Drug Uptake

Absorption: Oral: ~75%

Onset of action: ~1 hour

Serum half-life, elimination: 6 hours

Time to peak serum concentration: 2 hours

Pregnancy Risk Factor C

Breast-feeding Considerations No data reported

Dosage Forms Tablet, as hydrochloride: 50 mg

Generic Available No

Comments Literature reports suggest that the efficacy of tramadol in oral surgery pain is equivalent to the combination of aspirin and codeine. One study (Olson et al 1990) showed acetaminophen and dextropropoxyphene combination to be superior to tramadol and another study (Mehlisch et al, 1990) showed tramadol to be superior to acetaminophen and dextropropoxyphene combination. Tramadol appears to be at least equal to if not better than codeine alone. Recently, seizures have been reported with the use of tramadol.

Selected Readings

Collins M, Young I, Sweeney P, et al, "The Effect of Tramadol on Dento-Alveolar Surgical Pain," *Br J Oral Maxillofac Surg*, 1997, 35(1):54-8.

Kahn LH, Alderfer RJ, and Graham DJ, "Seizures Reported With Tramadol," *JAMA*, 1997, 278(20):1661.

Lewis KS and Han NH, "Tramadol: A New Centrally Acting Analgesic," *Am J Health Syst Pharm*, 1997, 54(6):643-52.

Mehlisch DR, Minn F, and Brown P, "Tramadol Hydrochloride: Efficacy Compared to Codeine Sulfate, Acetaminophen With Dextropropoxyphene and Placebo in Dental Extraction Pain," *Clin Pharmacol Ther*, 1992.

Olson NZ, Sunshine A, O'Neill, et al, *Tramadol Hydrochloride: Oral Efficacy in Postoperative Pain*, American Pain Society 9th Annual Scientific Meeting, St Louis, MO, October, 1990.

Sunshine A, "New Clinical Experience With Tramadol," *Drugs*, 1994, 47(Suppl 1):8-18.

Sunshine A, Olson NZ, Zighelboim I, et al, "Analgesic Oral Efficacy of Tramadol Hydrochloride in Postoperative Pain," *Clin Pharmacol Ther*, 1992; 51(6):740-6.

Voorhees F, Leibold DG, Stumpf, et al, "Tramadol Hydrochloride: Efficacy Compared to Codeine Sulfate, Aspirin With Codeine Phosphate, and Placebo in Dental Extraction Pain," *Clin Pharmacol Ther*, 1992, 51:122.

Wynn RL, "Tramadol (Ultram) -- A New Kind of Analgesic," *Gen Dent*, 1996, 44(3):216-8,220.

Trandate® *see* Labetalol *on page 537*

Trandolapril (tran DOE la pril)

Brand Names Mavik®

Therapeutic Category Angiotensin-Converting Enzyme (ACE) Inhibitors

Use Management of hypertension alone or in combination with other antihypertensive agents

Usual Dosage Adults:

Non-African-American patients: 0.5-1 mg for those not receiving diuretics; increase dose at 0.5-1 mg increments at 1- to 2-week intervals; maximum dose: 4 mg/day

Black patients: Initiate doses of 1-2 mg; maximum dose: 4 mg/day

Dosing adjustment in renal impairment: Cl_{cr} ≤30 mL/minute: Administer lowest doses

Mechanism of Action Trandolapril is an angiotensin-converting enzyme (ACE) inhibitor which prevents the formation of angiotensin II from angiotensin I. Trandolapril must undergo enzymatic hydrolysis, mainly in liver, to its biologically active metabolite, trandolaprilat. A CNS mechanism may also be involved in the hypotensive effect as angiotensin II increases adrenergic outflow from the CNS. Vasoactive kallikrein's may be decreased in conversion to active hormones by ACE inhibitors, thus, reducing blood pressure.

Local Anesthetic/Vasoconstrictor Precautions No information available to require special precautions

Effects on Dental Treatment No effects or complications reported

Other Adverse Effects

Cardiovascular: Tachycardia, chest pain, palpitations, orthostatic blood pressure changes, syncope, heart failure, hypotension, cardiogenic shock

Central nervous system: Headache, fatigue, dizziness, malaise, vertigo, drowsiness, ataxia, nervousness, insomnia, fever

Dermatologic: Rash, pruritus, alopecia, exfoliative dermatitis, urticaria, photosensitivity, angioedema

Endocrine & metabolic: Hyperkalemia, decreased libido

Gastrointestinal: Dysgeusia, abdominal pain, nausea, vomiting, diarrhea, anorexia, constipation, dry mouth, dysgeusia, glossitis

Genitourinary: Impotence

Hematologic: Neutropenia, agranulocytosis

Hepatic: Hepatitis

Neuromuscular & skeletal: Arthritis, arthralgia, myalgia, paresthesias

Ocular: Blurred vision

Otic: Tinnitus

Renal: Oliguria, Elevated BUN, elevated serum creatinine, proteinuria, worsening renal failure

Respiratory: Chest pain, chronic cough (nonproductive, persistent - more frequent in women)

Miscellaneous: Sweating

Warnings/Precautions Neutropenia, agranulocytosis, angioedema, decreased renal function (hypertension, renal artery stenosis, CHF), hepatic dysfunction (elimination, activation), proteinuria, first-dose hypotension (hypovolemia, CHF, dehydrated patients at risk, eg, diuretic use, elderly), elderly (due to renal function changes); use with caution and modify dosage in patients with renal impairment; use with caution in patients with collagen vascular disease, CHF, hypovolemia, valvular stenosis, hyperkalemia (>5.7 mEq/L), anesthesia

Drug Interactions

ACE inhibitors (trandolapril) and potassium-sparing diuretics → additive hyperkalemic effect

ACE inhibitors (trandolapril) and indomethacin or nonsteroidal anti-inflammatory agents → reduced antihypertensive response to ACE inhibitors (trandolapril)

Allopurinol and trandolapril → neutropenia

Antacids and ACE inhibitors → ↓ absorption of ACE inhibitors

Phenothiazines and ACE inhibitors → ↑ ACE inhibitor effect

Probenecid and ACE inhibitors (trandolapril) → ↑ ACE inhibitors (trandolapril) levels

(Continued)

Trandolapril *(Continued)*

Rifampin and ACE inhibitors (trandolapril) → ↓ ACE inhibitor effect
Digoxin and ACE inhibitors → ↑ serum digoxin levels
Lithium and ACE inhibitors → ↑ lithium serum levels
Tetracycline and ACE inhibitors (trandolapril) → ↓ tetracycline absorption (up to 37%)

Food decreases trandolapril absorption; rate, but not extent, of ramipril and fosinopril is reduced by concomitant administration with food; food does not reduce absorption of enalapril, lisinopril, or benazepril; trandolapril has a decreased rate and extent (25% to 30%) of absorption when taken with a high fat meal

Drug Uptake
Absorption: Rapid
Half-life: 24 hours
Pregnancy Risk Factor C (first trimester); D (second & third trimester)
Generic Available No
Comments Patients taking diuretics are at risk for developing hypotension on initial dosing; to prevent this, discontinue diuretics 2-3 days prior to initiating trandolapril; may restart diuretics if blood pressure is not controlled by trandolapril alone

Selected Readings

Bevan EG, McInnes GT, Aldigier JC, et al, "Effect of Renal Function on the Pharmacokinetics and Pharmacodynamics of Trandolapril," *Br J Clin Pharmacol*, 1993, 35(2):128-35.
Conen H and Brunner HR, "Pharmacologic Profile of Trandolapril, A New Angiotensin-Converting Enzyme Inhibitor," *Am J Heart*, 1993, 125(5 Pt 2):1524-31.
Zannad F, "Trandolapril. How Does It Differ From Other Angiotensin-Converting Enzyme Inhibitors?" *Drugs*, 1993, 46(Suppl 2):172-81.

Trandolapril and Verapamil *(tran DOE la pril & ver AP a mil)*
Brand Names Tarka®
Therapeutic Category Antihypertensive Agent, Combination
Use Combination drug for the treatment of hypertension
Local Anesthetic/Vasoconstrictor Precautions No information available to require special precautions
Effects on Dental Treatment No effects or complications reported
Dosage Forms Tablet:
Trandolapril 1 mg and verapamil hydrochloride 240 mg
Trandolapril 2 mg and verapamil hydrochloride 180 mg
Trandolapril 2 mg and verapamil hydrochloride 240 mg
Trandolapril 4 mg and verapamil hydrochloride 240 mg
Generic Available No

Tranexamic Acid *(tran eks AM ik AS id)*
Brand Names Cyklokapron® Injection; Cyklokapron® Oral
Therapeutic Category Antihemophilic Agent
Use Short-term use (2-8 days) in hemophilia patients during and following tooth extraction to reduce or prevent hemorrhage
Usual Dosage Children and Adults: I.V.: 10 mg/kg immediately before surgery, then 25 mg/kg/dose orally 3-4 times/day for 2-8 days

Alternatively:
Oral: 25 mg/kg 3-4 times/day beginning 1 day prior to surgery
I.V.: 10 mg/kg 3-4 times/day in patients who are unable to take oral
Mechanism of Action Forms a reversible complex that displaces plasminogen from fibrin resulting in inhibition of fibrinolysis; it also inhibits the proteolytic activity of plasmin
Local Anesthetic/Vasoconstrictor Precautions No information available to require special precautions
Effects on Dental Treatment No effects or complications reported
Other Adverse Effects
>10%: Gastrointestinal: Nausea, diarrhea, vomiting
1% to 10%:
Cardiovascular: Hypotension, thrombosis
Ocular: Blurred vision
<1%: Endocrine & metabolic: Unusual menstrual discomfort
Drug Uptake
Serum half-life: 2-10 hours
Pregnancy Risk Factor B
Generic Available No

Transdermal-NTG® *see* Nitroglycerin *on page 685*
Transderm-Nitro® *see* Nitroglycerin *on page 685*
Transderm Scop® Patch *see* Scopolamine *on page 858*

Trans-Ver-Sal® AdultPatch [OTC] *see* Salicylic Acid *on page 853*
Trans-Ver-Sal® PediaPatch [OTC] *see* Salicylic Acid *on page 853*
Trans-Ver-Sal® PlantarPatch [OTC] *see* Salicylic Acid *on page 853*
Tranxene® *see* Clorazepate *on page 251*

Tranylcypromine (tran il SIP roe meen)

Brand Names Parnate®
Therapeutic Category Antidepressant, Monoamine Oxidase Inhibitor
Use Symptomatic treatment of depressed patients refractory to or intolerant to tricyclic antidepressants or electroconvulsive therapy; has a more rapid onset of therapeutic effect than other MAO inhibitors, but causes more severe hypertensive reactions
Usual Dosage Adults: Oral: 10 mg twice daily, increase by 10 mg increments at 1- to 3-week intervals; maximum: 60 mg/day
Mechanism of Action Inhibits the enzymes monoamine oxidase A and B which are responsible for the intraneuronal metabolism of norepinephrine and serotonin and increasing their availability to postsynaptic neurons; decreased firing rate of the locus ceruleus, reducing norepinephrine concentration in the brain; agonist effects of serotonin
Local Anesthetic/Vasoconstrictor Precautions Attempts should be made to avoid use of vasoconstrictor due to possibility of hypertensive episodes with monoamine oxidase inhibitors
Effects on Dental Treatment Orthostatic hypotension in >10% of patients; meperidine should be avoided as an analgesic due to toxic reactions with MAO inhibitors
Other Adverse Effects
1% to 10%: Cardiovascular: Orthostatic hypotension
<1%:
Cardiovascular: Edema, hypertensive crises
Central nervous system: Drowsiness, hyperexcitability, headache
Dermatologic: Skin rash, photosensitivity
Gastrointestinal: Dry mouth, constipation
Genitourinary: Urinary retention
Hepatic: Hepatitis
Ocular: Blurred vision
Drug Interactions
Decreased effect of antihypertensives
Increased toxicity with disulfiram (seizures), fluoxetine and other serotonin-active agents (eg, paroxetine, sertraline), tricyclic antidepressants (cardiovascular instability), meperidine (cardiovascular instability), phenothiazine (hypertensive crisis), sympathomimetics (hypertensive crisis), sumatriptan (hypothetical), CNS depressants, levodopa (hypertensive crisis), tyramine-containing foods (eg, aged foods), dextroamphetamine (psychosis)
Drug Uptake
Onset of action: 2-3 weeks are required of continued dosing to obtain full therapeutic effect
Serum half-life: 90-190 minutes
Time to peak serum concentration: Within 2 hours
Pregnancy Risk Factor C
Generic Available No

Trasylol® *see* Aprotinin *on page 84*

Trazodone (TRAZ oh done)

Related Information
Vasoconstrictor Interactions With Antidepressants *on page 1226*
Brand Names Desyrel®
Therapeutic Category Antidepressant, Miscellaneous
Use Treatment of depression
Usual Dosage Oral: Therapeutic effects may take up to 4 weeks to occur; therapy is normally maintained for several months after optimum response is reached to prevent recurrence of depression

Children 6-18 years: Initial: 1.5-2 mg/kg/day in divided doses; increase gradually every 3-4 days as needed; maximum: 6 mg/kg/day in 3 divided doses
Adolescents: Initial: 25-50 mg/day; increase to 100-150 mg/day in divided doses
Adults: Initial: 150 mg/day in 3 divided doses (may increase by 50 mg/day every 3-7 days); maximum: 600 mg/day
Elderly: 25-50 mg at bedtime with 25-50 mg/day dose increase every 3 days for inpatients and weekly for outpatients, if tolerated; usual dose: 75-150 mg/day
Mechanism of Action Inhibits reuptake of serotonin and norepinephrine by the presynaptic neuronal membrane and desensitization of adenyl cyclase, down
(Continued)

Trazodone *(Continued)*

regulation of beta-adrenergic receptors, and down regulation of serotonin receptors

Local Anesthetic/Vasoconstrictor Precautions No information available to require special precautions

Effects on Dental Treatment >10% of patients will experience dry mouth; trazodone elicits anticholinergic effects, but occur much less frequently than with tricyclic antidepressants; more than 10% of patients will have significant dry mouth especially in the elderly which could contribute to periodontal diseases and oral discomfort

Other Adverse Effects

>10%:

Central nervous system: Dizziness, headache, confusion
Gastrointestinal: Nausea, bad taste in mouth
Neuromuscular & skeletal: Muscle tremors

1% to 10%:

Gastrointestinal: Diarrhea, constipation
Neuromuscular & skeletal: Weakness
Ocular: Blurred vision

<1%:

Cardiovascular: Hypotension, tachycardia, bradycardia
Central nervous system: Agitation, seizures, extrapyramidal reactions
Dermatologic: Skin rash
Genitourinary: Prolonged priapism, urinary retention
Hepatic: Hepatitis

Drug Interactions

Decreased effect: Clonidine, methyldopa, anticoagulants
Increased toxicity: Fluoxetine; increased effect/toxicity of phenytoin, CNS depressants, MAO inhibitors; digoxin serum levels increase

Drug Uptake

Onset of effect: Therapeutic effects take 1-3 weeks to appear
Serum half-life: 4-7.5 hours, 2 compartment kinetics
Time to peak serum concentration: Within 30-100 minutes, prolonged in the presence of food (up to 2.5 hours)

Pregnancy Risk Factor C

Generic Available Yes

Trecator®-SC *see* Ethionamide *on page 382*

Trental® *see* Pentoxifylline *on page 741*

Tretinoina (Mexico) *see* Tretinoin, Topical *on next page*

Tretinoin, Oral (TRET i noyn, oral)

Brand Names Vesanoid®

Therapeutic Category Antineoplastic Agent, Miscellaneous

Synonyms All-*trans*-Retinoic Acid

Use Acute promyelocytic leukemia (APL): Induction of remission in patients with APL, French American British (FAB) classification M3 (including the M3 variant), characterized by the presence of the t(15;17) translocation or the presence of the PML/RARα gene who are refractory to or who have relapsed from anthracycline chemotherapy, or for whom anthracycline-based chemotherapy is contraindicated. Tretinoin is for the induction of remission only. All patients should receive an accepted form of remission consolidation or maintenance therapy for APL after completion of induction therapy with tretinoin.

Mechanism of Action Retinoid that induces maturation of acute promyelocytic leukemia (APL) cells in cultures; induces cytodifferentiation and decreased proliferation of APL cells

Local Anesthetic/Vasoconstrictor Precautions No information available to require special precautions

Effects on Dental Treatment <1% of patients may have bleeding gums, dry mouth

Other Adverse Effects Virtually all patients experience some drug-related toxicity, especially headache, fever, weakness and fatigue. These adverse effects are seldom permanent or irreversible nor do they usually require therapy interruption

>10%:

Cardiovascular: Arrhythmias, flushing, hypotension, hypertension, peripheral edema, chest discomfort, edema
Central nervous system: Dizziness, anxiety, insomnia, depression, confusion, malaise, pain
Dermatologic: Burning, redness, cheilitis, inflammation of lips, dry skin, pruritus, photosensitivity

Endocrine & metabolic: Increased serum concentration of triglycerides

Gastrointestinal: GI hemorrhage, abdominal pain, other GI disorders, diarrhea, constipation, dyspepsia, abdominal distention, weight gain or loss, anorexia, xerostomia

Hematologic: Hemorrhage, disseminated intravascular coagulation

Local: Phlebitis, injection site reactions

Neuromuscular & skeletal: Bone pain, arthralgia, myalgia, paresthesia

Ocular: Itching of eye

Renal: Renal insufficiency

Respiratory: Upper respiratory tract disorders, dyspnea, respiratory insufficiency, pleural effusion, pneumonia, rales, expiratory wheezing, dry nose

Miscellaneous: Infections, shivering

1% to 10%:

Cardiovascular: Cardiac failure, cardiac arrest, myocardial infarction, enlarged heart, heart murmur, ischemia, stroke, myocarditis, pericarditis, pulmonary hypertension, secondary cardiomyopathy, cerebral hemorrhage, pallor

Central nervous system: Intracranial hypertension, agitation, hallucination, agnosia, aphasia, cerebellar edema, cerebellar disorders, convulsions, coma, CNS depression, encephalopathy, hypotaxia, no light reflex, neurologic reaction, spinal cord disorder, unconsciousness, dementia, forgetfulness, somnolence, slow speech, hypothermia

Dermatologic: Skin peeling on hands or soles of feet, rash, cellulitis

Endocrine & metabolic: Fluid imbalance, acidosis

Gastrointestinal: Hepatosplenomegaly, ulcer, unspecified liver disorder

Genitourinary: Dysuria, polyuria, enlarged prostate

Hepatic: Ascites, hepatitis

Neuromuscular & skeletal: Tremor, leg weakness, hyporeflexia, dysarthria, facial paralysis, hemiplegia, flank pain, asterixis, abnormal gait

Ocular: Dry eyes, photophobia

Renal: Acute renal failure, renal tubular necrosis

Respiratory: Lower respiratory tract disorders, pulmonary infiltration, bronchial asthma, pulmonary/larynx edema, unspecified pulmonary disease

Miscellaneous: Face edema, lymph disorders

Warnings/Precautions

Not to be used in women of childbearing potential unless woman is capable of complying with effective contraceptive measures; therapy is normally begun on the second or third day of next normal menstrual period; two reliable methods of effective contraception must be used during therapy and for 1 month after discontinuation of therapy, unless abstinence is the chosen method. Within one week prior to the institution of tretinoin therapy, the patient should have blood or urine collected for a serum or urine pregnancy test with a sensitivity of at least 50 mIU/L. When possible, delay tretinoin therapy until a negative result from this test is obtained. When a delay is not possible, place the patient on two reliable forms of contraception. Repeat pregnancy testing and contraception counseling monthly throughout the period of treatment.

Drug Interactions Metabolized by the hepatic cytochrome P-450 system: All drugs that induce or inhibit this system would be expected to interact with tretinoin cytochrome P-450 2C9 substrate

Increased toxicity: Ketoconazole increases the mean plasma AUC of tretinoin

Drug Uptake

Serum half-life, terminal: Parent drug: 0.5-2 hours

Time to peak serum concentration: Within 1-2 hours

Pregnancy Risk Factor D

Dosage Forms Capsule: 10 mg

Generic Available No

Tretinoin, Topical (TRET i noyn, TOP i kal)

Brand Names Avita® Topical; Retin-A™ Micro Topical; Retin-A™ Topical

Canadian/Mexican Brand Names Retisol-A® (Canada); Stieva-A® 0.025% (Mexico); Stieva-A® (Canada); Stieva-A Forte® (Canada); Stieva-A® (Mexico)

Therapeutic Category Acne Products; Retinoic Acid Derivative; Vitamin, Topical

Synonyms Tretinoina (Mexico)

Use Treatment of acne vulgaris, photodamaged skin, and some skin cancers

Mechanism of Action Keratinocytes in the sebaceous follicle become less adherent which allows for easy removal; decreases microcomedone formation

Local Anesthetic/Vasoconstrictor Precautions No information available to require special precautions

Effects on Dental Treatment No effects or complications reported

Other Adverse Effects 1% to 10%:

Cardiovascular: Edema

(Continued)

Tretinoin, Topical (Continued)

Dermatologic: Excessive dryness, erythema, scaling of the skin, hyperpigmentation or hypopigmentation, photosensitivity, initial acne flare-up

Local: Stinging, blistering

Drug Interactions Increased toxicity: Sulfur, benzoyl peroxide, salicylic acid, resorcinol (potentiates adverse reactions seen with tretinoin)

Drug Uptake Absorption: Topical: Minimum absorption occurs

Pregnancy Risk Factor C

Dosage Forms

Cream

Avita®: 0.025% (20 g, 45 g)

Retin-A™: 0.025% (20 g, 45 g); 0.05% (20 g, 45 g); 0.1% (20 g, 45 g)

Gel, topical (Retin-A™): 0.01% (15 g, 45 g); 0.025% (15 g, 45 g)

Gel, topical (Retin-A™ Micro): 0.1% (20 g, 45 g)

Liquid, topical (Retin-A™): 0.05% (28 mL)

Generic Available No

TRH see Protirelin on page 818

Triacet® see Triamcinolone on this page

Triacetin (trye a SEE tin)

Brand Names Ony-Clear® Nail

Therapeutic Category Antifungal Agent, Topical

Synonyms Glycerol Triacetate

Use Fungistat for athlete's foot and other superficial fungal infections

Local Anesthetic/Vasoconstrictor Precautions No information available to require special precautions

Effects on Dental Treatment No effects or complications reported

Generic Available No

Triacin-C® see Triprolidine, Pseudoephedrine, and Codeine on page 970

Triam-A® see Triamcinolone on this page

Triamcinolone (trye am SIN oh lone)

Related Information

Corticosteroid Equivalencies Comparison on page 1139

Corticosteroids, Topical Comparison on page 1140

Oral Nonviral Soft Tissue Ulcerations or Erosions on page 1070

Respiratory Diseases on page 1018

Brand Names Amcort®; Aristocort®; Aristocort® A; Aristocort® Forte; Aristocort® Intralesional; Aristospan® Intra-Articular; Aristospan® Intralesional; Atolone®; Azmacort™; Delta-Tritex®; Flutex®; Kenacort®; Kenaject-40®; Kenalog®; Kenalog-10®; Kenalog-40®; Kenalog® H; Kenalog® in Orabase®; Kenonel®; Nasacort®; Nasacort® AQ; Tac™-3; Tac™-40; Triacet®; Triam-A®; Triam Forte®; Triderm®; Tri-Kort®; Trilog®; Trilone®; Tristoject®

Canadian/Mexican Brand Names Kenacort® (Mexico); Ledercort® (Mexico); Zamacort® (Mexico)

Therapeutic Category Anti-inflammatory Agent; Corticosteroid, Inhalant; Corticosteroid, Systemic; Corticosteroid, Topical (Medium Potency)

Synonyms Triamcinolone Acetonide, Aerosol; Triamcinolone Acetonide, Parenteral; Triamcinolone Diacetate, Oral; Triamcinolone Diacetate, Parenteral; Triamcinolone Hexacetonide; Triamcinolone, Oral

Use Severe swelling or immunosuppression; nasal spray for symptoms of seasonal and perennial allergic rhinitis

Usual Dosage In general, single I.M. dose of 4-7 times oral dose will control patient from 4-7 days up to 3-4 weeks.

Children 6-12 years:

Oral inhalation: 1-2 inhalations 3-4 times/day, not to exceed 12 inhalations/day

I.M. (acetonide or hexacetonide): 0.03-0.2 mg/kg at 1- to 7-day intervals

Intra-articular, intrabursal, or tendon-sheath injection: 2.5-15 mg, repeated as needed

Children >12 years and Adults:

Intranasal: 2 sprays in each nostril once daily; may increase after 4-7 days up to 4 sprays once daily or 1 spray 4 times/day in each nostril

Topical: Apply a thin film 2-3 times/day

Oral: 4-48 mg/day

I.M.: Acetonide or hexacetonide: 60 mg (of 40 mg/mL), additional 20-100 mg doses (usual: 40-80 mg) may be given when signs and symptoms recur, best at 6-week intervals to minimize HPA suppression

Oral inhalation: 2 inhalations 3-4 times/day, not to exceed 16 inhalations/day

Intra-articular (hexacetonide): 2-20 mg every 3-4 weeks as hexacetonide salt

Intralesional (use 10 mg/mL) (diacetate or acetonide): 1 mg/injection site, may be repeated one or more times/week depending upon patients response; maximum; 30 mg at any one time; may use multiple injections if they are more than 1 cm apart

Intra-articular, intrasynovial, and soft-tissue injection (use 10 mg/mL or 40 mg/mL) (diacetate or acetonide): 2.5-40 mg depending upon location, size of joints, and degree of inflammation; repeat when signs and symptoms recur

Sublesional (as acetonide): Up to 1 mg per injection site and may be repeated one or more times weekly; multiple sites may be injected if they are 1 cm or more apart, not to exceed 30 mg

See table.

Triamcinolone Dosing

	Acetonide	Diacetate	Hexacetonide
Intrasynovial	2.5-40 mg	5-40 mg	
Intralesional	2.5-40 mg	5-48 mg	Up to 0.5 mg/sq inch affected area
Sublesional	1-30 mg		
Systemic I.M.	2.5-60 mg/d	~40 mg/wk	20-100 mg
Intra-articular		5-40 mg	2-20 mg average
large joints	5-15 mg		10-20 mg
small joints	2.5-5 mg		2-6 mg
Tendon sheaths	10-40 mg		
Intradermal	1 mg/site		

Mechanism of Action Decreases inflammation by suppression of migration of polymorphonuclear leukocytes and reversal of increased capillary permeability; suppresses the immune system by reducing activity and volume of the lymphatic system; suppresses adrenal function at high doses

Local Anesthetic/Vasoconstrictor Precautions No information available to require special precautions

Effects on Dental Treatment No effects or complications reported

Other Adverse Effects
>10%:
Central nervous system: Insomnia, nervousness
Gastrointestinal: Increased appetite, indigestion
1% to 10%:
Dermatologic: Hirsutism
Endocrine & metabolic: Diabetes mellitus
Neuromuscular & skeletal: Arthralgia
Ocular: Cataracts
Respiratory: Epistaxis
<1%:
Central nervous system: Seizures, mood swings, headache, delirium, hallucinations, euphoria
Dermatologic: Skin atrophy, bruising, hyperpigmentation, acne
Endocrine & metabolic: Amenorrhea, sodium and water retention, Cushing's syndrome, hyperglycemia
Gastrointestinal: Abdominal distention, ulcerative esophagitis, pancreatitis
Hematologic: Bone growth suppression
Neuromuscular & skeletal: Muscle wasting
Miscellaneous: Hypersensitivity reactions

Drug Uptake
Duration of action: Oral: 8-12 hours
Absorption: Topical: Systemic absorption may occur
Serum half-life, biologic: 18-36 hours
Time to peak: I.M.: Within 8-10 hours

Pregnancy Risk Factor C

Generic Available Yes

Comments Triamcinolone 16 mg is equivalent to cortisone 100 mg (no mineralocorticoid activity)

Triamcinolone Acetonide, Aerosol see Triamcinolone on previous page

Triamcinolone Acetonide Dental Paste
(trye am SIN oh lone a SEE toe nide DEN tal paste)
Brand Names Kenalog® in Orabase®
Canadian/Mexican Brand Names Oracort (Canada)
Therapeutic Category Anti-inflammatory Agent
(Continued)

Triamcinolone Acetonide Dental Paste *(Continued)*

Use
Dental: For adjunctive treatment and for the temporary relief of symptoms associated with oral inflammatory lesions and ulcerative lesions resulting from trauma
Medical: Localized inflammation responsive to steroids

Usual Dosage Press a small dab (about ¼ inch) to the lesion until a thin film develops. A larger quantity may be required for coverage of some lesions. For optimal results use only enough to coat the lesion with a thin film.

Mechanism of Action Decreases inflammation by suppression of migration of polymorphonuclear leukocytes and reversal of increased capillary permeability; suppresses the immune system by reducing activity and volume of the lymphatic system; suppresses adrenal function at high doses

Local Anesthetic/Vasoconstrictor Precautions No information available to require special precautions

Effects on Dental Treatment No effects or complications reported

Other Adverse Effects No data reported

Contraindications Known hypersensitivity to triamcinolone; contraindicated in the presence of fungal, viral, or bacterial infections of the mouth or throat

Warnings/Precautions Patients with tuberculosis, peptic ulcer or diabetes mellitus should not be treated with any corticosteroid preparation without the advice of the patient's physician. Normal immune responses of the oral tissues are depressed in patients receiving topical corticosteroid therapy. Virulent strains of oral microorganisms may multiply without producing the usual warning symptoms of oral infections. The small amount of steroid released from the topical preparation makes systemic effects very unlikely. If local irritation or sensitization should develop, the preparation should be discontinued. If significant regeneration or repair of oral tissues has not occurred in seven days, re-evaluation of the etiology of the oral lesion is advised.

Drug Interactions No data reported

Drug Uptake
Absorption: Topical: Systemic absorption may occur
Serum half-life: Biological: 18-36 hours

Pregnancy Risk Factor C

Breast-feeding Considerations No data reported

Dosage Forms Tubes: 5 g; each g provides 1 mg (0.1%) triamcinolone in emollient dental paste containing gelatin, pectin, and carboxymethylcellulose sodium in a polyethylene and mineral oil gel base

Generic Available Yes

Comments When applying to tissues, attempts to spread this preparation may result in a granular, gritty sensation and cause it to crumble. This preparation should be applied at bedtime to permit steroid contact with the lesion throughout the night.

Triamcinolone Acetonide, Parenteral *see* Triamcinolone *on page 954*

Triamcinolone Diacetate, Oral *see* Triamcinolone *on page 954*

Triamcinolone Diacetate, Parenteral *see* Triamcinolone *on page 954*

Triamcinolone Hexacetonide *see* Triamcinolone *on page 954*

Triamcinolone, Oral *see* Triamcinolone *on page 954*

Triam Forte® *see* Triamcinolone *on page 954*

Triaminic® Allergy Tablet [OTC] *see* Chlorpheniramine and Phenylpropanolamine *on page 219*

Triaminic® AM Decongestant Formula [OTC] *see* Pseudoephedrine *on page 820*

Triaminic® Cold Tablet [OTC] *see* Chlorpheniramine and Phenylpropanolamine *on page 219*

Triaminic® Expectorant [OTC] *see* Guaifenesin and Phenylpropanolamine *on page 454*

Triaminicol® Multi-Symptom Cold Syrup [OTC] *see* Chlorpheniramine, Phenylpropanolamine, and Dextromethorphan *on page 222*

Triaminic® Oral Infant Drops *see* Pheniramine, Phenylpropanolamine, and Pyrilamine *on page 747*

Triaminic® Syrup [OTC] *see* Chlorpheniramine and Phenylpropanolamine *on page 219*

Triamterene *(trye AM ter een)*
Related Information
Cardiovascular Diseases *on page 1010*
Brand Names Dyrenium®
Therapeutic Category Diuretic, Potassium Sparing
Synonyms Triamtereno (Mexico)

Use Alone or in combination with other diuretics to treat edema and hypertension; decreases potassium excretion caused by kaliuretic diuretics

Usual Dosage Oral:
Children: 2-4 mg/kg/day in 1-2 divided doses; maximum: 300 mg/day
Adults: 100-300 mg/day in 1-2 divided doses; maximum dose: 300 mg/day

Mechanism of Action Competes with aldosterone for receptor sites in the distal renal tubules, increasing sodium, chloride, and water excretion while conserving potassium and hydrogen ions; may block the effect of aldosterone on arteriolar smooth muscle as well

Local Anesthetic/Vasoconstrictor Precautions No information available to require special precautions

Effects on Dental Treatment No effects or complications reported

Other Adverse Effects
1% to 10%:
Cardiovascular: Hypotension, edema, congestive heart failure, bradycardia
Central nervous system: Dizziness, headache, fatigue
Dermatologic: Rash
Gastrointestinal: Constipation, nausea
Respiratory: Dyspnea
<1%:
Cardiovascular: Flushing
Endocrine & metabolic: Hyperkalemia, dehydration, hyponatremia, gynecomastia, hyperchloremic, metabolic acidosis, postmenopausal bleeding
Genitourinary: Inability to achieve or maintain an erection

Drug Interactions
Increased risk of hyperkalemia if given together with amiloride, spironolactone, angiotensin-converting enzyme (ACE) inhibitors
Increased toxicity of amantadine (possibly by decreasing its renal excretion)

Drug Uptake
Onset of action: Diuresis occurs within 2-4 hours
Duration: 7-9 hours
Absorption: Oral: Unreliable

Pregnancy Risk Factor D

Dosage Forms Capsule: 50 mg, 100 mg

Generic Available No

Triamtereno Hidroclorotiacida (Mexico) see Hydrochlorothiazide and Triamterene on page 478

Triamtereno (Mexico) see Triamterene on previous page

Triapin® see Butalbital Compound on page 154

Triapin® see Butalbital Compound and Acetaminophen on page 155

Triavil® see Amitriptyline and Perphenazine on page 62

Triazolam (trye AY zoe lam)

Related Information
Dental Drug Interactions: Update on Drug Combinations Requiring Special Considerations on page 1144
Patients Requiring Sedation on page 1081

Brand Names Halcion®

Canadian/Mexican Brand Names Apo®-Triazo (Canada); Gen-Triazolam® (Canada); Novo-Triolam (Canada); Nu-Triazo® (Canada)

Therapeutic Category Benzodiazepine; Hypnotic; Sedative

Use
Dental: Oral premedication before dental procedures
Medical: Short-term treatment of insomnia

Restrictions C-IV; Refillable up to 5 times in 6 months

Usual Dosage Oral:
Children <18 years: Dosage not established
Adults: 0.25 mg taken the evening before oral surgery; or 0.25 mg 1 hour before procedure

Mechanism of Action Depresses all levels of the CNS, including the limbic and reticular formation, probably through the increased action of gamma-aminobutyric acid (GABA), which is a major inhibitory neurotransmitter in the brain

Local Anesthetic/Vasoconstrictor Precautions No information available to require special precautions

Effects on Dental Treatment No effects or complications reported

Other Adverse Effects
>10%: Central nervous system: Drowsiness
1% to 10%:
Central nervous system: Headache, dizziness, nervousness, lightheadedness, coordination disorders, ataxia
Gastrointestinal: Nausea, vomiting

(Continued)

Triazolam *(Continued)*

<1%:

Cardiovascular: Tachycardia, chest pain

Central nervous system: Euphoria, tiredness, confusion, memory impairment, depression, insomnia, dreams/nightmares, amnesia

Dermatologic: Dermatitis

Gastrointestinal: Constipation, taste alteration, diarrhea, xerostomia

Ocular: Visual disturbances

Otic: Tinnitus

Contraindications Hypersensitivity to triazolam, or any component, cross-sensitivity with other benzodiazepines may occur; severe uncontrolled pain; pre-existing CNS depression; narrow-angle glaucoma; not to be used in pregnancy or lactation

Warnings/Precautions May cause drug dependency; avoid abrupt discontinuance in patients with prolonged therapy or seizure disorders; not considered a drug of choice in the elderly

Drug Interactions Decreased effect with phenytoin, phenobarbital; increased effect/toxicity with CNS depressants, cimetidine, erythromycin

Drug Uptake

Onset of hypnotic effect: Within 15-30 minutes

Duration: 6-7 hours

Serum half-life: 1.7-5 hours

Time to peak serum concentration: Oral: ~2 hours

Pregnancy Risk Factor X

Breast-feeding Considerations No data reported

Dosage Forms Tablet: 0.125 mg, 0.25 mg

Dietary Considerations No data reported

Generic Available Yes

Selected Readings

Berthold CW, Dionne RA, and Corey SE, "Comparison of Sublingually and Orally Administered Triazolam for Premedication Before Oral Surgery," *Oral Surg Oral Med Oral Pathol Oral Radiol Endod*, 1997, 84(2):119-24.

Berthold CW, Schneider A, and Dionne RA, "Using Triazolam to Reduce Dental Anxiety," *J Am Dent Assoc*, 1993, 124(11):58-64.

Kaufman E, Hargreaves KM, and Dionne RA, "Comparison of Oral Triazolam and Nitrous Oxide With Placebo and Intravenous Diazepam for Outpatient Premedication," *Oral Surg Oral Med Oral Pathol*, 1993, 75(2):156-64.

Kurzrock M, "Triazolam and Dental Anxiety," *J Am Dent Assoc*, 1994, 125(4):358, 360.

Lieblich SE and Horswell B, "Attenuation of Anxiety in Ambulatory Oral Surgery Patients With Oral Triazolam," *J Oral Maxillofac Surg*, 1991, 49(8):792-7.

Milgrom P, Quarnstrom FC, Longley A, et al, "The Efficacy and Memory Effects of Oral Triazolam Premedication in Highly Anxious Dental Patients," *Anesth Prog*, 1994, 41(3):70-6.

Triban® *see Trimethobenzamide on page 964*

Tribavirin *see Ribavirin on page 841*

Tri-Chlor® *see Trichloroacetic Acid on next page*

Trichlormethiazide *(trye klor meth EYE a zide)*

Related Information

Cardiovascular Diseases *on page 1010*

Brand Names Metahydrin®; Naqua®

Therapeutic Category Diuretic, Thiazide

Use Management of mild to moderate hypertension; treatment of edema in congestive heart failure and nephrotic syndrome

Usual Dosage Oral:

Children >6 months: 0.07 mg/kg/24 hours or 2 mg/m^2/24 hours

Adults: 1-4 mg/day

Mechanism of Action The diuretic mechanism of action of the thiazides is primarily inhibition of sodium, chloride, and water reabsorption in the renal distal tubules, thereby producing diuresis with a resultant reduction in plasma volume. The antihypertensive mechanism of action of the thiazides is unknown. It is known that doses of thiazides produce greater reduction in blood pressure than equivalent diuretic doses of loop diuretics. There has been speculation that the thiazides may have some influence on vascular tone mediated through sodium depletion, but this remains to be proven.

Local Anesthetic/Vasoconstrictor Precautions No information available to require special precautions

Effects on Dental Treatment No effects or complications reported

Other Adverse Effects

1% to 10%: Endocrine & metabolic: Hypokalemia

<1%:

Cardiovascular: Hypotension

Dermatologic: Photosensitivity

Endocrine & metabolic: Fluid and electrolyte imbalances (hypocalcemia, hypo-
magnesemia, hyponatremia); hyperglycemia
Hematologic: Rarely blood dyscrasias
Renal: Prerenal azotemia

Drug Interactions
Decreased effect of oral hypoglycemics; decreased absorption with cholestyra-
mine and colestipol
Increased effect with furosemide and other loop diuretics
Increased toxicity/levels of lithium

Drug Uptake
Onset of of diuretic effect: Within 2 hours
Peak: 4 hours
Duration: 12-24 hours

Pregnancy Risk Factor D
Generic Available Yes

Trichloroacetic Acid (trye klor oh a SEE tik AS id)
Brand Names Tri-Chlor®
Therapeutic Category Keratolytic Agent
Use Debride callous tissue
Local Anesthetic/Vasoconstrictor Precautions No information available to
require special precautions
Effects on Dental Treatment No effects or complications reported
Generic Available Yes

Tri-Clear® Expectorant [OTC] see Guaifenesin and Phenylpropanolamine on
page 454

Tricor® see Fenofibrate on page 396

Triderm® see Triamcinolone on page 954

Tridesilon® see Desonide on page 290

Tridihexethyl (trye dye heks ETH il)
Brand Names Pathilon®
Therapeutic Category Anticholinergic Agent; Antispasmodic Agent, Gastroin-
testinal
Use Adjunctive therapy in peptic ulcer treatment
Local Anesthetic/Vasoconstrictor Precautions No information available to
require special precautions
Effects on Dental Treatment >10% of patients experience dry mouth
Other Adverse Effects
>10%:
Dermatologic: Dry skin
Gastrointestinal: Constipation, dry throat
Respiratory: Dry nose
Miscellaneous: Decreased sweating
1% to 10%: Gastrointestinal: Dysphagia
<1%:
Dermatologic: Rash
Cardiovascular: Tachycardia
Central nervous system: Confusion, headache, loss of memory, nausea,
fatigue, drowsiness, nervousness, insomnia
Gastrointestinal: Bloated feeling, vomiting
Genitourinary: Urinary retention
Neuromuscular & skeletal: Weakness
Ocular: Increased intraocular pressure, blurred vision
Pregnancy Risk Factor C
Generic Available No

Tridil® see Nitroglycerin on page 685

Tridione® see Trimethadione on page 963

Triethanolamine Polypeptide Oleate-Condensate
(trye eth a NOLE a meen pol i PEP tide OH lee ate-KON den sate)
Brand Names Cerumenex®
Therapeutic Category Otic Agent, Cerumenolytic
Use Removal of ear wax (cerumen)
Usual Dosage Children and Adults: Otic: Fill ear canal, insert cotton plug; allow to
remain 15-30 minutes; flush ear with lukewarm water as a single treatment; if a
second application is needed for unusually hard impactions, repeat the proce-
dure
Mechanism of Action Emulsifies and disperses accumulated cerumen
(Continued)

959

Triethanolamine Polypeptide Oleate-Condensate
(Continued)

Local Anesthetic/Vasoconstrictor Precautions No information available to require special precautions

Effects on Dental Treatment No effects or complications reported

Other Adverse Effects <1%: Dermatologic: Mild erythema and pruritus, severe eczematoid reactions, localized dermatitis

Drug Interactions No data reported

Drug Uptake Onset of effect: Produces slight disintegration of very hard ear wax by 24 hours

Pregnancy Risk Factor C

Dosage Forms Solution, otic: 6 mL, 12 mL

Generic Available No

Triethanolamine Salicylate (trye eth a NOLE a meen sa LIS i late)
Brand Names Myoflex® [OTC]; Sportscreme® [OTC]

Therapeutic Category Analgesic, Topical

Use Relief of pain of muscular aches, rheumatism, neuralgia, sprains, arthritis on intact skin

Local Anesthetic/Vasoconstrictor Precautions No information available to require special precautions

Effects on Dental Treatment No effects or complications reported

Other Adverse Effects 1% to 10%:
Central nervous system: Confusion, drowsiness
Gastrointestinal: Nausea, vomiting, diarrhea
Respiratory: Hyperventilation

Generic Available No

Triethylenethiophosphoramide *see* Thiotepa *on page 928*

Trifed-C® *see* Triprolidine, Pseudoephedrine, and Codeine *on page 970*

Trifluoperacina, Clorhidrato De (Mexico) *see* Trifluoperazine *on this page*

Trifluoperazine (trye floo oh PER a zeen)
Brand Names Stelazine®

Canadian/Mexican Brand Names Flupazine® (Mexico)

Therapeutic Category Antipsychotic Agent; Phenothiazine Derivative

Synonyms Trifluoperacina, Clorhidrato De (Mexico)

Use Treatment of psychoses and management of nonpsychotic anxiety

Usual Dosage

Children 6-12 years: Psychoses:
Oral: Hospitalized or well supervised patients: Initial: 1 mg 1-2 times/day, gradually increase until symptoms are controlled or adverse effects become troublesome; maximum: 15 mg/day
I.M.: 1 mg twice daily

Adults:
Psychoses:
Outpatients: Oral: 1-2 mg twice daily
Hospitalized or well supervised patients: Initial: 2-5 mg twice daily with optimum response in the 15-20 mg/day range; do not exceed 40 mg/day
I.M.: 1-2 mg every 4-6 hours as needed up to 10 mg/24 hours maximum
Nonpsychotic anxiety: Oral: 1-2 mg twice daily; maximum: 6 mg/day; therapy for anxiety should not exceed 12 weeks; do not exceed 6 mg/day for longer than 12 weeks when treating anxiety; agitation, jitteriness, or insomnia may be confused with original neurotic or psychotic symptoms
Not dialyzable (0% to 5%)

Mechanism of Action Blocks postsynaptic mesolimbic dopaminergic receptors in the brain; exhibits a strong alpha-adrenergic blocking effect and depresses the release of hypothalamic and hypophyseal hormones

Local Anesthetic/Vasoconstrictor Precautions No information available to require special precautions

Effects on Dental Treatment Significant hypotension may occur, especially when the drug is administered parenterally; orthostatic hypotension is due to alpha-receptor blockade, the elderly are at greater risk for orthostatic hypotension

Tardive dyskinesia: Prevalence rate may be 40% in elderly; development of the syndrome and the irreversible nature are proportional to duration and total cumulative dose over time

Extrapyramidal reactions are more common in elderly with up to 50% developing these reactions after 60 years of age; drug-induced **Parkinson's syndrome** occurs often; **Akathisia** is the most common extrapyramidal reaction in elderly

Increased confusion, memory loss, psychotic behavior, and agitation frequently occur as a consequence of anticholinergic effects

Antipsychotic associated sedation in nonpsychotic patients is extremely unpleasant due to feelings of depersonalization, derealization, and dysphoria

Other Adverse Effects
>10%:
  Cardiovascular: Hypotension, orthostatic hypotension
  Central nervous system: Pseudoparkinsonism, akathisia, dystonias, tardive dyskinesia (persistent), dizziness
  Gastrointestinal: Constipation
  Ocular: Pigmentary retinopathy
  Respiratory: Nasal congestion
  Miscellaneous: Decreased sweating
1% to 10%:
  Dermatologic: Photosensitivity, skin rash
  Endocrine & metabolic: Changes in menstrual cycle, changes in libido, pain in breasts
  Gastrointestinal: Weight gain, nausea, vomiting, stomach pain
  Genitourinary: Dysuria, ejaculatory disturbances
  Neuromuscular & skeletal: Trembling of fingers
<1%:
  Central nervous system: Neuroleptic malignant syndrome (NMS), impairment of temperature regulation, lowering of seizures threshold
  Dermatologic: Discoloration of skin (blue-gray)
  Endocrine & metabolic: Galactorrhea
  Genitourinary: Priapism
  Hematologic: Agranulocytosis, leukopenia
  Hepatic: Cholestatic jaundice, hepatotoxicity
  Ocular: Cornea and lens changes

Drug Interactions
  Decreased effect of anticonvulsants (increases requirements), guanethidine, anticoagulants; decreased effect with anticholinergics
  Increased effect/toxicity with CNS depressants, metrizamide (increased seizures), propranolol, lithium (rare encephalopathy)

Drug Uptake
  Serum half-life: >24 hours with chronic use

Pregnancy Risk Factor C

Generic Available Yes

Triflupromazine (trye floo PROE ma zeen)

Brand Names Vesprin®

Therapeutic Category Phenothiazine Derivative

Use Treatment of psychoses, nausea, vomiting, and intractable hiccups

Local Anesthetic/Vasoconstrictor Precautions No information available to require special precautions

Effects on Dental Treatment Significant hypotension may occur, especially when the drug is administered parenterally; orthostatic hypotension is due to alpha-receptor blockade, the elderly are at greater risk for orthostatic hypotension

Tardive dyskinesia: Prevalence rate may be 40% in elderly; development of the syndrome and the irreversible nature are proportional to duration and total cumulative dose over time

Extrapyramidal reactions are more common in elderly with up to 50% developing these reactions after 60 years of age; drug-induced **Parkinson's syndrome** occurs often; **Akathisia** is the most common extrapyramidal reaction in elderly

Increased confusion, memory loss, psychotic behavior, and agitation frequently occur as a consequence of anticholinergic effects

Antipsychotic associated sedation in nonpsychotic patients is extremely unpleasant due to feelings of depersonalization, derealization, and dysphoria

Pregnancy Risk Factor C

Generic Available No

Trifluridine (trye FLURE i deen)

Related Information
  Systemic Viral Diseases *on page 1047*

Brand Names Viroptic®

Therapeutic Category Antiviral Agent, Ophthalmic
  (Continued)

Trifluridine *(Continued)*

Use Treatment of primary keratoconjunctivitis and recurrent epithelial keratitis caused by herpes simplex virus types I and II

Usual Dosage Adults: Instill 1 drop into affected eye every 2 hours while awake, to a maximum of 9 drops/day, until re-epithelialization of corneal ulcer occurs; then use 1 drop every 4 hours for another 7 days; do **not** exceed 21 days of treatment; if improvement has not taken place in 7-14 days, consider another form of therapy

Mechanism of Action Interferes with viral replication by incorporating into viral DNA in place of thymidine, inhibiting thymidylate synthetase resulting in the formation of defective proteins

Local Anesthetic/Vasoconstrictor Precautions No information available to require special precautions

Effects on Dental Treatment No effects or complications reported

Other Adverse Effects

1% to 10%: Ocular: Burning, stinging

<1%:
  Cardiovascular: Hyperemia
  Ocular: Palpebral edema, epithelial keratopathy, keratitis, stromal edema, increased intraocular pressure
  Miscellaneous: Hypersensitivity reactions

Drug Interactions No data reported

Drug Uptake Absorption: Ophthalmic instillation: Systemic absorption is negligible, while corneal penetration is adequate

Pregnancy Risk Factor C

Generic Available No

Triglycerides, Medium Chain *see* Medium Chain Triglycerides *on page 586*

Trihexifenidico (Mexico) *see* Trihexyphenidyl *on this page*

Trihexy® *see* Trihexyphenidyl *on this page*

Trihexyphenidyl *(trye heks ee FEN i dil)*

Brand Names Artane®; Trihexy®

Canadian/Mexican Brand Names Apo®-Trihex (Canada); Hipokinon® (Mexico); Novo-Hexidyl® (Canada); PMS-Trihexyphenidyl® (Canada); Trihexyphen® (Canada)

Therapeutic Category Anticholinergic Agent; Anti-Parkinson's Agent

Synonyms Trihexifenidico (Mexico)

Use Adjunctive treatment of Parkinson's disease; also used in treatment of drug-induced extrapyramidal effects and acute dystonic reactions

Usual Dosage Adults: Oral: Initial: 1-2 mg/day, increase by 2 mg increments at intervals of 3-5 days; usual dose: 5-15 mg/day in 3-4 divided doses

Mechanism of Action Thought to act by blocking excess acetylcholine at cerebral synapses; many of its effects are due to its pharmacologic similarities with atropine

Local Anesthetic/Vasoconstrictor Precautions No information available to require special precautions

Effects on Dental Treatment >10% of patients experience significant dry mouth; normal salivary flow will resume with cessation of drug therapy. Prolonged xerostomia may contribute to development of caries, periodontal disease, oral candidiasis and discomfort

Other Adverse Effects

>10%:
  Dermatologic: Dry skin
  Gastrointestinal: Constipation
  Respiratory: Dry nose, throat
  Miscellaneous: Decreased sweating

1% to 10%:
  Endocrine & metabolic: Decreased flow of breast milk
  Gastrointestinal: Dysphagia
  Ocular: Photosensitivity

<1%:
  Cardiovascular: Orthostatic hypotension, ventricular fibrillation, tachycardia, palpitations
  Central nervous system: Confusion, drowsiness, headache, loss of memory, fatigue, ataxia
  Dermatologic: Skin rash
  Gastrointestinal: Bloated feeling, nausea, vomiting
  Genitourinary: Dysuria
  Neuromuscular & skeletal: Weakness
  Ocular: Increased intraocular pain, blurred vision

Drug Interactions
Decreased effect of levodopa
Increased toxicity with narcotic analgesics, phenothiazines, TCAs, quinidine, levodopa, anticholinergics
Drug Uptake
Peak effect: Within 1 hour
Serum half-life: 3.3-4.1 hours
Time to peak serum concentration: Within 1-1.5 hours
Pregnancy Risk Factor C
Dosage Forms
Capsule, as hydrochloride, sustained release: 5 mg
Elixir, as hydrochloride: 2 mg/5 mL (480 mL)
Tablet, as hydrochloride: 2 mg, 5 mg
Generic Available Yes: Tablet

Tri-K® *see* Potassium Acetate, Potassium Bicarbonate, and Potassium Citrate *on page 776*

Tri-Kort® *see* Triamcinolone *on page 954*

Trilafon® *see* Perphenazine *on page 744*

Tri-Levlen® *see* Ethinyl Estradiol and Levonorgestrel *on page 377*

Trilisate® *see* Choline Magnesium Trisalicylate *on page 230*

Trilog® *see* Triamcinolone *on page 954*

Trilone® *see* Triamcinolone *on page 954*

Trimazide® *see* Trimethobenzamide *on next page*

Trimethadione (trye meth a DYE one)
Brand Names Tridione®
Therapeutic Category Anticonvulsant, Oxazolidinedione
Synonyms Troxidone
Use Control absence (petit mal) seizures refractory to other drugs
Local Anesthetic/Vasoconstrictor Precautions No information available to require special precautions
Effects on Dental Treatment No effects or complications reported
Other Adverse Effects
>10%:
Central nervous system: Dizziness, drowsiness, sedation, headache
Ocular: Diplopia, photophobia
1% to 10%:
Central nervous system: Insomnia
Dermatologic: Alopecia
Gastrointestinal: Anorexia, stomach upset
Miscellaneous: Hiccups
<1%:
Dermatologic: Exfoliative dermatitis
Hematologic: Aplastic anemia, agranulocytosis, thrombocytopenia, exacerbation of porphyria
Hepatic: Hepatitis
Neuromuscular & skeletal: Myasthenia gravis syndrome
Miscellaneous: Systemic lupus erythematosus (SLE), nephrosis
Pregnancy Risk Factor D
Generic Available No

Trimethaphan Camsylate (Discontinued 4/96)
(trye METH a fan KAM si late)
Brand Names Arfonad®
Therapeutic Category Adrenergic Blocking Agent; Anticholinergic Agent; Ganglionic Blocking Agent
Use Immediate and temporary reduction of blood pressure in patients with hypertensive emergencies; controlled hypotension during surgery
Mechanism of Action Blocks transmission in both adrenergic and cholinergic ganglia by blocking stimulation from presynaptic receptors to postsynaptic receptors mediated by acetylcholine; possesses direct peripheral vasodilatory activity and is a weak histamine releaser
Local Anesthetic/Vasoconstrictor Precautions No information available to require special precautions
Effects on Dental Treatment No effects or complications reported
Other Adverse Effects 1% to 10%:
Cardiovascular: Hypotension (especially orthostatic), tachycardia
Central nervous system: Restlessness
Dermatologic: Itching, urticaria
Endocrine & metabolic: Sodium and water retention
(Continued)

Trimethaphan Camsylate (Discontinued 4/96)
(Continued)

Gastrointestinal: Anorexia, nausea, vomiting, dry mouth, adynamic ileus
Genitourinary: Urinary retention
    Neuromuscular & skeletal: Weakness
Ocular: Mydriasis, cycloplegia
Respiratory: Apnea, respiratory arrest

Drug Interactions
Increased effect:
    Anesthetics, procainamide, diuretics, and other hypotensive agents may increase hypotensive effects of trimethaphan
    Effects of tubocurarine and succinylcholine may be prolonged by trimethaphan

Pregnancy Risk Factor C
Generic Available No

Trimethobenzamide (trye meth oh BEN za mide)

Brand Names Arrestin®; Pediatric Triban®; Tebamide®; T-Gen®; Ticon®; Tigan®; Triban®; Trimazide®

Therapeutic Category Antiemetic

Use Control of nausea and vomiting (especially for long-term antiemetic therapy); less effective than phenothiazines but may be associated with fewer side effects

Usual Dosage Rectal use is contraindicated in neonates and premature infants
Children:
    Rectal: <14 kg: 100 mg 3-4 times/day
    Oral, rectal: 14-40 kg: 100-200 mg 3-4 times/day
Adults:
    Oral: 250 mg 3-4 times/day
    I.M., rectal: 200 mg 3-4 times/day

Mechanism of Action Acts centrally to inhibit the medullary chemoreceptor trigger zone

Local Anesthetic/Vasoconstrictor Precautions No information available to require special precautions

Effects on Dental Treatment No effects or complications reported

Other Adverse Effects
>10%: Central nervous system: Drowsiness
1% to 10%:
    Cardiovascular: Hypotension
    Central nervous system: Dizziness, headache
    Gastrointestinal: Diarrhea
    Neuromuscular & skeletal: muscle cramps
<1%:
    Central nervous system: Mental depression, convulsions, opisthotonus
    Dermatologic: Hypersensitivity skin reactions
    Hematologic: Blood dyscrasias
    Hepatic: Hepatic impairment

Drug Interactions Antagonism of oral anticoagulants may occur

Drug Uptake
Onset of antiemetic effect:
    Oral: Within 10-40 minutes
    I.M.: Within 15-35 minutes
Duration: 3-4 hours
Absorption: Rectal: ~60%

Pregnancy Risk Factor C
Generic Available No

Trimethoprim (trye METH oh prim)

Brand Names Proloprim®; Trimpex®

Therapeutic Category Antibiotic, Miscellaneous

Synonyms Trimetoprima (Mexico)

Use Treatment of urinary tract infections; acute otitis media in children; acute exacerbations of chronic bronchitis in adults; in combination with other agents for treatment of toxoplasmosis, Pneumocystis carinii

Usual Dosage Oral:
Children: 4 mg/kg/day in divided doses every 12 hours
Adults: 100 mg every 12 hours or 200 mg every 24 hours

Mechanism of Action Inhibits folic acid reduction to tetrahydrofolate, and thereby inhibits microbial growth

Local Anesthetic/Vasoconstrictor Precautions No information available to require special precautions

Effects on Dental Treatment No effects or complications reported

Other Adverse Effects
>10%: Dermatologic: Rash, pruritus
1% to 10%: Hematologic: Megaloblastic anemia
<1%:
Central nervous system: Fever
Dermatologic: Exfoliative dermatitis
Gastrointestinal: Nausea, vomiting, epigastric distress
Hepatic: Cholestatic jaundice, elevated LFTs
Hematologic: Thrombocytopenia, neutropenia, leukopenia
Renal: Elevated BUN and serum creatinine
Drug Interactions Increased effect/toxicity/levels of phenytoin
Drug Uptake
Absorption: Oral: Readily and extensive
Serum half-life: 8-14 hours, prolonged with renal impairment
Time to peak serum concentration: Within 1-4 hours
Pregnancy Risk Factor C
Generic Available Yes

Trimethoprim and Polymyxin B
(trye METH oh prim & pol i MIKS in bee)
Brand Names Polytrim® Ophthalmic
Therapeutic Category Antibiotic, Ophthalmic
Synonyms Polymyxin B and Trimethoprim
Use Treatment of surface ocular bacterial conjunctivitis and blepharoconjunctivitis
Local Anesthetic/Vasoconstrictor Precautions No information available to require special precautions
Effects on Dental Treatment No effects or complications reported
Other Adverse Effects 1% to 10%: Local: Burning, stinging, itching, increased redness
Generic Available No

Trimethoprim and Sulfamethoxazole
(trye METH oh prim & sul fa meth OKS a zole)
Related Information
Animal and Human Bites Guidelines *on page 1093*
Brand Names Bactrim™; Bactrim™ DS; Cotrim®; Cotrim® DS; Septra®; Septra® DS; Sulfamethoprim®; Sulfatrim®; Sulfatrim® DS; Sulfoxaprim®; Sulfoxaprim® DS; Trisulfam®; Uroplus® DS; Uroplus® SS
Canadian/Mexican Brand Names Anitrim® (Mexico); Apo®-Sulfatrim (Canada); Bactelan® (Mexico); Batrizol® (Mexico); Ectaprim-F® (Mexico); Ectaprim® (Mexico); Enterobacticel® (Mexico); Esteprim® (Mexico); Isobac® (Mexico); Kelfiprim® (Mexico); Metoxiprim® (Mexico); Novo-Trimel® (Canada); Nu-Cotrimox® (Canada); Pro-Trin® (Canada); Roubac® (Canada); Syraprim® (Mexico); Trimesuxol® (Mexico); Trimetoger® (Mexico); Trimetox® (Mexico); Trimzol® (Mexico); Trisulfa® (Canada); Trisulfa-S® (Canada)
Therapeutic Category Antibiotic, Sulfonamide Derivative
Synonyms Co-trimoxazole; SMZ-TMP; Sulfamethoxazole and Trimethoprim; TMP-SMZ
Use
Oral treatment of urinary tract infections; acute otitis media in children; acute exacerbations of chronic bronchitis in adults; prophylaxis of *Pneumocystis carinii* pneumonitis (PCP)
I.V. treatment of documented PCP, empiric treatment of PCP in immune compromised patients; treatment of documented or suspected shigellosis, typhoid fever, *Nocardia asteroides* infection, or other infections caused by susceptible bacterial
Usual Dosage Dosage recommendations are based on the trimethoprim component

Children >2 months:
Mild to moderate infections: Oral, I.V.: 8 mg TMP/kg/day in divided doses every 12 hours
Serious infection/*Pneumocystis*: I.V.: 20 mg TMP/kg/day in divided doses every 6 hours
Urinary tract infection prophylaxis: Oral: 2 mg TMP/kg/dose daily
Prophylaxis of *Pneumocystis*: Oral, I.V.: 10 mg TMP/kg/day or 150 mg TMP/m²/day in divided doses every 12 hours for 3 days/week; dose should not exceed 320 mg trimethoprim and 1600 mg sulfamethoxazole 3 days/week
Adults:
Urinary tract infection/chronic bronchitis: Oral: 1 double strength tablet every 12 hours for 10-14 days
Sepsis: I.V.: 20 TMP/kg/day divided every 6 hours
(Continued)

Trimethoprim and Sulfamethoxazole *(Continued)*

Pneumocystis carinii:
Prophylaxis: Oral, I.V.: 10 mg TMP/kg/day divided every 12 hours for 3 days/week

Treatment: I.V.: 20 mg TMP/kg/day divided every 6 hours

Mechanism of Action Sulfamethoxazole interferes with bacterial folic acid synthesis and growth via inhibition of dihydrofolic acid formation from para-aminobenzoic acid; trimethoprim inhibits dihydrofolic acid reduction to tetrahydrofolate resulting in sequential inhibition of enzymes of the folic acid pathway

Local Anesthetic/Vasoconstrictor Precautions No information available to require special precautions

Effects on Dental Treatment No effects or complications reported

Other Adverse Effects
>10%:
Dermatologic: Allergic skin reactions including rashes and urticaria, photosensitivity
Gastrointestinal: Nausea, vomiting, anorexia
1% to 10%:
Dermatologic: Stevens-Johnson syndrome, toxic epidermal necrolysis
Hematologic: Blood dyscrasias
Hepatic: Hepatitis
<1%:
Central nervous system: Confusion, depression, hallucinations, seizures, fever, ataxia, kernicterus in neonates
Dermatologic: Erythema multiforme
Gastrointestinal: Stomatitis, diarrhea, pseudomembranous colitis
Hematologic: Thrombocytopenia, megaloblastic anemia, granulocytopenia, aplastic anemia, hemolysis (with G-6-PD deficiency)
Renal: Interstitial nephritis
Miscellaneous: Serum sickness

Drug Interactions Co-trimoxazole causes:
Decreased effect: Cyclosporines
Increased effect: Sulfonylureas and oral anticoagulants
Increased toxicity: Phenytoin, cyclosporines (nephrotoxicity), methotrexate (displaced from binding sites)

Drug Uptake
Absorption: Oral: 90% to 100%
Serum half-life:
SMX: 9 hours
TMP: 6-17 hours, both are prolonged in renal failure
Time to peak serum concentration: Within 1-4 hours

Pregnancy Risk Factor C

Dosage Forms The 5:1 ratio (SMX to TMP) remains constant in all dosage forms:
Injection: Sulfamethoxazole 80 mg and trimethoprim 16 mg per mL (5 mL, 10 mL, 20 mL, 30 mL, 50 mL)
Suspension, oral: Sulfamethoxazole 200 mg and trimethoprim 40 mg per 5 mL (20 mL, 100 mL, 150 mL, 200 mL, 480 mL)
Tablet: Sulfamethoxazole 400 mg and trimethoprim 80 mg
Tablet, double strength: Sulfamethoxazole 800 mg and trimethoprim 160 mg
Generic Available Yes

Trimetoprima (Mexico) *see* Trimethoprim *on page 964*

Trimetrexate Glucuronate (tri me TREKS ate gloo KYOOR oh nate)

Brand Names Neutrexin™

Therapeutic Category Antibiotic, Miscellaneous

Use Alternative therapy for the treatment of moderate-to-severe *Pneumocystis carinii* pneumonia (PCP) in immunocompromised patients, including patients with acquired immunodeficiency syndrome (AIDS), who are intolerant of, or are refractory to, co-trimoxazole therapy or for whom co-trimoxazole and pentamidine are contraindicated (concurrent folinic acid (leucovorin) must always be administered)

Usual Dosage Adults: I.V.: 45 mg/m^2 once daily over 60 minutes for 21 days; it is necessary to reduce the dose in patients with liver dysfunction, although no specific recommendations exist

Mechanism of Action Exerts an antimicrobial effect through potent inhibition of the enzyme dihydrofolate reductase (DHFR)

Local Anesthetic/Vasoconstrictor Precautions No information available to require special precautions

Effects on Dental Treatment No effects or complications reported

Other Adverse Effects 1% to 10%:
  Central nervous system: Seizures, fever
  Dermatologic: Rash
  Gastrointestinal: Stomatitis, nausea, vomiting
  Hematologic: Neutropenia, thrombocytopenia, anemia
  Hepatic: Elevated liver function tests
  Neuromuscular & skeletal: Peripheral neuropathy
  Renal: Elevated serum creatinine
  Miscellaneous: Flu-like illness, hypersensitivity reactions

Drug Interactions
  Decreased effect of pneumococcal vaccine
  Increased toxicity (infection rates) of yellow fever vaccine

Drug Uptake
  Serum half-life: 15-17 hours

Pregnancy Risk Factor D

Generic Available No

Trimipramine (trye MI pra meen)

Brand Names Surmontil®

Canadian/Mexican Brand Names Apo®-Trimip (Canada); Novo-Tripramine® (Canada); Nu-Trimipramine® (Canada); Rhotrimine® (Canada)

Therapeutic Category Antidepressant, Tricyclic

Use Treatment of various forms of depression, often in conjunction with psycho-therapy

Usual Dosage Adults: Oral: 50-150 mg/day as a single bedtime dose up to a maximum of 200 mg/day outpatient and 300 mg/day inpatient

Mechanism of Action Increases the synaptic concentration of serotonin and/or norepinephrine in the central nervous system by inhibition of their reuptake by the presynaptic neuronal membrane

Local Anesthetic/Vasoconstrictor Precautions Use with caution; epineph-rine, norepinephrine and levonordefrin have been shown to have an increased pressor response in combination with TCAs

Effects on Dental Treatment >10% of patients experience dry mouth; long-term treatment with TCAs such as trimipramine increases the risk of caries by reducing salivation and salivary buffer capacity

Other Adverse Effects
  >10%:
    Central nervous system: Dizziness, drowsiness, headache
    Gastrointestinal: Constipation, increased appetite, nausea, unpleasant taste, weight gain
    Neuromuscular & skeletal: Weakness
  1% to 10%:
    Cardiovascular: Arrhythmias, hypotension
    Central nervous system: Confusion, delirium, hallucinations, nervousness, restlessness, parkinsonian syndrome, insomnia
    Endocrine & metabolic: Sexual dysfunction
    Gastrointestinal: Diarrhea, heartburn
    Genitourinary: Dysuria
    Neuromuscular & skeletal: Fine muscle tremors
    Ocular: Blurred vision, eye pain
    Miscellaneous: Excessive sweating
  <1%:
    Central nervous system: Anxiety, seizures
    Dermatologic: Alopecia, photosensitivity
    Endocrine & metabolic: Breast enlargement, galactorrhea, SIADH
    Gastrointestinal: Trouble with gums, decreased lower esophageal sphincter tone may cause GE reflux
    Genitourinary: Testicular swelling
    Hematologic: Agranulocytosis, leukopenia, eosinophilia
    Hepatic: Cholestatic jaundice, elevated liver enzymes
    Ocular: Increased intraocular pressure
    Otic: Tinnitus
    Miscellaneous: Allergic reactions

Drug Interactions
  Decreased effect of guanethidine, clonidine; decreased effect with barbiturates, carbamazepine, phenytoin
  Increased effect/toxicity with MAO inhibitors (hyperpyretic crises), CNS depres-sants, alcohol (CNS depression), methylphenidate (increased levels), cimeti-dine (decreased clearance), anticholinergics

Drug Uptake
  Therapeutic plasma levels: Oral: Occurs within 6 hours
  Serum half-life: 20-26 hours
  (Continued)

967

Trimipramine *(Continued)*
Pregnancy Risk Factor C
Generic Available Yes

Trimox® *see Amoxicillin on page 68*
Trimpex® *see Trimethoprim on page 964*
Trinalin® *see Azatadine and Pseudoephedrine on page 102*
Tri-Nefrin® Extra Strength Tablet [OTC] *see Chlorpheniramine and Phenylpropanolamine on page 219*
Tri-Norinyl® *see Ethinyl Estradiol and Norethindrone on page 379*
Triofed® Syrup [OTC] *see Triprolidine and Pseudoephedrine on next page*
Triostat™ *see Liothyronine on page 558*
Triotann® Tablet *see Chlorpheniramine, Pyrilamine, and Phenylephrine on page 223*

Trioxsalen *(trye OKS a len)*
Brand Names Trisoralen®
Therapeutic Category Psoralen
Use In conjunction with controlled exposure to ultraviolet light or sunlight for repigmentation of idiopathic vitiligo; increasing tolerance to sunlight with albinism; enhance pigmentation
Usual Dosage Children >12 years and Adults: Oral: 10 mg/day as a single dose, 2-4 hours before controlled exposure to UVA (for 15-35 minutes) or sunlight; do not continue for longer than 14 days
Mechanism of Action Psoralens are thought to form covalent bonds with pyrimidine bases in DNA which inhibit the synthesis of DNA. This reaction involves excitation of the trioxsalen molecule by radiation in the long-wave ultraviolet light (UVA) resulting in transference of energy to the trioxsalen molecule producing an excited state. Binding of trioxsalen to DNA occurs only in the presence of ultraviolet light. The increase in skin pigmentation produced by trioxsalen and UVA radiation involves multiple changes in melanocytes and interaction between melanocytes and keratinocytes. In general, melanogenesis is stimulated but the size and distribution of melanocytes is unchanged.
Local Anesthetic/Vasoconstrictor Precautions No information available to require special precautions
Effects on Dental Treatment No effects or complications reported
Other Adverse Effects
>10%:
Dermatologic: Itching
Gastrointestinal: Nausea
1% to 10%:
Central nervous system: Dizziness, headache, mental depression, insomnia, nervousness
Dermatologic: Severe burns from excessive sunlight or ultraviolet exposure
Gastrointestinal: Gastric discomfort
Drug Interactions No data reported
Drug Uptake
Peak photosensitivity: 2 hours
Duration: Skin sensitivity to light remains for 8-12 hours
Absorption: Rapid
Serum half-life, elimination: ~2 hours
Pregnancy Risk Factor C
Generic Available No

Tripelennamine *(tri pel EN a meen)*
Brand Names PBZ®; PBZ-SR®
Therapeutic Category Antihistamine
Use Perennial and seasonal allergic rhinitis and other allergic symptoms including urticaria
Usual Dosage Oral:
Children: 5 mg/kg/day in 4-6 divided doses, up to 300 mg/day maximum
Adults: 25-50 mg every 4-6 hours, extended release tablets 100 mg morning and evening up to 100 mg every 8 hours
Mechanism of Action Competes with histamine for H_1-receptor sites on effector cells in the gastrointestinal tract, blood vessels, and respiratory tract
Local Anesthetic/Vasoconstrictor Precautions No information available to require special precautions
Effects on Dental Treatment Chronic use of antihistamines will inhibit salivary flow, particularly in elderly patients; this may contribute to periodontal disease and oral discomfort

Other Adverse Effects
>10%:
Central nervous system: Slight to moderate drowsiness
Respiratory: Thickening of bronchial secretions
1% to 10%:
Central nervous system: Headache, fatigue, nervousness, dizziness
Gastrointestinal: Appetite increase, weight gain, nausea, diarrhea, abdominal pain, dry mouth
Neuromuscular & skeletal: Arthralgia
Respiratory: Pharyngitis
<1%:
Cardiovascular: Edema, palpitations, hypotension
Central nervous system: Depression, sedation, paradoxical excitement, insomnia
Dermatologic: Angioedema, photosensitivity, rash
Genitourinary: Urinary retention
Hepatic: Hepatitis
Neuromuscular & skeletal: Myalgia, paresthesia, tremor
Ocular: Blurred vision
Respiratory: Bronchospasm, epistaxis
Drug Interactions Increased effect/toxicity with alcohol, CNS depressants, MAO inhibitors
Drug Uptake
Onset of antihistaminic effect: Within 15-30 minutes
Duration: 4-6 hours (up to 8 hours with PBZ-SR®)
Pregnancy Risk Factor B
Generic Available Yes

Triphasil® see Ethinyl Estradiol and Levonorgestrel on page 377

Tri-Phen-Chlor® see Chlorpheniramine, Phenyltoloxamine, Phenylpropanolamine, and Phenylephrine on page 222

Triphenyl® Expectorant [OTC] see Guaifenesin and Phenylpropanolamine on page 454

Triphenyl® Syrup [OTC] see Chlorpheniramine and Phenylpropanolamine on page 219

Triple Antibiotic® Topical see Bacitracin, Neomycin, and Polymyxin B on page 108

Triple X® Liquid [OTC] see Pyrethrins on page 824

Triposed® Syrup [OTC] see Triprolidine and Pseudoephedrine on this page

Triposed® Tablet [OTC] see Triprolidine and Pseudoephedrine on this page

Triprolidina y Pseudoefedrina (Mexico) see Triprolidine and Pseudoephedrine on this page

Triprolidine and Pseudoephedrine
(trye PROE li deen & soo doe e FED rin)
Brand Names Actagen® Syrup [OTC]; Actagen® Tablet [OTC]; Allercon® Tablet [OTC]; Allerfrin® Syrup [OTC]; Allerfrin® Tablet [OTC]; Allerphed Syrup [OTC]; Aprodine® Syrup [OTC]; Aprodine® Tablet [OTC]; Cenafed® Plus Tablet [OTC]; Genac® Tablet [OTC]; Silafed® Syrup [OTC]; Triofed® Syrup [OTC]; Triposed® Syrup [OTC]; Triposed® Tablet [OTC]
Therapeutic Category Antihistamine/Decongestant Combination
Synonyms Triprolidina y Pseudoefedrina (Mexico)
Use Temporary relief of nasal congestion, decongest sinus openings, running nose, sneezing, itching of nose or throat and itchy, watery eyes due to common cold, hay fever, or other upper respiratory allergies
Usual Dosage Oral:
Children:
Syrup:
4 months to 2 years: 1.25 mL 3-4 times/day
2-4 years: 2.5 mL 3-4 times/day
4-6 years: 3.75 mL 3-4 times/day
6-12 years: 5 mL every 4-6 hours; do not exceed 4 doses in 24 hours
Tablet: 1/2 every 4-6 hours; do not exceed 4 doses in 24 hours

Children >12 years and Adults:
Syrup: 10 mL every 4-6 hours; do not exceed 4 doses in 24 hours
Tablet: 1 every 4-6 hours; do not exceed 4 doses in 24 hours
Mechanism of Action Refer to Pseudoephedrine monograph
Triprolidine is a member of the propylamine (alkylamine) chemical class of H_1-antagonist antihistamines. As such, it is considered to be relatively less sedating than traditional antihistamines of the ethanolamine, phenothiazine, and ethylenediamine classes of antihistamines. Triprolidine has a shorter half-life and duration of action than most of the other alkylamine antihistamines.
(Continued)

Triprolidine and Pseudoephedrine *(Continued)*

Like all H₁-antagonist antihistamines, the mechanism of action of triprolidine is believed to involve competitive blockade of H₁-receptor sites resulting in the inability of histamine to combine with its receptor sites and exert its usual effects on target cells. Antihistamines do not interrupt any effects of histamine which have already occurred. Therefore, these agents are used more successfully in the prevention rather than the treatment of histamine-induced reactions.

Local Anesthetic/Vasoconstrictor Precautions Use with caution since pseudoephedrine is a sympathomimetic amine which could interact with epinephrine to cause a pressor response

Effects on Dental Treatment Chronic use of antihistamines will inhibit salivary flow, particularly in elderly patients; this may contribute to periodontal disease and oral discomfort

Other Adverse Effects

>10%:

Cardiovascular: Tachycardia

Central nervous system: Slight to moderate drowsiness, nervousness, insomnia, transient stimulation

Respiratory: Thickening of bronchial secretions

1% to 10%:

Central nervous system: Headache, fatigue, dizziness

Gastrointestinal: Appetite increase, weight gain, nausea, diarrhea, abdominal pain, dry mouth

Genitourinary: Dysuria

Neuromuscular & skeletal: Arthralgia, weakness

Respiratory: Pharyngitis

Miscellaneous: Sweating

<1%:

Central nervous system: Depression, hallucinations, convulsions, paradoxical excitement, sedation

Cardiovascular: Edema, palpitations, hypotension

Dermatologic: Angioedema, rash, photosensitivity

Genitourinary: Urinary retention

Hepatic: Hepatitis

Neuromuscular & skeletal: Myalgia, paresthesia, tremor

Ocular: Blurred vision

Respiratory: Bronchospasm, dyspnea, epistaxis

Drug Interactions

Decreased effect of guanethidine, reserpine, methyldopa

Increased toxicity with MAO inhibitors (hypertensive crisis), sympathomimetics, CNS depressants, alcohol (sedation)

Pregnancy Risk Factor C

Generic Available Yes

Triprolidine, Pseudoephedrine, and Codeine

(trye PROE li deen, soo doe e FED rin, & KOE deen)

Brand Names Actagen-C®; Actifed® With Codeine; Allerfrin® w/Codeine; Aprodine® w/C; Triacin-C®; Trifed-C®

Therapeutic Category Antihistamine/Decongestant Combination; Cough Preparation

Use Symptomatic relief of cough

Local Anesthetic/Vasoconstrictor Precautions Use with caution since pseudoephedrine is a sympathomimetic amine which could interact with epinephrine to cause a pressor response

Effects on Dental Treatment Up to 10% of patients could experience tachycardia, palpitations, and dry mouth; use vasoconstrictor with caution

Pregnancy Risk Factor C

Generic Available Yes

Tri-Tannate® Tablet *see* Chlorpheniramine, Pyrilamine, and Phenylephrine *on page 223*

Tritec® *see* Ranitidine Bismuth Citrate *on page 835*

Tri-Vi-Flor® *see* Vitamins, Multiple *on page 995*

Trobicin® *see* Spectinomycin *on page 880*

Trocaine® [OTC] *see* Benzocaine *on page 118*

Trocal® [OTC] *see* Dextromethorphan *on page 298*

Troglitazone (TROE gli to zone)

Brand Names Rezulin®

Therapeutic Category Antidiabetic Agent; Hypoglycemic Agent, Oral

Use Use in patients with type II diabetes currently on insulin therapy whose hyperglycemia is not controlled (HbA$_{1c}$ >8.5%) despite insulin therapy of over 30 units/day given as multiple infections

Usual Dosage Oral (take with meals):

Adults:

Continue the current insulin dose upon initiation of troglitazone therapy.

Initiate therapy at 200 mg once daily in patients on insulin therapy. For patients not responding adequately, increase the dose after 2-4 weeks. The usual dose is 400 mg/day; maximum recommended dose: 600 mg/day.

It is recommended that the insulin dose be decreased by 10% to 25% when fasting plasma glucose concentrations decrease to <120 mg/dL in patients receiving concomitant insulin and troglitazone. Individualize further adjustments based on glucose-lowering response.

Elderly: Steady-state pharmacokinetics of troglitazone and metabolites in healthy elderly subjects were comparable to those seen in young adults

Mechanism of Action Thiazolidinedione antidiabetic agent that lowers blood glucose by improving target cell response to insulin, without increasing pancreatic insulin secretion. It has a unique mechanism of action that is dependent on the presence of insulin for activity. Troglitazone decreases hepatic glucose output and increases insulin-dependent glucose disposal in skeletal muscle and possible liver and adipose tissue.

Local Anesthetic/Vasoconstrictor Precautions No information available to require special precautions

Effects on Dental Treatment Troglitazone-dependent diabetics should be appointed for dental treatment in morning in order to minimize chance of stress-induced hypoglycemia

Other Adverse Effects

>10%:

Central nervous system: Headache, pain

Miscellaneous: Infection

1% to 10%:

Cardiovascular: Peripheral edema

Central nervous system: Dizziness

Gastrointestinal: Nausea, diarrhea, pharyngitis

Genitourinary: Urinary tract infection

Neuromuscular & skeletal: Neck pain, weakness

Respiratory: Rhinitis

Warnings/Precautions Patients with New York Heart Association (NYHA) Class III and IV cardiac status were not studied during clinical trials. Heart enlargement without microscopic changes has been observed in rodents at exposures exceeding 14 times the AUC of the 400 mg human dose. Caution is advised during the administration of troglitazone to patients with NYHA Class III or IV cardiac status.

During all clinical studies, a total of 20 troglitazone-treated patients were withdrawn from treatment because of liver function test abnormalities. Two of the 20 patients developed reversible jaundice. Both had liver biopsies that were consistent with an idiosyncratic drug reaction.

Because of its mechanism of action, troglitazone is active only in the presence of insulin. Therefore, do not use in type I diabetes or for the treatment of diabetic ketoacidosis.

Patients receiving troglitazone in combination with insulin may be at risk for hypoglycemia, and a reduction in the dose of insulin may be necessary. Hypoglycemia has not been observed during the administration of troglitazone as monotherapy and would not be expected based on the mechanism of action.

Across all clinical studies, hemoglobin declined by 3% to 4% in troglitazone-treated patients compared with 1% to 2% with placebo. White blood cell counts also declined slightly in troglitazone-treated patients compared with those treated with placebo. These changes occurred within the first 4-8 weeks of therapy. Levels stabilized and remained unchanged for ≤ 2 years of continuing therapy. (Continued)

Troglitazone (Continued)

These changes may be due to the dilutional effects of increased plasma volume and have not been associated with any significant hematologic clinical effects.

Drug Interactions Cytochrome P-450 3A4 Enzyme Inducer

Decreased effects:

Cholestyramine: Concomitant administration of cholestyramine with troglitazone reduces the absorption of troglitazone by 70%; CO-ADMINISTRATION OF CHOLESTYRAMINE AND TROGLITAZONE IS NOT RECOMMENDED.

Oral contraceptives: Administration of troglitazone with an oral contraceptive containing ethinyl estradiol and norethindrone reduced the plasma concentrations of both by 30%. These changes could result in loss of contraception.

Terfenadine: Coadministration of troglitazone with terfenadine decreases plasma concentrations of terfenadine and its active metabolite by 50% to 70% and may reduce the effectiveness of terfenadine

Increased effects: Furosemide increased the metformin plasma and blood C_{max} without altering metformin renal clearance in a single dose study

Increased toxicity:

Sulfonylureas (glyburide): Co-administration of troglitazone with glyburide may further decrease plasma glucose levels

Drug Uptake

Half-life, plasma elimination: 16-34 hours

Time to peak plasma concentrations: 2-3 hours

Pregnancy Risk Factor B

Dosage Forms Tablet: 200 mg, 400 mg

Dietary Considerations Food increases absorption by 30% to 85%

Generic Available No

Troleandomycin (troe lee an doe MYE sin)

Brand Names Tao®

Therapeutic Category Antibiotic, Macrolide

Use Adjunct in the treatment of corticosteroid-dependent asthma due to its steroid-sparing properties; antibiotic with spectrum of activity similar to erythromycin

Usual Dosage Oral:

Children 7-13 years: 25-40 mg/kg/day divided every 6 hours (125-250 mg every 6 hours)

Adjunct in corticosteroid-dependent asthma: 14 mg/kg/day in divided doses every 6-12 hours not to exceed 250 mg every 6 hours; dose is tapered to once daily then alternate day dosing

Children >13 years and adults: 250-500 mg 4 times/day

Mechanism of Action Decreases methylprednisolone clearance from a linear first order decline to a nonlinear decline in plasma concentration. Tao® also has an undefined action independent of its effects on steroid elimination. Inhibits RNA-dependent protein synthesis at the chain elongation step; binds to the 50S ribosomal subunit resulting in blockage of transpeptidation.

Local Anesthetic/Vasoconstrictor Precautions No information available to require special precautions

Effects on Dental Treatment No effects or complications reported

Other Adverse Effects

>10%: Gastrointestinal: Abdominal cramping and discomfort

1% to 10%:

Dermatologic: Urticaria, skin rashes

Gastrointestinal: Nausea, vomiting, diarrhea

<1%:

Dermatologic: Rectal burning

Hepatic: Cholestatic jaundice

Drug Interactions Increased effect/toxicity/levels of astemizole, carbamazepine, ergot alkaloids, methylprednisolone, terfenadine, theophylline, and triazolam

Drug Uptake

Time to peak serum concentration: Within 2 hours

Pregnancy Risk Factor C

Generic Available No

Tromethamine (troe METH a meen)

Brand Names THAM-E® Injection; THAM® Injection

Therapeutic Category Alkalinizing Agent, Parenteral

Synonyms Tris Buffer; Tris(hydroxymethyl)aminomethane

Use Correction of metabolic acidosis associated with cardiac bypass surgery or cardiac arrest; to correct excess acidity of stored blood that is preserved with acid citrate dextrose (ACD); to prime the pump-oxygenator during cardiac bypass surgery; indicated in severe metabolic acidosis in patients in whom sodium or carbon dioxide elimination is restricted [eg, infants needing alkalinization after receiving maximum sodium bicarbonate (8-10 mEq/kg/24 hours)]

Usual Dosage Dose depends on buffer base deficit; when deficit is known: tromethamine (mL of 0.3 M solution) = body weight (kg) x base deficit (mEq/L); when base deficit is not known: 3-6 mL/kg/dose I.V. (1-2 mEq/kg/dose)

Metabolic acidosis with cardiac arrest:
    I.V.: 3.5-6 mL/kg (1-2 mEq/kg/dose) into large peripheral vein; 500-1000 mL if needed in adults
    I.V. continuous drip: Infuse slowly by syringe pump over 3-6 hours

Excess acidity of acid citrate dextrose priming blood: 14-70 mL of 0.3 molar solution added to each 500 mL of blood

Mechanism of Action Acts as a proton acceptor, which combines with hydrogen ions to form bicarbonate buffer, to correct acidosis

Local Anesthetic/Vasoconstrictor Precautions No information available to require special precautions

Effects on Dental Treatment No effects or complications reported

Other Adverse Effects
1% to 10%:
    Cardiovascular: Venospasm
    Local: Tissue irritation, necrosis with extravasation
<1%:
    Endocrine & metabolic: Hyperkalemia, hypoglycemia, hyperosmolality of serum
    Hematologic: Increased blood coagulation time
    Hepatic: Liver cell destruction from direct contact with THAM®
    Respiratory: Apnea, respiratory depression

Drug Uptake
Absorption: 30% of dose is not ionized

Pregnancy Risk Factor C

Generic Available No

Comments 1 mM = 120 mg = 3.3 mL = 1 mEq of THAM®

Tronolane® [OTC] *see* Pramoxine *on page 784*

Tropicacyl® *see* Tropicamide *on this page*

Tropicamide (troe PIK a mide)

Brand Names Mydriacyl®; Opticyl®; Tropicacyl®

Therapeutic Category Ophthalmic Agent, Mydriatic

Synonyms Bistropamide

Use Short-acting mydriatic used in diagnostic procedures; as well as preoperatively and postoperatively; treatment of some cases of acute iritis, iridocyclitis, and keratitis

Usual Dosage Children and Adults (individuals with heavily pigmented eyes may require larger doses):
Cycloplegia: Instill 1-2 drops (1%); may repeat in 5 minutes
    Exam must be performed within 30 minutes after the repeat dose; if the patient is not examined within 20-30 minutes, instill an additional drop
Mydriasis: Instill 1-2 drops (0.5%) 15-20 minutes before exam; may repeat every 30 minutes as needed

Mechanism of Action Prevents the sphincter muscle of the iris and the muscle of the ciliary body from responding to cholinergic stimulation

Local Anesthetic/Vasoconstrictor Precautions No information available to require special precautions

Effects on Dental Treatment No effects or complications reported

Other Adverse Effects 1% to 10%:
Cardiovascular: Tachycardia, vascular congestion, edema, parasympathetic stimulations
Central nervous system: Drowsiness, headache
Dermatologic: Eczematoid dermatitis
Gastrointestinal: Dryness of the mouth
Local: Transient stinging
Ocular: Blurred vision, photophobia with or without corneal staining, increased intraocular pressure, follicular conjunctivitis

Drug Uptake
Onset of mydriasis: ~20-40 minutes
    Duration: ~6-7 hours
Onset of cycloplegia: Within 30 minutes
    Duration: <6 hours

Pregnancy Risk Factor C

Generic Available Yes

Trovafloxacin/Alatrofloxacin

Brand Names Trovan™

Therapeutic Category Antibiotic, Quinolone

Synonyms CP-99,219-27

Use Treatment of pneumonia, bronchitis, meningitis, uncomplicated urinary tract, and skin and soft tissue infections

Usual Dosage Adults:

Oral: 100-200 mg/day; total duration of therapy and dose depend on indication

I.V. (alatrofloxacin): 300 mg followed by 200 mg/day

Dosing adjustment in renal impairment: No adjustment needed

Dosing adjustment in mild/moderate cirrhosis:

I.V.: In normal hepatic function, dose is 300 mg; in chronic hepatic disease, adjust dose to 200 mg

Oral or I.V.: In normal hepatic function, dose is 200 mg; in chronic hepatic disease, adjust dose to 100 mg

Mechanism of Action Trovafloxacin is a unique fluoroquinolone antibiotic with *in vitro* activity against atypical, Gram-negative, Gram-positive including penicillin-resistant pneumococci, intracellular and anaerobic pathogens. It is a fluoroquinolone with a 2-4-difluorophenyl substituent at the N-1 position and a fused pyrolidine substituent at the 7 position.

Local Anesthetic/Vasoconstrictor Precautions No information available to require special precautions

Effects on Dental Treatment No effects or complications reported

Other Adverse Effects The most frequent adverse effect is mild dizziness in about 10% of patients; other symptoms include nausea, headache, vomiting, vaginitis, and diarrhea

Drug Interactions

Decreased trovafloxacin absorption: Sucralfate, ferrous sulfate, antacids, omeprazole

No effect by trovafloxacin: Theophylline, warfarin, digoxin

Drug Uptake

Protein binding: ~70%

Serum half-life: ~10 hours

Peak plasma concentration: 0.3-10.1 mg/L

Time to peak plasma concentration: 1-3 hours

Pregnancy Risk Factor C

Dosage Forms

Injection, as mesylate (alatrofloxacin): 5 mg/mL (40 mL, 60 mL)

Tablet, as mesylate (trovafloxacin): 100 mg, 200 mg

Comments *In vitro* trovafloxacin was more active than sparfloxacin, ofloxacin, ciprofloxacin, ceftriaxone, erythromycin and vancomycin against *S. pneumoniae*. It was also more active against penicillin-resistant strains than ceftriaxone, erythromycin or vancomycin. Trovafloxacin is very effective in bronchitis and pneumonia. It has good activity against resistant organisms, and penetration of the cerebral spinal fluid giving potential in the treatment of central nervous system infections.

Trovan™ see Trovafloxacin/Alatrofloxacin *on this page*

Troxidone see Trimethadione *on page 963*

Truphylline® see Aminophylline *on page 56*

Trusopt® see Dorzolamide *on page 333*

Trypsin, Balsam Peru, and Castor Oil

(TRIP sin, BAL sam pe RUE, & KAS tor oyl)

Brand Names Granulex

Therapeutic Category Enzyme, Topical Debridement; Protectant, Topical; Topical Skin Product

Use Treatment of decubitus ulcers, varicose ulcers, debridement of eschar, dehiscent wounds and sunburn

Local Anesthetic/Vasoconstrictor Precautions No information available to require special precautions

Effects on Dental Treatment No effects or complications reported

Generic Available No

Trysul® see Sulfabenzamide, Sulfacetamide, and Sulfathiazole *on page 889*

TSPA see Thiotepa *on page 928*

TST see Tuberculin Purified Protein Derivative *on next page*

T-Stat® Topical see Erythromycin, Topical *on page 364*

Tuberculin Purified Protein Derivative

(too BER kyoo lin PURE eh fide PRO teen dah RIV ah tiv)

Brand Names Aplisol®; Aplitest®; Tine Test PPD; Tubersol®

Therapeutic Category Diagnostic Agent, Skin Test

Synonyms Mantoux; PPD; Tine Test; TST; Tuberculin Skin Test

Use Skin test in diagnosis of tuberculosis, to aid in assessment of cell-mediated immunity; routine tuberculin testing is recommended at 12 months of age and at every 1-2 years thereafter, before the measles vaccination

Usual Dosage Children and Adults: Intradermal: 0.1 mL about 4" below elbow; use ¼" to ½" or 26- or 27-gauge needle; significant reactions are ≥5 mm in diameter

Interpretation of induration of tuberculin skin test injections: Positive: ≥10 mm; inconclusive: 5-9 mm; negative: <5 mm

Interpretation of induration of Tine test injections: Positive: >2 mm and vesiculation present; inconclusive: <2 mm (give patient Mantoux test of 5 TU/0.1 mL - base decisions on results of Mantoux test); negative: <2 mm or erythema of any size (no need for retesting unless person is a contact of a patient with tuberculosis or there is clinical evidence suggestive of the disease)

Mechanism of Action Tuberculosis results in individuals becoming sensitized to certain antigenic components of the *M. tuberculosis* organism. Culture extracts called tuberculins are contained in tuberculin skin test preparations. Upon intracutaneous injection of these culture extracts, a classic delayed (cellular) hypersensitivity reaction occurs. This reaction is characteristic of a delayed course (peak occurs >24 hours after injection, induration of the skin secondary to cell infiltration, and occasional vesiculation and necrosis). Delayed hypersensitivity reactions to tuberculin may indicate infection with a variety of nontuberculosis mycobacteria, or vaccination with the live attenuated mycobacterial strain of *M. bovis* vaccine, BCG, in addition to previous natural infection with *M. tuberculosis*.

Local Anesthetic/Vasoconstrictor Precautions No information available to require special precautions

Effects on Dental Treatment No effects or complications reported

Other Adverse Effects 1% to 10%:

Central nervous system: Pain

Gastrointestinal: Ulceration

Dermatologic: Vesiculation

Miscellaneous: Necrosis

Drug Uptake

Onset of action: Delayed hypersensitivity reactions to tuberculin usually occur within 5-6 hours following injection

Peak effect: Become maximal at 48-72 hours

Duration: Reactions subside over a few days

Pregnancy Risk Factor C

Generic Available Yes

Comments Test dose: 0.1 mL intracutaneously; examine site at 48-72 hours after administration; whenever tuberculin is administered, a record should be made of the administration technique (Mantoux method, disposable multiple-puncture device), tuberculin used (OT or PPD), manufacturer and lot number of tuberculin used, date of administration, date of test reading, and the size of the reaction in millimeters (mm).

Tuberculin Skin Test *see* Tuberculin Purified Protein Derivative *on this page*

Tubersol® *see* Tuberculin Purified Protein Derivative *on this page*

Tuinal® *see* Amobarbital and Secobarbital *on page 66*

Tums® [OTC] *see* Calcium Carbonate *on page 162*

Tums® E-X Extra Strength Tablet [OTC] *see* Calcium Carbonate *on page 162*

Tums® Extra Strength Liquid [OTC] *see* Calcium Carbonate *on page 162*

Tusibron® [OTC] *see* Guaifenesin *on page 452*

Tusibron-DM® [OTC] *see* Guaifenesin and Dextromethorphan *on page 453*

Tussafed® Drops *see* Carbinoxamine, Pseudoephedrine, and Dextromethorphan *on page 177*

Tussafin® Expectorant *see* Hydrocodone, Pseudoephedrine, and Guaifenesin *on page 484*

Tuss-Allergine® Modified T.D. Capsule *see* Caramiphen and Phenylpropanolamine *on page 173*

Tussar® SF Syrup *see* Guaifenesin, Pseudoephedrine, and Codeine *on page 455*

Tuss-DM® [OTC] *see* Guaifenesin and Dextromethorphan *on page 453*

Tussigon® *see* Hydrocodone and Homatropine *on page 481*

Tussionex® *see* Hydrocodone and Chlorpheniramine *on page 481*

Tussi-Organidin® DM NR *see* Guaifenesin and Dextromethorphan *on page 453*

Tussi-Organidin® NR *see* Guaifenesin and Codeine *on page 452*

Tuss-LA® *see* Guaifenesin and Pseudoephedrine *on page 454*

Tussogest® Extended Release Capsule *see* Caramiphen and Phenylpropanolamine *on page 173*

Tusstat® Syrup *see* Diphenhydramine *on page 323*

Twice-A-Day® Nasal [OTC] *see* Oxymetazoline *on page 714*

Twilite® Oral [OTC] *see* Diphenhydramine *on page 323*

Twin-K® *see* Potassium Citrate and Potassium Gluconate *on page 780*

Two-Dyne® *see* Butalbital Compound *on page 154*

Two-Dyne® *see* Butalbital Compound and Acetaminophen *on page 155*

Tylenol® [OTC] *see* Acetaminophen *on page 20*

Tylenol® Cold Effervescent Medication Tablet [OTC] *see* Chlorpheniramine, Phenylpropanolamine, and Acetaminophen *on page 222*

Tylenol® Cold No Drowsiness [OTC] *see* Acetaminophen, Dextromethorphan, and Pseudoephedrine *on page 25*

Tylenol® Extended Relief [OTC] *see* Acetaminophen *on page 20*

Tylenol® Flu Maximum Strength [OTC] *see* Acetaminophen, Dextromethorphan, and Pseudoephedrine *on page 25*

Tylenol® Sinus, Maximum Strength [OTC] *see* Acetaminophen and Pseudoephedrine *on page 24*

Tylenol® With Codeine *see* Acetaminophen and Codeine *on page 21*

Tylox® *see* Oxycodone and Acetaminophen *on page 711*

Typhim Vi® *see* Typhoid Vaccine *on this page*

Typhoid Vaccine (TYE foid vak SEEN)

Brand Names Typhim Vi®; Vivotif Berna™ Oral

Therapeutic Category Vaccine, Inactivated Bacteria

Synonyms Typhoid Vaccine Live Oral Ty21a

Use Promotes active immunity to typhoid fever for patients exposed to typhoid carrier or foreign travel to typhoid fever endemic area

Usual Dosage

S.C.:

Children 6 months to 10 years: 0.25 mL; repeat in ≥4 weeks (total immunization is 2 doses)

Children >10 years and Adults: 0.5 mL; repeat dose in ≥4 weeks (total immunization is 2 doses)

Booster: 0.25 mL every 3 years for children 6 months to 10 years and 0.5 mL every 3 years for children >10 years and adults

Oral: Adults:

Primary immunization: 1 capsule on alternate days (day 1, 3, 5, and 7)

Booster immunization: Repeat full course of primary immunization every 5 years

Mechanism of Action Virulent strains of *Salmonella typhi* cause disease by penetrating the intestinal mucosa and entering the systemic circulation via the lymphatic vasculature. One possible mechanism of conferring immunity may be the provocation of a local immune response in the intestinal tract induced by oral ingesting of a live strain with subsequent aborted infection. The ability of *Salmonella typhi* to produce clinical disease (and to elicit an immune response) is dependent on the bacteria having a complete lipopolysaccharide. The live attenuate Ty21a strain lacks the enzyme UDP-4-galactose epimerase so that lipopolysaccharide is only synthesized under conditions that induce bacterial autolysis. Thus, the strain remains avirulent despite the production of sufficient lipopolysaccharide to evoke a protective immune response. Despite low levels of lipopolysaccharide synthesis, cells lyse before gaining a virulent phenotype due to the intracellular accumulation of metabolic intermediates.

Local Anesthetic/Vasoconstrictor Precautions No information available to require special precautions

Effects on Dental Treatment No effects or complications reported

Other Adverse Effects

Oral:

1% to 10%:

Dermatologic: Skin rash

Gastrointestinal: Abdominal discomfort, stomach cramps, diarrhea, nausea, vomiting

<1%: Miscellaneous: Anaphylactic reaction

Injection: >10%:

Dermatologic: Erythema

Local: Tenderness, induration

Neuromuscular & skeletal: Myalgia

Drug Uptake
Oral:
Onset of immunity to *Salmonella typhi*: Within about 1 week
Duration: ~5 years
Parenteral: Duration of immunity: ~3 years
Pregnancy Risk Factor C
Generic Available Yes: Injection only
Comments Inactivated bacteria vaccine; federal law requires that the date of administration, the vaccine manufacturer, lot number of vaccine, and the administering person's name, title and address be entered into the patient's permanent medical record

Typhoid Vaccine Live Oral Ty21a *see* Typhoid Vaccine *on previous page*

Tyzine® Nasal *see* Tetrahydrozoline *on page 916*

U-90152S *see* Delavirdine *on page 285*

UAD Otic® *see* Neomycin, Polymyxin B, and Hydrocortisone *on page 672*

UCB-P071 *see* Cetirizine *on page 205*

ULR-LA® *see* Guaifenesin and Phenylpropanolamine *on page 454*

Ultiva® *see* Remifentanil *on page 837*

Ultram® *see* Tramadol *on page 948*

Ultra Mide® *see* Urea *on this page*

Ultrase® MT12 *see* Pancrelipase *on page 722*

Ultrase® MT20 *see* Pancrelipase *on page 722*

Ultra Tears® Solution [OTC] *see* Artificial Tears *on page 87*

Ultravate™ *see* Halobetasol *on page 462*

Unasyn® *see* Ampicillin and Sulbactam *on page 75*

Undecylenic Acid and Derivatives
(un de sil EN ik AS id & dah RIV ah tivs)
Brand Names Caldesene® Topical [OTC]; Fungoid® AF Topical Solution [OTC]; Pedi-Pro Topical [OTC]
Therapeutic Category Antifungal Agent, Topical
Synonyms Zinc Undecylenate
Use Treatment of athlete's foot (tinea pedis), ringworm (except nails and scalp), prickly heat, jock itch (tinea cruris), diaper rash and other minor skin irritations due to superficial dermatophytes
Local Anesthetic/Vasoconstrictor Precautions No information available to require special precautions
Effects on Dental Treatment No effects or complications reported
Other Adverse Effects 1% to 10%: Dermatologic: Skin irritation, sensitization
Generic Available Yes
Comments Ointment should be applied at night, powder may be applied during the day or used alone when a drying effect is needed

Unguentine® [OTC] *see* Benzocaine *on page 118*

Uni-Ace® [OTC] *see* Acetaminophen *on page 20*

Uni-Bent® Cough Syrup *see* Diphenhydramine *on page 323*

Unicap® [OTC] *see* Vitamins, Multiple *on page 995*

Uni-Decon® *see* Chlorpheniramine, Phenyltoloxamine, Phenylpropanolamine, and Phenylephrine *on page 222*

Uni-Dur® *see* Theophylline *on page 917*

Unipen® *see* Nafcillin *on page 659*

Uniphyl® *see* Theophylline *on page 917*

Uniretic® *see* Moexipril and Hydrochlorothiazide *on page 645*

Unitrol® [OTC] *see* Phenylpropanolamine *on page 754*

Uni-tussin® [OTC] *see* Guaifenesin *on page 452*

Uni-tussin® DM [OTC] *see* Guaifenesin and Dextromethorphan *on page 453*

Univasc® *see* Moexipril *on page 645*

Unna's Boot *see* Zinc Gelatin *on page 1004*

Unna's Paste *see* Zinc Gelatin *on page 1004*

Uracel® *see* Sodium Salicylate *on page 875*

Urea (yoor EE a)
Brand Names Amino-Cerv™ Vaginal Cream; Aquacare® [OTC]; Carmol® [OTC]; Nutraplus® [OTC]; Rea-Lo® [OTC]; Ultra Mide®; Ureacin®-20 [OTC]; Ureacin®-40; Ureaphil®
Canadian/Mexican Brand Names Onyvul® (Canada); Uremol® (Canada); Urisec® (Canada); Velvelan® (Canada)
Therapeutic Category Diuretic, Osmotic; Topical Skin Product
(Continued)

Urea (Continued)

Use Reduces intracranial pressure and intraocular pressure; topically promotes hydration and removal of excess keratin in hyperkeratotic conditions and dry skin; mild cervicitis

Usual Dosage
Children: I.V. slow infusion:
<2 years: 0.1-0.5 g/kg
>2 years: 0.5-1.5 g/kg

Adults:
I.V. infusion: 1-1.5 g/kg by slow infusion (1-2$^1/_2$ hours); maximum: 120 g/24 hours
Topical: Apply 1-3 times/day
Vaginal: Insert 1 applicatorful in vagina at bedtime for 2-4 weeks

Mechanism of Action Elevates plasma osmolality by inhibiting tubular reabsorption of water, thus enhancing the flow of water into extracellular fluid

Local Anesthetic/Vasoconstrictor Precautions No information available to require special precautions

Effects on Dental Treatment No effects or complications reported

Other Adverse Effects
>10%: Gastrointestinal: Nausea, vomiting
1% to 10%:
Central nervous system: Headache
Local: Transient stinging, local irritation, tissue necrosis from extravasation of I.V. preparation
<1%: Endocrine & metabolic: Electrolyte imbalance

Drug Interactions Decreased effect/toxicity/levels of lithium

Drug Uptake
Onset of therapeutic effect: I.V.: Maximum effects within 1-2 hours
Duration: 3-6 hours (diuresis can continue for up to 10 hours)
Serum half-life: 1 hour

Pregnancy Risk Factor C

Generic Available Yes

Urea and Hydrocortisone (yoor EE a & hye droe KOR ti sone)

Brand Names Carmol-HC® Topical

Therapeutic Category Corticosteroid, Topical (Low Potency); Topical Skin Product

Synonyms Hydrocortisone and Urea

Use Inflammation of corticosteroid-responsive dermatoses

Local Anesthetic/Vasoconstrictor Precautions No information available to require special precautions

Effects on Dental Treatment No effects or complications reported

Pregnancy Risk Factor C

Generic Available No

Ureacin®-20 [OTC] see Urea on previous page

Ureacin®-40 see Urea on previous page

Ureaphil® see Urea on previous page

Urecholine® see Bethanechol on page 128

Urex® see Methenamine on page 610

Urised® see Methenamine on page 610

Urispas® see Flavoxate on page 406

Urobak® see Sulfamethoxazole on page 893

Urocit®-K see Potassium Citrate on page 779

Urodine® see Phenazopyridine on page 746

Urofolitropina (Mexico) see Urofollitropin on this page

Urofollitropin (yoor oh fol li TROE pin)

Brand Names Fertinex® Injection; Metrodin® Injection

Canadian/Mexican Brand Names Fertinorm® H.P. (Mexico)

Therapeutic Category Ovulation Stimulator

Synonyms Urofolitropina (Mexico)

Use Induction of ovulation in patients with polycystic ovarian disease and to stimulate the development of multiple oocytes

Usual Dosage Adults: Female: S.C.: 75 units/day for 7-12 days, used with hCG may repeat course of treatment 2 more times

Mechanism of Action Preparation of follicle-stimulating hormone 75 IU with <1 IU of luteinizing hormone (LH) which is isolated from the urine of postmenopausal women. Follicle-stimulating hormone plays a role in the development of follicles. Elevated FSH levels early in the normal menstrual cycle are thought to play a significant role in recruiting a cohort of follicles for maturation. A single follicle is enriched with FSH receptors and becomes dominant over the rest of the recruited follicles. The increased number of FSH receptors allows it to grow despite declining FSH levels. This dominant follicle secretes low levels of estrogen and inhibin which further reduces pituitary FSH output. The ovarian stroma, under the influence of luteinizing hormone, produces androgens which the dominant follicle uses as precursors for estrogens.

Local Anesthetic/Vasoconstrictor Precautions No information available to require special precautions

Effects on Dental Treatment No effects or complications reported

Other Adverse Effects

>10%:
Endocrine & metabolic: Ovarian enlargement
Local: Swelling at injection site, pain

1% to 10%:
Cardiovascular: Arterial thromboembolism
Central nervous system: Fever, chills
Dermatologic: Rash
Gastrointestinal: Nausea, vomiting, abdominal pain, diarrhea
Miscellaneous: Hyperstimulation syndrome

Drug Interactions No data reported

Drug Uptake
Serum half-life, elimination: 3.9 hours and 70.4 hours (FSH has two half-lives)

Pregnancy Risk Factor X

Generic Available No

Urogesic® *see* Phenazopyridine *on page 746*

Urokinase (yoor oh KIN ase)

Related Information
Cardiovascular Diseases *on page 1010*

Brand Names Abbokinase®

Canadian/Mexican Brand Names Ukidan® (Mexico)

Therapeutic Category Thrombolytic Agent

Synonyms Uroquinasa (Mexico)

Use Thrombolytic agent used in treatment of recent severe or massive deep vein thrombosis, pulmonary emboli, myocardial infarction, and occluded arteriovenous cannulas; more expensive than streptokinase; not useful on thrombi over 1 week old

Usual Dosage

Children and Adults: Deep vein thrombosis: I.V.: Loading: 4400 units/kg over 10 minutes, then 4400 units/kg/hour for 12 hours

Adults:
Myocardial infarction: Intracoronary: 750,000 units over 2 hours (6000 units/minute over up to 2 hours)

Occluded I.V. catheters:
5000 units (use only Abbokinase® Open Cath) in each lumen over 1-2 minutes, leave in lumen for 1-4 hours, then aspirate; may repeat with 10,000 units in each lumen if 5000 units fails to clear the catheter; **do not infuse into the patient**; volume to instill into catheter is equal to the volume of the catheter

I.V. infusion: 200 units/kg/hour in each lumen for 12-48 hours at a rate of at least 20 mL/hour

Dialysis patients: 5000 units is administered in each lumen over 1-2 minutes; leave urokinase in lumen for 1-2 days, then aspirate

Clot lysis (large vessel thrombi): Loading: I.V.: 4400 units/kg over 10 minutes, increase to 6000 units/kg/hour; maintenance: 4400-6000 units/kg/hour adjusted to achieve clot lysis or patency of affected vessel; doses up to 50,000 units/kg/hour have been used. **Note:** Therapy should be initiated as soon as possible after diagnosis of thrombi and continued until clot is dissolved (usually 24-72 hours).

Acute pulmonary embolism: Three treatment alternatives: 3 million unit dosage
Alternative 1: 12-hour infusion: 4400 units/kg (2000 units/lb) bolus over 10 minutes followed by 4400 units/kg/hour (2000 units/lb); begin heparin 1000 units/hour approximately 3-4 hours after completion of urokinase infusion or when PTT is <100 seconds
Alternative 2: 2-hour infusion: 1 million unit bolus over 10 minutes followed by 2 million units over 110 minutes; begin heparin 1000 units/hour approximately 3-4 hours after completion of urokinase infusion or when PTT is <100 seconds

(Continued)

Urokinase *(Continued)*

    Alternative 3: Bolus dose only: 15,000 units/kg over 10 minutes; begin heparin 1000 units/hour approximately 3-4 hours after completion of urokinase infusion or when PTT is <100 seconds

Mechanism of Action Promotes thrombolysis by directly activating plasminogen to plasmin, which degrades fibrin, fibrinogen, and other procoagulant plasma proteins

Local Anesthetic/Vasoconstrictor Precautions No information available to require special precautions

Effects on Dental Treatment No effects or complications reported

Other Adverse Effects

>10%:
    Cardiovascular: Hypotension, arrhythmias
    Dermatologic: Angioneurotic edema
    Hematologic: Bleeding at sites of percutaneous trauma
    Ocular: Periorbital swelling
    Respiratory: Bronchospasm
    Miscellaneous: Anaphylaxis

<1%:
    Central nervous system: Headache, chills
    Dermatologic: Rash
    Gastrointestinal: Nausea, vomiting
    Hematologic: Anemia
    Ocular: Eye hemorrhage
    Respiratory: Epistaxis
    Miscellaneous: Sweating

Drug Interactions Increased toxicity (increased bleeding) with anticoagulants, antiplatelet drugs, aspirin, indomethacin, dextran

Drug Uptake
Onset of action: I.V.: Fibrinolysis occurs rapidly
Duration: 4 or more hours
Serum half-life: 10-20 minutes

Pregnancy Risk Factor B

Generic Available No

Uro-KP-Neutral® *see* Potassium Phosphate and Sodium Phosphate *on page 783*

Uroplus® DS *see* Trimethoprim and Sulfamethoxazole *on page 965*

Uroplus® SS *see* Trimethoprim and Sulfamethoxazole *on page 965*

Uroquinasa (Mexico) *see* Urokinase *on previous page*

Ursodeoxycholic Acid *see* Ursodiol *on this page*

Ursodiol *(ER soe dye ole)*

Brand Names Actigall™

Canadian/Mexican Brand Names Ursofalk (Mexico)

Therapeutic Category Gallstone Dissolution Agent

Synonyms Ursodeoxycholic Acid

Use Gallbladder stone dissolution

Usual Dosage Adults: Oral: 8-10 mg/kg/day in 2-3 divided doses; use beyond 24 months is not established; obtain ultrasound images at 6-month intervals for the first year of therapy; 30% of patients have stone recurrence after dissolution

Mechanism of Action Decreases the cholesterol content of bile and bile stones by reducing the secretion of cholesterol from the liver and the fractional reabsorption of cholesterol by the intestines

Local Anesthetic/Vasoconstrictor Precautions No information available to require special precautions

Effects on Dental Treatment No effects or complications reported

Other Adverse Effects

1% to 10%: Gastrointestinal: Diarrhea
<1%:
    Central nervous system: Fatigue, headache
    Dermatologic: Rash, pruritus
    Gastrointestinal: Nausea, vomiting, dyspepsia, metallic taste, abdominal pain, biliary pain, constipation

Drug Uptake
Serum half-life: 100 hours

Pregnancy Risk Factor B

Generic Available No

Comments Use beyond 24 months is not established; obtain ultrasound images at 6-month intervals for the first year of therapy; 30% of patients have stone recurrence after dissolution

Utimox® *see* Amoxicillin *on page 68*
Vagistat® *see* Tioconazole *on page 936*
Vagitrol® *see* Sulfanilamide *on page 895*

Valacyclovir (val ay SYE kloe veer)
Related Information
Systemic Viral Diseases *on page 1047*
Brand Names Valtrex®
Therapeutic Category Antiviral Agent, Oral
Use Treatment of herpes zoster (shingles) in immunocompetent patients; episodic treatment of recurrent genital herpes in immunocompetent patients; for first episode genital herpes
Usual Dosage Oral: Adults:
Shingles: 1 g 3 times/day for 7 days
Genital herpes: 500 mg twice daily
Mechanism of Action Valacyclovir, the L-valyl ester of acyclovir, is rapidly converted to acyclovir before it exerts its antiviral activity against HSV-1, HSV-2, or VZV. It is most active against HSV-1 and least against VZV due to its varied affinity for thymidine kinase. Thymidine kinase converts it into acyclovir monophosphate; this is then converted into the diphosphate and triphosphate forms. Acyclovir triphosphate inhibits replication of herpes viral DNA via competitive inhibition of herpes viral DNA polymerase, incorporation and termination of the growing viral DNA chain, and inactivation of the viral DNA polymerase.
Local Anesthetic/Vasoconstrictor Precautions No information available to require special precautions
Effects on Dental Treatment No effects or complications reported
Other Adverse Effects
>10%: Gastrointestinal: Nausea
1% to 10%:
Central nervous system: Headache, dizziness
Gastrointestinal: Diarrhea, constipation, abdominal pain, anorexia
Neuromuscular & skeletal: Weakness
Drug Interactions Decreased toxicity: Cimetidine and/or probenecid has decreased the rate but not the extent of valacyclovir conversion to acyclovir
Drug Uptake
Absorption: Rapid and converted to acyclovir and L-valine by first-pass/hepatic metabolism
Serum half-life: Normal renal function: 2.5-3.3 hours
Pregnancy Risk Factor B
Dosage Forms Caplets: 500 mg
Generic Available No

Valergen® Injection *see* Estradiol *on page 365*
Valertest No.1® Injection *see* Estradiol and Testosterone *on page 366*
Valisone® *see* Betamethasone *on page 126*
Valium® *see* Diazepam *on page 300*
Valpin® 50 *see* Anisotropine *on page 78*

Valproic Acid and Derivatives
(val PROE ik AS id & dah RIV ah tives)
Brand Names Depacon®; Depakene®; Depakote®
Canadian/Mexican Brand Names Atemperator-S® (Mexico); Cryoval® (Mexico); Epival® (Mexico); Leptilan® (Mexico); Valprosid® (Mexico)
Therapeutic Category Anticonvulsant, Miscellaneous
Synonyms Valproico Acido (Mexico)
Use Management of simple and complex absence seizures; mixed seizure types; myoclonic and generalized tonic-clonic (grand mal) seizures; may be effective in partial seizures and infantile spasms
Usual Dosage Children and Adults:
Oral: Initial: 10-15 mg/kg/day in 1-3 divided doses; increase by 5-10 mg/kg/day at weekly intervals until therapeutic levels are achieved; maintenance: 30-60 mg/kg/day in 2-3 divided doses
Children receiving more than 1 anticonvulsant (ie, polytherapy) may require doses up to 100 mg/kg/day in 3-4 divided doses
Rectal: Dilute syrup 1:1 with water for use as a retention enema; loading dose: 17-20 mg/kg one time; maintenance: 10-15 mg/kg/dose every 8 hours
Not dialyzable (0% to 5%)
Dosing adjustment/comments in hepatic impairment: Reduce dose
Mechanism of Action Causes increased availability of gamma-aminobutyric acid (GABA), an inhibitory neurotransmitter, to brain neurons or may enhance the action of GABA or mimic its action at postsynaptic receptor sites
(Continued)

Valproic Acid and Derivatives *(Continued)*

Local Anesthetic/Vasoconstrictor Precautions No information available to require special precautions

Effects on Dental Treatment No effects or complications reported

Other Adverse Effects

1% to 10%:
  Endocrine & metabolic: Change in menstrual cycle
  Gastrointestinal: Abdominal cramps, anorexia, diarrhea, nausea, vomiting, weight gain

<1%:
  Central nervous system: Drowsiness, ataxia, irritability, confusion, restlessness, hyperactivity, headache, malaise
  Dermatologic: Alopecia, erythema multiforme
  Endocrine & metabolic: Hyperammonemia
  Gastrointestinal: Pancreatitis
  Hematologic: Thrombocytopenia, prolongation of bleeding time
  Hepatic: Transient elevated liver enzymes, liver failure
  Neuromuscular & skeletal: Tremor
  Ocular: Nystagmus, spots before eyes

Drug Interactions

Carbamazepine decreases the plasma concentrations of valproic acid

Cholestyramine decreases the gastrointestinal absorption of valproic acid

Erythromycin - in one patient, valproic acid plasma levels increased after erythromycin resulting in symptoms of valproic acid toxicity

Clozapine - valproic acid decreases the plasma concentrations of clozapine

Felbamate decreases the plasma levels of valproic acid

Isoniazid - valproic acid plasma levels have increased after isoniazid

Lamotrigine - valproic acid inhibits the metabolism of lamotrigine; lamotrigine stimulates the metabolism of valproic acid resulting in lower plasma concentrations

Phenobarbital - valproic acid increases the plasma levels of phenobarbital; phenobarbital toxicity (excessive sedation) may occur in some patients

Primidone - valproic acid may increase the plasma levels of phenobarbital that is produced from primidone; excessive phenobarbital response may occur

Other - alcohol and CNS depressants may potentiate the depressant effects of valproic acid; valproic acid may increase the risk of bleeding in patients receiving anticoagulants (ie, warfarin) and antithrombotics (ie, aspirin)

Drug Uptake

Serum half-life: Adults: 8-17 hours

Time to peak serum concentration: Within 1-4 hours; 3-5 hours after divalproex (enteric coated)

Pregnancy Risk Factor D

Generic Available Yes

Selected Readings
  Redington K, Wells C, and Petito F, "Erythromycin and Valproic Acid Interaction," *Ann Intern Med*, 1992, 116(10):877-8.

Valproico Acido (Mexico) *see* Valproic Acid and Derivatives *on previous page*

Valsartan *(val SAR tan)*

Brand Names Diovan®

Therapeutic Category Angiotensin II Antagonists

Use Treatment of hypertension alone or in combination with other antihypertensives

Usual Dosage Adults: 80 mg/day; may be increased to 160 mg if needed (maximal effects observed in 4-6 weeks)

Mechanism of Action As a prodrug, valsartan produces direct antagonism of the angiotensin II (AT2) receptors, unlike the angiotensin-converting enzyme inhibitors. It displaces angiotensin II from the AT1 receptor and produces its blood pressure lowering effects by antagonizing AT1-induced vasoconstriction, aldosterone release, catecholamine release, arginine vasopressin release, water intake, and hypertrophic responses. This action results in more efficient blockade of the cardiovascular effects of angiotensin II and fewer side effects than the ACE inhibitors.

Local Anesthetic/Vasoconstrictor Precautions No information available to require special precautions

Effects on Dental Treatment No effects or complications reported

Other Adverse Effects Similar incidence to placebo; independent of race, age, and gender

>1%:
  Central nervous system: Headache, dizziness, drowsiness, ataxia
  Endocrine & metabolic: Decreased libido

Gastrointestinal: Diarrhea, abdominal pain, nausea, abnormal taste
Genitourinary: Polyuria
Hematologic: Neutropenia
Hepatic: Increased LFTs
Neuromuscular & skeletal: Arthralgia
Respiratory: Cough, upper respiratory infection, rhinitis, sinusitis, pharyngitis
<1%:
Hematologic: Anemia
Renal: Increased Cr

Warnings/Precautions Use extreme caution with concurrent administration of potassium-sparing diuretics or potassium supplements, in patients with mild-moderate hepatic dysfunction (adjust dose), in those who may be sodium/water depleted (eg, on high-dose diuretics), and in the elderly; avoid use in patients with congestive heart failure, unilateral renal artery stenosis, aortic/mitral valve stenosis, coronary artery disease, or hypertrophic cardiomyopathy, if possible

Drug Interactions
Decreased effect: Phenobarbital, ketoconazole, troleandomycin, sulfaphenazole
Increased effect: Cimetidine, moxonidine

Drug Uptake
Serum half-life: 9 hours
Time to peak serum concentration: 2 hours (maximal effect: 4-6 hours)

Pregnancy Risk Factor C, first trimester. D, second and third trimesters

Valtrex® see Valacyclovir on page 981

Vancenase® see Beclomethasone on page 112

Vancenase® AQ see Beclomethasone on page 112

Vanceril® see Beclomethasone on page 112

Vancocin® see Vancomycin on this page

Vancoled® see Vancomycin on this page

Vancomycin (van koe MYE sin)
Related Information
Cardiovascular Diseases on page 1010
Brand Names Lyphocin®; Vancocin®; Vancoled®
Canadian/Mexican Brand Names Balcoran® (Mexico); Vancocin® CP (Canada); Vanmicina® (Mexico)
Therapeutic Category Antibiotic, Miscellaneous
Use
Treatment of patients with the following infections or conditions:
Infections due to documented or suspected methicillin-resistant *S. aureus* or beta-lactam resistant coagulase negative *Staphylococcus*
Serious or life-threatening infections (ie, endocarditis, meningitis) due to documented or suspected staphylococcal or streptococcal infections in patients who are allergic to penicillins and/or cephalosporins
Empiric therapy of infections associated with gram-positive organisms; used orally for staphylococcal enterocolitis or for antibiotic-associated pseudomembranous colitis produced by *C. difficile*

Usual Dosage Initial dosage recommendation: I.V.:
Infants >1 month and Children with staphylococcal central nervous system infection: 60 mg/kg/day in divided doses every 6 hours
Adults with normal renal function: 1 g every 12 hours
Antibiotic lock technique (for catheter infections): 2 mg/mL in SWI/NS or D_5W; instill 3-5 mL into catheter port as a flush solution instead of heparin lock **(Note:** Do not mix with any other solutions)
Intrathecal: Vancomycin is available as a powder for injection and may be diluted to 1-5 mg/mL concentration in preservative-free 0.9% sodium chloride for administration into the CSF
Children: 5-20 mg/day
Adults: 20 mg/day
Oral: Pseudomembranous colitis produced by *C. difficile*:
Children: 40 mg/kg/day in divided doses every 6-8 hours, added to fluids
Adults: 125 mg 4 times/day

Mechanism of Action Inhibits bacterial cell wall synthesis by blocking glycopeptide polymerization through binding tightly to D-alanyl-D-alanine portion of cell wall precursor

Local Anesthetic/Vasoconstrictor Precautions No information available to require special precautions

Effects on Dental Treatment No effects or complications reported

Other Adverse Effects
>10%: Cardiovascular: Hypotension accompanied by flushing and erythematous rash on face and upper body (red neck or red man syndrome)
(Continued)

Vancomycin *(Continued)*

1% to 10%:
Central nervous system: Chills, drug fever
Hematologic: Eosinophilia

Contraindications Hypersensitivity to vancomycin or any component; avoid in patients with previous severe hearing loss

Warnings/Precautions Use with caution in patients with renal impairment or those receiving other nephrotoxic or ototoxic drugs; dosage modification required in patients with impaired renal function (especially elderly)

Drug Interactions Increased toxicity with general anesthetic agents

Drug Uptake
Serum half-life (biphasic):
Children >3 years: 2.2-3 hours
Adults: 5-11 hours, prolonged significantly with reduced renal function
Time to peak serum concentration: I.V.: Within 45-65 minutes

Pregnancy Risk Factor C

Breast-feeding Considerations No data reported

Dosage Forms
Capsule, as hydrochloride: 125 mg, 250 mg
Powder for oral solution, as hydrochloride: 1 g, 10 g
Powder for injection, as hydrochloride: 500 mg, 1 g, 2 g, 5 g, 10 g

Generic Available Yes

Vanoxide® [OTC] *see Benzoyl Peroxide on page 120*

Vanoxide-HC® *see Benzoyl Peroxide and Hydrocortisone on page 121*

Van R Gingibraid® *see Epinephrine, Racemic and Aluminum Potassium Sulfate on page 354*

Vansil™ *see Oxamniquine on page 706*

Vantin® *see Cefpodoxime on page 194*

Vaponefrin® *see Epinephrine, Racemic on page 354*

Varicella-Zoster Immune Globulin (Human)

(var i SEL a- ZOS ter i MYUN GLOB yoo lin HYU man)

Therapeutic Category Immune Globulin

Synonyms VZIG

Use Passive immunization of susceptible immunodeficient patients after exposure to varicella; most effective if begun within 96 hours of exposure

VZIG supplies are limited, restrict administration to those meeting the following criteria:
One of the following underlying illnesses or conditions:
Neoplastic disease (eg, leukemia or lymphoma)
Congenital or acquired immunodeficiency
Immunosuppressive therapy with steroids, antimetabolites or other immunosuppressive treatment regimens
Newborn of mother who had onset of chickenpox within 5 days before delivery or within 48 hours after delivery
Premature (≥28 weeks gestation) whose mother has no history of chickenpox
Premature (<28 weeks gestation or ≤1000 g VZIG) regardless of maternal history
One of the following types of exposure to chickenpox or zoster patient(s):
Continuous household contact
Playmate contact (>1 hour play indoors)
Hospital contact (in same 2-4 bedroom or adjacent beds in a large ward or prolonged face-to-face contact with an infectious staff member or patient)
Susceptible to varicella-zoster
Age of <15 years; administer to immunocompromised adolescents and adults and to other older patients on an individual basis

An acceptable alternative to VZIG prophylaxis is to treat varicella, if it occurs, with high-dose I.V. acyclovir

VZIG Dose Based on Weight

Weight of Patient		Dose	
kg	lb	Units	No. of Vials
0-10	0-22	125	1
10.1-20	22.1-44	250	2
20.1-30	44.1-66	375	3
30.1-40	66.1-88	500	4
>40	>88	625	5

Usual Dosage High risk susceptible patients who are exposed again more than 3 weeks after a prior dose of VZIG should receive another full dose; there is no evidence VZIG modifies established varicella-zoster infections.

I.M.: Administer by deep injection in the gluteal muscle or in another large muscle mass. Inject 125 units/10 kg (22 lb); maximum dose: 625 units (5 vials); minimum dose: 125 units; do not give fractional doses. Do not inject I.V. See table.

Mechanism of Action The exact mechanism has not been clarified but the antibodies in varicella-zoster immune globulin most likely neutralize the varicella-zoster virus and prevent its pathological actions

Local Anesthetic/Vasoconstrictor Precautions No information available to require special precautions

Effects on Dental Treatment No effects or complications reported

Other Adverse Effects

1% to 10%: Local: Discomfort at the site of injection (pain, redness, swelling)

<1%:

Central nervous system: Headache, malaise

Dermatologic: Rash, angioedema

Gastrointestinal: GI symptoms

Respiratory: Respiratory symptoms

Miscellaneous: Anaphylactic shock

Pregnancy Risk Factor C

Generic Available No

Comments Should be administered within 96 hours of exposure

Vascor® see Bepridil on page 124

Vaseretic® 5-12.5 see Enalapril and Hydrochlorothiazide on page 348

Vaseretic® 10-25 see Enalapril and Hydrochlorothiazide on page 348

Vasocidin® Ophthalmic see Sulfacetamide Sodium and Prednisolone on page 891

VasoClear® Ophthalmic [OTC] see Naphazoline on page 664

Vasocon-A® [OTC] Ophthalmic see Naphazoline and Antazoline on page 665

Vasocon Regular® Ophthalmic see Naphazoline on page 664

Vasoconstrictor Interactions With Antidepressants see page 1226

Vasodilan® see Isoxsuprine on page 527

Vasopressin (vay soe PRES in)

Brand Names Pitressin®

Canadian/Mexican Brand Names Pressyn® (Canada)

Therapeutic Category Antidiuretic Hormone Analog; Hormone, Posterior Pituitary

Use Treatment of diabetes insipidus; prevention and treatment of postoperative abdominal distention; differential diagnosis of diabetes insipidus

Unlabeled use: Adjunct in the treatment of GI hemorrhage and esophageal varices

Usual Dosage

Diabetes insipidus (highly variable dosage; titrated based on serum and urine sodium and osmolality in addition to fluid balance and urine output):

Children: I.M., S.C.: 2.5-10 units 2-4 times/day as needed

Adults:

I.M., S.C.: 5-10 units 2-4 times/day as needed (dosage range 5-60 units/day)

Intranasal: Administer on cotton pledget or nasal spray

Abdominal distention: Adults: I.M.: 5 mg stat, 10 mg every 3-4 hours

GI hemorrhage: Children and Adults: Continuous I.V. infusion: 0.5 milliunit/kg/hour (0.0005 unit/kg/hour); double dosage as needed every 30 minutes to a maximum of 10 milliunits/kg/hour

Children: 0.01 units/kg/minute; continue at same dosage (if bleeding stops) for 12 hours, then taper off over 24-48 hours

Adults: I.V.: Initial: 0.2-0.4 unit/minute, then titrate dose as needed; if bleeding stops, continue at same dose for 12 hours, taper off over 24-48 hours

Mechanism of Action Increases cyclic adenosine monophosphate (cAMP) which increases water permeability at the renal tubule resulting in decreased urine volume and increased osmolality; causes peristalsis by directly stimulating the smooth muscle in the GI tract

Local Anesthetic/Vasoconstrictor Precautions No information available to require special precautions

Effects on Dental Treatment No effects or complications reported

(Continued)

Vasopressin (Continued)

Other Adverse Effects

1% to 10%:
 Cardiovascular: Hypertension, bradycardia, arrhythmias, venous thrombosis, vasoconstriction with higher doses, angina, circumoral pallor
 Central nervous system: Pounding in the head, fever, vertigo
 Dermatologic: Urticaria
 Gastrointestinal: Flatulence, abdominal cramps, nausea, vomiting
 Neuromuscular & skeletal: Tremor
 Miscellaneous: Sweating

<1%:
 Cardiovascular: Myocardial infarction
 Endocrine & metabolic: Water intoxication
 Miscellaneous: Allergic reaction

Drug Interactions

Decreased effect: Lithium, epinephrine, demeclocycline, heparin, and alcohol block antidiuretic activity to varying degrees
Increased effect: Chlorpropamide, phenformin, urea and fludrocortisone potentiate antidiuretic response

Drug Uptake

Nasal:
 Onset of action: 1 hour
 Duration: 3-8 hours
Parenteral: Duration of action: I.M., S.C.: 2-8 hours
Absorption: Destroyed by trypsin in GI tract, must be administered parenterally or intranasally

Nasal:
 Serum half-life: 15 minutes

Pregnancy Risk Factor B

Generic Available Yes

Vasosulf® Ophthalmic see Sulfacetamide Sodium and Phenylephrine on page 890

Vasotec® see Enalapril on page 346

V-Cillin K® see Penicillin V Potassium on page 734

VCR see Vincristine on page 990

V-Dec-M® see Guaifenesin and Pseudoephedrine on page 454

Veetids® see Penicillin V Potassium on page 734

Velban® see Vinblastine on page 989

Velosef® see Cephradine on page 203

Velosulin® Human see Insulin Preparations on page 509

Venlafaxine (VEN la faks een)

Related Information

Vasoconstrictor Interactions With Antidepressants on page 1226

Brand Names Effexor®

Therapeutic Category Antidepressant, Miscellaneous

Use Treatment of depression in adults; has demonstrated effectiveness for obsessive-compulsive disorder, although it has not been approved for this indication

Usual Dosage Adults: Oral: 75 mg/day, administered in 2 or 3 divided doses, taken with food; dose may be increased in 75 mg/day increments at intervals of at least 4 days, up to 225-375 mg/day

Mechanism of Action Venlafaxine and its active metabolite o-desmethylvenlafaxine (ODV) are potent inhibitors of neuronal serotonin and norepinephrine reuptake and weak inhibitors of dopamine reuptake; causes beta-receptor down regulation and reduces adenylcyclase coupled beta-adrenergic systems in the brain

Local Anesthetic/Vasoconstrictor Precautions No information available to require special precautions

Effects on Dental Treatment >10% of patients experience significant dry mouth which may contribute to oral discomfort, especially in older patients

Other Adverse Effects

≥10%:
 Central nervous system: Headache, somnolence, dizziness, insomnia, nervousness
 Gastrointestinal: Nausea, constipation
 Genitourinary: Abnormal ejaculation
 Neuromuscular & skeletal: Neck pain, weakness
 Miscellaneous: Sweating

1% to 10%:
 Cardiovascular: Palpitations, hypertension, sinus tachycardia

Central nervous system: Anxiety
Gastrointestinal: Weight loss, anorexia, vomiting, diarrhea, dysphagia
Genitourinary: Impotence
Neuromuscular & skeletal: Tremor
Ocular: Blurred vision
<1%:
Central nervous system: Seizures
Otic: Ear pain

Drug Interactions Increased toxicity: Cimetidine, MAO inhibitors (hyperpyrexic crisis); tricyclic antidepressants (TCAs), fluoxetine, sertraline, phenothiazine, class 1C antiarrhythmics, warfarin; venlafaxine is a weak inhibitor of cytochrome P-450-2D6, which is responsible for metabolizing antipsychotics, antiarrhythmics, TCAs, and beta-blockers. Therefore, interactions with these agents are possible, however, less likely than with more potent enzyme inhibitors.

Drug Uptake
Absorption: Oral: 92% to 100%
Serum half-life: 3-7 hours (venlafaxine) and 11-13 hours (ODV)

Pregnancy Risk Factor C

Generic Available No

Venoglobulin®-I see Immune Globulin, Intravenous on page 503

Venoglobulin®-S see Immune Globulin, Intravenous on page 503

Ventolin® see Albuterol on page 35

Ventolin® Rotocaps® see Albuterol on page 35

VePesid® Injection see Etoposide on page 388

VePesid® Oral see Etoposide on page 388

Verapamil (ver AP a mil)

Related Information
Calcium Channel Blockers & Gingival Hyperplasia on page 1132
Cardiovascular Diseases on page 1010

Brand Names Calan®; Calan® SR; Covera-HS®; Isoptin®; Isoptin® SR; Verelan®

Canadian/Mexican Brand Names Apo®-Verap (Canada); Dilacoran-HTA® (Mexico); Dilacoran® (Mexico); Dilacoran-Retard® (Mexico); Novo-Veramil® (Canada); Nu-Verap® (Canada); Veraken® (Mexico); Verdilac® (Mexico)

Therapeutic Category Antianginal Agent; Antiarrhythmic Agent, Class IV; Antiarrhythmic Agent (Supraventricular & Ventricular); Calcium Channel Blocker

Use Orally used for treatment of angina pectoris (vasospastic, chronic stable, unstable) and hypertension; I.V. for supraventricular tachyarrhythmias (PSVT, atrial fibrillation, atrial flutter)

Usual Dosage
Children: SVT:
I.V.:
<1 year: 0.1-0.2 mg/kg over 2 minutes; repeat every 30 minutes as needed
1-16 years: 0.1-0.3 mg/kg over 2 minutes; maximum: 5 mg/dose, may repeat dose in 15 minutes if adequate response not achieved; maximum for second dose: 10 mg/dose
Oral (dose not well established):
1-5 years: 4-8 mg/kg/day in 3 divided doses **or** 40-80 mg every 8 hours
>5 years: 80 mg every 6-8 hours
Adults:
SVT: I.V.: 5-10 mg (approximately 0.075-0.15 mg/kg), second dose of 10 mg (~0.15 mg/kg) may be given 15-30 minutes after the initial dose if patient tolerates, but does not respond to initial dose
Angina: Oral: Initial dose: 80-120 mg twice daily (elderly or small stature: 40 mg twice daily); range: 240-480 mg/day in 3-4 divided doses
Hypertension: Usual dose is 80 mg 3 times/day or 240 mg/day (sustained release); range 240-480 mg/day (no evidence of additional benefit in doses >360 mg/day)

Mechanism of Action Inhibits calcium ion from entering the "slow channels" or select voltage-sensitive areas of vascular smooth muscle and myocardium during depolarization; produces a relaxation of coronary vascular smooth muscle and coronary vasodilation; increases myocardial oxygen delivery in patients with vasospastic angina; slows automaticity and conduction of A-V node.

Local Anesthetic/Vasoconstrictor Precautions No information available to require special precautions

Effects on Dental Treatment Calcium channel blockers (CCB) have been reported to cause gingival hyperplasia (GH). Verapamil induced GH has appeared 11 months or more after subjects took daily doses of 240-360 mg. The severity of hyperplastic syndrome does not seem to be dose-dependent. Gingivectomy is only successful if CCB therapy is discontinued. GH regresses markedly one week after CCB discontinuance with all symptoms resolving in 2 (Continued)

Verapamil *(Continued)*

months. If a patient must continue CCB therapy, begin a program of professional cleaning and patient plaque control to minimize severity and growth rate of gingival tissue.

Other Adverse Effects

1% to 10%:

Cardiovascular: Bradycardia; first, second, or third degree A-V block; congestive heart failure; hypotension; peripheral edema

Central nervous system: Dizziness, lightheadedness, nausea, fatigue

Dermatologic: Skin rash

Gastrointestinal: Constipation

Neuromuscular & skeletal: Weakness

<1%:

Cardiovascular: Chest pain, hypotension (excessive), tachycardia, flushing

Endocrine & metabolic: Galactorrhea

Gastrointestinal: Gingival hyperplasia

Drug Interactions

H_2-blockers (such as cimetidine) cause increased plasma levels of verapamil

Beta-blockers cause increased cardiac depressant effects on A-V conduction in combination with verapamil

Verapamil may cause increases in blood levels of the following drugs: Carbamazepine, cyclosporin, digitalis, quinidine, and theophylline; toxicities to all the above drugs could result

Drug Uptake

Oral (nonsustained tablets):

Peak effect: 2 hours

Duration: 6-8 hours

I.V.:

Peak effect: 1-5 minutes

Duration: 10-20 minutes

Serum half-life:

Infants: 4.4-6.9 hours

Adults: Single dose: 2-8 hours, increased up to 12 hours with multiple dosing; increased half-life with hepatic cirrhosis

Pregnancy Risk Factor C

Generic Available Yes

Selected Readings

Wynn RL, "Update on Calcium Channel Blocker Induced Gingival Hyperplasia," *Gen Dent*, 1995, 43(3):218-22.

Verazinc® [OTC] *see* Zinc Supplements *on page 1005*

Verazinc® Oral [OTC] *see* Zinc Sulfate *on page 1005*

Vercyte® *see* Pipobroman *on page 766*

Verelan® *see* Verapamil *on previous page*

Vergon® [OTC] *see* Meclizine *on page 584*

Vermizine® *see* Piperazine *on page 765*

Vermox® *see* Mebendazole *on page 583*

Verr-Canth™ *see* Cantharidin *on page 169*

Verrex-C&M® *see* Podophyllin and Salicylic Acid *on page 769*

Versacaps® *see* Guaifenesin and Pseudoephedrine *on page 454*

Versed® *see* Midazolam *on page 636*

Vesanoid® *see* Tretinoin, Oral *on page 952*

Vesprin® *see* TrifluPromazine *on page 961*

Vexol® *see* Rimexolone *on page 845*

Vibramycin® *see* Doxycycline *on page 338*

Vibra-Tabs® *see* Doxycycline *on page 338*

Vicks® 44D Cough & Head Congestion *see* Pseudoephedrine and Dextromethorphan *on page 821*

Vicks® 44E [OTC] *see* Guaifenesin and Dextromethorphan *on page 453*

Vicks® 44 Non-Drowsy Cold & Cough Liqui-Caps [OTC] *see* Pseudoephedrine and Dextromethorphan *on page 821*

Vicks Children's Chloraseptic® [OTC] *see* Benzocaine *on page 118*

Vicks Chloraseptic® Sore Throat [OTC] *see* Benzocaine *on page 118*

Vicks® DayQuil® Allergy Relief 4 Hour Tablet [OTC] *see* Brompheniramine and Phenylpropanolamine *on page 143*

Vicks® DayQuil® Sinus Pressure & Congestion Relief [OTC] *see* Guaifenesin and Phenylpropanolamine *on page 454*

Vicks Formula 44® [OTC] *see* Dextromethorphan *on page 298*

Vicks Formula 44® Pediatric Formula [OTC] *see* Dextromethorphan *on page 298*

Vicks® Pediatric Formula 44E [OTC] *see* Guaifenesin and Dextromethorphan *on page 453*

Vicks Sinex® Nasal Solution [OTC] *see* Phenylephrine *on page 752*

Vicodin® [5/500] *see* Hydrocodone and Acetaminophen *on page 478*

Vicodin® ES [7.5/750] *see* Hydrocodone and Acetaminophen *on page 478*

Vicon-C® [OTC] *see* Vitamin B Complex With Vitamin C *on page 994*

Vicon Forte® *see* Vitamins, Multiple *on page 995*

Vicon® Plus [OTC] *see* Vitamins, Multiple *on page 995*

Vicoprofen® *see* Hydrocodone and Ibuprofen *on page 482*

Vidarabina (Mexico) *see* Vidarabine *on this page*

Vidarabine (vye DARE a been)

Related Information
Oral Viral Infections *on page 1066*
Systemic Viral Diseases *on page 1047*

Brand Names Vira-A®

Canadian/Mexican Brand Names Adena® a Ungena (Mexico)

Therapeutic Category Antiviral Agent, Ophthalmic

Synonyms Vidarabina (Mexico)

Use Treatment of acute keratoconjunctivitis and epithelial keratitis due to herpes simplex virus; herpes simplex conjunctivitis

Usual Dosage
Children and Adults: Ophthalmic: Keratoconjunctivitis: Place ½" of ointment in lower conjunctival sac 5 times/day every 3 hours while awake until complete re-epithelialization has occurred, then twice daily for an additional 7 days

Mechanism of Action Inhibits viral DNA synthesis by blocking DNA polymerase

Local Anesthetic/Vasoconstrictor Precautions No information available to require special precautions

Effects on Dental Treatment No effects or complications reported

Other Adverse Effects Ocular: Burning, lacrimation, keratitis, photophobia, foreign body sensation, uveitis

Drug Interactions No data reported

Pregnancy Risk Factor C

Generic Available No

Vi-Daylin® [OTC] *see* Vitamins, Multiple *on page 995*

Vi-Daylin/F® *see* Vitamins, Multiple *on page 995*

Videx® *see* Didanosine *on page 307*

Vinblastine (vin BLAS teen)

Brand Names Alkaban-AQ®; Velban®

Canadian/Mexican Brand Names Lemblastine (Mexico)

Therapeutic Category Antineoplastic Agent, Mitotic Inhibitor

Synonyms Vincaleukoblastine; VLB

Use Palliative treatment of Hodgkin's disease; advanced testicular germinal-cell cancers; non-Hodgkin's lymphoma, histiocytosis, and choriocarcinoma

Usual Dosage Refer to individual protocols. Varies depending upon clinical and hematological response. Give at intervals of at least 7 days and only after leukocyte count has returned to at least 4000/mm^3; maintenance therapy should be titrated according to leukocyte count. Dosage should be reduced in patients with recent exposure to radiation therapy or chemotherapy; single doses in these patients should not exceed 5.5 mg/m^2.

Children and Adults: I.V.: 4-20 mg/m^2 (0.1-0.5 mg/kg) every 7-10 days **or** 5-day continuous infusion of 1.4-1.8 mg/m^2/day **or** 0.1-0.5 mg/kg/week

Hemodialysis effects: Not removed by hemodialysis

Mechanism of Action VLB binds to tubulin and inhibits microtubule formation, therefore, arresting the cell at metaphase by disrupting the formation of the mitotic spindle; it is specific for the M and S phases; binds to microtubular protein of the mitotic spindle causing metaphase arrest

Local Anesthetic/Vasoconstrictor Precautions No information available to require special precautions

Effects on Dental Treatment No effects or complications reported

Other Adverse Effects
>10%:
Dermatologic: Alopecia
Hematologic: May cause severe bone marrow suppression and is the dose-limiting toxicity of vinblastine (unlike vincristine); severe granulocytopenia and thrombocytopenia may occur following the administration of vinblastine and nadir 7-10 days after treatment

(Continued)

Vinblastine *(Continued)*

1% to 10%:
Cardiovascular: Tachycardia, orthostatic hypotension
Central nervous system: Depression, malaise, seizures, headache
Dermatologic: Rash, photosensitivity
Endocrine & metabolic: Hyperuricemia
Gastrointestinal: Paralytic ileus, stomatitis, nausea and vomiting are most common and are easily controlled with standard antiemetics; constipation, diarrhea, abdominal cramps, anorexia, metallic taste
Emetic potential: Moderate (30% to 60%)
Genitourinary: Urinary retention
Local: Extravasation: Vinblastine is a vesicant and can cause tissue irritation and necrosis if infiltrated; if extravasation occurs, follow institutional policy, which may include hyaluronidase and hot compresses
Neuromuscular & skeletal: Jaw pain, weakness, myalgia; vinblastine rarely produces neurotoxicity at clinical doses; however, neurotoxicity may be seen, especially at high doses; if it occurs, symptoms are similar to vincristine toxicity: peripheral neuropathy, loss of deep tendon reflexes, and GI symptoms

<1%:
Central nervous system: Neurotoxicity, pain
Dermatologic: Dermatitis
Gastrointestinal: Hemorrhagic colitis
Neuromuscular & skeletal: Numbness, myalgia
Respiratory: Bronchospasm

Drug Uptake
Absorption: Not reliably absorbed from the GI tract and must be given I.V.
Serum half-life (biphasic):
Initial 0.164 hours
Terminal: 25 hours

Pregnancy Risk Factor D
Generic Available Yes

Vincaleukoblastine *see* Vinblastine *on previous page*
Vincasar® PFS™ Injection *see* Vincristine *on this page*

Vincristine *(vin KRIS teen)*

Brand Names Oncovin® Injection; Vincasar® PFS™ Injection
Canadian/Mexican Brand Names Citomid (Mexico)
Therapeutic Category Antineoplastic Agent, Mitotic Inhibitor
Synonyms LCR; Leurocristine; VCR
Use Treatment of leukemias, Hodgkin's disease, neuroblastoma, malignant lymphomas, Wilms' tumor, and rhabdomyosarcoma
Usual Dosage Refer to individual protocols as dosages vary with protocol used. Adjustments are made depending upon clinical and hematological response and upon adverse reactions

Children: I.V. (maximum single dose: 2 mg):
≤10 kg or BSA <1 m²: 0.05 mg/kg once weekly
2 mg/m²; may repeat every week

Adults: I.V.: 0.4-1.4 mg/m² (up to 2 mg maximum); may repeat every week
Mechanism of Action Binds to microtubular protein of the mitotic spindle causing metaphase arrest; cell-cycle phase specific in the M and S phases
Local Anesthetic/Vasoconstrictor Precautions No information available to require special precautions
Effects on Dental Treatment No effects or complications reported
Other Adverse Effects
>10%:
Dermatologic: Alopecia: Occurs in 20% to 70% of patients
Local: Extravasation: Vincristine is a vesicant and can cause tissue irritation and necrosis if infiltrated; if extravasation occurs, follow institutional policy, which may include hyaluronidase and hot compresses
1% to 10%:
Cardiovascular: Hypotension (orthostatic)
Central nervous system: Neurotoxicity, seizures, CNS depression, cranial nerve paralysis
Dermatologic: Skin rash
Endocrine & metabolic: Hyperuricemia, SIADH
Gastrointestinal: Weight loss, paralytic ileus, constipation and possible paralytic ileus secondary to neurologic toxicity; oral ulceration, nausea, diarrhea, vomiting, bloating, abdominal cramps, anorexia, metallic taste
Local: Phlebitis

Hematologic: Occasionally mild leukopenia and thrombocytopenia may occur

Neuromuscular & skeletal: Numbness, motor difficulties, jaw pain, leg pain, myalgias, cramping, weakness

<1%:

Cardiovascular: Hypertension, hypotension

Central nervous system: Headache, fever; alterations in mental status such as depression, confusion, or insomnia. Cranial nerve palsies, headaches, jaw pain, optic atrophy with blindness have been reported. Intrathecal administration of vincristine has uniformly caused death, vincristine should **never** be administered by this route. Neurologic effects of vincristine may be additive with those of other neurotoxic agents and spinal cord irradiation.

Dermatologic: Photophobia, rash

Endocrine & metabolic: SIADH: Rarely occurs, but may be related to the neurologic toxicity; may cause symptomatic hyponatremia with seizures; the increase in serum ADH concentration usually subsides within 2-3 days after onset

Gastrointestinal: Stomatitis, weight loss; constipation, paralytic ileus, and urinary tract disturbances may occur. All patients should be on a prophylactic bowel management regimen.

Neuromuscular & skeletal: Peripheral neuropathy: Frequently the dose-limiting toxicity of vincristine. Most frequent in patients >40 years of age; occurs usually after an average of 3 weekly doses, but may occur after just one dose. Manifested as loss of the deep tendon reflexes in the lower extremities, tingling, pain, paresthesias of the fingers and toes (stocking glove sensation), and "foot drop" or "wrist drop".

Drug Uptake

Absorption: Oral: Poor

Serum half-life: Terminal: 24 hours

Pregnancy Risk Factor D

Generic Available Yes

Vinorelbine (vi NOR el been)

Brand Names Navelbine®

Therapeutic Category Antineoplastic Agent, Mitotic Inhibitor

Use Treatment of nonsmall cell lung cancer (as a single agent or in combination with cisplatin)

Unlabeled use: Breast cancer, ovarian carcinoma (cisplatin-resistant), Hodgkin's disease

Usual Dosage Varies depending upon clinical and hematological response (refer to individual protocols)

Adults: I.V.: 30 mg/m^2 every 7 days

Mechanism of Action Semisynthetic *Vinca* alkaloid which binds to tubulin and inhibits microtubule formation, therefore, arresting the cell at metaphase by disrupting the formation of the mitotic spindle; it is specific for the M and S phases; binds to microtubular protein of the mitotic spindle causing metaphase arrest

Local Anesthetic/Vasoconstrictor Precautions No information available to require special precautions

Effects on Dental Treatment No effects or complications reported

Other Adverse Effects

1% to 10%:

Cardiovascular: Chest pain

Central nervous system: Fatigue

Endocrine & metabolic: SIADH

Gastrointestinal: Nausea, vomiting, constipation

Genitourinary: Hemorrhagic cystitis

Hematologic: Neutropenia, leukopenia (nadir 7-8 days with recovery by days 15-17), anemia

Hepatic: Transient elevation in liver enzymes

Local: Phlebitis at sight of infusion, vesicant with extravasation

Neuromuscular & skeletal: Decreased deep tendon reflexes, tumor pain, jaw pain, parasthesia

Respiratory: Acute reversible dyspnea, hypoxemia, interstitial pulmonary infiltrates

<1%:

Cardiovascular: Myocardial infarction

Dermatologic: Alopecia

Hematologic: Thrombocytopenia

Drug Uptake

Absorption: Not reliably absorbed from the GI tract and must be given I.V.

Serum half-life (triphasic): Terminal: 27.7-43.6 hours

(Continued)

Vinorelbine (Continued)

Pregnancy Risk Factor D
Generic Available No

Vioform® [OTC] *see* Clioquinol *on page 244*
Viokase® *see* Pancrelipase *on page 722*
Vira-A® *see* Vidarabine *on page 989*
Viracept® *see* Nelfinavir *on page 669*
Viractin® [OTC] *see* Tetracaine *on page 913*
Viramune® *see* Nevirapine *on page 675*
Virazole® Aerosol *see* Ribavirin *on page 841*
Virilon® *see* Methyltestosterone *on page 626*
Viroptic® *see* Trifluridine *on page 961*
Viscoat® *see* Chondroitin Sulfate-Sodium Hyaluronate *on page 231*
Visine® Extra Ophthalmic [OTC] *see* Tetrahydrozoline *on page 916*
Visine® L.R. Ophthalmic [OTC] *see* Oxymetazoline *on page 714*
Visken® *see* Pindolol *on page 763*
Vistacon® *see* Hydroxyzine *on page 491*
Vistaject-25® *see* Hydroxyzine *on page 491*
Vistaject-50® *see* Hydroxyzine *on page 491*
Vistaquel® *see* Hydroxyzine *on page 491*
Vistaril® *see* Hydroxyzine *on page 491*
Vistazine® *see* Hydroxyzine *on page 491*
Vistide® *see* Cidofovir *on page 233*
Vita-C® [OTC] *see* Ascorbic Acid *on page 88*
VitaCarn® Oral *see* Levocarnitine *on page 547*
Vital HN® [OTC] *see* Enteral Nutritional Products *on page 350*

Vitamin A (VYE ta min aye)

Brand Names Aquasol A® [OTC]
Canadian/Mexican Brand Names Arovit® (Mexico); A-Vicon® (Mexico); A-Vitex® (Mexico)
Therapeutic Category Vitamin, Fat Soluble
Synonyms Vitamina A (Mexico)
Use Dental and Medical: Treatment and prevention of vitamin A deficiency
Usual Dosage
  RDA:
    <1 year: 375 mcg
    1-3 years: 400 mcg
    4-6 years: 500 mcg*
    7-10 years: 700 mcg*
    >10 years: 800-1000 mcg*
    Male: 1000 mcg
    Female: 800 mcg
    *mcg retinol equivalent (0.3 mcg retinol = 1 unit vitamin A)

  Vitamin A supplementation in measles (recommendation of the World Health Organization): Children: Oral: Give as a single dose; repeat the next day and at 4 weeks for children with ophthalmologic evidence of vitamin A deficiency:
    6 months to 1 year: 100,000 units
    >1 year: 200,000 units
  Note: Use of vitamin A in measles is recommended only for patients 6 months to 2 years of age hospitalized with measles and its complications **or** patients >6 months of age who have any of the following risk factors and who are not already receiving vitamin A: immunodeficiency, ophthalmologic evidence of vitamin A deficiency including night blindness, Bitot's spots or evidence of xerophthalmia, impaired intestinal absorption, moderate to severe malnutrition including that associated with eating disorders, or recent immigration from areas where high mortality rates from measles have been observed
  Note: Monitor patients closely; dosages >25,000 units/kg have been associated with toxicity

  Severe deficiency with xerophthalmia: Oral:
    Children 1-8 years: 5000-10,000 units/kg/day for 5 days or until recovery occurs
    Children >8 years and Adults: 500,000 units/day for 3 days, then 50,000 units/day for 14 days, then 10,000-20,000 units/day for 2 months
  Deficiency (without corneal changes): Oral:
    Children 1-8 years: 200,000 units every 4-6 months
    Children >8 years and Adults: 100,000 units/day for 3 days then 50,000 units/day for 14 days

Malabsorption syndrome (prophylaxis): Children >8 years and Adults: Oral: 10,000-50,000 units/day of water miscible product

Dietary supplement: Oral:

Children:

6 months to 3 years: 1500-2000 units/day

4-6 years: 2500 units/day

7-10 years: 3300-3500 units/day

Children >10 years and Adults: 4000-5000 units/day

Mechanism of Action Needed for bone development, growth, visual adaptation to darkness, testicular and ovarian function, and as a cofactor in many biochemical processes

Local Anesthetic/Vasoconstrictor Precautions No information available to require special precautions

Effects on Dental Treatment No effects or complications reported

Other Adverse Effects 1% to 10%:

Central nervous system: Irritability, vertigo, lethargy, malaise, fever, headache

Dermatologic: Drying or cracking of skin

Endocrine & metabolic: Hypercalcemia

Gastrointestinal: Weight loss

Ocular: Visual changes

Miscellaneous: Hypervitaminosis A

Contraindications Hypervitaminosis A, hypersensitivity to vitamin A or any component

Warnings/Precautions Evaluate other sources of vitamin A while receiving this product; patients receiving >25,000 units/day should be closely monitored for toxicity

Drug Interactions

Decreased effect: Cholestyramine decreases absorption of vitamin A; neomycin and mineral oil may also interfere with vitamin A absorption

Increased toxicity: Retinoids may have additive adverse effects

Drug Uptake

Absorption: Vitamin A in dosages **not** exceeding physiologic replacement is well absorbed after oral administration; water miscible preparations are absorbed more rapidly than oil preparations; large oral doses, conditions of fat malabsorption, low protein intake, or hepatic or pancreatic disease reduces oral absorption

Pregnancy Risk Factor A (X if dose exceeds RDA recommendation)

Dosage Forms

Capsule: 10,000 units [OTC], 25,000 units, 50,000 units

Drops, oral (water miscible) [OTC]: 5000 units/0.1 mL (30 mL)

Injection: 50,000 units/mL (2 mL)

Tablet [OTC]: 5000 units

Generic Available Yes

Vitamina A (Mexico) see Vitamin A on previous page

Vitamin A and Vitamin D (VYE ta min aye & VYE ta min dee)

Brand Names A and D™ Ointment [OTC]

Therapeutic Category Protectant, Topical; Topical Skin Product

Use Temporary relief of discomfort due to chapped skin, diaper rash, minor burns, abrasions, as well as irritations associated with ostomy skin care

Local Anesthetic/Vasoconstrictor Precautions No information available to require special precautions

Effects on Dental Treatment No effects or complications reported

Other Adverse Effects Irritation

Pregnancy Risk Factor B

Generic Available Yes

Vitamin B₅ see Pantothenic Acid on page 722

Vitamin B Complex (VYE ta min bee KOM pleks)

Brand Names Apatate® [OTC]; Gevrabon® [OTC]; Lederplex® [OTC]; Lipovite® [OTC]; Mega B® [OTC]; Megaton™ [OTC]; Mucoplex® [OTC]; NeoVadrin® B Complex [OTC]; Orexin® [OTC]; Surbex® [OTC]

Therapeutic Category Vitamin, Water Soluble

Use Supportive nutritional supplementation in conditions in which water-soluble vitamins are required like GI disorders, chronic alcoholism, pregnancy, severe burns, and recovery from surgery

Local Anesthetic/Vasoconstrictor Precautions No information available to require special precautions

Effects on Dental Treatment No effects or complications reported

Generic Available Yes

Vitamin B Complex With Vitamin C
(VYE ta min bee KOM pleks with VYE ta min see)

Brand Names Allbee® With C [OTC]; Surbex-T® Filmtabs® [OTC]; Surbex® with C Filmtabs® [OTC]; Thera-Combex® H-P Kapseals® [OTC]; Vicon-C® [OTC]

Therapeutic Category Vitamin, Water Soluble

Use Supportive nutritional supplementation in conditions in which water-soluble vitamins are required like GI disorders, chronic alcoholism, pregnancy, severe burns, and recovery from surgery

Local Anesthetic/Vasoconstrictor Precautions No information available to require special precautions

Effects on Dental Treatment No effects or complications reported

Generic Available Yes

Vitamin B Complex With Vitamin C and Folic Acid
(VYE ta min bee KOM pleks with VYE ta min see & FOE lik AS id)

Brand Names Berocca®; Nephrocaps® [OTC]

Therapeutic Category Vitamin, Water Soluble

Use Supportive nutritional supplementation in conditions in which water-soluble vitamins are required like GI disorders, chronic alcoholism, pregnancy, severe burns, and recovery from surgery

Local Anesthetic/Vasoconstrictor Precautions No information available to require special precautions

Effects on Dental Treatment No effects or complications reported

Generic Available Yes

Vitamin E (VYE ta min ee)

Brand Names Amino-Opti-E® [OTC]; Aquasol E® [OTC]; E-Complex-600® [OTC]; E-Vitamin® [OTC]; Vita-Plus® E Softgels® [OTC]; Vitec® [OTC]; Vite E® Creme [OTC]

Therapeutic Category Vitamin, Fat Soluble

Use Dental and Medical: Prevention and treatment of hemolytic anemia secondary to vitamin E deficiency, dietary supplement

Usual Dosage One unit of vitamin E = 1 mg dl-alpha-tocopherol acetate. Oral:
Vitamin E deficiency:
Children (with malabsorption syndrome): 1 unit/kg/day of water miscible vitamin E (to raise plasma tocopherol concentrations to the normal range within 2 months and to maintain normal plasma concentrations)
Adults: 60-75 units/day
Prevention of vitamin E deficiency:
Adults: 30 units/day
Prevention of retinopathy of prematurity or BPD secondary to O_2 therapy: (American Academy of Pediatrics considers this use investigational and routine use is not recommended):
Retinopathy prophylaxis: 15-30 units/kg/day to maintain plasma levels between 1.5-2 µg/mL (may need as high as 100 units/kg/day)
Cystic fibrosis, beta-thalassemia, sickle cell anemia may require higher daily maintenance doses:
Cystic fibrosis: 100-400 units/day
Beta-thalassemia: 750 units/day
Sickle cell: 450 units/day
Recommended daily allowance:
Children:
1-3 years: 6 mg (9 units)
4-10 years: 7 mg (10.5 units)
Children >11 years and Adults:
Male: 10 mg (15 units)
Female: 8 mg (12 units)
Topical: Apply a thin layer over affected area

Mechanism of Action Prevents oxidation of vitamin A and C; protects polyunsaturated fatty acids in membranes from attack by free radicals and protects red blood cells against hemolysis

Local Anesthetic/Vasoconstrictor Precautions No information available to require special precautions

Effects on Dental Treatment No effects or complications reported

Other Adverse Effects <1%:
Central nervous system: Headache
Dermatologic: Contact dermatitis with topical preparation
Gastrointestinal: Nausea, diarrhea, intestinal cramps
Genitourinary: Gonadal dysfunction
Neuromuscular & skeletal: Weakness
Ocular: Blurred vision

Contraindications Hypersensitivity to drug or any components

Warnings/Precautions May induce vitamin K deficiency; necrotizing enterocolitis has been associated with oral administration of large dosages (eg, >200 units/day) of a hyperosmolar vitamin E preparation in low birth weight infants

Drug Interactions
Decreased absorption with mineral oil
Delayed absorption of iron
Increased effect of oral anticoagulants

Drug Uptake
Absorption: Oral: Depends upon the presence of bile; absorption is reduced in conditions of malabsorption, in low birth weight premature infants, and as dosage increases; water miscible preparations are better absorbed than oil preparations

Pregnancy Risk Factor A (C if dose exceeds RDA recommendation)

Dosage Forms
Capsule: 100 units, 200 units, 330 mg, 400 units, 500 units, 600 units, 1000 units
Capsule, water miscible: 73.5 mg, 147 mg, 165 mg, 330 mg, 400 units
Cream: 50 mg/g (15 g, 30 g, 60 g, 75 g, 120 g, 454 g)
Drops, oral: 50 mg/mL (12 mL, 30 mL)
Liquid, topical: 10 mL, 15 mL, 30 mL, 60 mL
Lotion: 120 mL
Oil: 15 mL, 30 mL, 60 mL
Ointment, topical: 30 mg/g (45 g, 60 g)
Tablet: 200 units, 400 units

Generic Available Yes

Vitamin, Multiple, Prenatal *see* Vitamins, Multiple *on this page*

Vitamin, Multiple, Therapeutic *see* Vitamins, Multiple *on this page*

Vitamin, Multiple With Iron *see* Vitamins, Multiple *on this page*

Vitamins, Multiple (VYE ta mins MUL ti pul)

Brand Names Adeflor®; Allbee® With C; Becotin® Pulvules®; Cefol® Filmtab®; Chromagen® OB [OTC]; Eldercaps® [OTC]; Filibon® [OTC]; Florvite®; LKV-Drops® [OTC]; Multi Vit® Drops [OTC]; M.V.I.®; M.V.I.®-12; M.V.I.® Concentrate; M.V.I.® Pediatric; Natabec® [OTC]; Natabec® FA [OTC]; Natabec® Rx; Natalins® [OTC]; Natalins® Rx; NeoVadrin® [OTC]; Niferex®-PN; Poly-Vi-Flor®; Poly-Vi-Sol® [OTC]; Pramet® FA; Pramilet® FA; Prenavite® [OTC]; Secran®; Stresstabs® 600 Advanced Formula Tablets [OTC]; Stuartnatal® 1 + 1; Stuart Prenatal® [OTC]; Therabid® [OTC]; Theragran® [OTC]; Theragran® Hematinic®; Theragran® Liquid [OTC]; Theragran-M® [OTC]; Tri-Vi-Flor®; Unicap® [OTC]; Vicon Forte®; Vicon® Plus [OTC]; Vi-Daylin® [OTC]; Vi-Daylin/F®

Canadian/Mexican Brand Names Clanda® (Mexico); Complan® (Mexico); Suplena® (Mexico); Vi-Syneral® (Mexico)

Therapeutic Category Vitamin

Synonyms B Complex; B Complex With C; Children's Vitamins; Hexavitamin; Multiple Vitamins; Multivitamins/Fluoride; Parenteral Multiple Vitamin; Prenatal Vitamins; Therapeutic Multivitamins; Vitamin, Multiple, Prenatal; Vitamin, Multiple, Therapeutic; Vitamin, Multiple With Iron

Use Dental and Medical: Dietary supplement

Usual Dosage
Infants 1.5-3 kg: I.V.: 3.25 mL/24 hours (M.V.I.® Pediatric)
Children:
Oral:
≤2 years: Drops: 1 mL/day (premature infants may get 0.5-1 mL/day)
>2 years: Chew 1 tablet/day
≥4 years: 5 mL/day liquid
I.V.: >3 kg and <11 years: 5 mL/24 hours (M.V.I.® Pediatric)
Adults:
Oral: 1 tablet/day or 5 mL/day liquid
I.V.: >11 years: 5 mL of vials 1 and 2 (M.V.I.®-12)/one TPN bag/day
I.V. solutions: 10 mL/24 hours (M.V.I.®-12)

Local Anesthetic/Vasoconstrictor Precautions No information available to require special precautions

Effects on Dental Treatment No effects or complications reported

Other Adverse Effects 1% to 10%: Miscellaneous: Hypervitaminosis; refer to individual vitamin entries for individual reactions

Contraindications Hypersensitivity to product components

Warnings/Precautions RDA values are not requirements, but are recommended daily intakes of certain essential nutrients; periodic dental exams should be performed to check for dental fluorosis; use with caution in patients with severe renal or liver failure

Drug Interactions No data reported
(Continued)

Multivitamin Products Available

Product	Content Given Per	A IU	D IU	E IU	C mg	FA mg	B₁ mg	B₂ mg	B₃ mg	B₆ mg	B₁₂ mcg	Other
Theragran®	5 mL liquid	10,000	400		200		10	10	100	4.1	5	B_5 21.4 mg
Vi-Daylin®	1 mL drops	1500	400	4.1	35		0.5	0.6	8	0.4	1.5	Alcohol <0.5%
Vi-Daylin® Iron	1 mL	1500	400	4.1	35		0.5	0.6	8	0.4		Fe 10 mg
Albee® with C	tablet				300		15	10.2		5		Niacinamide 50 mg, pantothenic acid 10 mg
Vitamin B complex	tablet					400 mcg	1.5	1.7		2	6	Niacinamide 20 mg
Hexavitamin	cap/tab	5000	400		75		2	3	20			
Iberet-Folic-500®	tablet				500	0.8	6	6	30	5	25	B_5 10 mg, Fe 105 mg
Stuartnatal® 1+1	tablet	4000	400	11	120	1	1.5	3	20	10	12	Cu, Zn 25 mg, Fe 65 mg, Ca 200 mg
Theragran-M®	tablet	5000	400	30	90	0.4	3	3.4	30	3	9	Cu, Cr, I, K, B_5 10 mg, Mg, Mn, Mo, P, Se, Zn 15 mg, Fe 27 mg, biotin 30 mcg, beta-carotene 1250 IU
Vi-Daylin®	tablet	2500	400	15	60	0.3	1.05	1.2	13.5	1.05	4.5	B_5 15 mg, biotin 60 mcg
M.V.I.®-12 injection	5 mL	3300	200	10	100	0.4	3	3.6	40	4	5	B_5 15 mg, biotin 60 mcg
M.V.I.®-12 unit vial	20 mL											
M.V.I.® pediatric powder	5 mL	2300	400	7	80	0.14	1.2	1.4	17	1	1	B_5 5 mg, biotin 20 mcg, vitamin K 200 mcg

Vitamins, Multiple *(Continued)*

Pregnancy Risk Factor A (C if used in doses above RDA recommendation)
Dosage Forms See table.
Generic Available Yes

Vitaneed™ [OTC] *see* Enteral Nutritional Products *on page 350*
Vita-Plus® E Softgels® [OTC] *see* Vitamin E *on page 994*
Vitec® [OTC] *see* Vitamin E *on page 994*
Vite E® Creme [OTC] *see* Vitamin E *on page 994*
Vitrasert® *see* Ganciclovir *on page 436*
Vivactil® *see* Protriptyline *on page 819*
Viva-Drops® Solution [OTC] *see* Artificial Tears *on page 87*
Vivelle™ Transdermal *see* Estradiol *on page 365*
Vivonex® [OTC] *see* Enteral Nutritional Products *on page 350*
Vivonex® T.E.N. [OTC] *see* Enteral Nutritional Products *on page 350*
Vivotif Berna™ Oral *see* Typhoid Vaccine *on page 976*
V-Lax® [OTC] *see* Psyllium *on page 822*
VLB *see* Vinblastine *on page 989*
VM-26 *see* Teniposide *on page 906*
Volmax® *see* Albuterol *on page 35*
Voltaren® Ophthalmic *see* Diclofenac *on page 304*
Voltaren® Oral *see* Diclofenac *on page 304*
Voltaren-XR® Oral *see* Diclofenac *on page 304*
Vontrol® *see* Diphenidol *on page 324*
VōSol® HC Otic *see* Acetic Acid, Propylene Glycol Diacetate, and Hydrocortisone *on page 27*
Vumon Injection *see* Teniposide *on page 906*
V.V.S.® *see* Sulfabenzamide, Sulfacetamide, and Sulfathiazole *on page 889*
Vytone® Topical *see* Iodoquinol and Hydrocortisone *on page 517*
VZIG *see* Varicella-Zoster Immune Globulin (Human) *on page 984*

Warfarin *(WAR far in)*

Related Information
Cardiovascular Diseases *on page 1010*
Dental Drug Interactions: Update on Drug Combinations Requiring Special Considerations *on page 1144*
Dicumarol *on page 306*
Brand Names Coumadin®
Canadian/Mexican Brand Names Warfilone® (Canada)
Therapeutic Category Anticoagulant
Use Prophylaxis and treatment of venous thrombosis, pulmonary embolism and thromboembolic disorders; atrial fibrillation with risk of embolism and as an adjunct in the prophylaxis of systemic embolism after myocardial infarction

Unlabeled use: Prevention of recurrent transient ischemic attacks and to reduce risk of recurrent myocardial infarction
Usual Dosage
Oral:
Children: 0.05-0.34 mg/kg/day; children <12 months of age may require doses at or near the high end of this range; consistent anticoagulation may be difficult to maintain in children <5 years of age
Adults: 5-15 mg/day for 2-5 days, then adjust dose according to results of prothrombin time; usual maintenance dose ranges from 2-10 mg/day
I.V. (administer as a slow bolus injection): 2-5 mg/day
Mechanism of Action Interferes with hepatic synthesis of vitamin K-dependent coagulation factors (II, VII, IX, X)
Local Anesthetic/Vasoconstrictor Precautions No information available to require special precautions
Effects on Dental Treatment Signs of warfarin overdose may first appear as bleeding from gingival tissue; consultation with prescribing physician is advisable prior to surgery to determine temporary dose reduction or withdrawal of medication
Other Adverse Effects
1% to 10%:
Dermatologic: Skin lesions, alopecia, skin necrosis
Gastrointestinal: Anorexia, nausea, vomiting, stomach cramps, diarrhea
Hematologic: Hemorrhage; leukopenia, unrecognized bleeding sites (eg, colon cancer) may be uncovered by anticoagulation
Respiratory: Hemoptysis

Warfarin *(Continued)*

<1%:
Central nervous system: Fever
Dermatologic: Skin rash, discolored toes (blue or purple)
Gastrointestinal: Mouth ulcers
Hematologic: Agranulocytosis
Hepatic: Hepatotoxicity
Renal: Renal damage

Drug Interactions See tables.

Drugs and Mechanisms Which Decrease Anticoagulant Effects of Warfarin

Induction of Enzymes		Increased Procoagulant Factors	Decreased Drug Absorption	Other
Barbiturates Carbamazepine Glutethimide Griseofulvin	Nafcillin Phenytoin Rifampin	Estrogens Oral contraceptives Vitamin K (including nutritional supplements)	Aluminum hydroxide Cholestyramine* Colestipol*	Ethchlorvynol Griseofulvin Spironolactone† Sucralfate

Decreased anticoagulant effect may occur when these drugs are administered with oral anticoagulants.

*Cholestyramine and colestipol may increase the anticoagulant effect by binding vitamin K in the gut; yet, the decreased drug absorption appears to be of more concern.

†Diuretic-induced hemoconcentration with subsequent concentration of clotting factors has been reported to decrease the effects of oral anticoagulants.

Drugs Which Increase Bleeding Tendency With Warfarin

Inhibit Platelet Aggregation	Inhibit Procoagulant Factors	Ulcerogenic Drugs
Cephalosporins Dipyridamole Indomethacin Oxyphenbutazone Penicillin, parenteral Phenylbutazone Salicylates Sulfinpyrazone	Antimetabolites Quinidine Quinine Salicylates	Adrenal corticosteroids Indomethacin Oxyphenbutazone Phenylbutazone Potassium products Salicylates

Use of these agents with oral anticoagulants may increase the chances of hemorrhage.

Drugs and Mechanisms Which Enhance Anticoagulant Effects of Warfarin

Decrease Vitamin K	Displace Anticoagulant	Inhibit Metabolism	Other
Oral antibiotics Can ↑ or ↓ an INR Check an INR 3 days after a patient begins antibiotics to see the INR value and adjust the warfarin dose accordingly	Chloral hydrate Clofibrate Diazoxide Ethacrynic acid Miconazole Nalidixic acid Phenylbutazone Salicylates Sulfonamides Sulfonylureas Triclofos	Alcohol (acute ingestion)* Allopurinol Amiodarone Chloramphenicol Chlorpropamide Cimetidine Co-trimoxazole Disulfiram Metronidazole Phenylbutazone Phenytoin Propoxyphene Sulfinpyrazone Sulfonamides Tolbutamide	Acetaminophen Anabolic steroids Clofibrate Danazol Erythromycin Gemfibrozil Glucagon Influenza vaccine Ketoconazole Propranolol Ranitidine Sulindac Thyroid drugs

* The hypoprothrombinemic effect of oral anticoagulants has been reported to be both increased and decreased during chronic and excessive alcohol ingestion. Data are insufficient to predict the direction of this interaction in alcoholic patients.

Drug Uptake

Onset of anticoagulation effect: Oral: Within 36-72 hours
Absorption: Oral: Rapid
Serum half-life: 42 hours, highly variable among individuals

Pregnancy Risk Factor D
Generic Available Yes: Tablet

Wart-Off® [OTC] *see* Salicylic Acid *on page 853*
4-Way® Long Acting Nasal Solution [OTC] *see* Oxymetazoline *on page 714*
Wellbutrin® *see* Bupropion *on page 151*
Wellbutrin® SR *see* Bupropion *on page 151*
Wellcovorin® *see* Leucovorin *on page 544*
Whitfield's Ointment [OTC] *see* Benzoic Acid and Salicylic Acid *on page 120*
Whole Root Rauwolfia *see* Rauwolfia Serpentina *on page 836*
Wigraine® *see* Ergotamine *on page 360*
40 Winks® [OTC] *see* Diphenhydramine *on page 323*
Winstrol® *see* Stanozolol *on page 882*
Wolfina® *see* Rauwolfia Serpentina *on page 836*
WR2721 *see* Amifostine *on page 52*
Wycillin® *see* Penicillin G Procaine *on page 733*
Wydase® Injection *see* Hyaluronidase *on page 474*
Wygesic® *see* Propoxyphene and Acetaminophen *on page 812*
Wymox® *see* Amoxicillin *on page 68*
Wytensin® *see* Guanabenz *on page 456*
Xalatan® *see* Latanoprost *on page 543*
Xanax® *see* Alprazolam *on page 43*
X-Prep® Liquid [OTC] *see* Senna *on page 862*
X-seb® T [OTC] *see* Coal Tar and Salicylic Acid *on page 255*
Xylocaine® *see* Lidocaine *on page 553*
Xylocaine® With Epinephrine *see* Lidocaine and Epinephrine *on page 554*

Xylometazoline (zye loe met AZ oh leen)
Brand Names Otrivin® [OTC]
Therapeutic Category Adrenergic Agonist Agent; Nasal Agent, Vasoconstrictor
Use Symptomatic relief of nasal and nasopharyngeal mucosal congestion
Usual Dosage
Children 2-12 years: Instill 2-3 drops (0.05%) in each nostril every 8-10 hours
Children >12 years and Adults: Instill 2-3 drops or sprays (0.1%) in each nostril every 8-10 hours
Mechanism of Action Stimulates alpha-adrenergic receptors in the arterioles of the conjunctiva and the nasal mucosa to produce vasoconstriction
Local Anesthetic/Vasoconstrictor Precautions No information available to require special precautions
Effects on Dental Treatment No effects or complications reported
Other Adverse Effects 1% to 10%:
Cardiovascular: Palpitations
Central nervous system: Drowsiness, dizziness, seizures, headache
Ocular: Blurred vision, ocular irritation, photophobia
Miscellaneous: Sweating
Drug Interactions No data reported
Drug Uptake
Onset of action: Intranasal: Local vasoconstriction occurs within 5-10 minutes
Duration: 5-6 hours
Pregnancy Risk Factor C
Generic Available Yes

Yellow Mercuric Oxide *see* Mercuric Oxide *on page 600*
Yocon® *see* Yohimbine *on this page*
Yodoxin® *see* Iodoquinol *on page 516*

Yohimbine (yo HIM bine)
Brand Names Aphrodyne™; Dayto Himbin®; Yocon®; Yohimex™
Therapeutic Category Impotency Agent
Use No FDA sanctioned indications
Usual Dosage Adults: Oral: Impotence: 5.4 mg 3 times/day
Mechanism of Action Derived from the bark of the yohimbe tree (Pausingstalia yohimbe), this indole alkaloid produces an alpha$_2$-adrenergic blockade; also is a weak MAO inhibitor; parasympathetic tone is also decreased
Local Anesthetic/Vasoconstrictor Precautions No information available to require special precautions
Effects on Dental Treatment No effects or complications reported
(Continued)

Yohimbine *(Continued)*

Other Adverse Effects

Cardiovascular: Tachycardia, bradycardia, hypertension, hypotension (ortho-static), flushing, shock, sinus tachycardia, vasodilation, sinus bradycardia

Central nervous system: Anxiety, mania, hallucinations, irritability, dizziness, psychosis, insomnia, headache, panic attacks

Gastrointestinal: Nausea, vomiting, anorexia

Hematologic: Neutropenia, agranulocytosis

Neuromuscular & skeletal: Tremors, paresthesia

Ocular: Lacrimation, mydriasis

Respiratory: Bronchospasm, sinusitis

Miscellaneous: Antidiuretic action, salivation, diaphoresis

Drug Interactions Antidepressants, other mood-modifying drugs

Drug Uptake

Absorption: Oral: 33%

Half-life: 0.6 hour

Generic Available Yes

Yohimex™ *see Yohimbine on previous page*

Yutopar® *see Ritodrine on page 846*

Zafirlukast *(za FIR loo kast)*

Brand Names Accolate®

Therapeutic Category Leukotriene Receptor Antagonist

Use Prophylaxis and chronic treatment of asthma in adults and children ≥12 years of age

Usual Dosage Oral:

Children <12 years: Safety and effectiveness has not been established

Adults: 20 mg twice daily

Elderly: The mean dose (mg/kg) normalized AUC and Cmax increase and plasma clearance decreases with increasing age. In patients >65 years of age, there is an 2-3 fold greater Cmax and AUC compared to younger adults.

Mechanism of Action Zafirlukast is a selectively and competitive leukotriene-receptor antagonist (LTRA) of leukotriene D4 and E4 (LTD4 and LTE4), components of slow-reacting substance of anaphylaxis (SRSA). Cysteinyl leukotriene production and receptor occupation have been correlated with the pathophysiology of asthma, including airway edema, smooth muscle constriction and altered cellular activity associated with the inflammatory process, which contribute to the signs and symptoms of asthma.

Local Anesthetic/Vasoconstrictor Precautions No information available to require special precautions

Effects on Dental Treatment No effects or complications reported

Other Adverse Effects

>10%: Central nervous system: Headache (12.9%)

1% to 10%:

Central nervous system: Dizziness, pain, fever

Gastrointestinal: Nausea, diarrhea, abdominal pain, vomiting, dyspepsia

Neuromuscular & skeletal: Myalgia, weakness

Drug Interactions Cytochrome P-450 2C9 and 3A4 isoenzyme inhibitor

Decreased effect:

Erythromycin: Coadministration of a single dose of zafirlukast with erythromycin to steady state results in decreased mean plasma levels of zafirlukast by 40% due to a decrease in zafirlukast bioavailability.

Theophylline: Coadministration of zafirlukast at steady state with a single dose of liquid theophylline preparations results in decreased mean plasma levels of zafirlukast by 30%, but no effects on plasma theophylline levels were observed.

Increased effect: Aspirin: Coadministration of zafirlukast with aspirin results in mean increased plasma levels of zafirlukast by 45%

Increased toxicity: Warfarin: Coadministration of zafirlukast with warfarin results in a clinically significant increase in prothrombin time (PT). Closely monitor prothrombin times of patients on oral warfarin anticoagulant therapy and zafirlukast, and adjust anticoagulant dose accordingly.

Drug Uptake

Absorption: Food reduces bioavailability by 40%

Serum half-life: 10 hours

Time to peak serum concentration: 3 hours

Pregnancy Risk Factor B

Dosage Forms Tablet: 20 mg

Zagam® *see Sparfloxacin on page 879*

Zalcitabina (Mexico) *see Zalcitabine on next page*

Zalcitabine (zal SITE a been)

Related Information
HIV Infection and AIDS *on page 1024*
Systemic Viral Diseases *on page 1047*

Brand Names Hivid®

Therapeutic Category Antiviral Agent, Oral

Synonyms Zalcitabina (Mexico)

Use The FDA has approved zalcitabine for use in the treatment of HIV infections only in combination with zidovudine in adult patients with advanced HIV disease demonstrating a significant clinical or immunological deterioration

Usual Dosage Safety and efficacy in children <13 years of age have not been established

Adults: Monotherapy: 0.75 mg every 8 hours (2.25 mg total daily dose)
Combination therapy: 0.75 mg every 8 hours, given together with 200 mg of zidovudine (ie, total daily dose: 2.25 mg of zalcitabine and 600 mg of zidovudine); if zalcitabine is permanently discontinued or interrupted due to toxicities, decrease zidovudine dose to 100 mg every 4 hours

Mechanism of Action
Purine nucleoside analogue, zalcitabine or 2',3'-dideoxycitidine (ddC) has been found to have *in vitro* activity and is reported to be successful against HIV in short term clinical trials

Intracellularly, ddc is converted to active metabolite ddCTP; lack the presence of the 3'-hydroxyl group necessary for phosphodiester linkages during DNA replication. As a result viral replication is prematurely terminated. ddCTP acts as a competitor for binding sites on the HIV-RNA dependent DNA polymerase (reverse transcriptase) to further contribute to inhibition of viral replication.

Local Anesthetic/Vasoconstrictor Precautions No information available to require special precautions

Effects on Dental Treatment Oral ulceration in >10% of patients

Other Adverse Effects
>10%: Gastrointestinal: Oral ulcers
1% to 10%:
Cardiovascular: Chest pain
Central nervous system: Headache, dizziness, fatigue
Dermatologic: Rash, pruritus
Gastrointestinal: Nausea, dysphagia, anorexia, abdominal pain, vomiting, diarrhea, weight loss
Neuromuscular & skeletal: Myalgia, foot pain
Respiratory: Pharyngitis
<1%:
Cardiovascular: Edema, hypertension, palpitations, syncope, atrial fibrillation, tachycardia, heart racing
Central nervous system: Night sweats, fever, pain, malaise
Endocrine & metabolic: Hyperglycemia, hypocalcemia
Gastrointestinal: Constipation, pancreatitis
Hepatic: Jaundice, hepatitis
Neuromuscular & skeletal: Myositis, peripheral neuropathy, weakness
Respiratory: Epistaxis

Drug Interactions
Increased toxicity:
Amphotericin, foscarnet, and aminoglycosides may potentiate the risk of developing peripheral neuropathy or other toxicities associated with zalcitabine by interfering with the renal elimination of zalcitabine
Other drugs associated with peripheral neuropathy include chloramphenicol, cisplatin, dapsone, disulfiram, ethionamide, glutethimide, gold hydralazine, iodoquinol, isoniazid, metronidazole, nitrofurantoin, phenytoin, ribavirin, and vincristine
Concomitant use of zalcitabine with didanosine is not recommended

Drug Uptake
Absorption: Food decreases absorption by 39%
Serum half-life: 2.9 hours

Pregnancy Risk Factor C
Generic Available No

Zeasorb-AF® Powder [OTC] *see Tolnaftate on page 943*

Zebeta® *see Bisoprolol on page 133*

Zefazone® *see Cefmetazole on page 190*

Zephiran® [OTC] *see Benzalkonium Chloride on page 118*

Zephrex® *see Guaifenesin and Pseudoephedrine on page 454*

Zephrex LA® *see Guaifenesin and Pseudoephedrine on page 454*

Zerit® *see Stavudine on page 883*

Zestoretic® *see Lisinopril and Hydrochlorothiazide on page 561*

Zestril® *see Lisinopril on page 560*

Zetar® [OTC] *see Coal Tar on page 254*

Ziac™ *see Bisoprolol and Hydrochlorothiazide on page 134*

Zidovudina (Mexico) *see Zidovudine on this page*

Zidovudine (zye DOE vyoo deen)

Related Information

HIV Infection and AIDS *on page 1024*
Systemic Viral Diseases *on page 1047*
Zidovudine and Lamivudine *on next page*

Brand Names Retrovir®

Canadian/Mexican Brand Names Apo®-Zidovudine (Canada); Dipedyne® (Mexico); Kenamil® (Mexico); Novo-AZT® (Canada); Retrovir-AZT® (Mexico)

Therapeutic Category Antiviral Agent, Oral; Antiviral Agent, Parenteral

Synonyms Zidovudina (Mexico)

Use Management of patients with HIV infections who have had at least one episode of *Pneumocystis carinii* pneumonia or who have CD4 cell counts of ≤500/mm³; patients who have HIV-related symptoms or who are asymptomatic with abnormal laboratory values indicating HIV-related immunosuppression; does not reduce risk of transmitting HIV infections

Usual Dosage

Prevention of maternal-fetal HIV transmission:

Neonatal: Oral: 2 mg/kg/dose every 6 hours for 6 weeks beginning 8-12 hours after birth; infants unable to receive oral dosing may receive 1.5 mg/kg I.V. infused over 30 minutes every 6 hours

Maternal (>14 weeks gestation): Oral: 100 mg 5 times/day until the start of labor; during labor and delivery, administer zidovudine I.V. at 2 mg/kg over 1 hour followed by a continuous I.V. infusion of 1 mg/kg/hour until the umbilical cord is clamped

Asymptomatic/symptomatic HIV infection:

Children 3 months to 12 years:

Oral: 90-180 mg/m²/dose every 6 hours; maximum: 200 mg every 6 hours

I.V.: 1-2 mg/kg/dose (infused over 1 hour) administered every 4 hours around-the-clock (6 doses/day)

Adults:

Asymptomatic HIV infection: Oral: 100 mg every 4 hours while awake (500 mg/day)

Symptomatic HIV infection

Oral: Initial: 200 mg every 4 hours (1200 mg/day), then after 1 month, 100 mg every 4 hours (600 mg/day)

I.V.: 1-2 mg/kg/dose (infused over 1 hour) administered every 4 hours around-the-clock (6 doses/day)

Patients should receive I.V. therapy only until oral therapy can be administered

Combination therapy with zalcitabine: Oral: 200 mg with zalcitabine 0.75 mg every 8 hours

Mechanism of Action Zidovudine is a thymidine analog which interferes with the HIV viral RNA dependent DNA polymerase resulting in inhibition of viral replication

Local Anesthetic/Vasoconstrictor Precautions No information available to require special precautions

Effects on Dental Treatment No effects or complications reported

Other Adverse Effects

>10%:

Central nervous system: Severe headache, insomnia

Gastrointestinal: Nausea

Hematologic: Anemia, leukopenia, neutropenia

1% to 10%:

Dermatologic: Rash, hyperpigmentation of nails (bluish-brown)

Hematologic: Changes in platelet count

<1%:

Central nervous system: Neurotoxicity, confusion, mania, seizures

Gastrointestinal: Anorexia

Hematologic: Bone marrow suppression, granulocytopenia, thrombocytopenia, pancytopenia

Hepatic: Hepatotoxicity, cholestatic jaundice

Local: Tenderness

Neuromuscular & skeletal: Myopathy, weakness

Drug Interactions Increased toxicity: Coadministration with drugs that are nephrotoxic (amphotericin B), cytotoxic (flucytosine, vincristine, vinblastine, doxorubicin, interferon), inhibit glucuronidation or excretion (acetaminophen, cimetidine, indomethacin, lorazepam, probenecid, aspirin), or interfere with RBC/WBC number or function (acyclovir, ganciclovir, pentamidine, dapsone)

Drug Uptake

Absorption: Oral: Well absorbed (66% to 70%)

Serum half-life: Terminal: 60 minutes

Time to peak serum concentration: Within 30-90 minutes

Pregnancy Risk Factor C

Generic Available No

Zidovudine and Lamivudine

Related Information

HIV Infection and AIDS *on page 1024*

Brand Names Combivir®

Therapeutic Category Antiviral Agent, Oral

Synonyms AZT + 3TC

Use Treatment of HIV infection when therapy is warranted based on clinical and/or immunological evidence of disease progression. Combivir® given twice daily, provides an alternative regimen to lamivudine 150 mg twice daily plus zidovudine 600 mg/day in divided doses; this drug form reduces capsule/tablet intake for these two drugs to 2 per day instead of up to 8.

Local Anesthetic/Vasoconstrictor Precautions No information available to require special precautions

Effects on Dental Treatment No effects or complications reported

Other Adverse Effects See individual agents

Drug Interactions See individual agents

Dosage Forms Tablet: Zidovudine 300 mg and lamivudine 150 mg

Zilactin-B® Medicated [OTC] *see* Benzocaine *on page 118*

ZilaDent® [OTC] *see* Benzocaine *on page 118*

Zileuton (zye LOO ton)

Brand Names Zyflo®

Therapeutic Category 5-Lipoxygenase Inhibitor

Use Prophylaxis and chronic treatment of asthma in adults and children ≥12 years of age

Usual Dosage Oral:

Adults: 600 mg 4 times/day with meals and at bedtime

Elderly: Zileuton pharmacokinetics were similar in healthy elderly subjects (>65 years) compared with healthy younger adults (18-40 years)

Mechanism of Action Specific inhibitor of 5-lipoxygenase and thus inhibits leukotriene (LTB1, LTC1, LTD1 and LTE1) formation. Leukotrienes are substances that induce numerous biological effects including augmentation of neutrophil and eosinophil migration, neutrophil and monocyte aggregation, leukocyte adhesion, increased capillary permeability and smooth muscle contraction.

Local Anesthetic/Vasoconstrictor Precautions No information available to require special precautions

Effects on Dental Treatment No effects or complications reported

Other Adverse Effects

>10%:

Central nervous system: Headache (24.6%)

Hepatic: ALT elevation (12%)

1% to 10%:

Cardiovascular: Chest pain

Central nervous system: Pain, dizziness, fever, insomnia, malaise, nervousness, somnolence

Gastrointestinal: Dyspepsia, nausea, abdominal pain, constipation, flatulence

Hematologic: Low white blood cell count

Neuromuscular & skeletal: Myalgia, arthralgia, weakness

Ocular: Conjunctivitis

Warnings/Precautions Elevations of one or more liver function tests may occur during therapy. These laboratory abnormalities may progress, remain unchanged or resolve with continued therapy. Use with caution in patients who consume substantial quantities of alcohol or have a past history of liver disease. Zileuton is (Continued)

Zileuton *(Continued)*

not indicated for use in the reversal of bronchospasm in acute asthma attacks, including status asthmaticus. Zileuton can be continued during acute exacerbations of asthma.

Drug Interactions Cytochrome P-450 1A2, 2C9 and 3A4 enzyme substrate
Increased toxicity:

Propranolol: Doubling of propranolol AUC and consequent increased beta-blocker activity

Terfenadine: Decrease in clearance of terfenadine leading to increase in AUC

Theophylline: Doubling of serum theophylline concentrations - reduce theophylline dose and monitor serum theophylline concentrations closely.

Warfarin: Clinically significant increases in prothrombin time (PT) - monitor PT closely

Drug Uptake
Absorption: Oral: Rapidly absorbed
Serum half-life: 2.5 hours
Time to peak serum concentration: 1.7 hours

Pregnancy Risk Factor C
Generic Available No

Zinacef® *see* Cefuroxime *on page 199*
Zinc *see* Trace Metals *on page 948*
Zinc Acetate *see* Zinc Supplements *on next page*
Zinca-Pak® *see* Trace Metals *on page 948*
Zincate® *see* Zinc Supplements *on next page*
Zincate® Oral *see* Zinc Sulfate *on next page*

Zinc Chloride *(zingk KLOR ide)*

Therapeutic Category Trace Element, Parenteral
Use Cofactor for replacement therapy to different enzymes helps maintain normal growth rates, normal skin hydration and senses of taste and smell
Local Anesthetic/Vasoconstrictor Precautions No information available to require special precautions
Effects on Dental Treatment No effects or complications reported
Other Adverse Effects <1%:
Cardiovascular: Hypotension
Gastrointestinal: Indigestion, nausea, vomiting
Hematologic: Neutropenia, leukopenia
Hepatic: Jaundice
Respiratory: Pulmonary edema
Pregnancy Risk Factor C
Generic Available Yes
Comments Clinical response may not occur for up to 6-8 weeks

Zincfrin® Ophthalmic [OTC] *see* Phenylephrine and Zinc Sulfate *on page 754*

Zinc Gelatin *(zingk JEL ah tin)*

Brand Names Gelucast®
Therapeutic Category Protectant, Topical
Synonyms Dome Paste Bandage; Unna's Boot; Unna's Paste; Zinc Gelatin Boot
Use Protectant and to support varicosities and similar lesions of the lower limbs
Usual Dosage Apply externally as an occlusive boot
Local Anesthetic/Vasoconstrictor Precautions No information available to require special precautions
Effects on Dental Treatment No effects or complications reported
Other Adverse Effects 1% to 10%: Local: Irritation
Dosage Forms Bandage: 3" x 10 yards, 4" x 10 yards
Generic Available Yes

Zinc Gelatin Boot *see* Zinc Gelatin *on this page*
Zincon® Shampoo [OTC] *see* Pyrithione Zinc *on page 826*

Zinc Oxide *(zingk OKS ide)*

Therapeutic Category Topical Skin Product
Synonyms Base Ointment; Lassar's Zinc Paste
Use Protective coating for mild skin irritations and abrasions; soothing and protective ointment to promote healing of chapped skin, diaper rash
Usual Dosage Children and Adults: Topical: Apply as required for affected areas several times daily
Mechanism of Action Mild astringent with weak antiseptic properties
Local Anesthetic/Vasoconstrictor Precautions No information available to require special precautions

Effects on Dental Treatment No effects or complications reported
Other Adverse Effects 1% to 10%:
Dermatologic: Skin sensitivity
Local: Irritation
Generic Available Yes

Zinc Oxide, Cod Liver Oil, and Talc
(zingk OKS ide, kod LIV er oyl, & talk)
Brand Names Desitin® Topical [OTC]
Therapeutic Category Protectant, Topical
Use Relief of diaper rash, superficial wounds and burns, and other minor skin irritations
Usual Dosage Topical: Apply thin layer as needed
Local Anesthetic/Vasoconstrictor Precautions No information available to require special precautions
Effects on Dental Treatment No effects or complications reported
Other Adverse Effects 1% to 10%: Local: Skin sensitivity, irritation
Dosage Forms Ointment, topical: Zinc oxide, cod liver oil and talc in a petrolatum and lanolin base (30 g, 60 g, 120 g, 240 g, 270 g)
Generic Available Yes

Zinc Sulfate (zingk SUL fate)
Brand Names Eye-Sed® Ophthalmic [OTC]; Orazinc® Oral [OTC]; Verazinc® Oral [OTC]; Zincate® Oral
Therapeutic Category Electrolyte Supplement
Use Zinc supplement (oral and parenteral); may improve wound healing in those who are deficient
Usual Dosage
RDA: Oral:
Birth to 6 months: 3 mg elemental zinc/day
6-12 months: 5 mg elemental zinc/day
1-10 years: 10 mg elemental zinc/day
≥11 years: 15 mg elemental zinc/day

Zinc deficiency: Oral:
Infants and Children: 0.5-1 mg elemental zinc/kg/day divided 1-3 times/day; somewhat larger quantities may be needed if there is impaired intestinal absorption or an excessive loss of zinc
Adults: 110-220 mg zinc sulfate (25-50 mg elemental zinc)/dose 3 times/day
Local Anesthetic/Vasoconstrictor Precautions No information available to require special precautions
Effects on Dental Treatment No effects or complications reported
Pregnancy Risk Factor C
Dosage Forms
Capsule: 110 mg [elemental zinc 25 mg]; 220 mg [elemental zinc 50 mg]
Injection: 1 mg/mL (10 mL, 30 mL); 4 mg/mL (10 mL); 5 mg/mL (5 mL, 10 mL, 50 mL)
Tablet: 66 mg [elemental zinc 15 mg]; 200 mg [elemental zinc 46 mg]
Dietary Considerations May be administered with food if GI upset occurs; avoid foods high in calcium or phosphorus
Generic Available Yes

Zinc Sulfate *see* Zinc Supplements *on this page*

Zinc Supplements (zink)
Brand Names Eye-Sed® [OTC]; Orazinc® [OTC]; Verazinc® [OTC]; Zincate®
Therapeutic Category Mineral, Oral; Mineral, Parenteral; Trace Element
Synonyms Zinc Acetate; Zinc Sulfate
Use Cofactor for replacement therapy to different enzymes helps maintain normal growth rates, normal skin hydration and senses of taste and smell; zinc supplement (oral and parenteral); may improve wound healing in those who are deficient. May be useful to promote wound healing in patients with pressure sores.
Mechanism of Action Provides for normal growth and tissue repair, is a cofactor for more than 70 enzymes; ophthalmic astringent and weak antiseptic due to precipitation of protein and clearing mucus from outer surface of the eye
Local Anesthetic/Vasoconstrictor Precautions No information available to require special precautions
Effects on Dental Treatment No effects or complications reported
Other Adverse Effects <1%:
Cardiovascular: Hypotension
Gastrointestinal: Indigestion, nausea, vomiting
Hematologic: Neutropenia, leukopenia
(Continued)

Zinc Supplements *(Continued)*

Hepatic: Jaundice
Respiratory: Pulmonary edema

Drug Interactions
Decreased effect of zinc with dairy products; bran products and iron reduce absorption of zinc from GI tract
Zinc appears to inhibit the absorption of ciprofloxacin and tetracyclines by binding in GI tract. The absorption of doxycycline (Vibramycin®) is not affected by zinc.

Pregnancy Risk Factor C

Zinc Undecylenate *see* Undecylenic Acid and Derivatives *on page 977*

Zinecard® *see* Dexrazoxane *on page 295*

Zithromax™ *see* Azithromycin *on page 104*

ZNP® Bar [OTC] *see* Pyrithione Zinc *on page 826*

Zocor® *see* Simvastatin *on page 866*

Zofran™ *see* Ondansetron *on page 700*

Zoladex® Implant *see* Goserelin *on page 449*

Zolicef® *see* Cefazolin *on page 188*

Zolmitriptan *(zohl mi TRIP tan)*

Brand Names Zomig®
Therapeutic Category Antimigraine Agent; Serotonin Agonist
Synonyms 311C90
Use Acute treatment of adult migraine, with or without auras.
Usual Dosage Adults: Oral: Single doses of 1, 2.5 or 5 mg are effective in reducing symptoms of a migraine attack. Patients should be started at a dose of 2.5 mg or lower since the incidence of side effects increases somewhat with dose. If the headache returns, the dose may be repeated after 2 hours but NOT TO EXCEED 10 mg within a 24-hour period.
Mechanism of Action A selective 5-hydroxytryptamine (5-HT 1B/1D) receptor agonist. The drug binds tightly and specifically to this receptor. The current theory of migraine headaches suggests that symptoms are due to local cranial vasodilation or to the release of sensory neuropeptides through nerve endings in the trigeminal system. The activity of zolmitriptan can most likely be attributed to its agonist effects at the 5-HT 1B/1D receptors in intracranial blood vessels and sensory nerves, which results in cranial vessel constriction and the inhibition of pro-inflammatory neuropeptide release.
Local Anesthetic/Vasoconstrictor Precautions No information available to require special precautions
Effects on Dental Treatment No effects or complications reported
Dosage Forms Tablet: 2.5 mg, 5 mg
Comments Not intended for the prophylactic therapy of migraine or for use in the management of hemiplegic or basilar migraine. The safety and effectiveness of zolmitriptan for the treatment of cluster headache, have not been confirmed.

Zoloft™ *see* Sertraline *on page 863*

Zolpidem *(zole PI dem)*

Brand Names Ambien™
Therapeutic Category Hypnotic; Sedative
Use Short-term treatment of insomnia
Usual Dosage Duration of therapy should be limited to 7-10 days
Adults: Oral: 10 mg immediately before bedtime; maximum dose: 10 mg
Elderly: 5 mg immediately before bedtime

Not dialyzable
Dosing adjustment in hepatic impairment: Decrease dose to 5 mg
Mechanism of Action Structurally dissimilar to benzodiazepine, however, has much or all of its actions explained by its effects on benzodiazepine (BZD) receptors, especially the omega-1 receptor; retains hypnotic and much of the anxiolytic properties of the BZD, but has reduced effects on skeletal muscle and seizure threshold.
Local Anesthetic/Vasoconstrictor Precautions No information available to require special precautions
Effects on Dental Treatment No effects or complications reported
Other Adverse Effects
1% to 10%:
Central nervous system: Headache, drowsiness, dizziness
Gastrointestinal: Nausea, diarrhea
Neuromuscular & skeletal: Myalgia
<1%:
Central nervous system: Amnesia, confusion

Gastrointestinal: Vomiting
Neuromuscular & skeletal: Falls, tremor
Drug Interactions Increased effect/toxicity with alcohol, CNS depressants
Drug Uptake
Onset of action: 30 minutes
Duration: 6-8 hours
Absorption: Rapid
Serum half-life: 2-2.6 hours, in cirrhosis increased to 9.9 hours
Pregnancy Risk Factor B
Dosage Forms Tablet, as tartrate: 5 mg, 10 mg
Generic Available No

ORAL MEDICINE TOPICS

PART I.

DENTAL MANAGEMENT AND THERAPEUTIC
CONSIDERATIONS IN
MEDICALLY COMPROMISED PATIENTS

This section focuses on common medical conditions and their associated drug therapies with which the dentist must be familiar. Patient profiles with commonly associated drug regimens are described.

TABLE OF CONTENTS

CARDIOVASCULAR DISEASES

Cardiovascular disease is the most prevalent human disease affecting over 60 million Americans and this group of diseases accounts for more than 50% of all deaths in the United States. Surgical and pharmacologic therapy have resulted in many cardiovascular patients living healthy and profitable lives. Consequently, patients presenting to the dental office may require treatment planning modifications related to the medical management of their cardiovascular disease. For the purposes of this text, we will cover ischemic heart disease including angina pectoris and myocardial infarction, cardiac arrhythmias, congestive heart failure, and hypertension.

ISCHEMIC HEART DISEASE

Any long-term decrease in the delivery of oxygen to the heart muscle can lead to the condition ischemic heart disease. Often arteriosclerosis and atherosclerosis result in a narrowing of the coronary vessels' lumina and are the most common causes of vascular ischemic heart disease. Other causes such as previous infarct, mitral valve regurgitation, and ruptured septa may also lead to ischemia in the heart muscle. The two most common major conditions that result from ischemic heart disease are angina pectoris and myocardial infarction. Sudden death, a third category, can likewise result from ischemia.

To the physician, the most common presenting sign or symptom of ischemic heart disease is chest pain. This chest pain can be of a transient nature as in angina pectoris or the result of a myocardial infarction. It is now believed that sudden death represents a separate occurrence that essentially involves the development of a lethal cardiac arrhythmia or coronary artery spasm leading to an acute shutdown of the heart muscle blood supply. Risk factors in patients for coronary atherosclerosis include cigarette smoking, elevated blood lipids, hypertension, as well as diabetes mellitus, age, and gender (male).

Lipid-lowering and cholesterol-lowering drugs including atorvastatin, cholestyramine, colestipol, fluvastatin, gemfibrozil, lovastatin, nicotinic acid, pravastatin, probucol, and simvastatin (seen in the following list) have become standard treatments for patients with developing atherosclerosis in an attempt to lower blood cholesterol and thereby, indirectly reduce the risk of ischemia heart disease.

Lipid-Lowering Drugs

Cholestyramine Resin (Prevalite®, Questran®) *on page 229*
Clofibrate (Atromid-S®) *on page 246*
Colestipol (Colestid®) *on page 258*
Dextrothyroxine (Choloxin®) *on page 299*
Fenofibrate (Lipidil®, Tricor®) *on page 396*
Gemfibrozil (Lopid®) *on page 439*
Niacin (Nicotinic Acid) *on page 676*
Probucol (Lorelco®) *on page 796*

HMG-CoA Reductase Inhibitors

Atorvastatin (Lipitor®) *on page 97*
Cerivastatin (Baycol®) *on page 204*
Fluvastatin (Lescol®) *on page 425*
Lovastatin (Mevacor®) *on page 570*
Pravastatin (Pravachol®) *on page 785*
Simvastatin (Zocor™) *on page 866*

ANGINA PECTORIS

Angina pectoris is a symptomatic manifestation of ischemic heart disease characterized by thoracic pain resulting from oxygen deprivation to the heart muscle. Often metabolites build up in the vessels and the muscle tissue leading to the pain. Occasionally, the pain can radiate to the left arm or to the jaw. The pain is often midsternal and usually described as an extreme pressure sensation, not unlike an elephant sitting on one's chest (which we have all undoubtedly experienced). Three forms of angina pectoris are usually recognized. Stable angina includes chest pain that predictably is precipitated by overexertion, cold, or overactivity. Unstable angina pectoris usually is defined as a recent change in pattern of occurrence, usually a decreased threshold of stimulus and an unpredictable response to the major drug of choice, nitroglycerin. Prinzmetal's angina or variant angina often occurs due to spasm in a single large coronary artery and may have a cardiac dysrhythmia associated with it. Regardless of the type of angina pectoris, treatment includes control of risk factors, reducing oxygen demand to the myocardium, and increasing coronary blood flow.

The most common antianginal drugs fall into three categories. Nitrates are first-line drugs in the management of angina and include oral nitrate tablets or capsules. Nitrates can also be available as transcutaneous patches and are available in solution for I.V. administration. Beta-adrenergic blockers, the second category, are often used when a patient's angina responds poorly to nitrates.

Calcium channel blockers are also indicated for angina related to coronary vessel spasm with or without atherosclerosis. These drugs inhibit calcium ion passage through the slow channels of cell membranes. They tend to be used alone or in combination with nitrates and beta-blockers.

Selected antianginal drugs include:

Nitrates

> Erythrityl Tetranitrate (Cardilate®) *on page 361*
> Isosorbide Dinitrate (Dilitrate®-SR; Isordil®; Sorbitrate®) *on page 525*
> Isosorbide Mononitrate (Imdur®; Ismo™; Monoket®) *on page 526*
> Nitroglycerin (various products) *on page 685*
> Pentaerythritol Tetranitrate (Duotrate®; Peritrate®) *on page 735*

Beta-Adrenergic Blockers

> Atenolol (Tenormin®) *on page 95*
> Betaxolol (Betoptic®, Kerlone®) *on page 127*
> Bisoprolol (Zebeta®) *on page 133*
> Carteolol (Cartrol®; Ocupress®) *on page 182*
> Nadolol (Corgard®) *on page 657*
> Propranolol (Betachron E-R®; Inderal®) *on page 814*
> Sotalol (Betapace®) *on page 878*
> Timolol (Blocadren®) *on page 935*

Calcium Channel Blockers

> Amlodipine (Norvasc®) *on page 63*
> Bepridil (Vascor®) *on page 124*
> Diltiazem (Cardizem®, Dilacor™ XR) *on page 318*
> Nicardipine (Cardene®) *on page 677*
> Nifedipine (Adalat®; Procardia®) *on page 680*
> Verapamil (Calan®; Covera-HS®; Isoptin®; Verelan®) *on page 987*

The dental management of the patient with angina pectoris may include: sedation techniques for complicated procedures (see "Patients Requiring Sedation" *on page 1081*), to limit the extent of procedures, and to limit the use of local anesthesia containing 1:100,000 epinephrine to two carpules. Anesthesia without vasoconstrictor might also be selected. The appropriate use of vasoconstrictor in anesthesia, however, should be weighed against the necessity to maximize anesthesia. Please see "Management of Office Emergencies" *on page 1103*. Complete history and appropriate referral and consultation with the patient's physician for those patients who are known to be at risk for angina pectoris is recommended.

MYOCARDIAL INFARCTION

Myocardial infarction is the leading cause of death in the United States. It is an acute irreversible ischemic event that produces an area of myocardial necrosis in the heart tissue. If a patient has a previous history of myocardial infarction, he/she may be taking a variety of drugs (ie, antihypertensives, lipid lowering drugs, ACE inhibitors, and antianginal medications) to not only prevent a second infarct, but to treat the long-term associated ischemic heart disease. Postmyocardial infarction patients are often taking anticoagulants such as warfarin and antiplatelet agents such as aspirin. Consultation with the prescribing physician by the dentist is necessary prior to invasive procedures. Temporary dose reduction may allow the dentist to proceed with most procedures.

> Aspirin (various products) *on page 90*
> Warfarin (Coumadin®) *on page 997*

Thrombolytic drugs, that might dissolve hemostatic plugs, may also be given on a short-term basis immediately following an infarct and include:

> Alteplase (Activase®) *on page 45*
> Anistreplase (Eminase®) *on page 79*
> Streptokinase (Kabikinase®; Streptase®) *on page 884*
> Urokinase (Abbokinase®) *on page 979*

CARDIOVASCULAR DISEASES *(Continued)*

Alteplase is also currently in use for acute myocardial infarction. Following myocardial infarction and rehabilitation, outpatients may be placed on anticoagulants (such as coumadin), diuretics, beta-adrenergic blockers, ACE inhibitors to reduce blood pressure, and calcium-channel blockers. Depending on the presence or absence of continued angina pectoris, patients may also be taking nitrates, beta-blockers, or calcium-channel blockers as indicated for treatment of angina.

BETA-ADRENERGIC BLOCKING AGENTS CATEGORIZED ACCORDING TO SPECIFIC PROPERTIES

Alpha-Adrenergic Blocking Activity
Labetalol (Normodyne®, Trandate®) *on page 537*

Intrinsic Sympathomimetic Activity
Acebutolol (Sectral®) *on page 19*
Pindolol (Visken®) *on page 763*

Long Duration of Action and Fewer CNS Effects
Acebutolol (Sectral®) *on page 19*
Atenolol (Tenormin®) *on page 95*
Betaxolol (Kerlone®) *on page 127*
Nadolol (Corgard®) *on page 657*

Beta$_1$-Receptor Selectivity
Acebutolol (Sectral®) *on page 19*
Atenolol (Tenormin®) *on page 95*
Metoprolol (Lopressor®, Toprol XL®) *on page 629*

Non-Selective (blocks both beta$_1$ and beta$_2$ receptors)
Betaxolol (Kerlone®) *on page 127*
Labetalol (Normodyne®, Trandate®) *on page 537*
Nadolol (Corgard®) *on page 657*
Pindolol (Visken®) *on page 763*
Propranolol (Inderal®) *on page 814*
Timolol (Blocadren®) *on page 935*

ARRHYTHMIAS

Abnormal cardiac rhythm can develop spontaneously and survivors of a myocardial infarction are often left with an arrhythmia. An arrhythmia is any alteration or disturbance in the normal rate, rhythm, or conduction through the cardiac tissue. This is known as a cardiac arrhythmia. Abnormalities in rhythm can occur in either the atria or the ventricles. Various valvular deformities, drug effects, and chemical derangements can initiate arrhythmias. These arrhythmias can be a slowing of the heart rate (<60 beats/minute) as defined in bradycardia or tachycardia resulting in a rapid heart beat (usually >150 beats/minute). The dentist will encounter a variety of treatments for management of arrhythmias. Usually, underlying causes such as reduced cardiac output, hypertension, and irregular ventricular beats will require treatment. Pacemaker therapy is also sometimes used. Indwelling pacemakers may require supplementation with antibiotics, and consultation with the physician is certainly appropriate. Sinus tachycardia is often treated with drugs such as:

Propranolol (Betachron ER®; Inderal®) *on page 814*
Quinidine (Cardioquin®; Quinaglute®; Quinalan®; Quinidex®;
Quinora®) *on page 830*

Beta-blockers are often used to slow cardiac rate and diazepam may be helpful when anxiety is a contributing factor in arrhythmia. When atrial flutter and atrial fibrillation are diagnosed, digitalis preparations such as digitoxin and digoxin are the drugs of choice.

Digitoxin (Crystodigin®) *on page 312*
Digoxin (Lanoxin®) *on page 313*

ANTICOAGULANT THERAPY

Patients postmyocardial infarction and those with atrial fibrillation are also frequently placed on anticoagulants such as Coumadin®. (See Myocardial Infarction Section on previous page.)

Large numbers of patients are receiving oral anticoagulation therapy. The dental clinician is often faced with the decision as to how to manage these patients prior to invasive dental procedures. Key factors regarding the patient receiving anticoagulant therapy include: what is the bleeding risk of the procedure planned? what are the clotting risks (ie, can the medication management be safely altered?) and what is the patient's current anticoagulant therapy level in terms of bleeding measurements (ie, laboratory evaluations) and their prognosis?

Most patients receiving anticoagulant therapy are on one of two regimens. Warfarin, under the name Coumadin®, is the most common long-term outpatient anticoagulant given. Many patients, however, are also on aspirin products to achieve some level of anticoagulation. The mechanisms of the action of these two drugs are different and it is important that the clinician be aware of the appropriate tests and the appropriate time relative to treatment selection.

Partial thromboplastin time and bleeding time (IVY) are appropriate measures for platelet dysfunction. Aspirin and the new drug Clopidogrel (Plavix®) are actually considered antiplatelet drugs, whereas oral Coumadin® is considered an oral anticoagulant. Aspirin works by inhibiting cyclo-oxygenase which is an enzyme involved in the platelet system associated with clot formation. As little as one aspirin (300 mg dose) can result in an alteration in this enzyme pathway. Although aspirin is cleared from the circulation very quickly (within 15-30 minutes), the effect on the life of the platelet may last for up to 7-10 days. Therefore, the clinician planning an invasive procedure on patients with antiplatelet therapy may wish to consider a change prior to one week before the invasive treatment.

The effects of Coumadin® on the coagulation within patients, occur by way of the vitamin K-dependent clotting mechanism and are generally monitored by measuring the prothrombin time known as the PT. Often to prevent venous thrombosis, a patient will be maintained at approximately 1.5 times their normal prothrombin time. Other anticoagulant goals such as prevention of arterial thromboembolism, as in patients with artificial heart valves, may require 2-2.5 times the normal prothrombin time. It is important for the clinician to obtain not only the accurate PT but also the International Normalized Ratio (INR) for the patient. This ratio is calculated by dividing the patient's PT by the mean normal PT for the laboratory, which is determined by using the International Sensitivity Index (ISI) to adjust for the lab's reagents.

The response to oral anticoagulants varies greatly in patients and should be monitored regularly. The dental clinician planning an invasive procedure should consider not only what the patient can tell them from a historical point-of-view, but also when the last monitoring test was performed. In general, most dental procedures can be performed in patients that are 1.5 times normal or less. Some textbooks even suggest that 2 times normal would pose little risk in most dental patients and procedures, but these values may be misleading unless the INR is also determined. When in doubt, the prudent dental clinician would consult with the patients physician and obtain current prothrombin time in order to evaluate fully and plan for his patients. The clinician is referred to the excellent review: Herman WW, Konzelman JL, and Sutley SH, "Current Perspectives on Dental Patients Receiving Coumadin Anticoagulant Therapy," *J Am Dent Assoc*, 1997, 128:327-35.

Aspirin (various products) *on page 90*
Clopidogrel (Plavix®) *on page 251*
Warfarin (Coumadin®) *on page 997*

The basis for anticoagulation therapy is that mitral stenosis may be the result of the long-term arrhythmia and there is concern over the possibility of stroke. Ventricular dysrhythmias are often treated with drugs such as quinidine, procainamide, lidocaine, beta-adrenergic agents, and calcium channel blockers. Quinidine is used for selected arrhythmias. Lidocaine is often used when there are ventricular dysrhythmias. Procainamide (Pronestyl®) or flecainide (Tambocor®) are alternative agents.

CLASSIFICATION OF ANTIARRHYTHMIC DRUGS

Supraventricular

Digitoxin (digitalis) (Crystodigin®) *on page 312*
Digoxin (Lanoxin®) *on page 313*

Supraventricular and Ventricular

Acebutolol (Sectral®) *on page 19*
Adenosine (Adenocard®) *on page 33*
Amiodarone (Cordarone®) *on page 58*
Atenolol (Tenormin®) *on page 95*
Bepridil (Vascor®) *on page 124*

CARDIOVASCULAR DISEASES *(Continued)*

Bisoprolol (Zebeta®) *on page 133*
Bretylium (Bretylol®) *on page 138*
Diltiazem (Cardizem®; Dilacor™ XR) *on page 318*
Disopyramide (Norpace®) *on page 327*
Encainide (Enkaid®) *on page 348*
Flecainide (Tambocor®) *on page 407*
Lidocaine (Xylocaine®) *on page 553*
Mexiletine (Mexitil®) *on page 633*
Moricizine (Ethmozine®) *on page 648*
Nicardipine (Cardene®) *on page 677*
Phenytoin (Dilantin®) *on page 756*
Procainamide (Pronestyl®) *on page 796*
Propafenone (Rythmol®) *on page 806*
Propranolol (Inderal®) *on page 814*
Quinidine (Cardioquin®; Quinaglute®; Quinalan®; Quinidex®;
Quinora®) *on page 830*
Sotalol (Betapace®) *on page 878*
Tocainide (Tonocard®) *on page 939*
Verapamil (Calan®, Isoptin®) *on page 987*

Treatment of arrhythmias often can result in oral manifestations including oral ulcerations with drugs such as procainamide, lupus-like lesions, as well as xerostomia.

CONGESTIVE HEART FAILURE

Congestive heart failure is a clinical disease that occurs when the heart muscle gradually fails to deliver adequate oxygenated blood to the tissues. The chronically failing heart will attempt to compensate by three physiologic mechanisms: enlargement, increased heart rate, or dilatation. As the congestive heart failure becomes more profound, myocardial contractility diminishes and sodium and water retention increase leading to edema in the peripheral extremities. Edema is commonly seen in the patient with congestive heart failure. The failure of the heart may be right sided, left sided, or both. The treatment of congestive heart failure is usually rest with increased oxygenation.

The long-term treatment is to attempt to increase the strength and efficiency of the heart contractions, to avoid arrhythmias, and to reduce retention of water and sodium. Digitalis is one of the primary drugs used in treatment of congestive heart failure. It is usually prescribed in small doses and is coupled with diuretics and/or angiotensin-converting enzyme (ACE) inhibitors to decrease water retention. Nitrates and hydralazine are often given to patients with acute heart failure. The dentist may find that the patient is well compensated; however, treatment of CHF represents a complicated pharmacologic pattern necessary to be analyzed. Consultation with the managing physician regarding the patient's stability is recommended. Clinical signs of congestive heart failure might include distended neck veins, peripheral edema, and a ruddy complexion. Beta-blockers are now being approved for CHF, as well as hypertension

Digitoxin (Crystodigin®) *on page 312*
Digoxin (Lanoxin®) *on page 313*

Angiotensin-Converting Enzyme Inhibitors

Captopril (Capoten®) *on page 170*
Enalapril (Vasotec®) *on page 346*
Fosinopril (Monopril®) *on page 431*
Lisinopril (Prinivil®) *on page 560*
Quinapril (Accupril®) *on page 827*
Ramipril (Altace™) *on page 834*
Trandolapril (Mavik®) *on page 949*

Combined Alpha- and Beta-Adrenergic Blocking Agent

Carvedilol (Coreg®) *on page 183*

Direct-Acting Vasodilators

Hydralazine (Apresoline®) *on page 475*

Nitrates

Erythrityl Tetranitrate (Cardilate®) *on page 361*
Isosorbide Dinitrate (Dilitrate®-SR, Isordil®, Sorbitrate®) *on page 525*
Isosorbide Mononitrate (Imdur®; Ismo™; Monoket®) *on page 526*
Nitroglycerin (various products) *on page 685*
Pentaerythritol Tetranitrate (Duotrate®; Peritrate®) *on page 735*

HYPERTENSION

Adult blood pressure is usually measured in millimeters of mercury and represents systolic pressure that is exerted as the blood flows through the artery during a beat of the heart and the diastolic pressure when the blood is at rest between heart beats. Pulse pressure is a term commonly used and refers to the pressure difference between systolic and diastolic. Hypertension is a sustained elevated systolic or diastolic blood pressure (SBP and DBP). The definitions of elevated blood pressure and a referral scheme can be found in the following tables.

CLASSIFICATION OF BLOOD PRESSURE FOR ADULTS ≥18 YEARS OF AGE

Average DBP mm Hg	Average SBP mm Hg			
	<120	120-129	130-139	≥140
<80	Optimal*	Normal	High Normal	High
80-84	Normal	Normal	High Normal	High
85-89	High Normal	High Normal	High Normal	High
≥90	High	High	High	High

*Optimal blood pressure, with regard to cardiovascular risk, is SBP <120 mm Hg and DBP <80 mm Hg. However, unusually low readings should be evaluated for clinical significance.

Adapted from the *Joint National Committee Report*, October, 1992.

Category	Systolic (mm Hg)	Diastolic (mm Hg)	Category
Isolated systolic hypertension	>160	>120	Severe hypertension
Borderline systolic hypertension	140-159	105-120	Moderate hypertension
		90-104	Mild hypertension
Normal	<140	<90	Normal

Diastolic		
<85	Recheck at recall (within 2 years)	No restriction
85-89	Recheck at recall (within 1 year)	No restrictions
90-99	Recheck within 2 months; if still elevated, refer to physician promptly	No restrictions
100-109	Refer promptly to physician (within 1 month)	Limited elective care or emergency care
110-119	Refer promptly to physician (within 1 week)	Limited elective care or emergency care
≥120	Immediate referral to physician	Emergency care only
Systolic		
<140	Recheck at recall (within 2 years)	No restrictions
140-199	Recheck within 2 months; if still elevated, refer to physician promptly (within 2 months)	No restrictions
≥200	Refer promptly to physician	Limited elective care or emergency care

Generally, peripheral vascular resistance, intravascular fluid volume, and cardiac output determine the blood pressure of a patient. Selection of therapies for patients being treated for prolonged elevated blood pressure is generally dependent upon the severity of the condition, age, and the pharmacological stability related to other cardiac diseases. Nonpharmacologic management of the patient with elevated sustained blood pressure begins with diet restriction, avoidance of fatty foods, an exercise program, reduction in sodium intake, and cessation of smoking. If there is an inadequate response, pharmacologic management usually begins with a diuretic or a beta-adrenergic receptor blocker.

ACE inhibitors, calcium channel blockers, alpha-adrenergic blockers are currently gaining popularity as early treatment modalities, however, data on these agents reducing long-term morbidity and mortality are only now being published. If there is an inadequate response to these drugs, practitioners often increase drug dosage, substitute another drug, or add a second agent from a different class. If there is still

CARDIOVASCULAR DISEASES *(Continued)*

inadequate response, a second or third agent can be added, along with a diuretic if one has not already been utilized. Different combinations of drugs are often used in treating African-American patients.

When given in combination, these drugs can create not only side effects including xerostomia and oral ulcerations, but profound reduction in blood pressure. The new drug classifications Angiotensin Receptor Antagonists and T-type Calcium Channel Blockers are having new drugs approved regularly and are showing promise as alternative therapies. The 1992 Report of the Joint National Commission on Detection, Evaluation, and Treatment of High Blood Pressure is being re-evaluated and it is hopeful that new guidelines will be released in a 1997 or early 1998 Commission Report.

CLASSIFICATION OF ANTIHYPERTENSIVES

DIURETICS

Thiazide-Type

Bendroflumethiazide (Naturetin®) *on page 116*
Benzthiazide (Exna®) *on page 122*
Chlorothiazide (Diurigen®, Diuril®) *on page 215*
Chlorthalidone (Hygroton®) *on page 227*
Hydrochlorothiazide (Esidrix®) *on page 476*
Hydroflumethiazide (Diucardin®; Saluron®) *on page 485*
Indapamide (Lozol®) *on page 504*
Methyclothiazide (Aquatensen®, Enduron®) *on page 620*
Metolazone (Mykrox®, Zaroxolyn®) *on page 629*
Polythiazide (Renese®) *on page 773*
Quinethazone (Hydromox®) *on page 829*
Trichlormethiazide (Metahydrin®; Naqua®) *on page 958*

Loop

Bumetanide (Bumex®) *on page 147*
Ethacrynic Acid (Edecrin®) *on page 371*
Furosemide (Lasix®) *on page 434*
Torsemide (Demadex®) *on page 946*

Potassium-Sparing

Amiloride (Midamor®) *on page 53*
Spironolactone (Aldactone®) *on page 881*
Triamterene (Dyrenium®) *on page 956*

Potassium-Sparing Combinations

Hydrochlorothiazide and Spironolactone (Aldactazide®; Alazide®; Spironazide®; Spirozide®) *on page 477*
Hydrochlorothiazide and Triamterene (Dyazide®; Maxzide®) *on page 478*

ADRENERGIC INHIBITORS

Noncardioselective Beta-Adrenergic Blockers

Carteolol (Cartrol®, Ocupress®) *on page 182*
Carvedilol (Coreg®) *on page 183*
Nadolol (Corgard®) *on page 657*
Penbutolol (Levatol®) *on page 729*
Pindolol (Visken®) *on page 763*
Propranolol (Inderal®) *on page 814*
Timolol (Blocadren®) *on page 935*

Cardioselective Beta-Adrenergic Blockers

Acebutolol (Sectral®) *on page 19*
Atenolol (Tenormin®) *on page 95*
Betaxolol (Kerlone®) *on page 127*
Bisoprolol (Zebeta™) *on page 133*
Metoprolol (Lopressor®, Toprol XL®) *on page 629*
Sotalol (Betapace®) *on page 878*

Combined Alpha- and Beta-Adrenergic Blockers

Carvedilol (Coreg®) *on page 183*
Labetalol (Normodyne®, Trandate®) *on page 537*

Alpha-Adrenergic Blockers - Peripheral-Acting (Alpha₁-Blockers)

Doxazosin (Cardura®) *on page 334*
Guanadrel (Hylorel®) *on page 457*

Alpha-Adrenergic Blockers - Central-Acting (Alpha$_2$-Agonists)

VASODILATORS

Direct-Acting

Angiotensin-Converting Enzyme Inhibitors

Angiotensin-Converting Enzyme Inhibitors Combinations

Calcium Channel Blockers

T-Type Calcium Channel Blockers

Angiotensin Receptor Antagonists

The most common oral side effects of the management of the hypertensive patient are related to the antihypertensive drug therapy. A dry sore mouth can be caused by diuretics and central-acting adrenergic inhibitors. Occasionally, lichenoid reactions can occur in patients taking quinidine and methyldopa. The thiazides are occasionally also implicated. Lupus-like face rashes can be seen in patients taking calcium channel blockers as well as documented gingival hyperplasia in Appendix; see listing below.

Calcium Channel Blockers & Gingival Hyperplasia *on page 1132*

RESPIRATORY DISEASES

Diseases of the respiratory system put dental patients at increased risk in the dental office because of their decreased pulmonary reserve, the medications they may be taking, drug interactions between these medications, medications the dentist may prescribe, and in some patients with infectious respiratory diseases, a risk of disease transmission.

The respiratory system consists of the nasal cavity, the nasopharynx, the trachea, and the components of the lung including, of course, the bronchi, the bronchioles, and the alveoli. The diseases that affect the lungs and the respiratory system can be separated by location of affected tissue. Diseases that affect the lower respiratory tract are often chronic, although infections can also occur. Three major diseases that affect the lower respiratory tract are often encountered in the medical history for dental patients. These include chronic bronchitis, emphysema, and asthma. Diseases that affect the upper respiratory tract are usually of the infectious nature and include sinusitis and the common cold. The upper respiratory tract infections may also include a wide variety of nonspecific infections, most of which are also caused by viruses. Influenza produces upper respiratory type symptoms and is often caused by orthomyxoviruses. Herpangina is caused by the Coxsackie type viruses and results in upper respiratory infections in addition to pharyngitis or sore throat. One serious condition, known as croup, has been associated with *Haemophilus influenzae* infections. Other more serious infections might include respiratory syncytial virus, adenoviruses, and parainfluenza viruses.

The respiratory symptoms that are often encountered in both upper respiratory and lower respiratory disorders include cough, dyspnea (difficulty in breathing), the production of sputum, hemoptysis (coughing up blood), a wheeze, and occasionally chest pain. One additional symptom, orthopnea (difficulty in breathing when lying down) is often used by the dentist to assist in evaluating the patient with the condition, pulmonary edema. This condition results from either respiratory disease or congestive heart failure.

No effective drug treatments are available for the management of many of the upper respiratory tract viral infections. However, amantadine (sold under the brand name Symmetrel®) is a synthetic drug given orally (200 mg/day) and has been found to be effective against some strains of influenza. Treatment other than for influenza includes supportive care products available over the counter. These might include antihistamines for symptomatic relief of the upper respiratory congestion, antibiotics to combat secondary bacterial infections, and in severe cases, fluids when patients have become dehydrated during the illness (see Therapeutic Category Index for selection). The treatment of herpangina may include management of the painful ulcerations of the oropharynx. The dentist may become involved in managing these lesions in a similar way to those seen in other acute viral infections (see Viral Infection section).

SINUSITIS

Sinusitis also represents an upper respiratory infection that often comes under the purview of the practicing dentist. Acute sinusitis characterized by nasal obstruction, fever, chills, and midface head pain may be encountered by the dentist and discovered as part of a differential work-up for other facial or dental pain. Chronic sinusitis may likewise produce similar dental symptoms. Dental drugs of choice may include ephedrine or nasal drops, antihistamines, and analgesics. These drugs sometimes require supplementation with antibiotics. Most commonly, broad spectrum antibiotics, such as ampicillin, are prescribed. These are often combined with antral lavage to re-establish drainage from the sinus area. Surgical intervention such as a Caldwell-Luc procedure opening into the sinus is rarely necessary and many of the second generation antibiotics such as cephalosporins are used successfully in treating the acute and chronic sinusitis patient (see "Antibiotic Prophylaxis" *on page 1034*).

LOWER RESPIRATORY DISEASES

Lower respiratory tract diseases, including asthma, chronic bronchitis, and emphysema are often identified in dental patients. Asthma is an intermittent respiratory disorder that produces recurrent bronchial smooth muscle spasm, inflammation, swelling of the bronchial mucosa, and hypersecretion of mucus. The incidence of childhood asthma appears to be increasing and may be related to the presence of pollutants such as sulfur dioxide and indoor cigarette smoke. The end result is widespread narrowing of the airways and decreased ventilation with increased airway resistance, especially to expiration. Asthmatic patients often suffer from asthmatic attacks when stimulated by respiratory tract infections, exercise, and cold air. Medications such as aspirin and some nonsteroidal anti-inflammatory agents as well as cholinergic and beta-adrenergic blocking drugs, can also trigger asthmatic attacks in addition to chemicals, smoke, and emotional anxiety.

The classical chronic obstructive pulmonary diseases (COPD) of chronic bronchitis and emphysema are both characterized by chronic airflow obstructions during normal ventilatory efforts. They often occur in combination in the same patient and their treatment is similar. One common finding is that the patient is often a smoker. The dentist can play a role in reinforcement of smoking cessation in patients with chronic respiratory diseases.

Treatments include a variety of drugs depending on the severity of the symptoms and the respiratory compromise upon full respiratory evaluation. Patients who are having acute and chronic obstructive pulmonary attacks may be susceptible to infection and antibiotics such as penicillin, ampicillin, tetracycline, or trimethoprim-sulfamethoxazole are often used to eradicate susceptible infective organisms. Corticosteroids, as well as a wide variety of respiratory stimulants, are available in inhalant and/or oral forms. In patients using inhalant medication, oral candidiasis is occasionally encountered.

Amantadine (Symmetrel®) *on page 50*
Analgesics *on page 1231*
Antibiotics *on page 1236*
Antihistamines *on page 1242*
Decongestants *on page 1252*
Epinephrine (Dental) (Sus-Phrine®) *on page 353*

SPECIFIC DRUGS USED IN THE TREATMENT OF CHRONIC RESPIRATORY CONDITIONS

Beta$_2$-Selective

Albuterol (Proventil®,Ventolin®) *on page 35*
Bitolterol (Tornalate®) *on page 134*
Isoetharine (Bronkosol®, Bronkometer®) *on page 521*
Metaproterenol (Alupent®) *on page 605*
Pirbuterol (Maxair™) *on page 766*
Salmeterol (Serevent®) *on page 854*
Terbutaline (Brethine®, Brethaire®) *on page 908*

Methylxanthines

Aminophylline (Somophylline®) *on page 56*
Oxtriphylline (Choledyl®) *on page 708*
Theophylline (Theo-Dur®, Slo-Bid®) *on page 917*

Mast Cell Stabilizer

Cromolyn Sodium (Intal®) *on page 264*
Nedocromil Sodium (Tilade®) *on page 668*

Corticosteroids

Beclomethasone (Beclovent®, Vanceril®) *on page 112*
Dexamethasone (Decadron® phosphate Respihaler®) *on page 291*
Flunisolide (AeroBid®; Nasarel®) *on page 413*
Fluticasone (Flovent®) *on page 424*
Mometasone Furoate (Nasonex®) *on page 646*
Prednisone (Deltasone®; Liquid Pred®; Meticorten®; Prednicen-M®; Sterapred®) *on page 789*
Triamcinolone (Azmacort™) *on page 954*

Anticholinergics

Ipratropium (Atrovent®) *on page 517*

Leukotriene Receptor Antagonists

Zafirlukast (Accolate®) *on page 1000*

5-Lipoxygenase Inhibitors

Zileuton (Zyflo®) *on page 1003*

Other respiratory diseases include tuberculosis and sarcoidosis which are considered to be restrictive granulomatous respiratory diseases. Tuberculosis is covered in "Nonviral Infectious Diseases" *on page 1032*. Sarcoidosis is a condition that at one time was thought to be similar to tuberculosis, however, it is a multisystem disorder of unknown origin which has as a characteristic lymphocytic and mononuclear phagocytic accumulation in epithelioid granulomas within the lung. It occurs worldwide but shows a slight increased prevalence in temperate climates. The

RESPIRATORY DISEASES *(Continued)*

treatment of sarcoidosis is usually one that corresponds to its usually benign course, however, many patients are placed on corticosteroids at the level of 40-60 mg of prednisone daily. This treatment is continued for a protracted period of time. As in any disease requiring steroid therapy, consideration of adrenal suppression is necessary. Alteration of steroid dosage prior to stressful dental procedures may be necessary, usually increasing the steroid dosage prior to and during the stressful procedures and then gradually returning the patient to the original dosage over several days. Even in the absence of evidence of adrenal suppression, consultation with the prescribing physician for appropriate dosing and timing of procedures is advisable.

Prednisone *on page 789*

RELATIVE POTENCY OF ENDOGENOUS AND SYNTHETIC CORTICOSTEROIDS

Agent	Equivalent Dose (mg)
Short-Acting (8-12 h)	
Cortisol	20
Cortisone	25
Intermediate-Acting (18-36 h)	
Prednisolone	5
Prednisone	5
Methylprednisolone	4
Triamcinolone	4
Long-Acting (36-54 h)	
Betamethasone	0.75
Dexamethasone	0.75

Potential drug interactions for the respiratory disease patient exist. An acute sensitivity to aspirin-containing drugs and some of the nonsteroidal anti-inflammatory drugs is a threat for the asthmatic patient. Barbiturates and narcotics may occasionally precipitate asthmatic attacks as well. Erythromycin, clarithromycin, and ketoconazole are contraindicated in patients who are taking theophylline due to potential enhancement of theophylline toxicity. Patients that are taking steroid preparations as part of their respiratory therapy may require alteration in dosing prior to stressful dental procedures. The physician should be consulted.

Barbiturates *on page 1248*
Clarithromycin *on page 241*
Erythromycin *on page 361*
Ketoconazole *on page 533*

ENDOCRINE DISORDERS & PREGNANCY

The human endocrine system manages metabolism and homeostasis. Numerous glandular tissues produce hormones that act in broad reactions with tissues throughout the body. Cells in various organ systems may be sensitive to the hormone, or they release, in reaction to the hormone, a second hormone that acts directly on another organ. Diseases of the endocrine system may have importance in dentistry. For the purposes of this section, we will limit our discussion to diseases of the thyroid tissues, diabetes mellitus, and conditions requiring the administration of synthetic hormones, and pregnancy.

THYROID

Thyroid diseases can be classified into conditions that cause the thyroid to be overactive (hyperthyroidism) and those that cause the thyroid to be underactive (hypothyroidism). Clinical signs and symptoms associated with hyperthyroidism may include goiter, heat intolerance, tremor, weight loss, diarrhea, and hyperactivity. Thyroid hormone production can be tested by TSH levels and additional screens may include radioactive iodine uptake or a pre-T_4 (tetraiodothyronine, thyroxine) assay or iodine index or total serum T_3 (triiodothyronine). The results of thyroid function tests may be altered by ingestion of antithyroid drugs such as propylthiouracil, estrogen-containing drugs, and organic and inorganic iodides. When a diagnosis of hyperthyroidism has been made, treatment usually begins with antithyroid drugs which may include propranolol coupled with radioactive iodides as well as surgical procedures to reduce thyroid tissue. Generally, the beta-blockers are used to control cardiovascular effects of excessive T_4. Propylthiouracil or methimazole are the most common antithyroid drugs used. The dentist should be aware that epinephrine is definitely contraindicated in patients with uncontrolled hyperthyroidism.

Diseases and conditions associated with hypothyroidism may include bradycardia, drowsiness, cold intolerance, thick dry skin, and constipation. Treatment of hypothyroidism is generally with replacement thyroid hormone until a euthyroid state is achieved. Various preparations are available, the most common is levothyroxine, commonly known as Synthroid® or Levothroid® and is generally the drug of choice for thyroid replacement therapy.

Drugs to Treat Hypothyroidism

> Levothyroxine (Levothroid®, Synthroid®) *on page 552*
> Liothyronine (Cytomel®, Triostat™) *on page 558*
> Liotrix (Thyrolar®) *on page 559*
> Thyroid (Armour® Thyroid, S-P-T, Thyrar®, Thyroid Strong®) *on page 930*

Drugs to Treat Hyperthyroidism

> Methimazole (Tapazole®) *on page 612*
> Potassium Iodide (Pima®, SSKI®, Thyro-Block®) *on page 781*
> Propranolol (Betachron E-R®, Inderal®) *on page 814*
> Propylthiouracil *on page 816*

DIABETES

Diabetes mellitus refers to a condition of prolonged hyperglycemia associated with either abnormal production or lack of production of insulin. Commonly known as Type 1 diabetes, insulin-dependent diabetes (IDDM) is a condition where there are absent or deficient levels of circulating insulin therefore triggering tissue reactions associated with prolonged hyperglycemia. The kidney's attempt to excrete the excess glucose and the organs that do not receive adequate glucose essentially are damaged. Small vessels and arterial vessels in the eye, kidney, and brain are usually at the greatest risk. Generally, blood sugar levels between 70-120 mg/dL are considered to be normal. Inadequate insulin levels allow glucose to rise to greater than the renal threshold which is 180 mg/dL, and such elevations prolonged lead to organ damage.

The goals of treatment of the diabetic are to maintain metabolic control of the blood glucose levels and to reduce the morbid effects of periodic hyperglycemia. Insulin therapy is the primary mechanism to attain management of consistent insulin levels. Insulin preparations are categorized according to their duration of action. Generally, NPH or intermediate-acting insulin and long-acting insulin can be used in combination with short-acting or regular insulin to maintain levels consistent throughout the day.

ENDOCRINE DISORDERS & PREGNANCY *(Continued)*

In Type 2 or noninsulin-dependent diabetes (NIDDM), the receptor for insulin in the tissues is generally down regulated and the glucose, therefore, is not utilized at an appropriate rate. There is perhaps a stronger genetic basis for noninsulin-dependent diabetes than for Type 1. Treatment of the diabetes Type 2 patient is generally directed toward early nonpharmacologic intervention, mainly weight reduction, moderate exercise, and lower plasma-glucose concentrations. Oral hypoglycemic agents as seen in the list below are often used to maintain blood sugar levels. Often 30% of Type 2 diabetics require insulin as well as oral hypoglycemics in order to manage their diabetes. Generally, the two classes of oral hypoglycemics are the sulfonylureas and the biguanides. The sulfonylureas are prescribed more frequently and they stimulate beta cell production of insulin, increased glucose utilization, and tend to normalize glucose metabolism in the liver. The uncontrolled diabetic may represent a challenge to the dental practitioner.

Insulin Preparations (various products) *on page 509*

TYPES OF INSULIN

Type	Action	Duration (h)
Regular	Rapid	5-7
Semilente	Rapid	10-14
Lispro	Rapid	3.5 h
NPH	Intermediate	18-24
Lente	Intermediate	14-20
Ultralente	Prolonged	>36

Oral Hypoglycemic Agents

Acarbose (Precose®) *on page 18*
Acetohexamide (Dymelor®) *on page 27*
Chlorpropamide (Diabinese®) *on page 225*
Glimepiride (Amaryl®) *on page 442*
Glipizide (Glucotrol®) *on page 443*
Glyburide (Diaβeta; Glynase™, PresTab™, Micronase®) *on page 445*
Metformin (Glucophage®) *on page 607*
Miglitol (Glyset®) *on page 638*
Repaglinide (Prandin®) *on page 838*
Tolazamide (Tolinase®) *on page 940*
Tolbutamide (Orinase®) *on page 941*
Troglitazone (Rezulin®) *on page 971*

Adjunct Therapy

Cisapride (Propulsid®) *on page 237*
Metoclopramide (Clopra®, Maxolon®, Octamide®, Reglan®) *on page 627*

Oral manifestations of uncontrolled diabetes might include abnormal neutrophil function resulting in a poor response to periodontal pathogens. Increased risk of gingivitis and periodontitis in these patients is common. Candidiasis is a frequent occurrence. Denture sore mouth may be more prominent and poor wound healing following extractions may be one of the complications encountered.

HORMONAL THERAPY

Two uses of hormonal supplementation include oral contraceptives and estrogen replacement therapy. Drugs used for contraception interfere with fertility by inhibiting release of follicle stimulating hormone, luteinizing hormone, and by preventing ovulation. There are few oral side effects; however, moderate gingivitis, similar to that seen during pregnancy, has been reported. The dentist should be aware that decreased effect of oral contraceptives has been reported with most antibiotics. See individual monographs for specific details. Drugs commonly encountered include:

Estradiol (various products) *on page 365*
Ethinyl Estradiol and Ethynodiol Diacetate (Demulen®) *on page 375*
Ethinyl Estradiol and Levonorgestrel (Levlen®, Nordette®, Levora®, Tri-Levlen®, Triphasil™) *on page 377*

Estrogens or derivatives are usually prescribed as replacement therapy following menopause or cyclic irregularities and to inhibit osteoporosis. The following list of drugs may interact with antidepressants and barbiturates. New tissue-specific estrogens like Evista® may help with the problem of osteoporosis.

PREGNANCY

Normal endocrine and physiologic functions are altered during pregnancy. Endogenous estrogens and progesterone increase and placental hormones are secreted. Thyroid stimulating hormone and growth hormone also increase. Cardiovascular changes can result and increased blood volume can lead to blood pressure elevations and transient heart murmurs. Generally, in a normal pregnancy, oral gingival changes will be limited to gingivitis. Alteration of treatment plans might include limiting administration of all drugs to emergency procedures only during the first and third trimesters and medical consultation regarding the patients' status for all elective procedures. Limiting dental care throughout pregnancy to preventive procedures is not unreasonable.

HIV INFECTION AND AIDS

Human immunodeficiency virus (HIV) represents agents HIV-1 and HIV-2 that produce a devastating systemic disease. The virus causes disease by leading to elevated risk of infections in patients and, from our experience over the last 18 years, there clearly are oral manifestations associated with these patients. Also, there has been a revolution in infection control in our dental offices over the last two decades due to our expanding knowledge of this infectious agent. Infection control practices (see "Infectious Disease Information" on page 1151) have been elevated to include all of the infectious agents with which dentists often come into contact. These might include in addition to HIV, hepatitis viruses (of which the serotypes include A, B, C, D, E, F, and G) , the herpes viruses; sexually transmitted diseases such as syphilis, gonorrhea, papillomavirus, all of which are covered elsewhere in this book.

Acquired immunodeficiency syndrome (AIDS) has been recognized since early 1981 as a unique clinical syndrome manifest by opportunistic infections or by neoplasms complicating the underlying defect in the cellular immune system. These defects are now known to be brought on by infection and pathogenesis with human immunodeficiency virus 1 or 2 (HIV-1 is the predominant serotype identified). The major cellular defect brought on by infection with HIV is a depletion of T-cells, primarily the sub-type, T-helper cells, known as CD4+ cells. Over these years, our knowledge regarding HIV infection and the oral manifestations often associated with patients with HIV or AIDS, has increased dramatically. Populations of individuals known to be at high risk of HIV transmission include homosexuals, intravenous drug abuse patients, transfusion recipients, patients with other sexually transmitted diseases, and patients practicing promiscuous sex.

The definitions of AIDS have also evolved over this period of time. The natural history of HIV infection along with some of the oral manifestations can be reviewed in Table 1. The risk of developing these opportunistic infections increases as the patient progresses to AIDS.

Table 1.
NATURAL HISTORY OF HIV INFECTION/ORAL MANIFESTATIONS

Time From Transmission (Average)	Observation	CD4 Cell Count
0	Viral transmissions	Normal: 1000 ($\pm$500/mm^3)
2-4 weeks	Self-limited infectious mononucleosis-like illness with fever, rash, leukopenia, mucocutaneous ulcerations (mouth, genitals, etc), thrush	Transient decrease
6-12 weeks	Seroconversion (rarely requires $\geq$3 months for seroconversion)	Normal
0-8 years	Healthy/asymptomatic HIV infection; peripheral/persistent generalized lymphadenopathy; HPV, thrush, OHL; RAU, periodontal diseases, salivary gland diseases; dermatitis	$\geq$500/mm^3 gradual reduction with average decrease of 50-80/mm^3/year
4-8 years	Early symptomatic HIV infection previously called (AIDS-related complex): Thrush, vaginal candidiasis (persistent, frequent and/or severe), cervical dysplasia/CA Hodgkin's lymphoma, B-cell lymphoma, oral hairy leukoplakia, salivary gland diseases, ITP, xerostomia, dermatitis, shingles; RAU, herpes simplex, HPV, bacterial infections, periodontal diseases, molluscum contagiosum, other physical symptoms: fever, weight loss, fatigue	$\geq$300-500/mm^3
6-10 years	AIDS: Wasting syndrome, *Candida* esophagitis, Kaposi's sarcoma, HIV-associated dementia, disseminated *M. avium*, Hodgkin's or B-cell lymphoma, herpes simplex >30 days; PCP; cryptococcal meningitis, other systemic fungal infections; CMV	<200/mm^3

Natural history indicates course of HIV infection in absence of antiretroviral treatment. Adapted from Bartlett JG, "A Guide to HIV Care from the AIDS Care Program of the Johns Hopkins Medical Institutions," 2nd ed.

PCP - *Pneumocystis carinii* pneumonia; ITP - idiopathic thrombocytopenia purpura; HPV - human papilloma virus; OHL - oral hairy leukoplakia; RAU - recurrent aphthous ulcer

Patients with HIV infection and/or AIDS are seen in dental offices throughout the country. In general, it is the dentist's obligation to treat HIV individuals including patients of record and other patients who may seek treatment when the office is accepting new patients. These patients are protected under the Americans with Disabilities Act and the dentist has an obligation as described. Two excellent publications, one by the American Dental Association and the other by the American Academy of Oral Medicine, outline the dentist's responsibility as well as a very detailed explanation of dental management protocols for HIV patients. These protocols, however, are evolving just as our knowledge of HIV has evolved. New drugs and their interactions (see Dental Drug Interactions *on page 1144* in Appendix) present the dentist with continuous need for updates regarding the appropriate management of HIV patients. Diagnostic tests, including determining viral load in combination with the CD4 status, now are used to modify a patient's treatment in ways that allow them to remain relatively illness-free for longer periods of time. This places more of a responsibility on the dental practice team to be aware of drug changes, of new drugs, and of the appropriate oral management in such patients.

Our knowledge of AIDS allows us to properly treat these patients while protecting ourselves, our staff, and other patients in the office. All types of infectious disease require consistent practices in our dental offices known as Universal Precautions (see Infectious Disease Information *on page 1151* in Appendix). The office team that utilizes these precautions appropriately is well protected against passage of infectious agents. These agents include sexually transmitted disease agents, the highly virulent hepatitis viruses, and the less virulent but always worrisome HIV. In general, an office that is practicing universal precautions is one that is considered safe for patients and staff. Throughout this spectrum, HIV is placed somewhere in the middle in terms of infection risk in the dental office. Other sexually transmitted diseases and infectious diseases such as tuberculosis represent a greater threat to the dentist than HIV itself. However, due to the grave danger of HIV infection, many of our precautions have been instituted to assist the dentist in protecting himself, his staff, and other patients in situations where the office may be involved in treating a patient that is HIV positive.

As in the management of all medically compromised patients, the appropriate care of HIV patients begins with a complete and thorough history. This history must allow the dentist to identify risk factors in the development of HIV as well as identify those patients known to be HIV positive. Knowledge of all medications prescribed to patients at risk is also important. Some of the antiviral drugs commonly used are listed in Table 2. The newer drugs, protease inhibitors, non-nucleoside analogs and combination require constant updating of our knowledge.

The presence of other infections are an important part of the health history. Appropriate medical consultation may be mandated after a health history in order to accomplish a complete evaluation of the patients at risk. Uniformity in the taking of a history from a patient is the dentist's best plan for all patients so that no selectivity or discrimination can be implicated.

Table 2.
ANTIVIRAL DRUGS COMMONLY USED

Viral Infection	Drug
Human immunodeficiency virus-1 AIDS, Asymptomatic, CD4 <500	Delavirdine *on page 285* Didanosine *on page 307* Indinavir *on page 505* Lamivudine *on page 541* Nelfinavir *on page 669* Ritonavir *on page 847* Saquinavir Mesylate *on page 856* Stavudine *on page 883* Zalcitabine *on page 1001* Zidovudine *on page 1002* Zidovudine and Lamivudine *on page 1003*

An appropriate review of symptoms may also identify oral and systemic conditions that may be present in aggressive HIV disease. Medical physical examination may reveal pre-existing or developing intra- or extra-oral signs/symptoms of progressive disease. Aggressive herpes simplex, herpes zoster, papillomavirus, Kaposi's sarcoma or lymphoma are among the disorders that might be identified. In addition to these, intra-oral examination may raise suspicion regarding fungal infections, angular cheilitis, squamous cell carcinoma, and recurrent aphthous ulcers. The dentist should be vigilant in all patients regardless of HIV risk.

It will always be up to the dental practitioner to determine whether testing for HIV should be recommended following the history and physical examination of a new

HIV INFECTION AND AIDS (Continued)

patient. Because of the severe psychological implications of learning of HIV positivity for a patient, the dentist should be aware that there are appropriate referral sites where psychological counseling and appropriate discrete testing for the patient is available. The dentist's office should have these sites available for referral should the patient be interested. Candid discussions, however, with the patient regarding risk factors and/or other signs or symptoms in their history and physical condition that may indicate a higher HIV risk than the normal population, should be an area the dentist feels comfortable in broaching with any new patient. Oftentimes, it is appropriate to recommend testing for other infectious diseases should risk factors be present. For example, testing for hepatitis B may be appropriate for the patient and along with this the dentist could recommend that the patient consider HIV testing. Because of the legal issues involved, anonymity for HIV testing may be appropriate and it is always up to the patient to follow the doctor's recommendations.

When a patient has either given a positive history of knowing that they are HIV positive or it has been determined after referral for consultation, the dentist should be aware of the AIDS-defining illnesses. Of course, current medical status and drug therapy that the patient may be undergoing is of equal importance. The dentist, through medical consultation and regular follow-up with the patient's physician, should be made aware of the CD4 count (Table 3), the viral load, and the drugs that the patient is taking. The presence of other AIDS-defining illnesses as well as complications, such as higher risk of endocarditis and the risk of other systemic infections such as tuberculosis, are extremely important for the dentist. These may make an impact on the dental treatment plan in terms of the selection of preprocedural antibiotics or the use of oral medications to treat opportunistic infections in or around the oral cavity.

Table 3.
CD4+ LYMPHOCYTE COUNT AND PERCENTAGE AS RELATED TO THE RISK OF OPPORTUNISTIC INFECTION

CD4+ Cells/mm³	CD4+ Percentage*	Risk of Opportunistic Infection
>600	32-60	No increased risk
400-500	<29	Initial immune suppression
200-400	14-28	Appearance of opportunistic infections, some may be major
<200	<14	Severe immune suppression. AIDS diagnosis. Major opportunistic infections. Although variable, prognosis for surviving more than 3 years is poor.
<50	—	Although variable, prognosis for surviving more than 1 year is poor

*Several studies have suggested that the CD4+ percentage demonstrates less variability between measurements, as compared to the absolute CD4+ cell count. CD4+ percentages may therefore give a clearer impression of the course of disease.

AIDS-defining illnesses such as candidiasis, recurrent pneumonia, or lymphoma are clearly important to the dentist. Chemotherapy that might be being given to the patient for treatment for any or all of these disorders can have implications in terms of the patient's response to simple dental procedures.

Drug therapies have become complex in the treatment of HIV/AIDS. Because of the moderate successes with protease inhibitors and the drug combination therapies, more patients are living longer and receiving more dental care throughout their lives. Drug therapies are often tailored to the current CD4 count in combination with the viral load. In general, patients with high CD4 counts are usually at lower risk for complications in the dental office than patients with low CD4 counts. However, the presence of a high viral load with or without a stable CD4 count may be indicative or a more rapid progression of the HIV/AIDS disease process than had previously been thought. Patients with a high viral load and a declining CD4 count are considered to have the greatest risk and the poorest prognosis of all the groups.

Other organ damage, such as liver compromise potentially leading to bleeding disorders, can be found as the disease progresses to AIDS. Liver dysfunction may be related to pre-existing hepatic diseases due to previous infection with a hepatitis virus such as hepatitis B or other drug toxicities associated with the treatment of AIDS. The dentist must have available current prothrombin and partial thromboplastin times (PT and PTT) in order to accurately evaluate any risk of bleeding abnormality. Platelet count and liver function studies are also important. Potential drug interactions include some antibiotics, as well as any anticoagulating drugs, which may be contraindicated in such patients. It may be necessary to avoid nonsteroidal anti-inflammatory drugs as well as aspirin. (See the introductory text "Pharmacology of Drug Metabolism and Interactions" *on page 11*).

The use of preprocedural antibiotics is another issue in the HIV patient. As the absolute neutrophil count declines during the progression of AIDS, the use of antibiotics as a preprocedural step prior to dental care may be necessary. If protracted treatment plans are necessary, the dentist should receive updated information as the patient receives such from their physician. It is always important that the dentist have current CD4 counts, viral load assay, as well as liver function studies, AST and ALT, and bleeding indicators including platelet count, PT, and PTT. If any other existing conditions such as cardiac involvement or joint prostheses are involved, antibiotic coverage may also be necessary. However, these determinations are no different than in the non-HIV population and this subject is covered in "Preprocedural Antibiotic Prophylaxis Guidelines for Dental Patients" *on page 1034*. See Table 4 for normal blood values as general guidelines for provision of dental care.

Table 4.
NORMAL BLOOD VALUES

Test	Range of Normal Values
Complete blood count (CBC)	
White blood cells	4,500-11,000
Red blood cells (male)	$4.6\text{-}6.2 \times 10^6$ μL
Red blood cells (female)	$4.2\text{-}5.4 \times 10^6$ μL
Platelets	150,000-450,000
Hematocrit (male)	40% to 54%
Hematocrit (female)	38% to 47%
Hemoglobin (male)	13.5-18 g/dL
Hemoglobin (female)	12-16 g/dL
Mean corpuscular volume (MCV)	80-96 μm^3
Mean corpuscular hemoglobin (MCH)	27-31 pg
Mean corpuscular hemoglobin concentration (MCHC)	32% to 36%
Differential white blood cell count (%)	
Segmented neutrophils	56
Bands	3.0
Eosinophils	2.7
Basophils	0.3
Lymphocytes	34.0
Monocytes	4.0
Hemostasis	
Bleeding time (BT)	2-8 minutes
Prothrombin time (PT)	10-13 seconds
Activated partial thromboplastin time (aPTT)	25-35 seconds
Serum chemistry	
Glucose (fasting)	70-110 mg/dL
Blood urea nitrogen (BUN)	8-23 mg/dL
Creatinine (male)	0.1-0.4 mg/dL
Creatinine (female)	0.2-0.7 mg/dL
Bilirubin, indirect (unconjugated)	0.3 mg/dL
Bilirubin, direct (conjugated)	0.1-1 mg/dL
Calcium	9.2-11 mg/dL
Magnesium	1.8-3 mg/dL
Phosphorus	2.3-4.7 mg/dL
Serum electrolytes	
Sodium (Na$^+$)	136-142 mEq/L
Potassium (K$^+$)	3.8-5 mEq/L
Chloride (Cl$^-$)	95-103 mEq/L
Bicarbonate (HCO$_3^-$)	21-28 mmol/L
Serum enzymes	
Alkaline phosphatase	20-130 IU/L
Alanine aminotransferase (ALT) (formerly called SGPT)	4-36 units/L
Aspartate aminotransferase (AST) (formerly called SGOT)	8-33 units/L
Amylase	16-120 Somogyi units/dL
Creatine kinase (CK) (male)	55-170 units/L
Creatine kinase (CK) (female)	30-135 units/L

The consideration of current blood values is important in long-term care of any medically compromised patient and in particular the HIV-positive patient. Preventive

HIV INFECTION AND AIDS *(Continued)*

dental care is likewise valuable in these patients, however, the dentist's approach should be no different than as with all patients. See Table 5 for oral lesions commonly associated with HIV disease and a brief description of their usual treatment. The clinician is referred to other sections of the text for more detailed descriptions of these common oral lesions. Other important parts of the text that may be useful for the dentist include the Office Protocol for Universal Precautions *on page 1151* and the Frequently Asked Questions at the end of this chapter. The clinician should also be aware that several of the protease inhibitors have now been associated with drug interactions. Some of these drug interactions include therapies that the dentist may be utilizing. The basis for these drug interactions with the protease inhibitors is the inhibition of cytochrome P-450 isoforms which are important in the normal liver function and metabolism of drugs. A detailed description of the mechanisms of inhibition can be found in the section "Pharmacology of Drug Metabolism and Interactions" *on page 11*, as well as a table illustrating some of the known drug interactions with antiviral therapy and drugs commonly prescribed in the dental office. The metabolism of these drugs could be affected by the patient's antiviral therapy. Please see the section on selected references for more information on management of HIV patients.

Table 5.
ORAL LESIONS COMMONLY SEEN IN HIV/AIDS

Condition	Management
Oral candidiasis	See "Oral Fungal Infections" *on page 1063*
Angular cheilitis	See "Oral Fungal Infections" *on page 1063*
Oral hairy leukoplakia	See "Systemic Viral Diseases" *on page 1047*

Periodontal diseases
  Linear gingivitis
  Ulcerative periodontitis
	See "Oral Bacterial Infections" *on page 1059*

Herpes simplex	Acyclovir - see "Systemic Viral Diseases" *on page 1047*
Herpes zoster	Acyclovir - see "Systemic Viral Diseases" *on page 1047*
Chronic aphthous ulceration	Palliation / Thalidomide (likely to be approved for these patients in the near future)
Salivary gland disease	Referral
Human papillomavirus	Laser / Surgical excision
Kaposi's sarcoma	See "Antibiotic Prophylaxis" *on page 1034*; Biopsy / Laser
Kaposi's lymphoma	Biopsy / Referral
Tuberculosis	Referral

Dapsone (Avlosulfon®) *on page 281*

Delavirdine (Rescriptor™) *on page 285*

Didanosine (Videx®) *on page 307*

Indinavir (Crixivan®) *on page 505*

Lamivudine (Epivir®) *on page 541*

Nelfinavir (Viracept®) *on page 669*

Ritonavir (Norvir®) *on page 847*

Stavudine (Zerit®) *on page 883*

Zalcitabine (Hivid®) *on page 1001*

Zidovudine (Retrovir®) *on page 1002*

Zidovudine and Lamivudine (Combivir®) *on page 1003*

FREQUENTLY ASKED QUESTIONS

How does one get AIDS, aside from having unprotected sex?

Our current knowledge about the immunodeficiency virus is that it is carried via semen, contaminated needles, blood products, transfusion products, if indeed the transfusion products have not been tested, and potentially in other fluids of the body. Patients at highest risk would include I.V. drug abuse patients, patients receiving multiple transfusions with blood that has not been screened for HIV, or patients practicing unprotected sex with multiple partners where the history of the partner may not be as clear as the patient would like.

Are patients safe from AIDS or HIV infection when they present to the dentist office?

Our current knowledge indicates that the answer is an unequivocal yes. The patient is protected because the dental offices are practicing universal precautions using antimicrobial hand-washing agents, gloves, face masks, eye protection, special clothing, aerosol control, and instrument soaking and autoclaving. All of these procedures stop the potential transmission to a new patient as well as allow for easy disposal of contaminated office supplies for elimination of microbes by an antimicrobial technique should they be contaminated through the treatment of another patient. These precautions are mandated by the OSHA requirements and are covered in Universal Precautions in the Appendix.

What is the most common opportunistic infection that HIV-positive patients suffer that may be important in dentistry?

The most common opportunistic infection important to dentistry is oral candidiasis. This disease can present as white plaques, red areas, or angular cheilitis occurring at the corners of the mouth. Management of such lesions is appropriate by the dentist and is described in this handbook (see Oral Fungal Infections *on page 1063*). Other oral complications would include HIV-associated periodontal disease, as well as the other conditions outlined in Table 5. Of great concern to the dentist is the risk of tuberculosis. In many HIV-positive patients, tuberculosis has become a serious life-threatening opportunistic infection. The dentist should be aware that appropriate referral for anyone showing such respiratory signs and symptoms would be prudent.

Can one patient infect another through unprotected sex if the other patient has tested negative for HIV?

Yes, there is always the possibility that a sexual partner may be in the early window of time when plasma viremia is not at a detectable level. The antibody response to that plasma viremia may be slightly delayed and diagnostic testing may not indicate HIV positivity. This window of time represents a period when the patient may be infectious but yet not show up on normal diagnostic testing.

Can HIV be passed by oral fluids?

As our knowledge about HIV has evolved, we have thought that HIV is inactivated in saliva by an agent possibly associated with secretory leukocyte protease inhibitors known as SLPI. There is, however, a current resurgence in our interest in oral transmission because of some research that indicates that in moderate to advanced periodontal lesions or in other oral lesions where there is tissue damage, then the presence of a serous exudate may increase the risk of transmission. The dentist should be aware of this ongoing research and attempt to renew knowledge regularly so that any future breakthroughs will be noted.

RHEUMATOID ARTHRITIS AND OSTEOARTHRITIS

Arthritis and its variations represent the most common chronic musculoskeletal disorders of man. The conditions can essentially be divided into rheumatoid, osteoarthritic, and polyarthritic presentations. Differences in age of onset and joint involvement exist and it is now currently believed that the diagnosis of each may be less clear than previously thought. These autoinflammatory diseases have now been shown to affect young and old alike. Criteria for a diagnosis of rheumatoid arthritis include a positive serologic test for rheumatoid factor, subcutaneous nodules, affected joints on opposite sides of the body, and clear radiographic changes. The hematologic picture includes moderate normocytic hypochromic anemia, mild leukocytosis, and mild thrombocytopenia. During acute inflammatory periods, C-reactive protein is elevated and IgG and IgM (rheumatoid factors) can be detected. Osteoarthritis lacks these diagnostic features.

Other systemic conditions, such as systemic lupus erythematosus and Sjögren's syndrome, are often found simultaneously with some of the arthritic conditions. The treatment of arthritis includes the use of slow-acting and rapid-acting anti-inflammatory agents ranging from the gold salts to aspirin (see following listings). Long-term usage of these drugs can lead to numerous adverse effects including bone marrow suppression, platelet suppression, and oral ulcerations. The dentist should be aware that steroids (usually prednisone) are often prescribed along with the listed drugs and are often used in dosages sufficient to induce adrenal suppression. Adjustment of dosing prior to invasive dental procedures may be indicated along with consultation with the managing physician. Alteration of steroid dosage prior to stressful dental procedures may be necessary, usually increasing the steroid dosage prior to and during the stressful procedures and then gradually returning the patient to the original dosage over several days. Even in the absence of evidence of adrenal suppression, consultation with the prescribing physician for appropriate dosing and timing of procedures is advisable.

Gold Salts

Auranofin (Ridaura®) *on page 99*
Aurothioglucose (Solganol®) *on page 100*

Metabolic Inhibitor

Methotrexate *on page 615*

Nonsteroidal Anti-inflammatory Agents

Aminosalicylate Sodium (Sodium P.A.S.) *on page 58*
Bromfenac (Duract™) *on page 139*
Choline Magnesium Trisalicylate (Trilisate®) *on page 230*
Choline Salicylate (Arthropan®) *on page 230*
Diclofenac (Cataflam®, Voltaren®) *on page 304*
Diflunisal (Dolobid®) *on page 311*
Etodolac (Lodine®) *on page 387*
Fenoprofen (Nalfon®) *on page 398*
Flurbiprofen (Ansaid®) *on page 423*
Ibuprofen (various products) *on page 495*
Indomethacin (Indocin®) *on page 506*
Ketoprofen (Orudis®) *on page 534*
Ketorolac (Toradol®) *on page 535*
Magnesium Salicylate (Doan's®, Magan®, Mobidin®) *on page 577*
Meclofenamate (Meclomen®) *on page 585*
Mefenamic Acid (Ponstel®) *on page 588*
Nabumetone (Relafen®) *on page 656*
Naproxen (Naprosyn®) *on page 665*
Oxaprozin (Daypro™) *on page 706*
Oxyphenbutazone *on page 716*
Piroxicam (Feldene®) *on page 767*
Salsalate (various products) *on page 855*
Sulindac (Clinoril®) *on page 898*
Tolmetin (Tolectin®) *on page 943*

Combination NSAID Product to Prevent GI Distress

Diclofenac and Misoprostol (Arthrotec®) *on page 305*

Salicylates

Other

ANTI-INFLAMMATORY AGENTS USED IN THE TREATMENT OF RHEUMATOID ARTHRITIS AND OSTEOARTHRITIS

Drug	Adverse Effects
SLOW-ACTING	
GOLD SALTS	
Aurothioglucose I.M. parenteral injection (Myochrysine®); Auranofin (Ridaura®)	GI intolerance, diarrhea; leukopenia, thrombocytopenia, and/or anemia; skin and oral eruptions; possible nephrotoxicity and hepatotoxicity
METABOLIC INHIBITOR	
Methotrexate	Oral ulcerations, leukopenia
OTHER	
Hydroxychloroquine (Plaquenil®)	Usually mild and reversible; ophthalmic complications
Prednisone	Insomnia, nervousness, indigestion, increased appetite
RAPID-ACTING	
SALICYLATES	
Aspirin	Inhibition of platelet aggregation; gastrointestinal (GI) irritation, ulceration, and bleeding; tinnitus; teratogenicity
Choline magnesium salicylate (Trilisate®)	GI irritation and ulceration, weakness, skin rash, hemolytic anemia, troubled breathing
Salsalate	
OTHER NONSTEROIDAL ANTI-INFLAMMATORY DRUGS	
Diclofenac (Cataflam®, Voltaren®); Diflunisal (Dolobid®); Etodolac (Lodine®); Fenoprofen calcium (Nalfon®); Flurbiprofen sodium (Ansaid®); Ibuprofen (Motrin®); Indomethacin (Indocin®); Ketoprofen (Orudis®); Ketorolac tromethamine (Toradol®); Meclofenamate (Meclomen®); Nabumetone (Relafen®); Naproxen (Naprosyn®); Oxaprozin (Daypro™); Phenylbutazone; Piroxicam (Feldene®); Salsalate (Argesic®-SA, Artha-G®, Disalcid®, Mono-Gesic®, Salflex®, Salgesic®, Salsitab®); Sulindac (Clinoril®); Tolmetin (Tolectin®)	GI irritation, ulceration, and bleeding; inhibition of platelet aggregation; displacement of protein-bound drugs (eg, oral anticoagulants, sulfonamides, and sulfonylureas); headache; vertigo; mucocutaneous rash or ulceration; parotid enlargement
COMBINATION NSAID PRODUCT TO PREVENT GI DISTRESS	
Diclofenac and Misoprostol (Arthrotec®)	Inhibition of platelet aggregation; displacement of protein-bound drugs (eg, oral anticoagulants, sulfonamides, and sulfonylureas); headache; vertigo; mucocutaneous rash or ulceration; parotid enlargement; diarrhea

NONVIRAL INFECTIOUS DISEASES

Nonviral infectious diseases are numerous. For the purposes of this text, discussion will be limited to tuberculosis, gonorrhea, and syphilis.

TUBERCULOSIS

Tuberculosis is caused by the organism *Mycobacterium tuberculosis* as well as a variety of other mycobacteria including *M. bovis*, *M. avium-intracellulare*, and *M. kansasii*. Diagnosis of tuberculosis can be made from a skin test and a positive chest x-ray as well as acid-fast smears of cultures from respiratory secretions. Nucleic acid probes and polymerase chain reaction (PCR) to identify nucleic acid of *M. tuberculosis* have recently become useful.

The treatment of tuberculosis is based on the general principle that multiple drugs should reduce infectivity within 2 weeks and that failures in therapy may be due to noncompliance with the long-term regimens necessary. General treatment regimens last 6-12 months.

Isoniazid-resistant and multidrug-resistant mycobacterial infections have become an increasingly significant problem in recent years. TB as an opportunistic disease in HIV-positive patients has also risen. Combination drug therapy has always been popular in TB management and the advent of new antibiotics has not diminished this need.

ANTITUBERCULOSIS DRUGS

Bactericidal Agents

Capreomycin (Capastat®) *on page 169*
*Isoniazid (INH™, Laniazid®, Nydrazid®) *on page 522*
Kanamycin (Kantrex®) *on page 531*
*Pyrazinamide *on page 823*
Rifabutin (Mycobutin®) *on page 842*
*Rifampin (Rifadin®, Rimactane®) *on page 842*
*Streptomycin *on page 885*

Bacteriostatic Agents

Cycloserine (Seromycin® Pulvules®) *on page 271*
*Ethambutol (Myambutol®) *on page 372*
Ethionamide (Trecator®-SC) *on page 382*
Para-Aminosalicylate Sodium *on page 723*

*Drugs of Choice

SEXUALLY TRANSMITTED DISEASES

Sexually transmitted diseases (STDs) represent a group of infectious diseases that include bacterial, fungal, and viral etiologies. Several related infections are covered elsewhere. Gonorrhea and syphilis will be covered here.

The management of a patient with a STD begins with identification. Paramount to the correct management of patients with a history of gonorrhea or syphilis is when the condition was diagnosed, how and with what agent it was treated, did the condition recur, and are there any residual signs and symptoms potentially indicating active or recurrent disease. With universal precautions, the patient with *Neisseria gonorrhoea* or *Treponema pallidum* infection pose little threat to the dentist; however, diagnosis of oral lesions may be problematic. Gonococcal pharyngitis, primary syphilitic lesions (chancre), secondary syphilitic lesions (mucous patch), and tertiary lesions (gumma) may be identified by the dentist.

Drugs used in treatment of gonorrhea/syphilis include:

Cefixime (Suprax®) *on page 189*
Ceftriaxone (Rocephin®) *on page 197*
Ciprofloxacin (Cipro™) *on page 236*
Doxycycline (alternate) (Doryx®, Doxy®, Doxychel®, Vibramycin®, Vibra-Tabs®) *on page 338*
Ofloxacin (Floxin®, Ocuflox™) *on page 697*
Penicillin G Benzathine (Bicillin® L-A; Permapen®) *on page 731*
Penicillin G, Parenteral, Aqueous (Pfizerpen®) *on page 732*
Spectinomycin (alternate) (Trobicin®) *on page 880*

The drugs listed above are often used alone or in stepped regimens, particularly when there is concomitant *Chlamydia* infection or when there is evidence of disseminated disease. The proper treatment for syphilis depends on the state of the disease.

Current treatment regimens for syphilis include:

1°, 2°, early latent (<1 y)	Benzathine penicillin G
	I.M.: 2-4 million units x 1 (alternate doxycycline)
Latent (>1 y), gumma, or cardiovascular	As above but once weekly for 3 weeks
Neurosyphilis	Aqueous penicillin G
	I.V.: 12-24 million units/day for 14 days

ANTIBIOTIC PROPHYLAXIS
PREPROCEDURAL GUIDELINES FOR DENTAL PATIENTS

INTRODUCTION

In dental practice the clinician is often confronted with a decision to prescribe antibiotics. The focus of this chapter is on the use of antibiotics as a preprocedural treatment in the prevention of adverse infectious sequelae in the two most commonly encountered situations: prevention of endocarditis and prosthetic implants.

The criteria for preprocedural decisions begins with patient evaluation. An accurate and complete medical history is always the initial basis for any prescriptive treatments on the part of the dentist. These prescriptive treatments can include ordering appropriate laboratory tests, referral to the patient's physician for consultation, or immediate decision to prescribe preprocedural antibiotics. The dentist should also be aware that antibiotic coverage of the patient might be appropriate due to diseases that are covered elsewhere in this text, such as human immunodeficiency virus, cavernous thrombosis, undiagnosed or uncontrolled diabetes, lupus, renal failure, and periods of neutropenia as are often associated with cancer chemotherapy. In these instances, medical consultation is almost always necessary in making antibiotic decisions in order to tailor the treatment and dosing to the individual patient's needs.

All tables or figures in this chapter were adapted from the ADA Advisory Statement: "Antibiotic Prophylaxis for Dental Patients With Total Joint Replacement," *J Am Dent Assoc*, 1997, 128:1004-8 or from Dajani AS, Taubert KA, Wilson W, et al, "Prevention of Bacterial Endocarditis. Recommendations by the American Heart Association," *JAMA*, 1997, 277(22):1794-801.

PREVENTION OF BACTERIAL ENDOCARDITIS

Guidelines for the prevention of bacterial endocarditis have been updated by the American Heart Association with approval by the Council of Scientific Affairs of the American Dental Association.[1] These guidelines supercede those issued and published in 1990.[2] They were developed to more clearly define the situations of antibiotic use, to reduce costs to the patient, to reduce gastrointestinal adverse effects, and to improve patient compliance. Highlights of the current recommendations are shown in Table 1 and the specific antibiotic regimens are listed in Table 2 and further illustrated in Figure 1 found at the end of this chapter. Amoxicillin at a dose of 2 g 1 hour before the procedure is the suggested regimen for standard general prophylaxis. A follow-up dose is no longer necessary. This dose of amoxicillin is lower than the previous dosing regimen of 3 g 1 hour before the procedure and then 1.5 g 6 hours after the initial dose. Dajani, et al,[1] stated that the 2 g dose of amoxicillin resulted in adequate serum levels for several hours. They also stated that a second dose is not necessary, both because of a prolonged serum level of amoxicillin above the minimal inhibitory concentration for oral streptococci and an inhibitory activity of 6-14 hours by amoxicillin against streptococci.[3,4] The new pediatric dose is 50 mg/kg orally 1 hour before the procedure and not to exceed the adult dose. Amoxicillin is an amino-type penicillin with an extended spectrum of antibacterial action compared to penicillin VK. Amoxicillin is available in capsules (500 mg), liquid suspension (250 mg/5 mL) and chewable tablets (250 mg). The approximate retail cost of a 500 mg generic capsule is $1.80. The pharmacology of amoxicillin as a dental antibiotic has been reviewed previously in *General Dentistry*.[5]

Table 1.
HIGHLIGHTS OF THE NEWEST GUIDELINES FOR ENDOCARDITIS PREVENTION

No.	Change From Old Guidelines
1.	Oral initial dosing for amoxicillin reduced to 2 g
2.	Follow-up antibiotic dose is no longer recommended
3.	Erythromycin is no longer recommended for penicillin-allergic patients
4.	Clindamycin and other alternatives have been recommended to replace the erythromycin regimens
5.	Clearer guidelines for prophylaxis decisions for patients with mitral valve prolapse have been developed

For individuals unable to take oral medications, intramuscular or intravenous ampicillin is recommended for both adults and children (Table 2). It is to be given 30 minutes before the procedure at the same doses used for the oral amoxicillin medication. Ampicillin is also an amino-type penicillin having an antibacterial spectrum similar to amoxicillin. Ampicillin is not absorbed from the gastrointestinal tract as effectively as amoxicillin and, therefore, is not recommended for oral use.

Table 2.
PROPHYLACTIC REGIMENS FOR BACTERIAL ENDOCARDITIS FOR DENTAL PROCEDURES

Situation	Agent	Regimen*
Standard general prophylaxis	Amoxicillin *on page 68*	Adults: 2 g orally 1 hour before procedure Children: 50 mg/kg orally 1 hour before procedure
Unable to take oral medications	Ampicillin *on page 73*	Adults: 2 g I.M. or I.V. within 30 min before procedure Children: 50 mg/kg I.M. or I.V. within 30 min before procedure
Allergic to penicillin	Clindamycin *on page 243* or	Adults: 600 mg orally 1 hour before procedure Children: 20 mg/kg orally 1 hour before procedure
	Cephalexin *on page 201* or Cefadroxil *on page 186*	Adults: 2 g orally 1 hour before procedure Children: 50 mg/kg orally 1 hour before procedure
	Azithromycin *on page 104* or Clarithromycin *on page 241*	Adults: 500 mg orally 1 hour before procedure Children: 15 mg/kg orally 1 hour before procedure
Allergic to penicillin and unable to take oral medications	Clindamycin *on page 243* or	Adults: 600 mg I.V. within 30 min before procedure Children: 20 mg/kg I.V. within 30 min before procedure
	Cefazolin *on page 188*	Adults: 1 g I.M. or I.V. within 30 min before procedure Children: 25 mg/kg I.M. or I.V. within 30 min before procedure

*Total children's dose should not exceed adult dose.

Note: Cephalosporins should not be used in individuals with immediate-type hypersensitivity reaction (urticaria, angioedema, or anaphylaxis) to penicillins

Individuals who are allergic to the penicillins such as amoxicillin or ampicillin should be treated with an alternate antibiotic. The new guidelines have suggested a number of alternate agents including clindamycin, cephalosporins, azithromycin, and clarithromycin. Clindamycin (Cleocin®) occupies an important niche in dentistry as a useful and effective antibiotic and it was a recommended alternative agent for the prevention of bacterial endocarditis in the previous guidelines.[2] In the new guidelines, the oral adult dose is 600 mg 1 hour before the procedure. A follow-up dose is not necessary. Clindamycin is available as 300 mg capsules; thus 2 capsules will provide the recommended dose. The children's oral dose for clindamycin is 20 mg/kg 1 hour before the procedure. Clindamycin is available as pediatric-flavored granules for oral solution. When reconstituted with water, each bottle yields a solution containing 75 mg/

ANTIBIOTIC PROPHYLAXIS (Continued)

5 mL. Intravenous clindamycin is recommended in adults and children who are allergic to penicillin and unable to take oral medications. Refer to Table 2 for the intravenous doses of clindamycin.

Clindamycin was developed in the 1960s as a semisynthetic derivative of lincomycin which was found in the soil organism, *Streptomyces lincolnensis*, near Lincoln, Nebraska. It is commercially available as the hydrochloride salt to improve solubility in the gastrointestinal tract. Clindamycin is antibacterial against most aerobic gram-positive cocci including staphylococci and streptococci, and against many types of anaerobic gram-negative and gram-positive organisms. It has been used over the years in dentistry as an alternative to penicillin and erythromycins for the treatment of oral-facial infections. For a review, see Wynn and Bergman.[6]

The mechanism of antibacterial action of clindamycin is the same as erythromycin. It inhibits protein synthesis in susceptible bacteria resulting in the inhibition of bacterial growth and replication. Following oral administration of a single dose of clindamycin (150 mg, 300 mg, or 600 mg) on an empty stomach, 90% of the dose is rapidly absorbed into the bloodstream and peak serum concentrations are attained within 45-80 minutes. Administration with food does not markedly impair absorption into the bloodstream. Clindamycin serum levels exceed the minimum inhibitory concentration (MIC) for bacterial growth for at least 6 hours after the recommended dose of 600 mg. The serum half-life is 2-3 hours.

Adverse effects of clindamycin after a single dose are virtually nonexistent. Although it is estimated that 1% of patients taking clindamycin will develop symptoms of pseudomembranous colitis, these symptoms usually develop after 9-14 days of clindamycin therapy. These symptoms have never been reported in patients taking an acute dose for the prevention of endocarditis.

In lieu of clindamycin, penicillin-allergic individuals may receive cephalexin (Keflex®) or cefadroxil (Duricef®) provided that they have not had an immediate-type sensitivity reaction such as anaphylaxis, urticaria, or angioedema to penicillins. These antibiotics are first-generation cephalosporins having an antibacterial spectrum of action similar to amoxicillin and ampicillin. They elicit a bactericidal action by inhibiting cell wall synthesis in susceptible bacteria. The recommended adult prophylaxis dose for either of these drugs is 2 g 1 hour before the procedure. Again, no follow-up dose is needed. Cephalexin is supplied as 500 mg capsules and 500 mg tablets. Cefadroxil is supplied as 500 mg capsules and 1 g tablets. The children's oral dose for cephalexin and cefadroxil is 50 mg/kg 1 hour before the procedure. Both antibiotics are available in the form of oral suspension at concentrations of 125 mg, 250 mg, and 500 mg/5 mL.

For those individuals (adults and children) allergic to penicillin and unable to take oral medicines, parenteral cefazolin (Ancef®) may be used provided that they do not have the sensitivities described previously and footnoted in Table 2. Cefazolin is also a first-generation cephalosporin. Please note that the parenteral cefazolin can be given I.M. or I.V. Refer to Table 2 for the adult and children's doses of parenteral cefazolin.

Azithromycin (Zithromax®) and clarithromycin (Biaxin™) are members of the erythromycin-class of antibiotics known as the macrolides. The pharmacology of these drugs has been reviewed previously in *General Dentistry*.[7] The erythromycins have been available for use in dentistry and medicine since the mid 1950s. Azithromycin and clarithromycin represent the first additions to this class in over 40 years. The adult prophylactic dose for either drug is 500 mg 1 hour before the procedure with no follow-up dose. Azithromycin is well absorbed from the gastrointestinal tract and is extensively taken up from the circulation into tissues with a slow release from those tissues. It reaches peak serum levels in 2-4 hours. The serum half-life of azithromycin is 68 hours. Although the erythromycin family of drugs are known to inhibit the hepatic metabolism of theophylline and carbamazepine to enhance their effects, azithromycin has not been shown to affect the liver metabolism of these drugs.[8,9] Azithromycin is available under the brand name of Zithromax® and is not available generically as of this report. It is supplied as 250 mg capsules at a cost of $406 per 50 capsules.

Clarithromycin achieves peak plasma concentrations in 3 hours and maintains effective serum concentrations over a 12-hour period. Reports indicate that clarithromycin probably interacts with theophylline and carbamazepine by elevating the plasma concentrations of the two drugs.[7] Clarithromycin is available under the brand name of Biaxin® and is not available generically as of this report. Clarithromycin is supplied as 250 mg and 500 mg tablets at a cost of approximately $300 per 100 tablets. The pediatric prophylactic dose of azithromycin and clarithromycin is 15 mg/kg orally 1 hour before the procedure. Clarithromycin (Biaxin®) is available as powder for reconstitution to final concentrations of 125 mg and 500 mg per 5 mL. Azithromycin (Zithromax®) for oral suspension is supplied as single-dose packets containing 1 g of drug in each packet.

Amoxicillin (Amoxil®, Biomox®, Larotid®, Polymox®, Trimox®, Utimox®, Wymox®) *on page 68*

Ampicillin (Amcill®, Marcillin®, Omnipen®, Polycillin®, Principen®, Totacillin®) *on page 73*

Azithromycin (Zithromax™) *on page 104*

Cefadroxil (Duricef®, Ultracef®) *on page 186*

Cefazolin (Ancef®) *on page 188*

Cephalexin (Keflex®) *on page 201*

Clarithromycin (Biaxin™) *on page 241*

Clindamycin (Cleocin®) *on page 243*

Clinical Considerations for Dentistry

See Algorithm Figure 1 at the end of this chapter

The clinician should review carefully those detailed dental procedures in Table 3 to determine those treatment conditions where prophylaxis is, or is not, recommended. In general, in patients with cardiac conditions where prophylaxis is recommended (Table 4), invasive dental procedures where bleeding is likely to be induced from hard or soft tissues (Table 3) should be preceded by antibiotic coverage (Table 2). Clearly, the production of significant bacteremia during a dental procedure is the major risk factor. Patients with a suspicious history of a cardiac condition who are in need of an immediate dental procedure should be prophylaxed with an appropriate antibiotic prior to the procedure(s) until medical evaluation has been completed and the risk level determined. If unanticipated bleeding develops during a procedure in an at-risk patient, appropriate antibiotics should be given immediately. The efficacy of this action is based on animal studies and is possibly effective up to 2 hours after the bacteremia.[10]

Table 3.
DENTAL PROCEDURES AND PREPROCEDURAL ANTIBIOTICS

Endocarditis or Prosthesis Prophylaxis Recommended Due to Likely Significant Bacteremia
Dental extractions
Periodontal procedures including surgery, subgingival placement of antibiotic fibers/strips, scaling and root planing, probing, recall maintenance
Dental implant placement and reimplantation of avulsed teeth
Endodontic (root canal) instrumentation or surgery only beyond the apex
Initial placement of orthodontic bands but not brackets
Intraligamentary local anesthetic injections
Prophylactic cleaning of teeth or implants where bleeding is anticipated
Endocarditis Prophylaxis Not Recommended Due to Usually Insignificant Bacteremia
Restorative dentistry (operative and prosthodontic) with or without retraction cord**
Local anesthetic injections (nonintraligamentary)
Intracanal endodontic treatment; postplacement and build-up*
Placement of rubber dam*
Postoperative suture removal
Placement of removable prosthodontic/orthodontic appliances
Oral impressions*
Fluoride treatments
Taking of oral radiographs
Orthodontic appliance adjustment
Shedding of primary teeth
In general, the presence of moderate to severe gingival inflammation may elevate these procedures to a higher risk of bacteremia.

*Prophylaxis is recommended for patients with high- and moderate-risk cardiac as well as high-risk prosthesis conditions

This includes restoration of decayed teeth and replacement of missing teeth

**Clinical judgment may indicate antibiotic use in any circumstances that may create significant bleeding.

Patients with moderate to advanced gingival inflammatory disease and/or periodontitis should be considered at greater risk of bacteremia. However, the ongoing daily risk of self-induced bacteremia in these patients is currently thought to be minimal as compared to the bacteremia during dental procedures. The clinician may wish to consider the use of a preprocedural antimicrobial rinse in addition to antibiotic prophylaxis and, of course, efforts should always focus on improving periodontal health

ANTIBIOTIC PROPHYLAXIS *(Continued)*

during dental care. If a series of dental procedures is planned, the clinician must judge whether an interval between procedures, requiring prophylaxis, should be scheduled. The literature supports 9- to 14-day intervals as ideal to minimize the risk of emergence of resistant organisms.[11,12] Since serum levels of the standard amoxicillin dose may be adequate for 6-14 hours depending on the specific organism challenge, the clinician may have to consider the efficacy of a second dose if multiple procedures are planned over the course of a single day.

Table 4.
CARDIAC CONDITIONS PREDISPOSING TO ENDOCARDITIS

Endocarditis Prophylaxis Recommended
High-Risk Category
Prosthetic cardiac valves, including bioprosthetic and homograft valves
Previous bacterial endocarditis
Complex cyanotic congenital heart disease (eg, single ventricle states, transposition of the great arteries, tetralogy of Fallot)
Surgically constructed systemic pulmonary shunts or conduits
Moderate-Risk Category
Most other congenital cardiac malformations (other than above and below)
Acquired valvar dysfunction (eg, rheumatic heart disease)
Hypertrophic cardiomyopathy
Mitral valve prolapse with valvar regurgitation and/or thickened leaflets*

Endocarditis Prophylaxis Not Recommended
Negligible-Risk Category (no greater risk than the general population)
Isolated secundum atrial septal defect
Surgical repair of atrial septal defect, ventricular septal defect, or patent ductus arteriosus (without residual defects beyond 6 mo)
Previous coronary artery bypass graft surgery
Mitral valve prolapse without valvar regurgitation
Physiologic, functional, or innocent heart murmurs
Previous Kawasaki disease without valvar dysfunction
Previous rheumatic fever without valvar dysfunction
Cardiac pacemakers (intravascular and epicardial) and implanted defibrillators
Specific risk for patients with a history of fenfluramine or dexfenfluramine (fen-phen or Redux®) use, has not been determined. Such patients should have medical evaluation for potential cardiac damage, as currently recommended by the FDA.

For patients with suspected or confirmed mitral valve prolapse (MVP), the risk of infection as well as other complications such as tachycardia, syncope, congestive heart failure, or progressive regurgitation are variable. The risk depends on age and severity of MVP. The decision to recommend prophylaxis in such patients is oftentimes controversial but it is generally agreed that the determination of regurgitation is the most predictive (see Algorithm Figure 2 at the end of this chapter). Therefore, patients with MVP with mitral regurgitation require prophylaxis. If the regurgitation is undetermined and the patient is in need of an immediate procedure, then prophylaxis should be given in any case and the patient referred for further evaluation. If echocardiographic or Doppler studies demonstrate regurgitation, then prophylaxis would be recommended routinely. If no regurgitation can be demonstrated by these studies, then MVP alone does not require prophylaxis.

PREPROCEDURAL ANTIBIOTICS FOR PROSTHETIC IMPLANTS

A significant number of dental patients have had total joint replacements or other implanted prosthetic devices.[13] Prior to performing dental procedures that might induce bacteremia, the dentist must consider the use of antibiotic prophylaxis in these patients. Until recently, only the American Heart Association had taken a formal stance on implanted devices by suggesting guidelines for the use of antibiotic prophylaxis in patients with prosthetic heart valves.[1,2] These guidelines and the recent guidelines for prevention of bacterial endocarditis have been published in *General Dentistry*.[14]

The use of antibiotics in patients with other prosthetic devices, including total joint replacements has remained controversial because of several issues. Late infections of implanted prosthetic devices have rarely been associated with microbial organisms of oral origin.[15] Secondly, since late infections in such patients are often not reported, data is lacking to substantiate or refute this potential.[16] Also, there is general acceptance that patients with acute infections at distant sites such as the oral cavity may be at greater risk of infection of an implanted prosthetic device. Periodontal disease has been implicated as a distant site infection.[15] Since antibiotics are associated with allergies and other adverse reactions, and because the frequent use of antibiotics may lead to emergence of resistant organisms,[13] any perceived benefit of antibiotic prophylaxis must always be weighed against known risks of toxicity, allergy, or potential microbial resistance.

Recently, an advisory group made up of representatives from the American Dental Association and the American Academy of Orthopedic Surgeons published a statement in the *Journal of the American Dental Association* on the use of antibiotics prior to dental procedures in patients with total joint replacements.[17] The statement concluded that antibiotic prophylaxis should not be prescribed routinely for most dental patients with total joint replacements or for any patients with pins, plates, and screws. However, in an attempt to base the guidelines on available scientific evidence, the advisory group stated that certain patients may be potential risks for joint infection thus justifying the use of prophylactic antibiotics. Those conditions considered by the advisory group to be associated with potential elevated risk of joint infections are listed in Table 5.[18,22] The dentist should carefully review the patient's history to ensure identification of those medical problems leading to potential elevated risks of joint infections as listed in Table 5. Where appropriate, medical consultation with the patient's internist or orthopedist may be prudent to assist in this determination. The orthopedist should be queried specifically, as to the status of the joint prosthesis itself.

Table 5.
PATIENTS WITH POTENTIAL ELEVATED RISK OF JOINT INFECTION

Inflammatory arthropathies: Rheumatoid arthritis, systemic lupus erythematosus
Disease-, drug-, or radiation-induced immunosuppression
Insulin-dependent diabetes
First 2 years following joint replacement
Previous prosthetic joint infections
Patients with acute infections at a distant site
Hemophilia

Patients who present with elevated risks of joint infections, in which the dentist is going to perform any procedures associated with a high risk of bacteremia, need to receive preprocedural antibiotics. Those dental procedures associated with high risk of bacteremia are listed in Table 3. Patients undergoing dental procedures involving low risk of bacteremia, probably do not require premedication even though the patient may be in the category of elevated risk of joint infections. Patients with an acute oral infection or moderate to severe gingival inflammation and/or periodontitis must be considered at higher risk for bacteremia during dental procedures than those without active dental disease. In these patients, as in all patients, the dental clinician should aggressively treat these oral conditions striving for optimum oral health. The listing of low bacteremia risks in Table 3 may need to be reconsidered, depending on the patient's oral health.

ANTIBIOTIC REGIMENS

The antibiotic prophylaxis regimens as suggested by the advisory panel are listed in Table 6. These regimens are not exactly the same as those listed in Table 2 (for prevention of endocarditis) and must be reviewed carefully to avoid confusion. Cephalexin, cephradine, or amoxicillin may be used in patients not allergic to penicillin. The selected antibiotic is given as a single 2 g dose 1 hour before the procedure. A follow-up dose is not recommended. Cephalexin (Keflex®) and amoxicillin have been described earlier in this chapter. Cephradine (Velosef®) is a first-generation cephalosporin-type antibiotic effective against anaerobic bacteria and aerobic gram-positive bacteria. It is used in medicine predominantly to treat infections of the bones and joints, infections of the lower respiratory tract, urinary tract, and skin and soft tissues.

Parenteral cefazolin (Ancef®) or ampicillin are the recommended antibiotics for those patients unable to take oral medications; see Table 6 for doses. Cefazolin is a first-generation cephalosporin effective against anaerobes and aerobic gram-positive bacteria. Ampicillin is an aminopenicillin described earlier. For patients allergic to penicillin, clindamycin is the recommended antibiotic of choice. Clindamycin is active against aerobic and anaerobic streptococci, most staphylococci, the *Bacteroides*, and the *Actinomyces* families of bacteria. The recommended oral and parenteral doses of clindamycin in the joint prosthetic patient are listed in Table 6.

ANTIBIOTIC PROPHYLAXIS *(Continued)*

Table 6.
ANTIBIOTIC REGIMENS FOR PATIENTS WITH PROSTHETIC IMPLANTS

Patients not allergic to penicillin: Cephalexin, cephradine, or amoxicillin

 2 g orally 1 hour prior to dental procedure

Patients not allergic to penicillin and unable to take oral medications: Cefazolin or ampicillin

 Cefazolin 1 g or ampicillin 2 g I.M. or I.V. 1 hour prior to the procedure

Patients allergic to penicillin: Clindamycin

 600 mg orally 1 hour prior to dental procedure

Patients allergic to penicillin and unable to take oral medications: Clindamycin

 600 mg I.V. 1 hour prior to the procedure

Amoxicillin (Amoxil®, Biomox®, Larotid®, Polymox®, Trimox®, Utimox®, Wymox®) *on page 68*

Ampicillin (Amcill®, Marcillin®, Omnipen®, Polycillin®, Principen®, Totacillin®) *on page 73*

Cefazolin (Ancef®) *on page 188*

Cephalexin (Keflex®) *on page 201*

Cephradine (Velosef®) *on page 203*

Clindamycin (Cleocin®) *on page 243*

Clinical Considerations for Dentistry

See Algorithm Figure 3 at the end of this chapter.

The frequency of postinsertion infections in patients who have undergone total joint replacement or prosthetic device placement is variable. The most common cause of infection with all devices is found to be from contamination at the time of surgical insertions.[18,23] The presence of an acute distant infection at a site other than the joint, however, appears to be a risk factor for late infection of these devices. The rationale by the American Dental Association and the American Academy of Orthopedic Surgeons in their advisory statement[17] has been to provide guidelines to minimize the use of antibiotics to the first 2 years following total joint replacement. As more data are collected, these recommendations may be revised. However, it is thought to be prudent for the dental clinician to fully evaluate all patients with respect to history and or physical findings prior to determining the risk.

If a procedure considered to be low risk for bacteremia is performed in a patient at risk for joint complications, and inadvertent bleeding occurs, then an appropriate antibiotic should be given immediately. Although this is not ideal, animal studies suggest that it may be useful.[10] Likewise, in patients where concern exists over joint complications and a medical consultation cannot be immediately obtained, the patient should be treated as though antibiotic coverage is necessary until such time that an appropriate consultation can be completed. The presence of an acute oral infection, in addition to any pre-existing dental conditions, may increase the risk of late infection at the prosthetic joint. Even though most late joint infections are caused by *Staphylococcus* sp, the risk of bacteremia involving another organism, predominant in an acute infection, may increase the risk of joint infection.[13,18,23-25]

The dentist may also need to consider the question of multiple procedures over a period of time. Procedures planned over a period of several days would best be rescheduled at intervals of 9-14 days. The risk of emergence of resistant organisms in patients receiving multiple short-term doses of antibiotics has been shown to be greater than those receiving antibiotics over longer intervals of time.[11,12]

FREQUENTLY ASKED QUESTIONS

Can erythromycin still be used to prevent bacterial endocarditis in dental patients?

 If the clinician has successfully used erythromycin in the past, this form of prophylaxis can be continued using the regimen included in the recommendation of 1990.[2] Erythromycin has, however, been excluded for the vast majority of patients due to gastric upset.

If the patient is presently taking antibiotics for some other ailment, is prophylaxis still necessary?

 If a patient is already taking antibiotics for another condition, prophylaxis should be accomplished with a drug from another class. For example, in the patient who is not allergic to penicillin who is taking erythromycin for a medical condition such as mycoplasma infection, amoxicillin would be the drug of choice for prophylaxis. Also, in the penicillin-allergic patient taking clindamycin, prophylaxis would best be accomplished with azithromycin or clarithromycin. The new guidelines[1] restated the position that doses of antibiotics for prevention of recurrence of rheumatic fever are thought to be inadequate to prevent bacterial endocarditis and prophylaxis should be accomplished with the full dose of a drug from another class.

Can clindamycin be used safely in patients with gastrointestinal disorders?

If a patient has a history of inflammatory bowel disease and is allergic to penicillin, azithromycin or clarithromycin should be selected over clindamycin. In patients with a negative history of inflammatory bowel disease, clindamycin has not been shown to induce colitis following a single-dose administration.

Why do the suggested drug regimens for patients with joint prostheses resemble so closely the regimens for the prevention of bacterial endocarditis?

Bacteremia is the predisposing risk factor for the development of endocarditis in those patients at risk due to a cardiac condition. Likewise, the potential of bacteremia during dental procedures is considered to be the risk factor in some late joint prostheses infections, even though this risk is presumed to be much lower.

How do we determine those patients who have had joint replacement complications?

Patients who have had complications during the initial placement of a total joint would be those who had infection following placement, those with recurrent pain, or those who have had previous joint replacement failures. If the patient reports even minor complications, a medical consultation with the orthopedist would be the most appropriate action for the dentist.

Is prophylaxis required in patients with pins, screws, or plates often used in orthopedic repairs?

There is currently no evidence supporting use of antibiotics following the placement of pins, plates, or screws. Breast implants, dental implants, and implanted lenses in the eye following cataract surgery are also all thought to be at minimal risk for infection following dental procedures. Therefore, no antibiotic prophylaxis is recommended in these situations. There is, however, some evidence indicating elevated risk of infection following some types of penile implants and some vascular access devices, used during chemotherapy.[13] It is recommended that the dentist discuss such patients with the physician prior to determining the need for antibiotics.

What should I do if medical consultation results in a recommendation that differs from the published guidelines endorsed by the American Dental Association?

The dentist is ultimately responsible for treatment recommendations. Ideally, by communicating with the physician, a consensus can be achieved that is either in agreement with the guidelines or is based on other established medical reasoning.

What is the best antibiotic modality for treating dental infections?

Penicillin is still the drug of choice for treatment of infections in and around the oral cavity. Phenoxy-methyl penicillin (Pen VK®) has long been the most commonly selected antibiotic. In penicillin-allergic individuals, erythromycin may be an appropriate consideration. If another drug is sought, clindamycin prescribed 300 mg as a loading dose followed by 150 mg 4 times a day would be an appropriate regimen for a dental infection. In general, if there is no response to Pen VK®, then Augmentin® may be a good alternative in the nonpenicillin-allergic patient because of its slightly altered spectrum. Recommendations would include that the patient should take the drug with food.

Is there cross-allergenicity between the cephalosporins and penicillin?

The incidence of cross-allergenicity is 5% to 8% in the overall population. If a patient has demonstrated a Type I hypersensitivity reaction to penicillin, namely urticaria or anaphylaxis, then this incidence would increase to 20%.

Is there definitely an interaction between contraception agents and antibiotics?

There are well founded interactions between contraceptives and antibiotics. The best instructions that a patient could be given by their dentist are that should an antibiotic be necessary and the dentist is aware that the patient is on contraceptives, and if the patient is using chemical contraceptives, the patient should seriously consider alternative means of contraception during the antibiotic management.

Are antibiotic necessary in diabetic patients?

In the management of diabetes, control of the diabetic status is the key factor relative to all morbidity issues. If a patient is well controlled, then antibiotics will

ANTIBIOTIC PROPHYLAXIS *(Continued)*

likely not be necessary. However, in patients where the control is questionable or where they have recently been given a different drug regimen for their diabetes or if they are being titrated to an appropriate level of either insulin or oral hypoglycemic agents during these periods of time, the dentist might consider preprocedural antibiotics to be efficacious.

Do nonsteroidal anti-inflammatory drugs interfere with blood pressure medication?

At the current time there is no clear evidence that NSAIDs interfere with any of the blood pressure medications that are currently in use.

Is a patient who has taken phentermine at risk for cardiac problems just like a patient who took "fen-phen"?

No, there is often confusion with these drug names. "Fen-phen" referred to a combined use of fenfluramine and phentermine and it is this combination that has led to the FDA statement (see Table 4). The single drug phentermine has not been implicated in this current concern over cardiac complications.

Figure 1
Preprocedural Dental Action Plan for Patients With a History Indicative of Elevated Endocarditis Risk

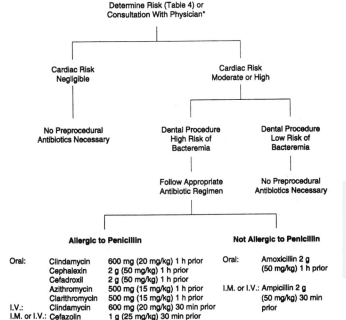

Child dosages in parentheses and should never exceed adult dose. Cephalasporins should be avoided in patients with previous Type I hypersensitivity reactions to penicillin due to some evidence of cross allergenicity.

* For Emergency Dental Care the clinician should attempt phone consultation. If unable to contact patient's physician or determine risk, the patient should be treated as though there is moderate or high risk of cardiac complication and follow the algorithm.

ANTIBIOTIC PROPHYLAXIS *(Continued)*

Figure 2
Patient With Suspected Mitral Valve Prolapse

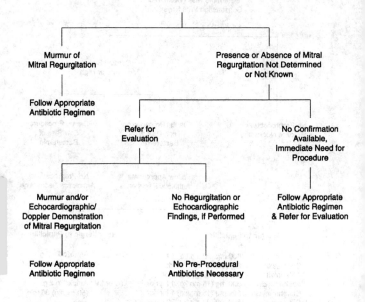

Figure 3
Preprocedural Dental Action Plan for
Patients With Prosthetic Implants

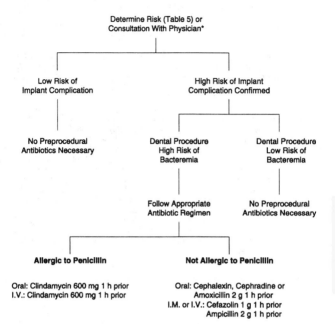

Cephalosporins should be avoided in patients with previous Type I hypersensitivity reactions to penicillin due to some evidence of cross allergenicity.

*For Emergency Dental Care the clinician should attempt phone consultation. If unable to contact patient's physician or determine risk, the patient should be treated as though there is high risk of implant complication and follow the algorithm.

ANTIBIOTIC PROPHYLAXIS *(Continued)*

REFERENCES

1. Dajani AS, Taubert KA, Wilson W, et al, "Prevention of Bacterial Endocarditis. Recommendations by the American Heart Association," *JAMA*, 1997, 277(22):1794-801.

2. Dajani AS, Bisno AI, Chung KJ, et al, "Prevention of Bacterial Endocarditis. Recommendations by the American Heart Association," *JAMA*, 1990, 264(22): 2919-22.

3. Dajani AS, Bawdon RE, and Berry MC, "Oral Amoxicillin as Prophylaxis for Endocarditis: What Is the Optimal Dose?" *Clin Infect Dis*, 1994, 18(2):157-60.

4. Fluckiger U, Francioli P, Blaser J, et al, "Role of Amoxicillin Serum Levels for Successful Prophylaxis of Experimental Endocarditis Due to Tolerant Streptococci," *J Infect Dis*, 1994, 169(6):1397-400.

5. Wynn RL, "Amoxicillin Update," *Gen Dent*, 1991, 39(5):322, 324, 326.

6. Wynn RL and Bergman SA, "Antibiotics and Their Use in the Treatment of Orofacial Infections, Part I," *Gen Dent*, 1994, 42(5): 398, 400, 402.

7. Wynn RL, "New Erythromycins," *Gen Dent*, 1996, 44(4):304-7.

8. Clauzel AM, Visier S, and Michel FB, "Efficacy and Safety of Azithromycin in Lower Respiratory Tract Infections," *Eur Respir J*, 1990, 3(Suppl 10):89S.

9. Rapeport WG, Dewland PM, Muirhead DC, et al, "Lack of Interaction Between Azithromycin and Carbamazepine," *Br J Clin Pharmacol*, 1992, 30:551P.

10. Berney P and Francioli P, "Successful Prophylaxis of Experimental Streptococcal Endocarditis With Single-Dose Amoxicillin Administered After Bacterial Challenge," *J Infect Dis*, 1990, 161(2):281-5.

11. Leviner E, Tzukert AA, Benoliel R, et al, "Development Resistant Oral Viridans Streptococci After Administration of Prophylactic Antibiotics: Time Management in the Dental Treatment of Patients Susceptible to Infective Endocarditis," *Oral Surg Oral Med Oral Pathol*, 1987, 64:417-20.

12. Simmons NA, Cawson RA, Clark CA, et al, "Prophylaxis of Infective Endocarditis," *Lancet*, 1986, 1(8492):1267.

13. Little JW, Falace DA, Miller CS, et al, "Prosthetic Implants," *Dental Management of the Medically Compromised Patient*, 5th ed, Mosby, St Louis: MO, 1997, 602-17.

14. Wynn RL, Meiller TF, and Crossley HL, "New Guidelines for the Prevention of Bacterial Endocarditis," *Gen Dent*, 1997. 45:426-34.

15. Bartzokas CA, Johnson R, Jane M, et al, "Relation Between Mouth and Haematogenous Infection in Total Joint Replacements," *BMJ*, 1994, 309(6953):506-8.

16. Hopkins CC, "Recognition of Endemic and Epidemic Prosthetic Device Infections: The Role of Surveillance, the Hospital Infection Control Practitioner, and the Hospital Epidemiologist," *Infect Dis Clin North Am*, 1989, 3(2):211-20.

17. "Advisory Statement for Dental Patients With Total Joint Replacement," *J Am Dent Assoc*, 1997, 128:1004-8.

18. Ching DW, Gould IM, Rennie JA, et al, "Prevention of Late Haematogenous Infection in Major Prosthetic Joints," *J Antimicrob Chemother*, 1989, 23(5):676-80.

19. Brause BD, "Infections Associated With Prosthetic Joints," *Clin Rheum Dis*, 1986, 12(2):523-36.

20. Johnson DP and Bannister GC, "The Outcome of Infected Arthroplasty of the Knee," *J Bone Joint Surg (Br)*, 1986, 68(2):289-91.

21. Jacobson JJ, Millard HD, Plezia R, et al, "Dental Treatment and Late Prosthetic Joint Infections," *Oral Surg Oral Med Oral Pathol*, 1986, 61(4):413-7.

22. Jacobson JJ, Patel B, Asher G, et al, "Oral Staphylococcus in Older Subjects With Rheumatoid Arthritis," *J Am Geriatr Soc*, 1997, 45(5):590-3.

23. Hansen AD, Osmon DR, and Nelson CL, "Prevention of Deep Prosthetic Joint Infection," *J Bone Joint Surg*, 1996, 78:458-71.

24. Skiest DJ and Coykendall AL, "Prosthetic Hip Infection Related to a Dental Procedure Despite Antibiotic Prophylaxis," *Oral Surg Oral Med Oral Pathol Oral Radiol Endod*, 1995, 79(5):661-3.

25. Wahl M, "Myths of Dental-Induced Prosthetic Joint Infections," *Clin Infect Dis*, 1995, 20:1420-5.

SYSTEMIC VIRAL DISEASES

HEPATITIS

The hepatitis viruses are a group of DNA and RNA viruses that produce symptoms associated with inflammation of the liver. Currently, hepatitis A through G have been identified by immunological testing; however, hepatitis A through E have received most attention in terms of disease identification. Recently, however, there has been increased interest in hepatitis viruses F and G, particularly as relate to healthcare professionals. Our knowledge is expanding rapidly in this area and the clinician should be alert to changes in the literature that might update their knowledge. Hepatitis F, for instance, remains a diagnosis of exclusion effectively being non-A, B, C, D, E, or G. Whereas, hepatitis G has serologic testing available, however, not commercially at this time. Research evaluations of various antibody and RT-PCR tests for hepatitis G are under development at this time.

Signs and symptoms of viral hepatitis in general are quite variable. Patients infected may range from asymptomatic to experiencing flu-like symptoms only. In addition, fever, nausea, joint muscle pain, jaundice, and hepatomegaly along with abdominal pain can result from infection with one of the hepatitis viruses. The virus also can create an acute or chronic infection. Usually following these early symptoms or the asymptomatic period, the patient may recover or may go on to develop chronic liver dysfunction. Liver dysfunction may be represented primarily by changes in liver function tests known as LFTs and these primarily include aspartate aminotransferase known as AST and alanine aminotransferase known as ALT. In addition, for A, B, C, D, and E there are serologic tests for either antigen, antibody, or both. Of hepatitis A through G, five forms have both acute and chronic forms whereas A and E appear to only create acute disease. There are differences in the way clinicians may approach a known postexposure to one of the hepatitis viruses. In many instances, gamma globulin may be used, however, the indications for gamma globulin as a drug limit their use to several of the viruses only. The dental clinician should be aware that the gastroenterologist may choose to give gamma globulin off-label.

Hepatitis A virus is an enteric virus that is a member of the Picornavirus family along with Coxsackie viruses and poliovirus. Previously known as infectious hepatitis, hepatitis A has been detected in humans for centuries. It causes acute hepatitis, often transmitted by oral-fecal contamination and having an incubation period of approximately 30 days. Typically, constitutional symptoms are present and jaundice may occur. Drug therapy that the dentist may encounter in a patient being treated for hepatitis A would primarily include immunoglobulin.

Hepatitis B virus is previously known as serum hepatitis and has particular trophism for liver cells. Hepatitis B virus causes both acute and chronic disease in suscep-tible patients. The incubation period is often long and the diagnosis might be made by serologic markers even in the absence of symptoms. No drug therapy for acute hepatitis B is known; however, chronic hepatitis has recently been successfully treated with alfa-interferon. There are vaccines available for hepatitis A and B. Hepatitis C virus was described in 1988 and has been formerly classified as non-A/non-B. It is clear that hepatitis C represents a high percentage of the transfusion-associated hepatitis that is seen. Treatment of acute hepatitis C infection is gener-ally supportive. Interferon Alfa-2a therapy has been used with some success recently and interferon-alfa may be beneficial with hepatitis C related chronic hepa-titis. Hepatitis D is previously known as the delta agent and is a virus that is incomplete in that it requires previous infection with hepatitis B in order to be manifested. Currently, no antiviral therapy is effective against hepatitis D. Hepatitis E virus is an RNA virus that represents a proportion of the previously classified non-A/non-B diagnoses. There is currently no antiviral therapy against hepatitis E.

Hepatitis F, as was mentioned, remains a diagnosis of exclusion. There are no known immunological tests available for identification of hepatitis F at present and currently the Centers for Disease Control have not come out with specific guidelines or recommendations. It is thought, however, that hepatitis F is a bloodborne virus and it has been used as a diagnosis in several cases of post-transfusion hepatitis. Hepatitis G virus (HGV), is the newest hepatitis and is also assumed to be a bloodborne virus. Similar in family to hepatitis C, it is thought to occur concomitantly with hepatitis C and appears to be even more prevalent in some blood donors than hepatitis C. Occupational transmission of HGV is currently under study (see the references for updated information) and currently there are no specific CDC recom-mendations for postexposure to an HGV individual as the testing for identification remains experimental.

SYSTEMIC VIRAL DISEASES *(Continued)*

PRE-EXPOSURE PROPHYLAXIS FOR HEPATITIS B

Health care workers*

Special patient groups (eg. adolescents, infants born to HB$_s$Ag–positive mothers, military personnel, etc)

   Hemodialysis patients†

   Recipients of certain blood products‡

Lifestyle factors

   Homosexual and bisexual men

   Intravenous drug abusers

   Heterosexually active persons with multiple sexual partners or recently acquired sexually transmitted diseases

Environmental factors

   Household and sexual contacts of HBV carriers

   Prison inmates

   Clients and staff of institutions for the mentally handicapped

   Residents, immigrants and refugees from areas with endemic HBV infection

   International travelers at increased risk of acquiring HBV infection

*The risk of hepatitis B virus (HBV) infection for health care workers varies both between hospitals and within hospitals. Hepatitis B vaccination is recommended for all health care workers with blood exposure.

†Hemodialysis patients often respond poorly to hepatitis B vaccination; higher vaccine doses or increased number of doses are required. A special formulation of one vaccine is now available for such persons (Recombivax HB®, 40 mcg/mL). The anti-HB$_s$ (antibody to hepatitis B surface antigen) response of such persons should be tested after they are vaccinated, and those who have not responded should be revaccinated with 1-3 additional doses.

Patients with chronic renal disease should be vaccinated as early as possible, ideally before they require hemodialysis. In addition, their anti- HB$_s$ levels should be monitored at 6- to 12-month intervals to assess the need for revaccination.

‡Patients with hemophilia should be immunized subcutaneously, not intramuscularly.

POSTEXPOSURE PROPHYLAXIS FOR HEPATITIS B*

Exposure	Hepatitis B Immune Globulin	Hepatitis B Vaccine
Perinatal	0.5 mL I.M. within 12 h of birth	0.5 mL† I.M. within 12 h of birth (no later than 7 d), and at 1 and 6 mo‡; test for HB$_s$Ag and anti-HB$_s$ at 12-15 mo
Sexual	0.06 mL/kg I.M. within 14 d of sexual contact; a second dose should be given if the index patient remains HB$_s$Ag-positive after 3 mo and hepatitis B vaccine was not given initially	1 mL I.M. at 0, 1, and 6 mo for homosexual and bisexual men and regular sexual contacts of persons with acute and chronic hepatitis B
Percutaneous; exposed person unvaccinated		
Source known HB$_s$Ag-positive	0.06 mL/kg I.M. within 24 h	1 mL I.M. within 7 d, and at 1 and 6 mo§
Source known, HB$_s$Ag status not known	Test source for HB$_s$Ag; if source is positive, give exposed person 0.06 mL/kg I.M. once within 7 d	1 mL I.M. within 7 d, and at 1 and 6 mo§
Source not tested or unknown	Nothing required	1 mL I.M. within 7 d, and at 1 and 6 mo
Percutaneous; exposed person vaccinated		
Source known HB$_s$Ag-positive	Test exposed person for anti-HB$_s$¶. If titer is protective, nothing is required; if titer is not protective, give 0.06 mL/kg within 24 h.	Review vaccination status#
Source known, HB$_s$Ag status not known	Test source for HB$_s$Ag and exposed person for anti-HB$_s$. If source is HB$_s$Ag-negative, or if source is HB$_s$Ag-positive but anti-HB$_s$ titer is protective, nothing is required. If source is HB$_s$Ag-positive and anti-HB$_s$ titer is not protective or if exposed person is a known nonresponder, give 0.06 mL/kg I.M. within 24 h. A second dose of hepatitis B immune globulin can be given 1 mo later if a booster dose of hepatitis B vaccine is not given.	Review vaccination status#
Source not tested or unknown	Test exposed person for anti-HB$_s$. If anti-HB$_s$ titer is protective, nothing is required. If anti-HB$_s$ titer is not protective, 0.06 mL/kg may be given along with a booster dose of hepatitis B vaccine.	Review vaccination status#

*HB$_s$Ag = hepatitis B surface antigen; anti-HB$_s$ = antibody to hepatitis B surface antigen; I.M. = intramuscularly; SRU = standard ratio units.

†Each 0.5 mL dose of plasma-derived hepatitis B vaccine contains 10 mcg of HB$_s$Ag; each 0.5 mL dose of recombinant hepatitis B vaccine contains 5 mcg or 10 mcg of HB$_s$Ag.

‡If hepatitis B immune globulin and hepatitis B vaccine are given simultaneously, they should be given at separate sites.

§If hepatitis B vaccine is not given, a second dose of hepatitis B immune globulin should be given 1 month later.

¶Anti-HB$_s$ titers <10 SRU by radioimmunoassay or negative by enzyme immunoassay indicate lack of protection. Testing the exposed person for anti-HB$_s$ is not necessary if a protective level of antibody has been shown within the previous 24 months.

#If the exposed person has not completed a three-dose series of hepatitis B vaccine, the series should be completed. Test the exposed person for anti-HB$_s$. If the antibody level is protective, nothing is required. If an adequate antibody response in the past is shown on retesting to have declined to an inadequate level, a booster dose (1 mL) of hepatitis B vaccine should be given. If the exposed person has inadequate antibody or is a known nonresponder to vaccination, a booster dose can be given along with one dose of hepatitis B immune globulin.

SYSTEMIC VIRAL DISEASES (Continued)

TYPES OF HEPATITIS VIRUS

Features	A	B	C	D	E	F	G
Incubation Period	2-6 wks	8-24 wks	2-52 wks	3-13 wks	3-6 wks	Unknown	Unknown
Onset	Abrupt	Insidious	Insidious	Abrupt	Abrupt	Insidious	Insidious
Symptoms							
Jaundice	Adults: 70% to 80%; Children: 10%	25%	25%	Varies	Unknown	Unknown	Unknown
Asymptomatic Patients	Adults: 50%; Children: Most	~75%	~75%	Rare	Rare	Common	Common
Routes of Transmission							
Fecal/Oral	Yes	No	No	No	Yes	Unknown	Unknown
Parenteral	Rare	Yes	Yes	Yes	No		
Sexual	No	Yes	Possible	Yes	No		
Perinatal	No	Yes	Possible	Possible	No		
Water/Food	Yes	No	No	No	Yes		
Sequelae (% of patients)							
Chronic state	No	Adults: 6% to 10%; Children: 25% to 50%; Infants: 70% to 90%	>75%	10% to 15%	No	Unknown	Likely
Case-Fatality Rate	0.6%	1.4%	1% to 2%	30%	1% to 2%; Pregnant women: 20%	Unknown	Unknown

Hepatitis A Vaccine (Havrix®) *on page 467*
Hepatitis B Immune Globulin (H-BIG®, HyperHep®) *on page 468*
Hepatitis B Vaccine (Engerix-B®, Recombivax HB®) *on page 468*
Immune Globulin, Intramuscular (Gamastan®, Gammar®) *on page 502*
Immune Globulin, Intravenous (Gamimune® N, Gammagard®, Gammagard® S/D, Gammar®-P, Polygam®, Polygam® S/D, Sandoglobulin®, Venoglobulin®-I, Venoglobulin®-S) *on page 503*
Interferon Alfa-2a (Roferon-A®) *on page 510*
Interferon Alfa-2b (Intron® A) *on page 511*

HERPES

The herpes viruses not only represent a topic of specific interest to the dentist due to oral manifestations, but are widespread as systemic infections. Herpes simplex virus is also of interest because of its central nervous system infections and its relationship as one of the viral infections commonly found in AIDS patients. Oral herpes infections will be covered elsewhere. Treatment of herpes simplex primary infection includes acyclovir. Ganciclovir is an alternative drug and foscarnet is also occasionally used. Epstein-Barr virus is a member of the herpesvirus family and produces syndromes important in dentistry, including infectious mononucleosis with the commonly found oral pharyngitis and petechial hemorrhages, as well as being the causative agent of Burkitt's lymphoma. The relationship between Epstein-Barr virus to oral hairy leukoplakia in AIDS patients has not been shown to be one of cause and effect; however, the presence of Epstein-Barr in these lesions is consistent. Currently, there is no accepted treatment for Epstein-Barr virus, although acyclovir has been shown in *in vitro* studies to have some efficacy. Varicella-zoster virus is another member of the herpesvirus family and is the causative agent of two clinical entities, chickenpox and shingles or herpes zoster. Oral manifestations of both chickenpox and herpes zoster include vesicular eruptions often leading to confluent mucosal ulcerations. Acyclovir is the drug of choice for treatment of herpes zoster infections.

There are other herpes viruses that produce disease in man and animals. These viruses have no specific treatment, therefore, incidence is thought to be less common than those mentioned and the specific treatment is not determined at present. The role of some of these viruses in concomitant infection with the HIV and other coinfection viruses is still under study.

ANTIVIRALS

ANTIVIRAL AGENTS OF ESTABLISHED THERAPEUTIC EFFECTIVENESS

Viral Infection	Drug
Cytomegalovirus	
Retinitis	Ganciclovir
	Foscarnet
Pneumonia	Ganciclovir
Hepatitis viruses	
Chronic hepatitis C	Interferon Alfa-2a
Chronic hepatitis B	Interferon Alfa-2b
Herpes simplex virus	
Orofacial herpes	
First episode	Acyclovir
Recurrence	Acyclovir
	Penciclovir
Genital herpes	
First episode	Acyclovir
Recurrence	Acyclovir
Suppression	Acyclovir
Encephalitis	Acyclovir
Mucocutaneous disease in immunocompromised	Acyclovir
Neonatal	Acyclovir
Keratoconjunctivitis	Trifluridine
	Vidarabine
Influenza A virus	Amantadine
	Rimantadine
Papillomavirus	
Condyloma acuminatum	Interferon Alfa-2b
	Imiquimod (Aldara®):
	(use for oral lesions is under
	study)
Respiratory syncytial virus	Ribavirin
Varicella-zoster virus	
Varicella in normal children	Acyclovir
Varicella in immunocompromised	Acyclovir
Herpes zoster in immunocompromised	Acyclovir
Herpes zoster in normal hosts	Acyclovir
	Famciclovir

Acyclovir (Zovirax®) *on page 31*
Amantadine (Symmetrel®) *on page 50*
Atovaquone (Mepron™) *on page 97*
Cidofovir (Vistide®) *on page 233*
Famciclovir (Famvir™) *on page 392*
Foscarnet (Foscavir®) *on page 429*
Ganciclovir (Cytovene®, Vitrasert®) *on page 436*
Hepatitis B Immune Globulin (H-BIG®, HyperHep®) *on page 468*
Imiquimod (Aldara®) *on page 502*
Immune Globulin, Intramuscular (Gamastan®, Gammar®) *on page 502*
Interferon Alfa-2a (Roferon-A®) *on page 510*
Interferon Alfa-2b (Intron® A) *on page 511*
Interferon Alfa-N3 (Alferon® N) *on page 513*
Penciclovir (Denavir®) *on page 729*
Rifabutin (Mycobutin®) *on page 842*
Rimantadine (Flumadine®) *on page 845*
Trifluridine (Viroptic®) *on page 961*
Valacyclovir (Valtrex®) *on page 981*
Vidarabine (Vira-A®) *on page 989*

PART II.
DENTAL MANAGEMENT AND THERAPEUTIC CONSIDERATIONS IN PATIENTS WITH SPECIFIC ORAL CONDITIONS AND OTHER MEDICINE TOPICS

This second part of the text focuses on therapies the dentist may choose to prescribe for patients suffering from oral disease or are in need of special care. Some overlap between these sections has resulted from systemic conditions that have oral manifestations and vice-versa. Cross-references to the descriptions and the monographs for individual drugs described elsewhere in this handbook allow for easy retrieval of information. Example prescriptions of selected drug therapies for each condition are presented so that the clinician can evaluate alternate approaches to treatment. Seldom is there a single drug of choice.

Those drug prescriptions listed represent prototype drugs and popular prescriptions and are examples only. The therapeutic index is available for cross-referencing if alternatives and additional drugs are sought.

TABLE OF CONTENTS

ORAL PAIN

PAIN PREVENTION

For the dental patient, the prevention of pain aids in relieving anxiety and reduces the probability of stress during dental care. For the practitioner, dental procedures can be accomplished more efficiently in a "painless" situation. Appropriate selection and use of local anesthetics is one of the foundations for success in this arena. Local anesthetics listed below include drugs for the most commonly confronted dental procedures. Ester anesthetics have a higher incidence of allergic manifestations due to the formation of the metabolic by-product, para-aminobenzoic acid. The amides have an almost negligible allergic rate, however, at least one well documented case of amide allergy was reported by Seng, et al.

The selection of a vasoconstrictor with the local anesthetic must be based on the length of the procedure to be performed, the patient's medical status (epinephrine is contraindicated in patients with uncontrolled hyperthyroidism), and the need for hemorrhage control. The following table lists some of the common drugs with their duration of action. Transoral patches with lidocaine are now available (Dentipatch®) and the new long-acting amide injectable, Ropivacaine (Naropin®) may be useful for postoperative pain management.

ORAL PAIN (Continued)

DENTAL ANESTHETICS
(Average Duration by Route)

Product	Infiltration	Inferior Alveolar Block
Marcaine® HCl 0.5% with epinephrine 1:200,000 (bupivacaine and epinephrine)	60 minutes	5-7 hours
Carbocaine® HCl 3% (mepivacaine)	20 minutes	40 minutes
Carbocaine® HCl 2% with Neo-Cobefrin® 1:20,000 (mepivacaine HCl and levonordefrin)	50 minutes	60-75 minutes
Duranest® Injection (etidocaine)	5-10 hours	5-10 hours
Citanest® Plain 4% (prilocaine)	20 minutes	2.5 hours
Citanest Forte® with Epinephrine (prilocaine with epinephrine)	2.25 hours	3 hours
Lidocaine HCl 2% and epinephrine 1:100,000 (lidocaine and epinephrine)	60 minutes	90 minutes

The use of preinjection topical anesthetics can assist in pain prevention (see also "Oral Viral Infections" *on page 1066* and "Oral Nonviral Soft Tissue Ulcerations or Erosions" *on page 1070*). Some clinicians are also using EMLA® (eutectic mixture of local anesthetic with lidocaine and prilocaine) as a topical. Skin patch available by Astra not currently approved for oral use.

Benzocaine (Hurricaine®, Numzident®, various other products) *on page 118*

Lidocaine (Dilocaine®, Duo-Trach®, Nervocaine®, Octocaine®, Xylocaine®) *on page 553*

Lidocaine Transoral (Dentipatch®) *on page 556*

Tetracaine (Pontocaine®, Viractin®) *on page 913*

PAIN MANAGEMENT

The patient with existing acute or chronic oral pain requires appropriate treatment and sensitivity on the part of the dentist, all for the purpose of achieving relief from the oral source of pain. Pain can be divided into mild, moderate, and severe levels and requires a subjective assessment by the dentist based on knowledge of the dental procedures to be performed, the presenting signs and symptoms of the patient, and the realization that most dental procedures are invasive often leading to pain once the patient has left the dental office. The practitioner must be aware that the treatment of the source of the pain is usually the best management. If infection is present, treatment of the infection will directly alleviate the patient's discomfort. However, a patient who is not in pain tends to heal better and it is wise to adequately cover the patient for any residual or recurrent discomfort suffered. Likewise, many of the procedures that the dentist performs have pain associated with them. Much of this pain occurs after leaving the dentist office due to an inflammatory process or a healing process that has been initiated. It is difficult to assign specific pain levels (mild, moderate, or severe) for specific procedures; however, the dentist should use his or her prescribing capacity judiciously so that overmedication is avoided.

The following categories of drugs and appropriate example prescriptions for each follow. These include management of mild pain with aspirin products, acetaminophen, and some of the nonsteroidal noninflammatory agents. Management of moderate pain includes codeine, Vicodin®, Vicodin ES®, Lorcet® 10/650; and Motrin® in the 800 mg dosage. Severe pain may require treatment with Percodan®, Percocet®, or Demerol®. All prescription pain preparations should be closely monitored for efficacy and discontinued if the pain persists or requires a higher level formulation.

The chronic pain patient represents a particular challenge for the practitioner. Some additional drugs that may be useful in managing the patient with chronic pain are covered in the temporomandibular dysfunction section of this text. It is always incumbent on the practitioner to reevaluate the diagnosis, source of pain, and treatment, whenever prolonged use of analgesics (narcotic or non-narcotic) is contemplated. Drugs such as Dilaudid® are not recommended for management of dental pain in most states.

Narcotic analgesics can be used on a short-term basis or intermittently in combination with non-narcotic therapy in the chronic pain patient. Judicious prescribing, monitoring, and maintenance by the practitioner is imperative, particularly whenever considering the use of a narcotic analgesic due to the abuse and addiction liabilities.

MILD PAIN

Acetaminophen (various products) *on page 20*

Aspirin (various products) *on page 90*

Diflunisal (Dolobid®) *on page 311*

Ibuprofen (various products) *on page 495*

Ketoprofen (Actron®, Orudis®, Orudis KT®, Oruvail®) *on page 534*

Naproxen (Aleve®, Anaprox®, Naprosyn®) *on page 665*

OVER-THE-COUNTER PRESCRIPTION EXAMPLES

Rx

Aspirin 325 mg

Disp

Sig: Take 2-3 tablets every 4 hours

Rx

Ibuprofen 200 mg

Disp

Sig: Take 2-3 tablets every 4 hours, up to 3200 mg (16 tablets)/ day

---

Note: Ibuprofen is available over-the-counter as Motrin IB®, Advil®, Nuprin®, and many other brands in 200 mg tablets.

Note: NSAIDs should never be taken together, nor should they be combined with aspirin. NSAIDs have anti-inflammatory effects as well as analgesics. An allergy to aspirin constitutes a contradiction to all the new NSAIDs. Aspirin and the NSAIDs may increase post-treatment bleeding.

Rx

Acetaminophen 325 mg

Disp

Sig: Take 2-3 tablets every 4 hours

Products include: Tylenol®, Datril®, Anacin® 3, and many others

---

Note: Acetaminophen can be given if patient has allergy, bleeding problems, or stomach upset secondary to aspirin or NSAIDs.

Rx

Aleve® 220 mg

Disp

Sig: 1-2 tablets every 8 hours

Ingredient: Naproxen

Rx

Orudis KT® 12.5 mg

Disp

Sig: 1-2 tablets every 8 hours

Ingredient: Ketoprofen

ORAL PAIN *(Continued)*

PRESCRIPTION ONLY EXAMPLES

Rx

Ketoprofen 25 mg

Disp

Sig: 1-2 tablets every 8 hours

Rx

Dolobid® 500 mg

Disp 16 tablets

Sig: Take 2 tablets initially, then 1 tablet every 8-12 hours for pain

---

Ingredient: Diflunisal

MODERATE/MODERATELY SEVERE PAIN

Aspirin and Codeine (Empirin® with Codeine) *on page 92*

Bromfenac (Duract™) *on page 139*

Dihydrocodeine Compound (Synalgos® DC) *on page 315*

Hydrocodone and Acetaminophen (Lortab®, Vicodin®, various products) *on page 478*

Ibuprofen (various products) *on page 495*

The following is a guideline to use when prescribing codeine with either aspirin or acetaminophen (Tylenol®):

Codeine No. 2 = codeine 15 mg

Codeine No. 3 = codeine 30 mg

Codeine No. 4 = codeine 60 mg

Example: ASA No. 3 = aspirin 325 mg + codeine 30 mg

PRESCRIPTION EXAMPLES

Rx

Duract™ 25 mg

Disp 24 tablets

Sig: Take 1 tablet every 6-8 hours as needed for pain*

Ingredients: Bromfenac

*Use should be limited to <10 days and avoided in patients with liver compromise

---

Rx

Motrin® 800 mg*

Disp 16 tablets

Sig: Take 1 tablet 3 times/day

Ingredient: Ibuprofen

Note: For more severe pain, Motrin® (800 mg) can be given up to 4 times/day.

*Note: Also available as 600 mg

Rx

Tylenol® No. 3*

Disp 16 (sixteen) tablets

Sig: Take 1 tablet every 4 hours as needed for pain

Ingredients: Acetaminophen and codeine

*Note: Also available as #2 and #4

Rx

Synalgos® DC

Disp 16 (sixteen) capsules

Sig: Take 1 capsule every 4 hours as needed for pain

Ingredients: Dihydrocodeine 16 mg, aspirin 356.4 mg, and caffeine 30 mg

---

Rx

Vicodin®

Disp 16 (sixteen) tablets

Sig: Take 1 tablet every 4 hours for pain

Ingredients: Hydrocodone 5 mg and acetaminophen 500 mg

Note: Available as Vicodin ES® for use 1 tablet every 8-12 hours

---

Rx

Lortab® 5 mg*

Disp 16 (sixteen) tablets

Sig: Take 1 or 2 tablets every 4 hours for pain (do not exceed 8 tablets in 24 hours)

Ingredients: Hydrocodone 5 mg and acetaminophen 500 mg

*Note: Available under other brand names with varying dosages and strengths

SEVERE PAIN

Hydrocodone and Ibuprofen (Vicoprofen®) *on page 482*

Meperidine (Demerol®) *on page 592*

Oxycodone (OxyContin®, OxyIR®, Roxicodone™) *on page 710*

Oxycodone and Acetaminophen (Percocet®, Roxicet®, Roxilox®, Tylox®) *on page 711*

Oxycodone and Aspirin (Codoxy®, Percodan®, Roxiprin®) *on page 712*

PRESCRIPTION EXAMPLES

Rx

Vicoprofen®

Disp 16 (sixteen) tablets

Sig: Take 1-2 tablets every 4-6 hours for pain   No Refills

Ingredients: Hydrocodone 7.5 mg and ibuprofen 200 mg

ORAL PAIN *(Continued)*

Rx

Demerol® 50 mg*

Disp 16 (sixteen) tablets

Sig: Take 1 tablet every 4 hours for pain   No Refills

Ingredients: Meperidine

*Triplicate prescription required in some states

Rx

Roxicodone™ 5 mg

Disp 24 tablets

Sig: Take 1 tablet every 6 hours for pain   No Refills

Ingredients: Oxycodone

Some formulations available as controlled release

Rx

Percodan®*

Disp 16 (sixteen) tablets

Sig: Take 1 tablet every 4 hours for pain   No Refills

Ingredients: Oxycodone 4.88 mg and aspirin 325 mg

*Triplicate prescription required in some states

Rx

Percocet® tablets or Tylox® capsules*

Disp 16 (sixteen) tablets or capsules

Sig: Take 1 tablet every 4 hours for pain   No Refills

Ingredients: Oxycodone 5 mg and acetaminophen 325 mg
(Tylox® contains acetaminophen 500 mg)

*Triplicate prescription required in some states

ORAL BACTERIAL INFECTIONS

Dental infection can occur for any number of reasons, primarily involving pulpal and periodontal infections. Secondary infections of the soft tissues as well as sinus infections pose special treatment challenges. The drugs of choice in treating most oral infections have been selected because of their efficacy in providing adequate blood levels for delivery to the oral tissues and their proven usefulness in managing dental infections. Penicillin and erythromycin remain the two primary drugs for treatment of dental infections of pulpal origin. The management of soft tissue infections may require the use of additional drugs.

SINUS INFECTION TREATMENT

Sinus infections represent a common condition which may present with confounding dental complaints. Treatment is sometimes instituted by the dentist, but due to the often chronic and recurrent nature of sinus infections, early involvement of an otolaryngologist is advised. These infections may require antibiotics of varying spectrum as well as requiring the management of sinus congestion. Although amoxicillin is usually adequate, many otolaryngologists go directly to Augmentin®. Second generation cephalosporins and clarithromycin are sometimes used depending on the chronicity of the problem.

Amoxicillin and Clavulanate Potassium (Augmentin®) *on page 69*
Amoxicillin Trihydrate (various products) *on page 68*
Ceftibuten (Cedax®) *on page 196*
Chlorpheniramine (Chlor-Trimeton®, various products) *on page 217*
Clarithromycin (Biaxin™) *on page 241*
Loratadine and Pseudoephedrine (Claritin-D®) *on page 567*
Oxymetazoline (Afrin®, various products) *on page 714*
Pseudoephedrine (Sudafed®, various products) *on page 820*

PRESCRIPTION EXAMPLES

Rx
Amoxicillin 500 mg Disp 21 capsules Sig: Take 1 capsule 3 times/day

Rx
Augmentin® 500 Disp 30 tablets Sig: Take 1 tablet 3 times/day

Ingredients: Amoxicillin 500 mg and clavulanate potassium 125 mg

The selected antibiotic should be used with a nasal decongestant and possibly an antihistamine.

Rx
Afrin® Nasal Spray (OTC) Disp 15 mL Sig: Spray 1 time in each nostril every 6-8 hours for no more than 3 days

Ingredient: Oxymetazoline

OR

Rx
Sudafed® 60 mg tablets (OTC) Disp 30 tablets Sig: Take 1 tablet every 4-6 hours as needed for congestion

Ingredient: Pseudoephedrine

ORAL BACTERIAL INFECTIONS *(Continued)*

Rx

Chlor-Trimeton® 4 mg (OTC)

Disp 14 tablets

Sig: Take 1 tablet 2 times/day

Ingredient: Chlorpheniramine

PULPAL AND PERIODONTAL INFECTIONS

Regardless of the condition to be treated, consideration should always be given to managing and monitoring the course of the infection with observations at 24 and 72 hours to ensure efficacy of the drug selected. Due to the usual multiorganism etiology of most pulpal and periodontal dental infections, culture and sensitivity studies may not be pertinent. Penicillin, clindamycin, and erythromycin are first-line drugs of choice for most dental infections. Some periodontal infections respond well to tetracyclines and metronidazole. Although culturing oral infections is not always necessary, a complete listing of the spectrum of antibiotics available can be found in the Appendix. Oral antimicrobial rinses may be useful in periodontal infections.

THE CLINICIAN AND PULPAL INFECTIONS

The clinician should be aware that the management of oral infections may require the use of a loading dose of the drug usually in the case of penicillin VK one gram instead of the 500 mg constant dose or the use of 300 mg of clindamycin prior to the onset of the regular regimen as outlined. The clinician should also be aware that some infections may be refractory to this initial therapy and broader spectrum antibiotics such as Augmentin® may be necessary to assist in the management of the acute infection.

Common Oral-Facial Infections and Antibiotics for Treatment *on page 1197*

Amoxicillin and Clavulanate Potassium (Augmentin®) *on page 69*
Amoxicillin Trihydrate (various products) *on page 68*
Cephalexin (Biocef®, Cefanex®, Keflet®, Keflex®, Keftab®) *on page 201*
Chlorhexidine (Peridex®, PerioGard®) *on page 211*
Clindamycin (Cleocin®) *on page 243*
Dicloxacillin (Dycill®, Dynapen®, Pathocil®) *on page 305*
Erythromycin (various products) *on page 361*
Metronidazole (Flagyl®, MetroGel®, Protostat®) *on page 631*
Mouthwash, Antiseptic (Listerine®) *on page 650*
Penicillin V Potassium (various products) *on page 734*
Tetracycline (Achromycin®, Sumycin®, Tetracyn®) *on page 914*

Note: Often penicillins are prescribed with a double or triple loading dose initially, then followed by the course described below.

PRESCRIPTION EXAMPLES

Rx

Penicillin V potassium 500 mg

Disp 28 tablets

Sig: Take 1 tablet 4 times/day

Rx

Augmentin® 500 mg

Disp 28 tablets

Sig: Take 1 tablet 4 times/day

Rx

Erythromycin base 250 mg

Disp 28 (enteric coated) tablets

Sig: Take 1 tablet 4 times/day

Rx

Cephalexin 250 mg

Disp 28 capsules

Sig: Take 1 capsule 4 times/day

Rx

Dicloxacillin 250 mg

Disp 28 capsules

Sig: Take 2 capsules once every 6 hours

Rx

Clindamycin 300 mg (Cleocin®)

Disp 14 capsules

Sig: Take 1 capsule every 6 hours

Rx

Metronidazole 250 mg (Flagyl®)

Disp 40 tablets

Sig: Take 1 tablet 4 times/day

Rx

Chlorhexidine Gluconate 0.12% (Peridex® and PerioGard®)

Disp 1 bottle

Sig: 20 mL for 30 seconds 3 times/day

Rx

Listerine® (OTC)

Disp 1 bottle

Sig: 20 mL for 30 seconds twice daily

ORAL BACTERIAL INFECTIONS (Continued)

FREQUENTLY ASKED QUESTIONS

What is the best antibiotic modality for treating dental infections?

Penicillin is still the drug of choice for treatment of infections in and around the oral cavity. Phenoxy-methyl penicillin (Pen VK®) long has been the most commonly selected antibiotic. In penicillin-allergic individuals, erythromycin may be an appropriate consideration. If another drug is sought, clindamycin prescribed 300 mg as a loading dose followed by 150 mg 4 times/day would be an appropriate regimen for a dental infection. In general, if there is no response to Pen VK®, then Augmentin® may be a good alternative in the nonpenicillin-allergic patient because of its slightly altered spectrum. Recommendations would include that the patient should take the drug with food.

Is there cross-allergenicity between the cephalosporins and penicillin?

The incidence of cross-allergenicity is 5% to 8% in the overall population. If a patient has demonstrated a Type I hypersensitivity reaction to penicillin, namely urticaria or anaphylaxis, then this incidence would increase to 20%.

Is there definitely an interaction between contraception agents and antibiotics?

There are well founded interactions between contraceptives and antibiotics. The best instructions that a patient could be given by their dentist are that should an antibiotic be necessary and the dentist is aware that the patient is on contraceptives, and if the patient is using chemical contraceptives, the patient should seriously consider alternative means of contraception during the antibiotic management.

Are antibiotics necessary in diabetic patients?

In the management of diabetes, control of the diabetic status is the key factor relative to all morbidity issues. If a patient is well controlled, then antibiotics will likely not be necessary. However, in patients where the control is questionable or where they have recently been given a different drug regimen for their diabetes or if they are being titrated to an appropriate level of either insulin or oral hypoglycemic agents during these periods of time, the dentist might consider preprocedural antibiotics to be efficacious.

Do nonsteroidal anti-inflammatory drugs interfere with blood pressure medication?

At the current time there is no clear evidence that NSAIDs interfere with any of the blood pressure medications that are currently in usage.

ORAL FUNGAL INFECTIONS

Oral fungal infections can result from alteration in oral flora, immunosuppression, and underlying systemic diseases that may allow the overgrowth of these opportunistic organisms. These systemic conditions might include diabetes, long-term xerostomia, adrenal suppression, anemia, and chemotherapy-induced myelosuppression for the management of cancer. Drugs of choice in treating fungal infections are amphotericin B, ciclopirox olamine, clotrimazole, itraconazole, ketoconazole, fluconazole, naftifine hydrochloride, nystatin, and oxiconazole. Patients being treated for fungal skin infections may also be using topical antifungal preparations coupled with a steroid such as triamcinolone. Clinical presentation might include pseudomembranous, atrophic, and hyperkeratotic forms. Fungus has also been implicated in denture stomatitis and symptomatic geographic tongue.

Nystatin (Mycostatin®) is effective topically in the treatment of candidal infections of the skin and mucous membrane. The drug is extremely well tolerated and appears to be nonsensitizing. In persons with denture stomatitis in which monilial organisms play at least a contributory role, it is important to soak the prosthesis overnight in a nystatin suspension. Nystatin ointment can be placed in the denture during the daytime much like a denture adhesive. Medication should be continued for at least 48 hours after disappearance of clinical signs in order to prevent relapse. Patients must be re-evaluated after 14 days of therapy. Predisposing systemic factors must be reconsidered if the oral fungal infection persists. Topical applications rely on contact of the drug with the lesions. Therefore, 4-5 times daily with a dissolving troche or pastille is appropriate. Concern over the presence of sugar in the troches and pastilles has led practitioners to sometimes prescribe the vaginal suppository formulation.

Amphotericin B (Fungizone®) *on page 71*
Clotrimazole (Mycelex®) troches *on page 252*
Fluconazole (Diflucan®) *on page 408*
Itraconazole (Sporanox®) *on page 529*
Ketoconazole (Nizoral®) *on page 533*
Nystatin (Mycostatin®) ointment or cream *on page 695*
Nystatin (Mycostatin®) oral suspension *on page 695*
Nystatin (Mycostatin®) pastilles *on page 695*
Nystatin (Mycostatin®) powder *on page 695*
Nystatin and Triamcinolone (Mycolog®) cream *on page 695*

Note: Consider Peridex® oral rinse, or Listerine® antiseptic oral rinse for long-term control in immunosuppressed patients.

PRESCRIPTION EXAMPLES

Rx

Mycostatin® pastilles

Disp 70 pastilles

Sig: Dissolve 1 tablet in mouth until gone, 4-5 times/day for 14 days

---

Ingredients: 200,000 units of nystatin per tablet

Special indications: Pastille is more effective than oral suspension due to prolonged contact

---

Rx

Mycostatin® oral suspension

Disp 60 mL (4 oz)

Sig: Use 1 teaspoonful 4-5 times/day; rinse and hold in mouth as long as possible before swallowing or spitting out (2 minutes); do not eat or drink for 30 minutes following application

---

Ingredients: Nystatin 100,000 units/mL; vehicle contains 50% sucrose and not more than 1% alcohol

ORAL FUNGAL INFECTIONS *(Continued)*

Rx

Mycostatin® ointment or cream

Disp 15 g or 30 g tube

Sig: Apply liberally to affected areas 4-5 times/day; do not eat or drink for 30 minutes after application

---

Note: Denture wearers should apply to dentures prior to each insertion; for edentulous patients, we can also prescribe Mycostatin® powder (15 g) to be sprinkled on denture

Ingredients:

Cream: 100,000 units nystatin per g, aqueous vanishing cream base

Ointment: 100,000 units nystatin per g, polyethylene and mineral oil gel base

OR

Rx

Mycelex® troche 10 mg

Disp 70 tablets

Sig: Dissolve 1 tablet in mouth 5 times/day

Ingredients: Clotrimazole

Note: Tablets contain sucrose, risk of caries with prolonged use (>3 months); care must be exercised in diabetic patients

---

Rx

Fungizone® oral suspension

Disp 50 mL

Sig: 1 mL, swish and swallow 4 times/day between meals

MANAGEMENT OF FUNGAL INFECTIONS REQUIRING SYSTEMIC MEDICATION

If the patient is refractory to topical treatment, consideration of a systemic route might include Diflucan® or Nizoral®. Also, when the patient cannot tolerate topical therapy, ketoconazole (Nizoral®) is an effective, well tolerated, systematic drug for mucocutaneous candidiasis. Concern over liver function and possible drug interactions must be considered.

PRESCRIPTION EXAMPLES

Rx

Nizoral® 200 mg

Disp 10 or 28 tablets

Sig: Take 1 tablet daily for 10-14 days

Ingredients: Ketoconazole

Note: To be used if *Candida* infection does not respond to mycostatin; potential for liver toxicity; liver function should be monitored with long-term use (>3 weeks)

Rx

Diflucan® 100 mg

Disp 15 tablets

Sig: Take 2 tablets the first day and 1 tablet a day for 10-14 days

---

Ingredients: Fluconazole

MANAGEMENT OF ANGULAR CHEILITIS

Angular cheilitis may represent the clinical manifestation of a multitude of etiologic factors. Cheilitis-like lesions may result from local habits, from a decrease in the intermaxillary space, or from nutritional deficiency. More commonly, angular cheilitis represents a mixed infection coupled with an inflammatory response involving *Candida albicans* and other organisms. The drug of choice is now formulated to contain nystatin and triamcinolone and the effect is excellent.

PRESCRIPTION EXAMPLE

Rx

Mycolog® cream

Disp 15 g tube

Sig: Apply to affected area after each meal and before bedtime

ORAL VIRAL INFECTIONS

Oral viral infections are most commonly caused by herpes simplex viruses and Coxsackie viruses. Oral pharyngeal infections and upper respiratory infections are commonly caused by the Coxsackie group A viruses. Soft tissue viral infections, on the other hand, are most often caused by the herpes simplex viruses. Herpes zoster or varicella-zoster virus, which is one of the herpes family of viruses, can likewise cause similar viral eruptions involving the mucosa.

The diagnosis of an acute viral infection is one that begins by ruling out bacterial etiology and having an awareness of the presenting signs and symptoms associated with viral infection. Acute onset and vesicular eruption on the soft tissues generally favors a diagnosis of viral infection. Unfortunately, vesicles do not remain for a great length of time in the oral cavity; therefore, the short-lived vesicles rupture leaving ulcerated bases as the only indication of their presence. These ulcers, however, are generally small in size and only when left unmanaged do they coalesce to form larger, irregular ulcerations. Distinction should be made between the commonly occurring intraoral ulcers (aphthous ulcerations) which do not have a viral etiology and the lesions associated with intraoral herpes. The management of an oral viral infection may be palliative for the most part; however, with the advent of acyclovir we now have a drug that can assist us in managing primary and secondary infection. Human *Papillomavirus* is implicated in a number of oral lesions, the most common of which is *Condyloma acuminatum*. Recently, Aldara® has been approved for genital warts; oral use is under study.

It should be noted that herpes can present as, a primary infection (gingivostomatitis), recurrent lip lesions (herpes labialis), and intraoral ulcers (recurrent intraoral herpes), three primary forms involving the oral and perioral tissues. Primary infection is one that is generally a systemic infection that leads to acute gingivostomatitis involving multiple tissues of the buccal mucosa, lips, tongue, floor of the mouth, and the gingiva. Treatment of primary infections utilizes acyclovir in combination with supportive care. Dyclonine 0.5%, a topical anesthetic used in combination with Benadryl® 0.5% in a saline vehicle, are found to be effective oral rinses in the symptomatic treatment of primary herpetic gingivostomatitis. Other agents available for symptomatic and supportive treatment include commercially available elixir of Benadryl®, Xylocaine® viscous, Ora-Jel® (OTC), Camphophenique® (OTC), and antibiotics to prevent secondary infections. Systemic supportive therapy should include forced fluids, high concentration protein, vitamin and mineral food supplements, and rest.

Antivirals

Supportive Therapy

**Antibiotics for Prevention of
Secondary Bacterial Infection**

PRIMARY INFECTION

PRESCRIPTION EXAMPLE

Rx
Zovirax® 200 mg
Disp 70 capsules
Sig: Take 1 capsule every 4 hours (maximum: 5/day) for 2 weeks

Ingredient: Acyclovir

SUPPORTIVE CARE FOR PAIN AND PREVENTION OF SECONDARY INFECTION

Primary infections often become secondarily infected with bacteria, requiring antibiotics. Dietary supplement may be necessary. Options are presented due to variability in patient compliance and response.

PRESCRIPTION EXAMPLE

Rx

Benadryl® powder 0.5% with dyclonine 0.5% in saline

Disp 8 oz

Sig: Rinse with 1 teaspoonful every 2 hours

Ingredient: Diphenhydramine and dyclonine

Rx

Benadryl® elixir 12.5 mg/5 mL

Disp 4 oz bottle

Sig: Rinse with 1 teaspoonful for 2 minutes before each meal

Ingredient: Diphenhydramine

Rx

Benadryl® elixir 12.5 mg/5 mL with Kaopectate®, 50% mixture by volume

Disp 8 oz

Sig: Rinse with 1 teaspoonful every 2 hours

Ingredients: Diphenhydramine and attapulgite

Rx

Xylocaine® viscous 2%

Disp 450 mL bottle

Sig: Swish with 1 tablespoon 4 times/day and spit out

Ingredient: Lidocaine

Rx

Penicillin V 250 mg tablets

Disp 40 tablets

Sig: 1 tablet 4 times/day

Rx

Erythromycin 250 mg tablets

Disp 40 tablets

Sig: 1 tablet 4 times/day

Rx

Meritene®

Disp 1 lb can (plain, chocolate, eggnog flavors)

Sig: Take 3 servings daily; prepare as indicated on can

Ingredients: Protein-vitamin-mineral food supplement

ORAL VIRAL INFECTIONS *(Continued)*

RECURRENT HERPETIC INFECTIONS

Following this primary infection, the herpesvirus remains latent until such time as it has the opportunity to recur. The etiology of this latent period and the degree of viral shedding present during latency is currently under study; however, it is thought that some trigger in the mucosa or the skin causes the virus to begin to replicate. This process may involve Langerhans cells which are immunocompetent antigen-presenting cells resident in all epidermal surfaces. The virus replication then leads to eruptions in tissues surrounding the mouth. The most common form of recurrence is the lip lesion or herpes labialis, however, intraoral recurrent herpes also occurs with some frequency. Prevention of recurrences has been attempted with drugs such as Lysine® (500-1000 mg/day). Response has been variable. Pain management during intraoral recurrences can be utilized as in primary infections.

Water-soluble bioflavonoid-ascorbic acid complex, now available as Peridin-C®, may be helpful in reducing the signs and symptoms associated with recurrent herpes simplex virus infections. As with all agents used, the therapy is more effective when instituted in the early prodromal stage of the disease process.

PRESCRIPTION EXAMPLE

Rx
Citrus bioflavonoids and ascorbic acid tablets 400 mg (Peridin-C®)   Disp 10 tablets   Sig: Take 2 tablets at once, then 1 tablet tid for 3 days

PREVENTION

Where a recurrence is usually precipitated by exposure to sunlight, the lesion may be prevented by the application to the area of a sunscreen, with a high skin protection factor (SPF) in the range of 10-15.

PRESCRIPTION EXAMPLE

Rx
PreSun® (OTC) 15 sunscreen lotion   Disp 4 fluid oz   Sig: Apply to susceptible area 1 hour before sun exposure

TREATMENT

Vidarabine (Vira-A®) possesses antiviral activity against herpes simplex types 1 and 2. The ophthalmic ointment may be used topically to treat recurrent mucosal and skin lesions. In the 3% strength, it does not penetrate well on the skin lesions thereby providing questionable relief of symptoms. If recommended, its use should be closely monitored. Penciclovir, an active metabolite of famciclovir, has been recently approved in a cream for treatment of recurrent herpes lesions. The drug is to be released in the near future; prescribing information will be available at that time.

PRESCRIPTION EXAMPLES

Rx
Vira-A® ophthalmic ointment 3%   Disp 3.5 g tube   Sig: Apply to affected area 4 times/day

Ingredient: Vidarabine

Rx

Zovirax® ointment 5% (3%)

Disp 15 g

Sig: Apply thin layer to lesions 6 times/day for 7 days

Ingredient: Acyclovir

Rx

Zovirax® 200 mg

Disp 70 capsules

Sig: Take 1 capsule every 4 hours (maximum: 5/day) for 2 weeks

Ingredient: Acyclovir

ORAL NONVIRAL SOFT TISSUE ULCERATIONS OR EROSIONS

RECURRENT APHTHOUS STOMATITIS

Kenalog® in Orabase is indicated for the temporary relief of symptoms associated with infrequent recurrences of minor aphthous lesions and ulcerative lesions resulting from trauma. More severe forms of recurrent aphthous stomatitis may be treated with an oral suspension of tetracycline. The agent appears to reduce the duration of symptoms and decrease the rate of recurrence by reducing secondary bacterial infection. Its use is contraindicated during the last half of pregnancy, infancy, and childhood to the age of 8 years. *Lactobacillus acidophilus* preparations (Bacid®, Lactinex®) are occasionally effective for reducing the frequency and severity of the lesions. Patients with long-standing history of recurrent aphthous stomatitis should be evaluated for iron, folic acid, and vitamin B$_{12}$ deficiencies. Regular use of Listerine® antiseptic has been shown in clinical trials to reduce the severity, duration, and frequency of aphthous stomatitis. Chlorhexidine oral rinses 20 mL x 30 sec bid or tid have also demonstrated efficacy in reducing the duration of aphthae. With both of these products, however, patient intolerance of the burning from the alcohol content is of concern. Viractin® has recently been approved for symptomatic relief. Immunocompromised patients such as those with AIDS may have severe ulcer recurrences and the drug thalidomide is likely to be approved for these patients.

Amlexanox (Aphthasol®) *on page 63*
Attapulgite (Diasorb®, Kaopectate®, Rheaban®) *on page 99*
Chlorhexidine (Peridex®, PerioGard®) *on page 211*
Clobetasol (Temovate®) *on page 245*
Dexamethasone (Decadron®) *on page 291*
Diphenhydramine (Benadryl®, various products) *on page 323*
Fluocinonide (Lidex®) ointment with Orabase *on page 415*
Lactobacillus acidophilus and *Lactobacillus bulgaricus* (Bacid®, Lactinex®) *on page 539*
Metronidazole (Flagyl®) *on page 631*
Mouthwash, Antiseptic (Listerine®) *on page 650*
Prednisone (various products) *on page 789*
Tetracaine (Pontocaine®, Viractin®) *on page 913*
Tetracycline liquid *on page 914*
Triamcinolone (Kenalog®) Acetonide Dental Paste *on page 955*

PRESCRIPTION EXAMPLES

Rx
Listerine® antiseptic (OTC)
20 mL x 30 sec bid

Rx
Peridex® oral rinse
Disp 1 bottle
Sig: 20 mL x 30 sec tid

Rx
PerioGard® oral rinse
Disp 1 bottle
Sig: 20 mL x 30 sec tid

Rx

Tetracycline capsules 250 mg

Disp 40 capsules

Sig: Suspend contents of 1 capsule in a teaspoonful of water; rinse for 2 minutes 4 times/day and swallow

Note: This comes as liquid 125 mg/5 mL which is convenient to use

Sig: Swish 5 mL for 2 minutes 4 times/day

Rx

Kenalog® in Orabase 0.1%

Disp 5 g tube

Sig: Coat the lesion with a film after each meal and at bedtime

BURNING TONGUE SYNDROME, GEOGRAPHIC TONGUE, MILD FORMS OF ORAL LICHEN PLANUS

Elixir of Benadryl®, a potent antihistamine, is used in the oral cavity primarily as a mild topical anesthetic agent for the symptomatic relief of certain allergic deficiencies which should be ruled out as possible etiologies for the oral condition under treatment. It is often used alone as well as in solutions with agents such as Kaopectate® or Maalox® to assist in coating the oral mucosa. Benadryl® can also be used in capsule form.

PRESCRIPTION EXAMPLE

Rx

Benadryl® elixir 12.5 mg/5 mL

Disp 4 oz bottle

Sig: Rinse with 1 teaspoonful for 2 minutes before each meal and swallow

Ingredient: Diphenhydramine

EROSIVE LICHEN PLANUS AND MAJOR APHTHAE

Elixir of dexamethasone (Decadron®), a potent anti-inflammatory agent, is used topically in the management of acute episodes of erosive lichen planus and major aphthae. Continued supervision of the patient during treatment is essential.

PRESCRIPTION EXAMPLE

Rx

Decadron® elixir 0.5 mg/5 mL

Disp 100 mL bottle

Sig: Rinse with 1 teaspoonful for 2 minutes 4 times/day; do not swallow

Ingredient: Dexamethasone

ORAL NONVIRAL SOFT TISSUE ULCERATIONS OR EROSIONS *(Continued)*

For severe cases and when the oropharynx is involved, some practitioners have the patient swallow after a 2-minute rinse.

Allergy	Benadryl®
Aphthous	Benadryl®/Maalox® (compounded prescription)
	Benadryl®/Kaopectate® (compounded prescription)
	Lidex® in Orabase (compounded prescription)
	Kenalog® in Orabase
	Tetracycline mouth rinse
Oral inflammatory disease	Lidex® in Orabase (compounded prescription)
	Kenalog® in Orabase
	Prednisone
	Temovate® cream

The use of long-term steroids is always of concern due to possible adrenal suppression. If systemic steroids are contemplated for a protracted time, medical consultation is advisable.

PRESCRIPTION EXAMPLES

Rx

Benadryl® 50 mg

Disp 16 capsules

Sig: 3-4 times/day

Ingredient: Diphenhydramine hydrochloride

Special considerations: Use 3-4 times/day for 4 days depending on the duration of the allergic reaction; may cause drowsiness

---

Rx

Benadryl® syrup (mix 50/50) with Kaopectate®*

Disp 8 oz total

Sig: Use 2 teaspoons as rinse as needed to relieve pain or burning (use after meals)

---

*Note: Benadryl can be mixed with Maalox® if constipation is a problem

---

Rx

Kenalog® in Orabase®

Disp 5 mg

Sig: Apply thin layer to affected area 3 times/day

Rx

Lidex® ointment mixed 50/50 with Orabase®

Disp 30 g total

Sig: Apply thin layer to oral lesions 4-6 times/day

Ingredient: Fluocinonide 0.05%

Note: To be used for oral inflammatory lesions that do not respond to Kenalog® in Orabase®

Ingredient: Triamcinolone acetonide

Systemic steroids may be considered:

Rx

        Prednisone 5 mg

        Disp 60 tablets

        Sig: Take 4 tablets in morning and 4 tablets at noon for 4 days; then decrease the total number of tablets by 1 each day until down to zero

---

Caution: Take medication with food

For a high potency corticosteroid:

Rx

        Temovate® cream 0.05%

        Disp 15 g tube

        Sig: Apply locally 4-6 times/day

And for secondary infections:

Rx

        Tetracycline liquid 125 mg/5 mL

        Disp 100 mL

        Sig: Rinse 1 tablespoonful in mouth 4 times/day then spit out; do not eat or drink for 30 minutes after using

---

Note: Tetracycline rinse is effective in approximately 33% of the patients with aphthous ulcers

NECROTIZING ULCERATING PERIODONTITIS (HIV Periodontal Disease)

Initial Treatment (In-Office)
    Betadine rinse *on page 783*
Ensure patient has no iodine allergies
Gentle debridement

At-Home
Listerine® rinses
    Peridex® rinse *on page 211*
    Metronidazole (Flagyl®) 7-10 days *on page 631*

Follow-Up Therapy
    Proper dental cleaning including scaling and root planing (repeat as needed)
    Continue Peridex® rinse (indefinite) *on page 211*
    Listerine® antiseptic rinse (20 mL for 30 seconds twice daily)

DENTIN HYPERSENSITIVITY; HIGH CARIES INDEX; XEROSTOMIA

DENTIN HYPERSENSITIVITY

Suggested steps in resolving dentin hypersensitivity (a thorough exam had ruled any other source for the problem).

Treatment Steps

- Home treatment with a desensitizing toothpaste containing potassium nitrate (used to brush teeth as well as a thin layer applied, each night for 2 weeks)
- If needed, in office potassium oxalate (Protect® by Butler) and/or in office fluoride iontophoresis
- If sensitivity is still not tolerable to the patient, consider pumice then dentin adhesive and unfilled resin or composite restoration overlaying a glass ionomer base

Home Products: All contain nitrate as active ingredient

Promise®
Denquel®
Sensodyne®

Dentifrice Products *on page 1172*

ANTICARIES AGENTS

Fluoride gel 0.4%, rinse 0.05% *on page 415*

New toothpastes with triclosan such as Colgate Total® show promise for combined treatment/prevention of caries, plaque, and gingivitis.

FLUORIDE GELS

Oral Rinse Products *on page 1187*

Used for the prevention of demineralization of the tooth structure secondary to xerostomia. For patients with long-term or permanent xerostomia, daily application is accomplished using custom gel applicator trays. Patients with porcelain crowns should use a neutral pH fluoride.

1.1% neutral pH sodium fluoride
Thera-Flur-N® or Prevident®
0.4% stannous fluoride
Gel-Kam® unflavored

REMINERALIZING GEL

In addition to fluoride gel to remineralize enamel breakdown in severely xerostomic patients, applicator trays may be used.

Revive®

Note: Many preparations are available over-the-counter so prescriptions sometimes are not required. If caries is severe, use fluoride gel in custom tray once daily as long as needed (years).

ANTIPLAQUE AGENTS

PRESCRIPTION EXAMPLES

Rx
Listerine® antiseptic (OTC)
20 mL for 30 seconds twice daily

Rx
Peridex® oral rinse 0.12%
Disp 3 times 16 oz
Sig: ½ oz, swish for 30 seconds 2-3 times/day

Rx

PerioGard® oral rinse

Disp 3 times 16 oz

Sig: ½ oz, swish for 30 seconds 2-3 times/day

Ingredient: Chlorhexidine

Peridex may:

- Stain teeth yellow to brown (can be removed with dental cleaning)

- Alter taste (temporary)

- Increase the deposition of calculus (reversible)

    Chlorhexidine (Peridex®) *on page 211*

XEROSTOMIA

Dry mouth associated with radiation therapy, drug therapy, aging, and Sjögren's disease may be managed by rinsing with a solution of sodium carboxymethylcellulose. It is a nonirritating agent that moistens and lubricates the oral tissues and may be used for prolonged periods of time without adverse effects. Salagen® was recently indicated for these patients. For dentulous patients, fluoride and electrolytes have been added to this solution to reduce caries susceptibility (Xero-Lube®). Consideration of alternative medical drug regimens in consult with the physician may assist in management. Numerous patients being treated for anxiety or depression are often susceptible to chronic xerostomia due to medications selected; see table on following page.

Pilocarpine (Dental) (Salagen®) *on page 761*

Saliva Substitute (Moi-Stir®; MouthKote®; Optimoist®; Salivart®; Xero-Lube®) *on page 854*

DENTIN HYPERSENSITIVITY; HIGH CARIES INDEX;
XEROSTOMIA *(Continued)*

OTHER DRUGS IMPLICATED IN XEROSTOMIA

>10%	1% to 10%
Alprazolam	Acrivastine and Pseudoephedrine
Amitriptyline hydrochloride	Albuterol
Amoxapine	Amantadine hydrochloride
Anisotropine methylbromide	Amphetamine sulfate
Atropine sulfate	Astemizole
Belladonna and Opium	Azatadine maleate
Benztropine mesylate	Beclomethasone dipropionate
Bupropion	Bepridil hydrochloride
Chlordiazepoxide	Bitolterol mesylate
Clomipramine hydrochloride	Brompheniramine maleate
Clonazepam	Carbinoxamine and Pseudoephedrine
Clonidine	Chlorpheniramine maleate
Clorazepate dipotassium	Clemastine fumarate
Cyclobenzaprine	Clozapine
Desipramine hydrochloride	Cromolyn sodium
Diazepam	Cyproheptadine hydrochloride
Dicyclomine hydrochloride	Dexchlorpheniramine maleate
Diphenoxylate and Atropine	Dextroamphetamine sulfate
Doxepin hydrochloride	Dimenhydrinate
Ergotamine	Diphenhydramine hydrochloride
Estazolam	Disopyramide phosphate
Flavoxate	Doxazosin
Flurazepam hydrochloride	Dronabinol
Glycopyrrolate	Ephedrine sulfate
Guanabenz acetate	Flumazenil
Guanfacine hydrochloride	Fluvoxamine
Hyoscyamine sulfate	Gabapentin
Interferon Alfa-2a	Guaifenesin and Codeine
Interferon Alfa-2b	Guanadrel sulfate
Interferon Alfa-N3	Guanethidine sulfate
Ipratropium bromide	Hydroxyzine
Isoproterenol	Hyoscyamine, Atropine, Scopolamine, and Phenobarbital
Isotretinoin	Imipramine
Loratadine	Isoetharine
Lorazepam	Levocabastine hydrochloride
Loxapine	Levodopa
Maprotiline hydrochloride	Levodopa and Carbidopa
Methscopolamine bromide	Levorphanol tartrate
Molindone hydrochloride	Meclizine hydrochloride
Nabilone	Meperidine hydrochloride
Nefazodone	Methadone hydrochloride
Oxybutynin chloride	Methamphetamine hydrochloride
Oxazepam	Methyldopa
Paroxetine	Metoclopramide
Phenelzine sulfate	Morphine sulfate
Prochlorperazine	Nortriptyline hydrochloride
Propafenone hydrochloride	Ondansetron
Protriptyline hydrochloride	Oxycodone and Acetaminophen
Quazepam	Oxycodone and Aspirin
Reserpine	Pentazocine
Selegiline hydrochloride	Phenylpropanolamine hydrochloride
Temazepam	Prazosin hydrochloride
Thiethylperazine maleate	Promethazine hydrochloride
Trihexyphenidyl hydrochloride	Propoxyphene
Trimipramine maleate	Pseudoephedrine
Venlafaxine	Risperidone
	Sertraline hydrochloride
	Terazosin
	Terbutaline sulfate

PRESCRIPTION EXAMPLES

Rx

Sodium carboxymethylcellulose (Baker) 0.5% aqueous solution

Disp 8 oz

Sig: Use as a rinse frequently as needed to relieve symptoms of
dry mouth

Rx

Xero-Lube®*

Disp 1 bottle

Sig: Apply several drops or sprays to mouth as necessary for
dryness

Note: Consider topical treatment in custom trays for those patients
with severe xerostomia

*Note: Alternatives: Moi-Stir®; MouthKote®; Optimoist®; Salivart®

Systemic stimulation of saliva has been achieved in some patients using pilocarpine.

Rx

Salagen® 5 mg

Disp 120 tablets

Sig: 1 tablet 3-4 times/day, not top exceed 30 mg/day

Note: Patients should be treated for a minimum of 90 days to
achieve clinical effects.

TEMPOROMANDIBULAR DYSFUNCTION (TMD)

Temporomandibular dysfunction comprises a broad spectrum of signs and symptoms. Although TMD presents in patterns, diagnosis is often difficult. Evaluation and treatment is time-intensive and no single therapy or drug regimen has been shown to be universally beneficial.

The thorough diagnostician should perform a screening examination for the temporomandibular joint on all patients. Ideally, a base line maximum mandibular opening along with lateral and protrusive movement evaluation should be performed. Secondly, the joint area should be palpated and an adequate exam of the muscles of mastication and the muscles of the neck and shoulders should be made. These muscle would include the elevators of the mandible (masseter, internal pterygoid, and temporalis); the depressors of the mandible (including the external pterygoid and digastric); etrusive muscles (including the temporalis and digastric), and protrusive muscles (including the external and internal pterygoids). These muscles also account for lateral movement of the mandible. The clinician should also be alert to indicators of dysfunction, primarily a history of pain with jaw function, chronic history of joint noise (although this can often be misinterpreted), pain in the muscles of the neck, limited jaw movement, pain in the actual muscles of mastication, and headache or even earache. The signs and symptoms are extremely variable and the clinician should be alert for any or all of these areas of interest. Because of the complexity of both evaluation and diagnosis, the general dentist often finds it too time consuming to spend the countless hours evaluating and treating the temporomandibular dysfunction patient. Therefore, oral medicine specialists trained in temporomandibular evaluation and treatment often accept referrals for the management of these complicated patients.

The Oral Medicine specialist in TMD management, the physical therapist interested in head and neck pain, and the Oral and Maxillofacial surgeon will all work together with the referring general dentist to accomplish successful patient treatment. Table 1 lists the wide variety of treatment alternatives available to the team. Depending on the diagnosis, one or more of the therapies might be selected. For organic diseases of the joint not responding to nonsurgical approaches, a wide variety of surgical techniques are available (Table 2).

ACUTE TMD

Acute TMD oftentimes presents alone or as an episode during a chronic pattern of signs and symptoms. Trauma such as a blow to the chin or the side of the face can result in acute TMD. Occasionally, similar symptoms will follow a lengthy wide open mouth dental procedure.

The condition usually presents as continuous deep pain in the TMJ. If edema is present in the joint, the condyle sometimes can be displaced which will cause abnormal occlusion of the posterior teeth on the affected side. The diagnosis is usually based on the history and clinical presentation. Management of the patient includes:

1. Restriction of all mandibular movement to function in a pain-free range of motion
2. Soft diet
3. NSAIDs (eg, Anaprox® DS 1 tablet every 12 hours for 7-10 days)
4. Moist heat applications to the affected area for 15-20 minutes, 4-6 times/day

Additional therapies could include referral to a physical therapist for ultrasound therapy 2-4 times/week and a single injection of steroid in the joint space. A team approach with an oral maxillofacial surgeon for this procedure may be helpful. Spray and stretch with Fluori-methane® is often helpful for rapid relief of trismus.

Dichlorodifluoromethane and Trichloromonofluoromethane (Fluori-methane®) *on page 303*

Nonsteroidal Anti-inflammatory Agent (NSAID), Oral *on page 1259*

CHRONIC TMD

Following diagnosis which is often problematic, the most common therapeutic modalities include:

- Explaining the problem to the patient
- Recommending a soft diet:
  - avoid chewing gum, salads, biting into large sandwiches, biting into hard fruit
  - diet should consist of soft foods such as eggs, yogurt, casseroles, soup, ground meat

- Reducing stress; moist heat application 4-6 times daily for 15-20 minutes coupled with a monitored exercise program will be beneficial. Usually, working with a physical therapist is ideal.
- Medications include analgesics, anti-inflammatories, tranquilizers, and muscle relaxants

MEDICATION OPTIONS

Most commonly used medication (NSAIDs):

Aminosalicylate Sodium (Sodium P.A.S.) *on page 58*

Bromfenac (Duract™) *on page 139*

Choline Magnesium Trisalicylate (Trilisate®) *on page 230*

Choline Salicylate (Arthropan®) *on page 230*

Diclofenac (Cataflam®, Voltaren®) *on page 304*

Diflunisal (Dolobid®) *on page 311*

Etodolac (Lodine®) *on page 387*

Fenoprofen (Nalfon®) *on page 398*

Flurbiprofen (Ansaid®) *on page 423*

Ibuprofen (various products) *on page 495*

Indomethacin (Indocin®) *on page 506*

Ketoprofen (Orudis®) *on page 534*

Ketorolac (Toradol®) *on page 535*

Magnesium Salicylate (Doan's®, Magan®, Mobidin®) *on page 577*

Meclofenamate (Meclomen®) *on page 585*

Mefenamic Acid (Ponstel®) *on page 588*

Nabumetone (Relafen®) *on page 656*

Naproxen (Naprosyn®) *on page 665*

Oxaprozin (Daypro™) *on page 706*

Oxyphenbutazone *on page 716*

Piroxicam (Feldene®) *on page 767*

Salsalate (various products) *on page 855*

Sulindac (Clinoril®) *on page 898*

Tolmetin (Tolectin®) *on page 943*

Tranquilizers and muscle relaxants when used appropriately can provide excellent adjunctive therapy. These drugs should be primarily used for a short period of time to manage acute pain. In low dosages, amitriptyline is often used to treat chronic pain and occasionally migraine headache.

Common minor tranquilizers include:

Alprazolam (Xanax®) *on page 43*

Diazepam (Valium®) *on page 300*

Lorazepam (Ativan®) *on page 567*

Common muscle relaxants include:

Chlorzoxazone (Parafon® Forte DSC) *on page 228*

Methocarbamol (Robaxin®) *on page 613*

Orphenadrine (Norgesic® Forte) *on page 704*

Cyclobenzaprine (Flexeril®) *on page 268*

Muscle relaxants and tranquilizers should generally be prescribed with an analgesic or NSAID to relieve pain as well

Narcotic analgesics can be used on a short-term basis or intermittently in combination with non-narcotic therapy in the chronic pain patient. Judicious prescribing, monitoring, and maintenance by the practitioner is imperative whenever considering the use of narcotic analgesics due to the abuse and addiction liabilities.

TEMPOROMANDIBULAR DYSFUNCTION (TMD) *(Continued)*

Table 1.
TMD - NONSURGICAL THERAPIES

1. Moist heat and cold spray
2. Injections in muscle trigger areas (procaine)
3. Exercises (passive, active)
4. Medications
   a. Muscle relaxants
   b. Minerals
   c. Multiple vitamins (Ca, B_6, B_{12})
5. Orthopedic craniomandibular respositioning appliance (splints)
6. Biofeedback, acupuncture
7. Physiotherapy: TMJ muscle therapy
8. Myofunctional therapy
9. TENS (transcutaneous electrical neural stimulation), Myo-Monitor
10. Dental therapy
    a. Equilibration (coronoplasty)
    b. Restoring occlusion to proper vertical dimension of maxilla to mandible by orthodontics, dental restorative procedures, orthognathic surgery, permanent splint, or any combination of these

Table 2.
TMD - SURGICAL THERAPIES

1. Cortisone injection into joint (with local anesthetic)
2. Bony and/or fibrous ankylosis: requires surgery (osteoarthrotomy with prosthetic appliance)
3. Chronic subluxation: requires surgery, depending on problem (possibly eminectomy and/or prosthetic implant)
4. Osteoarthritis: requires surgery, depending on problem
   a. Arthroplasty with implant
   b. Meniscectomy with implant
   c. Arthroplasty with repair of disc and/or implant
   d. Implant with Silastic insert
5. Rheumatoid arthritis
   a. Arthroplasty with implant with Silastic insert
   b. "Total" TMJ replacement
6. Tumors: require osteoarthrotomy — removal of tumor and restoring of joint when possible
7. Chronic disc displacement: requires repair of disc and possible removal of bone from condyle

PATIENTS REQUIRING SEDATION

Anxiety constitutes the most frequently found psychiatric problem in the general population. Anxiety can range from simple phobias to severe debilitating anxiety disorders. Functional results of this anxiety can, therefore, range from simple avoidance of dental procedures to panic attacks when confronting stressful situations such as seen in some patients regarding dental visits. Many patients claim to be anxious over dental care when in reality they simply have not been managed with modern techniques of local anesthesia, the availability of sedation, or the caring dental practitioner.

The dentist may detect anxiety in patients during the treatment planning evaluation phase of the care. The anxious person may appear overly alert, may lean forward in the dental chair during conversation or may appear concerned over time, possibly using this as a guise to require that they cut short their dental visit. Anxious persons may also show signs of being nervous by demonstrating sweating, tension in their muscles including their temporomandibular musculature, or they may complain of being tired due to an inability to obtain an adequate night's sleep.

The management of such patients requires a methodical approach to relaxing the patient, discussing their dental needs, and then planning, along with the patient the best way to accomplish dental treatment in the presence of their fears, both real or imagined. Consideration may be given to sedation to assist with managing the patient. This sedation can be oral or parenteral, or inhalation in the case of nitrous oxide. The dentist must be adequately trained in administering the sedative of choice, as well as in monitoring the patient during the sedated procedures. Numerous medications are available to achieve the level of sedation usually necessary in the dental office: Valium®, Ativan®, Xanax®, Vistaril®, Serax®, and BuSpar® represent a few. BuSpar® is soon to be available as a transdermal patch. These oral sedatives can be given prior to dental visits as outlined in the following prescriptions. They have the advantage of allowing the patient a good night's sleep prior to the day of the procedures and providing on the spot sedation during the procedures. Nitrous oxide represents an in the office administered sedative that is relatively safe, but requires additional training and carefully planned monitoring protocols of any auxiliary personnel during the inhalation procedures. Both the oral and the inhalation techniques can, however, be applied in a very useful manner to manage the anxious patient in the dental office.

Alprazolam (Xanax®) on page 43
Buspirone (BuSpar®) on page 152
Diazepam (Valium®) on page 300
Hexobarbital (Pre-Sed®) on page 470
Hydroxyzine (Vistaril®, various products) on page 491
Lorazepam (Ativan®) on page 567
Nitrous Oxide on page 687
Oxazepam (Serax®) on page 707
Triazolam (Halcion®) on page 957

PRESCRIPTION EXAMPLES

Rx

Valium® 5 mg*

Disp 6 (six) tablets

Sig: Take 1 tablet in evening before going to bed and 1 tablet 1
hour before your appointment

Ingredient: Diazepam

*Note: Also available as 2 mg and 10 mg

Rx

Ativan® 1 mg*

Disp 4 (four) tablets

Sig: Take 2 tablets in evening before going to bed and take 2
tablets 1 hour before your appointment

Ingredient: Lorazepam

*Note: Also available as 0.5 mg and 2 mg

PATIENTS REQUIRING SEDATION *(Continued)*

Rx

Xanax® 0.5 mg

Disp 4 (four) tablets

Sig: Take 1 tablet in evening before going to bed and 1 tablet 1
hour before your appointment

Ingredient: Alprazolam

Rx

Pre-Sed® 260 mg

Disp 6 (six) tablets

Sig: Take 1 tablet* 1 hour prior to dental appointment

Ingredient: Hexobarbital
*Dose may be 2 tablets 1 hour prior

Rx

Vistaril® 25 mg

Disp 16 capsules

Sig: Take 2 capsules in evening before going to bed and 2
capsules 1 hour before your appointment

Ingredient: Hydroxyzine

Rx

Halcion® 0.25 mg

Disp 4 (four) tablets

Sig: Take 1 tablet in evening before going to bed and 1 tablet 1
hour before your appointment

Ingredient: Triazolam

Rx

Serax® 10 mg

Disp 2 (two) capsules

Sig: Take 1 capsule before bed and 1 capsule 30 minutes before
your appointment.

Ingredient: Oxazepam

PATIENTS UNDERGOING CANCER THERAPY

The statistics released by the American Cancer Society for projections of cancer trends in 1998 are indeed encouraging. Due to re-evaluation of the incidence of prostate cancer diagnoses, as well as decreases in other cancer categories, there has been a 9% decrease in the adjusted estimate for cancer rates. As healthcare practitioners, the reduction in cancer occurrence cannot be thought to be an end in itself. Other efforts in early detection and identification by the dental team as well as the management of oral complications associated with cancer treatment as outlined in this chapter are ever important for the dental practitioner. Treatment projections for new cancer cases also have shown signs of improvement. Although prostate cancer still leads as the site diagnosed by sex for the most prevalence, there have been reductions in lung and bronchial cancer and the success in treating prostate cancer as measured by estimated cancer deaths is also down.

The dental management recommendations for patients undergoing chemotherapy, bone marrow transplantation, and/or radiation therapy for the treatment of cancer are based primarily on clinical observations. The following protocols will provide a conservative, consistent approach to the dental management of patients undergoing chemotherapy or bone marrow transplantation. Many of the cancer chemotherapy drugs produce oral side effects including mucositis, oral ulceration, dry mouth, acute infections, and taste aberrations. Cancer drugs include antibiotics, alkylating agents, antimetabolites, DNA inhibitors, hormones, and cytokines (see "Cancer Chemotherapy Regimens" *on page 1133*).

DENTAL PROTOCOL

All patients undergoing chemotherapy or bone marrow transplantation for malignant disease should have the following baseline:

A. Panoramic radiograph
B. Dental consultation and examination
C. Dental prophylaxis and cleaning (if the neutrophil count is >1500/mm^3 and the platelet count is >50,000/mm^3

  - Prophylaxis and cleaning will be deferred if the patient's neutrophil count is <1500 and the platelet count is <50,000. Oral hygiene recommendations will be made.

D. Oral Hygiene. Patients should be encouraged to follow normal hygiene procedures. Addition of a chlorhexidine mouth rinse such as Peridex® or PerioGard® is usually helpful. If patient develops oral mucositis, tolerance of such alcohol-based products may be limited.

E. If the patient develops mucositis, bacterial, viral, and fungal cultures should be obtained. Sucralfate suspension in either a pharmacy prepared form or Carafate® suspension as well as Benadryl® or Xylocaine® viscous can assist in helping the patient to tolerate food. Patients may also require systemic analgesics for pain relief depending on the presence of mucositis. Positive fungal cultures may require a nystatin swish and swallow prescription.

F. The determination of performing dental procedures must be based on the goal of preventing infection during periods of neutropenia. Timing of procedures must be coordinated with the patient's hematologic status.

G. If oral surgery is required, at least 7-10 days of healing should be allowed before the anticipated date of bone marrow suppression (eg, ANC of <1000/mm^3 and/or platelet count of 50,000/mm^3).

H. Daily use of topical fluorides is recommended for those who have received radiation therapy to the head-neck region involving salivary glands. Any patients with prolonged xerostomia subsequent to graft versus host disease and/or chemotherapy can also be considered for fluoride supplement. Use the fluoride-containing mouthwashes (Act®, Fluorigard®, etc) each night before going to sleep; swish, hold 1-2 minutes, spit out or use prescription fluorides (gels or rinses); apply them daily for 3-4 minutes as directed; if the mouth is sore (mucositis), use flavorless/colorless gels (Thera-Flur®, Gel-Kam®). Improvement in salivary flow following radiation therapy to the head and neck has been noted with Salagen®. See "Oral Rinse Products" *on page 1187* .

Benzonatate (Tessalon® Perles) *on page 120*

Chlorhexidine (Peridex®, PerioGard®) *on page 211*

Diphenhydramine (Benadryl® elixir) *on page 323*

PATIENTS UNDERGOING CANCER THERAPY *(Continued)*

Lidocaine (Xylocaine®) *on page 553*

Pilocarpine (Dental) (Salagen®) *on page 761*

Povidone-Iodine (Betadine®) *on page 783*

Sucralfate (Carafate®) *on page 887*

PRESCRIPTION EXAMPLES

Rx

Peridex® or PerioGard® oral rinse

Disp 3 bottles

Sig: 20 mL x 30 sec tid; swish and expectorate

Ingredient: Chlorhexidine

Rx

Xylocaine® viscous 2%

Disp 450 mL bottles

Sig: Swish with 1 tablespoonful 4 times/day

Ingredient: Lidocaine

Rx

Betadine® mouthwash 0.8%

Disp 6 oz bottle

Sig: Rinse with 1 tablespoonful 4 times/day; do not swallow

Ingredient: Povidone-Iodine

Rx

Mycostatin® oral suspension 100,000 units/mL

Disp 60 mL bottle

Sig: 2 mL 4 times/day; hold in mouth for 2 minutes and swallow

---

Ingredient: Nystatin

When the oral mucous membranes are especially sensitive, nystatin "popsicles" can be made by adding 2 mL of nystatin oral suspension to the water in ice cube trays. Tessalon Perles® have been used ad lib to provide relief in painful mucositis.

Rx

Tessalon Perles®

Disp 50

Sig: Squeeze contents of capsule and apply to lesion

Ingredient: Benzonatate

ORAL CARE PRODUCTS

BACTERIAL PLAQUE CONTROL

Patients should use an extra soft bristle toothbrush and dental floss for removal of plaque. Sponge/foam sticks and lemon-glycerine swabs do not adequately remove bacterial plaque.

PRESCRIPTION EXAMPLE

Rx

Ultra Suave® toothbrush

Biotene Supersoft® toothbrush

Chlorhexidine 0.12% (Peridex® or other preparations available in Canada and Europe) may be used to assist with bacterial plaque control.

SALIVA SUBSTITUTES

Carboxymethylcellulose or mucopolysaccharide*-based sprays for temporary relief from xerostomia include:

Glandosane® *on page 854*
Moi-Stir® *on page 854*
*Mouth-Kote® *on page 854*
Optimoist® *on page 854*
Salivart® *on page 854*
Xerolube® *on page 854*

FLUORIDE GELS

Oral Rinse Products *on page 1187*

Used for the prevention of demineralization of the tooth structure secondary to xerostomia. For patients with long-term or permanent xerostomia, daily application is accomplished using custom gel applicator trays. Patients with porcelain crowns should use a neutral pH fluoride.

1.1% neutral pH sodium fluoride
Thera-Flur-N® or PreviDent® *on page 415*
0.4% stannous fluoride
Gel-Kam® unflavored *on page 415*

REMINERALIZING GEL

In addition to fluoride gel to remineralize enamel breakdown in severely xerostomic patients, applicator trays may be used.

Revive®

ORAL AND LIP MOISTURIZERS/LUBRICANTS

Mouth Pain, Cold Sore, Canker Sore Products *on page 1183*

Water-based gels should first be used to provide moisture to dry oral tissues.

Surgi-Lube®
K-Y Jelly®
Oral Balance®
Mouth Moisturizer®

PALLIATION OF PAIN

Mouth Pain, Cold Sore, Canker Sore Products *on page 1183*

Palliative pain preparations should be monitored for efficacy.

- For relief of pain associated with isolated ulcerations, topical anesthetic and protective preparations may be used.

  Orabase-B® with 20% benzocaine *on page 118*
  Oratect Gel® with 15% benzocaine and protective film *on page 118*
  ZilaDent® with 6% benzocaine and protective film *on page 118*

- For generalized oral pain:

  Chloraseptic Spray® (OTC) anesthetic spray without alcohol *on page 749*
  Ulcer-Ease® anesthetic/analgesic mouthrinse
  Xylocaine® 2% viscous *on page 553*
  May anesthetize swallowing mechanism and cause aspiration of food; caution patient against using too close to eating; lack of sensation may also allow patient to damage intact mucosa

PATIENTS UNDERGOING CANCER THERAPY *(Continued)*

Tantum Mouthrinse® (benzydamine hydrochloride); available
only in Canada and Europe; may be diluted as required

PATIENT PREPARED PALLIATIVE MIXTURES

Coating agents:

Maalox® *on page 48*

Mylanta® *on page 49*

Gelusil® *on page 49*

Kaopectate® *on page 99*

These products can be mixed with Benadryl® elixir 50:50

Diphenhydramine (Benadryl®) *on page 323*

Mouth Pain, Cold Sore, Canker Sore Products *on page 1183*

Topical anesthetics (diphenhydramine chloride)

Benadryl® elixir or Benylin® cough syrup *on page 323*

Choose product with lowest alcohol and sucrose contents; ask
pharmacist for assistance

PHARMACY PREPARATIONS

A Pharmacist may also prepare the following solutions for relief of
generalized oral pain:

Benadryl-Lidocaine Solution

Diphenhydramine injectable 1.5 mL (50 mg/mL) *on
page 323*

Xylocaine viscous 2% (45 mL) *on page 553*

Magnesium aluminum hydroxide solution (45 mL)

Swish and hold 1 teaspoonful in mouth for 30 seconds

Do not use too close to eating

Rx

Carafate suspension 1 g/10 mL

Disp 420 mL

Sig: Swish and hold 1 teaspoonful in mouth for 30 seconds

CHEMICAL DEPENDENCY AND SMOKING CESSATION

INTRODUCTION

As long as history has been recorded, every society has used drugs that alter mood, thought, and feeling. In addition, pharmacological advances sometimes have been paralleled by physical as well as unfortunate behavioral dependence on agents initially consumed for therapeutic purposes.

In 1986, the American Dental Association passed a policy statement recognizing chemical dependency as a disease. In recognizing this disease, the Association mandated that dentists have a responsibility to include questions relating to a history of chemical dependency or more broadly substance abused in their health history questionnaire. A positive response may require the dentist to alter the treatment plan for the patient's dental care. This includes patients who are actively abusing alcohol, drugs, or patients who are in recovery. The use and abuse of drugs is not a topic that is usually found in the dental curriculum. Information about substance abuse is usually gleaned from newspapers, magazines, or just hearsay.

This chapter reviews street drugs, where they come from, signs and symptoms of the drug abuser, and some of the dental implications of treating patients actively using or in recovery from these substances. There are many books devoted to this topic that provide greater detail. The intent is to provide an overview of some of the most prevalent drugs, how patients abusing these drugs may influence dental treatment, and how to recognize some signs and symptoms of use and withdrawal.

Street drugs, like other drugs, can come from various sources. They may be derived from natural sources (ie, morphine and codeine). They may be semisynthetic, that is a natural product is chemically modified to produce another molecule (ie, morphine conversion to heroin). Street drugs may also be synthetic with no natural origin.

BENZODIAZEPINES AND OTHER NONALCOHOL SEDATIVES

Benzodiazepines are the most commonly prescribed drugs worldwide. These drugs are used mainly for treatment of anxiety disorders and, in some instances, insomnia. Even though they are used in high quantities throughout the world, intentional abuse is not that common. These drugs, however, have the ability to induce a strong physical dependency on the use of the medication. As tolerance builds up to the drug, the physical dependency increases dramatically. Unlike the street drugs where addiction is a primary consideration, the overuse of benzodiazepine lies in its ability to induce this physical dependency. When these drugs are taken for several weeks, there is relatively little tolerance induced. However, after several months, the proportion of patients who become tolerant increases and reducing the dose or stopping the medication produces severe withdrawal symptoms.

Benzodiazepine Withdrawal Symptoms
Craving for benzodiazepines
Irritability
Anxiety
Sleep disturbances

It is extremely difficult for the physician to distinguish between the withdrawal symptoms and the reappearance of the myriad anxiety symptoms that cause the drug to be prescribed initially. Many patients increase their dose over time because tolerance develops to at least the sedative effects of the drug. The antianxiety benefits of the benzodiazepines continue to occur long after tolerance to the sedating effects. Patients often take these drugs for many years with relatively few ill effects other than the risk of withdrawal. The dentist should be keenly aware of the signs and symptoms and the historical pattern in patients taking benzodiazepines.

CHEMICAL DEPENDENCY AND SMOKING CESSATION
(Continued)

BARBITURATES AND NON-BENZODIAZEPINE SEDATIVES

The use of barbiturates as sedative medications has declined over the years due to the increased safety and efficacy of benzodiazepines. Abuse problems with barbiturates resemble those with the benzodiazepines in many ways. Drugs in this category are frequently prescribed as hypnotics for patients complaining of insomnia. The physician should, therefore, be aware of the problems that can develop when the hypnotic agent is withdrawn. The underlying problem that has lead to the insomnia is not treated directly by the use of barbiturates and the patient seeking a sleep medication may have altered ability to sleep normally because of the medication. The withdrawal symptoms for the barbiturates are similar to the benzodiazepine sedatives.

ALCOHOL

The chronic use of alcohol as well as that of other sedatives is associated with the development of depression. The risk of suicide among alcoholics is one of the highest of any diagnostic category. Cognitive deficits have been reported in alcoholics tested while sober. These deficits usually improve after weeks to months of abstinence. More severe recent memory impairment is associated with specific brain damage caused by nutritional deficiencies common in alcoholics.

Alcohol is toxic to many organ systems. As a result, the medical complications of alcohol abuse and dependence include liver disease, cardiovascular disease, endocrine and gastrointestinal effects, and malnutrition, in addition to CNS dysfunctions. Ethanol readily crosses the placental barrier, producing the *fetal alcohol syndrome*, a major cause of mental retardation.

Alcohol Withdrawal Syndrome Signs and Symptoms
Alcohol craving
Tremor, irritability
Nausea
Sleep disturbance
Tachycardia
Hypertension
Sweating
Perceptual distortion
Seizures (12-48 hours after last drink)
Delirium tremens (rare in uncomplicated withdrawal):
Severe agitation
Confusion
Visual hallucinations
Fever, profuse sweating
Tachycardia
Nausea, diarrhea
Dilated pupils

NICOTINE

Cigarette (nicotine) addiction is influenced by multiple variables. Nicotine itself produces reinforcement; users compare nicotine to stimulants such as cocaine or amphetamine, although its effects are of lower magnitude.

Nicotine is absorbed readily through the skin, mucous membranes, and of course, through the lungs. The pulmonary route produces discernible central nervous system effects in as little as 7 seconds. Thus, each puff produces some discrete reinforcement. With 10 puffs per cigarette, the 1 pack per day smoker reinforces the habit 200 times daily. The timing, setting, situation, and preparation all become associated repetitively with the effects of nicotine.

Nicotine has both stimulant and depressant actions. The smoker feels alert, yet there is some muscle relaxation. Nicotine activates the nucleus accumbens reward system in the brain. Increased extracellular dopamine has been found in this region after nicotine injections in rats. Nicotine affects other systems as well, including the release of endogenous opioids and glucocorticoids.

Nicotine Withdrawal Syndrome Signs and Symptoms
Irritability, impatience, hostility
Anxiety
Dysphoric or depressed mood
Difficulty concentrating
Restlessness
Decreased heart rate
Increased appetite or weight gain

Medications to assist users in breaking a nicotine habit are available.

Bupropion (Zyban®) *on page 151*

Nicotine (Habitrol®, Nicoderm®, Nicorette® (polacrilex gum - OTC),
Nicotrol® (OTC), ProStep®) *on page 678*

SMOKING CESSATION PRODUCTS

Several years ago, the journal *Science* stated that about 80% of smokers say they want to quit, but each year fewer than 1 in 10 actually succeed. Nicotine transdermal delivery preparations (or nicotine patches) were approved by the U.S. Food and Drug Administration in 1992 as aids to smoking cessation for the relief of nicotine withdrawal symptoms. Four preparations were approved simultaneously: Habitrol®, Nicoderm®, Nicotrol®, and Prostep®. These products differ in how much nicotine is released and whether they provide a 24-hour or 16-hour release time.

Studies are still being reported on the effectiveness of nicotine patches on smoking cessation. Most previous studies had good entry criteria including definition of the Fagerstrom score. Dr Fred Cowan of Oregon Health Sciences University described these Fagerstrom criteria in a previous report on nicotine substitutes in AGD *Impact*. Abstinence of smoking cessation has usually been assessed by self-report, measurement of carbon monoxide in breath, and plasma or urine nicotine products.

In numerous protocols, percentages of study subjects who abstained from smoking after 3-10 weeks of patch treatment with nicotine compared to placebo, have never exceeded 40%. After the initial assessment, six studies continued to follow the study subjects through 24-52 weeks of patch treatment. The results were even poorer with less than 25% sustained success. A review of these and additional studies, reveals some general conclusions regarding the effectiveness of nicotine patches in smoking cessation. In every study, many smokers abstained after treatment with placebo patches; nicotine treatment was initially more effective than placebo; and improved abstinence rates were more marked in the short term (10 weeks) than in the long term (52 weeks). Subjects undergoing smoking cessation trails tended to gain weight irrespective of whether placebo or nicotine patches were worn. Patients often favor the nicotine polacrilex gum (Nicorette®) which releases nicotine into the blood stream via the oral mucosa.

Data are now available from smoking cessation studies carried out in general medical practices. The effectiveness of nicotine patch substitution under these conditions is similar to the results described above. Most patch systems and gum are now available as over-the-counter products; only Habitrol® remains prescription. Practitioners and patients should remain skeptical since these aids appear to work best only when supplemented with psychological counseling and a single-minded effort on the part of the patient. New products such as Zyban® are now also being marketed as smoking cessation aids. These drugs are norepinephrine serotonin reuptake inhibitors and their action directly affects the craving for tobacco.

OPIATES

The opiates are most often called narcotics. The most common opiate found on the street is heroin. Heroin is the diacetyl derivative of morphine which is extracted from opium. Although commercial production of morphine involves extraction from the dried opium plant which grows in many parts of the world, some areas still harvest opium by making slits in the unripened seed pod. The pod secretes a white, viscous material which upon contact with the air turns a blackish-brown color. It is this off-white material that is called opium. The opium is then dried and smoked or processed to yield morphine and codeine. Actually, the raw opium contains several chemicals that are used medicinally or commercially. Much (it has been estimated that 50%) of the morphine is converted chemically into heroin which finds its way into the United States and then on the street. Heroin is a Schedule I drug and as

CHEMICAL DEPENDENCY AND SMOKING CESSATION
(Continued)

such has no acceptable use in the United States today. In fact, possession is a violation of the Controlled Substances Act of 1970. The majority of the heroin found on the streets is from Southeast Asia and can be as concentrated as 100%.

The heroin user goes through many phases once the drug has been administered. When administered intravenously, the user initially feels a "rush" often described as an "orgasmic rush". This initial feeling is most likely due to the release of histamine resulting in cutaneous vasodilation, itching, and a flushed appearance. Shortly after this "rush" the user becomes euphoric. This euphoric stage often called "stoned" or being "high" lasts approximately 3-4 hours. During this stage, the user is lethargic, slow to react to stimuli, speech is slurred, pain reaction threshold is elevated, exhibits xerostomia, slowed heart rate, and the pupils may be constricted. Following the "high", the abuser is "straight" for about 2 hours, with no tell-tale signs of abuse. Approximately 6-8 hours following the last injection of heroin, the user begins to experience a runny nose, lacrimation, and abdominal muscle cramps as they begin the withdrawal from the drug. During this stage and the one that follows, the person may become agitated as they develop anxiety about where they are going to get their next "hit". The withdrawal signs and symptoms become more intense. For the next 3 days, the abuser begins to sweat profusely in combination with cutaneous vasoconstriction. The skin becomes cold and clammy, hence the term "cold turkey". Tachycardia, pupillary dilation, diarrhea, and salivation occur for the 3 days following the last injection. Withdrawal signs and symptoms may last longer than the average of 3 days or they may be more abrupt.

Opioid Withdrawal Signs and Symptoms

Symptoms	Signs
Regular Withdrawal	
Craving for opioids	Pupillary dilation
Restlessness, irritability	Sweating
Increased sensitivity to pain	Piloerection ("gooseflesh")
Nausea, cramps	Tachycardia
Muscle aches	Vomiting, diarrhea
Dysphoric mood	Increased blood pressure
Insomnia, anxiety	Yawning
	Fever
Protracted Withdrawal	
Anxiety	Cyclic changes in weight, pupil size, respiratory center sensitivity
Insomnia	
Drug craving	

Many of these patients who have been abusing opiates for any length of time will exhibit multiple carious lesions, particularly class V lesions. This increased caries rate is probably a result of the heroin-induced xerostomia, high intake of sweets, and lack of daily oral hygiene. Patients who are recovering from heroin or any opiate addiction should not be given any kind of opiate analgesic, whether it be for sedation or as a postoperative analgesic because of the increased chance of relapse. The nonsteroidal anti-inflammatory drugs (NSAIDs) should be used to control any postoperative discomfort. Patients who admit to a past history of intravenous heroin use or any intravenous drug for that matter, are at higher risk for subacute bacterial endocarditis (SBE), HIV disease, and hepatitis but with the exception of postoperative analgesia should present no special problem for dental care.

MARIJUANA

The number one most abused illegal drug by high school students today is marijuana. Marijuana is a plant that grows throughout the world, but is particularly suited for a warm, humid environment. There are three species of plant but the two most frequently cited are *Cannabis sativa* and *Cannabis indica*. All species possess a female and male plant. Although approximately 450 chemicals have been isolated from the plant, the major psychoactive ingredient is delta-9-tetrahydrocannabinol (THC). Of these 450 chemicals, there are about 23 psychoactive chemicals, THC being the most abundant. The highest concentration of THC is found in the bud of the female plant. The concentration of THC varies according to growing conditions and location on the plant but has increased from about 2% to 3% in marijuana sold in the 50s to about 30% sold on the streets today. Marijuana can be smoked in cigarettes (joints), pipes, water pipes (bongs), or baked in brownies, cakes, etc, and then ingested. However, smoking marijuana is more efficient and the "high" has a quicker onset. Marijuana is a Schedule I drug but has been promoted as a medicinal for the treatment of glaucoma, for increasing appetite in patients who have HIV disease, and to prevent the nausea associated with cancer chemotherapy. In response to this request, the FDA approved dronabinol (Marinol®), a synthetic THC and placed this drug in Schedule II to be prescribed by physicians for the indicated medical conditions.

Dronabinol (Marinol®) *on page 340*

An individual under the influence of marijuana may exhibit no signs or symptoms of intoxication. The pharmacologic effects are dose-dependent and depend to a large extent on the set and setting of the intoxicated individual. As the dose of THC increases, the person experiences euphoria or a state of well-being, often referred to as "mellowing out". Everything becomes comical, problems disappear, and their appetite for snack foods increases. This is called the "munchies". The marijuana produces time and spatial distortion, which contribute, as the dose increases, to a dysphoria characterized by paranoia and fear. Although there has never been a death reported from marijuana overdose, certainly the higher doses may produce such bizarre circumstances as to increase the chances of accidental death. THC is fat soluble. Daily consumption of marijuana will result in THC being stored in body fat which will result in detectable amounts of THC being found in the urine for as long as 60 days in some cases.

Marijuana Withdrawal Syndrome Signs and Symptoms
Restlessness
Irritability
Mild agitation
Insomnia
Restlessness
Sleep EEG disturbance
Nausea, cramping

Because of anxiety associated with dental visits, marijuana would be the most likely drug, after alcohol, to be used when coming to the dental office. But, unlike alcohol, marijuana may not produce any detectable odor on the breath nor any signs of intoxication. Fortunately, local anesthetics, analgesics, and antibiotics used by the general dentist do not interact with marijuana. The major concern with the marijuana intoxicated patient is a failure to follow directions while in the chair, and the inability to follow postoperative instructions.

COCAINE

Cocaine, referred to on the street as "snow", "nose candy", "girl", and many other euphemisms, has created an epidemic. This drug is like no other local anesthetic. Known for about the last two thousand years, cocaine has been used and abused by politicians, scientists, farmers, warriors, and of course, on the street. Cocaine is derived from the leaves of a plant called *Erythroxylon coca* which grows in South America. Ninety percent of the world's supply of cocaine originates in Peru, Bolivia, and Colombia. At last estimate, the United States consumes 75% of the world's supply. The plant grows to a height of approximately four feet and produces a red berry. Farmers go through the fields stripping the leaves from the plant three times a year. During the working day the farmers chew the coca leaves to suppress appetite and fight the fatigue of working the fields. The leaves are transported to a laboratory site where the cocaine is extracted by a process called maceration. It takes approximately 7-8 pounds of leaves to produce one ounce of cocaine.

On the streets of the United States, cocaine can be found in two forms. One form is as the hydrochloride salt. In this form, the cocaine can be "snorted" or it can be dissolved in water and injected intravenously. The other form of cocaine is as the free base. The free base form can be smoked. The free base form is sometimes referred to as "crack", "rock", or "free base". It is called crack because it cracks or pops when large pieces are smoked. It is called rock because it is so hard and difficult to break into smaller pieces. The most popular method of administration of cocaine is "snorting." In this method, small amounts of cocaine hydrochloride are divided into segments or "lines". The person uses any straw-like device to inhale one or more lines of the cocaine into their nose. Although the cocaine does not reach the lungs, enough cocaine is absorbed through the nasal mucosa to provide a "high" within 3-5 minutes. Rock or crack on the other hand is heated

CHEMICAL DEPENDENCY AND SMOKING CESSATION
(Continued)

and inhaled from any device available. This form of cocaine does reach the lungs and provides a much faster onset of action as well as a more intense stimulation. There are dangers to the user with any form of cocaine. Undoubtedly the most dangerous form, though, is the intravenous route.

Cocaine Withdrawal Signs and Symptoms
Dysphoria, depression
Sleepiness, fatigue
Cocaine craving
Bradycardia

The cocaine user, regardless of how the cocaine was administered, presents the potential of a life-threatening situation in the dental operatory. The patient under the influence of cocaine could be compared to a car going 100 miles per hour. Blood pressure is elevated and heart rate is likely increased. The use of a local anesthetic with epinephrine in such a patient may result in a medical emergency. Such patients can be identified by their jitteriness, irritability, talkativeness, tremors, and short abrupt speech patterns. These same signs and symptoms may also be seen in a normal dental patient with preoperative dental anxiety; therefore, the dentist must be particularly alert in order to identify the potential cocaine abuser. If a patient is suspected, they should never be given a local anesthetic with vasoconstrictor for fear of exacerbating the cocaine-induced sympathetic response. Life-threatening episodes of cardiac arrhythmias and hypertensive crises have been reported when local anesthetic with vasoconstrictor was administered to a patient under the influence of cocaine. No local anesthetic used by any dentist can interfere with, nor test positive for cocaine in any urine testing screen. Therefore, the dentist needn't be concerned with any false drug use accusations associated with dental anesthesia.

PSYCHEDELIC AGENTS

Perceptual distortions that include hallucinations, illusions, and disorders of thinking such as paranoia can be produced by toxic doses of many drugs. These phenomena also may be seen during toxic withdrawal from sedatives such as alcohol. There are, however, certain drugs that have as their primary effect the production of perception, thought, or mood disturbances at low doses with minimal effects on memory and orientation. These are commonly called *hallucinogenic drugs*, but their use does not always result in frank hallucinations.

LSD: LSD is the most potent hallucinogenic drug and produces significant psychedelic effects with a total dose of as little as 25-50 mcg. This drug is over 3000 times more potent than mescaline. LSD is sold on the illicit market in a variety of forms. A popular contemporary system involves postage stamp-sized papers impregnated with varying doses of LSD (50-300 mcg or more). A majority of street samples sold as LSD actually contain LSD. In contrast, the samples of mushrooms and other botanicals sold as sources of psilocybin and other psychedelics have a low probability of containing the advertised hallucinogenics.

Phencyclidine (PCP): PCP deserves special mention because of its widespread availability and because its pharmacological effects are different from LSD. PCP was originally developed as an anesthetic in the 1950s and later abandoned because of a high frequency of postoperative delirium with hallucinations. It was classed as a dissociative anesthetic because, in the anesthetized state, the patient remains conscious with staring gaze, flat facies, and rigid muscles. It was discovered as a drug of abuse in the 1970s, first in an oral form and then in a smoked version enabling a better control over the dose.

INHALANTS

Anesthetic gases such as nitrous oxide or halothane are sometimes used as intoxicants by medical personnel. Nitrous oxide also is abused by food service employees because it is supplied for use as a propellant in disposable aluminum minitanks for whipping cream canisters. Nitrous oxide produces euphoria and analgesia and then loss of consciousness. Compulsive use and chronic toxicity rarely are reported, but there are obvious risks of overdose associated with the abuse of this anesthetic. Chronic use has been reported to cause peripheral neuropathy.

The dental team should be alert to the signs and symptoms of drug abuse and withdrawal. Further reading is recommended.

ANIMAL AND HUMAN BITES GUIDELINES

The dentist is often confronted with early management of animal and human bites. The following protocols may assist in appropriate care and referral.

WOUND MANAGEMENT

Irrigation: Critically important; irrigate all penetration wounds using 20 mL syringe, 19-gauge needle and >250 mL 1% povidone iodine solution. This method will reduce wound infection by a factor of 20. When there is high risk of rabies, use viricidal 1% benzalkonium chloride in addition to the 1% povidone iodine. Irrigate wound with normal saline after antiseptic irrigation.

Debridement: Remove all crushed or devitalized tissue remaining after irrigation; minimize removal on face and over thin skin areas or anywhere you would create a worse situation than the bite itself already has; do not extend puncture wounds surgically — rather, manage them with irrigation and antibiotics.

Suturing: Close most dog bites if <8 hours (<12 hours on face); do not routinely close puncture wounds, or deep or severe bites on the hands or feet, as these are at highest risk for infection. Cat and human bites should not be sutured unless cosmetically important. Wound edge freshening, where feasible, reduces infection; minimize sutures in the wound and use monofilament on the surface.

Immobilization: Critical in all hand wounds; important for infected extremities.

Hospitalization/I.V. Antibiotics: Admit for I.V. antibiotics all significant human bites to the hand, especially closed fist injuries, and bites involving penetration of the bone or joint (a high index of suspicion is needed). Consider I.V. antibiotics for significant established wound infections with cellulitis or lymphangitis, any infected bite on the hand, any infected cat bite, and any infection in an immunocompromised or asplenic patient. Outpatient treatment with I.V. antibiotics may be possible in selected cases by consulting with infectious disease.

LABORATORY ASSESSMENT

Gram's Stain: Not useful prior to onset of clinically apparent infection; examination of purulent material may show a predominant organism in established infection, aiding antibiotic selection; not warranted unless results will change your treatment.

Culture: Not useful or cost-effective prior to onset of clinically apparent infection.

X-ray: Whenever you suspect bony involvement, especially in craniofacial dog bites in very small children or severe bite/crush in an extremity; cat bites with their long needle like teeth may cause osteomyelitis or a septic joint, especially in the hand or wrist.

IMMUNIZATIONS

Tetanus: All bite wounds are contaminated. If not immunized in last 5 years, or if not current in a child, give DPT, DT, Td, or TT as indicated. For absent or incomplete primary immunization, give 250 units tetanus immune globulin (TIG) in addition.

Rabies: In the U.S. 30,000 persons are treated each year in an attempt to prevent 1-5 cases. Domestic animals should be quarantined for 10 days to prove need for prophylaxis. High risk animal bites (85% of cases = bat, skunk, raccoon) usually receive treatment consisting of:
- human rabies immune globulin (HRIG): 20 units/kg I.M. (unless previously immunized with HDCV)
- human diploid cell vaccine (HDCV): 1 mL I.M. on days 0, 3, 7, 14, and 28 (unless previously immunized with HDCV - then give only first 2 doses)

Rabies Immune Globulin, Human *on page 832*
Rabies Virus Vaccine *on page 832*
Tetanus Immune Globulin, Human *on page 911*

BITE WOUNDS AND PROPHYLACTIC ANTIBIOTICS

Parenteral vs Oral: If warranted, consider an initial I.V. dose to rapidly establish effective serum levels, especially if high risk, delayed treatment, or if patient reliability is poor.

ANIMAL AND HUMAN BITES GUIDELINES *(Continued)*

Dog Bite:

1. Rarely get infected (~5%)

2. Infecting organisms: Staph coag negative, staph coag positive, alpha strep, diphtheroids, beta strep, *Pseudomonas aeruginosa*, gamma strep, *Pasteurella multocida*

3. Prophylactic antibiotics are seldom indicated. Consider for high risk wounds such as distal extremity puncture wounds, severe crush injury, bites occurring in cosmetically sensitive areas (eg, face), or in immunocompromised or asplenic patients.

Cat Bite:

1. Often get infected (~25% to 50%)

2. Infecting organisms: *Pasteurella multocida* (first 24 hours), coag positive staph, anaerobic cocci (after first 24 hours)

3. Prophylactic antibiotics are indicated in all cases.

Human Bite:

1. Intermediate infection rate (~15% to 20%)

2. Infecting organisms: Coag positive staph α, β, γ strep, *Haemophilus*, *Eikenella corrodens*, anaerobic streptococci, *Fusobacterium*, *Veillonella*, bacteroides.

3. Prophylactic antibiotics are indicated in almost all cases except superficial injuries.

Amoxicillin (various products) *on page 68*

Amoxicillin and Clavulanate Potassium (Augmentin®) *on page 69*

Cefazolin (Ancef®; Kefzol®; Zolicef®) *on page 188*

Cefotetan (Cefotan®) *on page 193*

Ceftriaxone (Rocephin®) *on page 197*

Clindamycin (Cleocin®) *on page 243*

Doxycycline (various products) *on page 338*

Imipenem/Cilastatin (Primaxin®) *on page 500*

Trimethoprim and Sulfamethoxazole (various products) *on page 965*

BITE WOUND ANTIBIOTIC REGIMENS

	Dog Bite	Cat Bite	Human Bite
Prophylactic Antibiotics			
Prophylaxis	No routine prophylaxis, consider if involves face or hand, or immunosuppressed or asplenic patients	Routine prophylaxis	Routine prophylaxis
Prophylactic antibiotic	Amoxicillin	Amoxicillin	Amoxicillin
Penicillin allergy	Doxycycline if >10 y or co-trimoxazole	Doxycycline if >10 y or co-trimoxazole	Doxycycline if >10 y or erythromycin and cephalexin*
Outpatient Oral Antibiotic Treatment (mild to moderate infection)			
Established infection	Amoxicillin and clavulanic acid	Amoxicillin and clavulanic acid	Amoxicillin and clavulanic acid
Penicillin allergy (mild infection only)	Doxycycline if >10 y	Doxycycline if >10 y	Cephalexin* or clindamycin
Outpatient Parenteral Antibiotic Treatment (moderate infections — single drug regimens)			
	Ceftriaxone	Ceftriaxone	Cefotetan
Inpatient Parenteral Antibiotic Treatment			
Established infection	Ampicillin + cefazolin	Ampicillin + cefazolin	Ampicillin + clindamycin
Penicillin allergy	Cefazolin*	Ceftriaxone*	Cefotetan* or imipenem
Duration of Prophylactic and Treatment Regimens			
Prophylaxis: 5 days			
Treatment: 10-14 days			

*Contraindicated if history of immediate hypersensitivity reaction (anaphylaxis) to penicillin.

NATURAL PRODUCTS, HERBALS, AND DIETARY SUPPLEMENTS

Medical problem: " I have a toothache."

2000 BC response: "Here, eat this root."

1000 AD: "That root is heathen; here, say this prayer."

1850 AD: "That prayer is superstitious; here, drink this potion."

1940 AD: "That potion is snake oil; here, swallow this pill."

1985 AD: "That pill is ineffective; here, take this new antibiotic."

2000 AD: "That antibiotic is artificial; here, eat this root."

Adapted from an anonymous Internet communication.

INTRODUCTION

For centuries, Eastern and Western civilizations have attributed a large number of medical uses to plants and herbs. Over time, modern scientific methodologies have emerged from some of these remedies. Conversely, some of these agents have fallen into less popularity as more medical knowledge has evolved. In spite of this dichotomy, herbal and natural therapies for treatment of common medical ailments have become exceedingly popular. In America, people consistently seek out natural products that may be able to offset some perceived ailment of may assist in the prevention of an ailment. One area that has consistently drawn patients interested in herbal or natural remedies has been the area of weight loss. There are numerous systemic considerations when some of the natural products that have been attributed weight loss powers are utilized. Many of these products are sold under the blanket of dietary supplements and, therefore, avoid some of the more stringent Food and Drug Administration legislation. In 1994, that legislation was modified to include herbs, vitamins, minerals, and amino acids that may be taken as dietary supplements and that information must be available to patients taking them. The real concern, however, lies in the fact that health claims need not be approved by the FDA, but the advertisements must include a disclaimer saying that the product has not yet been fully evaluated. Claims of medicinal use/value are often drawn from popular use, not necessarily from scientific studies. The safety, however, when these agents are taken in combination with other prescription drugs is of concern and medical risk might result. Many of these natural products may have real medicinal value but caution on the part of the dental clinician is prudent. It is impossible within this chapter to cover all of the popular natural products. The chapter, therefore, has been limited to brief reviews of some of the most popular dietary supplements, herbs, and natural remedies currently being used by patients you might treat and what we know about the effects of some of these agents on the body's various systems. An extensive reading list is provided.

TOP 20 MOST POPULAR NATURAL PRODUCTS

ALFALFA

Alfalfa has been touted as a natural laxative, an antifungal, a liver detoxifier, a diuretic, and a food additive useful in treating kidney stones and urinary infections. Alfalfa is an important animal feed worldwide and its chemical constituents are well known. However, studies have concluded that alfalfa contains nothing of significant therapeutic value in the amounts generally recommended. The seed contains L-canabanine which has been implicated in pancytopenia in humans and may induce systemic lupus in monkeys. Allergic reactions have been provoked in some users.

ALOE VERA

Products derived from this plant have been used for centuries. Aloe is popularly used as a cure-all and it has been advertised for use in treating acne, burns, and minor wounds. Although the FDA does not recognize the uses of aloe for the treatment of any specific condition, there is evidence to suggest that fresh aloe gel is an effective agent in wound healing. Data to support these claims are inconclusive, however, and the use of aloe by patients should not interfere with dental care.

BILBERRY

Bilberry, also known as blueberry, is recommended by herbalists for use in connection with vascular and blood disorders and in treating varicose veins, thromboses, diarrhea, and angina. Preliminary studies have indicated that bilberry may have some benefit in aiding visual acuity, however, there is little clinical evidence to support the widespread usage. Potential interactions with over-the-counter prescription medications are unknown at this time.

CAYENNE

Most cooks know of the chemical cayenne that is the active ingredient in chili pepper and lends itself to the strong taste of this herb. Cayenne has been known for many years to stimulate digestion and to promote sweating; sometimes assisting, therefore, in reducing fever. Cayenne contains an ingredient known as capsaicin which is the active ingredient in many over-the-counter and prescription forms of cream to treat arthritis. Capsaicin appears to alter the action of the compound associated with pain, the mechanism of which has not been completely studied.

CHAMOMILE

This agent is often found in the form of dried leaves that can be used to create a tea. The tea is taken internally and has been recommended by naturalists as a cure for stomach pain, menstrual discomfort, and stress. Chamomile teas appear to have some unknown mechanism of immune activation, perhaps due to the presence of flavonoids in the compound.

CRANBERRY

Cranberry has been used for centuries as an agent to assist in treatment of urinary tract infections. Cranberry juices contain pH-altering chemical which may be of use in treating these infections. It is now thought that the cranberry actually prevents bacteria from adhering to the lining of the bladder and urinary tract. Again, this agent is rich in flavonoids, citric acids, and vitamin C.

ECHINACEA

Echinacea is reported to have uses for treatment of colds, flu, bacterial and fungal infections, and even cancer. AIDS patients are sometimes advised by their peers to take echinacea. To date, pharmacological components and their actions on the human body are unclear. However, complex polysaccharides are found in the agent and seem to hold some promise as compounds for immunostimulation. In general, echinacea appears to be relatively safe but clinical information is lacking.

EPHEDRA

Also known as ma-huang, ephedra has been used in China for more than 4000 years to treat symptoms of upper respiratory infections and asthma. Ephedra can be used as a nasal decongestant and has recently gained new popularity as a weight loss product. This agent, when used in combination with St John's Wort, apparently has effects on serotonin levels similar to the drug fenfluramine which was recently taken off the market. This combination of drugs has been known as natural fen-phen. Ephedra has also been recommended as an aphrodisiac.

FEVERFEW

Feverfew has a long history of use in traditional and cult medicine as a treatment for fever, headache, and menstrual irregularities. More recently, it has been suggested for migraine headaches, arthritis, and insect bites. The dentist should be aware that patients may self-medicate with feverfew in an effort to treat migraine headaches. One study of commercially available feverfew products has found that there is a lactone present that appears to have some activity. However, there are no long-term toxicology studies to indicate or refute this claim.

GARLIC

Garlic and related products have been used for thousands of years. It is generally considered by herbalists and naturalists as a cure-all. When garlic is crushed, it produces allicin which possesses some antibiotic, antiplatelet, anticholesterol properties. In addition, other sulfur-containing compounds are found in garlic and these produce some antithrombotic properties. For the most part, the consumption of moderate amounts of garlic is harmless. Large doses, however, are likely to stimulate heartburn and gastric or intestinal disorders.

GINGER

Ginger has been taken for centuries due to its calming effects on an upset stomach. The stem of the rhizome from a tropical plant has been used to make the ginger root. Today it is widely used for morning sickness, seasickness, and motion sickness. Ginger may have some effect on cholesterol levels although further study is necessary. The presence of essential oils in ginger may be the active ingredients in this agent.

GINKGO BILOBA

Ginkgo supplements are claimed by herbalists to help with the aging process and with mental acuity. The most popular of these agents is used as an extract to promote improved blood flow to a portion of the body. Clinical research has not proven that these claims are or are not true.

GINSENG

Ginseng is commonly used as a substance to support general good health and has also been marketed in some countries as an aphrodisiac. As with the majority of herbal agents, there are few clinical studies. However, commercial products vary

NATURAL PRODUCTS, HERBALS, AND DIETARY SUPPLEMENTS *(Continued)*

widely and the clinician may be aware that ginseng could produce some side effects.

GREEN TEA

Green tea has been widely used in Asia to treat numerous ailments. This tea is derived from leaves and delicate leaf buds of an evergreen bush. It is thought that green tea has some antioxidant effect, as well as containing compounds and flavonoids as with many of the other herbs.

KAVA

Kava is one of the most popular herbs on today's market. It is extracted from a root and is used to promote sleep and relaxation in anxious patients. This agent appears to be extremely safe, however, the full effect of the active ingredient know as kavalactones, is unknown. They appear to have an effect on the neural transmitter activity in the central nervous system.

LICORICE

Licorice has been used for centuries to treat intestinal disorders and stomach distress. There appears to be some activity of licorice on patients who suffer from mild preulcerous conditions in the GI tract. Again, the flavonoids appear to be an active component.

PSYLLIUM

Psyllium has been used by herbalists and natural product advocates to promote regular intestinal function, primarily as an agent to assist in constipation and in GI distress.

ST JOHN'S WORT

St John's wort has become popular in the treatment of depression, anxiety, and even in AIDS. While some of the constituents seem to show a minimal amount of antidepressant activity, other components may suggest that St John's wort is ineffective in treating these illnesses.

SAW PALMETTO

Saw palmetto was an official drug used for a variety of ailments, mainly associated with urogenital disorders. It has actually been shown to have some efficacy in managing benign prostate hypertrophy. The drug, however, has not yet passed any of the rigid FDA requirements prior to being able to substantiate this claim.

VALERIAN

Valerian has, for centuries, made claims of being a natural tranquilizer, a relaxant for pain and muscle spasms, as well as promoting restful sleep. The dentist should be aware that some patients may be drawn to use valerian in an effort to reduce TMD dysfunction or muscle pain.

Herbalists have often used these natural products singularly or in combination to achieve a therapeutic effect. Some of the natural agents have been combined for assisted weight loss or for reduction of more serious ailments such as high blood pressure or cardiovascular disease. One such combination recommends ephedra and St John's wort as a "natural fen-phen". These agents are not directly related to fenfluramine, but are thought to also act on serotonin levels in the brain. The dentist should be aware that there are some known interactions of these agents with drug therapies that the dentist may be using. However, our knowledge is extremely limited in this extent. The dentist is referred for additional readings so that a personal opinion can be formed.

EFFECTS ON VARIOUS SYSTEMS

CENTRAL NERVOUS SYSTEM

(Aconite, Ginseng, Xanthine derivatives)

Aconite and hawthorn have potentially sedating effects, and aconite also contains various alkaloids and traces of ephedrine. Some documented central nervous system (CNS) effects of aconite include sedation, vertigo, and incoordination. Hawthorn has been reported to exert a depressive effect on the CNS leading to sedation.

Ginseng, ma-huang, and xanthine derivatives can exert a stimulant effect on the central nervous system. Some of the CNS effects of ginseng include nervousness, insomnia, and euphoria. The action of ma-huang is due to the presence of ephedrine and pseudoephedrine. Ma-huang exerts a stimulant action on the CNS similar to decongestant/weight loss products (Dexatrim®, etc) thus causing nervousness, insomnia, and anxiety. Kola nut, green tea, guarana, and yerba mate contain varying amounts of caffeine, a xanthine derivative. Stimulant properties exerted by these herbs are expected to be comparable to those of caffeine, including insomnia, nervousness, and anxiety.

Products containing aconite and hawthorn should be used with caution in patients with known history of depression, vertigo, or syncope. Ginseng or xanthine derivatives should be avoided in patients with history of insomnia or anxiety. Use of natural products with these components may contribute to a worsening of a patient's pre-existing medical condition. Patients taking CNS-active medications should avoid or use extreme caution when using preparations containing any of the above components. These components may interact directly or indirectly with CNS-active medications causing an increase or decrease in overall effect.

CARDIOVASCULAR SYSTEM

CONGESTIVE HEART FAILURE

(Diuretics, Xanthine derivatives, Licorice, Ginseng, Aconite)

Alisma plantago, bearberry (*Arctostaphylos uva-ursi*), buchu (*Barosma betulina*), couch grass, dandelion, horsetail rush, juniper, licorice, and xanthine derivatives exert varying degrees of diuretic action. Many patients with congestive heart failure (CHF) are already taking a diuretic medication. By taking products containing one or more of these components, patients already on diuretic medications may increase their risk for dehydration.

Ginseng and licorice can potentially worsen congestive heart failure and edema by causing fluid retention. Aconite has varying effects on the heart that itself could lead to heart failure. Patients with CHF should be advised to consult with their healthcare provider before using products containing any of these components.

HYPERTENSION/HYPOTENSION

(Diuretics, Ginkgo biloba, Ginseng, Hawthorn, Ma-huang, Xanthine derivatives)

The stimulant properties of ginseng and ma-huang could worsen pre-existing hypertension. Elevated blood pressure has been reported as a side effect of ginseng. Although ma-huang contains ephedrine, a known vasoconstrictor, ma-huang's effect on blood pressure varies between individuals. Ma-huang can cause hypotension or hypertension. Due to its unpredictable effects, patients with pre-existing hypertension should use caution when using natural products containing ma-huang. Providers should caution patients with labile hypertension against the use of ginseng.

The diuretic effect of xanthine derivatives and other diuretic components could increase the effects of antihypertensive medications, increasing the risk for hypotension. Hawthorn and ginkgo biloba can cause vasodilation increasing the hypotensive effects of antihypertensive medication. Patients susceptible to hypotension or patients taking antihypertensive medication should use caution when taking products containing xanthine derivatives or diuretics. Patients with pre-existing hypertension or hypotension who wish to use products containing these components should be closely monitored by a healthcare professional for changes in blood pressure control.

ARRHYTHMIAS

(Ginseng)

It has been reported that ginseng may increase the risk of arrhythmias, although it is unclear whether this effect is due to the actual ingredient (ginseng) or other possible impurities. Patients at risk for arrhythmias should be cautioned against the use of products containing ginseng without first consulting with their healthcare provider.

GASTROINTESTINAL SYSTEM

PEPTIC ULCER DISEASE

(Betaine Hydrochloride, White Willow)

Betaine hydrochloride is a source of hydrochloric acid. The acid released from betaine hydrochloride could aggravate an existing ulcer. White willow, like aspirin, contains salicylates.

Aspirin has been known to induce gastric damage by direct irritation on the gastric mucosa and by an indirect systemic effect. As a result, patients with a history of peptic ulcer disease or gastritis are informed to avoid use of aspirin and other salicylate derivatives. These precautions should also apply to white willow. Patients

NATURAL PRODUCTS, HERBALS, AND DIETARY SUPPLEMENTS *(Continued)*

with a history of peptic ulcer disease or gastritis should not use products containing white willow or betaine hydrochloride as either could exacerbate ulcers.

INFLAMMATORY BOWEL DISEASE

(Cascara Sagrada, Senna, Dandelion)

Cascara sagrada and senna are stimulant laxatives. Their laxative effect is exerted by stimulation of peristalsis in the colon and by inhibition of water and electrolyte secretion. The laxative effect produced by these herbs could induce an exacerbation of inflammatory bowel disease. Patients with a history of inflammatory bowel disease should avoid using products containing cascara sagrada or senna, and use caution when taking products containing dandelion which may also have a laxative effect.

OBSTRUCTION/ILEUS

(Glucomannan, Kelp, Psyllium)

Glucomannan, kelp, and psyllium act as bulk laxatives. In the presence of water, bulk laxatives swell or form a viscous solution adding extra bulk in the gastrointestinal tract. The resulting mass is thought to stimulate peristalsis. In the presence of an ileus, these laxatives could cause an obstruction.

If sufficient water is not consumed when taking a bulk laxative, a semisolid mass can form resulting in an obstruction. Any patient who wishes to take a natural product containing kelp, psyllium, or glucomannan should drink sufficient water to decrease the risk of obstruction. This may be of concern in particular disease states such as CHF or other cases where excess fluid intake may influence the existing disease presentation. Patients with a suspected obstruction or ileus should avoid using products containing kelp, psyllium, or glucomannan without consent of their primary healthcare provider.

HEMATOLOGIC SYSTEM

ANTICOAGULATION THERAPY & COAGULATION DISORDERS

(Horsetail Rush, Ginseng, Ginkgo Biloba, Guarana, White Willow)

Horsetail rush, ginseng, ginkgo biloba, guarana, and white willow can potentially affect platelet aggregation and bleeding time. Ginkgo biloba, ginseng, guarana, and white willow inhibit platelet aggregation resulting in an increase in bleeding time. Horsetail rush, on the other hand, may decrease bleeding time. Patients with coagulation disorders or patients on anticoagulation therapy may be sensitive to the effects on coagulation by these components and should, therefore, avoid use of products containing any of these components.

ENDOCRINE SYSTEM

DIABETES MELLITUS

(Chromium, Glucomannan, Ginseng, Hawthorn, Ma-huang, Periploca, Spirulina)

Ma-huang and spirulina both may increase glucose levels. This could cause a decrease in glucose control, thereby, increasing a patient's risk for hyperglycemia. Patients with diabetes or glucose intolerance should avoid using ma-huang and spirulina containing products.

Chromium, ginseng, glucomannan, periploca *(gymneme sylvestre)*, and hawthorn should be used with caution in patients being treated for diabetes. These ingredients may reduce glucose levels increasing the risk for hypoglycemia in patients who are already taking a hypoglycemic agent. Patients with diabetes who wish to use products containing these ingredients should be closely monitored for fluctuations in blood glucose levels.

OTHER

PHENYLKETONURIA

(Aspartame, Spirulina)

Patients with phenylketonuria should not use products containing aspartame or spirulina. Aspartame, a common artificial sweetener, is metabolized to phenylalanine, while spirulina contains phenylalanine.

GOUT

(Diuretics, White Willow)

Patients with a history of gout should avoid using natural products containing components with diuretic action or white willow. By increasing urine output, ingredients with diuretic action may concentrate uric acid in the blood increasing the risk of gout in these patients. White willow, like aspirin, may inhibit excretion of urate resulting in an increase in uric acid concentration. The increase in urate levels could cause precipitation of uric acid resulting in an exacerbation of gout.

SELECTED NATURAL PRODUCTS SOLD FOR WEIGHT LOSS

Product (Distributor)	Other Ingredients
24 hour Diet Herbal Tea® (GNC)	Papaya (carcia papaya), moon daisy (leucanthemum vulgare), parsley (petroselinum hortense), citrus peel (citrus aurantium), spices, natural flavor, althaea
24 hour Diet Shake® (GNC)	Soy protein isolate, sodium/calcium caseinate, whey, corn syrup solids, fiber blend, Dutch cocoa, herbal blend (dahlulin, chickweed, schizandra, L-selenomethionate, inosine, CoQ10), sunflower oil, calcium blend
24 hour Diet Shake	Potassium chloride, natural/artificial flavors, magnesium oxide, soy lecithin, vitamin C, vitamin E, d-alpha tocopherol, vitamin A palmitate, niacinamide, zinc oxide, iron, copper gluconate, d-calcium panthenate
24 hour Diet Shake	Vitamin D_3, pyridoxine hydrochloride, riboflavin, thiamine mononitrate, cyanocobalamin, folate, biotin, potassium iodide
24 hour Dietgel: Energy for Dieters® (GNC)	Cayenne powder, cranberry concentrate, gotu kola
Chroma Plus Slim® (Richardson Labs)	L-carnitine USP, choline bitartrate, inositol, DL-methionine, potassium chloride, pantothenic acid, vitamin B_6, peppermint, bromelain
Chroma Slim for Men® (Richardson Labs)	L-carnitine USP, choline bitartrate, inositol, DL-methionine, pantothenic acid, vitamin B_6, peppermint, saw palmetto berries, cayenne, mustard seed powder, cinnamon, ginger root extract
Chroma Slim Plus Complete® (Richardson Labs)	Hydroxycitric acid, vanadyl sulfate, CoQ10, inositol, folate, potassium chloride, magnesium oxide, B_5 (cal d-pantothenate), niacin, whole food blend, mustard seed, cayenne
Citralean® (Advanced Research)	Hydroxycitric acid, vanadyl sulfate
Diet Fuel: Thermogenic Formula® (Twin Lab)	Hydroxycitric acid, L-carnitine, potassium phosphate, magnesium phosphate, citrus, bioflavonoids, ginger root powder, cayenne powder
Diet Max: Fat Control® (Kal, Inc)	Lotus leaf, cinnamon bark, stephania, rhapontica, L-carnitine tartrate, niacin, choline bitartrate, pantothenic acid, vitamin B_6, capsicum powder, mustard powder, magnesium oxide/citrate, potassium citrate
Diet Max: Sweet Balance® (Kal, Inc)	Bittermelon, bay leaf powder, cinnamon powder, niacin, magnesium citrate/oxide, medium chain triglycerides, lecithin, oleic acid, natural mixed tocopherols
Excel: Fat Burner Formula® (Human Energy Co)	Garcinia cambogia, (hydroxycitric acid), cayenne
Fat Burners® (Action Labs, Inc)	Choline, inositol, methionine, vitamin B_6, bromelain (pineapple), potassium citrate, calcium ascorbate, L-carnitine, pantothine, corn silk, alfalfa
Fat Fighters® (Only Natural, Inc)	Oat bran, rice brain, apple pectin, carrot fiber, beef fiber, L-acidophilus, lecithin, choline bitartrate, inositol, L-carnitine, aloe vera, bromelain, CoQ10, calcium carbonate, magnesium hydroxide, potassium citrate

NATURAL PRODUCTS, HERBALS, AND DIETARY SUPPLEMENTS *(Continued)*

SELECTED NATURAL PRODUCTS SOLD FOR WEIGHT LOSS
(continued)

Product (Distributor)	Other Ingredients
Ginseng Trim Maxx® (Body Breakthrough)	Locust plant (cassia augustifolia), gynostermma (pentaphyllum), lycii berry leaf
Metabo Lift Thermogenic Formula® (Twin Lab)	Cayenne
Slim Max® (USA Sports Labs)	Potassium, L-carnitine complex, vitamin B_6, bromelain
Super Diet Max With Chromium® (Natural Max Co)	Mustard seed powder, garcinia cambogia, schizandra extract
Super Dieters Tea® (Laci Le Beau)	Citrus reticulate (orange peel), carcia papaya, lonicera japonica (honeysuckle), chrysanthemum officinalis (German chamomile), spice, natural flavor, althaea officinalis
Thermachrome 5000	L-carnitine, ginger, boron proteinate, gotu kola, saw palmetto
Ultra Lean Herbal® (Schiff)	Garcinia cambogia extract, cayenne, iodine, potassium (glycerophosphate), magnesium (glycinate), cellulose, vegetable stearates
Ultra Lean Tablet® (Schiff)	Cayenne, iodine, potassium (glycerophosphate), magnesium (glycinate), vanadyl sulfate, cellulose, vegetable stearates, brindall berry extract (garcinia cambogia)

Adapted from Mistry MG and Mays DA, "Precautions Against Global Use of Natural Products for Weight Loss: A Review of Active Ingredients and Issues Concerning Concomitant Disease States," *Therapeutic Perspectives*, 1996, 10(1):2.

DENTAL OFFICE EMERGENCIES

Protocols should be established for most Office Emergencies. Recognition and rapid diagnosis lead to appropriate management. Major drugs discussed under the various headings are listed below.

Ammonia Spirit, Aromatic *on page 64*

Atropine *on page 98*

Dexamethasone (Decadron®) *on page 291*

Diazepam (Valium®) *on page 300*

Diphenhydramine (Benadryl®) *on page 323*

Epinephrine *on page 353*

Hydrocortisone *on page 484*

Isoproterenol *on page 523*

Naloxone (Narcan®) *on page 662*

Meperidine (Demerol®) *on page 592*

Methohexital (Brevital®) *on page 614*

Morphine *on page 648*

Theophylline *on page 917*

SYNCOPE (Fainting)

Cause: Decreased circulation of blood to the brain

Symptoms:

- Pallor
- Anxiety
- Nausea
- Diaphoresis
- Rapid pulse (tachycardia)
- Loss of consciousness
- Decreased blood pressure
- Dilatation of pupils

Treatment:

- Place patient in supine position, with feet slightly elevated
- Maintain airway
- Monitor vital signs
- Administer oxygen
- Place crushed ammonia carpule under nose
- Apply cold compress to face and neck
- Reassure and comfort patient

POSTURAL HYPOTENSION - ORTHOSTATIC HYPOTENSION (Syncope in Moving From the Supine to Upright Position)

Treatment:

- Place patient in supine position
- Maintain airway; check breathing
- Oxygen (as needed)
- Monitor vital signs
- Reposition patient slowly, after stable

DENTAL OFFICE EMERGENCIES (Continued)

AIRWAY OBSTRUCTION

Cause: Foreign body in larynx and pharynx

Symptoms:

- Choking
- Gagging
- Violent expiratory effort
- Substernal notch retraction
- Cyanosis
- Labored breathing
- Rapid pulse initially, then decreased pulse
- Cardiac arrest

Treatment:

- Place patient in supine position
- Tilt head backward
- Clear airway manually of debris (suction oral cavity)
- Check for respiratory sounds; ventilate if necessary
- Administer oxygen
- Perform Heimlich maneuver, if needed
- Place oropharyngeal or nasopharyngeal airway, if obstruction is visible, try to dislodge
- Perform cricothyrotomy, if unable to clear airway
- If foreign body passes, refer immediately for radiographic examination
- Child: Small child may be held upside down and four sharp blows delivered between shoulder blades

HYPERVENTILATION SYNDROME

Cause: Excessive loss of carbon dioxide, producing respiratory alkalosis

Symptoms:

- Rapid, shallow breathing
- Confusion
- Vertigo (dizziness)
- Paresthesia (numbness or tingling of extremities)
- Carpo-pedal spasm

Treatment:

- Position patient semi-reclining
- Calm and reassure patient vocally
- Instruct patient to breathe carbon dioxide enriched air through rebreathing bag
- Do **not** administer oxygen
- Administer medication to calm patient, if needed

BRONCHIAL ASTHMA

Cause: Spasm and constriction of the bronchi

Symptoms:

- Labored breathing
- Wheezing
- Anxiety
- Cyanosis

Treatment:

- Position patient semi-reclining
- Administer bronchodilator-mistometer
- Administer oxygen
- Administer parenteral medications:
  - Adult: I.M. epinephrine 1:1000 0.3 mL, repeat if necessary
  - Children: I.M. epinephrine 1:1000 0.1 mL, repeat if necessary
- I.V. medication optional:
  - Aminophylline: 250 mg (slowly)
  - Hydrocortisone sodium succinate: 100 mg

DRUG OVERDOSE

LOCAL ANESTHETIC

Cause: Drug overdose

> **Symptoms:** Excitement of central nervous system followed by depression

- Apprehension
- Anxiety
- Restlessness
- Confusion
- Tremors
- Rapid breathing
- Rapid heart rate

Treatment:

Mild Reaction:

- Administer oxygen, if needed
- Monitor vital signs
- Administer anticonvulsant drug, if needed (ie, Valium® - I.V.)
- Medical consult, if necessary

Severe Reaction:

- Place patient in supine position
- Suction mouth and throat
- Manage seizures
- Provide basic life support
- Monitor vital signs
- Administer anticonvulsant drug, if needed
- Manage postseizure depression

EPINEPHRINE OVERDOSE

Treatment:

- Position patient semi-reclining
- Monitor vital signs
- Administer oxygen, if necessary (except during hyperventilation syndrome)
- Reassure patient

SEDATIVE-HYPNOTIC OVERDOSE

Treatment:

- Place patient in supine position
- Maintain airway
- Monitor vital signs
- Administer oxygen and artificially ventilate, if necessary
- Administer Vasoxyl®, 20 mg I.V., for low blood pressure

NARCOTIC-ANALGESIC OVERDOSE

Treatment:

- Place patient in supine position
- Maintain airway
- Check ventilation
- Artificial ventilation and oxygen, as needed
- Administer Narcan® (naloxone) 0.4 mg I.M. or I.V.

DRUG REACTIONS - ALLERGY

URTICARIA OR PRURITUS

Cause: Allergy

> **Symptoms:**

- Urticaria: Red eruption of face, neck, hands, and arms

DENTAL OFFICE EMERGENCIES *(Continued)*

- Pruritus: Itching of above areas

Treatment:

Immediate:

- Administer epinephrine 0.3 mL of 1:1000 I.M. or I.V.
- Administer antihistamine
- Prescribe for oral antihistamine
- Withdraw drug in question

Delayed:

- Administer Benadryl® (diphenhydramine hydrochloride) 50 mg orally or I.M. every 6-8 hours
- If severe, administer Benadryl® 10-50 mg I.V. initially
- Withdraw drug in question

ANGIONEUROTIC EDEMA

Cause: Allergic reaction

Symptoms:

- Single localized sealing of lips, eyelids, cheeks, pharynx, and larynx
- Pruritus, urticaria, hoarseness, stridor, cyanosis

Treatment:

- Administer Benadryl® 10-50 mg I.M. or I.V.
- Administer epinephrine 0.2-0.5 mL, 1:1000 I.M. or S.C.
- Inject Solu-Cortef® 100 mg I.M. or Decadron® 4 mg I.V.
- Administer oxygen
- Give aminophylline 250 mg I.V., slowly
- Withdraw drug in question

ANAPHYLACTIC SHOCK

Cause: Allergic reaction

Symptoms:

- Progressive respiratory and circulatory failure
- Itching of nose and hands
- Flushed face
- Feeling of substernal depression
- Labored breathing, stridor
- Coughing
- Sudden hypotension
- Cyanosis
- Loss of consciousness
- Incontinence

Treatment:

- Place patient in supine position
- Clear airway
- Monitor vital signs
- Administer oxygen and ventilate manually, if necessary
- Administer aqueous epinephrine 1:1000, 0.2-0.5 mL I.M. or S.C. (Children: 0.125-0.25 mL I.V.)
- Give Decadron® 4 mg I.V., if necessary
- Start I.V. fluids (1000 mL or 500 mL of D_5W or Ringer's lactate)
- Give aminophylline 250 mg I.V. very slowly
- Apply tourniquet to injection site (if injection is in extremity)
- Transfer patient to hospital

SEIZURE DISORDERS

Cause:

- Intermittent disorder of nervous system caused by sudden discharge of cerebral neurons
- Idiosyncracy to drug

Symptoms:

- Excitement, tremor, followed by clonic-tonic convulsions

- Trance-like state

Treatment:

- Place patient on floor
- Loosen clothing and ensure safety of patient
- Maintain airway
- Administer Valium® 5-20 mg I.V. or Brevital® I.V. (Children: 5 mg I.V.) until cessation of seizure
- Be prepared for postseizure depression; support respiration

CEREBRAL VASCULAR ACCIDENTS

Cause: Obstruction of blood vessel of brain

Symptoms:

- Weakness
- Confusion
- Headache
- Dizziness
- Dysphagia
- Vital signs usually satisfactory
- Aphasia
- Nausea
- Paralysis
- Loss of consciousness

Treatment:

Transient Ischemic Attack

- Monitor vital signs
- Obtain medical consult with physician

CVA (Conscious Patient)

- Position patient semi-reclining
- Monitor vital signs
- Seek medical assistance

CVA (Unconscious Patient)

- Place patient in supine position
- Record vital signs
- Provide basic life support
- Transfer to hospital

RESPIRATORY ARREST

Cause:

- Respiratory obstruction
- Drug overdose
- Allergic reaction
- Cessation of breathing

Symptoms:

- Change in pattern of breathing to possible cessation of respirations
- Patient unable to breathe
- Cyanosis

Treatment:

- Place patient in supine position with firm back support
- Maintain airway
- Give oxygen and artificially ventilate
- Administer Narcan® 1 mL if due to narcotic depression
- Give CPR, if necessary
- Transfer to hospital

ANGINA PECTORIS

Cause:

- Insufficient blood supply to cardiac muscle

DENTAL OFFICE EMERGENCIES (*Continued*)

- May be precipitated by stress and anxiety

Symptoms:

- Pain in chest
- Vital signs satisfactory
- Patient history of angina; pain persists 3-5 minutes

Treatment:

- Position patient semi-reclining
- Administer oxygen
- Administer nitroglycerine 1/150 gr sublingually (may be repeated in 5 minutes)
- Reassure patient
- If history of angina or pain does not subside, suspect myocardial infarction

MYOCARDIAL INFARCTION

Cause: Occlusion of coronary vessels

Symptoms:

- Severe pain in chest which may radiate to neck, shoulder, and jaws
- Palpitations, tachycardia
- Dyspnea
- Cyanosis
- Diaphoresis
- Weakness
- Feeling of impending doom
- Pulse thready

Treatment:

- Position patient semi-reclining with firm back support
- Administer oxygen
- Reassure patient
- Inject morphine sulfate 10-15 mg I.M. or Demerol® 75-100 mg for pain
- Start I.V. fluids 1000 D₅W or Ringer's lactate
- Transfer to hospital

Management of Special Complications

- Arrhythmias: Do not administer drugs unless EKG is on site
- Sudden death: Administer CPR
- Transfer to hospital; accompany patient in ambulance

CARDIAC ARREST

A sudden emergency due to either actual standstill (asystole) or ventricular fibrillation with ineffective contractions; respiratory arrest may follow

Signs & symptoms:

- Collapse of blood pressure
- Dilated pupils
- Ashen skin
- No peripheral pulse
- Possible loss of respiration

* No heart sounds

Treatment: CPR

* Slap anterior left chest briskly, only if you witness the arrest
* Place patient in supine position with firm back support
* Make sure airway is open; suction mouth and pharynx; intubate, if necessary
* Closed chest cardiac massage 60/minute (CPR - adult)
* Give oxygen under positive pressure with AMBU resuscitator up to 8 L/minute
* If no AMBU or tracheal tube available, give 4 breaths (mouth to mouth); then start closed chest cardiac compression (60/minute)
* Start I.V. sodium bicarbonate I.V. 44.6 mEq (children: half the dose)
* Monitor EKG
* If in ventricular fibrillation: Defibrillate 200-400 watt/second (start at 200, if no result, move up to higher voltage)
* Keep patient warm
* Epinephrine 0.5 mL I.V. 1:1000 in 10 mL of saline
* Repeat sodium bicarbonate unless blood is pH normal
* May need other drugs (ie, $CaCl_2$, atropine, etc)

Transvenous pacemaker may be needed to reinitiate heartbeat
Possible open chest massage (very few indications and may not be any more effective than closed massage)

INSULIN SHOCK

Cause: Hypoglycemia or hyperinsulinism
Symptoms:

* Nervousness
* Confusion
* Profuse sweating
* Sudden onset
* Drooling from mouth
* Full and bounding pulse
* Convulsions
* Moist, pale skin
* Coma

Treatment:

* Administer oral sugar with orange juice
* If unconscious, administer 50% dextrose I.V.

DIABETIC ACIDOSIS

Cause: Hyperglycemia, insufficient insulin in the body to metabolize carbohydrates and fats, acidosis
Symptoms:

* Gradual onset
* Dry, flushed skin
* Dry mouth, intense thirst
* Exaggerated respirations (Kussmaul)
* Confusion
* Disoriented
* Stuporous
* Sweet breath
* Coma

Treatment:

* Call for medical assistance
* Position patient semi-reclining
* Maintain airway, administer oxygen
* Start I.V. and administer lactated Ringer's
* Keep warm
* Administer basic life support
* Transfer to hospital

DENTAL OFFICE EMERGENCIES *(Continued)*

ADRENAL INSUFFICIENCY

Cause: Insufficient corticosteroid output during a stimulus such as a stressful dental situation or infection

Symptoms:
- Weakness
- Pallor
- Cardiovascular attack
- Perspiration
- Thready, rapid pulse

Treatment:
- Administer oxygen
- Send for medical assistance
- Administer Decadron® 4 mg I.V. to adults, 1-4 mg I.V. to children

SUGGESTED READINGS

ANTIBIOTIC PROPHYLAXIS

See listing at the back of the chapter.

CANCER

American Cancer Society, *Cancer Facts and Figures* 1995, Atlanta, GA.

American Cancer Society, *Cancer Manual,* 8th ed, American Cancer Society, Boston, MA Division, 1990.

Barasch A, Gofa A, Krutchkoff DJ, et al, "Squamous Cell Carcinoma of the Gingiva. A Case Series Analysis," *Oral Surg Oral Med Oral Pathol Oral Radiol Endod,,* 1995, 80(2):183-7.

Carl W, "Oral Complications of Local and Systemic Cancer Treatment," *Curr Opin Oncol,* 1995, 7(4):320-4.

Chambers MS, Toth BB, Martin JW, et al, "Oral and Dental Management of the Cancer Patient: Prevention and Treatment of Complications," *Support Care Cancer,* 1995, 3(3):168-75.

Hobson RS and Clark JD, "Management of the Orthodontic Patient 'At Risk' From Infective Endocarditis," *Br Dent J,* 1995, 179(2):48.

Jullien JA, Downer MC, Zakrzewska JM, et al, "Evaluation of a Screening Test for the Early Detection of Oral Cancer and Precancer," *Community Dent Health,* 1995, 12(1):3-7.

Messer NC, Yant WR, and Archer RD, "Developing Provider Partnerships in the Detection of Oral Cancer and the Prevention of Smokeless Tobacco Use," *Md Med J,* 1995, 44(10):788-91.

National Institutes of Health, Consensus Development Conference on Oral Complications of Cancer Therapies: Diagnosis, Prevention, and Treatment. NCI Monograph No. 9 U.S. Public Health Service, Washington, DC: U.S. Government Printing Office, 1990.

National Institutes of Health, Consensus Development Conference on Oral Complications of Cancer Therapies: Diagnosis, Prevention, and Treatment. (Final Conference Statement and Recommendations), *J Am Dent Assoc,* 1989, 119(1):179-83.

Partridge M and Langdon JD, "Oral Cancer: A Serious and Growing Problem," *Ann R Coll Surg Engl,* 1995, 77(5):321-2.

Peterson DE and Sonis ST, eds, *Oral Complications of Cancer Chemotherapy,* Boston, MA: Martinus and Nijhoff, 1983.

Peterson DE, Elias EG, and Sonis ST, eds, *Head and Neck Management of the Cancer Patient,* Boston, MA: Martinus and Nijhoff Publishers, 1986.

Sandmann BJ, Sokol SA, and Buck GW, "Formulation and Stability of an Oral Mouthwash to Treat Symptoms of Mucositis," *Int Pharm Abstracts,* 1996, 33(1).

Shaffer J and Wexler LF, "Reducing Low-Density Lipoprotein Cholesterol Levels in an Ambulatory Care System. Results of Multidisciplinary Collaborative Practice Lipid Clinic Compared With Traditional Physician-Based Care," *Arch Int Med,* 1995, 155(21):2330-5.

Silverman S, *Oral Cancer,* 3rd ed, Atlanta, GA: American Cancer Society, 1990.

Takinami S, Yahata H, Kanoshima A, et al, "Hepatocellular Carcinoma Metastatic to the Mandible," *Oral Surg Oral Med Oral Pathol Oral Radiol Endod,* 1995, 79(5):649-54.

Vigneswaran N, Tilashalski K, Rodu B, et al, "Tobacco Use and Cancer. A Reappraisal," *Oral Surg Oral Med Oral Pathol Oral Radiol Endod,* 1995, 80(2):178-82.

SUGGESTED READINGS *(Continued)*

CARDIOVASCULAR

American Dental Association: *ADA Oral Health Care Guidelines: Patients With Cardiovascular Disease,* Chicago, IL: American Dental Association, 1989.

American Heart Association, *Textbook of Advanced Cardiac Life Support,* 2nd ed, American Heart Association, Dallas, TX, 1990.

Assael LA, "Acute Cardiac Care in Dental Practice," *Dent Clin N Am,* 1995, 39(3):555-65.

Dajani AS, Bisno AL, Chung KJ, et al, "Prevention of Bacterial Endocarditis. Recommendations by the American Heart Association," *JAMA,* 1990, 264(22):2919-22.

Giuliani ER, Gersh BJ, McGoon MD, et al, *Mayo Clinic Practice of Cardiology,* 3rd ed, St Louis, MO: Mosby-Year Book, Inc, 1996, 1698-814.

Gorgia H, et al, "Prevention of Tolerance to Hemodynamic Effects of Nitrates With Concomitant Use of Hydralazine in Patients With Chronic Heart Failure," *J Am Coll Cardiol,* 1995, 26(1):1575-80.

Grey AB, Stapleton JP, Evans MC, et al, "The Effect of the Anti-Estrogen Tamoxifen on Cardiovascular Risk Factors in Normal Postmenopausal Women," *J Clin Endocrinol Metab,* 1995, 80(11):3191-5.

Henning RJ and Grenvik A, *Critical Care Cardiology,* New York, NY: Churchill Livingston, 1989, 233.

Kerpen SJ, Kerpen HO, and Sachs SA, "Mitral Valve Prolapse: A Significant Cardiac Defect in the Development of Infective Endocarditis," *Spec Care Dentist,* 1984, 4(4):158-9.

McDonald CC, Alexander FE, Whyte BW, et al, "Cardiac and Vascular Morbidity in Women Receiving Adjuvant Tamoxifen for Breast Cancer in a Randomised Trial. The Scottish Cancer Trials Breast Group," *BMJ,* 1995, 311(7011):977-80.

Murgatroyd FD and Camm AJ, "Atrial Arrhythmias," *Lancet,* 1993, 341(8856):1317-22.

Naegeli B, Osswald S, Deola M, et al, "Intermittent Pacemaker Dysfunction Caused by Digital Mobile Telephones," *J Am Coll Cardiol,* 1996, 27(6):1471-7.

Pabor M, et al , "Risk of Gastrointestinal Haemorrhage With Calcium Antagonists in Hypertensive Persons Over 67 Years Old," *Lancet,* 1996, 347(20):1061-5.

Pieper SJ and Stanton MS, "Narrow QRS Complex Tachycardias," *Mayo Clin Proc,* 1995, 70(4):371-5.

Pritchett EL, "Management of Atrial Fibrillation," *N Engl J Med,* 1992, 326(19):1264-71.

Textbook of Advanced Cardiac Life Support, 2nd ed, Dallas, TX: American Heart Association, 1990.

The Fifth Report of the Joint National Committee on Detection, Evaluation, and Treatment of High Blood Pressure (JNC V), *Arch Intern Med,* 1993, 153(2):154-83.

Tierney LM, McPhee SJ, Papadakis MA, et al, *Current Medical Diagnosis and Treatment,* East Norwalk, CT: Appleton & Lange, 1993.

Williams GH, "Hypertensive Vascular Disease," *Harrison's Principles in Internal Medicine,* 13th ed, Isselbacher KJ, et al, eds, New York, NY: McGraw-Hill, 1994, 1116-31.

CHEMICAL DEPENDENCY AND SMOKING CESSATION

Abelin T, et al, "Controlled Trial of Transdermal Nicotine Patch in Tobacco Withdrawal," *Lancet,* 1989, 1(1):7-10.

Alterman AI, Droba M, Antelo RE, et al, "Amantadine May Facilitate Detoxification of Cocaine Addicts," *Drug Alcohol Depend,* 1992, 31(1):19-29.

Benowitz NL, Porchet H, Sheiner L, et al, "Nicotine Absorption and Cardiovascular Effects With Smokeless Tobacco Use: Comparison With Cigarettes and Nicotine Gum," *Clin Pharmacol Ther,* 1988, 44(1):23-8.

Buchkremer G, Bents H, Horstmann M, et al, "Combination of Behavioral Smoking Cessation and Transdermal Nicotine Substitution," *Addict Behav,* 1989, 14(2):229-38.

Ciancio SG, ed, *ADA Guide to Dental Therapeutics,* 1st ed, Chicago, IL: ADA Publishing Co, 1998.

Cowan FF, "Dentists Prescribe Nicotine Substitutes, in Just the Right Dose," *AGD Impact,* 1993, 12(2):11.

Daughton DM, Heatley SA, Prendergast JJ, et al, "Effect of Transdermal Nicotine Delivery as an Adjunct to Low-Intervention Smoking Cessation Therapy," *Arch Int Med,* 1991, 151(4):749-52.

DSM IV, *Diagnostic and Statistical Manual of Mental Disorders,* 4th ed, Washington DC: American Psychiatric Association, 1994.

Fagerstrom KO, "Measuring Degree of Physical Dependence to Tobacco Smoking With Reference to Individualization of Treatment," *Addict Behav,* 1978, 3(3-4):235-41.

Fiester S, Goldstein M, Resnick M, et al, "Practice Guideline for the Treatment of Patients With Nicotine Dependence," *Am J Psych,* 1996, 15(10):Supplement 31.

Gariti P, Auriacombe M, Incmikoski R, et al, "A Randomized Double-Blind Study of Neuroelectric Therapy in Opiate and Cocaine Detoxification," *J Subst Abuse,* 1992, 4(3):299-308.

Henningfield JE, "Nicotine Medications for Smoking Cessation," *N Engl J Med,* 1995, 333(18):1196-203.

Herkenham MA, "Localization of Cannabinoid Receptors in Brain: Relationship to Motor and Reward Systems," *Biological Basis of Substance Abuse,* Korenman SG and Barchas JD, eds, New York, NY: Oxford University Press, 1993, 187-200.

Higgins ST, Budney AJ, Bickel WK, et al, "Outpatient Behavioral Treatment for Cocaine Dependence: One-Year Outcome," Problems of Drug Dependence Symposium, College. 1994.

Hurt RD, Finlayson RE, Morse RM, et al, "Nicotine-Replacement Therapy With Use of a Transdermal Nicotine Patch - A Randomized Double-Blind Placebo Controlled Trial," *Mayo Clin Proc,* 1990, 65(12):1529-37.

Kreek MJ, "Rationale for Maintenance Pharmacotherapy of Opiate Dependence," O'Brien CP and Barchas JD, eds, *Addictive States,* New York, NY: Raven Press, 1992, 205-30.

Krumpe P, "Efficacy of Transdermal Nicotine Administration as an Adjunct for Smoking Cessation in Heavily Nicotine Addicted Smokers," *Am Rev Respir Dis,* 1989, 139(1):A377.

Leshnitz AI, "Molecular Mechanisms of Cocaine Addiction," *N Engl J Med,* 1996, 335(2):128-9.

Li Wan Po A, "Transdermal Nicotine in Smoking Cessation: A Meta-analysis" *Eur J Clin Pharmacol,* 1993, 45(6):519-28.

Mendelson JH and Mello NK, "Management of Cocaine Abuse and Dependence," *N Engl J Med,* 1996, 334(15):965-72.

Mulligan SC, Masterson JG, Devane JG, et al, "Clinical and Pharmacokinetic Properties of a Transdermal Nicotine Patch," *Clin Pharmacol Ther,* 1990, 47(3):331-7.

Nowak R, "Nicotine Scrutinized as FDA Seeks to Regulate Cigarettes," *Science,* 1994, 263(5153):1555-6.

SUGGESTED READINGS *(Continued)*

O'Brien CP, "Drug Addiction and Drug Abuse," *The Pharmacological Basis of Therapeutics,* 9th ed, Molinoff PB and Ruddon R, eds, New York, NY: McGraw-Hill, 1996, 557-77.

O'Brien CP, "Treatment of Alcoholism as a Chronic Disorder," *Toward a Molecular Basis of Alcohol Use and Abuse,* Jansson B, Jornvall H, Rydberg U, et al, eds, Basel, Switzerland: Birkhauser Verlag, 1994, Vol 71, EXS, 349-59.

Ostrowski DJ and DeNelsky GY, "Pharmacologic Management of Patients Using Smoking Cessation Aids," *Dental Clin North Am,* 1996, 40(3):779-801.

Rose JE, Levin ED, Behm FM, et al, "Transdermal Nicotine Facilitates Smoking Cessation," *Clin Pharmacol Ther,* 1990, 47(3):323-30.

Sachs DPL, et al, "Effectiveness of a 16-Hour Transdermal Nicotine Patch in a Medical Practice Setting Without Intensive Group Counseling," *Arch Intern Med,* 1993, 153(1):1881-90.

Schneider NG, Olmstead R, Nilsson F, et al, "Efficacy of a Nicotine Inhaler in Smoking Cessation: A Double-Blind, Placebo-Controlled Trial," *Addiction,* 1996, 91(9):1293-306.

Self DW, Barnhart WJ, Lehman DA, et al, "Opposite Modulation of Cocaine-Seeking Behavior by D1- and D2-Like Dopamine Receptor Agonists," *Science,* 1996, 271(5255):1586-9.

The Smoking Cessation Clinical Practice Guideline Panel and Staff, The Agency for Health Care Policy and Research Smoking Cessation Clinical Practice Guideline, *JAMA,* 1996, 275(1):1270-80.

Tonnesen P, Norregaard J, Simonsen K, et al, "A Double-Blind Trial of a 16-Hour Transdermal Nicotine Patch in Smoking Cessation," *N Engl J Med,* 1991, 325(5):311-5.

Transdermal Nicotine Group, "Transdermal Nicotine for Smoking Cessation. Six-Month Results From Two Multicenter Controlled Clinical Trials," *JAMA,* 1991, 266(22):3133-8.

DIAGNOSIS AND MANAGEMENT OF PAIN

Beckett D, "Topical Guanethidine Relieves Dental Hypersensitivity and Pain," *J R Soc Med,* 1995, 88(1):60.

Berthold CW, Schneider A, and Dionne RA, "Using Triazolam to Reduce Dental Anxiety," *J Am Dent Assoc,* 1993, 124(11):58-64.

Brown RS, Hinderstein B, Reynolds DC, et al, "Using Anesthetic Localization to Diagnose Oral and Dental Pain," *J Am Dent Assoc,* 1995, 126(5):633-4, 637-41.

Coderre TJ, Katz J, Vaccarino AL, et al, "Contribution of Central Neuroplasticity to Pathological Pain: Review of Clinical and Experimental Evidence," *Pain,* 1993, 52(3):259-85.

Delcanho RE and Graff-Radford SB, "Chronic Paroxysmal Hemicrania Presenting as Toothache," *J Orofacial Pain,* 1993, 7:300.

Denson DD and Katz JA, "Nonsteroidal Anti-inflammatory Agents," *Practical Management of Pain,* 2nd ed, PP Raj, ed, St Louis, MO: Mosby Year Book, 1992.

Forbes JA, Butterworth GA, Burchfield WH, et al, "Evaluation of Ketorolac, Aspirin, and an Acetaminophen-Codeine Combination in Postoperative Oral Surgery Pain," *Pharmacotherapy,* 1990, 10(6 Pt 2):77S-93S.

Graff-Radford SB, "Headache Problems That Can Present as Toothache," *Dent Clin North Am,* 1991, 35(1):155-70.

Harvey M and Elliott M, "Transcutaneous Electrical Nerve Stimulation (TENS) for Pain Management During Cavity Preparations in Pediatric Patients," *ASDC J Dent Child,* 1995, 62(1):49-51.

Henry G, "Postoperative Pain Experience With Flurbiprofen and Acetaminophen With Codeine," *J Dent Res*, 1992, 71:952.

Jaffe JH and Martin WR, "Opioid Analgesic and Antagonists," *The Pharmacological Basis of Therapeutics*, 8th ed, Gilman AG, Rall TW, Nies AD, et al, eds, New York, NY: Maxwell Pergamon MacMillan Publishing, 1990.

Kalso E and Vainio A, "Morphine and Oxycodone Hydrochloride in the Management of Cancer Pain," *Clin Pharmacol Ther*, 1990, 47(5):639-46.

Lee AG, "A Case Report. Jaw Claudication: A Sign of Giant Cell Arteritis," *J Am Dent Assoc*, 1995, 126(7):1028-9.

McQuay H, Carroll D, Jadad AR, et al, "Anticonvulsant Drugs for Management of Pain: A Systemic Review," *BMJ*, 1995, 311(7012):1047-52.

Olin BR, Hebel SK, Connell SI, et al, *Drug Facts and Comparisons*, 1993, St Louis, MO: Facts and Comparisons, Inc.

Pendeville PE, Van Boven MJ, Contreras V, et al, "Ketorolac Tromethamine for Postoperative Analgesia in Oral Surgery," *Acta Anaesthesiol Belg*, 1995, 46(1):25-30.

Robertson S, Goodell H, and Wolff HG, "The Teeth as a Source of Headache and Other Pain," *Arch Neurol Psychiatry*, 1947, 57:277.

Sandler NA, Ziccardi V, and Ochs M, "Differential Diagnosis of Jaw Pain in the Elderly," *J Am Dent Assoc* 1995, 126(9):1263-72.

Scully C, Eveson JW, and Porter SR, "Munchausen's Syndrome: Oral Presentations," *Br Dent J*, 1995, 178(2):65-7.

Seng GF, Kraus K, Cartwright G, et al, "Confirmed Allergic Reactions to Amide Local Anesthetics," *Gen Dent*, 1996, 44(1):52-4.

Ship JA, Grushka M, Lipton JA, et al, "Burning Mouth Syndrome: An Update" *J Am Dent Assoc*, 1995, 126(7):842-53.

Wright EF and Schiffman EL, "Treatment Alternatives for Patients With Masticatory Myofascial Pain," *J Am Dent Assoc*, 1995, 126(7):1030-9.

HIV INFECTION AND AIDS

Borrow P, Lewicki H, Hahn BH, et al, "Virus-Specific CD8+ Cytotoxic T-Lymphocyte Activity Associated With Control of Viremia in Primary Human Immunodeficiency Virus Type I Infection," *J Virol*, 1994, 68(9):6103-9.

Brookmeyer R and Gail MH, "AIDS Epidemiology: A Quantitative Approach," New York, NY: Oxford Press, 1994.

Center for Disease Control (CDC), CfDC. "Update: AIDS Cases in Males Who Have Sex With Males," *MMWR Morb Mortal Wkly Rep*, 1995, 44(29):401-2.

Center for Disease Control (CDC), CfDC. "First 500,000 AIDS Cases," *MMWR Morb Mortal Wkly Rep*, 1995, 44(46):849-53.

Center for Disease Control (CDC), CfDC. "Update: HIV Exposures in HCWs," *MMWR Morb Mortal Wkly Rep*, 1995, 44(50):929.

Center for Disease Control (CDC), CfDCaP. "Recommended Infection-Control Practices for Dentistry," *MMWR Morb Mortal Wkly Rep*, 1993, 42(RR-8).

Center for Disease Control (CDC), CfDCaP. "Revised Classification System for HIV Infection and Expanded Surveillance Case Definition for AIDS Among Adolescents and Adults," *MMWR Morb Mortal Wkly Rep*, 1993, 41(RR-17).

Council on Dental Materials I, and Equipment, Therapeutics CoD, Research CoD, Practice CoD, "Infection Control Recommendations for the Dental Office and the Dental Laboratory," *J Am Dent Assoc*, 1992, 123(8).

El-Sadr W, Oleske JM, Agins BD, et al, "Evaluation and Management of Early HIV Infection," Agency for Health Care Policy and Research, Public Health Service, US Department of Health and Human Services, 1994

SUGGESTED READINGS *(Continued)*

Clinical Practice Guideline No. 7, ACHPR Publication No. 94-0572, Rockville, MD.

Glick M, *Dental Management of Patients With HIV*, Chicago, IL: Quintessence Publishing Co, 1994.

Glick M and Silverman S, "Dental Management of HIV-Infected Patients," *J Am Dent Assoc* (Supplement to Reviewers), 1995.

Glick M, *Clinicians Guide to Treatment of HIV-Infected Patients*, Academy of Oral Medicine, 1996.

Greenspan D, Greenspan JS, Schiodt M, et al, *AIDS and the Mouth*, Munksgaard, Copenhagen, 1990.

Greenspan JS and Greenspan D, "Oral Manifestations of HIV Infection," *The Proceedings of the Second International Workshop*, Chicago, IL: Quintessence Publishing Co, 1995.

"Oral Health Care for Adults With HIV Infection," New York, NY: AIDS Institute, New York State Department of Health, 1993.

Little JW, Melnick SL, Rhame FS, et al, "Prevalence of Oral Lesions in Symptomatic and Asymptomatic HIV Patients," *Gen Dent*, 1994, 42(5):446-50.

Silverman S, *Color Atlas of Oral Manifestations of AIDS*, 2nd ed, St Louis, MO: Mosby, 1996.

Travers K, Souleymane M, Mrlink R, et al, "Natural Protection Against HIV-1 Provided by HIV-2," *Science*, 1995, 268(5219):1833.

Weiss R, "The Virus and Its Target Cells," Broder S, Merigan T, Bolognesis D, eds, *Textbook of AIDS Medicine*, Baltimore, MD: Williams & Wilkins, 1994.

Zeitlin S and Shaha A, "Parotid Manifestations of HIV Infection," *J Surg Oncol*, 1991, 47(4):230-2.

NATURAL PRODUCTS, HERBALS, AND DIETARY SUPPLEMENTS

1995 Martindale - The Extra Pharmacopoeia, Vol 86, Roy Pharm Soc, GB, 1996.

Castleman M, *The Healing Herbs: The Ultimate Guide to the Curative Power of Nature's Medicines*, Rodale Press, Emmaus, 1991.

Lust J, *The Herb Book*, New York, NY: Benedict Lust Publications, 1974.

Mistry MG and Mays DA, "Precautions Against Global Use of Natural Products for Weight Loss: A Review of Active Ingredients and Issues Concerning Concomitant Disease States," *Therapeutic Perspectives*, 1996, 10(1):2.

Murray M and Pizzorno J, *Encyclopedia of Natural Medicine*, Prima Publishing, 1991.

Olin BR, Hebel SK, Connell SI, et al, *Drug Facts and Comparisons*, St Louis, MO: Facts and Comparisons, Inc, 1993.

Polunin M and Robbins C, *The Natural Pharmacy*, New York, NY: MacMillan Publishing, 1992.

Tyler VF, *The Honest Herbal: A Sensible Guide to the Use of Herbs and Related Remedies*, Birmingham, AL: The Hawthorn Press, Inc, 1993.

ORAL INFECTIONS

Baron EJ and Finegold SM, eds, "Gram-Negative Cocci (*Neisseria* and *Branhamella*)," Bailey and Scott's Diagnostic Microbiology, St Louis, MO: Mosby Year Book, 1990.

Borssen E and Sundquist G, "Actinomycosis of Infected Dental Root Canals," *Oral Surg Oral Med Oral Pathol*, 1981, 51(1):643-7.

1993 Sexually Transmitted Diseases Treatment Guidelines, Centers for Disease Control and Prevention, *MMWR Morb Mortal Wkly Rep,* 1993, 42(RR-14):1-102.

Chow AW, "Infections of the Oral Cavity, Neck, and Head," *Principles and Practice of Infectious Diseases,* 4th ed, Mandell GL, Bennett JE, Dolin R, eds, New York, NY: Churchill Livingstone, 1995, 593-605.

Crockett DN, O'Grady JF, and Reade PC, "*Candida* Species and *Candida albicans* Morphotypes in Erythematous Candidiasis, "*Oral Surg Oral Med Oral Pathol,* 1992, 73(5):559-63.

Dajani A, Taubert K, Ferrieri P, et al, "Treatment of Acute Streptococcal Pharyngitis and Prevention of Rheumatic Fever: A Statement for Health Professionals," *Pediatrics,* 1995, 96(4):758-64.

Diz Dios P, Ocampo Hermida A, Miralles Alvarez C, et al, "Fluconazole-Resistant Oral Candidiasis in HIV-Infected Patients," *AIDS,* 1995, 9(7):809-10.

Dobson RL, "Antimicrobial Therapy for Cutaneous Infections," *J Am Acad Dermatol,* 1990, 22(5):871-3.

Ferris DG, Litaker MS, Woodward L, et al, "Treatment of Bacterial Vaginosis: A Comparison of Oral Metronidazole, Metronidazole Vaginal Gel, and Clindamycin Vaginal Cream," *J Fam Pract,* 1995, 41(5):443-9.

Fox RI, Luppi M, Kang HI, et al, "Reactivation of Epstein-Barr Virus in Sjögren's Syndrome," *Springer Semin Immunopathol,* 1991, 13(2):217-31.

Giunta JL and Fiumara NJ, "Facts About Gonorrhea and Dentistry," *Oral Surg Oral Med Oral Pathol,* 1986, 62(5):529-31.

Goldberg MH and Topazian R, "Odontogenic Infections and Deep Facial Space Infections of Dental Origin," *Oral and Maxillofacial Infections,* 3rd ed, Philadelphia, PA: WB Saunders, 1994, 232-6.

Goulden V and Goodfield MJ, "Treatment of Childhood Dermatophyte Infections With Oral Terbinafine," *Pediatr Dermatol,* 1995, 12(1):53-4.

"Cefadroxil in the Management of Facial Cellulitis of Odontogenic Origin," *Oral Surg Oral Med Oral Pathol,* 1991, 71(4):496-8.

Hook EW 3d and Marra CM, "Acquired Syphilis in Adults," *N Engl J Med,* 1992, 326(16):1060-9.

Larsen PE, "Alveolar Osteitis After Surgical Removal of Impacted Mandibular Third Molars. Identification of the Patient at Risk," *Oral Surg Oral Med Oral Pathol,* 1992, 73(4):393-7.

Lewis MA, Parkhurst CL, Douglas CW, et al, "Prevalence of Penicillin Resistant Bacteria in Acute Suppurative Oral Infection," *J Antimicrob Chemother,* 1995, 35(6):785-91.

Musher DM, Hamill RJ, and Baughn RE, "Effect of Human Immunodeficiency Virus (HIV) Infection on the Course of Syphilis and on the Response to Treatment," *Ann Intern Med,* 1990, 113(11):872-81.

Muzyka BC and Glick M, "A Review of Oral Fungal Infections and Appropriate Therapy," *J Am Dent Assoc,* 1995, 126(1):63-72.

Namavar F, Roosendaal R, Kuipers EJ, et al, "Presence of *Helicobacter pylori* in the Oral Cavity, Oesophagus, Stomach and Faeces of Patients With Gastritis," *Eur J Clin Microbiol Infect Dis* 1995, 14(4):234-7.

Nguyen AM, el-Zaatari FA, and Graham DY, "*Helicobacter pylori* in the Oral Cavity. A Critical Review of the Literature," *Oral Surg Oral Med Oral Pathol Oral Radiol Endod,* 1995, 79(6):705-9.

Pogrel MA, "Complications of Third Molar Surgery," *J Oral Maxillofac Surg,* 1990, 2(1):441-8.

Schiodt M, "HIV-Associated Salivary Gland Disease: A Review," *Oral Surg Oral Med Oral Pathol,* 1992, 73(2):164-7.

SUGGESTED READINGS (Continued)

Sjögren U, Figdor L, Spangberg, et al, "The Antimicrobial Effect of Calcium Hydroxide as a Short-Term Intracanal Dressing," *Int Endod,* 1991, 24(3):119-24.

Talal N, Dauphinee MJ, Dang H, et al, "Detection of Serum Antibodies to Retroviral Proteins in Patients With Primary Sjögren's Syndrome (Autoimmune Exocrinopathy)," *Arthritis Rheum,* 1990, 33(6):774-81.

Torabinejad M, Kettering JD, McGraw JC, et al, "Factors Associated With Endodontic Interappointment Emergencies of Teeth With Necrotic Pulps," *J Endod,* 1988, 14(5):261-6.

Walton R and Fouad A, "Endodontic Interappointment Flare-Ups: A Prospective Study of Incidence and Related Factors," *J Endod,* 1992, 18(4):172-7.

Wheeler TT, Alberts MA, Dolan TA, et al, "Dental, Visual, Auditory and Olfactory Complications in Paget's Disease of Bone," *J Am Geriatr Soc,* 1995, 43(12):1384-91.

Williams JW Jr, Holleman DR Jr, Samsa GP, et al, "Randomized Controlled Trial of 3 vs 10 Days of Trimethoprim/Sulfamethoxazole for Acute Maxillary Sinusitis," *JAMA,* 1995, 273(13):1015-21.

Wormser GP, "Lyme Disease: Insights Into the Use of Antimicrobials for Prevention and Treatment in the Context of Experience With Other Spirochetal Infections," *Mt Sinai J Med,* 1995, 62(3):188-95.

ORAL LEUKOPLAKIA

Barker JN, Mitra RS, Griffiths CE, et al, "Keratinocytes as Initiators of Inflammation," *Lancet,* 1991, 337(8735):211-4.

Belton CM and Eversole LR, "Oral Hairy Leukoplakia: Ultrastructural Features," *J Oral Pathol,* 1986, 15(9):493-9.

Boehncke WH, Kellner I, Konter U, et al, "Differential Expression of Adhesion Molecules on Infiltrating Cells in Inflammatory Dermatoses," *J Am Acad Dermatol,* 1992, 26(6):907-13.

Chou MJ and Daniels TE, "Langerhans Cells Expressing HLA-DQ, HLA-DR, and T6 Antigens in Normal Oral Mucosa and Lichen Planus," *J Oral Pathol Med,* 1989, 18(10):573-6.

Corso B, Eversole LR, and Hutt-Fletcher L, "Hairy Leukoplakia: Epstein-Barr Virus Receptors on Oral Keratinocyte Plasma Membranes," *Oral Surg Oral Med Oral Pathol,* 1989, 67(4):416-21.

Eisen D, Ellis CN, Duell EA, et al, "Effect of Topical Cyclosporine Rinse on Oral Lichen Planus. A Double-Blind Analysis," *N Engl J Med,* 1990, 323(5):290-4.

Greenspan D, Greenspan JS, Overby G, et al, "Risk Factors for Rapid Progression From Hairy Leukoplakia to AIDS: A Nested Case-Control Study, *J Acquir Immune Defic Syndr,* 1991, 4(7):652-8.

Regezi JA, Stewart JC, Lloyd RV, et al, "Immunohistochemical Staining of Langerhans Cells and Macrophages in Oral Lichen Planus," *Oral Surg Oral Med Oral Pathol,* 1985, 60(4):396-402.

Sciubba JJ, "Oral Leukoplakia," *Crit Rev Oral Biol Med,* 1995, 6(2):147-60.

ORAL SOFT TISSUE DISEASES

Anhalt GJ, "Pemphigoid: Bullous and Cicatricial," *Dermatol Clin,* 1990, 8(4):701-16.

Berk MA and Lorincz AL, "The Treatment of Bullous Pemphigoid With Tetracycline and Niacinamide. A Preliminary Report," *Arch Dermatol,* 1986, 122(6):670-4.

Den Besten P and Giambro N, "Treatment of Fluorosed and White-Spot Human Enamel With Calcium Sucrose Phosphate *in vitro,*"*Pediatr Dent* 1995, 17(5):340-5.

Firth NA and Reade PC, "Angiotensin-Converting Enzyme Inhibitors Implicated in Oral Mucosal Lichenoid Reactions," *Oral Surg Oral Med Oral Pathol,* 1989, 67(1):41-4.

Fritz KA and Weston WL, "Topical Glucocorticosteroids," *Ann Allergy,* 1983, 50(2):68-76.

Gallant C and Kenny P, "Oral Glucocorticoids and Their Complications. A Review," *J Am Acad Dermatol,* 1986, 14(2):161-77.

Goupil MT, "Occupational Health and Safety Emergencies," *Dent Clin North Am,* 1995, 39(3):637-47.

Grady D, Ernster VL, Stillman L, et al, "Smokeless Tobacco Use Prevents Aphthous Stomatitis," *Oral Surg Oral Med Oral Pathol,* 1992, 74(4):463-5.

Hamuryudan V, Yurdakul S, Serdaroglu S, et al, "Topical Alpha Interferon in the Treatment of Oral Ulcers in Behcet's Syndrome: A Preliminary Report," *Clin Exp Rheumatol,* 1990, 8(1):51-4.

Hoover CI, Olson JA, and Greenspan JS, "Humoral Responses and Cross-Reactivity to Viridans Streptococci in Recurrent Aphthous Ulceration," *J Dent Res,* 1986, 65(8):1101-4.

Jungell P, "Oral Lichen Planus: A Review," *Int J Oral Maxillofac Surg,* 1991, 20(3):129-35.

Lindemann RA, Riviere GR, and Sapp JP, "Oral Mucosal Antigen Reactivity During Exacerbation and Remission Phases of Recurrent Aphthous Ulceration," *Oral Surg Oral Med Oral Pathol,* 1985, 60(3):281-4.

MacPhail LA, Greenspan D, Greenspan JS, et al, "Recurrent Aphthous Ulcers in Association With HIV Infection. Diagnosis and Treatment," *Oral Surg Oral Med Oral Pathol,* 1992, 73(3):283-8.

Meiller TF, Kutcher MJ, Overholser CD, et al, "Effect of an Antimicrobial Mouthrinse on Recurrent Aphthous Ulcerations," *Oral Surg Oral Med Oral Pathol,* 1991, 72(4):425-9.

Moncarz V, Ulmansky M, and Lustmann J, "Lichen Planus: Exploring Its Malignant Potential," *J Am Dent Assoc,* 1993, 124(3):102-8.

Pederson A, Klausen B, Hougen P, et al, "T-Lymphocyte Subsets in Recurrent Aphthous Ulceration," *J Oral Pathol Med,* 1989, 18(1):59-60.

Porter SR, Scully C, and Flint S, "Hematological Status in Recurrent Aphthous Stomatitis Compared With Other Oral Disease," *Oral Surg Oral Med Oral Pathol,* 1988, 66(1):41-4.

Porter SR, Scully C, and Midda M, "Adult Linear Immunoglobulin, A Disease Manifesting as Desquamative Gingivitis," *Oral Surg Oral Med Oral Pathol,* 1990, 70(4):450-3.

Rodu B and Mattingly G, "Oral Mucosal Ulcers: Diagnosis and Management," *J Am Dent Assoc,* 1992, 123(10):83-6.

Rothman KJ, "Teratogenicity of High Vitamin A Intake," *N Engl J Med,* 1995, 333(21):1414-5.

Savage NW, "Oral Ulceration. Assessment of Treatment of Commonly Encountered Oral Ulcerative Disease," *Aust Fam Physician,* 1988, 17(4):247-50.

Schiodt M, Holmstrup P, Dabelsteen E, et al, "Deposits of Immunoglobulins, Complement, and Fibrinogen in Oral Lupus Erythematosus, Lichen Planus, and Leukoplakia," *Oral Surg Oral Med Oral Pathol,* 1981, 51(6):603-8.

Scully C and Porter S, "Recurrent Aphthous Stomatitis: Current Concepts of Etiology, Pathogenesis, and Management," *J Oral Pathol Med,* 1989, 18(1):21-7.

Shiohara T, Moriya N, Mochizuki T, et al, "Lichenoid Tissue Reaction (LTR) Induced by Local Transfer of Ia-Reactive T-cell Clones: LTR by Epidermal Invasion of Cytotoxic Lymphokine-Producing Autoreactive T Cells," *J Invest Dermatol,* 1987, 89(1):8-14.

SUGGESTED READINGS *(Continued)*

Shohat-Zabarski R, Kalderon S, Klein T, et al, "Close Association of HLA-B51 in Persons With Recurrent Aphthous Stomatitis," *Oral Surg Oral Med Oral Pathol,* 1992, 74(4):455-8.

Van Dis ML and Vincent SD, "Diagnosis and Management of Autoimmune and Idiopathic Mucosal Diseases," *Dent Clin North Am,* 1992, 36(4):897-917.

Vincent SD and Lilly GE, "Clinical, Historic, and Therapeutic Features of Aphthous Stomatitis. Literature Review and Open Clinical Trial Employing Steroids," *Oral Surg, Oral Med, Oral Pathol,* 1992, 74(1):79-86.

ORAL VIRAL DISEASES

Ades AE, Peckham CS, Dale GE, et al, "Prevalence of Antibodies to Herpes Simplex Virus Types 1 and 2 in Pregnant Women, and Estimated Rates of Infection," *J Epidemiol Community Health,* 1989, 43(1):53-60.

Amsterdam JD, Maislin G, and Rybakowski J, "A Possible Antiviral Action of Lithium Carbonate in Herpes Simplex Virus Infections," *Biol Psychiatry,* 1990, 27(4):447-53.

Balfour HH, Rotbart HA, Feldman S, et al, "Acyclovir Treatment of Varicella in Otherwise Healthy Adolescents. The Collaborative Acyclovir Varicella Study Group," *J Pediatr,* 1992, 120(4):627-33.

Carey WD and Patel G, "Viral Hepatitis in the 1990s, Part III, Hepatitis C, Hepatitis E, and Other Viruses," *Cleve Clin J Med,* 1992, 59(6):595-601.

Chang Y, et al, "Identification of Herpesvirus-Like DNA Sequences in AIDS-Associated Kaposi's Sarcoma," *Science,* 1994, 266(5192):1865-9.

Corey L and Spear PG, "Infections With Herpes Simplex Viruses," *N Engl J Med,* 1986, 314(11):686-91, 749-57.

Dolin R, "Antiviral Chemotherapy and Chemoprophylaxis," *Science,* 1985, 227(4692):1296-303.

Ficarra G and Shillitoe EJ, "HIV-Related Infections of the Oral Cavity," *Oral Biol Med,* 1992, 3(3):207-31.

Fiddian AP and Ivanyi L, "Topical Acyclovir in the Management of Recurrent *Herpes labialis,*" *Br J Dermatol* 1983, 109(3):321-6.

Gupta S, Govindarajan S, Cassidy WM, et al, "Acute Delta Hepatitis: Sero-logical Diagnosis With Particular Reference to Hepatitis Delta Virus RNA," *Am J Gastroenterol,* 1991, 86(9):1227-31.

Huff JC, Bean B, Balfour HH Jr, et al, "Therapy of Herpes Zoster With Oral Acyclovir ," *Am J Med,* 1988, 85(2A):84-9.

Johnson RJ, Gretch DR, and Yamabe H, "Membranoproliferative Glomerulo-nephritis Associated With Hepatitis C Virus Infection," *N Engl J Med,* 1993, 328(7):505-6.

Markowitz M, et al, "A Preliminary Study of Ritonavir, an Inhibitor of HIV-1 Protease, to Treat HIV-1 Infection," *N Engl J Med,* 1995, 333(23):1534-9.

McCreary C, Bergin C, Pilkington R, et al, "Clinical Parameters Associated With Recalcitrant Oral Candidiasis in HIV Infection: A Preliminary Study," *Int J STD AIDS,* 1995, 6(3):204-7.

Robinson WS, "Hepatitis B Virus and Hepatitis D Virus," *Principles and Practice of Infectious Disease,* 4th ed, 1995, New York, NY: Churchill Livingstone. 1995.

Roizman B and Sears AE, "An Inquiry Into the Mechanisms of Herpes Simplex Virus Latency," *Annu Rev in Microbiol,* 1987, 41:543-71.

Rooney JF, Bryson Y, Mannix ML, et al, "Prevention of Ultraviolet Light-Induced *Herpes labialis* by Sunscreen," *Lancet* 1991, 338(8780):1419-22.

Snijders PJ, Schulten EA, Mullink H, et al, "Detection of Human Papillomavirus and Epstein-Barr Virus DNA Sequences in Oral Mucosa of HIV-Infected

Patients by the Polymerase Chain Reaction," *Am J Pathol,* 1990, 137(3):659-66.

Spruance SL, Stewart JC, Rowe NH, et al, "Treatment of Recurrent Herpes Simplex Labialis With Oral Acyclovir," *J Infect Dis,* 1990, 161(2):185-90.

Whitley RJ, Soong SJ, Dolin R, et al, "Early Vidarabine Therapy to Control the Complications of Herpes Zoster in Immunosuppressed Patients," *N Engl J Med,* 1982, 307(16):971-5.

PERIODONTOLOGY

Barak S, Engelberg IS, and Hiss J, "Gingival Hyperplasia Caused by Nifedipine. Histopathologic Findings," *J Periodontol,* 1987, 58(9):639-42.

Carson HG and Rainone AD, "Occult Periodontal Disease With Heat Sensitivity: A Different Diagnostic Problem," *Gen Dent,* 1992, 23(3):191-5.

Checchi L, Trombelli L, and Nonato M, "Postoperative Infections and Tetracycline Prophylaxis in Periodontal Surgery: A Retrospective Study," *Quintessence Int,* 1992, 23(3):191-5.

Creath CJ, Steinmetz S, and Roebuck R, "A Case Report. Gingival Swelling Due to a Fingernail-Biting Habit," *J Am Dent Assoc,* 1995, 126(7):1019-21.

Crow HC and Ship JA, "Are Gingival and Periodontal Conditions Related to Salivary Gland Flow Rates in Healthy Individuals?" *J Am Dent Assoc,* 1995, 126(11):1514-20.

Dens F, Boute P, Otten J, et al, "Dental Caries, Gingival Health, and Oral Hygiene of Long-Term Survivors of Paediatric Malignant Diseases," *Arch Dis Child,* 1995, 72(2):129-32.

Harel-Raviv M, Ekler M, Lalani K, et al, "Nifedipine-Induced Gingival Hyperplasia. A Comprehensive Review and Analysis," *Oral Surg Oral Med Oral Pathol,* 1995, 79(6):715-22.

Holt RD, Wilson M, and Musa S, "Mycoplasmas in Plaque and Saliva of Children and Their Relationship to Gingivitis," *J Periodontol,* 1995, 66(2):97-101.

Lareau DE, Herzberg MC, and Nelson RD, "Human Neutrophil Migration Under Agarose to Bacteria Associated With the Development of Gingivitis," *J Periodontol,* 1984, 55(9):540-9.

Listgarten MA, "Pathogenesis of Periodontitis," *J Clin Periodontol,* 1986, 13(5):418-30.

Listgarten MA, Lindhe J, and Hellden L, "Effect of Tetracycline and/or Scaling on Human Periodontal Disease. Clinical, Microbiological, and Histological Observations," *J Clin Periodontol,* 1978, 5(4):246-71.

Loesche WJ, Syed SA, Laughon BE, et al, "The Bacteriology of Acute Necrotizing Ulcerative Gingivitis," *J Periodontol,* 1982, 53(4):223-30.

McLoughlin P, Newman L, and Brown A, "Oral Squamous Cell Carcinoma Arising in Phenytoin-Induced Hyperplasia," *Br Dent J,* 1995, 178(5):183-4.

Moghadam BK and Gier RE, "Common and Less Common Gingival Overgrowth Conditions," *Cutis,* 1995, 56(1):46-8.

Mombelli A, Buser D, Lang NP, et al, "Suspected Periodontopathogens in Erupting Third Molar Sites of Periodontally Healthy Individuals," *J Clin Periodontol,* 1990, 17(1):48-54.

Moore LV, Moore WE, Cato EP, et al, "Bacteriology of Human Gingivitis," *J Dent Res,* 1987, 66(5):989-95.

Navazesh M and Mulligan R, "Systemic Dissemination as a Result of Oral Infection in Individuals 50 Years of Age and Older," *Spec Care Dentist,* 1995, 15(1):11-9.

Nery EB, Edson RG, Lee KK, et al, "Prevalence of Nifedipine-Induced Gingival Hyperplasia," *J Periodontol,* 1995, 66(7):572-8.

SUGGESTED READINGS *(Continued)*

Nickoloff BJ, Griffiths CE, and Barker JN, "The Role of Adhesion Molecules, Chemotactic Factors, and Cytokines in Inflammatory and Neoplastic Skin Disease," *J Invest Dermatol*, 1990, 94(Suppl 6):151S-7S.

Pinson M, Hoffman WH, Garnick JJ, et al, "Periodontal Disease and Type I Diabetes Mellitus in Children and Adolescents," *J Clin Periodontol*, 1995, 22(2):118-23.

Preber H and Bergstrom J, "Effect of Cigarette Smoking on Periodontal Healing Following Surgical Therapy," *J Clin Periodontol*, 1990, 17(5):324-8.

Ramfjord SP and Ash MM, "Periodontology and Periodontics: Modern Theory and Practice," St Louis, MO: Ishryalar Euro-America, 1989.

Ramsdale DR, Morris JL, and Hardy P,"Gingival Hyperplasia With Nifedipine," *Br Heart J*, 1995, 73(2):115.

Ransier A, Epstein JB, Lunn R, et al, "A Combined Analysis of a Toothbrush, Foam Brush, and a Chlorhexidine-Soaked Foam Brush in Maintaining Oral Hygiene," *Cancer Nurs*, 1995, 18(5):393-6.

Robertson PB and Greenspan JS, *Perspectives on Oral Manifestations of AIDS: Diagnosis and Management of HIV-Associated Infection,* Littleton, MA: PSG Publishing Co, 1988.

Wahlstrom E, Zamora JU, and Teichman S, "Improvement in Cyclosporine-Associated Gingival Hyperplasia With Azithromycin Therapy," *N Engl J Med*, 1995, 332(11):753-4.

RESPIRATORY DISEASES

"Asthma Mortality and Hospitalization Among Children and Young Adults - United States, 1980-1993," *Morb Mortal Wkly Rep*, 1996, 45(17):350-3.

Barnes PF and Barrows SA, "Tuberculosis in the 1990s," *Ann Intern Med*, 1993, 119(5):400-10.

Snider DE, Jr and Roper WL, "The New Tuberculosis," *N Engl J Med*, 1992, 326(10):703-5.

Cohen C, Krutchkoff D, and Eisenberg E, "Systemic Sarcoidosis: Report of Two Cases With Oral Lesions," *J Oral Surg*, 1981, 39(8):613-8.

DeLuke DM and Sciubba JJ, "Oral Manifestations of Sarvoidosis: Report of a Case Masquerading as a Neoplasm," *Oral Surg Oral Med Oral Pathol*, 1985, 59(2):184-8.

Drosos AA, Constantopoulos SH, Psychos D, et al, "The Forgotten Cause of Sicca Complex: Sarcoidosis," *J Rheumatol*, 1989, 16(12):1548-51.

Egman DH and Christiani DC, *Respiratory Disorders in Occupational Health: Recognizing and Preventing Work-Related Disease,* 2nd ed, Levy BS and Wegman DH, eds, Boston, MA: Little-Brown, 1988, 319-44.

Frieden TR, Sterling T, Pablos-Mendez A, et al, "The Emergence of Drug Resistant Tuberculosis in New York City," *N Engl J Med*, 1993, 328(8):521-6.

Murciano D, Auclair MH, Pariente R, et al, "A Randomized Controlled Trial of Theophylline in Patients With Severe Chronic Obstructive Pulmonary Disease," *N Engl J Med*, 1989, 320(23):1521-5.

Bass JB, Farer LS, Hopewell PC, et al, "Treatment of Tuberculosis and Tuberculosis Infection in Adults and Children. American Thoracic Society and the Centers for Disease Control and Prevention," *Am J Respir Crit Care Med*, 1994, 149(5):1359-74.

TEMPOROMANDIBULAR DYSFUNCTION

Becker IM, "Occlusion as a Causative Factor in TMD. Scientific Basis to Occlusal Therapy, *NY State Dent J*, 1995, 61(9):54-7.

Bell WE, et al, *Temporomandibular Disorders: Classification Diagnosis, Management,* 3rd ed, Chicago, IL: Year Book Medical Publishers, 1990.

Bloch M, Riba H, Redensky D, et al, "Cranio-Mandibular Disorder in Children," *NY State Dent J,* 1995, 61(3):48-50.

Canavan D and Gratt BM, "Electronic Thermography for the Assessment of Mild and Moderate Temporomandibular Joint Dysfunction," *Oral Surg Oral Med Oral Pathol Oral Radiol Endod,* 1995, 79(6):778-86.

Carlson CR, Okeson JP, Falace DA, et al, "Comparison of Psychologic and Physiologic Functioning Between Patients With Masticatory Muscle Pain and Matched Controls," *J Orofacial Pain,* 1993, 7(1):15-22.

Clark GT and Takeuchi H, "Temporomandibular Dysfunction, Chromic Orofacial Pain and Oral Motor Disorders in the 21st Century," *J Calif Dent Assoc,* 1995, 23(4):44-6, 48-50.

Clayton JA, "Occlusion and Prosthodontics," *Dent Clin North Am,* 1995, 39(2):313-33.

Dos Santos J Jr, "Supportive Conservative Therapies for Temporomandibular Disorders," *Dent Clin North Am,* 1995, 39(2):459-77.

Kai S, Kai H, Nakayama E, et al, "Clinical Symptoms of Open Lock Position of the Condyle. Relation to Anterior Dislocation of the Temporomandibular Joint," *Oral Surg Oral Med Oral Pathol,* 1992, 74(2):143-8.

Lund JP, Donga R, Widmer CG, et al, "The Pain-Adaptation Model: A Discussion of the Relationship Between Chronic Musculoskeletal Pain and Motor Activity," *Can J Physiol Pharmacol,* 1991, 69(5):683-94.

Okeson JP, "Occlusion and Functional Disorders of the Masticatory System," *Dent Clin North Am,* 1995, 39(2):285-300.

Okeson JP, *The Management of Temporomandibular Disorders and Occlusion,* 3rd ed, St Louis, MO: Mosby Year Book, 1993.

Quinn JH, "Mandibular Exercises to Control Bruxism and Deviation Problems," *Cranio,* 1995, 13(1):30-4.

Schiffman E, Haley D, Baker C, et al, "Diagnostic Criteria for Screening Headache Patients for Temporomandibular Disorders," *Headache,* 1995, 35(3):121-4.

"Temporomandibular Disorder Prosthodontics: Treatment and Management Goals. Report of the Committee on Temporomandibular Disorders of the American College of Prosthodontics," *J Prosthodontology,* 1995, 4(1):58-64.

Widmark G, Kahnberg KE, Haraldson T, et al, "Evaluation of TMJ Surgery in Cases Not Responding to Conservative Treatment," *Cranio,* 1995, 13(1):44-9.

APPENDIX TABLE OF CONTENTS

COMMON SYMBOLS & ABBREVIATIONS

μg	microgram
°C	degrees Celsius (Centigrade)
<	less than
>	greater than
≤	less than or equal to
≥	greater than or equal to
ABG	arterial blood gas
ACE	angiotensin-converting enzyme
ACLS	adult cardiac life support
ADH	antidiuretic hormone
AED	antiepileptic drug
ALL	acute lymphoblastic leukemia
ALT	alanine aminotransferase (was SGPT)
AML	acute myeloblastic leukemia
ANA	antinuclear antibodies
ANC	absolute neutrophil count
ANL	acute nonlymphoblastic leukemia
APTT	activated partial thromboplastin time
ASA (class I-IV)	classification of surgical patients according to their baseline health (eg, healthy ASA I and II or increased severity of illness ASA III or IV)
AST	aspartate aminotransferase (was SGOT)
A-V	atrial-ventricular
BMT	bone marrow transplant
BUN	blood urea nitrogen
cAMP	cyclic adenosine monophosphate
CBC	complete blood count
CHF	congestive heart failure
CI	cardiac index
Cl_{cr}	creatinine clearance
CNS	central nervous system
COPD	chronic obstructive pulmonary disease
CSF	cerebral spinal fluid
CT	computed tomography
CVA	cerebral vascular accident
CVP	central venous pressure
d	day
D_5W	dextrose 5% in water
$D_5/_{0.45}$ NaCl	dextrose 5% in sodium chloride 0.45%
$D_{10}W$	dextrose 10% in water
DIC	disseminated intravascular coagulation
DNA	deoxyribonucleic acid
DVT	deep vein thrombosis
EEG	electroencephalogram
EKG	electrocardiogram
ESR	erythrocyte sedimentation rate
E.T.	endotracheal
FEV_1	forced expiratory volume
FVC	forced vital capacity
g	gram
G-6-PD	glucose-6-phosphate dehydrogenase
GA	gestational age
GABA	gamma-aminobutyric acid
GE	gastroesophageal
GI	gastrointestinal
GU	genitourinary
h	hour
HIV	human immunodeficiency virus
HPLC	high performance liquid chromatography
IBW	ideal body weight
ICP	intracranial pressure
IgG	immune globulin G
I.M.	intramuscular
INR	international normalized ratio
I.O.	intraosseous
I.V.	intravenous

(continued)

IVH	intraventricular hemorrhage
IVP	intravenous push
I & O	input and output
IOP	intraocular pressure
I.T.	intrathecal
JRA	juvenile rheumatoid arthritis
kg	kilogram
L	liter
LDH	lactate dehydrogenase
LE	lupus erythematosus
LP	lumbar puncture
MAO	monoamine oxidase
MAP	mean arterial pressure
mcg	microgram
mg	milligram
MI	myocardial infarction
μmol	micromole
min	minute
mL	milliliter
mo	month
mOsm	milliosmoles
MRI	magnetic resonance image
ND	nasoduodenal
ng	nanogram
NG	nasogastric
NMDA	n-methyl-d-aspartate
nmol	nanomole
NPO	nothing per os (nothing by mouth)
NSAID	nonsteroidal anti-inflammatory drug
O.R.	operating room
OTC	over-the-counter (nonprescription)
PALS	pediatric advanced life support
PCA	postconceptional age
PCP	*Pneumocystis carinii* pneumonia
PCWP	pulmonary capillary wedge pressure
PDA	patent ductus arteriosus
PNA	postnatal age
PSVT	paroxysmal supraventricular tachycardia
PT	prothrombin time
PTT	partial thromboplastin time
PUD	peptic ulcer disease
PVC	premature ventricular contraction
qsad	add an amount sufficient to equal
RAP	right atrial pressure
RIA	radioimmunoassay
RNA	ribonucleic acid
S-A	sino-atrial
S.C.	subcutaneous
S_{cr}	serum creatinine
SIADH	syndrome of inappropriate antidiuretic hormone
S.L.	sublingual
SLE	systemic lupus erythematosus
SVR	systemic vascular resistance
SVT	supraventricular tachycardia
SWI	sterile water for injection
TT	thrombin time
UTI	urinary tract infection
V_d	volume of distribution
V_{dss}	volume of distribution at steady-state
y	year

*Other than drug synonyms

APOTHECARY/METRIC EQUIVALENTS

Approximate Liquid Measures

Basic equivalent: 1 fluid ounce = 30 mL

Examples:

1 gallon	3800 mL	1 gallon	128 fluid ounces
1 quart	960 mL	1 quart	32 fluid ounces
1 pint	480 mL	1 pint	16 fluid ounces
8 fluid oz	240 mL	15 minims	1 mL
4 fluid oz	120 mL	10 minims	0.6 mL

Approximate Household Equivalents

1 teaspoonful	5 mL	1 tablespoonful	15 mL

Weights

Basic equivalents:

1 oz	30 g	15 gr	1 g

Examples:

4 oz	120 g	1 gr	60 mg
2 oz	60 g	1/100 gr	600 mcg
10 gr	600 mg	1/150 gr	400 mcg
7½ gr	500 mg	1/200 gr	300 mcg
16 oz	1 lb		

Metric Conversions

Basic equivalents:

1 g	1000 mg	1 mg	1000 mcg

Examples:

5 g	5000 mg	5 mg	5000 mcg
0.5 g	500 mg	0.5 g	500 mcg
0.05 g	50 mg	0.05 mg	50 mcg

Exact Equivalents

1 g	=	15.43 gr		
1 mL	=	16.23 minims		
1 minim	=	0.06 mL		
1 gr	=	64.8 mg		
1 pint (pt)	=	473.2 mL		
1 oz	=	28.35 g		
1 lb	=	453.6 g		
1 kg	=	2.2 lbs		
1 qt	=	946.4 mL		

0.1 mg	=	1/600 gr
0.12 mg	=	1/500 gr
0.15 mg	=	1/400 gr
0.2 mg	=	1/300 gr
0.3 mg	=	1/200 gr
0.4 mg	=	1/150 gr
0.5 mg	=	1/120 gr
0.6 mg	=	1/100 gr
0.8 mg	=	1/80 gr
1 mg	=	1/65 gr

Solids*

¼ grain	=	15 mg
½ grain	=	30 mg
1 grain	=	60 mg
1½ grains	=	100 mg
5 grains	=	300 mg
10 grains	=	600 mg

*Use exact equivalents for compounding and calculations requiring a high degree of accuracy.

POUNDS-KILOGRAMS CONVERSION

1 pound = 0.45359 kilograms
1 kilogram = 2.2 pounds

lb	=	kg	lb	=	kg	lb	=	kg
1		0.45	70		31.75	140		63.50
5		2.27	75		34.02	145		65.77
10		4.54	80		36.29	150		68.04
15		6.80	85		38.56	155		70.31
20		9.07	90		40.82	160		72.58
25		11.34	95		43.09	165		74.84
30		13.61	100		45.36	170		77.11
35		15.88	105		47.63	175		79.38
40		18.14	110		49.90	180		81.65
45		20.41	115		52.16	185		83.92
50		22.68	120		54.43	190		86.18
55		24.95	125		56.70	195		88.45
60		27.22	130		58.91	200		90.72
65		29.48	135		61.24			

TEMPERATURE CONVERSION

Celsius to Fahrenheit = ($^\circ$C x 9/5) + 32 = $^\circ$F
Fahrenheit to Celsius = ($^\circ$F - 32) x 5/9 = $^\circ$C

°C	=	°F	°C	=	°F	°C	=	°F
100.0		212.0	39.0		102.2	36.8		98.2
50.0		122.0	38.8		101.8	36.6		97.9
41.0		105.8	38.6		101.5	36.4		97.5
40.8		105.4	38.4		101.1	36.2		97.2
40.6		105.1	38.2		100.8	36.0		96.8
40.4		104.7	38.0		100.4	35.8		96.4
40.2		104.4	37.8		100.1	35.6		96.1
40.0		104.0	37.6		99.7	35.4		95.7
39.8		103.6	37.4		99.3	35.2		95.4
39.6		103.3	37.2		99.0	35.0		95.0
39.4		102.9	37.0		98.6	0		32.0
39.2		102.6						

BODY SURFACE AREA OF ADULTS AND CHILDREN

Calculating Body Surface Area in Children

In a child of average size, find weight and corresponding surface area on the boxed scale to the left; or, use the nomogram to the right. Lay a straightedge on the correct height and weight points for the child, then read the intersecting point on the surface area scale.

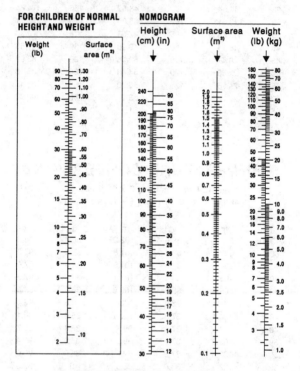

FOR CHILDREN OF NORMAL HEIGHT AND WEIGHT

NOMOGRAM

BODY SURFACE AREA FORMULA
(Adult and Pediatric)

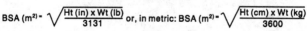

$$BSA\ (m^2) = \sqrt{\frac{Ht\ (in)\ x\ Wt\ (lb)}{3131}} \quad \text{or, in metric: } BSA\ (m^2) = \sqrt{\frac{Ht\ (cm)\ x\ Wt\ (kg)}{3600}}$$

References
Lam TK, Leung DT, *N Engl J Med*, 1988, 318:1130, (Letter).
Mosteller RD, "Simplified Calculation of Body Surface Area", *N Engl J Med*, 1987, 317:1098.

AVERAGE WEIGHTS AND SURFACE AREAS

Average Weight and Surface Area of Preterm Infants, Term Infants, and Children

Age	Average Weight (kg)*	Approximate Surface Area (m²)
Weeks Gestation		
26	0.9-1	0.1
30	1.3-1.5	0.12
32	1.6-2	0.15
38	2.9-3	0.2
40 (term infant at birth)	3.1-4	0.25
Months		
3	5	0.29
6	7	0.38
9	8	0.42
Year		
1	10	0.49
2	12	0.55
3	15	0.64
4	17	0.74
5	18	0.76
6	20	0.82
7	23	0.90
8	25	0.95
9	28	1.06
10	33	1.18
11	35	1.23
12	40	1.34
Adult	70	1.73

*Weights from age 3 months and older are rounded off to the nearest kilogram.

CALCIUM CHANNEL BLOCKERS & GINGIVAL HYPERPLASIA

Generic Preparation	FDA Approval	Cases Cited in Literature	Common Name
Amlodipine	1992	0	Norvasc®
Bepridil	1993	0	Vascor®
Diltiazem	1982	>20	Cardizem®; Dilacor®
Felodipine	1992	1	Plendil®
Isradipine	1991	0	DynaCirc®
Nicardipine	1989	0	Cardene®
Nifedipine	1982	>120	Adalat®; Procardia®
Nimodipine	1989	0	Nimotop®
Nitrendipine*		1	Baypress®
Verapamil	1982	7	Calan®; Isoptin®; Verelan®

*Not yet approved for use in the United States.

SOME GENERAL OBSERVATIONS OF CCB-INDUCED GH

Most of the reported cases listed in the Calcium Channel Blockers and Gingival Hyperplasia table have involved patients >50 years of age taking CCBs chronically for postmyocardial infarction syndrome, angina pain, essential hypertension, and Raynaud's syndrome. Nifedipine-induced GH has appeared between 1 and 9 months after a daily dose of 30-100 mg, verapamil-induced GH has appeared at 11 months or more after a daily dose of 240-360 mg, and diltiazem-induced GH has appeared between 1 and 24 months after a daily dose of 60-135 mg. As with phenytoin, there does not seem to be a dose-dependent effect of CCBs on the severity of the hyperplastic syndrome. Discontinuance of the CCB usually results in complete disappearance or marked regression of symptoms, with symptoms reappearing upon remediation. The time required after drug discontinuance for marked regression of GH has been one week. Complete disappearance of all symptoms usually takes two months. If gingivectomy is performed and the drug retained or resumed, the hyperplasia will usually recur. Only when the medication is discontinued or a switch to a non-CCB occurs will the gingivectomy usually be successful. One study of Nishikawa[1], et al, showed that if nifedipine could not be discontinued, hyperplasia did not recur after gingivectomy when extensive plaque control was carried out. If the CCB is changed to another class of cardiovascular agent, the gingival hyperplasia will probably regress and disappear. A switch to another CCB, however, will probably result in continued hyperplasia. For example, Giustiniani[2], et al, reported disappearance of symptoms within 15 days after discontinuance of verapamil, with the reoccurrence of symptoms after resumption with diltiazem. The reader is referred to the review of 1991[3] for descriptive clinical and histological findings of CCB-induced GH.

1. Nishikawa SI, Tada H, Hamasaki A, et al, "Nifedipine-Induced Gingival Hyperplasia: A Clinical and In Vitro Study," *J Periodontol*, 1991, 62(1):30-5.
2. Giustiniani S, Robestelli della Cuna F, and Marienei M, "Hyperplastic Gingivitis During Diltiazem Therapy," *Int J Cardiol*, 1987, 15(2):247-9.
3. Wynn RL, "Calcium Channel Blockers and Gingival Hyperplasia," *Gen Dent*, 1991, 240-3.

CANCER CHEMOTHERAPY REGIMENS

ADULT REGIMENS

Breast Cancer

AC

Doxorubicin (Adriamycin®, I.V., 45 mg/m², day 1
Cyclophosphamide, I.V., 500 mg/m², day 1

Repeat cycle every 21 days

ACe

Doxorubicin (Adriamycin®, I.V., 40 mg/m², day 1
Cyclophosphamide, P.O., 200 mg/m²/d, days 1-3 or 3-6

Repeat cycle every 21-28 days

CAF

Cyclophosphamide, P.O., 100 mg/m², days 1-14
Doxorubicin (Adriamycin®, I.V., 30 mg/m², days 1 & 8
Fluorouracil, I.V., 400-500 mg/m², days 1 & 8

Repeat cycle every 28 days

or

Cyclophosphamide, I.V., 500 mg/m², day 1
Doxorubicin (Adriamycin®, I.V., 50 mg/m², day 1
Fluorouracil, I.V., 500 mg/m², day 1

Repeat cycle every 21 days

or Dose Intensification of CAF*

Cyclophosphamide, I.V., 600 mg/m², day 1
Doxorubicin (Adriamycin®, I.V., 60 mg/m², day 1
Fluorouracil, I.V., 600 mg/m², day 1
G-CSF, I.V./S.C., 5 mcg/kg/dose

Repeat cycle every 21 days

*Preliminary data presented at ASCO (March, 1992) suggests better response with dose intensification.

CFM

Cyclophosphamide, I.V., 500 mg/m², day 1
Fluorouracil, I.V., 500 mg/m², day 1
Mitoxantrone, I.V., 10 mg/m², day 1

Repeat cycle every 21 days

CFPT

Cyclophosphamide, I.V., 150 mg/m², days 1-5
Fluorouracil, I.V., 300 mg/m², days 1-5
Prednisone, P.O., 10 mg tid, days 1-7
Tamoxifen, P.O., 10 mg bid, days 1-42

Repeat cycle every 42 days

CMF

Cyclophosphamide, P.O., 100 mg/m², days 1-14
Methotrexate, I.V., 40-60 mg/m², days 1 & 8
Fluorouracil, I.V., 400-600 mg/m², days 1 & 8

Repeat cycle every 28 days

or

Cyclophosphamide, I.V., 600 mg/m², days 1 & 8
Methotrexate, I.V., 40-60 mg/m², days 1 & 8
Fluorouracil, I.V., 400-600 mg/m², days 1 & 8

Repeat cycle every 28 days

CMFP

Cyclophosphamide, P.O., 100 mg/m², days 1-14
Methotrexate, I.V., 40-60 mg/m², days 1 & 8
Fluorouracil, I.V., 600-700 mg/m², days 1 & 8
Prednisone, P.O., 40 mg (first 3 cycles only), days 1-14

Repeat cycle every 28 days

CMFVP (Cooper's)

Cyclophosphamide, P.O., 2-2.5 mg/kg/d for 9 months
Methotrexate, I.V., 0.7 mg/kg/wk for 8 weeks then every other week for 7 months
Fluorouracil, I.V., 12 mg/kg/wk for 8 weeks then every other week for 7 months
Vincristine, I.V., 0.035 mg/kg (max 2 mg/wk) for 5 weeks then once monthly
Prednisone, P.O., 0.75 mg/kg/d, taper over next 40 days, discontinue, days 1-10

or

Cyclophosphamide, I.V., 400 mg/m², day 1
Methotrexate, I.V., 30 mg/m², days 1 & 8

CANCER CHEMOTHERAPY REGIMENS *(Continued)*

Fluorouracil, I.V., 400 mg/m², days 1 & 8
Vincristine, I.V., 1 mg, days 1 & 8
Prednisone, P.O., 20 mg qid, days 1-7

Repeat cycle every 28 days

FAC

Fluorouracil, I.V., 500 mg/m², days 1 & 8
Doxorubicin (Adriamycin®), I.V., 50 mg/m², day 1
Cyclophosphamide, I.V., 500 mg/m², day 1

Repeat cycle every 21 days

IMF

Ifosfamide, I.V., 1.5 g/m², days 1 & 8
Mesna, I.V., 20% of ifosfamide dose, give immediately before and 4
    and 8 hours after ifosfamide infusion, days 1 & 8
Methotrexate, I.V., 40 mg/m², days 1 & 8
Fluorouracil, I.V., 600 mg/m², days 1 & 8

Repeat cycle every 28 days

NFL

Mitoxantrone (Novantrone®), I.V., 12 mg/m², day 1
Fluorouracil, I.V., 350 mg/m², days 1-3, given after leucovorin calcium
Leucovorin calcium, I.V., 300 mg/m², days 1-3

or

Mitoxantrone (Novantrone®), I.V., 10 mg/m², day 1
Fluorouracil, I.V., 1000 mg/m² continuous infusion, given
after leucovorin calcium, days 1-3
Leucovorin calcium, I.V., 100 mg/m², days 1-3

Repeat cycle every 21 days

VATH

Vinblastine, I.V., 4.5 mg/m², day 1
Doxorubicin (Adriamycin®), I.V., 45 mg/m², day 1
Thiotepa, I.V., 12 mg/m², day 1
Fluoxymesterone (Halotestin®), P.O., 30 mg qd, days 1-21

Repeat cycle every 21 days

Single-Agent Regimens

Doxorubicin, I.V., 60 mg/m², every 3 weeks

or

Doxorubicin, I.V., 20 mg/m², every week

or

Doxorubicin, I.V., 20 mg/m² continuous infusion, days 1-3, every 3
    weeks

Mitomycin C, I.V., 8-10 mg/m², every 6-8 weeks

Paclitaxel, I.V., 175 mg/m² over 3-24 h, every 21 d
    Patient must be premedicated with:
    Dexamethasone 20 mg P.O., 12 and 6 h prior
    Diphenhydramine 50 mg I.V., 30 min prior
    Cimetidine 300 mg I.V., or ranitidine 50 mg I.V., 30 min prior

Vinblastine, I.V., 12 mg/m², every 3-4 weeks

Colon Cancer

F-CL

Fluorouracil, I.V., 375 mg/m², days 1-5
Calcium leucovorin, I.V., 200 mg/m², days 1-5

Repeat cycle every 28 days

or

Fluorouracil, I.V., 500 mg/m² weekly 1 h after initiating the calcium
    leucovorin infusion for 6 weeks
Calcium leucovorin, I.V., 500 mg/m², over 2 h, weekly for 6 weeks

Two-week break, then repeat cycle

FLe

Fluorouracil, I.V., 450 mg/m² for 5 days, then, after a pause of 4 weeks,
    450 mg/m², weekly for 48 weeks
Levamisole, P.O., 50 mg tid for 3 days, repeated every 2 weeks for 1
    year

FMV

Fluorouracil, I.V., 10 mg/kg/d, days 1-5
Methyl-CCNU, P.O., 175 mg/m², day 1
Vincristine, I.V., 1 mg/m² (max 2 mg), day 1

Repeat cycle every 35 days

FU/LV

Fluorouracil, I.V., 370-400 mg/m^2/d, days 1-5
Leucovorin calcium, I.V., 200 mg/m^2/d, commence infusion 15 min prior
to fluorouracil infusion, days 1-5

Repeat cycle every 21 days

or

Fluorouracil, I.V., 1000 mg/m^2/d by continuous infusion, days 1-4
Leucovorin calcium, I.V., 200 mg/m^2/d, days 1-4

Repeat cycle every 28 days

Weekly 5FU/LV

Fluorouracil, I.V., 600 mg/m^{2}over 1 h given after leucovorin, repeat
weekly x 6 then 2-week rest period = 1 cycle, days 1, 8, 15, 22,
29, 36
Leucovorin calcium, I.V., 500 mg/m^{2}over 2 h, days 1, 8, 15, 22, 29, 36

Repeat cycle every 56 days

5FU/LDLF

Fluorouracil, I.V., 370 mg/m^2/d, days 1-5
Leucovorin calcium, I.V., 20-25 mg/m^2/d, days 1-5

Repeat cycle every 28 days

Gastric Cancer

EAP

Etoposide, I.V., 120 mg/m^2, days 4, 5, 6
Doxorubicin (Adriamycin®), I.V., 20 mg/m^2, days 1, 7
Cisplatin (Platinol®), I.V., 40 mg/m^2, days 2, 8

Repeat cycle every 21 days

ELF

Etoposide, I.V., 120 mg/m^2, days 1-3
Leucovorin calcium, I.V., 300 mg/m^2, days 1-3
Fluorouracil, I.V., 500 mg/m^2, days 1-3

Repeat cycle every 21-28 days

FAM

Fluorouracil, I.V., 600 mg/m^2, days 1, 8, 29, & 36
Doxorubicin (Adriamycin®), I.V., 30 mg/m^2, days 1 & 29
Mitomycin C, I.V., 10 mg/m^2, day 1

Repeat cycle every 56 days

FAME

Fluorouracil, I.V., 350 mg/m^2, days 1-5, 36-40
Doxorubicin (Adriamycin®), I.V., 40 mg/m^2, days 1 & 36
Methyl-CCNU, P.O., 150 mg/m^2, day 1

Repeat cycle every 70 days

FAMTX

Methotrexate, IVPB, 1500 mg/m^2, day 1
Fluorouracil, IVPB, 1500 mg/m^{2}1 h after methotrexate, day 1
Leucovorin calcium, P.O., 15 mg/m^{2}q6h x 48 h 24 h after methotrexate,
day 2
Doxorubicin (Adriamycin®), IVPB, 30 mg/m^2, day 15

Repeat cycle every 28 days

FCE

Fluorouracil, I.V., 900 mg/m^2/d continuous infusion, days 1-5
Cisplatin, I.V., 20 mg/m^2, days 1-5
Etoposide, I.V., 90 mg/m^2, days 1, 3, & 5

Repeat cycle every 21 days

PFL

Cisplatin (Platinol®), I.V., 25 mg/m^{2}continuous infusion, days 1-5
Fluorouracil, I.V., 800 mg/m^{2}continuous infusion, days 2-5
Leucovorin calcium, I.V., 500 mg/m^{2}continuous infusion, days 1-5

Repeat cycle every 28 days

Genitourinary Cancer
Bladder

CAP

Cyclophosphamide, I.V., 400 mg/m^2, day 1
Doxorubicin (Adriamycin®), I.V., 40 mg/m^2, day 1
Cisplatin (Platinol®), I.V., 60 mg/m^2, day 1

Repeat cycle every 21 days

CANCER CHEMOTHERAPY REGIMENS *(Continued)*

CISCA

Cisplatin, I.V., 70-100 mg/m², day 2
Cyclophosphamide, I.V., 650 mg/m², day 1
Doxorubicin (Adriamycin®), I.V., 50 mg/m², day 1
Repeat cycle every 21-28 days

CMV

Cisplatin, I.V., 100 mg/m² over 4 h start 12 h after MTX, day 2
Methotrexate, I.V., 30 mg/m², days 1 & 8
Vinblastine, I.V., 4 mg/m², days 1 & 8
Repeat cycle every 21 days

m-PFL

Methotrexate, I.V., 60 mg/m², day 1
Cisplatin (Platinol®), I.V., 25 mg/m² continuous infusion, days 2-6
Fluorouracil, I.V., 800 mg/m² continuous infusion, days 2-6
Leucovorin calcium, I.V., 500 mg/m² continuous infusion, days 2-6
Repeat cycle every 28 days for 4 cycles

MVAC

Methotrexate, I.V., 30 mg/m², days 1, 15, 22
Vinblastine, I.V., 3 mg/m², days 2, 15, 22
Doxorubicin (Adriamycin®), I.V., 30 mg/m², day 2
Cisplatin, I.V., 70 mg/m², day 2
Repeat cycle every 28 days

Prostate

FL

Flutamide, P.O., 250 mg tid, days 1-28
Leuprolide acetate, S.C., 1 mg qd, days 1-28
Repeat cycle every 28 days

or

Flutamide, P.O., 250 mg tid, days 1-28
Leuprolide acetate depot, I.M., 7.5 mg, day 1
Repeat cycle every 28 days

FZ

Flutamide, P.O., 250 mg tid
Goserelin acetate (Zoladex®), S.C., 3.6 mg implant, every 28 days

L-VAM

Leuprolide acetate, S.C., 1 mg qd, days 1-28
Vinblastine, I.V., 1.5 mg/m²/d continuous infusion, days 2-7
Doxorubicin (Adriamycin®), I.V., 50 mg/m² continuous infusion, day 1
Mitomycin C, I.V., 10 mg/m², day 2
Repeat cycle every 28 days

Testicular, Induction, Good Risk

BEP

Bleomycin, I.V., 30 units, days 2, 9, 16
Etoposide, I.V., 100 mg/m², days 1-5
Cisplatin (Platinol®), I.V., 20 mg/m², days 1-5
Repeat cycle every 21 days

PE

Cisplatin (Platinol®), I.V., 20 mg/m², days 1-5
Etoposide, I.V., 100 mg/m², days 1-5
Repeat cycle every 21 days

PVB

Cisplatin (Platinol®), I.V., 20 mg/m², days 1-5
Vinblastine, I.V., 6 mg/m², days 1, 2
Bleomycin, I.V., 30 units, weekly
Repeat cycle every 21-28 days

Testicular, Induction, Poor Risk

VIP

Etoposide (VePesid®), I.V., 75 mg/m², days 1-5
Ifosfamide, I.V., 1.2 g/m², days 1-5
Cisplatin (Platinol®), I.V., 20 mg/m², days 1-5
Mesna, I.V., 120 mg/m² then 1200 mg/m²/d continuous infusion, days 1-5
Repeat cycle every 21 days

VIP (Einhorn)
> Vinblastine, I.V., 0.11 mg/kg, days 1-2
> Ifosfamide, I.V., 1200 mg/m², days 1-5
> Cisplatin (Platinol®), I.V., 20 mg/m², days 1-5
> Mesna, I.V., 120 mg/m², then 1200 mg/m²/d continuous infusion, days 1-5
>
> Repeat cycle every 21 days

Testicular, Induction, Salvage

VAB VI
> Vinblastine, I.V., 4 mg/m², day 1
> Dactinomycin (Actinomycin D), I.V., 1 mg/m², day 1
> Bleomycin, I.V., 30 units push day 1, then 20 units/m²/d continuous infusion, days 1-3
> Cisplatin, I.V., 120 mg/m², day 4
> Cyclophosphamide, I.V., 600 mg/m², day 1
>
> Repeat cycle every 21 days

VBP (PVB)
> Vinblastine, I.V., 6 mg/m², days 1 & 2
> Bleomycin, I.V., 30 units, days 1, 8, 15, (22)
> Cisplatin (Platinol®), I.V., 20 mg/m², days 1-5
>
> Repeat cycle every 21-28 days

Gestational Trophoblastic Cancer

DMC
> Dactinomycin, I.V., 0.37 mg/m², days 1-5
> Methotrexate, I.V., 11 mg/m², days 1-5
> Cyclophosphamide, I.V., 110 mg/m², days 1-5
>
> Repeat cycle every 21 days

Head and Neck Cancer

CAP
> Cyclophosphamide, I.V., 500 mg/m², day 1
> Doxorubicin (Adriamycin®), I.V., 50 mg/m², day 1
> Cisplatin (Platinol®), I.V., 50 mg/m², day 1
>
> Repeat cycle every 28 days

CF
> Cisplatin, I.V., 100 mg/m², day 1
> Fluorouracil, I.V., 1000 mg/m²/d continuous infusion, days 1-5
>
> Repeat cycle every 21-28 days

CF
> Carboplatin, I.V., 400 mg/m², day 1
> Fluorouracil, I.V., 1000 mg/m²/d continuous infusion, days 1-5
>
> Repeat cycle every 21-28 days

COB
> Cisplatin, I.V., 100 mg/m², day 1
> Vincristine (Oncovin®), I.V., 1 mg/m², days 2 & 5
> Bleomycin, I.V., 30 units/d continuous infusion, days 2-5
>
> Repeat cycle every 21 days

5-FU HURT
> Hydroxyurea, P.O., 1000 mg q12h x 11 doses; start PM of admission, give 2 hours prior to radiation therapy, days 0-5
> Fluorouracil, I.V., 800 mg/m²/d continuous infusion, start AM after admission, days 1-5
> Paclitaxel, I.V., 5-25 mg/m²/d continuous infusion, start AM after admission; dose escalation study — refer to protocol, days 1-5
> G-CSF, S.C., 5 mcg/kg/d, days 6-12, start ≥12 hours after completion of 5-FU infusion
>
> 5-7 cycles may be administered

MAP
> Mitomycin C, I.V., 8 mg/m², day 1
> Doxorubicin (Adriamycin®), I.V., 40 mg/m², day 1
> Cisplatin (Platinol®), I.V., 60 mg/m², day 1
>
> Repeat cycle every 28 days

MBC (MBD)
> Methotrexate, I.M./I.V., 40 mg/m², days 1 & 15
> Bleomycin, I.M./I.V., 10 units, days 1, 8, 15
> Cisplatin, I.V., 50 mg/m², day 4
>
> Repeat cycle every 21 days

CANCER CHEMOTHERAPY REGIMENS *(Continued)*

MF

Methotrexate, I.V., 125-250 mg/m^2, day 1
Fluorouracil, I.V., 600 mg/m^{2}beginning 1 h after methotrexate, day 1
Leucovorin calcium, I.V./P.O., 10 mg/m^{2}q6h x 5 doses beginning 24 h
  after methotrexate

Repeat cycle every 7 days

PFL

Cisplatin (Platinol®), I.V., 100 mg/m^2, day 1
Fluorouracil, I.V., 600-800 mg/m^2/d continuous infusion, days 1-5
Leucovorin calcium, I.V., 200-300 mg/m^2/d, days 1-5

Repeat cycle every 21 days

PFL+IFN

Cisplatin (Platinol®), I.V., 100 mg/m^2, day 1
Fluorouracil, I.V., 640 mg/m^2/d continuous infusion, days 1-5
Leucovorin calcium, P.O., 100 mg q4h, days 1-5

CORTICOSTEROID EQUIVALENCIES COMPARISON

Glucocorticoid	Approximate Equivalent Dose (mg)	Routes of Administration	Relative Anti-Inflammatory Potency	Relative Mineralocorticoid Potency	Half-life Plasma (min)	Half-life Biologic (h)
Short-Acting						
Cortisone	25	P.O., I.M.	0.8	2	30	8-12
Hydrocortisone	20	I.M., I.V.	1	2	80-118	
Intermediate-Acting						
Prednisone	5	P.O.	4	1	60	18-36
Prednisolone	5	P.O., I.M., I.V., intra-articular, intradermal, soft tissue injection	4	1	115-212	
Triamcinolone	4	P.O., I.M., intra-articular, intradermal, intrasynovial, soft tissue injection	5	0	200+	
Methylprednisolone	4	P.O., I.M., I.V.	5	0	78-188	
Long-Acting						
Dexamethasone	0.75	P.O., I.M., I.V., intra-articular, intradermal, soft tissue injection	25-30	0	110-210	36-54
Betamethasone	0.6-0.75	P.O., I.M., intra-articular, intradermal, intrasynovial, soft tissue injection	25	0	300+	

CORTICOSTEROIDS, TOPICAL COMPARISON

Steroid		Vehicle
Lowest Potency (may be ineffective for some indications)		
0.1%	Betamethasone	Cream
0.2%	Betamethasone (Celestone®)	Cream
0.05%	Desonide	Cream
0.04%	Dexamethasone (Hexadrol®)*	Cream
0.1%	Dexamethasone (Decadron® Phosphate, Decaderm®)*	Cream, gel
1%	Hydrocortisone	Cream, ointment, lotion
2.5%	Hydrocortisone	Cream, ointment
0.25%	Methylprednisolone acetate (Medrol®)	Ointment
1%	Methylprednisolone acetate (Medrol®)	Ointment
0.5%	Prednisolone (Meti-Derm®)	Cream
Low Potency		
0.01%	Betamethasone valerate (Valisone®, reduced strength)	Cream
0.1%	Clocortolone (Cloderm®)	Cream
0.03%	Flumethasone pivalate (Locorten®)	Cream
0.01%	Fluocinolone acetonide (Synalar®)*	Cream, solution
0.025%	Fluorometholone (Oxylone®)	Cream
0.025%	Flurandrenolide (Cordran®, Cordran® SP)*	Cream, ointment
0.2%	Hydrocortisone valerate (Westcort®)	Cream
0.025%	Triamcinolone acetonide (Kenalog®)*	Cream, ointment
Intermediate Potency		
0.025%	Betamethasone benzoate	Cream, gel, lotion
0.1%	Betamethasone valerate (Valisone®)*	Cream, ointment, lotion
0.05%	Desonide (Tridesilon®)	Cream, ointment
0.05%	Desoximetasone (Topicort® LP)	Cream
0.025%	Fluocinolone acetonide*	Cream, ointment
0.05%	Flurandrenolide (Cordran®, Cordran® SP)*	Cream, ointment, lotion
0.025%	Halcinonide (Halog®)	Cream, ointment
0.1%	Triamcinolone acetonide (Kenalog®)*	Cream, ointment
High Potency		
0.1%	Amcinonide (Cyclocort®)	Cream, ointment
0.05%	Betamethasone dipropionate (Diprosone®)	Cream, ointment, lotion
0.05%	Clobetasol dipropionate	Cream, ointment
0.25%	Desoximetasone (Topicort®)	Cream
0.05%	Diflorasone diacetate (Florone®, Maxiflor®)	Cream, ointment
0.2%	Fluocinolone (Synalar-HP®)	Cream
0.05%	Fluocinonide (Lidex®)*	Cream, ointment
0.1%	Halcinonide (Halog®)	Cream, ointment, solution
0.5%	Triamcinolone acetonide*	Cream, ointment

*Fluorinated.

NARCOTIC AGONISTS

Comparative Pharmacokinetics

Drug	Onset (min)	Peak (h)	Duration (h)	t ½ (h)	Average Dosing Interval (h)		Equianalgesic Doses* (mg)	
							I.M.	P.O.
Alfentanil	Immediate	ND	ND	1-2	—	—	ND	NA
Buprenorphine	15	1	4-8	2-3			0.4	—
Butorphanol	I.M.: 30-60 I.V.: 4-5	0.5-1	3-5	2.5-3.5	3	(3-6)	2	—
Codeine	P.O.: 30-60 I.M.: 10-30	0.5-1	4-6	3-4	3	(3-6)	120	200
Fentanyl	I.M.: 7-15 I.V.: Immediate	ND	1-2	1.5-6	1	(0.5-2)	0.1	NA
Hydrocodone	ND	ND	4-8	3.3-4.4	6	(4-8)	ND	ND
Hydromorphone	P.O.: 15-30	0.5-1	4-6	2-4	4	(3-6)	1.5	7.5
Levorphanol	P.O.: 10-60	0.5-1	4-8	12-16	6	(6-24)	2	4
Meperidine	P.O./I.M./ S.C.: 10-15 I.V.: ≤5	0.5-1	2-4	3-4	3	(2-4)	75	300
Methadone	P.O.: 30-60 I.V.: 10-20	0.5-1	4-6 (acute) >8 (chronic)	15-30	8	(6-12)	10	20
Morphine	P.O.: 15-60 I.V.: ≤5	P.O./I.M./ S.C.: 0.5-1 I.V.: 0.3	3-6	2-4	4	(3-6)	10	60# (acute) 30 (chronic)
Nalbuphine	I.M.: 30 I.V.: 1-3	1	3-6	5		—	10	—
Naloxone†	2-5	0.5-2	0.5-1	0.5-1.5		—	—	—
Oxycodone	P.O.: 10-15	0.5-1	4-6	3-4	4	(3-6)	NA	30
Oxymorphone	5-15	0.5-1	3-6				1	10‡
Pentazocine	15-20	0.25-1	3-4	2-3	3	(3-6)		
Propoxyphene	P.O.: 30-60	2-2.5	4-6	3.5-15	6	(4-8)	ND	130§- 200¶
Sufentanil	1.3-3	ND	ND	2.5-3	—	—	0.02	NA

ND = no data available. NA = not applicable.

*Based on acute, short-term use. Chronic administration may alter pharmacokinetics and decrease the oral parenteral dose ratio. The morphine oral-parenteral ratio decreases to ~1.5-2.5:1 upon chronic dosing.

#Extensive survey data suggest that the relative potency of I.M.:P.O. morphine of 1:6 changes to 1:2-3 with chronic dosing.

†Narcotic antagonist.

‡Rectal.

§HCl salt.

¶Napsylate salt.

NARCOTIC AGONISTS *(Continued)*

Comparative Pharmacology

Drug	Analge-sic	Antitus-sive	Constipa-tion	Respiratory Depression	Sedation	Nausea/Vomiting
Phenanthrenes						
Codeine	+	+++	+	+	+	+
Hydrocodone	+	+++		+		
Hydromorphone	++	+++	+	++	+	+
Levorphanol	++	++	++	++	++	+
Morphine	++	+++	++	++	++	++
Oxycodone	++	+++	++	++	++	++
Oxymorphone	++	+	++	+++		+++
Phenylpiper-idines						
Alfentanil	++					
Fentanyl	++			+		+
Meperidine	++	+	+	++		
Sufentanil	+++					
Diphenylheptanes						
Methadone	++	++	++	++	+	+
Propoxyphene	+			+	+	+
Agonist/Antagonist						
Buprenorphine	++	N/A	+++	+++	++	++
Butorphanol	++	N/A	+++	+++	++	+
Dezocine	++		+	++	+	++
Nalbuphine	++	N/A	+++	+++	++	++
Pentazocine	++	N/A	+	++	++ or stimula-tion	++

NONSTEROIDAL ANTI-INFLAMMATORY AGENTS, COMPARATIVE DOSAGES, AND PHARMACOKINETICS

Drug	Maximum Recommended Daily Dose (mg)	Time to Peak Levels (h)†	Half-life (h)
Propionic Acids			
Fenoprofen (Nalfon®)	3200	1-2	2-3
Flurbiprofen (Ansaid®)	300	1.5	5.7
Ibuprofen	3200	1-2	1.8-2.5
Ketoprofen (Orudis®)	300	0.5-2	2-4
Naproxen (Naprosyn®)	1500	2-4	12-15
Naproxen sodium (Anaprox®)	1375	1-2	12-13
Oxaprozin (Daypro™)	1800	2-4	40-50
Acetic Acids			
Diclofenac sodium delayed release (Voltaren®)	225	2-3	1-2
Diclofenac potassium immediate release (Cataflam®)	200	1	1-2
Etodolac (Lodine®)	1200	1-2	7.3
Indomethacin (Indocin®)	200	1-2	4.5
Indomethacin SR	150	2-4	4.5-6
Ketorolac (Toradol®)	I.M.: 120‡ P.O.: 40	0.5-1	3.8-8.6
Sulindac (Clinoril®)	400	2-4	7.8 (16.4)§
Tolmetin (Tolectin®)	2000	0.5-1	1-1.5
Fenamates (Anthranilic Acids)			
Meclofenamate (Meclomen®)	400	0.5-1	2 (3.3)¶
Mefenamic acid (Ponstel®)	1000	2-4	2-4
Nonacidic Agent			
Nabumetone (Relafen®)	2000	3-6	24
Oxicam			
Piroxicam (Feldene®)	20	3-5	30-86
Salicylic Acid Derivative			
Diflunisal (Dolobid®)	1500	2-3	8-12

Dosage is based on 70 kg adult with normal hepatic and renal function.

†Food decreases the rate of absorption and may delay the time to peak levels.

‡150 mg on the first day.

§Half-life of active sulfide metabolite.

¶Half-life with multiple doses.

DENTAL DRUG INTERACTIONS: UPDATE ON DRUG COMBINATIONS REQUIRING SPECIAL CONSIDERATIONS

This update discussion includes 16 drug interaction monographs describing clinically important drug combinations requiring special considerations in dental practice. The actions which have resulted from these combinations range from life-threatening adverse effects to attenuation of the therapeutic effects of the interacting drug. The monographs are organized according to the four major groups of drugs used in dentistry: antibiotics, nonsteroidal anti-inflammatory drugs (including aspirin), epinephrine (vasoconstrictors), and narcotic analgesics. An additional monograph on Valium® and alcohol is included.

ANTIBIOTICS - ORAL CONTRACEPTIVES

Description of the Interaction

Case reports suggest that antibiotics used in dentistry can reduce the effectiveness of oral contraceptives resulting in breakthrough ovulation and unplanned pregnancies.

Mechanism

Estrogens, which are components of oral contraceptives, are activated in the intestine by bacteria and reabsorbed into the blood stream as active compounds to inhibit ovulation. Antibiotics reduce the bacteria population in the intestine, which may result in less activated estrogen available to inhibit ovulation.

Background Reports

Tetracyclines: One report described a woman on an estrogen-type oral contraceptive who became pregnant after a 5-day course of tetracycline[1]. Also, several cases of unintended pregnancy and menstrual irregularities have been reported following concurrent use of tetracyclines and oral contraceptives[2,3].

Penicillins: Ampicillin has been shown to reduce estrogen levels in women not taking oral contraceptives and there are reports of unplanned pregnancies in women taking ampicillin with oral contraceptives[4,5]. Concomitant use of penicillin with estrogen-containing oral contraceptives decreased the efficacy of the contraceptive and increased the incidence of breakthrough bleeding[6,7]. Since amoxicillin is closely related to other penicillins, it may also interact with oral contraceptives.

Cephalosporins: Cephalexin (Keflex®) has been reported to interact with oral contraceptives resulting in an unplanned pregnancy[8].

Erythromycins: Unlike ampicillin and tetracyclines, erythromycins have been implicated in only a few cases of oral contraceptive failure over the last 15 years and it is questionable whether erythromycin was the cause of those reported failures[9].

Management

If antibiotics are prescribed to oral contraceptive users, it is suggested that the patients be advised to use additional methods of birth control during both 7 to 10 day dosing, and the two-dose prophylaxis regimens. Any additional method of birth control should be continued through the remaining oral contraceptive cycle.

1. Bacon JF and Shenfield GM, "Pregnancy Attributable to Interaction Between Tetracycline and Oral Contraceptives," *Br Med J,* 1980, 280(6210):293.
2. Orme MLE, "The Clinical Pharmacology of Oral Contraceptive Steroids," *Br J Clin Pharmacol,* 1982, 14:31.
3. Back DJ, Grimmer SF, Orme ML, et al, "Evaluation of Committee on Safety of Medicines Yellow Card Reports on Oral Contraceptive-Drug Interactions With Anticonvulsants and Antibiotics," *Br J Clin Pharmacol,* 1988, 25(5):527-32.
4. Trybuchowski H, "Effect of Ampicillin on the Urinary Output of Steroidal Hormones in Pregnant and Nonpregnant Women," *Clin Chim Acta,* 1973, 45:9-18.
5. Aldercreutz H, Martin F, Lehtinen T, et al, "Effect of Ampicillin Administration on Plasma Conjugated and Unconjugated Estrogen and Progesterone Levels in Pregnancy," *Am J Obstet Gynecol,* 1977, 128(3):266-71.
6. Proudfit CW, "Concurrent Oral Contraceptive and Antibiotic Therapy," *JAMA,* 1981, 246:2076.
7. True RJ, "Interactions Between Antibiotics and Oral Contraceptives," *JAMA,* 1982, 247(10):1408.
8. Bainton R, "Interaction Between Antibiotic Therapy and Contraceptive Medication," *Oral Surg Oral Med Oral Pathol,* 1986, 61(5):453-5.

TETRACYCLINES - ANTACIDS (Containing Divalent or Trivalent Ions)

Description of the Interaction

Concomitant therapy with a tetracycline and an antacid containing aluminum, calcium, or magnesium products can reduce serum concentration and the efficacy of the tetracycline.

Mechanism

Aluminum, calcium, and magnesium ions can combine with the tetracycline molecule in the gastrointestinal tract to form a larger ionized molecule unable to be absorbed into the blood stream.

Background

The interaction between tetracyclines and antacids containing aluminum, calcium, and magnesium is well documented. Foods and dairy products containing calcium will also impair the absorption of tetracyclines. Some reports suggest that doxycycline and minocycline are minimally affected by antacids and dairy products[1,2].

Management

Tetracyclines should be given as far apart as possible from antacids and dairy products.

1. Welling PG, Koch PA, Lau CC, et al, "Bioavailability of Tetracycline and Doxycycline in Fasted and Nonfasted Subjects," *Antimicrob Agents Chemother*, 1977, 11(3):462-9.
2. "Anti-Infective Drug Interactions," *Drug Interactions and Updates*, Hansten PD and Horn JR, eds, Malvern, PA: Lea and Febiger.

TETRACYCLINE - PENICILLIN

Description of the Interaction

Simultaneous tetracycline-penicillin therapy may impair the efficacy of penicillin.

Mechanism

Penicillin kills bacteria by inhibiting cell wall synthesis. Tetracycline inhibits protein synthesis in bacteria and this action has been shown to antagonize the cell wall inhibiting effect of penicillin.

Background

Most of the manufacturers product information contains warnings against using tetracyclines and penicillins together.

Management

Tetracycline-penicillin combination should never be used to treat oral infections. For penicillin two-dose prophylaxis, it would be prudent not to give to patients taking tetracycline. Reappoint if possible.

ERYTHROMYCIN - PENICILLIN

Description of the Interaction

Simultaneous erythromycin-penicillin therapy may impair the efficacy of penicillin.

Mechanism

Penicillin kills bacteria by inhibiting cell wall synthesis. Erythromycin inhibits protein synthesis in bacteria and this action may antagonize the cell wall inhibiting effect of penicillin.

Background

This interaction has not been sufficiently documented in clinical studies.

Management

Erythromycin-penicillin combination should not be used to treat oral infections. For penicillin two-dose prophylaxis, it would be prudent not to give to patients taking erythromycin. Reappoint if possible.

ERYTHROMYCIN - THEOPHYLLINE

Description of the Interaction

Erythromycins interact with theophylline, a bronchodilator, to result in symptoms suggestive of a relative overdose of theophylline. Resulting symptoms were nausea, vomiting, and seizures.

Mechanism

A recent study showed that erythromycin forms complexes with a specific enzyme that metabolizes theophylline and that this complex may explain the impairment of theophylline metabolic inactivation resulting in symptoms of theophylline overdose[1].

Background

An erythromycin regimen of 5 to 20 day daily dosing in theophylline patients caused increased blood levels, a longer half-life and decreased urinary clearance of the theophylline[2]. A more recent review indicated that many patients did not experience any interactions between the two drugs with 8 out of 22 studies reporting no change in theophylline kinetics after erythromycin dosing[3]. The interactions which have occurred have included all formulations of erythromycin. There have been no reported interactions between erythromycin and theophylline when using the prophylaxis dosing schedule.

DENTAL DRUG INTERACTIONS: UPDATE ON DRUG COMBINATIONS REQUIRING SPECIAL CONSIDERATIONS
(Continued)

Management

Patients taking theophylline and who may be at increased risk for theophylline toxicity should be given erythromycin with caution and only if there is absolutely no alternative to erythromycin. These patients should be monitored closely.

1. Delaforge M and Sartori E, "In Vivo Effects of Erythromycin, Oleandomycin, and Erythralosamine Derivatives on Hepatic Cytochrome P-450," *Biochem Pharmacol*, 1990, 40(2):223-8.
2. Cummins LH, et al, "Erythromycin's Effect on Theophylline Blood Levels. Correspondence," *Pediatrics*, 1977, 59:144-5.
3. Ludden TM, "Pharmacokinetic Interactions of the Macrolide Antibiotics," *Clin Pharmacokinet*, 1985, 10(1):63-79.

ERYTHROMYCIN - CARBAMAZEPINE (Tegretol®)

Description of the Interaction

Erythromycin has interacted with carbamazepine (Tegretol®), an antiepileptic, to cause increased blood levels resulting in carbamazepine toxicity[1]. Symptoms were drowsiness, dizziness, nausea, headache, and blurred vision.

Mechanism

This interaction is suggestive of an inhibition of the hepatic metabolizing enzymes by erythromycin which normally convert carbamazepine to inactive products.

Background

The increased blood levels of carbamazepine has occurred within one day of concomitant erythromycin therapy[1]. This effect has not been reported with the two-dose erythromycin, prophylaxis regimen.

Management

Patients taking carbamazepine and who may be at increased risk for carbamazepine toxicity should be given erythromycin with caution and only if there is absolutely no alternative to erythromycin. These patients should be monitored closely.

1. Ludden TM, "Pharmacokinetic Interactions of the Macrolide Antibiotics," *Clin Pharmacokinet*, 1985, 10(1):63.

ERYTHROMYCIN - TRIAZOLAM (Halcion®)

Description of the Interaction

Erythromycin has interacted with triazolam (Halcion®), a hypnotic type antianxiety agent, to cause increased blood levels resulting in triazolam toxicity. Resulting effects were psychomotor impairment and memory dysfunction.

Mechanism

This interaction is suggestive of an inhibition of the hepatic metabolizing enzymes by erythromycin which normally convert triazolam to inactive products.

Background

Erythromycin has caused significant increases in triazolam blood concentrations within 3 days after 333 mg erythromycin base 3 times/day and triazolam 0.5 mg daily[1].

Management

Patients taking triazolam should be given erythromycin with caution and only if there is absolutely no alternative to erythromycin. These patients should be closely monitored.

1. Phillips JP, "A Pharmacokinetic Drug Interaction Between Erythromycin and Triazolam," *J Clin Psychopharmacol*, 1986, 6(5):297-9.

IBUPROFEN (Motrin®, Advil®, Nuprin®) - ORAL ANTICOAGULANTS (Coumarins)

Description of the Interaction

Bleeding may occur when ibuprofen is administered to patients taking coumarin type anticoagulants.

Mechanism

Inhibition of prostaglandins by ibuprofen results in decreased platelet aggregation and interference with blood clotting, resulting in an enhancement of the anticoagulant effect of coumarins.

Background

Product information on ibuprofen in the 1995 edition of the *Physicians' Desk Reference* (PDR) states that Motrin® inhibits platelet aggregation, but the effect is quantitatively less and of shorter duration than aspirin. It goes on to state that bleeding has been reported when Motrin® had been administered to patients on coumarin-type anticoagulants and the clinician should use caution in these circumstances. Additional product information on naproxen, diflunisal, and flurbiprofen is listed in the same edition of the PDR. It advises caution when using naproxen with couma-rins since interactions have been seen with other NSAIDs of this class; it states that diflunisal, when given with warfarin, resulted in prolongation of prothrombin time; and it states that serious clinical bleeding has been reported in patients taking flurbiprofen together with coumarins. Product information for warfarin (Coumadin®) in the 1995 PDR states that ibuprofen, naproxen, and diflunisal may be responsible for increased prothrombin time response of the warfarin. Flurbiprofen was not mentioned.

Management

It is suggested that ibuprofen (Motrin®, Advil®, Nuprin®) and other dental NSAIDs such as naproxen (Naprosyn®), naproxen sodium (Anaprox®, Aleve®), diflunisal (Dolobid®), flurbiprofen (ANSAID®), and ketorolac (Toradol® Oral), be used with caution (if at all) in patients taking coumarin-type anticoagulants. Use of other analgesics is preferred.

IBUPROFEN (Motrin®, Advil®, Nuprin®) - LITHIUM

Description of the Interaction

Concurrent administration of ibuprofen with lithium produces symptoms of lithium toxicity including nausea, vomiting, slurred speech, and mental confusion.

Mechanism

Prostaglandins stimulate renal lithium tubular secretion. NSAIDs inhibit prosta-glandin-induced renal secretion of lithium, which increases lithium plasma levels and produces symptoms of lithium toxicity.

Background

Lithium is used for the treatment of acute mania and to prevent recurrent episodes of bipolar (manic-depressive) illness. The therapeutic lithium plasma concentration is extremely narrow (0.8-1.2 mEq/L) and drugs that cause lithium plasma levels to go outside this narrow therapeutic range will result in lithium toxicity. Of the four NSAIDs used in dentistry (ibuprofen, naproxen, diflunisal, and flurbiprofen) the former two have been well documented to interact with lithium. In 1980, Ragheb, et al, reported that a patient taking 2400 mg ibuprofen daily experienced nausea and drowsiness while stabilized on lithium[1]. The lithium plasma level increased from 0.8 to 1.0 mEq/L. Subsequently, in a study of 11 healthy volunteers, Kristoff, et al, observed that 400 mg of ibuprofen 4 times/day combined with 450 mg of lithium carbonate every 12 hours, increased lithium plasma levels within several days[2]. Decreased ability to concentrate, lightheadedness, and fatigue resulted from this interaction.

Ragheb reported that concomitant administration of lithium and ibuprofen (1.8 g/day) in nine patients with bipolar- or schizoid-type disorders resulted in significant increases (average 34%) in lithium plasma concentrations as well as decreases in lithium clearance[3]. Individual variations were observed, with increases in lithium levels ranging from 12% to 66% within 6 days of concomitant administration of ibuprofen. In this study, tremors occurred in three patients as a result of this interaction. Ragheb reported that patients older than 50 years were more suscep-tible to lithium toxicity. The 1993 edition of the *Physician's Desk Reference* (PDR) (in the monograph for Motrin®) warns that concomitant use of ibuprofen and lithium citrate or carbonate may elevate lithium plasma levels and reduce renal lithium clearance.

In a 1986 study by Ragheb and Powell, concomitant administration of naproxen and lithium has resulted in individual variations in plasma lithium levels (from increases of 0% to 42%[4]. In that study, lithium renal clearance decreased in patients who were taking daily doses of lithium (900 mg) and naproxen (750 mg) for 6 days. The monograph for Naprosyn® in the 1993 PDR cautions that concomitant use of naproxen and lithium could increase lithium plasma concentrations.

Interactions between diflunisal (Dolobid®) and lithium, and flurbiprofen (Ansaid®) and lithium have not been reported. Nor is any potential interaction between these two NSAIDs and lithium mentioned in the PDR. Interestingly, aspirin has been shown to affect plasma lithium levels in healthy subjects[5]. Lack of documentation about diflunisal and flurbiprofen does not mean these agents are safe to use in conjunction with lithium. NSAIDs should be used with caution by dental patients who are taking lithium. Substitution of NSAIDs with acetaminophen preparations may be warranted.

Management

Extreme caution is necessary in administering NSAIDs to lithium patients; use of analgesics other than NSAIDs is preferred.

1. Ragheb M, Ban TA, Buchanan D, et al, "Interaction of Indomethacin and Ibuprofen With Lithium in Manic Patients Under a Steady-State Lithium Level," *J Clin Psychiatry*, 1980, 41(11):397-8.

DENTAL DRUG INTERACTIONS: UPDATE ON DRUG COMBINATIONS REQUIRING SPECIAL CONSIDERATIONS
(Continued)

2. Kristoff CA, Hayes PE, Barr WH, et al, "Effect of Ibuprofen on Lithium Plasma and Red Blood Cell Concentrations," *Clin Pharm*, 1986, 5(1):51-5.
3. Ragheb M, "Ibuprofen Can Increase Serum Lithium Level in Lithium-Treated Patients," *J Clin Psychiatry*, 1987, 48(4):161-3.
4. Ragheb M and Powell AL, "Lithium Interaction With Sulindac and Naproxen," *J Clin Psychopharmacol*, 1986, 6(3):150-4.
5. Reimann IW, Diener U, and Frolich JC, "Indomethacin But Not Aspirin Increases Plasma Lithium Ion Levels," *Arch Gen Psychiatry*, 1983, 40(3):283-6.

ASPIRIN - ORAL ANTICOAGULANTS (Coumarins)

Description of the Interaction

Aspirin increases the risk of bleeding in patients taking oral anticoagulants.

Mechanism

Small doses of aspirin inhibit platelet function. Larger doses (>3 g/day) elicit a hypoprothrombinemic effect. Aspirin may also displace oral anticoagulants from plasma protein-binding sites. These actions of aspirin all contribute to increase the risk of bleeding in patients taking oral anticoagulants.

Background

There is much documentation in the literature confirming this interaction. One study using over 500 patients showed that excessive bleeding was about 3 times more common with warfarin (Coumadin®) plus aspirin (500 mg/day) than with warfarin alone[1]. Another study showed enhanced hypoprothrombinemia in warfarin patients during the first few days of aspirin therapy (1 g/day)[2]. There are other reports describing bleeding episodes due to concurrent therapy with aspirin and oral anticoagulants[3,4].

Management

Patients receiving oral anticoagulants should avoid aspirin and aspirin-containing products.

1. Chesebro JH, Fuster V, Elveback LR, et al, "Trial of Combined Warfarin Therapy Plus Dipyridamole or Aspirin Therapy in Prosthetic Heart Valve Replacement: Danger of Aspirin Compared With Dipyridamole," *Am J Cardiol*, 1983, 51(9):1537-41.
2. Donaldson DR, Sreeharan N, Crow MJ, et al, "Assessment of the Interaction of Warfarin With Aspirin and Dipyridamole," *Thromb Haemost*, 1982, 47(1):77.
3. Starr KJ and Petrie JC, "Drug Interactions in Patients on Long-Term Oral Anticoagulant and Antihypertensive Adrenergic Neuron-Blocking Drugs," *Br Med J*, 1972, 4(833):133-5.
4. Udall JA, "Drug Interference With Warfarin Therapy," *Clin Med*, 1970, 77:20.

ASPIRIN - PROBENECID (Benemid®)

Description of the Interaction

Aspirin inhibits the uricosuric action of probenecid.

Mechanism

Unknown

Background

The inhibition of probenecid-induced uricosuria by aspirin is dose-dependent. Doses of aspirin of 1 g or less do not appear to affect probenecid uricosuria. Larger doses, however, appear to considerably inhibit uricosuria. Conversely, probenecid appears to inhibit uricosuria following large doses of aspirin. Aspirin does not interfere with the actions of probenecid to inhibit the renal elimination of penicillins.

Management

It appears prudent to use a nonsalicylate-type analgesic (ie, acetaminophen or NSAID) in patients receiving probenecid as a uricosuric agent (treatment of gouty arthritis).

EPINEPHRINE (Vasoconstrictor) - TRICYCLIC ANTIDEPRESSANTS

Description of the Interaction

Use of epinephrine as vasoconstrictor in local anesthetic injections may cause a hypertensive interaction in patients taking tricyclic antidepressants.

Mechanism

Tricyclic antidepressants cause increases of norepinephrine in synaptic areas in the central nervous system and periphery. Epinephrine may add to the effects of norepinephrine resulting in vasoconstriction and transient hypertension.

Background

There is adequate information in the literature to confirm a hypertensive interaction between epinephrine, norepinephrine, and levonordefrin with TCAs. An I.V. infusion of epinephrine to healthy subjects receiving imipramine resulted in two- to four-fold increases in the pressor response to epinephrine[1,2]. Also cardiac dysrhythmias were reported. Although these effects were seen with I.V. infusions, these reports suggested that caution should certainly be exercised if epinephrine is administered by other routes. I.V. infusions of norepinephrine to healthy subjects receiving imipramine resulted in a four- to eight-fold increase in the pressor response to norepinephrine[1,2] and a later study showed a two-fold increase in pressor response to norepinephrine[3]. Other tricyclics were associated with a three-fold increase in pressor response to norepinephrine[4]. This increased pressor response was probably due to tricyclic antidepressant-induced inhibition of norepinephrine reuptake. Similar effects have been reported with levonordefrin[5].

Management

The use of epinephrine in patients taking tricyclic type antidepressants is potentially dangerous. Use minimum amounts of vasoconstrictor with caution in patients on tricyclic antidepressants.

1. Boakes AJ, Laurence DR, Teoh PC, et al, "Interactions Between Sympathomimetic Amines and Antidepressant Agents in Man," *Br Med J*, 1973, 1(849):311-5.
2. Svedmyr N, "The Influence of a Tricyclic Antidepressive Agent (Protriptyline) on Some of the Circulatory Effects of Noradrenaline and Adrenaline in Man," *Life Sci*, 1968, 7(1):77-84.
3. Larochelle P, Hamet P, and Enjalbert M, "Response to Tyramine and Norepinephrine After Imipramine and Trazodone," *Clin Pharmacol Ther*, 1979, 26(1):24-30.
4. Mitchell JR, Cavanaugh JH, Arias L, et al, "Guanethidine and Related Agents. III. Antagonism by Drugs Which Inhibit the Norepinephrine Pump in Man," *J Clin Invest*, 1970, 49(8):1596-604.
5. Jastak JT and Yagiela JA, "Vasoconstrictors and Local Anesthesia: A Review and Rationale for Use," *J Am Dent Assoc*, 1983, 107(4):623-30.

EPINEPHRINE (Vasoconstrictor) - MONOAMINE OXIDASE INHIBITORS

Description of the Interaction

Use of epinephrine as vasoconstrictor in local anesthetic injections may cause a hypertensive interaction in patients taking monoamine oxidase inhibitors.

Mechanism

Drugs which inhibit monoamine oxidase cause increases in the concentration of endogenous norepinephrine, serotonin, and dopamine in storage sites throughout the central nervous system. Epinephrine may add to the effects of norepinephrine resulting in vasoconstriction and transient hypertension.

Background

One study reported on four healthy subjects taking MAOIs and given I.V. epinephrine. There was no significant effect on heart rate or blood pressure[1]. This same study also showed a lack of interaction with norepinephrine and MAOI> Nevertheless, it is advisable that vasoconstrictors be used with caution in these patients. Hansten and Horn[2] report that MAOIs may slightly increase the pressor response to norepinephrine and epinephrine, an action which appeared to be due to receptor sensitivity by the MAOI.

Management

There is a potential for unexpected increases in blood pressure when using epinephrine vasoconstrictor in patients taking monoamine oxidase inhibitors. Use vasoconstrictor with caution in these patients.

1. Boakes AJ, Laurence DR, Teoh PC, et al, "Interactions Between Sympathomimetic Amines and Antidepressant Agents in Man," *Br Med J*, 1973, 1(849):311-5.
2. Hansten PD and Horn JR, eds, "Monoamine Oxidase Inhibitor Interactions," *Drug Interactions and Updates*, Malvern, PA: Lea and Febiger, 1990, 387-8.

NARCOTIC ANALGESICS - CIMETIDINE (Tagamet®)

Description of the Interaction

Cimetidine may increase the adverse effects of narcotic analgesics.

Mechanism

The hepatic metabolism of narcotic analgesics to inactive products may be inhibited by cimetidine. The central nervous system effects of narcotic analgesics and cimetidine may be additive.

Background

One study reported that cimetidine, when given to patients taking meperidine (Demerol®), reduced the rate of renal excretion of the narcotic, resulting in increased sedation and an increase in respiratory depression[1]. Additional studies showed that cimetidine may inhibit the liver metabolism of meperidine and fentanyl, another narcotic analgesic thus exacerbating the sedative effects of both of these narcotics[2,3].

Management

Although the side effects of cimetidine on codeine, hydrocodone, and oxycodone are unknown, it is advised to use caution in prescribing these narcotic analgesics in

DENTAL DRUG INTERACTIONS: UPDATE ON DRUG COMBINATIONS REQUIRING SPECIAL CONSIDERATIONS
(Continued)

dental patients taking cimetidine. Ranitidine (Zantac®) is probably less likely to interact with narcotic analgesics.

1. Guay DR, Meatherall RC, Chalmers JL, et al, "Cimetidine Alters Pethidine Disposition in Man," *Br J Clin Pharmacol*, 1984, 18(6):907-14.
2. Knodell RG, Holtzman JL, Crankshaw DL, et al, "Drug Metabolism by Rat and Human Hepatic Microsomes in Response to Interaction With H_2-Receptor Antagonists," *Gastroenterology*, 1982, 82(1):84-8.
3. Lee HR, et al, "Effect of Histamine H_2-Receptors on Fentanyl Metabolism," *Pharmacologist*, 1982, 24:145.

BENZODIAZEPINES - Diazepam (Valium®) - ALCOHOL
Description of the Interaction

Alcohol may enhance the adverse psychomotor effects of benzodiazepines such as Valium®. Combined use may result in dangerous inebriation, ataxia, and respiratory depression.

Mechanism

Alcohol and benzodiazepines have additive central nervous system depressant activity. Also, alcohol may increase the gastrointestinal absorption of diazepam[1,2] leading to symptoms of diazepam overdose.

Background

There is much documentation in the literature to confirm the serious interaction between alcohol and benzodiazepines. Many controlled studies have shown that benzodiazepines such as diazepam enhance the detrimental effects of alcohol on simulated driving, reaction times, and other psychomotor skills[3-6].

Management

Patients receiving benzodiazepines such as diazepam (Valium®) should be warned against taking any alcohol until the benzodiazepine is cleared from the body. This is usually 48-72 hours after the last dose. This interaction has been unpredictable and significant CNS depression and ataxia has occurred with only a single dose of diazepam (5 mg) along with a moderate amount of alcohol.

1. Hayes SL, Pablo G, Radomski T, et al, "Ethanol and Oral Diazepam Absorption," *N Engl J Med*, 1977, 296(4)-186-9.
2. MacLeod SM, Giles HG, Parzalek G, et al, "Diazepam Actions and Plasma Concentrations Following Ethanol Ingestion," *Eur J Clin Pharmacol*, 1977, 11(5):345-9.
3. Linnoila M and Hakkinen S, "Effects of Diazepam and Codeine, Alone and in Combination With Alcohol, on Simulated Driving," *Clin Pharmacol Ther*, 1974, 15(4):368-73.
4. Linnoila M, "Effects of Diazepam, Chlordiazepoxide, Thioridazine, Haloperidol, Flupenthixole, and Alcohol on Psychomotor Skills Related to Driving," *Ann Med Exp Biol Fenn*, 1973, 51(3):125-32.
5. Linnoila M, "Drug Interaction on Psychomotor Skills Related to Driving: Diazepam and Alcohol," *Eur J Clin Pharmacol*, 1973, 5:186.
6. Morland J, Setekleiv J, Haffner JF, et al, "Combined Effects of Diazepam and Ethanol on Psycho-motor Functions," *Acta Pharmacol Toxicol*, 1975, 34(1):5-15.

OCCUPATIONAL EXPOSURE TO BLOODBORNE PATHOGENS (UNIVERSAL PRECAUTIONS)

OVERVIEW AND REGULATORY CONSIDERATIONS

Every healthcare employee, from nurse to housekeeper, has some (albeit small) risk of exposure to HIV and other viral agents such as hepatitis B and Jakob-Creutzfeldt agent. The incidence of HIV-1 transmission associated with a percutaneous exposure to blood from an HIV-1 infected patient is approximately 0.3% per exposure.[1] In 1989, it was estimated that 12,000 United States healthcare workers acquired hepatitis B annually.[2] An understanding of the appropriate procedures, responsibilities, and risks inherent in the collection and handling of patient specimens is necessary for safe practice and is required by Occupational Safety and Health Administration (OSHA) regulations.

The Occupational Safety and Health Administration published its "Final Rule on Occupational Exposure to Bloodborne Pathogens" in the Federal Register on December 6, 1991. OSHA has chosen to follow the Center for Disease Control (CDC) definition of universal precautions. The Final Rule provides full legal force to universal precautions and requires employers and employees to treat blood and certain body fluids as if they were infectious. The Final Rule mandates that healthcare workers must avoid parenteral contact and must avoid splattering blood or other potentially infectious material on their skin, hair, eyes, mouth, mucous membranes, or on their personal clothing. Hazard abatement strategies must be used to protect the workers. Such plans typically include, but are not limited to, the following:

- safe handling of sharp items ("sharps") and disposal of such into puncture resistant containers
- gloves required for employees handling items soiled with blood or equipment contaminated by blood or other body fluids
- provisions of protective clothing when more extensive contact with blood or body fluids may be anticipated (eg, surgery, autopsy, or deliveries)
- resuscitation equipment to reduce necessity for mouth to mouth resuscitation
- restriction of HIV- or hepatitis B-exposed employees to noninvasive procedures

OSHA has specifically defined the following terms: **Occupational exposure** means reasonably anticipated skin, eye mucous membrane, or parenteral contact with blood or other potentially infectious materials that may result from the performance of an employee's duties. **Other potentially infectious materials** are human body fluids including semen, vaginal secretions, cerebrospinal fluid, synovial fluid, pleural fluid, pericardial fluid, peritoneal fluid, amniotic fluid, saliva in dental procedures, and body fluids that are visibly contaminated with blood, and all body fluids in situations where it is difficult or impossible to differentiate between body fluids; any unfixed tissue or organ (other than intact skin) from a human (living or dead); and HIV-containing cell or tissue cultures, organ cultures, and HIV- or HBV-containing culture medium or other solutions, and blood, organs, or other tissues from experimental animals infected with HIV or HBV. An **exposure incident** involves specific eye, mouth, other mucous membrane, nonintact skin, or parenteral contact with blood or other potentially infectious materials that results from the performance of an employee's duties.[3] It is important to understand that some exposures may go unrecognized despite the strictest precautions.

A written Exposure Control Plan is required. Employers must provide copies of the plan to employees and to OSHA upon request. Compliance with OSHA rules may be accomplished by the following methods.

- **Universal precautions (UPs)** means that all human blood and certain body fluids are treated as if known to be infectious for HIV, HBV, and other bloodborne pathogens. UPs do not apply to feces, nasal secretions, saliva, sputum, sweat, tears, urine, or vomitus unless they contain visible blood.
- **Engineering controls (ECs)** are physical devices which reduce or remove hazards from the workplace by eliminating or minimizing hazards or by isolating the worker from exposure. Engineering control devices include sharps disposal containers, self-resheathing syringes, etc.
- **Work practice controls (WPCs)** are practices and procedures that reduce the likelihood of exposure to hazards by altering the way in which a task is performed. Specific examples are the prohibition of two-handed recapping of needles, prohibition of storing food alongside potentially contaminated material, discouragement of pipetting fluids by mouth, encouraging handwashing after removal of gloves, safe handling of contaminated sharps, and appropriate use of sharps containers.
- **Personal protective equipment (PPE)** is specialized clothing or equipment worn to provide protection from occupational exposure. PPE includes gloves, gowns, laboratory coats (the type and characteristics will depend upon the task and degree of exposure anticipated), face shields or masks, and eye protection. Surgical caps or hoods and/or shoe covers or boots are required in instances in which gross contamination can reasonably be anticipated (eg, autopsies, orthopedic surgery). If PPE is penetrated by blood or any contaminated material, the item must be removed immediately or as soon as feasible.

OCCUPATIONAL EXPOSURE TO BLOODBORNE PATHOGENS (UNIVERSAL PRECAUTIONS) *(Continued)*

The employer must provide and launder or dispose of all PPE at no cost to the employee. Gloves must be worn when there is a reasonable anticipation of hand contact with potentially infectious material, including a patient's mucous membranes or nonintact skin. Disposable gloves must be changed as soon as possible after they become torn or punctured. Hands must be washed after gloves are removed. OSHA has revised the PPE standards, effective July 5, 1994, to include the requirement that the employer certify in writing that it has conducted a hazard assessment of the workplace to determine whether hazards are present that will necessitate the use of PPE. Also, verification that the employee has received and understood the PPE training is required.[4]

Housekeeping protocols: OSHA requires that all bins, cans, and similar receptacles, intended for reuse which have a reasonable likelihood for becoming contaminated, be inspected and decontaminated immediately or as soon as feasible upon visible contamination and on a regularly scheduled basis. Broken glass that may be contaminated must not be picked up directly with the hands. Mechanical means (eg, brush, dust pan, tongs, or forceps) must be used. Broken glass must be placed in a proper sharps container.

Employers are responsible for teaching appropriate clean-up procedures for the work area and personal protective equipment. A 1:10 dilution of household bleach is a popular and effective disinfectant. It is prudent for employers to maintain signatures or initials of employees who have been properly educated. If one does not have written proof of education of universal precautions teaching, then by OSHA standards, such education never happened.

Pre-exposure and postexposure protocols: OSHA's Final Rule includes the provision that employees, who are exposed to contamination, be offered the hepatitis B vaccine at no cost to the employee. Employees may decline; however, a declination form must be signed. The employee must be offered free vaccine if he/she changes his/her mind. Vaccination to prevent the transmission of hepatitis B in the healthcare setting is widely regarded as sound practice.[5] In the event of exposure, a confidential medical evaluation and follow-up must be offered at no cost to the employee. Follow-up must include collection and testing of blood from the source individual for HBV and HIV if permitted by state law if a blood sample is available. If a postexposure specimen must be specially drawn, the individual's consent is usually required. Some states may not require consent for testing of patient blood after accidental exposure. One must refer to state and/or local guidelines for proper guidance.

The employee follow-up must also include appropriate postexposure prophylaxis, counseling, and evaluation of reported illnesses. The employee has the right to decline baseline blood collection and/or testing. If the employee gives consent for the collection but not the testing, the sample must be preserved for 90 days in the event that the employee changes his/her mind within that time. Confidentiality related to blood testing must be ensured. **The employer does not have the right to know the results** of the testing of either the source individual or the exposed employee.

MANAGEMENT OF OCCUPATIONAL EXPOSURE TO HIV IN THE WORKPLACE[6]

1. Likelihood of transmission of HIV-1 from occupational exposure is 0.2% per parenteral exposure (eg, needlestick) to blood from HIV infected patients.
2. Factors that increase risk for occupational transmission include advanced stages of HIV in source patient, hollow bore needle puncture, a poor state of health or inexperience of healthcare worker (HCW).
3. Immediate actions an exposed healthcare worker should take include aggressive first aid at the puncture site (eg, scrubbing site with povidone-iodine solution for 10 minutes) or at mucus membrane site (eg, saline irrigation of eye for 15 minutes). Then immediate reporting to the hospital's occupational medical service. The authors indicate that there is no direct evidence for the efficacy of their recommendations. Other institutions suggest rigorous scrubbing with soap.
4. After first aid is initiated, the healthcare worker should report exposure to a supervisor and to the institution's occupational medical service for evaluation.
5. Occupational medicine should perform a thorough investigation including identifying the HIV and hepatitis B status of the source, type of exposure, volume of inoculum, timing of exposure, extent of injury, appropriateness of first aid, as well as psychological status of the healthcare worker. HIV serologies should be performed on the healthcare worker. HIV risk counselling should begin at this point.
6. All parenteral exposures should be treated equally until they can be evaluated by the occupational medicine service, who will then determine the actual risk of exposure. Follow-up counselling sessions may be necessary.
7. Although the data are not clear, antiviral prophylaxis may be offered to healthcare workers who are parenterally or mucous membrane exposed. If used, antiretroviral prophylaxis should be initiated within 1-2 hours after exposure.
8. Counselling regarding risk of exposure, antiviral prophylaxis, plans for follow up, exposure prevention, sexual activity, and providing emotional support and

response to concerns are necessary to support the exposed healthcare worker. Follow-up should consist of periodic serologic evaluation and blood chemistries and counts if antiretroviral prophylaxis is initiated. Additional information should be provided to healthcare workers who are pregnant or planning to become pregnant.

HAZARDOUS COMMUNICATION

Communication regarding the dangers of bloodborne infections through the use of labels, signs, information, and education is required. Storage locations (eg, refrigerators and freezers, waste containers) that are used to store, dispose of, transport, or ship blood or other potentially infectious materials require labels. The label background must be red or bright orange with the biohazard design and the word biohazard in a contrasting color. The label must be part of the container or affixed to the container by permanent means.

Education provided by a qualified and knowledgeable instructor is mandated. The sessions for employees must include:

- accessible copies of the regulation
- general epidemiology of bloodborne diseases
- modes of bloodborne pathogen transmission
- an explanation of the exposure control plan and a means to obtain copies of the written plan
- an explanation of the tasks and activities that may involve exposure
- the use of exposure prevention methods and their limitations (eg, engineering controls, work practices, personal protective equipment)
- information on the types, proper use, location, removal, handling, decontamination, and disposal of personal protective equipment)
- an explanation of the basis for selection of personal protective equipment
- information on the HBV vaccine, including information on its efficacy, safety, and method of administration and the benefits of being vaccinated (ie, the employee must understand that the vaccine and vaccination will be offered free of charge)
- information on the appropriate actions to take and persons to contact in an emergency involving exposure to blood or other potentially infectious materials
- an explanation of the procedure to follow if an exposure incident occurs, including the method of reporting the incident
- information on the postexposure evaluation and follow-up that the employer is required to provide for the employee following an exposure incident
- an explanation of the signs, labels, and color coding
- an interactive question-and-answer period

RECORD KEEPING

The OSHA Final Rule requires that the employer maintain both education and medical records. The medical records must be kept confidential and be maintained for the duration of employment plus 30 years. They must contain a copy of the employee's HBV vaccination status and postexposure incident information. Education records must be maintained for 3 years from the date the program was given.

OSHA has the authority to conduct inspections without notice. Penalties for cited violation may be assessed as follows.

Serious violations. In this situation, there is a substantial probability of death or serious physical harm, and the employer knew, or should have known, of the hazard. A violation of this type carries a mandatory penalty of up to $7000 for each violation.

Other-than-serious violations. The violation is unlikely to result in death or serious physical harm. This type of violation carries a discretionary penalty of up to $7000 for each violation.

Willful violations. These are violations committed knowingly or intentionally by the employer and have penalties of up to $70,000 per violation with a minimum of $5000 per violation. If an employee dies as a result of a willful violation, the responsible party, if convicted, may receive a personal fine of up to $250,000 and/or a 6-month jail term. A corporation may be fined $500,000.

Large fines frequently follow visits to laboratories, physicians' offices, and healthcare facilities by OSHA Compliance Safety and Health Offices (CSHOS). Regulations are vigorously enforced. A working knowledge of the final rule and implementation of appropriate policies and practices is imperative for all those involved in the collection and analysis of medical specimens.

Effectiveness of universal precautions in averting exposure to potentially infectious materials has been documented.[7] Compliance with appropriate rules, procedures, and policies, including reporting exposure incidents, is a matter of personal professionalism and prudent self-preservation.

Footnotes
1. Henderson DK, Fahey BJ, Willy M, et al, "Risk for Occupational Transmission of Human Immunodeficiency Virus Type 1 (HIV-1) Associated With Clinical Exposures. A Prospective Evaluation," *Ann Intern Med*, 1990, 113(10):740-6.
2. Niu MT and Margolis HS, "Moving Into a New Era of Government Regulation: Provisions for Hepatitis B Vaccine in the Workplace, *Clin Lab Manage Rev*, 1989, 3:336-40.

OCCUPATIONAL EXPOSURE TO BLOODBORNE PATHOGENS (UNIVERSAL PRECAUTIONS) *(Continued)*

3. Bruning LM, "The Bloodborne Pathogens Final Rule — Understanding the Regulation," *AORN Journal*, 1993, 57(2):439-40.
4. "Rules and Regulations," *Federal Register*, 1994, 59(66):16360-3.
5. Schaffner W, Gardner P, and Gross PA, "Hepatitis B Immunization Strategies: Expanding the Target," *Ann Intern Med*, 1993, 118(4):308-9.
6. Fahey BJ, Beekmann SE, Schmitt JM, et al, "Managing Occupational Exposures to HIV-1 in the Health-care Workplace," *Infect Control Hosp Epidemiol*, 1993, 14(7):405-12.
7. Wong ES, Stotka JL, Chinchilli VM, et al, "Are Universal Precautions Effective in Reducing the Number of Occupational Exposures Among Healthcare Workers?" *JAMA*, 1991, 265(9):1123-8.

References

Buehler JW and Ward JW, "A New Definition for AIDS Surveillance," *Ann Intern Med*, 1993, 118(5):390-2.

Brown JW and Blackwell H, "Complying With the New OSHA Regs, Part 1: Teaching Your Staff About Biosafety," *MLO*, 1992, 24(4)24-8. Part 2: "Safety Protocols No Lab Can Ignore," 1992, 24(5):27-9. Part 3: "Compiling Employee Safety Records That Will Satisfy OSHA," 1992, 24(6):45-8.

Department of Labor, Occupational Safety and Health Administration, "Occupational Exposure to Blood-borne Pathogens; Final Rule (29 CFR Part 1910.1030), "*Federal Register*, December 6, 1991, 64004-182.

Gold JW, "HIV-1 Infection: Diagnosis and Management," *Med Clin North Am*, 1992, 76(1):1-18.

"Hepatitis B Virus: A Comprehensive Strategy for Eliminating Transmission in the United States Through Universal Childhood Vaccination," Recommendations of the Immunization Practices Advisory Committee (ACIP), *MMWR Morb Mortal Wkly Rep*, 1991, 40(RR-13):1-25.

"Mortality Attributable to HIV Infection/AIDS — United States", *MMWR Morb Mortal Wkly Rep*, 1991, 40(3):41-4.

National Committee for Clinical Laboratory Standards, "Protection of Laboratory Workers From Infectious Disease Transmitted by Blood, Body Fluids, and Tissue," NCCLS Document M29-T, Villanova, PA: NCCLS, 1989, 9(1).

"Nosocomial Transmission of Hepatitis B Virus Associated With a Spring-Loaded Fingerstick Device — California," *MMWR Morb Mortal Wkly Rep*, 1990, 39(35):610-3.

Polish LB, Shapiro CN, Bauer F, et al, "Nosocomial Transmission of Hepatitis B Virus Associated With the Use of a Spring-Loaded Fingerstick Device," *N Engl J Med*, 1992, 326(11):721-5.

"Recommendations for Preventing Transmission of Human Immunodeficiency Virus and Hepatitis B Virus to Patients During Exposure-Prone Invasive Procedures," *MMWR Morb Mortal Wkly Rep*, 1991, 40(RR-8):1-9.

"Update: Acquired Immunodeficiency Syndrome — United States," *MMWR Morb Mortal Wkly Rep*, 1992, 41(26):463-8.

"Update: Transmission of HIV Infection During an Invasive Dental Procedure — Florida," *MMWR Morb Mortal Wkly Rep*, 1991, 40(2):21-7, 33.

"Update: Universal Precautions for Prevention of Transmission of Human Immunodeficiency Virus, Hepatitis B Virus, and Other Bloodborne Pathogens in Healthcare Settings," *MMWR Morb Mortal Wkly Rep*, 1988, 37(24):377-82, 387-8.

Penicillins, Penicillin-Related Antibiotics & Other Antibiotics

KEY TO TABLE

- **A** Recommended drug therapy
- **B** Alternate drug therapy
- **C** Organism is usually or always sensitive to this agent
- **D** Organism portrays variable sensitivity to this agent
- (Blank) This drug should not be used for this organism or insufficient data is available

GRAM-POSITIVE AEROBES

Class	Drug	Listeria monocytogenes	Corynebacterium jeikeium	Corynebacterium sp.	Streptococcus, Viridans Group	Streptococcus pneumoniae	Streptococcus bovis (Group D)	Enterococcus sp. (Group D)	Streptococcus agalactiae (Group B)	Streptococcus pyogenes (Group A)	Staph. epidermidis: Methicillin-Resistant	Staph. epidermidis: Methicillin-Susceptible	Staph. aureus: Methicillin-Resistant	Staph. aureus: Methicillin-Susceptible
Penicillins	Amoxicillin				C	C	C		C	C				
Penicillins	Ampicillin	A			C	C	C	A	C	C				
Penicillins	Penicillin G	A	B	B	A	A	A	A	A	A				
Penicillins	Penicillin V				C	C	C	C	C	C				
Penicillins	Azlocillin													
Penicillins	Mezlocillin				D	C	D	D	C	C				
Penicillins	Piperacillin				D	C	D	C	C	C				
Penicillins	Ticarcillin				D	C	D		C	C				
Penicillins	Cloxacillin				D						D	A		A
Penicillins	Dicloxacillin				D						D	A		A
Penicillins	Methicillin				D						D	A		A
Penicillins	Nafcillin				D						D	A		A
Penicillins	Oxacillin				D						D	A		A
Penicillin-Related Antibiotics	Amoxicillin/Clavulanate	C			C	C	C	C	C	C		C		C
Penicillin-Related Antibiotics	Ampicillin/Sulbactam	C			C	C	C	C	C	C		C		C
Penicillin-Related Antibiotics	Ticarcillin/Clavulanate				C	C	C	D	C	C		C		C
Penicillin-Related Antibiotics	Aztreonam													
Penicillin-Related Antibiotics	Imipenem/Cilastatin				C	C	C	D	C	C		C		C
Penicillin-Related Antibiotics	Piperacillin/Tazobactam				C	C	C	C	C	C		C		C
Other Antibiotics	Chloramphenicol	C				B		D						
Other Antibiotics	Clindamycin			D	D	C	D		C	C		B		B
Other Antibiotics	Co-trimoxazole	B				C					B	C	B	C
Other Antibiotics	Metronidazole													
Other Antibiotics	Rifampin			D							A	C	A	C
Other Antibiotics	Sulfonamides													
Other Antibiotics	Tetracyclines	C			C	C			C				A	D
Other Antibiotics	Vancomycin	D	A		B	B	B	B	B	B	B	A	B	A
UTI Agents	Indanyl Carbenicillin							D						
UTI Agents	Nitrofurantoin							D						

Penicillins, Penicillin-Related Antibiotics & Other Antibiotics

KEY TO TABLE

- **A** Recommended drug therapy
- **B** Alternate drug therapy
- **C** Organism is usually or always sensitive to this agent
- **D** Organism portrays variable sensitivity to this agent
- (Blank) This drug should not be used for this organism or insufficient data is available

		GRAM-NEGATIVE AEROBES — Enteric bacilli										Cocci		
Class	Drug	Yersinia enterocolitica	Shigella sp.	Serratia sp.	Salmonella sp.	Providencia sp.	Proteus mirabilis	Klebsiella pneumoniae	Escherichia coli	Enterobacter sp.[1]	Citrobacter sp.[1]	Neisseria meningitidis	Neisseria gonorrhoeae	Moraxella (Branhamella) catarrhalis
Penicillin	Amoxicillin				B		A		C				C	D
	Ampicillin		A		B		A		A				C	D
	Penicillin G												A	D
	Penicillin V													D
	Azlocillin													
	Mezlocillin			A		B	B	C	B	C	A	A		D
	Piperacillin			A		B	B	C	B	C	A	A		D
	Ticarcillin			A		B	B	C	D	C	A	A		D
	Cloxacillin													
	Dicloxacillin													
	Methicillin													
	Nafcillin													
	Oxacillin													
Penicillin-Related Antibiotics	Amoxicillin/Clavulanate			C			C	C	C			C	C	A
	Ampicillin/Sulbactam		C	C			C	C	C			C	C	C
	Ticarcillin/Clavulanate	C	A	C	C	C	B	C	B	C	A	A	C	C
	Aztreonam	C	B	C	C	C	C	C	B	C	A	C	C	C
	Imipenem/Cilastatin	B	B	C	B	B	C	B	C	B	B	D	C	C
	Piperacillin/Tazobactam	C	A	C	B	C	B	C	B	C	A	A	C	C
Other Antibiotics	Chloramphenicol	C			B				C			B		
	Clindamycin													
	Co-trimoxazole	C	A	C	B	A	C	B	C	A	C	C		A
	Metronidazole													
	Rifampin											D		
	Sulfonamides			C	C		C	C	C			D		
	Tetracyclines	C	C					C	C	D		C	B	C
	Vancomycin													
UTI Agents	Indanyl Carbenicillin			C		C	C	C	C	C	C			
	Nitrofurantoin							C	C	C	C			

[1] *Citrobacter freundii, Citrobacter diversus, Enterobacter cloacae* and *Enterobacter aerogenes* often have significantly different antibiotic sensitivity patterns. Speciation and susceptibility testing are particularly important

Penicillins, Penicillin-Related Antibiotics & Other Antibiotics

KEY TO TABLE

- **A** Recommended drug therapy
- **B** Alternate drug therapy
- **C** Organism is usually or always sensitive to this agent
- **D** Organism portrays variable sensitivity to this agent
- (Blank) This drug should not be used for this organism or insufficient data is available

GRAM-NEGATIVE AEROBES — Other bacilli

Class	Drug	Vibrio cholerae	Xanthomonas maltophilia	Pseudomonas aeruginosa	Pasteurella multocida	Legionella pneumophila	Haemophilus influenzae	Haemophilus ducreyi	Gardnerella vaginalis	Francisella tularensis	Campylobacter jejuni	Brucella sp.	Bordetella pertussis	Alcaligenes	Acinetobacter sp.
Penicillin	Amoxicillin				C		B		C						
	Ampicillin				C		B		B		D				
	Penicillin G				A										
	Penicillin V				C										
	Azlocillin														
	Mezlocillin			A	C		D								A
	Piperacillin			A	C		D								A
	Ticarcillin			A	C		D								A
	Cloxacillin														
	Dicloxacillin														
	Methicillin														
	Nafcillin														
	Oxacillin														
Penicillin-Related Antibiotics	Amoxicillin/Clavulanate				B		B	B	C						C
	Ampicillin/Sulbactam				B		C	C	C						C
	Ticarcillin/Clavulanate		B	A	C		C								A
	Aztreonam			C			C								B
	Imipenem/Cilastatin			A			C								B
	Piperacillin/Tazobactam			A	C		C								A
Other Antibiotics	Chloramphenicol		C		C		B			A	C	C			
	Clindamycin								C		C				
	Co-trimoxazole	A	A				A	B				B	A		
	Metronidazole								A						
	Rifampin					A	D				D	A			
	Sulfonamides				C				C			C			
	Tetracyclines	A			C			C	C	B	A	C			
	Vancomycin														
UTI Agents	Indanyl Carbenicillin			D											C
	Nitrofurantoin														

(Continued)

Penicillins, Penicillin-Related Antibiotics & Other Antibiotics

KEY TO TABLE

- **A** Recommended drug therapy
- **B** Alternate drug therapy
- **C** Organism is usually or always sensitive to this agent
- **D** Organism portrays variable sensitivity to this agent
- ☐ (Blank) This drug should not be used for this organism or insufficient data is available

	Drug	Treponema pallidum	Leptospira sp.	Borrelia burgdorferi (Lyme disease)	Rickettsia sp.	Mycoplasma pneumoniae	Ureaplasma urealyticum	Chlamydia trachomatis	Chlamydia pneumoniae (TWAR)	Chlamydia psittaci	Bacteroides sp. (Gram −)	Streptococcus, anaerobic (Gram +)	Clostridium perfringens	Clostridium difficile [2]
Penicillin	Amoxicillin			B								D	C	D
	Ampicillin			B								C	C	D
	Penicillin G	A	A	B								C	A	A
	Penicillin V	C	C	B								C	C	C
	Azlocillin													
	Mezlocillin											C	C	C
	Piperacillin											C	C	C
	Ticarcillin											C	C	C
	Cloxacillin													
	Dicloxacillin													
	Methicillin													
	Nafcillin													
	Oxacillin													
Penicillin-Related Antibiotics	Amoxicillin/Clavulanate											C	C	C
	Ampicillin/Sulbactam											C	C	C
	Ticarcillin/Clavulanate											C	C	C
	Aztreonam													
	Imipenem/Cilastatin											C	C	B
	Piperacillin/Tazobactam											C	C	C
Other Antibiotics	Chloramphenicol				A						C	C	C	D
	Clindamycin										A	B	B	
	Co-trimoxazole													
	Metronidazole										A	D	A	A
	Rifampin													
	Sulfonamides							D						
	Tetracyclines	B	B	A	A	A	A	A	A	B	B	D	C	C
	Vancomycin											B		B
UTI Agents	Indanyl Carbenicillin													
	Nitrofurantoin													

[2] Vancomycin is effective orally only.

Cephalosporins, Aminoglycosides, Macrolides & Quinolones

KEY TO TABLE

- **A** Recommended drug therapy
- **B** Alternate drug therapy
- **C** Organism is usually or always sensitive to this agent
- **D** Organism portrays variable sensitivity to this agent
- (Blank) This drug should not be used for this organism or insufficient data is available

GRAM-POSITIVE AEROBES

Class	Drug	Listeria monocytogenes	Corynebacterium jeikeium	Corynebacterium sp.	Streptococcus, Viridans Group	Streptococcus pneumoniae	Streptococcus bovis (Group D)	Enterococcus sp. (Group D)	Streptococcus agalactiae (Group B)	Streptococcus pyogenes (Group A)	Staph. epidermidis: Methicillin-Susceptible	Staph. epidermidis: Methicillin-Resistant	Staph. aureus: Methicillin-Susceptible	Staph. aureus: Methicillin-Resistant
1st Generation	Cefadroxil				B	B	C		B	B	B		B	
	Cefazolin				B	B	C		B	B	B		B	
	Cephalexin				B	B	C		B	B	B		B	
	Cephalothin				B	B	C		B	B	B		B	
	Cephapirin				B	B	C		B	B	B		B	
	Cephradine				B	B	C		B	B	B		B	
2nd Generation and others	Cefaclor				C	C	C		C	C	D		D	
	Cefamandole				C	C	C		C	C	C		C	
	Cefmetazole				C	C	C		C	C	D		D	
	Cefonicid				C	C	C		C	C	D		D	
	Cefotetan				C	C	C		C	C	D		D	
	Cefoxitin				C	C	C		C	C	D		D	
	Cefpodoxime Proxetil				C	C	C		C	C	D		D	
	Cefprozil				C	C	D		C	C			D	
	Cefuroxime				C	C	C		C	C	D		D	
	Cefuroxime Axetil				C	C			C	C	C		C	
	Loracarbef				C	C	D		C	C	C		C	
3rd Generation	Cefixime				D	D			C	C				
	Cefoperazone				D	D	C		C	C	D		D	
	Cefotaxime				D	D	C		C	C	D		D	
	Ceftazidime				D		D		D	D				
	Ceftizoxime				D	D	C		C	C	D		D	
	Ceftriaxone				C	C	C		C	C	D		D	
Aminoglycosides	Amikacin	C	C				D	D						
	Gentamicin	A	B		A		D	A			A	D	A	D
	Netilmicin	C	C					C						
	Streptomycin						D	C						
	Tobramycin	C	C				D							D
Macrolides	Azithromycin	C			C	C			C	C				C
	Clarithromycin	C			C	C			C	C				C
	Erythromycin	C	C	A	C	B			B	B				C
Quinolones	Lomefloxacin		D				D	D	D	D	D	D	D	D
	Ciprofloxacin		D			D	D	D	D	D	D	D	D	D
	Norfloxacin						D	D						
	Ofloxacin		D			D	D	D	D	D	D	D	D	D

(Continued)

Cephalosporins, Aminoglycosides, Macrolides & Quinolones

KEY TO TABLE

- **A** Recommended drug therapy
- **B** Alternate drug therapy
- **C** Organism is usually or always sensitive to this agent
- **D** Organism portrays variable sensitivity to this agent
- (Blank) This drug should not be used for this organism or insufficient data is available

All organism columns below are **GRAM-NEGATIVE AEROBES**. Columns 1–11 are **Enteric bacilli**; columns 12–14 are **Cocci**.

Class	Drug	Yersinia enterocolitica	Shigella sp.	Serratia sp.	Salmonella sp.	Providencia sp.	Proteus sp.	Proteus mirabilis	Klebsiella pneumoniae	Escherichia coli	Enterobacter sp.[1]	Citrobacter sp.[1]	Neisseria meningitidis	Neisseria gonorrhoeae	Moraxella (Branhamella) catarrhalis
1st Generation	Cefadroxil								A	A	B				D
1st Generation	Cefazolin								A	A	B				D
1st Generation	Cephalexin								A	A	B				D
1st Generation	Cephalothin								A	A	B				D
1st Generation	Cephapirin								A	A	B				D
1st Generation	Cephradine								A	A	B				D
2nd Generation and others	Cefaclor								C	A	B			C	B
2nd Generation and others	Cefamandole							D	C	A	B			C	B
2nd Generation and others	Cefmetazole	D	C	C			C	D	C	A	B			C	B
2nd Generation and others	Cefonicid								C	A	B			C	B
2nd Generation and others	Cefotetan	C	C	C			C	D	C	A	B			C	B
2nd Generation and others	Cefoxitin			D			C	D	C	A	B			C	B
2nd Generation and others	Cefpodoxime Proxetil								C	A	B			C	B
2nd Generation and others	Cefprozil		C						C	D	B			C	B
2nd Generation and others	Ceftibuten														
2nd Generation and others	Cefuroxime	C	C					D	C	A	B			C	B
2nd Generation and others	Cefuroxime Axetil								C	A	B		C	C	B
2nd Generation and others	Loracarbef								C	C	B			C	B
3rd Generation	Cefepime							A							
3rd Generation	Cefixime	C	C				C	C	A	A				C	B
3rd Generation	Cefoperazone		B	A	A	A	A	C	A	A	A	A			B
3rd Generation	Cefotaxime	A	B	A	A	A	A	C	A	A	A	A	B	C	B
3rd Generation	Ceftazidime		B	A		A	A	C	A	A	A	A			B
3rd Generation	Ceftizoxime	A	B	A	A	A	A	C	A	A	A	A	B	C	B
3rd Generation	Ceftriaxone	A	B	A	A	A	A	C	A	A	A	A	B	A	B
Aminoglycosides	Amikacin	A		C		C	C	C	C	C	C	C			
Aminoglycosides	Gentamicin	A	D	C	D	D	C	C	C	C	C	C			
Aminoglycosides	Netilmicin	A	D	C	D	D	C	C	C	C	C	C			
Aminoglycosides	Streptomycin				D										
Aminoglycosides	Tobramycin	A		C	D	D	C	C	C	C	C	C			
Macrolides	Azithromycin													C	C
Macrolides	Clarithromycin													C	C
Macrolides	Dirithromycin														
Macrolides	Erythromycin													D	C
Quinolones	Lomefloxacin	C	C	C	C	C	C	C	C	C	C	D	C	C	C
Quinolones	Ciprofloxacin	C	B	C	B	C	C	C	C	C	C	C	C	A	C
Quinolones	Norfloxacin	C	C	C	C	C	C	C	C	C	C	C		C	
Quinolones	Ofloxacin	C	C	C	C	C	C	C	C	C	C	C	C	A	C

[1] Citrobacter freundii, Citrobacter diversus, Enterobacter cloacae and Enterobacter aerogenes often have significantly different antibiotic sensitivity patterns. Speciation and susceptibility testing are particularly important

Cephalosporins, Aminoglycosides, Macrolides & Quinolones

KEY TO TABLE

- **A** Recommended drug therapy
- **B** Alternate drug therapy
- **C** Organism is usually or always sensitive to this agent
- **D** Organism portrays variable sensitivity to this agent
- ☐ (Blank) This drug should not be used for this organism or insufficient data is available

GRAM-NEGATIVE AEROBES — Other bacilli

	Drug	Vibrio cholerae	Xanthomonas maltophilia	Pseudomonas aeruginosa	Pasteurella multocida	Legionella pneumophila	Haemophilus influenzae	Haemophilus ducreyi	Gardnerella vaginalis	Campylobacter jejuni	Brucella sp.	Bordetella pertussis	Acinetobacter sp.
1st Generation	Cefadroxil						D						
	Cefazolin						D						
	Cephalexin						D						
	Cephalothin						D						
	Cephapirin						D						
	Cephradine						D						
2nd Generation and others	Cefaclor						B						
	Cefamandole				C		B						
	Cefmetazole				D		C						
	Cefonicid						C						
	Cefotetan				D		C						
	Cefoxitin				D		C						
	Cefpodoxime Proxetil						B						
	Cefprozil						B						
	Cefuroxime						B						
	Cefuroxime Axetil				D		B						
	Loracarbef						B						
3rd Generation	Cefixime						A						D
	Cefoperazone		D	D	C		A	C					D
	Cefotaxime		D		C		C						A
	Ceftazidime		D	A			C						A
	Ceftizoxime		D		C		C						A
	Ceftriaxone		D		C		A						A
Aminoglycosides	Amikacin		C	A			C		C				C
	Gentamicin		C	A			C		C	C			C
	Netilmicin		C	A			C		C			C	
	Streptomycin										C		
	Tobramycin		C	A			C		C				C
Macrolides	Azithromycin				D	B	C	C		C		C	
	Clarithromycin				D	B	C			C		C	
	Erythromycin				D	A		C		A		A	
Quinolones	Lomefloxacin	C	C	D	C		C	C	D	B	C		D
	Ciprofloxacin	C	B	A	C	B	C	B	C	B	C		C
	Norfloxacin			C						B			D
	Ofloxacin	C	B	D	C	C	C	C	C	B	C		C

(Continued)

Cephalosporins, Aminoglycosides, Macrolides & Quinolones

KEY TO TABLE

A — Recommended drug therapy

B — Alternate drug therapy

C — Organism is usually or always sensitive to this agent

D — Organism portrays variable sensitivity to this agent

(Blank) — This drug should not be used for this organism or insufficient data is available

	Treponema pallidum	Leptospira sp.	Borrelia burgdorferi (Lyme disease)	Rickettsia sp.	Ureaplasma urealyticum	Mycoplasma pneumoniae	Chlamydia trachomatis	Chlamydia psittaci	Chlamydia pneumoniae (TWAR)	Bacteroides sp.	Streptococcus, anaerobic	Clostridium perfringens	Clostridium difficile [2]
1st Generation													
Cefadroxil											B		
Cefazolin											B		
Cephalexin											B		
Cephalothin											B		
Cephapirin											B		
Cephradine											B		
2nd Generation and others													
Cefaclor													
Cefamandole													
Cefmetazole										C	C	C	
Cefonicid													
Cefotetan										B	C	C	
Cefoxitin										B	C	C	
Cefpodoxime Proxetil													
Cefprozil													
Cefuroxime											C	C	
Cefuroxime Axetil													
Loracarbef													
3rd Generation													
Cefixime													
Cefoperazone												D	
Cefotaxime			C							D	C	C	
Ceftazidime												D	
Ceftizoxime			C							D	C	C	
Ceftriaxone	C	A									C		
Aminoglycosides													
Amikacin													
Gentamicin													
Netilmicin													
Streptomycin													
Tobramycin													
Macrolides													
Azithromycin	D	C		B	C	C	C	C			D	D	
Clarithromycin	D	D		B	C	C	C	C			D	D	
Erythromycin	D	C		A	A	A	A	A			D	D	
Quinolones													
Lomefloxacin						D	D	D					
Ciprofloxacin					D	D	D	D					
Norfloxacin													
Ofloxacin						D	D	D	C				

[2] Vancomycin is effective orally only.

ANTIMICROBIAL PROPHYLAXIS IN SURGICAL PATIENTS

Nature of Operation	Likely Pathogens	Recommended Drugs	Adult Dosage Before Surgery*
CLEAN			
Cardiac			
Prosthetic valve and other open-heart surgery	S. epidermidis, S. aureus, Corynebacterium, enteric gram-negative bacilli	Cefazolin or vancomycin‡	1 g I.V.
Vascular			
Arterial surgery involving the abdominal aorta, a prosthesis, or a groin incision	S. aureus, S. epidermidis, enteric gram-negative bacilli	Cefazolin or vancomycin‡	1 g I.V.
Lower extremity amputation for ischemia	S. aureus, S. epidermidis, enteric gram-negative bacilli, clostridia	Cefazolin or vancomycin‡	1 g I.V.
Neurosurgery			
Craniotomy	S. aureus, S. epidermidis	Cefazolin or vancomycin‡	1 g I.V.
Orthopedic			
Total joint replacement, internal fixation of fractures	S. aureus, S. epidermidis	Cefazolin or vancomycin‡	1 g I.V.
Ocular§	S. aureus, S. epidermidis, streptococci, enteric gram-negative bacilli, Pseudomonas	Gentamicin or tobramycin or combination of neomycin, gramicidin, and polymyxin B,	Multiple drops topically over 2-24 h
		cefazolin	100 mg subconjunctivally at end of procedure
CLEAN-CONTAMINATED			
Head and neck			
Entering oral cavity or pharynx	S. aureus, streptococci, oral anaerobes	Cefazolin or	2 g I.V.¶
		clindamycin	600 mg I.V.
Gastroduodenal			
High risk, gastric bypass, or percutaneous endoscopic gastrostomy only	Enteric gram-negative bacilli, gram-positive cocci	Cefazolin	1 g I.V.
Biliary tract			
High risk only	Enteric gram-negative bacilli, enterococci, clostridia	Cefazolin	1 g I.V.
Colorectal	Enteric gram-negative bacilli, anaerobes	Oral:	
		Neomycin plus erythromycin base	1 g of each at 1 PM, 2 PM, and 11 PM the day before the operation#
		Parenteral: Cefoxitin or	1 g I.V.¶
		cefotetan	1 g I.V.
Appendectomy	Enteric gram-negative bacilli, anaerobes	Cefoxitin or	1 g I.V.¶
		cefotetan	1 g I.V.
Vaginal or abdominal hysterectomy	Enteric gram-negative bacilli, anaerobes, group B streptococci, enterococci	Cefazolin or Cefoxitin or	1 g I.V.¶
		cefotetan	1 g I.V.
Cesarean section	Same as for hysterectomy	High risk only: Cefazolin	1 g I.V. after cord clamping
Abortion	Same as for hysterectomy	First trimester in patients with previous pelvic inflammatory disease:	

ANTIMICROBIAL PROPHYLAXIS IN SURGICAL PATIENTS
(Continued)

Nature of Operation	Likely Pathogens	Recommended Drugs	Adult Dosage Before Surgery*
		Aqueous penicillin G or	1 million units I.V.
		doxycycline	100 mg P.O. 1 hour before abortion, then 200 mg P.O. 30 minutes after abortion
		Second trimester: Cefazolin	1 g I.V.
DIRTY			
Ruptured viscus	Enteric gram-negative bacilli, anaerobes, enterococci	Cefoxitin or clindamycin plus gentamicin	1 g I.V.
		cefotetan with or without gentamicin or	1 g I.V. 1.5 mg/kg q8h I.V.
		clindamycin plus gentamicin	600 mg I.V. q6h 1.5 mg/kg q8h I.V.
Traumatic wound•	*S. aureus*, group A streptococci, clostridia	Cefazolin	1 g q8h I.V.

*Parenteral prophylactic antimicrobials for clean and clean-contaminated surgery can be given as a single intravenous dose just before the operation. Cefazolin can also be given intramuscularly. For prolonged operations, additional intraoperative doses should be given every 4-8 hours for the duration of the procedure. For "dirty" surgery, therapy should usually be continued for 5-10 days.

‡For hospitals in which methicillin-resistant *S. aureus* and *S. epidermidis* frequently cause wound infection, or for patients allergic to penicillins or cephalosporin.

§In addition, at the end of the operation many ophthalmologists give a subconjunctival injection of an aminoglycoside such as gentamicin (10-20 mg), with or without a cephalosporin such as cefazolin (100 mg).

¶In controlled studies, 2 g were effective, while 0.5 g was not (JT Johnson and VL Yu, *Ann Surg*, 1988, 207:108).

#After appropriate diet and catharsis.

•For bite wounds, in which likely pathogens may also include oral anaerobes, *Eikenella corrodens* (humans), and *Pasteurella multocida* (dog and cat), some *Medical Letter* consultants recommend use of amoxicillin-clavulanic acid (Augmentin®) or ampicillin/sulbactam (Unasyn®).

ORGANISMS ISOLATED IN HEAD & NECK INFECTIONS

Organisms	Percentage Infections
Alpha hemolytic streptococci	41
Staphylococci aureas	27
Staphylococci epidermidis	23
Bacteroides sp	17
Streptococcus intermedius	7
Klebsiella pneumoniae	7
Beta hemolytic streptococci	7
Non-A, Non-B, Non-D	7
Group A	7
Group B	5
Peptostreptococcus sp	6
Fungi	6
Mycobacteria tuberculosis	6
Actinobacter	5
Other anaerobic gram-negative rods	5
Proteus	3
Enterobacter	3
Anaerobic gram-negative cocci	3
Neisseria	3
Bacillus sp	3
Actinomyces	3
Other Klebsiella sp	3
Streptococcus pneumoniae	3
Bifidobacterium	3
Microaerophilic streptococci	3
Propionibacterium sp	3
Pseudomonas	1
Escherichia coli	1

PREDOMINANT CULTIVABLE MICROORGANISMS OF THE ORAL CAVITY

Type	Predominant Genus or Family
Aerobic or Facultative	
Gram-positive cocci	*Streptococcus* sp
	S. mutans
	S. sanguis
	S. mitior
	S. salivarius
Gram-positive rods	*Lactobacillus* sp
	Corynebacterium sp
Gram-negative cocci	*Moraxella* sp
Gram-negative rods	*Enterobacteriaceae* sp
Anaerobic	
Gram-positive cocci	*Peptostreptococcus* sp
Gram-positive rods	*Actinomyces* sp
	Eubacterium sp
	Lactobacillus sp
	Leptotrichia sp
Gram-negative cocci	*Veillonella* sp
Gram-negative rods	*Actinobacillus* sp
	Fusobacterium sp
	Prevotella sp
	Porphyromonas sp
	Bacteroides sp
	Campylobacter sp
Spirochetes	*Treponema* sp
Fungi	*Candida* sp

REFERENCE VALUES FOR ADULTS

Automated Chemistry (CHEMISTRY A)

Test	Values	Remarks
SERUM PLASMA		
Acetone	Negative	
Albumin	3.2-5 g/dL	
Alcohol, ethyl	Negative	
Aldolase	1.2-7.6 IU/L	
Ammonia	20-70 mcg/dL	Specimen to be placed on ice as soon as collected
Amylase	30-110 units/L	
Bilirubin, direct	0-0.3 mg/dL	
Bilirubin, total	0.1-1.2 mg/dL	
Calcium	8.6-10.3 mg/dL	
Calcium, ionized	2.24-2.46 mEq/L	
Chloride	95-108 mEq/L	
Cholesterol, total	$\leq$220 mg/dL	Fasted blood required – normal value affected by dietary habits. This reference range is for a general adult population
HDL cholesterol	40-60 mg/dL	Fasted blood required – normal value affected by dietary habits
LDL cholesterol	65-170 mg/dL	LDLC calculated by Friewald formula... which has certain inaccuracies and is invalid at trig levels >300 mg/dL
CO_2	23-30 mEq/L	
Creatine kinase (CK) isoenzymes		
CK-BB	0%	
CK-MB	0%-3.9%	
CK-MM	96%-100%	
CK-MB levels must be both $\geq$4% and 10 IU/L to meet diagnostic criteria for CK-MB positive result consistent with myocardial injury.		
Creatine phosphokinase (CPK)	8-150 IU/L	
Creatinine	0.5-1.4 mg/dL	
Ferritin	13-300 ng/mL	
Folate	3.6-20 ng/dL	
GGT (gamma-glutamyltranspeptidase)		
male	11-63 IU/L	
female	8-35 IU/L	
GLDH	To be determined	
Glucose (2-h postprandial)	Up to 140 mg/dL	
Glucose, fasting	60-110 mg/dL	
Glucose, nonfasting (2-h postprandial)	60-140 mg/dL	
Hemoglobin A_{1c}	8	
Hemoglobin, plasma free	<2.5 mg/100 mL	
Hemoglobin, total glycosolated (Hb A_1)	4%-8%	
Iron	65-150 mcg/dL	
Iron binding capacity, total (TIBC)	250-420 mcg/dL	
Lactic acid	0.7-2.1 mEq/L	Specimen to be kept on ice and sent to lab as soon as possible
Lactate dehydrogenase (LDH)	56-194 IU/L	
Lactate dehydrogenase (LDH) isoenzymes		
LD_1	20%-34%	
LD_2	29%-41%	
LD_3	15%-25%	
LD_4	1%-12%	
LD_5	1%-15%	

REFERENCE VALUES FOR ADULTS (Continued)

Automated Chemistry (CHEMISTRY A) (continued)

Test	Values	Remarks
Flipped LD$_1$/LD$_2$ ratios (>1 may be consistent with myocardial injury) particularly when considered in combination with a recent CK-MB positive result		
Lipase	23-208 units/L	
Magnesium	1.6-2.5 mg/dL	Increased by slight hemolysis
Osmolality	289-308 mOsm/kg	
Phosphatase, alkaline		
adults 25-60 y	33-131 IU/L	
adults 61 y or older	51-153 IU/L	
infancy-adolescence	Values range up to 3-5 times higher than adults	
Phosphate, inorganic	2.8-4.2 mg/dL	
Potassium	3.5-5.2 mEq/L	Increased by slight hemolysis
Prealbumin	>15 mg/dL	
Protein, total	6.5-7.9 g/dL	
SGOT (AST)	<35 IU/L	
SGPT (ALT)	<35 IU/L	
Sodium	134-149 mEq/L	
Transferrin	>200 mg/dL	
Triglycerides	45-155 mg/dL	Fasted blood required
Urea nitrogen (BUN)	7-20 mg/dL	
Uric acid		
male	2.0-8.0 mg/dL	
female	2.0-7.5 mg/dL	

CEREBROSPINAL FLUID

Glucose	50-70 mg/dL	
Protein		
adults and children	15-45 mg/dL	CSF obtained by lumbar puncture
newborn infants	60-90 mg/dL	

On CSF obtained by cisternal puncture: About 25 mg/dL
On CSF obtained by ventricular puncture: About 10 mg/dL

Note: Bloody specimen gives erroneously high value due to contamination with blood proteins

URINE
(24-hour specimen is required for all these tests unless specified)

Amylase	32-641 units/L	The value is in units/L and not calculated for total volume
Amylase, fluid (random samples)		Interpretation of value left for physician, depends on the nature of fluid
Calcium	Depends upon dietary intake	
Creatine		
male	150 mg/24 h	Higher value on children and during pregnancy
female	250 mg/24 h	
Creatinine	1000-2000 mg/24 h	
Creatinine clearance (endogenous)		
male	85-125 mL/min	A blood sample must accompany urine specimen
female	75-115 mL/min	
Glucose	1 g/24 h	
5-hydroxyindoleacetic acid	2-8 mg/24 h	
Iron	0.15 mg/24 h	Acid washed container required
Magnesium	146-209 mg/24 h	
Osmolality	500-800 mOsm/kg	With normal fluid intake
Oxalate	10-40 mg/24 h	
Phosphate	400-1300 mg/24 h	

Automated Chemistry (CHEMISTRY A) *(continued)*

Test	Values	Remarks
Potassium	25-120 mEq/24 h	Varies with diet; the interpretation of urine electrolytes and osmolality should be left for the physician
Sodium	40-220 mEq/24 h	
Porphobilinogen, qualitative	Negative	
Porphyrins, qualitative	Negative	
Proteins	0.05-0.1 g/24 h	
Salicylate	Negative	
Urea clearance	60-95 mL/min	A blood sample must accompany specimen
Urea N	10-40 g/24 h	Dependent on protein intake
Uric acid	250-750 mg/24 h	Dependent on diet and therapy
Urobilinogen	0.5-3.5 mg/24 h	For qualitative determination on random urine, send sample to urinalysis section in Hematology Lab
Xylose absorption test		
children	16%-33% of ingested xylose	
adults	>4 g in 5 h	
FECES		
Fat, 3-day collection	<5 g/d	Value depends on fat intake of 100 g/d for 3 days preceding and during collection
GASTRIC ACIDITY		
Acidity, total, 12 h	10-60 mEq/L	Titrated at pH 7

BLOOD GASES

	Arterial	Capillary	Venous
pH	7.35-7.45	7.35-7.45	7.32-7.42
pCO_2 (mm Hg)	35-45	35-45	38-52
pO_2 (mm Hg)	70-100	60-80	24-48
HCO_3 (mEq/L)	19-25	19-25	19-25
TCO_2 (mEq/L)	19-29	19-29	23-33
O_2 saturation (%)	90-95	90-95	40-70
Base excess (mEq/L)	-5 to +5	-5 to +5	-5 to +5

REFERENCE VALUES FOR ADULTS (Continued)

HEMATOLOGY
Complete Blood Count

Age	Hgb (g/dL)	Hct (%)	RBC (mill/mm³)	RDW
0-3 d	15.0-20.0	45-61	4.0-5.9	<18
1-2 wk	12.5-18.5	39-57	3.6-5.5	<17
1-6 mo	10.0-13.0	29-42	3.1-4.3	<16.5
7 mo to 2 y	10.5-13.0	33-38	3.7-4.9	<16
2-5 y	11.5-13.0	34-39	3.9-5.0	<15
5-8 y	11.5-14.5	35-42	4.0-4.9	<15
13-18 y	12.0-15.2	36-47	4.5-5.1	<14.5
Adult male	13.5-16.5	41-50	4.5-5.5	<14.5
Adult female	12.0-15.0	36-44	4.0-4.9	<14.5

Age	MCV (fL)	MCH (pg)	MCHC (%)	PLTS (x 10³/mm³)
0-3 d	95-115	31-37	29-37	250-450
1-2 wk	86-110	28-36	28-38	250-450
1-6 mo	74-96	25-35	30-36	300-700
7 mo to 2 y	70-84	23-30	31-37	250-600
2-5 y	75-87	24-30	31-37	250-550
5-8 y	77-95	25-33	31-37	250-550
13-18 y	78-96	25-35	31-37	150-450
Adult male	80-100	26-34	31-37	150-450
Adult female	80-100	26-34	31-37	150-450

WBC and Diff

Age	WBC (x 10³/mm³)	Segs	Bands	Lymphs	Monos
0-3 d	9.0-35.0	32-62	10-18	19-29	5-7
1-2 wk	5.0-20.0	14-34	6-14	36-45	6-10
1-6 mo	6.0-17.5	13-33	4-12	41-71	4-7
7 mo to 2 y	6.0-17.0	15-35	5-11	45-76	3-6
2-5 y	5.5-15.5	23-45	5-11	35-65	3-6
5-8 y	5.0-14.5	32-54	5-11	28-48	3-6
13-18 y	4.5-13.0	34-64	5-11	25-45	3-6
Adults	4.5-11.0	35-66	5-11	24-44	3-6

Age	Eosinophils	Basophils	Atypical Lymphs	No. of NRBCs
0-3 d	0-2	0-1	0-8	0-2
1-2 wk	0-2	0-1	0-8	0
1-6 mo	0-3	0-1	0-8	0
7 mo to 2 y	0-3	0-1	0-8	0
2-5 y	0-3	0-1	0-8	0
5-8 y	0-3	0-1	0-8	0
13-18 y	0-3	0-1	0-8	0
Adults	0-3	0-1	0-8	0

Segs = segmented neutrophils
Bands = band neutrophils

Lymps = lymphocytes
Monos = monocytes

Erythrocyte Sedimentation Rates and Reticulocyte Counts

Sedimentation rate, Westergren	Children	0-20 mm/hour
	Adult male	0-15 mm/hour
	Adult female	0-20 mm/hour
Sedimentation rate, Wintrobe	Children	0-13 mm/hour
	Adult male	0-10 mm/hour
	Adult female	0-15 mm/hour
Reticulocyte count	Newborns	2%-6%
	1-6 mo	0%-2.8%
	Adults	0.5%-1.5%

ARTIFICIAL SALIVA PRODUCTS

Product	Dosage Form	Ingredients
Glandosane	Spray	Sodium carboxymethylcellulose, sorbitol, sodium chloride, potassium chloride, calcium chloride dihydrate, magnesium chloride hexahydrate, dipotassium hydrogen phosphate
Moi-Stir 10[a]	Pump spray	Sodium carboxymethylcellulose, potassium chloride, dibasic sodium phosphate, methylparaben, propylparaben
Moi-Stir Mouth Moistening	Pump spray	Carboxymethylcellulose
Moi-Stir Oral Swabsticks[a]	Swab	Carboxymethylcellulose
MouthKote	Spray	Water, xylitol, sorbitol, yerba santa, citric acid, flavor, ascorbic acid, sodium benzoate, sodium saccharin
Optimoist	Liquid	Citric acid, calcium phosphate, sodium monofluorophosphate, preservative, sweetener, xylitol, polysorbate 20, flavor, hydroxyethylcellulose, sodium hydroxide
Saliva Substitute[a]	Spray	Sorbitol, sodium carboxymethylcellulose, methylparaben
Salivart Synthetic Saliva[a]	Aerosol spray	Sorbitol 3%, sodium carboxymethylcellulose 1%, potassium chloride 0.12%, sodium chloride 0.084%, calcium chloride dihydrate, magnesium chloride hexahydrate, potassium phosphate dibasic, nitrogen (as propellant)

[a]Carries American Dental Association (ADA) seal indicating safety and efficacy.

Reprinted with permission from *Handbook of Nonprescription Drugs*, 10th ed, *Product Updates*, Washington, DC, American Pharmaceutical Association, 1995, 272.

DENTIFRICE PRODUCTS

Product	Abrasive Ingredient	Therapeutic Ingredient	Foaming Agent
Aim AntiTartar Gel Formula with Fluoride	Hydrated silica	Sodium monofluorophosphate 0.79% (fluoride 0.15%)	Sodium lauryl sulfate
	Other Ingredients: Sorbitol and related polyols, water, glycerin, zinc citrate trihydrate, SD alcohol 38B, flavor, cellulose gum, sodium saccharin, sodium benzoate, blue #1, yellow #10		
Aim Baking Soda Gel with Fluoride	Hydrated silica	Sodium monofluorophosphate 0.79% (fluoride 0.15%)	Sodium lauryl sulfate
	Other Ingredients: Sorbitol and related polyols, water, glycerin, SD alcohol 38B, flavor, sodium bicarbonate, cellulose gum, sodium saccharin, sodium benzoate, blue #1, yellow #10		
Aim Regular Strength Gel with Fluoride	Hydrated silica	Sodium monofluorophosphate 0.79% (fluoride 0.15%)	Sodium lauryl sulfate
	Other Ingredients: Sorbitol and other related polyols, water, glycerin, SD alcohol 38B, flavor, cellulose gum, sodium saccharin, sodium benzoate, blue #1, yellow #10		
Aquafresh Baking Soda Toothpaste	Calcium carbonate, hydrated silica	Sodium monofluorophosphate	Sodium lauryl sulfate
	Other Ingredients: Calcium carrageenan, cellulose gum, colors, flavor, glycerin, PEG-8, sodium benzoate, sodium bicarbonate, sodium saccharin, sorbitol, titanium dioxide, water		
Aquafresh Extra Fresh Toothpaste[a]	Hydrated silica, calcium carbonate	Sodium monofluorophosphate	Sodium lauryl sulfate
	Other Ingredients: Sorbitol, water, glycerin, PEG-8, titanium dioxide, cellulose gum, flavor, sodium saccharin, sodium benzoate, calcium carrageenan, colors		
Aquafresh for Kids Toothpaste[a]	Hydrated silica, calcium carbonate	Sodium monofluorophosphate	Sodium lauryl sulfate
	Other Ingredients: Sorbitol, water, glycerin, PEG-8, titanium dioxide, cellulose gum, flavor, sodium saccharin, calcium carrageenan, sodium benzoate, colors		
Aquafresh Sensitive Toothpaste	Hydrated silica	Potassium nitrate, sodium fluoride	Sodium lauryl sulfate
	Other Ingredients: Colors, flavors, glycerin, sodium benzoate, sodium saccharin, sorbitol, titanium dioxide, water, xanthan gum		
Aquafresh Tartar Control Toothpaste[a]	Hydrated silica	Sodium fluoride	Sodium lauryl sulfate
	Other Ingredients: Tetrapotassium, pyrophosphate, tetrasodium pyrophosphate, sorbitol, glycerin, PEG-8, flavor, xanthan gum, sodium saccharin, sodium benzoate, D&C red #30 lake, FD&C blue #1, D&C yellow #10, titanium dioxide, water		
Aquafresh Triple Protection Toothpaste[a]	Hydrated silica, calcium carbonate	Sodium monofluorophosphate	Sodium lauryl sulfate
	Other Ingredients: PEG-8, sorbitol, cellulose gum, sodium benzoate, titanium dioxide, calcium, carrageenan, flavor, sodium saccharin, colors, water		
Aquafresh Whitening Toothpaste	Hydrated silica	Sodium fluoride	Sodium lauryl sulfate
	Other Ingredients: D&C yellow #10, FD&C blue #1, flavor, glycerin, PEG-8, sodium benzoate, sodium hydroxide, sodium saccharin, sodium tripolyphosphate, sorbitol, titanium dioxide, water, xanthan gum		
Arm & Hammer Dental Care Baking Soda Tartar Control Toothpaste	Sodium bicarbonate	Sodium fluoride	Sodium lauryl sulfate
	Other Ingredients: Water, glycerin, sodium pyrophosphates, sodium saccharin, PEG-8, flavor blend, sodium phosphates, cellulose gum, sodium lauroyl sarcosinate		

Product	Abrasive Ingredient	Therapeutic Ingredient	Foaming Agent
Arm & Hammer Dental Care Baking Soda Gel	Hydrated silica, sodium bicarbonate	Sodium fluoride	Sodium lauryl sulfate
	Other Ingredients: Sorbitol, water, glycerin, PEG-8, flavor blend, cellulose gum, sodium lauroyl sarcosinate, sodium saccharin, FD&C blue #1, D&C yellow #10		
Arm & Hammer Dental Care Baking Soda Tartar Control Gel	Sodium bicarbonate, hydrated silica	Sodium fluoride	Sodium lauryl sulfate
	Other Ingredients: Water, sorbitol, glycerin, sodium pyrophosphates, PEG-8, flavor, cellulose gum, sodium saccharin, sodium lauroyl sarcosinate, FD&C blue #1, D&C yellow #10		
Arm & Hammer Dental Care Baking Soda Tooth Powder	Sodium bicarbonate	Sodium fluoride	
	Other Ingredients: Mint flavor, sodium saccharin, trisodium saccharin, trisodium magnesium oxide, PEG-8		
Arm & Hammer Dental Care Baking Soda Toothpaste	Sodium bicarbonate	Sodium fluoride	Sodium lauryl sulfate
	Other Ingredients: Water, glycerin, sodium saccharin, PEG-8, flavor blend, cellulose gum, sodium lauroyl sarcosinate		
Arm & Hammer PerioxiCare Toothpaste	Sodium bicarbonate, silica	Sodium fluoride	Sodium carbonate peroxide, sodium lauryl sulfate
	Other Ingredients: PEG-8, poloxamer 338, flavor, water, sodium saccharin, sodium lauroyl sarconsinate		
Caffree Anti-Stain Fluoride Toothpaste[a]		Sodium monofluorophosphate	Sodium lauryl sulfate
	Other Ingredients: Water, diatomaceous earth, glycerin, sorbitol, aluminum silicate, titanium dioxide, hydroxyethylcellulose, flavor, sodium saccharin, methylparaben, propylparaben		
Close-Up Anti-Plaque Gel	Hydrated silica	Stannous fluoride 0.41%	Sodium lauryl sulfate
	Other Ingredients: Sorbitol, water, PEG-32, SD alcohol 38B, flavor, zinc citrate trihydrate, cellulose gum, sodium saccharin, sodium benzoate, sodium hydroxide, blue #1		
Close-Up Crystal Clear Mint Gel	Hydrated silica	Sodium monofluorophosphate 0.79% (fluoride 0.15%)	Sodium lauryl sulfate
	Other Ingredients: Sorbitol, water, glycerin, SD alcohol 38B, flavor, cellulose gum, sodium saccharin, polysorbate 20, sodium benzoate, sodium chloride, blue #1, mica, red #33, titanium dioxide		
Close-Up Original Gel	Hydrated silica	Sodium monofluorophosphate 0.79% (fluoride 0.15%)	Sodium lauryl sulfate
	Other Ingredients: Sorbitol, water, glycerin, SD alcohol 38B, flavor, cellulose gum, sodium saccharin, sodium benzoate, sodium chloride, red #33, red #40		
Close-Up Tartar Control Gel	Hydrated silica	Sodium monofluorophosphate 0.79% (fluoride 0.15%)	Sodium lauryl sulfate
	Other Ingredients: Sorbitol and related polyols, water, glycerin, zinc citrate trihydrate, SD alcohol 38B, flavor, cellulose gum, sodium saccharin, sodium benzoate, sodium chloride, red #33, red #40		
Close-Up with Baking Soda Toothpaste	Hydrated silica	Sodium monofluorophosphate 0.79% (fluoride 0.15%)	Sodium lauryl sulfate

DENTIFRICE PRODUCTS *(Continued)*

Product	Abrasive Ingredient	Therapeutic Ingredient	Foaming Agent
	Other Ingredients: Sorbitol and related polyols, water, glycerin, SD alcohol 38B, flavor, sodium bicarbonate, cellulose gum, sodium saccharin, sodium benzoate, red #33, red #40, titanium dioxide		
Colgate Baking Soda Gel[a]	Hydrated silica	Sodium fluoride 0.243%	Sodium lauryl sulfate
	Other Ingredients: Glycerin, PEG-12, cellulose gum, flavor, sodium saccharin, FD&C blue #1, D&C yellow #10		
Colgate Baking Soda Tartar Control Gel or Toothpaste	Hydrated silica, sodium bicarbonate	Sodium fluoride 0.243%	Sodium lauryl sulfate
	Other Ingredients: Glycerin, tetrasodium pyrophosphate, PVM/MA copolymer, cellulose gum, flavor, sodium saccharin, sodium hydroxide, titanium dioxide (paste), FD&C blue #1, D& C yellow #10 (gel)		
Colgate Baking Soda Toothpaste[a]	Hydrated silica, sodium bicarbonate	Sodium fluoride 0.243%	Sodium lauryl sulfate
	Other Ingredients: Glycerin, cellulose gum, flavor, sodium saccharin, titanium dioxide		
Colgate Junior Gel[a]	Hydrated silica	Sodium fluoride 0.243%	Sodium lauryl sulfate
	Other Ingredients: Sorbitol, PEG-12, flavor, tetrasodium pyrophosphate, cellulose gum, sodium saccharin, mica, titanium dioxide, FD&C blue #1, D&C yellow #10		
Colgate Micro Cleansing Tartar Control Gel or Toothpaste[a]	Synthetic amorphous silica 27%, hydrated amorphous silica 3%	Sodium fluoride 0.243%	Sodium lauryl sulfate
	Other Ingredients: Water, sorbitol, glycerin, PEG-12, tetrasodium pyrophosphate, PVM/MA copolymer, cellulose gum, flavor, sodium hydroxide, titanium dioxide (Paste), sodium saccharin, carrageenan, FD&C blue #1 (gel)		
Colgate Peak Toothpaste	Hydrated silica, sodium bicarbonate, precipitated calcium carbonate		Sodium lauryl sulfate
	Other Ingredients: Glycerin, cellulose gum, flavor, sodium saccharin, titanium dioxide, sodium benzoate		
Colgate Toothpaste[a]	Dicalcium phosphate dihydrate	Sodium monofluorophosphate 0.76%	Sodium lauryl sulfate
	Other Ingredients: Glycerin, cellulose gum, tetrasodium pyrophosphate, sodium saccharin, flavor		
Colgate Winterfresh Gel[a]	Hydrated silica	Sodium fluoride 0.243%	Sodium lauryl sulfate
	Other Ingredients: Sorbitol, glycerin, PEG-12, flavor, tetrasodium pyrophosphate, cellulose gum, sodium saccharin, FD&C blue #1		
Crest Baking Soda Gel or Toothpaste[a] (mint)	Hydrated silica	Sodium fluoride	Sodium lauryl sulfate
	Other Ingredients: Sorbitol, water, sodium bicarbonate, glycerin, sodium carbonate, flavor, cellulose gum, sodium saccharin, titanium dioxide (paste), FD&C blue #1 (gel)		
Crest Baking Soda Tartar Control Gel or Toothpaste[a] (mint)	Hydrated silica	Sodium fluoride	Sodium lauryl sulfate
	Other Ingredients: Water, sodium bicarbonate, glycerin, sorbitol, tetrasodium pyrophosphate, PEG-6, sodium carbonate, flavor, cellulose gum, sodium saccharin, titanium dioxide (paste), FD&C blue #1 (gel)		
Crest Cavity Fighting Gel[a] (cool mint)	Hydrated silica	Sodium fluoride	Sodium lauryl sulfate

Product	Abrasive Ingredient	Therapeutic Ingredient	Foaming Agent
	Other Ingredients: Sorbitol, water, trisodium phosphate, flavor, sodium phosphate, xanthan gum, sodium saccharin, carbomer 956, FD&C blue #1		
Crest Cavity Fighting Toothpaste[a] (icy mint or regular flavor)	Hydrated silica	Sodium fluoride	Sodium lauryl sulfate
	Other Ingredients: Sorbitol, water, glycerin, mint, trisodium phosphate, flavor, sodium phosphate, cellulose gum (mint), xanthan gum (regular), sodium saccharin, carbomer 956, titanium dioxide, FD&C blue #1		
Crest for Kids, Sparkle Fun Gel[a]	Hydrated silica	Sodium fluoride	Sodium lauryl sulfate
	Other Ingredients: Sorbitol, water, trisodium phosphate, sodium phosphate, xanthan gum, flavor, sodium saccharin, carbomer 956, mica, titanium dioxide, FD&C blue #1		
Crest Sensitivity Protection Toothpaste[a] (mild mint)	Hydrated silica	Potassium nitrate, sodium fluoride	Sodium lauryl sulfate
	Other Ingredients: Water, glycerin, sorbitol, trisodium phosphate, cellulose gum, flavor, xanthan gum, sodium saccharin, titanium dioxide		
Crest Tartar Control Gel[a] (fresh mint or smooth mint)	Hydrated silica	Sodium fluoride	Sodium lauryl sulfate
	Other Ingredients: Water, sorbitol, glycerin, tetrapotassium pyrophosphate, PEG-6, disodium pyrophosphate, tetrasodium pyrophosphate, flavor, xanthan gum, sodium saccharin, carbomer 956, FD&C blue #1, (fresh mint & smooth mint), FD&C yellow #5 (smooth mint)		
Crest Tartar Control Toothpaste[a] (original flavor)	Hydrated silica	Sodium fluoride	Sodium lauryl sulfate
	Other Ingredients: Water, sorbitol, glycerin, tetrapotassium pyrophosphate, PEG-6, disodium pyrophosphate, tetrasodium pyrophosphate, flavor, xanthan gum, sodium saccharin, carbomer 956, titanium dioxide, FD&C blue #1		
Dentagard Toothpaste[a]	Hydrated silica	Sodium monofluorophosphate 0.76%	Sodium lauryl sulfate
	Other Ingredients: Sorbitol, glycerin, PEG-12, flavor, sodium benzoate, titanium dioxide, cellulose gum, sodium saccharin, FD&C red #40		
Gleem Toothpaste	Hydrated silica	Sodium fluoride	Sodium lauryl sulfate
	Other Ingredients: Sorbitol, water, trisodium phosphate, flavor, sodium phosphate, xanthan gum, sodium saccharin, carbomer 956, titanium dioxide		
Interplak Toothpaste with Fluoride	Hydrated silica	Sodium fluoride	Sodium lauryl sulfate
	Other Ingredients: Purified water, poloxamer 407, sorbitol, glycerin, flavor, dibasic sodium phosphate, sodium saccharin, monobasic sodium phosphate, sodium benzoate, D&C yellow #10		
Mentadent Fluoride Toothpaste with Baking Soda & Peroxide[a]	Hydrated silica, sodium bicarbonate	Sodium fluoride 0.24% (fluoride 0.15%)	Sodium lauryl sulfate, hydrogen peroxide
	Other Ingredients: Water, sorbitol, glycerin, poloxamer 407, PEG-32, SD alcohol 38B, flavor, cellulose gum, sodium saccharin, phosphoric acid, blue #1, titanium dioxide		
Oral-B Sensitive Toothpaste with Fluoride	Hydrated silica	Potassium nitrate 5%, sodium fluoride 0.225%	Sodium lauryl sulfate
	Other Ingredients: Water, glycerin, cellulose gum, PEG-8, sodium saccharin, methylparaben, propylparaben, flavor		

DENTIFRICE PRODUCTS *(Continued)*

Product	Abrasive Ingredient	Therapeutic Ingredient	Foaming Agent
Oral-B Sesame Street Toothpaste, Bubblegum, or Fruity[a]	Hydrated silica	Sodium fluoride 0.248%	Sodium lauryl sulfate
Other Ingredients: Water, sorbitol, glycerin, xanthan gum, acesulfame K, carbomer 980, sodium hydroxide, FD&C red #3, methylparaben, propylparaben			
Oral-B Tooth and Gum Care Toothpaste	Calcium pyrophosphate	Stannous fluoride 0.4%	
Other Ingredients: Water, glycerin, sorbitol, PEG-8, sodium saccharin, methylparaben, propylparaben, zinc citrate, flavor, PVM/MA copolymer			
Pearl Drops Baking Soda Whitening Toothpaste Tartar Control	Hydrated silica, sodium bicarbonate	Sodium fluoride	Sodium lauryl sulfate
Other Ingredients: Sorbitol, glycerin, tetrapotassium pyrophosphate, tetrasodium pyrophosphate, PEG-12, titanium dioxide, flavor, sodium saccharin, cellulose gum			
Pearl Drops Extra Strength Whitening Toothpaste	Hydrated silica, calcium pyrophosphate, dicalcium phosphate	Sodium monofluorophosphate	Sodium lauryl sulfate
Other Ingredients: Sorbitol, glycerin, PEG-12, flavor, titanium dioxide, cellulose gum, trisodium phosphate, sodium phosphate, sodium saccharin			
Pearl Drops Whitening Gel or Paste, Tartar Control w/Fluoride	Hydrated silica	Sodium fluoride	Sodium lauryl sulfate
Other Ingredients: Sorbitol, glycerin, tetrapotassium pyrophosphate, tetrasodium pyrophosphate, PEG-12, flavor, titanium dioxide (paste), cellulose gum, sodium saccharin, FD&C blue #1 (gel), FD&C yellow #10 (gel)			
Pearl Drops Whitening Toothpolish Gel	Hydrated silica	Sodium monofluorophosphate	Sodium lauryl sulfate
Other Ingredients: Sorbitol, glycerin, PEG-12, flavor, cellulose gum, trisodium phosphate, sodium phosphate, sodium saccharin, FD&C blue #1			
Pearl Drops Whitening Toothpolish (regular or spearmint)	Aluminum hydroxide, hydrated silica	Sodium monofluorophosphate	Sodium lauryl sulfate
Other Ingredients: Sorbitol, glycerin, PEG-12, flavor, titanium dioxide, cellulose gum, trisodium phosphate, sodium phosphate, sodium saccharin			
Pepsodent Baking Soda Toothpaste	Hydrated silica	Sodium fluoride 0.24%	Sodium lauryl sulfate
Other Ingredients: Sorbitol, water, sodium bicarbonate, PEG-32, SD alcohol 38B, flavor, cellulose gum, sodium saccharin, titanium dioxide			
Pepsodent Original Fluoride Toothpaste	Hydrated silica	Sodium monofluorophosphate 0.79% (fluoride 0.15%)	Sodium lauryl sulfate
Other Ingredients: Sorbitol and related polyols, water, glycerin, SD alcohol 38B, flavor, cellulose gum, sodium saccharin, sodium benzoate, titanium dioxide			
PeriGel Toothpaste System	Sodium bicarbonate 59%	Sodium fluoride	Hydrogen peroxide 3%
Platinum Whitening Toothpaste with Fluoride		Sodium monofluorophosphate 0.76%	

Product	Abrasive Ingredient	Therapeutic Ingredient	Foaming Agent
Promise Toothpaste	Silica	Potassium nitrate, sodium monofluorophosphate	Sodium lauryl sulfate
Other Ingredients: Water, dicalcium phosphate, hydroxyethylcellulose, flavor, sodium saccharin, methylparaben, propylparaben, D&C yellow #10, FD&C blue #1			
Pycopay Tooth Powder	Sodium bicarbonate, calcium carbonate, tricalcium phosphate, magnesium carbonate		
Other Ingredients: Sodium chloride, eugenol, methyl salicylate			
Rembrandt Brushing Gel with Peroxide		Sodium monofluorophosphate	Carbamide peroxide, sodium lauryl sulfate
Other Ingredients: Glycerin, sodium citrate, carbomer, titanium dioxide, flavor, triethanolamine			
Rembrandt Whitening Sensitive Toothpaste		Sodium monofluorophosphate 0.76%, potassium nitrate	Sodium lauryl sulfate
Other Ingredients: Dicalcium phosphate dihydrate, glycerin, sorbitol, water, alumina, papain, sodium citrate, flavor, sodium carboxymethylcellulose, sodium saccharin, methylparaben, citric acid, FD&C red #40			
Rembrandt Whitening Toothpaste (mint or regular)		Sodium monofluorophosphate 0.76%	Sodium lauryl sulfate
Other Ingredients: Dicalcium phosphate dihydrate, water, glycerin, sorbitol, alumina, papain, sodium citrate, flavor, sodium carrageenan, sodium saccharin, methylparaben, citric acid, FD&C blue #1			
Revelation Toothpowder	Calcium carbonate		Vegetable soap powder
Other Ingredients: Methyl salicylate, menthol			
Sensodyne Baking Soda Toothpaste	Sodium bicarbonate, hydrated silica, silica	Potassium nitrate, sodium fluoride	Sodium lauryl sulfate
Other Ingredients: Water, glycerin, sorbitol, flavor, hydroxyethylcellulose, titanium dioxide, sodium saccharin			
Sensodyne Gel (cool mint)	Hydrated silica, silica	Potassium nitrate, sodium fluoride	
Other Ingredients: Water, sorbitol, glycerin, sodium carboxymethylcellulose, sodium methyl cocoyl taurate, flavor, guar gum, sodium saccharin, methylparaben, propylparaben, sodium hydroxide, FD&C blue #1			
Sensodyne Toothpaste[a] (fresh mint)	Silica	Potassium nitrate, sodium monofluorophosphate	Sodium lauryl sulfate
Other Ingredients: Water, dicalcium phosphate dihydrate, glycerin, sorbitol, dicalcium phosphate, hydroxyethylcellulose, flavor, sodium saccharin, methylparaben, propylparaben, D&C yellow #10, FD&C blue #1			
Sensodyne-SC Toothpaste[a]	Calcium carbonate, silica	Strontium chloride hexahydrate 10%	
Other Ingredients: Water, glycerin, sorbitol, hydroxyethylcellulose, sodium methyl cocoyl taurate, flavor, PEG-40, stearate, titanium dioxide, sodium saccharin, methylparaben, propylparaben, D&C red #28			
Thermodent Toothpaste	Diatomaceous earth, silica	Strontium chloride hexahydrate	Sodium methyl cocoyl taurate
Other Ingredients: Sorbitol, glycerin, titanium dioxide, hydroxyethylcellulose, flavor, preservative			

DENTIFRICE PRODUCTS *(Continued)*

Product	Abrasive Ingredient	Therapeutic Ingredient	Foaming Agent
Tom's Natural Baking Soda Toothpaste with Fluoride	Calcium carbonate, sodium bicarbonate	Sodium monofluorophosphate	Sodium lauryl sulfate
	Other Ingredients: Glycerin, carrageenan, xylitol, peppermint oil		
Tom's Natural Toothpaste for Children with Fluoride	Calcium carbonate, hydrated silica	Sodium monofluorophosphate	Sodium lauryl sulfate
	Other Ingredients: Glycerin, fruit extracts, carrageenan		
Tom's Natural Toothpaste with Calcium and Fluoride	Calcium carbonate	Sodium monofluorophosphate	Sodium lauryl sulfate
	Other Ingredients: Glycerin, carrageenan, xylitol, spearmint and peppermint oil		
Tom's Natural Toothpaste with Propolis and Myrrh	Calcium carbonate		Sodium lauryl sulfate
	Other Ingredients: Glycerin, carrageenan, oil of spearmint, peppermint, cassia, or fennel, propolis, myrrh		
Toothpaste Booster			Hydrogen peroxide, sodium lauryl sulfate
	Other Ingredients: Deionized water, cornstarch, sorbitol, propylene glycol, carbomer 940, menthol, sodium benzoate, potassium sorbate		
Topol Gel[a] (spearmint)	Hydrated silica	Sodium monofluorophosphate	Sodium lauryl sulfate
	Other Ingredients: Sorbitol, deionized water, glycerin, PEG-6, flavor, xanthan gum, sodium saccharin, methylparaben, propylparaben, zirconium silicate, FD&C blue #1, FD&C yellow #5		
Topol Plus Baking Soda Whitening Gel or Toothpaste	Hydrated silica	Sodium monofluorophosphate	Sodium lauryl sulfate
	Other Ingredients: Water, sorbitol (gel), glycerin, calcium carbonate (gel), sorbitol, PEG-6, disodium phosphate, flavor, xanthan gum, sodium saccharin, titanium dioxide, methylparaben, propylparaben, FD&C blue #1 (gel)		
Topol Toothpaste[a] (peppermint)	Hydrated silica, sodium bicarbonate	Sodium monofluorophosphate	Sodium lauryl sulfate
	Other Ingredients: Sorbitol, deionized water, glycerin, PEG-6, flavor, xanthan gum, titanium dioxide, sodium saccharin, methylparaben, propylparaben, zirconium silicate		
Triplex Toothpaste	Hydrated silica, sodium bicarbonate	Sodium fluoride	Calcium peroxide, sodium lauryl sulfate
	Other Ingredients: Glycerin, sorbitol, urea, flavor, titanium dioxide, carbomer, sodium saccharin, ethyl cellulose, sodium benzoate		
Ultra Brite Baking Soda Toothpaste	Hydrated silica, sodium bicarbonate, alumina	Sodium monofluorophosphate 0.76%	Sodium lauryl sulfate
	Other Ingredients: Glycerin, tetrasodium pyrophosphate, cellulose gum, flavor, sodium saccharin, titanium dioxide		
Ultra Brite Gel[a]	Hydrated silica	Sodium monofluorophosphate 0.76%	Sodium lauryl sulfate
	Other Ingredients: Sorbitol, PEG-12, flavor, cellulose gum, sodium saccharin, glycerin, FD&C blue #1, D&C red #33		
Ultra Brite Toothpaste	Hydrated silica, alumina	Sodium monofluorophosphate 0.76%	Sodium lauryl sulfate

Product	Abrasive Ingredient	Therapeutic Ingredient	Foaming Agent
	Other Ingredients: Glycerin, cellulose gum, carrageenan gum, sodium benzoate, titanium dioxide, sodium saccharin, flavor		
Viadent Fluoride Gel	Hydrated silica	Sodium monofluorophosphate 0.8%, sanguinaria extract 0.075%	Sodium lauryl sulfate
	Other Ingredients: Sodium saccharin, zinc chloride, teaberry flavor, sodium carboxymethylcellulose, sorbitol		
Viadent Fluoride Toothpaste	Hydrated silica	Sodium monofluorophosphate 0.8%, sanguinaria extract 0.075%	Sodium lauryl sulfate
	Other Ingredients: Sorbitol, titanium dioxide, carboxymethylcellulose, flavor, sodium saccharin, citric acid, zinc chloride		
Viadent Original Toothpaste	Dicalcium phosphate	Sanguinaria extract 0.075%	Sodium lauryl sulfate
	Other Ingredients: Glycerin, sorbitol, titanium dioxide, zinc chloride, carrageenan, flavor, sodium saccharin, citric acid		

[a]Carries American Dental Association (ADA) seal indicating safety and efficacy.

[b]Topical fluoride rinse

Reprinted with permission from *Handbook of Nonprescription Drugs*, 10th ed, *Product Updates*, Washington, DC, American Pharmaceutical Association, 1995, 265-71.

DENTURE ADHESIVE PRODUCTS

Product	Dosage Form	Ingredients
Confident (Block Drug)	Cream	Carboxymethylcellulose gum 32%, ethylene oxide polymer 13%, petrolatum, liquid petrolatum, propylparaben
Corega	Powder	Karaya gum 94.6%, water-soluble ethylene oxide polymer 5%, flavor
Dentrol	Liquid	Carboxymethylcellulose sodium, ethylene oxide polymer, mineral oil, polyethylene, flavor, propylparaben
Denturite	Liquid, powder	Liquid: Butyl phthalyl butyl glycolate, vinyl acetate, SDA alcohol Powder: Polyethyl methacrylate polymer
Effergrip[a]	Cream	Carboxymethylcellulose sodium 24.8%, calcium sodium mixed salt of methyl vinyl ether-maleic anhydride 29.8%, preservatives, red lake blend
Ezo Cushions	Pad	Paraffin wax, cotton
Fasteeth	Powder	Calcium/zinc poly (vinyl methyl ether maleate), sodium carboxymethylcellulose, cornstarch, silicon dioxide, peppermint oil, rectified
Fasteeth Extra Hold	Powder	Calcium/zinc poly (vinyl methyl ether maleate), sodium carboxymethylcellulose, silicon dioxide, peppermint oil, rectified
Fixodent	Cream	Calcium/zinc poly (vinyl methyl ether maleate), sodium carboxymethylcellulose, mineral oil, petrolatum, silicon dioxide, color
Fixodent Fresh	Cream	Calcium/zinc poly (vinyl methyl ether maleate), sodium carboxymethylcellulose, mineral oil, petrolatum, silicon dioxide, color, peppermint flavor, methyl lactate, menthol
Orafix	Cream	Karaya gum 51%, petrolatum 30%, mineral oil 13%, peppermint oil 0.08%
Orafix Special[a]	Cream	Gantrez MS955, sodium carboxymethylcellulose type 7H4XF, povidone K-90, white petrolatum, mineral oil, heavy, isopropyl palmitate, isopropyl myristate, flavors, colors
Plasti-Liner	Strip	Polyethyl metacrylate polymer, butyl phthalyl butyl glycolate, triacetin
Poli-Grip	Cream	Karaya gum 51%, petrolatum 36.7%, liquid petrolatum, magnesium oxide, propylparaben, flavor
Poly-Grip Super	Cream	Carboxymethylcellulose sodium, ethylene oxide polymer, petrolatum, mineral oil flavor, propylparaben
Poli-Grip Super	Powder	Calcium sodium methyl vinyl ether-maleic copolymer, carboxymethylcellulose sodium, flavor
Polident Dentu-Grip	Cream	Carboxymethylcellulose gum 49%, ethylene oxide polymer 21%, flavor
Quik-Fix	Liquid, powder	Liquid: Methyl methacrylate monomer, hydroxyethyl metacylate monomer, colorstable concentrate, triacetin; Powder: Polyethyl methacrylate polymer

(continued)

Product	Dosage Form	Ingredients
Rigident	Powder	Acacia gum, karaya gum, sodium borate
Rigident[a]	Cream	Carboxymethylcellulose sodium, calcium sodium salts of methyl vinyl ether maleic anhydride copolymer, petrolatum, mineral oil, talc, flavor, propylparaben, D&C red #27 aluminum lake
Sea-Bond	Pad	Ethylene oxide polymer, sodium alginate
Wernet's	Cream	Carboxymethylcellulose gum 32%, petrolatum, mineral oil, ethylene oxide polymer 13%, propylparaben, flavor 0.5%
Wernet's	Powder	Karaya gum 94.6%, water-soluble ethylene oxide polymer 5%, flavor 0.4%

[a]Carries American Dental Association (ADA) seal indicating safety and efficacy.

Reprinted with permission from *Handbook of Nonprescription Drugs*, 10th ed, *Product Updates*, Washington, DC, American Pharmaceutical Association, 1995, 277.

DENTURE CLEANSER PRODUCTS

Product	Dosage Form	Ingredients
Ban-A-Stain**	Liquid	Phosphoric acid 25%, deionized water, imidurea, methylparaben, xanthan gum, alkyl phenoxy polyethoxy ethanol, oil of cassis, FD&C red #40
Complete[a]	Paste	Calcium carbonate, water, glycerin, sorbitol, cellulose gum, sodium lauryl sulfate, silica, flavor, magnesium aluminum silicate, sodium saccharin, methylparaben, propylparaben
Dentu-Creme	Paste	Dicalcium phosphate dihydrate, propylene glycol, calcium carbonate, silica, sodium lauryl sulfate, glycerin, hydroxyethylcellulose, flavor, magnesium aluminum silicate, sodium saccharin, methylparaben, propylparaben
Efferdent Antibacterial[a]	Tablet	Potassium monopersulfate, sodium perborate monohydrate, sodium carbonate, sodium lauryl sulfoacetate, sodium bicarbonate, citric acid, magnesium stearate, flavor
Efferdent, 2 Layer	Tablet	Sodium bicarbonate, sodium carbonate, citric acid, potassium monopersulfate, sodium perborate monohydrate, sodium lauryl sulfoacetate, flavor
Polident	Tablet, powder	Potassium monopersulfate, sodium perborate monohydrate, sodium carbonate, surfactant, chelating agents (tablet), proteolytic enzyme (tablet), sodium acid pyrophosphate (powder), sodium bicarbonate, citric acid (tablet), fragrance
Rembrandt Daily Denture Renewal	Gel	Citroxain
Smokers' Polident	Tablet	Sodium carbonate, potassium monopersulfate, citric acid, sodium bicarbonate, sodium perborate monohydrate, surfactant, chelating agents, proteolytic enzyme, fragrance

[a]Carries American Dental Association (ADA) seal indicating safety and efficacy.

Reprinted with permission from *Handbook of Nonprescription Drugs*, 10th ed, *Product Updates*, Washington, DC, American Pharmaceutical Association, 1995, 276.

MOUTH PAIN, COLD SORE, CANKER SORE PRODUCTS

Product	Anesthetic/ Analgesic	Other Ingredients
Amosan Powder		Sodium peroxyborate monohydrate, sodium bitartrate, saccharin, peppermint, menthol, and vanilla flavors
Anbesol Baby Gel (grape or original)	Benzocaine 7.5%	Benzoic acid (grape), carbomer 934P, D&C red #33, disodium EDTA, FD&C blue #1 (grape), flavor, glycerin, methylparaben (grape), PEG-8, propylparaben (grape), saccharin, water
Anbesol Gel	Benzocaine 6.3%, phenol 0.5%, camphor	Alcohol 70%, carbomer 934P, D&C red #33, D&C yellow #10, FD&C blue #1, FD&C yellow #6, flavor, glycerin
Anbesol Liquid	Benzocaine 6.3%, phenol 0.5%, camphor, menthol	Alcohol 70%, glycerin, potassium iodide, povidone iodine
Anbesol Maximum Strength Gel	Benzocaine 20%	Alcohol 60%, carbomer 934P, D&C yellow #10, FD&C red #40, flavor, PEG-12, saccharin
Anbesol Maximum Strength Liquid	Benzocaine 20%	Alcohol 60%, D&C yellow #10, FD&C blue #1, FD&C red #40, flavor, PEG-8, saccharin
Babee Teething Lotion	Benzocaine 2.5%, menthol, camphor	Alcohol 20%, witch hazel
Benzodent Denture Analgesic Ointment[a]	Benzocaine 20%, eugenol	8-hydroxyquinoline sulfate, petrolatum, sodium CMC, color
Betadine Mouthwash/ Gargle		Povidone-iodine 0.5%, alcohol 8.8%
Blistex Medicated Lip Ointment	Menthol 0.6%, camphor 0.5%, phenol 0.5%	Allantoin 1%
Blistex Lip Medex Ointment	Camphor 1%, menthol 1%, phenol 0.5%	Petrolatum, cocoa butter, flavor, lanolin, mixed waxes, oil of cloves
Campho-Phenique Antiseptic Gel	Camphor 10.8%, phenol 4.7%	Eucalyptus oil
Campho-Phenique Cold Sore Gel[b]	Camphor 10.8%, phenol 4.7%	Eucalyptus oil
Campho-Phenique Liquid	Camphor 10.8%, phenol 4.7%	Eucalyptus oil
Chap Stick Medicated Lip Balm (jar or squeeze tube)	Camphor 1%, menthol 0.6%, phenol 0.5%	Petrolatum 60% (jar), petrolatum 67% (squeeze tube), microcrystalline wax, mineral oil, cocoa butter, lanolin, paraffin wax (jar)
Chap Stick Medicated Lip Balm Stick	Camphor 1%, menthol 0.6%, phenol 0.5%	Petrolatum 41%, paraffin wax, mineral oil, cocoa butter, 2-octyl dodecanol, arachadyl propionate, polyphenylmethylsiloxane 556, white wax, isopropyl lanolate, carnauba wax, isopropyl myristate, lanolin, fragrance, methylparaben, propylparaben, oleyl alcohol, cetyl alcohol
Cold Sore Lotion[b]	Camphor, menthol	Alcohol 85%, gum benzoin 7%, thymol, eucalyptol
Curasore Liquid		Ethyl ether, ethyl alcohol
Dent's 3 in 1 Toothache Relief (gel, gum, drops)	Benzocaine 20%	Alcohol 74% (drops), chlorobutanol anhydrous 0.09% (drops), eugenol

MOUTH PAIN, COLD SORE, CANKER SORE PRODUCTS
(Continued)

Product	Anesthetic/Analgesic	Other Ingredients
Dent's Double-Action Kit (tablets, drops)	Benzocaine 20% (drops)	Denatured alcohol 74%, chlorobutanol 0.09%, acetaminophen 325 mg (tablet), eugenol
Dent's Extra Strength Toothache Gum	Benzocaine 20%	Petrolatum, cotton and wax base, beeswax, FD&C red #40 aluminum lake, eugenol
Dent's Maxi-Strength Toothache Treatment Drops	Benzocaine 20%	Alcohol 74%, chlorobutanol 0.09%, propylene glycol, FD&C red #40, eugenol
Dent-Zel-Ite Oral Mucosal Analgesic Liquid	Benzocaine 5%, camphor	Alcohol 81%, wintergreen, glycerin
Dent-Zel-Ite Temporary Dental Filling Liquid	Camphor	Alcohol 55%, sandarac gum, methyl salicylate
Dent-Zel-Ite Toothache Relief Drops	Eugenol 85%, camphor	Alcohol 13.5%, wintergreen
GargleAid Granular Effervescent	Dyclonine HCl 69 mg	Sucrose, salt, sodium bicarbonate, citric acid, natural lemon flavor, sodium ascorbate
HDA Toothache Gel	Benzocaine 6.5%	Clove oil
Herpecin-L Stick[b]		Allantoin, padimate O, titanium dioxide
Hurricaine Aerosol (wild cherry)	Benzocaine	Polyethylene glycol, saccharin, flavoring
Hurricaine Gel (wild cherry, pina colada, or watermelon)	Benzocaine	Polyethylene glycol, saccharin, flavoring
Hurricaine Liquid (wild cherry or pina colada)	Benzocaine	Polyethylene glycol, saccharin, flavoring
Isodettes Spray	Phenol 1.4%	Propylene glycol 10%, artificial and sodium hydroxide 0.0047%, natural wild cherry flavor 0.5%, artificial and natural eucalyptus flavor, FD&C red #40, water
Kank-A-Professional Strength Liquid[a]	Benzocaine 20%, benzyl alcohol	Benzoin tincture compound 0.5%, cetylpyridinium chloride, ethylcellulose, SD alcohol, dimethyl isosorbide, castor oil, flavor, tannic acid, propylene glycol, saccharin
Lip Medex Ointment	Camphor 1.0%, menthol 0.5%, phenol 0.5%	Petrolatum 73.7%
Lotion-Jel	Benzocaine	Distilled water, methylparaben, propylparaben, propylene glycol, carbopol 934-P, methyl salicylate, FD&C red #40, 2.2' iminodiethanol
Medadyne Liquid	Benzocaine 10%, menthol, camphor	Benzalkonium chloride, tannic acid, flavors, SD alcohol, benzyl alcohol, thymol
Mouth Kote-PR Ointment	Benzyl alcohol 3.5%, diphenhydramine 1.25%	PEG 8, cellulose gum, PEG 75, poloxamer 407, yerba santa, flavor
Mouth Kote-PR Solution	Diphenhydramine 1.25%, benzyl alcohol 1%	Water, cetylpyridinium chloride, disodium EDTA flavor, sodium benzoate, sodium hydroxide, sodium saccharin, yerba santa
Mouth Kote-OR Solution	Benzyl alcohol 1%, menthol	Water, sorbitol, sodium chloride, yerba santa, flavor, poloxamer 407, sodium saccharin, cetylpyridinium chloride, disodium EDTA

(continued)

Product	Anesthetic/ Analgesic	Other Ingredients
Numzident (Adult Strength) Gel	Benzocaine 10%	PEG 400 47.86%, glycerin 30%, PEG 3350 10%, sodium saccharin 1%, purified water 0.75%, cherry vanilla flavor 0.4%
Numzit Teething Gel	Benzocaine 7.5%	PEG 400 66.2%, PEG 3350 26.1%, sodium saccharin 0.036%, clove oil 0.09%, peppermint oil 0.018%, purified water 0.056%
Numzit Teething Lotion	Benzocaine 0.2%	Alcohol 12.1%, glycerin 2%, kelgin MV 0.5%, sodium saccharin 0.02%, methylparaben 0.1%, FD&C red #40 0.1%, FD&C blue #1 0.009%
Orabase Baby Gel[a]	Benzocaine 7.5%	Glycerin, PEG, carbopol, preservative, sweetener, flavor
Orabase Gel	Benzocaine 15%	Ethanol, PEG, hydroxyethyl chloride, tannic acid, salicylic acid, flavor, sodium saccharin
Orabase Lip Cream	Benzocaine 5%, menthol 0.5%, camphor, phenol	Allantoin 1%, sodium carboxymethylcellulose, veegum, Tween 80, phenonip, PEG, biopure, talc, kaolin, lanolin, petrolatum, oil of clove, aerosil
Orabase Plain Paste[a]		Pectin, gelatin, carboxymethylcellulose sodium, polyethylene, mineral oil, flavors, preservative, guar, tragacanth
Orabase-B with Benzocaine Paste[a]	Benzocaine 20%	Plasticized hydrocarbon gel, guar, carboxymethylcellulose, tragacanth, pectin, preservatives, flavors
Orajel Baby Gel	Benzocaine 7.5%	FD&C red #40, flavor, glycerin, polyethylene glycols, sodium saccharin, sorbic acid, sorbitol
Orajel Baby Nighttime Formula Gel	Benzocaine 10%	FD&C red #40, flavor, glycerin, polyethylene glycols, sodium saccharin, sorbic acid, sorbitol
Orajel Denture Gel	Benzocaine 10%, eugenol	Chlorothymol, FD&C red #40, flavor, polyethylene glycols, purified water, sodium saccharin, sorbic acid
Orajel Maximum Strength Gel	Benzocaine 20%	Clove oil, flavor, polyethylene glycols, sodium saccharin, sorbic acid
Orajel Mouth-Aid Gel	Benzocaine 20%	Zinc chloride 0.1%, benzalkonium chloride 0.02%. allantoin, carbomer, edetate disodium, peppermint oil, polyethylene glycol, polysorbate 60, propyl gallate, polysorbate 60, glycol, purified water, povidone sodium saccharin propylene, sorbic acid, stearyl alcohol
Orajel Mouth-Aid Liquid	Benzocaine 20%	Cetylpyridinium chloride 0.1%, ethylcellulose
Orajel Regular Strength Gel	Benzocaine 10%	Clove oil, flavor, polyethylene glycols, sodium saccharin, sorbic acid
Orasol Liquid	Benzocaine 6.3%, phenol 0.5%	Alcohol 70%
Painalay Sore Throat Gargle & Spray	Phenol 0.5%	
Probax Ointment[b]		Propolis 2%, petrolatum, mineral oil
Red Cross Toothache Medication Drops	Eugenol 85%	Sesame oil

MOUTH PAIN, COLD SORE, CANKER SORE PRODUCTS
(Continued)

Product	Anesthetic/ Analgesic	Other Ingredients
SensoGARD Gel[b]	Benzocaine 20%	Methylparaben, polycarbophil, polyethylene glycol, propylparaben, sorbitan monooleate
Sore Throat Spray (cherry, menthol, or mint)	Phenol 1.4%	
Tanac Liquid	Benzocaine 10%	Benzalkonium chloride 0.125%, saccharin
Tanac Medicated Gel	Dyclonine HCl 1.0%	Allantoin 0.5%
Tanac Roll-On Lotion	Benzocaine 5%	Benzalkonium chloride 0.12%, sodium saccharin, glycerin, polyethylene glycol, tannic acid
Tanac Stick	Benzocaine 7.5%	Benzalkonium chloride 0.125%
Throtoceptic Pump Spray	Phenol 1.4%	Alum 0.5%, flavor
Tisol Solution	Benzyl alcohol 1%	Water, sorbitol, sodium chloride, yerba santa, poloxamer 407, menthol, saccharin, cetylpyridinium chloride, disodium EDTA
Vaseline Lip Therapy Ointment	Camphor 0.8%, menthol 0.8%, phenol 0.5%	White petrolatum 92.8%, allantoin 1%
Viractin	Tetracaine 2%	
Vicks Chloraseptic Advanced Formula Sore Throat Spray	Phenol 1.4%	Colors, flavors, glycerin, purified water, saccharin, sodium
Vicks Chloraseptic Sore Throat Spray, Childrens	Phenol 0.5%	FD&C blue #1, FD&C red #40, flavor, glycerin, purified water, saccharin sodium, sorbitol
Vicks Chloraseptic Sore Throat Gargle, Menthol	Phenol 1.4%	D&C green #5, D&C yellow #10, FD&C green #3, flavor, glycerin, water, saccharin sodium
Zilactin Medicated Gel	Benzyl alcohol 10%	Tannic acid, hydroxypropyl cellulose filmformer
Zilactin-L Liquid	Lidocaine 2.5%	

[a]Carries American Dental Association (ADA) seal indicating safety and efficacy.
[b]For cold sore treatment only.

Reprinted with permission from *Handbook of Nonprescription Drugs*, 10th ed, *Product Updates*, Washington, DC, American Pharmaceutical Association, 1995, 278-81.

ORAL RINSE PRODUCTS

Product	Antiseptic	Other Ingredients
Act[b]	Cetylpyridinium chloride, menthol, methyl salicylate	Sodium fluoride 0.05%, edetate calcium disodium, FD&C green #3, FD&C yellow #5, flavor, glycerin, monobasic sodium phosphate, dibasic sodium phosphate, poloxamer 407, polysorbate-20, potassium sorbate, propylene glycol, sodium benzoate, sodium saccharin, water
Act for Kids[ab]	Cetylpyridinium chloride	Sodium fluoride 0.05%, D&C red #33, dibasic sodium phosphate, edetate calcium disodium, flavors, glycerin, monobasic sodium phosphate, poloxamer 407, polysorbate-80, propylene glycol, sodium benzoate, sodium saccharin, water
Astring-O-Sol	SD alcohol 38-B, 75.6%, methyl salicylate	Water, myrrh extract, zinc chloride, citric acid
Cankaid	Carbamide peroxide 10%	Citric acid monohydrate, sodium citrate dihydrate, edetate disodium
Cepacol Mouthwash/Gargle	Alcohol 14%, cetylpyridinium chloride 0.05%	Edetate disodium, colors, flavors, glycerin, polysorbate 80, saccharin, sodium B phosphate, sodium phosphate, water
Cepacol Mouthwash/Gargle, Mint	Alcohol 14.5%, cetylpyridinium chloride 0.5%	Colors, flavors, glucono delta-lactone, glycerin, poloxamer-407, sodium saccharin, sodium gluconate, water
Clear Choice	Cetylpyridinium chloride	Glycerin, sodium phosphate, poloxamer 338, flavor, sodium saccharin, domiphen bromide
Fluorigard Anti-Cavity Fluoride Rinse[ab]		Sodium fluoride 0.05%
Gly-Oxide[c]	Carbamide peroxide 10%	Citric acid, flavor, glycerin, propylene glycol, sodium stannate, water
Lavoris	SD Alcohol 38-B	Water, glycerin, citric acid, poloxamer 407, water, saccharin, clove oil, polysorbate 80, zinc chloride, zinc oxide, sodium hydroxide, flavors, colors
Lavoris Crystal Fresh	SD Alcohol 38-B	Purified water, glycerin, poloxamer 407, citric acid, zinc oxide, sodium hydroxide, saccharin, polysorbate 80, flavors
Listerine[a] Topical Fluoride Rinse	Alcohol 26.9%, menthol, methyl salicylate, eucalyptol, thymol	
Listerine, Coolmint[a]	Alcohol 21.6%, menthol, methyl salicylate, eucalyptol, thymol	Anetmole
Listerine, Freshburst[a]	Alcohol 21.6%, eucalyptol, menthol, methyl salicylate, thymol	Glycerin, benzoic acid, poloxamer 407, sodium saccharin, sodium citrate, FD&C green #3, D&C yellow #10

ORAL RINSE PRODUCTS *(Continued)*

Product	Antiseptic	Other Ingredients
Listermint with Fluoride	Alcohol 6.65%	Sodium fluoride 0.02%, zinc chloride, glycerin, poloxamer 407, sodium lauryl sulfate, sodium citrate, flavor, sodium saccharin, citric acid, D&C yellow #10, FD&C green #3
Mouth Wash Antiseptic	Alcohol 26.9%, eucalyptol 0.09%, thymol 0.06%, methyl salicylate 0.06%, menthol 0.04%	
MouthKote-FR		Sodium fluoride 0.04%, benzyl alcohol, menthol, water, xylitol, sorbitol, sodium chloride, yerba santa, poloxamer 407, cetylpyridinium chloride, disodium EDTA
Orajel Perioseptic[c]	Carbamide peroxide 15%	Citric acid, edetate disodium, propylene glycol, purified water, sodium chloride, sodium, flavor, methylparaben saccharin
Oral-B Anti-Cavity Rinse Alcohol Free[b]	Cetylpyridinium chloride monohydrate	Sodium fluoride 0.05%, water, glycerin, cremophor RH40, flavor, methylparaben, sodium saccharin, sodium benzoate, propylparaben, FD&C blue #1
Oral-B Anti-Cavity Rinse[ab]		Sodium fluoride 0.05%, water, sodium benzoate, potassium sorbate, sodium saccharin, glycerin, PEG-40, FD&C blue #1, phosphoric acid
Oral-B Anti-Plaque Rinse	Alcohol 8%, cetylpyridinium chloride	Water, glycerin, sodium saccharin, methylparaben, propylparaben, FD&C blue #1, D&C yellow #10, poloxamer 407
Oral-B Anti-Plaque Rinse Alcohol Free	Cetylpyridinium chloride 0.05%	Water, glycerin, flavor, polysorbate 20, methylparaben, sodium saccharin, propylparaben, sodium benzoate, FD&C blue #1, D&C yellow #10
Peroxyl Hygienic Dental Rinse[c]	Alcohol 5%, hydrogen peroxide 1.5%	Pluronic F108, sorbitol, sodium saccharin, dye, polysorbate 20, mint flavor
Peroxyl Oral Spot Treatment Gel[c]	Hydrogen Peroxide 1.5%	Mint flavor, ethyl alcohol 5%, pluronic F108, polysorbate 20, sorbitol, sodium saccharin, dye, pluronic F127
Plax Advanced Formula, Clear Peppermint	Alcohol 8.5%	Water, glycerin, tetrasodium pyrophosphate, benzoic acid, sodium lauryl sulfate, sodium benzoate, polomer 407, flavor, xanthan gum
Plax Advanced Formula, Original Flavor	Alcohol 8.5%	Sodium lauryl sulfate, water, glycerin, sodium benzoate, tetrasodium pyrophosphate, benzoic acid, poloxamer 407, saccharin, flavor, xanthan gum

(continued)

Product	Antiseptic	Other Ingredients
Plax Advanced Formula, Softmint	Alcohol 8.5%	Sodium lauryl sulfate, water, glycerin, sodium benzoate, tetrasodium pyrophosphate, benzoic acid, poloxamer 407, saccharin, flavor, xanthan gum, flavor enhancer, FD&C blue #1, FD&C yellow #5
Scope Baking Soda Clean Mint	SD alcohol 38-F 9.9%, cetylpyridinium chloride, domiphen bromide	Water, sorbitol, sodium bicarbonate, poloxamer 407, polysorbate 80, sodium saccharin, flavor
Scope Original, Mint	SD alcohol 38-F 18.9%, cetylpyridinium chloride, domiphen bromide	Purified water, glycerin, sodium saccharin, sodium benzoate, flavor, benzoic acid, FD&C blue #1, FD&C yellow #5
Scope, Peppermint	SD alcohol 38-F 14%, cetylpyridinium chloride, domiphen bromide	Purified water, glycerin, poloxamer 407, sodium saccharin, sodium benzoate, N-ethylmethylcarboxamide, benzoic acid, FD&C blue #1
Targo		
Tech 2000	Cetylpyridinium chloride	Water, glycerin, poloxamer 407, flavor, FD&C blue #1, FD&C yellow #5, nutritive dextrose or sucrose and/or calcium saccharin
Tom's of Maine Mouthwash	Menthol	Water, glycerin, aloe vera juice, witch hazel, poloxamer 335, spearmint oil, ascorbic acid
Viadent Oral Rinse	Alcohol 10%	Sanguinaria extract, glycerin, polysorbate 80, flavor, sodium saccharin, poloxamer 237, citric acid, zinc chloride 0.2%

[a]Carries American Dental Association (ADA) seal indicating safety and efficacy.

[b]Topical fluoride rinse

[c]Oral debriding agent/wound cleanser

Reprinted with permission from *Handbook of Nonprescription Drugs*, 10th ed, *Product Updates*, Washington, DC, American Pharmaceutical Association, 1995, 273-5.

SUGAR-FREE LIQUID PHARMACEUTICALS

The following sugar-free liquid preparations are listed by therapeutic category and alphabetically within each category. Please note that product formulations are subject to change by the manufacturer. Some of these products may contain sorbitol, xylitol, or other sweeteners which may be partially metabolized to provide calories.

Analgesics

Acetaminophen Elixir (various)
APAP/APAP Plus
Aspirin/Buffered Aspirin (Medique®)
Bufferin® A/F Nite Time
Children's Anacin-3® Infants Drops
Children's Myapap® Elixir
Children's Panadol® Drops, Liquid, and Chewable Tablets
Children's Tylenol® Chewable Tablets
Conex® Liquid
Conex® With Codeine Liquid
Dolanex® Elixir
Extra Strength Tylenol® PM
Febrol® and Febrol® EX
I-Prin®
Methadone Hydrochloride Intensol
MS-Aid®
Myapap® Drops
No Drowsiness Tylenol®
Pain-Off®
Paregoric USP
Sep-A-Soothe® II
St Joseph® Aspirin-Free Liquid and Drops
Tempra® Chewable Tablets
Tylenol® Drops

Antacids/Antiflatulents

Alcalak®
Aldroxicon®
Almag® Suspension
Aludrox® Suspension
Aluminum Hydroxide Suspension
Calglycine® Tablets
Camalox® Suspension
Citrocarbonate® Granules
Creamalin® Suspension
Delcid®
Di-Gel® Liquid (mint, lemon & orange flavored)
Digestamic®
Dimacid®
Gaviscon® Liquid
Gelusil® II
Gelusil® Liquid
Gelusil® Liquid Flavor Pack
Gelusil-M® Liquid
Kolantyl® Gel
Maalox® Plus Suspension
Maalox® Suspension
Maalox® Therapeutic Concentrate
Magnatril® Suspension
Magnesia and Alumina Oral Suspension USP
Mallamint® Chewable Tablets
Marblen® Suspension and Tablets
Medi-Seltzer®/Plus
Milk of Bismuth
Milk of Magnesia USP
Mylanta® Liquid
Mylanta®-II Liquid
Mylicon® Drops
Nephrox® Suspension
Nutrajel®
Nutramag®
Pepto-Bismol® Liquid and Tablets
Phosphaljel® Suspension
Riopan Plus®
Riopan® Suspension

Silain-Gel® Liquid
Trisogel®
Titralac® Liquid
Titralac® Plus Liquid
WinGel® Liquid and Tablets

Antiasthmatics

Aerolate® Liquid
Alupent® Syrup
Choledyl® Pediatric Syrup
Droxine®
Elixophyllin® Elixir
Elixophyllin®-GG Liquid
Lanophyllin® Elixir
Lixolin® Liquid
Lufyllin® Elixir
Metaprel® Syrup
Mucomyst®-10
Mucomyst®-20
Mudrane® GG Elixir
Neothylline® Elixir
Neothylline® G
Organidin® Solution
Slo-Phyllin® 80 Syrup
Somophyllin® Oral Liquid
Somophyllin®-DF Oral Liquid
Tedral® Elixir and Suspension
Theolair™ 80 Syrup
Theolixir®
Theon® Syrup
Theo-Organidin® Elixir
Theophylline Elixir

Antidepressants

Sinequan® Oral Concentrate

Antidiarrheals

Corrective Mixture With Paregoric
Diasorb® Liquid and Tablets
Di-Gon® II
Diotame®
Donnagel®
Infantol® Pink
Kalicon® Suspension
Kaolin Mixture With Pectin NF
Kaolin-Pectin Suspension
Konsyl® Powder
Lomanate®
Lomotil® Liquid
Paregoric USP (various)
Parepectolin® (various)
Pepto-Bismol®
St Joseph® Antidiarrheal

Antiepileptics

Mysoline® Suspension
Paradione® Solution

Antihistamine-Decongestants

Actifed® With Codeine
Actifed® Syrup
Actidil® Syrup
Bromphen® Elixir
Dimetane® Decongestant Elixir
Dimetapp® Elixir
Hay-Febrol® Liquid
Isoclor® Liquid and Capsules
Naldecon® Pediatric Drops and Syrup
Naldecon® Syrup
Novahistine® Elixir
Phenergan® Fortis Syrup
Phenergan® Syrup
Rondec® DM Drops
Ryna® Liquid
S-T® Forte® Liquid
Tavist® Syrup
Trind® Liquid
Veltap® Elixir
Vistaril® Oral Suspension

SUGAR-FREE LIQUID PHARMACEUTICALS *(Continued)*

Anti-Infectives
Augmentin® Suspension
Furadantin® Oral Suspension
Furoxone® Suspension
Humatin®
Mandelamine® Suspension/Forte®
Minocin® Suspension
Mycifradin® Sulfate Oral Solution
NegGram® Suspension
Proklar® Suspension
Sulfamethoxazole and Trimethoprim Suspension
Vibramycin® Syrup

Antiparkinsonism Agents
Artane® Elixir

Antispasmodics
Antrocol® Elixir
Spasmophen® Elixir

Corticosteroids
Decadron® Elixir
Dexamethasone Solution (Roxane)
Dexamethasone Intensol Solution
Pediapred® Oral Liquid

Cough Medicines
Anatuss® With Codeine Syrup
Anatuss® Syrup
Brown Mixture NF (Lannett)
CCP® Caffeine Free
CCP® Cough/Cold Tablets
Cerose-DM®
Chlorgest-HD®
Codagest® Expectorant
Codiclear® DH Syrup
Codimal® DM
Colrex® Compound Elixir
Colrex® Expectorant
Conar® Syrup
Conar® Expectorant Syrup
Conex® Liquid
Conex® With Codeine Syrup
Contac Jr® Liquid
Day-Night Comtrex®
Decoral® Forte®
Dexafed® Cough Syrup
Dimetane®-DC Cough Syrup
Dimetane®-DX Cough Syrup
Entuss® Expectorant Liquid
Fedahist® Expectorant Syrup and Pediatric Drops
Guaificon®-DMS
Histafed® Pediatric Liquid
Hycomine® Syrup and Pediatric Syrup
Lanatuss® Expectorant
Medicon® D
Medi-Synal®
Naldecon-DX® Pediatric Drops and Syrup
Naldecon-DX® Adult Liquid
Non-Drowsy Comtrex®
Noratuss®-II Expectorant and Liquid
Organidin® Solution
Potassium Iodide Solution (various)
Prunicodeine®
Queltuss® Tablets
Robitussin-CF® Liquid
Robitussin® Night Relief Liquid
Rondec®-DM Drops
Rondec®-DM Syrup
Ryna® Liquid
Ryna-C® Liquid
Ryna-CX® Liquid
Scot-Tussin® DM Syrup
Scot-Tussin® Expectorant
Scot-Tussin® DM Cough Chasers
Silexin® Cough Syrup

Sorbutuss®
S-T® Expectorant, SF/D-F
S-T® Forte®, Sugar-Free
Sudodrin®/Sudodrin® Forte®
Terpin® Hydrate With Codeine Elixir (various)
Toclonol® Expectorant
Toclonol® Expectorant With Codeine
Tolu-Sed® Cough Syrup
Tolu-Sed® DM
Tricodene® Liquid
Trind-DM® Liquid
Tuss-Ornade®
Tussar® SF
Tussionex® Extended Release Suspension
Tussi-Organidin® Liquid
Tussirex® Sugar-Free

Dental Preparations and Fluoride Preparations
Cepacol® Mouthwash
Cepastat® Mouthwash and Gargle
Chloraseptic® Mouthwash and Gargle
Fluorigard® Mouthrinse
Fluorinse®
Flura-Drops®
Flura-Loz®
Flura® Tablets
Gel-Kam®
Karigel®
Karigel® N
Luride® Drops
Luride® SF Lozi-Tabs
Luride® 0.25 and 0.5 Lozi-Tabs
Luride® Lozi-Tabs
Pediaflor® Drops
Phos-Flur® Rinse/Supplement
Point-Two® Mouthrinse
Prevident® Disclosing Drops
Thera-Flur® Gel and Drops

Diagnostic Agents
Gastrografin®

Dietary Substitutes
Co-Salt®

Iron Preparations/Blood Modifiers
Amicar® Syrup
Beminal® Stress Plus With Iron
Chel-Iron® Drops
Chel-Iron® Liquid
Geritol® Complete Tablets
Geritonic™ Liquid
Hemo-Vite® Liquid
Iberet® Liquid
Iberet®-500 Liquid
Incremin® With Iron Syrup
Kovitonic® Liquid
Niferex®
Nu-Iron® Elixir
Vita-Plus H® Half Strength, Sugar-Free
Vita-Plus H®, Sugar-Free

Laxatives
Agoral® (plain, marshmallow, and raspberry)
Aromatic Cascara Fluidextract USP
Castor Oil
Castor Oil (flavored)
Castor Oil USP
Colace®, Liquid
Cologel®
Disonate™ Liquid
Doxinate® Solution
Emulsoil®
Fiberall® Powder
Haley's MO®
Hydrocil® Instant Powder
Hypaque® Oral Powder
Kondremul®
Kondremul® With Cascara

SUGAR-FREE LIQUID PHARMACEUTICALS *(Continued)*

Konsyl® Powder
Liqui-Doss®
Magnesium Citrate Solution NF
Metamucil® Instant Mix (lemon-lime or orange)
Metamucil® SF Powder
Milk of Magnesia
Milk of Magnesia/Cascara Suspension
Milk of Magnesia/Mineral Oil Emulsion (various)
Milkinol® Liquid
Mineral Oil (various)
Neoloid® Liquid
Nu-LYTELY®
Phospho-Soda®
Sodium Phosphate & Biphosphate Oral Solution USP
Zymenol® Emulsion

Potassium Products
Cena-K® Solution
EM-K®-10% Liquid
K-G® Elixir
Kaochlor-Eff® Tablets for Solution
Kaochlor® S-F Solution
Kaon® Elixir (grape and lemon-lime flavor)
Kaon-Cl® 20% Liquid
Kay Ciel® Elixir
Kay Ciel® Powder
Kaylixir®
Klor-Con®/25 Powder
Klor-Con® EF Tablets
Klor-Con® Liquid 20%
Klor-Con® Powder
Klorvess® Effervescent Tablets
Klorvess® Granules
Kolyum® Liquid and Powder
Potachlor® 10% and 20% Liquid
Potasalan® Elixir
Potassine® Liquid
Potassium Chloride Oral Solution USP 5%, 10%, and 20% (various)
Potassium Gluconate Elixir NF
Rum-K® Solution
Tri-K® Liquid
Trikates® Solution

Sedatives-Tranquilizers-Antipsychotics
Butabarbital Sodium Elixir
Butisol Sodium® Elixir
Haldol® Concentrate
Loxitane® C Drops
Mellaril® Concentrate
Serentil® Concentrate
Thorazine® Concentrate

Vitamin Preparations-Nutritionals
Aquasol A® Drops
BioCal® Tablets
Bugs Bunny™ Chewable Tablets
Bugs Bunny™ Plus Iron Chewable Tablets
Bugs Bunny™ With Extra C Chewable Tablets
Bugs Bunny™ Plus Minerals Chewable Tablets
Calciferol™ Drops
Caltrate® 600 Tablets
Ce-Vi-Sol® Drops
Cod Liver Oil (various)
Decagen® Tablets
DHT™ Intensol Solution (Roxane)
Drisdol® in Propylene Glycol
Flintstones™ Complete Chewable Tablets
Flintstones™ With Extra C Chewable Tablets
Flintstones™ Plus Iron Chewable Tablets
Incremin® With Iron Liquid
Kandium® Drops Tablets
Lanoplex® Elixir
Lycolan® Elixir
Oyst-Cal® 500 Tablets
Pediaflor®
PMS® Relief

Poly-Vi-Flor® Drops
Poly-Vi-Flor®/Iron Drops
Poly-Vi-Sol® Drops
Poly-Vi-Sol®/Iron Drops
Posture® Tablets
Spiderman™ Children's Chewable Vitamin Tablets
Spiderman™ Children's Plus Iron Tablets
Theragran® Jr Children's Chewable Tablets
Tri-Vi-Flor® Drops
Tri-Vi-Sol® Drops
Tri-Vi-Sol®/Iron Drops
Vi-Daylin® ADC Drops
Vi-Daylin® ADC/Fluoride Drops
Vi-Daylin® ADC Plus Iron Drops
Vi-Daylin® Drops
Vi-Daylin®/Fluoride Drops
Vi-Daylin® Plus Iron Drops
Vitalize®

Miscellaneous

Altace™ Capsules
Bicitra® Solution
Cibalith-S® Syrup
Colestid® Granules
Dayto® Himbin® Liquid
Digoxin® Elixir
Duvoid®
Glandosane®
Lipomul®
Lithium Citrate Syrup
Nicorette® Chewing Gum
Polycitra®-K Solution
Polycitra®-LC Solution
Tagamet® Liquid

References:
Hill EM, Flaitz CM, and Frost GR, "Sweetener Content of Common Pediatric Oral Liquid Medications," *Am J Hosp Pharm*, 1988, 45(1):135-42.
Kumar A, Rawlings RD, and Beaman DC, "The Mystery Ingredients: Sweeteners, Flavorings, Dyes, and Preservatives in Analgesic/Antipyretic, Antihistamine/Decongestant, Cough and Cold, Antidiarrheal, and Liquid Theophylline Preparations," *Pediatrics*, 1993, 91(5):927-33.
"Sugar Free Products," *Drug Topics Red Book*, 1992, 17-8.

ALLERGIC SKIN REACTIONS TO DRUGS

Skin eruptions are the most common clinically observed form of drug "allergy." Cutaneous manifestations of hypersensitivity may include pruritus, urticaria, and angioedema; maculopapular, morbilliform, or erythematous rashes; erythema multiforme; eczema; erythema nodosum; photosensitivity reactions; and fixed drug eruptions. The most severe drug-related reactions are exfoliative dermatitis and vesiculobullous eruptions such as the Stevens-Johnson syndrome and toxic epidermal necrolysis (Lyell's syndrome). This table lists the incidence of drugs associated with cutaneous manifestations reported in 22,227 consecutive medical inpatients in the Boston Collaborative Drug Surveillance Program.

Drug	Reaction per 1000 Recipients
Sulfamethoxazole and trimethoprim	59
Ampicillin	52
Semisynthetic penicillins	36
Blood, whole human	35
Corticotropin	28
Erythromycin	23
Sulfisoxazole	17
Penicillin G	16
Gentamicin sulfate	16
Practolol	16
Cephalosporins	13
Quinidine	13
Plasma protein fraction	12
Dipyrone	11
Mercurial diuretics	9.5
Nitrofurantoin	9.1
Packed RBCs	8.1
Heparin	7.7
Chloramphenicol	6.8
Trimethobenzamide	6.6
Phenazopyridine	6.5
Methenamine	6.4
Nitrazepam	6.3
Barbiturates	4.7
Glutethimide	4.5
Indomethacin	4.4
Chlordiazepoxide	4.2
Metoclopramide	4.0
Diazepam	3.8
Propoxyphene	3.4
Isoniazid	3.0
Guaifenesin and theophylline	2.9
Nystatin	2.9
Chlorothiazide	2.8
Furosemide	2.6
Isophane insulin suspension	1.3
Phenytoin	1.1
Phytonadione	0.9
Flurazepam	0.5
Chloral hydrate	0.2

Reference:
Patterson R and Anderson J, "Allergic Reactions to Drugs and Biologic Agents," *JAMA*, 1982, 248:2637-45.

COMMON ORAL-FACIAL INFECTIONS AND ANTIBIOTICS FOR TREATMENT

Pathogens	Infections	Antibiotics
Aerobic gram-positive cocci	Cellulitis	Primary
	Periapical abscess	
	Periodontal abscess	Penicillin VK
and	Acute suppurative pulpitis	
	Oral-nasal fistulas	Alternates
Anaerobes	Pericorinitis	
	Osteitis	Erythromycin
	Osteomyelitis	
	Postsurgical and post-traumatic infection	Clindamycin

CONTROLLED SUBSTANCES

Schedule I = C-I

The drugs and other substances in this schedule have no legal medical uses except research. They have a **high** potential for abuse. They include selected opiates such as heroin, opium derivatives, and hallucinogens.

Schedule II = C-II

The drugs and other substances in this schedule have legal medical uses and a **high** abuse potential which may lead to severe dependence. They include former "Class A" narcotics, amphetamines, barbiturates, and other drugs.

Schedule III = C-III

The drugs and other substances in this schedule have legal medical uses and a **lesser** degree of abuse potential which may lead to **moderate** dependence. They include former "Class B" narcotics and other drugs.

Schedule IV = C-IV

The drugs and other substances in this schedule have legal medial uses and **low** abuse potential which may lead to **moderate** dependence. They include barbiturates, benzodiazepines, propoxyphenes, and other drugs.

Schedule V = C-V

The drugs and other substances in this schedule have legal medical uses and **low** abuse potential which may lead to **moderate** dependence. They include narcotic cough preparations, diarrhea preparations, and other drugs.

Note: These are federal classifications. Your individual state may place a substance into a more restricted category. When this occurs, the more restricted category applies. Consult your state law.

DRUGS ASSOCIATED WITH ADVERSE HEMATOLOGIC EFFECTS

Drug	Red Cell Aplasia	Thrombo-cytopenia	Neutro-penia	Pancyto-penia	Hemolysis
Acetazolamide		+	+	+	
Allopurinol			+		
Amiodarone	+				
Amphotericin B				+	
Amrinone		++			
Asparaginase		+++	+++	+++	++
Barbiturates		+		+	
Benzocaine					++
Captopril			++		+
Carbamazepine		++	+		
Cephalosporins			+		++
Chloramphenicol		+	++	+++	
Chlordiazepoxide			+	+	
Chloroquine		+			
Chlorothiazides		++			
Chlorpropamide	+	++	+	++	+
Chlortetracycline				+	
Chlorthalidone			+		
Cimetidine		+	++	+	
Codeine		+			
Colchicine				+	
Cyclophosphamide		+++	+++	+++	+
Dapsone					+++
Desipramine		++			
Digitalis		+			
Digitoxin		++			
Erythromycin		+			
Estrogen		+		+	
Ethacrynic acid			+		
Fluorouracil		+++	+++	+++	+
Furosemide		+	+		
Gold salts	+	+++	+++	+++	
Heparin		++			+
Ibuprofen			+		
Imipramine			++		
Indomethacin		+	++	+	
Isoniazid		+		+	
Isosorbide dinitrate					+
Levodopa					++
Meperidine		+			
Meprobamate		+	+	+	
Methimazole			++		
Methyldopa		++			+++
Methotrexate		+++	+++	+++	++
Methylene blue					+
Metronidazole			+		
Nalidixic acid					+
Naproxen				+	
Nitrofurantoin			++		+
Nitroglycerine		+			
Penicillamine		++	+		
Penicillins		+	++	+	+++
Phenazopyridine					+++
Phenothiazines		+	++	+++	+
Phenylbutazone		+	++	+++	+
Phenytoin		++	++	++	+
Potassium iodide		+			
Prednisone		+			
Primaquine					+++
Procainamide			+		
Procarbazine		+	++	++	+
Propylthiouracil		+	++	+	+
Quinidine		+++	+		

DRUGS ASSOCIATED WITH
ADVERSE HEMATOLOGIC EFFECTS *(Continued)*

Drug	Red Cell Aplasia	Thrombo-cytopenia	Neutro-penia	Pancyto-penia	Hemolysis
Quinine		+++	+		
Reserpine		+			
Rifampicin		++	+		+++
Spironolactone			+		
Streptomycin		+		+	
Sulfamethoxazole with trimethoprim			+		
Sulfonamides	+	++	++	++	++
Sulindac	+	+	+	+	
Tetracyclines		+			+
Thioridazine			++		
Tolbutamide		++	+	++	
Triamterene					+
Valproate	+				
Vancomycin			+		

+ = rare or single reports.

++ = occasional reports.

+++ = substantial number of reports.

Adapted from D'Arcy PF and Griffin JP, eds, *Iatrogenic Diseases*, New York, NY: Oxford University Press, 1986, 128-30.

HERBAL MEDICINES

CHEMICAL ANALYSIS OF SELECTED PRODUCTS

Herb		Main Components	Pharmacological Claim
Latin Name	Chinese Name		
Ledebouriella seseloides	Fang feng	Essential oils, alcohol derivatives, organic acids	Dispels "wind", antipyretic, analgesic antibacterial
Potentilla chinensis	Wei ling cai	Vitamin C, tannin, proteins, Ca++ salts	Antibacterial (antituberculosis) muscle relaxant, removes toxic "heats"
Akebia clematidie	Chuan mu tong	Aristolochic acid, akebin saponin	Reduces "heat", diuretic, antibacterial myocardial stimulant
Rehmannia glutinosa	Sheng di huang	Sterol, campesterol, rehmannin, alkaloids	Cardiotonic, diuretic, aids blood coagulation, anti-inflammatory
Paeonia lactiflora	Chi shao	Glycosides (eg, paeoninflorin), essential oils	Increases leucocyte cell count, removes "heat", eliminates blood stasis
Lophatherum gracile	Dan zhu ye	Arundoin, cylindrin, frieldelin	Diuretic, removes "heat", reduces "wind", antipyretic, antibacterial
Dictamnus dasycarpus	Bai xian pi	Dictamnine, alkaloids, psoralen, essential oils	Removes "damp heat", dispels "wind", antifungal
Tribulus terrestris	Ci ji li	Harmane, harmine	Hypotensive, diuretic, suppresses hyperactivity of liver, promotes blood circulation
Glycyrrhiza uralensis	Gan cao	Glycyrrhizin	Strengthens spleen and stomach, removes "heat" and toxins
Schizonepeta tenuifolia	Jing jie sui	Essential oils, D-methone, Di-limonene	Expels "wind", induces diaphoresis, reduces bleeding time

HERBAL MEDICINES (Continued)

HERBS AND COMMON NATURAL AGENTS

The authors have chosen to include this list of natural products and proposed medical claims. However, due to limited scientific investigation to support these claims, this list is not intended to imply that these claims have been scientifically proven.

PROPOSED MEDICINAL CLAIMS

Herb	Medicinal Claim
Agrimony	Digestive disorders
Alfalfa	Source of carotene (vitamin A); contains natural fluoride
Allspice	General health
Aloe	Healing agent
Angelica root	Diseases of the lungs and heart; distaste for alcoholic beverages
Anise seed	Prevent gas
Arthritis tea	Treat osteoarthritis
Astragalus	Enhance energy reserves; used with ginseng
Barberry bark	Treat halitosis
Basil leaf	Remedy to inhibit vomiting
Bayberry bark	Relieve and prevent varicose veins
Bay leaf	Relieves cramps
Bee pollen	Renewal of enzymes, hormones, vitamins, amino acids, and others
Bergamot herb	Calming effect
Bilberry leaf	Increases night vision, reduces eye fatigue
Birch bark	Treat urinary problems; used for rheumatism
Blackberry leaf	Treat diarrhea
Black cohosh	Relieves menstrual cramps; same effects as estrogen
Blessed thistle (Holy thistle)	Aids circulation to the brain
Blueberry leaf	General medicinal
Blue Cohosh	Regulate menstrual flow; emergency remedy for allergic reactions to bee stings
Blue flag	Useful in the treatment of skin diseases and constipation
Blue violet	Relieves severe headaches
Boldo leaf	Stimulates digestion; treatment of gallstones
Boneset	Treatment of colds and flu
Borage leaf	Reduces high fevers
Bromelain	Fat melting enzyme; stimulates the metabolism
Buchu leaf	Diuretic; treatment of acute and chronic bladder and kidney disorders
Buckthorn bark	Expels worms and will remove warts
Burdock leaf and root	Treatment of severe skin problems and cases of arthritis
Butternut bark	Works well for constipation
Calamus root	General medicinal
Calendula flower	Mending and healing of cuts or wounds
Capsicum (Cayenne)	Normalizes blood pressure; stops bleeding on contact
Caraway seed	Aids digestion
Cascara sagrada bark	Remedies for chronic constipation and gallstones
Catnip	Benefits gas or cramps
Celery leaf and seed	Incontinence of urine
Centaury	Stimulates the salivary gland
Chamomile flower	Excellent for a nervous stomach; relieves cramping associated with the menstrual cycle
Chervil	Stimulant, mild diuretic, lowers blood pressure
Chickweed	Rich in vitamin C and minerals (calcium, magnesium, and potassium)
Chicory root	Effective in disorders of the kidneys, liver, and urinary canal

PROPOSED MEDICINAL CLAIMS *(continued)*

Herb	Medicinal Claim
Cinnamon bark	Prevents infection and indigestion; helps break down fats during digestion
Cleavers	Treatment of kidney and bladder disorders; useful in obstructions of the urinary organ
Cloves	General medicinal
Colombo root	Colon trouble
Coltsfoot herb and flower	Useful for asthma, bronchitis, and spasmodic cough
Coriander seed	Stomach tonic
Cornsilk	Prostate gland
Cranberry	Bladder or kidney infection
Cubeb berry	Chronic bladder trouble; increases flow of urine
Damiana leaf	Sexual impotency
Dandelion leaf and root	Detoxify poisons in the liver; beneficial in lowering blood pressure
Dill weed	General medicinal
Dong Quai root	Female troubles
Echinacea root	Treat strep throat, lymph glands
Eucalyptus leaf	General medicinal
Elder	General medicinal
Elecampane root	General medicinal
Eyebright herb	General medicinal
Fennel seed	Remedies for gas and acid stomach
Fenugreek seed	Allergies, coughs, digestion, emphysema, headaches, migraines, intestinal inflammation, ulcers, lungs, mucous membranes, and sore throat
Feverfew herb	Migraines; helps reduce inflammation in arthritis joints
Garlic capsules	"Nature's antibiotic"
Gentian	Digestive organs and increase circulation
Ginger root	Remedy for sore throat
Ginkgo biloba	Improves blood circulation to the brain
Ginseng root, Siberian	Resistance against stress; slows the aging process
Goldenseal	Treatment of bladder infections, cankers, mouth sores, mucous membranes, and ulcers
Gota kola	"Memory herb"; nerve tonic
Gravelroot (Queen of the Meadow)	Remedy for stones in the kidney and bladder
Green barley	Excellent antioxidant
Hawthorn	Strengthens and regulates the heart; relieves insomnia
Henna	External use only
Hibiscus flower	Stimulant for the intestines and kidneys
Holy thistle (Blessed thistle)	Remedy for migraine headaches
Hops flower	Insomnia; used to decrease the desire for alcohol
Horehound	Acute or chronic sore throat and coughs
Horsetail (Shavegrass)	Rich in minerals, especially silica; used to develop strong fingernails and hair, good for split ends
Ho shou wu	Rejuvenator
Hydrangea root	Backaches
Hyssop	Asthma
Juniper berry	Kidney ailments
Kava kava root	Induce sleep and help calm nervousness
Kelp	High contents of natural plant iodine, for proper function of the thyroid; high levels of natural calcium, potassium, and magnesium
Lavender flower	Flavor moderator
Lecithin	Break up cholesterol; prevent arteriosclerosis
Licorice root	Mild laxative
Ma-huang	Cleanses respiratory system

HERBAL MEDICINES (Continued)

PROPOSED MEDICINAL CLAIMS (continued)

Herb	Medicinal Claim
Malva flower	Soothes inflammation in the mouth and throat; helpful for earaches
Marjoram	Beneficial for a sour stomach or loss of appetite
Marshmallow leaf	Inflammation
Milk thistle herb	Liver detoxifier
Motherwort	Chest cold, nervousness
Mugwort	Used for rheumatism and gout
Mullein leaf	High in iron, magnesium, and potassium; sinuses; relieves swollen joints
Mustard seed	General medicinal
Myrrh gum	Removes bad breath; sinus problems
Nettle leaf	In combination with seawrack, will bring splendid results in weight loss; remedy for dandruff
Nutmeg	Gas
Oregano leaf	Settles the stomach after meals; helps treat colds
Oregon grape root	Useful in rheumatism
Papaya leaf	Digestive stimulant; contains the enzyme papain
Paprika (sweet)	Stimulates the appetite and gastric secretions
Parsley leaf	High in iron
Passion flower	Mild sedative
Patchouli leaf	Excellent seasoning
Pau d'arco	Protects immune system
Pennyroyal	Relieves high fevers and brings on perspiration
Peppermint leaf	Excellent for headaches
Plantain leaf	Useful for infection, hemorrhoids, and inflammation
Pleurisy root	Break up a cold
Poppy seed blue	Excellent in the making of breads and desserts
Prickly ash bark	Increases circulation
Prince's pine	Diuretic; for rheumatism and chronic kidney problems
Psyllium seed	Lubricant to the intestinal tract
Red clover	Purify the blood
Red raspberry leaf	Eases menstrual cramps
Rhubarb root	Powerful laxative
Rose hips	High content of vitamin C
Safflower	Eliminates buildup of uric and lactic acid in the body, the leading cause of gout
Saffron	Natural digestive aid
Sanicle	Cleansing herb
Sarsaparilla root	Remedy for rheumatism and gout; acts as a diuretic; same effects on the body as the male hormone testosterone
Sassafras leaf and root	Stimulates the action of the liver to clear toxins from the body
Saw palmetto berry	Mucus in the head and nose
Scullcap	Nerve sedative; hangover remedy
Seawrack (Bladderwrack)	Combat obesity
Senna leaf	Splendid laxative
Shepherd's purse	Remedy for diarrhea
Sheep sorrel	Remedy for kidney trouble
Slippery elm bark	Normalize bowel movement; beneficial for hemorrhoids and constipation
Solomon's seal root	Poultice for bruises
Speedwell	Used as a gargle for mouth and throat sores
Spikenard	Skin ailments such as acne, pimples, blackheads, rashes, and general skin problems
Star anise	Promotes appetite and relieves flatulence

PROPOSED MEDICINAL CLAIMS *(continued)*

Herb	Medicinal Claim
St John's wort	Correct irregular menstruation
Strawberry leaf	Prevents diarrhea
Sumac berry and bark	Sores and cankers in the mouth
Summer savory leaf	Treats diarrhea, upset stomach, and sore throat
Thyme leaf	Relief of migraine headaches
Uva-ursi leaf	Digestive stimulant
Valerian root	Promotes sleep
Vervain	Remedy for fevers
White oak bark	Strong astringent
White willow bark	Used for minor aches and pains in the body
Wild alum root	Powerful astringent; used as rinse for sores in mouth and bleeding gums
Wild cherry	Asthma
Wild Oregon grape root	Chronic skin disease
Wild yam root	Helps expel gas
Wintergreen leaf	Valuable for colic and gas in the bowels
Witch hazel bark and leaf	Restores circulation; for stiff joints
Wood betony	Relieves pain in the face and head
Woodruff	Insomnia and hysteria
Wormwood	Aids bruises and sprains
Yarrow root	Unsurpasses for flue and fevers
Yellow dock root	Good in all skin problems
Yerba santa	Bronchial congestion
Yohimbe	Natural aphrodisiac
Yucca root	Reduces inflammation of the joints

POISON INFORMATION CENTERS

Updated from "Poisoning Hotlines," *Emergency Medicine*, 1994, 26:96-102; and American Association of Poison Control Centers, *Vet Hum Toxicol*, 1994, 36:484-6.

*Denotes certified Regional Poison Control Centers by the American Association of Poison Control Centers (April, 1997)

Centers in each state are listed alphabetically by city.

ALABAMA

Regional Poison Control Center*
The Children's Hospital of Alabama
1600 7th Ave, S
Birmingham, AL 35233
(800) 292-6678 (Alabama only)
(205) 933-4050
(205) 939-9201
(205) 939-9202

The Alabama Poison Center*
408-A Paul Bryant Dr
Tuscaloosa, AL 35401
(800) 462-0800 (Alabama only)
(205) 345-0600

ALASKA

Anchorage Poison Control Center
Providence Hospital Pharmacy
3600 Providence Dr
PO Box 196604
Anchorage, AK 99516
(800) 478-3193 (Alaska only)
(907) 271-3193 (Anchorage only)
(907) 261-3633

ARIZONA

Samaritan Regional Poison Center*
Good Samaritan Regional Medical Center
1111 E McDowell Rd
Phoenix, AZ 85006
(602) 253-3334
(800) 362-0101 (Arizona only)

Arizona Poison and Drug Information Center*
University of Arizona
Arizona Health Sciences Center
1501 N Campbell Ave, Rm 1156
Tucson, AZ 85724
(800) 362-0101 (Arizona only)
(602) 626-6016

ARKANSAS

Arkansas Poison and Drug Information Center
University of Arkansas for Medical Sciences
College of Pharmacy
Slot 522 (internal mailing)
4301 W Markham St
Little Rock, AR 72205
(800) 376-4766 (MDs and hospitals; Arkansas only)
(501) 661-6161
(501) 666-5532 (MDs and hospitals)

CALIFORNIA

California Poison Control System – Fresno Division*
Valley Children's Hospital
3151 N Milbrook
Fresno, CA 93703
(209) 445-1222
(800) 876-4766 (Central California only)

Los Angeles County Regional Drug and Poison Information Center
1200 N State St, Rm 1107A and B
Los Angeles, CA 90033
(800) 777-6476 (Los Angeles, Santa Barbara, and Ventura counties only)
(213) 222-3212
(213) 222-8086 (MDs and hospitals)

Chevron Emergency Information Center
100 Chevron Way
Richmond, CA 94802
(800)231-0623
(510)231-0149

California Poison Control System – Sacramento Division*
2315 Stockton Blvd, Room 1024, house staff facility
Sacramento, CA 95817
(800) 876-4766 (Northern California only)
(916) 734-3692

California Poison Control System – San Diego Division*
UCSD Medical Center
200 West Arbor Dr
San Diego, CA 92103
(800) 876-4766
(619) 543-6000

California Poison Control System – San Francisco Division
San Francisco General Hospital
1001 Potrero Ave, Building 80, Rm 230
San Francisco, CA 94110
(800) 876-4766

Santa Clara Valley Regional Poison Center
Valley Health Center
750 S Bascom Ave, Suite 310
San Jose, CA 95128
(800) 662-9886 (CA only)
(408) 885-6000

COLORADO

Rocky Mountain Poison and Drug Center*
8802 E 9th Ave
Denver, CO 80220
(303) 629-1123
(800) 332-3073 (Colorado only)
(800) 446-6179 (Las Vegas, Idaho only)
(800) 525-5042 (Montana only)

CONNECTICUT

Connecticut Poison Control Center*
University of Connecticut Health Center
263 Farmington Ave
Farmington, CT 06030
(800) 343-2722 (Connecticut only)
(203) 679-3473 (Administration)
(203) 679-4346 (TDD)

DELAWARE

Interstate Centers
The Poison Control Center*
3600 Science Center, Suite 220
Philadelphia, PA
(800) 722-7112
(215) 386-2100

DISTRICT OF COLUMBIA

National Capital Poison Center*
George Washington University Medical Center

POISON INFORMATION CENTERS *(Continued)*

3201 New Mexico Ave, NW, Suite 310
Washington, DC 20016
(202) 625-3333
(202) 362-8563 (TTY)

FLORIDA

Florida Poison Information Center – Jacksonville*
University Medical Center
University of Florida Health Science Center-Jacksonville
655 W 8th St
Jacksonville, FL 32209
(800) 282-3171 (Florida only)
(305) 585-5253

Florida Poison Information Center – Miami*
University of Miami School of Medicine
Department of Pediatrics
PO Box 016960 (R-131)
Miami, FL 33101
(800) 282-3171
(305) 585-5250
(305) 585-5253

Tallahassee Memorial Regional Medical Center
1300 Miccosukee Road
Tallahassee, FL 32308
(904)681-5411

Florida Poison Information Center – Tampa*
Tampa General Hospital
PO Box 1289
Tampa, FL 33601
(800) 282-3171 (Florida only)
(813) 253-4444 (Tampa)

GEORGIA

Georgia Poison Center*
Grady Memorial Hospital
80 Butler St, SE
Box 26066
Atlanta, GA 30335
(800) 282-5846 (Georgia only)
(404) 616-9000

HAWAII

Hawaii Poison Center
Kapiolani Women's and Children's Medical Center
1319 Punahou St
Honolulu, HI 96826
(800) 362-3585 (outer islands of Hawaii only)
(800) 362-3586
(808) 941-4411

IDAHO

Idaho Poison Center
1055 North Curtis Road
Boise, ID 83706
(800) 860-0620 (Idaho only)

ILLINOIS

Illinois Poison Center
222 Riverside Plaza, Suite 1900
Chicago, IL 60606
(800) 942-5969 (Illinois only)
(312) 942-5969
(312) 942-7064

INDIANA

Indiana Poison Center*
Methodist Hospital of Indiana
I-65 and 21st Street
PO Box 1367
Indianapolis, IN 46206

(800) 382-9097 (Indiana only)
(317) 929-2323

Interstate Centers
Kentucky Regional Poison Center of Kosair Children's Hospital*
Louisville, KY
(502) 589-8222 (Southern Indiana only)

IOWA

Variety Club Poison and Drug Information Center
Iowa Methodist Medical Center
1200 Pleasant St
Des Moines, IA 50309
(800) 362-2327 (Iowa only)
(515) 241-6254

St Luke's Poison Center
St Luke's Regional Medical Center
2720 Stone Park Blvd
Sioux City, IA 51104
(800) 352-2222 (Western Iowa, Northeastern Nebraska, and Southern South
Dakota only)
(712) 277-2222

Interstate Centers
McKennan Hospital Poison Center
PO Box 5045
Sioux Falls, SD
(800) 952-0123
(605) 322-3894

KANSAS

Mid-America Poison Control Center*
University of Kansas Medical Center
3901 Rainbow, Rm B-400
Kansas City, KS 66160
(800) 332-6633 (Kansas only)
(913) 588-6633

Stormont-Vail Regional Medical Center Emergency Department
1500 West 10th St
Topeka, KS 66604
(913) 354-6106

HCA Wesley Poison Control Center Medical Center
550 N Hillside Ave
Wichita, KS 67214
(316) 688-2277

KENTUCKY

Kentucky Regional Poison Center of Kosair Children's Hospital*
Medical Towers South, Ste 572
PO Box 35070
Louisville, KY 40232
(800) 722-5725 (Kentucky only)
(502) 629-7275
(502) 589-8222

LOUISIANA

Louisiana Drug and Poison Information Center*
Northeast Louisiana University School of Pharmacy
Sugar Hall
Monroe, LA 71209
(800) 256-9822 (Louisiana only)
(318) 362-5393

MAINE

Maine Poison Control Center
Maine Medical Center
22 Bramhall St
Portland, ME 04102
(800) 442-6305 (Maine only)
(207) 871-2950

POISON INFORMATION CENTERS *(Continued)*

MARYLAND

Maryland Poison Center*
University of Maryland School of Pharmacy
20 N Pine St
Baltimore, MD 21201
(800) 492-2414 (Maryland only)
(410) 706-7701

Interstate Centers
National Capital Poison Center*
3201 New Mexico Ave, NW, Suite 310
Washington, DC 20016
(202) 625-3333 (DC suburbs only)
(202) 362-8563 (TTY)

MASSACHUSETTS

Massachusetts Poison Control System*
300 Longwood Ave
Boston, MA 02115
(800) 682-9211 (Massachusetts only)
(617) 355-6609 (Administration)
(617) 232-2120 (Boston)

MICHIGAN

Children's Hospital of Michigan Poison Control Center*
4160 John R, Ste 425
Detroit, MI 48201
(313) 745-5711
(800) 764-7661 (Michigan only)

Blodgett Regional Poison Center*
Blodgett Memorial Medical Center
1840 Wealthy St, SE
Grand Rapids, MI 49506
(800) 764-7661 (Michigan only)
(800) 356-3232 (TTY)
(616) 774-7851 (Administration)

MINNESOTA

Hennepin Regional Poison Center*
Hennepin County Medical Center
701 Park Ave
Minneapolis, MN 55415
(612) 347-3141
(612) 337-7474 (TDD)
(612) 337-7387 (Petline)

Minnesota Regional Poison Center*
St Paul-Ramsey Medical Center
8100 34th Ave, S
Minneapolis, MN 55440-1309
(800) 222-1222 (Minnesota only)
(612) 221-2113

MISSISSIPPI

Mississippi Regional Poison Control Center
University Medical Center
2500 N State St
Jackson, MS 39216
(601) 354-7660

MISSOURI

Children's Mercy Hospital
2401 Gillham Rd
Kansas City, MO 64108
(816) 234-3430

Cardinal Glennon Children's Hospital Regional Poison Center*
1465 S Grand Blvd
St Louis, MO 63104

(800) 366-8888
(314) 772-5200

MONTANA

Interstate Centers
Rocky Mountain Poison and Drug Center*
8802 E 9th Ave
Denver, CO 80204
(303) 629-1123

NEBRASKA

The Poison Center*
Childrens Memorial Hospital
8301 Dodge St
Omaha, NE 68114
(800) 955-9119 (Nebraska and Wyoming only)
(402) 354-5555

NEVADA

Interstate Centers
Rocky Mountain Poison and Drug Center*
645 Bannock St
Denver, CO 80204
(800) 446-6179 (Las Vegas only)
(303) 629-1123

Poison Center
Humana Hospital Sunrise
3186 Maryland Pkwy
Las Vegas, NV 89109
(800) 446-6179 (Clark and Nye County only)

Poison Center
Washoe Medical Center
77 Pringle Way
Reno, NV 89520
(702) 328-4144
(702) 328-4100
(702) 328-4129

NEW HAMPSHIRE

New Hampshire Poison Information Center
Dartmouth Hitchcock Memorial Hospital
1 Medical Center Dr
Lebanon, NH 03756
(800) 562-8236 (New Hampshire only)
(603) 650-5000 (New Hampshire and bordering towns in Maine, Massachusetts, and Vermont only)

NEW JERSEY

New Jersey Poison Information and Education System*
Newark Beth Israel Medical Center
201 Lyons Ave
Newark, NJ 07112
(800) 764-7661
(201) 926-8008 (TTY)

Warren Hospital Poison Control Center
185 Roseberry St
Phillipsburg, NJ 08865
(800) 962-1253
(908) 859-6767

NEW MEXICO

New Mexico Poison and Drug Information Center*
University of New Mexico
Health Sciences Library, Rm 125
Albuquerque, NM 87131
(800) 432-6866 (New Mexico only)
(505) 272-2222

NEW YORK

Western New York Regional Poison Control Center
Children's Hospital of Buffalo
219 Bryant St

POISON INFORMATION CENTERS *(Continued)*

Buffalo, NY 14222
(716) 878-7654
(716) 878-7655

Long Island Regional Poison Control Center*
Winthrop-University Hospital
259 First St
Mineola, NY 11501
(516) 542-2323
(516) 542-6315
(516) 542-6316
(516) 542-6317

New York City Poison Control Center*
New York City Department of Health
455 First Ave, Rm 123
New York, NY 10016
(212) 340-4494
(212) POISONS (764-7667)
(212) 689-9014 (TDD)

Hudson Valley Regional Poison Center*
Phelps Memorial Hospital Center
701 N Broadway
Sleepy Hollow, NY 10591
(800) 336-6997 (New York only)
(914) 366-3030

Finger Lakes Poison Center*
University of Rochester Medical Center
Box 321
601 Elmwood Ave
Rochester, NY 14642
(800) 333-0542
(716) 275-3232
(716) 275-2700 (TTY)

Central New York Regional Poison Control Center*
SUNY Health Science Center at University Hospital
750 E Adams St
Syracuse, NY 13210
(800) 252-5655 (New York only)
(315) 476-4766

NORTH CAROLINA

Western NC Poison Control Center
St Joseph's Hospital
428 Biltmore Ave, Box 60
Asheville, NC 28801
(800) 542-4225 (North Carolina only)
(704) 255-4490

Carolinas Poison Center*
1012 S Kings Drive, Ste 206
PO Box 32861
Charlotte, NC 28232
(800) 84-TOXIN (848-6946)
(704) 355-4000

Triad Poison Center at Moses H Cone Memorial Hospital
1200 N Elm St
Greensboro, NC 27401
(800) 953-4001 (Alamance, Forsyth, Guilford, Rockingham, and Randolph
counties only)
(910) 574-8105

NORTH DAKOTA

North Dakota Poison Information Center*
MeritCare Medical Center
720 Fourth St, N
Fargo, ND 58122
(800) 732-2200 (North Dakota, Minnesota only)
(701) 234-5575 (local)

OHIO

Akron Regional Poison Center
1 Perkins Square
Akron, OH 44308
(800) 362-9922 (Ohio only)
(330) 379-8562
(330) 379-8446 (TTY)

Cincinnati Drug & Poison Information Center and Regional Poison Control System*
PO Box 670144
Cincinnati, OH 45267-0144
(800) 872-5111 (Ohio only)
(513) 558-5111

Greater Cleveland Poison Control Center
11100 Euclid Ave
Cleveland, OH 44106
(216) 231-4455
(888) 234-4455

Central Ohio Poison Center*
700 Children's Dr
Columbus, OH 43205-2696
(800) 682-7625 (Ohio only)
(614) 461-2012
(614) 228-1323
(614) 228-2272 (TTY)

Firelands Community Hospital Poison Information Center
1101 Decatur St
Sandusky, OH 44870
(419) 626-7423

Poison and Drug Information Center of Northwest Ohio
Medical College of Ohio
3000 Arlington Ave
Toledo, OH 43614
(800) 589-3897 (Ohio only)
(419) 381-3897

Bethesda Poison Control Center
2951 Maple Ave
Zanesville, OH 43701
(614) 454-4000
(800) 682-7625

OKLAHOMA

Oklahoma Poison Control Center
Children's Hospital of Oklahoma
940 NE 13 St
Oklahoma City, OK 73104
(800) 764-7661 (Oklahoma only)
(405) 271-5454

OREGON

Oregon Poison Center*
Oregon Health Sciences University
3181 SW Sam Jackson Park Rd, CB550
Portland, OR 97201
(800) 452-7165 (Oregon only)
(503) 494-8968

PENNSYLVANIA

Regional Poison Prevention Education Center
Mercy Regional Health System
2500 7th Ave
Altoona, PA 16602
(814) 949-4197

Central Pennsylvania Poison Center*
Milton S Hershey Medical Center
University Dr, PO Box 850
Hershey, PA 17033
(800) 521-6110
(717) 531-6111

POISON INFORMATION CENTERS *(Continued)*

St Joseph Hospital and Health Care Center
250 College Ave
PO Box 3509
Lancaster, PA 17604
(717) 299-4546
(717) 291-8314
(717) 291-8425

The Poison Control Center*
3600 Sciences Center, Ste 220
Philadelphia, PA 19104-2641
(800) 722-7112
(215) 386-2100

Pittsburgh Poison Center*
Children's Hospital of Pittsburgh
1 Children's Pl
3705 Fifth Ave
Pittsburgh, PA 15213
(412) 681-6669

RHODE ISLAND

Rhode Island Poison Center
Rhode Island Hospital
593 Eddy St
Providence, RI 02903
(401) 444-5727

SOUTH CAROLINA

Palmetto Poison Center
University of South Carolina
College of Pharmacy
Columbia, SC 29208
(800) 922-1117 (South Carolina only)
(803) 777-1117 (Columbia area only)

SOUTH DAKOTA

McKennan Poison Control Center
McKennan Hospital
800 E 21 St
PO Box 5045
Sioux Falls, SD 57117
(800) 952-0123 (South Dakota only)
(800) 843-0505 (Iowa, Minnesota, North Dakota, and Nebraska only)
(605) 336-3894

TENNESSEE

Southern Poison Center, Inc
847 Monroe Ave, Suite 230
Memphis, TN 38163
(901) 528-6048 (East Arkansas)
(901) 448-6800
(800) 288-9999 (Tennessee)

Middle Tennessee Regional Poison Center*
The Center for Clinical Toxicology
1161 21st Ave S
501 Oxford House
Nashville, TN 37232-4632
(800) 288-9999
(615) 936-2034

TEXAS

Texas Panhandle Poison Center
PO Box 1110
15012 Coulter
Amarillo, TX 79175
(800) 764-7661 (Texas only)

North Texas Poison Center*
Parkland Hospital
5201 Harry Hines Blvd
PO Box 35926

Dallas, TX 75235
(800) 764-7661 (Northern Texas only)
(214) 590-5000

West Texas Poison Control Center
RE Thomason General Hospital
4815 Alameda Ave
El Paso, TX 79905
(800) 764-7661
(915) 521-7661

Southeast Texas Poison Center*
University of Texas Medical Branch
301 University Ave
Galveston, TX 77550-2780
(800) 764-7661
(409) 765-1420 (Galveston only)
(713) 654-1701 (Houston)

South Texas Poison Center
University of Texas Health Science Center at San Antonio
Forensic Science Building, Room 146
7703 Floyd Curl Drive
San Antonio, TX 78284
(800) 764-7661
(210) 764-7661

Central Texas Poison Center at Scott and White
2401 S 31st St
Temple, TX 76508
(800) 764-7661
(817) 724-7401

UTAH

Utah Poison Control Center*
410 Chipeta Way, Ste 230
Salt Lake City, UT 84108
(800) 456-7707 (Utah only)
(801) 581-2151

VERMONT

Vermont Poison Center
Medical Center Hospital of Vermont
111 Colchester Ave
Burlington, VT 05401
(802) 658-3456

VIRGINIA

Blue Ridge Poison Center*
University of Virginia Health Sciences Center
Blue Ridge Hospital
Box 67
Charlottesville, VA 22901
(800) 451-1428
(804) 924-5543

Virginia Poison Center
Virginia Commonwealth University
MCV Station, Box 980522
401 N 12th St
Richmond, VA 23298
(800) 552-6337 (Virginia only)
(804) 828-4780

Interstate Centers
National Capital Poison Center* (Northern VA only)
3201 New Mexico Ave, NW, Ste 310
Washington, DC 20016
(202) 625-3333
(202) 362-8563 (TTY)

WASHINGTON

Washington Poison Center*
155 NE 100th St, Ste 400
Seattle, WA 98125
(800) 732-6985

POISON INFORMATION CENTERS *(Continued)*

(800) 572-0638 (TDD)
(206) 526-2121
(206) 517-2394 (TDD)

WEST VIRGINIA

West Virginia Poison Center*
West Virginia University
Robert C. Byrd Health Sciences Center/Charleston Division
3110 MacCorkle Ave, SE
Charleston, WV 25304
(800) 642-3625 (West Virginia only)
(304) 348-4211

WISCONSIN

Regional Poison Control Center
University of Wisconsin Hospital and Clinics
600 Highland Ave
Madison, WI 53792
(800) 815-8855
(608) 262-3702 (also TDD)

Milwaukee Poison Center
Children's Hospital of Wisconsin
9000 W Wisconsin Ave
PO Box 1997
Milwaukee, WI 53201
(800) 815-8855
(414) 266-2222

WYOMING

Interstate Centers
The Poison Center*
8301 Dodge St
Omaha, NE 68114
(800) 955-9119 (Wyoming only)
(402) 390-5555 (Omaha)

FOREIGN

†Denotes American Association of Poison Control Centers:
Canadian Poison Center members.

CANADA

Alberta

PADIS (Poison and Drug Information Service)†
Foothills Provincial General Hospital
1403 29th St, NW
Calgary, Alberta T2N 2T9
(403) 670-1414

British Columbia

BC Drug and Poison Information Centre†
St Paul's Hospital
1081 Burrard St
Vancouver, BC V6Z 1Y6
(604) 682-5050

Manitoba

Poison Control Centre†
Children's Hospital
685 Bannatyne Ave
Winnipeg, Manitoba R3E OW1
(204) 787-2444

Nova Scotia

Izaak Walton Killan Children's Hospital
PO Box 3070
Halifax, Nova Scotia B3J 3G9

(800) 565-8161 (Prince Edward Island)
(902) 428-8161 (Nova Scotia)

Ontario

Provincial Regional Poison Control Centre
Children's Hospital
Eastern Ontario
401 Smyth Rd
Ottawa, Ontario K1H 8L1
(800) 267-1373
(613) 737-1100

Ontario Regional Poison Centre†
Hospital for Sick Children
555 University Ave
Toronto, Ontario M5G 1X8
(800) 268-9017
(416) 813-5900

Quebec

Quebec Poison Control Center†
Centre Hospitalier de l'Universite Laval
2705 Boulevard Laurier; J-782
Sainte-Foy Quebec
Canada GIV 4G2
(418) 656-8090
(418) 654-2731

COSTA RICA

Centro Nacional de Control de Intoxicaciones
Hospital Nacional de Ninos
"Dr Carlos Saenz Herrera"
Apartado 1654
San Jose, Costa Rica
(506) 23-10-28

MEXICO

Centro Panamerico de Ecologia Humana y
Salud — Toxicologia
Rancho Guadalupe
Metepec, Edo de Mexico
Apartado 37-473
06696 Mexico, DF
52-(91-721)
6-44-04
6-43-44

PUERTO RICO

University of Puerto Rico
College of Pharmacy
GPO Box 5067
San Juan, Puerto Rico
(809) 758-2525 ext 1516
(809) 763-0196

PRESCRIPTION WRITING

Doctor's Name
Address
Phone Number

Patient's Name/Date
Patient's Address/Age

Rx

Drug Name/Dosage Size

Disp: Number of tablets, capsules, ounces to be dispensed (roman numerals added as precaution for abused drugs)

Sig: Direction on how drug is to be taken

Doctor's signature

State license number

DEA number (if required)

PRESCRIPTION REQUIREMENTS

1. Date
2. Full name and address of patient
3. Name and address of prescriber
4. Signature of prescriber

If Class II drug, Drug Enforcement Agency (DEA) number necessary.

If Class II and Class III narcotic, a triplicate prescription form (in the state of California) is necessary and it must be handwritten by the prescriber.

Please turn to appropriate oral medicine chapters for examples of prescriptions.

ABBREVIATIONS COMMONLY USED IN MEDICAL ORDERS

Abbreviation	From	Meaning
aa, aa	ana	of each
ac	ante cibum	before meals or food
ad	ad	to, up to
a.d.	aurio dextra	right ear
ad lib	ad libitum	at pleasure
a.l.	aurio laeva	left ear
AM	ante meridiem	morning
amp		ampul
amt		amount
aq	aqua	water
aq. dest.	aqua destillata	distilled water
a.s.	aurio sinister	left ear
ASAP		as soon as possible
a.u.	aures utrae	each ear
bid	bis in die	twice daily
bm		bowel movement
bp		blood pressure
BSA		body surface area
c̄	cong	a gallon
c̄	cum	with
cal		calorie
cap	capsula	capsule
cc		cubic centimeter
cm		centimeter
comp	compositus	compound
cont		continue
d	dies	day

(continued)

Abbreviation	From	Meaning
d/c		discontinue
dil	dilue	dilute
disp	dispensa	dispense
div	divide	divide
dtd	dentur tales doses	give of such a dose
elix, el	elixir	elixir
emp		as directed
et	et	and
ex aq		in water
f, ft	fac, fiat, fiant	make, let be made
FDA		Food and Drug Administration
g	gramma	gram
gr	granum	grain
gtt	gutta	a drop
h	hora	hour
hs	hora somni	at bedtime
I.M.		intramuscular
I.V.		intravenous
kcal		kilocalorie
kg		kilogram
L		liter
liq	liquor	a liquor, solution
mcg		microgram
mEq		milliequivalent
mg		milligram
mixt	mixtura	a mixture
mL		milliliter
mm		millimeter
M	misce	mix
m. dict	more dictor	as directed
NF		National Formulary
no.	numerus	number
noc	nocturnal	in the night
non rep	non repetatur	do not repeat, no refills
NPO		nothing by mouth
O, Oct	octarius	a pint
o.d.	oculus dexter	right eye
o.l.	oculus laevus	left eye
o.s.	oculus sinister	left eye
o.u.	oculo uterque	each eye
pc, post cib	post cibos	after meals
per		through or by
PM	post meridiem	afternoon or evening
P.O.	per os	by mouth
P.R.	per rectum	rectally
prn	pro re nata	as needed
pulv	pulvis	a powder
q		every
qad	quoque alternis die	every other day
qd		every day
qh	quiaque hora	every hour
qid	quater in die	four times a day
qod		every other day
qs	quantum sufficiat	a sufficient quantity
qs ad		a sufficient quantity to make
qty		quantity

PRESCRIPTION WRITING *(Continued)*

Abbreviation	From	Meaning
qv	quam volueris	as much as you wish
Rx	recipe	take, a recipe
rep	repetatur	let it be repeated
s̄	sine	without
sa	secundum artem	according to art
sat	sataratus	saturated
S.C.		subcutaneous
sig	signa	label, or let it be printed
sol	solutio	solution
solv		dissolve
ss	semis	one-half
sos	si opus sit	if there is need
stat	statim	at once, immediately
supp	suppositorium	suppository
syr	syrupus	syrup
tab	tabella	tablet
tal		such
tid	ter in die	three times a day
tr, tinct	tincture	tincture
trit		triturate
tsp		teaspoonful
ung	unguentum	ointment
USAN		United States Adopted Names
USP		United States Pharmacopeia
u.d., ut dict	ut dictum	as directed
v.o.		verbal order
w.a.		while awake
x3		3 times
x4		4 times

SAFE WRITING PRACTICES

Health professionals and their support personnel frequently produce handwritten copies of information they see in print; therefore, such information is subjected to even greater possibilities for error or misinterpretation on the part of others. Thus, particular care must be given to how drug names and strengths are expressed when creating written healthcare documents.

The following are a few examples of safe writing rules suggested by the Institute for Safe Medication Practices, Inc.*

1. There should be a space between a number and its units as it is easier to read. There should be no periods after the abbreviations mg or mL.

Correct	Incorrect
10 mg	10mg
100 mg	100mg

2. Never place a decimal and a zero after a whole number (2 mg is correct and 2.0 mg is incorrect). If the decimal point is not seen because it falls on a line or because individuals are working from copies where the decimal point is not seen, this causes a tenfold overdose.

3. Just the opposite is true for numbers less than one. Always place a zero before a naked decimal (0.5 mL is correct, .5 mL is **in** correct).

4. Never abbreviate the word unit. The handwritten U or u, looks like a 0 (zero) and may cause a tenfold overdose error to be made.

5. Q.D. is not a safe abbreviation for once daily, as when the Q is followed by a sloppy dot, it looks like QID which means 4 times daily.

6. O.D. is not a safe abbreviation for once daily, as it is properly interpreted as meaning "right eye" and has caused liquid medications such as saturated solution of potassium iodide and Lugol's solution to be administered incorrectly. There is no safe abbreviation for once daily. It must be written out in full.

7. Do not use chemical names such as 6-mercaptopurine or 6-thioguanine, as sixfold overdoses have been given when these were not recognized as chemical names. The proper names of these drugs are mercaptopurine or thioguanine.

8. Do not abbreviate drug names (5FC, 6MP, 5-ASA, MTX, HCTZ CPZ, PBZ, etc) as they are misinterpreted and cause error.

9. Do not use the apothecary system or symbols.

10. Do not abbreviate microgram as µg; instead use mcg as there is less likelihood of misinterpretation.

11. When writing an outpatient prescription, write a complete prescription. A complete prescription can prevent the prescriber, the pharmacist, and/or the patient from making a mistake and can eliminate the need for further clarification.

    The legible prescriptions should contain:
    a. patient's full name
    b. for pediatric or geriatric patients: their age (or weight where applicable)
    c. drug name, dosage form and strength; if a drug is new or rarely prescribed, print this information
    d. number or amount to be dispensed
    e. complete instructions for the patient, including the purpose of the medication
    f. when there are recognized contraindications for a prescribed drug, indicate to the pharmacist that you are aware of this fact (ie, when prescribing a potassium salt for a patient receiving an ACE inhibitor, write "K serum leveling being monitored")

*From "Safe Writing" by Davis NM, PharmD and Cohen MR, MS, Lecturers and Consultants for Safe Medication Practices, 1143 Wright Drive, Huntingdon Valley, PA 19006. Phone: (215) 947-7566.

TOP 200 PRESCRIBED DRUGS IN 1997

Product	Generic Name
1. Trimox	Co-trimoxazole
2. Premarin Tablets	Conjugated estrogens
3. Synthroid	Levothyroxine
4. Hydrocodone/APAP	Hydrocodone
5. Prozac	Fluoxetine
6. Lanoxin	Digoxin
7. Prilosec	Omeprazole
8. Vasotec	Enalapril
9. Zithromax	Azithromycin
10. Norvasc	Amlodipine
11. Zoloft	Sertraline
12. Claritin	Loratadine
13. Coumadin Tabs	Warfarin
14. Augmentin	Amoxicillin & clavulanate acid
15. Zocor	Simvastatin
16. Furosemide Oral	Furosemide
17. Paxil	Paroxetine
18. Albuterol areosol	Albuterol
19. Zantac	Ranitidine
20. Zestril	Lisinopril
21. Procardia XL	Nifedipine
22. Prempro	Conjugated estrogen & medroxyprogesterone
23. Cardizem CD	Diltiazem
24. Biaxin	Clarithromycin
25. Amoxil	Amoxicillin
26. Trimethoprim & sulfamethoxazole	Trimethoprim & sulfamethoxazole
27. Cephalexin	Cephalexin
28. Acetaminophen with codeine	Acetaminophen with codeine
29. Glucophage	Metformin
30. Cipro	Ciprofloxacin
31. Propoxyphene-N & APAP	Propoxyphene-N & APAP
32. Veetids	Penicillin V potassium
33. Amoxicillin	Amoxicillin
34. Pravachol	Pravastatin
35. Triamterene & hydrochlorothiazide	Triamterene & hydrochlorothiazide
36. Ultram	Tramadol
37. Ibuprofen	Ibuprofen
38. Hytrin	Terazosin
39. Ambien	Zolpidem
40. Levoxyl	Levothyroxine
41. Ortho-Novum 7/7/7	Norethindrone & ethinyl estradiol
42. K-Dur 20	Potassium chloride
43. Accupril	Quinapril
44. Triphasil	Levonorgestrel & ethinyl estradiol
45. Relafen	Nabumetone
46. Amitriptyline	Amitriptyline
47. Claritin D - 12-Hour	Loratadine & pseudoephedrine
48. Humulin N	Human insulin
49. Dilantin Kapseals	Phenytoin
50. Pepcid	Famotidine
51. Glucotrol XL	Glipizide
52. Lotensin	Benazepril
53. Prinivil	Lisinopril
54. Cephalexin	Cephalexin
55. Acetaminophen with codeine	Acetaminophen with codeine

(continued)

Product	Generic Name
56. Cardura	Doxazosin
57. Mevacor	Lovastatin
58. Cefzil	Cefprozil
59. Alprazolam	Alprazolam
60. Prednisone Oral	Prednisone Oral
61. Atenolol	Atenolol
62. Lipitor	Atorvastatin
63. Propulsid	Cisapride
64. Lorazepam	Lorazepam
65. Diflucan	Fluconazole
66. Atrovent	Ipratropium bromide
67. Depakote	Divalproex
68. Hydrochlorothiazide	Hydrochlorothiazide
69. /adalat CC	Nifedipine
70. Prevacid	Lansoprazole
71. Glyburide	Glyburide
72. Ceftin	Cefuroxime axetil
73. Toprol XL	Metoprolol
74. Propoxyphene N w/APAP	Propoxyphene N w/APAP
75. Pondimen	Fenfluramine
76. Zyrtec	Cetirizine
77. Lescol	Fluvastatin
78. Daypro	Oxaprozin
79. Ortho Tri-Cyclen	Norgestimate & ethinyl estradiol
80. Albuterol nebulizing solution	Albuterol
81. Flonase	Fluticasone
82. Ery-Tab	Erythromycin
83. Imdur	Isosorbide mononitrate
84. Verapamil SR	Verapamil
85. Imitrex	Sumatriptan
86. Nitrostat	Nitroglycerin
87. Clonazepam	Clonazepam
88. Cycrin	Medroxyprogesteron
89. BuSpar	Buspirone
90. Allegra	Fexofenadine
91. Humulin	Human insulin
92. Axid	Nizatadine
93. Vancenase AQ	Beclomethsone
94. Atenolol	Atenolol
95. Lotrisone	Clotrimoxazole
96. Naproxen	Naproxen
97. Hydrocodone with APAP	Hydrocodone with APAP
98. Phentermine	Phentermine
99. Lorazepam	Lorazepam
100. Cozaar	Losartan
101. Azmacort	Triamcinolone
102. Fosamax	Alendronate
103. Desogen	Desogestrel
104. Alprazolam	Alprazolam
105. Lo/Ovral 28	Ethinyl estradiol & Norgestrel
106. Roxicet	Oxycodone & acetaminophen
107. Albuterol aerosol	Albuterol
108. Proventil aerosol	Albuterol
109. Atenolol	Atenolol
110. Metoprolol tartrate	Metoprolol tartrate
111. Klor-Con	Potassium chloride

TOP 200 PRESCRIBED DRUGS IN 1997 *(Continued)*

Product	Generic Name
112. Medroxyprogesterone tablets	Medroxyprogesterone
113. Serevent	Salmeterol
114. Cyclobenzaprine	Cyclobenzaprine
115. Deltasone	Prednisone
116. Methylphenidate	Methylphenidate
117. Triamterene with hydrochlorothiazide	Triamterene with hydrochlorothiazide
118. Provera	Medroxyprogesterone
119. Monopril	Fosinopril
120. Tri-Levlen	Levonorgestrel & ethinyl estradiol
121. Ziac	Bisoprolol
122. Neomycin/polymyxin/hydrocortisone	Neomycin/polymyxin/hydrocortisone
123. Carisoprodol	Carisoprodol
124. Estrace tablets	Estradiol
125. Ortho-Cyclen	Norgestimate & ethinyl estradiol
126. Ibuprofen	Ibuprofen
127. Diazepam	Diazepam
128. Macrobid	Nitrofurantoin
129. Ortho-Cept	Desonorgestrel & ethinyl estradiol
130. Bactroban	Mupirocin
131. Cimetidine	Cimetidine
132. Claritin D 24-Hour	Loratadine & pseudoephedrine
133. Effexor	Venlafaxine
134. Methylprednisone tablets	Methylprednisone
135. Loestrin FE 1.5/30	Norethindrone & ethinyl estradiol
136. Redux	Dexfenfluamine
137. Guaifenesin & phenylpropanolamine	Guaifenesin & phenylpropanolamine
138. Risperdal	Risperidone
139. Cefaclor	Cefaclor
140. Temazepam	Temazepam
141. Glyburide	Glyburide
142. Lorabid	Loracarbef
143. Propacet 100	Propoxyphene & acetaminophen
144. Endocet	Oxycodone & acetaminophen
145. Retin-A	Tretinoin
146. Calan SR	Verapamil
147. Alprazolam	Alprazolam
148. Gemfibrozil	Gemfibrozil
149. Potassium chloride	Potassium chloride
150. Lasix Oral	Furosemide
151. Atenolol	Atenolol
152. Phenergan suppositories	Promethazine
153. Lodine	Etodolac
154. Dyazide	Triamterene & hydrochlorothiazide
155. Xalatan	Latanoprost
156. Glipizide	Glipizide
157. Clonidine	Clonidine
158. Naproxen	Naproxen
159. Hydrocodone & APAP	Hydrocodone & APAP
160. Humulin R	Regular human insulin
161. Floxin	Ofloxacin
162. Ventolin aerosol	Albuterol
163. Vanceril	Beclomethasone

(continued)

Product	Generic Name
164. Zovirax	Acyclovir
165. Glynase prestab	Glyburide
166. Estradiol oral	Estradiol
167. Guaifenesin & phenylpropanolamine	Guaifenesin & phenylpropanolamine
168. Doxycycline	Doxycycline
169. Elocon	Mometasone
170. Alprazolam	Alprazolam
171. Serzone	Nefazadone
172. Zestoretic	Lisinopril & hydrochlorothiazide
173. Loestrin Fe 1/20	Ethinyl estradiol & Norethindrone w/FE
174. Furosemide oral	Furosemide
175. Ibuprofen	Ibuprofen
176. TruSopt	Dorzolamide
177. TobraDex	Tobramycin & dexamethasone
178. Altace	Rampiril
179. Darvocet-N 100	Propoxyphene & acetaminophen
180. Cyclobenzaprine	Cyclobenzaprine
181. Dicyclomine	Dicyclomine
182. Hydrochlorothiazide	Hydrochlorothiazide
183. Metoprolol	Metoprolol
184. Amoxicillin	Amoxicillin
185. Promethazine & codeine	Promethazine & codeine
186. Klonopin	Clonazepam
187. Ortho-Novum 1/35	Norethindrone
188. Trazodone	Trazodone
189. Neurontin	Gabapentin
190. Nitro-Dur	Nitroglycerin
191. Tamoxifen	Tamoxifen
192. Biaxin suspension	Clarithromycin
193. Rhinocort	Budesonide
194. Estraderm	Estradiol
195. Genora 1/35	Norethindrone & ethinyl estradiol
196. Suprax	Cefixime
197. Xanax	Alprazolam
198. Timoptic XE	Timolol maleate
199. Demulen 1/35	Ethynodiol diacetate & ethinyl estradiol
200. Albuterol oral liquid	Albuterol

VASOCONSTRICTOR INTERACTIONS WITH ANTIDEPRESSANTS

Antidepressant	Effects With Epinephrine, Norepinephrine, Levonordefrin	Contraindicated	Recommendation
Bupropion (Wellbutrin®)	No adverse interactions reported	No	No precautions appear to be necessary
Fluoxetine (Prozac®)	No adverse interactions reported	No	No precautions appear to be necessary
Maprotiline (Ludiomil®)	Potential for inc pressor response	No	Same precaution as TCAs since it has similar pharmacology
Paroxetine (Paxil®)	No adverse interactions reported	No	No precautions appear to be necessary
Sertraline (Zoloft®)	No adverse interactions reported	No	No precautions appear to be necessary
TCAs	epi = inc pressor response; cardiac dysrhythmias; ne = inc pressor response; levo = inc pressor response	No	Potentially dangerous; use minimal amounts with caution in local anesthetics
Trazodone (Desyrel®)	No adverse interactions reported	No	No precautions appear to be necessary
Venlafaxine (Effexor®)	No adverse interactions reported	No	No precautions appear to be necessary

Reference: Wynn RL, "Antidepressant Medications", *Gen Dent*, 1992, 40(3):192-7.

WHAT'S NEW

New Drugs Introduced or Approved by the FDA in 1997/98

Brand Name	Generic Name	Use
Accolate®	zafirlukast	Asthma
Agrylin®	anagrelide	Thrombocythemia
Aldara®	imiquimod	External genital warts
Alphagan®	brimonidine	Glaucoma
Amaryl®	glimepiride	Type II diabetes
Amerge®	naratriptan	Migraine
Antizol®	fomepizole	Antifreeze antidote
Anzemet®	dolasetron	Nausea/vomiting
Aphthasol®	amlexanox	Aphthous ulcers
Aricept®	donepezil	Alzheimer's disease
Arthrotec®	diclofenac and misoprostol	Osteoarthritis
Astelin®	azelastine	Antihistamine (allergic rhinitis)
Avapro®	irbesartan	Hypertension
Baycol®	cerivastatin	High cholesterol
Combivir®	zidovudine and lamivudine	HIV infection
Copaxone®	glatiramer acetate	Multiple sclerosis
Cystadane®	betaine anhydrous	Homocystinuria
Denavir®	penciclovir	Cold sores
Diovan®	valsartan	Hypertension
Dostinex®	cabergoline	Hyperprolactinemia
Duract®	bromfenac	Acute pain
Elmiron®	pentosan polysulfate sodium	Interstitial cystitis
Ethyol®	amifostine	Reduction of cumulative renal toxicity associated with administration of cisplatin
Evista®	raloxifene	Osteoporosis
Fareston®	toremifene	Breast cancer
Flomax™	tamsulosin	Benign prostatic hyperplasia (BPH)
Gabitril®	tiagabine	Seizures
Glyset®	miglitol	Type II diabetes
IvyBlock®	bentoquatam	Poison ivy
Levaquin®	levofloxacin	Bacterial respiratory tract infection
Lexxel®	enalapril and felodipine	Hypertension
Lipidil®	fenofibrate	High triglyceride
Lipitor®	atorvastatin	High cholesterol
Mentax®	butenafine	Ringworm and other topical fungi
Meridia™	sibutramine	Obesity
Mirapex®	pramipexole	Parkinson's disease
Monurol™	fosfomycin	Urinary tract infections
Naropin™	ropivacaine	Anesthetic (infiltration)
Nilandron™	nilutamide	Prostate cancer
Normiflo®	ardeparin	Deep vein thrombosis
Norvir®	ritonavir	HIV infection
Orgaran®	danaparoid	Deep vein thrombosis
Patanol™	olopatadine	Allergic conjunctivitis
Plavix®	clopidogrel	Atherosclerosis
Posicor®	mibefradil	Hypertension
Prandin®	repaglinide	Diabetes
ProAmatine®	midodrine	Orthostatic hypotension
Raxar®	grepafloxacin	Quinolong antibiotic
Regranex®	becaplermin	Diabetic foot/leg ulcers
Requip®	ropinirole	Parkinson's disease
Rescriptor™	delavirdine	HIV infection
Retavase®	reteplase	Acute myocardial infarction

WHAT'S NEW (Continued)

Brand Name	Generic Name	Use
Rezulin®	troglitazone	Type II diabetes
Rituxan®	rituximab	Non-Hodgkin's lymphoma
Seroquel®	quetiapine	Antipsychotic
Singulair®	montelukast	Asthma
Skelid®	tiludronate	Paget's disease of the bone
Stromectol®	ivermectin	Intestinal parasites (worms)
Tarka®	trandolapril and verapamil	Hypertension
Tasmar®	tolcapone	Parkinson's disease
Tazorac®	tazarotene	Psoriasis, acne vulgaris
Teczem®	enalapril and diltiazem	Hypertension
Teveten®	eprosartan	Hypertension
Topamax®	topiramate	Seizures
Trovan™ I.V.	alatrofloxacin	Quinolone antibiotic
Trovan™ Oral	trovafloxacin	Quinolone antibiotic
Viracept®	nelfinavir	HIV infection
Zagam®	sparfloxacin	Community-acquired pneumonia
Zanaflex®	tizanidine	Multiple sclerosis, spinal cord injury
Zomig®	zolmitriptan	Migraine
Zyflo®	zileuton	Asthma
PENDING DRUGS OR DRUGS IN CLINICAL TRIALS		
Alredase®	tolrestat	Controlling late complications of diabetes
Arkin-Z®	vesnarinone	Congestive heart failure agent
Baypress®	nitrendipine	Calcium channel blocker for hypertension
Berotec®	fenoterol	Beta-2 agonist for asthma
Catatrol®	viloxazine	Bicyclic antidepressant
Cipralan®	cifenline succinate	Antiarrhythmic agent
Decabid®	indecainide hydrochloride	Antiarrhythmic agent
Delaprem®	hexoprenaline sulfate	Tocolytic agent
Dirame®	propiram	Opioid analgesic
Eldisine®	vindesine sulfate	Antineoplastic
Enable®	tenidap sodium	Arthritis
Fareston®	toremifene citrate	Antiestrogen for breast cancer
Freedox®	triliazad mesylate	Prevents progressive neuronal degeneration
Frisium®	clobazam	Benzodiazepine
Gastrozepine®	pirenzepine	Antiulcer drug
Inhibace®	cilazapril	ACE inhibitor
Isoprinosine®	inosiplex	Immunomodulating drug
Lacipil®	lacidipine	Hypertension
Maxicam®	isoxicam	NSAID
Mentane®	velnacrine	Alzheimer's disease agent
Micturin®	terodiline hydrochloride	Agent for urinary incontinence
Mogadon®	nitrazepam	Benzodiazepine
Motilium®	domperidone	Antiemetic
Napa®	acecainide	Antiarrhythmic agent
Pindac®	pinacidil	Antihypertensive
Prothiaden®	dothiepin hydrochloride	Tricyclic antidepressant
Rimadyl®	caprofen	NSAID
Roxiam®	remoxipride	Antipsychotic agent
Sabril®	vigabatrin	Anticonvulsant
Selecor®	celiprolol hydrochloride	Beta-adrenergic blocker
Soriatane®	acitretin	Recalcitrant psoriasis
Spexil®	trospectomycin	Antibiotic, a spectinomycin analog
Targocoid®	teicoplanin	Antibiotic, similar to vancomycin
Unicard®	dilevalol	Beta-adrenergic blocker
Zaditen®	ketotifen	Antiasthmatic

THERAPEUTIC CATEGORY INDEX

ANTIANGINAL AGENT *(Continued)*

ANTIANXIETY AGENT

ANTIARRHYTHMIC AGENT, CLASS I

ANTIARRHYTHMIC AGENT, CLASS I-A

ANTIARRHYTHMIC AGENT, CLASS I-B

ANTIARRHYTHMIC AGENT, CLASS I-C

ANTIARRHYTHMIC AGENT, CLASS II

ANTIARRHYTHMIC AGENT, CLASS III

ANTIARRHYTHMIC AGENT, CLASS IV

ANTIARRHYTHMIC AGENT (SUPRAVENTRICULAR)

ANTIARRHYTHMIC AGENT (SUPRAVENTRICULAR & VENTRICULAR)

ANTIBIOTIC, SULFONAMIDE DERIVATIVE

ANTIBIOTIC, SULFONE

ANTIBIOTIC, TETRACYCLINE DERIVATIVE

ANTIBIOTIC, TOPICAL

ANTIBIOTIC, URINARY IRRIGATION

ANTIBIOTIC, VAGINAL

ANTIBIOTIC, MISCELLANEOUS

(Continued)

ANTIHYPERTENSIVE

ANTIHYPERTENSIVE AGENT, COMBINATION

ANTIHYPOGLYCEMIC AGENT

ANTI-INFECTIVE AGENT, ORAL

ANTI-INFLAMMATORY AGENT

(Continued)

ANTI-PARKINSON'S AGENT *(Continued)*

ANTIPLAQUE AGENT

ANTIPLATELET AGENT

ANTIPROTOZOAL

ANTIPRURITIC, TOPICAL

ANTIPSORIATIC AGENT, SYSTEMIC

ANTIPSORIATIC AGENT, TOPICAL

ANTIPSYCHOTIC AGENT

ANTIPYRETIC

ANTISEBORRHEIC AGENT, TOPICAL

ANTISECRETORY AGENT

ANTISPASMODIC AGENT, GASTROINTESTINAL

ANTISPASMODIC AGENT, URINARY

ANTITHYROID AGENT

ANTITRYPSIN DEFICIENCY AGENT

ANTITUBERCULAR AGENT

ANTITUSSIVE

ANTIUROLITHIC

ANTIVIRAL AGENT, INHALATION THERAPY

ANTIVIRAL AGENT, OPHTHALMIC

ANTIVIRAL AGENT, ORAL

(Continued)

(Continued)

FOLIC ACID DERIVATIVE

FLUORIDE

GALLSTONE DISSOLUTION AGENT

GANGLIONIC BLOCKING AGENT

GASTRIC ACID SECRETION INHIBITOR

GASTROINTESTINAL AGENT, PROKINETIC

GASTROINTESTINAL AGENT, STIMULANT

GASTROINTESTINAL AGENT, MISCELLANEOUS

GENERAL ANESTHETIC, INTRAVENOUS

GENITOURINARY IRRIGANT

GLUCOCORTICOID

GOLD COMPOUND

GONADOTROPIN

GONADOTROPIN RELEASING HORMONE ANALOG

GROWTH HORMONE

HEMOPHILIC AGENT

HEMOSTATIC AGENT
(Continued)

HEMOSTATIC AGENT *(Continued)*

HISTAMINE H₂ ANTAGONIST

HMG-COA REDUCTASE INHIBITOR

HORMONE, POSTERIOR PITUITARY

H. PYLORI AGENT

HYPERTHERMIA, TREATMENT

HYPNOTIC

HYPOGLYCEMIC AGENT, ORAL

IMMUNE GLOBULIN

IMMUNE MODULATOR

IMMUNE RESPONSE MODIFIER

IMMUNOSUPPRESSANT AGENT

ALPHABETICAL INDEX

ALPHABETICAL INDEX

ALPHABETICAL INDEX

ALPHABETICAL INDEX

ALPHABETICAL INDEX

ALPHABETICAL INDEX

NOTES

NOTES

NOTES

NOTES

"Lexi-Comp's Clinical Reference Library™ (CRL) has established the new standard for quick reference information"

Lexi-Comp offers the Clinical Reference Library™ (CRL™), a series of clinical databases, as portable handbooks or integrated as part of a CD-ROM that also includes clinical decision support modules. CRL™ is delivered with a powerful search engine on a single CD-ROM and can be used with Microsoft® Windows™ release 3.1 or higher. In addition to our CD-ROM for Windows™, Lexi-Comp's databases can also be licensed for distribution on your Intranet, or used with your palmtop, Newton, or Windows™ CE device.

NEW titles targeted for release in print and on CD-ROM will include:

- *Drug Information Handbook for Nursing*
- *Drug Information Handbook for Cancer*
- *Drug Information Handbook for the Criminal Justice Professional*
- *Drug Information Handbook for Psychiatry*

Other titles offered by Lexi-Comp . . .

DRUG INFORMATION HANDBOOK 6th Edition 98/99

by Charles Lacy, PharmD; Lora L. Armstrong, BSPharm; Naomi Ingrim, PharmD; and Leonard L. Lance, BSPharm

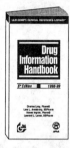

Specifically compiled and designed for the healthcare professional requiring quick access to concisely stated comprehensive data concerning clinical use of medications.

The Drug Information Handbook is an ideal portable drug information resource, containing 1100 drug monographs. Each monograph typically provides the reader with up to 29 key points of data concerning clinical use and dosing of the medication. Material provided in the Appendix section is recognized by many users to be, by itself, well worth the purchase of the handbook.

DRUG INFORMATION HANDBOOK POCKET 98/99

by Charles Lacy, PharmD; Lora L. Armstrong, BSPharm; Naomi Ingrim, PharmD; and Leonard L. Lance, BSPharm

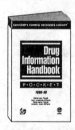

All medications found in the Drug Information Handbook, 6th Edition are included in this abridged pocket edition. It is specifically compiled and designed for the healthcare professional requiring quick access to concisely stated comprehensive data concerning clinical use of medications.

The outstanding cross-referencing allows the user to quickly locate the brand name, generic name, synonym, and related information found in the Appendix making this a useful quick reference for medical professionals at any level of training or experience.

ANESTHESIOLOGY & CRITICAL CARE DRUG HANDBOOK 98/99

by Andrew J. Donnelly, PharmD; Francesca E. Cunningham, PharmD; and Verna L. Baughman, MD

New!

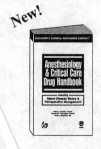

Contains over 450 generic medications with up to 25 fields of information presented in each monograph. It also contains the following Special Issues and Topics: Allergic Reaction, Anesthesia for Cardiac Patients in Noncardiac Surgery, Anesthesia for Obstetric Patients in Nonobstetric Surgery, Anesthesia for Patients With Liver Disease, Chronic Pain Management, Chronic Renal Failure, Conscious Sedation, Perioperative Management of Patients on Antiseizure Medication, Substance Abuse and Anesthesia.

The Appendix contains over 140 pages of useful and valuable information including: Abbreviations & Measurements, Anesthesiology Information, Assessment of Liver & Renal Function, Comparative Drug Charts, Infectious Disease-Prophylaxis & Treatment, Laboratory Values, Therapy Recommendation, Toxicology, *and much more . . .*

PEDIATRIC DOSAGE HANDBOOK 5th Edition 98/99

by Carol K. Taketomo, PharmD; Jane Hurlburt Hodding, PharmD; and Donna M. Kraus, PharmD

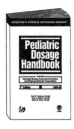

Special considerations must frequently be taken into account when dosing medications for the pediatric patient. This highly regarded quick reference handbook is a compilation of recommended pediatric doses based on current literature as well as the practical experience of the authors and their many colleagues who work every day in the pediatric clinical setting.

The Pediatric Dosage Handbook 5th Edition includes neonatal dosing, drug administration, and extemporaneous preparations for 619 medications used in pediatric medicine.

GERIATRIC DOSAGE HANDBOOK 4th Edition 98/99

by Todd P. Semla, PharmD; Judith L. Beizer, PharmD; and Martin D. Higbee, PharmD

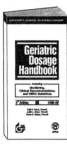

Many physiologic changes occur with aging, some of which affect the pharmacokinetics or pharmacodynamics of medications. Strong consideration should also be given to the effect of decreased renal or hepatic functions in the elderly as well as the probability of the geriatric patient being on multiple drug regimens.

Healthcare professionals working with nursing homes and assisted living facilities will find the 745 drug monographs contained in this handbook to be an invaluable source of helpful information.

DRUG INFORMATION HANDBOOK FOR THE ALLIED HEALTH PROFESSIONAL 5th Edition 98/99

by Leonard L. Lance, BSPharm; Charles Lacy, PharmD; and Morton P. Goldman, PharmD

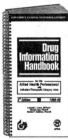

Working with clinical pharmacists, hospital pharmacy and therapeutics committees, and hospital drug information centers, the authors have assisted hundreds of hospitals in developing institution specific formulary reference documentation.

The most current basic drug and medication data from those clinical settings have been reviewed, coalesced, and cross-referenced to create this unique handbook. The handbook offers quick access to abbreviated monographs for 1441 generic drugs.

This is a great tool for physician assistants, medical records personnel, medical transcriptionists and secretaries, pharmacy technicians, and other allied health professionals.

INFECTIOUS DISEASES HANDBOOK 2nd Edition 97/98

by Carlos M. Isada MD; Bernard L. Kasten Jr. MD; Morton P. Goldman PharmD; Larry D. Gray PhD; and Judith A. Aberg MD

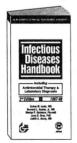

This four-in-one quick reference is concerned with the identification and treatment of infectious diseases. A unique feature of the handbook is that entries in each of the four sections of the book (164 disease syndromes, 143 organisms, 231 laboratory tests, and 222 antimicrobials) contain related information and cross-referencing to one or more of the other three sections.

The disease syndrome section provides straight-forward information on the clinical presentation, differential diagnosis, diagnostic tests, and drug therapy recommended for treatment of more common infectious diseases. The organism section presents discussion of the microbiology, epidemiology,

diagnosis, and treatment of each organism. The laboratory diagnosis section describes performance of specific tests and procedures. The antimicrobial therapy section presents important facts and considerations regarding each drug recommended for specific diseases of organisms.

POISONING & TOXICOLOGY COMPENDIUM 98/99 (New 8½ x 11 Size!)
by Jerrold B. Leikin, MD and Frank P. Paloucek, PharmD

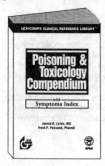

A six-in-one reference wherein each major entry contains information relative to one or more of the other sections. This handbook offers comprehensive concisely-stated monographs covering 645 medicinal agents, 256 nonmedicinal agents, 273 biological agents, 49 herbal agents, 254 laboratory tests, 79 antidotes, and 222 pages of exceptionally useful appendix material.

A truly unique reference that presents signs and symptoms of acute overdose along with considerations for overdose treatment. Ideal reference for emergency situations.

LABORATORY TEST HANDBOOK - CONCISE (New!)
by David S. Jacobs, MD, FACP, FCAP; Wayne R. DeMott, MD, FCAP; Harold J. Grady, PhD; Rebecca T. Horvat, PhD; Douglas W. Huestis, MD; Bernard L. Kasten Jr., MD, FCAP

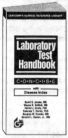

The authors of Lexi-Comp's highly regarded Laboratory Test Handbook have selected and extracted key information for presentation in this portable abridged version. It contains more than 800 test entries for quick reference and is ideal for residents, nurses, and medical students or technologists requiring information concerning patient preparation, specimen collection and handling, and test result interpretation.

LABORATORY TEST HANDBOOK 4th Edition 1996
by David S. Jacobs MD, FACP; Wayne R. DeMott, MD, FACP; Harold J. Grady, PhD; Rebecca T. Horvat, PhD; Douglas W. Huestis, MD; and Bernard L. Kasten Jr., MD, FACP

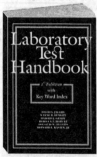

This is a single reference source that contains difficult to find general and interpretive information pertinent to the use of over 900 clinical laboratory tests.

Includes sections on Molecular Pathology and Trace Elements and each test entry in a section is complete in itself providing the user with the test name, synonyms, patient care recommendations, specimen requirements, reference ranges, methodology, footnotes, and references. Updated CPT and ICD-9 coding is also provided. This handbook delivers answers to many typical questions posed about laboratory tests. An extremely useful reference for practitioners and other healthcare professionals.

DIAGNOSTIC PROCEDURE HANDBOOK by Joseph A. Golish, MD

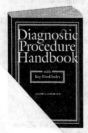

An ideal companion to the Laboratory Test Handbook this publication details 295 diagnostic procedures including: Allergy, Immunology/Rheumotology, Infectious Disease, Cardiology, Critical Care, Gastroenterology, Nephrology, Urology, Hematology, Neurology, Ophthalmology, Pulmonary Function, Pulmonary Medicine, Computed Tomography, Diagnostic Radiology, Invasive Radiology, Magnetic Resonance Imaging, Nuclear Medicine, and Ultrasound. A great reference handbook for healthcare professionals at any level of training and experience.